AF319058

PRINCIPLES OF RESPIRATORY MEDICINE

PRINCIPLES OF RESPIRATORY MEDICINE

Second Edition

Editors

Farokh Erach Udwadia
MD FRCP (London & Edinburgh) Master FCCP FAMS FCPS DSc
Emeritus Professor of Medicine
Grant Medical College and JJ Group of Hospitals, Mumbai
Consultant Physician and Director in Charge of the ICU
Breach Candy Hospital, Mumbai
Consultant Physician, Parsee General Hospital
Mumbai, Maharashtra, India

Zarir F Udwadia
MD DNB FRCP (London) FCCP (USA)
Consultant Chest Physician, Hinduja Hospital, Mumbai
Consultant Physician, Breach Candy Hospital and Parsee General Hospital
Mumbai, Maharashtra, India

Anirudh F Kohli
MD DNB DMRD
Head of Imaging, Breach Candy Hospital, Mumbai
Consultant Radiologist, Jaslok Hospital
Mumbai, Maharashtra, India

Khyati Shah
MBBS
Consultant Physician and Research Officer
Breach Candy Hospital
Mumbai, Maharashtra, India

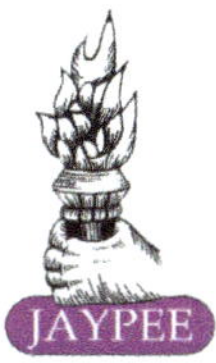

JAYPEE BROTHERS MEDICAL PUBLISHERS
The Health Sciences Publisher
New Delhi | London

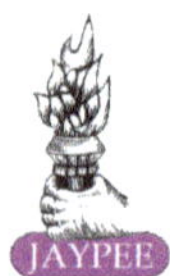 **Jaypee Brothers Medical Publishers (P) Ltd**

Headquarters
Jaypee Brothers Medical Publishers (P) Ltd.
4838/24, Ansari Road, Daryaganj
New Delhi 110 002, India
Phone: +91-11-43574357
Fax: +91-11-43574314
E-mail: jaypee@jaypeebrothers.com

Overseas Office
JP Medical Ltd.
83 Victoria Street, London
SW1H 0HW (UK)
Phone: +44-20 3170 8910
Fax: +44(0)20 3008 6180
E-mail: info@jpmedpub.com

Website: www.jaypeebrothers.com
Website: www.jaypeedigital.com

Principles of Respiratory Medicine

First Edition: 2010
Second Edition: 2020

ISBN: 978-93-88958-58-5

Dedicated to

Vera, Gool, Malavika, Vanaiya, and our children for their love and support

Preface to the Second Edition

The first edition of this landmark book, *Principles of Respiratory Medicine*, not only in India but also in Southeast Asia, has been extremely well received. A second edition is both warranted and has been eagerly awaited. This second edition has been thoroughly revised and brought up-to-date.

The revision extends to the generally accepted description of respiratory diseases common to the affluent West and the poor tropical countries. However, the revised and updated epidemiology of these diseases, their subtle variations in clinical presentation, and natural history as observed in India and Southeast Asia have merited special emphasis. The epidemiological study of respiratory diseases in these countries remains unfortunately poor and our task is therefore beset with considerable difficulty.

Respiratory diseases peculiar to India and other tropical countries have been revised wherever necessary. The chapter on Dengue has been extensively revised and we have newly included the complications of Scrub Typhus. For obvious reasons, respiratory diseases peculiar to the tropics have been given more attention than have been given by western authors. This continues to be a very important feature of this book.

Every section and most chapters of this book have been updated. Prevailing concepts in lung cancer, asthma, interstitial lung disease, and several other diseases have been discussed at length with special reference to India and Southeast Asia.

As in the first edition, the highlight of this book is the section on tuberculosis (TB). Pulmonary TB exists on an epic scale—a killer that stalks millions of Indians, not only killing many, but impoverishing many more. India accounts for more than one-third of the TB burden of the world; TB causes one death per minute in this country and over a million deaths annually. Every aspect of this disease has been revised with special regard to epidemiology, MDR-TB, XDR-TB, the relation between TB and human immunodeficiency virus (HIV) infection, the drug regimes in use, and the newer drugs available in treatment. The section on newer diagnostic aids now available, chiefly involving genetic and molecular biology, has been extensively revised.

Another noteworthy feature of this book is the large number of excellent images that illustrate the text. Every chapter of every section is illustrated wherever necessary with high-quality images contributing to a better understanding of the text.

As in the first edition to ensure conformity in content, form, and style, we did not invite contributions from colleagues working in different parts of the country. There were two exceptions—Dr Thirumali Rajgopal who contributed chapters on "Common Occupational Disease and Environmental Pollution" and Dr Camila Rodrigues who contributed a chapter on "Antibiotic Resistance and its Management". Dr Rajgopal is the Medical Advisor to Hindustan Lever and Lever Brothers and Dr Rodrigues is the senior consultant and Head of Microbiology at the Hinduja Hospital, Mumbai, Maharashtra, India. We are extremely grateful to both these colleagues for their contribution.

What makes this book different from similar works written by Western authors is the emphasis on respiratory diseases as practiced in India, Southeast Asia, and other tropical countries.

This edition will continue to be useful to medical registrars, registrars in pulmonary medicine, postgraduate students, medical practitioners, consultants in general medicine, and pulmonologists not only in India and Southeast Asia but also to an extent in Africa and South America. It will also be of interest to our western colleagues, as in a shrinking world and the ease of travel, an awareness of different diseases in different parts of the world becomes necessary.

We have included one more author in this second edition—Dr Khyati Shah, the research officer at Breach Candy Hospital, Mumbai, Maharashtra, India. She has been responsible for the organization of the numerous sections and chapters, the corrections and repeated revisions, the numerous references in each section and chapter, the insertion of the many images at the appropriate places throughout the volume, the correction of page proofs again and again and the meticulous attention to detail in the production of this work. Without her devotion, diligence, cheerful disposition, and invaluable help, this book would not have been possible.

We owe a great deal of gratitude to Mr Sanjiv Mehta, CEO of Hindustan Lever, India, who has been kind enough to give an extraordinarily generous subsidy toward the publication of this work. The price of this book has thereby been substantially reduced so as to bring it within the reach of all students and colleagues in this profession.

We also thank Mrs Vera F Udwadia for her help in correcting the page proof. We also thank Mr Neeraj Chawan for helping to type the manuscript. We thank the various authors whose works we have consulted in the preparation of this book and to those publishers who have granted permission to use some figures, images, and tables from their books/ journals.

Finally, we thank Jaypee Brothers Medical Publisher (P) Ltd. for their unstinted help and cooperation in publishing this book.

Farokh Erach Udwadia
Zarir F Udwadia
Anirudh F Kohli

Preface to the First Edition

The prime reason for writing a book on pulmonary medicine is our firm conviction that a description of respiratory diseases occurring in India is best written by experienced physicians working for decades in the same country. The contents of such a text we felt would also by and large be applicable to other developing and poor countries of the world. Considering the fact that far more people live in the underprivileged regions of the world compared to the affluent West, the raison d'être for such a text seemed unquestionable.

We knew that our task was indeed daunting and we made it doubly so by deciding not to invite contributions from colleagues working in various regions of the country. We were determined to accomplish the work by ourselves, so as to finish the task quickly, and to ensure a uniformity of style, language, content and a focussed dedication, all so essential to achieve what we set out to do. The work started in the spring of 2009 and was submitted for publication by August 2010. We however allowed for two exceptions when we invited Dr Thirumalai Rajgopal to contribute two chapters on 'Common Occupational Lung Diseases' and 'Environmental Pollution' and Dr Camilla Rodrigues to write on 'Antibiotic Resistance and its Management'.

In India we encounter almost all the respiratory diseases found in the West. In addition, we live among respiratory diseases which are peculiar only to India and other developing tropical countries, that are uncommon in the West. It is therefore important that physicians practising in these countries are trained in the understanding, diagnosis, and management of both these groups of diseases. The authors sincerely hope that this book achieves this objective. We have not compromised on the generally accepted description of respiratory diseases common to both the affluent West and to poor tropical countries. However, the epidemiology of these diseases, their often subtle variations in clinical presentation, and natural history as observed in the Indian and Southeast Asian context have been clearly emphasized.

Respiratory disorders peculiar to India and other tropical countries have, for obvious reasons, been dealt with in considerable detail. For example, pulmonary infections in the tropics, together with pulmonary complications of tropical diseases is a subject that deserves far more attention than what has been accorded by western authors. Parasitic infections of the lungs, the lung in fulminant malaria, in amoebic infection, in salmonellosis, leptospirosis, dengue, in other fulminant, and not so fulminant infections in the tropics, have been discussed in special detail because they are both frequent and important.

The increasing menace of lung cancer in India has been given special emphasis; with a comparison of recent epidemiological data on lung cancer in various parts of India vis-à-vis Southeast Asia, China, and several other countries of the world.

Both chronic obstructive pulmonary disease as well as asthma have a significant morbidity and mortality rate in India, Southeast Asia, and also in the West. These topics have been discussed at length with special reference to India and Southeast Asia.

A highlight of the book is a discussion on the threat of pulmonary tuberculosis and its unsolved challenges. Pulmonary tuberculosis dominates medicine in India and other developing countries. It exists on an epic scale with India accounting for a third of the world's TB burden. Every aspect of this disease has been dealt with, including a detailed epidemiological description, MDR and XDR tuberculosis, tuberculosis in relation to the HIV epidemic, the new diagnostic aids involving the use of genetics and molecular biology, and also the future needs to counter the unsolved challenges of this disease.

We have also included, among others, sections on basic 'Lung Physiology', 'Clinical Approach to Respiratory Disease-Symptoms and Signs', 'Occupational and Environmental Lung Diseases', 'Infectious Diseases' and a section on 'HIV and the Lung'.

The volume begins with the section 'Imaging Techniques and Imaging of the Chest'. Of all the recent discoveries in respiratory medicine, the most iconic is the discovery of spiral computed tomography in the 1990s. Continuing technological advances have further enhanced the imaging of the microarchitecture of the lung and have enabled a reconstruction of images that allow a three-dimensional view of a lung pathology and of pathologies involving the mediastinum. The advent of virtual bronchoscopy permits a view of the whole bronchial tree and its surrounding structures. These, together with the use of ultrasonography, ventilation-perfusion lung scans, magnetic resonance imaging (MRI), and positron emission tomography (PET scans) in respiratory medicine have been briefly described with suitable illustrations in this section. What is more, every single chapter of every section is illustrated wherever necessary with high-quality images that contribute to the further understanding of different respiratory diseases. We feel that the visual image is as important as the written word and often is longer lasting in the mind's eye.

Principles of Respiratory Medicine is a book written by clinicians for clinicians, and though not encyclopedic in content, is comprehensive in its scope. The varying emphasis given to different respiratory diseases is related to respiratory medicine as observed and practiced in India and to an extent in Southeast Asia and other tropical countries. In this respect, the book differs significantly from many others written by western authors.

This is a landmark book not only in India but probably also in Southeast Asia. It will prove to be of considerable benefit to medical registrars, registrars in pulmonary medicine, postgraduate students, medical practitioners, consultants in general medicine, and to pulmonologists practising in these countries as well as to some extent in Africa and South America. It will also be of interest to our colleagues in the West, for surely they would be keen to know the pattern of respiratory diseases in the other half of the world—in the teaming populations of poor tropical countries. Also, ours is a shrinking world and the frequency and the ease of travel from one continent to another has increasingly resulted in the need for a global awareness—an awareness of different diseases in different parts of the world.

We have based this book on current knowledge, evidence, experience, and recent advances, all perhaps in equal measure. Yet it behoves the reader to bear in mind that what is true today may not be true tomorrow, for the history of medicine, including respiratory medicine, is a chronicle of change. We leave the reader with the words of Sir Francis Bacon… 'Read not to contradict and confute, nor to believe and take for granted, nor to find talk and discourse, but to weigh and consider'.

We owe a great deal of gratitude to a number of individuals, some of whom deserve special mention. We owe an immense debt of gratitude to Mr Shreyas Doshi of Shrenuj and Company who has been kind enough to give an extraordinarily generous subsidy towards the publication of this work. The price of the book has thereby been substantially reduced to bring it within the reach of all students and colleagues in the profession.

Our sincerest thanks above all to Dr Khyati Mehta, our research assistant, without whose devotion, diligence, cheerful disposition, and invaluable help this book would never have been possible. She has been largely responsible for the organization of the numerous sections and chapters, the insertion of so many images and illustrations at appropriate places throughout the volume and meticulous attention to detail in the production of this work. Her help with the page-proofs, with the huge number of references, and her cordial liaison with our publishers have been of immense help. She indeed is as much a part of the book as the authors inscribed on the cover.

Our sincerest thanks to Dr Thirumalai Rajgopal for his chapters on 'Common Occupational Lung Diseases' and 'Environmental Pollution'. We also thank Dr Camilla Rodrigues for her chapter on 'Antibiotic Resistance and its Management'.

We are grateful to AV Graphic Designers Pvt Ltd (Mumbai) for creating excellent illustrations and tables that have been used throughout the book. Their cooperation and punctuality during the production of this work was outstanding. Our thanks to Dr Maansi Parekh for her help with the images and to Ms Kinni Makwana who has provided us with four special illustrations.

We thank Mrs Vera F Udwadia for her help in the correction of the page-proofs. We also thank Mr Neeraj Chavan for his help in typing the manuscript. We thank the many authors whose work we have consulted during the preparation of this book, in particular the text on *Clinical Respiratory Medicine* edited by Albert RK, Spiro SC and Jett R. We would also like to extend our thanks to those publishers and authors who have granted permission for some figures, images, and tables from their books/journals.

Finally, our sincerest thanks to the team at Oxford University Press in Delhi and Mumbai for their unstinted help and cooperation in publishing this work.

Farokh Erach Udwadia

Contents

Section 20 Drug-induced Lung Injuries

Section 21 Trauma and Chest Wall Disorders

Section 22 Sleep-related Breathing Disorders

Imaging Techniques and Imaging of the Chest

CHAPTER 1

Imaging Techniques and Imaging of the Chest

INTRODUCTION

The chest radiograph remains the primary imaging investigation in the evaluation of diseases of the respiratory system. It is a low-radiation, cheap and easily available imaging technique, providing invaluable information regarding the lung parenchyma, pleura, mediastinum and chest wall. It has its share of limitations being a projectional two-dimensional (2D) imaging modality. Computed tomography (CT), a cross-sectional imaging modality provides excellent detail of the lung, pleura, mediastinum as well as chest wall to compensate for the limitations of chest X-ray. The chest X-ray as well as the CT scan suffice for all imaging needs in the chest. Ultrasonography (USG)/ magnetic resonance imaging (MRI)/positron emission tomography (PET) have complementary roles in the evaluation of chest diseases.

CHEST RADIOGRAPHS

Even after 100 years of technological developments, the chest X-ray remains the primary imaging modality for diseases of the chest. It is obtained with the patient erect, facing the cassette, with the X-ray beam directed from behind the patient, from a distance of 6 feet to avoid magnification of mediastinal structures **(Figs. 1 and 2)**. The X-ray is obtained at deep inspiration. A film obtained in expiration will result in alteration of the mediastinal contour as well as a misleading appearance of diffuse lung disease **(Figs. 3A and B)**. It is important to position the patient well such that he or she is not rotated. A well-centered X-ray will demonstrate the medial ends of the clavicles to be equidistant from the spinous processes of the vertebrae. Rotation to the left results in the manubrium sternum, superior vena cava (SVC) and great vessels

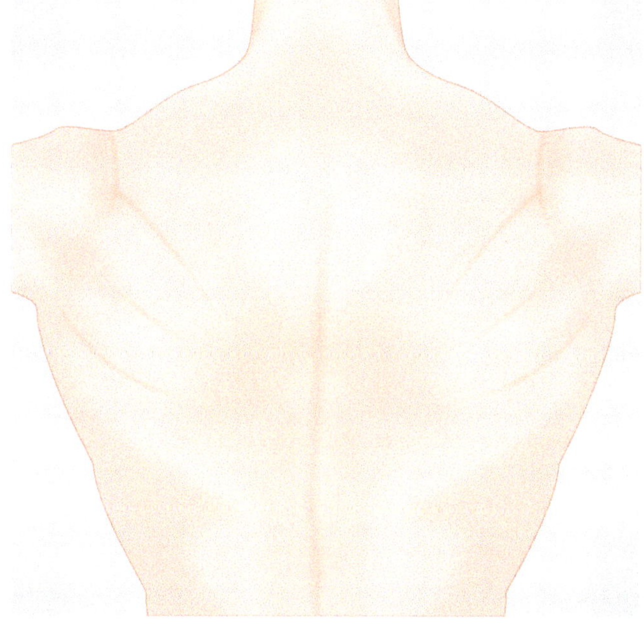

Fig. 1: PA view of the chest: Positioning for a PA view of the chest with patient facing the cassette and arms rotated forward to take the scapulae off the film.

appearing prominent—this may simulate a mediastinal mass **(Figs. 4A and B)**. Rotation may also result in one lung appearing more or less translucent **(Figs. 5A to C)**. To minimize the shadow of the scapula on the lungs, the arms are placed on the sides and shoulders rotated forward so as to rotate the scapula laterally.

A large part of the lungs on a frontal radiograph are obscured by the bony rib cage. To be able to visualize larger areas of lung parenchyma free from significant obscuration by the ribs, high kVp (peak kilovoltage) techniques are used. As the coefficient of X-ray absorption of soft tissue and bone approach each other at high kVp, the bony rib cage no longer obscures the lungs to the same extent as on lower kVp films. The mediastinum is also penetrated better in high-kVp films, thereby allowing more details to be viewed of the mediastinum and large airways **(Fig. 6)**. Scattered radiation is higher at high kVp, causing significant degradation of image quality. To minimize this effect a grid or an air gap of 15 cm between the patient and cassette is used, thereby improving image quality. If an air gap is used, the distance between patient and X-ray beam is increased to 12 feet to avoid magnification of the mediastinum. A drawback of high kVp is a lack of demonstration of calcified lesions and small pulmonary nodules. Low-kVp films have the advantage of providing excellent detail in the unobscured lung, as there is excellent contrast resolution between vessels and aerated lung.

Digital chest radiography has now nearly totally replaced analog radiography modalities. There have been compelling reasons for this shift. The availability of data in an electronic form makes it possible to postprocess the image data so as to present optimal image quality, view the images on large high-resolution workstations, archive as well as distribute images across a hospital network or to any remote location. Computed radiography or CR, the first commercially available digital X-ray imaging technique is still the most popular digital imaging technique available today. In this technique, conventional X-ray film is replaced by a phosphor plate. This phosphor plate when exposed to X-rays, stores the X-ray radiation as energy. This phosphor plate is read by a laser beam which releases the energy stored on the phosphor plate as light, producing an image. Recently, flat panel detectors have been introduced.

These do away with the need to have a cassette containing the phosphor plate. The images are instantly available as soon as the X-ray is exposed. The image quality

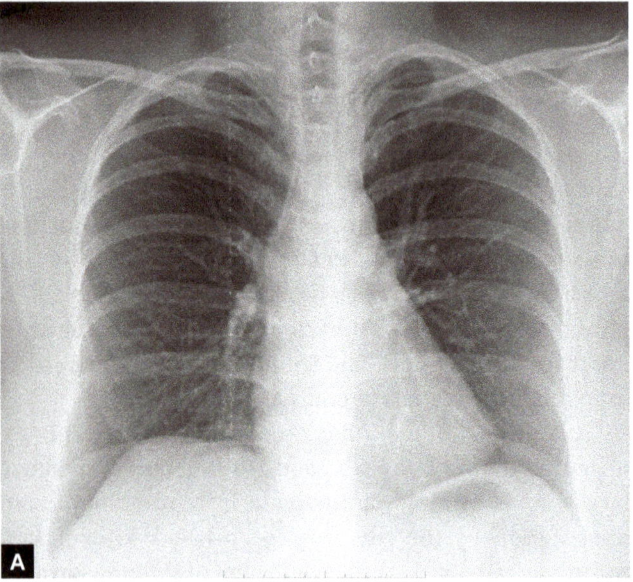

Fig. 2: PA view of the chest: Normal chest X-ray, note scapulae have been rotated off the chest so as to avoid obscuration of lung parenchyma.

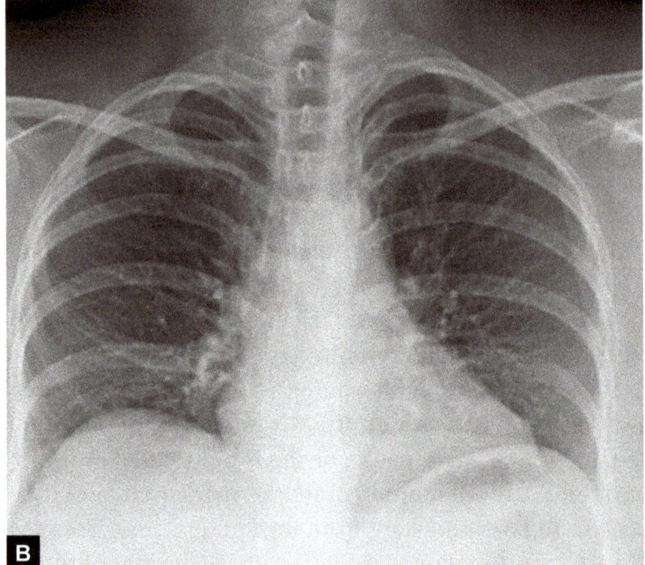

Figs. 3A and B: Inspiratory and expiratory views: PA view of the chest in inspiration (A) and in expiration (B) of same patient. Note change in mediastinal contour as well as diffuse haziness in both lung bases on expiratory view simulating interstitial lung disease.

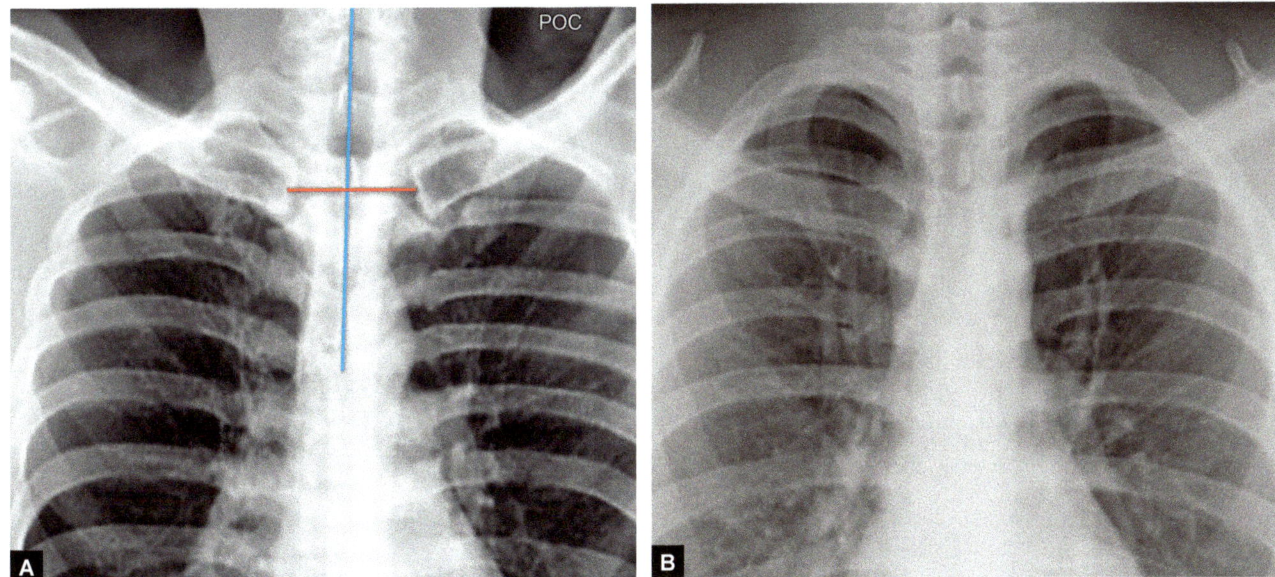

Figs. 4A and B: Rotation: (A) To check for rotation on a PA view, a vertical line is drawn along the spinous processes of the vertebrae (blue). Horizontal line is drawn between the medial ends of the clavicles so as to cut the vertical line. The medial ends of the clavicles should be equidistant when there is no rotation (B) Note rotation to left as medial end of right clavicles rotates further away this results in a right paratracheal opacity representing SVC shadow. This opacity may simulate a mass or adenopathy.

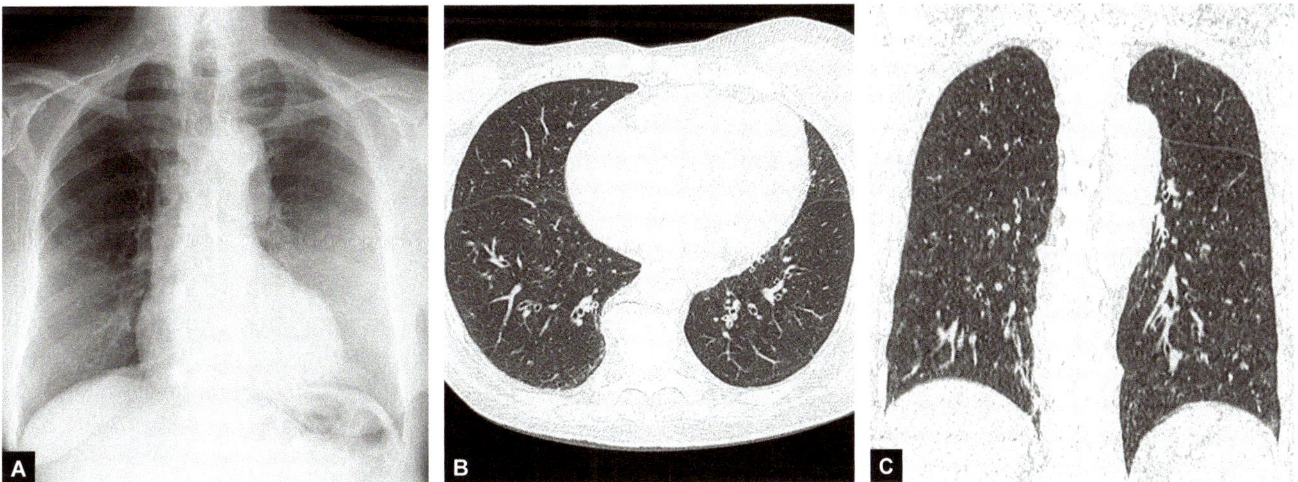

Figs. 5A to C: (A) Chest X-ray reveals haziness in the left mid and lower zones. (B and C) Axial and coronal CT sections revealed absence of any pathology. Left sided haziness in the X-ray was due to the rotation to the left.

is superior and as no cassette is involved, the work flow is much faster.

◼ ADDITIONAL VIEWS

Lateral

The utility of this view is to check whether an equivocal frontal chest X-ray shadow is actually present, to position an abnormality seen on a frontal X-ray, and define as to which lobe it is located in. The patient stands perpendicular to the cassette with arms held high and well away from the thorax. The lateral chest X-ray is not of much use in evaluating the apices, as the shoulders overlap this region (**Figs. 7 to 10**).

Lateral Decubitus

Lateral decubitus is a useful view to demonstrate a small pleural effusion which is not visible on the PA view, or differentiate a free pleural effusion from loculated pleural

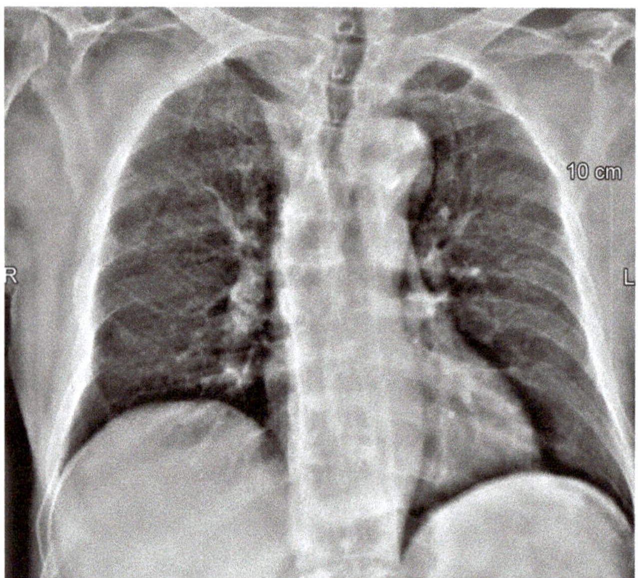

Fig. 6: High-kVp X-ray demonstrates the lung fields well, the opacity of overlying ribs is reduced considerably; note the detail of the mediastinum and trachea. A disadvantage of this technique is a lower detection rate of pulmonary nodules and calcified granulomas as compared to low-kVp X-ray.

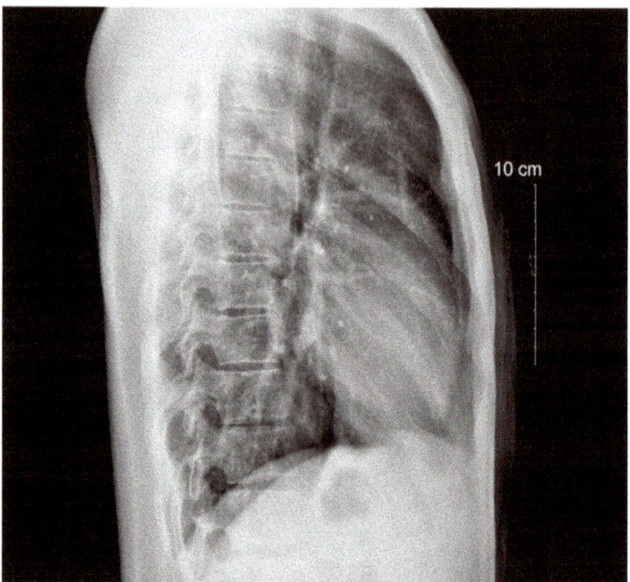

Fig. 8: Lateral X-ray of chest: A normal lateral X-ray of the chest. Important points to note are: (1) Increasing lucency of the descending dorsal vertebrae. Loss of this progressive lucency is indicative of a pathological process in this location. (2) Homogenous cardiac opacity as well as aerated retrosternal region. Loss of homogeneity in this region would indicate the presence of a pathological process.

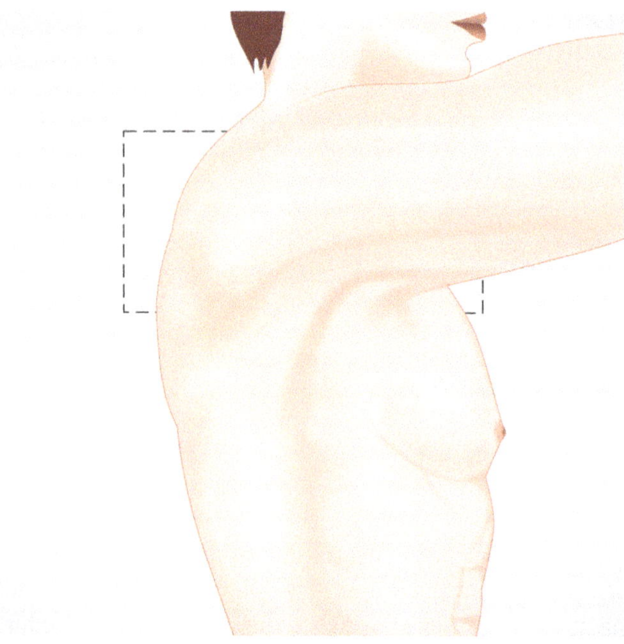

Fig. 7: Lateral view of chest and positioning for a lateral view: Left side of chest is in contact with the cassette, this reduces cardiac magnification as compared to right side; arms are held up.

fluid or pleural thickening **(Fig. 11)**. A frontal radiograph is obtained with the patient lying in a decubitus position with the side suspected to have pleural effusion down. Free fluid gravitates along the dependent chest wall between the lungs and chest wall.

Lateral Shoot Through

This view is useful to demonstrate a small anterior pneumothorax in a supine patient. The X-ray beam is directed horizontally from one lateral chest wall and the cassette is placed along the other lateral chest wall.

Lateral Oblique

This view is used to demonstrate rib fractures and rib lesions. The axillary course of a rib is obscured on a frontal radiograph; on oblique view these are well visualized. The patient is rotated by 45° and a frontal radiograph is obtained.

Lordotic View

On a frontal radiograph the apices are often obscured by the clavicle and first rib thereby obscuring a lesion in this location. Subtle tubercular lesions hidden beneath the first rib/clavicle can be well-demonstrated on this view

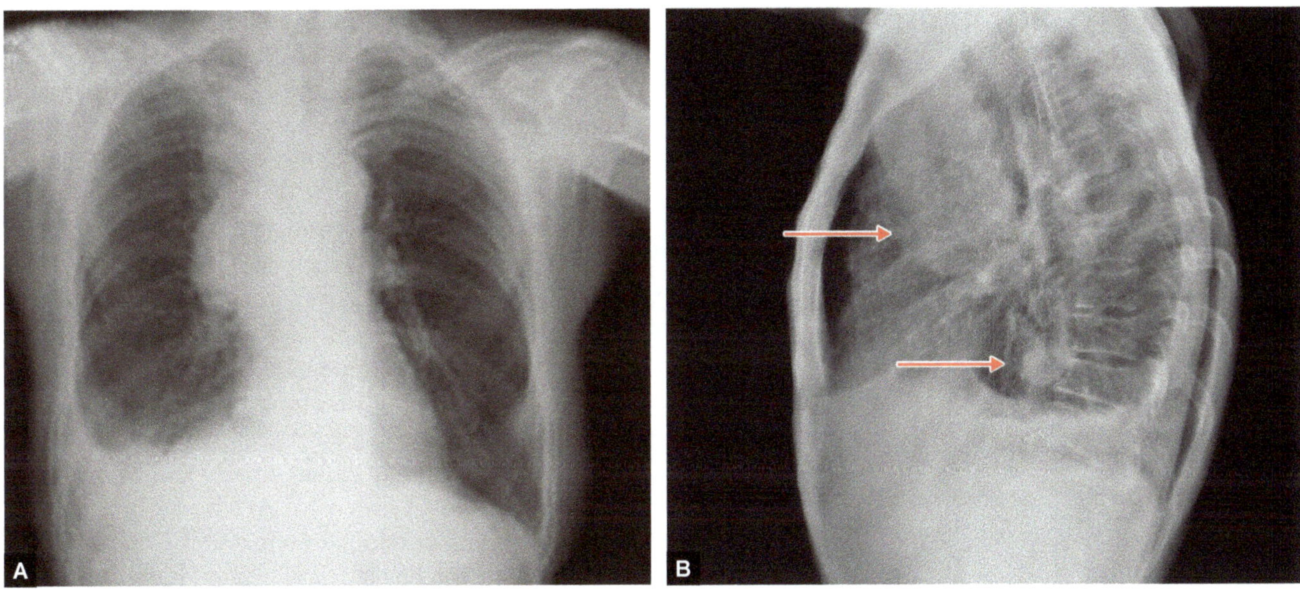

Figs. 9A and B: (A) PA view of the chest demonstrates a large mass lesion in the right upper and middle zone, silhouetting the right mediastinal border, with a small right pleural effusion; (B) Lateral X-ray demonstrates the large opacity overlying the upper cardiac silhouette as well as partly obliterating the retrosternal air space. The translucency over the lower dorsal vertebrae is lost due to presence of pleural fluid. Note well-defined lower zone pulmonary nodule overlying anterior end of lower dorsal vertebra. This lesion was not appreciated on the PA view.

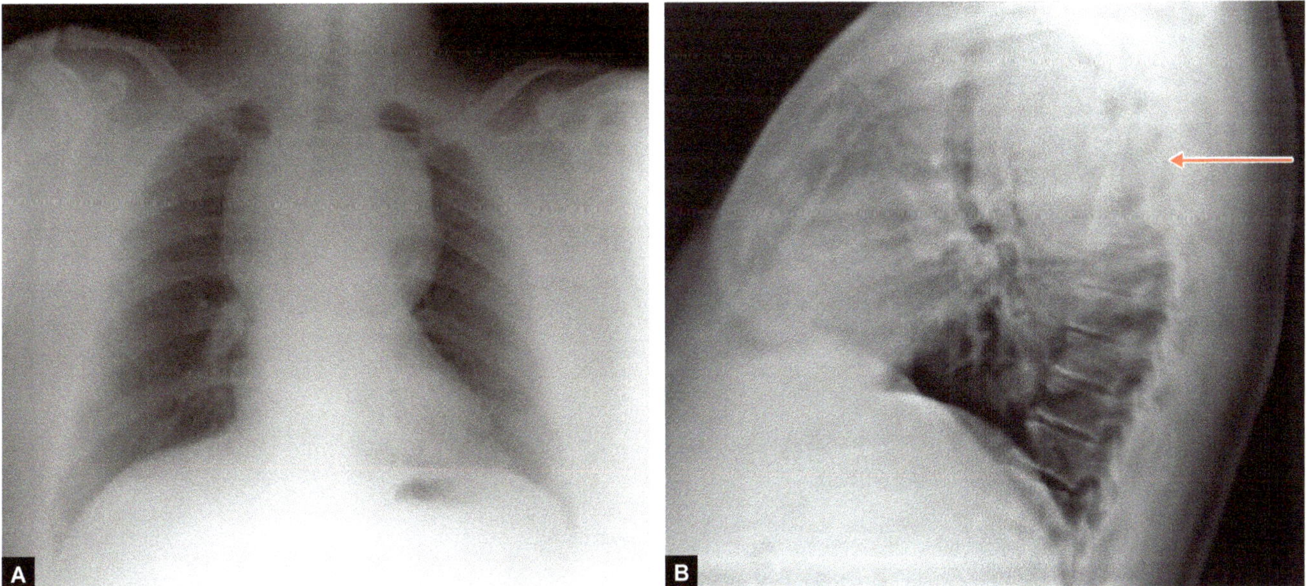

Figs. 10A and B: Posterior mediastinal mass: (A) PA view of the chest reveals a large mass lesion occupying and extending beyond the confines of the mediastinum; (B) Lateral view localizes the mass to the posterior mediastinum. The mass lesion is seen as a homogenous opacity posterior to the trachea as well as displacing the trachea anteriorly.

(Figs. 12A and B). Additionally, on a PA view it may be difficult to discern between a fibrotic tubercular lesion and costochondral cartilage; a lordotic view would be able to differentiate the two. The patient is positioned upright and the X-ray beam is angled 15° upward or alternatively the X-ray beam is kept horizontal and the patient arched backward resembling the posture of a "lord" **(Figs. 13A and B)**.

PORTABLE RADIOGRAPHS

These are extremely useful as they are performed at the patient's bedside. They do have their share of limitations. Due to the shorter tube focus distance, there is mediastinal magnification. High-kVp techniques are not possible as the output of these machines is limited, the exposure time is longer, so that patients may be unable to hold their breath, resulting in motion artifacts. The positioning of these patients is also a challenge as they are often half

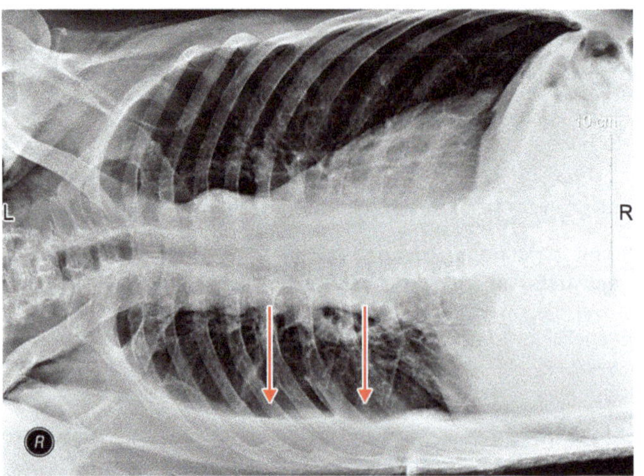

Fig. 11: Lateral decubitus: PA view of the chest had demonstrated a right basal opacity, ? collapse consolidation, ? pleural fluid. X-ray taken with patient lying on his right side; there is fluid layering along the chest wall indicating a free pleural effusion.

upright or rotated. Patients also find it difficult to take a deep breath in a semi-erect position. Digital X-rays have fortunately helped considerably to improve image quality of portable X-rays. Similar to X-rays taken in the imaging department using CR, the same CR cassettes can be used in the intensive care unit (ICU), and processed in the same readers available in the imaging department. DR or digital radiography units which do not require a cassette and which are available for an imaging department are also available for portable radiography **(Figs. 14A and B)**. These have a great advantage; they provide an instant image, thereby saving precious time—time taken to transport a cassette to the imaging department, process it, archive the image and transport it back. These however at present are extremely expensive. As a bridge, portable CR readers are being developed, so that at the bedside itself the CR cassette can be read, producing a quick image.

There are newer novel applications developing in digital radiography—*Dual Energy, Tomosynthesis and Temporal Subtraction.*

Dual-energy Subtraction Imaging

The absorption of X-ray by tissues depends upon the kilovoltage (kV) used, as well as on the consistency of the tissues. When kV is varied the response of tissues changes; as a result tissues can be separated from each other at different kVs. In the chest, bone and soft tissue

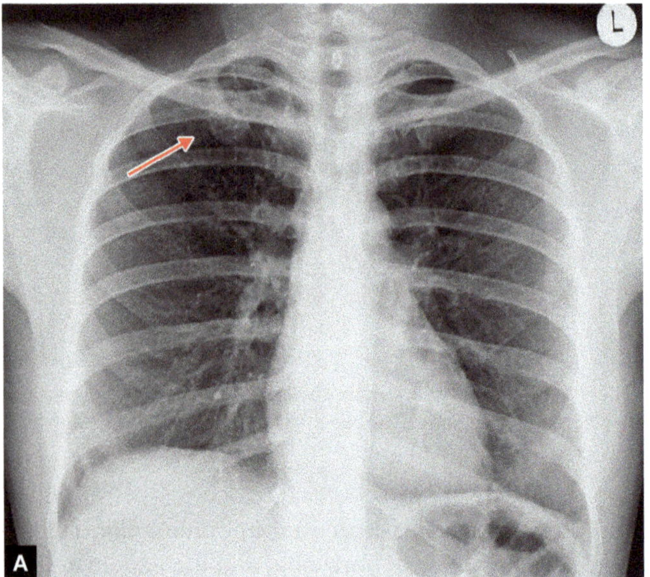

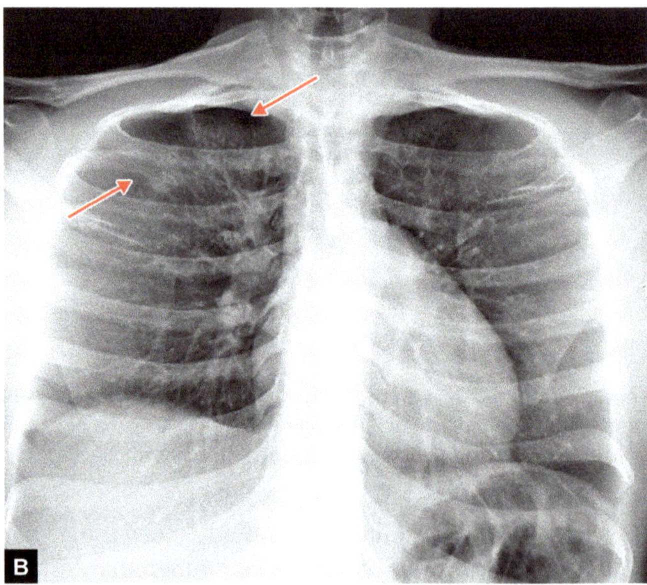

Figs. 12A and B: Lordotic view: (A) PA view of the chest reveals a questionable opacity underlying the first rib on the right side; (B) Lordotic view uncovers the first rib demonstrating ill-defined soft opacities in the right apex due to active tuberculous infection.

both appear bright on low kV, so that a pulmonary nodule underlying a rib will be obscured due to their similar densities. At higher kV the attenuation of calcium and soft tissue to X-rays differs. This principle is used to generate images using different kVs. The images are subtracted to provide images with only soft tissue. This helps to improve detection of a solitary pulmonary nodule as only soft tissue is seen and no bone.

Digital Tomosynthesis

Digital tomosynthesis is a technique where images of a certain depth in the chest are obtained. The tissues above and below this level are blurred, only tissue at that depth is visualized. This is similar to tomography of the olden days, now using digital techniques to enhance the evaluation.

Temporal Subtraction

This technique utilizes subtraction of a previous image from the present image. If there is any interval change it will be demonstrated. Inaccuracies do occur in terms of positioning as well as differences in breathhold.

Computer-aided Diagnosis

This is a technique which relies on a pattern recognition approach using artificial intelligence to help detect lesions which may be missed by radiologists. The main applications being evaluated at present are detection of pulmonary nodules, as well as pulmonary emboli (**Fig. 15**). These techniques are yet to become popular, as there is a high rate of false-positive detection; also the detection rate is similar to that observed by radiologists.

■ LIMITATIONS OF CHEST X-RAY

The limitations of a chest X-ray relate essentially to the fact that the chest X-ray is a 2D modality, imaging a

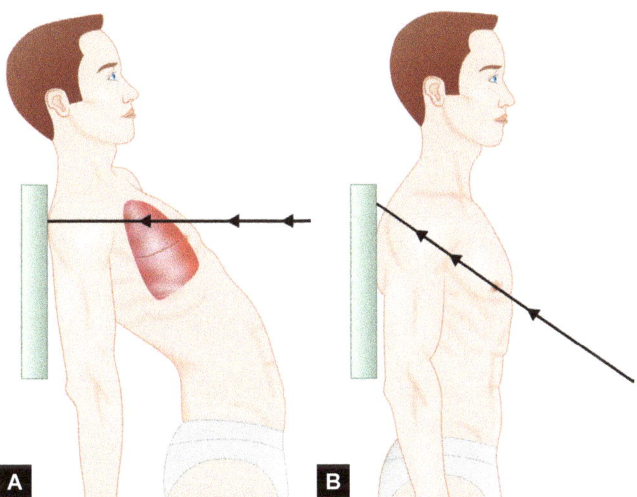

Figs. 13A and B: Lordotic X-rays demonstrate two methods of demonstration of the apices without overlap of first rib, in (A) the X-ray beam is horizontal, the patient is arched back simulating a "lord". In the other method (B) the X-ray beam is angled upwards by 15° to the apex, the patient stands straight with back to the cassette.

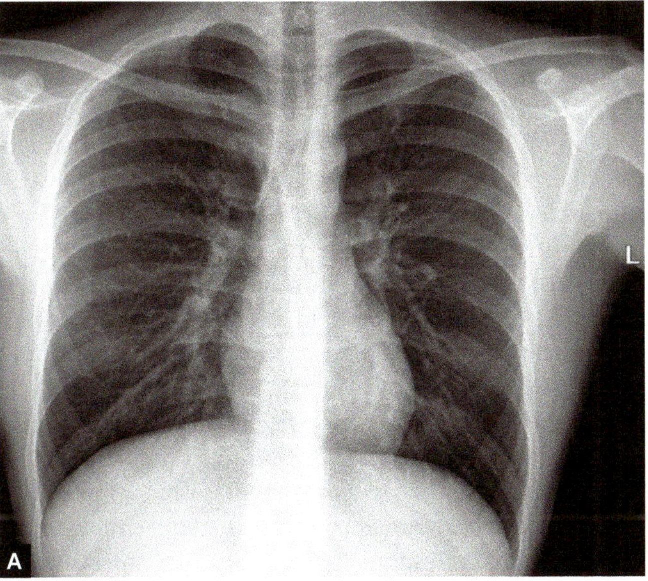
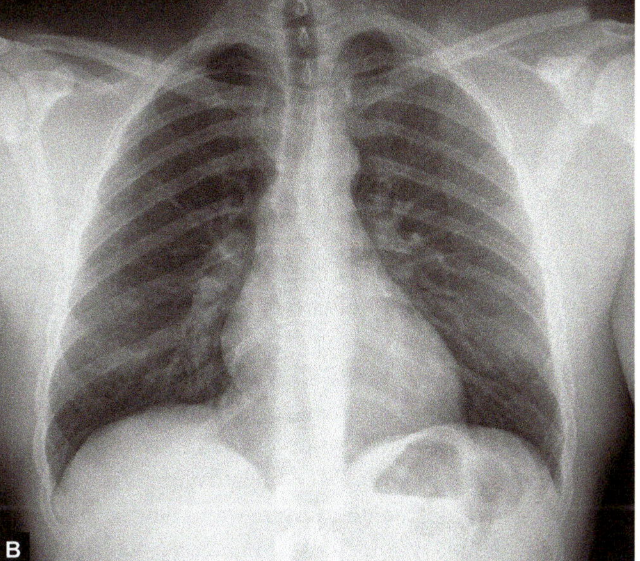

Figs. 14A and B: Portable chest radiograph: (A) PA view and (B) portable AP view of the chest. Note the change in cardiac outline between a PA view and an AP view. Commenting on cardiomegaly on an AP view may be hazardous.

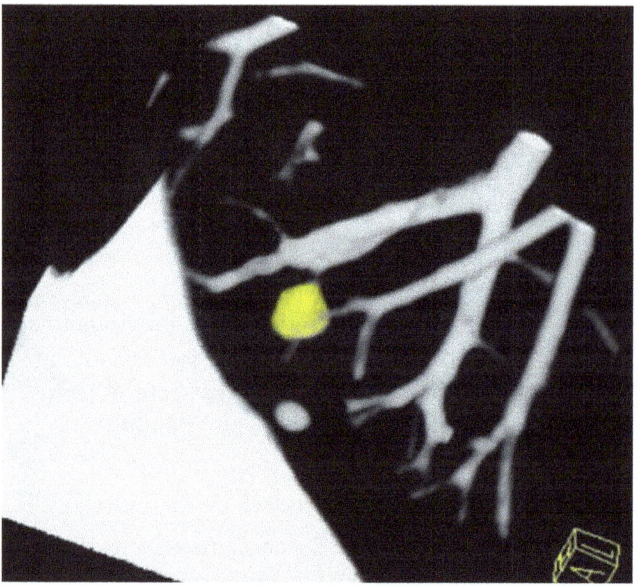

Fig. 15: Computer-aided diagnosis (CAD): CAD demonstrates a pulmonary nodule colored in yellow, separate from adjacent vessels. The volume of this nodule can be easily determined. The nodule can be followed up on subsequent examinations to determine rate of growth. CAD helps in detecting lesions which may have been missed by radiologists; at present CAD has a high false-positive detection rate; however, it is extremely useful for volume measurements.

three-dimensional (3D) structure. Nearly 75% of the lungs are covered by ribs, mediastinum and diaphragm; as a result a number of anatomical structures are superimposed reducing the detectability of lesions. From a technical aspect since the chest is a large region to be imaged, approximately 40 cm, as the whole of this area has to be radiated, there is significant scatter radiation resulting in degradation of image quality.

■ COMPUTED TOMOGRAPHY

CT has been heralded as the greatest discovery in medicine following the discovery of X-rays. The history of the development of the CT scanner is extremely unique. Electrical and musical industries (EMI) became famous in the 1960s as they were the record label for the Beatles. At their Abbey Road studios they recorded enough Vinyl for the Beatles to go around the earth's circumference. They became a cash-rich company. Godfrey Hounsfield, an eminent scientist with EMI who had already developed the first all-transistor computer, was keen to develop a product which would more effectively evaluate the attenuation of X-rays through soft tissues. This research was funded directly by profits from the Beatles. In 1972,

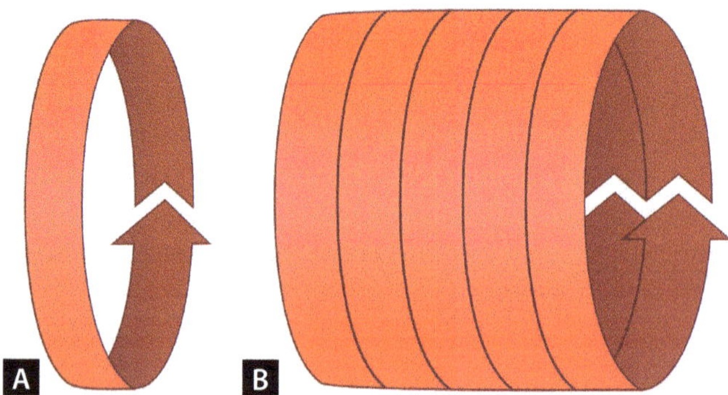

Figs. 16A and B: Helical CT: (A) Demonstrates a conventional CT which obtained slices one by one; (B) Demonstrates a helical CT, all slices are obtained simultaneously in one breathhold.

Godfrey Hounsfield unveiled the first CT scanner to the world named as EMI. That scanner took 4 minutes to acquire a single slice and a further 7 minutes to reconstruct the image. CT has come a long way since those days with the entire thorax being scanned with a dual-source CT in under a second in 2010. Not only did the Beatles spawn an entire shift in musical tastes, outlook, physical appearance and hairstyles for nearly the entire globe, they contributed to one of the greatest advances in medicine since the discovery of X-rays.

CT scanners are based on the same principles as X-ray. Tissues attenuate X-rays differently depending on their composition, i.e. atomic number; thereby a CT scanner is able to detect minute differences in attenuation by tissues, providing extremely high anatomical detail. A CT scanner consists of an X-ray tube which emits X-rays, and a detector opposite to the X-ray tube. This combined assembly rotates 360° around the patient acquiring data. Data from one 360° rotation produces a single image. Present-day scanners are helical scanners; data is acquired simultaneously with the table moving and X-ray tube rotating during a single breathhold. This technique has significant advantages over the previous nonhelical scanners. As scans are acquired in a single breathhold, the possibility of missing a pulmonary nodule due to respiratory misregistration does not arise **(Figs. 16 and 17)**. Data is acquired as a volume and therefore can be reconstructed at any slice thickness as well as in any plane which is desired. Additionally, as the scan time is shorter, less intravenous contrast medium is required. Helical scanners have advanced technologically from being single-detector to multidetector scanners (MDCT) **(Figs. 18A and B)**. These MDCT scanners may have from 2 rows to 64 rows of detectors. Increasing the

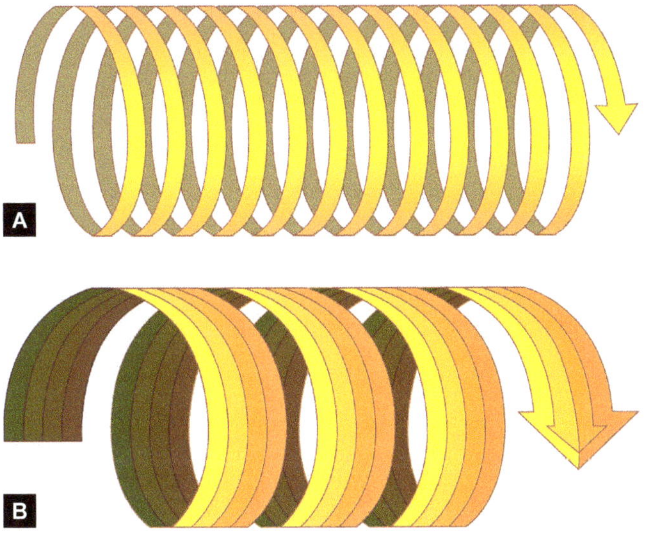

Figs. 17A and B: Multidetector CT: (A) Demonstrates a single-slice helical CT rotation; (B) Demonstrates a multidetector helical CT rotation.

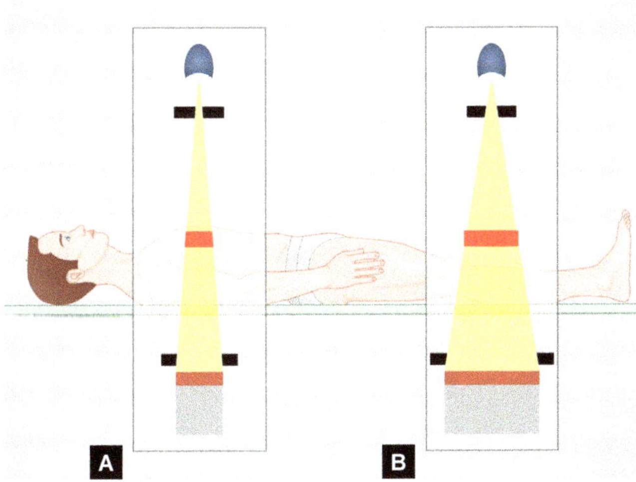

Figs. 18A and B: Multidetector CT: Comparison between a single-detector CT and a multidetector CT. (A) Single-detector (B) Multidetector CT. Note the increased coverage in a single rotation with a multidetector CT allowing for large volume coverage in shorter time with thinner slices.

number of rows of detectors enables faster scans, reducing respiratory and motion artifacts. Angiographic images may be obtained as well as larger volumes may be covered, with thinner sections obtained. A CT image is a 2D image, but there is a third dimension, depth or slice thickness. A thick slice contains different tissues within the section, which will be averaged to produce the final image. To obtain a high degree of anatomical detail as with high-resolution CT (HRCT) very thin sections are required, 1 mm or less,

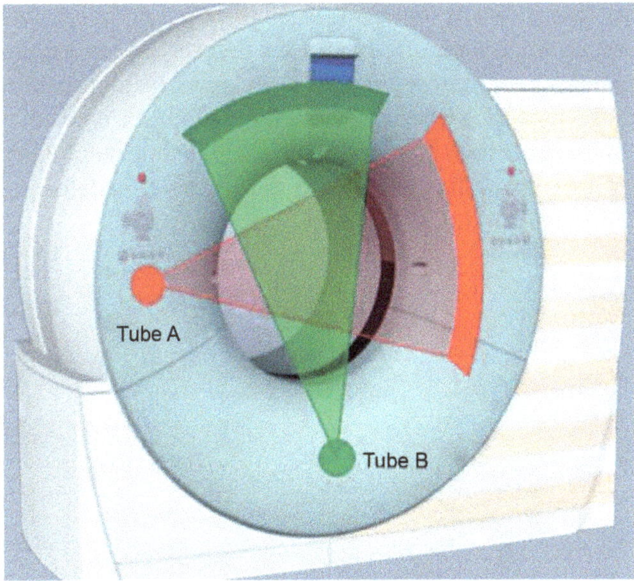

Fig. 19: Dual-source CT: New generation of CT scanners with two CT tubes, providing faster scans and higher temporal resolution, of particular value in coronary angiograms as there is no need of beta-blockers, and images are of higher resolution.

so that there is no averaging of tissues. These scanners have further revolutionized the diagnostic potential of CT, especially the 16, 64 slice scanners, as these produce thin slices (0.6–0.75 mm) which are isotropic, i.e. reconstruction of these slices in any plane results in no loss of resolution. These scanners have essentially converted CT from an axial cross-sectional technique to a true 3D technique allowing arbitrary selection of scan planes, and volumetric display of data. Newer scanners with 128 rows, 256 rows, 360 rows and dual-source CT have been introduced essentially to facilitate CT coronary angiography. The dual-source CT houses two CT scanners in one CT gantry. The advantage of this is in the performance of CT coronary angiograms without the need to use beta-blockers. As dual-source CT scanners have two X-ray tubes, they can fire at different energies resulting in dual-energy scans **(Figs. 19 and 20)**. This is useful in obtaining lung perfusion scans. These help in the detection of pulmonary embolism. Segmental and subsegmental emboli may only be detected by demonstrating a perfusion defect on dual-energy scans **(Figs. 21A and B)**.

Respiratory Misregistration

Conventional CT scanned the chest slice by slice. With every slice, the patient was asked to hold his or her breath, the table then moved to the next table position and another slice was obtained. The illustration demonstrates respiratory misregistration. In the first section, due to an increased inspiratory effort the nodule goes below the slice; in the next slice where the nodule should be visualized, it is not, as the patient has taken only a moderate inspiratory effort. This resulted in a lower accuracy for CT in detecting pulmonary nodules **(Fig. 22)**.

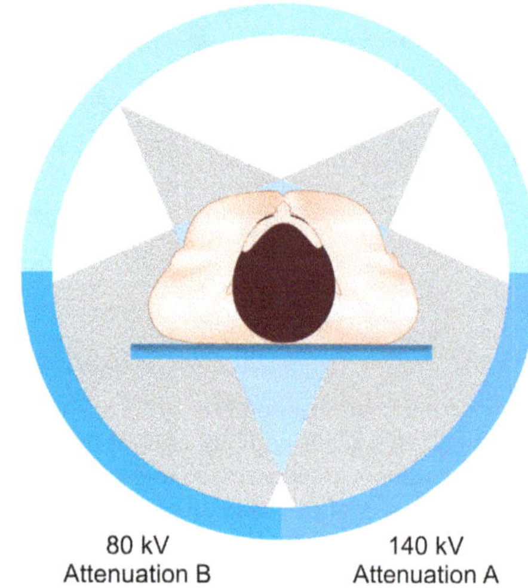

Fig. 20: Dual-energy CT: Schematic diagram of a dual-energy CT scan, two tubes firing at different kVs, one at 80 kV and other at 140 kV simultaneously.

Multiplanar reconstructions (MPR) allow reconstruction of images in any plane such as the coronal, sagittal or any oblique plane **(Figs. 23A to D)**. Curved multiplanar reconstructions are also possible where a curved structure such as a vessel or airway may be straightened out; its diameter as well as extent of stenosis may be quantified **(Figs. 24 and 25)**.

Volume-rendering techniques (VRTs) are 3D techniques which provide a rendering of the surface of the organ. These are useful for demonstrating the tracheobronchial tree, as well as vasculature, especially the aorta and coronary arteries. An adaptation of this technique is virtual bronchoscopy. A 3D volume of the tracheobronchial tree is obtained, utilizing a fly-through software. The internal contents of the tracheobronchial tree can be visualized similar to an optical bronchoscopy, the advantages of a virtual bronchoscopy being the ability to demonstrate tracheobronchial stenosis, extrinsic compression, intraluminal masses, foreign bodies or intraluminal extension of extrinsic lesions. Internal measurements of the tracheobronchial tree are also possible **(Figs. 26 to 31)**. This helps to determine the length and size of stents required in planning surgery. The main disadvantage is the inability to obtain biopsies and lavages.

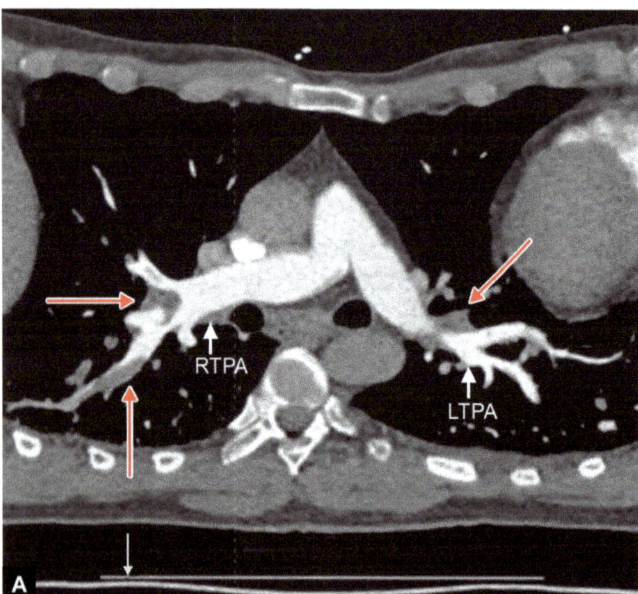

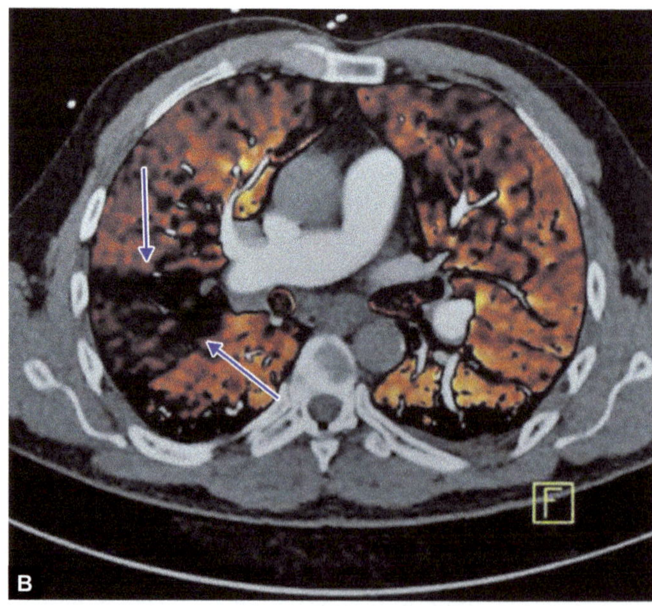

Figs. 21A and B: Dual-energy CT: CT pulmonary angiogram (A) demonstrates bilateral pulmonary emboli, particularly on the right side. Dual-energy CT (B) demonstrates perfusion defects, particularly wedge-shaped defect in right mid-zone. Dual-energy CT provides a CT angiography with a perfusion scan, thereby increasing accuracy in detection of pulmonary embolism, especially subsegmental emboli. CT data in MDCT scanners is acquired as a data volume; this data can be postprocessed to provide a variety of different images
(RTPA: Right pulmonary artery; LTPA: Left pulmonary artery).

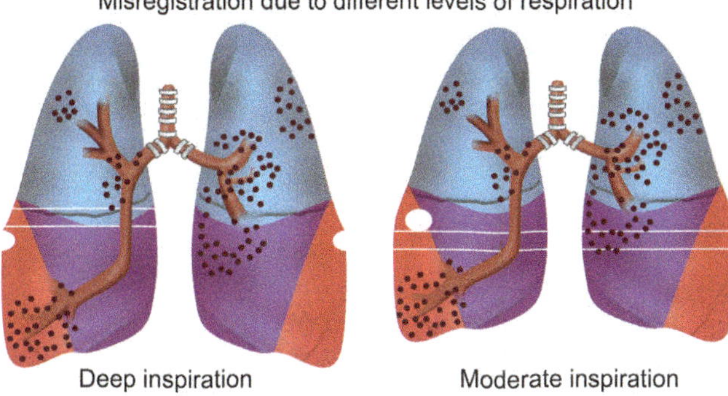

Fig. 22: Problems of conventional CT scan.

Maximum Intensity Projections

The disadvantage of thin-section CT is the inability to differentiate small nodules from vessels. On thicker sections it is possible to differentiate these as the branching appearance of vessels is easily appreciated. Maximum intensity projections (MIPs) create a thicker slab of tissue and highlight structures with high intensity such as vessels and nodules. As the slab is thicker, the branching nature of the vessels is well-appreciated, the detection of nodules is much easier **(Figs. 32A and B)**. The ideal thickness is 3 mm; an additional benefit beyond

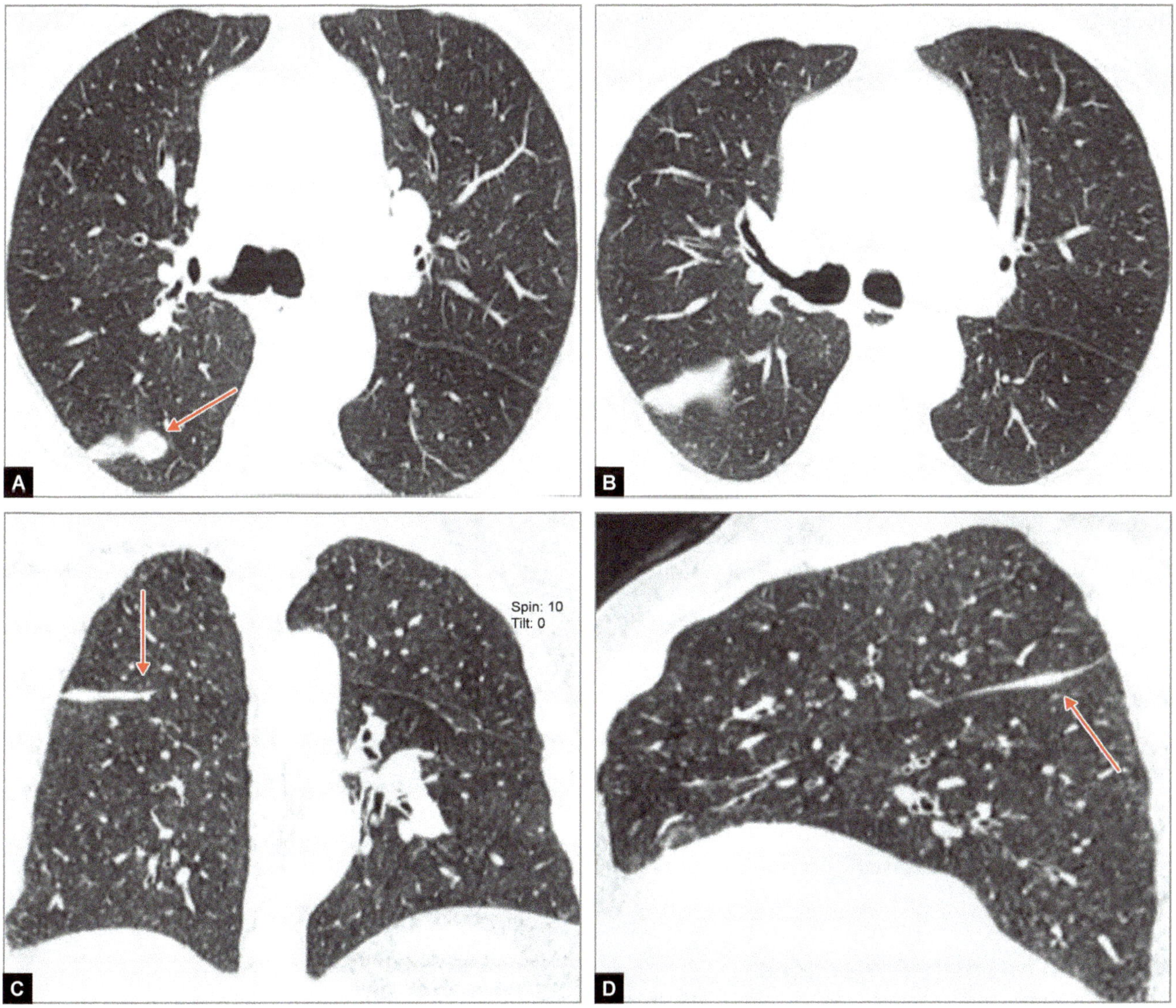

Figs. 23A to D: (A and B) Axial CT scans reveal an opacity in the right upper lobe. On the axial scans it is difficult to determine the etiology of the lesion; (C and D) Coronal and sagittal reconstructions demonstrate that the opacity represents fluid in the interlobar fissure. An example of how visualization of an abnormality in multiple planes may help establish the location, extent and etiology of the lesion.

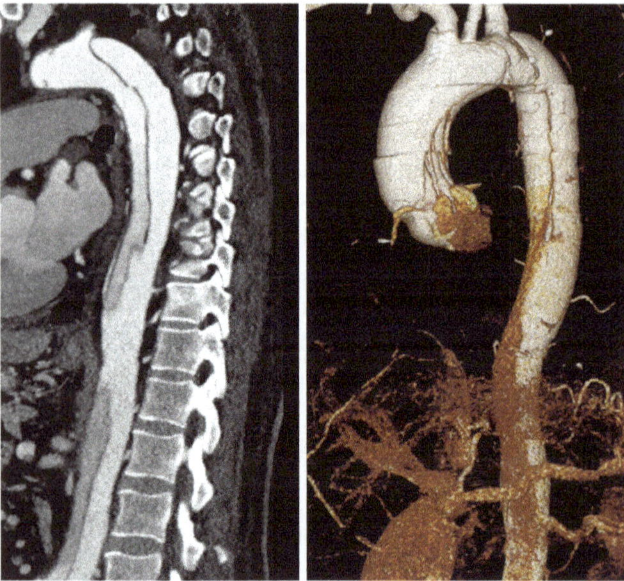

Fig. 24: Curved multiplanar reconstruction (MPR): Curved MPR of aorta demonstrates displaced intimal flap separating true from false lumen, this is also well depicted on the volume rendering technique (VRT) image. The advantage of curved MPR is that a curvilinear structure can be straightened out.

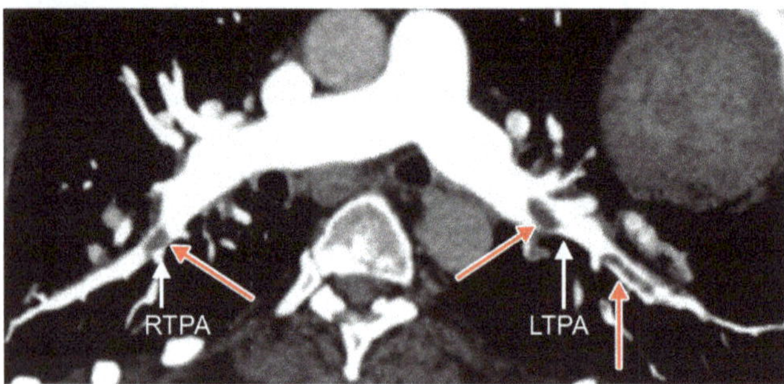

Fig. 25: Curved multiplanar reconstruction (MPR) of pulmonary arteries: Curved MPR demonstrates main pulmonary artery and both right and left pulmonary arteries in one image. Note multiple pulmonary emboli in right and left pulmonary arteries. The advantage of a curved MPR is that the main, right and left pulmonary arteries can be demonstrated in a single image.
(RTPA: Right pulmonary artery; LTPA: Left pulmonary artery)

precise detection is an accurate characterization of the location of the nodules in relation to the vessels—whether centrilobular or perivascular. For detection of miliary nodules or pulmonary metastatic deposits this technique is ideal.

Minimum Intensity Projections

In emphysema, bronchiolitis obliterans, the contrast between normal and low-attenuation lung parenchyma may be subtle on inspiratory HRCT. Such subtle regional

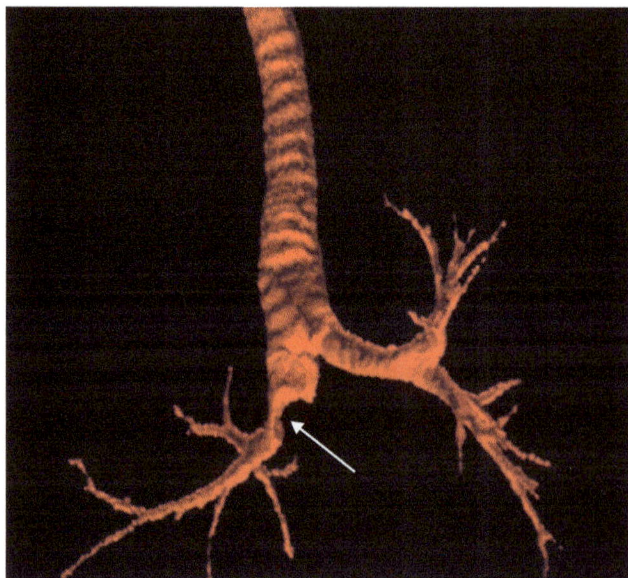

Fig. 26: Volume rendering technique (VRT) of trachea: Volume-rendered image of the trachea demonstrates an extrinsic mass lesion indenting the right main bronchus, causing significant narrowing of its lumen.

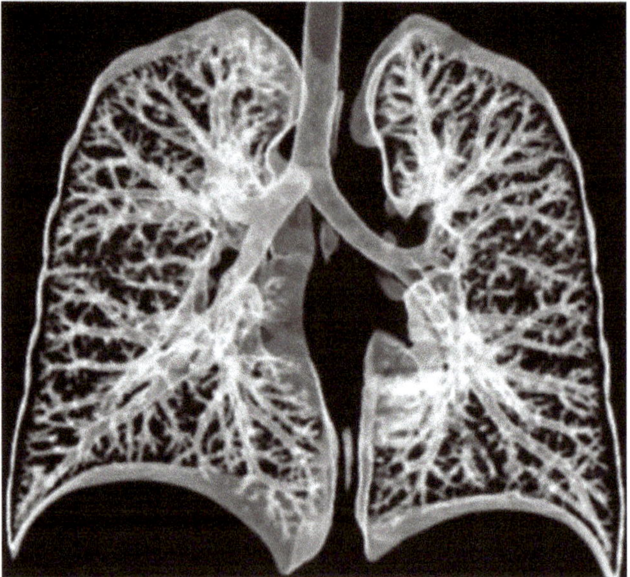

Fig. 27: Volume rendering technique (VRT) tracheobronchial tree. Volume-rendered 3D image of the tracheobronchial tree, no abnormality was detected. Note the visualization of not only the tracheobronchial tree, but also segmental and subsegmental bronchi.

density differences can be highlighted by minimum intensity projections (MinIPs) **(Figs. 33 and 34)**. MinIPs correlate excellently with pulmonary function tests. Another useful application of MinIP is demonstration

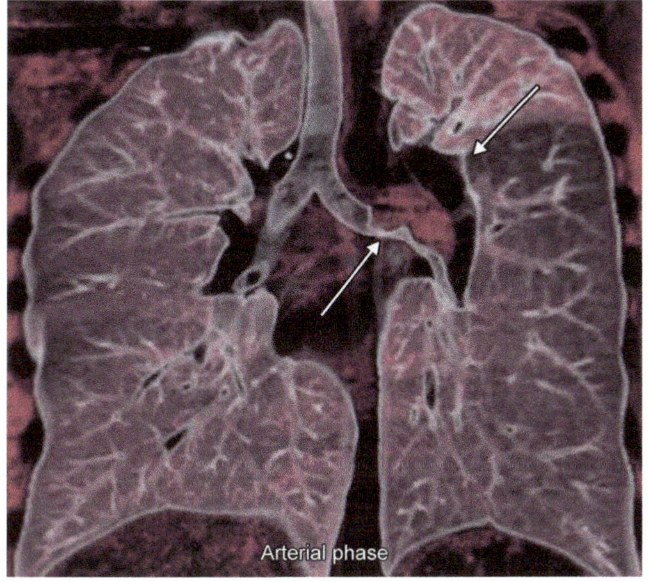

Fig. 28: Volume rendering technique (VRT) tracheobronchial tree: Volume-rendered image of tracheobronchial tree and lung parenchyma. Mass lesion seen in left upper lobe infiltrates the left upper lobe bronchus causing significant narrowing of its lumen.

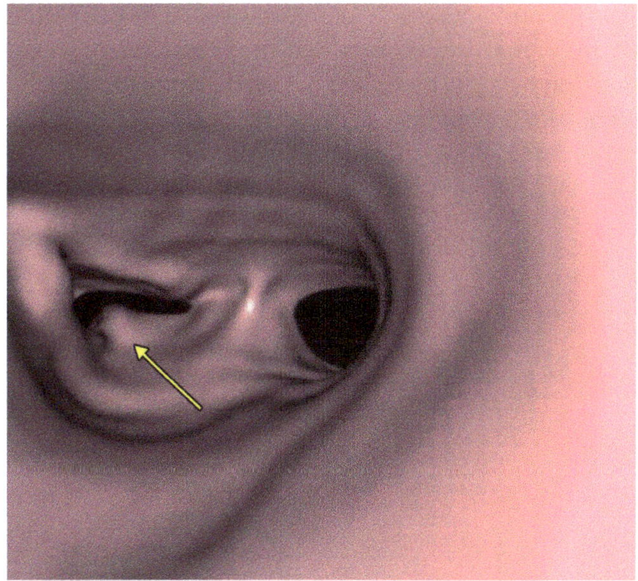

Fig. 29: Virtual bronchoscopy. Virtual bronchoscopy at the level of the carina reveals marked irregularity and narrowing of the right main bronchus due to a bronchogenic carcinoma.

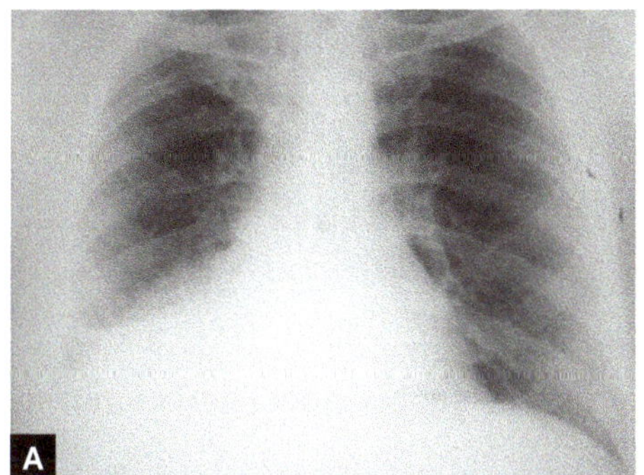
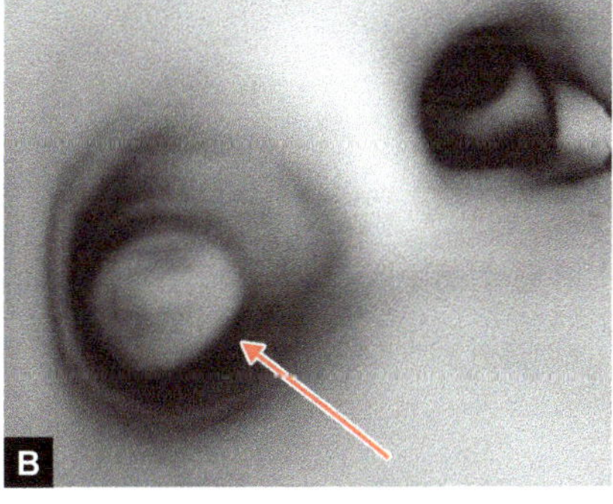
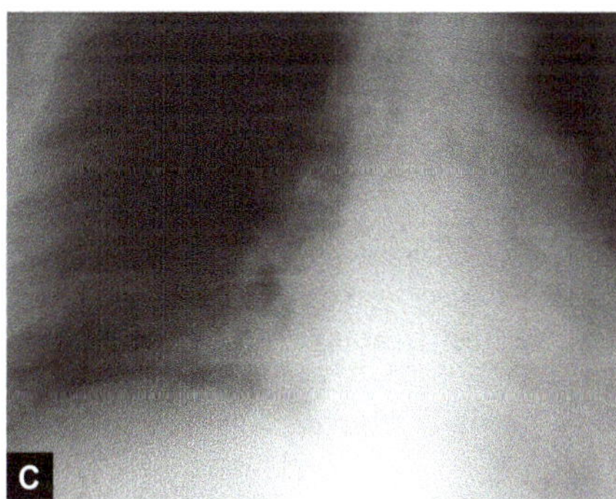

Figs. 30A to C: Virtual bronchoscopy: (A) Chest X-ray reveals an area of collapse consolidation in right lower zone. (B) Virtual bronchoscopy reveals a well-defined foreign body in the right bronchus. (C) Post procedure, chest X-ray reveals clearing of collapse consolidation.

of tracheobronchial tree stenosis/occlusions **(Fig. 35)**. A window width of 350–500 HU and a window level of –750 to –900 HU is ideal **(Fig. 36)**.

Window Settings

To visualize body structures the CT images are "windowed". Two variables are used to select the densities to be viewed: window width and window level. CT density is measured in HU values. Arbitrarily, water is considered as zero and air as –1,000. Window width determines the number of Hounsfield units to be demonstrated. Any densities greater than the upper limit of the window width are displayed as white and any below are displayed as black.

Between these two levels all densities are demonstrated in shades of gray.

■ CONTRAST MEDIA

Intravenous contrast enhancement is required to enhance mediastinal vasculature and separate vessels from mediastinal masses as well as demonstrate enhancement within mass lesions. Ionic contrast mediums which had a significant incidence of mild, moderate as well as severe reactions have now been nearly universally replaced by nonionic contrast media which are far safer. Other than anaphylactic reactions, contrast-induced nephropathy (CIN) is an important adverse event.

Contrast-induced nephropathy is an exacerbation of previously demonstrated impairment in renal function occurring within 3 days following intravascular administration of contrast medium. This is in the absence of an alternative etiology for the deteriorating renal function. An increase in serum creatinine of more than 0.5 mg/dL or 25% above the baseline serum creatinine is considered the criterion to determine the presence of contrast-induced nephropathy. CIN is by no means uncommon. It is the third most common cause of acute renal failure in patients admitted to hospital. The incidence is estimated to be 1% with intravenous contrast medium, and 2–7% with intra-arterial contrast medium. In diabetics with normal renal function it rises to 16%. In patients with preexisting renal insufficiency prior to receiving contrast media, the incidence of developing CIN is 33%. Diabetics with associated renal insufficiency are at the greatest risk for developing CIN. Other risk factors for developing CIN are dehydration, hypotension, nephrotic syndrome, multiple myeloma, use of higher dose of contrast media, repeated doses of contrast media within 48 hours, use of higher osmolar contrast media and concurrent use of nephrotoxic drugs.

To minimize the risk of CIN, universal use of nonionic contrast media, a volume expansion and the use of N-acetyl cystine are recommended. If the serum creatinine is greater than 1.4 mg/dL the possibility of another imaging modality should be considered. If a CT with contrast is considered imperative, the risk-benefit ratio should decide the issue.

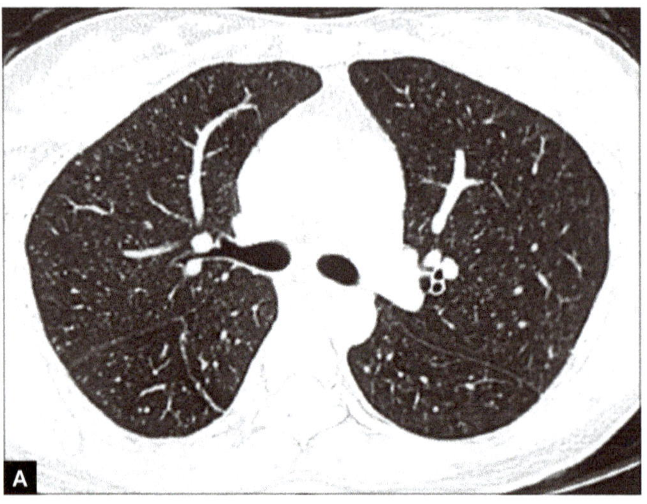

Fig. 31: Virtual bronchoscopy: Virtual bronchoscopy in an individual with carcinoma esophagus. The esophageal mass indents the posterior surface of the trachea as well as infiltrates into the lower trachea. Seen as nodular lesions projecting into the distal aspect of the trachea. This is an excellent non-invasive technique to determine local extension into the tracheobronchial tree.

SUPPORTIVE IMAGING TECHNIQUES

Sonography

This is a very useful imaging modality to demonstrate pleural fluid, especially at the bedside. Fluid manifests

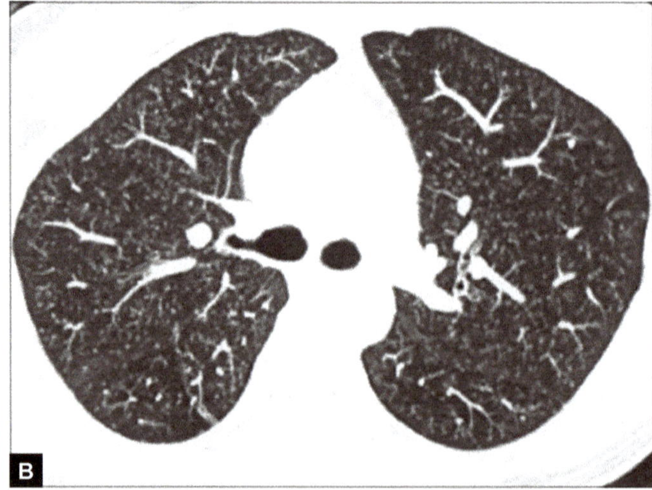

Figs. 32A and B: Maximum intensity projection (MIP): (A) Routine high-resolution computed tomography (HRCT) reveals suspicious small nodules in the lung parenchyma. As the slice thickness is very thin, it is difficult to be certain whether these represent nodules or vessels. (B) MIP demonstrates vessels very well as branching structures. The fine nodules are seen well-separate from the vessels. This technique is very useful in detecting subtle miliary nodules.

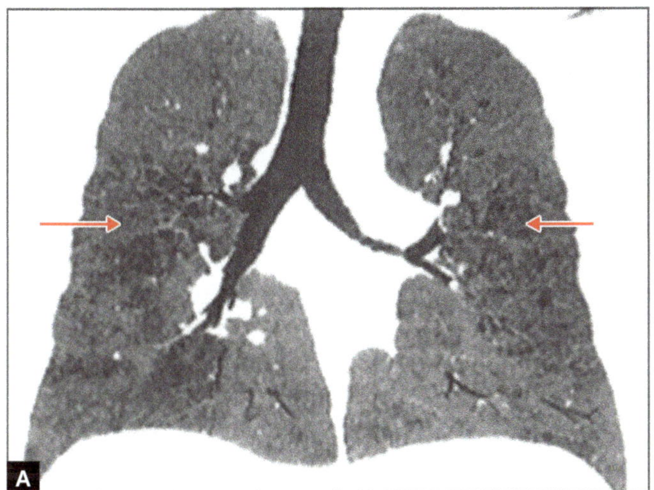

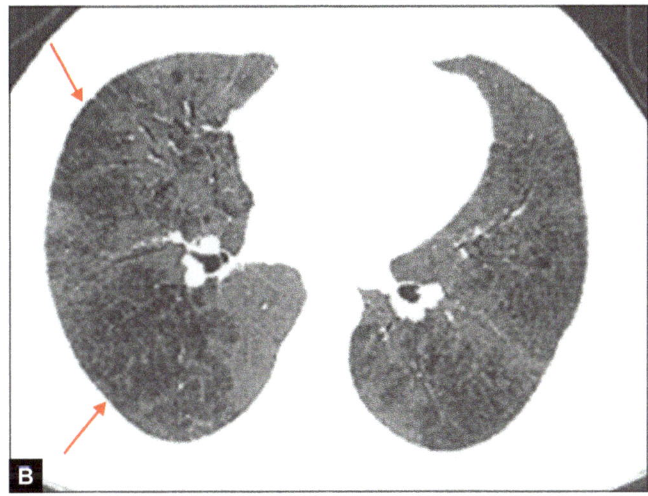

Figs. 33A and B: Minimum intensity projection: (A) coronal and (B) axial minimum intensity projections demonstrate ill-defined areas of decreased attenuation in the lung fields representing areas of emphysema.

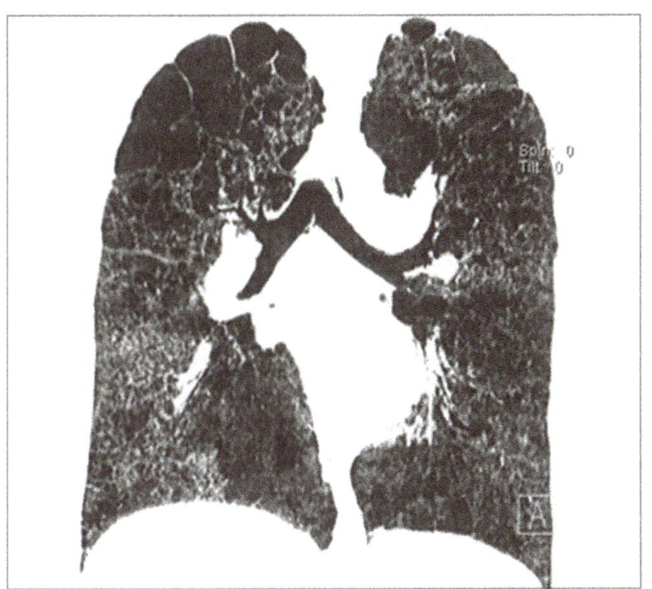

Fig. 34: Minimum intensity projections: High-resolution computed tomography (HRCT) demonstrates extensive emphysema; narrow window settings demonstrate emphysematous changes very well. Minimum intensity projections demonstrate the involvement extremely well, providing a global view.

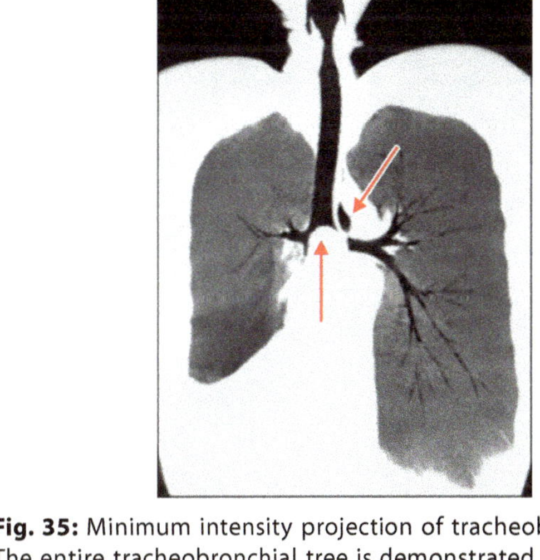

Fig. 35: Minimum intensity projection of tracheobronchial tree. The entire tracheobronchial tree is demonstrated from the level of the pharynx. There is a mass lesion at the carina indenting the carina, extending to engulf the right lower lobe bronchus with resultant right lower lobe collapse; there is extension to the left to encase the left main bronchus narrowing and obliterating the left main bronchus. Note right lower lobe collapse with elevation of diaphragm.

as an anechoic area separating the echogenic margin of lung and diaphragm. The contents of pleural fluid can also be estimated depending upon its echogenicity. Pleural fluid is usually anechoic; exudates are also anechoic but usually have internal septae **(Fig. 37)**. Empyemas have echoes within and a hemothorax has echogenic fluid. Sonography is very useful to determine whether a basal opacity on an X-ray is due to pleural fluid or collapse consolidation.

Sonography is also an excellent guide for thoracocentesis, reducing the incidence of postaspiration pneumothorax.

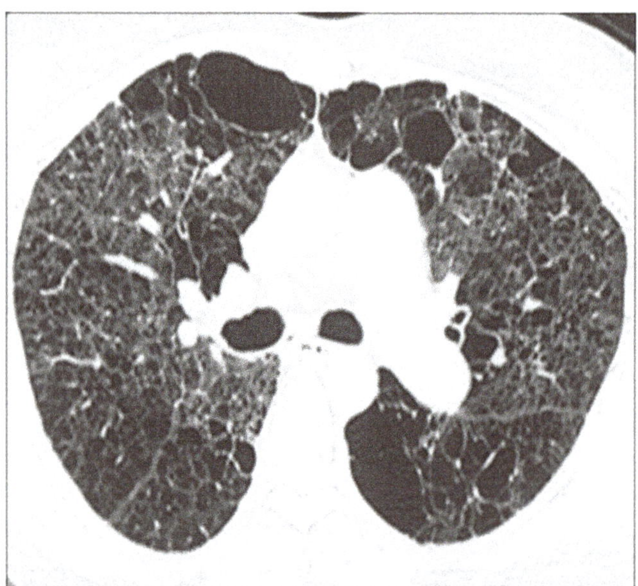

Fig. 36: Ideal window settings displaying emphysema.

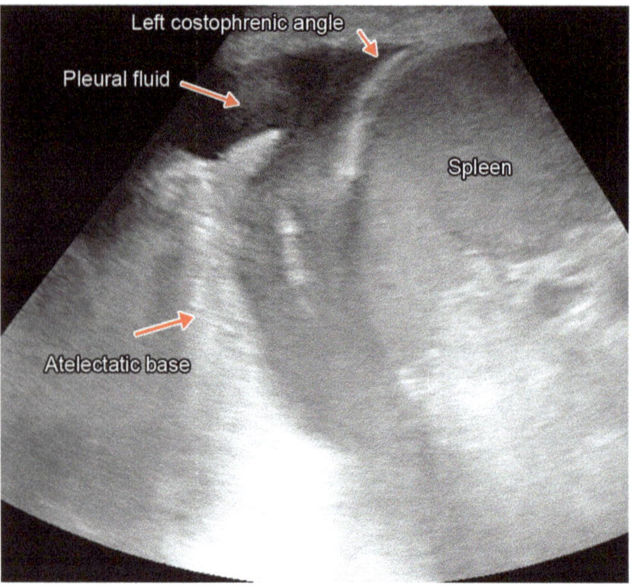

Fig. 37: Ultrasonography (USG) of the chest demonstrates a hypoechoic area representing a pleural effusion.

◾ RADIONUCLIDE IMAGING

The main utility of radionuclide imaging in the respiratory system is in the detection of pulmonary embolism. Ventilation/Perfusion scans also known as V/Q scans simultaneously image the pulmonary blood flow as well as alveolar ventilation.

Perfusion imaging is performed by intravenous injection of microparticles or human protein-labeled technetium (Tc-99). These are trapped in the pulmonary capillaries on their first pass. In patients with a right to left shunt there is a small possibility of the particles occluding systemic vessels with resultant tissue ischemia/necrosis. Similarly, in patients with pulmonary hypertension there is a risk of further occlusion of an already depleted vascular bed. In both these situations the quantum of radiotracer particles injected should be reduced, though there is usually a wide safety margin. The radiotracer has a half-life of 6–8 hours; by 24 hours, most of the activity is only visible in the kidneys and gut. The radiotracer is injected with the patient in the supine position; this limits the effect of gravity on regional blood flow. The particles mix in the heart and consequently are trapped by pulmonary precapillary arterioles. The distribution of the particles is proportional to the regional blood flow. At least six views are obtained—anterior, posterior, right lateral, left lateral, right posterior oblique, left posterior oblique. Additionally, right anterior oblique and left anterior oblique views may be obtained, if required. Even though multiple projections are obtained, perfusion scans underestimate perfusion abnormalities. For example, the medial basal segment of the right lower lobe is completely surrounded by normal lung; consequently, a perfusion defect is not detected on planar perfusion imaging.

All parenchymal diseases cause a reduction in pulmonary blood flow in the affected lung zone. In pulmonary embolism, perfusion is reduced whereas ventilation is preserved. Parenchymal lung diseases cause both a ventilation defect and a perfusion defect. Tc-99m radio-labeled aerosols are used for ventilation scans. Approximately 30 mCi of radiotracer in 3 mL of saline is placed within a nebulizer. Oxygen is forced through the nebulizer at high pressure to form aerosolized droplets which are inhaled by the patient via a mouthpiece. The distribution of the radiotracer is proportional to regional ventilation. Images are obtained in multiple planes similar to perfusion imaging.

In pulmonary embolism there are perfusion defects which may be subsegmental, segmental or even involve an entire lobe or lung **(Figs. 38 and 39)**. The ventilation scan in these patients is normal; thereby there are mismatched defects. In patients who have pulmonary embolism with infarcts there would also be a ventilation defect; however, the ventilation defect is smaller in size than the perfusion defect. Matched defects occur in chronic obstructive pulmonary disease (COPD) as there is a ventilation defect as well as reflex hypoperfusion.

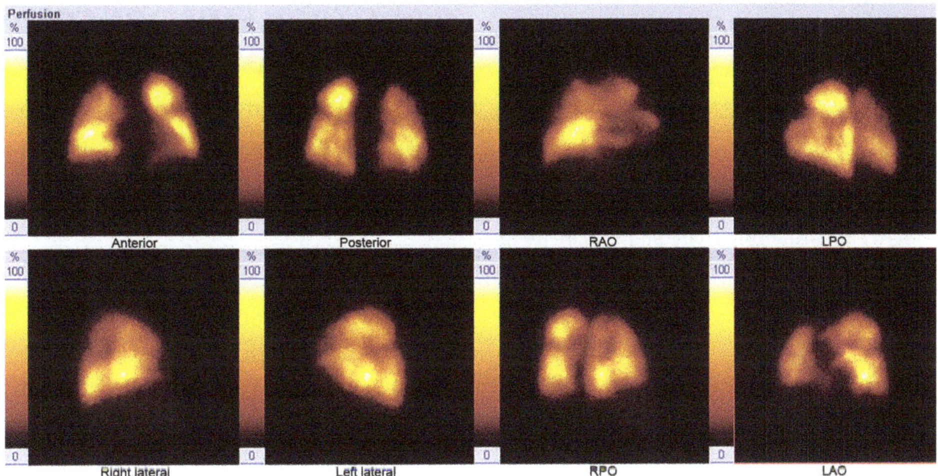

Fig. 38: Perfusion scan: Perfusions scans demonstrate multiple perfusion defects bilaterally, ventilation scan revealed no abnormality, indicative of ventilation-perfusion mismatch due to pulmonary embolism.

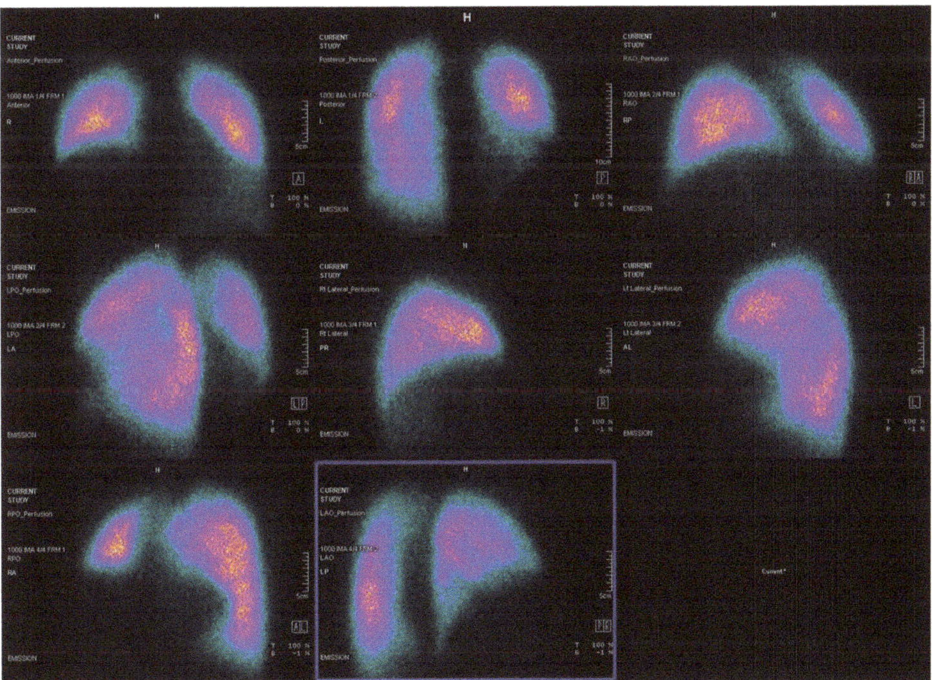

Fig. 39: Perfusion scan: Perfusion scan demonstrates no evidence of perfusion defect. A normal perfusion scan virtually rules out the possibility of a pulmonary embolism.

CT angiography has virtually replaced ventilation-perfusion scans as the modality of choice in the detection of pulmonary embolism **(Table 1)**.

CT angiography has additional advantages. It is available at most institutions round the clock; many institutions may not have nuclear medicine facilities. Clinical mimics of pulmonary embolism such as aortic dissection and pneumonia can be detected by CT. Concurrent venous imaging to detect lower limb/pelvic venous thrombosis is possible with CT angiography, increasing the sensitivity of CT angiography, though at the cost of a higher radiation dose. The requirement to use contrast in CT angiography is a potential disadvantage, especially in individuals with renal impairment or in

Table 1: Differences between V/Q scan and CT angiography.

	V/Q scan	*CT angiography*
Nondiagnostic	26.5%	6%
Sensitivity, specificity	77%, 98%	83%, 96%
Definitive diagnosis	74%	94%

Source: Acute pulmonary embolism: sensitivity and specificity of ventilation-perfusion scintigraphy in PIOPED II study; Dirk Sostman: Radiology. 2008;246(3):941-6.

patients with a history of anaphylaxis to nonionic contrast media. Another debatable issue is the quantum of radiation dose in these two modalities. CT angiography has a higher radiation dose ranging from 2.7 mSev to 10.2 mSev depending on the type of scanner and technique used, as compared to radiation dose in V/Q, ranging from 1.2 mSev to 6.8 mSev. The newer dual-source CT scanners utilize a much lower radiation dose, 1.9–2.7 mSev, similar to the radiation dose of V/Q scan. In pregnancy the radiation dose to the fetus in V/Q scans is 0.1–0.8 mGy as compared to CT angiography, 0.01–0.6 mGy. CT angiography is thus preferred over V/Q scan in pregnancy. The dose to maternal breasts is much higher using CT angiography than V/Q scan; however, this can easily be minimized by using bismuth breast shields. In view of these significant advantages with a positive benefit over risk ratio, CT angiography is the preferred modality.

■ MAGNETIC RESONANCE IMAGING

Magnetic resonance imaging (MRI) is making rapid strides in the evaluation of the abdominal pathologies. Its utility in imaging the brain, spine, musculoskeletal system and pelvis is well established. Evaluation for pulmonary pathologies is limited by a number of factors—the lower proton density of lung, and by cardiac and respiratory motion. These limitations are magnified with increasing field strength; the recent shift to 3T by institutions has not helped. Outside the lung parenchyma, MRI can be a useful alternative to CT, especially when intravenous (IV) contrast is contraindicated such as in patients with renal failure or history of anaphylaxis to contrast media. MRI is useful in the evaluation of the chest wall and mediastinum, to detect mass lesions, as well as demonstrate their local extension **(Figs. 40A to D)**. It is also useful to evaluate the pulmonary arteries, aorta and heart **(Fig. 41)**. IV contrast may be used if serum creatinine is not elevated. Advances are occurring rapidly using newer sequences as well as experimenting with gases for ventilation scans.

■ POSITRON EMISSION TOMOGRAPHY-COMPUTED TOMOGRAPHY

Positron emission tomography-computed tomography (PET-CT) combines a PET scanner and a CT scanner in one gantry. Images acquired from both devices can be obtained sequentially in the same session and images superimposed in a single image.

Positron emission tomography imaging is based on the fact that metabolically active cells take up glucose. PET-CT fuses anatomical and functional data to provide an excellent correlation of anatomic and metabolic information. A radionuclide-labeled glucose analog Fluorine 18-deoxyglucose (FDG) is taken up by malignant tumors, inflammation/infection and active tissue repair. Sixty minutes after IV FDG, a CT is acquired over approximately 30 seconds, followed by a slow transit of the patient through the bore of the PET. This data acquisition takes 30–40 minutes. Standard uptake values can be calculated from the PET data. This is useful as a value above 2.5 SUV is considered significant. The main utilities of PET-CT in respiratory medicine are in the staging of neoplastic processes, including lymphoma and mesothelioma. It is also useful in the detection of inflammatory processes which are not detected by other imaging modalities **(Figs. 42 and 43)**.

■ PULMONARY ANGIOGRAPHY

Pulmonary angiography is considered to be the gold standard in the evaluation of pulmonary thrombo-embolism. This is an invasive procedure with an incidence of 1.5% serious complications. Acute pulmonary emboli are demonstrated as intraluminal filling defects, peripheral occlusion of pulmonary vessels and/or wedge-shaped perfusion defects **(Fig. 44)**. To improve the detection of small pulmonary emboli, dedicated techniques are now available, such as cine angiography, balloon occlusion angiography and superselective angiography.

Many studies using spiral CT angiography have demonstrated a sensitivity and specificity for spiral CT angiogram to match that of pulmonary angiogram. The limitations of both spiral CT angiography and pulmonary angiography are also comparable. It is reported that 10% of spiral CT examinations will be inconclusive compared to 12% for pulmonary angiograms. Three percent of spiral CT angiograms will be technically inadequate compared to 4% for pulmonary angiograms. In view of the less invasiveness

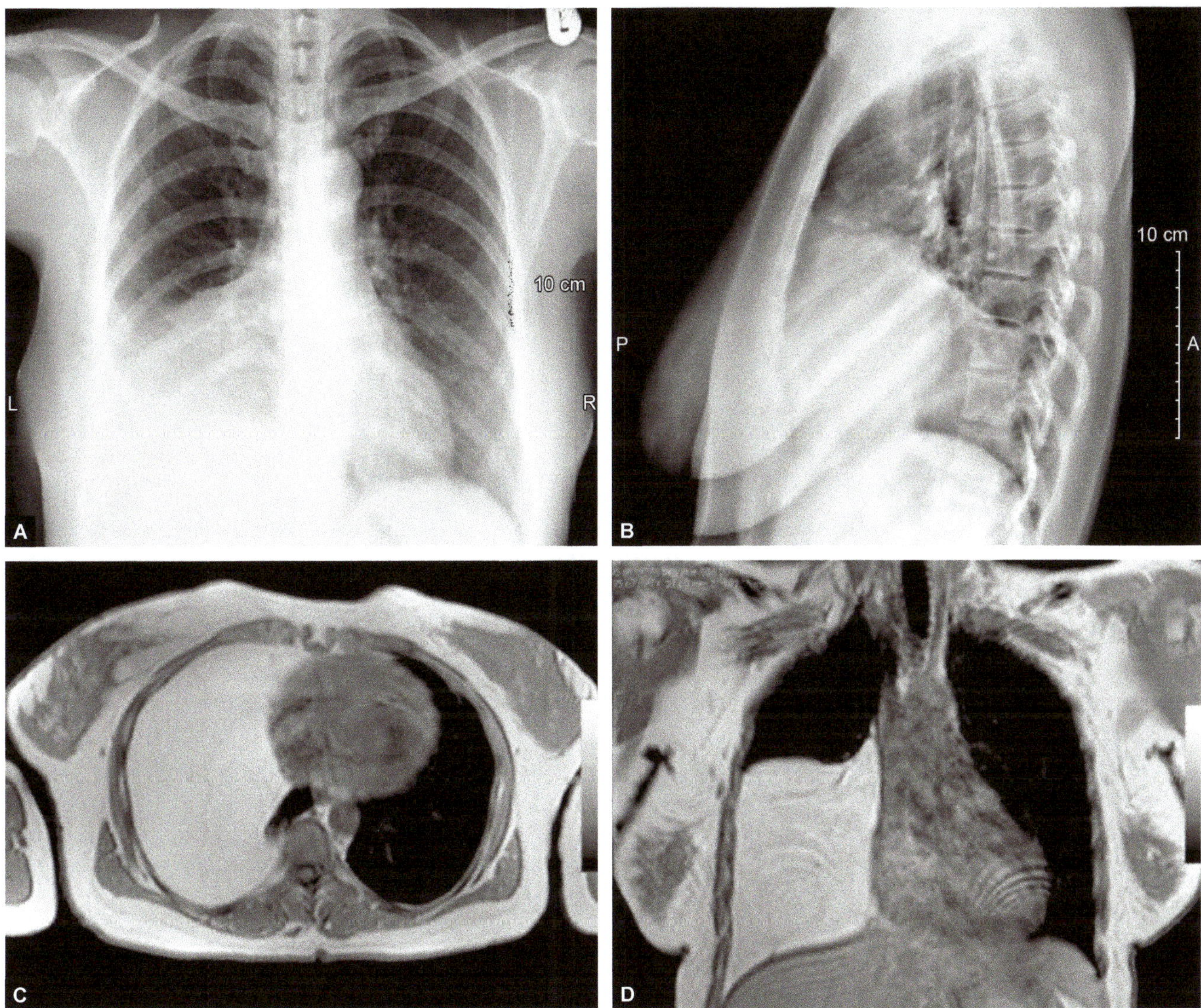

Figs. 40A to D: Lipoma: (A) Chest X-ray demonstrates a large homogenous mass in the right lower zone with no shift of the mediastinum; (B) Lateral X-ray demonstrates opacity in an anterior location; (C and D) MRI characterizes the lesion as a lipoma, as the mass is of fat intensity.

and similar sensitivity and specificity of spiral CT angiogram as compared to pulmonary angiograms, spiral CT angiograms have by and large replaced pulmonary angiograms in the detection of pulmonary emboli **(Fig. 44)**.

BRONCHIAL ARTERY EMBOLIZATION

Bronchial artery embolization is performed to stop massive hemoptysis. The bronchial arteries arise from the intercostobronchial trunk which arises from the aorta at T5. There is a single bronchial artery on the right side and two on the left side. As with most anatomical structures there are variations in the anatomy of the bronchial arteries. These vessels are selectively cannulated and if on angiography, there is extravasation of the dye from an artery or its branch, that vessel is selectively embolized using polyvinyl alcohol or gel foam **(Figs. 45A and B)**. Serious complications following bronchial artery embolization are rare. Patients mainly complain of occasional hemoptysis, transient fever and chest pain.

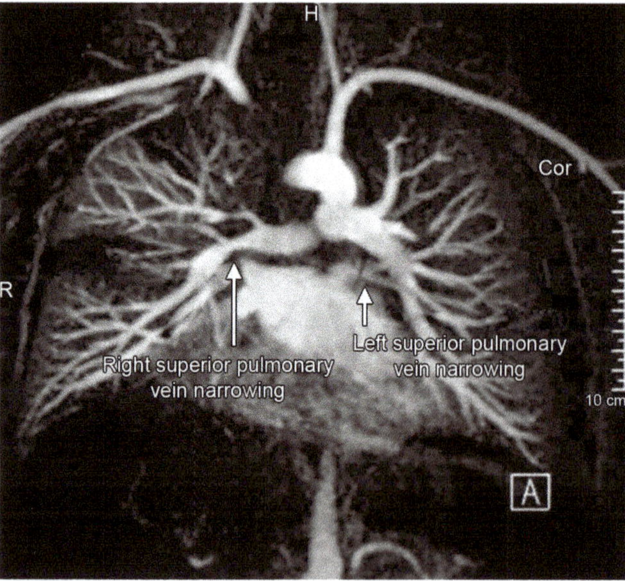

Fig. 41: Mediastinal fibrosis: Contrast-enhanced MRI reveals bilateral superior pulmonary vein narrowing due to mediastinal fibrosis.

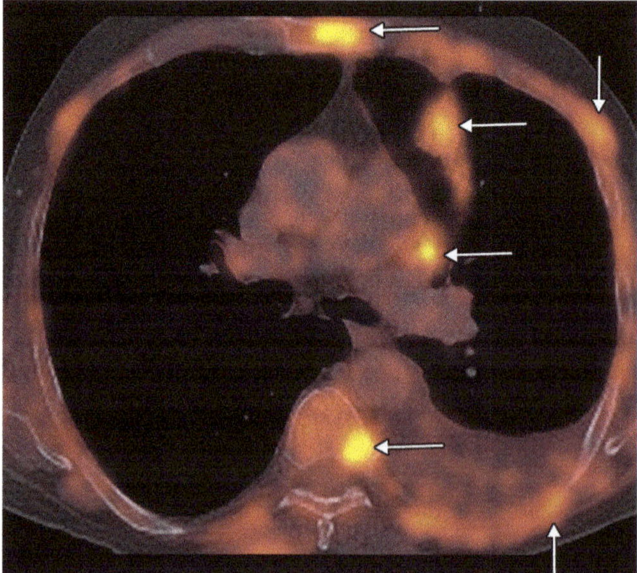

Fig. 43: Positron emission tomography-computed tomography (PET-CT) demonstrates a lesion in the left lingula with multiple bony lesions in sternum, ribs, vertebral body and soft tissue lesions in the spleen and left costal pleura representing a primary lung neoplasm with metastatic deposits.

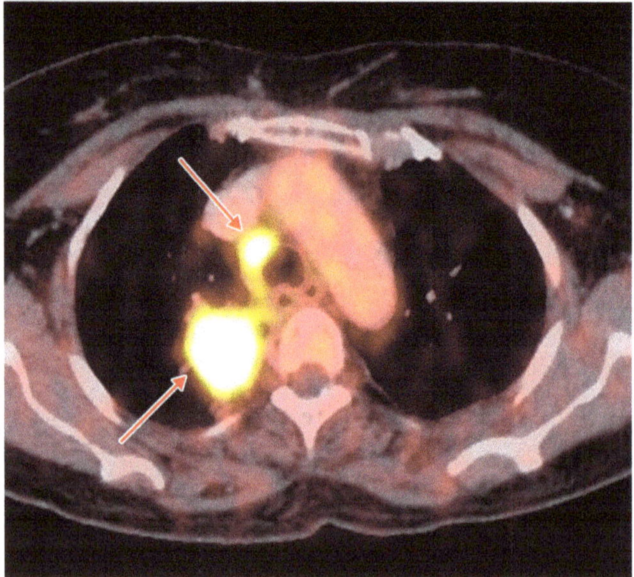

Fig. 42: Positron emission tomography-computed tomography (PET-CT) examination demonstrates uptake in right upper lobe mass lesion and in right paratracheal lymph node representing primary lung neoplasm with nodal spread.

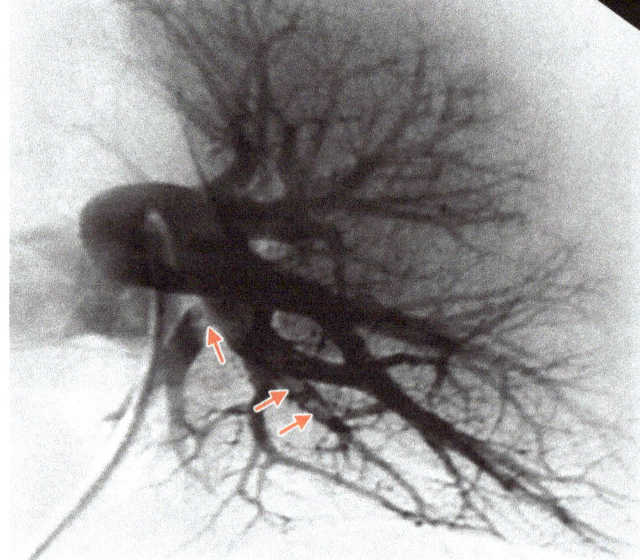

Fig. 44: Pulmonary angiogram: Selective injection of left pulmonary artery demonstrates multiple filling defects in lower branch pulmonary arteries.

■ APPEARANCES OF A NORMAL CHEST RADIOGRAPH

Lung Parenchyma

The lung markings seen on a chest X-ray represent vascular shadows. Occasionally, an accompanying bronchus may be visualized along with the vessels as an air-filled thin tube. Bronchi are best demonstrated end on with the accompanying vessel. In the erect position, the vascular markings are more prominent in the lower zones as the diameters of vessels are larger in the lower zones. In the supine position there is an equalization of the diameters of

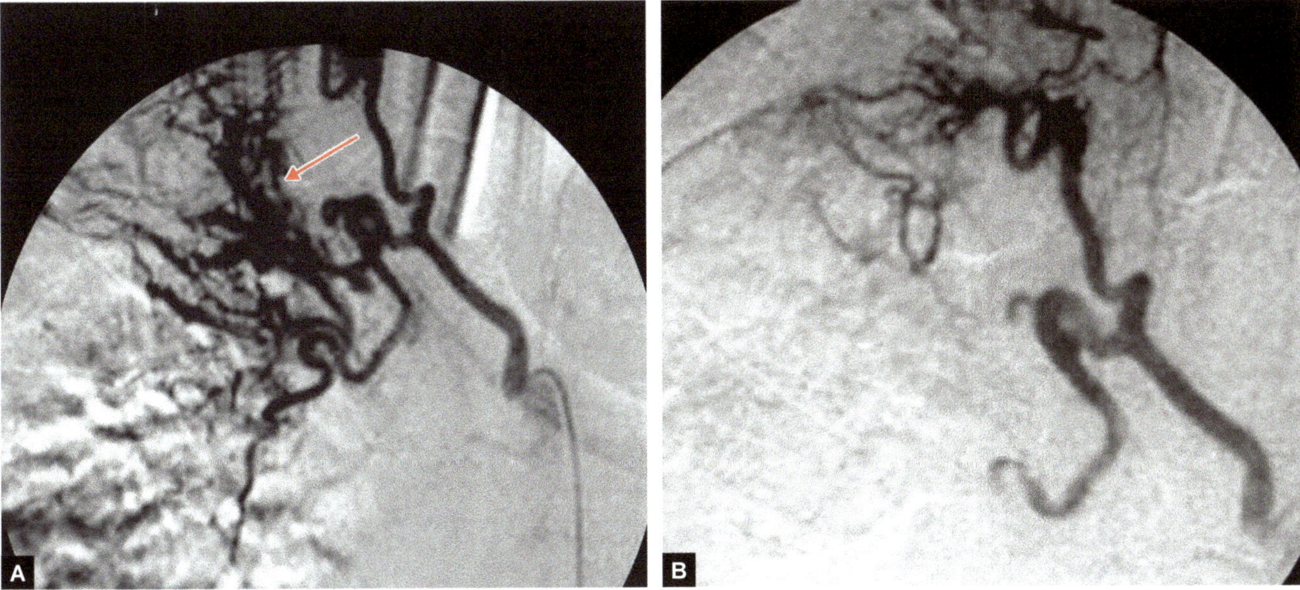

Figs. 45A and B: Bronchial artery angiogram: A patient with active tuberculosis presented with massive hemoptysis. Bronchial arteriogram (A) demonstrates large feeding vessels with extravasation of contrast, indicative of bleeding vessel; (B) The large feeder vessel was occluded with coils to stop the bleeding.

the vessels in the apices and bases. The vascular markings are a combination of pulmonary arteries and veins. In the upper zones it is not possible to differentiate these as they course similarly in a curvilinear fashion; in the lower zones they may be separated as veins course horizontally and arteries more vertically.

Trachea

The trachea enters the thorax 1–3 cm above the level of the suprasternal notch, the intrathoracic portion is 6–9 cm in length. The trachea contains 16–20 incomplete or horseshoe-shaped cartilage rings giving the trachea a corrugated outline—calcification of the cartilage rings occurs after the age of 40 years. The trachea deviates mildly to the right to accommodate the left-sided aortic arch. With unfolding and ectasia of the aorta the trachea deviates more to the right.

The trachea divides into the two mainstem bronchi at the carina, approximately at the level of the T5. The left main bronchus extends up to twice as far as the right main bronchus before giving off its upper lobe division. The right main bronchus is approximately 25 mm long; the left main bronchus is approximately 50 mm long. In children the angles between the bronchi are symmetric, but in adults the right mainstem bronchus has a steeper angle than the left. The segmental bronchi are not well

demonstrated on the X-ray unless seen end on; they are well-demonstrated on CT.

Hilum

The hilar opacity is mainly due to pulmonary arteries and to a lesser extent due to the pulmonary veins. There is a small contribution by adenopathy, fat and bronchial walls. The left hilum is higher in position than the right hilum; this is because the left pulmonary artery arches over the left bronchus and descends posterior to the left bronchus while the right pulmonary artery extends directly inferiorly, anterior to the right bronchus. In 5% of individuals they may be at the same level. If the left hilum is found to be lower than the right hilum, it is useful to evaluate for left lower lobe collapse or a right upper lobe collapse. There is usually a wide variation in size of the hilum in normal individuals. If there is prominence of a hilar shadow, the possibility that this is due to a technical factor such as rotation or scoliosis should be first excluded. The margins of the hilum are usually smooth; if there is a lobulated contour a mass should be suspected.

The pulmonary arteries descend vertically downwards; the size of the descending vessels is relatively equal to a little finger. If the descending pulmonary artery is not visualized on the right side, always check for right lower lobe collapse. A mass lesion at the hilum in contact with the hilar vessels will result in a loss of the hilar silhouette. If the hilum is well-visualized through a mass lesion then the mass has not silhouetted the hilum, indicating that the mass is anterior or posterior to the hilum.

Diaphragm

The right dome is normally at the level of the sixth rib anteriorly. The left dome is usually about 1.5–2.5 cm below the right dome. There may be variations in the position of the diaphragm; they may be one interspace higher or lower, they may be at the same level or occasionally, the left is higher than the right but not more than 1 cm. During a respiratory cycle the diaphragm may move between 2.5 cm and 8.0 cm.

Nipples

These may be visualized as bilaterally symmetric dense well-defined spherical shadows with a sharp and a non-sharp margin **(Fig. 46)**. If they are asymmetric they may be mistaken for a pulmonary nodule **(Fig. 47)**. To clarify whether a shadow is a nipple or a pulmonary nodule, a marker may be placed on the nipple **(Fig. 48)**, or in a female the breasts are manually elevated. If a nipple casts a shadow, the marker will be on the opacity; if the breasts have been elevated, the nipple will move up, the pulmonary nodule will remain in the same location.

Fissures

Major fissures are present bilaterally and separate the upper from the lower lobes. The fissures run obliquely forward and downward crossing the hilum. They arise from the fifth thoracic vertebrae and end at the diaphragm approximately 3 cm behind the sternum. On a lateral radiograph, often parts or the whole of a fissure may be visualized. On a frontal radiograph the major fissures are rarely visualized.

A minor fissure is present on the right side dividing the upper and middle lobes **(Fig. 49)**. The fissure extends from the hilum anteriorly and laterally. On a frontal radiograph it is seen in nearly 50% of individuals, contacting the lateral chest wall at or near the axillary portion of the sixth rib. It is also seen on the lateral chest radiograph in approximately 50% of individuals extending anteriorly from the hilum.

Azygous Lobe Fissure

This fissure develops due to failure of the azygous vein to migrate from the chest wall through the lung into its location at the tracheobronchial angle. The invaginated visceral and parietal pleura persist to form a fissure, at the bottom of which lies the azygous vein **(Fig. 50)**. This may be occasionally seen on the left side with the left superior intercostal vein occupying the bottom of the fissure.

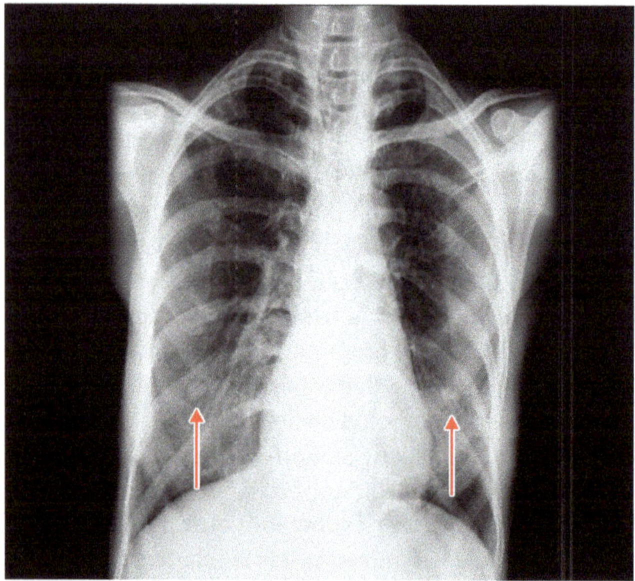

Fig. 46: PA view of the chest demonstrates bilaterally symmetric dense well-defined rounded shadows with a sharp and a non sharp margin in the lower zones. These represent bilateral nipple shadows.

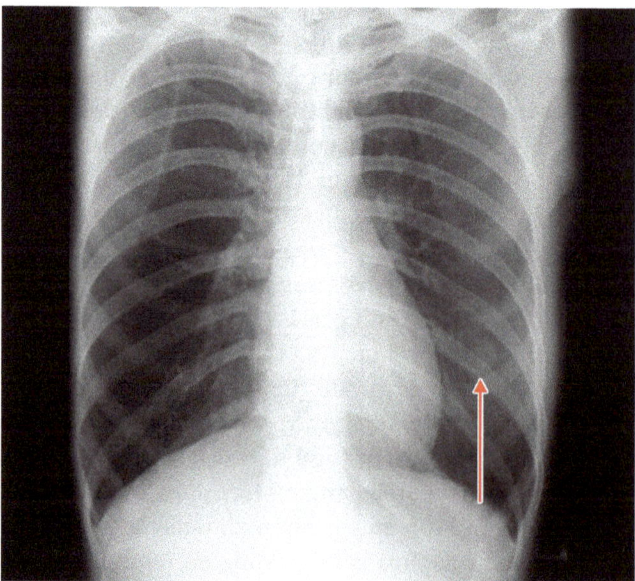

Fig. 47: Nipple shadow: PA view of the chest demonstrates a well-defined nodular lesion in the left lower zone, this may represent a nipple shadow or a nodular lesion.

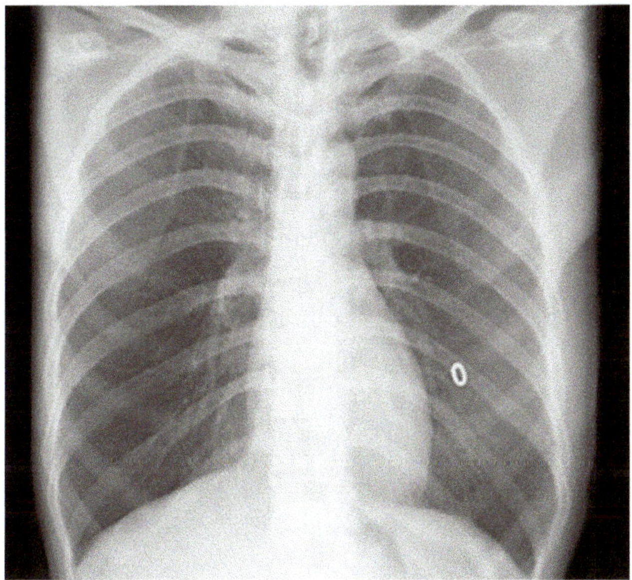

Fig. 48: Nipple shadow: PA view of the chest shows a nipple marker coinciding with nodular lesion indicating that the shadow was a nipple.

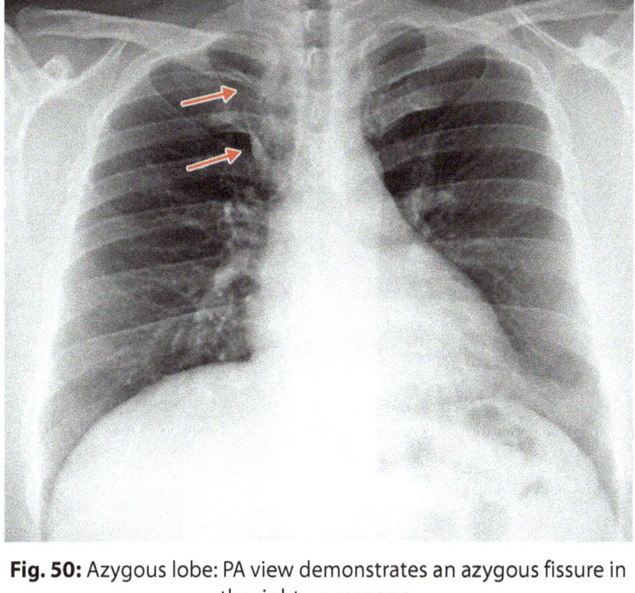

Fig. 50: Azygous lobe: PA view demonstrates an azygous fissure in the right upper zone.

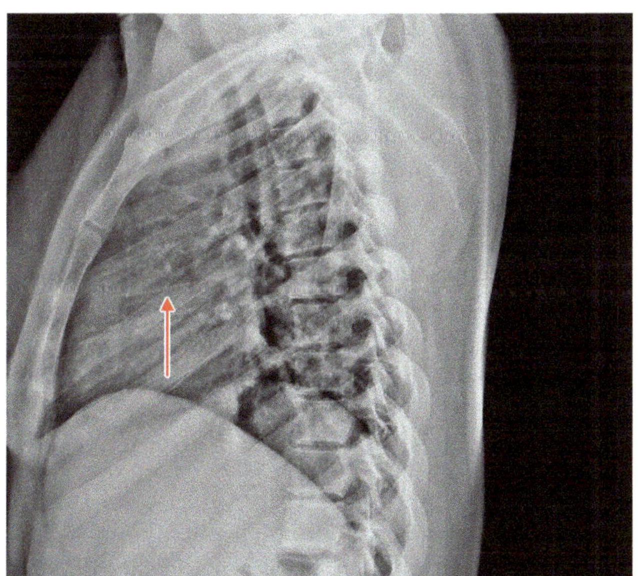

Fig. 49: Minor fissure: Lateral view of chest reveals minor fissure as a horizontal line extending from the hilum anteriorly.

Mediastinum

The left mediastinal border above the level of the aortic arch is constituted by the left subclavian and carotid arteries. The left wall of the trachea is not visualized as it is in contact with the vessels. From the level of the aortic arch inferiorly the border is constituted by the aorta, main pulmonary artery, and heart **(Fig. 51A)**. A small nodular well-defined opacity may be seen just below the aortic knuckle; this represents the left superior intercostal vein as it arches around the aorta before entering the left brachiocephalic vein. This should not be misinterpreted for a lymph node. The left border of the descending aorta is visualized through the main pulmonary artery and heart down to the aortic hiatus in the diaphragm.

The right mediastinal border is formed by the right brachiocephalic vein, SVC and right atrium. The right paratracheal stripe consisting of the tracheal wall and adjacent fat is seen through the brachiocephalic vein and SVC as the lung is in contact with the posterior wall of the trachea. The presence of this stripe excludes the possibility of a paratracheal mass lesion. This stripe is visible in two-thirds of individuals. At the lower end of this stripe is the azygous vein in the tracheobronchial angle.

Lateral View

On the lateral view there are three zones to observe. The vertebrae, each thoracic vertebra appears more translucent than the one above. The cardiac shadow is visualized as a homogenous opacity. The retrosternal space is well-aerated, any alteration in this pattern indicates an abnormality **(Fig. 51B)**.

The two domes of the diaphragm overlap each other. It is fairly easy to separate the two. The right is visualized all the way from front to back. The left is only seen from

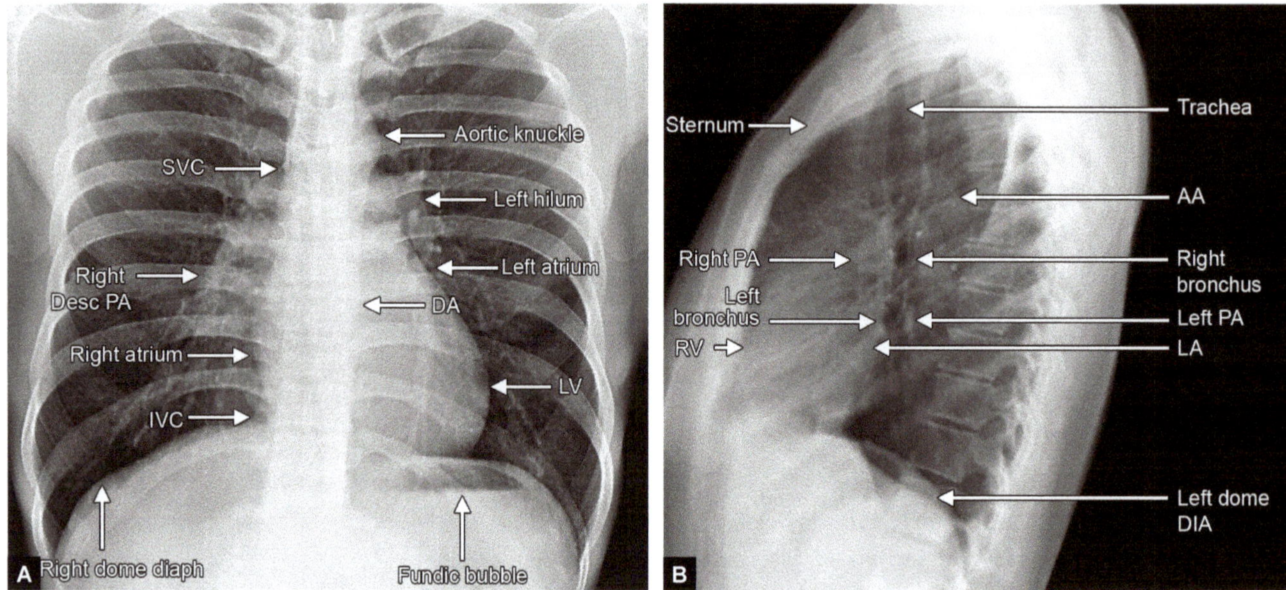

Figs. 51A and B: (A) PA and (B) lateral views of chest demonstrating anatomy.
(PA: Pulmonary artery; AA: Arch of aorta; DA: Descending aorta; LA: Left atrium; RV: Right ventricle; LV: Left ventricle; SVC: Superior venacava; Desc: Descending; IVC: Inferior venacava; Diaph/DIA: Diaphragm)

the costophrenic recess posteriorly to the point where it meets the cardiac silhouette. Anterior to this point, it is not visualized as the lung/diaphragm interface is obliterated by the cardiac silhouette. Occasionally, it may be difficult to separate the two domes as they totally overlap. If the diaphragm silhouette is lost, an abnormality in the lower lobes should be suspected.

It is difficult to differentiate the right from the left hilum as they totally overlap each other. The right pulmonary artery traverses anterior to the right bronchus and the left pulmonary artery hooks over and is posterior to the left bronchus. The bronchi are seen end on, the higher ring is the right and the lower the left bronchus. If the hilum is considerably prominent, large in size and lobulated in contour, a hilar mass should be suspected.

The mediastinal opacity is occupied by the heart. The portion behind the hila is the left atrium; the posterior border below the hilum is constituted by the left ventricle, the anterior surface of the shadow constitutes the right ventricle. If the cardiac silhouette does not appear to be homogenous, the possibility of a superimposed pulmonary pathology may be considered.

The aortic arch is well-visualized with the brachiocephalic artery often being visualized arising and extending anterior to the trachea. The left and right brachiocephalic veins are often visualized as an extrapleural bulge beneath the manubrium sternum and

should not be mistaken for a sternal/chest wall mass. Similarly, in the inferior part of the chest, the anterior paracardiac fat may simulate a mass lesion posterior to the chest wall. This is because the two lungs do not meet in the midline, the heart and paracardiac fat being interposed.

The horizontal fissure is seen on most lateral chest X-rays. Oblique fissures appear like the blades of a propeller. The right oblique fissure at its most posterior position lies 4–5 cm behind the sternum, the left oblique is positioned slightly more superior **(Figs. 49 and 52)**.

The IVC may be visible as a well-defined vertical line which meets the posterior and inferior aspect of the heart.

Interpreting Chest Radiographs

A systematic approach to the interpretation of a chest radiograph is very important. This is particularly so when an obvious abnormality is present. The PA view of the chest is printed as if the patient is facing the interpreter, with the right side facing the interpreter's left side. It is important first to evaluate the radiograph from a technical quality perspective. Important factors to evaluate are **(Fig. 53)**.

Exposure: In a well-exposed radiograph the dorsal intervertebral disks should just be visible through the cardiac shadow. In an overexposed X-ray the vertebral bodies are well-outlined, the lung fields are darkened. The risk of overexposure is that parenchymal lung lesions may

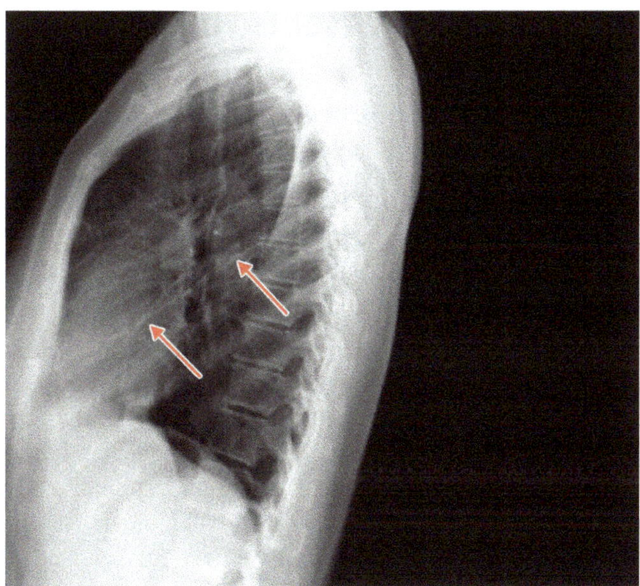

Fig. 52: Lateral view of chest demonstrates the normal oblique fissures extending from the fifth dorsal vertebra posteriorly to the cardiophrenic angle crossing the hilum.

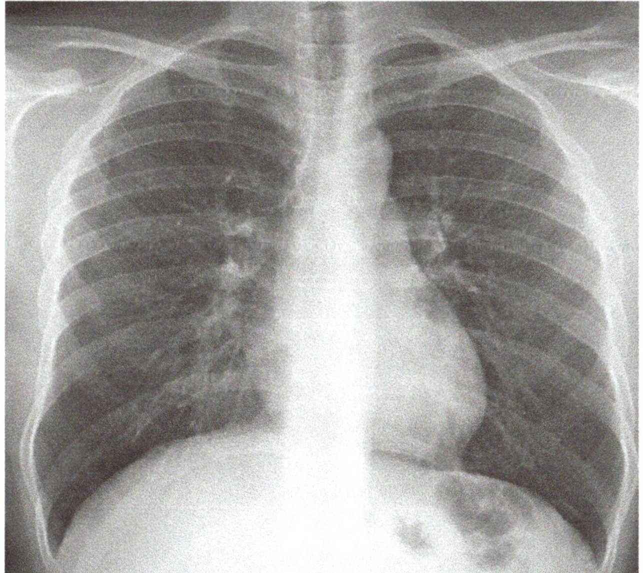

Fig. 53: Normal chest X-ray: A perfectly exposed X-ray as the dorsal interspaces are just visualized. There is no rotation as the clavicles are equidistant from the cervical spinous processes; the inspiratory effort is adequate, as the anterior ends of the sixth ribs are at the mid-diaphragmatic level.

not be visible, though the retrocardiac regions are well-visualized. In an underexposed X-ray the mediastinum appears brighter than usual; also, there is no visualization of the dorsal intervertebral disks.

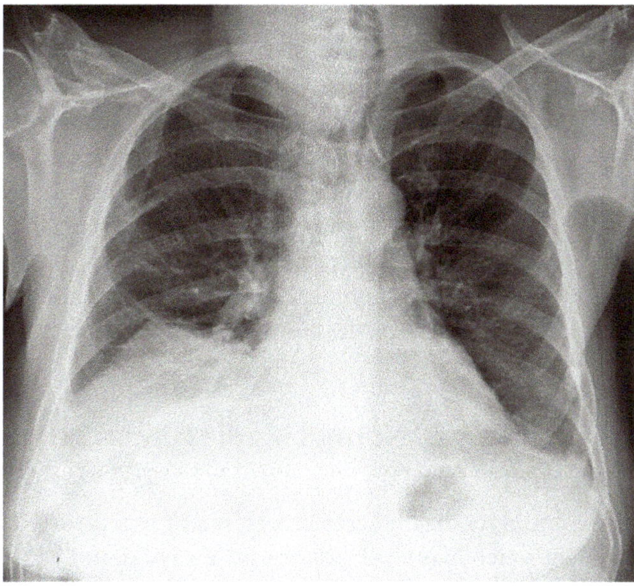

Fig. 54: Tracheal deviation: PA view of the chest demonstrates tracheal deviation as a result of mass lesion in the neck arising from the thyroid causing significant displacement and compression to the left.

Inspiratory effort: Chest X-rays are obtained in deep inspiration; the midpoint of the right hemidiaphragm should be at the anterior end of the sixth rib.

Rotation: The medial ends of the clavicle should be equidistant from the spinous processes of the cervical vertebrae.

Evaluation of Different Structures on a Chest X-ray

Start with the trachea, note its position, mass effect, deviation and caliber **(Fig. 54)**. Then evaluate the mediastinal silhouette, the right border, then the left border from above downwards. Note any loss of silhouette, cardiomegaly. Next evaluate the hilum, again one at a time, position of hilum, right in relation to left, equality in size and density. If a hilum appears larger or denser, a lateral view is very useful to confirm or exclude a mass lesion. For example, if the right hilum is prominent, presence of a mass will be seen on the lateral view as being posterior to the trachea, since the right pulmonary artery is anterior to the trachea. For the left, it is converse as the left pulmonary artery is posterior to the trachea. The lower lobe pulmonary vessels are well-visualized on a radiograph. Absence of this leash of vessels on a well-centered X-ray is a useful clue to lobar collapse. Evaluate the diaphragms for position, contour any loss of silhouette. Now evaluate the lungs. A useful method is to examine them in a zigzag fashion from below upward. Evaluate each zone from a size, transradiancy perspective. The position of the horizontal fissure if visible should be noted, as this may also be a clue toward lobar collapse. Finally, evaluate the ribs and chest wall. Before concluding, pitfall areas where abnormalities may lurk should be evaluated. These include the central mediastinum, lungs behind the diaphragm and heart, lung apices, lung and pleura along the inner surface of the chest wall.

CT Anatomy of Normal Mediastinum and the Lung

The normal mediastinal structures, heart, blood vessels, tracheobronchial tree, esophagus are always identified on cross-sectional imaging **(Figs. 55A to D)**.

■ MEDIASTINAL VASCULATURE

The vertical portions of the ascending and descending aorta are well-visualized as spherical tubes, the diameter of the ascending aorta is 3.5 cm and of the descending aorta 2.5 cm. The descending aorta descends to the left of the vertebrae and then takes a more midline course to enter the abdomen anterior to the vertebrae. The arch of the aorta is seen in cross-section traversing from the ascending aorta to the descending aorta right to left, anterior to the trachea. Above the level of the aortic arch the great vessels are well-visualized in an arc anterior and to the left of the trachea. The left common carotid artery lies to the left of the trachea, left subclavian artery to the left or posterior to the trachea. The brachiocephalic artery is larger than the left common carotid and left subclavian artery. In 0.5% of the population the right subclavian artery has an anomalous origin arising distal to the left

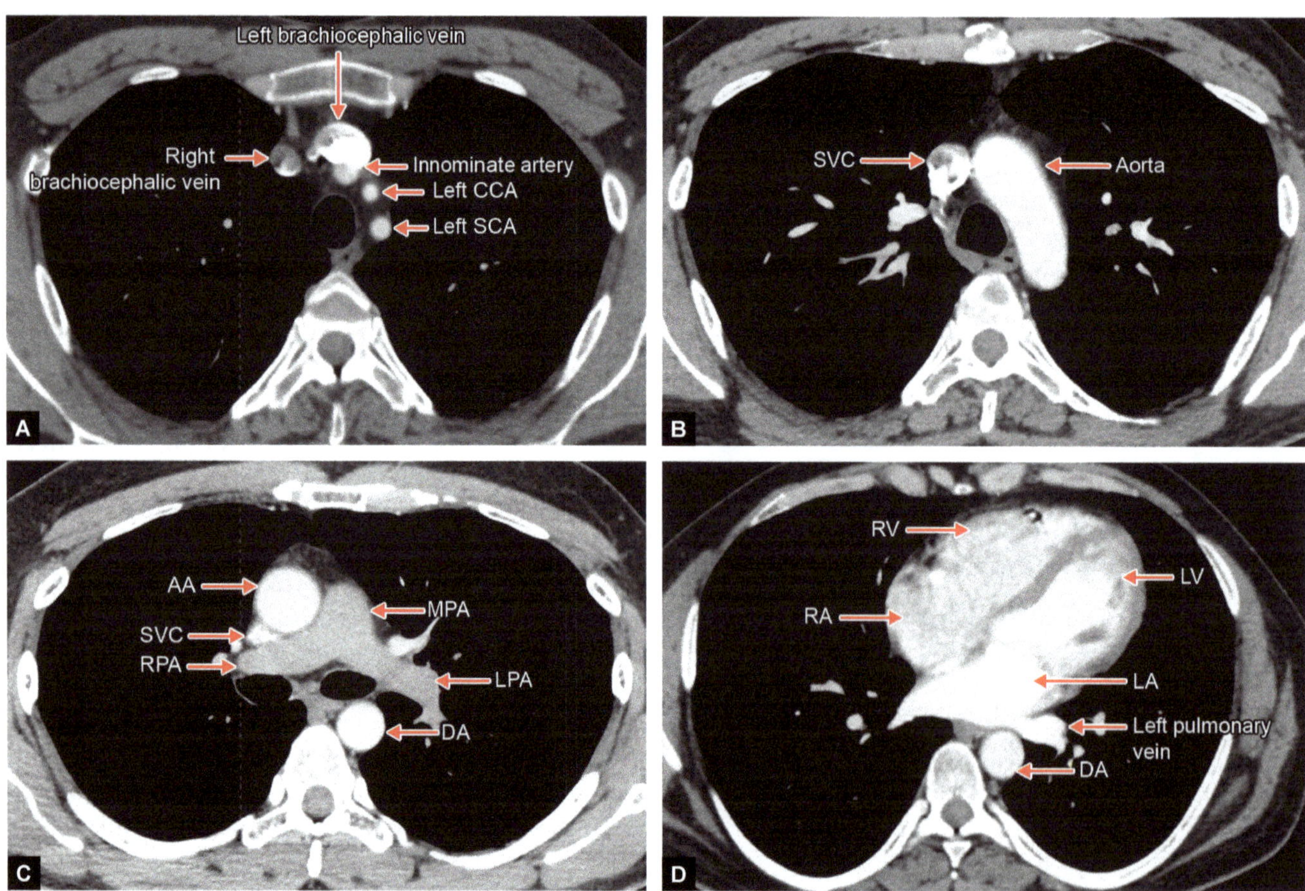

Figs. 55A to D: CT anatomy of normal mediastinal structures.
(CCA: Common carotid artery; SCA: Subclavian artery; SVC: Superior venacava; AA: Ascending aorta; DA: Descending aorta; MPA: Main pulmonary artery; RPA: Right pulmonary artery; LPA: Left pulmonary artery; RA: Right atrium; RV: Right ventricle; LV: Left ventricle; LA: Left atrium)

subclavian artery. It courses from left to right, posterior to the esophagus at the level of the aortic arch; it then ascends in the right paravertebral space to the root of the neck. The brachiocephalic in this situation becomes the right common carotid artery, with a size similar to that of the left common carotid artery. A barium swallow will demonstrate the posterior indentation of the esophagus caused by the anomalous right subclavian artery **(Figs. 56A and B)**. Pressure on the esophagus by this artery may cause dysphagia.

The right subclavian and jugular vein unite to form the right brachiocephalic vein, which descends vertically in the mediastinum to continue as the superior vena cava (SVC) following its union with the left brachiocephalic vein. The SVC is usually half to two-thirds the diameter of the ascending aorta. The left brachiocephalic vein courses through the mediastinum from the left to the right, anterior to the great vessels. In 0.3–0.5% of the population a left SVC is present. This is more commonly seen in individuals with congenital heart disease. The left SVC is formed by the union of the left jugular and subclavian veins, and descends vertically in the left mediastinum to open into the coronary sinus. Due to the increased blood flow, the coronary sinus is increased in size in this situation.

The azygous vein ascends from the diaphragm in the prevertebral space to the right or posterior to the esophagus; it arches over the right main bronchus to open into the posterior wall of the SVC. In 1% of individuals the azygous penetrates the lung as it arches over the bronchus resulting in an azygous lobe. Occasionally, the IVC does not develop, the azygous becomes the conduit to drain blood back to the heart, and is then termed as the azygous continuation of the IVC. The hepatic veins then open directly into the right atrium and the azygous vein dilates. Variants in vascular anatomy such as left-sided SVC, azygous continuation of IVC, left superior intercostal vein, may be mistaken for a mass lesion or adenopathy on an unenhanced scan or chest X-ray. The hemiazygous and accessory hemiazygous veins ascend posterior to the descending aorta. The accessory hemiazygous may cross to the right to open into the azygous or open into the left superior intercostal vein. The left superior intercostal vein is a small vein, which arches around the aorta at the level of the arch and descending aorta to open into the left brachiocephalic vein. It is only occasionally identified on X-ray/CT.

Pulmonary Artery

The main pulmonary artery runs backward and upward obliquely to the left of the ascending aorta **(Fig. 57)**. The right branch travels horizontally to the right between the ascending aorta and tracheobronchial tree; it then descends anterior to the right bronchus. The left branch curves upward and posteriorly over the left main bronchus and descends posterior to the left main bronchus. The main pulmonary artery diameter is approximately 2.8 cm. A main pulmonary artery/aortic ratio greater than 1 indicates pulmonary hypertension. The pulmonary artery branches are two-thirds the diameter of the main pulmonary artery.

Thymus

The thymus is best visualized in a section at the level of the aortic arch, anterior to the aorta and pulmonary artery,

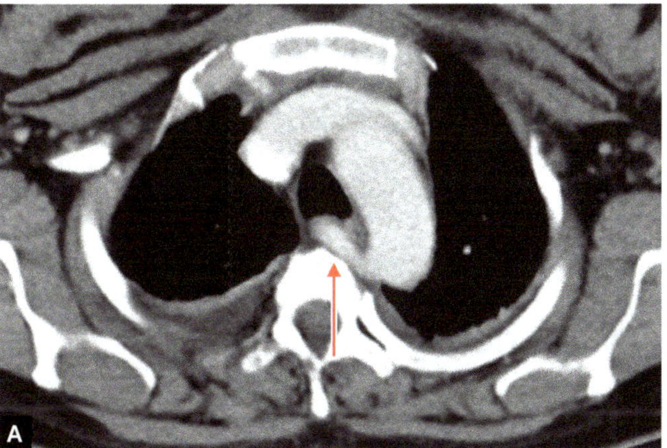
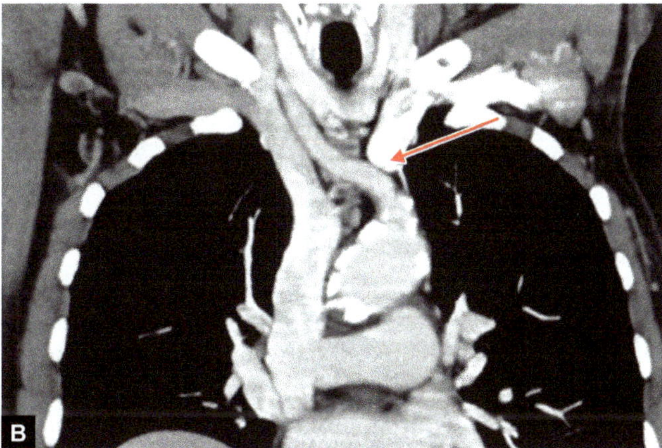

Figs. 56A and B: Aberrant right subclavian artery: CECT chest demonstrates right subclavian artery arising distal to the left subclavian and courses from left to right, posterior to the trachea and esophagus.
(CECT: Contrast enhanced computed tomography)

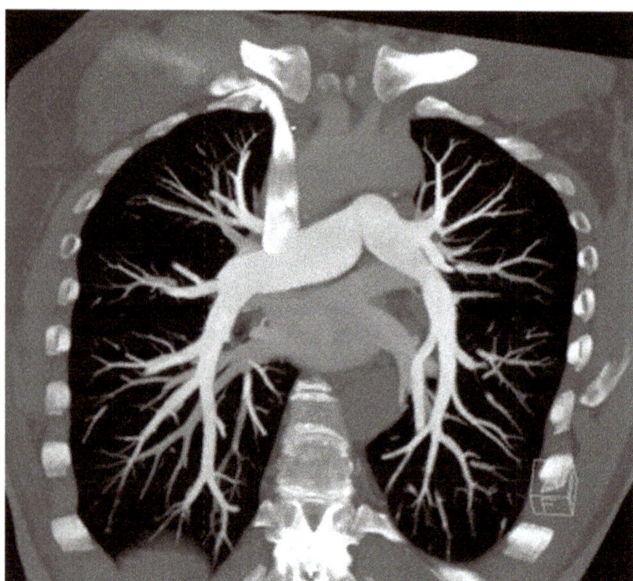

Fig. 57: Computed tomography (CT) pulmonary angiogram demonstrates a normal pulmonary angiography.

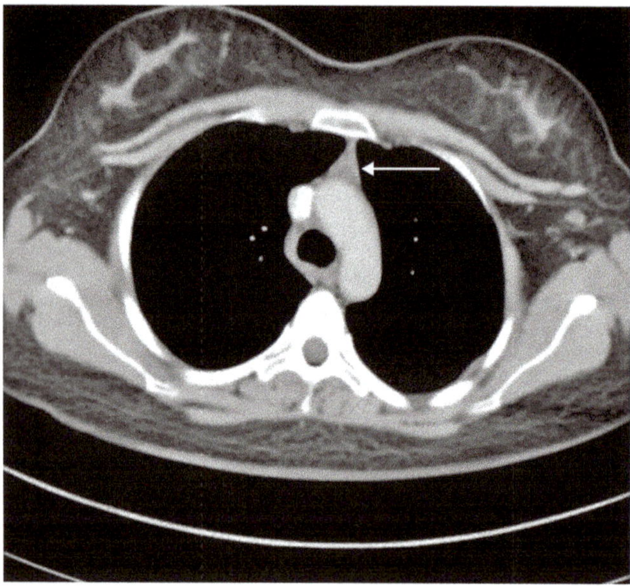

Fig. 58: Thymus: CT scan chest demonstrates a normal thymus. Seen as a triangular well-defined soft-tissue density with internal fat densities.

inferior to the left brachiocephalic vein, and superior to the right pulmonary artery **(Fig. 58)**. Till puberty the thymus occupies most of the anterior mediastinum with a density of soft tissue. After puberty the gland starts to get replaced by fatty tissue; by 40 the gland is not visualized as it is replaced by fatty tissue. In individuals on chemotherapy the thymus may be visualized in adults, termed as thymic rebound.

Mediastinal Lymph Nodes

Ninety-five percent of normal mediastinal lymph nodes measure less than 10 mm in short axis diameter. Mediastinal lymph nodes are chiefly located in the paratracheal, prevascular, pretracheal, subcarinal and aortopulmonary regions.

Trachea

In cross-section, the trachea is round or oval with a flattened posterior margin formed by the fibromuscular membrane. On expiration there is a significant change in the diameter of the trachea. This is due to forward motion of the posterior wall of the trachea; there is consequent reduction in the AP diameter of the trachea.

The trachea divides into the two mainstem bronchi at the carina, approximately at the level of T5. The left main bronchus extends up to twice as far as the right main bronchus before giving off its upper lobe division. The right main bronchus is approximately 25 mm long, the left main bronchus is approximately 50 mm long. In children the angles between the bronchi are symmetric, but in adults the right mainstem bronchus has a steeper angle than the left. The segmental bronchi are well-demonstrated on CT.

The right upper lobe bronchus divides into the right apical, posterior and anterior segmental upper lobe bronchi **(Fig. 59)**.

The right lower lobe bronchus divides into right lower lobe superior segment bronchus, (middle lobe medial and lateral) segmental bronchi and anterior, lateral, posterior and medial lower lobe segmental bronchi.

On the left side the upper lobe bronchus divides into apicoposterior and anterior upper lobe segmental bronchi as well as the lingular superior and inferior segmental bronchi. The left lower lobe bronchus divides into superior segmental and anterior medial basal, posterior and lateral basal segmental bronchi.

■ VARIATIONS

- Common origin of right upper/middle bronchus
- Tracheal bronchus—either a segmental or the entire right upper lobe bronchus arises from the trachea; there may be a displaced or supernumerary bronchus **(Figs. 60A and B)**

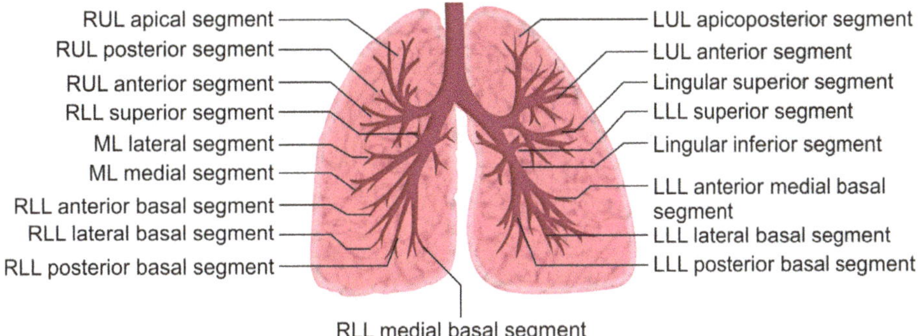

Fig. 59: Anatomy of tracheobronchial tree: AP view of branches of airways beyond the segmental bronchi.
(LUL: Left upper lobe; RUL: Right upper lobe; RLL: Right lower lobe; ML: Middle lobe; LLL: Left lower lobe)

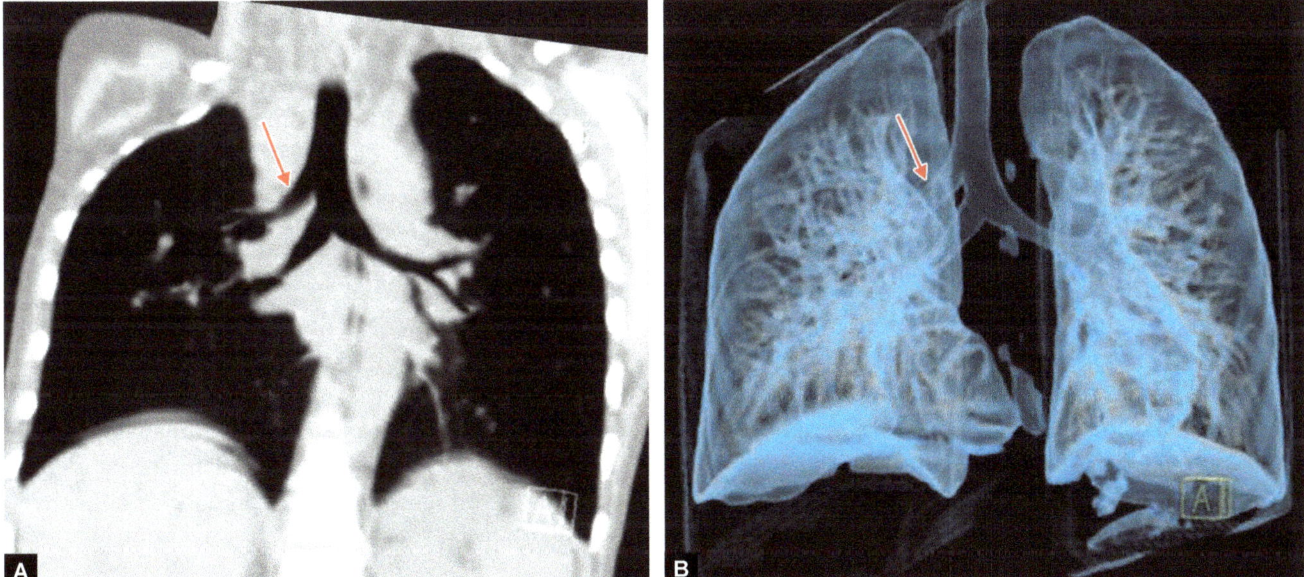

Figs. 60A and B: Tracheal bronchus: (A) Minimum intensity projection and (B) Volume-rendered images of the tracheobronchial tree demonstrate a tracheal bronchus. The right upper lobe bronchus is seen to arise directly from the trachea.

- Accessory cardiac bronchus arising from the medial aspect of the right main bronchus, usually blind-ended but may supply a small lobule
- Lateral inversion of right and left-sided airways in "*situs inversus*"
- *Situs ambiguus*—airway has either bilateral right-sided or left-sided configuration
- Bridging bronchus—right lower lobe bronchus arises from the left main bronchus, crosses the mediastinum to reach the right lung.

The segmental bronchi divide progressively into smaller airways till after 6–20 divisions become bronchioles which further divide till terminal bronchioles. These are the last of the conducting airways. Beyond the terminal bronchioles lie the gas exchange units, the acini. The anatomy of the secondary lobule is discussed under the HRCT section of this chapter.

Diaphragm

The diaphragm consists of a large dome-shaped central tendon with radiating striated muscle attached to the xiphisternum and to the 7th to 12th ribs. The two crura arise from the first three lumbar vertebrae forming the lateral walls of the aortic hiatus. The aorta, azygous, hemiazygous veins and thoracic duct pass through this hiatus. There are two more hiatuses anterior to the aortic hiatus in the diaphragm—the esophageal hiatus through which pass the esophagus, esophageal arteries and vagus nerve, and the hiatus for the IVC.

Fissures

The major fissures are well-visualized as thin white lines traversing from posterior to anterior and from cephalad to caudal. The minor fissure lies in the plane of the scanning, therefore, the fissure per se is not visualized. Its position can be inferred as there is an avascular zone in the subpleural regions **(Figs. 61A and B)**.

An avascular zone in the right middle lobe points to the site of the minor fissure.

Interstitium: Normal HRCT Anatomy

The lung is supported by a network of connective tissue fibers known as the interstitium of the lung. The interstitium is divided into three components, the axial interstitium, the peripheral interstitium and the intralobular interstitium which communicates between the axial and peripheral interstitium. The peripheral interstitium is located beneath the visceral pleura; it envelops the lung like a fibrous sac from which connective tissue septae penetrate into the lung parenchyma. Between each interlobular septa lies a secondary lobule. The axial interstitium consists of the peribronchovascular interstitium which is strong connective tissue encasing the central bronchi and arteries. This interstitium extends from the level of the pulmonary hila to the periphery of the lung, encasing the centrilobular arteries and bronchioles in the secondary lobules **(Fig. 62)**. The secondary lobule is the smallest unit of lung structure varying in size from 1 cm to 2.5 cm containing 10–12 acini. It is polygonal in shape, with its apex pointing to the hilum and base toward the pleural surface. Each is supplied by a small bronchiole and pulmonary arterial branch—centrilobular artery. This is visualized on HRCT sections as a small dot; however, the bronchus is not visualized as it is below the resolution of present-day HRCT scans **(Fig. 63)**. The interlobular septae which marginate the secondary lobules contain pulmonary veins and lymphatics. At the level of the secondary lobule all three connective tissue systems are present.

Anatomy of Bronchi and Pulmonary Vessels

The bronchi and pulmonary arteries run parallel to each other. Their appearances depend upon the scan plane they are sectioned in. If the scan plane is perpendicular to their course they will appear as well-defined round structures adjacent to each other. If sectioned in the same plane, they will appear as tubular structures running parallel to each other. The artery is seen as a well-defined round homogenous white structure. The accompanying bronchus has a thin well-defined wall with a lucent center containing air resembling a pipe with air in its lumen. The outer surface of these structures is smooth. The inner diameter of the bronchus to accompanying arterial diameter is usually 0.65/0.7:1. A bronchoarterial ratio of 1:1 is considered normal; greater than this is considered as bronchiectasis **(Fig. 64)**. An increased bronchoarterial

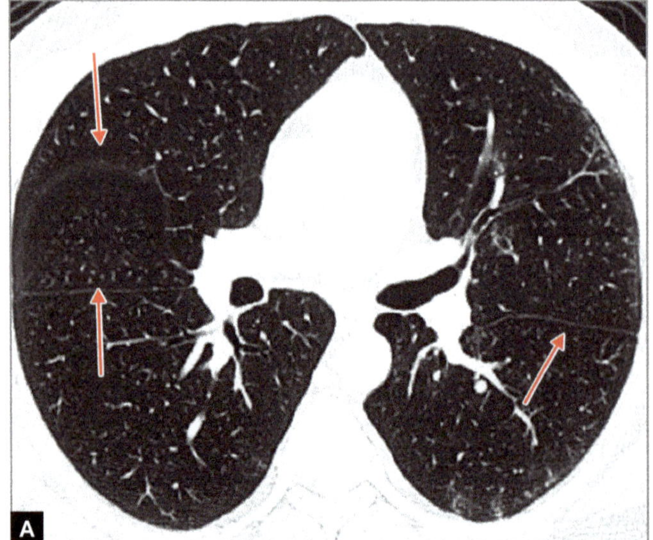 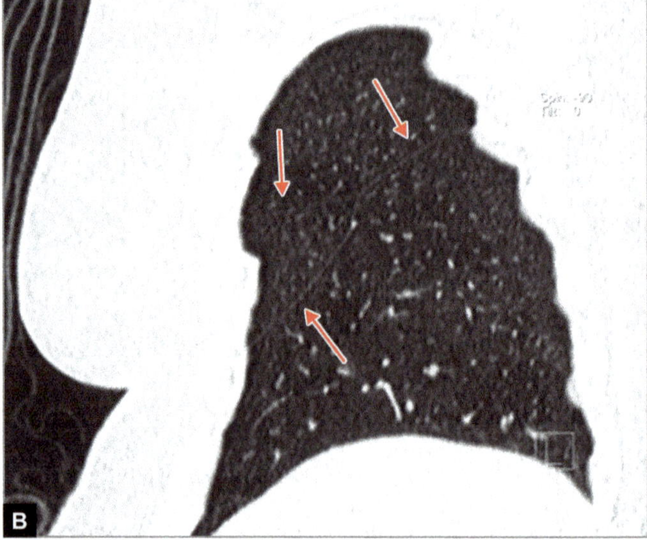

Figs. 61A and B: Fissures: (A) Axial and (B) sagittal reconstructions demonstrate major interlobar fissures. The minor fissure is not seen on the axial scan as it is in the same plane as the slices. The position of this fissure is inferred on the axial images as a zone of avascularity.

ratio greater than 1 may be seen in patients who reside at a high altitude; the mild hypoxemia induces mild bronchial dilatation as well as vasoconstriction, resulting in an altered bronchoarterial ratio. Bronchi are visualized till the peripheral 2 cm of the lung. It is rare to see normal bronchi in the peripheral 2 cm of the lung. Normal bronchi may extend till 1 cm of the mediastinal surface.

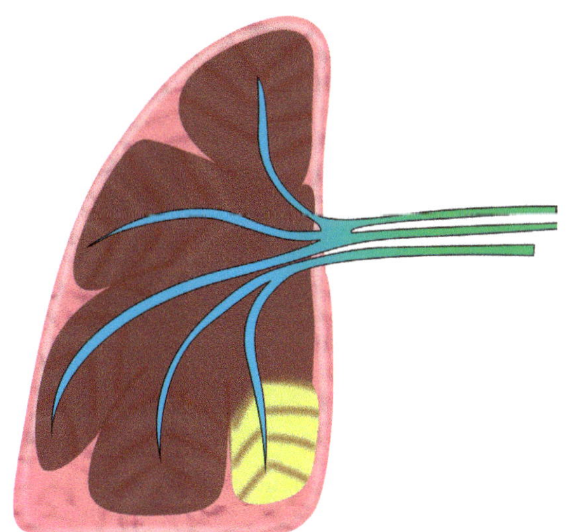

Fig. 62: Normal anatomy of interstitium: Schematic diagram demonstrates peribronchovascular interstitium in green extending to the secondary lobules. In secondary lobules it forms centrilobular interstitium (blue). The periphery of the secondary lobule is bounded by the interlobular interstitium (yellow). Within the secondary lobule the fine bands in brown represent the intralobular interstitium.

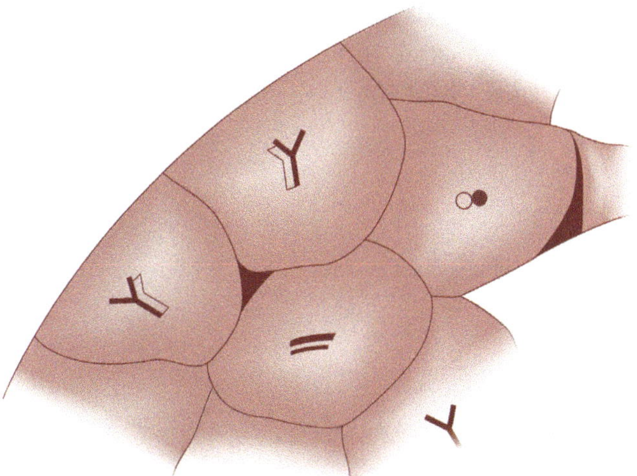

Fig. 63: Anatomy of secondary lobule—schematic diagram demonstrates polygonal secondary lobules. The secondary lobules share common walls with lymphatics and pulmonary veins in their walls. The center of the secondary lobule contains the centrilobular artery and bronchus.

■ RADIOGRAPHIC PATTERNS OF DISEASE PROCESSES

The most important aspects of imaging are to determine the anatomic location of a lesion, whether in the lungs, mediastinum, pleura or chest wall as well as the nature of the lesion. The most common abnormality visualized on a radiograph is a pulmonary opacity **(Table 2)**. An opacity is often ill-defined and is more opaque than the surrounding lung. It is useful to categorize the patterns of pulmonary opacities as it helps to narrow the differential diagnostic possibilities.

Consolidation/Air-space Opacities

Air-space opacities represent one or more ill-defined areas of increased density in the lung parenchyma. When they abut the pleura they have a sharp margin. Vascular shadows are obscured by the air-space opacity, as the air-filled dark lung does not contrast with the

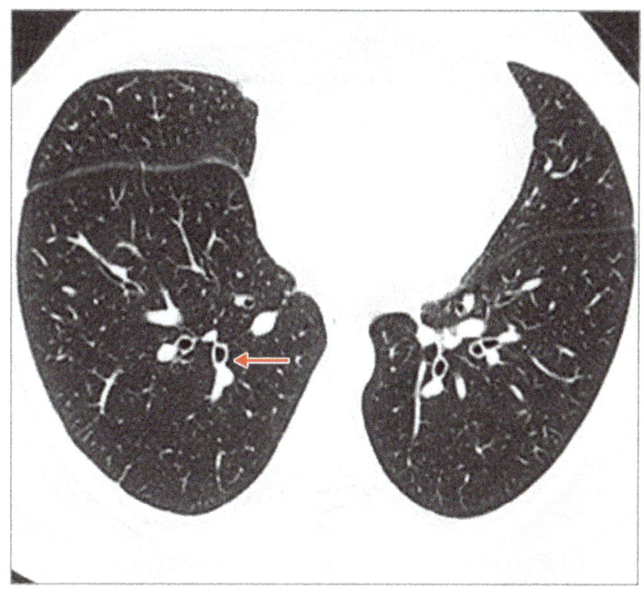

Fig. 64: CT chest showing the normal bronchoarterial ratio.

Table 2: Patterns of pulmonary opacities.
• Consolidation or air-space opacities
• Atelectasis
• Linear/band-like opacities
• Nodular/reticulonodular opacities
• Nodules/masses
• Cavitations
• Cysts/bullae/honeycombing
• Calcifications

soft tissue density of vessels. Similarly, intrapulmonary airways are rarely visible on chest X-rays. With air-space opacification the air in the airways contrasts with the air-space opacity, so that the airways become visible. This appearance is known as an air bronchogram sign. It also confirms the opacity is intrapulmonary. Another useful sign is the silhouette sign. The borders of the heart and domes of the diaphragm are well-visualized as they are contrasted by the interface with the dark lung. If a pulmonary opacity is in contact with the margins of the heart/diaphragm there is an interruption of the margins resulting in a loss of silhouette. This helps in detecting and localizing the abnormality. Conversely, presence of an opacity with preservations of the silhouette would indicate that the pulmonary abnormality is not in contact with the heart border or diaphragmatic surface. Cavitation may occur within air-space opacities. The cavity results following expulsion or drainage of necrotic contents via the bronchial tree. A gas-filled space with or without an air-fluid level is seen in the air-space opacity. CT is more sensitive in detection of air-space opacities; it may detect opacities even when the chest X-ray is normal. The causes of air-space opacities are numerous; any pathological process which results in filling of alveoli will result in an air-space opacity. The differential diagnosis of air-space opacities includes pneumonia, atelectasis, infarction, hemorrhage, neoplasm, and edema (**Figs. 65 to 74**).

Important points which may help in the differential diagnosis of air-space opacities:

- Opacities over half a lobe with no loss of lung volume are virtually diagnostic of pneumonia.
- Widespread pneumonia is invariably accompanied by cough and fever.
- Lobar consolidation with lobar expansion causing bulging of the fissure is most often seen in infection due to *Klebsiella pneumoniae*. It is also occasionally seen following infection with *Streptococcus pneumoniae*, staphylococcus, and other gram-negative bacteria.
- Neoplastic obstruction of a lobar bronchus usually causes some degree of atelectasis. However, bronchoalveolar carcinoma and lymphoma may appear as lobar pneumonia with no evidence of atelectasis, as the neoplastic process spreads in the alveolar spaces without involvement of the bronchi.
- Aspiration should be suspected with a history of alcoholism, seizures, unconscious state. Air-space opacities with evidence of associated loss of volume

are seen in patients with aspiration pneumonia. Air-space opacities with well-marked hemoptysis may occur in intrapulmonary hemorrhage.

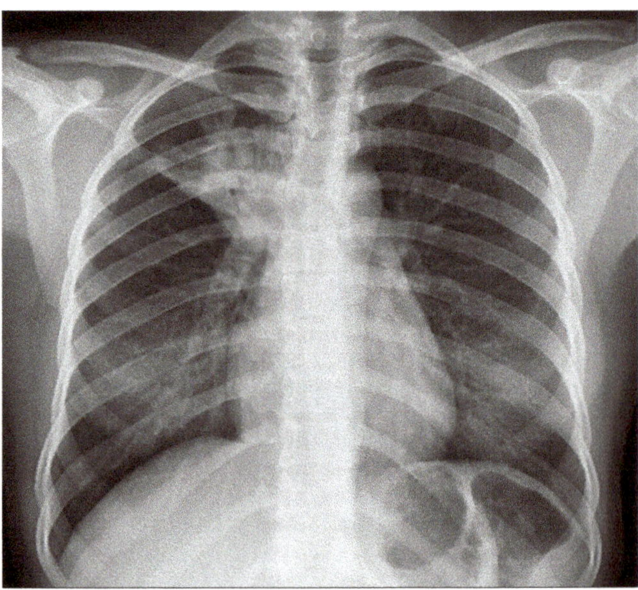

Fig. 65: Right upper lobe pneumonia: PA view of the chest demonstrates a consolidation in the right upper zone with loss of silhouette of right aortic border. Note there is no loss of volume and silhouette of right cardiac border. There is no shift of mediastinal structures. This is a feature of pneumonia.

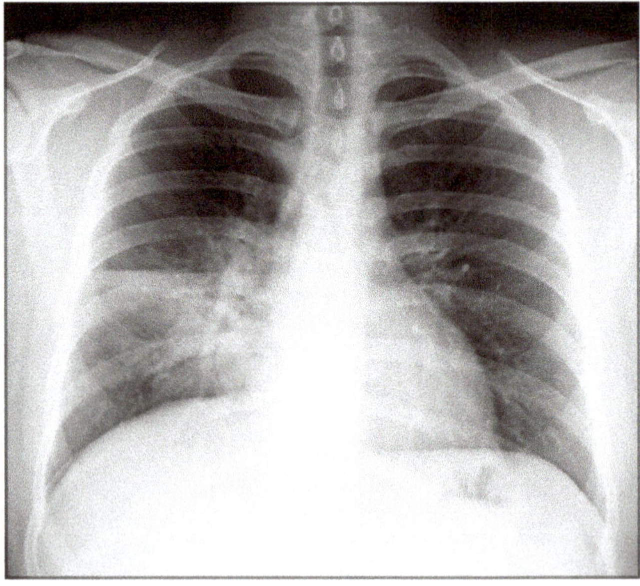

Fig. 66: Right middle lobe pneumonia: PA view of the chest demonstrates ill-defined air space opacities in the right lower zone which has an ill-defined inferior margin and sharp superior margin. Air space opacities are ill-defined, however, when they about the pleura in this case, they have a sharp margin. Note there is loss of silhouette of right cardiac border but silhouette of right aortic border is preserved.

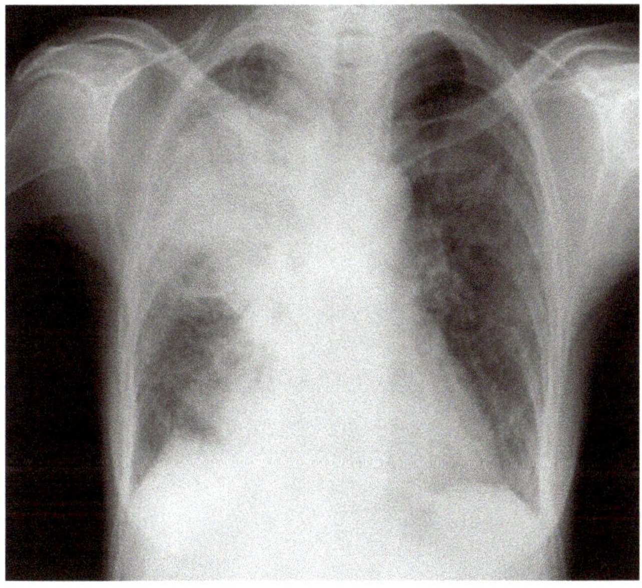

Fig. 67: Right upper and middle lobe pneumonia: Large area of consolidation is seen in the right lung with loss of silhouettes of both right cardiac and right aortic borders and with subtle bronchograms within; note there is no evidence of loss of volume or mediastinal shift.

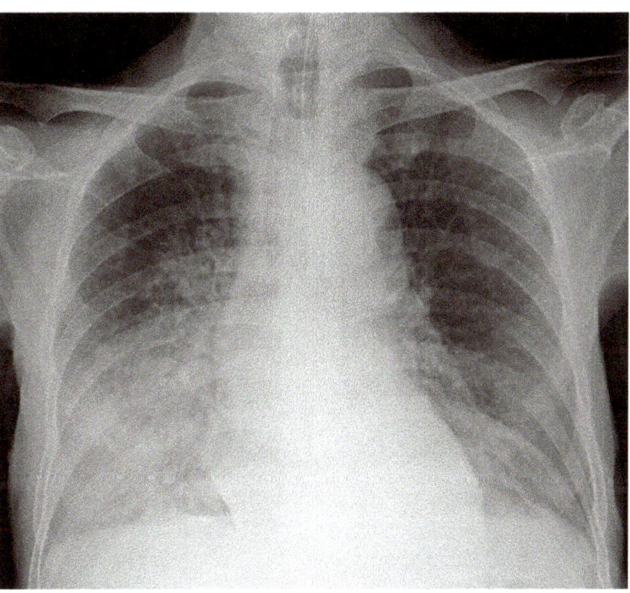

Fig. 69: Right lower lobe pneumonia. PA view of the chest demonstrates an ill-defined area of consolidation in the right lower zone; there is no loss of the silhouette of the cardiac as well as diaphragmatic surface indicating this consolidation is not in contact with either the diaphragm or cardiac surface.

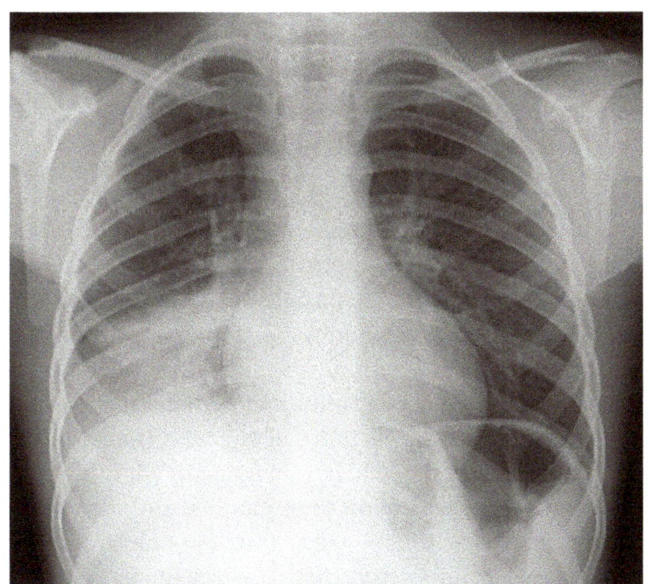

Fig. 68: Right lower lobe pneumonia. PA view of the chest demonstrates an ill-defined consolidation in the right lower zone preserving silhouette with cardiac margin but loss of silhouette with diaphragm.

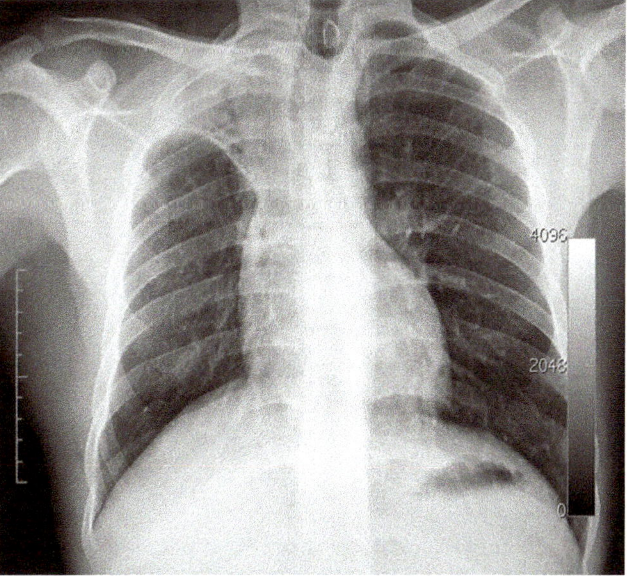

Fig. 70: Right upper lobe pneumonia with collapse consolidation: PA view of the chest reveals a triangular shaped consolidation with air bronchograms in the right upper zone associated with elevation of the minor fissure and mild deviation of trachea to the right representing a right upper lobe consolidation with partial collapse.

- Cavitation within a consolidated lobe could represent tuberculosis or a necrotizing pneumonia **(Fig. 72)**. The latter is commonly caused by *Klebsiella (Kl.) pneumoniae,*

Pseudomonas (Ps.) aeruginosa, Staphylococcus aureus and anaerobic bacteria. Cavitation could also arise in relation to noninfectious etiologies such as Wegener's

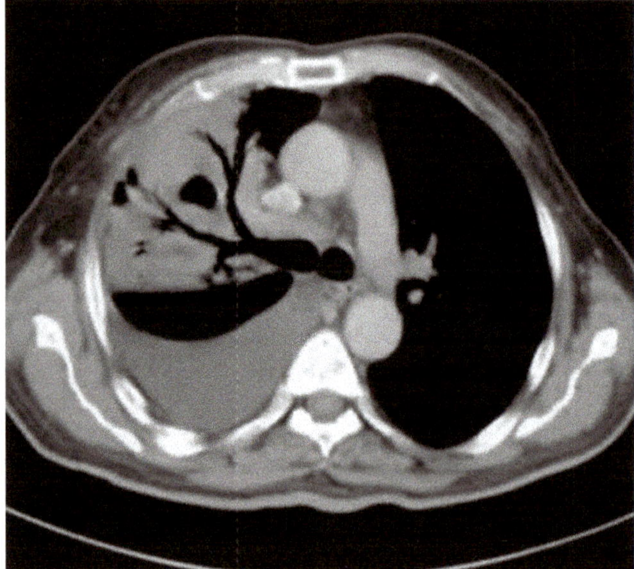

Fig. 71: Consolidation. CT chest demonstrates a large consolidation in the right middle lobe with an air bronchogram pattern. There is an associated pleural effusion.

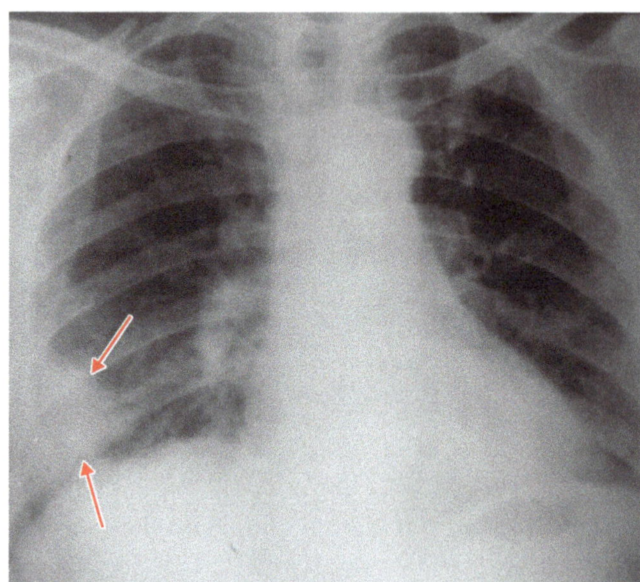

Fig. 73: Pulmonary infarct. PA view of the chest reveals a wedge-shaped area of consolidation in the right lower zone abutting the pleura. The appearance of a wedge-shaped consolidation should raise the possibility of a pulmonary infarct.

- Rib or vertebral body destruction in the absence of a mass points to a metastatic lesion, though tuberculosis or fungal infections can also present similarly, as destructive bone lesions.

■ BAT WING PATTERN OF PULMONARY OPACITY

This is a term used to describe diffuse parahilar opacities which have ill-defined margins. These may be symmetric or asymmetric, being larger on one side. The most common cause for this opacity is pulmonary edema, especially if associated with cardiomegaly/pleural effusion/Kerly A/B lines. Another feature of pulmonary edema is the rapid appearance and disappearance of opacities **(Figs. 78 and 79)**. Other conditions which may present with this type of opacities are aspiration pneumonias, and inhalation exposure to noxious gases. Immunocompromised patients, especially *Pneumocystis jirovecii* pneumonia can have a similar appearance **(Fig. 80)**. Bat wing opacities unchanged over a long period of time with nonspecific symptoms, suggest the possibility of alveolar proteinosis **(Fig. 81)** or a neoplastic process such as lymphangitic carcinomatosis.

Peripheral air-space consolidations are considered as a photographic negative of pulmonary edema as the opacities are in the lung periphery. Especially when

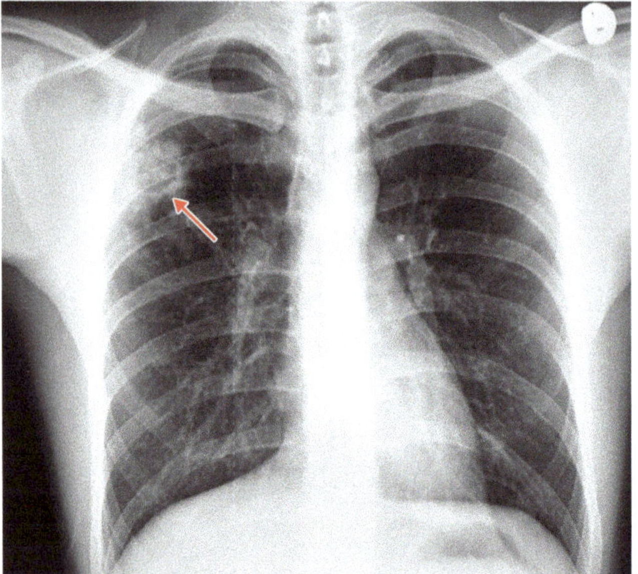

Fig. 72: Consolidation with cavitation: PA view of the chest reveals ill-defined area of consolidation with cavitation in the right upper zone. Causative organism—*Staphylococcus aureus*.

granulomatosis, other forms of vasculitis and in neoplasms **(Figs. 75 to 77)**.

- Lucencies seen within an air-space opacity could be due to overlying uninvolved lung, areas of centrilobular emphysema within the abnormal lung, necrosis of tissue with cavitation, pneumatoceles.

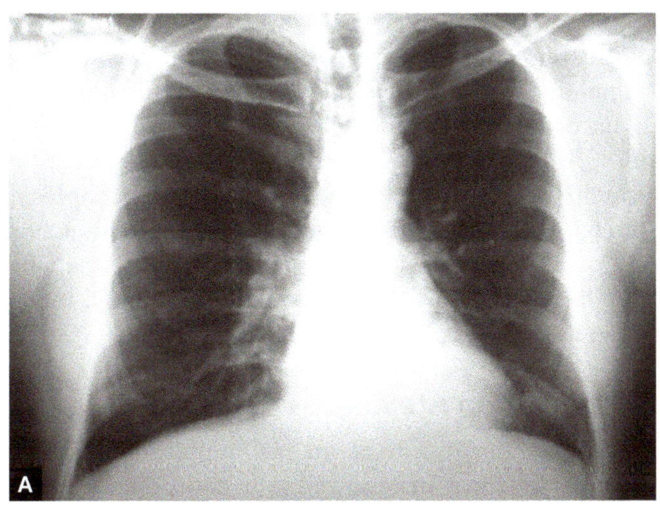

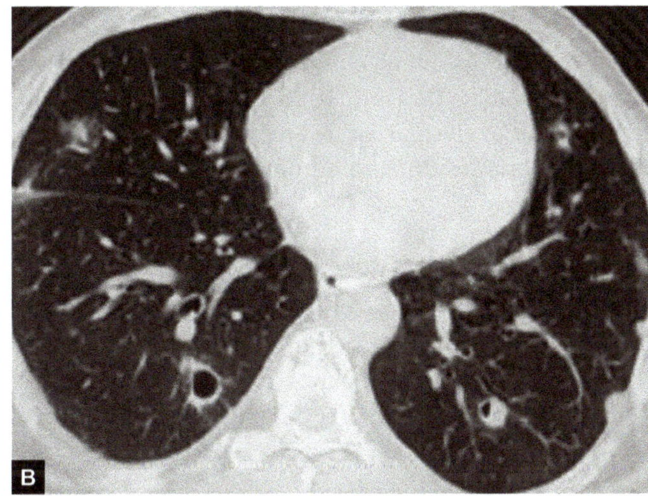

Figs. 74A and B: (A) X-ray chest in a febrile patient demonstrates no abnormality; (B) CT chest reveals multiple bilateral cavitating and subpleural nodular lesions. CT is more sensitive than chest X-rays in detection of focal lesions, as well as demonstrating internal morphology of focal lesions, such as cavitation, necrosis, calcification, and air bronchograms.

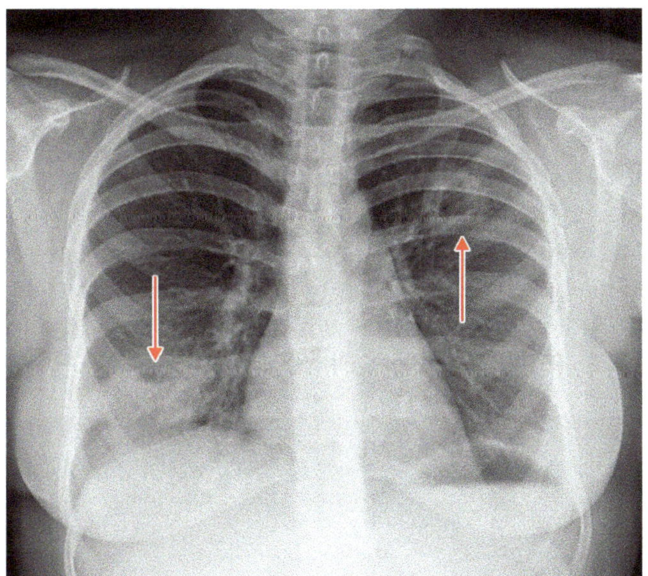

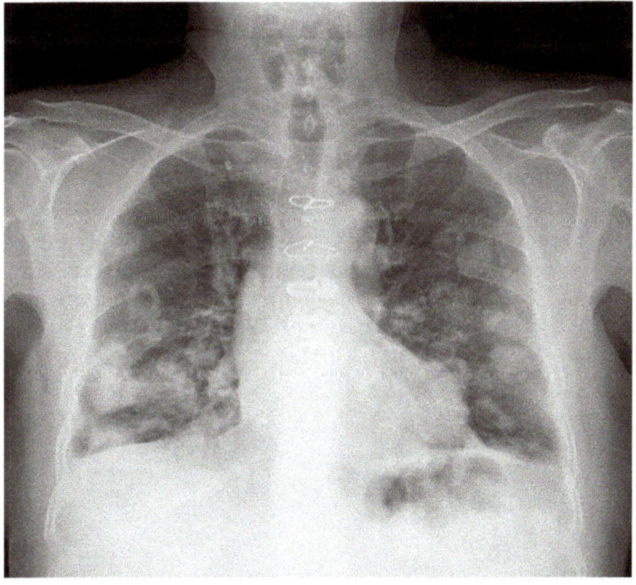

Fig. 75: Lung abscess: PA view of chest reveals thick-walled cavitatory lesions with air-fluid level in the left upper zone as well as in the right lower zone. These lesions represent lung abscesses.

Fig. 76: Wegener's granulomatosis: PA view of the chest X-ray reveals multiple well-defined rounded nodular lesions in both the mid and lower zones. Some appear solid, some cavitatory and some with air-fluid levels. c-ANCA was strongly positive in this patient confirming Wegener's granulomatosis.

present in the upper zones the most common possibility is chronic eosinophilic pneumonia. If the opacities are not predominantly in the upper zones, the possibilities include cryptogenic organizing pneumonia, viral pneumonia or a mycoplasmal pneumonia. Fleeting shadows, shadows which come and go, or appear in different regions of the lungs, raise the possibilities of pulmonary edema, eosinophilic pneumonia, asthma, ABPA and vasculitis **(Figs. 82A to D)**.

White-out lungs are typical for acute respiratory distress syndrome (ARDS), especially with associated air bronchograms **(Fig. 83)**. Sarcoid may present with patchy opacities in the lungs which may be spherical and have associated mediastinal adenopathy.

■ COLLAPSE/ATELECTASIS

Often the words collapse and consolidation are used interchangeably. Consolidation is essentially due to replacement of alveolar air by an exudate, transudate or cellular debris resulting in a homogenous opacity with no loss of volume. Atelectasis or its synonym "collapse" indicates volume loss. The atelectatic/collapsed segment or lobe of the lung will therefore demonstrate a homogenous opacity with accompanying volume loss. Atelectasis is caused by bronchial obstruction which is either due to an intrabronchial pathology, foreign body or extrinsic compression of the bronchus (**Figs. 84A and B**). Compression atelectasis can be due to compression of adjacent lung by tumor, bulla, pneumothorax or pleural effusion.

Cicatrization Atelectasis

Following resolution of an inflammatory/infective process there may be localized atelectasis. This is due to either direct destruction of lung parenchyma or fibrotic contraction, termed as cicatrization fibrosis. This is commonly seen in tuberculosis, radiation fibrosis, interstitial pulmonary fibrosis, and bronchostenosis (**Figs. 85 and 86**).

Pulmonary fibrosis can cause significant loss of volume due to fibrotic contraction of lung parenchyma.

Plate or Discoid Atelectasis

This is a form of atelectasis, which is due to hypoventilation, leading to alveolar collapse. The alveoli in the lung bases as well as posterior aspects of the lung fields are the most prone to collapse. These appear as linear plate or disk-like opacities in the lower zones,

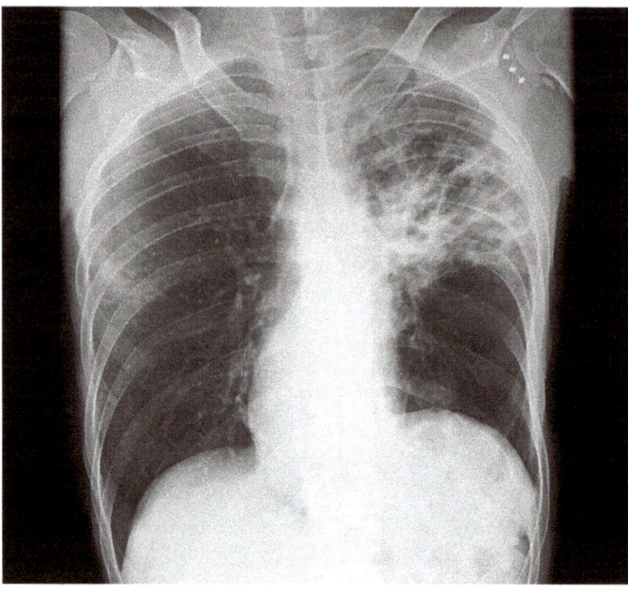

Fig. 77: Tuberculosis: PA view of the chest reveals ill-defined fibrocavitatory lesion in left upper and mid zones as well as patchy nodular consolidation with cavitation in right mid zone. Incidentally note is dextrocradia. The presence of upper/mid zone cavitation in the Indian subcontinent favors the diagnosis of tuberculosis.

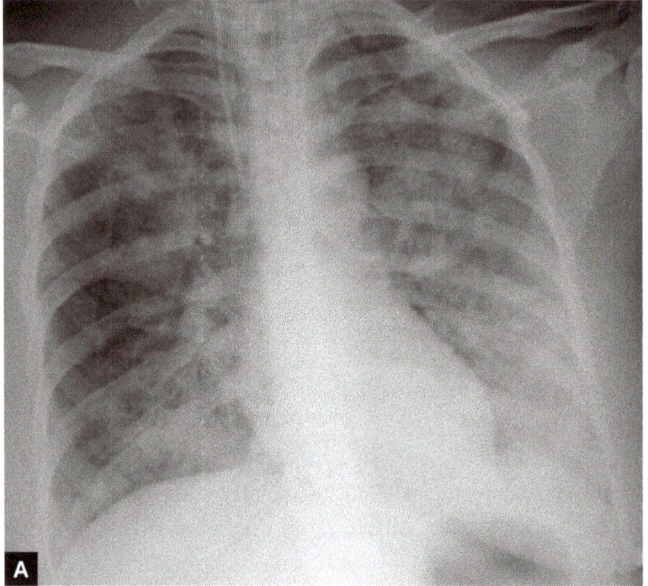

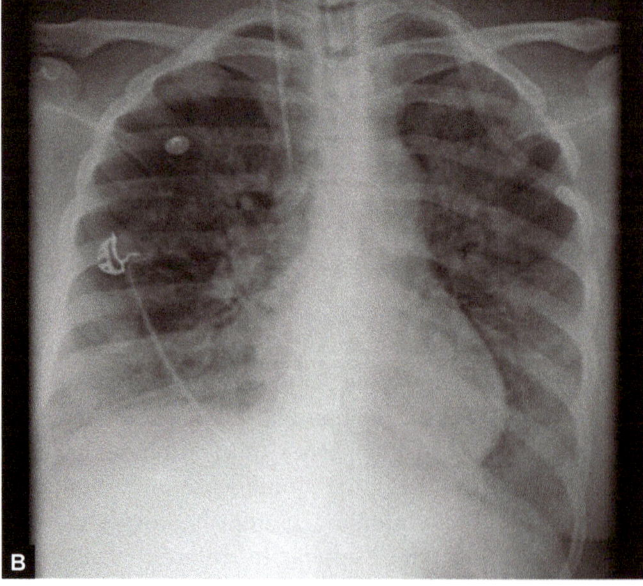

Figs. 78A and B: Pulmonary edema. AP view portable X-ray. (A) demonstrates ill-defined fluffy opacities in both lung fields; within a few hours, on a follow-up X-ray; (B) the opacities regressed.

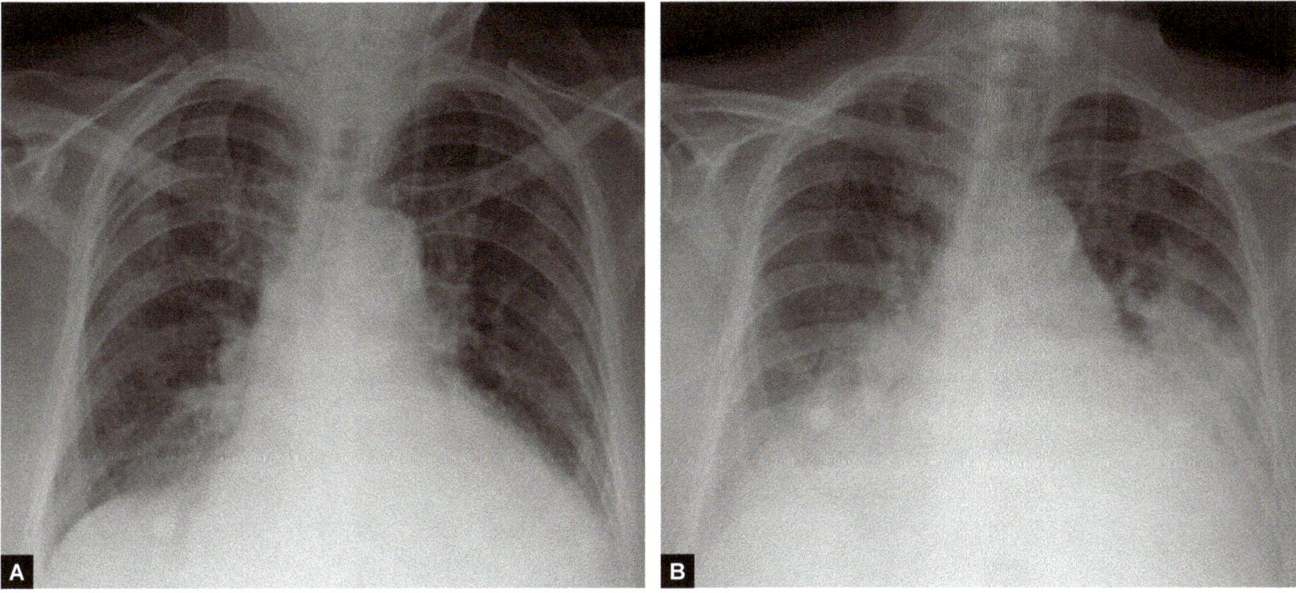

Figs. 79A and B: Pulmonary edema. Portable chest X-rays in a patient with left centralvenous catheter *in situ*. X-ray (A) reveals an ill-defined opacity in the right lower zone; (B) subsequent X-ray a few hours later reveals increasing opacities in the both lungs. This feature of rapidly appearing and disappearing shadows is highly suggestive of pulmonary edema.

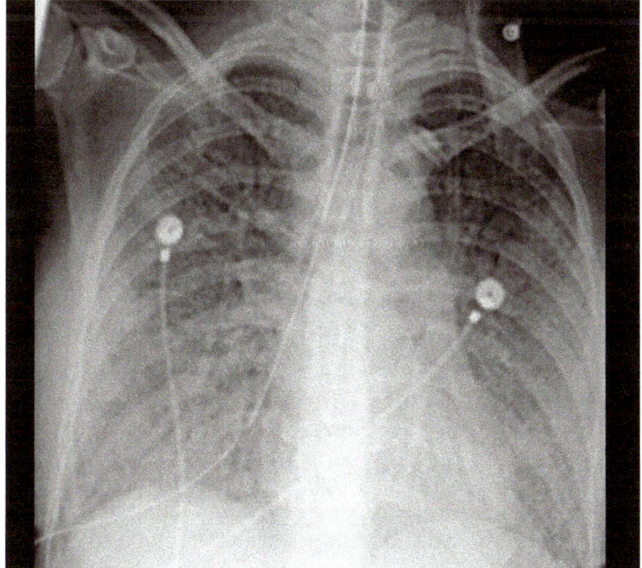

Fig. 80: *Pneumocystis jirovecii* pneumonia (PCP): Immuno-compromised patient with diffuse ill-defined air-space opacities. In the setting of immunocompromise, the most likely etiology would be *Pneumocystis jirovecii* pneumonia.

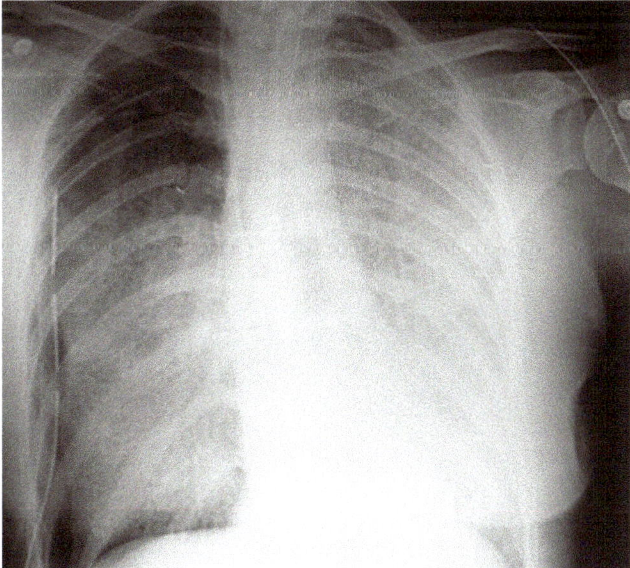

Fig. 81: Alveolar proteinosis. PA view of the chest demonstrates ill-defined airspace opacities in both lung fields sparing the right upper lobe. Intercostal drainage (ICD) seen in situ following thoracoscopic biopsy which revealed pulmonary alveolar proteinosis. Patient presented with cough, fever and mild dyspnea over 3 months. This is an example of bilateral white-out lungs with subacute to chronic symptoms.

occasionally extending across the whole breadth of the lower lobe **(Fig. 87)**. As these are due to hypoventilation they are seen mainly in hospitalized patients, post general anesthesia and in patients with an acute abdomen where the diaphragm is splinted, resulting in reduced respiratory excursion.

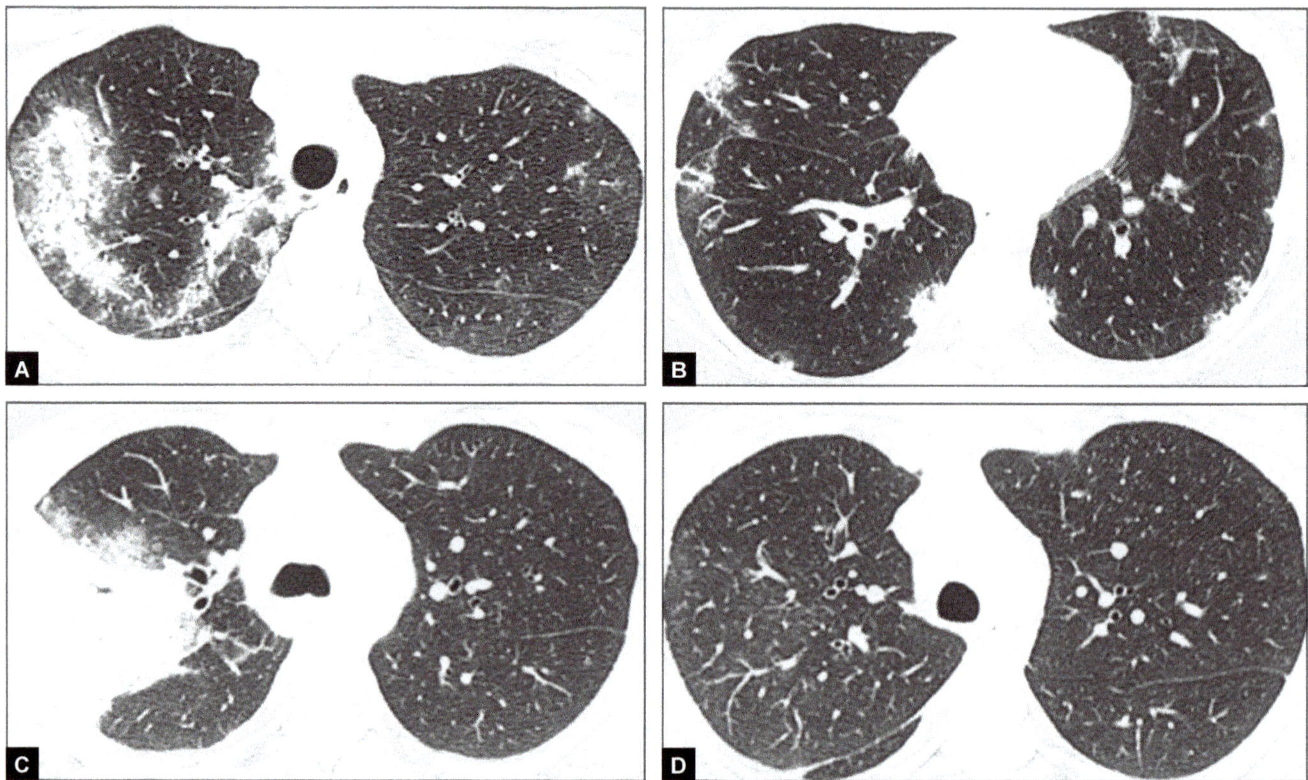

Figs. 82A to D: Fleeting opacities. Serial high-resolution computed tomography (HRCT) chest performed in 30-year-old patient with blood eosinophilia reveal (A) multiple ill-defined areas of consolidation seen in right upper lobe on 30/8/13. (B) resolution of previously seen consolidation with reappearance of lesions of less severe extent on 25/11/13. (C) ill-defined areas of peribronchovascular and subpleural consolidation with air bronchogram and adjacent areas of ground-glass attenuation involving right upper and middle lobes on 17/09/18. (D) regression in the right lung consolidation on 27/09/18. CT-guided biopsy performed on 30/08/13 revealed Churg-Strauss syndrome with vasculitis.

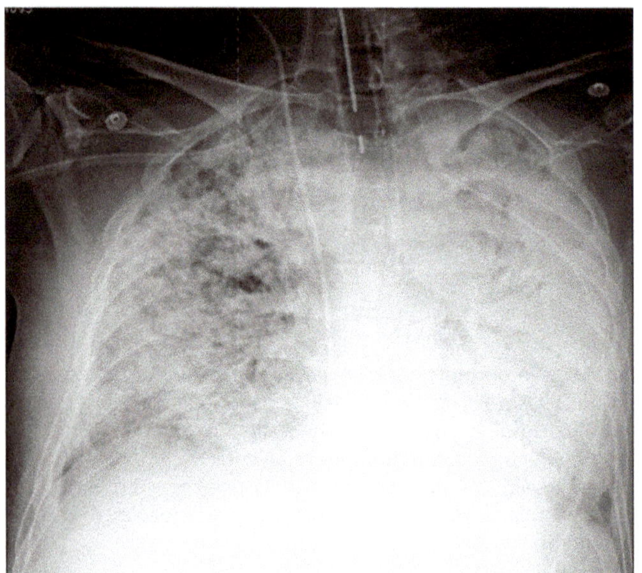

Fig. 83: Acute lung injury: Typical white-out lung appearance seen in acute lung injury.

Lobar Collapse/Atelectasis

The imaging features of lobar collapse are a pulmonary opacity with evidence of volume loss. The pulmonary opacity is due to loss of air in the alveoli of the collapsed segment/lobe and/or due to retained mucous secretions. The loss of volume is demonstrated by a shift of normal structures such as the hilum, interlobar fissures, mediastinum, with crowding of ribs, and of bronchovascular structures and elevation of the dome of the diaphragm. There is hypertranslucency of the normal ipsilateral lung due to compensatory overexpansion, with pulmonary vessels within it being more widely separated when compared to the opposite lung. It is important to note that when there is severe/total collapse of a lobe it may not always be possible to demonstrate the shadow of the lobar collapse on an X-ray, as the signs are too subtle. A shift of the hilum, fissure or the mediastinum should always suggest an underlying atelectasis.

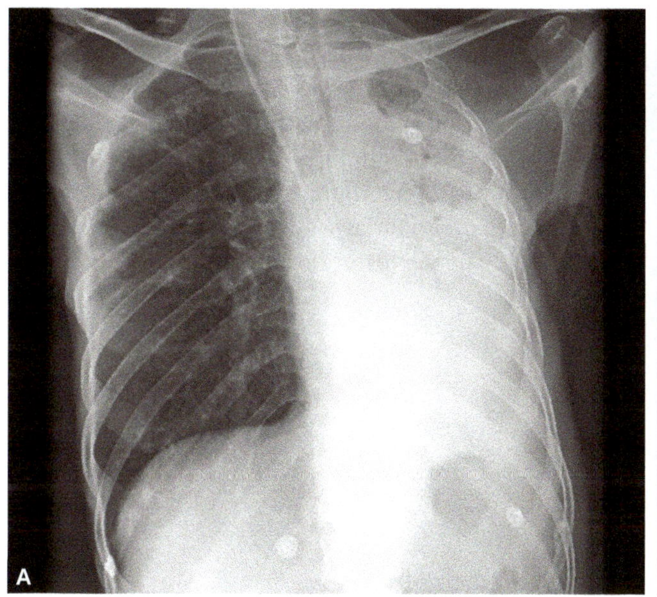

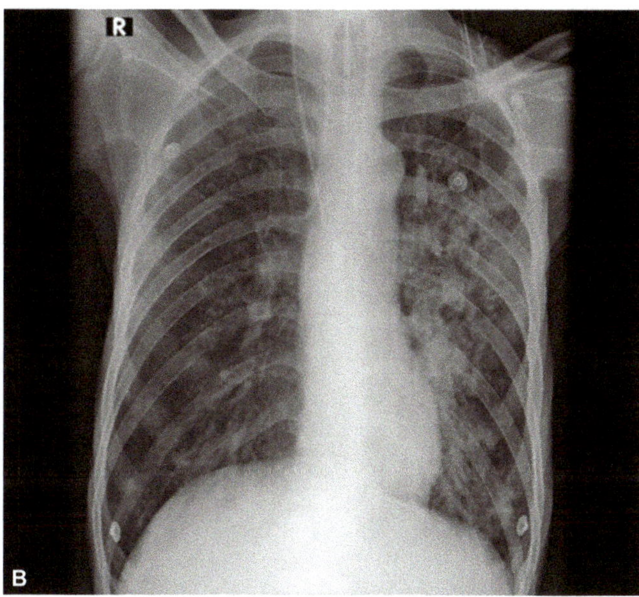

Figs. 84A and B: Obstructive atelectasis. Chest X-ray (A) demonstrates an opaque left hemithorax with a shift of the mediastinum to the left indicative collapse of left lung. The most likely cause would be an obstruction to the left main bronchus. Bronchoscopy revealed a mucus plug obstructing the left main bronchus; (B) after aspirating the mucus plug the lung expanded with few residual opacities.

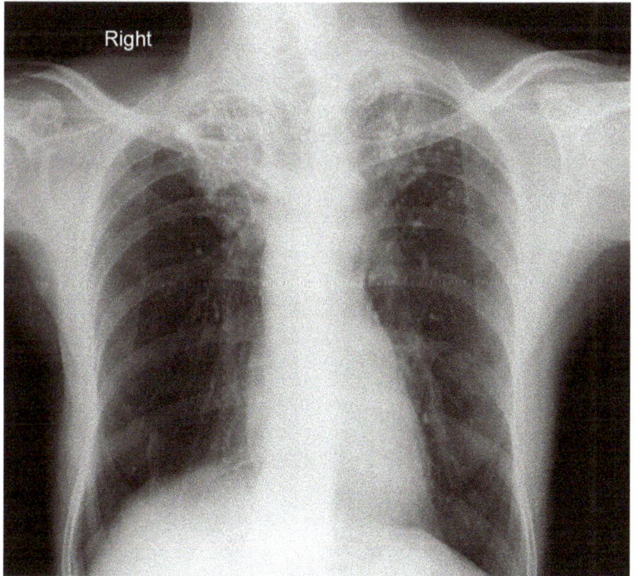

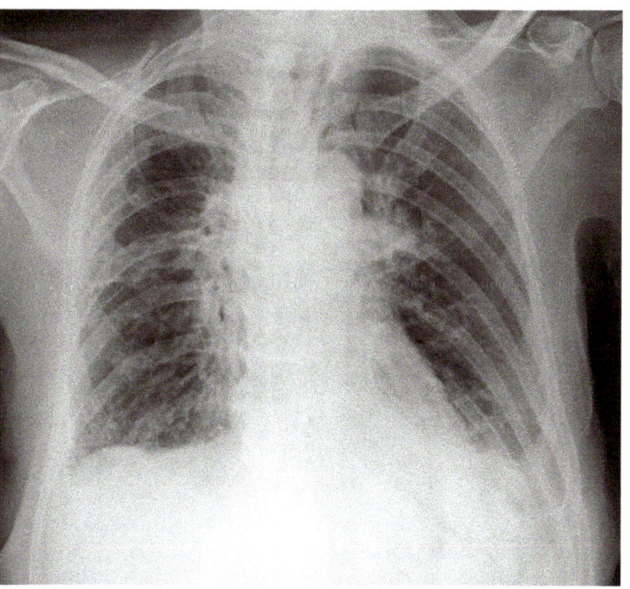

Fig. 85: Fibrocalcareous tuberculosis (TB). PA view of the chest reveals bilateral apical fibrotic lesions with calcified nodular lesions in both apices. These features of reticular opacities with calcified nodules and loss of volume are typical of old healed tuberculosis.

Fig. 86: Radiation fibrosis. PA view of the chest reveals an ill-defined opacity in the right apical region with associated loss of volume, shift of trachea to the right, with the right hilum pulled up. Patient had received radiation for cancer of the esophagus with resultant radiation fibrosis.

■ GOLDEN S-SIGN

When there is obstructive collapse by a central neoplasm with consequent peripheral collapse—the shape of the fissure assumes an "S" shape, as the fissure is concave peripherally and convex centrally.

Lower Lobe Atelectasis

The appearances of right and left lower lobe atelectasis are similar. The lobes collapse posteromedially in the lower part of the chest. Left lower lobe atelectasis is often difficult to detect as the collapsed lobe is hidden by the cardiac silhouette **(Fig. 88)**. A penetrated X-ray would reveal the opacity of the collapsed lower lobe **(Figs. 89A and B)**. As the lobe collapses posteromedially, the oblique fissure rotates backward and medially, the upper portion of the oblique fissure swinging downward. The collapsed lobe is seen as a triangular opacity lying against the mediastinum. On the right side the medial aspect of the diaphragm is obscured, the lateral margin of the adjacent vertebrae is effaced, the ipsilateral hilum is depressed and the ipsilateral lower lobe pulmonary artery is not visualized **(Figs. 90 and 91)**. Lower lobe atelectasis is better demonstrated on a lateral view **(Fig. 92)**. The lung collapses posteriorly, therefore is seen as an opacity overlying the vertebrae. Normally, the vertebrae on a lateral view demonstrate increasing transradiancy of the lower dorsal vertebrae. On CT the

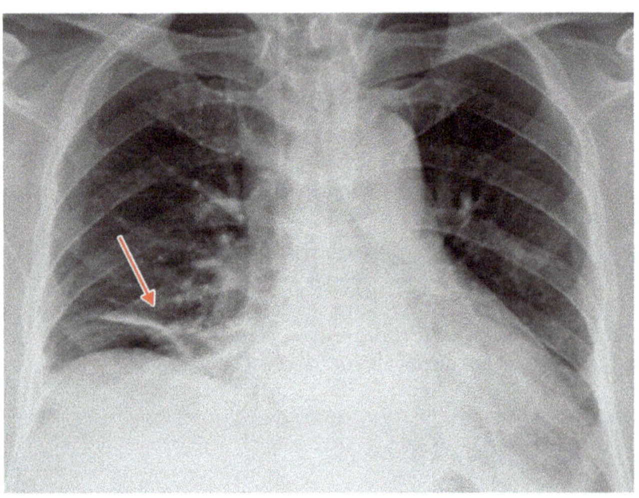

Fig. 87: Plate atelectasis. PA view of the chest in a postoperative patient reveals a central line in situ. Plate atelectasis is seen in the left lower zone with evidence of loss of volume as evidenced by elevation of left dome of diaphragm.

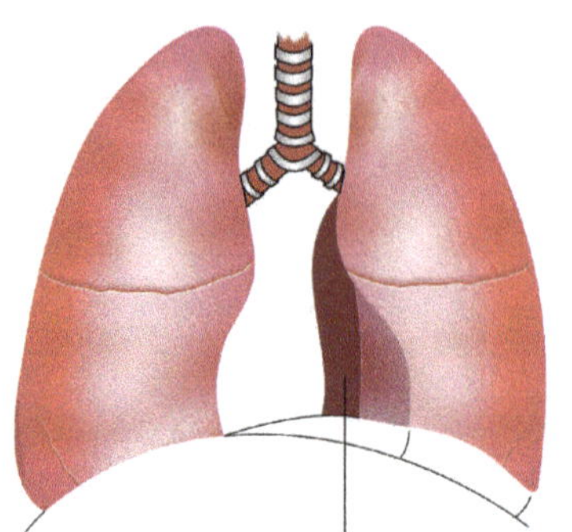
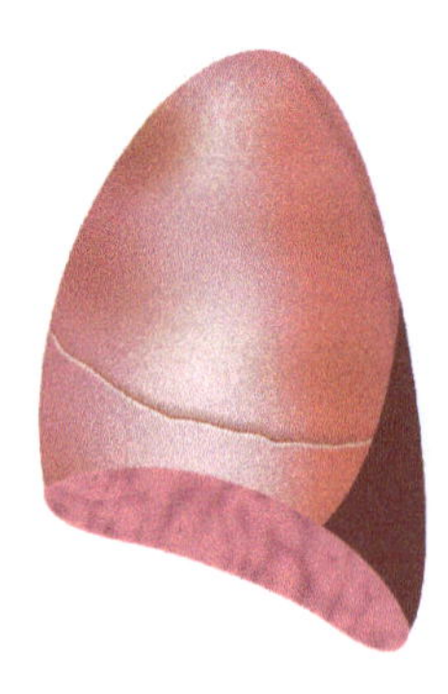
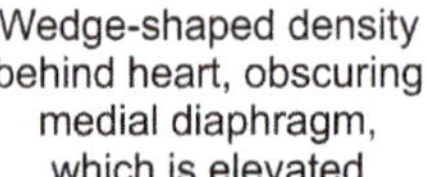

Fig. 88: Lower lobe collapse: Schematic diagram of left lower lobe collapse. The lower lobe collapses behind the cardiac silhouette on the PA view. The diaphragm is mildly elevated and the left lung volume is reduced. The diagram of the lateral view demonstrates the posterior collapse of the lower lobe, and a shift of the oblique fissure posteriorly.

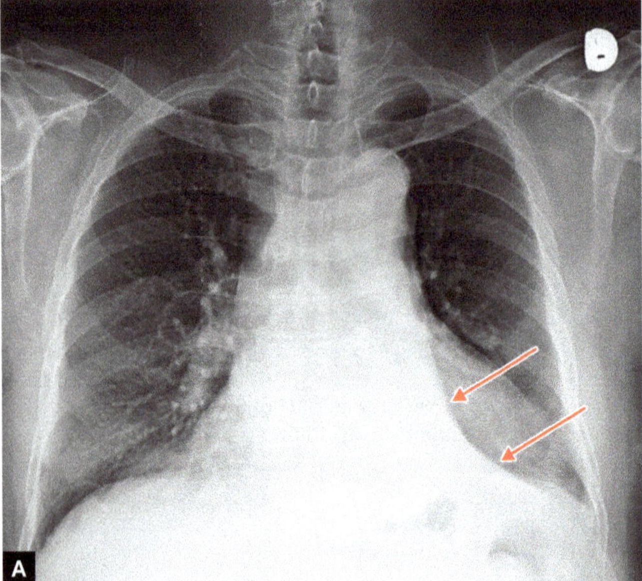

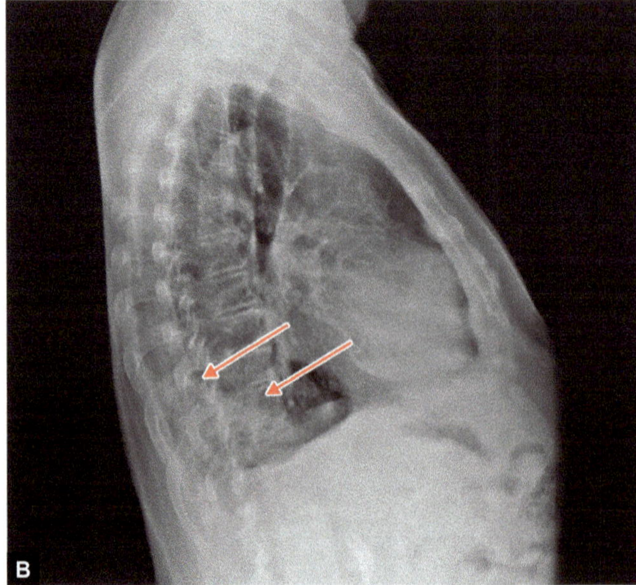

Figs. 89A and B: Left lower lobe collapse. (A) PA view of the chest demonstrates a homogenous opacity with a smooth margin behind the cardiac silhouette due to the collapse of left lower lobe. Note the evidence of volume loss in the left lung. (B) Lateral view of the chest demonstrates obscuration of the density of lower dorsal vertebral bodies due to the posteriorly collapsed left lower lobe.

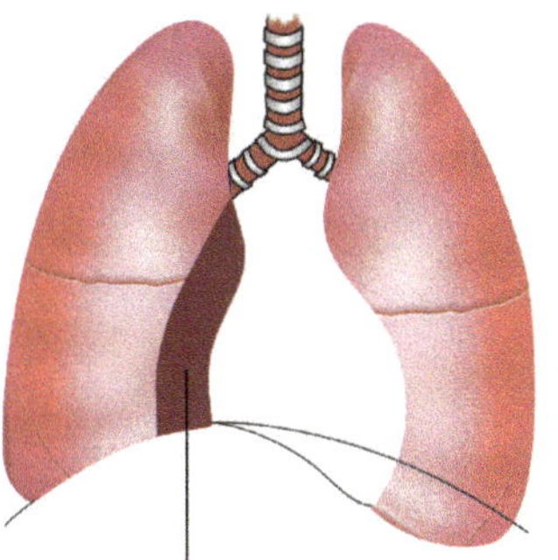
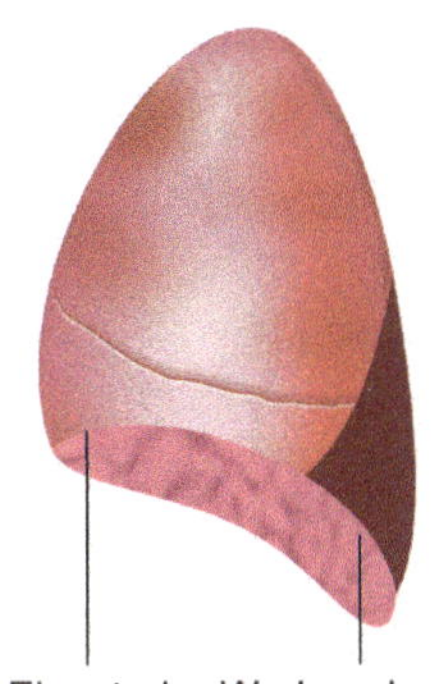

Fig. 90: Right lower lobe collapse: Schematic diagram—PA view demonstrates collapsed segment along the right heart border abutting the diaphragm. There is elevation of the right dome of diaphragm, loss of volume in the right lung and a shift of mediastinum to the right. Lateral view reveals the collapsed lung posteriorly with shift of the oblique fissure posteriorly.

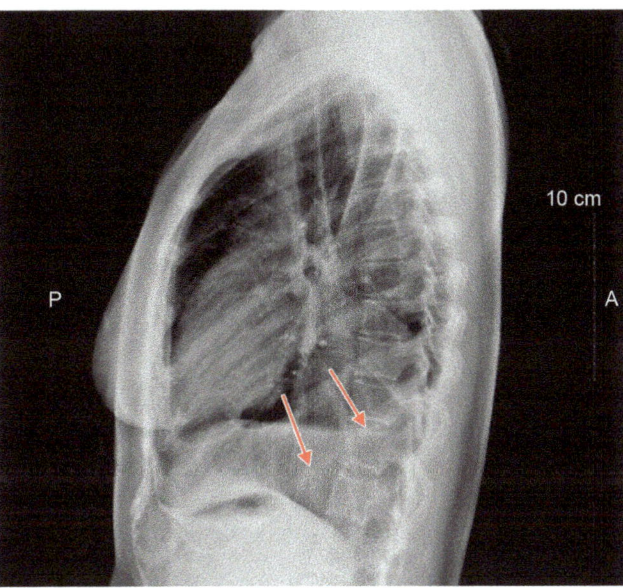

Fig. 92: Right lower lobe collapse. Lateral view demonstrates an ill-defined haze overlying the lower dorsal vertebrae. There is loss of normal increasing translucency of lower dorsal vertebrae due to the collapsed right lower lobe opacity overlapping the vertebrae. Note the elevated right dome of the diaphragm.

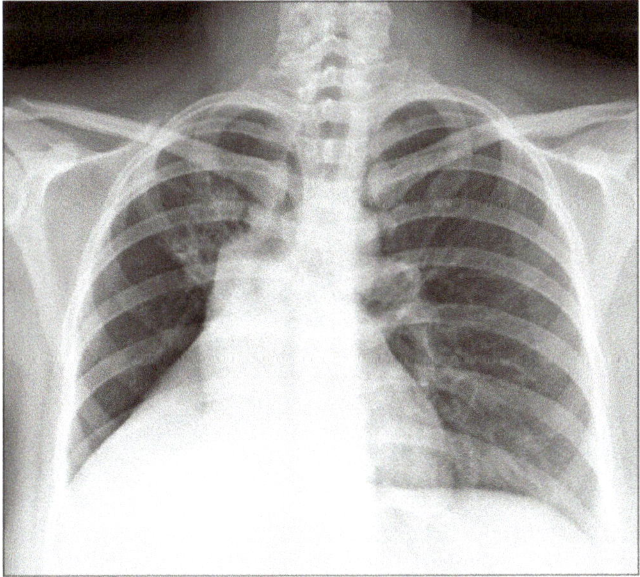

Fig. 91: Right lower lobe collapse. PA view of the chest demonstrates a homogenous opacity in the right paracardiac region with loss of the cardiac and diaphragmatic silhouette. There is evidence of loss of volume, as the right dome of the diaphragm is elevated and the right lung is smaller in size as compared to the left.

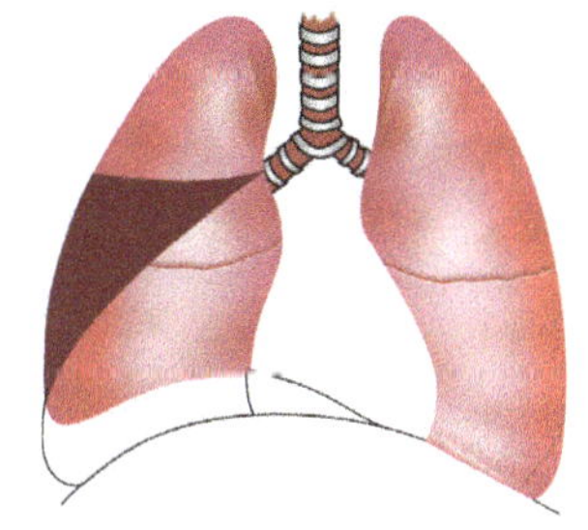
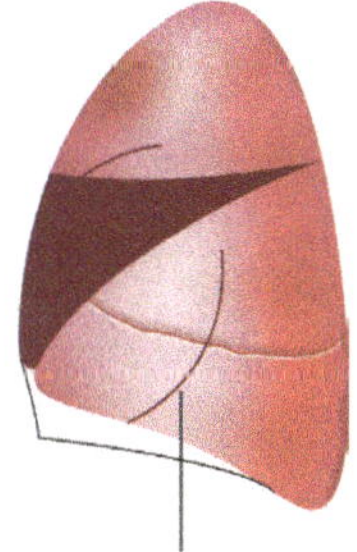

Fig. 93: Right middle lobe collapse. Schematic diagram demonstrates right lower zone opacity abutting the cardiac silhouette with elevation of the diaphragm, and reduction in right lung volume. Lateral view demonstrates minor and major fissure approximate with each other, with a triangular opacity representing the collapsed middle lobe within.

collapsed lobe is seen plastered along the vertebral column in a posteromedial location. The major fissure rotates to lie obliquely.

Right Middle Lobe Atelectasis

The atelectatic right middle lobe on a chest X-ray is seen as an opacity along the right heart border resulting in a loss of the silhouette of the right cardiac border **(Figs. 93 and 94A)**. There is no significant change in the vasculature; the right hilum does not change in position. Right middle lobe atelectasis is best demonstrated on a lateral view as the horizontal fissure descends with increasing atelectasis **(Fig. 94B)**. The atelectatic lobe is seen as an opaque wedge extending from the hilum anteriorly. Occasionally,

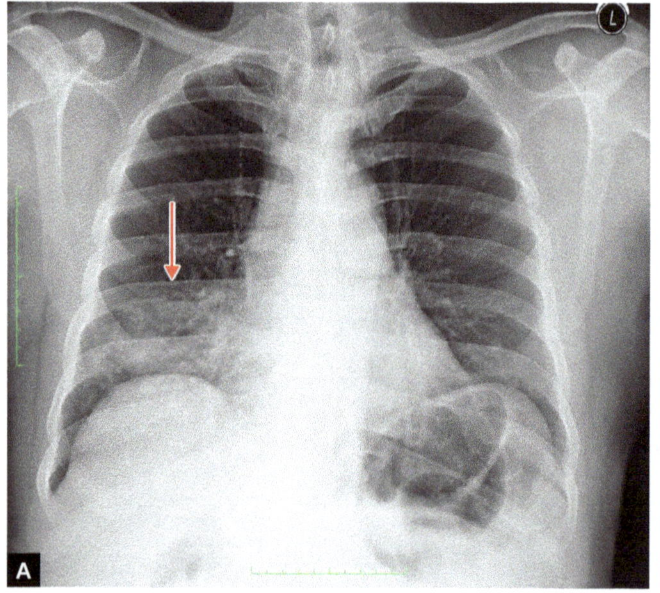

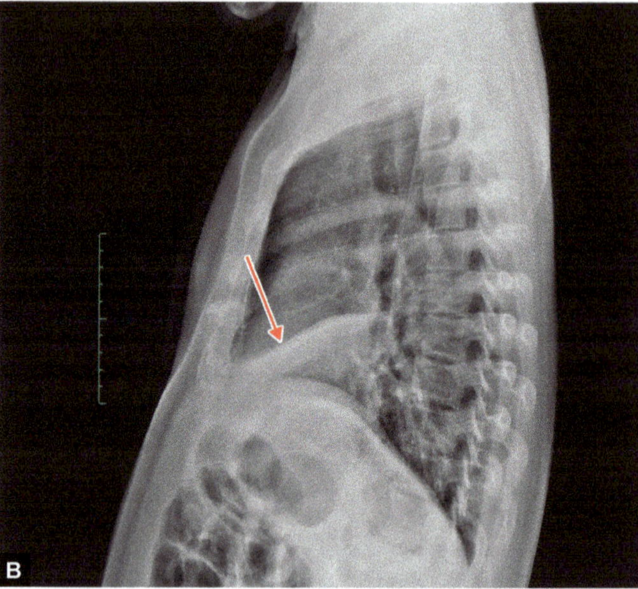

Figs. 94A and B: Right middle lobe collapse. (A) PA view demonstrates an ill-defined opacity in the right lower zone; (B) Lateral view of the chest reveals a homogenous opacity overlying the cardiac silhouette bounded by the interlobar fissures representing right middle lobe collapse. Note the marked downward shift of the lesser fissure.

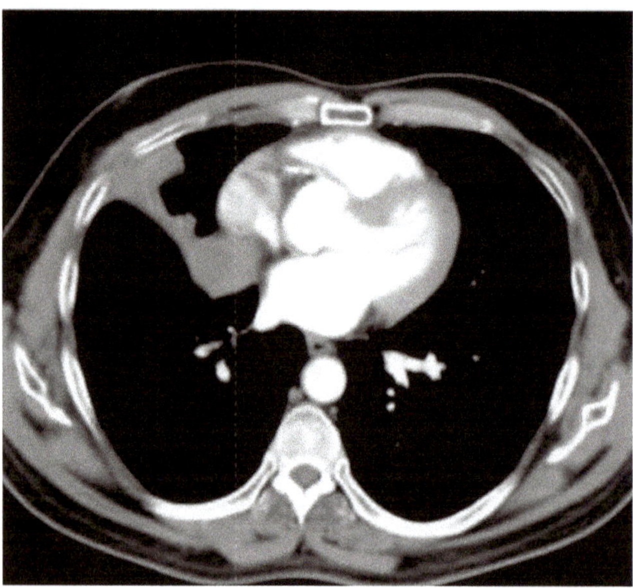

Fig. 95: Collapse of the lateral segment of the right middle lobe. CT chest reveals a mass lesion in the right hilum causing collapse of the lateral segment of the right middle lobe, seen as a band-like shadow in the right middle lobe.

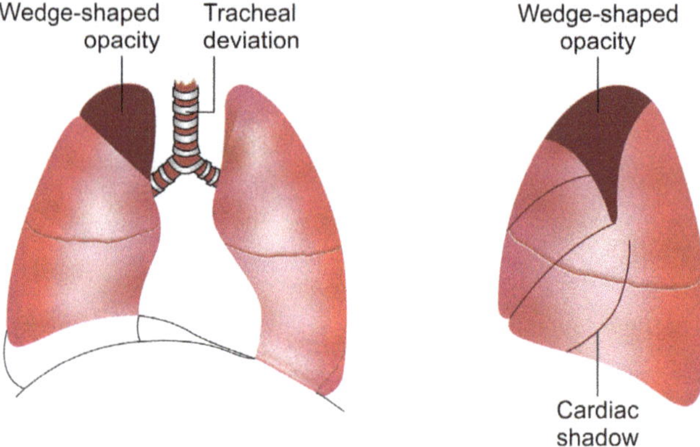

Fig. 96: Right upper lobe collapse: Schematic diagram demonstrates on PA view right upper lobe opacity, elevation of minor fissure, right hilum and right dome of diaphragm. Lateral view demonstrates elevation and backward rotation of minor fissure with collapsed right upper lobe opacity within the two fissures.

when the atelectasis is very severe the appearances may resemble a thickened fissure. On CT, right middle lobe atelectasis is seen as a triangular wedge atelectatic lung, bound by the major fissure posteriorly and minor fissure anteriorly **(Fig. 95)**.

Right Upper Lobe Collapse

The right upper lobe collapses against the mediastinum and lung apex **(Fig. 96)**. As the lobe collapses the silhouette of the superior vena cava is lost. When there is total collapse a wedge of tissue is seen in the right upper zone along the mediastinum **(Fig. 97)**. The right middle and lower lobes demonstrate compensatory expansion and there is elevation of the right hilum. The major and minor fissures move upward and toward each other. This is well seen on the lateral view. The collapsed lobe on the lateral view silhouettes the ascending aorta. On CT, the collapsed right upper lobe appears as a triangular soft tissue density lying against the mediastinum and anterior chest wall.

Left Upper Lobe Atelectasis

The pattern of collapse is complex, as there is no horizontal fissure. As the lobe collapses it pulls the major

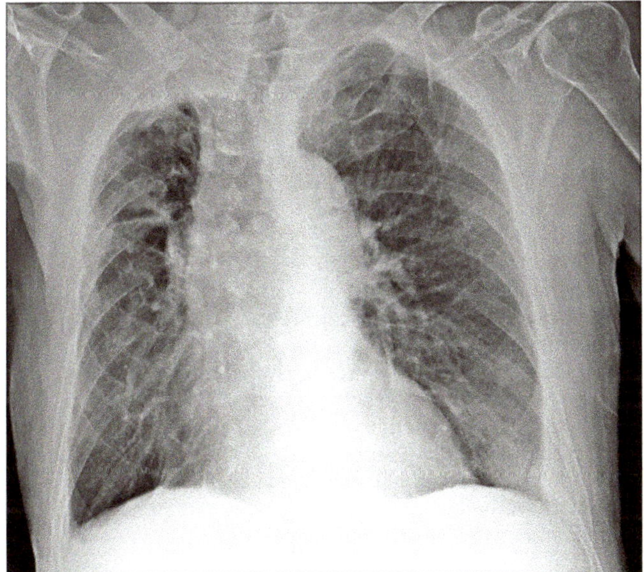

Fig. 97: Right upper lobe collapse: PA view of the chest demonstrates triangular opacity in the right apical region with the deviation of the trachea to the right and loss of volume in right hemithorax. This is due to the right upper lobe collapse.

fissure forward and the lower lobe expands posterior to the major fissure **(Figs. 98A to C)**. As the left lower lobe expands posterior to the collapsing left upper lobe, on PA radiographs the atelectatic left upper lobe appears as a diffuse haze overlying the left hilum often extending to the lung apex, but fading inferiorly and laterally **(Figs. 99A and B)**. The left cardiac and mediastinal silhouette is lost. As the lower lobe expands the aortic knuckle may be visible and consequently the left apex and upper mediastinum may be visible as the expanded lung occupies these regions.

On the lateral view the collapsed lung is seen anteriorly with the major fissure moving anteriorly to be relatively parallel to the chest wall. As the lower lobe overexpands air may be seen between the sternum and the atelectatic lung. The appearances on CT are very similar to those seen with right upper lobe atelectasis **(Fig. 99C)**.

Right Middle and Lower Lobe Atelectasis

This type of atelectasis is rare considering the distance between the two bronchi. It may however occur due to separate occlusions of the right middle and lower lobe bronchi. The appearances resemble a right lower lobe atelectasis; the extent of involvement is more extensive, extending to the lateral costophrenic angle on the PA view and to anterior chest wall on the lateral view.

Linear and Band-like Opacities

Linear opacities are linear densities less than 5 mm and bands are considered to be linear densities more than

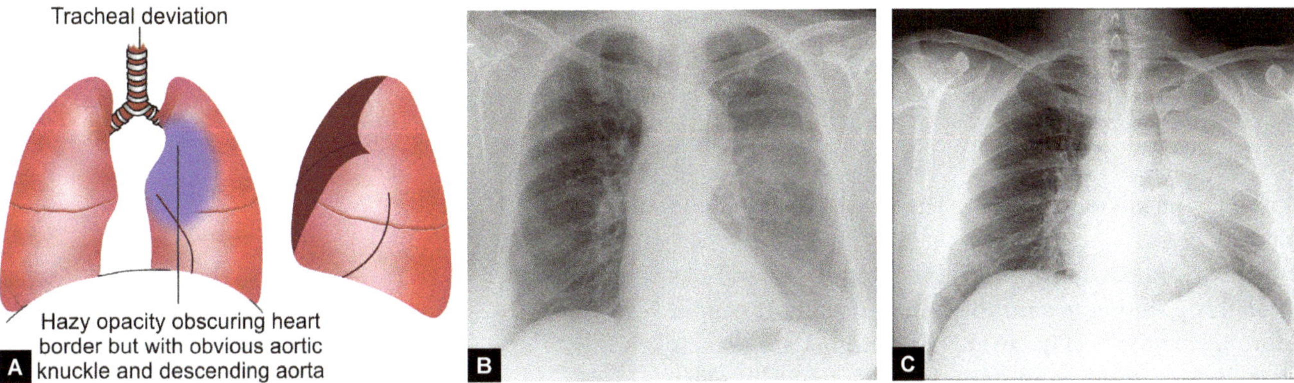

Figs. 98A to C: Left upper lobe collapse (A) Schematic diagram (B and C) PA views demonstrate an ill-defined haze overlying the left upper lobe. A homogenous opacity is not seen as in other lobar collapses as the compensatory expansion of the left lower lobe occurs posterior to the collapsed left upper lobe. These opacities are summated on a PA view resulting in only a hazy opacity. On the lateral view the opacity of the collapsed left upper lobe is better visualized, though with marked expansion of the lower lobe, the expanded lower lobe may intersperse between the sternum and collapsed left upper lobe. Note the major fissure has moved anteriorly parallel to the anterior chest wall.

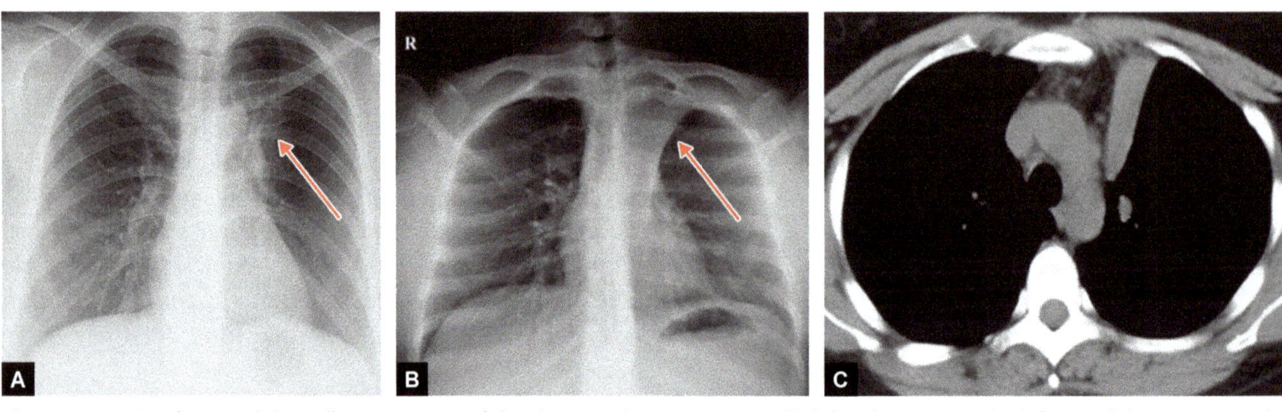

Figs. 99A to C: Left upper lobe collapse. PA view of the chest (A) demonstrates an ill-defined opacity in the left suprahilar region. Lordotic view (B) demonstrates a well-defined opacity plastered against the mediastinum. CT chest (C) demonstrates collapsed lobe abutting mediastinum.

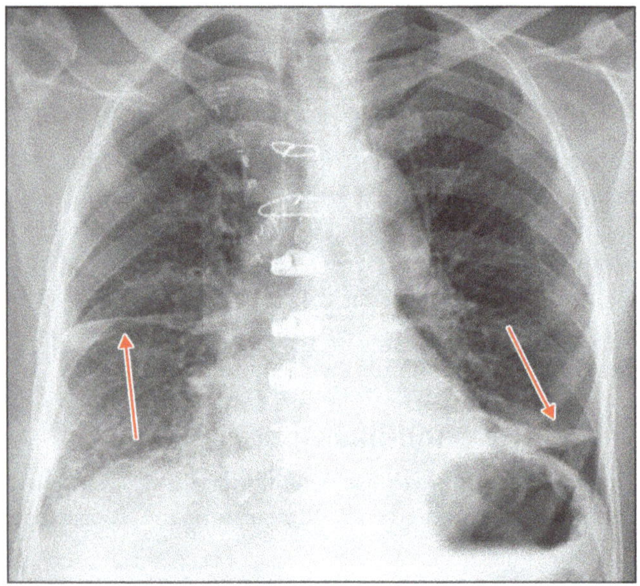

Fig. 100: Plate or Discoid atelectasis. PA view of the chest reveals linear bands in the right mid and left lower zone due to plate atelectasis, following general anesthesia.

Table 3: Causes of linear opacities.
• Clothing, tubes, etc.
• Wall of a bleb or pneumatocele
• Bronchocele (mucoid impaction)
• Parenchymal or pleuroparenchymal scar
• Discoid atelectasis
• Organizing pneumonia (presenting with a band-like pattern)
• Anomalous blood vessels or feeding and draining vessels to arteriovenous malformations
• Thickening of pleural fissures
• Pleural tail associated with pulmonary nodule
• Septal lines (Kerley lines) as in pulmonary edema, neoplastic infiltration, lymphangitis carcinomatosis

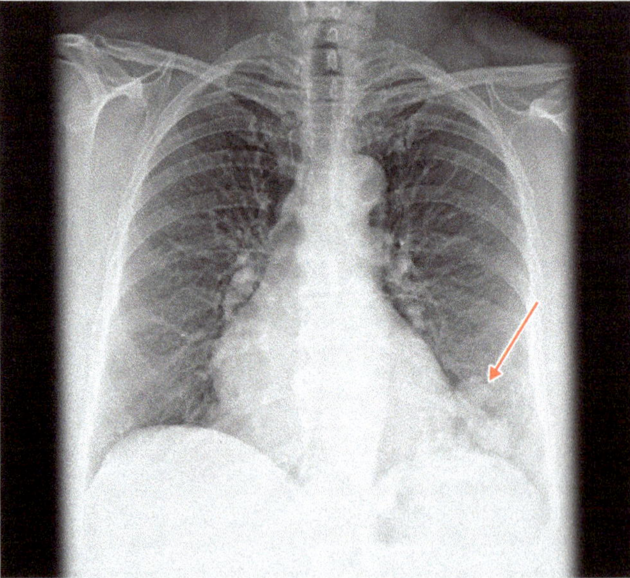

Fig. 101: Mucoid impaction chest X-ray reveals well-defined nodular opacities in left lower zone. CT demonstrated the nodular opacities to be due to mucoid impaction. The nodular opacities seen on X-ray are due to end on dilated bronchi with mucoid impaction.

5 mm in thickness **(Fig. 100)**. The causes are tabled in **Table 3**.

Mucoid impaction appears as one or more band-like opacities pointing toward the hilum, usually 1.0 cm or more in diameter **(Fig. 101)**. The margins are usually sharply demarcated and smooth with a finger-in-glove appearance. This appearance is mainly seen in ABPA but may also be seen as a result of bronchial obstruction in bronchial carcinoid, lung Ca, bronchostenosis, broncholithiasis, and bronchial atresia. If the lung distal to the obstructed segment is consolidated or collapses, the linear bands of mucoid impaction will not be visualized as they are now silhouetted by the collapse/consolidation.

Septal Lines

Interlobular septa of normal lungs are not visible on chest radiographs or even HRCT. When septa become thickened they become visible. Kerley first described septal lines especially in pulmonary edema. They were named ABC, "A" referred to septal lines which ranged up to 4.0 cm radiating from the hila into the central portions of the lung, more visible in the upper/mid zones of lung. These are now referred to as deep septa. The "B" lines are short, less than 1.0 cm in length, are parallel to each other and at right angles to the pleura. They are referred to as peripheral interlobular septa, and are seen most frequently in the lung bases. Kerley "C" lines have been dropped, as they actually represent many B lines superimposed on each other. It is important to differentiate septal lines from vascular shadows. Kerley B lines are essentially visualized in the last 1 cm of lung parenchyma; lung vessels are not seen in the last 1 cm of the lung. Kerley A lines are differentiated from lung vessels as they are much thinner and do not branch **(Figs. 102A and B)**.

Reticular and Reticulonodular Opacities (Table 4) (Figs. 103 to 110)

Table 4: Reticular and reticulonodular opacities.

- Interstitial lung disease
- Pulmonary edema or pneumonia
- Fever with reticular opacities—mycoplasmic or viral pneumonia
- Lymphangitis carcinomatosis—unilateral reticular opacities
- Tuberculosis, rarer causes include fungal disease (histoplasmosis), chronic hypersensitivity pneumonitis, ankylosing spondylitis
- Sarcoidosis
- Pneumoconiosis
- Calcified opacities in both lung fields—miliary metastases due to thyroid carcinoma, osteogenic sarcoma, tuberculosis
- High-density miliary nodules are observed in silicosis, baritosis, microlithiasis
- Cloud-like punctate calcification is typically seen in alveolar microlithiasis
- Conglomerate opacities with fibrosis and miliary nodules—progressive massive fibrosis with pneumoconiosis

Unilateral Transradiancy of the Lung

The causes for unilateral transradiancy of the lung are:

- *Radiographic artifact*: The radiographic output is usually adjusted to increase the output in the region of the bases as compared to the apices. This is known as a heel-toe effect. If this heel-toe effect is horizontally oriented rather than vertically, it will result in one

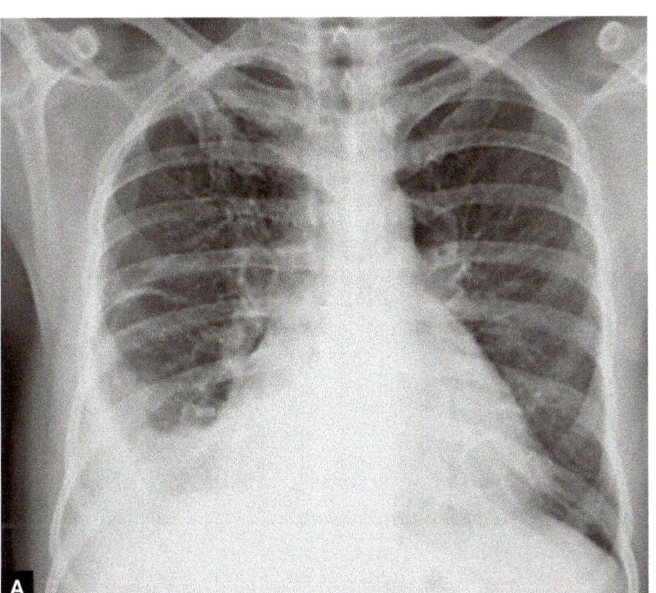

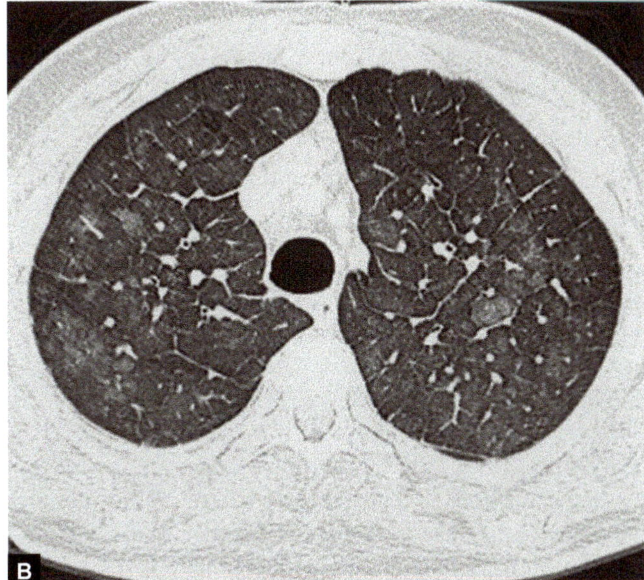

Figs. 102A and B: Septal lines: (A) Chest X-ray demonstrates cardiomegaly, right pleural effusion and prominent lung markings; (B) CT chest demonstrates smooth septal thickening with ground-glass densities due to pulmonary edema secondary to congestive cardiac failure.

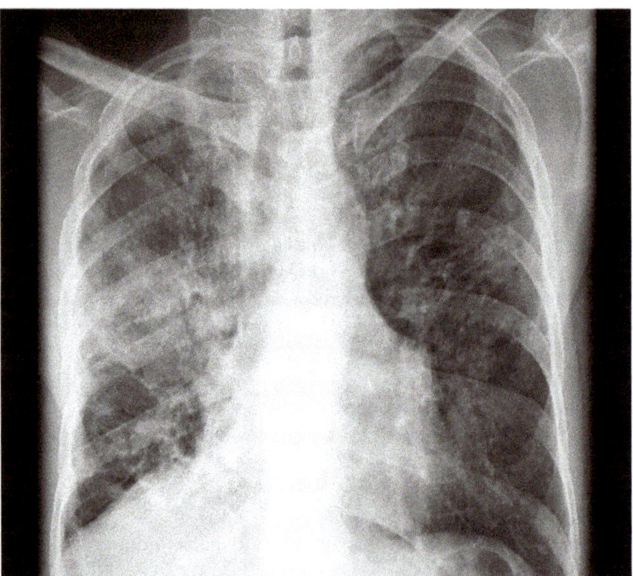

Fig. 103: Interstitial pneumonia: Chest X-ray reveals extensive reticular opacities and ill-defined areas of consolidation more on right mid zone as result of an interstitial pneumonia.

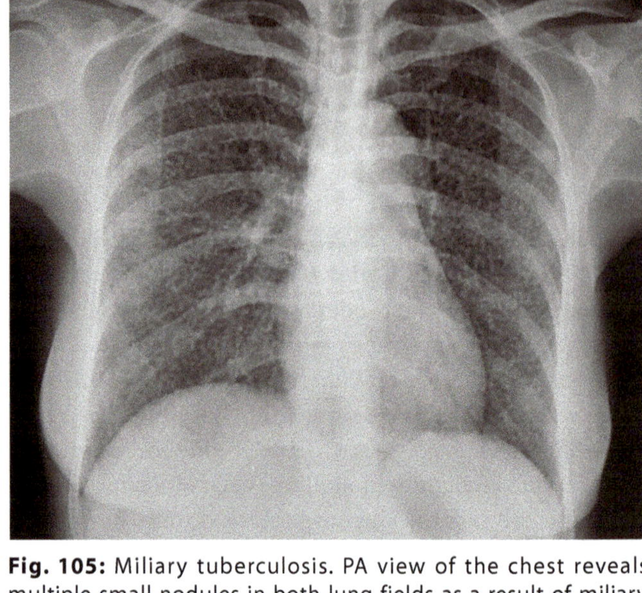

Fig. 105: Miliary tuberculosis. PA view of the chest reveals multiple small nodules in both lung fields as a result of miliary tuberculosis.

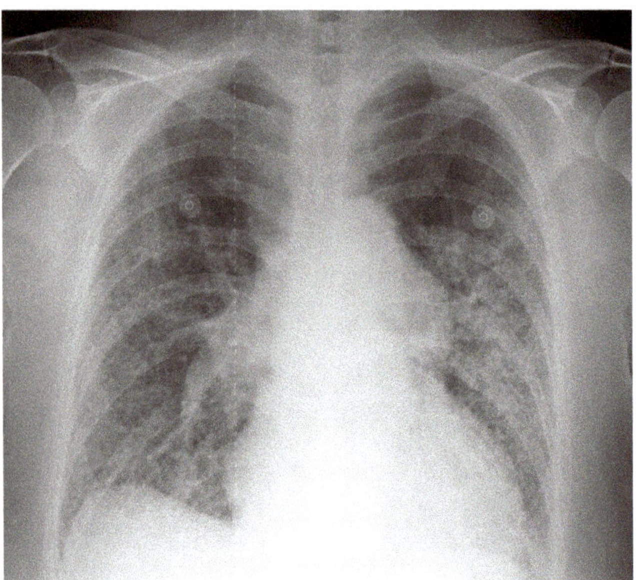

Fig. 104: Sarcoidosis: There is evidence of large bilateral hilar adenopathy as well as multiple small nodular lesions in both the mid and lower zones (left>right). These represent mediastinal adenopathy and interstitial lesions of sarcoidosis (Stage 2).

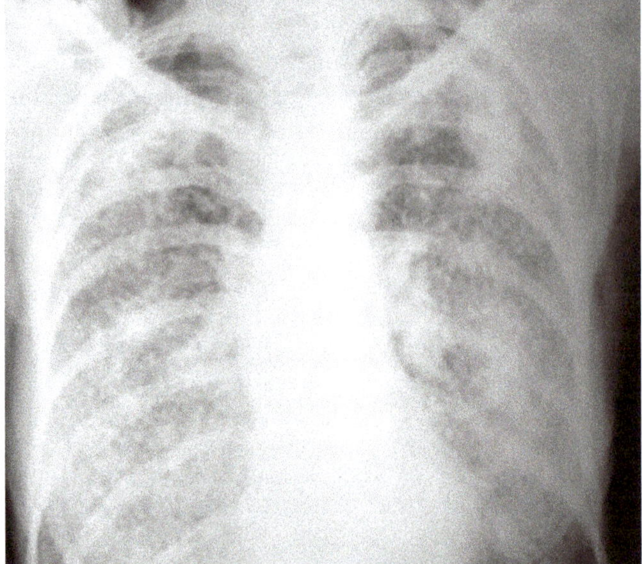

Fig. 106: Alveolar microlithiasis. PA view of chest reveals extensive small nodular high densities in both lung fields. The very high density is typical of microlithiasis.

hemithorax being overpenetrated. A similar effect occurs when the patient is rotated. This can be detected by observing the soft tissue in relation to the shoulders; the penetration will be different.

- *Thoracic wall and soft tissue abnormalities*: Unilateral mastectomy or congenital absence of pectoralis muscle (Poland syndrome) **(Fig. 111)**.

- Overexpansion or increased translucency of one lung:
    - Obstructive emphysema due to a foreign body, or intrabronchial mass lesion
    - Compensatory emphysema due to severe lobar collapse or lobectomy
    - Pulmonary embolism involving one major pulmonary artery

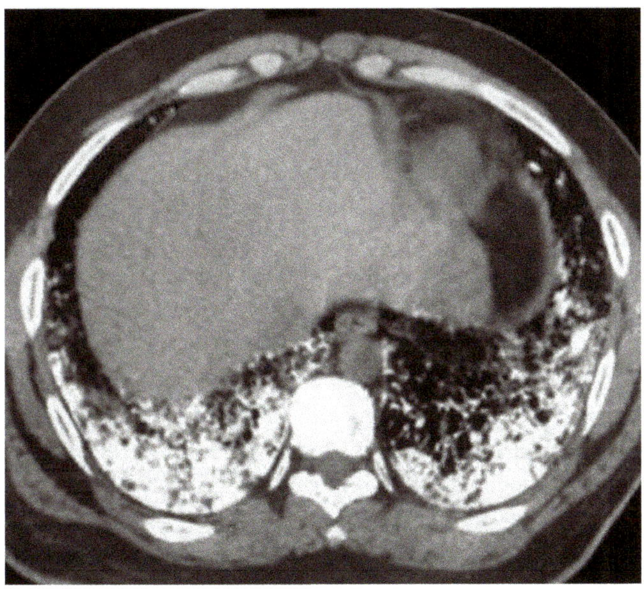

Fig. 107: Alveolar microlithiasis: CT chest in a relatively asymptomatic patient reveals extensive small nodular high-density calcified lesions in both lung fields as a result of alveolar microlithiasis.

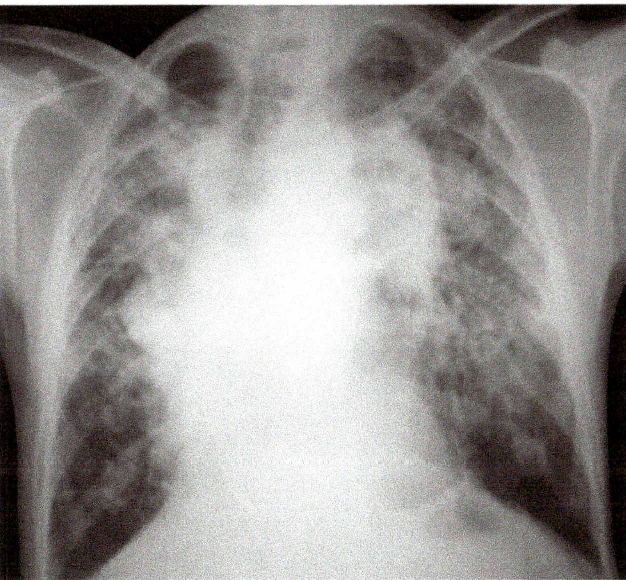

Fig. 109: Progressive massive fibrosis: PA view of the chest reveals bilateral ill-defined parahilar mass lesions with multiple small ill-defined nodular lesions along the periphery of the lesion.

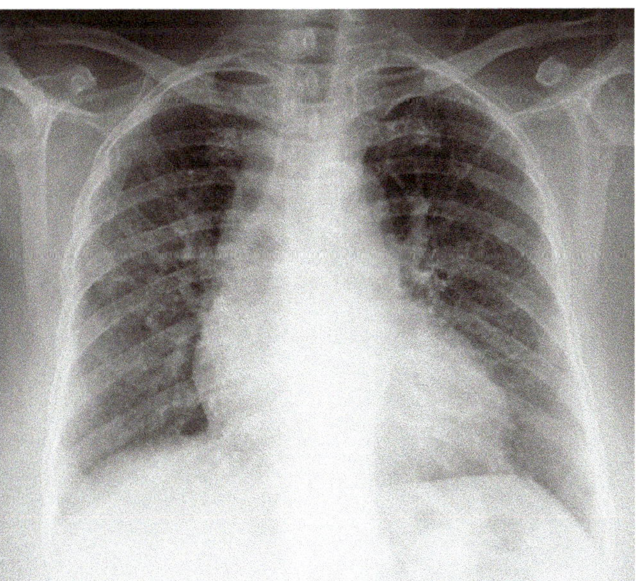

Fig. 108: Reticular opacities: PA view of chest reveals reticular opacities in both lung fields particularly lung bases. HRCT revealed interstitial pulmonary fibrosis.

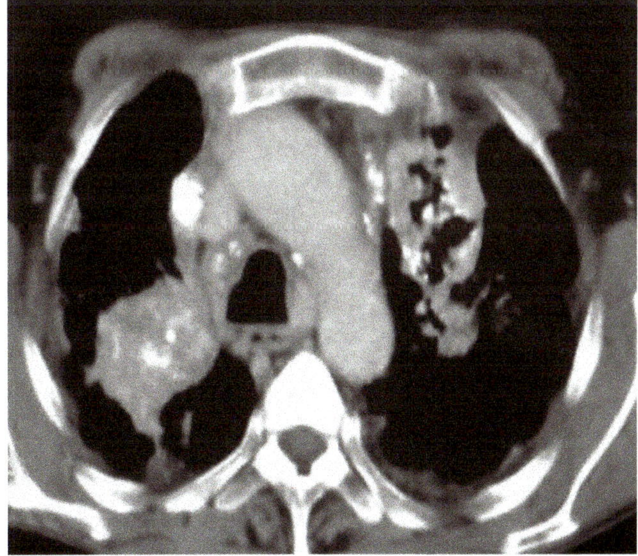

Fig. 110: Progressive massive fibrosis: CT chest reveals ill-defined soft tissue mass lesions with internal calcification and cavitation in a patient with progressive massive fibrosis secondary to silicosis.

- – Pleural effusion in a supine patient, causing an ipsilateral increase in density of the hemithorax, consequently the opposite hemithorax appears to be hypertranslucent **(Fig. 112)**
- – Macleod's or Swyer-James syndrome.

- • Increased translucency of both lungs:
  - – Widespread transradiancy of both lungs may be seen in airway disease such as constrictive bronchiolitis, asthma and emphysema
  - – Obstruction of flow from right side of heart with a right to left cardiac shunt such as Fallot's tetralogy,

Eisenmenger's syndrome, severe widespread pulmonary arterial stenosis and massive pulmonary embolism.

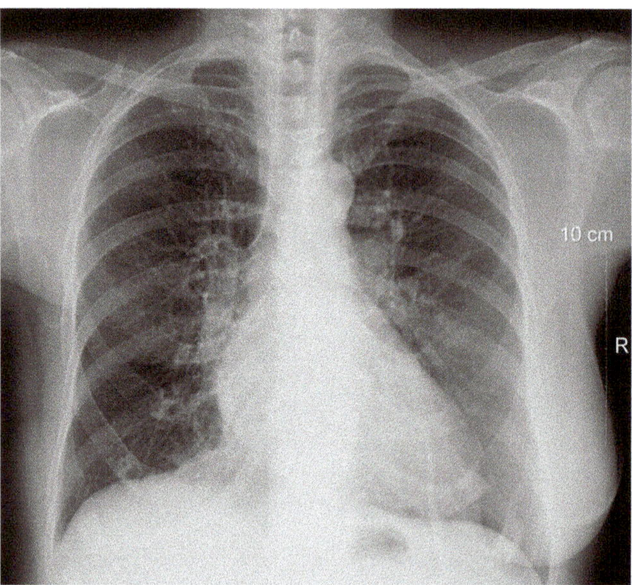

Fig. 111: Unilateral mastectomy: PA view of the chest, note right lung appears more translucent than left lung. This is due to mastectomy on the right side.

Solitary Pulmonary Nodule

A pulmonary nodule is referred to as a spherical opacity with relatively well-defined margins with a diameter of up to 3 cm **(Fig. 113)**. Lesions more than 3 cm in size are considered as mass lesions. A well-defined spherical opacity below 1 cm in diameter is referred to as a small SPN.

With increasing use of MDCT and its high spatial resolution, small nodules are being detected with an increasing frequency. Though most are benign in etiology, it is important to remember that 20–30% of lung cancers present as a solitary pulmonary nodule. One of the primary roles of imaging, beyond detection is to accurately differentiate malignant from benign lesions. It is important to obtain 3/5 mm sections as well as thin 1-mm sections through the lung on CT. The thinner sections help to reduce partial volume averaging so as to provide an accurate assessment of the internal contents and margins of the nodule. The thicker 3/5 mm sections are important as it is difficult to differentiate small SPN from vessels in thin 1 mm sections.

The first step in the radiological evaluation is to determine whether the nodule is pulmonary or extrapulmonary, as the chest X-ray gives a 2D image.

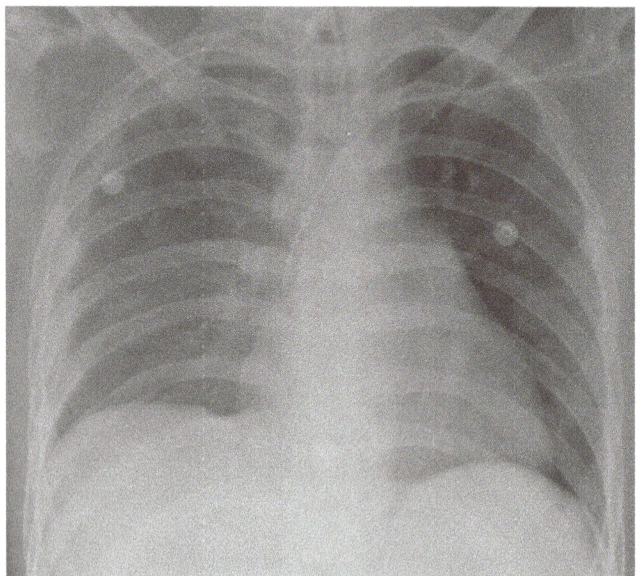

Fig. 112: Unilateral translucency: Frontal chest X-ray in supine position reveals uniform haziness of right hemithorax with transradiancy of left hemithorax. This is due to a right pleural effusion layering along the chest wall contributing to the right hemithorax opacity and consequent transradiancy of left hemithorax.

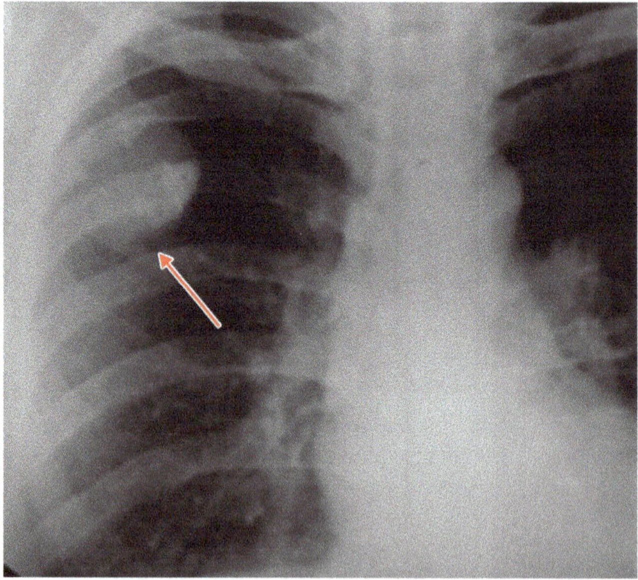

Fig. 113: Solitary pulmonary nodule: Chest X-ray demonstrates a well-defined nodular lesion with calcification along its medial aspect in the right upper zone. The lateral margins of the lesion appear to have obtuse angles with the chest wall, a sign suggesting that the lesion is extrapulmonary.

Skin, pleural or rib lesions can appear as an intrathoracic lesion. Lateral, oblique X-rays or a CT scan would help to localize the lesion **(Figs. 114 to 116)**. Once the lesion is confirmed to be intrapulmonary, the possibilities would essentially be an infective lesion, benign lesion or a malignant lesion. There is a significant overlap in the imaging appearances. To help differentiate, it is useful to look at the clinical and morphological features.

Nodule Morphology

Calcification: Presence of calcification in a pulmonary nodule is a useful sign to differentiate benign from malignant nodules. However, 13% of all lung carcinomas demonstrate calcification; only 2% less than 3 cm in size demonstrate calcification. The different types of calcification which may be visualized in a pulmonary nodule are—concentric, popcorn, punctate/eccentric and uniform.

Concentric: The calcification occupies the entire SPN or the entire periphery of the SPN in a laminated manner. This calcification is mainly seen in tuberculous and fungal infections.

Popcorn calcification: Multiple small rings or nodules of calcification which overlap are seen in hamartomas/cartilage tumors **(Fig. 117)**.

Punctate/Eccentric calcification: Punctate/Eccentric calcification is suspicious as it may be seen in infections and malignancies. A malignancy may engulf a calcified focus representing an old-healed granuloma, with

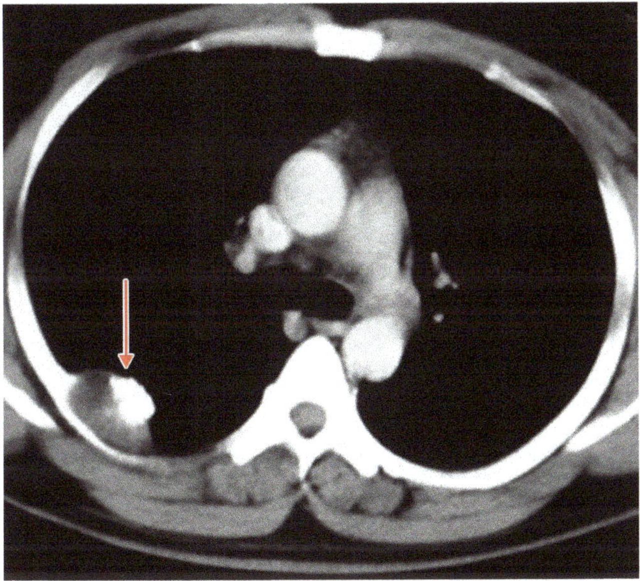

Fig. 114: Solitary pulmonary nodule: CT demonstrates that the nodule demonstrated on the chest X-ray is not intrapulmonary. It arose from the posterior end of the rib with calcification along its anterior aspect. The histopathology revealed an enchondroma.

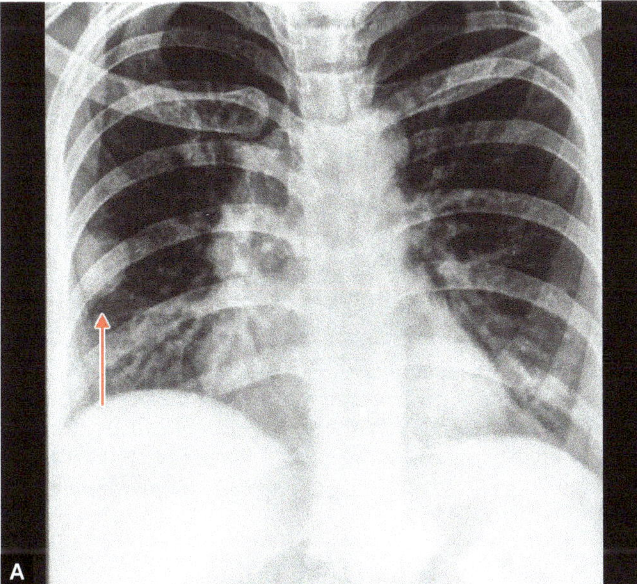

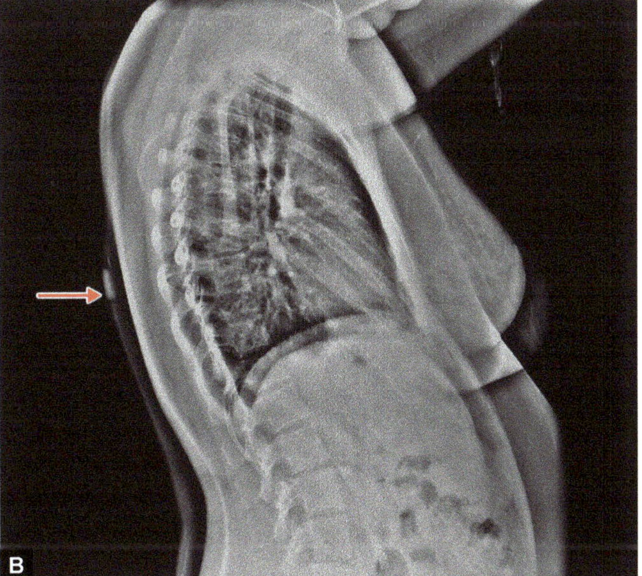

Figs. 115A and B: Solitary pulmonary nodule (A) PA view demonstrates a solitary pulmonary nodule in right lower zone; (B) lateral view demonstrates nodule is subcutaneous (arrow). This case demonstrates the paramount importance of a lateral X-ray of the chest in determining the location of a nodular opacity.

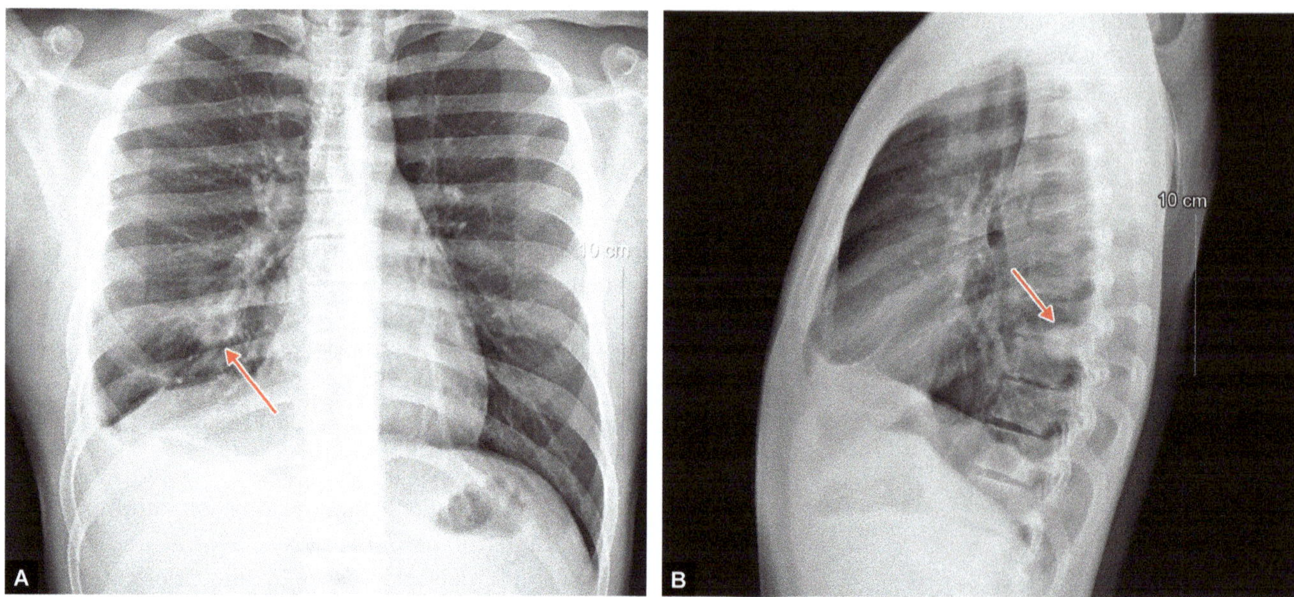

Figs. 116A and B: (A) Chest X-ray reveals solitary pulmonary nodule in right lower zone. (B) Lateral view demonstrates nodule in posterior, pleural base with a wide pleural attachment and with obtuse angles against the chest wall. These features favor pleural/extrapleural mass lesion rather than an intrapulmonary lesion.

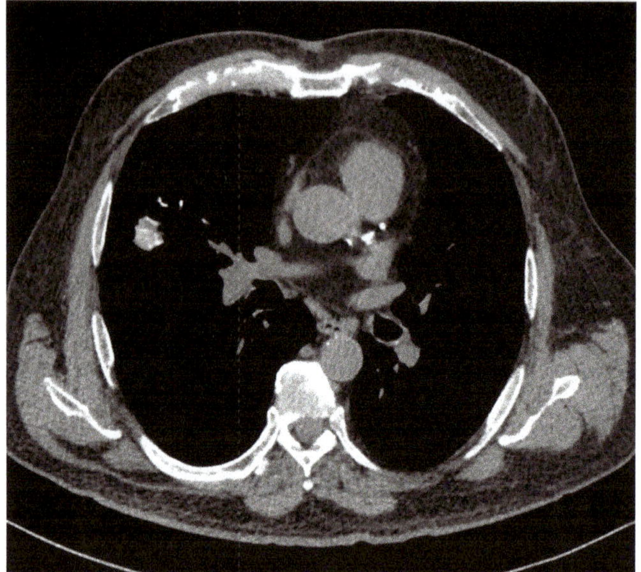

Fig. 117: Solitary pulmonary nodule: CT chest demonstrates a well-defined nodule in the right upper lobe. There is a popcorn type of distribution of calcification typical of a hamartoma.

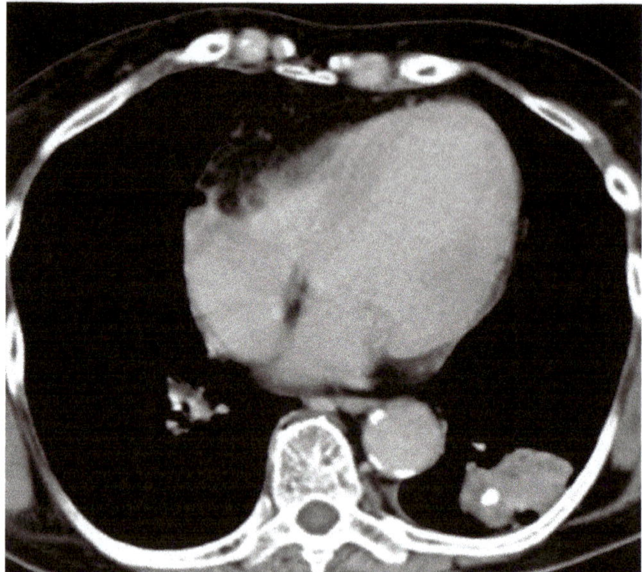

Fig. 118: Solitary pulmonary nodule: CT chest reveals a nodular mass lesion in the left lower lobe with a calcific speck along its periphery, an example of an eccentric type of calcification. CT-guided biopsy revealed an adenocarcinoma. The calcific density represented an old granuloma which healed with calcification and was engulfed by the neoplasm.

calcification appearing on the periphery of the lesion **(Fig. 118)**.

Uniform calcification: The entire SPN is calcified; this is typical of calcified granulomas **(Fig. 119)**.

Size

Most malignant nodules are larger than 2 cm in size, however 40% are less than 2 cm, 15% are less than 1 cm, 1% of malignant lesions are less than 7 mm in size. Most lesions above 3 cm are likely to be either bronchogenic carcinoma, lung abscess, Wegener's granulomatosis, lymphoma, round atelectasis, focal pneumonia, or hydatid cysts. It is difficult to detect a lesion less than 5 mm in diameter on a chest X-ray. If a lesion which is 5 mm or less is seen on a chest X-ray, it is invariably calcified.

Shape

A spiculated margin is very suggestive of carcinoma; the spicules represent spread into the interstitium of the lung **(Figs. 120 and 121)**. Lobulation and notching which indicate unequal growth are suggestive signs for malignancy but may be seen in inflammatory lesions. There is considerable overlap in the findings between benign and malignant. A spiculated lesion though has a predictive value of 90% to be a malignant lesion. An inflammatory lesion with fibrosis may however have a similar appearance. Benign lesions usually have smooth margins. Conversely 20% of primary lung tumors have smooth margins; most metastatic lesions also have smooth margins.

Cavitation

Cavitation occurs in inflammatory as well as primary and metastatic tumors. Benign lesions tend to have thinner and smoother walls as compared to malignant lesions, which have thicker and irregular walls **(Figs. 122 and 123)**.

Fat

Demonstration of fat within a solitary pulmonary nodule is pathognomonic of a hamartoma, (50% of hamartomas demonstrate fat in the lesion) **(Fig. 124)**. Rarely, lipoid pneumonia/metastatic liposarcoma or renal cell carcinoma metastasis may demonstrate fat densities.

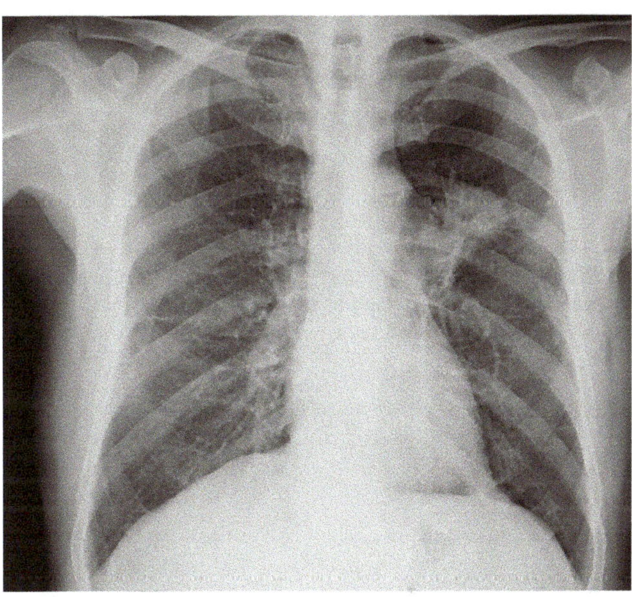

Fig. 120: Solitary pulmonary nodule: Chest X-ray demonstrates a nodule in the left upper lobe. Note its spiculated margin, a relatively specific sign to indicate malignancy.

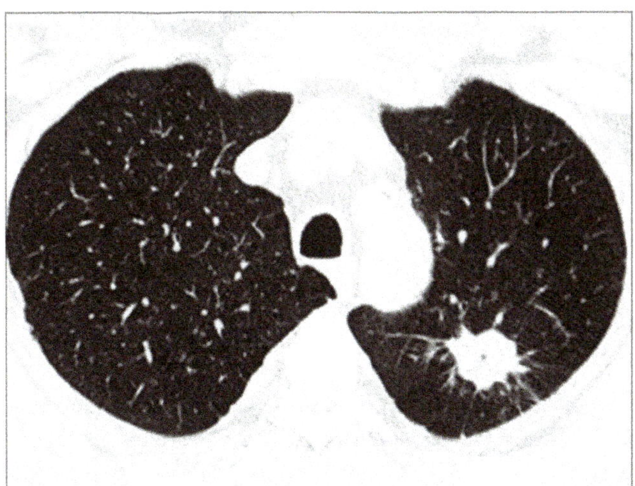

Fig. 121: Solitary pulmonary nodule: CT chest demonstrates a nodular lesion in the left apex. There are multiple radiating bands arising from the surface of the nodule resulting in a spiculated appearance. This is typical of a malignant lesion. Rarely, an inflammatory lesion may demonstrate spiculation.

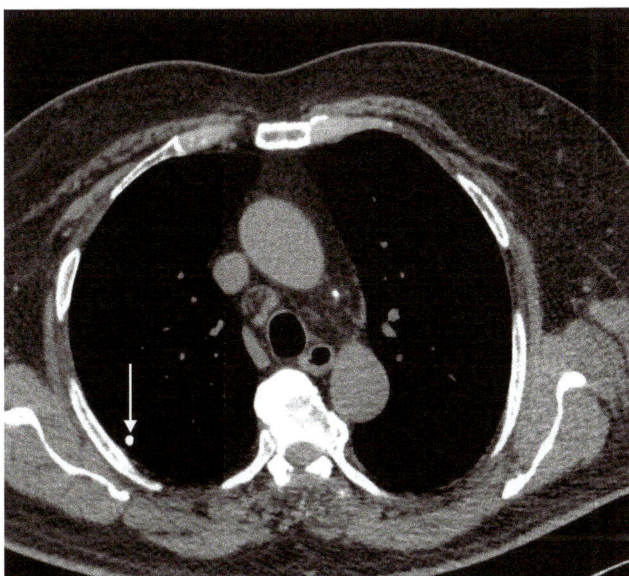

Fig. 119: Solitary pulmonary nodule: CT chest demonstrates a well-defined pulmonary nodule in the right upper lobe. The nodule is densely calcified, representing a uniform type of calcification, indicating with certainty that the nodule is benign.

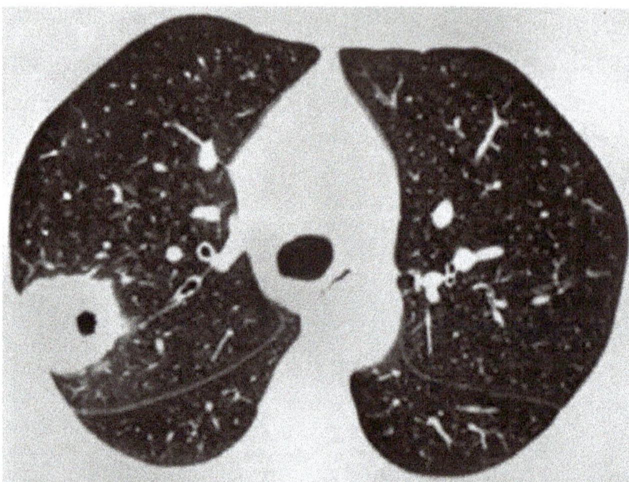

Fig. 122: Solitary pulmonary nodule: CT chest reveals a well-defined nodular lesion in the right upper lobe abutting the pleura with internal cavitation, the margins of which are smooth. CT-guided biopsy revealed this lesion to be due to *Mycobacterium tuberculosis*.

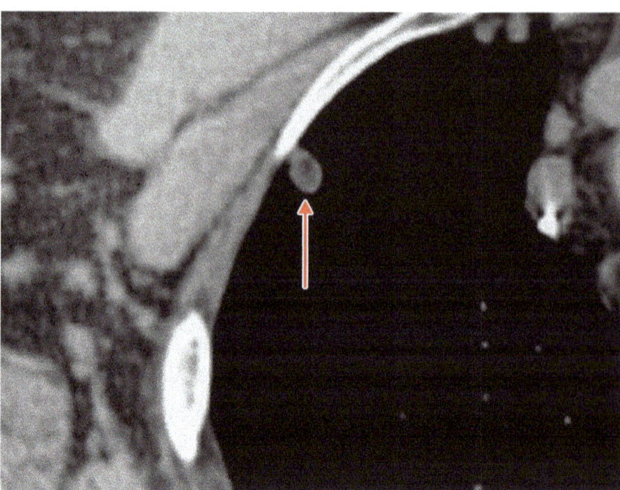

Fig. 124: Solitary pulmonary nodule: CT chest reveals a small pulmonary nodule in the right chest anteriorly. There is a fat density within the lesion; this is typical of a hamartoma.

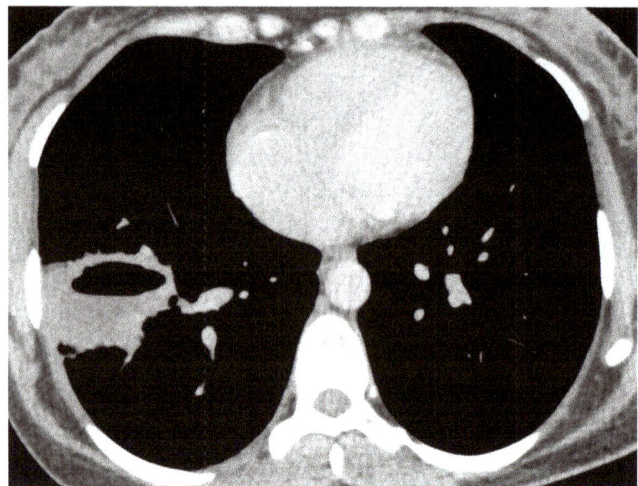

Fig. 123: Solitary pulmonary nodule: CT chest reveals a large nodular lesion with internal necrosis and cavitation in the right lower lobe. The inner margins of the cavitation are irregular: CT-guided biopsy revealed a squamous carcinoma.

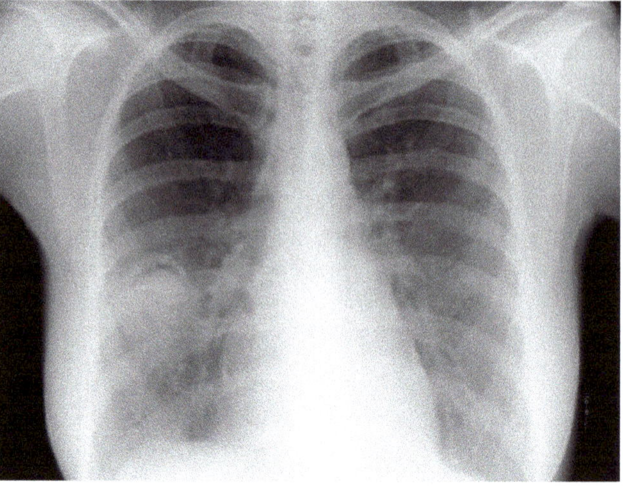

Fig. 125: Solitary pulmonary nodule: Well-defined solitary pulmonary nodule in right mid-zone with an air crescent along superior surface of nodule. The air crescent indicates that the nodule represents a fungal ball in a cavity—aspergilloma.

Satellite Nodules

Multiple small peripheral nodules around an SPN are very useful signs indicating a benign lesion, especially inflammatory in etiology. It has a positive predictive value of 90%.

Air Bronchogram

Presence of an air bronchogram does not exclude a neoplasm as this may be seen in a bronchoalveolar carcinoma or in lymphoma. Presence of an air crescent is useful to diagnose an aspergilloma **(Fig. 125)**.

CT Halo Sign

Lung cancers can have a halo around them, though such halos may also be seen in inflammatory lesions, especially in invasive aspergillosis **(Fig. 126)**.

Rate of Growth

Lung cancers take from 1 month to 18 months to double in volume, the average time being 4.2–7.3 months. Volume doubling faster than 1 month suggests an infection/infarction/aggressive lymphoma. Doubling after 18 months is seen in granuloma/hamartoma/carcinoid/round atelectasis. A lesion which has not grown or has reduced in size in 2 years is likely to be benign. For a nodule to double in volume, the change in nodule diameter is approximately 26% **(Figs. 127A and B)**. A 4 mm nodule which increases to 5 mm would have doubled in volume. Thus accurate measurements are critical in deciding doubling time. There is significant

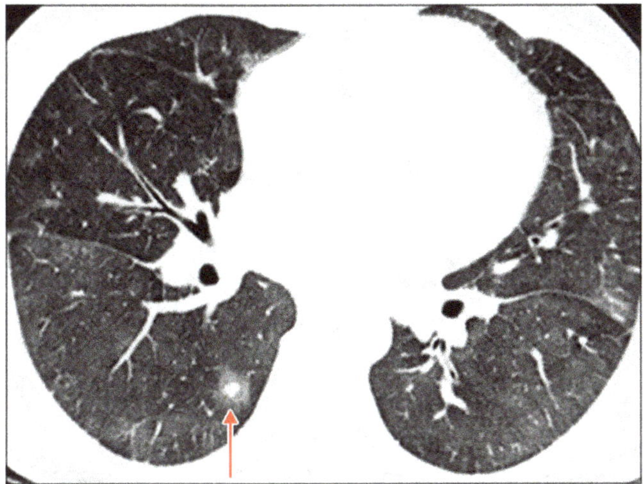

Fig. 126: Solitary pulmonary nodule: High-resolution computed tomography (HRCT) demonstrates a well-defined nodule in the apical segment of the right lower lobe with an ill-defined halo of ground-glass around the nodule. This appearance is seen in invasive aspergillosis.

inter- and intraobserver variation in measurements, especially in spiculated lesions. The ideal method to evaluate growth is to evaluate volume, as an irregular-shaped structure is being measured. Automated volume measuring techniques are very useful in this setting. The problems of inter-/intraobserver variations are minimized, as all spiculated and irregular margins are taken into consideration for measurements. Most modern CT workstations have automated software that enables accurate measurements.

Nodule Enhancement and Metabolism

There are numerous reports in Western literature on the utility of contrast enhancement to differentiate between benign and malignant SPN. If the enhancement of a nodule following contrast enhancement exceeds 20 HU then it is most likely malignant, whereas if less than 15 HU it is most likely benign. Enhancement is determined by measuring HU values, postcontrast after 1, 2, 3, 4 minutes. The peak HU value is subtracted from the precontrast HU value. Sensitivities of 98%, specificity of 73%, positive predictive value of 77%, and negative predictive value of 98% have been reported. However, these findings do not apply to patients in the Indian subcontinent as the most likely differential diagnosis of a malignant SPN is an inflammatory lesion (in particular a tuberculous lesion). A tuberculoma will enhance to a similar extent as a malignant

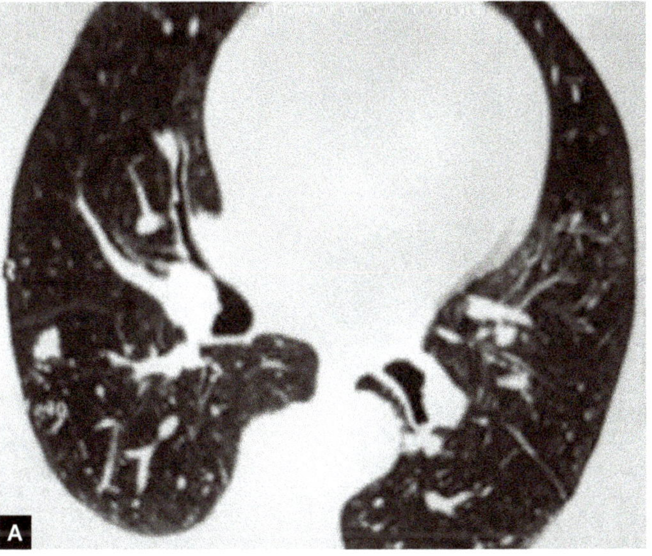
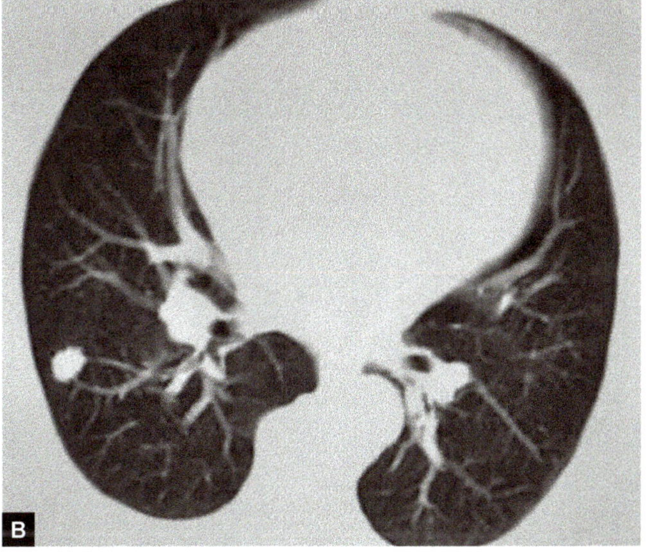

Figs. 127A and B: Solitary pulmonary nodule: CT chest studies done 6 months apart reveal progression in size of nodule. CT-guided fine-needle aspiration cytology (FNAC) of lesion revealed a non-small-cell cancer; this is the most important sign in the evaluation of a pulmonary nodule (its progression in a short-period of time). It indicates the need for further intervention, FNAC, biopsy or surgical excision.

nodule. For the same reason the FDG PET is insensitive in differentiating a malignant from a tuberculous or other inflammatory pathology. Further, PET can be quite insensitive in detecting pulmonary nodules, especially metastatic nodules, less than 1 cm in diameter.

High-resolution Computed Tomography Patterns of Diffuse Lung Disease

The detection and diagnosis of diffuse lung diseases is based on the demonstration and recognition of specific abnormal findings. These findings can be classified into essentially two groups, those with increased lung attenuation and those with decreased lung attenuation. Those with increased lung attenuation can be further subdivided into reticular opacities, nodular opacities and parenchymal opacification. Those with decreased lung attenuation can be subdivided into cystic lesions, emphysema, bronchiectasis, mosaic perfusion/ attenuation and air trapping.

■ RETICULAR OPACITIES

Thickening of the interstitial fiber network of the lung by inflammation, fluid, fibrous tissue or neoplastic infiltration results in linear/reticular opacities. Thickening of the axial interstitium results in thickening of the interstitium along the walls of the bronchovascular structures **(Fig. 128)**. Since bronchial walls and vessels have similar densities,

it is difficult to differentiate the interstitial thickening from the underlying bronchovascular structures. Consequently, the appearances are of thickening of the bronchial wall and an increase in the vessel diameter.

Thickening of the peripheral interstitium is easy to demonstrate, as septal thickening is seen in the subpleural regions, marginating the secondary pulmonary nodule, and interlobular interstitium. This is manifested as radiating bands extending perpendicular to the pleural surface **(Figs. 129 and 130)**.

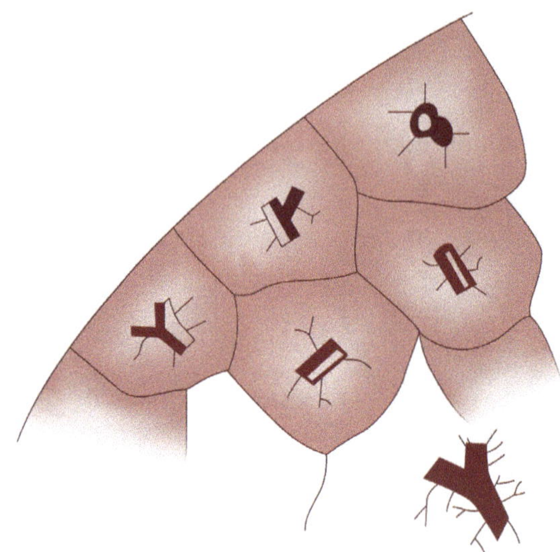

Fig. 129: Interlobular interstitial thickening: Schematic diagram of secondary lobules demonstrates thickening of walls of secondary lobule as well as centrilobular interstitium.

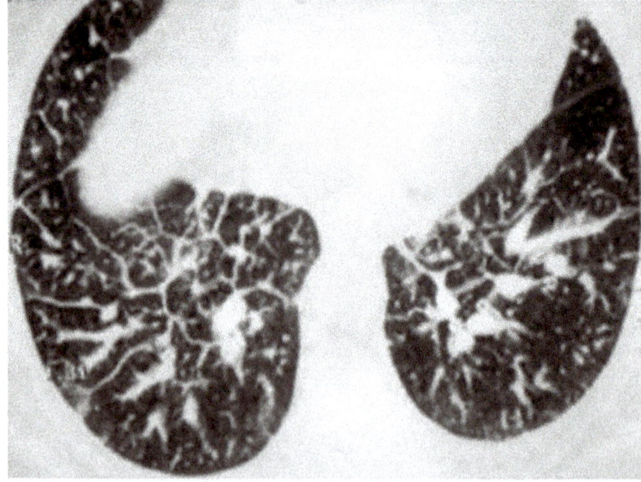

Fig. 128: Peribronchovascular interstitial thickening: The vessels appear to be prominent in size with irregular surfaces. This is due to peribronchovascular interstitial thickening. There is extension of the interstitial thickening peripherally into the subpleural regions.

Fig. 130: Interlobular interstitial thickening: HRCT in a patient with lymphangitis carcinomatosis reveals smooth thickening of the interlobar interstitium. The walls of the secondary lobule are thickened, and the internal architecture is preserved, demonstrating the anatomy of the secondary lobule very well.

Thickening of the intralobular interstitium, which lies within the secondary lobule, is seen as a fine haze of linear opacities or may appear as ground-glass opacities **(Fig. 131)**.

The interstitial thickening may be smooth, nodular or irregular. Smooth thickening is seen in pulmonary edema, lymphangitis carcinomatosis **(Figs. 132A and B)**. Nodular thickening is seen in lymphangitis carcinomatosis, sarcoidosis. Irregular septal thickening

is seen mainly in patients with lung fibrosis **(Fig. 133)**. Extensive peribronchovascular fibrosis can result in large conglomerate masses of fibrous tissue as seen in sarcoidosis, silicosis, tuberculosis and talcosis. Subtle peribronchovascular interstitial thickening may be difficult to detect.

Involvement of the peribronchovascular interstitium predominantly is seen in nonspecific interstitial pneumonias (NSIPs) **(Figs. 134A and B)** as compared to predominantly subpleural interstitial thickening seen in usual interstitial pneumonia. Another differentiating feature is the lack of honeycombing, seen typically in UIP. Also in UIP, there are no significant ground-glass densities and parenchymal opacification which are seen in the cellular variety of NSIP **(Fig. 135)**.

Axial Interstitium

In patients with irregular interstitial thickening, fibrotic tissue along the bronchial walls causes traction resulting in "traction bronchiectasis" **(Figs. 136 and 137)**. A similar involvement of the peripheral bronchioles is termed traction bronchiolectasis. The dilated bronchi have a varicose or a corkscrew appearance.

When there is involvement of the terminal bronchioles, the bronchioles may dilate to occupy the entire secondary lobule, resulting in honeycomb cysts. On HRCT, honeycomb cysts are usually 1.0 cm

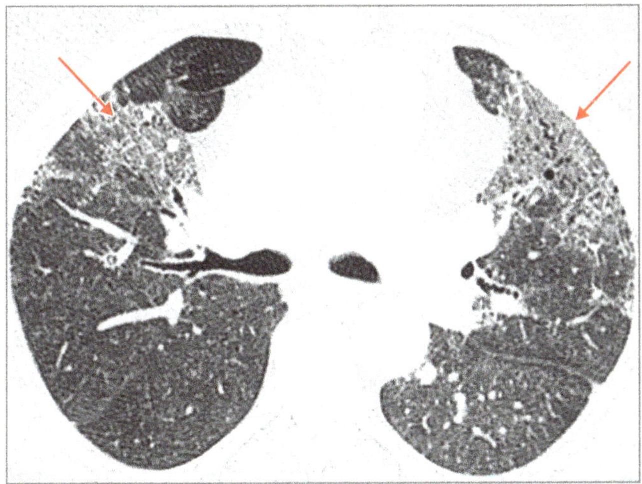

Fig. 131: Intralobular interstitium: HRCT demonstrates ill-defined reticular ground-glass densities in the right middle lobe and left lingula associated with traction bronchiectasis. These features are due to intralobular interstitial thickening.

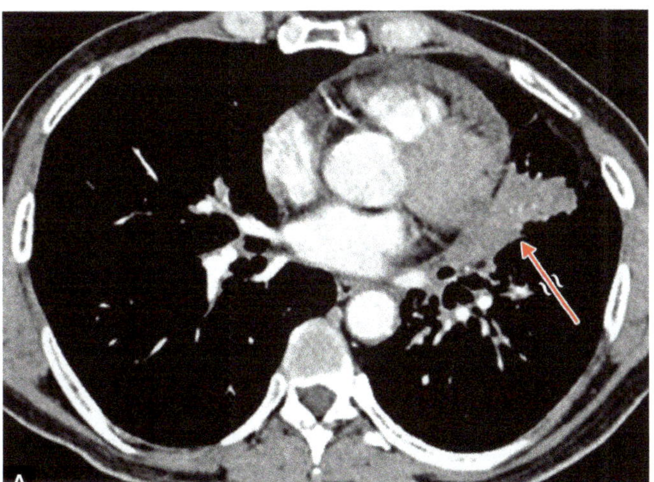

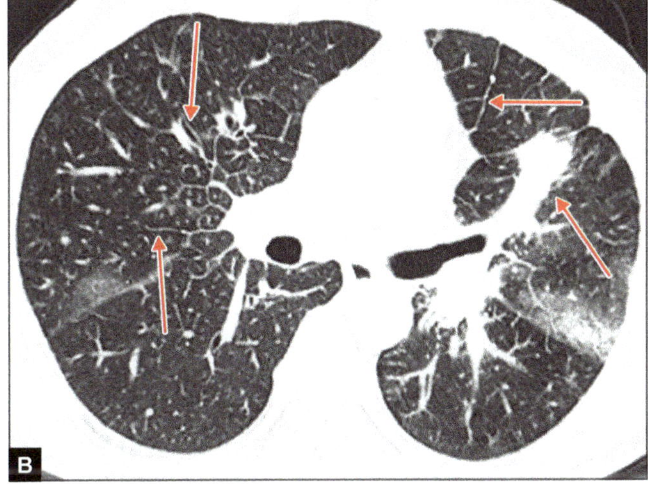

Figs. 132A and B: Smooth interstitial thickening: CT chest (A) demonstrates an ill-defined mass lesion in the lingula flush with the pericardium. CT-guided fine-needle aspiration cytology (FNAC) revealed an adenocarcinoma. HRCT (B) reveals smooth septal thickening from the surface of the mass lesion, this represents lymphatic infiltration by the mass lesion. Smooth septal thickening is also present in the right middle lobe with preservation of the secondary lobule. This is due to lymphangitis carcinomatosis secondary to hematogenous spread.

or more in diameter with thin walls in the subpleural regions. These honeycomb cysts share their walls and occur in several contiguous layers **(Figs. 138 and 139)**. Honeycombing indicates end-stage lung disease. The location of honeycombing is important in the differential diagnosis of chronic ILD. If the honeycombing is basal and posterior with associated significant fibrosis and architectural distortion, the diagnosis is UIP. If honeycomb cysts are seen in the upper zones the possibility of sarcoid should be considered; if in the mid-zone with a patchy distribution, the diagnosis of chronic hypersensitivity pneumonitis should be entertained. Anterior honeycomb cysts with fibrosis are seen in ARDS since the posterior portions of the lungs are protected by collapse/consolidation and are therefore not exposed to the deleterious effects of mechanical ventilation.

Nodular Opacities

A nodule is defined as a rounded opacity which can be well- or ill-defined. A small nodule is one which is less than 1.0 cm; a large nodule varies in size between 1.0 cm and 3.0 cm; nodules above 3.0 cm are termed as masses.

Small nodules are of two types: (1) interstitial and (2) air-space. Interstitial nodules are well-defined and discrete, as seen in sarcoidosis, miliary tuberculosis, silicosis and metastatic lesions. Air-space nodules tend to be ill-defined and conglomerative. Airspace nodules may have a soft tissue density or demonstrate a diffuse ground-glass haze. Examples of air-space nodules are seen in exudative bronchiolitis. Despite these differences in appearance, it is often difficult to differentiate interstitial from air-space nodules on HRCT. The distribution of nodules is extremely useful in establishing the differential diagnosis. Nodules may be perilymphatic, random or centrilobular in distribution. Perilymphatic nodules occur in relation to the lymphatics/interstitium **(Figs. 140 and 141)**, i.e. in relation to the perihilar bronchovascular interstitium,

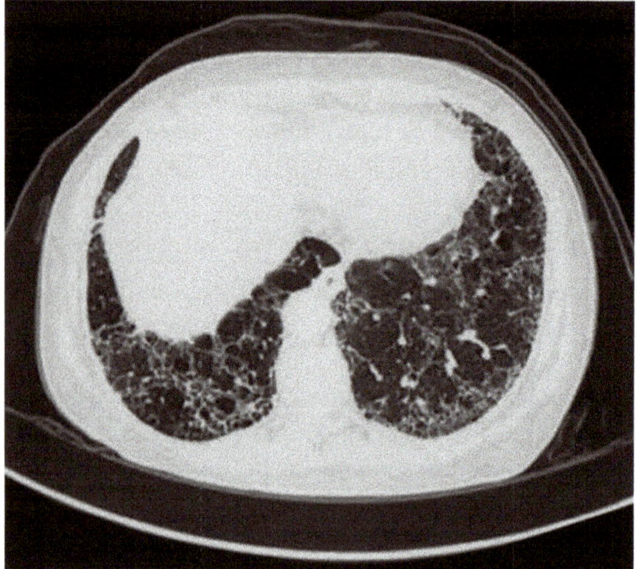

Fig. 133: Irregular septal thickening: HRCT demonstrates irregular interstitial thickening in both lung bases posteriorly in a subpleural and peribronchovascular location as seen in usual interstitial pneumonia.

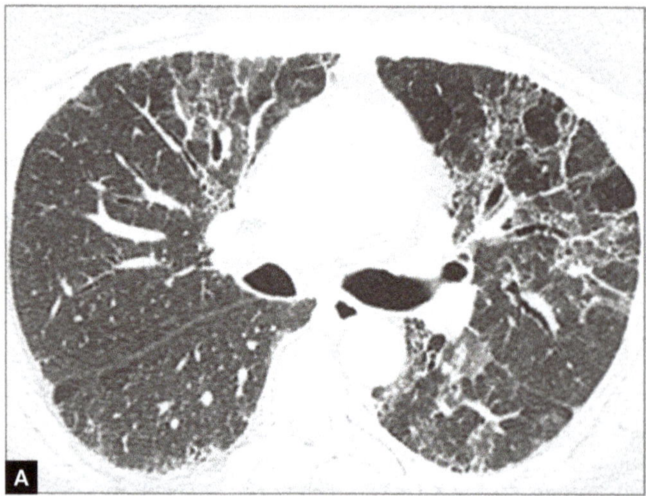

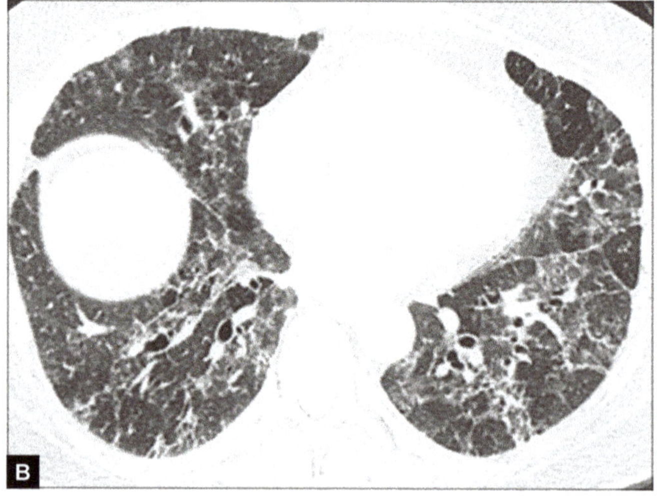

Figs. 134A and B: Fibrotic nonspecific interstitial pneumonia (NSIP): Extensive interstitial thickening in the lungs anteriorly in the upper lobes and posteriorly in the lung bases. The predominant interstitial thickening is in the peribronchovascular interstitium and not in the subpleural regions.

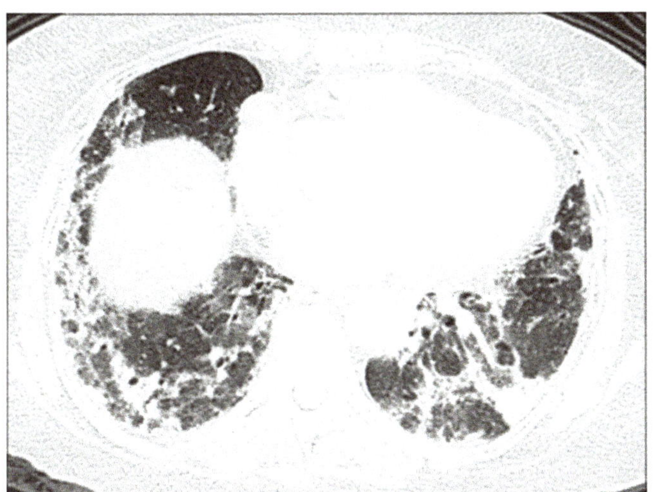

Fig. 135: Cellular nonspecific interstitial pneumonia (NSIP): HRCT demonstrates ill-defined areas of air-space opacification in the peribronchovascular and subpleural regions of both lung bases. There are no honeycomb changes. In view of the parenchymal opacification, lack of honeycomb changes, and significant fibrotic lesions this would represent the cellular variety of nonspecific interstitial pneumonia.

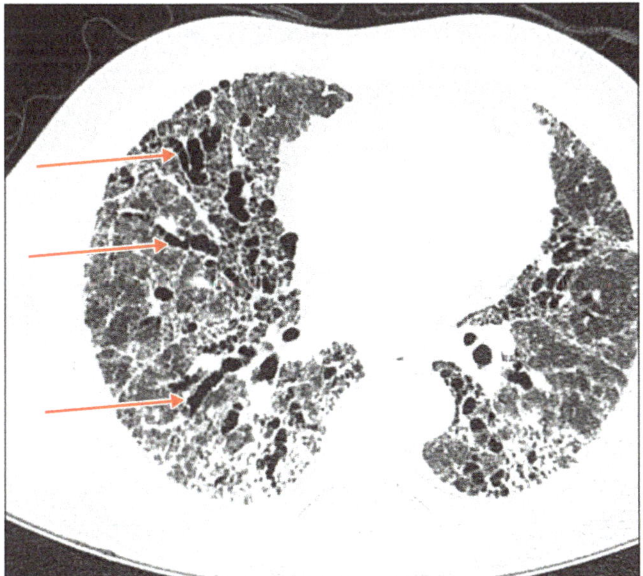

Fig. 136: Traction bronchiectasis: HRCT demonstrates peribronchovascular interstitial thickening as evidenced by thickening and irregularity of the vessel and bronchial wall. There is dilatation and irregularity secondary to peribronchial interstitial thickening, representing traction bronchiectasis.

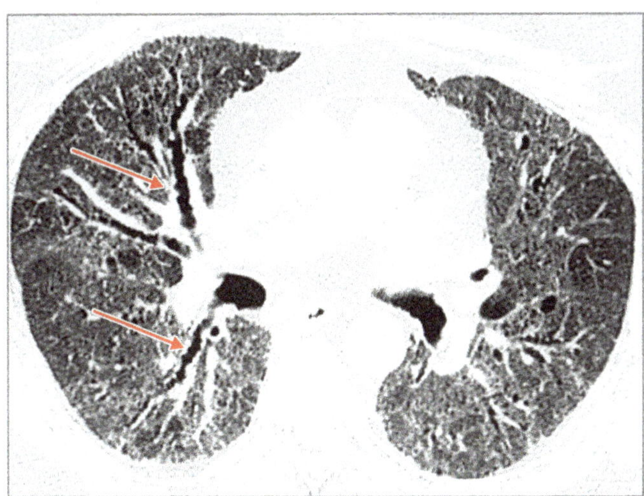

Fig. 137: Traction bronchiectasis: HRCT demonstrates peribronchovascular interstitial thickening with consequent traction bronchiectasis and multiple ground-glass opacities.

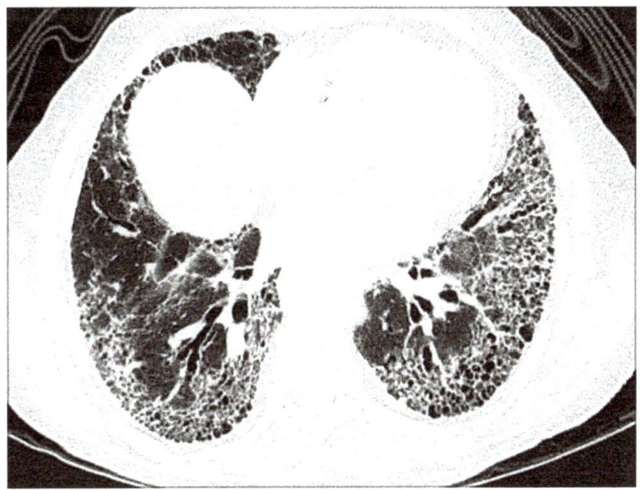

Fig. 138: Honeycomb cysts: Extensive honeycomb cysts are seen in both lung fields especially the left.

interlobular septae, subpleural interstitium. The subpleural distribution of nodules is best demonstrated in relation to fissures. These small nodules in the subpleural regions may coalesce to form pseudoplaques along the pleura. These nodules may also coalesce to form large conglomerative masses. Satellite nodules may be seen in relation to these conglomerative masses giving the appearance of a galaxy **(Fig. 142)**. This pattern is seen in sarcoidosis, silicosis/coal workers pneumoconiosis, lymphangitic carcinomatosis, lymphoproliferative disorders. These diseases demonstrate different patterns of perilymphatic involvement, allowing a distinction.

Sarcoidosis

Nodules are seen essentially in relation to the peribronchovascular interstitium and subpleural regions.

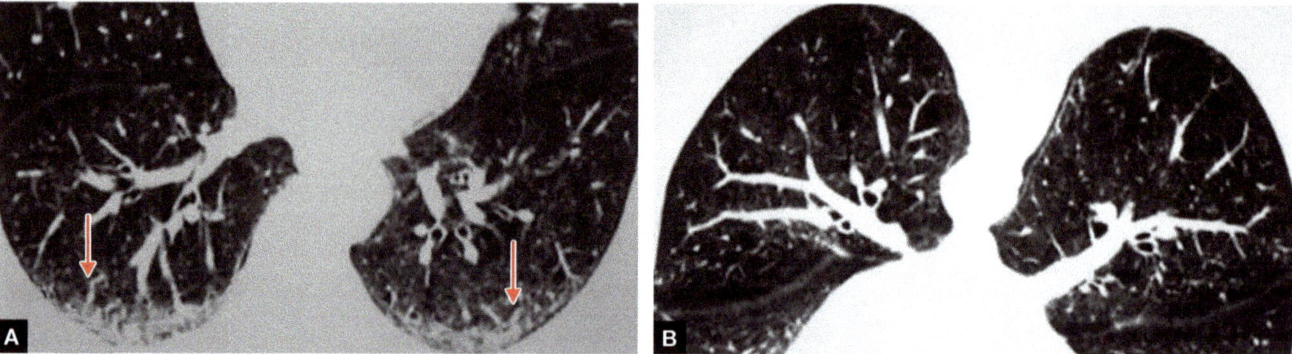

Figs. 139A and B: Dependent densities: Supine HRCT reveals ill-defined opacities in the lung bases posteriorly. (A) These appear as reticular opacities due to interstitial fibrosis. Prone scans at the same level; (B) demonstrate that the opacities have resolved. These opacities in the lung base on a supine scan represent basal atelectasis. It is important to obtain prone scans in all patients with basal posterior opacities to exclude basal atelectasis.

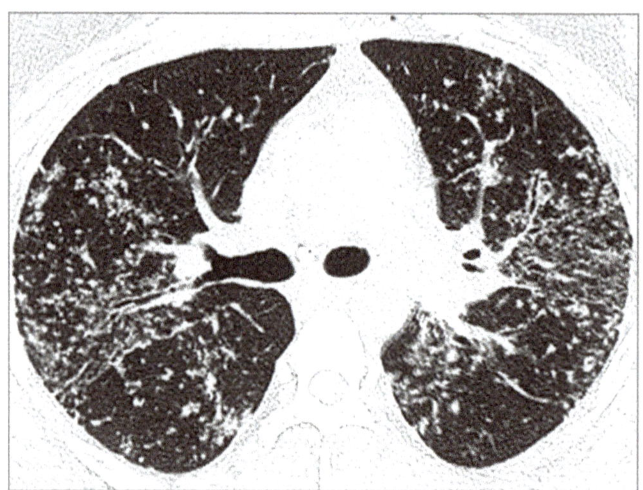

Fig. 140: Perilymphatic nodules: HRCT demonstrates extensive nodules in a peribronchovascular location along the vascular surfaces as well as the fissures. As the vessels are white and the nodular areas also white, the appearance is of a nodular surface of the vessels.

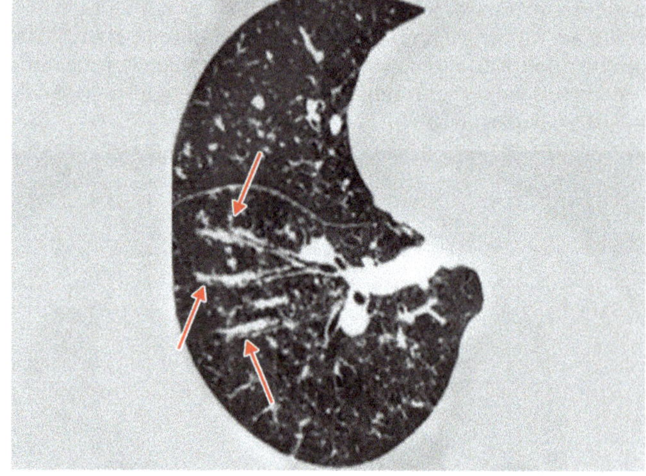

Fig. 141: Perilymphatic nodules: HRCT demonstrates multiple small well-defined nodules along the surface of the bronchi and vessels. The vessels have a beaded appearance. These represent interstitial nodules along the peribronchovascular interstitium.

The central bronchovascular structures and fissures have a nodular appearance. An upper lobe preponderance is common, with the lung involved in a patchy asymmetric fashion, groups of nodules occurring in one region, normal lung in other regions.

Silicosis/CWP

Nodules are distributed in a subpleural and centrilobular location, rarely in a peribronchovascular location as compared to sarcoidosis. Nodules tend to be more evenly distributed as compared to sarcoidosis **(Fig. 143)**.

Lymphangitic Carcinomatosis

There is smooth thickening of the peribronchovascular and interlobular interstitium. Nodules are seen in relation to these thickened septae. The involvement may be unilateral, patchy or bilateral and symmetric.

Patterns of Distribution of Nodules

Random

The distribution is uniform with no predilection for any anatomic structures, bilateral and symmetric as seen in

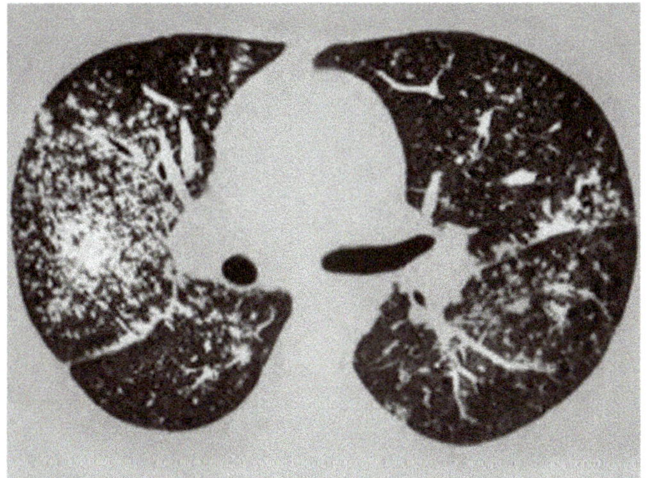

Fig. 142: Sarcoidosis: HRCT demonstrates multiple small nodules in an interstitial location, along the fissures, vessels and bronchi as well as in the subpleural regions. The distribution is asymmetric and essentially perilymphatic. The nodules are seen to conglomerate in the right middle lobe with a number of satellite nodules resulting in an appearance akin to a galaxy. This distribution pattern is typical of sarcoidosis.

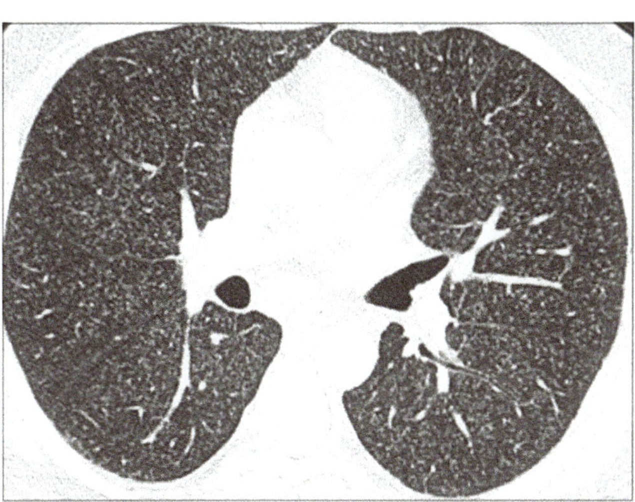

Fig. 144: Miliary tuberculosis: HRCT demonstrates multiple small nodules in a random distribution. There is no predilection for any anatomic structure; the distribution is uniform. This is typically seen in the miliary tuberculosis.

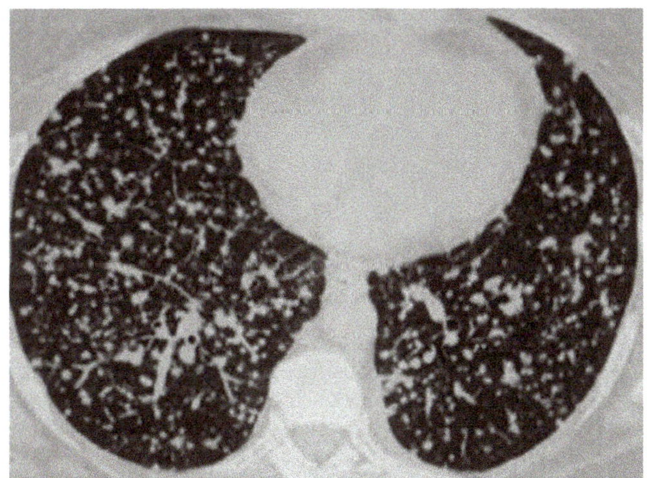

Fig. 143: Silicosis: HRCT demonstrates multiple small well-defined nodules distributed evenly in both lung fields. These nodules are along the vessels, fissures and in the subpleural regions, i.e. perilymphatic in location. As compared to the asymmetric distribution of nodules in sarcoidosis the distribution is uniform in silicosis.

miliary tuberculosis (**Fig. 144**), hematogenous metastasis, and fungal infection.

Centrilobular

Ill-defined small nodules are centered on the centrilobular structures of the secondary pulmonary lobule.

Nodules which are predominantly centrilobular in location are most likely secondary to bronchiolar/peribronchiolar inflammation resulting in infiltration or fibrosis of the surrounding interstitium and alveoli (**Figs. 145A and B**). Angiocentric diseases may also manifest as centrilobular nodules. Bronchiolar diseases manifesting as centrilobular nodules are endobronchial spread of tuberculosis, nontuberculous mycobacterial infections, granulomatous infections, bronchopneumonia, panbronchiolitis, bronchiectasis, ABPA, hypersensitivity pneumonitis (**Fig. 146**), Langerhans' cell histiocytosis, respiratory bronchiolitis (**Fig. 147**), endobronchial spread of neoplasm. Angiocentric nodules are due to pulmonary edema and pulmonary hemorrhage.

Centrilobular nodules due to bronchiolar inflammation may have a tree-in-bud appearance; as the bronchioles dilate and are filled with inspissated mucus, a branching pattern is visualized (**Figs. 145A and B**).

Parenchymal Opacification

Diffuse or multifocal increase in lung attenuation is a common finding on HRCT in patients with chronic lung disease. Increased lung opacity may be ground-glass or consolidation. These represent varying degrees of parenchymal opacification, depending upon whether the vessels are obscured or not by the parenchymal

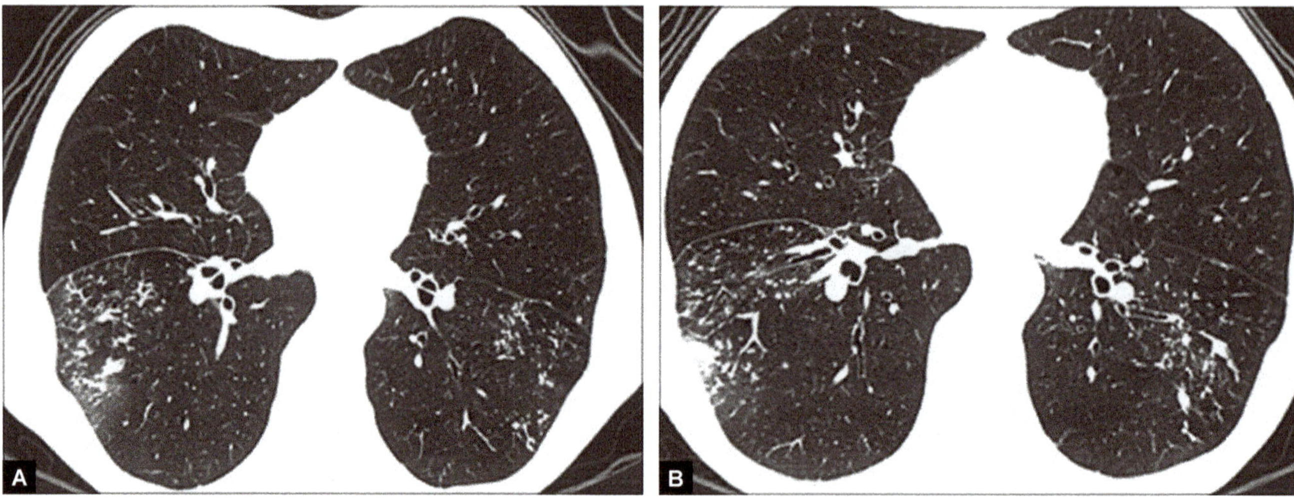

Figs. 145A and B: Centrilobular nodules: HRCT demonstrates multiple small ill-defined nodular lesions in centrilobular location.

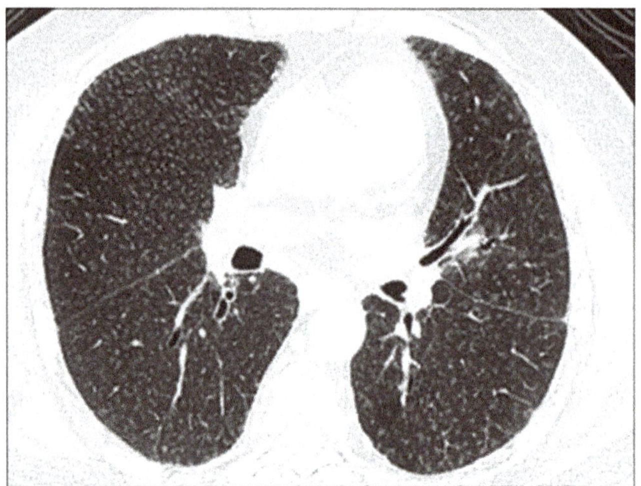

Fig. 146: Hypersensitivity pneumonitis: HRCT demonstrates multiple small nodules in both lung fields distributed uniformly, evenly spaced, representing centrilobular nodules due to hypersensitivity pneumonitis.

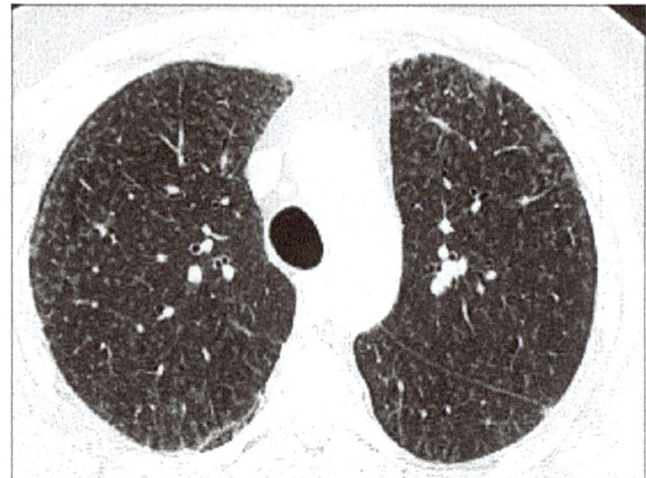

Fig. 147: Respiratory bronchiolitis: HRCT demonstrates multiple small pulmonary nodules in both lung fields. These nodules are evenly spaced at the centers of the secondary lobule. These represented nodules due to respiratory bronchiolitis.

opacification. Ground-glass opacity is an area of parenchymal opacification not associated with obscuration of the underlying vessels **(Fig. 148)**. Parenchymal consolidation obscures the vessels **(Fig. 149)**.

Ground-glass opacity results from either fluid, inflammatory material within the alveoli/interstitium or the presence of fine interstitial fibrosis in the intralobular interstitium of the secondary lobule. The distribution is usually geographic with areas of spared lung interspersed with areas of affected lung. Detection of ground-glass opacity is of significance as this indicates an ongoing active as well as potentially treatable process. Since

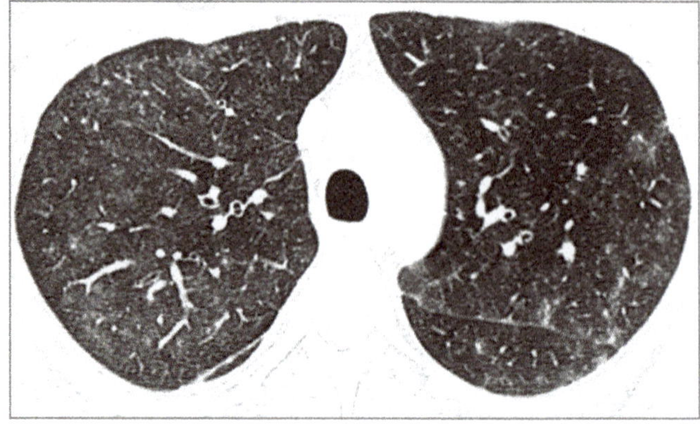

Fig. 148: Ground-glass pattern of parenchymal opacification.

ground-glass opacity may also be a manifestation of intralobular interstitial thickening, presence of significant areas of fibrosis/lung destruction in other regions would indicate that the ground-glass densities are more likely due to intralobular fibrosis.

Pitfalls in Diagnosis of Ground-Glass Opacity

There is a reduction in the amount of air in the alveoli during expiration; consequently there is an increase in lung attenuation, mimicking the appearance of ground-glass

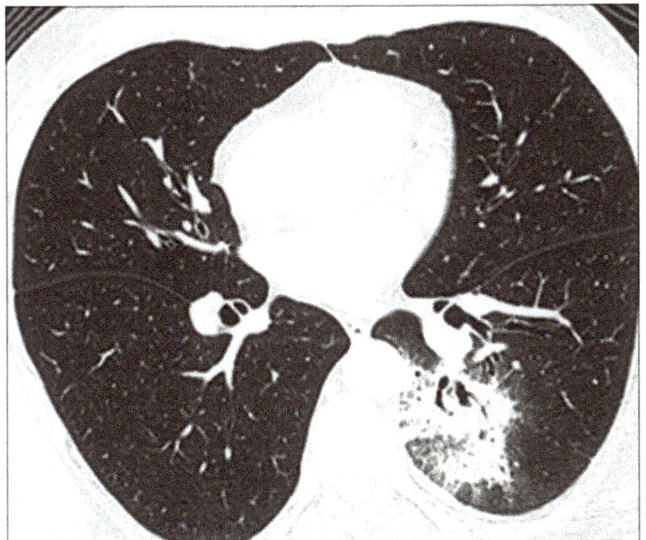

Fig. 149: Computed tomography (CT) chest showing consolidation in the left lower lobe with air bronchogram.

densities. It is useful to check the shape of the trachea to determine whether the scan has an adequate inspiratory effort. If the posterior tracheal surface is seen to bulge into the tracheal lumen, it is an expiratory scan rather than inspiratory **(Figs. 150A and B)**. The diagnosis of ground-glass opacity is essentially subjective, based on quantitative assessment of lung attenuation. It is important to maintain consistent window settings. Using too low a window mean with a narrow window width may give an appearance of ground-glass densities. Similar appearances may occur with a wider window width without changing the window mean. A useful tip is to see the air in the trachea or bronchi. If the air appears gray rather than black, the apparent increase in attenuation of lung parenchyma is usually not genuine. In patients with patchy areas of emphysema or air-trapping, normal lung regions may appear as areas of increased attenuation due to the contrast with darker areas. This can be avoided by using consistent window settings. Additionally in regions of normal lung attenuation, air bronchograms are not visualized as seen in areas of ground-glass density. Expiratory images are also useful in confirming lucent areas to represent areas of emphysema or air-trapping **(Figs. 151A and B)**.

Differential Diagnosis of Ground-Glass Densities

A large number of diseases may be associated with ground-glass opacities on HRCT as the pathological processes in the early stages are similar **(Fig. 152)**. These disease

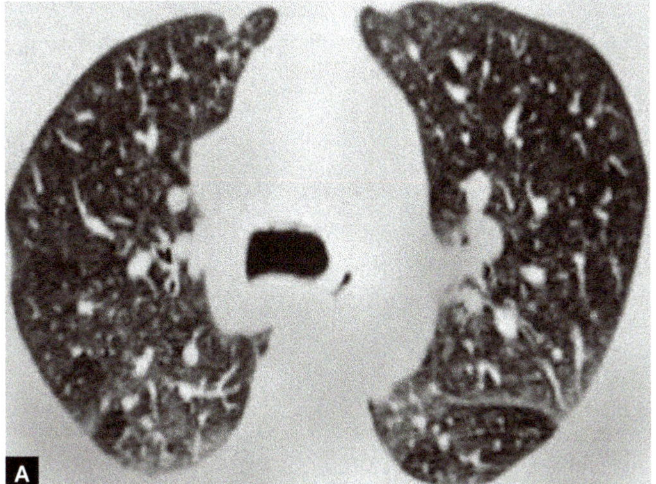
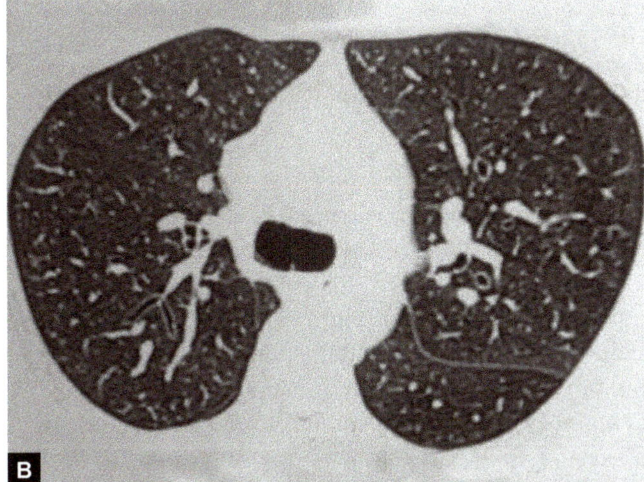

Figs. 150A and B: Pitfall in diagnosis: HRCT (A) reveals ill-defined ground-glass densities in both lung fields. Note shape of trachea; the posterior wall is bulging inwards showing that this is an expiratory scan; (B) HRCT in deep inspiration in same patient at same level. Note trachea is well-distended and there are no ground-glass densities.

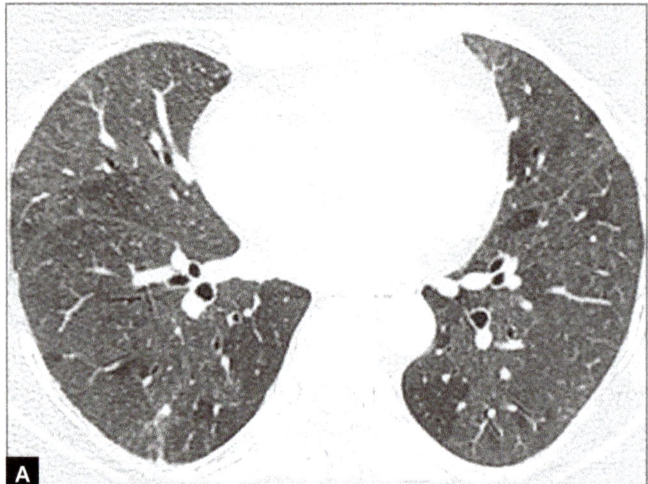
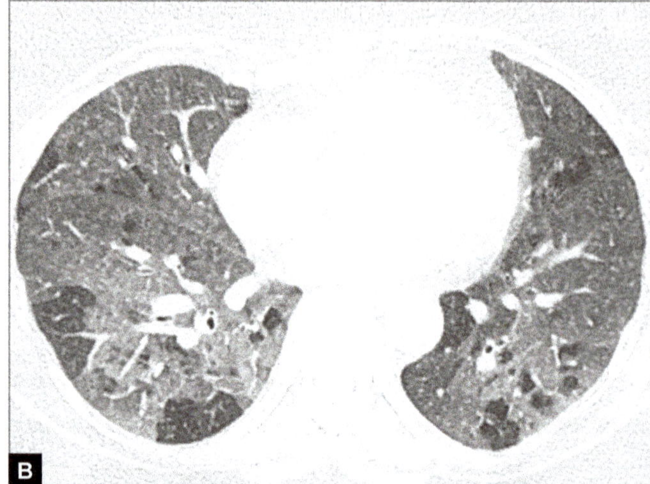

Fig. 151A and B: Hypersensitivity pneumonitis: HRCT reveals ill-defined areas of ground-glass densities in the inspiratory (A) and expiratory phases (B). Note the accentuation of air trapping in the expiratory phase.

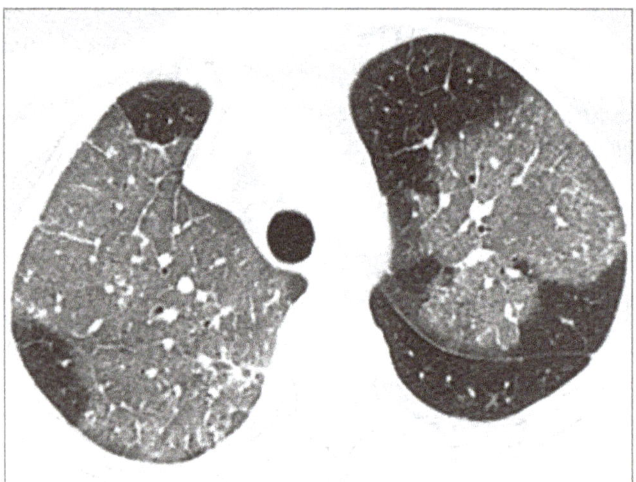
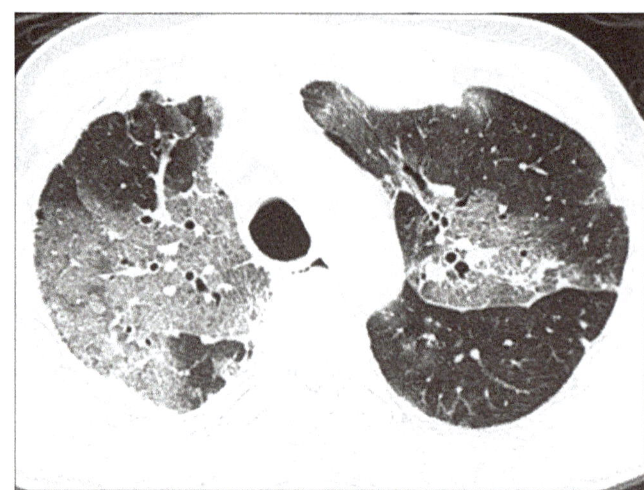

Fig. 152: *Pneumocystis jirovecii* pneumonia (PCP): Seropositive patient presented with fever and dyspnea. HRCT revealed diffuse ground-glass densities indicative of PCP. confirmed on bronchoalveolar lavage.

Figs. 153: Acute interstitial pneumonia: HRCT chest demonstrates ill-defined areas of increased lung attenuation in an acutely breathless patient.

processes may be acute, subacute or chronic. Acute disease processes manifesting as ground-glass densities include acute interstitial pneumonia **(Figs. 153 and 154)**, diffuse alveolar damage **(Fig. 155)**, pulmonary edema, ARDS, pulmonary hemorrhage **(Fig. 156)**, pneumonia and early radiation fibrosis. Subacute/chronic disease processes include interstitial pneumonias, especially NSIP, DIP **(Fig. 157)**, respiratory bronchiolitis, interstitial lung disease, hypersensitivity pneumonitis, drug reactions, chronic eosinophilic pneumonia, Churg Strauss syndrome, lupoid pneumonia, sarcoidosis and alveolar proteinosis **(Fig. 158)**.

Decreased Lung Attenuation

Pathological processes with decreased lung attenuation may be due to lung cysts, emphysema, bronchiectasis, mosaic attenuation or air-trapping.

Emphysema

This is a result of permanent abnormal enlargement of air-spaces with destruction of their walls distal to terminal bronchioles. On HRCT emphysema appears as focal or diffuse areas of decreased attenuation compared to normal lung parenchyma. By modifying the window settings of

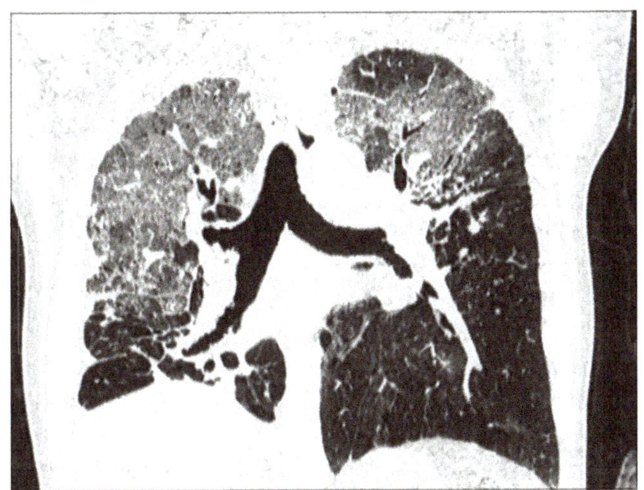

Fig. 154: Acute interstitial pneumonia: HRCT of the chest with coronal reconstruction in an acutely breathless patient demonstrates ill-defined areas of ground-glass opacification and consolidation.

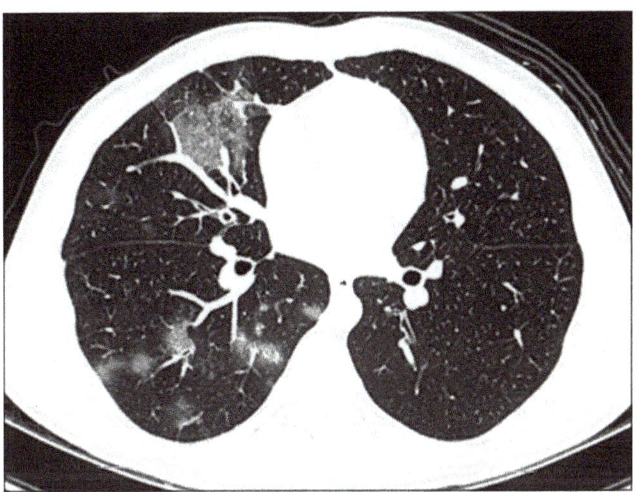

Fig. 156: Alveolar hemorrhage: HRCT in a patient with hemoptysis demonstrates ill-defined areas of ground-glass density in right middle lobe as well as right lower lobe. The ground-glass densities were due to alveolar hemorrhage.

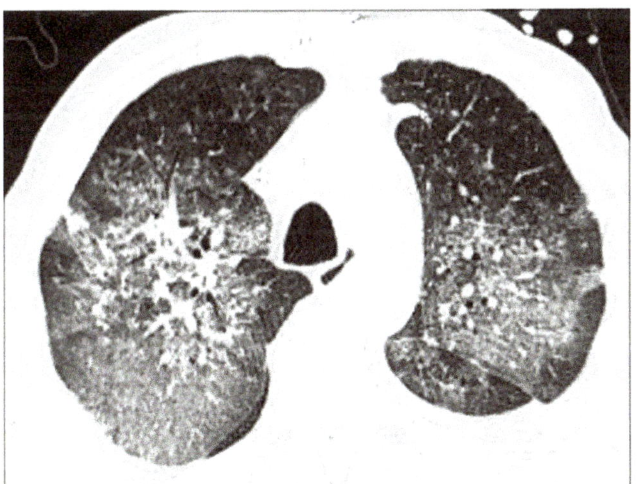

Fig. 155: Diffuse alveolar damage: Drug-induced diffuse alveolar damage seen on HRCT as diffuse ill-defined areas of increased lung attenuation in both lung fields.

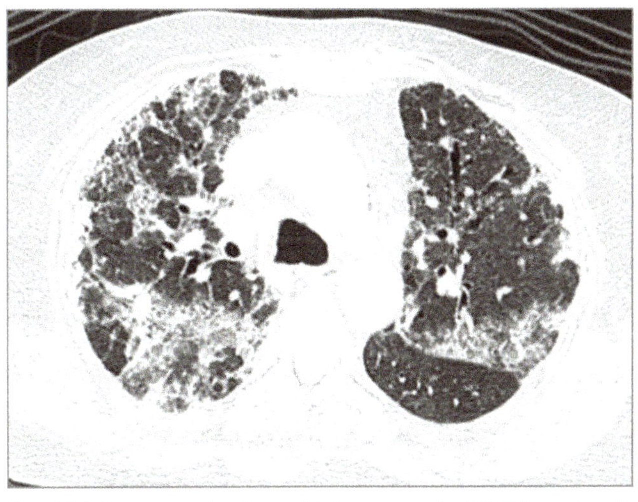

Fig. 157: Desquamative interstitial pneumonia: HRCT in a chronic smoker reveals ill-defined areas of parenchymal opacification in the subpleural and peribronchovascular regions. Thoracoscopic biopsy revealed desquamative interstitial pneumonia.

HRCT (600–800 window mean) emphysema can be very well-demonstrated **(Figs. 156 and 158)**. Emphysema is essentially of four types:

1. *Centrilobular*: This occurs predominantly in the upper lobes with lung destruction around the centrilobular arterial branches resulting in lucencies grouped around the centers of the secondary pulmonary lobule. With more severe destruction the appearances resemble panlobular emphysema. Centrilobular emphysema occurs in cigarette smokers due to enzymatic destruction of lung parenchyma as there is an imbalance between lung proteases and antiproteases **(Figs. 159 and 160)**.

2. *Panlobular emphysema*: This is characterized by uniform destruction of the pulmonary lobule leading to widespread areas of low attenuation. The pulmonary vessels appear fewer and thinner in appearance, termed as a diffuse simplification of lung architecture. Panlobular emphysema occurs in individuals with alpha-protease inhibitor deficiency

and as an extension of centrilobular emphysema in cigarette smokers **(Figs. 161A and B)**.

3. *Paraseptal emphysema*: The area of destruction involves the alveolar ducts and alveolar sacs marginated by the interlobular septa. On HRCT there are subpleural cysts which share thin walls. These cysts may become fairly large and reach up to a size of 1.0 cm. Paraseptal emphysema may be confused with honeycomb cysts, as both are in a subpleural location. Honeycomb cysts tend to be in several contiguous layers as compared to paraseptal emphysema which tends to occur in a single layer. Additionally, lung fibrosis usually accompanies honeycomb cysts, whereas other forms of emphysema such as centrilobular and panacinar may be present with paraseptal emphysema. Honeycomb cysts tend to be in the lung bases as compared to paraseptal emphysema which tends to be in the upper lobes.

4. *Bullous emphysema* is characterized by large bullae, often associated with centrilobular/paraseptal emphysema **(Fig. 162)**.

Bulla represents a sharply demarcated area of emphysema measuring 1.0 cm or more in diameter with a thin wall not more than 1 mm. They may range up to 20 cm in diameter but generally range between 2 cm and 8 cm in diameter **(Fig. 163)**.

Bleb—Bleb refers to a gas-containing space within the visceral pleura.

Pneumatocele is a thin-walled gas-filled space within the lung, occurring from lung necrosis and bronchiolar obstruction. It usually occurs in an acute setting following an acute pneumonia and is often transient. Pneumatocele has a similar appearance to lung cyst or bulla.

Differential Diagnosis of Cystic Lesions

The differential diagnosis of diffuse cystic lung diseases includes pulmonary Langerhans' cell histiocytosis, usual interstitial pneumonia, and centrilobular emphysema. Langerhans' cell histiocytosis chiefly involves the upper lobes and also shows the presence of nodules **(Fig. 164)**. UIP chiefly involves the lower lobes with cysts subpleural in location. The cystic spaces in centrilobular emphysema do not have well-defined walls. Lymphangioleiomyomatosis

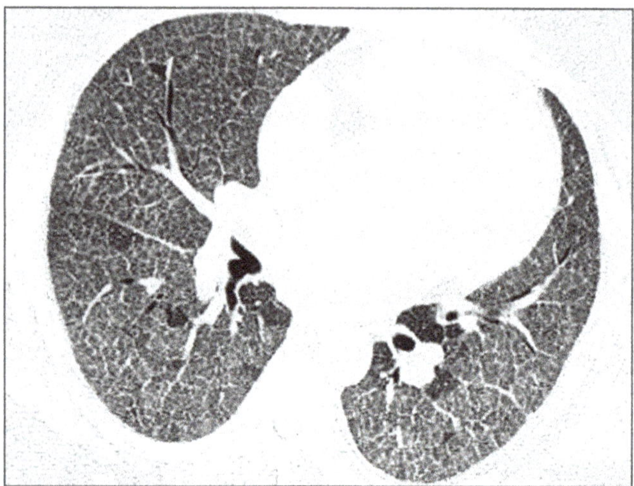

Fig. 158: Alveolar proteinosis: HRCT reveals ill-defined ground-glass densities in both lung fields with a background of septal thickening. This appearance simulates a crazy pavement appearance, most commonly seen in alveolar proteinosis.

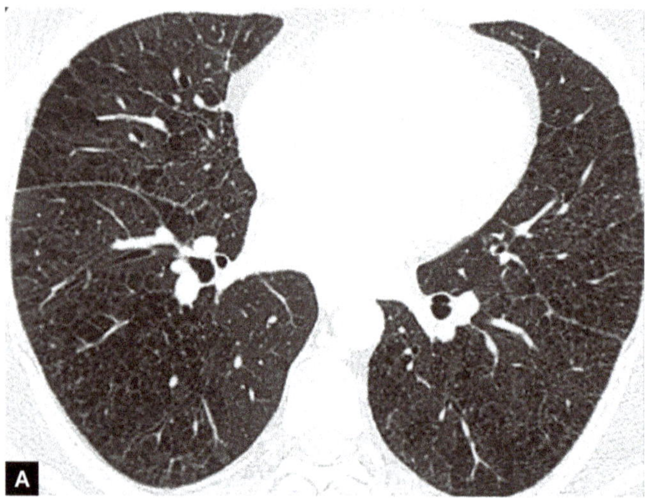

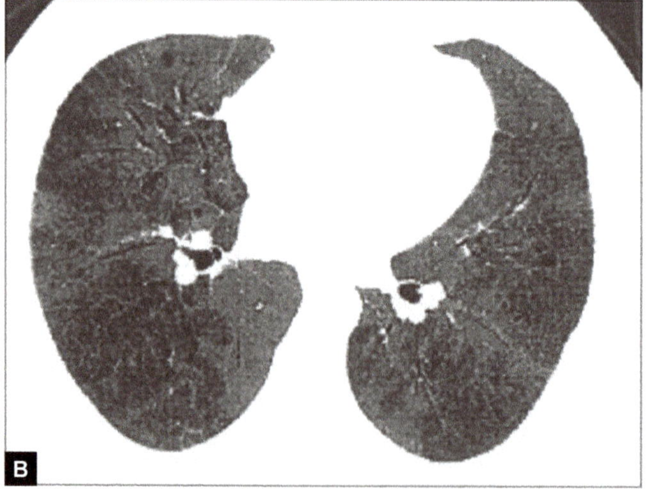

Figs. 159A and B: Centrilobular emphysema: (A) multiple thin-walled air spaces in both lung fields due to centrilobular emphysema (B) These are well-demonstrated on minimum intensity projection.

occurs in young females with evenly distributed cysts in both lung fields. Cystic bronchiectasis may also enter into the differential diagnosis and is generally easily identified.

Mosaic Attenuation

The lung may have an inhomogenous attenuation pattern with ill-defined areas of increased and decreased lung attenuation intermixed. This may be due to infiltrative diseases with areas of ground-glass density, increased lung attenuation with areas of normal lung attenuation intermixed **(Figs. 165A and B)**.

Mosaic perfusion is characterized by areas of decreased lung attenuation with areas of normal lung attenuation. Lung density is partially determined by the amount of blood present in lung tissue. Regional perfusion differences may occur due to airway abnormalities or vascular abnormalities. If there is reduced ventilation of a portion of the lung due to narrowing of the airways, there is reflex vasoconstriction resulting in hypoperfusion of the hypoventilated region. This is seen in bronchiolitis obliterans, bronchiolitis, bronchiectasis, and cystic fibrosis. If there is vascular obstruction there would be areas of hypoperfusion resulting in areas of low attenuation as seen in acute and chronic pulmonary thromboembolism.

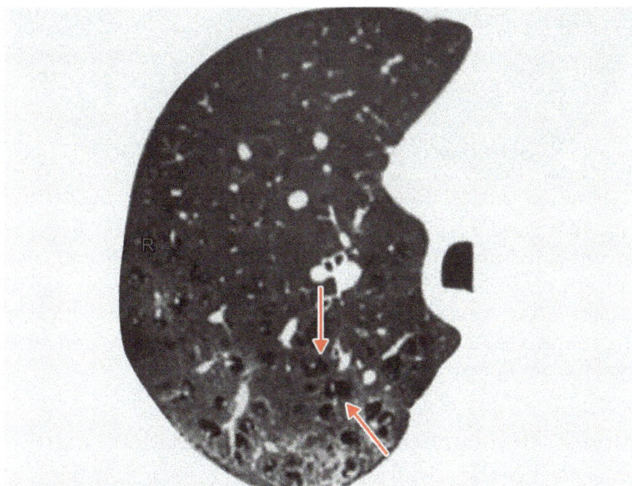

Fig. 160: Centrilobular emphysema: Multiple well-defined air spaces are seen with a central vessel within. These findings are typical for centrilobular emphysema. Lung destruction is seen to be occurring around the centrilobular vessel.

Airway Diseases

Upper Airways Obstruction

Tracheal stenosis: Tracheal stenosis can be related to inflammatory or neoplastic causes and is sometimes due to Wegener's granulomatosis. The lesion may occur anywhere within the trachea and may involve the major bronchi also **(Figs. 166A and B)**.

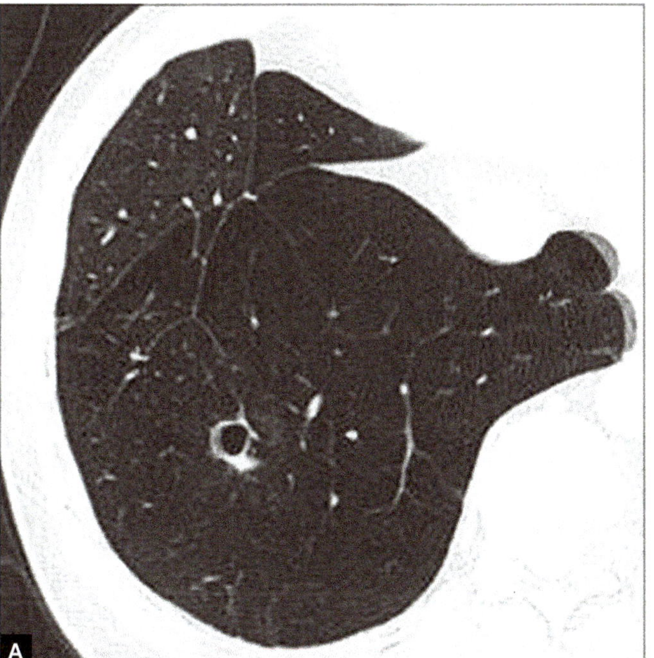

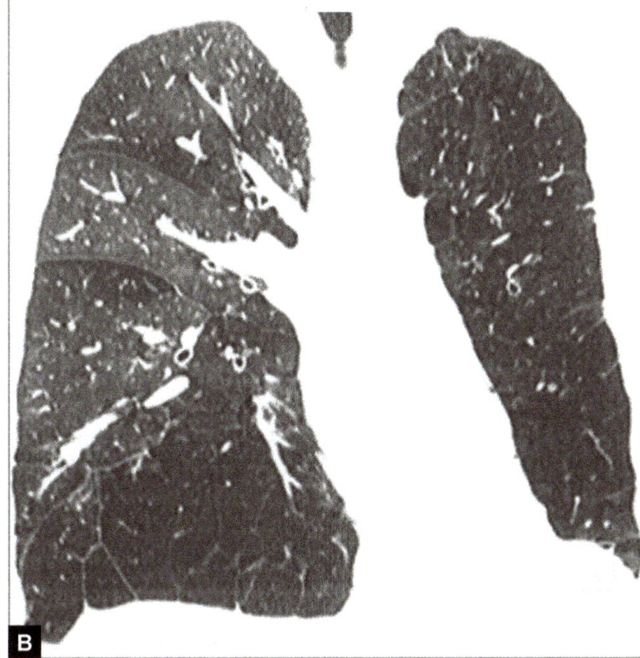

Figs. 161A and B: Panacinar emphysema: (A) Axial and (B) coronal HRCT images demonstrate large area of lung destruction seen in right lower zone. The density of the lung parenchyma is reduced and there is considerable thinning and separation of the vessels.

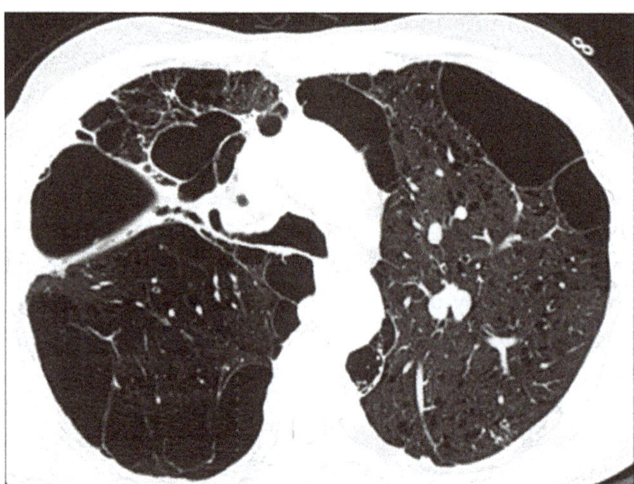

Fig. 162: Bullous emphysema: HRCT demonstrates extensive bullae in both lung fields, especially right with consequent compression of the lung parenchyma. There is extensive centrilobular emphysema in both lung fields.

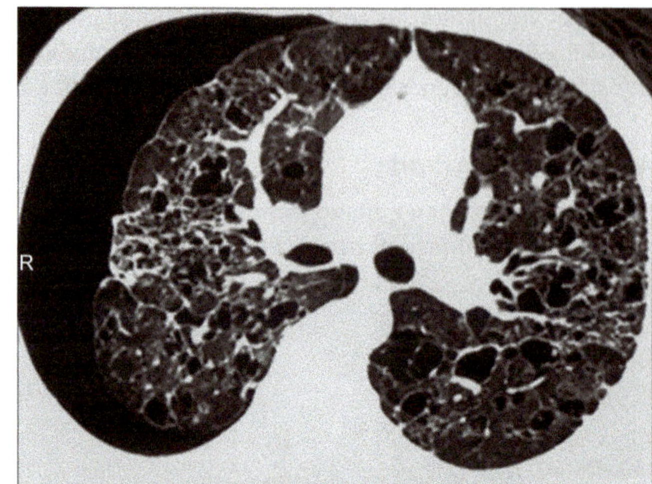

Fig. 164: Pulmonary Langerhans' cell histiocytosis: HRCT reveals a right-sided pneumothorax with multiple bizarre-shaped cysts in both lung fields. The bizarre shape of the cysts as well as history of exposure to cigarette smoke helps to differentiate from the thin-walled smooth cysts seen predominantly in females in lymphangioleiomyomatosis.

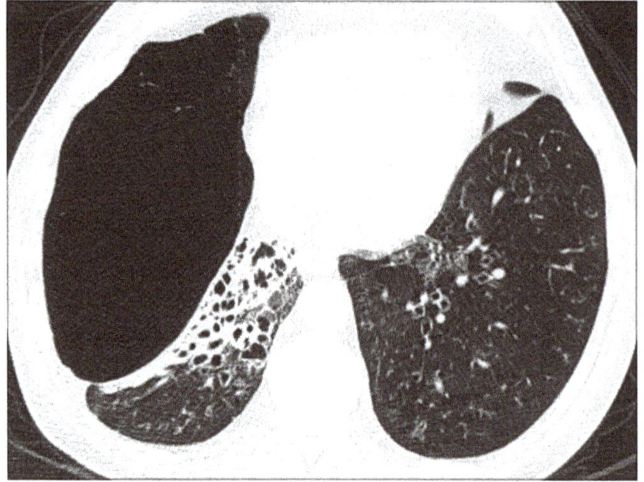

Fig. 163: Bulla: HRCT demonstrates a huge thin-walled air space in the right lung field representing a bulla. Also noted are the bronchiectatic changes in the superior segments of both lower lobes.

Clinical features include breathlessness, sometimes accompanied by a wheeze. A stridor is often observed when the obstruction is subglottic or if it involves the main trachea. This condition is often mistaken for asthma because of the presence of a wheeze. Even if the wheeze is present, as for example in a patient with obstruction to the right or left bronchus, it is monophonic in nature and not polyphonic as seen in patients with asthma. Flow volume loop confirms the diagnosis. Initially there is flattening of the inspiratory loop but later a flattening of both inspiratory and expiratory loops of the flow volume curve is observed.

Bronchiectasis: Bronchiectasis is defined as localized irreversible dilatation of the bronchial tree. There are a wide variety of causes. It is usually as a result of acute, chronic or recurrent infection. Bronchiectasis is classified on the basis of its severity as cylindrical (the walls of the bronchi are dilated but parallel), varicose (there is dilatation of the bronchi with focal constrictions, thereby giving a varicose appearance), and cystic, where the bronchi are ballooned (**Figs. 167 to 170**).

On HRCT, the dilated bronchi are visualized depending on the plane they are traversing in. If perpendicular to the plane of CT, i.e. running vertically down, they are visualized in cross-section. This appearance has been likened to a signet ring appearance—the dilated bronchus as the ring and the accompanying pulmonary artery as the jewel on the ring. If the bronchi are running parallel to the scan plane, i.e. horizontal they are visualized as tram tracks or parallel lines. There may be associated atelectasis resulting in the bronchi being bunched up, this gives an appearance of multiple cysts. Bronchial wall thickening may also be seen as well as air-fluid levels, especially in cystic bronchiectasis.

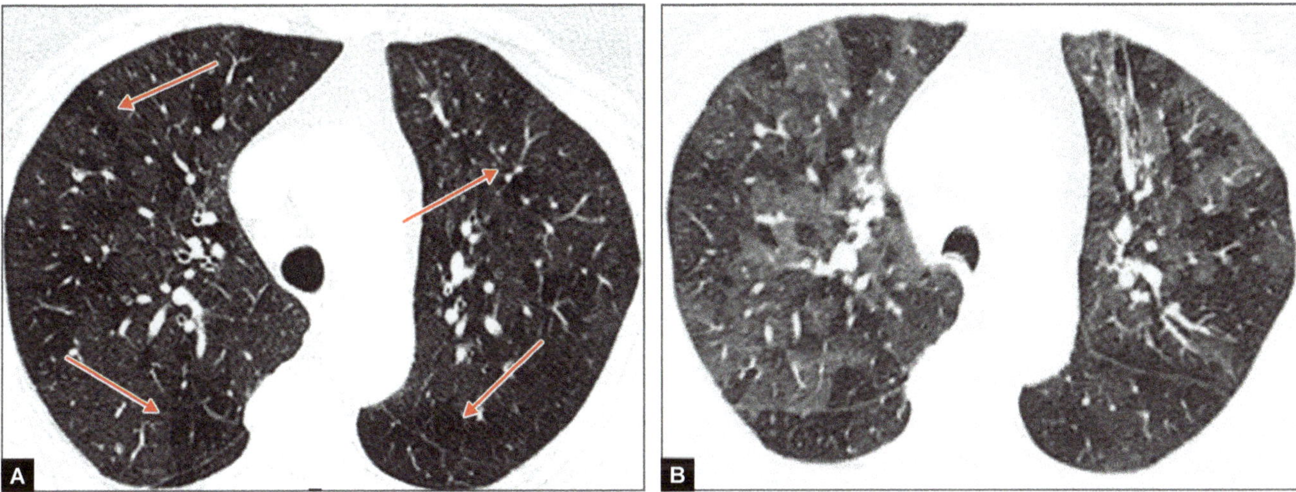

Figs. 165A and B: (A) HRCT demonstrates subtle inhomogenous areas of attenuation in both lung fields on inspiratory scan. On expiratory scans (B) there is accentuation of the inhomogenous areas of altered attenuation. Focal areas are seen to be darker and focal areas are brighter. The vessels within the areas which are darker are sparse in distribution and thinner in caliber, representing air-trapping. Mosaic attenuation was due to constrictive bronchiolitis.

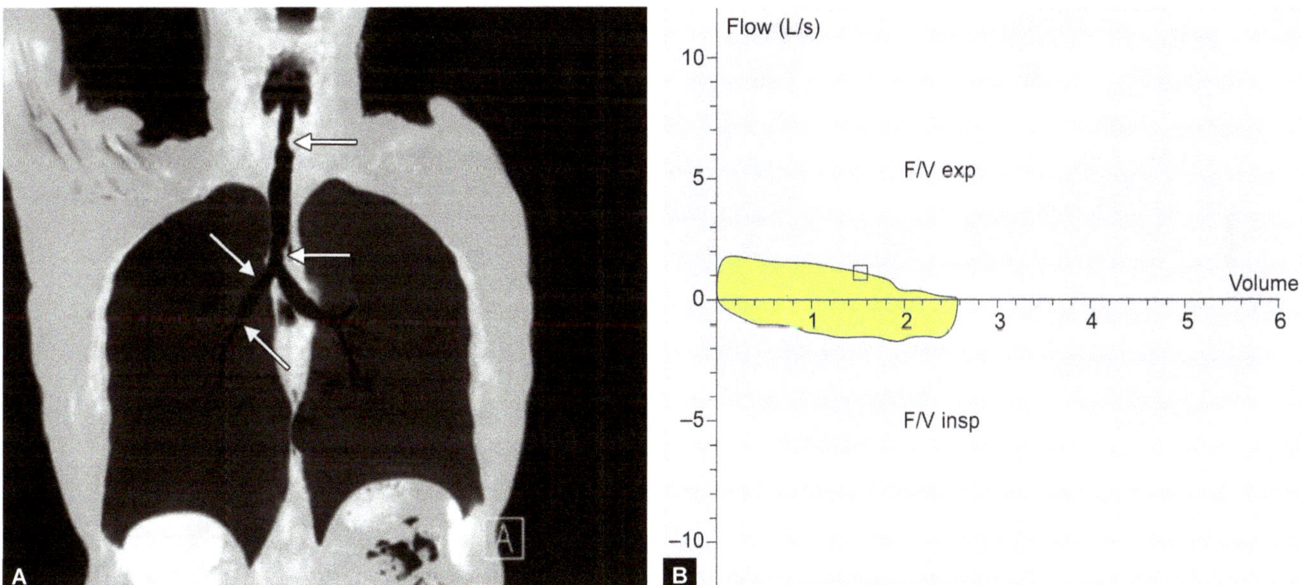

Figs. 166A and B: (A) Coronal CT section shows tracheal stenosis at two sites—an upper and a lower one, just above the carina. This patient was a young 23-year-old lady diagnosed as having asthma because of difficulty in breathing and a wheeze on auscultation. Clinical examination revealed noisy breathing, often amounting to a stridor. Auscultation revealed a monophonic wheeze; (B) The flow volume loop demonstrated a marked flattening of the inspiratory and expiratory curve. Surgical correction of this disorder was successfully done. The etiology of this tracheal stenosis was uncertain. It was probably related to Wegener's granulomatosis.

Small Airway Diseases: Bronchiolar Diseases

HRCT has revolutionized our ability to diagnose small airway disease. The HRCT findings can be divided into two groups based on the imaging findings:

1. Constrictive bronchiolitis
2. Exudative bronchiolitis.

1. *Constrictive bronchiolitis:* Constrictive bronchiolitis is concentric fibrosis involving the submucosal and peri-bronchial tissues of the terminal bronchioles resulting in

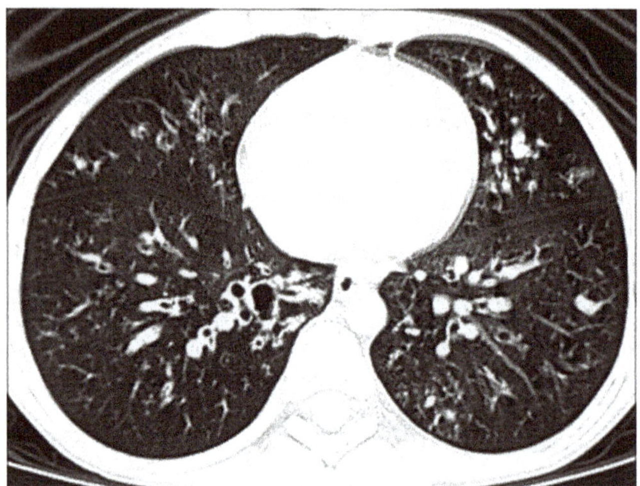

Fig. 167: Bronchiectasis: HRCT chest demonstrates dilated bronchi representing bronchiectasis.

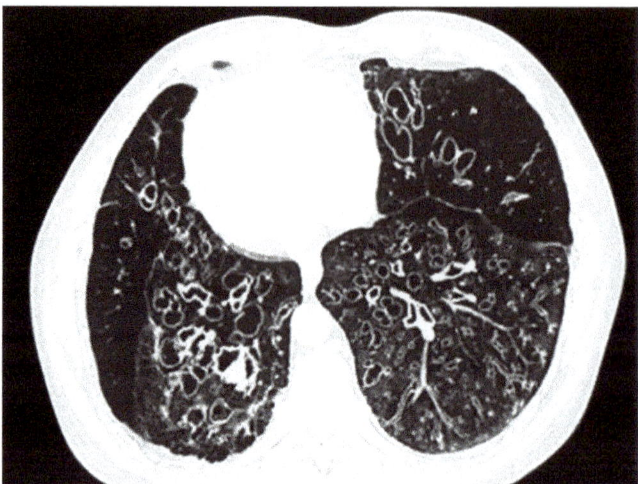

Fig. 169: Bronchiectasis: HRCT demonstrates dilated bronchi in both lung fields, note dextrocardia in a case of Kartagener's syndrome.

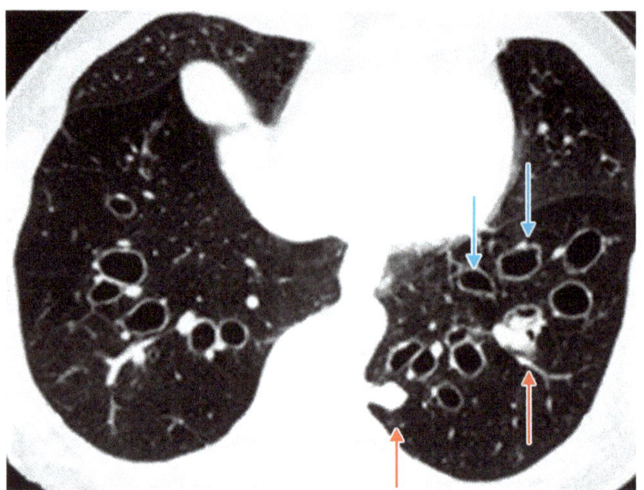

Fig. 168: Bronchiectasis: HRCT demonstrates dilated bronchi (blue arrows) in both lung bases. Note marked difference in the diameter of the bronchus and accompanying artery. A few dilated bronchi in the left lower lobe demonstrate soft-tissue within their lumen representing mucoid impaction (red arrows).

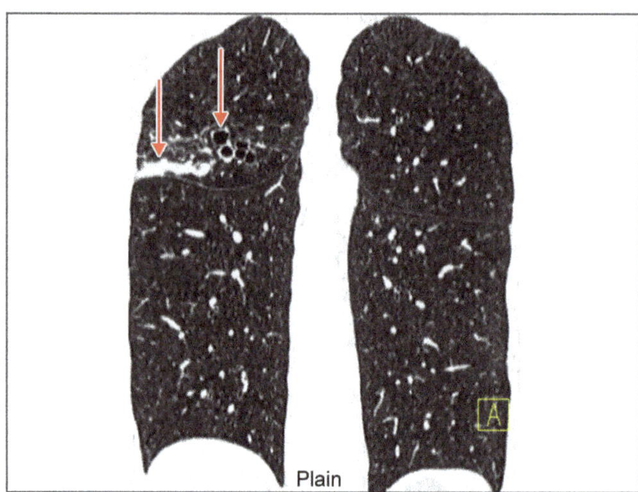

Fig. 170: Bronchiectasis: Coronal HRCT demonstrates dilated bronchi in the right upper lobe. There is a linear well-defined tubular opacity extending to the subpleural region representing mucoid impaction in dilated bronchus.

bronchial narrowing and obliteration **(Figs. 171A and B)**. The HRCT findings reflect the pathophysiology that causes airflow limitation. There is both hypoventilation of the involved segments of the lung and air-trapping. This is seen as areas of mosaic attenuation. The affected segments are dark and demonstrate air-trapping on expiratory scans. Hypoventilation of the involved areas of the lung results in reflex hypoperfusion so that vessels in the involved segments appear attenuated and sparse. The airways in

these segments may also demonstrate abnormalities in the form of focal bronchial dilatation and wall thickening.

2. *Exudative bronchiolitis:* There is mucoid impaction in the terminal bronchioles. On chest X-ray these are seen as numerous small (5 mm) ill-defined nodules **(Figs. 172 and 173)**. On HRCT the areas of mucoid impaction are seen as tubular branching structures in the peripheral lung parenchyma resembling toy jacks also termed as

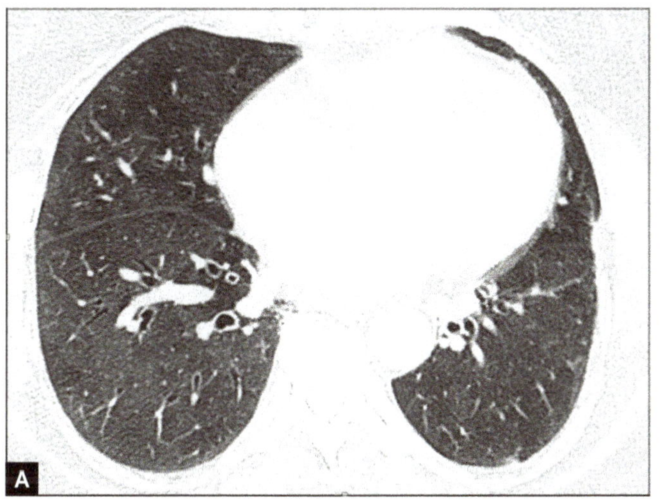

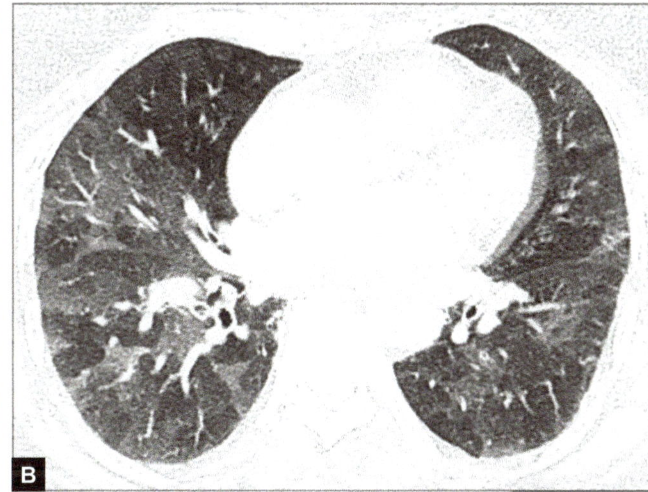

Figs. 171A and B: Constrictive bronchiolitis: (A) Inspiratory CT chest: areas of inhomogenous attenuation with areas of increased and decreased attenuation; (B) Expiratory scans reveal air-trapping as the areas of decreased attenuation retain their attenuation whereas the areas of increased attenuation become brighter: the air-trapping indicates small-airway disease.

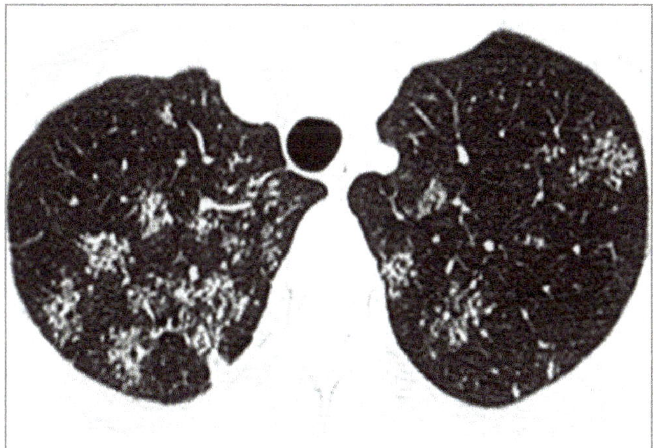

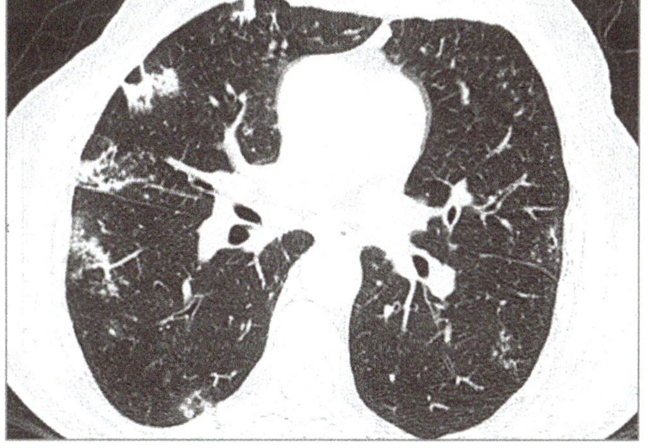

Fig. 172: Exudative bronchiolitis: HRCT demonstrates multiple small conglomerated nodular lesions representing mucoid impaction in terminal bronchioles as a result of exudative bronchiolitis.

Fig. 173: Exudative bronchiolitis: HRCT demonstrates multiple small conglomerated nodular lesions representing mucoid impaction in terminal bronchioles with associated ground-glass densities as a result of exudative bronchiolitis with peribronchiolar inflammation.

tree-in-bud appearance. When seen in cross-section they appear as centrilobular nodules.

Swyer-James Syndrome (Fig. 174)

This condition is usually caused by a viral infection to the immature lung, before it has completed development (below eight years of age). There is obliterative bronchiolitis involving the distal airways. Usually, an entire lung is involved, occasionally segments are spared. There is hypoplasia of the lung together with hypoplasia of the pulmonary artery to the involved lung.

On the chest X-ray there is unilateral transradiancy, the opposite lung appears to be plethoric. The ipsilateral hilum may be small chiefly because of a hypoplastic pulmonary artery supplying the involved lung.

■ IMPORTANT CONGENITAL MALFORMATIONS AND ANOMALIES

Pulmonary Arteriovenous Malformations

Nearly 70% of cases with pulmonary arteriovenous malformations (PAVM) are associated with hereditary hemorrhagic telangiectasia (HHT or Rendu-Osler-Weber disease). This is an autosomal dominant disorder characterized by the triad of telangiectasia, recurrent epistaxis and a family history of the disease. There is a wide spectrum of presentations. Patients may be asymptomatic, lesions being detected incidentally on a

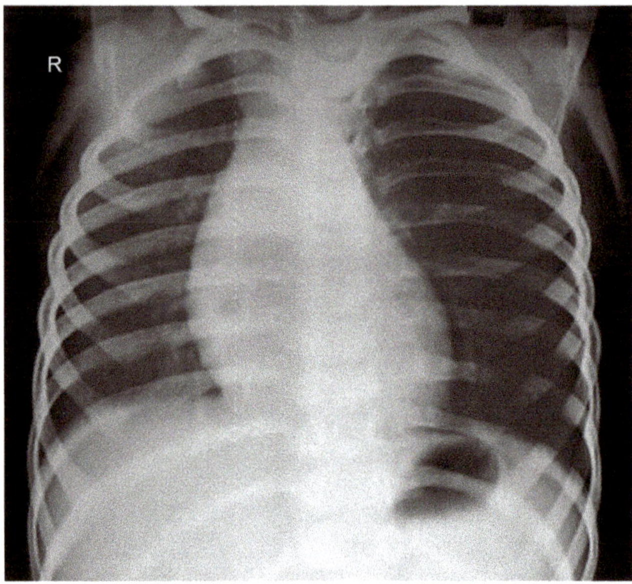

Fig. 174: Swyer-James syndrome: Chest X-ray demonstrates unilateral transradiancy on the left side due to infantile bronchiolitis resulting in a Swyer-James syndrome.

chest X-ray. If the AVM is large enough to cause a marked right to left shunt, the patient may present with cyanosis, dyspnea, clubbing, hemoptysis, and cardiac failure. Usually, in these cases a distinct bruit is heard over the hemithorax. Patients may also present with cerebral abscesses and cerebral infarction due to paradoxical embolism. An important clinical finding in PAVMs is orthodeoxia—there is a drop in oxygen saturation from the supine to erect position. This is because PAVMs are mainly in the lower zones; this results in an increased right to left shunting of blood within the lungs in the erect position **(Figs. 175 and 176)**.

On chest radiographs AVMs are seen as well-defined nodules ranging in size from 1 cm to more than 1 cm. Peripheral AVMs usually demonstrate feeding arteries and draining veins as curvilinear structures. The more central AVMs are more difficult to detect as they may be overlapped by the hilum; the feeding draining vessels may not be visualized as they traverse a short distance.

CT is extremely sensitive and specific in demonstrating pulmonary AVMs. It is able to demonstrate feeding as well as draining vessels. There is intense enhancement of these lesions; CT scans are also able to detect the presence of multiple lesions. Remy Jardin and colleagues in fact found CT more sensitive than pulmonary angiograms, which have been considered the gold standard for the diagnosis of AVMs. CT detected AVMs in 98% of cases compared to

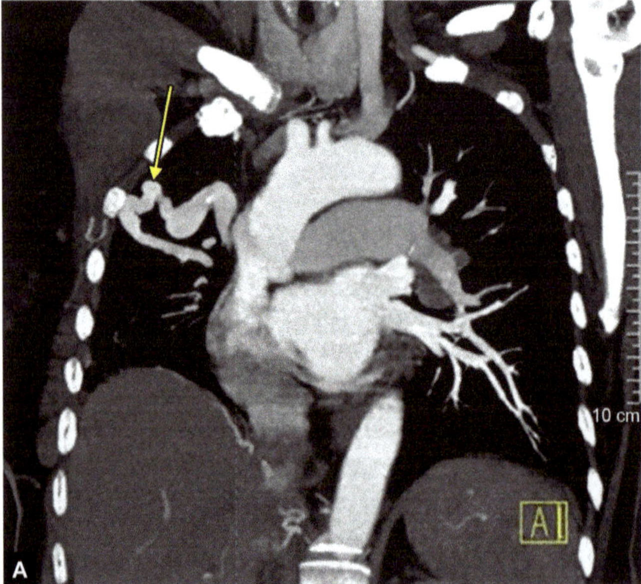
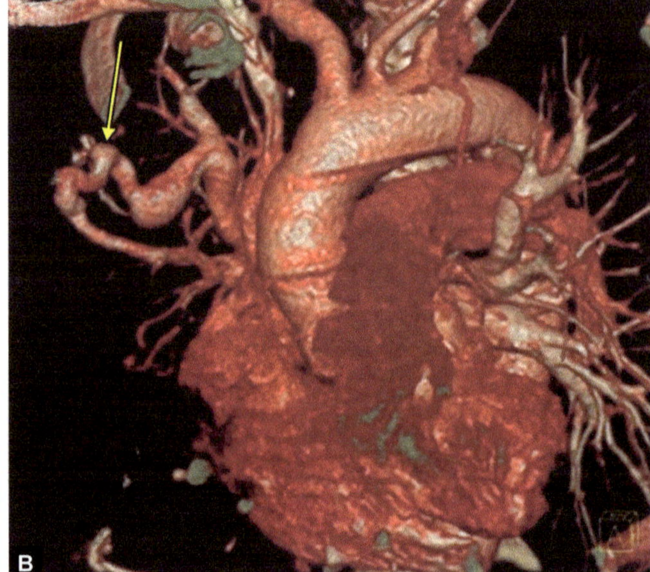

Figs. 175A and B: Pulmonary arteriovenous malformation: (A) Maximum intensity projection (MIP) and (B) Volume rendering technique (VRT) images of CT angiography demonstrate an arteriovenous malformation in the right upper zone with feeding arteries and draining veins.

pulmonary angiograms, which detected AVMs in 60%. CT additionally assists in deciding further management of these lesions. Using 2D and 3D reconstructions the feeding arteries can be demonstrated. Feeding arteries greater than 3 mm in diameter are embolized interventionally using coils, detachable balloons, to decrease the right to left shunting. Contrast echocardiography can be used to demonstrate complex angioarchitecture as well as provide a road map of the extent of the right to left shunt. MRI is useful in demonstrating larger PAVMs but smaller PAVMs may not be as well detected as in a CT.

Congenital Diaphragmatic Hernia

The classical congenital diaphragmatic hernia results from failure of the pleuroperitoneal cavity to close with resultant herniation of abdominal contents into the thorax. The incidence is 1:2,400 births, and is most commonly left-sided (90%). In the neonatal period these present as respiratory distress, as the herniated abdominal contents cause compressive effects on the lung and mediastinum. The diagnosis is fairly easy on the chest X-ray as there is evidence of soft tissue and air-filled bowel loops in the left hemithorax. When the stomach is included in the hernial sac, the nasogastric tube rather than descending in the abdomen is seen to take a turn upwards into the thorax from the gastroesophageal junction **(Figs. 177 and 178)**.

Hernias on the right side may be difficult to detect as there is usually herniation of liver; the chest radiograph demonstrates a soft tissue opacity in the lower right hemithorax.

Bochdalek Hernia

These result from herniation through a posterior diaphragmatic defect close to the crura. They tend to manifest later in life and may be bilateral and symmetric.

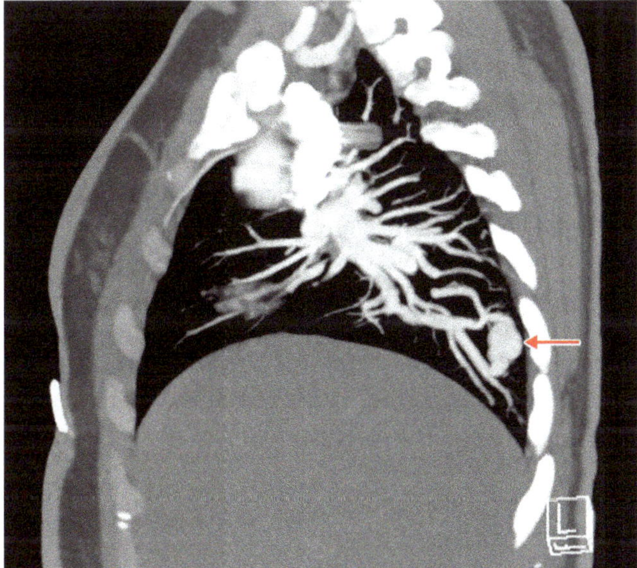

Fig. 176: Pulmonary arteriovenous malformation: Sagittal multiplanar reconstruction (MPR) demonstrates feeding arteries and draining vein of pulmonary arteriovenous malformation.

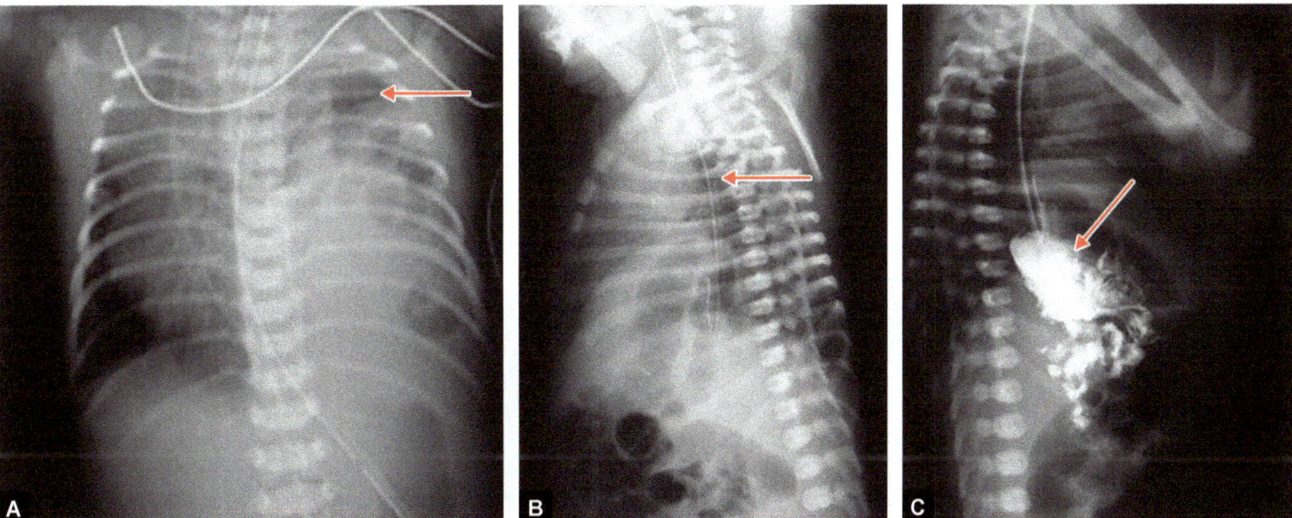

Figs. 177A to C: Diaphragmatic hernia: (A) AP and (B) oblique views demonstrate soft-tissue opacity and bowel loops in the left hemithorax with shift of the mediastinum to the right; (C) Barium study confirms bowel loops in the hemithorax.

The liver prevents herniation on the right side. Occasionally, kidney and/or stomach may herniate on the left side.

Morgagni's Hernia

These are due to herniation between sternal and costal attachments usually developing in the right anterior cardiophrenic sulcus. On the left herniation is impeded by the heart. Visual contents of the hernia are liver and omentum, occasionally transverse colon. On chest X-ray herniation of liver and omentum is visualized as a paracardiac mass with a D/D of pericardial cyst, paracardiac fat pad or a pleural/pulmonary mass (**Figs. 179A and B**). When there is herniation of colon, the presence of a gas-filled viscus makes the diagnosis easy. A lateral view of the chest helps to localize the hernia anteriorly. CT is diagnostic as CT demonstrates the herniation of liver/omentum and bowel (**Figs. 180 and 181**).

■ ABSENCE OF LUNG OR LOBES OF LUNGS

Unilateral agenesis is a rare congenital anomaly presenting with minimal clinical problems. It is frequently associated with other congenital anomalies particularly tracheoesophageal fistula and the VACTERL association (non-random association of birth defects). When the bronchus is absent, it is termed as "agenesis".

When the bronchus is present but rudimentary, it is termed aplasia. The ipsilateral pulmonary artery develops but is usually hypoplastic.

Agenesis of the right lung is often accompanied by esophageal atresia and is twice as common as left lung agenesis (**Figs. 182A and B**). Left lung agenesis is often accompanied by tracheoesophageal fistula. On imaging there is loss of aeration and volume on the ipsilateral side as evidenced by elevation of the diaphragm, shift of

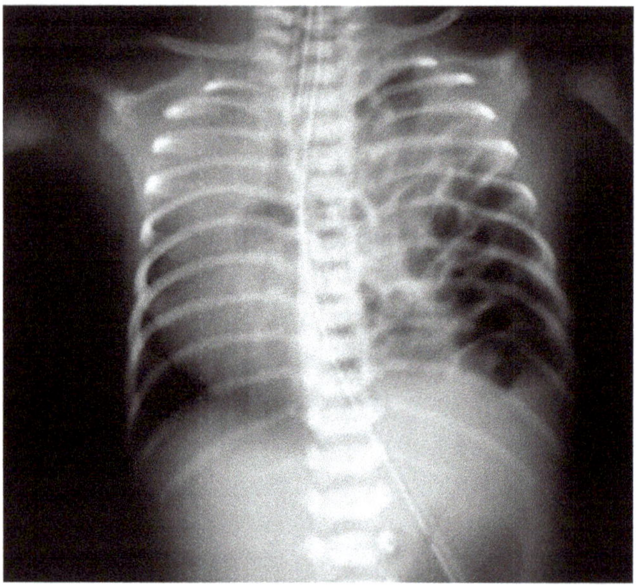

Fig. 178: Diaphragmatic hernia: Chest X-ray in a neonate reveals ill-defined opacities in the left hemithorax with multiple air-filled loops representing a diaphragmatic hernia. There is consequently a shift of the mediastinum to the right.

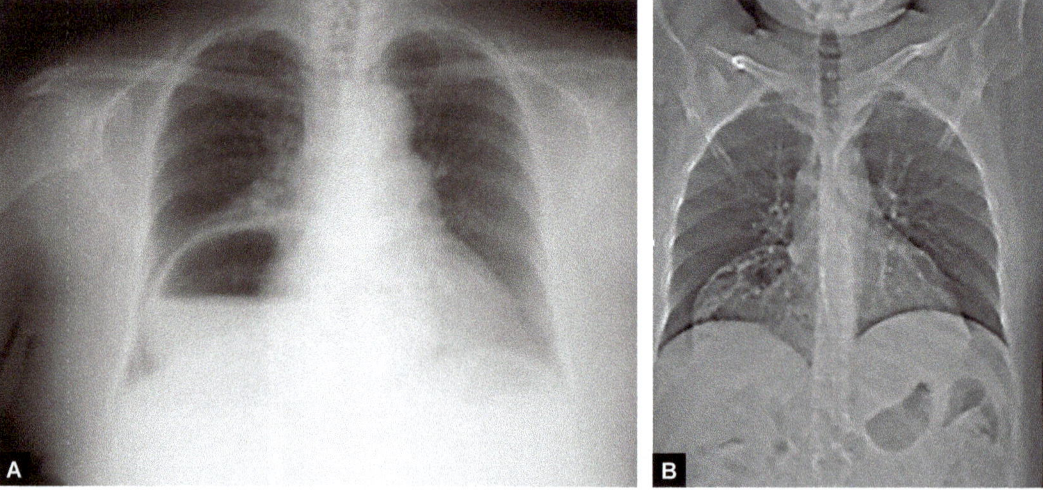

Figs. 179A and B: Morgagni's hernia: (A) PA view and (B) topogram of the chest reveals a bowel loop with an air-fluid level in the right hemithorax.

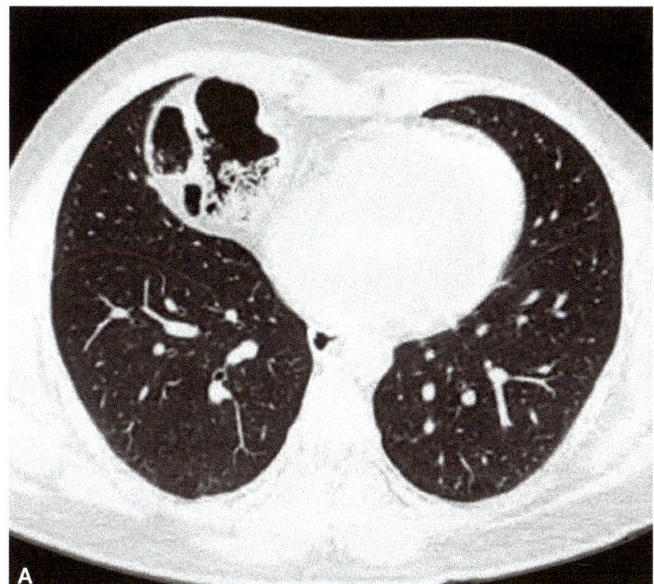

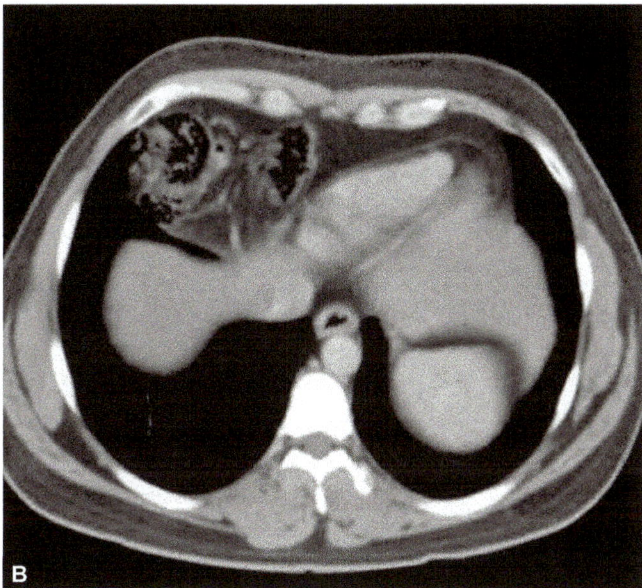

Figs. 180A and B: Morgagni's hernia: CT scans show herniation of colon through an anterior abdominal wall defect into the anterior hemithorax, representing a Morgagni's hernia.

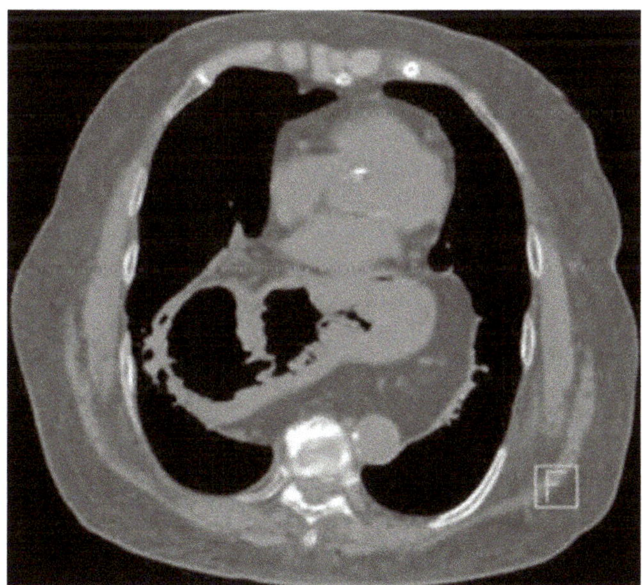

Fig. 181: Hiatus hernia: CT demonstrates a huge hiatus hernia with the stomach extending into the thoracic cavity.

the mediastinum to the ipsilateral side and increase in extrapleural fat to fill the space due to congenital hypoplasia.

Absence of individual lobes is a form of hypoplastic lung syndrome. When there is absence of a lobe there is compensatory expansion of the rest of the lung, distorting bronchovascular structures. This overexpansion is never adequate to revert the lung to normal size. The size of the ipsilateral lung is always smaller, similar to what is seen in pulmonary hypoplasia. The difference is easily determined on CT as a bronchus is absent, whereas in hypoplasia all segments are present but the tracheobronchial tree is stunted and underdeveloped.

Tracheoesophageal Fistula

Tracheoesophageal fistulas are associated with esophageal atresia and are usually diagnosed in the neonatal period. Rarely, tracheoesophageal fistulas are not diagnosed till later in life as the symptoms may be nonspecific. These fistulas are of the "H" type—a short horizontal communication between the trachea and esophagus— the horizontal communication being represented by the H bar. Symptoms are due to recurrent aspiration, paroxysmal cough, feeding difficulties and recurrent pneumonia. The appearances on chest radiographs are of aspiration, excessive air may also pass from the trachea into the esophagus as well as into the gut. This may be visualized also on an X-ray as air in the esophagus and/or gaseous distension of the bowel. An obvious tracheoesophageal fistula is fairly easy to demonstrate. A small tracheoesophageal fistula, especially the "H" variety is best demonstrated in the prone position using a feeding tube which is slowly withdrawn while a nonionic water

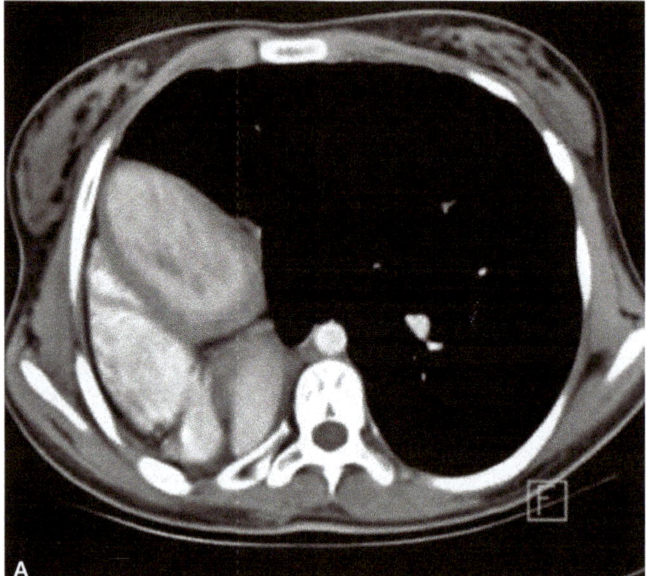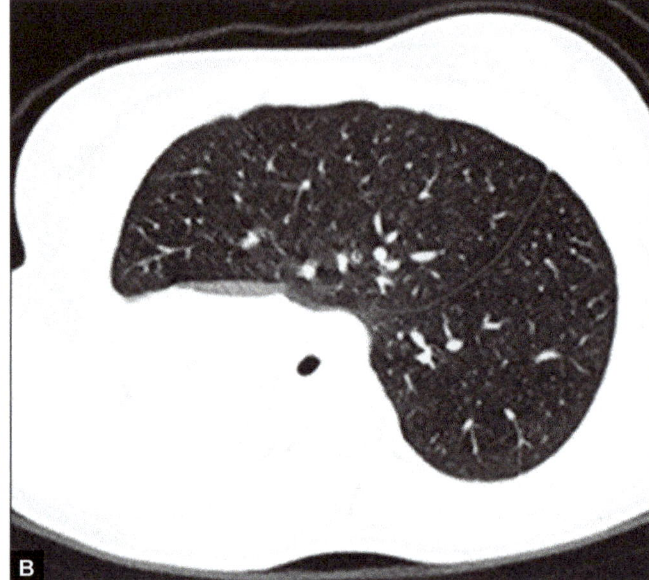

Figs. 182A and B: Agenesis of right lung: (A) CT chest reveals a marked shift of mediastinum to the right with no lung tissue seen in right hemithorax; (B) there is compensatory expansion of left lung. The right pulmonary artery was absent.

soluble contrast is injected to demonstrate the fistulous communication. The "H" type of tracheoesophageal fistulas is usually associated with other congenital anomalies—these have been designated by acronyms: VATER—vertebral, anal, tracheoesophageal, renal; VACTEL—vertebral, anal, cardiac, tracheoesophageal and limb. Pulmonary hypoplasia, tracheal stenosis and pulmonary sequestration may also be associated.

Bronchial Atresia

There is a short segment of atresia involving a segment or subsegmental bronchus. There is consequently dilatation of the bronchus distal to the atresia, resulting in accumulation of mucus in the dilated bronchus. This mucocele is seen on imaging as a mass-like structure; there may be a branching configuration which helps establish the diagnosis. The surrounding lung in the affected segment is hypertranslucent as the lung beyond the atretic segment is aerated by collateral drift and because there is reflex hypoperfusion of the vessels in the affected segment. The vessels appear thinner and less is number in the affected segment. Most patients are asymptomatic. Bronchial atresia has limited clinical significance; the only issue is that it may be mistaken for a mass. CT very effectively demonstrates the central mucous-filled mass, atresia of the segmental bronchus, and the hypertranslucent lung segment.

Pulmonary Sequestration

Pulmonary sequestration is characterized by the presence of pulmonary tissue which does not communicate with the central airways through a normal bronchial connection and receives its blood supply via an anomalous systemic artery. Pulmonary sequestration is divided into intralobar and extralobar varieties, based on venous drainage. If the venous drainage is to the pulmonary veins, it is termed "intralobar sequestration" **(Figs. 183A and B)**. If the drainage is to the systemic veins, it is termed "extralobar sequestration".

Extralobar sequestrations are congenital abnormalities usually associated with other congenital abnormalities, such as congenital heart disease, diaphragmatic hernia, or cystic adenomatoid malformation. They are asymptomatic and therefore discovered incidentally on antenatal ultrasound, chest X-ray, sonography, CT, angiography or during surgical repair of a congenital diaphragmatic hernia with which they are commonly associated. An extralobar sequestration has a complete serosal covering; it may have a narrow vascular pedicle as it is separate from the normal lung. Extralobar sequestrations in 90% of cases occur on the left side. Torsion is a complication and this may result in a tension hydrothorax.

Extralobar sequestrations are seen on imaging as mass lesions of homogenous density. They have well-defined

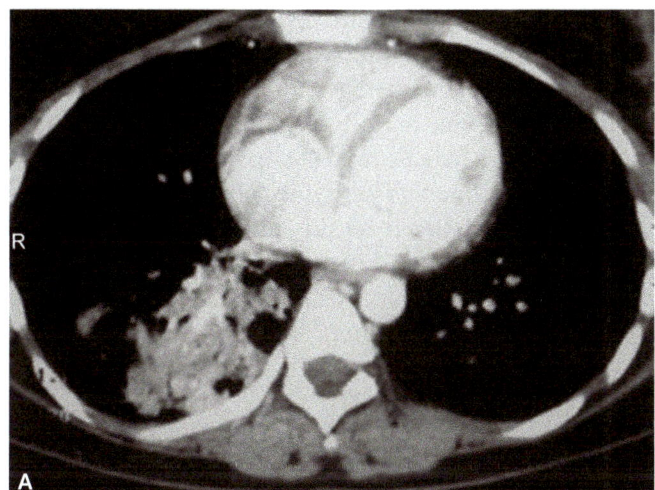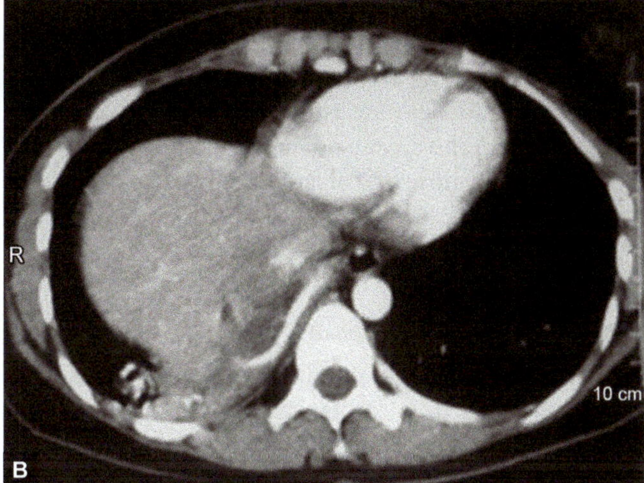

Figs. 183A and B: Pulmonary sequestration: (A) CT scan demonstrates an ill-defined consolidation; (B) CT angiography demonstrates arterial branch arising from aorta feeding the consolidation representing an intralobar sequestration.

margins, in particular the lateral margin which is covered by pleura. The medial margin may be difficult to discern as it abuts the mediastinum, often giving the appearance of a mediastinal mass. Sequestration may be seen in relation to the pericardium, diaphragm, and the retroperitoneum, occasionally communicating with the esophagus or stomach, which can be demonstrated by barium studies.

As compared to extralobar sequestration which is a congenital abnormality, intralobar sequestration is being considered to be more likely an acquired lesion rather than a congenital abnormality. Chronic bronchial obstruction due to foreign body, carcinoid tumor and postobstructive pneumonia are considered to be causes of intralobar sequestration. The chronic inflammatory process "parasites" its blood supply from the systemic circulation, often a branch from the descending aorta or branches from the inferior pulmonary ligament. Therefore, 98% of all sequestrations occur in the lower lobes. As compared to extralobar sequestrations which are asymptomatic, intralobar sequestrations present as an infective lesion or sequelae of an infective lesion. On imaging they appear as round, oval, lobulated mass lesions simulating an intrapulmonary mass lesion. Air and air-fluid levels may be seen within these masses due to communication with bronchi secondary to episodes of infection. CT appearances are similar to those of a chest X-ray; however, CT more frequently detects air, air-fluid levels, and the presence of emphysema adjacent to the sequestration. The emphysema occurs due to impaired ventilation secondary to chronic obstruction

with consequent collateral air drift and air-trapping. Occasionally, a pure cystic form of sequestration is detected with air-trapping, focal emphysema and bulla formation. The key in differentiating from other cystic masses is the demonstration of a systemic arterial supply. CT angiography on MDCT scanner has replaced the need for invasive angiography to demonstrate systemic arterial supply, the key to the diagnosis of sequestration. The differential diagnosis of sequestration encompasses infective lesions, pulmonary masses, mediastinal and pleural masses. The clue to the correct diagnosis is location, arterial supply, venous drainage, and a history of repeated infections.

Congenital Lobar Overinflation

Previously known as congenital lobar emphysema, it is now termed as congenital lobar overinflation (CLO). The pathophysiology of this condition is characterized by overinflation of normal alveoli most likely due to central airway obstruction, presumably due to aplasia, hypoplasia or dysplasia of the bronchial support structures. A clinically similar condition is polyalveolar lobe—the lobe contains four to five times the number of alveoli normally present, resulting in a large lobe having all the compressive effects seen in CLO. CLO manifests in the neonatal period with respiratory distress. On chest X-ray there is hyperexpansion of a lobe of the lung, usually upper or middle lobe. Involvement of more than one lobe or the lower lobe is extremely rare. The hyperexpanded lobe causes mass effect on the adjacent structures, heart, mediastinum and diaphragm **(Fig. 184)**. The main differential diagnosis is obstruction to the bronchus by a foreign body, mucous plug, endobronchial mass, extrinsic compression of the airway or a localized pneumothorax. CT is useful to confirm the diagnosis of hyperinflation of a lobe. CT angiography differentiates CLO from other forms of pulmonary hypoplasia.

Pulmonary Hypoplasia

Primary unilateral pulmonary hypoplasia is usually associated with the scimitar syndrome or with other vascular malformations. Patients present with repeated episodes of wheezing and pneumonia. The affected lung is small in size, the mediastinum is displaced toward the ipsilateral hemithorax and the pulmonary vasculature is reduced in size. On the lateral chest X-ray, a sharply marginated opacity is seen behind and parallel to the sternum. This is due to the displacement of the heart and mediastinum into the ipsilateral thorax. Primary bilateral pulmonary hypoplasia is very rare. Chest X-ray reveals bilateral small lungs with a normal-sized abdominal cavity, presenting a bell-shaped appearance of the chest and abdomen.

Unilateral Absence of Pulmonary Artery

This is a rare anomaly characterized by the absence of a short segment or atresia of the proximal left or right

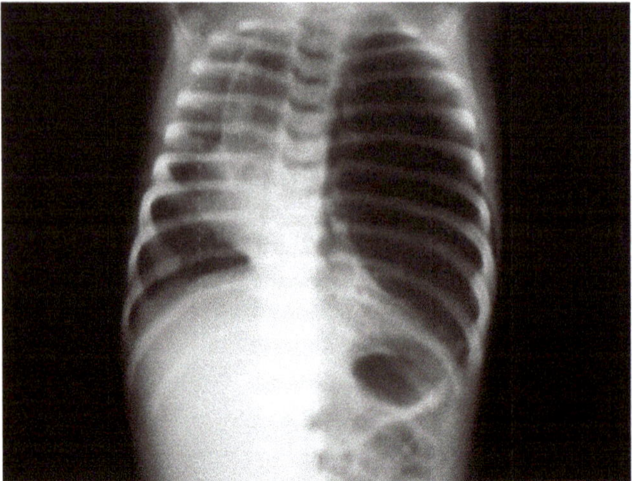

Fig. 184: Congenital lobar overinflation (CLO). Chest X-ray demonstrates marked overinflation of the left upper lobe causing a shift of the mediastinum to the right and collapse of the left lower lobe. Collapsed left lower lobe is seen along the left cardiac border.

pulmonary artery; the more distal segments are usually present. Chest radiographs demonstrate reduction in lung volume, shift of mediastinum, small-sized or absent pulmonary hilum; peripheral pulmonary perfusion is reduced. There may be reticular opacities in the affected lung due to pulmonary-systemic collaterals. The normal lung may be plethoric as the entire cardiac output is shunted through the lung. CT will demonstrate the absence of the pulmonary artery and the presence of systemic pulmonary collaterals.

Scimitar Syndrome

This is a condition involving essentially the right lung which is hypoplastic, with underdevelopment of the airways as well as vasculature. The characteristic finding which in turn contributes to its name is anomalous pulmonary drainage. A large anomalous pulmonary vein descends vertically inferiorly to open into the inferior vena cava above or below the diaphragm. The vein broadens as it curves medially to enter into the vena cava, thereby simulating the appearance of a Turkish sword—scimitar. The anomalous vein may also drain into the coronary sinus, right atrium, or rarely into hepatic veins. The scimitar syndrome may be associated with other congenital anomalies such as septal defects, eventration, Bochdalek hernia, bronchiectasis and tracheal diverticuli. On a chest radiograph, the key feature is the presence of the anomalous draining vein. Additional features are a small-sized right lung, shift of the mediastinum to the right and a small ipsilateral pulmonary artery **(Fig. 185)**. CT is useful to confirm the diagnosis, demonstrating the anomalous draining vessel and its termination, tracheobronchial anomalies, small ipsilateral pulmonary artery, as well as associated abnormalities such as tracheal diverticuli and bronchiectasis.

Imaging of Pleura

Pleural Effusions

Free pleural effusions tend to gravitate to the most dependent portions of the pleural cavity. On erect chest X-rays these are seen as homogenous densities in the lower zone with a typical concave or upward-sloping contour **(Figs. 186 and 187)**, the lateral margin being higher than the medial margin. Fluid collects in the subpulmonic space **(Fig. 188)** then spills into the posterior and finally lateral costophrenic sulcus. The posterior costophrenic (CP)

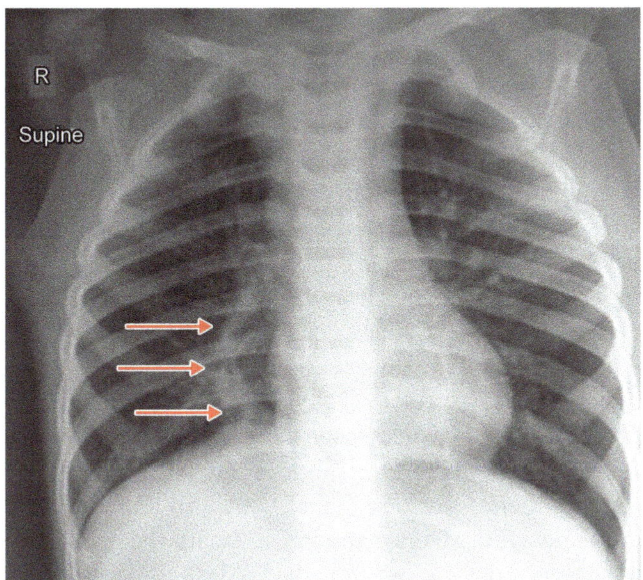

Fig. 185: Scimitar syndrome: AP view demonstrates typical curvilinear vascular opacity in right paracardiac region.

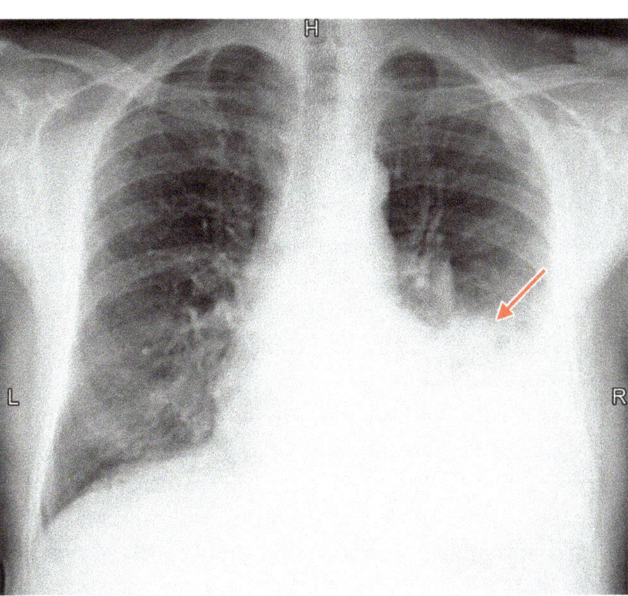

Fig. 187: Pleural effusion: PA view of chest reveals a left-sided pleural effusion. There is also an underlying spiculated mass which on biopsy was proven to be an adenocarcinoma of lung.

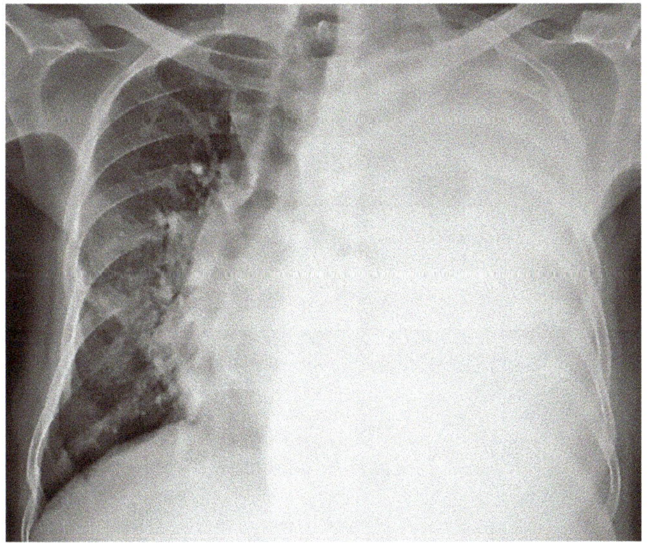

Fig. 186: Pleural effusion: Chest X-ray reveals a large homogenous opacity in left hemithorax and there is mediastinal shift to the right. This is diagnostic of a pleural effusion.

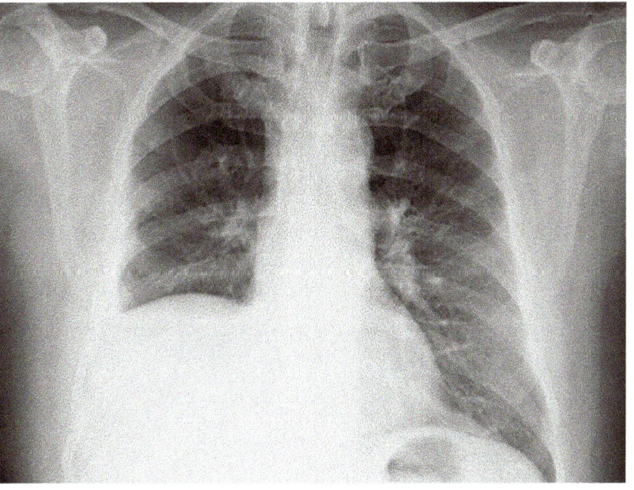

Fig. 188: Subpulmonic pleural effusion: PA view of the chest demonstrates a homogenous opacity in the right lower zone, appearing as an elevated flattened dome of the diaphragm. This appearance is suggestive of a subpulmonic pleural effusion. Sonography confirmed the presence of a pleural effusion.

sulcus is the deepest portion of the pleura. This is the site where the fluid tends to first accumulate. Radiologically, this is seen as blunting of the costophrenic angle on the lateral view.

At least 200 mL of fluid is required to cause obliteration of the CP angle on a PA view of the chest, though in some cases there is no blunting of the angle even when 500 mL of fluid is present. The lateral decubitus view is the most sensitive X-ray to demonstrate free fluid. Fluid is seen layering the dependent part of the chest wall as a thin uniform opacity. This view however may be technically difficult to obtain in a patient who is critically ill. In patients who are too critically ill to sit erect, a diagnosis of pleural effusion has to be made on a supine X-ray chest.

The findings in moderate-sized or large effusions are a homogenous opacity of the affected hemithorax with absence of the vascular markings. This is because the fluid is layering posteriorly along the chest wall. Fluid also tends to accumulate along the apex, like an apical pleural cap, and in the base, as these are the most dependent areas on a supine film. Small pleural effusions can be easily missed on a supine radiograph. In fact only 67% sensitivity and 70% specificity have been reported for the detection of a pleural effusion on supine chest X-ray as opposed to a lateral decubitus view.

In critically ill patients who cannot be positioned for a lateral decubitus view, or if a supine radiograph shows equivocal or negative findings, sonography is an excellent means for demonstrating pleural fluid. This imaging modality is portable and can be easily performed at the bedside. Pleural fluid is seen as an anechoic area separating the echogenic line of the diaphragm and the echogenic inferior margin of the lung **(Figs. 189 and 190)**. Sonography is also useful in differentiating a pleural effusion from atelectasis/consolidation which may simulate an effusion on the chest X-ray. Further, it is an excellent guide for thoracocentesis, markedly reducing the incidence of iatrogenic pneumothorax.

Occasionally, free pleural fluid may accumulate in a subpulmonic location between the lung and diaphragm, with the lung floating on the fluid. The upper margin of the fluid may then take the appearance of the diaphragm.

There is however a subtle difference from the normal appearance of the diaphragm in a subpulmonic effusion **(*see* Fig. 188)**. The peak of the diaphragm is more lateral, the medial aspect has a more gradual slope and the lateral aspect a steeper slope. On a lateral X-ray the posterior costophrenic sulcus is obliterated. Left-sided subpulmonic effusions may be detected by noting the wide distance between the stomach air bubble and diaphragm. On the right side differentiation from an enlarged liver pushing the diaphragm upwards may be difficult. In these cases either a lateral decubitus view or sonography is useful to clinch the diagnosis. A loculated effusion may occur when there are adhesions between the visceral and parietal pleura, as a result of which the fluid does not shift with change of the patient's position **(Figs. 191A and B)**. Empyema and hemothorax may appear as loculated effusions. Sonography will demonstrate the fluid is echogenic rather than anechoic in empyemas/hemothorax.

CT is extremely sensitive in detecting even small pleural fluid collections **(Fig. 192)**. With the patient supine, free fluid accumulates posteriorly as a hypodense layer conforming to the contour of the chest wall. The presence of septae in the pleural fluid (denoting a likely exudate) is however brought out by a sonographic study rather than by a CT scan. Acute hemorrhage in the pleural space can be well-identified by the hyperdensity of blood **(Fig. 193)**. CT is also useful in the assessment of the site, extent and wall thickening of loculated effusions

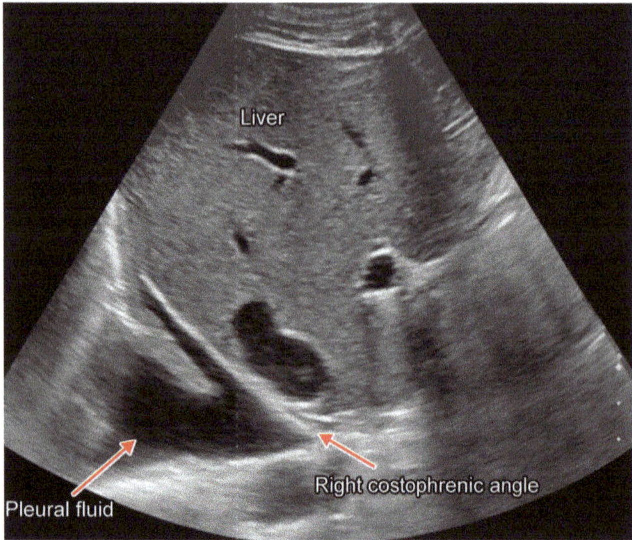

Fig. 189: Pleural effusion: Sonography demonstrates a hypoechoic appearance of pleural fluid layering above diaphragm.

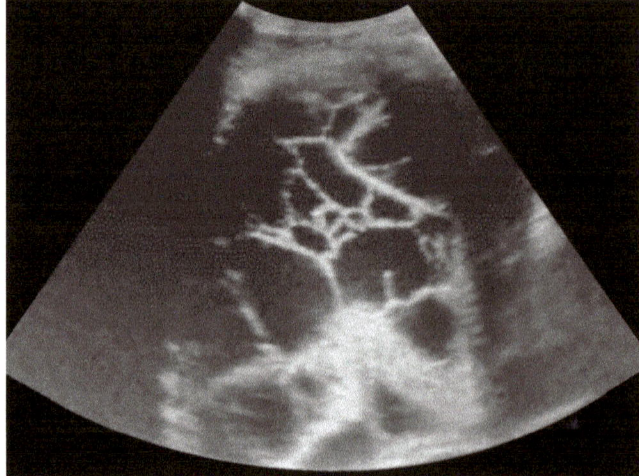

Fig. 190: Pleural effusion: Sonography demonstrates pleural effusion as an echoic fluid collection. There are multiple linear bands within this fluid collection; these represent septae. Presence of septae is highly suggestive of the effusion being an exudate.

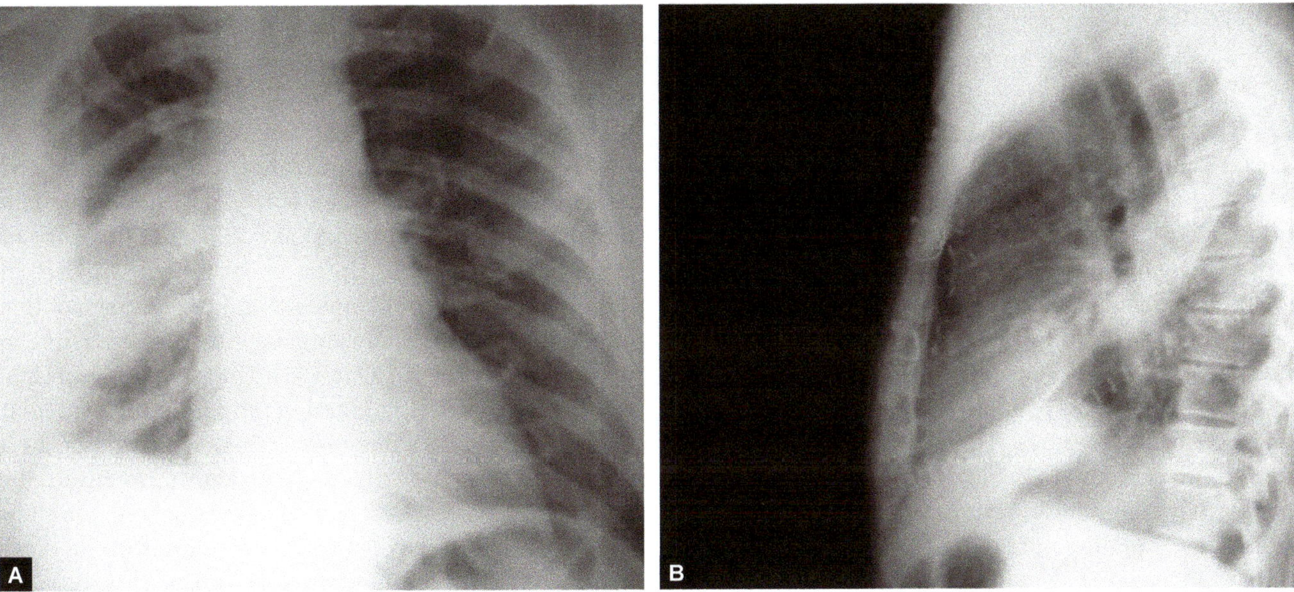

Figs. 191A and B: Interlobar effusion: (A) PA view demonstrates a well-defined opacity in the right mid-zone (B) Lateral view demonstrates the homogenous opacity seen on the PA view, represents loculated fluid in the major interlobar fissure. The inferior part of the fissure as well as the minor fissure is mildly thickened. The homogenous appearance on the PA view of an opacity in the location of the fissure would suggest the need for a lateral view to localize the lesion.

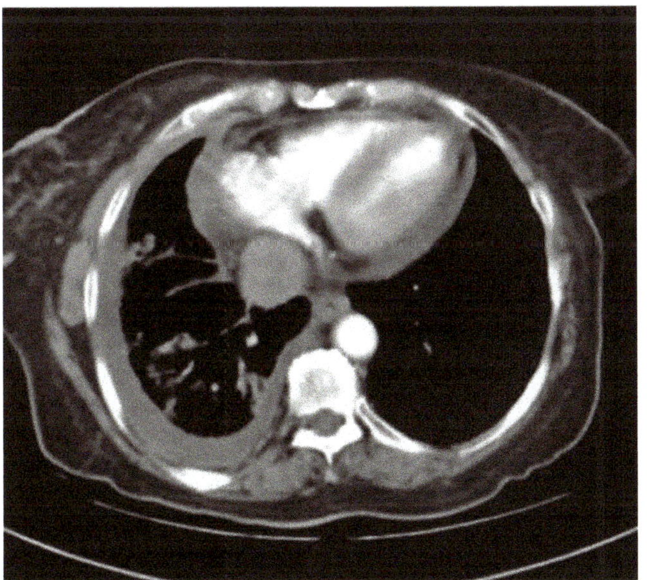

Fig. 192: Pleural effusion: CT is extremely sensitive in detecting small pleural and pericardial effusion.

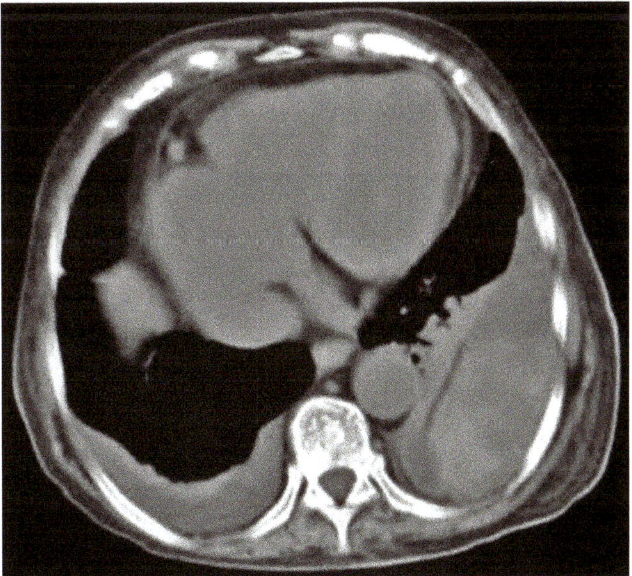

Fig. 193: Hemorrhagic pleural effusion: CT chest without IV contrast reveals a thin pleural effusion on the right side and a moderate-sized pleural fluid collection on the left. The pleural fluid collection on the left is hyperdense indicating hemorrhage and the right side hypodense indicating fluid. CT is useful in differentiating pleural effusion from a hemothorax.

(Fig. 194), and for loculated interlobar effusions. These may simulate a mass lesion on plain X-ray but can easily be differentiated on CT. CT with intravenous contrast medium is very useful in differentiating parenchymal from pleural lesions, especially when a plain radiograph has not been helpful.

Empyema

On a chest radiograph an empyema is usually seen as a loculated fluid collection. It tends to be lenticular in shape as compared to a lung abscess which is rounded **(Figs. 195 and 196A)**. Further, an empyema usually forms an obtuse angle with the chest wall while a lung abscess forms an acute angle. CT is very useful in the diagnosis and management of empyema. On CT an empyema appears as a well-defined fluid collection with enhancing parietal and visceral pleura **(Fig. 196B)**. This sign of separation of the pleura is known as the split pleura sign.

Traditionally, empyemas have been treated with insertion of chest tubes. The success rate with chest tube drainage is 35–71%. However, 35% of all patients treated with conventional chest tubes are found to subsequently require either open chest tube drainage or decortication. Several studies have estimated the success rate of fluoroscopy, sonography and CT in image-guided percutaneous insertion of chest tubes to be between 70% and 90%. Under imaging guidance, the chest tube can be placed accurately in the fluid collection. In fact image-guided percutaneous drainage of empyemas is advocated as the primary method of treating empyemas. Patients who show inadequate drainage or progressive persistent pleural thickening may finally require decortication.

Pneumothorax

Pneumothorax may be spontaneous, either primary or secondary. A rupture of an apical pleural bleb is the most likely cause for a primary spontaneous pneumothorax.

The radiographic appearances depend upon the patient's position (air is seen in the most nondependent portion of the pleural cavity) as well as the presence or absence of loculations. In an erect patient, air rises in the pleural space to the apicolateral regions, separating lung from chest wall, allowing the visceral pleural line to become visible **(Figs. 197 to 199)**. The visceral pleural line separates the vessel-containing lung from the avascular pneumothorax. This line remains parallel with the chest wall; therefore, in a shallow pneumothorax it may be difficult to separate the visceral pleural line from the chest wall, especially if covered by ribs. To demonstrate these questionable or subtle pneumothoraxes an expiratory film is very useful **(Figs. 200A and B)**. This increases the volume of the pneumothorax as well as changes the orientation of the ribs.

There are a number of mimics of a pneumothorax on a chest X-ray. Any curvilinear shadow projected over the lung, especially the apex, may mimic a visceral pleural line. Skin folds, tubes, vascular lines, clothing, scapulae, walls of bulla/cavities all may mimic a visceral pleural line. One

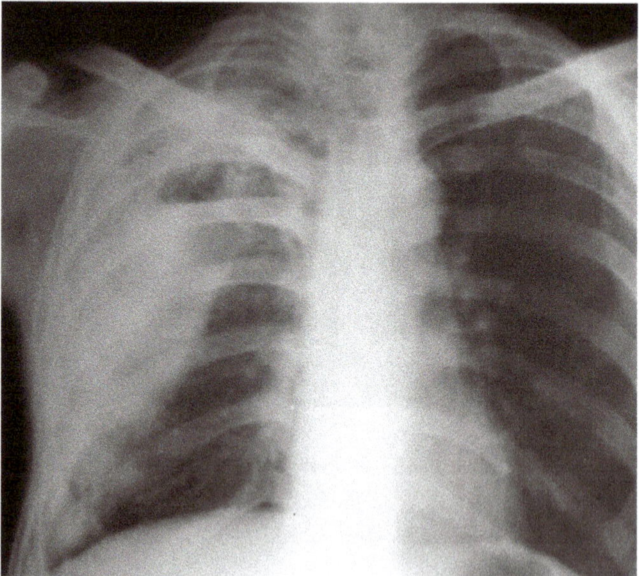

Fig. 194: Loculated pleural effusion: CT chest demonstrates pleural fluid in the right hemithorax loculated along the right lateral chest wall with multiple loculations.

Fig. 195: Empyema: PA view of the chest demonstrates a homogenous lenticular fluid collection along right lateral chest wall with an air-fluid level. Sonography confirmed the homogenous opacity was fluid with internal echoes. An aspiration revealed an empyema.

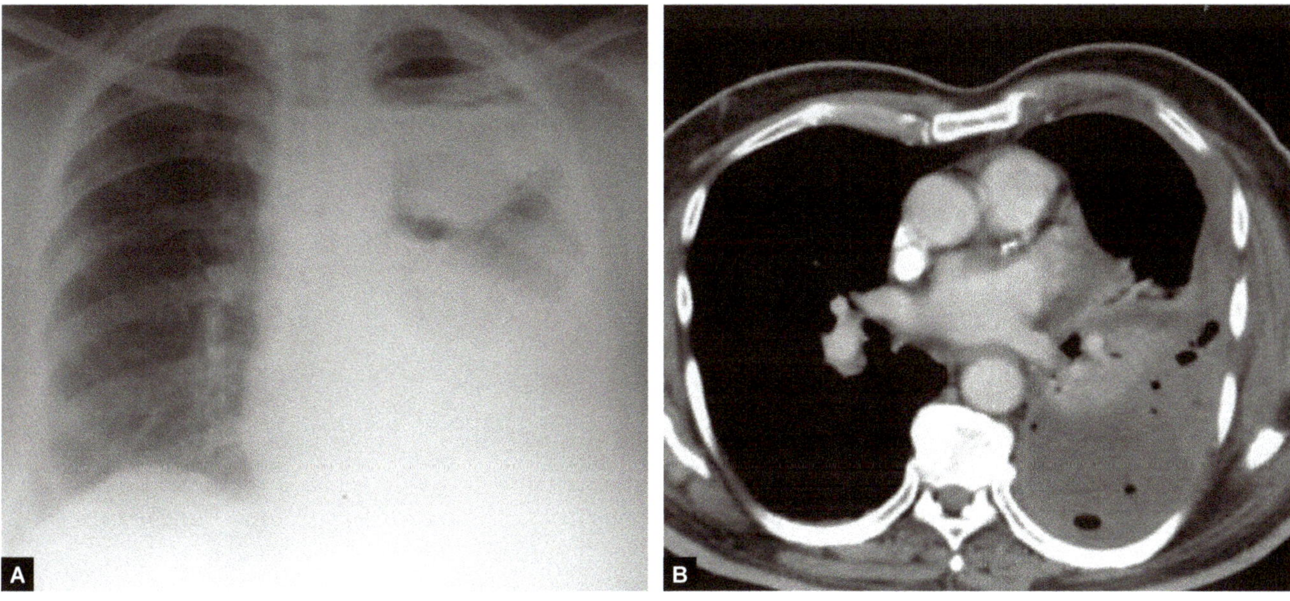

Figs. 196A and B: Empyema: Chest X-ray and CT chest demonstrate a loculated fluid collection in the left hemithorax. There are multiple specks of air in the fluid collection. The presence of air in a pleural collection is highly suggestive of infection in the pleural fluid. Air may also be present in pleural fluid if it has been inadvertently introduced during aspiration of the fluid.

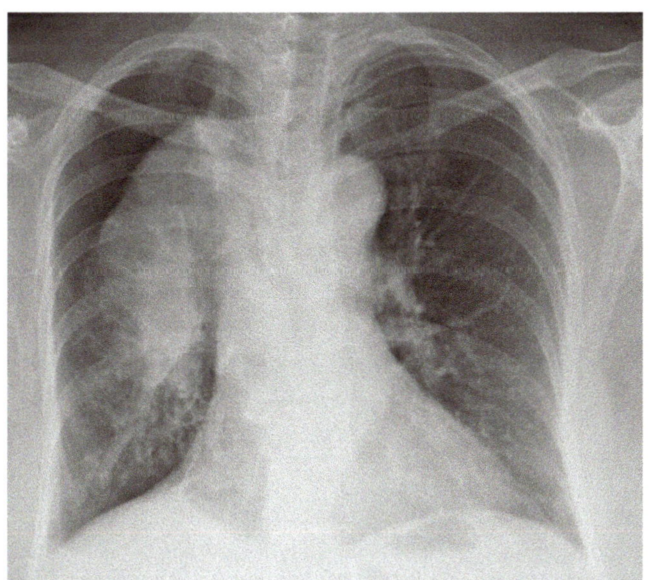

Fig. 197: Pneumothorax: PA view of chest demonstrates a right sided pneumothorax with underlying partial collapse of right upper lobe.

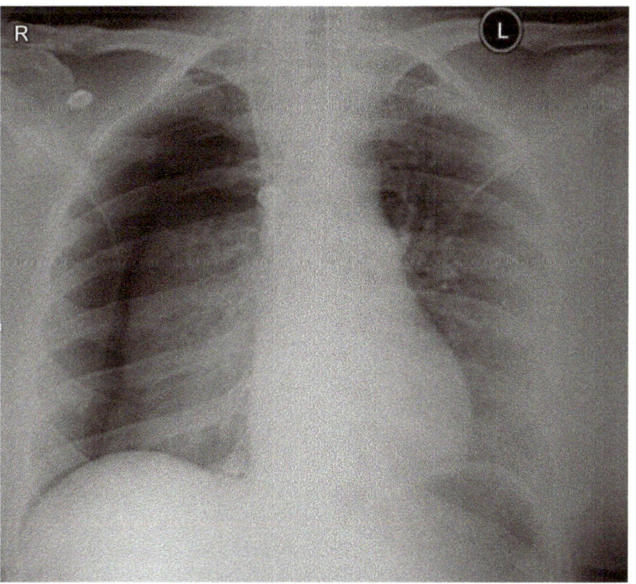

Fig. 198: Pneumothorax: AP portable erect X-ray reveals a large pneumothorax on the right side with partial collapse of right lung. A central line is seen in situ on the right side. The pneumothorax occurred following placement of the central line.

of the most helpful differentiators is to follow the so-called visceral pleural line beyond the margins of the chest wall. Other helpful differentiators are when the orientation of the line is not in the orientation of the collapsed lung, or vessels are seen beyond the line. The above circumstances negate the diagnosis of a pneumothorax.

Skin folds appear as thick linear bands with a sharp outer margin and a fading medial margin. The outer

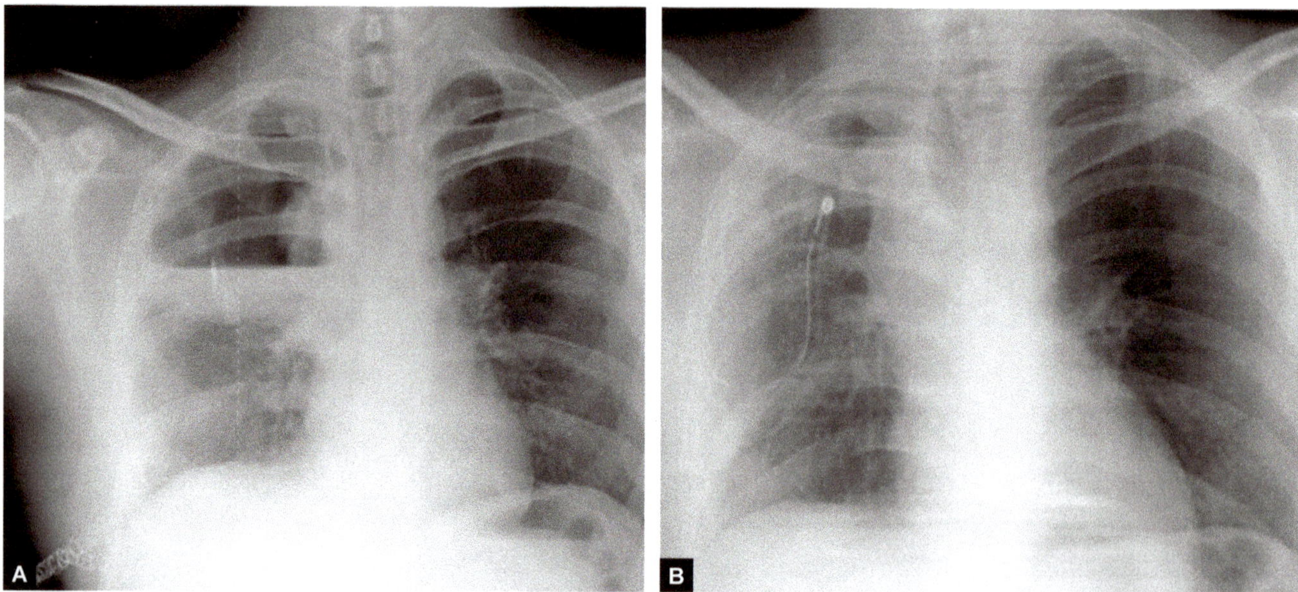

Figs. 199A and B: Hydropneumothorax: (A) Chest X-ray demonstrates a right upper zone pneumothorax with an air-fluid level representing a hydropneumothorax. Intercostal drainage (ICD) was placed to drain the hydropneumothorax; (B) Chest X-ray demonstrates total evacuation of hydropneumothorax.

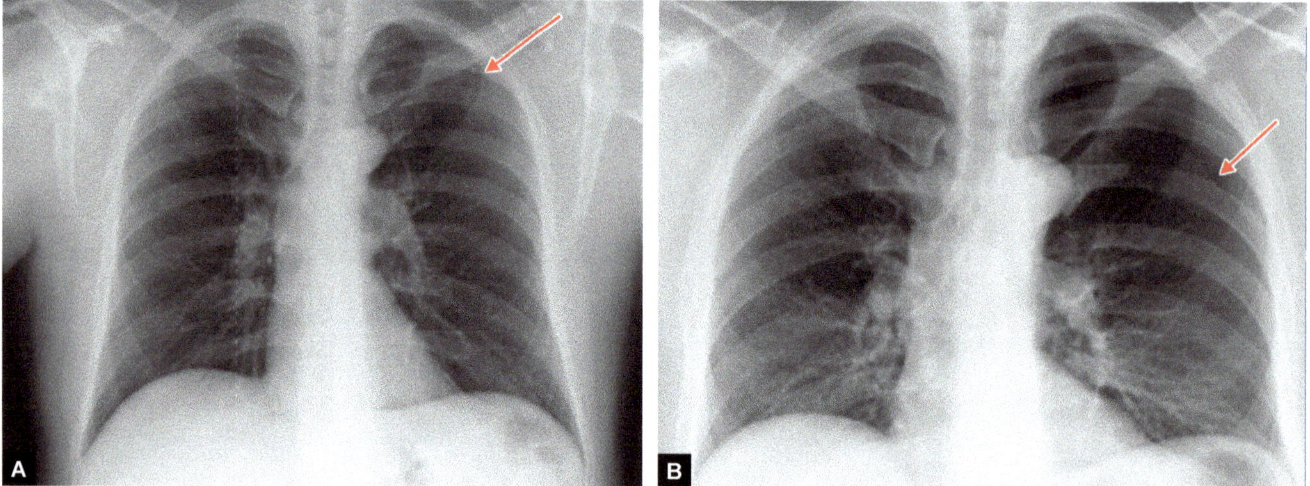

Figs. 200A and B: Pneumothorax: (A) Chest X-ray inspiratory PA view demonstrates a suspicious thin visceral pleural line at the left apex. (B) Expiratory PA view demonstrates a large pneumothorax with a well-defined visceral pleural line. Expiratory chest X-rays are very useful to demonstrate a suspicious pneumothorax as well as the extent of the pneumothorax.

margin is transradiant due to air trapped between skin fold and skin **(Fig. 201)**. The scapula edge is a common mimic and must be looked out for. Extrapleural dissection of air from a pneumomediastinum may also be mistaken for a pneumothorax, the linear abnormality is confined to the lung apex and does not progress in size. The most difficult to differentiate are bullae as they appear translucent/avascular, and have thin well-defined margins. One

differentiating feature is that the inner margin of a bulla is concave as compared to a pneumothorax, which would be convex, in line with the chest wall. CT is very helpful in excluding these mimics of a pneumothorax **(Figs. 202 and 203)**.

As the pneumothorax increases in size and the lung collapses, the density of the underlying lung increases, till finally in total collapse it appears like a

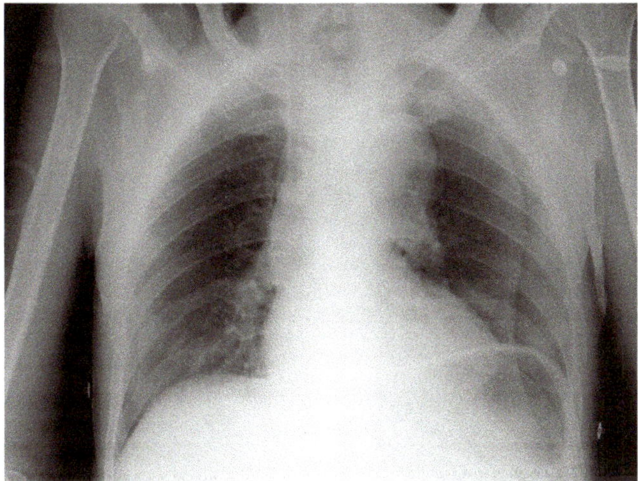

Fig. 201: PA view of the chest revealed a well-defined line in the left hemithorax simulating a pneumothorax. This, however, is a skin fold resembling a pneumothorax as the line is seen to extend beyond the confines of the thorax into the abdomen.

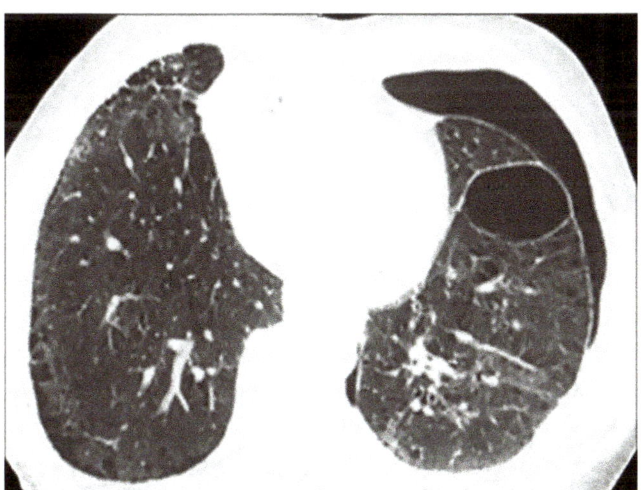

Fig. 202: Pneumothorax: CT lung window demonstrates a left pneumothorax with a large thin-walled bulla in the left lingula.

fist-like opacity overlying the hilum. As the density of the collapsing lung increases it becomes easier to detect etiological causes for the pneumothorax. For this reason, apical pleural blebs, the most common cause of a primary spontaneous pneumothorax are visible only on 15% of chest X-rays at the time of the pneumothorax. These blebs are best seen on a CT scan, being detected in 85% of cases. On both X-rays and CT scans other causes such as cysts/bullae/bronchiectasis, etc. should also be looked for. It is also important from a management

perspective to estimate the size of a pneumothorax. A simple method is to measure hemithorax distance, interpleural distance.

$$\% \text{ of pneumothorax} = 100 - \frac{(\text{Hemithorax} - \text{interpleural distance})^3}{\text{Hemithorax distance}^3} \times 100$$

For example, if the hemithorax distance is 10 cm and the interpleural distance is 2 cm, the size of the pneumothorax is 50%, an indication that the pneumothorax is much larger than what might be apparent on an X-ray chest.

Pneumothorax in a Supine Patient

In a number of patients in a critical care setting X-rays can only be done in a supine position. It is important to recognize the signs of a pneumothorax in a supine patient. Air collects in the highest portion of the pleural cavity which in the supine position is anterior or anteriomedially at the base. The displaced visceral pleural line is difficult to demonstrate on a supine X-ray. In the absence of this specific sign, other signs to demonstrate the collection of air are important. As air collects in the anterior costophrenic sulcus there is transradiancy in the hypochondrial region overlying the diaphragm. There is increased sharpness of the adjacent mediastinal margin and diaphragm. The costophrenic sulcus becomes deep with a well-defined margin. The inferior edge of collapsed lung becomes visible. The ipsilateral hemidiaphragm is depressed. Cardiac margins become sharp and pericardial fat pads become well-outlined.

A pneumothorax suspected on a supine film can be confirmed on a cross-table lateral view or lateral decubitus with suspect side uppermost. If there is any doubt a CT will be very useful, as it would be confirmatory **(Figs. 204 and 205)**.

Tension pneumothorax is an absolute emergency and if untreated results in death. A tension pneumothorax occurs when air enters during inspiration but cannot exit during expiration due to a check valve mechanism **(Figs. 206 and 207)**. On a chest X-ray, the entire hemithorax is hypertranslucent, the mediastinum is shifted to the opposite side and the ipsilateral lung is compressed. In addition the diaphragm on the affected side may be deeply inverted.

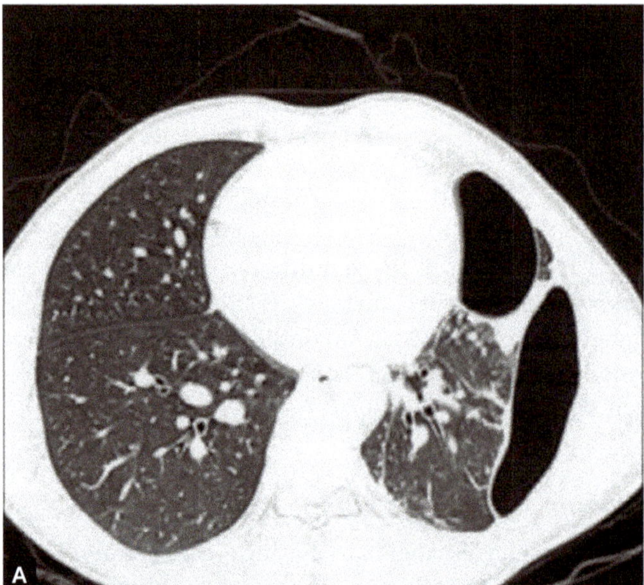
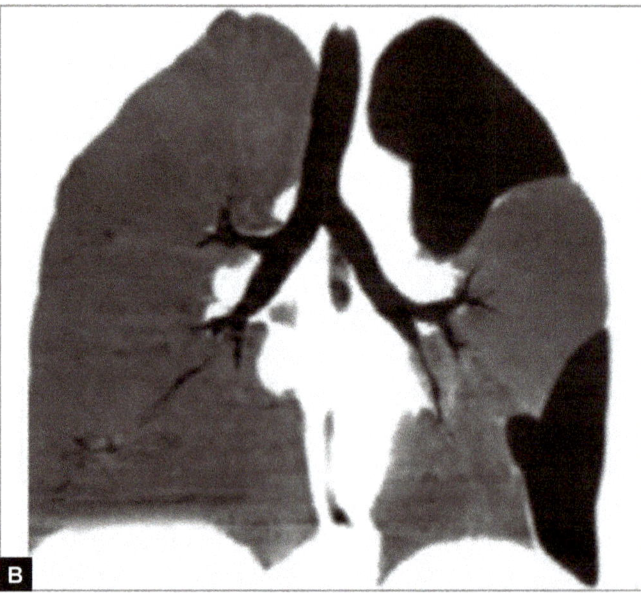

Figs. 203A and B: Pneumothorax: (A) CT lung window and (B) minimum intensity projection demonstrate a loculated pneumothorax with adhesions along the left anterior lateral parietal pleura.

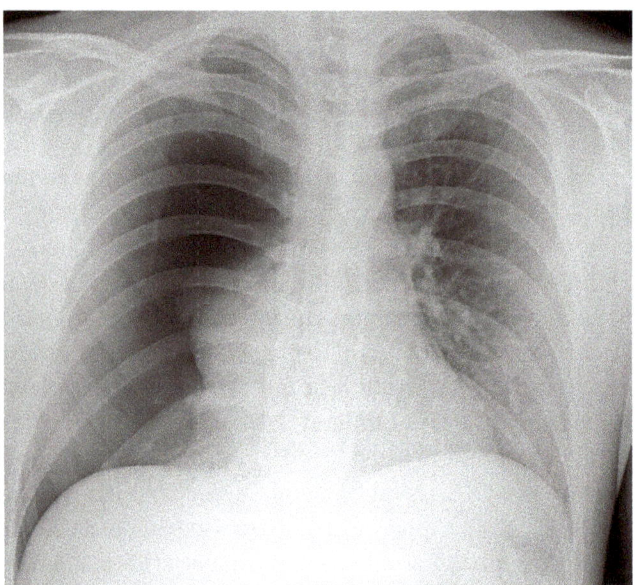
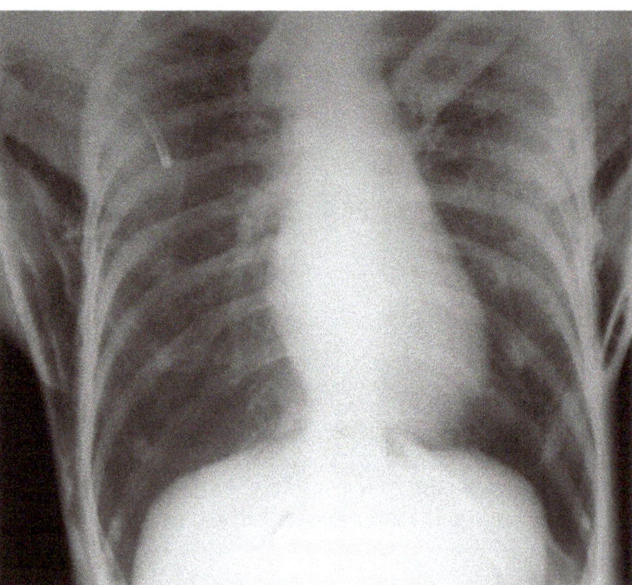

Fig. 204: Pneumothorax: Supine AP view in a patient who was hemodynamically unstable; an erect view was not possible. The costophrenic and cardiophrenic recess on the right side are deep and well-outlined. The right dome of the diaphragm is well-outlined as compared to the left. These are all features of a pneumothorax in a supine patient.

Fig. 205: Pneumothorax: Supine AP view reveals bilateral pneumothorax as evidenced by a sharp diaphragmatic contour and sharp deep bilateral costophrenic sulci. There is extensive surgical emphysema.

Management of Pneumothorax

Not every pneumothorax requires drainage. An asymptomatic pneumothorax with interpleural distance less than 2.0 cm may be successfully managed by observation with or without oxygen therapy. Larger symptomatic pneumothoraces may resolve if the air is totally aspirated and the two pleural surfaces appose each other.

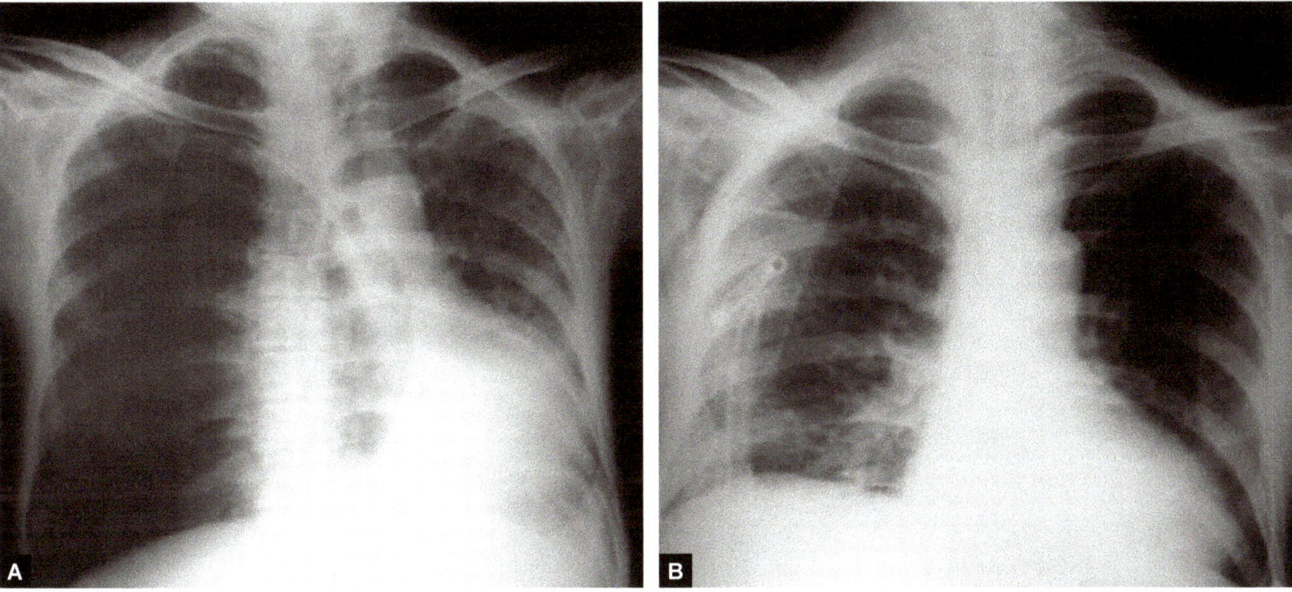

Figs. 206A and B: Tension pneumothorax: (A) Chest PA view reveals a translucency in left hemithorax due to a large pneumothorax. There is a mediastinal shift to right. These are features of a tension pneumothorax; (B) After intercostal drainage (ICD) tube insertion there is expansion of lung with return of mediastinal structures to their normal position.

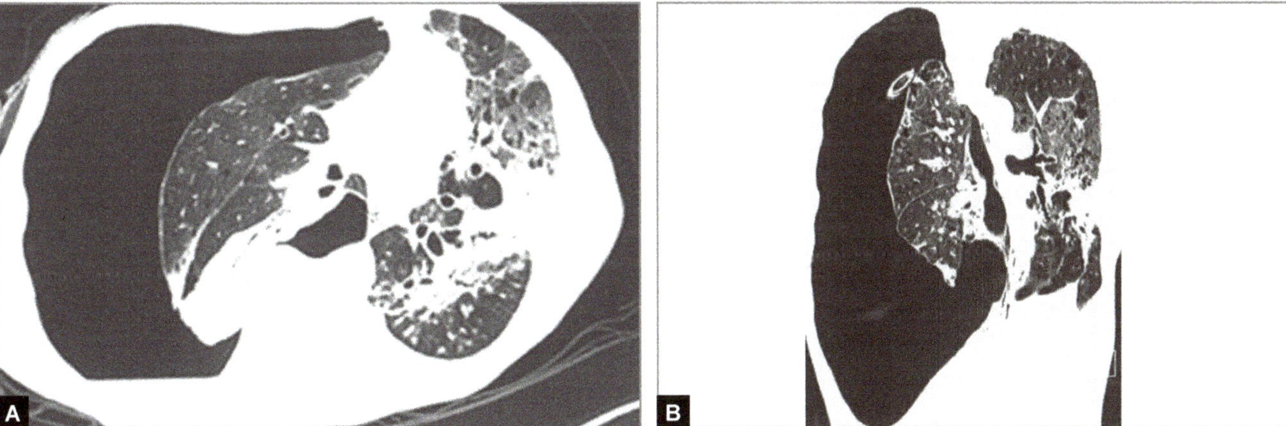

Figs. 207A and B: Tension pneumothorax: (A) Axial and (B) coronal CT demonstrate a large pneumothorax on the right side. The pneumothorax is under tension as evidenced by inversion of the right dome of the diaphragm and displacement of the mediastinum. Extensive centrilobular emphysema is seen in both lung fields.

Bronchopleural Fistula

A bronchopleural fistula may be central when the communication is between the bronchus and pleura. A peripheral BPF exists when the communication is between lung parenchyma or a peripheral bronchus and the pleura. The chest radiography signs of a bronchopleural fistula are an increase in air in a pneumonectomy space, with a loss of normal mediastinal shift toward the operated side. Occasionally, the only sign is a persistence of air following pneumonectomy. CT is useful to demonstrate the bronchopleural fistula, but may do so in only 30–50% of cases **(Figs. 208 to 210)**.

Pleural Thickening

Pleural thickening is seen as a veil-like opacity along the inner margins of the chest wall, sharply marginated along its inner aspect and fading into the chest wall along its lateral aspect. Pleural thickening involving the costophrenic angle is seen as an angular opacity differentiating it from pleural fluid which is seen as a smooth curvilinear

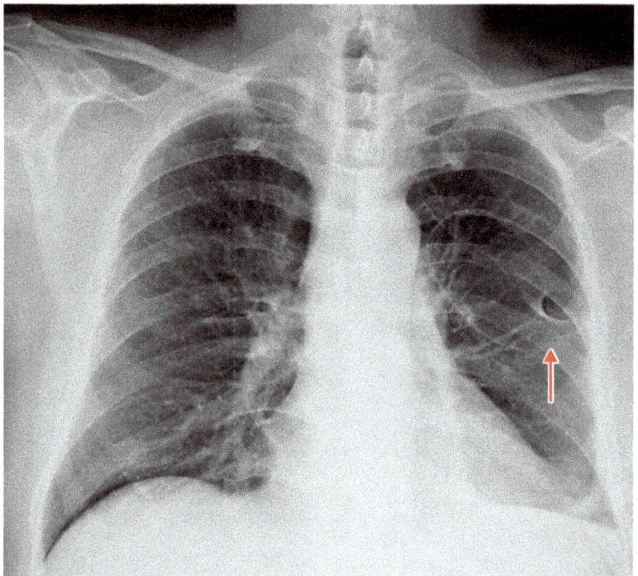

Fig. 208: Bronchopleural fistula: PA view of the chest reveals well-defined walled rounded air-space in the left mid zone with an associated another small more lucent air-space along its lateral aspect.

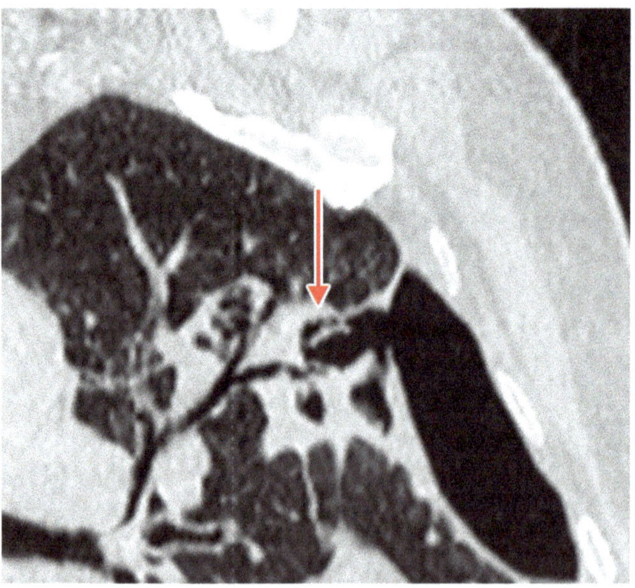

Fig. 209: Bronchopleural fistula: CT chest with multiplanar reconstruction demonstrates a dilated bronchus communicating with a loculated pneumothorax. The thin-walled large air-space seen on the X-ray represents the located pneumothorax seen on the CT scan. The well-defined smaller lucent air-space along the lateral aspect represents a dilated bronchus communicating with the loculated pneumothorax. These are seen end on the X-ray.

margin **(Figs. 211A and B)**. In cases of difficulty, a lateral decubitus or ultrasound would help in differentiation. CT is very sensitive in the detection of pleural thickening.

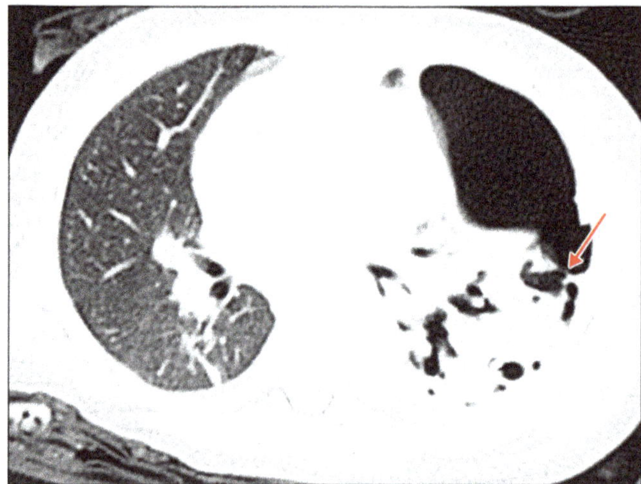

Fig. 210: Bronchopleural fistula: In a case of pneumothorax, air bronchograms are seen to communicate with the left pleural cavity indicating a peripheral bronchopleural fistula.

Extrapleural fat can mimic pleural thickening; this is also well-differentiated on CT.

Pleural Calcification

Pleural calcification is visualized as a sheet of calcification. When visualized en face, it appears as a veil-like opacity; when visualized in profile it is seen as a linear dense band parallel to the inner chest wall **(Fig. 212)**. Following resolution of an empyema, calcification may be seen as a double layer due to calcification of visceral and parietal pleura. This is well-appreciated on CT.

Mesothelioma

On imaging, there are plaques/nodules on visceral/parietal pleura forming a lobular sheet of tumor up to several centimeters thick encasing the lung and growing into the interlobar fissure. Invasion of the mediastinum, diaphragm, lung may occur, though late. An important sign is the loss of lung volume on the ipsilateral side, because the mesothelioma grows as a sheet entrapping the lung **(Figs. 213 and 214)**. These appearances are very well demonstrated on a CT, which is useful for detection, as also for demonstration of chest wall and or mediastinal invasion. Occasionally, the only finding may be pleural thickening with a small-sized ipsilateral hemithorax. The pleural masses are seen to creep along the pleural surfaces. MRI is also useful for demonstrating chest wall and mediastinal involvement.

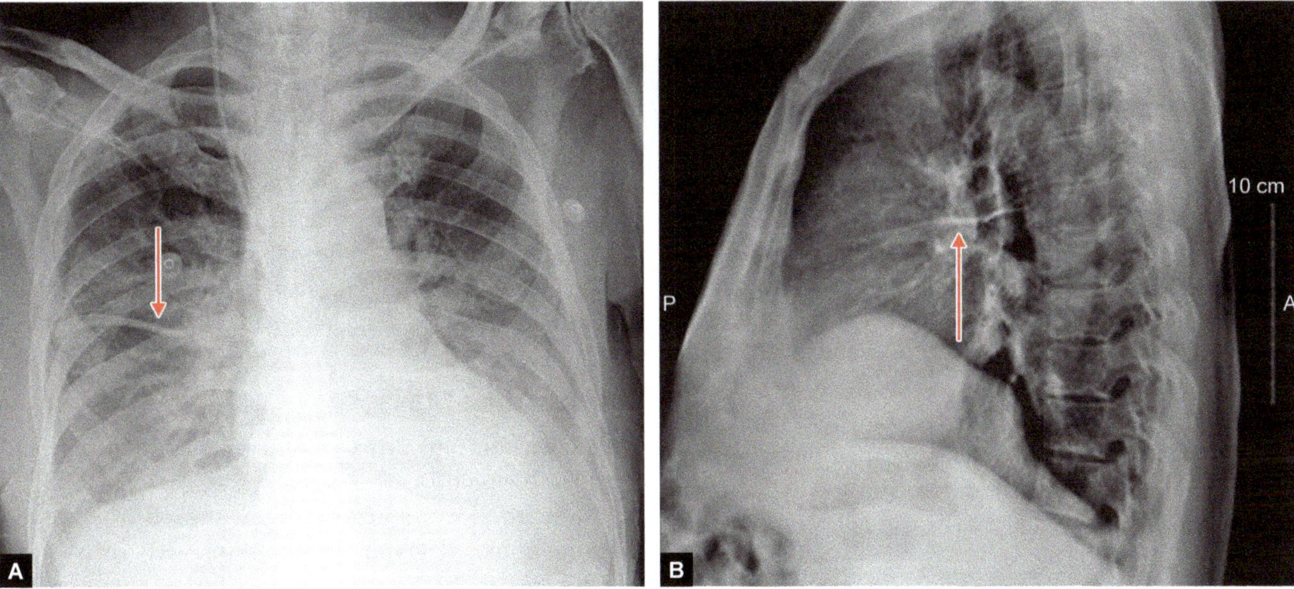

Figs. 211A and B: Pleural thickening: (A) PA and (B) lateral views demonstrate thickening of the minor fissure following resolution of an interlobar effusion.

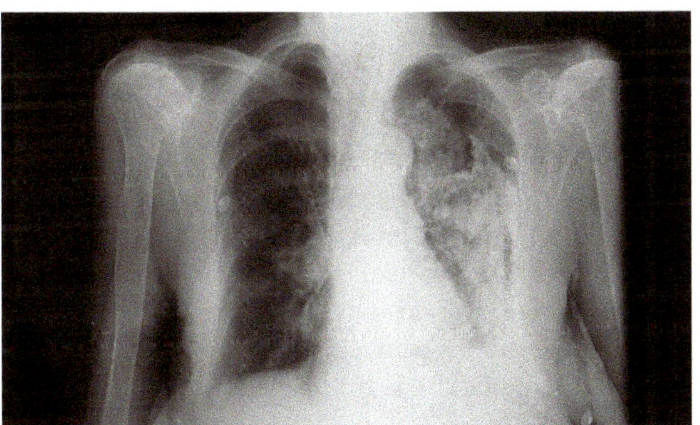

Fig. 212: Pleural calcification: AP view of chest reveals veil-like calcification in the left hemithorax.

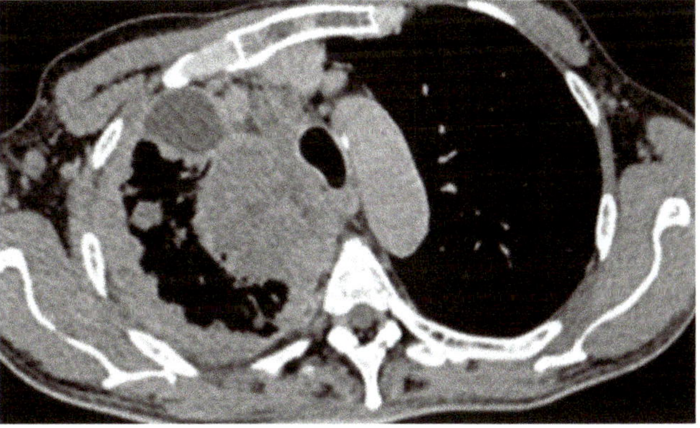

Fig. 213: Pleural mesothelioma: CT chest shows presence of multiple lobulated enhancing lesions along the entire right pleural surface.

■ MEDIASTINUM

The chest radiograph is usually the first investigation performed for a suspected mediastinal/hilar mass lesion. Mediastinal masses may also be detected incidentally on X-rays done for other reasons. If a mediastinal pathology is suspected and the chest X-ray reveals no abnormality, a cross-sectional imaging technique, ideally a CT scan is required. Mediastinal pathology may be obscured by mediastinal vasculature on an X-ray. A CT scan is very useful to characterize the mass lesion; it also serves as a guide for biopsy of a mediastinal mass. Mediastinal masses appear on chest X-rays as projections from the mediastinal silhouette. Hilar masses are visualized as prominence and or enlargement of the hilum. The first step in the differential diagnosis is to determine if the lesion arises from the mediastinum or lung. A spiculated mass lesion will nearly always be of pulmonary origin. Homogenous masses which project beyond the confines of the mediastinum, have a broad base and form obtuse angles with the mediastinum, arise from the mediastinum or mediastinal pleura. The differential diagnosis of mediastinal masses is based on their location and internal morphology.

■ LOCATION

Prevascular Masses

Prevascular masses are located anterior to the ascending aorta and its branches. These are most commonly thymic masses, thyroid masses, germ cell tumors or lymphadenopathy. Thyroid masses are easy to diagnose as they are seen in the superior mediastinum contiguous with the thyroid in the neck. On unenhanced scans they are of a higher attenuation than adjacent skeletal muscle in view of their iodine content. Internally, thyroid masses are heterogeneous with calcific densities and cysts. Thyroid masses are the most common lesions to cause deviation of the trachea. Thymic and germ cell tumors appear similar on imaging; their differentiation is based on clinical and laboratory features. Thymomas may be clinically associated with myasthenia gravis, red cell

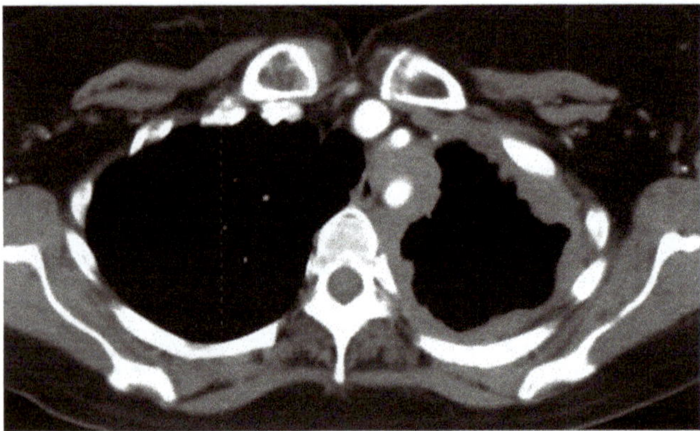

Fig. 214: Mesothelioma: CT chest reveals plaque-like thickening of pleural surface with nodularity of surface in left apical region. Biopsy revealed a mesothelioma. Note vascular encasement of the great vessels by the mesothelioma.

aplasia, and hypogammaglobulinemia. An elevated HCG or alpha fetoprotein levels are indicative of a germ cell tumor. Thymoma, germ cell tumors may demonstrate calcification. Presence of fat, cartilaginous calcification, teeth or a fat-fluid level are indicative of a mature teratoma.

Unusual causes of prevascular masses are parathyroid adenoma (usually evidence of hyperparathyroidism). Lymphangioma (cystic with multiple internal septations). Cystic hygroma should be considered when a cystic mass is seen extending from the neck into the mediastinum.

Paracardiac Masses

Chiefly include pericardial cyst, diaphragmatic hernia and lymphadenopathy.

Pericardial cysts are easily diagnosed as they are homogenous, of water attenuation, with thin walls. Diaphragmatic hernias (Morgagni's hernia) are due to a defect in the diaphragm with herniation of a pad of fat and or bowel loops into the thorax. Occasionally, germ cell tumors and thymomas may be visualized in a paracardiac location.

Paratracheal, Subcarinal and Paraesophageal Masses

These are considered together as they are contained in one fascial sheath. The group includes lymphadenopathy **(Figs. 215 to 219)**, foregut malformations, esophageal tumors, thyroid mass lesions, hiatus hernia, aneurysms, vascular anomalies and pancreatic pseudocyst. The most common of these is lymphadenopathy. Esophageal

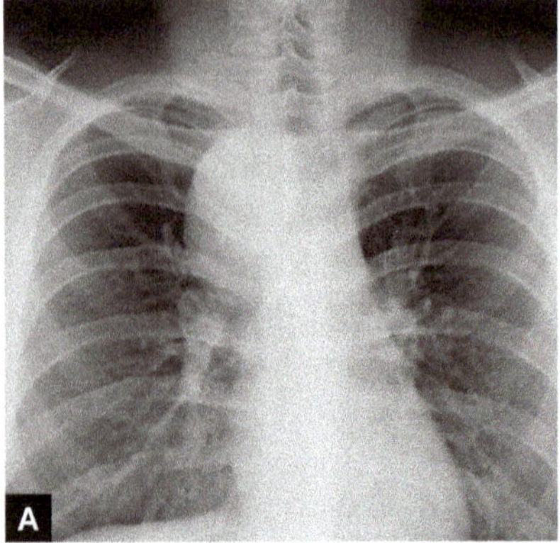
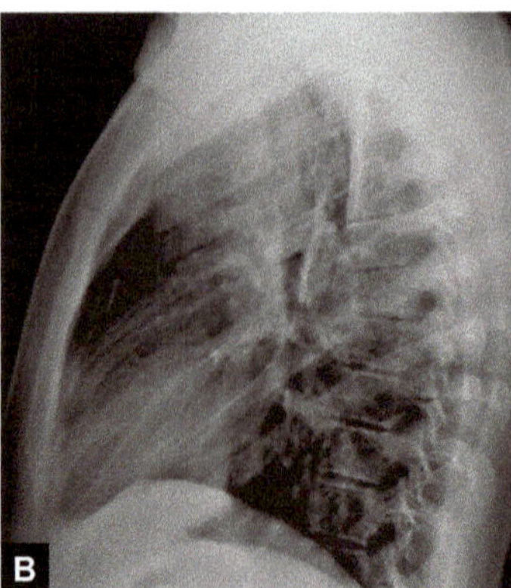
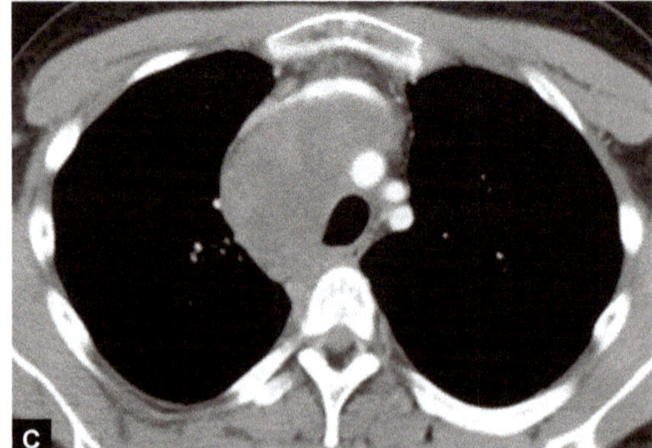

Figs. 215A to C: Mediastinal adeuopathy: Chest X-ray (A) reveals a large right paratracheal mass lesion. Note it is homogenous with a wide mediastinal base and obtuse angles with the lung indicating a mediastinal mass lesion. Lateral view (B) demonstrates the mass lesion to be anterior mediastinum. CT chest (C) confirms that the mass lesion is a large necrotic adenopathy. CT-guided aspiration confirmed the adenopathy to be of tubercular origin.

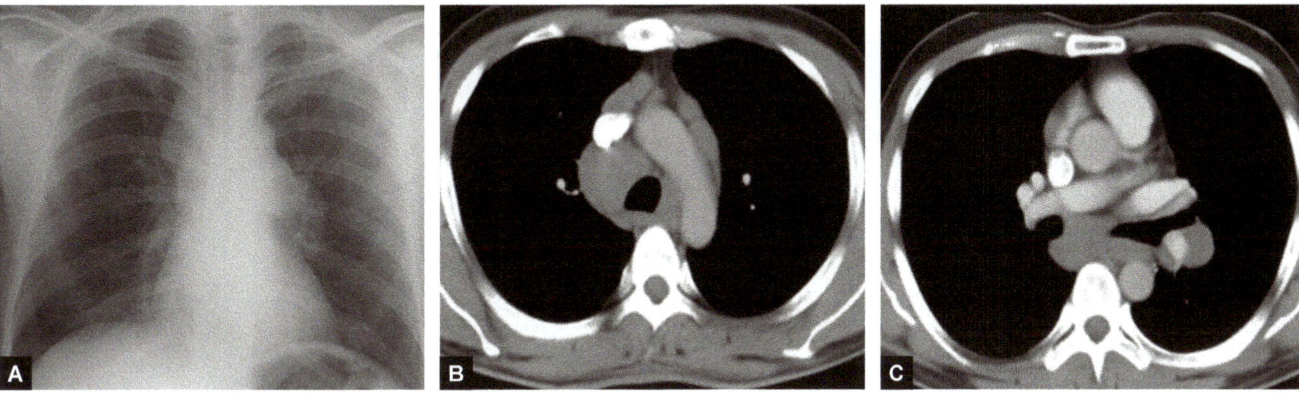

Figs. 216A to C: Mediastinal adenopathy: (A) Chest X-ray reveals right paratracheal and left hilar adenopathy (B and C) CT chest confirms adenopathy as well as demonstrates small left prevascular adenopathy and large subcarinal adenopathy, not detected on the X-ray as these were covered by the mediastinum.

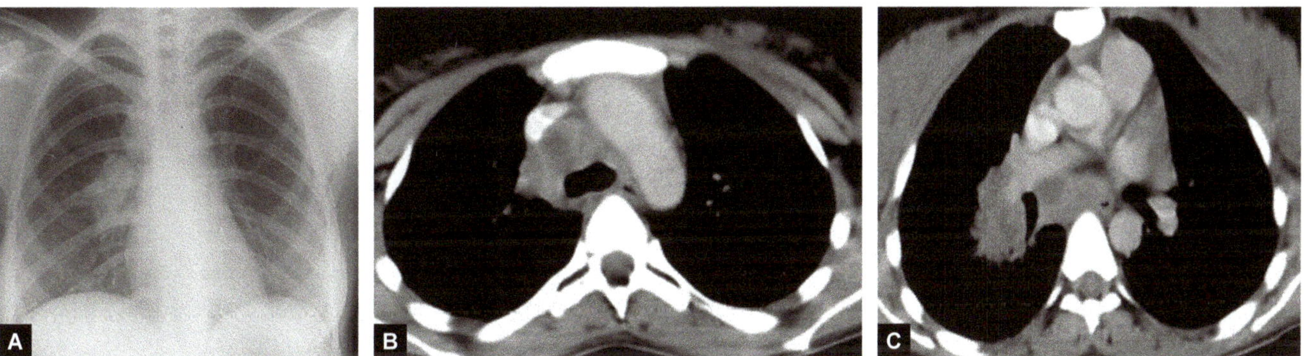

Figs. 217A to C: Mediastinal adenopathy: (A) Chest X-ray demonstrates large right paratracheal and hilar adenopathy; (B) CT chest; (C) confirms adenopathy, which are necrotic, indicating tuberculosis.

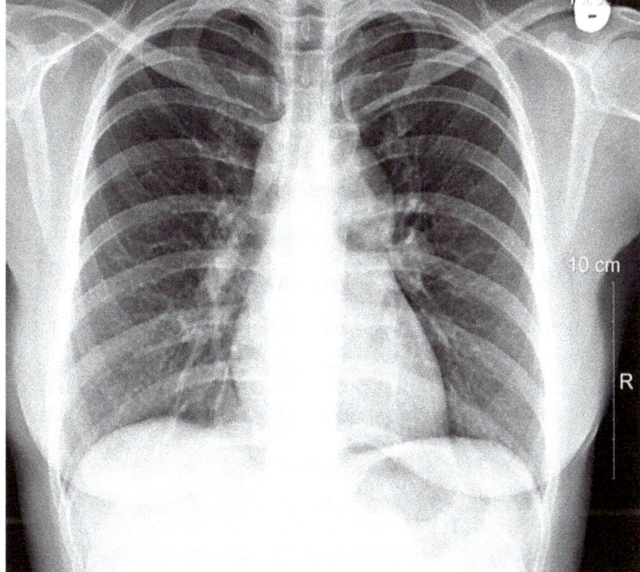

Fig. 218: Mediastinal adenopathy: Chest X-ray demonstrates large hilar and right paratracheal mass lesions representing adenopathy.

carcinoma presents early as dysphagia and generally results in a small mass lesion. Vascular anomalies and aneurysms are visualized as homogenous enhancing structures. Foregut malformations are fluid-filled well-defined lesions in relation to the vertebrae, esophagus or tracheobronchial tree.

Prevertebral Masses

These are most commonly neurogenic tumors, or lymph gland masses. Other pathologies include mesenchymal tumors, lesions arising from the pharynx, or vertebra. A paraspinal abscess and an aneurysm of the descending aorta are also observed in the prevertebral location.

Imaging studies of prevascular masses, of paracardiac masses, of paratracheal, subcarinal, paraesophageal masses and of prevertebral masses have been amply illustrated in the chapter on Diseases of the Mediastinum and therefore do not bear repetition.

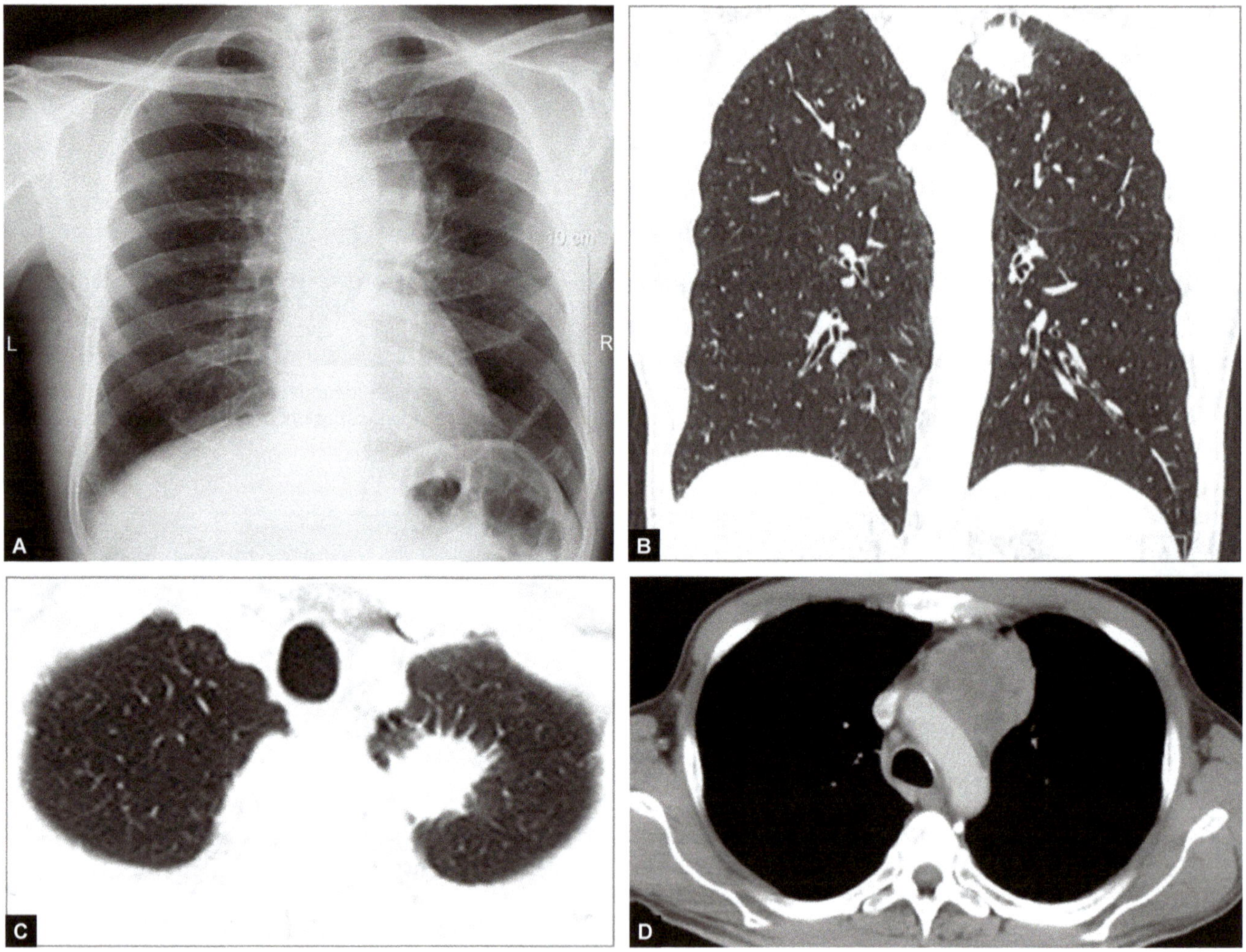

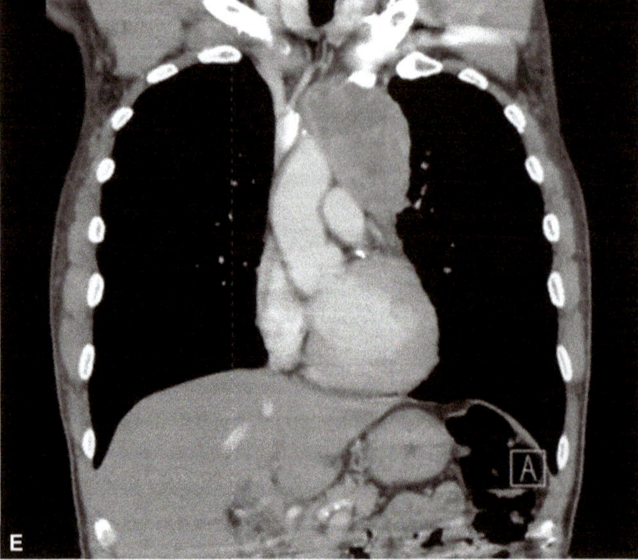

Figs. 219A to E: Metastatic mediastinal adenopathy: (A) Chest X-ray reveals an opacity in the left para-aortic region, however, not silhouetting the aorta; (B) Coronal CT demonstrates a spiculated mass lesion in the left apex; (C) axial CT demonstrates spiculated apical mass lesion very well. CT-guided fine-needle aspiration cytology (FNAC) revealed mass to be squamous cell carcinoma; (D) axial post-contrast CT reveals large anterior mediastinal mass lesion representing metastatic adenopathy; (E) coronal reconstruction demonstrates large anterior mediastinal adenopathy.

■ SUGGESTED READING

1. David MH, Peter A, David L, et al. Imaging of the Diseases of the Chest, 4th edition. Philadelphia: Elsevier Mosby; 2005.
2. Grenier PA. Imaging of airway diseases. Radiol Clin North Am. 2009;47.
3. Sanjiv B. Thoracic MDCT comes of age. Radiol Clin North Am. 2010;48.
4. Webb R, Muller NL, Naidich DP. High Resolution CT of the Lung, 4th edition. Philadelphia: Lippincott Williams and Wilkins; 2008.

Section 2

Lung Physiology

CHAPTER 2

Mechanics of Ventilation

■ INTRODUCTION

This chapter starts by describing lung volumes and then deals with the basic action of respiratory muscles. It goes on to explain the physical properties of the lung and chest wall and the interaction between the two that influences the movement of air in and out of the lungs during the cyclic process of ventilation. Next, the chapter explains the regional differences in ventilation, airway resistance and its measurement and the physiological factors that affect airway resistance. It goes on to explain the dynamic compression of the airways during a forced expiration and finally considers the work required to move the lung and chest wall during ventilation.

■ LUNG VOLUMES

The total gas-containing capacities can be partitioned into different volumes which when combined give lung capacities.

Total lung capacity (TLC) is the largest amount of air held within the lungs at maximum inspiration. The residual volume (RV) is the amount of air left within the lung after a maximal forced expiration. The greatest volume of air that can be inspired or expired is the vital capacity (VC). The VC is therefore the difference between the TLC and RV.

Tidal volume (TV) is the inspiratory or expiratory volume during normal breathing at rest. It constitutes about 10% of the VC. TV increases with strenuous exercise, but even so does not exceed 50–60% of VC. The volume of air contained in the lung at end-expiratory position is termed the functional residual capacity (FRC). The FRC is roughly about 50% of the TLC. The FRC consists of the expiratory reserve volume plus RV. The volume of air that can be maximally inspired from the resting end-inspiratory level is the inspiratory reserve volume (IRV). The maximal volume of air inspired from the end-expiratory level is the inspiratory capacity (IC). Lung volumes and capacities are defined in **Table 1** and are depicted schematically in **Figure 1** and which have been obtained using a spirometer.

■ RESPIRATORY MUSCLES

Inspiration

The most important muscle of inspiration is the diaphragm, which is a dome-shaped sheet of muscle attached to the lower ribs. The diaphragm contracts on inspiration, pushing the abdominal contents downward and forward (the upper abdominal wall in the supine posture is seen to bulge upward on inspiration) and also increasing the vertical dimension of the chest cavity. In addition, the rib margins are lifted upward and outward thereby increasing the transverse diameter of the chest wall.

The diaphragm is supplied by the phrenic nerve from cervical segments 3, 4, and 5. When the diaphragm is paralyzed, it is drawn upward during inspiration because of the increased negativity of the intrapleural pressure. This is termed a *paradoxical movement*. It can be diagnosed at the bedside when the upper abdomen moves inward rather than outward on inspiration. Diaphragmatic paralysis is best proven by the "sniff test" (a sharp inspiratory sniff through the nostrils with the mouth closed). Fluoroscopic examination during the sniff shows paradoxical upward movement of the diaphragm instead of the usual downward movement. Patients with diaphragmatic paralysis are unable to lie down flat; they become breathless and hypoxic. Substantial relief is observed on sitting or standing.

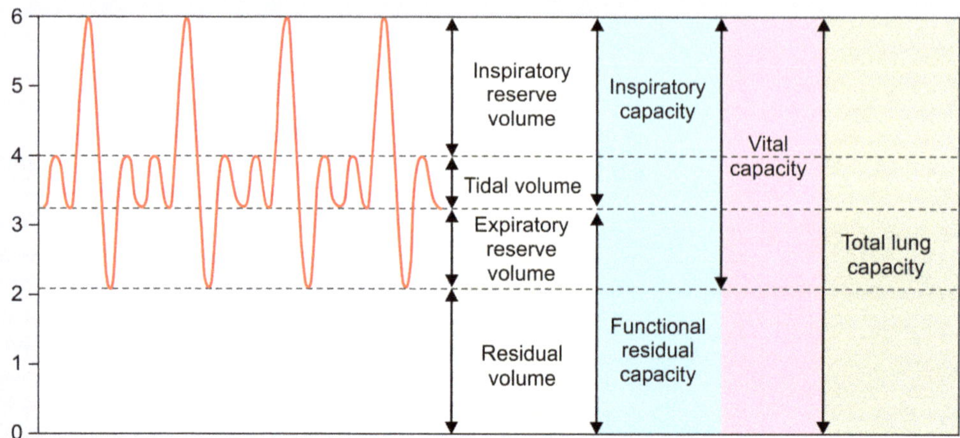

Fig. 1: Lung volumes and capacities as recorded by a spirometer.
The definitions of these subdivisions are found in Table 1.

Table 1: Glossary for static lung volumes and capacities.

Term	Abbreviation	Definition
Volumes		
Residual volume	RV	Volume of air remaining in the lungs after maximal expiration
Expiratory reserve volume	ERV	Maximal volume of air expired from the resting end-expiratory level
Tidal volume	TV	Volume of air expired or inspired with each breath during normal breathing
Inspiratory reserve volume	IRV	Maximal volume of air inspired from the resting end-inspiratory level
Capacities		
Inspiratory capacity	IC	Maximal volume of air inspired from the end-expiratory level
Vital capacity	VC	Maximal volume of air expired from the maximal inspiration
Functional residual capacity	FRC	Volume of air remaining in the lung at the end-expiratory level
Total lung capacity	TLC	Volume of air in the lungs after maximal inspiration

The external intercostal muscles also help with inspiration. They slope downward and forward and on contraction pull the ribs upward and forward increasing both the transverse and the anteroposterior diameter of the chest. The lateral expansion of the chest is due to a "bucket-handle" movement of the ribs. The intercostal muscles are supplied by the intercostal nerves arising from the spinal cord segments at the same level.

Expiration

Expiration is a passive process during quiet breathing. Expiration becomes active during exercise and during purposeful hyperventilation. The most important muscles of expiration are those of the abdominal wall, the rectus, the external and internal oblique and the transversalis. Contraction of these muscles raises the intra-abdominal pressure and pushes the diaphragm upward. These muscles are also involved in the forced expiratory movements that accompany coughing, sneezing or vomiting.

The internal intercostal muscles help in expiration by pulling the ribs downward and inward thereby decreasing the thoracic volume. Their active contraction also prevents the intercostal spaces from bulging, particularly during straining or during any act involving forceful expiration.

ELASTIC PROPERTIES OF THE LUNG AND CHEST WALL SYSTEM

Elastic Properties of the Lung

The lung is a structure with inherent elasticity so that it tends to recoil to a volume equal to (in fact a little less than) RV. To increase the volume of the lung from this resting state requires a force that should distend the lung. This force, termed the transpulmonary pressure, is the difference between the alveolar pressure and the pressure surrounding the lung which is the intrapleural pressure. The relation between lung volume and transmural pressure is illustrated in **Figure 2**. The graph illustrates the elastic properties of the lung and its tendency to recoil. This graph is applicable to an excised lung inflated by a pump, to an in vivo lung inflated by a ventilator or to a normal lung inflated by a normal physiological inspiration. In each case, the graph of volume versus transpulmonary pressure remains the same.

The slope of the pressure-volume curve is a measure of the compliance of the lung. Compliance is defined as the change in volume per unit change in pressure.

$$C = \Delta V / \Delta P$$

In the normal range (intrapleural pressure –5 to –10 cm of H_2O), the lung is markedly compliant or distensible. The compliance of the normal human lung is 200 mL/cm H_2O. The compliance as seen from the graph is more at the beginning of the curve and decreases with greater distending pressure when lung volume approaches TLC.

Compliance is obviously dependent on the lung size, so that the small lungs of a child are less compliant than those of an adult. A patient living on one lung following a pneumonectomy will obviously have a lower compliance (half of normal) even though the lung is perfectly healthy. For this reason, compliance is often divided by lung volume to give the volume-independent specific compliance.

Compliance of the lung is reduced in pulmonary fibrosis, pulmonary edema, atelectasis and consolidation. Compliance also falls if the lung remains poorly ventilated for a long time, presumably due to an increase in the stiffness of elastic tissue within the lung and due to diffuse air-space atelectasis. An increased compliance is present in emphysema and in the normal aging lung.

It should be noted that the pressure surrounding the lung (i.e. the intrapleural pressure) is less than atmospheric pressure because of the elastic recoil of the lung. The tendency of the lung to return or rather recoil to its resting volume is related to the presence of elastic tissue (elastin) visible on histological studies in alveolar walls and around bronchi and vessels. West believes that the elastic behavior of the lung has less to do with simple elongation of these fibers than it does with their geometric arrangement.

The **Figure 2** illustrates the pressure-volume curve during inspiration. **Figure 3** shows the pressure-volume curves during inspiration and expiration. It will be noted that the curves which the lung follows are different in inspiration and expiration or during inflation and deflation. This phenomenon is termed hysteresis. It is also noted that for any given pressure the lung volume is more

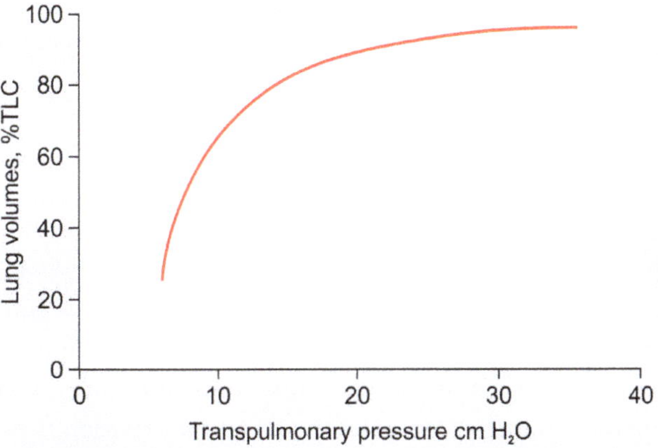

Fig. 2: Pressure-volume curve of the lung during inspiration.

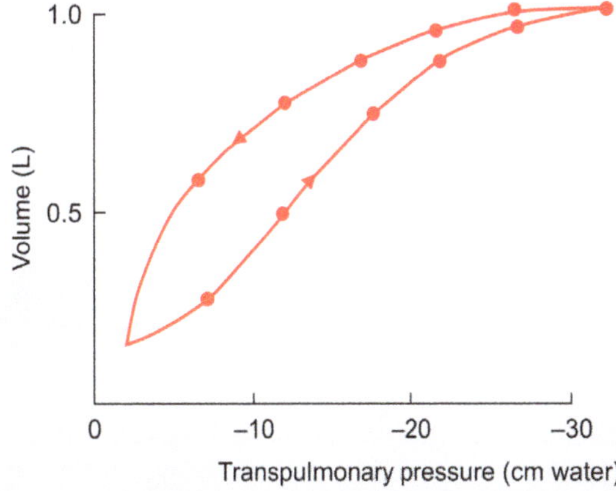

Fig. 3: Curves which the lung follows during inflation and deflation are different. This behavior is known as hysteresis.

in expiration or deflation than in inspiration or inflation. The curve further shows that even without any expanding pressure, the lung has some air within it.

Surface Tension

The elastic properties of the lung seen in pressure-volume curves are influenced by the surface tension of the liquid lining the alveolar walls. Surface tension is produced because the attractive forces between the adjacent molecules of the liquid lining the alveolar walls are much greater than those between liquid and gas. The liquid area as a result shrinks and becomes small. A lung filled with saline so that surface tension forces are thereby abolished will have a different pressure-volume curve reflecting only the tissue properties of the lung **(Fig. 4)**. The saline-filled curve is shifted to the left showing that the lung can be distended with much less pressure. The air-containing lung requires greater pressure for distention and as remarked earlier shows hysteresis—the volume curve during deflation following a different course than that observed during inflation. Also, the deflation curve of the air-filled lung is close to the volume curve of the saline-filled lung at low volumes, indicating that the pressure within alveoli from surface tension is reduced at low volumes. This seems paradoxical for according to Laplace's law, pressure

within a sphere should increase if the radius is reduced, P = 2T/r. This paradox is explained by the presence of a unique fluid lining the alveoli, termed surfactant. Surfactant is responsible for reducing surface tension in a volume-dependent manner so that as the volume of the alveoli decreases, surface tension also decreases, the surface tension being almost absent at RV.

The role of surfactant in the alveoli of the lung is important for the following reasons:

- It prevents collapse and ensures stability of the alveoli. If pressure within alveoli with smaller volume were to increase as per Laplace's law, they would empty into interconnecting larger alveoli with lower pressure. Surfactant prevents this by paradoxically reducing the pressure within the low-volume alveoli through reduction of surface tension.
- A low surface tension in the alveoli increases the compliance of the lung and reduces the work of breathing.
- The force of surface tension at the corners of the alveoli tends to draw fluid inward into the alveoli from outside capillaries and the interstitium. Surfactant, by lowering surface tension, prevents pulmonary edema.

Surfactant is secreted by type II alveolar epithelial cells. These are compact cells which on electron microscopy show lamellar bodies. These bodies are extruded into the alveolar lining fluid as tubular myelin which spreads as a thin layer at the air-liquid interface. The component of the surfactant known to produce a surface tension-lowering effect is dipalmitoylphosphatidylcholine (DPPC). DPPC is synthesized within the lungs from fatty acids that are either extracted from the blood or synthesized within the lung itself. DPPC has a rapid turnover and is synthesized quickly. Surfactant is produced late in fetal life. Babies born without surfactant develop severe respiratory distress and may die if the condition is not recognized and adequately treated.

The molecules of DPPC are hydrophobic at one end and hydrophilic at the other. When these molecules align themselves on the surface, the intermolecular repulsive forces counter the attracting forces between the liquid surface molecules responsible for surface tension. The action of surfactant is even more marked in alveoli with smaller volumes. The reduction in surface tension is even greater when the film of surfactant is compressed, because the DPPC molecules are crowded together repelling each other to a greater extent.

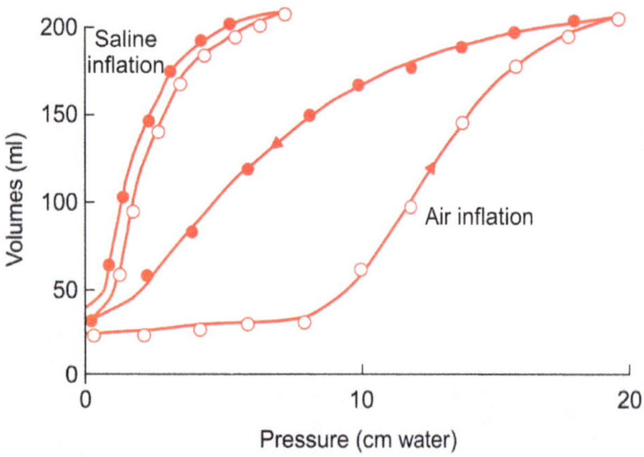

Fig. 4: Comparison of pressure-volume curves of air-filled and saline-filled lung (cat). Open circles, inflation; closed circles, deflation. Note that the saline-filled lung has a higher compliance and also much less hysteresis than the air-filled lung.
Source: Adapted with permission from West JB. Respiratory Physiology: The Essentials, 7th edition. Philadelphia: Lippincott Williams and Wilkins. 2007.

Elastic Properties of the Chest Wall and of the Lung plus Chest Wall

The thoracic cage, like the lung, is also an elastic structure. The recoil pressure for the relaxed chest wall equals pleural pressure (Ppl) minus the atmospheric pressure (Patm).

$$\text{Elastic recoil of chest wall} = \text{Ppl} - \text{Patm}$$

Since Patm is taken as zero, elastic recoil of the chest wall equals the Ppl. When the recoil pressure of the chest wall is zero, the chest wall moves outward so that its "unstressed" volume is quite high. This is illustrated in **Figure 5** when a pneumothorax is produced by introducing air into the pleural space raising the pleural pressure to the atmospheric. The lung is then observed to collapse and moves inward and the chest wall moves outward. It follows that under conditions of equilibrium, the chest wall is pulled inward and the lung pulled outward, the two pulling forces balancing each other.

Figure 6 shows the pressure-volume curve of the lung alone, the chest wall alone and the lung plus chest wall together. The pressure-volume curve of the lung alone is similar to that illustrated in **Figure 4**, only for clarity no hysteresis is shown. The curve shows the airway pressure determined at different volumes. The chest wall pressure-volume curve is for the chest wall only and one has to imagine a normal chest wall with no lung within! It is noted that at FRC the recoil pressure is negative (about $-5\,\text{cm}\,\text{H}_2\text{O}$)

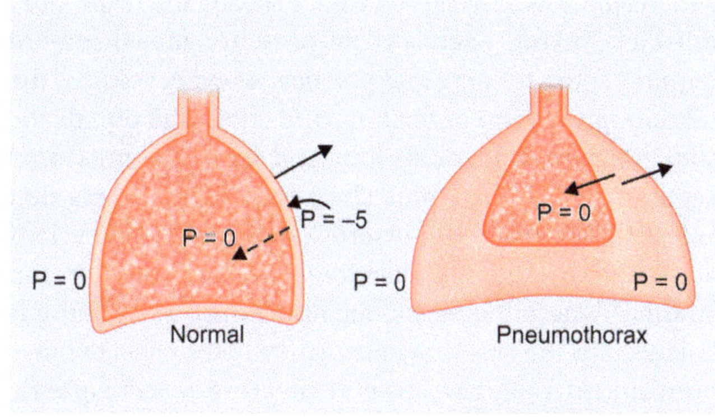

Fig. 5: The tendency of the lung to recoil to its deflated volume is balanced by the tendency of the rib cage to bow out. As a result, the intrapleural pressure is subatmospheric. Pneumothorax allows the lung to collapse and the thorax to spring out.

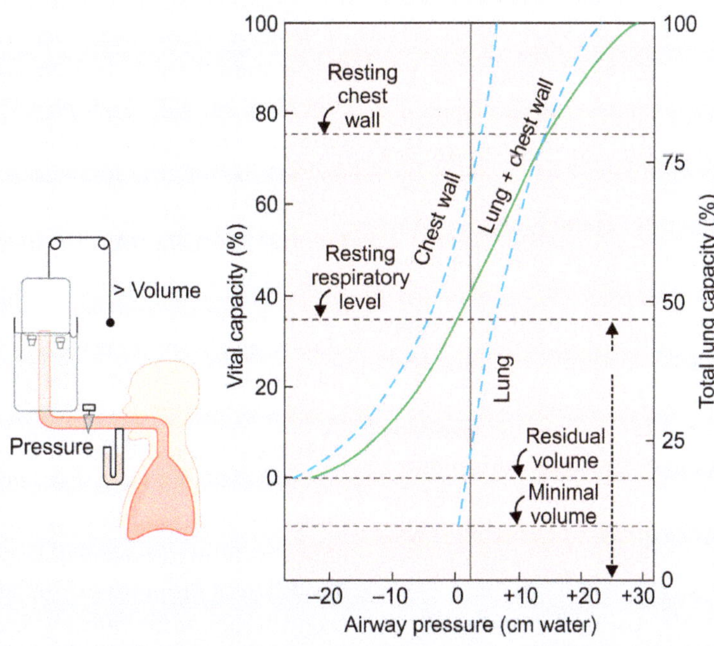

Fig. 6: The graph in this figure gives the pressure-volume curves of the lung, chest wall and the lung plus chest wall taken as one unit. The lung plus chest wall curve is obtained by the individuals inspiring a certain volume from the spirometer the pressure at that volume being measured with the respiratory muscles relaxed. The recoil pressure of the lung plus chest wall acting as one is equal to the sum of the recoil pressure of the lung and of the chest wall measured separately.
Source: Adapted with permission from West JB. Respiratory Physiology: The Essentials, 7th edition. Philadelphia: Lippincott Williams and Wilkins; 2007.

so that the chest wall would tend to move outward. It is only when the volume of the chest wall has increased to 75% of the VC that the recoil pressure is atmospheric.

The pressure-volume curve of the combined lung and chest wall is of considerable interest. For this curve, the individual inspires or expires from a spirometer and for each individual volume the airway pressure is measured with respiratory muscles relaxed. Relaxing the respiratory muscles during each airway pressure measurement requires some training and practice. At every volume, the relaxation pressure of the lung and chest wall equals the sum of the pressure of the lung and chest wall measured separately. The lung plus chest wall curve shows that at FRC the relaxation pressure, i.e. the recoil pressure is atmospheric (i.e. zero). Therefore, FRC is the "equilibrium volume" where the elastic recoil pressure of the lung is balanced by the elastic recoil pressure of the chest to move outward. At FRC, the alveolar pressure = atmospheric pressure = zero. The pleural pressure is roughly –5 cm H_2O.

Thus, lung recoil pressure at FRC = Alveolar pressure – Pleural pressure

$$= 0 - (-5) = 5 \text{ cm } H_2O$$

Chest wall recoil pressure = Pleural pressure – Atmospheric pressure

$$= -5 - 0$$
$$= -5 \text{ cm } H_2O$$

It is seen how the inward recoil of lung is balanced by the outward recoil of the chest wall. A few further features are worthy of note.

- The negative opposing pressure of the lung and chest wall produces a subatmospheric (negative) intrapleural pressure (–5 cm H_2O).
- It is this negative intrapleural pressure which counters or opposes both lung recoil inward and chest wall recoil outward.
- Since pressure at a particular volume is inversely proportional to compliance, the total compliance of the lung plus chest wall is equal to the sum of the reciprocal of the compliance of the lung and chest wall measured separately.

$$1/C_{(lung + chest \, wall)} = 1/C_{lung} + 1/C_{chest \, wall}$$

It will be noted from **Figure 6** that at FRC the lung is distended above its low unstressed volume and the chest wall is held distended below its relatively high unstressed volume. Any change in the unstressed volume or compliance of either lung or chest wall will lead to a new

FRC. Thus, emphysema leads to both an increase in lung compliance together with increase in unstressed volume of the lung, thereby leading to a higher FRC. Obesity on the other hand reduces the unstressed volume of the chest wall and thereby leads to a reduced FRC.

Recoil pressure of lung, chest wall and lung-chest wall combined. Recoil pressure (transmural pressure) of:

Lungs	$= (P_A) - (Ppl)$
Chest wall	$= (Ppl) - (Patm)$
	$= (Ppl)$, since Patm is zero
Lungs + chest wall	$= (P_A - Ppl) + (Ppl - Patm)$
	$= P_A - Patm$

where P_A = alveolar pressure, Ppl = intrapleural pressure, Patm = atmospheric pressure.

■ AIRWAY RESISTANCE

Airflow during expiration from alveoli will depend on the driving pressure (i.e. pressure difference between alveoli and the atmosphere) and the airway resistance.

$$\text{Airflow} = \dot{V} = \frac{\text{Pressure difference between alveoli and atmosphere } (\Delta P)}{\text{Resistance } (R_{aw})}$$

Normal airway resistance (R_{aw}) during quiet breathing is less than 2 cm ELO/L/second. If air flows through a tube (and the airways approximate to tubes), the pressure difference depends on the rate and the pattern of flow. If the flow rate is slow, the stream of air flowing through the tube is parallel to the sides of the wall. This pattern is termed as *laminar* flow **(Fig. 7A)**. A rather unique feature of laminar flow is that the gas in the center of the flow moves twice as fast as the average velocity. There is therefore a "spike" of moving gas along the axis of the tube. This change in velocity across the diameter of the tube is termed the *velocity profile*. If the flow rate increases, eddies tend to form particularly at the branching of the tubes and the pattern is termed *transitional* flow **(Fig. 7C)**. At high flow rates, the stream of flow is disorganized and the pattern of flow is termed *turbulent* flow **(Fig. 7B)**. Turbulent flow has different properties from laminar flow. Pressure is not proportional to the flow but is approximately equal to its square. Pressure (P) = kV^2, where k is a constant. Also, turbulent flow does not have the high central or axial flow velocity observed in laminar flow.

In the rapidly branching bronchial tree, laminar flow is probably to be found only in the terminal bronchioles.

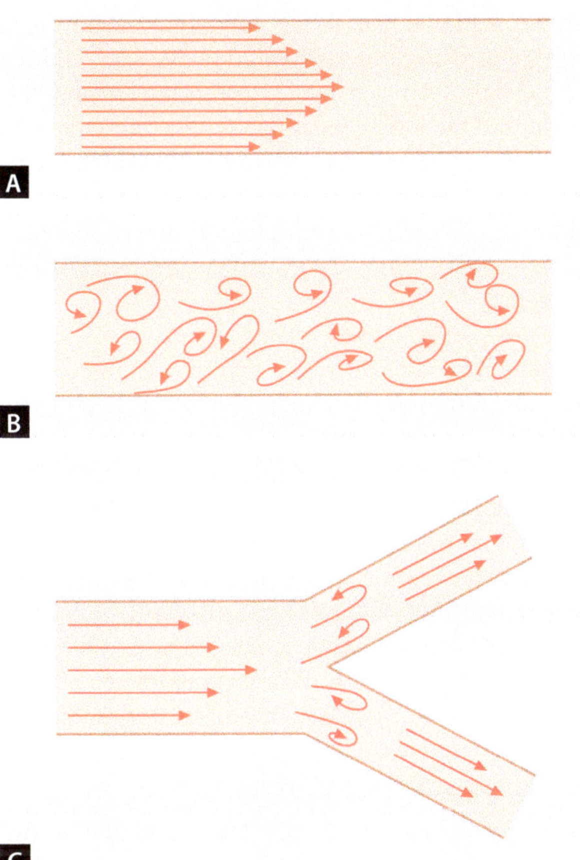

Figs. 7A to C: Patterns of airflow. (A) Laminar flow; (B) Turbulent flow; (C) Transition flow.

In most of the other bronchi, the flow pattern is transitional. Turbulent flow may occur in the trachea, particularly with high flow rates as with exercise.

Airway resistance is inversely proportional to flow rate, and the driving pressure is directly proportional to the flow rate. Airway resistance depends on:

- Caliber of the bronchial tube which is again dependent on the position of the bronchial tube in the lung.
- On the length of airways. R_{aw} is directly proportional to the length, so that doubling the length doubles the resistance.
- Radius of the airways. R_{aw} is proportional to $1/r^4$. Therefore, reducing the radius of a breathing tube by half causes a 16-fold increase in R_{aw}.
- Viscosity and density of inhaled gas—the higher the viscosity and density, the greater the resistance.

Of all these factors, change in caliber or the radius of the breathing tubes determines airway resistance to the maximum extent. Factors that affect change in caliber are:

- Lung volume—smaller lung volumes are associated with a smaller caliber of breathing tubes.
- Bronchial muscle tone which is under the control of the autonomic nervous system and is also directly affected by histamine and other-related substances.
- Secretions partially blocking the breathing tube.
- Pressure across the airway wall.

The last point is of importance and needs further explanation. **Figures 8A to D** schematically shows the forces acting across an airway within the lung. Just before inspiration at FRC, the alveolar pressure = atmospheric pressure (at the mouth) = zero. Airway pressure all along is also zero. Because intrapleural pressure is –5 cm H_2O, there is a pressure of +5 cm H_2O that keeps the airways open **(Fig. 8A)**.

During quiet inspiration, there is an increase in the negativity of the intrapleural pressure and the alveolar pressure (by say 5 cm H_2O) so that air flows from the mouth to the alveoli. If the pressure in the airways is –2 cm H_2O, there is pressure of +8 cm H_2O keeping the airway open **(Fig. 8B)**. At end inspiration, alveolar pressure and airway pressure are equal to atmospheric pressure = zero. The intrapleural pressure is say –12 cm H_2O and the airway is kept open by a pressure 12 cm H_2O **(Fig. 8C)**.

In passive expiration, the intrapleural pressure is less negative but a positive alveolar pressure is caused by elastic recoil.

In forced expiration, the alveolar pressure is high because of the alveolar recoil pressure (taken at 12 cm H_2O in **Fig. 8D**) plus the very positive intrapleural pressure (+25 cm H_2O in **Fig. 8D**). This high pressure (25 + 12 = 37 cm H_2O) drives flow downstream toward the mouth. However, once the intraluminal pressure within the airways falls below the high intrapleural pressure (equal pressure point) there is a dynamic compression of the airways, and airflow becomes limited. Further effort increases alveolar pressure but again increases the force of compression so that flow remains limited however strong the effort **(Fig. 8D)**.

Maximum airflow rates can be directly measured by recording a flow-volume loop through a spirometer. Maximum flow rates for any volume except at the highest volume at the very start of exhalation remain the same even with submaximal effort and cannot increase with increased effort **(Fig. 9)**. The mechanism for flow

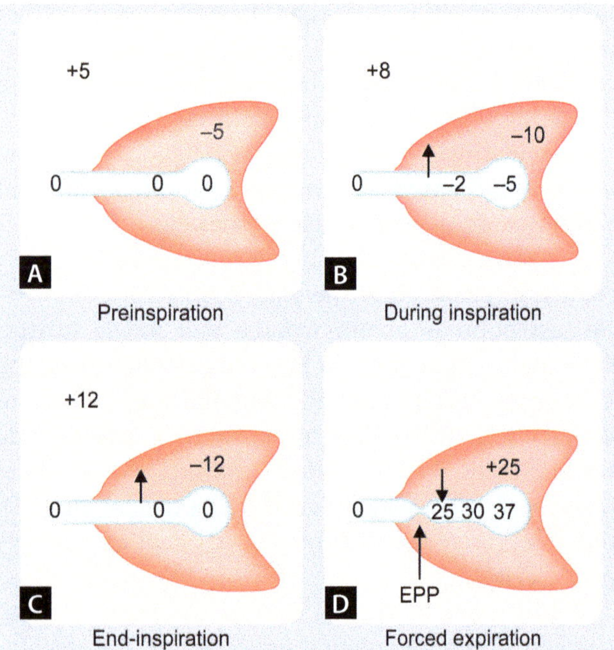

Figs. 8A to D: Scheme showing airways compression during forced expiration. Note that the pressure difference across the airways is holding it open, except during a forced expiration (see text). (EPP: Equal pressure point)

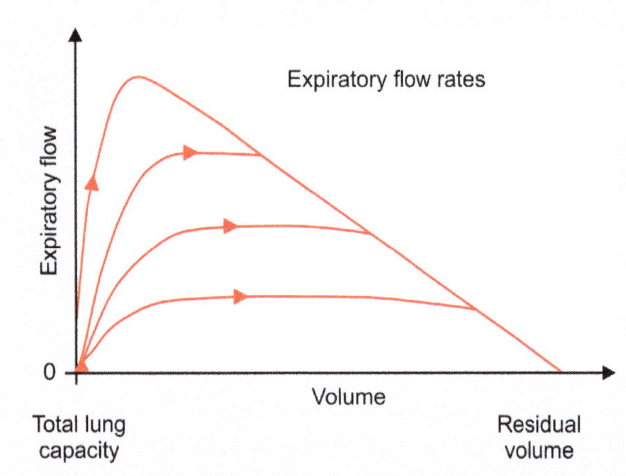

Fig. 9: Flow-volume curves at different levels of effort. Note that at submaximal efforts the descending portion of the flow-volume curve takes the same path.

limitation is dynamic compression of the airways as explained above. This compression as already explained occurs just beyond the point where the pressure within the airways is just below the intrapleural pressure. The driving pressure up to this point is the difference between the intra-alveolar pressure and the pleural pressure:

P_A – Ppl, i.e. 37 cm H_2O – 25 cm H_2O **(Fig. 8D)** which equals 12 cm H_2O. This is equal to the elastic recoil pressure of the lung in the illustrative diagram, and the elastic recoil pressure is related to volume of the lung and not to effort. If the individual doubles his expiratory effort so that the intrapleural pressure is 50 cm H_2O at the same lung volume, the driving pressure will be 62 cm H_2O (in the alveoli) – 50 cm H_2O (intrapleural pressure) which still remains at 12 cm H_2O so that the flow rate remains unchanged.

There are certain points worth stressing:

- Maximal flow rates decrease with lung volume as the pressure difference between alveolar pressure and intrapleural pressure decreases.
- An increase in resistance of peripheral airways leads to an increase in the magnitude of the pressure drop within the lumen of the airways during forced expiration with a sharper decrease in intraluminal pressure, thereby exaggerating the flow-limiting mechanism.
- Loss of or impaired elastic recoil coupled with loss of support to the alveolar walls as in emphysema reduces the driving pressure and leads to early airflow limitation.

Major Sites of Airways Resistance

The airways, to start with, are large but divide and subdivide into narrow and narrower tubes ultimately ending into numerous respiratory bronchioles. Resistance as mentioned earlier is most influenced by caliber of the breathing tubes so that halving the radius of the breathing tube increases the resistance 16-fold. It used to be thought till recent times that the maximum resistance was in the very small airways. It has however been shown by actual measurement that the major site of resistance is in the medium-sized bronchi and that the very small bronchioles or airways contribute comparatively little to resistance. In fact, the small airways contribute not more than 20% of the total airways resistance. This is of clinical importance because there can be fairly extensive and significant disease in the small airways of the lung without it being detected clinically or on routine lung function tests. For this reason, the small airways of the lung are often referred to as the silent zone within the lung.

■ WORK OF BREATHING

Work is necessary to move the chest wall and the lungs during inspiration. Work performed is best equated to pressure × volume.

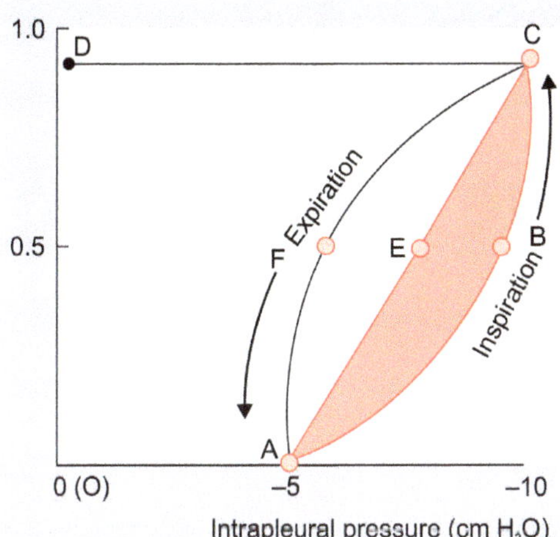

Fig. 10: Pressure-volume curve of the lung showing the inspiratory work done overcoming elastic forces (area OAECDO) and viscous forces (colored area ABCEA).

In the pressure-volume curve **(Fig. 10)**, the intrapleural pressure during inspiration follows the curve ABC and the work during inspiration is given by the area OABCDO. Of this area, the quadrilateral OAECDO represents the work done to overcome the elastic forces and the colored area ABCEA represents the work done to overcome airway and tissue resistance. If the airway resistance was to increase, the colored areas would increase in size due to an associated increase in the negative intrapleural pressure.

On expiration, the area AECFA is the work required to overcome airways resistance. This however is encompassed within the area of the trapezoid OAECDO. Therefore, this work can be done by the energy stored in the expanded elastic structure which is released during expiration. The difference between the areas OAECDO and AECFA represents the work dissipated as heat.

Increase in the frequency of respiration leads to increased flow rates leading to increased resistive work with increase in the area ABCEA. Increase in TV would lead to increase in elastic work, with a corresponding increase in the area OACDO.

Patients with interstitial pulmonary fibrosis who have lowered compliance and stiff lungs tend to have an increased respiratory rate, while patients with airways obstruction tend to breathe slowly. These patterns of breathing reduce the workload on the lung.

■ SUGGESTED READING

1. Bachofen H, Hildebrandt J, Bachofen M. Pressure-volume curves of air- and liquid-filled excised lungs-surface tension in situ. J Appl Physiol. 1970;29(4):422-31.
2. De Troyer A. The respiratory muscles. In: Crystal RG, West JB, Barnes PJ, Weibel ER (Eds). The Lung: Scientific Foundations, 2nd edition. New York: Lippincott-Raven Press; 1997.
3. Hyatt RE, Black LF. The flow-volume curve: a current perspective. Am Rev Respir Dis. 1973;107:191-9.
4. Orton C, Ward S, Jordan S, et al. Flow-volume loop: window to a smooth diagnosis? Thorax. 2015;70(3):302, 304.
5. Otis AB. The work of breathing. Physiol Rev. 1954;34:449-58.
6. Sterner JB, Morris MJ, Still JM, et al. Inspiratory flow-volume curve evaluation for detecting upper airway disease. Respir. Care. 2009;54(4):461-6.
7. West JB. Mechanics of breathing. In: West JB. Respiratory Physiology: The Essentials, 9th edition. Lippincott Williams and Wilkins; 2012.

CHAPTER 3

Gas Exchange in the Lung

■ INTRODUCTION

The basic function of the lung is to provide oxygen and remove carbon dioxide from the blood perfusing the lung. This involves efficient gas exchange, the oxygen reaching the alveoli from the inspired air being transferred to the capillaries perfusing them and carbon dioxide from the capillaries around the alveoli being transferred to the alveoli and then to the outside air during expiration. This gas exchange occurs during each cycle of ventilation—inspiration and expiration, and the basic principles of the exchange will be described below.

■ ANATOMY OF THE GAS EXCHANGE AREA OF THE LUNG

The lung can be divided into two zones: a conducting zone which merely serves to conduct or transport inspired and expired gas in and out of the lungs, and a gas exchange zone where oxygen from the outside air reaching the gas exchange zone is transferred to blood perfusing the lungs and carbon dioxide from the blood reaching the gas exchange zone is expired into the outside air.

The conducting zone of the lung consists of the upper respiratory tract, the trachea, the bronchi, the subdivisions of the bronchi, the bronchioles which again divide, right up to the terminal bronchioles. These conducting passages take no part in gas exchange.

The terminal bronchioles divide into two to five generations of respiratory bronchioles, which have increasing number of alveoli on their walls. The respiratory bronchioles divide further into alveolar ducts which also have alveoli on their walls; the alveolar ducts open into large air spaces called alveoli. The gas exchange unit therefore extends only from the respiratory bronchioles to the alveoli. The unit of lung supplied by one terminal bronchiole is termed the acinus. Several acini close to each other form a lung lobule. There is a collateral flow of gas and blood within the lobules and to a lesser extent between lobules. The main gas exchange occurs in the alveoli which are irregular spaces about 250 μm in diameter. There are over 300 million alveoli within the lungs and if they were to be stretched out would cover the size of a tennis court. Eighty-five to ninety percent of the total alveolar surface is covered by capillaries providing an excellent surface area of 70 m^2 for gas exchange between the alveolar surface and the blood (**Fig. 1**).

The alveolar surface is covered by epithelial cells; these are of two types—Type I and Type II. The alveolar cells are attached directly to a thin basement membrane. The alveoli are perfused by capillaries which surround them. The capillaries are lined by endothelial cells and again rest on the basement membrane. Over the greater part of the gas exchange area the basement membrane of the alveolar cells and the basement membrane of capillary endothelial cells are fused with no intervening space between them. For oxygen exchange, oxygen from the alveolus needs to go through the alveolar wall, the basement membranes (of both alveoli and capillary walls), the endothelial lining of the capillaries into their lumen where oxygen is taken up by the hemoglobin of the blood perfusing the capillaries. Carbon dioxide has a reverse process going from the capillaries through the basement membrane, alveolar walls into the alveolus to be expired to the outside.

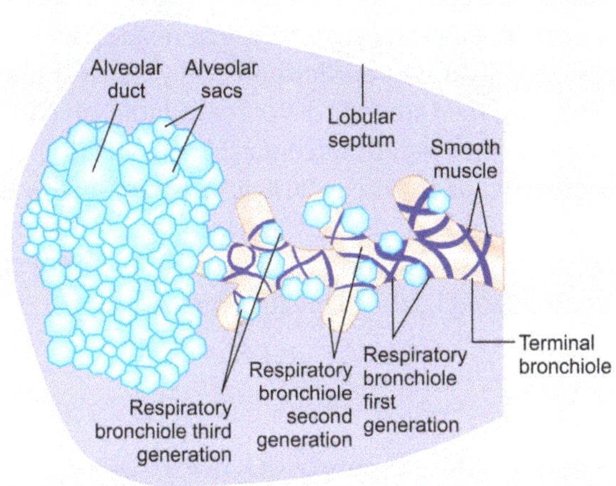

Fig. 1: Gas exchange zone of the lung.

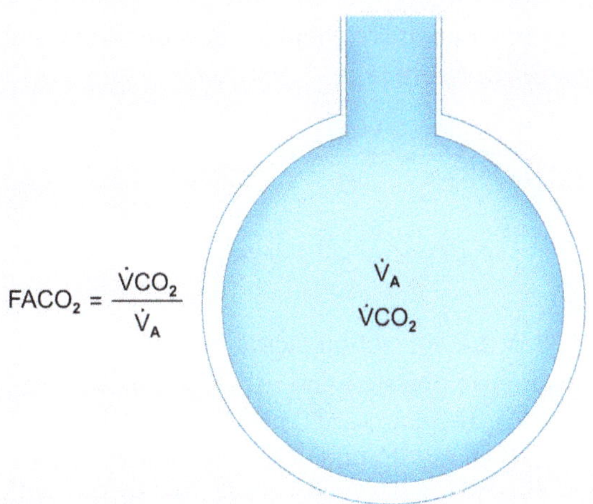

Fig. 2: Concept of alveolar ventilation.

PHYSIOLOGIC CONCEPT

The volume of air breathed in and out during quiet resting respiration is termed the tidal volume. If, for example, the tidal volume is taken as 500 mL and the individual breathes 14 breaths/min, the minute ventilation is $500 \times 14 = 7$ L. It is important to realize that not all 500 mL of air inhaled in one breath participates in gas exchange. Only that portion of air reaching perfused alveoli does so. Alveolar ventilation is therefore related to that portion of inspired air or gas reaching perfused alveoli and taking part in gas exchange. This takes us to the concept of dead space which is dealt with just a little later.

Efficient gas exchange in the lungs requires:

- Adequate alveolar ventilation evenly distributed to both lungs
- Even ventilation-perfusion ratios of 0.8 to 1. Uneven ventilation-perfusion ratios or ventilation-perfusion mismatch is an important cause of hypoxia or poor arterial oxygenation. A ventilation-perfusion mismatch is characterized clinically and physiologically by two features: (1) An increase in dead space—ventilation of unperfused or poorly perfused alveoli which are hyperventilated in relation to the blood perfusing them; (2) an increase in venous admixture, i.e. perfusion of atelectatic alveoli causing a true right to left shunt. Alveoli which are hypoventilated in relation to blood perfusing them, also contribute to a shunt effect.
- Diffusion of oxygen across the alveolar wall into the capillaries perfusing the alveoli, and of carbon dioxide from the capillaries out into the alveolar space.

A severe diffusion defect may contribute to a low partial pressure of oxygen in arterial blood (PaO_2) but is hardly ever its sole cause. Most pathologies producing a diffusion defect also lead to an uneven compliance within the lungs and thereby to a ventilation-perfusion mismatch.

ALVEOLAR VENTILATION

The partial pressure of carbon dioxide in arterial blood ($PaCO_2$) is the best indicator of alveolar ventilation. This basic fact in respiratory physiology is explained below. Consider for purposes of illustration an alveolus of volume $\dot{V}_A$ **(Fig. 2)**. It contains a volume of CO_2, i.e. $\dot{V}CO_2$. The fractional concentration of CO_2 in this alveolus ($FACO_2$) is given by the volume of CO_2 divided by the volume of the alveolus ($\dot{V}_A$).

$$FACO_2 = \frac{\dot{V}CO_2}{\dot{V}_A}$$

The CO_2 released into the alveolus from the blood perfusing it, will be cleared from the alveolus by ventilation; the greater the ventilation the lower the concentration of CO_2 in the alveolus. The alveolar concentration will be a balance between the alveolar ventilation and the rate at which the CO_2 is evolved ($\dot{V}CO_2$). Let us again consider the equation:

$$FACO_2 = \frac{\dot{V}CO_2}{\dot{V}_A}$$

The fractional concentration of CO_2, $FACO_2$ (0.05–0.06), exerts a pressure equal to the same fraction of the barometric pressure (P_B).

$$\frac{P_A CO_2}{P_B} = \frac{\dot{V}CO_2}{\dot{V}_A}$$

$$P_A CO_2 = \frac{\dot{V}CO_2}{\dot{V}_A} \times 0.863$$

0.863 is the correction factor that takes into account the barometric pressure and the different units in which $\dot{V}CO_2$ and $\dot{V}_A$ are expressed. This is the alveolar ventilation equation. It shows that the $P_A CO_2$ is directly proportional to the CO_2 produced, and inversely proportional to alveolar ventilation ($\dot{V}_A$). If $\dot{V}CO_2$ is constant, then $P_A CO_2$ is inversely proportional to $\dot{V}_A$.

$$P_A CO_2 \propto \frac{1}{\dot{V}_A}$$

There is good evidence to show that $PaCO_2$ (arterial PCO_2) is very close to the average alveolar PCO_2, i.e. $P_A CO_2$. Thus,

$$P_A CO_2 = PaCO_2 = \frac{\dot{V}CO_2}{\dot{V}_A} \times 0.863$$

The $PaCO_2$ is thus inversely related to $\dot{V}_A$. A high $PaCO_2$ (>48 mm Hg) denotes hypoventilation; a low $PaCO_2$ (<35 mm Hg) denotes hyperventilation; a normal $PaCO_2$ (35–45 mm Hg) denotes normal alveolar ventilation. It should be evident from the above equation that if the normal $PaCO_2$ of 40 mm Hg is doubled to 80 mm Hg, it means that the alveolar ventilation is just half of what is normally necessary to deal with the CO_2 produced by the body. It is to be also noted that the $PaCO_2$ may rise if the $\dot{V}CO_2$ rises and if the patient for some reason cannot increase his alveolar ventilation to get rid of the extra CO_2.

CONCEPT OF DEAD SPACE

The anatomical dead space is that constituted by the trachea and the bronchi right up to, but not including, the gas exchange unit of the lung. It is the volume of inspired air which fills the airways and is breathed out unchanged. Air entering alveoli which have no blood perfusing them, also does not take part in gas exchange and is breathed out unchanged. This is wasted ventilation and constitutes alveolar dead space. The sum of the anatomical dead space and the alveolar dead space is termed the physiological dead space, though admittedly there is nothing physiological about this dead space. **Figure 3** illustrates the concept of anatomical and alveolar dead space.

Effective alveolar ventilation is only that ventilation entering perfused alveoli. Hyperventilated alveoli will contribute to the overall concept of alveolar dead space.

Ordinarily, as much as 30% of tidal volume is dead space ventilation. This may increase considerably in patients with diseased lungs. The quantum of dead space can be calculated by the following equation:

$$\frac{\dot{V}_D}{\dot{V}_T} = \frac{PaCO_2 - P_E CO_2}{PaCO_2}$$

where $P_E CO_2$ is the pressure of CO_2 in expired gas.

ALVEOLAR OXYGEN

Fresh oxygen from inspired gas enters alveoli during ventilation; the oxygen diffuses through the alveolar wall into the blood perfusing the alveoli. For any given concentration of oxygen in inspired gas (FiO_2), the alveolar concentration of oxygen (FAO_2) will be a balance between alveolar ventilation ($\dot{V}_A$) and the oxygen taken up ($\dot{V}O_2$) by the blood perfusing ventilated alveoli.

$$FiO_2 - F_A O_2 = \frac{\dot{V}O_2}{\dot{V}_A}$$

In terms of partial pressure,

$$PIO_2 - P_A O_2 = \frac{\dot{V}O_2}{\dot{V}_A} \times 0.863$$

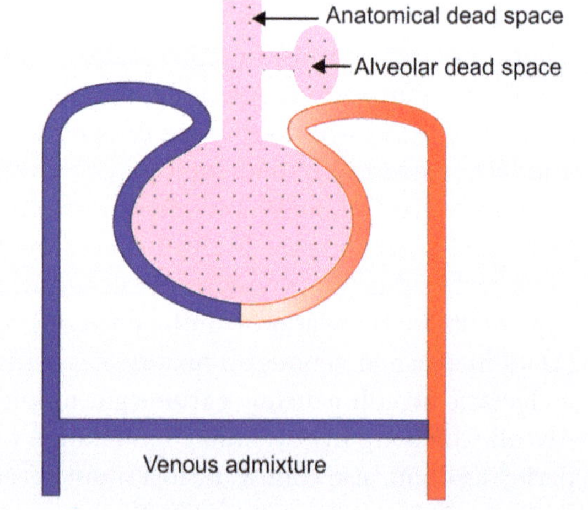

Fig. 3: Concept of anatomical and alveolar dead space and venous admixture (right to left shunt within the lungs).
Source: From Udwadia FE. Principles of Critical Care Medicine, 3rd edition. New Delhi: Jaypee Brothers Medical Publishers; 2014.

We have already defined $\dot{V}_A$ (under alveolar ventilation) in terms of $PaCO_2$.

$$P_AO_2 = PIO_2 - P_ACO_2 = \frac{\dot{V}O_2}{\dot{V}CO_2} \times 0.863$$

The ratio $\dot{V}CO_2/\dot{V}O_2$ is in fact the respiratory exchange ratio R, and R in a steady state equals the metabolic respiratory quotient. Thus, $P_AO_2 = PIO_2 - PaCO_2 \times 1/R$.

If carbohydrates are preponderantly burnt as fuel, R = 1; if fats are burnt as fuel R = 0.7; if carbohydrates and fats are both burnt as fuel, as is usually the case, R = 0.8.

The above equation is a simplified form of the alveolar air equation. It is of great use because:

(a) It allows a quick determination of alveolar oxygen pressure (P_AO_2) if the PIO_2 and the $PaCO_2$ are known.

(b) If the P_AO_2 is known and the PaO_2 is available through an arterial blood gas measurement, the alveolar-arterial oxygen gradient can be calculated as the difference between P_AO_2 and PaO_2. The upper normal of this gradient is 15 to at the most 20 mm Hg. In most normal individuals it averages 10 mm Hg.

(c) The alveolar equation points to a linear relationship between P_AO_2 and $PaCO_2$. The O_2–CO_2 diagram **(Fig. 4)** or line is further elaborated upon in the chapter on Acute Respiratory Failure in Adults. From this diagram one can quickly plot the expected P_AO_2 if the $PaCO_2$ is known for any given inspired oxygen concentration. If the alveolar arterial oxygen gradient is taken as 10–15 mm Hg, then for any given $PaCO_2$ one can read off the PaO_2. This is true provided the alveolar-arterial oxygen gradient is not abnormally increased.

(d) A consideration of the alveolar air equation shows that at a given inspired oxygen concentration and a given respiratory quotient, the alveolar PO_2 is dependent on alveolar ventilation. A lower alveolar ventilation would thus lead to a lowered alveolar PO_2, and hence a lowered arterial PO_2.

(e) The alveolar air equation helps the physician to check on blood gas measurements. If the value of the measured $PaCO_2$ is taken as correct, the alveolar equation allows one to compute the P_AO_2. If the PaO_2 reported by the laboratory is higher than the P_AO_2, it is obviously incorrect.

■ ALVEOLAR-ARTERIAL OXYGEN GRADIENT

The normal range of the alveolar-arterial oxygen gradient has already been mentioned. An increased

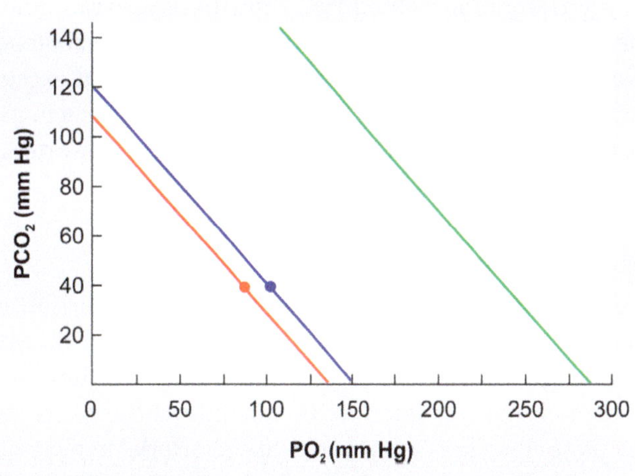

Fig. 4: O_2–CO_2 diagram.
The blue line represents the relationship between alveolar PO_2 and alveolar PCO_2 with a RQ of 0.8 and when breathing air (PIO_2) = 149 mm Hg. The circle marked on this line presents the normal P_AO_2 and P_ACO_2.
The green line illustrates the PO_2–PCO_2 relationship with an RQ of 0.8 when breathing 40% oxygen (PIO_2 = 285 mm Hg).
The red line gives the relationship between arterial PaO_2 and arterial carbon dioxide pressure $PaCO_2$ provided the alveolar arterial gradient is normal (10–15 mm Hg). Therefore from the above diagram if the P_AO_2 is known the expected PaO_2 and the corresponding P_ACO_2 can also be determined.
Source: From Udwadia FE. Principles of Critical Care Medicine, 3rd edition. New Delhi: Jaypee Brothers Medical Publishers; 2014.

alveolar-arterial oxygen gradient denotes an impairment of gas exchange across the alveolar capillary membrane. When, however, a low PaO_2 is due to hypoventilation, or is related to breathing at high altitudes then there is no increase in the alveolar-arterial oxygen gradient since the P_AO_2 is also proportionately low. A lowered PaO_2 from any other cause (V/Q mismatch, increased shunt, impaired diffusion) is always associated with an increased alveolar-arterial oxygen gradient. Also, the greater the alveolar-arterial oxygen gradient, the greater the disturbance in gas exchange within the lungs. This observation should however be viewed in its proper perspective. Thus an alveolar-arterial gradient of 20 mm Hg (upper limit of normal), occurring on the steep part of the oxygen dissociation curve will denote a gross disturbance in pulmonary gas exchange. Let us consider a patient with chronic bronchitis in severe hypercapnic respiratory failure. If the P_AO_2 of this patient is 50 mm Hg and the PaO_2 is 30 mm Hg, the gradient of just 20 mm Hg (upper limit of normal) would suggest that the hypoxia is chiefly due to alveolar hypoventilation. However at a PO_2 of 50 mm Hg the oxygen saturation is 85%; at a PO_2 of 30 mm Hg the oxygen saturation is about 55%. Thus, the oxygen saturation has fallen 30% between the alveoli and the arterial blood. Normally, the fall in oxygen saturation does not exceed 2%. It is evident that there is a serious disturbance in gas exchange in this patient, even though the alveolar-arterial oxygen gradient is not unduly increased.

■ VENOUS ADMIXTURE

Venous admixture **(Figs. 5 A to C)** is that portion of the cardiac output which does not take part in the gas exchange within the alveoli and which is therefore returned unoxygenated to the left side of the heart. An increase in venous admixture leads to arterial hypoxemia and is one of the chief causes of respiratory failure. A number of unrelated pathological conditions involving the lung can lead to an increase in venous admixture resulting in arterial hypoxemia and respiratory failure. The total venous admixture or shunt may be contributed to by—(1) anatomical shunt and (2) intrapulmonary capillary shunt.

1. *Anatomical shunt*: Normally this is constituted by the bronchial veins, pleural veins and Thebesian veins; it generally does not cause shunting to a degree exceeding 2%. Only in the presence of large pathological arteriovenous communication, arteriovenous aneurysms or a substantial right to left cardiac shunt will an anatomical shunt give rise to a marked increase in venous admixture so as to cause arterial hypoxemia.

2. *Intrapulmonary capillary shunt*: The respiratory physician is more concerned with venous admixture due to an intrapulmonary capillary shunt. If unoxygenated blood perfuses atelectatic alveoli, the oxygen content of the blood leaving the atelectatic alveoli will be less than that leaving alveoli which are normally ventilated and perfused. This constitutes the concept of venous admixture. Venous admixture at the bedside has two components—(i) a true right to left shunt due to perfusion of totally atelectatic alveoli, and (ii) a shunt effect observed in alveoli which are hypoventilated in relation to the blood perfusing them, i.e. alveoli with low ventilation-perfusion ratios. This is not a true right to left shunt (as with atelectasis), but it is assumed for conceptual reasons that the portion of the blood which remains unoxygenated after perfusing these alveoli behaves in a way similar to an equivalent amount of blood shunted from the right to left. The total venous admixture consists of both (i) and (ii). Some would also include the small anatomical shunt in total venous admixture. Ordinarily, the anatomical shunt as mentioned above is negligible.

A true right to left shunt (also called a true venous admixture) is unchanged by increasing inspired

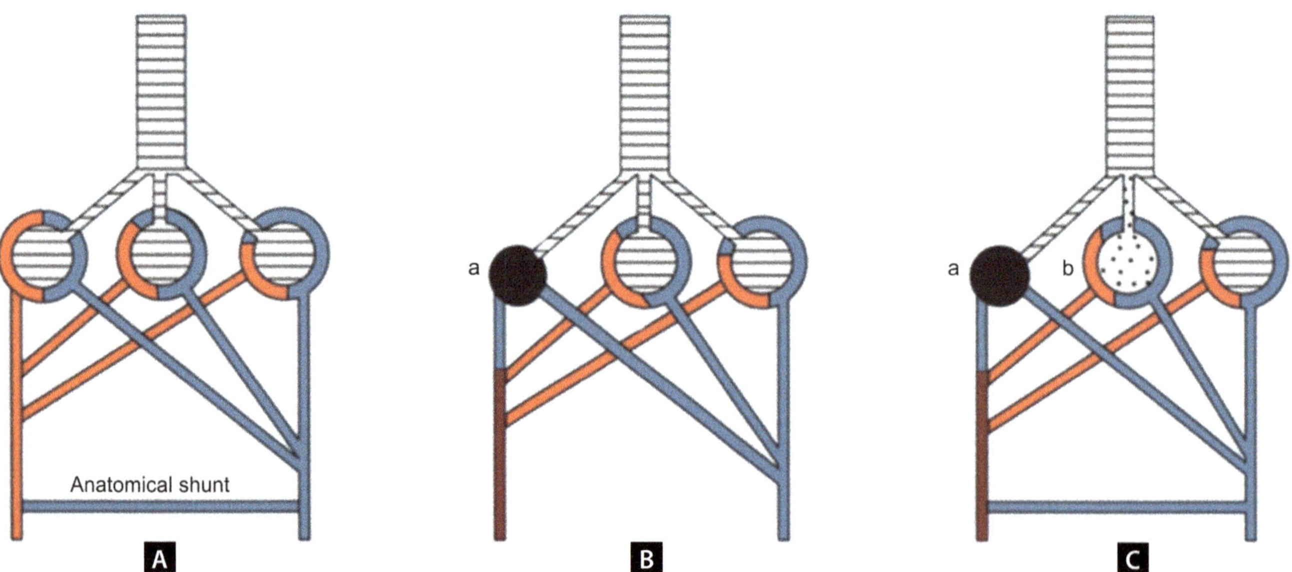

Figs. 5A to C: (A) Anatomical shunt (portion of cardiac output bypassing pulmonary capillaries). (B) True right to left shunt in the lungs caused by perfusion of atelectatic alveoli (Alveolus a). (C) An overall shunt due to perfusion of atelectatic alveoli (Alveolus a) to a lowered ventilation/perfusion ratio causing a shunt effect (Alveolus b) and the anatomical shunt.
Source: From Udwadia FE. *Principles of Critical Care Medicine*, 3rd edition. New Delhi: Jaypee Brothers Medical Publishers; 2014.

concentration of oxygen. In other words, the PaO_2 does not rise to any appreciable extent even with a significant increase in the inspired oxygen concentration. The shunt effect produced by alveoli with lowered ventilation-perfusion ratios will however be abolished, so that the PaO_2 rises sharply on increasing the inspired oxygen concentration. The simple bedside test of noting the degree of rise in PaO_2 with 100% inspired oxygen, thus distinguishes between a true right to left shunt within the lungs, and a shunt effect produced by ventilation-perfusion inequalities. More often than not, a right to left shunt as also ventilation-perfusion inequalities are present in the same patient. This is further elaborated upon in the chapter on Acute Respiratory Failure. The mathematical calculation of the venous admixture or shunt is given by the following equation:

$$\frac{Q_S}{Q_T} = \frac{C_cO_2 - CaO_2}{C_cO_2 - C_vO_2}$$

where Qs is the shunt fraction, Q_T the cardiac output, C_cO_2 the capillary oxygen content, CaO_2 the arterial oxygen content and C_vO_2 the mixed venous oxygen content.

In practice, end-capillary oxygen content is calculated from the alveolar PO_2 by assuming that P_AO_2 is equal to end-capillary PO_2. Arterial oxygen content is either derived from the PaO_2, or estimated by an oximeter. Mixed venous oxygen content is obtained by sampling blood from the pulmonary artery through a Swan-Ganz catheter.

The normal Q_S/Q_T is generally not more than 5%. A shunt fraction exceeding 30% is serious, and a shunt fraction approaching 50% indicates a gross degree of venous admixture, and carries a grim prognosis.

■ REGIONAL GAS EXCHANGE IN THE LUNG

Ventilation-perfusion ratios are not exactly identical in all parts of the lung. In a standing individual, ventilation increases slowly from top to bottom of the lung whereas blood flow increases from top to bottom more rapidly. As a result, ventilation blood flow ratios are very high at the top of the lung (blood flow very less) and much lowered at the base of the lung (blood flow more in proportion to the ventilation). The ventilation-perfusion differences can be plotted on an O_2–CO_2 diagram to illustrate the resulting difference in gas exchange.

The lung in a standing individual (**Fig. 6**) *divided into horizontal sections, each of which is located on the ventilation-perfusion line (i.e. the O_2–CO_2 diagram) determined by its own ventilation-perfusion ratio.* This ratio is high at the apex so that the V/Q point is to the right of the line. The ratio is comparatively low at the bottom so that the V/Q point is to the left.

Effects on Arterial Blood Gases in Patients with Well-marked Ventilation-Perfusion Inequality

When there are a number of alveoli with low V/Q ratios, the blood leaving these alveoli will have a low oxygen concentration and a low PaO_2. Even if there are other remaining alveoli which hyperventilate (as compensation) they cannot compensate for low PaO_2 of alveoli with a low V/Q ratio. This is because even if the hyperventilated alveoli have comparatively high PaO_2 (say 110 mm Hg), the hemoglobin (Hb) in the blood is already fully saturated at a PaO_2 of 100 mm Hg so increasing PaO_2 pressure further cannot increase O_2 saturation. On the other hand the high $PaCO_2$ present in blood leaving alveoli with low V/Q ratios (i.e. hypoventilated alveoli) can be compensated for by other hyperventilating alveoli. Hyperventilation is induced by stimulation of the chemoreceptors by the raised $PaCO_2$. It ceases once the $PaCO_2$ is within normal limits.

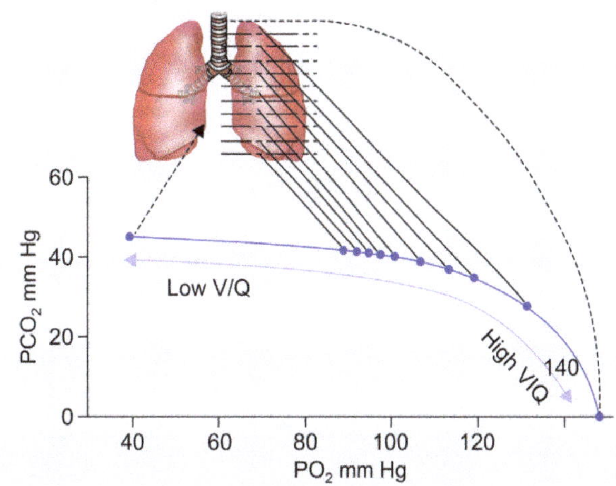

Fig. 6: High ventilation-perfusion ratio at the apex results in a high PaO_2 and low $PaCO_2$. The low ventilation-perfusion ratio at base result in low PaO_2.
Source: With permission from Respiratory Physiology: The Essentials by John B. West, 7th edition. Philadelphia: Lippincott Williams and Wilkins.

■ DISTRIBUTIONS OF VENTILATION-PERFUSION RATIOS

The distribution of ventilation-perfusion ratios in patients with lung disease can be measured by infusing inert dissolved gases with varying solubilities and measuring the concentration of these gases in arterial blood and expired gas. A distribution of ventilation and blood flow plotted against ventilation-perfusion ratios with 50 compartments equally spaced on a log scale is obtained.

Figure 7 illustrates the V/Q ratios with regard to distribution of ventilation and perfusion in a normal adult. The V/Q ratios are close to 1.0 and there is no blood flow to unventilated areas.

Figure 8 shows the same distribution curves in a patient with chronic bronchitis and emphysema. It is noted that there is an increased blood flow to poorly ventilated or nonventilated units leading to decreased V/Q ratios.

■ CONCEPT OF OXYGEN CONTENT AND OXYGEN TRANSPORT

The heart-lung combine working in unison ensures oxygenation of arterial blood. But this is not enough. Blood should have adequate oxygen content, and what is more the oxygen within the blood should be efficiently delivered or transported to tissue cells all over the body. This principle should never lose sight in the management of critically ill patients in the ICU.

■ OXYGEN CONTENT

1 g of Hb combines with 1.39 mL of oxygen at full saturation:

$$O_2 \text{ content} = 1.39 \times Hb \times (\% \text{ saturation}/100) + 0.003 \times PO_2$$

Where, the solubility coefficient of oxygen at 37°C is 0.003 mL/100 mL blood/mm Hg.

The percent saturation of Hb in arterial blood is related to the PaO_2. Oxygen content thus depends on Hb concentration and the PaO_2. The amount of oxygen in solution in plasma is very low (0.3 mL) due to its relative insolubility. Anemia will decrease O_2 content in a linear fashion so that a reduction in Hb from 15 g to 7.5 g/100 mL will reduce arterial oxygen content by one half—i.e. from 21 mL to 10.5 mL. However, a fall in PaO_2 from 90 mm Hg to 45 mm Hg, i.e. by 50% results in just a 20% reduction in the arterial oxygen content. It is evident that significant changes in hemoglobin concentration have a greater influence on CaO_2 than changes in PaO_2.

It is mentioned above that the PaO_2 has an important influence on arterial Hb saturation. There are two other situations (rare though they be) that can also influence Hb saturation. In methemoglobinemia, the iron in the Hb molecule is oxidized to its ferric state; reversible oxygen binding is not possible and Hb is unavailable for oxygen transport. Again, in carbon monoxide poisoning, the Hb molecule avidly binds to carbon monoxide, and can neither bind to oxygen nor offer effective transport.

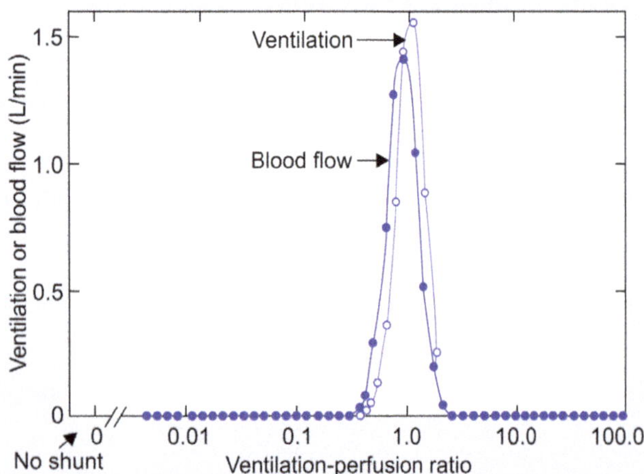

Fig. 7: Distribution of ventilation-perfusion ratios in a young normal subject.
Source: Adapted from Respiratory Physiology: The Essentials by John B. West, 7th edition. Philadelphia: Lippincott Williams and Wilkins.

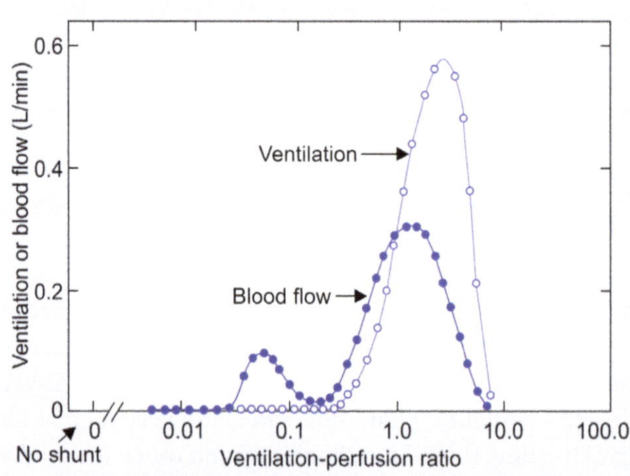

Fig. 8: Distribution of ventilation-perfusion ratios in a patient with chronic bronchitis and emphysema.
Source: Adapted from Respiratory Physiology: The Essentials by John B. West, 7th edition. Philadelphia: Lippincott Williams and Wilkins.

Both these situations are characterized by a normal Hb, a normal PaO_2, but lowered percent of Hb saturation with oxygen, a poor oxygen content and transport.

OXYGEN TRANSPORT

Transport of oxygen to tissues is a vital function of the cardiorespiratory system. A normal arterial oxygenation or oxygen content does not ensure adequate oxygen transport. The latter is crucially dependent on cardiac output.

$$\text{Oxygen transport } (DO_2) = \text{Cardiac output } (Q)$$
$$\times \text{Arterial oxygen content } (CaO_2)$$
$$DO_2 = Q\, CaO_2$$
$$= Q \times (1.39 \times Hb\, SaO_2) \times 10$$

It is to be noted that the dissolved oxygen component is removed and that the factor 10 converts the result to mL/min. If the cardiac index (cardiac output/body surface area) is used instead of the cardiac output, the DO_2 is expressed as $mL/min/m^2$. The normal range for DO_2 is 520–570 $mL/min/m^2$.

It is obvious that both a good cardiac output and satisfactory CaO_2 are necessary for adequate oxygen transport.

FICK PRINCIPLE

The interrelationship between oxygen transport and oxygen utilization ($\dot{V}O_2$) was described by Fick in 1872.

$$\dot{V}O_2 = Q_T \times C\,(a-v)O_2$$

i.e. oxygen consumption = cardiac output × arteriovenous oxygen content difference.

The normal range for $\dot{V}O_2$ is 110–160 $mL/min/m^2$.

An increase in oxygen consumption ($\dot{V}O_2$) by the tissues is brought about by an increase in the Q_T, so that the arteriovenous oxygen content difference remains the same (normally about 4–5 mL). If for some reason the cardiac output does not increase appropriately, then the step-up in $\dot{V}O_2$ is met by an increase in oxygen extraction by the tissues, i.e. by an increase in the arteriovenous oxygen content difference. The equation in Fick's principle thus remains unaltered, and well balanced. A widened arteriovenous oxygen content difference (i.e. a lowered PvO_2 and SvO_2) occurs in the following conditions in critical care medicine.

- An inadequate cardiac output for tissue needs.
- Very low arterial oxygen content, as with severe anemia.

- When tissue demands for oxygen are so great that the normal circulatory system cannot keep pace with excessive tissue demands. This could happen for example in patients with uncontrolled seizures in fulminant tetanus.

As mentioned above, the increased extraction of oxygen by tissues from the blood, leads to a lowered PvO_2 and SvO_2. The normal PvO_2 is 35–40 mm Hg, and the SvO_2 is 75%. There is a reserve which allows for a fall in PvO_2 to about 20 mm Hg, and the SvO_2 to 25–30%, in conditions characterized by a very low cardiac output, while still enabling diffusion of oxygen at a level that prevents cellular death **(Fig. 9)**.

In critical care settings, the PvO_2 and the SvO_2 can thus act as indicators for adequacy or inadequacy of cardiac output and tissue perfusion **(Table 1)**.

Underlying Fick's principle is the concept that VO_2 is governed by tissue needs and not by oxygen delivery

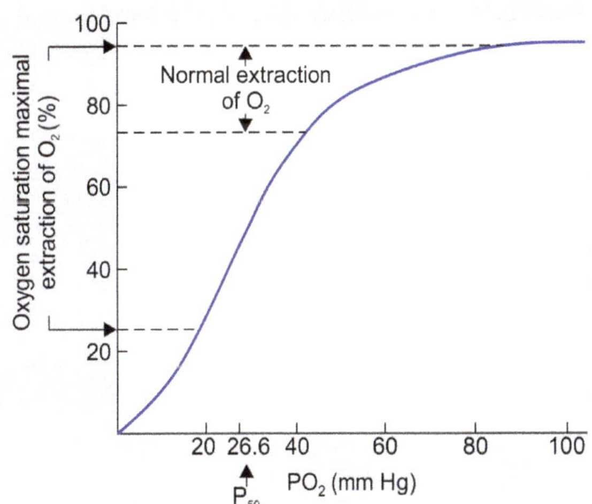

Fig. 9: The normal oxyhemoglobin dissociation curve ($P_{50} = 26.6$ mm Hg). At a normal PaO_2, O_2 saturation is close to 100%. At a PaO_2 of 40 mm Hg (venous blood), O_2 saturation is about 75%. Maximum O_2 extraction allows a reserve down to about 25%, corresponding to a PaO_2 about 20 mm Hg.
Source: From Udwadia FE. Principles of Critical Care Medicine, 3rd edition. New Delhi: Jaypee Brothers Medical Publishers; 2014.

Table 1: PvO_2 and SvO_2 as indicators of cardiac output and tissue perfusion adequacy.

PvO_2 (mm Hg)	SvO_2 (%)	Clinical state
36–42	71–79	Normal range
>45	>80	Septic shock
<30	<50	Lactic acidosis
<17	<20	Neural damage

(DO_2). However, below a critical level of oxygen delivery, $\dot{V}O_2$ *does* depend on oxygen supply. It was earlier believed that in certain pathological states like sepsis, septic shock, acute respiratory distress syndrome, $\dot{V}O_2$ was dependent on DO_2 at all levels of oxygen delivery. The current though not universal consensus is that this is not really so. Nevertheless, the importance of ensuring adequate oxygen transport in the management of critically ill patients cannot be overemphasized.

■ OXYGEN EXTRACTION RATIO (O_2 ER)

The oxygen extraction ratio (O_2 ER) is the ratio of oxygen uptake to oxygen delivery ($\dot{V}O_2/DO_2$). It signifies the fraction of oxygen taken up by the tissues; the normal O_2 ER is 0.2–0.3, i.e. 20–30%. Oxygen extraction can vary. It increases when the increased demand for oxygen by tissue is not met by an increase in cardiac output. In trained athletes the O_2 ER may be as high as 0.8 at maximal exercise. In diseased states like severe sepsis, multiple organ dysfunctions, acute respiratory distress syndrome, oxygen extraction by tissue cells can be poor in spite of adequate oxygen supply.

■ SUGGESTED READING

1. Hsia CC, Hyde DM, Weibel ER, et al. Lung structure and the intrinsic challenges of gas exchange. Compr Physiol. 2016;6(2):827-95.
2. Petersson J, Glenny RW. Gas exchange and ventilation-perfusion relationships in the lung. Eur Respir J. 2014;44(4):1023-41.
3. Udwadia FE. Basic cardiorespiratory physiology in the intensive care unit. In: Udwadia FE (Ed). Principles of Critical Care, 3rd edition. New Delhi: Oxford University Press; 2005.
4. West JB. Gas transport by the blood in "Respiratory Physiology: The Essentials", 9th edition. Philadelphia: Lippincott Williams and Wilkins; 2006.
5. West JB. Ventilation/Blood Flow and Gas Exchange, 7th edition. Oxford: Blackwell, UK; 1990.
6. West JB. Ventilation-Perfusion Relationship in "Respiratory Physiology: The Essentials", 9th edition. Philadelphia: Lippincott Williams and Wilkins; 2006.

CHAPTER 4

Acid-base Balance and Control of Ventilation

■ GENERAL CONSIDERATIONS

The maintenance of normal acid-base balance (pH 7.35–7.45) in the blood is of crucial importance and is a vital homeostatic function of the body. Any variation from the normal constitutes an emergency in that a significant change in the H^+ ion concentration of the plasma or the extracellular fluid is incompatible with life; a pH < 7, or a pH > 7.8 spells imminent danger and death.

Acid-base disturbances occur very frequently in patients who are critically ill. It is of vital importance to bear in mind the fact that in patients with respiratory disease, acid-base disturbances and changes in pH may not solely be related to respiratory failure and adverse alterations in lung function. Many of these patients, particularly when critically ill, have associated metabolic problems as also problems associated with other organ systems that can independently influence and alter acid-base equilibrium. These independent alterations in acid-base balance may at times worsen alterations produced by respiratory disease, yet at times may counter them. Hence the great importance for respiratory physicians to have an overall perspective of acid-base disturbances rather than a mere awareness of changes seen in respiratory failure and respiratory disease. This chapter first deals with the basic physiology underlying acid-base balance. It then goes on to briefly describe acid-base disturbances with special reference to those caused by respiratory diseases. It then gives a brief discussion based on illustrative case studies on mixed acid-base disturbances often encountered in patients with respiratory disease and respiratory failure.

The manifestations of an altered acid-base homeostasis in such patients are often subtle, virtually impossible to clinically detect, and are often masked by the clinical features of the illness. There are no barriers to these disturbances; they are encountered in all fields and all specialties of medicine and surgery. Not uncommonly, the realization that sudden clinical deterioration or death in a particular patient may have been related to acid-base disturbances dawns on the physician a trifle too late. An early diagnosis of a change in acid-base equilibrium demands a sharp clinical acumen, a grasp of the physiopathology underlying these changes, and an intelligent interpretation of laboratory data.

No satisfactory assessment of the presence and degree of acid-base disturbances can be made without measuring the pH of the blood by the pH electrode. It is imperative that the importance of pH and acid-base measurements through a blood gas machine using the Astrup technique is universally recognized in all developing countries. Today, though many critical care units in the large metropolitan cities of India provide this very necessary facility, most critical care units in smaller cities lack this basic amenity. It is also unfortunate that many doctors are unable to correctly appreciate the results provided by this technique. Most students and doctors are taught to interpret arterial blood gases and acid-base disturbances by rule of the thumb or by reference to standard charts and graphs which allow a prompt solution for the basic problem. This may be satisfactory—but only to a point. Correct interpretation of blood gases and acid-base disturbances necessitates a familiarity with the basic physiology in this field. Then only can altered physiology be better understood. Intelligent and in-depth interpretation leads to a more rational management of the patient as a whole.

■ BASIC CONCEPTS

Concept of an Acid

An acid is a potential H^+ ion or proton donor. Conversely a base is a potential proton acceptor.

The strength of an acid (HA) is measured by the extent to which it dissociates in an aqueous solution.

$$HA \rightleftharpoons [H^+] + [A^-]$$

When the above reaction is in equilibrium, for a strong acid $(H^+) + (A^-)$ will be in a greater concentration than HA in the undissociated form. Also, at equilibrium, the product of the concentration on one side of the equation will bear a constant relationship to the product of concentration on the other.

$$Ka = \frac{[H^+]\,[A^-]}{[HA]}$$

where, Ka is the acid dissociation constant. Strong acids have a high Ka. Similar equations would apply to the dissociation of a base.

Concept of pH

The acidity of an aqueous solution is measured by its hydrogen (H^+) ion concentration or activity. The H^+ activity is expressed as pH. This terminology was introduced to simplify the expression of a wide range of H ions found in various fluids within the body. A quantification of H ions in various fluids in moles would have been cumbersome and difficult. The notation pH is the negative logarithm of H ion concentration. This allows a large range of H^+ concentrations to be simply expressed and measured. Thus,

$$pH = \frac{1}{[H^+]}$$
$$= -\log 10\,[H^+]$$
$$= \text{Negative exponent of an expression of}$$
$$[H^+] \text{ to the power 10}$$

Thus, a pH of $7.4 = (H^+) \times 10^{-7.4}$

The normal H^+ ion concentration of blood is 40 nanomoles/L or 40×10^{-9} moles/L. This is equivalent to a pH of 7.4. Changes in acid-base balance can be looked upon either as changes in the H ion concentration or changes in pH. **Table 1** given below shows the H ion concentration in relation to the corresponding pH values.

Table 1: Correlation between H^+ ion concentration and pH values.

H ion concentration (nmoles/l)	pH
10	8.00
20	7.70
30	7.52
40	7.40
50	7.30
60	7.22
70	7.15
80	7.10
90	7.05
100	7.00

The Henderson-Hasselbalch Equation

In the earlier section on the concept of an acid, it has been noted that:

$$Ka = \frac{[H^+]\,[A^-]}{[HA]}$$

If we wish to express H ion concentration (H^+) as pH (log 1/H), we may rewrite the above:

$$[H^+] = Ka \frac{[HA]}{[A^-]}$$

Taking reciprocals,

$$\frac{1}{[H^+]} = \frac{1}{Ka} \times \frac{[A^-]}{[HA]}$$

Taking logs,

$$\log \frac{1}{[H^+]} = \log \frac{1}{Ka} + \log \frac{[A^-]}{[HA]}$$

i.e.

$$pH = pKa + \log \frac{[A^-]}{[HA]}$$

where, pKa is the negative logarithm of the dissociation constant Ka. The above is the Henderson-Hasselbalch equation.

Buffers

Buffers are substances which react with an acid or base and thereby minimize changes in pH. The metabolic processes within the body add a daily load of H ions to the body. These H ions if not properly dealt with within the body would produce a disastrous rise in H ion concentration, and a catastrophic fall in the pH. The homeostasis of acid-base balance however remains unchanged because of the buffering systems within the body and due to the role of the kidneys.

The main buffer systems of the body are:

- Hemoglobin and to a much lesser extent organic phosphates within the red blood cells.
- Bicarbonates and inorganic phosphates within the blood.
- Plasma proteins
- Tissue proteins
- Minerals (phosphates, carbonates) within the bones.

It is only possible in this chapter to deal with the bicarbonate-carbonic acid buffer systems. The reader is referred to a standard textbook on Physiology for a more thorough understanding of the subject.

The bicarbonate-carbonic acid reaction is important in regulating acid-base balance. It constitutes a weak buffer system which can be used as a measure or reflection of all acid-base reactions within the body, because buffer systems are in dynamic equilibrium, and carbon dioxide diffuses freely across all tissues and membranes. Also, these chemical reactions occur very rapidly.

The carbon dioxide (CO_2) produced by tissue metabolism diffuses into plasma and the red blood cells (RBCs). The enzyme carbonic anhydrase within the RBCs catalyzes the formation of carbonic acid:

$$H_2O + CO_2 = H_2CO_3$$

The carbonic acid within the RBCs is dissociated thus:

$$H_2CO_3 \rightleftharpoons H^+ + HCO_3^-$$

The bicarbonate within the RBCs diffuses out into the plasma, while the H ions are mopped up by the hemoglobin which acts as a buffer base. The loss of one ion from the cell has to be compensated by the entry of an equivalent ion. Thus chloride ions (Cl^-) from the plasma enter the red blood cells in place of the bicarbonate ions which have diffused out into the plasma.

When the blood reaches the lungs, the chloride shift is reversed and bicarbonate enters the red blood cells. The bicarbonate within the RBCs breaks down into H_2O and CO_2. The CO_2 diffuses out through the capillaries into the alveoli, and is washed out into the outside air.

The bicarbonate-carbonic reaction can be looked at from another angle as regards the role it plays in controlling acid-base balance. Thus, when H^+ enters tissue fluids:

$$H^+ + HCO_3^- \rightleftharpoons H_2CO_3 \rightleftharpoons CO_2 + H_2O$$

The CO_2 is rapidly washed out via the lungs leading to a rapid control of H ion production, but of course at the expense of a fall in (HCO_3).

The Henderson-Hasselbalch equation for the bicarbonate-carbonic acid reaction aptly illustrates the role played by this reaction in regulating acid-base balance.

$$pH = pK + \log \frac{HCO_3^-}{H_2CO_3}$$

$$= 6.1 + \log \frac{HCO_3^-}{H_2CO_3}$$

$$= 6.1 + \log \frac{HCO_3^-}{0.03 \times PCO_2}$$

where, 0.03 is the solubility of CO_2 in plasma, and PCO_2 the partial pressure of CO_2 in plasma.

If instead of pH one considers the H ion concentration, then the following modification of the Henderson-Hasselbalch equation can be used.

$$[H^+] = 24 \times \frac{PCO_2}{HCO_3} \text{ nmol/L}$$

Normally, (H^+) = $24 \times 40/24$ = 40 nmol/L (pH 7.4).

The Henderson–Hasselbalch equation expresses the relationship between three reactants—H^+, HCO_3^- and PCO_2, and can be used as an expression of acid-base balance within the body.

■ ROLE OF THE KIDNEYS IN ACID-BASE BALANCE

The kidneys play a crucial role in H ion regulation. They do so in the following ways:

- Regulating excretion and reabsorption of bicarbonate (HCO^-). Bicarbonate is filtered by the glomerulus, the quantity of bicarbonate in the filtrate being dependent on the plasma bicarbonate, and the glomerular filtration rate. The bicarbonate is then dealt with as follows:
  - Reabsorption of bicarbonate in the proximal renal tubules at a rate which is dependent on the PCO_2. The higher the PCO_2, the greater the degree of bicarbonate reabsorption; the lower the PCO_2, the lesser the degree of reabsorption of bicarbonate, and the greater its excretion. This enables respiratory acidosis (due to a high $PaCO_2$) to be compensated through retention of bicarbonate, and respiratory alkalosis (due to a low $PaCO_2$) to be compensated by an increased excretion

of bicarbonate (*see* subsections on Respiratory Acidosis and Respiratory Alkalosis).

– In metabolic acidosis, H ions are excreted into the urine. The enzyme carbonic anhydrase catalyzes the reaction:

$$H^+ + HCO_3^- \rightleftharpoons H_2CO_3 \rightleftharpoons H_2O + CO_2$$

The CO_2 is reabsorbed and is excreted through the lungs. This is an important means by which the pH is controlled.

- *Use of buffering systems*: H ions can be mopped up by phosphate buffers, thus tending to increase the pH, while at the same time conserving bicarbonate.

Thus, under the influence of carbonic anhydrase,

$$H^+ + HCO_3^- \rightleftharpoons H_2CO_3 (\text{in the tubular cells})$$

$$H_2CO_3 \rightleftharpoons HCO_3^- + H^+$$

The bicarbonate ion is reabsorbed. The H ion is mopped up by $NaHPO_4$ thus—

$$H^+ + NaHPO_4 \rightleftharpoons NaH_2PO_4$$

which is excreted via the urine.

- Ammonia. NH_4^+ is formed in the tubular cells by conversion of glutamine to glutamate. Thus,

$$
\begin{array}{ccc}
CONH_2 & & COO^- \\
| & & | \\
(CH_2)_2 & & (CH_2)_2 \\
| & +H_2O \rightleftharpoons NH_4^+ + & | \\
CHNH_3 & & CHNH_3 \\
| & & | \\
COO^- & & COO^- \\
\text{GLUTAMINE} & & \text{GLUTAMATE}
\end{array}
$$

NH_4^+ combines with chloride and is excreted via the urine, the reaction being controlled by the enzyme glutaminase. NH_4^+ excretion to be fully operative takes time. It is however an extremely important mechanism for pH control, as excretion of ammonia allows the excretion of a significantly large quantity of H ions via the kidney.

- *Reabsorption of sodium*: The active reabsorption of sodium from the filtrate into tubule cells causes a potential gradient across the cell membrane. The positively charged H ion within the tubule cell thus passes across the membrane into the filtrate, and is buffered within the filtrate by a phosphate buffer.

$$H^+ + NaHPO_4 \rightleftharpoons NaH_2PO_4$$

In summary, the kidneys help to maintain acid-base balance in the following ways:

- Retention of bicarbonate when the PCO_2 increases.
- Excretion of bicarbonate when the PCO_2 falls.
- Reabsorption of bicarbonate when there is accumulation of H ions in the blood.
- Excretion of titratable acid and NH_4 to counter an increase of H ions in the blood.
- Excretion of H ions when there is a primary loss of bicarbonate.
- Increased bicarbonate excretion in the urine, together with a loss of K^+ in the urine, when there is a primary increase in plasma bicarbonate.

■ DISTURBANCES IN ACID-BASE BALANCE

Terminology

Terms used: Acidemia, alkalemia, acidosis, alkalosis.

The normal pH of arterial blood is maintained within the range of 7.35 to 7.45.

Acidemia exists when the pH of arterial blood is below the normal range, i.e. less than 7.35.

Alkalemia is the state in which pH of arterial blood is above the normal range, i.e. greater than 7.45.

Acidosis is an abnormal state leading to an increase in the acid in the body.

Alkalosis is an abnormal state leading to a fall in acid or an increase in the alkali in the body.

When acidosis induces compensatory changes in the body so that pH remains within the normal range, it is termed compensatory acidosis. When acidosis produces a fall in pH below 7.35, it is termed uncompensated acidosis. Uncompensated acidosis and acidemia are thus synonymous.

Similarly, alkalosis can be compensated or uncompensated, and alkalemia is synonymous with the latter.

Acidosis and alkalosis (as also acidemia and alkalemia) may result from primary respiratory or metabolic disturbances so that we have respiratory acidosis and metabolic acidosis, as also respiratory alkalosis and metabolic alkalosis.

Respiratory acidosis and respiratory acidemia (uncompensated respiratory acidosis) result from alveolar hypoventilation which leads to hypercapnia.

Respiratory alkalosis and respiratory alkalemia (uncompensated respiratory alkalosis) result from alveolar hyperventilation which causes hypocapnia.

Metabolic acidosis and metabolic acidemia are caused by either accumulation of acid or loss of base from the body.

Metabolic alkalosis and metabolic alkalemia are due to accumulation of base or loss of acid from the body.

Mixed acid-base disturbances are caused by a combination of respiratory and metabolic factors.

■ LABORATORY DIAGNOSIS OF DISTURBANCES IN ACID-BASE EQUILIBRIUM

Estimation of Serum Electrolytes

This is mandatory in every patient with acid-base disturbances, as electrolyte abnormalities are frequently seen and are often inseparable from changes in acid-base balance.

Interpretation of pH and Acid-base Measurements by the Astrup Technique

In this technique, the pH and PCO_2 of the blood are measured by a sensitive instrument (radiometer). The values of standard bicarbonate, actual bicarbonate, CO_2 content, and base excess or deficit are then read from a standard nomogram. These concepts are briefly explained below.

The standard bicarbonate is the bicarbonate content in the plasma of blood which has been equilibrated at a PCO_2 of 40 mm Hg, as also with oxygen so as to saturate it with oxygen. The standard bicarbonate is a measure of the nonrespiratory bicarbonate. It is the most active, mobile, rapidly reacting fraction of the total buffer potential, and its rate of excretion and retention is governed by the kidneys. A fall in the standard bicarbonate therefore indicates a metabolic acidosis; conversely a rise in the standard bicarbonate indicates a metabolic alkalosis. Normal standard bicarbonate indicates metabolic equilibrium.

The actual bicarbonate content is the bicarbonate concentration in mEq or mmoles/L in the plasma. It is not directly estimated; its value is derived from a nomogram in the Astrup technique, or from the CO_2 content of blood which can be estimated by the Van Slyke apparatus.

The CO_2 content of plasma is the actual bicarbonate content + dissolved CO_2. As stated above, it can be estimated by gasometry (Van Slyke apparatus), or is derived from a nomogram if the pH and $PaCO_2$ are known.

Base excess defines the presence in blood of excess or deficit of base, the physiological range being ± 2.3 mEq/L. It denotes the amount of strong acid or base per liter of blood, which has been added as a consequence of a metabolic disturbance. It is an in vitro concept, and is again derived from a nomogram if the pH and $PaCO_2$ are known.

Some of the terms described above are apt to prove confusing to the resident training in respiratory medicine. For purposes of simplification, acid-base changes are best interpreted by a consideration of the Henderson–Hasselbalch equation:

$$pH = pK + \log \frac{HCO_3^-}{PCO_2 \times 0.03}$$

In other words, pH is the "balance" between the respiratory parameter represented by $PaCO_2$ (controlled by the lungs) and the metabolic parameter represented by bicarbonate (controlled by the kidneys). This is most simply illustrated in **Figure 1**. The PO_2 ($PaCO_2$) in this illustration and in subsequent illustrations is in mm Hg and the bicarbonate is in mEq/L.

A primary change in the respiratory parameter (partial pressure of carbon dioxide in arterial blood, $PaCO_2$) disturbs the "balance" illustrated in **Figure 1** to produce respiratory acid-base disturbances; a primary change in the metabolic parameter (bicarbonate) disturbs the balance and produces metabolic acid-base disturbances.

A rise in $PaCO_2$ primarily due to alveolar hypoventilation causes respiratory acidosis, and when this acidosis

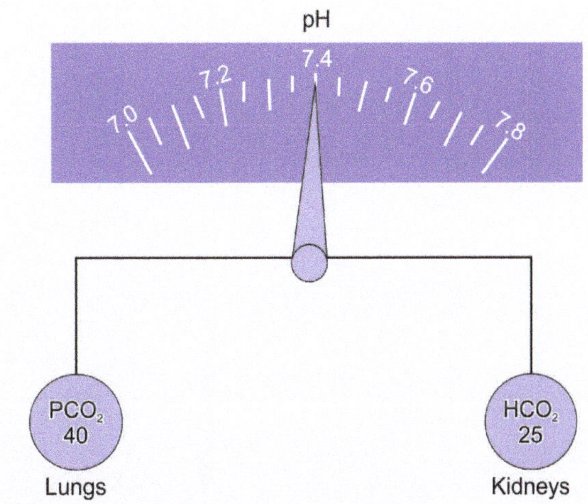

Fig. 1: Normal acid-base balance.

lowers the pH to less than 7.35, respiratory acidemia results. A fall in $PaCO_2$ produced by hyperventilation induces respiratory alkalosis and if the pH rises to greater than 7.45, respiratory alkalemia results.

Homeostasis demands that primary changes in $PaCO_2$ lead to secondary changes in the plasma bicarbonate, so that the pH is kept within the normal range as far as possible. An acute rise in $PaCO_2$ (due to sudden hypoventilation following poisoning or a near respiratory arrest), will lead to a very small rise in the plasma bicarbonate (*see* earlier description on bicarbonate-carbonic acid reaction). The degree of retention of plasma bicarbonate is just 0.1 mmole or 0.1 mEq per 1 mm Hg rise in $PaCO_2$. The standard bicarbonate will remain unchanged. This can produce a gross imbalance between the respiratory and metabolic parameters, and can lead to a sharp and dangerous fall in pH. This is illustrated in **Figure 2**.

On the other hand, a slow or chronic rise in $PaCO_2$ (so frequently observed in patients with chronic airways obstruction) allows renal compensation to come into play. The kidneys retain bicarbonate—3 to 4 mEq or mmoles/L being retained for every 10 mm Hg rise in $PaCO_2$. Significant bicarbonate retention thus compensates for the chronic rise in $PaCO_2$, and helps to preserve the "balance". Retention of bicarbonate by the kidneys takes time; it probably starts 4-6 hours after the rise in $PaCO_2$, and is complete after 1-3 days. Compensation however can only occur up to a point—a rise in $PaCO_2$ > 65-70 mm Hg is generally associated with a fall in pH below normal in spite of bicarbonate retention. The degree of rise in bicarbonate enables one to determine whether in a given patient the respiratory acidosis is acute or chronic. Uncompensated respiratory acidosis and compensated respiratory acidosis (respiratory acidemia) are illustrated in **Figures 2 and 3** respectively.

Comparison of degrees of rise in bicarbonate in vivo due to acute and chronic rise in $PaCO_2$ is illustrated in **Figure 4**.

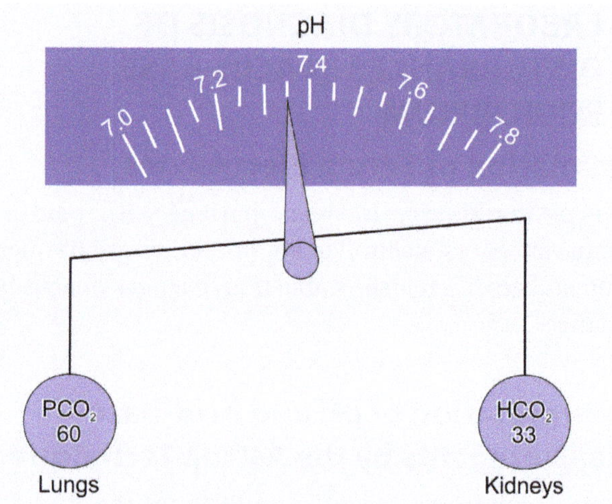

Fig. 3: Compensated respiratory acidosis.

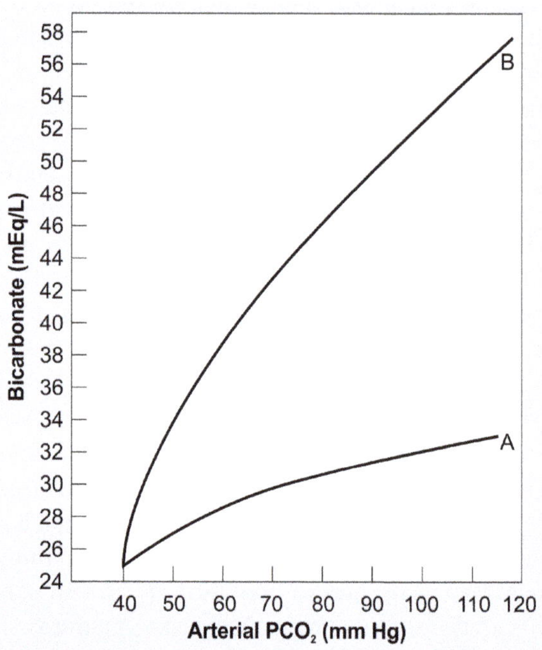

Fig. 4: Comparison curves showing rise in bicarbonate levels in vivo chronic and acute hypercapnia. A = rise in acute hypercapnia. B = rise in chronic hypercapnia, because of retention of bicarbonate by the kidney.

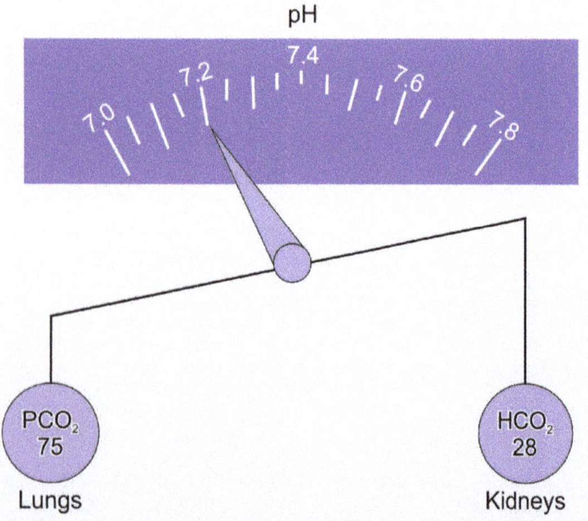

Fig. 2: Uncompensated respiratory acidosis and acidemia.

A fall in $PaCO_2$ primarily due to alveolar hyperventilation leads to a compensatory fall in plasma bicarbonate, the degree of fall approximating 0.1–0.3 mmoles/L for 1 mm Hg fall in $PaCO_2$. Acid-base balance in acute, uncompensated respiratory alkalosis is illustrated in **Figure 5**.

When primary metabolic problems produce a fall in bicarbonate, metabolic acidosis results. When the pH falls to less than 7.35, metabolic acidemia results.

Metabolic alkalosis results following retention of bicarbonate due to metabolic causes; metabolic alkalemia ensues when the pH rises to greater than 7.45.

Primary metabolic changes in bicarbonate result in secondary changes in $PaCO_2$, thus minimizing changes in the pH. Thus metabolic acidosis stimulates the respiratory center, and the resulting hyperventilation reduces the $PaCO_2$. The degree of compensatory fall in $PaCO_2$ roughly equals 1.2 mm Hg for every 1 mmole or mEq/L fall in bicarbonate (or roughly equals 1.5 × bicarbonate content + 8). On the other hand, metabolic alkalosis depresses the respiratory center and produces a compensatory rise in $PaCO_2$, the degree of rise being 0.6–1 mm Hg for 1 mmole or mEq/L rise in bicarbonate. The expected $PaCO_2$ can also be considered as = 0.7 × $(HCO_3) + 20$ (±1.5). **Figures 6 and 7** illustrate compensated metabolic acid-base disturbances.

Mixed Acid-base Disturbances

Acid-base disturbances in critically ill patients are often due to both respiratory and metabolic problems occurring independently. They are often observed in patients with both acute and chronic respiratory failure. A consideration of the clinical picture, the pH, $PaCO_2$ and bicarbonate, invariably clarifies the diagnosis. The degree of compensation present in relation to bicarbonate in primary respiratory disturbances, and the degree of compensation present in relation to $PaCO_2$ in primary metabolic problems, enables one to judge whether acid-base disturbances are due to mixed causes. The examples briefly quoted below help to give a more practical understanding of the problems involved.

A patient with chronic bronchitis emphysema deteriorated over a period of weeks, and was admitted to

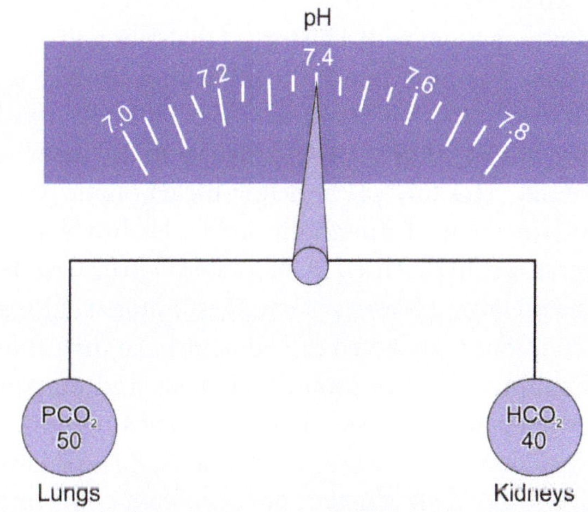

Fig. 6: Compensated metabolic alkalosis.

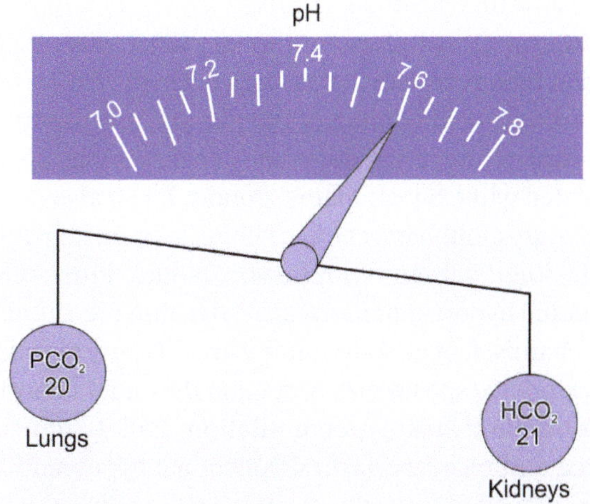

Fig. 5: Acute uncompensated respiratory alkalosis.

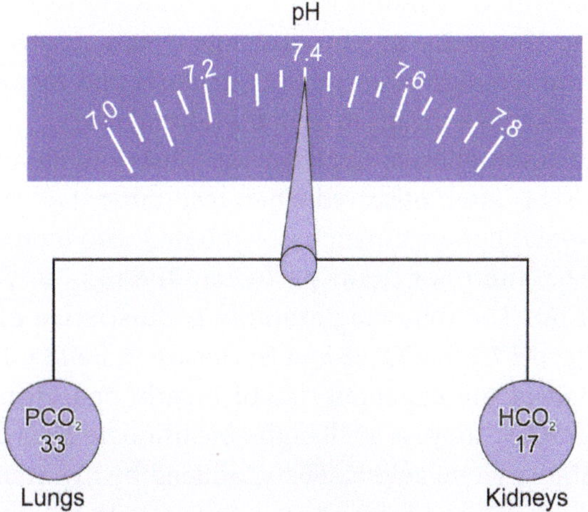

Fig. 7: Compensated metabolic acidosis.

hospital in a critically ill condition with acute respiratory failure. The $PaCO_2$ was 82 mm Hg, PaO_2 34 mm Hg, pH 7.15, bicarbonate 26 mEq/L. This patient obviously had respiratory acidosis ($PaCO_2$ 82 mm Hg). However, in a slowly deteriorating respiratory problem the rise in $PaCO_2$ should have been offset by a rise in plasma bicarbonate at a rate of 4 mEq/L for every 10 mm Hg rise in $PaCO_2$, i.e. approximately 40 mEq/L. Even in severe acute respiratory failure, the bicarbonate should increase at a rate of 1 mEq/L for every 10 mm Hg rise in $PaCO_2$. The low bicarbonate associated with the high $PaCO_2$ seen in this patient, is therefore due to an associated metabolic acidosis, possibly due to severe hypoxemia inducing a lactic acid acidosis. The combination of respiratory acidosis and metabolic acidosis was responsible for the sharp fall in pH to 7.15.

Another patient with a history of diabetes and chronic bronchitis was admitted to hospital in a drowsy state. His pH was 7.21, $PaCO_2$ 42 mm Hg, PaO_2 50 mm Hg, bicarbonate 14 mEq/L. He had ketosis in the urine with ketonemia. The low pH and low bicarbonate pointed to the presence of metabolic acidosis; however, the comparatively high $PaCO_2$ (it should ordinarily have been 28 mm Hg) indicates an associated respiratory acidosis.

A frequently observed mixed acid-base disturbance is a combination of respiratory acidosis and metabolic alkalosis in patients with chronic airways obstruction, who are hypokalemic due to the use of diuretics. The following example in a patient with the above problem is illustrative: pH 7.44; $PaCO_2$ 60 mm Hg; bicarbonate 38 mEq/L; serum K^+ 3 mEq/L. A $PaCO_2$ of 60 mm Hg points to respiratory acidosis. However, the rise in the bicarbonate significantly exceeds the maximum of 0.4 mEq/mm Hg rise in the $PaCO_2$. This is due to a hypokalemic metabolic alkalosis. The combination of respiratory acidosis and metabolic alkalosis allows the pH to be in the normal range.

A combination of respiratory acidosis and metabolic acidosis is often observed when respiratory failure due to alveolar hypoventilation is combined with increasing hypoxia and poor tissue perfusion due to poor pump function. The following example is illustrative of this profile: pH 7.1; $PaCO_2$ 55 mm Hg; bicarbonate 15 mEq/L. Instead of the expected rise in bicarbonate due to a high $PaCO_2$, there is a fall in the bicarbonate because of metabolic lactic acid acidosis induced by hypotension and poor tissue perfusion in a patient with respiratory failure.

A combination of respiratory alkalosis and metabolic alkalosis is at times observed in hepatic failure. The latter causes tachypnea with respiratory alkalosis. If there is associated vomiting, or there is aspiration of gastric contents through a nasogastric tube, the loss of H ions, K^+ and chloride leads to an associated metabolic alkalosis. The following example is illustrative: pH 7.61; $PaCO_2$ 25 mm Hg; bicarbonate 34 mEq/L.

A combination of respiratory alkalosis and metabolic acidosis may occur in septic shock and also in terminal acute liver cell failure. Both these conditions can cause tachypnea with respiratory alkalosis. The metabolic (lactic acid) acidosis is related to shock and poor tissue perfusion. The same combination is often observed in patients who are hyperventilated on mechanical ventilation (with resulting respiratory alkalosis), and who are hypotensive from shock or poor pump function (which causes lactic acid acidosis).

Arterial pH of blood gases and bicarbonate levels should always be interpreted with reference to the history, clinical findings, and other investigations in every individual problem. Occasionally, the complexity of an acid-base disturbance is only apparent on a follow-up of the patient.

Clinical Features and Management of Acid-Base Disturbances

The clinical features and management of metabolic acidosis and metabolic alkalosis are not considered in this chapter. The respiratory physician should however be fully conversant with these metabolic disturbances.

Respiratory acidosis is discussed in the chapter on Acute Respiratory Failure. Respiratory alkalosis results from alveolar hyperventilation causing a fall in the $PaCO_2$ and in the carbonic acid content of the plasma. It is observed in hysterical or functional states and in patients who are over-ventilated while on ventilator support. It can also occur in pulmonary embolism, cardiac failure, in brainstem lesions and in some patients with hepatic failure. Purposeful or functional hyperventilation can lead to tingling, numbness of the hands, feet and circumoral area. Tetany manifested by carpopedal spasm may occur and the patient may faint. Fainting abolishes hyperventilation; $PaCO_2$ returns to normal and recovery ensues. Functional hyperventilation is best managed by asking the patients to rebreathe into a paper bag, and by reassurance.

CONTROL OF VENTILATION

The main function of the lung is to ensure efficient gas exchange of oxygen and carbon dioxide so as to maintain normal levels of PaO_2 and $PaCO_2$. This holds true not only with a subject at rest but in numerous conditions with varying demands of oxygen uptake and CO_2 output made by the body. The maintenance of gas exchange under varying conditions is only possible because of a fine control over ventilation.

Ventilation control has three elements:

1. A sensory system which feeds sensory inputs to a central controlling mechanism.
2. A central controlling mechanism in the brainstem which receives these sensory inputs and then sends out coordinated nervous impulses to the effector system.
3. *Effector system*: This system consists of respiratory muscles which effect ventilation.

CENTRAL CONTROLLING SYSTEM

The central controlling system is the respiratory center in the brainstem. This center consists of loosely arranged groups of neurons. It has three components, i.e. three groups of neurons exerting ventilation control—the medullary center, the apneustic center in the lower pons and the pneumotaxic center in the upper pons.

Medullary Respiratory Center

This center lies in the reticular formation of the brainstem, beneath the floor of the fourth ventricle. The dorsal group of neurons controls inspiration and the ventral group expiration. It is believed that the medullary respiratory center has an inherent intrinsic rhythm which enables it to fire repetitive nervous impulses to the effector system (the diaphragm and inspiratory muscles). The medullary center is responsible for the basic rhythm of ventilation and this rhythm persists even when all afferent stimuli to the center are abolished.

The intrinsic rhythmicity of the medullary center is characterized by a latent period followed by a progressive increase in the discharge of action potentials causing neuronal impulses to reach the muscle of inspiration. During this progressive increase in neuronal discharge from the center, there follows a progressive increase in the strength of contraction of the inspiratory muscles. Then the action potential from the center to the inspiratory muscles

is turned off and expiration begins. In normal resting conditions, expiration consists of a passive relaxation of the chest wall to a position of equilibrium which is at functional residual capacity (FRC) level. However, active expiration as for example in exercise is related to action potentials discharged from the ventral group of nuclei beneath the floor of the fourth ventricles.

Apneustic Center

The apneustic center consists of loosely grouped neurons in the lower pons. The center is so named because if a transection of the brain is made above this center in experimental animals, respiration is characterized by prolonged respiratory efforts or gasps (apneuses) interrupted by transient respiratory efforts. It appears that this center influences the dorsal neurons in the medulla controlling inspiration, tending to prolong the progressively increasing action potentials arising in this medullary center. It is uncertain whether the apneustic center plays a role in control of ventilation. However, lesions in the pons are known to produce the breathing (apneustic breathing) described above.

Pneumotaxic Center

Pneumotaxic center is in the upper pons. This center has the ability to terminate the inspiratory action potential of the inspiratory medullary center, thereby regulating the volume and rate of ventilation. It is believed to "fine-tune" the inspiratory center in the medulla.

Cortex

The cortex can exert voluntary control over ventilation to an extent, overriding the brainstem centers. This is evident when one considers voluntary hyperventilation which can be powerful enough to substantially reduce the $PaCO_2$. Voluntary hypoventilation is also possible though not to the same extent as hyperventilation, probably because of the effects of a lowered PaO_2 and an increased $PaCO_2$.

Influence of centers in the cerebrum other than the cortex is evinced by changes in ventilation produced by emotion, fear, rage which probably are related to the limbic system and the hypothalamus.

Sensory System

Sensory receptors which on stimulation relay afferent nervous impulses to the regulating center in the brainstem consist of central chemoreceptors, peripheral chemoreceptors and lung receptors.

Central Chemoreceptors

Central chemoreceptors respond to changes in the chemical composition or the pH of the fluid or blood around them. They are situated below the ventral surface of the fourth ventricle in close proximity to the medullary respiratory center and are of crucial importance in control of ventilation. The central chemoreceptors are bathed in the extracellular fluid of the brain, the composition of which is determined by local blood supply, local metabolism and the cerebrospinal fluid (CSF). The CSF is the most important governing factor. It is separated from the blood by the blood-brain barrier, which is comparatively impermeable to H^+ ions and HCO_3 ions but easily permeable to CO_2. When the PCO_2 rises, CO_2 diffuses through the blood-brain barrier into the CSF; H^+ ions are liberated and these H^+ ions stimulate the chemoreceptors. A rise in PCO_2 in the blood therefore chiefly stimulates ventilation through its effect on the H^+ ions and pH of the CSF. The increased ventilation serves to reduce the PCO_2 in the blood and thereby also reduce the CO_2 and H^+ ions' concentration in the CSF.

It should be noted that the change in CSF pH for a given increase in PCO_2 is much greater than the pH change in blood, because the CSF has much lower buffering capacity compared to blood. If pH in the CSF is lowered for a prolonged period, compensation takes place by diffusion of HCO_3 through the blood-brain barrier into the CSF. The restoration of pH occurs far more promptly in the CSF as compared to restoration of the pH in the blood through renal compensation which may take over 2 days. Since CSF pH returns toward normal more quickly than blood pH, CSF pH exerts a more important effect in the control over ventilation.

Peripheral Chemoreceptors

Peripheral chemoreceptors are in the carotid bodies at the bifurcation of the common carotid artery and the aortic bodies above and below the aortic arch. The carotid body is the predominant chemoreceptor and consists of glomus cells which are of two types. Type I cells contain a store of dopamine and show an intense fluorescent stain. These cells are in close apposition to the nerve endings of the carotid sinus nerve. The Type II cells have a rich

capillary supply. Changes in pH, PaO_2, $PaCO_2$ or other chemical changes in blood are sensed by glomus cells which are the site of chemoreceptors. This leads to release of neurotransmitters which influence the discharge rate of the afferent nerve fibers in the carotid body. Impulses reach the central nervous system through the carotid sinus nerve. The peripheral chemoreceptors in the carotid bodies are stimulated by a fall in arterial PaO_2, a rise in arterial $PaCO_2$ and a fall in pH. The carotid bodies have a large blood supply compared to their size as also a small arteriovenous oxygen difference. They respond to change in arterial PO_2 rather than venous PO_2. Their response to a fall in PaO_2 and a rise in $PaCO_2$ is extremely fast, even small cyclic changes in blood gases during breathing elicit a response from the carotid bodies.

Arterial hypoxemia therefore exerts a stimulant effect on the chemoreceptors within the carotid body leading to an increase in ventilation. In fact the increase in ventilation induced by hypoxemia is solely related to carotid body stimulation. Bilateral carotid body removal in an individual abolishes the increased ventilatory drive normally induced by hypoxemia. In fact in such patients arterial hypoxemia is noted to depress ventilation.

The response of the carotid body to change in $PaCO_2$ is less compared to change in PaO_2. Around 20% of the increased ventilatory response observed following a rise in $PaCO_2$ is believed to be related to stimulation of carotid body chemoreceptors. A lowered arterial pH also increases ventilation through stimulation of carotid body chemoreceptors. A combination of arterial hypoxemia, hypercapnia and a lowered pH has the maximal stimulatory effect on the central chemoreceptors.

Lung Receptors

- *Pulmonary stretch receptors*: Pulmonary stretch receptors are slowly-adapting stretch receptors situated within airways smooth muscle. They are stimulated during lung inflation and their activity is sustained during inflation, showing little adaptation. The impulse from these stretch receptors travels via the vagus nerves to the medullary center inhibiting inspiratory muscle activity. During deflation the opposite effect is observed, the lungs tending to initiate inspiration. This results in a self-regulating mechanism of negative feedback.

The reflex described through stimulation of the slow adaptive stretch receptors is termed the Hering Breuer inflation reflex. The stimulation of this reflex results in a slowing of the respiratory rate due to increase in expiratory time. The Hering Breuer reflex authenticated in animal experiments was believed to play a major role in humans as well, with regard to regulating the depth and rate of respiration. However, recent work suggests that this reflex plays little role in the control of ventilation unless the tidal volume is more than one liter, or in exercise.

- *Irritant receptors*: Irritant receptors are believed to be rapidly-adapting pulmonary stretch receptors situated between airways epithelial cells. They are stimulated by noxious stimuli like cigarette smoke, dust, and noxious gases as also by inhalation of cold air. Impulses from these receptors travel up the vagus nerve in myelinated fibers causing reflex bronchoconstriction and hyperpnea. They are rapidly-adapting receptors and may play a role in the bronchoconstriction of asthma, through their response to noxious stimuli.
- *J receptors*: J receptors were discovered by Prof Paintal working at the Patel Chest Institute in New Delhi, first in the cat and then in the human being. These receptors are in the alveolar walls close to the capillaries. Impulses arising through stimulation of J receptors travel up the slow conducing unmyelinated fibers of the vagus nerves, resulting in reflex rapid shallow breathing. Interstitial edema from any cause stimulates the J receptors. The rapid shallow breathing in patients with left ventricular failure is due to stimulation of J receptors. The tachypnea associated with interstitial lung disease is also related to the stimulation of these receptors.
- *Bronchial C fibers*: These are close to the bronchial circulation. Their stimulation results in reflex rapid shallow breathing, bronchoconstriction and increased mucous secretion.

Besides central chemoreceptors, peripheral chemoreceptors and pulmonary receptors, ventilation can be reflexly influenced by other peripheral receptors. These are:

Nose and Upper Airways Receptors

Receptors present in the nose, nasopharynx, larynx, and trachea respond to mechanical and chemical stimuli producing various reflex responses such as sneezing, coughing, bronchoconstriction and laryngeal spasm.

Receptors within Intercostal Muscles and Diaphragm

The intercostal muscles and diaphragm contain receptors in muscle spindles which sense muscle stretch. The stretch sensed by these receptors is used to reflexly control the strength of respiratory muscle contraction. Excessive stimulation of these receptors may be responsible for uncomfortable awareness of breathing that characterizes dyspnea. This could be of particular relevance in patients with *chronic obstructive pulmonary disease* (COPD) who need extra respiratory muscle effort to meet the marked increase in resistive load.

Arterial Baroreceptors

An increase in arterial blood pressure particularly, when sudden, can cause reflex hypoventilation through stimulation of the carotid and aortic baroreceptors. Conversely, hypotension can lead to hyperventilation. The reflex pathways involved in these reflexes are unknown.

Receptors in Muscles and Joints

Impulses arising through receptors in muscles and joints are believed to reflexly activate ventilation during exercise, particularly in the early phase.

An integrated response from the central controlling system in the medulla results following the processing of various sensory inputs mentioned above; the exact nature of this integration and its mechanism continues to be a subject of active research. It needs to be restressed that ventilation is most influenced by changes in $PaCO_2$, PaO_2 and pH of arterial blood. Experimental work shows that ventilation increases by as much as 1–2 L/min for each 1 mm Hg rise in $PaCO_2$. Lowering the PaO_2 results in even higher ventilation for a given $PaCO_2$. As mentioned earlier most of the increase in ventilation caused by an increased $PaCO_2$ is through central chemoreceptors but peripheral chemoreceptors also come into play with a faster response.

The ventilatory response to a rise in PCO_2 is reduced when the respiratory center is depressed by various drugs such as narcotics and sedatives. Interestingly, the ventilator response to CO_2 is also decreased if the work of breathing is increased. Perhaps this may be one of the reasons for the reduced ventilatory response to CO_2 and for CO_2 retention in some patients of COPD. However the main reason for CO_2 retention in these patients is the inability of the respiratory muscles to produce the effort necessary to meet the markedly increased resistive load.

The PaO_2 exerts negligible control over ventilation under normoxic conditions. PaO_2 as seen in hypoxic conditions is however an important cause of increased ventilation. Only peripheral chemoreceptors are involved in causing reflex increase in ventilation.

A lowered pH as in any form of metabolic acidosis induces an increase in ventilation and this effect is independent of the $PaCO_2$. A fall in pH acts chiefly through peripheral chemoreceptors. Central chemoreceptors and the respiratory center itself may to a lesser extent also be stimulated with a fall in pH.

■ VENTILATORY RESPONSE TO EXERCISE

Ventilation increases within some seconds of starting exercise. With maximal exercise, a fit young subject can increase the minute ventilation to 150 L which is close to 16 times the minute ventilation at rest. There is a corresponding increase in oxygen consumption to 4 L/min and an increase in carbon dioxide output. The reason for this marked increase in ventilatory response to exercise is not understood.

The $PaCO_2$ does not change during exercise; in fact with a very high workload it may fall just a little. The PaO_2 remains constant; with maximal exercise there may be a slight fall but not at all enough to be responsible for the marked increase in minute ventilation. The pH of arterial blood remains constant except with very heavy workloads when there is a slight fall in the pH due to lactic acid production in the muscles and anaerobic glycolysis.

Several hypotheses have been put forward to explain the ventilatory response to exercise. Perhaps the very prompt rise (within 10 to 15 seconds) in ventilation may be explained by stimulation of receptors in joints and muscles of the limbs which cause a reflex increase in ventilation. Evidently, changes in PaO_2, $PaCO_2$ and pH are not sufficient to explain the ventilatory response. One hypothesis states that it is the oscillation in arterial PaO_2 and $PaCO_2$ which stimulates peripheral chemoreceptors even though the mean PaO_2 and $PaCO_2$ remain unchanged. Another hypothesis is that the central chemoreceptors stimulate the respiratory center to increase ventilation, so as to keep the $PaCO_2$ constant by a sort of servomechanism, acting very similar to a thermostat that keeps a constant temperature. A third hypothesis states that the increased ventilatory response is related to the high content of CO_2 presented to the lungs in the mixed venous blood. This has been shown to occur in animal experiments, ventilation increasing pari passu with increasing infusion of CO_2 into venous blood. Yet receptors which could initiate this increase in ventilation have not been found. Perhaps some increase in ventilation may be related to impulses from the cortex, the medullary respiratory center, as also to a slight rise in body temperature during heavy exercise. None of the hypotheses stated above provide a satisfactory explanation for the ventilatory response during exercise.

■ SUGGESTED READING

1. Adrogué HJ, Madias NE. Secondary responses to altered acid-base status: the rules of engagement. J Am Soc Nephrol. 2010;21:920-3.
2. Morgan TJ. Clinical review: the meaning of acid-base abnormalities in the intensive care—effects of fluid administration. Crit Care. 2005;9:204-11.
3. Morgan TJ. The meaning of acid-base abnormalities in the intensive care unit: part III—effects of fluid administration. Crit Care. 2005;9(2):204-11.
4. Oh YK. Acid-base disorders in ICU patients. Electrolytes and blood pressure: E & BP. 2010;8(2):66-71.
5. Story DA. Bench to bedside review: a brief history of clinical acid-base. Crit Care. 2004;8:253-8.
6. Udwadia FE. Acid-base Disturbances in the Critically Ill. In: Udwadia FE (Ed). Principles of Critical Care, 2nd edition. New Delhi: Oxford University Press; 2005.
7. West JB. Control of ventilation. In: West JB (Ed). Respiratory Physiology: The Essentials, 6th edition. Philadelphia: Lippincott Williams and Wilkins; 2006.

CHAPTER 5

Pulmonary Circulation

■ INTRODUCTION

The pulmonary artery arises from the right ventricle. It then divides into right and left branches. Each of these divides further and further into smaller branches. These vessels accompany the airways as far as the terminal bronchioles and then break up to form a vast capillary bed perfusing the millions of alveoli in the lungs. The capillary network is both profuse and rich; many physiologists regard the capillary bed as a sheet of blood to which oxygen is added from within the alveoli and from which carbon dioxide diffuses into the alveoli. The oxygenated blood is collected by small veins, which merge to form four large veins (two on either side superior and inferior). These veins open into the left atrium thereby providing the left heart with oxygenated blood. The pulmonary circulation extends from the start of the pulmonary artery to the opening of the pulmonary veins into the left atrium.

■ HEMODYNAMICS OF THE PULMONARY CIRCULATION

The pulmonary circulation constitutes a low-pressure, high-flow, high-volume circuit. It carries a volume of blood equal to that carried by the systemic circulation but manages to do so with a far less driving pressure thus reducing the stress on the right ventricle. The right ventricle is not structured to handle "load" (in contrast to the left ventricle), but fortunately can handle volume effectively. The systolic pressure of the pulmonary artery is 20–25 mm Hg and the diastolic 8 mm Hg with a mean pulmonary artery pressure of around 15 mm Hg. In contrast systolic and diastolic pressure in the systemic circulation are 120 mm Hg and 80 mm Hg respectively, the mean arterial blood pressure being about 100 mm Hg—more than six times the mean pulmonary artery pressure. Pressures in the right atrium are around 2–5 mm Hg and in the left atrium 5–10 mm Hg. The pressure difference in the pulmonary circulation is 15 – 5 mm Hg = 10 mm Hg. In the systemic circulation it is 100 – 2 mm Hg = 98 mm Hg; which is close to 10 times that in the pulmonary circulation.

The walls of the pulmonary arteries and their branches are thin and contain relatively less smooth muscle, probably related to the low pressures within the whole system. The reason for the difference between the pulmonary and systemic circulation is largely related to much greater work required of the left ventricle to supply blood to various organ systems of the body, including structures above the level of the heart. In contrast, the right heart through the pulmonary circulation pumps the whole cardiac output solely to the lungs. It has less work to do and does so by maintaining lower pressure in the pulmonary circuit, enough however to allow efficient gas exchange within the lungs.

Though the mean pressure in the pulmonary artery is 15 mm Hg, the pressure in the pulmonary capillaries is uncertain. It is probably mid-way between the pressure in the pulmonary artery and veins. Studies suggest that there seems to be a gradual symmetrical drop of pressure in the pulmonary vessels toward the capillaries. In contrast, most of the pressure drop in the systemic circulation is just above the capillary level. However, it must be noted that the pressure within the pulmonary capillaries is not the same throughout the lung; it varies in different parts of the lung because of their exposure to different hydrostatic pressures. This aspect has been explained later in this chapter.

The thin-walled capillaries adjoin the alveoli, which they perfuse. The blood in the capillaries is separated from the air in the alveoli by the thin endothelial lining of the capillary wall, the fused basement membrane of the capillary wall plus alveolar wall, and the epithelial cells lining the alveoli. The pulmonary capillaries are therefore strongly influenced by the pressure within the alveoli and are likely to expand if alveolar pressure is low and collapse if the pressure is high. The alveolar pressure is atmospheric at end of expiration of a tidal volume breath. It is also atmospheric at end-inspiration with the mouth open. By and large therefore under ordinary circumstances, the pressure around pulmonary capillaries is close to the alveolar pressure. Overinflation of alveoli compresses capillaries; under-inflation allows them to dilate.

The pressure around the larger pulmonary vessels and veins is, however, considerably less than alveolar pressure. This is because these vessels are kept open by the radial traction of the elastic lung parenchyma surrounding them, so that these vessels increase their caliber with lung expansion. Consequently, the effective pressure around them is low.

To summarize, whereas the caliber of the pulmonary capillaries (or alveolar vessels) is influenced by alveolar pressure and the intraluminal pressure within them, the caliber of the large vessels (extra-alveolar vessels) is influenced by lung volume rather than alveolar pressure. The large vessels at the hilum are outside the lung and are influenced by the intrapleural pressure.

■ PULMONARY VASCULAR RESISTANCE

Vascular resistance in a vessel = Input pressure – output pressure/blood flow

Pulmonary vascular resistance = 15 – 5/5 to 6 = 1.7–2 mm Hg/L/min.

Where 15 mm Hg is the mean pulmonary artery pressure, 5 mm Hg is the pressure in the left atrium and the pulmonary blood flow is 5–6 L/min. The pulmonary vascular resistance is thus markedly low, well-nigh 10 times lower than the systemic vascular resistance. The high systemic vascular resistance is related to muscular arterioles regulating blood flow to various organ systems. The pulmonary vascular system has thin vessels walls with low resistance enabling a widespread distribution of a thin film of blood along the alveolar walls, ensuring efficient gas exchange.

Remarkably, this low pulmonary vascular resistance is capable of falling further if the pulmonary artery pressure is raised. There are two mechanisms responsible for this capability:

1. *Recruitment*: Normally (under resting conditions) some capillaries have no blood flowing through them. When pulmonary artery pressure is raised these vessels open up and have blood flowing through them thereby reducing overall pulmonary vascular resistance. This mechanism is termed recruitment.

2. *Dilatation*: A rise in pulmonary artery pressure leads to dilatation with a rounding of the normally flattened pulmonary capillaries, resulting again in a fall in pulmonary vascular resistance. The distension or dilatation of the capillaries is possible because of the very thin membrane separating the capillaries from the alveolar wall. Dilatation or distension is the chief mechanism for lowering pulmonary vascular resistance in the presence of significantly increased pulmonary vascular pressures. Both recruitment and distension may occur together to produce the same effect **(Fig. 1)**.

Lung volume is another important determinant of pulmonary vascular resistance. It has been mentioned earlier that the walls of the extra-alveolar vessels on inspiration are pulled apart thereby reducing their vascular resistance at large lung volumes. The walls of

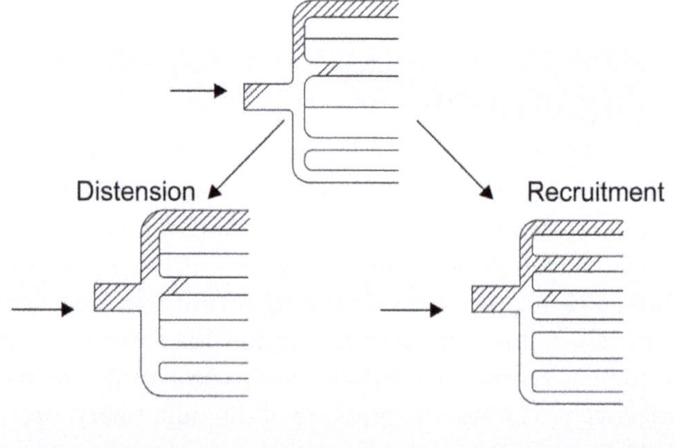

Fig. 1: Recruitment and distension. These are the two mechanisms for the decrease in pulmonary vascular resistance that occurs as vascular pressures are raised.
Source: Adapted from Respiratory Physiology: The Essentials by John B West, 7th edition. Philadelphia: Lippincott Williams and Wilkins.

these extra-alveolar vessels contain smooth muscle, which resists distension and tends to reduce their caliber. Therefore, when the lung volume is low, these vessels have an increased resistance. If a lobe or lung is completely atelectatic, the resistance of these extra-alveolar vessels is so high that the pulmonary artery pressure must be raised markedly above the normal before flow occurs at all. In other words, the critical opening pressure that enables blood to flow is significantly raised. Lung volumes also affect pulmonary capillary pressure. They do so in two ways:

1. If the intra-alveolar pressure is high as compared to the luminal pressure within the capillaries (i.e. an increase in transmural pressure) the capillaries are constricted and the pulmonary vascular resistance increases.
2. If the alveoli are distended for any reason even if there is no increase in intra-alveolar pressure, the distension of the alveoli squeezes the adjoining pulmonary capillaries and increases the pulmonary vascular resistance.

In summary both increase and decrease in lung volumes can increase pulmonary vascular resistance.

The extra-alveolar vessels have smooth muscle within their walls. Drugs, which act on smooth muscle, can thereby influence pulmonary vascular resistance. Norepinephrine and histamine contract smooth muscle and increase pulmonary vascular resistance. Isoproterenol is a drug, which relaxes smooth muscle and this decreases pulmonary vascular resistance. Hypoxia is a strong constrictor of pulmonary capillaries and produces pulmonary hypertension. Hypercapnia normally causes vasodilatation of systemic vessels but constricts pulmonary vessels leading to pulmonary hypertension.

■ MEASUREMENT OF PULMONARY BLOOD FLOW

Pulmonary blood flow can be measured by the Fick Principle:

$$\dot{V}O_2 = Q\,(CaO_2 - CvO_2)$$
$$Q = \dot{V}O_2/CaO_2 - CvO_2$$

Where $\dot{V}O_2$ is the oxygen consumption per minute, CaO_2 is the arterial oxygen content, CvO_2 is the mixed venous oxygen content, and Q is the blood flow through the lungs.

$\dot{V}O_2$ is measured by collecting the expired gas in a large spirometer over a minute and measuring the oxygen concentration.

CaO_2 is estimated from blood withdrawn through the radial artery. CvO_2 is estimated by collecting a mixed venous blood sample from the pulmonary artery via a pulmonary artery catheter.

Pulmonary blood flow can also be measured by the indicator dilution technique in which a dye or other indicator is injected into the venous circulation and its concentration in the arterial blood is recorded.

■ DISTRIBUTION OF PULMONARY FLOW IN THE LUNG

Blood flow through the lungs is not uniformly distributed. In fact, there is considerable inequality of blood flow in the human lung. In the upright standing posture, blood flow decreases from the bottom or base of the lung to the top or apex in an almost linear fashion. In the supine position, the blood flow at the apex increases but the basal flow is unchanged so that the blood flow is more uniformly distributed from the apex to the base. However, the flow in the posterior or dependent portion of the lung is more than in the anterior portion. On exercise both upper and lower zones have an increased blood flow, the difference between the two being less marked than at rest **(Fig. 2)**.

The inequality in the distribution of blood flow within the lungs can be explained by differences in hydrostatic pressure from top to bottom. The difference in hydrostatic

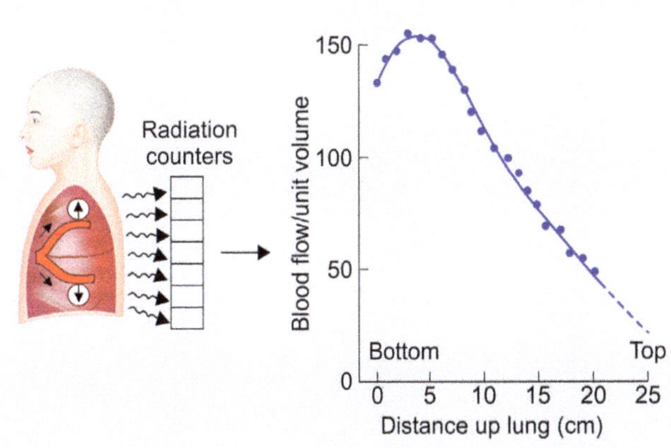

Fig. 2: Measurement of the distribution of blood flow in the upright human lung using radioactive xenon. The dissolved xenon is evolved into alveolar gas from the pulmonary capillaries. The units of blood flow are such that if flow were uniform, all values would be 100.
Source: Adapted with permission from Respiratory Physiology: The Essentials by John B West, 7th edition. Philadelphia: Lippincott Williams and Wilkins.

pressure from the apex of the lung to the bottom can be as high as 30 cm of H_2O. This large difference in hydrostatic pressure significantly affects regional blood flow in the existing low-pressure pulmonary circulation.

The lung can be looked upon as consisting of three zones **(Fig. 3)**. In the upper zone (Zone I), there may be regions where the pulmonary artery pressure falls well below the alveolar pressure (which is close to atmospheric pressure). If this does occur, the pulmonary capillaries are squeezed shut and no blood flow occurs through them. This does not happen normally as the pulmonary artery pressure is just sufficient to raise blood right up to the apex of the lung. But it could well occur if the pulmonary artery pressure falls as after hemorrhage or hypovolemia from any cause, or if the intra-alveolar pressure in Zone I is increased as in a patient on positive pressure ventilator support. If this transpires, the alveolar pressure squeezes the capillaries shut and this portion of the lung cannot take part in gas exchange.

In Zone II (further down the lung), the hydrostatic effect causes an increase in the pulmonary artery pressure. The pulmonary artery pressure now is more than the alveolar pressure. The pulmonary venous pressure is, however, still low. The blood flow in this zone is not determined by the usual arteriovenous pressure difference but by the difference between the pulmonary arterial pressure and alveolar pressure. Venous pressure has no influence on blood flow unless it exceeds alveolar pressure.

In Zone III (which includes the base of the lung), there is increased blood flow and dilatation of capillaries due to hydrostatic forces. The venous pressure now exceeds alveolar pressure so that blood flow in Zone III is governed by the usual arteriovenous pressure difference. In this zone, therefore, the pulmonary artery pressure is greater than the pulmonary venous pressure, which in turn is greater than the pulmonary alveolar pressure. As one goes down toward the base of the lung, there is increased blood flow through the capillaries while the alveolar pressure remains constant. The transmural pressure (between capillary and alveolar pressure) rises and the capillaries are more dilated.

Finally, one must consider pulmonary flow at low lung volumes. At low volumes there is (as has been already explained) an increased resistance of the extra-alveolar vessels. This assumes importance as there is a resultant reduction in the regional blood flow starting first at the base of the lung, which is less expanded. This region of reduced blood flow is sometimes termed Zone IV and results from a narrowing of the extra-alveolar vessels when the lung around them is partially atelectatic and poorly inflated.

West, in his excellent book on *Respiratory Physiology*, mentions other possible causes of inequality of blood flow. These include possible higher vascular resistance in some regions of the lung, perhaps a reduced blood flow to peripheral parts of the lung compared to the central areas. The random arrangements of blood vessels and capillaries may to some extent contribute to the inequality of pulmonary blood flow.

FACTORS INFLUENCING PULMONARY CIRCULATION

The hemodynamic factors determining blood flow, vascular resistance and pressure in the pulmonary circuit have already been discussed.

An extremely important influencing factor is a fall in the PO_2 of alveolar gas (a low P_AO_2). This results in hypoxic vasoconstriction of the pulmonary arterioles due to active contraction of smooth muscle within the pulmonary arteriolar walls. Almost certainly, it is the hypoxia itself which is responsible for this vasoconstrictive effect. Neurogenic factors are not involved. Equally important, experiments suggest that it is the low PO_2 of the alveolar gas and not a low PO_2 in the pulmonary arterial blood, which is responsible for this vasoconstrictive response.

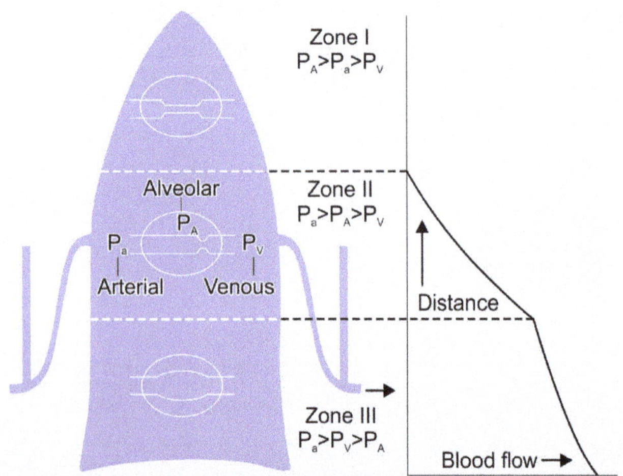

Fig. 3: Uneven distribution of blood in the lung, based on the pressure affecting the capillaries. P_a is pulmonary artery pressure. P_A is alveolar pressure, P_V is venous pressure.
Source: Adapted from Respiratory Physiology: The Essentials by John B West, 7th edition. Philadelphia: Lippincott Williams and Wilkins.

This can be proved by perfusing a lung with a high PO_2 while keeping the alveolar PO_2 low. The vasoconstrictive response is still observed. It is noted that when the alveolar PO_2 is altered in the region above 100 mm Hg, there is no change in the vascular response. It is only when the alveolar PO_2 is reduced below 70 mm Hg, that vasoconstriction occurs. Vasoconstriction increases with further lowering of alveolar PO_2. At very low alveolar PO_2, local blood flow almost ceases.

The exact mechanism of hypoxic vasoconstriction is unknown. Recent studies suggest that the effect may be induced by inhibition of voltage-gated potassium channels and membrane depolarization leading to accumulation of calcium within the cytoplasm of cells within the arteriolar wall. An increase in calcium within the cytoplasm could lead to smooth muscle contraction. Hypoxic vasoconstriction helps to divert pulmonary blood flow from hypoxic alveoli to better or normally ventilated alveoli. This improves overall gas exchange. A low alveolar PO_2 is found in hypoventilation from any cause, when a bronchus to an area of the lung is obstructed by secretions or by an intraluminal growth or from extrinsic obstruction.

At high altitude, there is a generalized pulmonary vasoconstriction because of a low alveolar O_2 pressure throughout all alveoli in the lungs. The severe pulmonary hypertension is chiefly responsible for pulmonary edema.

During fetal life, the pulmonary vascular resistance is very high because of hypoxic pulmonary vasoconstriction. When the baby is born, the first breath oxygenates the alveoli; the alveolar O_2 rises, the pulmonary vascular resistance falls and pulmonary blood flow (which in fetal life amounts only to 20% of the cardiac output) rises dramatically.

A rise in the $PaCO_2$ also causes pulmonary vasoconstriction though this is not as strong a stimulus as hypoxia. Remarkably, a rise in $PaCO_2$ causes vasodilatation in all vessels except the pulmonary vessels where it causes vasoconstriction. A fall in the pH, particularly in the presence of hypoxia also causes vasoconstriction. An increase in sympathetic vascular resistance probably also leads to some degree of increased pulmonary vascular resistance.

■ FLUID EXCHANGE ACROSS THE ALVEOLAR CAPILLARY MEMBRANE

The alveoli must be kept free of fluid if proper gas exchange is to be maintained, particularly so since just 0.3 um of tissue separates capillary blood from alveolar air. Fluid exchange along the alveolar-capillary membrane obeys Starling's law. The filtration force tending to push fluid from the capillaries into the alveoli is the capillary hydrostatic pressure (P_C) minus the hydrostatic pressure in the interstitial fluid (P_I), i.e. $P_C - P_I$. The force tending to pull fluid into the capillaries is the osmotic pressure of the plasma protein in the blood (Πc) minus the osmotic pressure of fluid in the interstitial space ($\Pi c - H$). This force is dependent on the coefficient α, which indicates the efficiency of the capillary wall to prevent passage of proteins through it. Therefore, fluid exchange across the alveolar capillary membrane is governed by the following equation:

$$K\,[(P_C - P_I) - \alpha\,(\Pi_C - \Pi_I)]$$

where, K is the constant called the filtration coefficient.

The capillary hydrostatic pressure (filtration pressure) is around 35 mm Hg being higher at the base of the lung compared to the top. The colloid osmotic pressure in the capillaries is 25–28 mm Hg. The colloid interstitial pressure is not known but it is about 20 mm Hg in the lung lymph. The interstitial hydrostatic pressure is not known but is probably subatmospheric. It is likely that the net balance as per Starling's equation is to push a little fluid out of the capillaries into the interstitial space causing thereby a small lymph flow of about 20 mL/hour under normal resting conditions. This fluid tracks through the interstitial space into the perivascular and peribronchial space toward the hilar glands via the numerous perivascular and peribronchial lymphatics. The pressure in the perivascular and peribronchial space is low; this helps in drawing and draining the fluid toward the hilar glands.

Pulmonary edema occurs when more fluid is filtered through the capillaries. Early pulmonary edema is interstitial. Later the edema fluid crosses the alveolar epithelium into the alveolar spaces. This probably occurs when the fluid filtered through the capillaries into the interstitium exceeds considerably the maximum drainage rate of the fluid within the interstitium. Fluid reaching the alveoli is actively pumped out by a sodium potassium ATPase pump in alveolar epithelial cells. But this is ineffective in the presence of significant alveolar edema. Alveolar edema interferes with gas exchange and leads to increasing hypoxia.

Pulmonary edema in clinical medicine is related to one or more of the following three factors—increased capillary hydrostatic pressure as in left ventricular failure, a marked decrease in plasma osmotic pressure as is seen with any condition causing marked hypoproteinemia and in particular hypoalbuminemia, and finally increased capillary permeability, classically seen in the acute respiratory distress syndrome.

■ METABOLIC FUNCTION OF THE LUNG

Gas exchange is the prime and most important function of the lung. The lung also has a metabolic function. A brief account of the metabolic function of the lung is given below.

Like the heart, the lung is the only other organ to receive the whole circulatory output and, therefore, is aptly placed to metabolize or modify blood-borne substances. The lung is responsible for the biological activation of angiotensin I to angiotensin II. This conversion is catalyzed by the angiotensin-converting enzyme (ACE). Angiotensin II is 50 times more potent than angiotensin I and is unaffected by passage through the lung.

Many vasoactive substances are partially or completely inactivated after passage through the lungs. These include norepinephrine and prostaglandin E_1, E_2, E_3. Serotonin is removed through increased uptake and storage within platelets. Bradykinin is inactivated by ACE. Some vasoactive substances pass through the lung unchanged; these include epinephrine, vasopressin and prostaglandin A_1, A_2.

A few vasoactive substances are metabolized in the lung and are released into the circulation under certain circumstances. Good examples are the arachidonic acid metabolites. Arachidonic acid is derived from membrane-bound phospholipid through the action of phospholipase A_2. The further metabolism of arachidonic acid is along two pathways—one catalyzed by lipoxygenase and the other by cyclooxygenase. The first catalytic reaction leads to the production of leukotrienes. These cause airways obstruction and play a role in bronchial asthma. Other leukotrienes are mediators of inflammatory processes. The second catalytic reaction leads to the production of prostaglandins and thromboxaneA_2. Prostaglandins are potent vasoconstrictors or vasodilators. Prostaglandins affect platelet aggregation and play an active role in the kallikrein-kinin clotting cascade. They also mediate bronchoconstriction in patients with bronchial asthma.

The lung has plenty of heparin-containing mast cells within the interstitium, which may perhaps have a role in the clotting mechanism of blood. The lung also has an important immunological function because it secretes the immunoglobulin A_2 in the bronchial mucus. This immunoglobulin enhances the local immune response within the lung to infection.

Among the synthetic functions of the lung is the production of phospholipids such as dipalmitoyl phosphoacetylcholine, which is the important component of surfactant synthesized by alveolar Type II epithelial cells. Protein synthesis is probably important because collagen and elastin form the framework of the lung. Finally, the lung has a role in carbohydrate metabolism, as it elaborates mucopolysaccharides of bronchial mucus.

■ SUGGESTED READING

1. Von Euler C. Neural organization and rhythm generation. In: Crystal RG, West JB, Barnes PJ, Weibel ER (Eds). The Lung: Scientific Foundations, 2nd edition. Philadelphia: Lippincott-Raven Press; 1997.
2. West JB. Control of ventilation. In: West JB (Ed). Respiratory Physiology: The Essentials, 6th edition. Philadelphia: Lippincott Williams and Wilkins; 2006.
3. Widdicombe JG. Reflexes from the upper respiratory tract. In: Cherniack NS, Widdicombe JG (Eds). Handbook of Physiology, Sec. 3, The Respiratory System Vol. II: Control of Breathing, Part I. Bethesda, Maryland: The American Physiological Society; 1986. pp. 363-94.
4. Yuan JX, Morrell NW, Harikrishnan S, et al. Pulmonary circulation: a new venue for communicating your findings, ideas and perspectives. Pulm Circ. 2011;1(1):1-2.

CHAPTER 6

Respiratory Muscle Function Testing

■ INTRODUCTION

When muscles contract they develop force and shorten. In the respiratory system, the force of muscle contraction is estimated by measurement of the pressure and the shortening caused by contraction by change in volume. Quantifying pressure and volume changes is a measure of respiratory muscle function.

Respiratory muscle weakness is characterized by a fall in vital capacity (VC). A fall in VC is, however, not specific for respiratory muscle weakness. It is a fairly early feature in restrictive lung and chest wall disease and also occurs in well-marked obstructive airways disease. The clinician needs to take this into account and rule out the above-mentioned diseases before attributing a fall in VC to respiratory muscle weakness. A marked fall (>30%) in VC in the supine posture compared to the sitting or standing posture is indicative of severe bilateral diaphragmatic weakness.

■ MEASUREMENT OF MAXIMAL STATIC INSPIRATORY AND EXPIRATORY PRESSURES

Inspiratory and expiratory muscle strength can be estimated easily by measuring the maximum static inspiratory (PImax) and expiratory (PEmax) pressure that a subject can generate at the mouth. The pressure is measured at the side port of a mouthpiece that is closed at one end. The maximum pressure sustained for 1 second is recorded **(Figs. 1 A and B)**. The pressure recorded at the mouth in these tests is a measure of pressure developed in the respiratory muscles plus the elastic recoil pressure of the lung and chest wall. At residual volume (RV) where PImax is usually measured, the elastic recoil pressure of the lung and chest wall may be as high as 30 cm H_2O. Similarly, when PEmax is measured, which is at total lung capacity (TLC), the elastic recoil pressure of the lung and chest wall can be as high as 40 cm H_2O.

PImax = Pressure generated by respiratory muscles + elastic recoil pressure of lung and chest wall.

PEmax = Pressure generated by respiratory muscles + elastic recoil pressure of lung and chest wall.

Clinical measurements of PImax and PEmax do not consider elastic recoil pressure of lung and chest wall, which ideally should be subtracted from the record of static maximum inspiratory and expiratory pressures measured at the mouth to assess solely the pressure generated by the respiratory muscles.

The normal range of PImax and PEmax is wide and, therefore, difficult in a particular individual to relate to the presence and degree of respiratory muscle weakness. Values less negative than the ones stated above are difficult to interpret. A low PImax with a normal PEmax suggests diaphragmatic weakness. The predicted equations and lower limits of PImax and PEmax are given below in **Table 1**.

Transdiaphragmatic Pressure

If the previous test suggests inspiratory muscle weakness one needs to determine whether this is related to the diaphragm or not. The integrity and strength of the diaphragm is estimated by the measurement of the maximum transdiaphragmatic pressure (Pdi, max). The Pdi, max is the difference between the gastric pressure (which reflects intra-abdominal pressure) and the

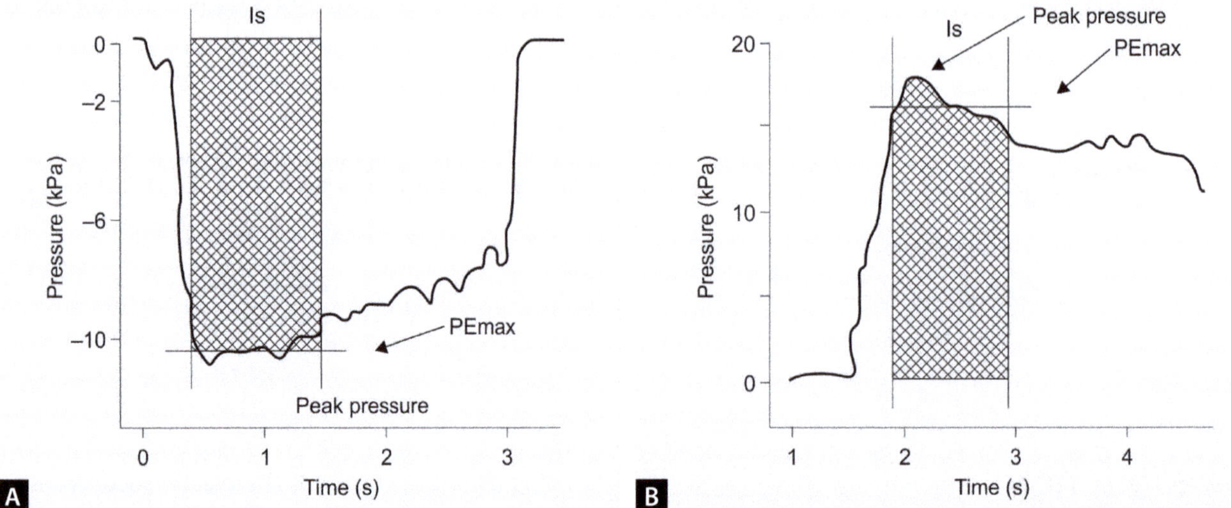

Figs. 1A and B: (A) Pressure tracing from a subject performing a maximum inspiratory maneuver (PImax). A peak pressure is seen and the 1 second average is determined by calculating the shaded area. (B) Typical pressure tracing from a subject performing a maximum expiratory maneuver (PEmax).
Source: Adapted from ATS/ERS: Statement on Respiratory Muscles Testing. Am J Res Crit Care Med. 2002;166:518-624.

Table 1: Lower limits of normal and predicted equations for PImax and PEmax.

	$PImax\ cm\ H_2O$		$PEmax\ cm\ H_2O$	
	Lower limit of normal	*Predicted mean*	*Lower limit of normal*	*Predicted mean*
Male	71	143 – (0.55 × age)	111	268 – (1.03 × age)
Female	39	104 – (0.51 × age)	88	170 – (0.53 × age)

Source: Equations and lower of normal from Black LF, Hyatt RE. Maximal respiratory pressures: normal values and relationship to age and sex. Am Rev Respir Dis. 1969;99:696-702.

esophageal pressure (which reflects intrapleural pressure) on a maximum inspiratory effort made from residual volume (RV). The gastric pressure is measured during this maneuver by a balloon catheter in the stomach and the esophageal pressure by a balloon catheter in the esophagus.

Sniff Pressure

A sniff is a short sharp inspiratory effort made from functional residual capacity (FRC) through one or both unoccluded nostrils with the mouth closed. It causes a rapid coordinated contraction of both the diaphragm and other inspiratory muscles. The transdiaphragmatic pressure measured during a short sniff reflects the strength of the diaphragm, and the pressure recorded by the balloon catheter in the esophagus represents the overall combined pressure of the inspiratory muscles on the lungs. It is not necessary to have a balloon catheter inserted into the esophagus for measuring the intraesophageal pressure reading. Pressures measured in one nostril approximate the intraesophageal pressure. Pressure is measured by wedging a catheter in one nostril using foam to hold it in place. The patient sniffs through the other open nostril. There is a wide range of normal values with regard to the maximum transdiaphragmatic pressure (Pdi, max) in the sniff test. However, if the Pdi, max in the sniff test is greater than 100 cm H_2O in males and 80 cm H_2O in females, there can be no clinically significant diaphragmatic weakness. Also, if the maximal nasal or esophageal sniff pressure is greater than 70 cm H_2O in males and 60 cm H_2O in females, there can be no significant inspiratory muscle weakness. It is to be remembered that these values reflect overall integrated pressure of all inspiratory muscles. Weakness of small muscles' groups could be missed but again this would not be of clinical significance.

■ ELECTROPHYSIOLOGICAL TESTING

If the preceding test reveals weakness of the diaphragm, the next step would be to determine whether this is related to impaired transmission of nervous impulses in the nerve or neuromuscular junction or whether it is related to weakness of diaphragmatic muscle. Electrophysiological studies could determine this. However, in clinical practice this is indeed rarely necessary, because a good history, a careful clinical examination almost always will determine the correct issue. Electrophysiological testing is, therefore, of academic and research value to the clinician. The basic principles underlying this test will only be stated. The test involves measurement of Pdi following bilateral submaximal electric or magnetic stimulation of the phrenic nerves with simultaneous recording of the electromyography (EMG) of the diaphragm with either surface or esophageal electrodes. If the phrenic nerve is stimulated, the diaphragm contracts and this contraction is termed as a *twitch*. For physiological and technical reasons, the transdiaphragmatic pressure developed in response to a single supramaximal phrenic nerve stimulation at 1 Hz called the twitch Pdi is measured. The result is independent of patient effort and also allows for the measurement of phrenic nerve conduction time. A prolonged conduction time points to phrenic nerve involvement.

■ CONCEPT OF LOAD VERSUS EFFORT, AND OF ENERGY DEMAND VERSUS ENERGY SUPPLY IN SPONTANEOUS BREATHING

In spontaneous breathing, the inspiratory muscles must generate force, which is sufficient to overcome the elastic recoil of the lung and chest wall (elastic load), as also to overcome airway and tissue resistance (resistive load). To do so necessitates an intact neural discharge from the center to the muscles of inspiration, normal neuromuscular transmission of nervous impulses, an intact chest wall and normal strength of the inspiratory muscles. We have, therefore, "load" on the one hand and "effort" of the neuromuscular apparatus to meet this load on the other. Ordinarily, not only does "effort" meet the "load" but there is sufficient reserve in the "effort" that enables an upward adjustment of the minute ventilation in the event of an increased load, so as to maintain adequate gas exchange. "Effort" as outlined above will be dependent on energy stores within the inspiratory muscles, the ability of the muscles to extract and utilize this energy source, oxygen saturation, and adequate blood flow to the inspiratory muscles.

Inspiratory muscle fatigue sets in when, for any reason, the "effort" fails to meet the "load". In disease, this usually is due to an excessive increase in the "load" that cannot be met by "effort". Increase in load occurs through an increase in "the elastic load of the lung and/or chest wall (elastic load), or an increase in airways resistance (resistive load) or due to an increase in both the elastic and resistive load". To give an example, in chronic obstructive pulmonary disease (COPD) for various reasons (discussed under COPD) the "load" is markedly increased. If there is a proportionate increase in "effort" to meet this load, ventilation continues without muscle fatigue and gas exchange is maintained. If, however, a stage comes when the "load" is far too excessive and the "effort" fails to meet it, gas exchange suffers and in due course of time muscle fatigue sets in. The question that needs an answer is the reason why effort of the inspiratory muscles cannot meet the excessive load. "Effort" depends on energy supply to inspiratory muscles; it is when energy supplied to inspiratory muscles is less than the energy demand imposed by the excessive increase in load that effort fails to meet the load. One can, therefore, look upon load as being related to energy demand and "effort" being related and dependent on energy supply. Inspiratory muscle fatigue occurs, when energy demand exceeds energy supply.

There are certain respiratory parameters which enable us to assess increase in load, which can be translated to mean an increase in energy demand. Load (i.e. energy demand) increases proportionately with the mean pressure developed by the inspiratory muscle per breath (P_I) expressed as a fraction of the maximum pressure developed by the respiratory muscles (P_I/PImax), minute ventilation (V_E), V_T/T_I which is the mean inspiratory flow (Tidal volume/Inspiratory time), T_I/T_{TOT}, i.e. inspiratory duty cycle (fraction of inspiration to total breathing cycle duration).

The product of T_I/T_{TOT} and the mean diaphragmatic pressure expressed as a fraction of maximal (Pdi/Pdimax) is defined as the "tension-time index" (TTIdi), which is related to the endurance time (i.e. the time that the diaphragm can meet the load imposed on it). Whenever, TTIdi is less than 0.15–0.18, the load can be sustained for a limited time, i.e. the endurance time. The TTIdi is inversely related to the endurance time. The concept underlying tension time index is applicable not only to the diaphragm but to all inspiratory muscles, so that

$$\text{TTI} = \frac{P_I}{\text{PImax}} \times \frac{T_I}{T_{TOT}}$$

Obviously, an increase in either P_I/PImax or T_I/T_{TOT} will increase the TTI value, which means an increase in load or an increase in energy demand.

To summarize, spontaneous breathing without respiratory muscle fatigue is possible when "effort" required by the inspiratory muscles is adequate (in fact more than adequate) to meet the "load" imposed on them. "Effort" is related to energy supply and load dictates energy demand. Therefore, when effort is inadequate for the load imposed (as when there is an excessive increase in load), or energy supply to inspiratory muscles does not meet their energy demands, both inadequate gas exchange and muscle fatigue set in. Parameters to assess increased load (whether increase in elastic load or resistive load) have been mentioned above. The concept of tension time index in relation to muscle fatigue is of considerable interest.

■ MUSCLE FATIGUE

"Fatigue is defined as the loss of capacity to develop force and/or velocity in response to a load that is reversible by rest". Muscle fatigue should be distinguished from weakness in which the loss of capacity to develop force in response to a load is not reversed by rest. Where is the site of muscle fatigue located? Voluntary muscle contraction depends on a chain of events starting from the brain, "traveling" through nerves, nerve endings, and neuromuscular junctions, to the final contractile end organ—the muscle. Researchers, in this field, have classified fatigue into central fatigue, peripheral high-frequency fatigue, and peripheral low-frequency fatigue.

Central Fatigue

Central muscle fatigue is said to exist when maximum voluntary contraction generates less force than that induced by maximal electrical stimulation. If maximal electrical stimulation given during maximal voluntary contraction potentiates the force and strength of the muscle contraction, an element of central fatigue exists. A number of experiments suggest that when there is excessive load (increased energy demands) there occurs a form of central diaphragmatic fatigue. A significant part of the reduction of force during diaphragmatic contraction at such times is related to the failure of the central nervous system to fully activate the diaphragm. This could be related to a decrease in the central drive, decrease in motor units recruited by the central drive, or decrease in discharge rates of the motor units or a combination of the above factors. A decrease in discharge rate may well be an adaptive mechanism to help preserve for a longer time the strength of the diaphragmatic muscle.

Peripheral Fatigue

Peripheral fatigue exists when the force of muscle contraction falls in response to direct electrical stimulation. The fault may lie at the neuromuscular junction, the muscle surface membrane or may result from impaired excitation-contraction coupling or may be related to a defect within the muscle itself—perhaps an alteration in the contractile protein for unclear reasons.

Peripheral fatigue can be high-frequency fatigue, which is a lowered force of contraction in response to high-frequency stimulation (50–100 Hz) and low-frequency fatigue, which is characterized by reduction in force of contraction at low-frequency stimulation (1–20 Hz). The force of contraction in the latter situation is, however, not affected or reduced by high-frequency stimulation.

The site of high-frequency fatigue may be located presynaptically or postsynaptically. The block in transmission of the nerve impulses may again be an adaptive mechanism to prevent the muscle from using up all its stores of adenosine triphosphate (ATP).

The mechanism of low-frequency fatigue is not known. It is probably related either to the low availability of calcium, to lowered concentration of calcium in the muscle fibers or perhaps a lessened sensitivity of muscle fibers to calcium.

Whereas high-frequency fatigue resolves quickly when the work load is sharply reduced, low-frequency fatigue takes long to recover.

One must conclude by mentioning that respiratory muscle fatigue which has clinical relevance can be generally determined at the bedside by a careful clinical examination. The clinical features of respiratory muscle fatigue at the bedside have been detailed later in more than one section of the book. Admittedly the measurements required to objectively assess muscle fatigue are by and large not possible in critically ill patients where fatigue is most likely to arise or be actively present. Therefore, the relevance of these measurements in respiratory medicine at this point in time is unfortunately poor.

■ INFLAMMATORY CHANGES IN RESPIRATORY MUSCLES

Strenuous diaphragmatic contraction over long periods of time against an increased "load" as in COPD can excite an inflammatory reaction within the diaphragmatic muscle. The inflammation is related to cytokines produced within the diaphragm itself due to excessive diaphragmatic activity. This results an ultrastructural injury to the diaphragmatic muscle. The exact mechanism of injury is not known. Besides cytokines induction, an influx of inflammatory cells, upregulation of adhesion molecules, and formation of reactive oxygen radicals may all play a role.

ADAPTIVE CHANGES IN RESPIRATORY MUSCLES TO "LOAD"

Compensatory adaptive changes occur in respiratory muscles when they are required to cope with increasing "load" over long periods of time as for example in COPD. The main adaptation observed is a change in the type of muscle fiber of the respiratory muscles. Muscles fibers are classified either as Type I or Type II depending on the myosin heavy chain component of the myosin molecule. Myosin heavy chains exist in various isoforms. In increasing order of maximum shortening velocity there is myosin heavy chain (MHC) I, MHC II A, and MHC II B; the MHC II B fibers show both maximum speed and maximum shortening during contraction. The diaphragm in healthy individuals consists of 50% Type I fibers, 25% II A, and 25% II B fibers. The Type I fibers have a slower speed of contraction and are fatigue-resistant in comparison to Type II fibers. In COPD, there is a transformation of Type II fibers into Type I fatigue-resistant fibers. This increases resistance to fatigue which is a decided advantage considering the increased load the respiratory muscles need to cope with. However, the transformation of Type II to Type I fibers also reduces the diaphragm's contractile strength and force-generating capacity.

Another adaptation of the respiratory muscles in COPD, which is observed in animal models of COPD, and perhaps also occurs in COPD in humans, is a decrease in the number and length of sarcomeres. This adaptation results in a leftward shift of the length-tension curve, so that the muscle adapts to the shorter operating length caused by overinflation of the lungs, as also to an increase in the AP diameter of the chest with more horizontally placed ribs. To an extent, this reduces the mechanical disadvantage of the diaphragm and the inspiratory muscles of the chest caused by hyper-inflated lungs.

The adaptation of respiratory muscles to increased load has as its counterpart a different form of adaptation when they are rendered inactive, as for example during prolonged mechanical ventilation. Inactivity and the unloading of work normally performed by the diaphragm can lead to atrophy of the diaphragmatic muscle and a reduction of its force-generating capacity. This ventilator-induced diaphragmatic dysfunction (VIDD) becomes apparent when the patient is weaned off ventilator support. VIDD is one reason for difficulty in weaning of some patients who have been on prolonged ventilator support. The reasons for diaphragmatic dysfunction following inactivity are unclear. Dysfunction could be partly related to muscle atrophy, structural injury, and perhaps to muscle fiber remodeling.

SUGGESTED READING

1. American Thoracic Society/European Respiratory Society Task Force. Statement on Respiratory Muscle Testing. Am J Respir Crit Care Med. 2002;166:518-624.
2. Black LF, Hyatt RE. Equations and lower of normal from—maximal respiratory pressures: normal values and relationship to age and sex. Am Rev Respir Dis. 1969;99:696-702.
3. Black LF, Hyatt RE. Maximal static respiratory pressure in generalized neuromuscular disease. Am Rev Respir Dis. 1971;103:641.
4. Laghi F, Tobin M. Disorders of respiratory muscles. Am J Respir Crit Care Med. 2003;168:10-48.
5. Levi OM. Structure and function of the respiratory muscles in patients with COPD: impairment of adaptation? Eur Respir J. 2003;22(Suppl 46):41s-51s.
6. Vincken GH, Cosio MG. Maximal static respiratory pressure in adults: normal values and their relationship to determine of respiratory function. Bull Eur Physiopathol Respir. 1987;23:435.

Pulmonary Function Testing

INTRODUCTION

Pulmonary function tests (PFTs) characterize respiratory physiology and, therefore, enable a physician to determine the nature of disturbance in lung function in a patient with respiratory complaints or respiratory disease. They provide an objective, quantitative assessment of altered lung physiology allowing a correlation with symptoms, clinical examination, and radiography of the chest. The quantitative objective assessment of lung function done at periodic intervals helps to assess disease severity and the progress of disease in a given patient. This is particularly important when respiratory symptoms do not reflect disease severity or progression.

It must, however, be remembered that normal lung functions do not exclude lung disease. In fact, normal lung function can be associated with a serious lung pathology.

Disturbance in lung function often falls into specific patterns and recognition of these patterns by a clinician helps in the overall assessment of the patient. By themselves, lung function tests do not provide a specific diagnosis because specific patterns of disturbance in lung function are common to a number of diseases and there is often an overlap between the two basic patterns arising from disturbed lung function. It is the triad of history cum clinical examination, radiography of the chest, and lung function tests taken together and correlated that provides a specific diagnosis in most respiratory diseases.

OBJECTIVES OF PULMONARY FUNCTION TESTS

- To assess objectively and quantitatively the nature and degree of altered physiology in a patient with respiratory disease.
- To assess the effect of therapy on deranged lung function.
- To keep a longitudinal follow-up of patients with respiratory disease and help in the assessment of the natural history of the respiratory disease in a given patient.
- To allow surveillance in patients exposed to environmental insults, in patients who have received cytotoxic drugs or who have received radiotherapy to the lungs, mediastinum, or chest wall.
- To evaluate the effect of neuromuscular or cardiovascular disease on the respiratory system.
- To identify presymptomatic lung disease in smokers.

The National Health and Nutrition Examination Survey and Lung Health Study confirmed through PFTs the presence of abnormal lung function in asymptomatic smokers. This study also provided data to show that the presence of abnormal PFT in this group prompted smokers to seek medical advice and attempt stopping to smoke. Based on the above findings, the study recommended office-based spirometry for current smokers 45 years of age and for any smoker with respiratory symptoms.

SPIROMETRY

Spirometry allows basic lung function tests, which can be performed in the office. Spirometry measures the volume of air exhaled or inhaled by a subject as a function of time, so that both volume and flow rates are available.

A basic and useful spirometry test is the measurement of a single forced expiration. This requires the subject to forcefully expel air from the point of maximum inspiration (i.e. total lung capacity—TLC) as hard and as completely as possible—i.e. to the point of maximal expiration (residual volume—RV). The total volume exhaled is termed the forced vital capacity (FVC) and the volume exhaled in the 1st second is termed the forced expiratory volume in the first second (FEV_1). Normally, the FEV_1 is 80% of the FVC, i.e. $FEV_1/FVC = 80\%$. The FVC and FEV_1/FVC are the most important values obtained from the forced expiration maneuver. When during the forced expiratory maneuver, expelled volume is charted against time, FEV_1 is easily obtained. A number of other functional measurements are provided, if during the forced expiratory maneuver, volume expelled is charted against the flow rate. **Table 1** lists the measurements possible when volume is charted against time and against the flow rate. **Figure 1A** shows

expiratory volume plotted against time and **Figure 1B** is flow plotted against the volume.

Significant information can be derived from measurements of FVC and FEV_1. In pulmonary disease, two patterns are generally distinguished. In obstructive lung disease, the FEV_1 is reduced giving a low $FEV_1/FVC\%$. In restrictive lung disease, as for example in pulmonary fibrosis, both FVC and FEV_1 are reduced but the $FEV_1/FVC\%$ remains normal or is even increased. However, many respiratory diseases may be associated with mixed restrictive and obstructive patterns.

Though most laboratories measure vital capacity (VC) through a forced expiratory maneuver, there are some who

Table 1: Commonly used spirometry parameters.		
Reported value	**Description**	**Interpretation**
VC	Vital capacity	Generally preserved in obstruction, but reduced in restriction
FVC	Forced vital capacity	Reduction in FVC is suggestive of restrictive lung disease or well marked airways obstruction, or a mixed pattern. Used to grade severity of restriction
FEV_1	Forced expiratory volume in 1 second	Reduced in restrictive as well as obstructive lung disease. Used to grade severity of obstruction
FEV_1/FVC	Ratio of FEV_1/FVC	Reduction is indicative of airways obstruction
FEF22-75	Mean expiratory flow rate in the middle of half of FVC (mid-expiratory flow rate)	Sensitive but nonspecific indicator of small airways obstruction
PEF	Peak expiratory flow	Worsening correlate with severity of asthma; PEF is also effort dependent
MVV	Maximum voluntary ventilation	Disproportionate reduction relative to FEV_1 may indicate upper airways obstruction, muscle weakness, or poor effort

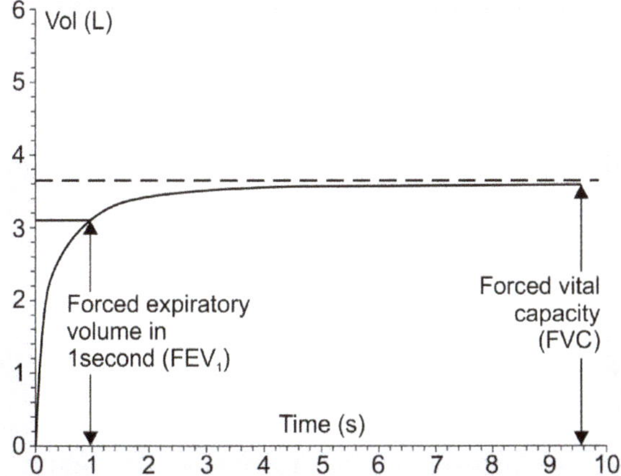

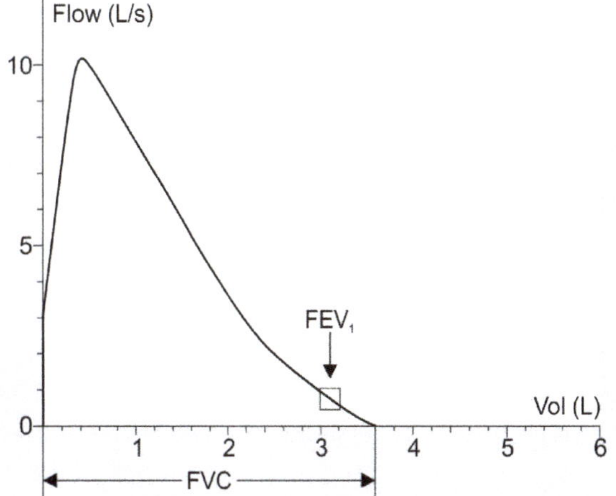

Fig. 1A: Normal forced expiratory spirogram plotted as exhaled volume versus time. The forced expiratory volume at 1 second (FEV_1) and forced vital capacity (FVC) are indicated by arrows. In above graph FVC = 3.6 L, FEV_1 = 3.1, and FEV_1/FVC ratio = 86.1%.

Fig. 1B: Normal expiratory flow-volume curve. The same forced expiratory time volume maneuver shown in 7.1A is plotted as a flow volume curve. The airflow rate reaches a peak early in the exhalation then decreases progressively until airflow ceases at residual volume. (FEV_1: Forced expiratory volume at 1 second)

prefer to measure VC following a relaxed or slow expiration maneuver. This is because the VC determined by forced expiration or maneuver may result in increased airways resistance compared to airway pressures produced during a relaxed expiratory maneuver. The increased airways resistance associated with the forced expiratory maneuver can lead to decreased flows in some patients. This has prompted both the American Thoracic Society (ATS) and the European Respiratory Society (ERS) to recommend the use of a slow or relaxed VC relative to the FEV_1 to establish the diagnosis of obstructive airways disease. However, relaxed or slow VC measurements are often greater than FVC measurements, so that FEV_1/VC may in this method overestimate the degree of airways obstruction.

In addition to FVC and FEV_1, a graphic representation of flow rate against forced expired volume gives expiratory flow rates between 25% and 75% of exhaled VC—the mid-expiratory flow rate. There are clinicians who believe that a reduction in mid-expiratory flow rate is indicative of small airways obstruction. The mid-expiratory flow rates show significant variability both within and between individuals. By and large they are not more sensitive in the detection of airflow limitation compared to the FEV_1/FVC ratio.

The peak expiratory flow rate is another measurement from a flow volume graph. The peak flow shows effort-to-effort variability even in the same individual. A peak flow measurement can also be measured by a handheld peak flow meter, a device often used by asthmatic patients at home to assess the degree of airways obstruction.

Bronchodilator Response

Spirometry is often done before and after the administration of an inhaled aerosolized bronchodilator like salbutamol. At times, particularly in patients with chronic obstructive pulmonary disease (COPD), bronchodilator response to ipratropium bromide or tiotropium is observed. For a bronchodilator response to be positive there should be an increase in either FEV_1 or FVC of 12% of the baseline value and an increase in the baseline value of FVC or FEV_1 more than 200 mL. A change in the FEV_1 more than 200 mL more closely relates to the reversibility of airways obstruction. At times, a patient may experience symptomatic relief with bronchodilators without the expected change in FVC and FEV_1. This must not be dismissed; a reduction in functional residual capacity (FRC) and RV may be responsible for symptomatic relief in the absence of a change in FVC and FEV_1. Also, bronchodilator response can vary over time,

a number of individuals (30–50%) changing over from positivity to negativity or vice-versa.

A positive bronchodilator response as in asthma is an obvious indication for bronchodilator therapy. A negative response does not necessarily mean that sustained use of a bronchodilator will be of no benefit. This is with particular reference to COPD patients. Finally, in some patients, the routine spirometry is normal yet there is significant increase in FVC and FEV_1 after use of an aerosolized bronchodilator, pointing to occult airflow limitation.

Bronchoprovocation Test

Spirometry performed before and after a bronchoprovocation challenge can help to identify bronchial hyper-reactivity. Methacholine and histamine are generally used as bronchoprovocative agents. A positive bronchoprovocation test is characterized by a 15–20% fall in FEV_1 after aerosolized inhalation of either one of these agents. Bronchoprovocation test is chiefly used to identify patients with occult asthma who have symptoms of cough or complain of breathlessness and yet have normal spirometry. Bronchoprovocation tests can be positive in patients with allergic rhinitis, COPD, and following viral upper respiratory tract infection. Patients with nasal allergy with no asthma may also show positive bronchoprovocation tests.

Flow-Volume Loop

Current lung function machines have microprocessors, which allow a flow-volume loop incorporating both inspiration followed by a forced expiration recording both FVC and flow rates. Flow rates at 50% and 75% of the exhaled volumes are processed and reported. Flow rates at 75% of exhaled volumes mean really flow rates at remaining 25% of VC. Normal flow-volume loop and flow-volume loops in obstructive and restrictive lung disease are illustrated in **Figures 2A to C**.

Maximum Voluntary Ventilation

Maximum voluntary ventilation (MVV) is measured through a maneuver that requires maximal inspiratory and expiratory effort over 12–15 seconds. This is extrapolated to 1 minute and is measured in liters. The MVV in any individual should be 30–40 times the baseline FEV_1. The MVV can be reduced in patients with COPD, upper airways obstruction, neuromuscular disease causing

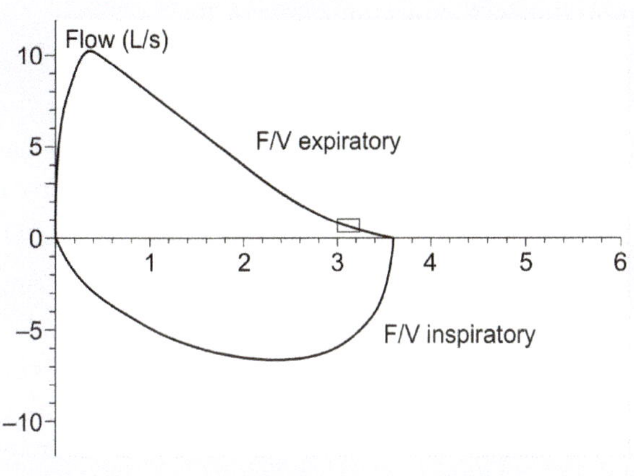

Fig. 2A: Normal flow-volume loop.

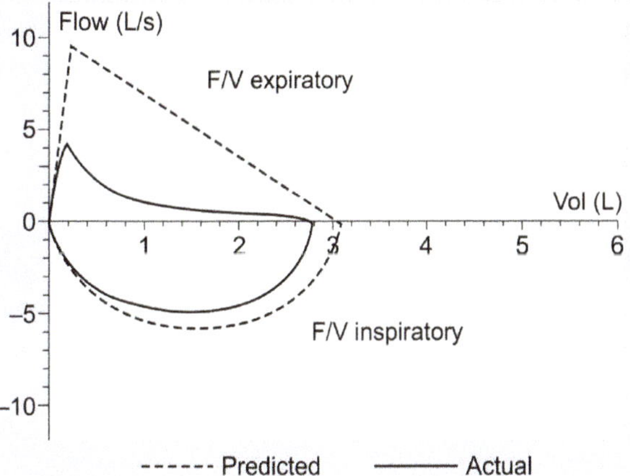

Fig. 2B: Obstructive flow-volume loop.

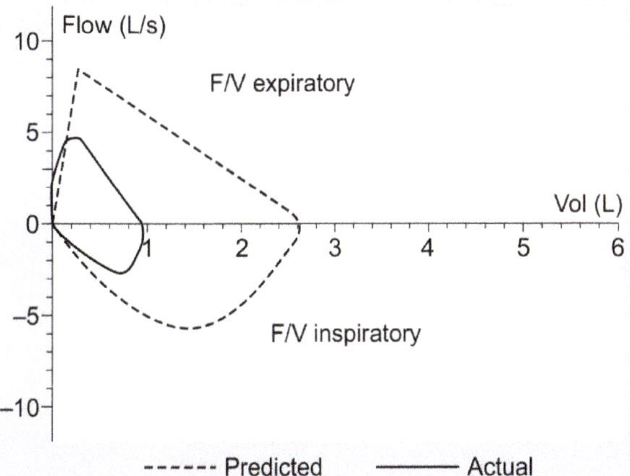

Fig. 2C: Restrictive flow-volume loop.

muscle weakness, and when there is poor performance of the test. The MVV is a nonspecific test but offers two valuable inferences:

1. A reduced MVV correlates well with the reduced exercise capacity and breathlessness on exertion
2. An MVV value below 40–45 L/min is a contraindication for pneumonectomy.

Reference Standards

Many lung function machines in India have norms related to Western standards. This is incorrect and leads to wrong inferences. The range of normal values is not only related to height, gender, age, but also to ethnicity. In fact, the range of normal values with regard to spirometric readings in Southern India is different from those in the North. The range observed in the city of Mumbai (in Western India) is not the same as in other parts of the country. This needs to be taken into account when interpreting both spirometric readings and lung volumes in different parts of the country.

■ LUNG VOLUMES

Spirometry allows volume measurement of inhaled and exhaled air. It cannot determine the total amount of air in the lung (which is the sum of VC and RV); nor can spirometry give the volume of air left in the lung after maximal expiration (RV), nor can it provide the volume of air present in the lung at the end of quiet expiration (FRC). The static lung volumes can be determined by any one of the following three methods—(1) inert gas dilution, (2) nitrogen washout, (3) body plethysmography.

Inert Gas Dilution Technique

The inert gas most often used is helium. The subject breathes from a spirometer containing a known volume and concentration of helium (10–15%). The breathing commences at the point of end-tidal expiration. Carbon dioxide is absorbed and oxygen is added during equilibration to make up for the oxygen consumed. The subject continues to breathe until a steady lower helium concentration is reached. The helium concentration in the spirometer and the lung are now the same. The unknown lung volume (FRC), which was added to the circuit (when the valve was turned allowing the patient to start breathing from the circuit) is calculated from the dilution of the initial helium concentration. FRC is thus calculated by direct measurement **(Figs. 3A and B)**. TLC is determined as FRC plus inspiratory capacity, and RV as TLC – FRC.

Helium dilution technique assumes even distribution of helium throughout the lung. But this may not happen in patients with COPD and in patients with noncommunicating air spaces or cavities. In such patients, the FRC may be underestimated.

$$V_1 C_1 = C_2 (V_1 + V_2)$$

V_1 = Volume of spirometer

C_1 = Original concentration of helium

V_2 = FRC

C_2 = Concentration of helium evenly distributed in the spirometer and lung.

Nitrogen Washout Test

The lung normally contains 80% nitrogen. Lung volumes are determined by washing out all nitrogen from the lungs. The subject is made to breathe 100% oxygen and the exhaled gas is collected by means of a one-way valve. The subject continues to breathe 100% oxygen till all the nitrogen from the lung is washed, the concentration of nitrogen reaching a fixed target value. The total collected expired nitrogen is then analyzed and knowledge of the original concentration is used to determine lung volume. This test has the same drawback as the helium dilution technique and is likely to underestimate FRC in patients with COPD. Nitrogen washout may need to be prolonged for a longer time—as long as 15–20 minutes. The normal washout time is 3–5 minutes.

Body Plethysmography

Plethysmographic measurement of lung volumes is based on Boyle's law, which states that at constant temperatures the product of pressure and volume of a gas remains constant.

$$P_1 V_1 = P_2 V_2.$$

Plethysmography measures mouth pressure changes during compression and rarefaction of intrathoracic air by a subject enclosed in a sealed box. This enables measurement of all static lung volumes. The patient in the box makes an inspiratory effort from end-tidal volume. If the pressure in the box before and after the inspiratory effort are P_1 and P_2 respectively and V_1 the volume of the box before inspiratory effort then $P_1 V_1 = P_2 (V_1 - \Delta V)$ where ΔV is the change in the volume of the box. The value of ΔV is then obtained. Now Boyle's law is applied to the gas in the lung $P_3 V_2 = P_4 (V_2 + \Delta V)$, where P_3 is the mouth pressure measured before the inspiratory effort, P_4 is the mouth pressure after inspiratory effort, and V_2 is the FRC **(Fig. 4)**.

Repeated measurements can be made quite easily unlike with the inert gas technique, which requires recalibration before repeating the test. Plethysmographic measurements take all intrathoracic air into account, including air in bullae, in large air spaces, and in noncommunicating air spaces. Lung volumes are, therefore, far more accurate, particularly in patients with emphysema.

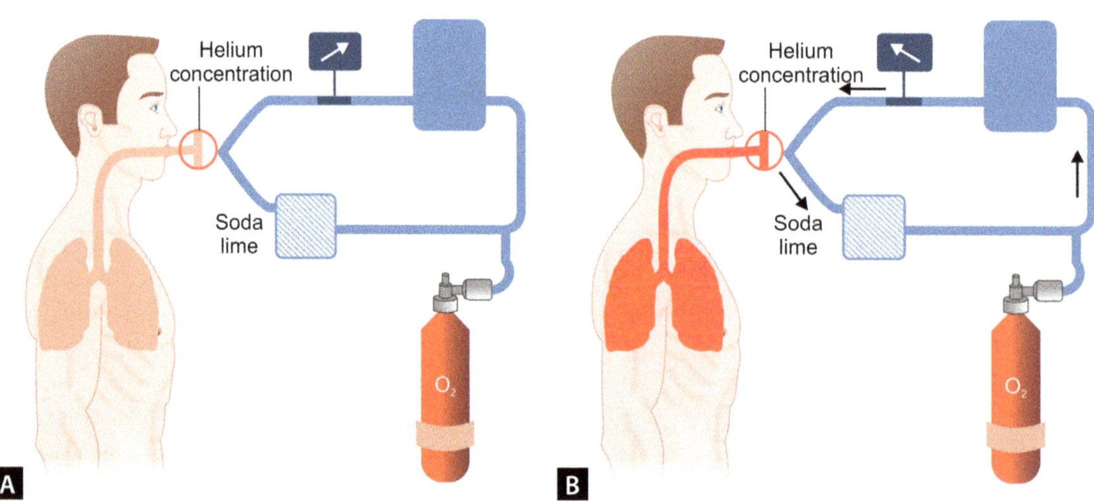

Figs. 3A and B: Lung volume measurement by helium dilution. (FRC: Functional residual capacity)

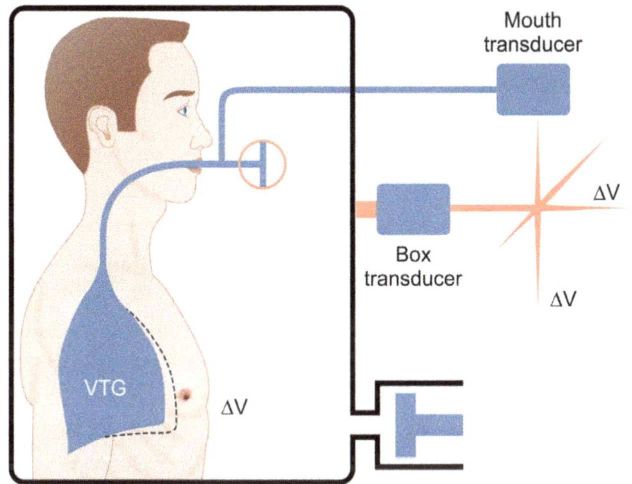

Fig. 4: Lung volume measurement by body plethysmography. (FRC: Functional residual capacity; VTG: Volume of thoracic gas; ΔV: Change in the volume of the box)

Lung Volume Changes in Obstructive and Restrictive Lung Disease

Obstructive Lung Disease

Airflow limitation and airflow obstruction during expiration causes early airway closure, so that expiration ceases at higher lung volumes. Loss of elastic recoil in emphysema is a contributing factor to early airway closure in expiration, so that these patients breathe at a higher FRC. There is an increase in RV, FRC, and a normal to high TLC. The RV increases to a greater extent than the TLC. The VC is lowered with increasing airways obstruction.

Restrictive Lung Disease

Parenchymal lung diseases, which lower compliance rendering the lung more stiff, cause a restrictive ventilatory pattern. This is characterized by a low TLC with a parallel reduction in FRC and RV. In some patients, a fall in the RV is noted early because increase in elastic recoil (a feature of restrictive lung disease) leads to delayed closure of the small airways.

Figures 5A to C illustrate flow volume loops in obstructive, restrictive, and mixed patterns.

■ DIFFUSING CAPACITY (FIG. 6)

The transfer of carbon monoxide (CO) is limited solely by diffusion. Hence, it is the gas ideally suited for measuring

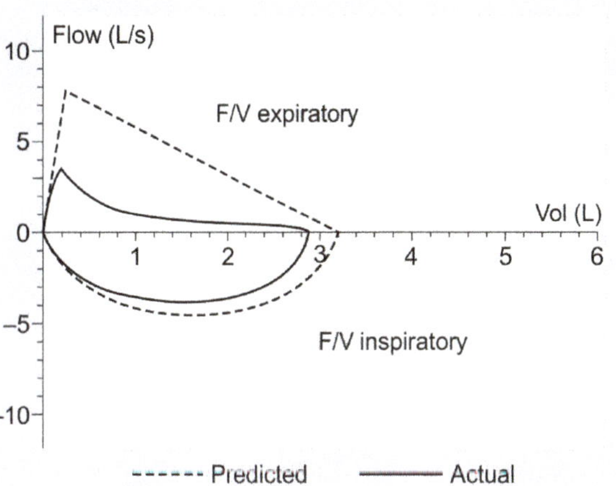

Fig. 5A: Obstructive flow-volume loop.

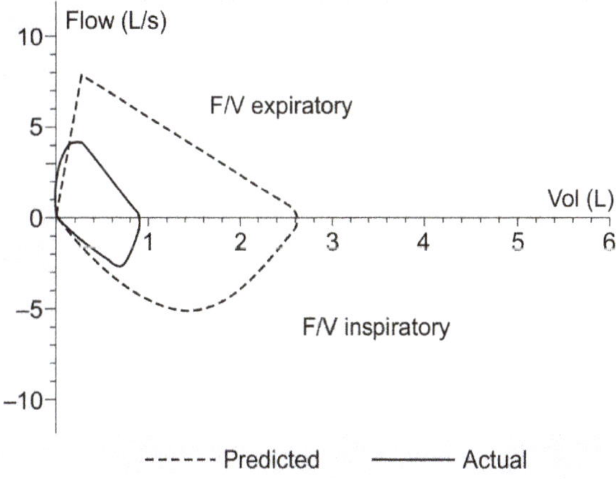

Fig. 5B: Restrictive flow-volume loop.

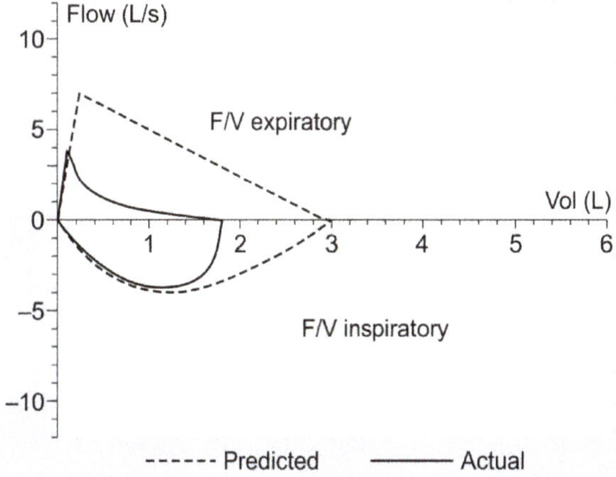

Fig. 5C: Restrictive + obstructive flow-volume loop.

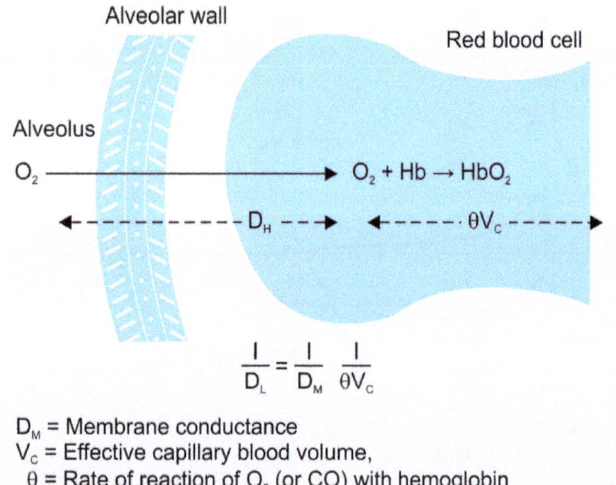

D_M = Membrane conductance
V_c = Effective capillary blood volume,
θ = Rate of reaction of O_2 (or CO) with hemoglobin

Fig. 6: The diffusion capacity of the lung (D_L) is made up of two components that due to diffusion process itself and that attributable to the time taken for oxygen (O_2).

the diffusing capacity of the lungs. The equation for diffusion of CO across the alveolar capillary membrane can be written, thus:

$$V_{CO} = D_L \times (P_1 - P_2)$$

Where V_{CO} is the gas transferred, D_L is the diffusion capacity of the lung, which includes the area, thickness, and diffusing properties of the alveolar capillary sheet and of the gas concerned, and where P_1 and P_2 are pressures of alveolar gas and capillary blood, respectively. The diffusion capacity of the lung for CO is:

$$D_L = V_{CO}/P_1 - P_2$$

However, the partial pressure of CO in capillary blood is extremely small and can be neglected. Hence,

$$D_L = V_{CO}/P_{ACO}$$

Thus, the diffusion capacity of the lung for carbon monoxide is the volume of carbon monoxide transferred in mL per minute per mm Hg of alveolar partial pressure. The normal value of the diffusion capacity of CO at rest is about 25 mL/min/mm Hg. This increases to three times the resting volume following exercise because of recruitment of blood-filled capillaries.

The usual method to measure the diffusing capacity of the lung is the single breath method. The subject exhales to RV and then takes a maximal inhalation (up to VC) of the test gas containing 0.3% CO and a diluent inert gas—10% helium. The rate of disappearance of CO during 10-second breath hold is estimated by an infrared analyzer, which measures the inspired and expired concentration of CO. Allowance is made for the fact that

concentration of CO is not constant during the breath-holding period.

A problem with the diffusing capacity measurement is that for various technical reasons the calculated values vary significantly, the published predicted values varying by 20% or more. It is, therefore, better for each laboratory to standardize its own values with the equipment it uses.

It is important to remember that diffusion is not just a measure of the thickness of the alveolar capillary membrane. A dominant factor is the capillary blood volume, which influences the surface area available for gas exchange as also the hemoglobin available to accept the CO. Therefore, exercise, left to right shunts within the heart, as also any hyperdynamic circulatory state that leads to an increased volume of blood in the capillaries of the lung wall increase the diffusing capacity. Extravasated blood as in pulmonary hematomas and intra-alveolar hemorrhage will also cause an increase in the diffusion capacity readings.

A fall in diffusing capacity is most consistently noted in patients with interstitial lung disease (particularly interstitial lung fibrosis) and in parenchymal lung disease.

It is, however, rare even in well-marked interstitial lung disease for the alveolar capillary wall to be so markedly thickened as to be solely responsible for a fall in diffusion capacity. Almost always, the main cause of a fall in CO diffusion is the ventilation perfusion inequality, which is always present in patients with severe interstitial lung disease. The diffusion capacity is also reduced in emphysema, again because of ventilation perfusion inequalities, which give rise to a considerable increase in dead space.

The diffusing capacity of the lung for CO, as mentioned earlier, is not just dependent on the area and thickness of the alveolar capillary membrane but is also affected by the distribution of diffusion properties, alveolar volume, and volume of capillary blood. The term transfer factor is sometimes used to emphasize that the measurement is not solely related to the diffusing properties of the lung. Many laboratories also report the diffusing capacity as a ratio to the alveolar volume D_L/V_A, termed the transfer coefficient (KCO). This is to imply that a loss of lung volume for whatever reason is associated with a fall in the diffusing capacity. In early interstitial lung disease, the D_L is reduced more than the D_L/V_A, which may even fall in the normal range. As the disease progresses, both D_L and D_L/V_A are reduced. In emphysema, both D_L and D_L/V_A are low because of loss of capillary surface area. The D_L and D_L/V_A are also low in patients with pulmonary vasculitis, in recurrent pulmonary embolism and pulmonary hypertension.

LUNG COMPLIANCE

Lung compliance is the volume change per unit change of pressure. In the normal range of respiration (–5 to –10 cm H_2O), the lung is remarkably compliant. The normal compliance is 200 mL per cm H_2O. At high expanding pressure, the compliance is reduced. In disease, low compliance is typically met with in interstitial lung disease, in particular interstitial pulmonary fibrosis. It is also reduced in diffuse bilateral inflammatory disease, in pulmonary edema, and in the adult respiratory distress syndrome. Lung compliance is increased in emphysema.

Measurement of compliance is technically difficult. A comparatively easy method of measuring compliance is to have a subject breathe out about 500 mL at a time from TLC into a spirometer and to measure the esophageal pressure through a balloon catheter within the esophagus. The glottis should be opened and the lung allowed to stabilize for a few seconds before a pressure reading is taken. After every 500 mL of air expired, esophageal pressure readings are taken and a pressure-volume curve is plotted. This curve represents the compliance of the lung **(Fig. 7)**. It is noted from the curve that the lung compliance will vary depending on what lung volume is used. Compliance by convention is reported in relation to the slope over a liter above FRC measured during deflation.

AIRWAY RESISTANCE (FIG. 8)

Airway resistance is the pressure difference between the alveoli and the mouth per unit of airflow. It is best measured in a body plethysmograph. Before inspiration, the box pressure is atmospheric. At inspiration, the increase in alveolar volume by AV is associated with a fall in alveolar pressure. The increased AV in the volume of the alveolar gas compresses the air in the body box; and from this change in pressure, AV can be calculated. If lung volume is known, AV can be converted into alveolar pressure using Boyle's law. Flow is simultaneously measured, so that airways resistance is obtained. The same measurement can be made during expiration.

Normal airway resistance is 2.5 cm H_2O/L/s. Factors influencing airways obstruction have been briefly discussed in the chapter Mechanics of Ventilation.

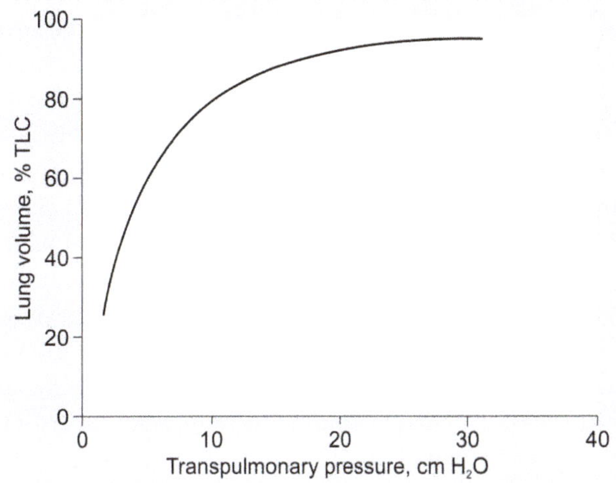

Fig. 7: Pressure-volume curve of the lung during inspiration.

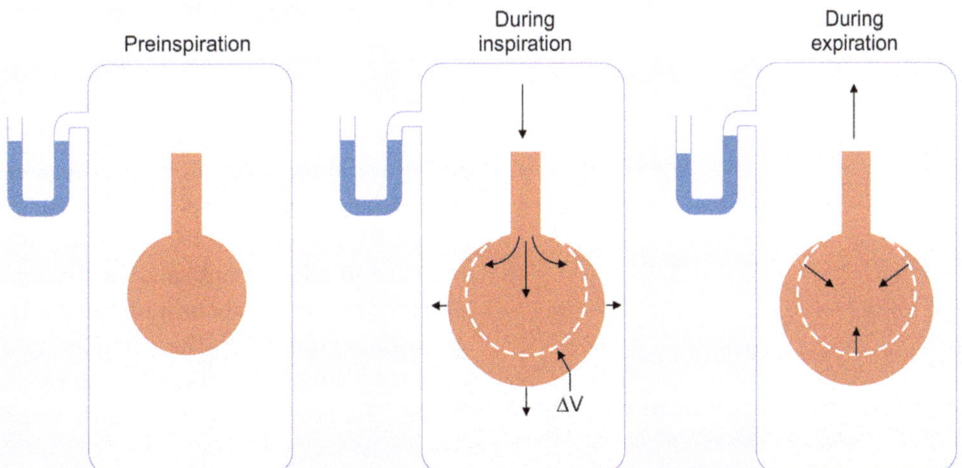

Fig. 8: Measurement of airways resistance with the body plethysmograph. During inspiration, the lung is expanded, and the box pressure rises. From this, alveolar pressure can be calculated. The difference between alveolar and mouth pressure divided by flow gives airway resistance.
Source: Adapted from West JB. Respiratory Physiology: The Essentials, 7th edition. Philadelphia: Lippincott Williams and Wilkins; 2004.

■ CLOSING VOLUME

Early disease of small airways as for example in smokers can be brought out by using the single-breath nitrogen washout test. This test consists of the subject taking a full inspiratory (up to VC) breath of 100% oxygen. During the subsequent exhalation, the nitrogen concentration is measured at the lips through a nitrogen meter. Four phases are observed:

Phase I: In this phase, only dead space air is exhaled.

Phase II: This phase consists of a mixture of dead space gas and alveolar gas.

Phase III: This phase consists of pure alveolar gas.

Phase IV: Towards the end of expiration, there is a sudden increase in nitrogen concentration.

This signals the closure of small airways at the base of the lung. The abrupt increase in nitrogen concentration is due to emptying of the alveoli air at the lung apex, which has a high nitrogen concentration. The reason for the higher concentration of nitrogen at the apex is because during maximum inspiration, the apex expands less (compared for example with mid-zones and bases) and is, therefore, less diluted with oxygen. The volume at which the small airways begin to close is the closing volume and is read off the nitrogen washout tracing **(Fig. 9)**. In a young healthy adult, the closing volume is about 10% of the VC. The closing volume increases with age, so that by the age of 70 years, the closing volume in as high as 40% of VC. Disease of the small airways in cigarette smokers leads to earlier closure of the small airways with an increase in closing volume. Changes in closing volume may precede changes in the FVC, FEV_1 and FEV_1/FVC ratio in patients with early small airways disease.

■ ARTERIAL BLOOD GAS ESTIMATION

The arterial potential of hydrogen (pH), partial pressure of oxygen (PaO_2), and partial pressure of carbon dioxide ($PaCO_2$) are measured as part of the lung function tests. The pH and $PaCO_2$ are directly measured and the bicarbonate concentration is calculated from the *Henderson–Hasselbalch* equation. Hypercapnia (increased $PaCO_2$ > 50 mm Hg) means alveolar hypoventilation. Hypoventilation can result from several causes. In COPD, hypoventilation and hypercapnia most commonly result from the inability of the respiratory muscles to meet the increased load necessitated by changes in the lung and in chest wall mechanics. Hypercapnia can also occur from a decreased central respiratory drive. Both mechanical impairment and poor central respiratory drive may operate in the same patient. A patient with an FEV_1 more than 1 liter rarely retains CO_2. The likelihood of CO_2 retention increases if the FEV_1 falls below 1 liter, though amazingly some patients with FEV_1 close to 0.5 liter still manage to breathe hard enough to prevent the CO_2 in the blood from unduly rising.

Most restrictive lung pathologies are associated with hyperventilation, so that the $PaCO_2$ may be even less than normal. Advanced restrictive disease with few functioning alveoli is associated with hypercapnia.

■ CARDIOPULMONARY EXERCISE TESTING

A stress test is of use to determine the presence and severity of coronary artery disease, though admittedly there are some false negative tests and occasionally even false positive tests (sensitivity and specificity of about 71.4% and 90.4% respectively). A significant increase in clinical information during exercise can be obtained by simultaneous measurement of the respiratory gas exchange through the use of a metabolic cart. This mode of testing is termed cardiopulmonary stress testing (CPX). The present section outlines its principles and its use.

The heart and the lungs together with the systemic and pulmonary circulation form a closely knit, inter-related

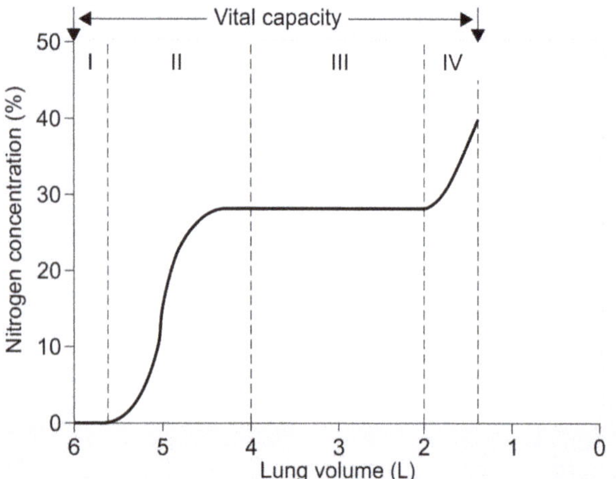

Fig. 9: Measurement of the closing volume. If a maximal inspiration of 100% oxygen (O_2) is followed by a full expiration, four phases in the nitrogen (N_2) concentration measured at the lips can be recognized (*see* text). The last is caused by preferential emptying of the apex of the lung after the lower zone airways have closed.

unit whose purpose is to supply oxygen and other nutrients to working muscles and remove carbon dioxide and other metabolites produced during exercise. In short the heart lung unit is responsible for the exchange of gases between the environment and man (cells within the body).

Graded exercise is done on a treadmill or a bicycle. In a steady state condition respiratory oxygen uptake ($\dot{V}O_2$) and carbon dioxide outflow ($\dot{V}CO_2$) measured at the mouth are equivalent to oxygen utilization (QO_2) and carbon dioxide production (QCO_2) respectively within the cells. Direct measurements can be made of $\dot{V}O_2$, $\dot{V}CO_2$, minute ventilation (VE), tidal volume, respiratory rate on a breath by breath basis using a nonrebreathing valve connected to a metabolic cart. The metabolic cart contains a gas analyzer, a computer and screen which continuously displays a 12 lead ECG, ST segment analysis, heart rate, blood pressure and a graphical display of the physiological changes as they occur during exercise. Expired air is typically assessed every 15 seconds and real time data obtained are given both in a tabulated form as also graphically. The oxygen saturation is also monitored and recorded through an oximeter. The above data is enough to derive and generate several metabolic parameters which have been listed in **Table 2**.

■ INDICATIONS FOR CPX

The American Thoracic Society and the American College of Chest Physician have given the following indications for cardiopulmonary exercise testing:

- Evaluation of exercise tolerance where the diagnosis is known or order to objectively evaluate functional capacity.
- Evaluation of undiagnosed exercise intolerance where cardiac and respiratory etiologies may coexist and the symptoms are disappropriate to results of resting investigations or the investigations are not diagnostic.
- Evaluation of patients with cardiovascular disease.
- Evaluation of patients with respiratory disease/symptoms.
- Preoperative evaluation.

Contraindications to cardiopulmonary testing:
- Acute myocardial infarction
- Acute coronary syndrome
- Acute myocarditis
- Severe valvular disease
- Uncontrolled heart failure
- Deep vein thrombosis

Table 2: Metabolic parameters measured or derived from CPX.

- *Peak oxygen uptake (PkVO₂)*: The highest $\dot{V}O_2$ achieved during the CPX and generally occurs at or near peak exercise. Reported as a weight-adjusted parameter in mL/kg per minute.
- *Maximal oxygen uptake (V̇O₂max)*: The value achieved when $\dot{V}O_2$ remains stable despite a progressive increase in the intensity of exercise. This is synonymous with peak aerobic capacity.
- *Breathing reserve (BR)*: The reserve capacity of the ventilatory system, calculated as 1 minus the ratio of peak exercise minute ventilation (V_E) to maximal voluntary ventilation. A normal value would be ≥30%.
- *Anaerobic threshold (AT)*: The highest oxygen uptake attained without a sustained increase in blood lactate concentration and lactate/pyruvate ratio. Reported as a weight-adjusted parameter in mL/kg per minute.
- *Respiratory exchange ratio (RER)*: Related but not equivalent to its cellular counterpart, the respiratory quotient, and is defined as the ratio of $\dot{V}CO_2$ to $\dot{V}O_2$.
- *Oxygen saturation (SpO₂)*: The percentage of hemoglobin that is saturated with oxygen. Typically measured by pulse oximetry.
- *O₂ pulse*: The amount of O_2 consumed from the volume of blood delivered to tissues by each heartbeat; is calculated as: O_2 pulse = $\dot{V}O_2$/heart rate.
- *Ventilation/carbon dioxide production ratio (VE/V̇CO₂)*: Also known as the ventilatory equivalent for CO_2, this represents a respiratory control function that reflects chemoreceptor sensitivity, acid-base balance, and ventilatory efficiency.
- *Peak V̇O₂ lean*: The peak oxygen uptake adjusted for lean body mass. Reported as a lean body weight-adjusted parameter in mL/kg per minute.

- Uncontrolled asthma
- Room air oxygen saturation < 85%
- Respiratory failure.

Metabolic Derangements in Disease

Metabolic derangements can occur at one or more sites along the circuitry involved in gas exchange. For example, it could occur in relation to ventilation with regard to oxygen uptake ($\dot{V}O_2$) and CO_2 output ($\dot{V}CO_2$), to gas exchange across the alveolar capillary membrane, to oxygen transport (dependent on cardiac output and oxygen content) and the utilization of oxygen by the mitochondria of cells. It could also depend on CO_2 produced by tissues and its transport via the venous system to the lungs and from the lungs to the outside environment. Knowing the site and extent of metabolic derangement helps in the evaluation of various problems in cardiopulmonary medicine.

Cardiopulmonary exercise testing is of great help for evaluating patients who present with breathlessness on exertion and easy fatigability. The common causes of these symptoms are related to cardiovascular disease or to pulmonary dysfunction or to both. Obesity and lack of exercise leading to deconditioning could also cause the same symptoms. Clinical examination and other standard diagnostic tests in the resting state may not be able to assess cardiac and pulmonary reserve, so that the true cause of the above symptoms may remain unidentified. Cardiopulmonary exercise testing may help the physicians to distinguish between overlapping etiologies.

The Value of Gas Exchange Parameters in Patients with Dyspnea (Flowchart 1)

A peak oxygen uptake PkVO$_2$ < 85% of the value predicted by age and gender is considered to be low. The normal anaerobic threshold (AT) is generally about 60% of the predicted PkVO$_2$. An anaerobic threshold (*see* definition of anaerobic threshold in **Table 2**) less than 40% of the predicted PkVO$_2$ is considered to be abnormal and indicative of circulatory insufficiency. A breathing reserve (*see* **Table 2** for definition of breathing reserve) less than 30% indicates ventilatory impairment particularly when this is accompanied by O$_2$ desaturation on exercise. Patients with dyspnea who have both combined cardiovascular and respiratory disease may have a reduction in both AT and BR. The one which show a greater degree of reduction would indicate the primary cause of the functional disability.

A respiratory exchange ratio of <1.1 without any metabolic abnormalities suggests poor effort, anxiety or mild disease.

Prognosis in Heart Failure

We need to briefly mention the use of CPX in estimating the prognosis of patients with heart failure. PkVO$_2$ is the single best parameter of survival. The mortality rate for patient with a PkVO$_2$ of ≤ 14.5 mL/kg/min was double that of patients who exceeded this value. If instead of using the weight adjusted figure of 14.5 mL/kg/min, it would be more appropriate to considered PkVO$_2$ in relation to lean body weight. It is then agreed upon that PkVO$_2$ cut off value would be 19 mL/kg/min. Using the lean adjusted peak oxygen uptake eliminates earlier observed disparities between genders and between obese and nonobese patients. There have also been reports of the usefulness of peak O$_2$ pulse values (cut-off 10 mL/beat) especially when corrected for lean body mass (cut-off value 11 mL/beat) in predicting prognosis in patients with chronic systolic heart failure.

Cardiopulmonary Exercise Testing for Preoperative Assessment

A PkVO$_2$ of < 11.5 mL/kg/min and an AT of α 11 mL/kg/min are associated with a high risk of perioperative complications in patients undergoing noncardiac surgery. It has been noted that patients with AT >11 mL/kg/min have less cardiovascular mortality and length of stay after major surgery.

In thoracic surgery, a $\dot{V}O_2$ < 15 mL/kg/min is associated with a high risk. Preoperative testing is advised in patients who after lung resection are expected to have an FEV$_1$ and a transfer factor (DLCO) < 40% of that predicted for age

Flowchart 1: Algorithm for the differential diagnosis of exertional dyspnea and fatigue.

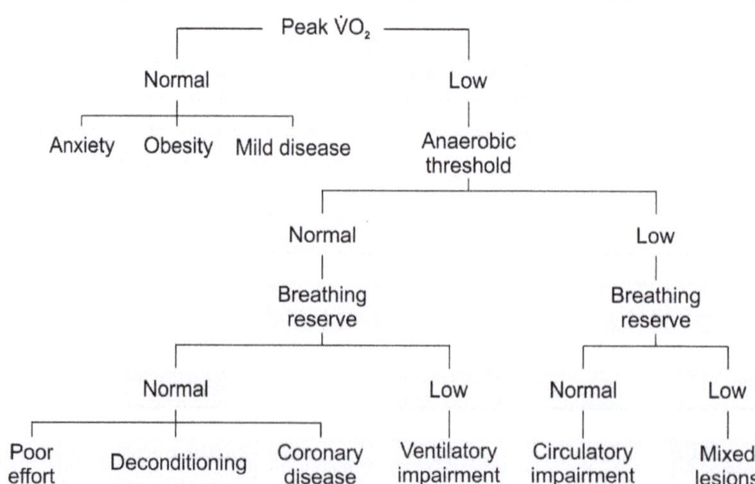

and gender. A $\dot{V}O_2$ of <15 mL/kg/min generally predicts a high risk of complications following lobectomy and an AT value of <10 mL/kg/min often predicts cardiovascular complications.

Functional Walk Tests

Functional walk tests utilize an activity which all patients are used to, requiring very little equipment, when the much comprehensive cardiopulmonary testing equipment is not available.

Either one of the two tests are commonly used:
- The Six Minute Walk Test (6MWT) ;
- The Incremental Shuttle Test (ISWT).

6MWT: In this test the patient walks for 6 minutes at his or her own maximum speed turning around cones placed 100 feet distances at each end. Median distance covered by healthy subjects is 500–600 meters. Measurements at the end of the 6 minute walk include the distance walked in meters, SpO_2, maximum heart rate and the Borg scale assessment for dyspnea and leg fatigue.

ISWT: Patients in this test walk around cones placed at a distance of 9 meters (going round then covers 10 meters) at speeds that increase every minute by 0.17 meter per second in time to audio signals. As the test progresses the time required to walk between shuttles decreases. Failure to reach the cone before the next 'beep', or exhaustion will stop the test and the total distance covered is recorded.

Distance walked in the both tests correlates well with $\dot{V}O_2$. The 6MWT is more frequently performed as the shuttle test is more difficult to administer. A patient with a 6MWT of less than 427 meters is likely to be at high postoperative risk and a patient with a negative 6MWT would be considered a low postoperative risk.

A fall in O_2 saturation is most marked in patients with interstitial lung disease. The greater the drop in O_2 after 6 minute walk test the greater the severity of the ILD.

■ SUGGESTED READING

1. Balady GJ, Arena R, Sietsema K, et al. Clinician's Guide to cardiopulmonary exercise testing in adults: a scientific statement from the American Heart Association. Circulation. 2010;122:191.
2. Casanova C, Celli BR, Barria P, et al. The 6-min walk distance in healthy subjects: reference standards from seven countries. Eur Respir J. 2011;37:150.
3. Clay RD, Iyer VN, Reddy DR, et al. The "Complex Restrictive" pulmonary function pattern: clinical and radiologic analysis of a common but previously undescribed restrictive pattern. Chest. 2017;152:1258.
4. Culver BH, Graham BL, Coates AL, et al. Recommendations for a Standardized Pulmonary Function Report. An Official American Thoracic Society Technical Statement. Am J Respir Crit Care Med. 2017;196:1463.
5. Macintyre N, Crapo RO, Viegi G, et al. Standardisation of the single-breath determination of carbon monoxide uptake in the lung. Eur Respir J. 2005;26:720-35.
6. Miller MR, Crapo R, Hankinson J, et al. General consideration for lung function testing. Eur Respir J. 2005;26:153-61.
7. Miller MR, Hankinson J, Brusasco V, et al. Standardisation of spirometry. Eur Respir J. 2005;26:319-38.
8. Pellengriino R, Viegi G, Brusasco V, et al. Interpretative strategies for lung function tests. Eur Respir J. 2005;26:948-68.
9. Probst VS, Hernandes NA, Teixeira DC, et al. Reference values for the incremental shuttle walking test. Respir Med. 2012;106:243.
10. Wanger J, Clausen JL, Coates A, et al. Standardisation of the measurement of lung volumes. Eur Respir J. 2005;26:511-22.

Section 3

Diagnostic and Therapeutic Procedures

CHAPTER 8

Diagnostic and Therapeutic Procedures

■ ENDOTRACHEAL INTUBATION

Endotracheal (ET) intubation can be performed orally or nasally through the larynx and into the trachea. The main indications for ET intubation are:

- Relief of airway obstruction, e.g. facial burns, smoke inhalation, epiglottitis, or vocal cord edema
- Protection of airway, e.g. prevention of aspiration, incoordination of swallowing muscles, obtunded and comatose patients
- Ventilatory support, e.g. acute respiratory failure, during general anesthesia, flail chest (also *see* chapter on Airway Management).

Oral Endotracheal Intubation

Intubation by mouth is preferred over nasal intubation as it allows a larger ET tube with less airflow resistance. However, oral intubation is less comfortable to the patient producing excessive secretions. Conscious patients find it difficult to tolerate the ET intubation and they may constantly gag or bite at the tube.

Instrument tray for oral ET intubation should include the following:

- Laryngoscope with both straight (Miller) and curved (Macintosh) blades, ranging from size 0 (neonates) to 4 (adults). It is vital to check that the blades attach to the handles well and that both batteries and the bulb are in place, so that it lights sharply (brightly) on snapping open the blades of the laryngoscope.
- Endotracheal tubes, which come in sizes ranging from 2 to 10. The size refers to the internal diameter (ID) of the tube in mm and it comes in 0.5 mm increments **(Table 1)**. Along the body of the tube, a radiopaque line runs lengthwise for the proper verification of tube

Table 1: Estimation of size of endotracheal (ET) tube.

Patient	Size
Neonates < 1,000 g	2.5 mm
Neonates 1,000–3,000 g	3.4 mm
Child 1–2 years	4–5 mm
Child 2–12 years	4.5 + (age/4) mm
Average adult female	7.5–8.5 mm
Average adult male	8–9 mm

placement on X-ray. Markings in mm are also shown along the body for easy determination of the depth of insertion. The distal end of the tube has a cuff, which is connected to a balloon at the proximal end, which is used to regulate volume of air in the cuff via a 10 mL or larger syringe.

Portex tubes are the most commonly used tubes, but stiff rubber ET tubes (Rush) should also be handy, as they may prove useful in difficult intubations.

- Syringes, lubricants, securing tape, flexible guiding stylet, topical anesthetic, McGill forceps, suction catheters, and an AMBU bag with proper connections should also be provided.

Procedure for Oral Intubation

After assessing the patient, clearing the mouth of any foreign body such as dentures and checking the ET tray and laryngoscope, place the patient in sniffing position by tilting the head back, so that the oral, pharyngeal, and laryngeal axes are aligned. This is usually achieved by resting the head by about 10 cm with pads under the occiput, while shoulders remain on the table **(Fig. 1)**. Always explain the procedure to the patient and reassure him if he is

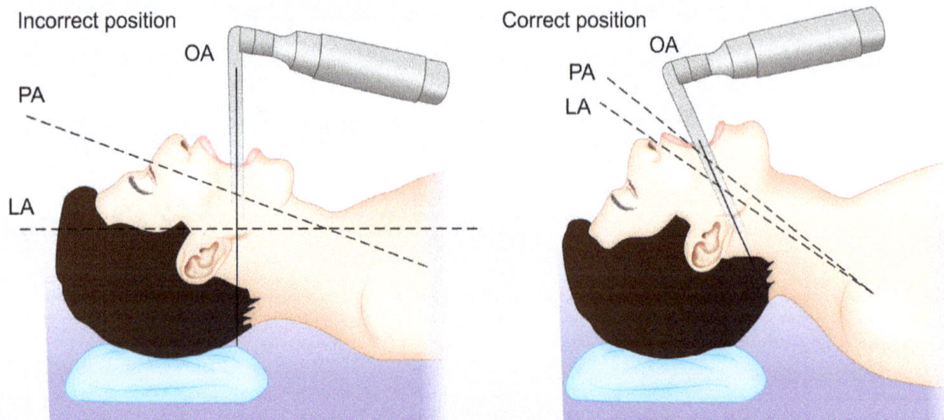

Fig. 1: The position of the head and neck for endotracheal intubation.
(OA: Oral axis; PA: Pharyngeal axis; LA: Laryngeal axis)

conscious. Next, lubricate the deflated cuff at the distal end of the ET. It is always best to ventilate and preoxygenate the patients with 100% O_2 using an AMBU bag and a face mask. If ET intubation is not successful in 30 seconds, ventilate the patient once again using 100% O_2. Now hold the laryngoscope handle with the left hand **(Fig. 1)** and insert the blade into the right side of the mouth, sliding the blade to the base of the tongue and simultaneously swapping the blade to the left. Maneuver the tip of the straight (Miller) blade underneath the epiglottis, or the tip of the curved Macintosh blade at the vallecula. Lift the handle and blade up anteriorly to display the tongue and attached soft tissues. You should now be able to locate the larynx and vocal cords and insert the ET under direct vision. Check for airflow at the proximal end and auscultate for breath sounds and then inflate the cuff. It is always best to confirm proper tube placement with X-ray chest.

Nasal Intubation

The initial preparations and head positioning are the same as for oral intubation. This is a blind technique and intubation is done by inserting the ET tube (size smaller than one would use for oral intubation) through a nostril. This should be advanced slowly and when the distal end can be seen through the mouth, it is laryngoscopically guided by McGill forceps into the trachea. In a fully conscious and cooperative patient, the tube may be advanced slowly during inspiratory efforts; and when the distal end approaches, the air movement in the trachea can be felt and heard through the tube. At this point, the tube is gently pushed into the trachea releasing a gush

of air almost audible through the tube. Tube placement should be immediately confirmed by ensuring bilateral breath sounds and later by an X-ray chest.

Common Problems and Errors of ET Intubation

The most common error is wrong placement of the tube. The tube could be wrongly pushed, so that its tip lies in a bronchus (usually the right bronchus) instead of the trachea (above the carina). If undetected and uncorrected, this could cause a disastrous collapse of the unventilated lung. The tube could also lie with its tip in the oropharynx, or pushed down into the esophagus instead of the trachea. This is immediately detected by the absence of breath sounds on manually ventilating the patient and the stomach getting distended. It is mandatory to always confirm correct tube placement by auscultating both lungs for good air entry and confirming the location of the tip by an X-ray of the chest. Measurement of the end-tidal CO_2 ($ETCO_2$) is also useful in confirming the placement of the ET tube.

The ET intubation should be *secured* firmly. Usually, an adhesive tape or a commercially made harness is used, but invariably moisture and secretions gather between the tape and skin and loosen the tape creating a risk of self-extubation. It is, hence, important to check the fit frequently and to use adhesive tapes of good material.

Ischemic injury and tissue necrosis may occur, if the *cuff pressure* is too high and exceeds the capillary perfusion pressure in the trachea. The ET pressure should be less than 25 cm H_2O to allow adequate capillary pressure;

and for patients with hypotension, it should be kept even lower. To ensure and monitor proper cuff pressure, a Posey Cufflator with an inbuilt manometer is available.

To avoid suction-induced hypoxia, the patient is preoxygenated and the suction time kept less than 15 seconds.

Certain specific problems can be encountered when using the laryngoscope, especially in oral intubation. A common mishap is aspiration of dentures, if one has forgotten to check and remove them. Trauma to the teeth and soft tissue can also occur. This can be avoided by being more gentle and careful during the procedure. Also, with experience, one can guide and maneuver the tube over the blade of laryngoscope with greater skill, especially in difficult intubations. Complications of ET intubation have been dealt with in the chapter on Airway Management.

The general criteria for extubation are listed in **Table 2**. For care of ET tube and extubation, *see* chapter on Airway Management.

◼ CRICOTHYROIDOTOMY

Cricothyroidotomy is a bedside surgical procedure, which can be lifesaving when performed for the correct indication.

Indications

Surgical cricothyroidotomy is indicated in all patients who require immediate intubation, which cannot be performed because of the following problems—(1) severe maxillofacial problems; (2) poor visualization of vocal cords due to local edema, blood, or abnormal anatomy; (3) cervical spine lesions requiring immobilization and where the neck cannot be manipulated.

Table 2: General criteria for extubation.

- *Rapid breathing test:*
  - *f/VT < 100 min/L*
    (VT is tidal volume in liters)
- *ABG:*
  - *Acceptable blood gases on FiO$_2$ less than 0.4 and spontaneous minute ventilation <10 L/mm*
  - *PaO$_2$/FiO$_2$ > 250 mm Hg*
- *Ventilatory pressure:*
  - *Maximum inspiratory pressure > –20 cm H$_2$O*
  - *VC > 15 mL/kg*
- *Cardiopulmonary assessment:*
  - *Stable cardiac and pulmonary status*

(ABG: Arterial blood gas; f: Respiratory frequency; FiO$_2$: Fraction of inspired oxygen; PaO$_2$: Partial pressure of oxygen; VC: Vital capacity)

Equipment

- Kelly or Crile clamp
- Scalpel
- Antiseptic solution and surgical gloves
- Tracheostomy tube; number 6 size.

Procedure

The most important part of the procedure is the correct identification of the cricothyroid membrane. The cricoid cartilage is the first small notch on sliding the index finger upwards in the midline from the sternal notch. The firm membrane between it and the thyroid cartilage (Adam's apple) is the cricothyroid membrane.

The patient should be supine with the neck in neutral position and the thumb and index finger of the nonoperating hand should stabilize the tracheal laryngeal complex by firmly fixing the thyroid cartilage as shown in **Figures 2A to D**. A 3–4 cm vertical or transverse incision should be made through the skin, dermis, and cricothyroid membrane. This should identify the cricothyroid space, which should be dissected and opened transversely by means of a sharp knife. In spontaneously breathing patients, a successful incision of the membrane should immediately be followed by a gush of air. The index finger should be immediately inserted in the space and a clamp is next inserted to spread the membrane and enlarge the space. Now by pulling the clamp upwards, the trachea is elevated and a number 6 tracheostomy tube is inserted under the clamp and the clamp is removed.

Complications

- Laceration of the anterior jugular veins is a potential complication because of their paramedian and superficial location, which is in close proximity to the incision. With a vertical incision, the likelihood of injury to the veins is less. However, in the event they are injured, the bleed can be stopped with manual pressure; or at worse, it may require suture ligation.
- Oropharyngeal injury is a major complication and can occur, if the scalpel penetrates the posterior wall of the trachea. This is avoided by dissecting the cricothyroid membrane with a finger or a blunt clamp but never by using a sharp and penetrating instrument like a knife. Observing proper fixation of the thyrolaryngeal complex and taking an adequate

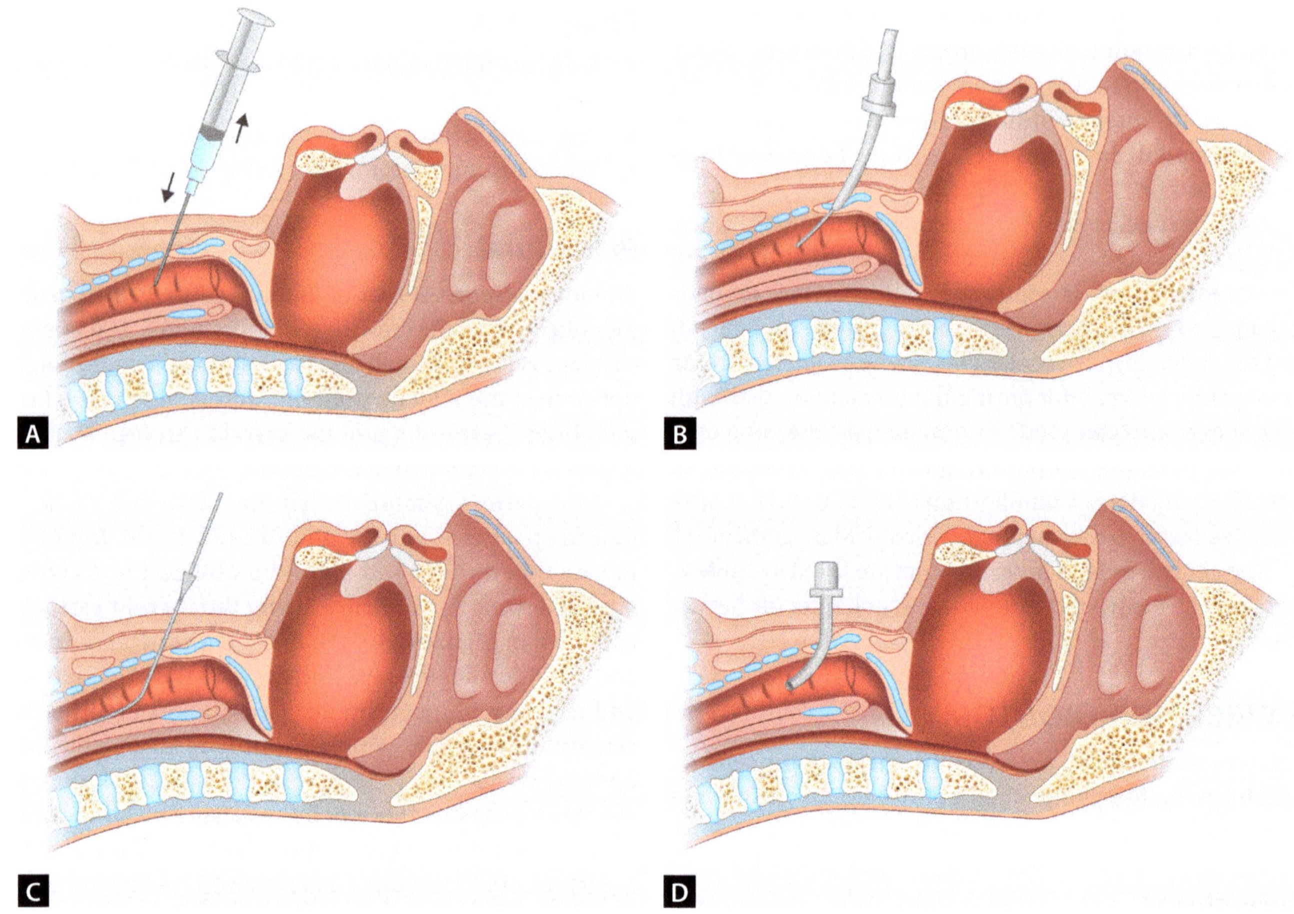

Figs. 2A to D: Procedure for cricothyroidotomy. (A) Pass needle through cricothyroid membrane; (B) Insert guidewire through the needle; (C) Jointly advance dilator and tracheostomy tube over guidewire; (D) Tracheostomy tube in place.

incision enabling good visualization of the thyroid and cricoid cartilage are very important in avoiding this mishap.

- Bleeding from adjacent structures is probably the most common problem but can be avoided or minimized by staying in the midline during the surgery.

PERCUTANEOUS DILATATIONAL TRACHEOSTOMY

Indications

- As an elective procedure when it is desirable to shift from ET intubation to a tracheostomy. In this situation, the ET tube is left in position and removed only at the appropriate time.
- To secure an airway in an emergency, when ET intubation fails or when ET intubation is not considered feasible for technical or anatomical reasons.

It is to be noted that though percutaneous dilatational tracheostomy (PDT) is perhaps more expedient than a formal tracheostomy in a dire emergency, it carries a greater risk of perioperative cardiopulmonary complications and death. It requires not only expertise but also experience. PDT should also be avoided in children and in obese patients.

Procedure

The two most commonly available kits for this procedure are:

1. Cook kit, or
2. Portex kit.

In an elective PDT, the ET tube is left in place throughout the procedure and removed only at the appropriate time. The procedure begins with a small 2 cm vertical incision made mid-way between the cricoid cartilage and sternal notch. After separating the pretracheal muscles, the trachea is palpated through the incision. Next a needle attached to a 10 mL syringe filled with saline is digitally guided and inserted in the midline through the second and third tracheal rings, with constant suction on the syringe while inserting. On entering the trachea bubbles of air are aspirated into the syringe and at this point, it is vital to hold the needle still and disconnect the syringe.

Once the needle is stabilized, a guidewire is gently passed through its lumen and the needle then withdrawn. A dilator is next passed over the guidewire to dilate the existing tract. After removing the dilator, a guiding catheter is passed over the guidewire and inserted into the trachea. Progressive dilatations are now done starting from 12 Fr dilator up to the largest 36 Fr and these are all done over the guidewire and the guiding catheter. Serial dilatations should be done at a correct angle and with minimal force to avoid injury to trachea or creating a false pretracheal passage. After the largest dilator is inserted and withdrawn, a digit is inserted through the incision into the trachea for palpating the ET. An assistant is asked to withdraw the ET slowly and stop withdrawal when the tip of the tube is right over the palpating finger. A number 8 Shiley tracheostomy tube fitted snugly with a 28 Fr dilator is now introduced over the guidewire and guiding catheter complex into the trachea. Once the tracheostomy tube is in place the guidewire, the guiding catheter and the 28 Fr dilator are all withdrawn. The balloon of the tracheostomy tube is inflated and the tube placement is confirmed by auscultation and only then the ET is removed.

Complications

- Incorrect placement of needle. This may be avoided by introducing the needle under digital guidance.
- Perforation of the posterior wall of the trachea by dilators. This can be avoided by not applying unnecessary force to the dilator while putting it into the trachea and placing the dilator at the correct angle.
- Bleeding into the trachea. This can occur with a low placement of the tube causing injury to the thoracic inlet vessels; though rare, the most lethal is an injury to the innominate artery. If such a complication occurs, direct pressure should be applied until the patient is moved to the OT for surgical repair.

The sophistication, ease, and safety of this technique have made it an increasingly popular approach, so that it can be performed by a trained intensivist at the bedside.

■ BRONCHOSCOPY

Bronchoscopy is an essential tool in the armory of the chest physician and is a field where technology continues to evolve at a rapid pace **(Figs. 3 and 4)**.

Indications

The indications for bronchoscopy are both diagnostic and therapeutic and are listed in **Table 3**.

Safety and Contraindications

The safety of bronchoscopy has been documented by several earlier multicenter studies. Several recent

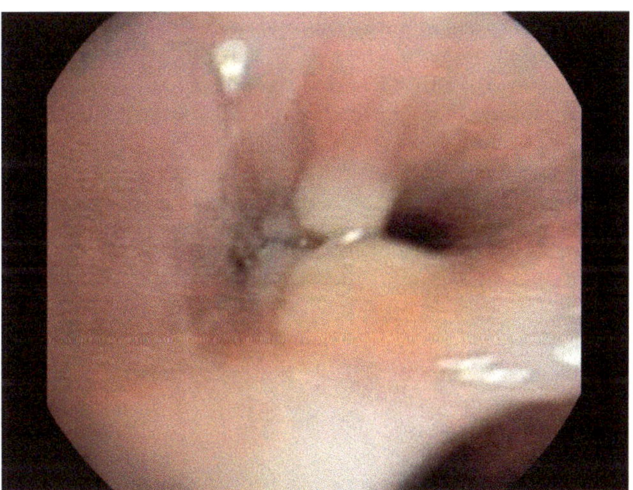

Fig. 3: Bronchoscopic view of a left upper lobe tumor.

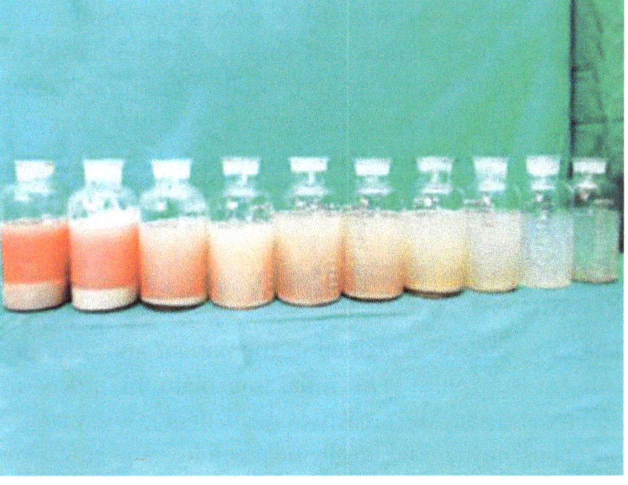

Fig. 4: Therapeutic bronchoscopy to obtain bronchoalveolar lavage (BAL) fluid in a patient of pulmonary alveolar proteinosis. Note the milky color of the BAL fluid.

Table 3: Indications for bronchoscopy.

Diagnostic:

- Cough
- Unexplained wheeze and stridor
- Hoarseness and vocal cord palsy
- Hemoptysis
- Unresolved consolidation or collapse
- Chemical and thermal burns of the tracheobronchial tree
- Suspected pulmonary infections
- Carcinoma of the lung
- Mediastinal masses
- Tracheobronchial strictures, stenosis, and fistula
- Assessment of endotracheal tube placement
- Diagnostic bronchoalveolar lavage
- Protected specimen brushing in ventilator acquired pneumonia
- Evaluation of ILD with transbronchial lung biopsy

Therapeutic:

- Retained secretions, mucus plugs, and clots
- Hemoptysis
- Strictures to be dilated by balloon bronchoplasty
- Obstructing tumors for bronchoscopic debulking
- Bronchopleural fistula
- Tracheoesophageal fistula
- Bronchogenic cysts
- Endotracheal intubation
- Therapeutic BAL in pulmonary alveolar proteinosis

Special procedures:

- Brachytherapy
- Laser therapy
- Photodynamic therapy
- Electrocautery
- Argon plasma cauterization
- Cryotherapy
- Bronchial thermoplasty in asthma

(BAL: Bronchoalveolar lavage; ILD: Interstitial lung disease)

Table 4: Contraindications to bronchoscopy.

- Refractory hypoxemia, which is likely to worsen during or after bronchoscopy
- Unstable cardiovascular status
- *Bleeding diathesis:* A low platelet count is a contraindication to biopsies but a BAL can still be safely performed
- *Uremia:* A creatinine > 3 mg/dL is a relative contraindication to biopsy because of probable platelet dysfunction

(BAL: Bronchoalveolar lavage)

surveys have confirmed very low rates of complications in experienced hands, but this should not result in complacency because major complications do still occur mainly in improperly selected patients and in the hands of inexperienced bronchoscopists.

The contraindications to bronchoscopy are listed in **Table 4**.

Procedure

The procedure is explained to the patient and informed consent is taken. It is essential to explain the procedure and try and allay the anxiety of the patient at every step. A bronchoscopy should ideally be a painless and stress-free procedure for every patient. If badly performed, however, it can be an extremely traumatic experience. We do not use any premedication except for a small dose of midazolam; 4% lignocaine sprayed at the back of the pharynx reduces cough during the procedure. We have also found transtracheal injection of 1–2 mL of 4% lignocaine to be very effective at suppressing cough during the procedure and permitting a smoother bronchoscopy. The nasal or the oral route can be used and it is important that the bronchoscopist be trained to introduce his scope via both routes. If the nasal approach is favored, the nose must be inspected for any obvious septal deviation or obvious obstruction and some lignocaine jelly on a swab stick be used to numb the nasal mucosa. It should be noted that the blood concentration of lignocaine after topical administration may be up to 50% of that obtained after rapid intravenous administration. Lignocaine toxicity after overliberal use of topical lignocaine at bronchoscopy has been reported; hence, the minimal dose should be used. If the upper airway has been well anesthetized, it is quite easy to pass through the vocal cords after carefully inspecting their movements. A careful study of the tracheobronchial tree can then be performed and bronchoalveolar lavage (BAL), endobronchial biopsy, and transbronchial biopsies can be taken as indicated.

Bronchoalveolar Lavage

Bronchoalveolar lavage is performed by wedging the tip of the bronchoscope in a segmental or subsegmental bronchus, which has been anesthetized by 2% lignocaine instilled through the bronchoscope. In the absence of local lung pathology, the right middle lobe or lingula is recommended for this procedure because they are both readily accessible and give a good return of lavage fluid. Sterile saline is introduced in aliquots of 20–60 mL through the biopsy channel of the bronchoscope to a total of around 100–200 mL. In normal subjects, BAL usually yields around 50% recovery of the instilled fluid. For diagnostic studies, instilling a total of 50–60 mL may be sufficient to obtain an adequate volume of returning fluid, which can then be sent for microbiological and cytological analysis. Larger BAL volumes are needed for research purposes when the yield of alveolar macrophages and lymphocytes needs to be higher. In normal individuals, BAL fluid comprises mainly of alveolar macrophages and a few lymphocytes. A study of the differential count of cells within the BAL fluid may help in the diagnosis of certain respiratory diseases.

Transbronchial Lung Biopsies

Both diffuse and localized lung lesions can be biopsied by passing the forceps beyond the visible bronchi into the adjacent alveolar tissue. We would recommend that this procedure always be performed with the aid of fluoroscopy, so the exact position of the forceps is confirmed prior to taking the biopsy. The two main complications of this procedure are bleeding and pneumothorax. Biopsies taken too proximally can cause bleeding from the pulmonary vessels, which are larger in this region. Those taken too peripherally can result in pneumothorax. To biopsy diffuse lung disease, the bronchoscope is wedged in the appropriate subsegmental bronchus and the forceps advanced into the periphery of the lung under fluoroscopic guidance. The forceps is opened and then advanced after the patient is made to hold his breath at the end of expiration. The forceps is removed with the accompanying tissue with firm but not excessive pressure and withdrawn from the bronchoscope. The sample is dropped into a test tube containing 10% formaldehyde for careful analysis. The overall diagnostic rate in diffuse lung disease is 35–65%. The yield is higher in bronchocentric diseases like sarcoidosis and extrinsic allergic alveolitis where the yield in our hands has consistently been around 70–80%. The diagnostic yield in opportunistic infection is in the region of 76–88%.

■ TRANSBRONCHIAL AND ESOPHAGEAL ULTRASOUND-GUIDED BIOPSY OF THE MEDIASTINUM

Mediastinal lymphadenopathy is generally due to infective pathologies or mitotic lesions. The most common infective pathology responsible for mediastinal adenopathy in our part of the world is tuberculosis. The most common mitotic lesion causing mediastinal adenopathy is involvement of the mediastinal glands in lung cancer—chiefly a nonsmall-cell lung cancer (NSCLC) or a small-cell lung cancer (SCLC). Metastasis to mediastinal lymph glands from a malignancy outside the chest is also an important consideration; finally, mediastinal adenopathy may be due to lymphoproliferative disease—chiefly Hodgkin's

disease, non-Hodgkin's lymphoma, or leukemia. There are numerous ways of sampling mediastinal lymph nodes. These include a computed tomography (CT)-guided biopsy whenever feasible, mediastinoscopy, thoracoscopy, mediastinotomy, a video-assisted thoracoscopy, and biopsy through a formal thoracotomy. The last four procedures involve expense, hospitalization, and carry a significant morbidity. Transbronchial and esophageal ultrasound-guided biopsy of a mediastinal pathology is a minimally invasive procedure that has less morbidity and is less risky when compared to most of the procedures listed above.

Indications for Transbronchial Ultrasound-guided Biopsy of the Mediastinum

- *Diagnosis*: This procedure helps to determine the cause of mediastinal adenopathy, which is of uncertain etiology.
- *Staging of NSCLC*: This is probably the most important indication for a transbronchial ultrasound-guided biopsy. Sampling enlarged mediastinal glands in patients with NSCLC allows staging of the disease, which in turn allows planned treatment. In countries where tuberculosis is prevalent, one occasionally finds a patient with NSCLC who has a mediastinal adenopathy unrelated to cancer, but due to tuberculosis. Without sampling the mediastinal nodes, such a patient would have been deemed inoperable.
- Diagnosis and staging of a wide range of other cancers originating outside the lungs.
- Accurate differentiation between lymphadenopathy due to infection, cancer, and lymphoma.

Endobronchial Ultrasound Miniprobes

For use within the central airways, a flexible catheter for the probes with a balloon at the tip allows circular contact for the ultrasound, providing a 360° image of the parabronchial and paratracheal structures. Thereby, structures at a distance of up to 4.0 cm can be visualized. The probes can be used with a flexible bronchoscope that has a biopsy channel of at least 2.6 mm.

Use in Early Lung Cancer

Small radiologically invisible tumors are in some units managed by endoscopic therapeutic interventions.

Tumors, a few millimeters in diameter, can be analyzed reliably by endobronchial ultrasound. They can be distinguished from benign lesions, and their extraluminal and intraluminal extent within the different layers of the bronchial wall determined. The use of EBUS with autofluorescence bronchoscopy has been evaluated in prospective studies and has become the basis for curative endobronchial treatment of very early malignancies in specialized institutions. Treatment involves the use of photodynamic therapy or brachytherapy or coagulation.

Use of EBUS in Advanced Cancer

- EBUS allows a detailed analysis of intraluminal, submucosal, and intramural tumor spread, features that are important for decisions on resection margins.
- EBUS is useful to demonstrate the involvement of the great vessels such as the aorta or pulmonary artery, or involvement of the wall of the esophagus by a mediastinal tumor. Studies have shown that EBUS is superior to CT in distinguishing compression of the tracheobronchial tree from infiltration of the tracheobronchial wall caused by a mediastinal tumor mass. The sensitivity of EBUS versus CT in this regard was 89% versus 25% and the specificity 100% versus 89%.

Scope of the EBUS-TBNA

The EBUS-TBNA can sample paratracheal nodes, as also nodes in the aortopulmonary window, pretracheal, subcarinal nodes, and hilar nodes.

The technique for fiberoptic bronchoscopy and the precautions during endoscopy have already been described. Images can be obtained by direct contact of the probe against the airway wall or by attaching a balloon to the probe tip and inflating it with saline. The balloon is designed not to overinflate, so that the central airway remains unoccluded. When the lesion is clearly outlined, a 21-G full-length steel needle is introduced through the biopsy channel of the bronchoscope. Doppler examination is used immediately before biopsy to avoid unintentional puncture and damage of vessels that may be present between the bronchus and the lesion. Under real-time ultrasound guidance, the needle is then placed within the lesion. Suction is applied through a syringe attached to the needle, while the needle is moved back and forth within

the lesion. The biopsy obtained is sent for staining and histopathology.

In a large trial in 502 patients with mediastinal lymphadenopathy EBUS-TBNA yielded a diagnosis in 94%.

A study has also reported sampling of mediastinal nodes less than a centimeter in size. A positive diagnosis of malignancy was confirmed by surgical biopsy or exploratory thoracotomy. In this study, the sensitivity of EBUS-TBNA for detecting malignancy was 92% and the specificity 100%. Thus, EBUS-TBNA can sample even small nodes with safety and help in the final staging procedure before thoracotomy in patients with NSCLC.

■ ENDOESOPHAGEAL ULTRASOUND

Endoesophageal ultrasound enables the endoscopist to obtain a view of not only the lumen and wall of the esophagus, but also of the surrounding structures. The target lesion outside the esophagus is punctured through the esophageal wall under ultrasound guidance. The material obtained in this way is available for cytological and polymerase chain reaction (PCR) analysis. For esophageal ultrasound-guided fine-needle biopsy, only a linear ultrasound probe is used.

Procedure

The patient is placed in the left lateral position, sedated with midazolam, and an endoscopy of the esophagus performed. The ultrasound probe is passed into the distal part of the esophagus until the left lobe of the liver is visualized. The left adrenal gland can also be visualized at this point of time.

The scope is then slowly withdrawn inch-by-inch while making circular movements to enable the endoscopist to view most parts of the mediastinum. Location, size, and echo features of any surrounding lesion are noted. Suspicious lesions or lymph glands can be punctured through the wall of the esophagus, a fine-needle aspiration biopsy being performed under real-time ultrasound guidance.

In our part of the world, caseous adenopathy due to tuberculous involvement of mediastinal glands posterior to the esophagus is not an uncommon observation. These glands cause dysphagia. A fine-needle puncture of these necrotic caseous glands under ultrasound guidance not only gives a diagnosis but is of therapeutic value. The caseous contents are discharged into the esophagus and the dysphagia is relieved.

■ CHEST TUBE DRAINAGE

Intercostal tubes are used to aspirate air or fluid from the intrapleural space. At times, as in a tension pneumothorax, intercostal drainage needs to be performed as an emergency procedure. This is basically a bedside procedure, which can be performed easily and safely in the intensive care unit (ICU), and all senior resident doctors looking after ICU patients should familiarize themselves with the technique of chest tube insertion.

Emergency Procedure

A tension pneumothorax can cause very rapid hemodynamic deterioration, leading to cardiopulmonary collapse and death, if not relieved immediately. Inserting a chest tube may be time consuming; therefore as an immediate emergency measure, a 16-G angiocath (catheter over needle device) is inserted in the second intercostal space, anteriorly, in the midclavicular line. Once the pleural space is entered, the air under tension is immediately released and the pneumothorax is decompressed. At this point, the needle is removed and leaving the catheter in the pleural space. The catheter hub is connected to a long tubing, the other end of which is placed under a water seal. This is however a temporary procedure and preparation for an immediate chest tube placement must be made for more efficient decompression of the pneumothorax.

Drainage System

A conventional two- or three-bottle system is commonly used for evacuation of intrapleural air and fluid as shown in **Figure 5**. Each bottle is placed in a series. The first is the trap bottle, which collects the fluid from the pleural space and at the same time allows air to pass through to the next bottle, i.e. the water seal bottle. This second bottle acts as a one-way valve and allowing air to escape from the pleural space, but preventing atmospheric air from entering the pleural space when negative pleural pressure is created during inspiration. The inlet tube in the second bottle is placed underwater, thereby creating a back pressure on the pleural space, which is equal to the submerged depth of the inlet tube. This back pressure, called the water seal pressure, is usually 1–2 cm of H_2O, and should ideally suffice to reinflate the lung. Further negative pressure, if

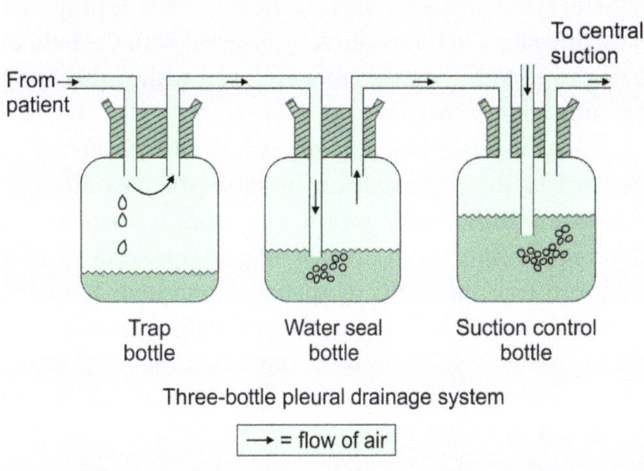

Fig. 5: Three-bottle pleural drainage system.

required, can be provided by applying a central suction. However, for reasons of safety, a third bottle called the "suction control bottle" is added in the series. This bottle has an underwater tube, which is open to the atmosphere, as shown in **Figure 5**.

Procedure for Chest Tube Insertion

A chest tube tray containing sterile drapes, local anesthetic, medium and large Kelly clamps, and other material such as sutures, antiseptic solution, and dressing materials should be kept ready. Chest tubes of various sizes are available from 12 Fr to 42 Fr. Larger sized tubes are used for traumatic hemothorax or hemopneumothorax, whereas smaller tubes ranging from 12 Fr to 22 Fr may be used for spontaneous pneumothorax. The tube itself is made of a transparent material with multiple side holes over the distal third of its length; there is also a radiopaque strip at the distal end of the tube to mark its placement in the pleural space. These tubes are available with a trocar for tunneling through the intercostal space. In case these special tubes are not available, a simple Malecot's catheter may be used.

The patient should lie flat with the involved side elevated by a pillow and arms flexed over the head. After infiltrating the skin with lidocaine (1% or 2% solution), a skin incision is made at the appropriate site of tube insertion, which is usually in the fifth or sixth intercostal space in the anterior axillary line. Some operators prefer the second intercostal space in the midclavicular line, but the penetration of muscles and breast tissue is more difficult at this site. After incising the skin at the appropriate puncture site, the tube is directly inserted with the help of a trocar. Rotating movements are used while advancing the tube with the trocar.

Once the pleural space is entered, the tube is advanced upward in the direction of the apex for treatment of a pneumothorax and toward a postbasal position for drainage of fluid, with the last side hole inserted 2 mm or 3 mm into the chest to ensure dependent drainage. Prior to insertion, the approximate length of the tube that should lie within the thoracic cage is estimated, and the position where the tube should emerge from the chest wall is marked with a silk tie.

Once the tube is properly placed in the pleural space, it is fastened to the skin with 1-0 or 2-0 silk sutures, using a mattress stitch. Before fixing the tube, it is ascertained that the last side hole is in the pleural space. The ends of the suture are not cut, but are wrapped around the tube and secured with a tape, so that they can be used later to close the wound after the tube is removed.

Throughout the procedure, the proximal end of the tube is kept clamped and is opened only when the tube is finally connected to the drainage system. The placement is confirmed by the drainage of fluid or by the bubbling of air in the drainage bottle.

Precautions

There is no absolute contraindication for inserting a chest tube. Coagulation abnormalities should however be corrected before insertion of the tube.

A chest tube should never be inserted at the bedside for the purpose of draining a massive hemothorax. Accumulated blood in a massive hemothorax acts as a seal preventing further bleeding from the source, and insertion of a chest tube may precipitate catastrophic hemorrhage. Hence, a massive hemothorax should always be drained in the operation theater where facilities for controlling such a bleed, if necessary with an open thoracotomy, are available.

Complications

Common complications of chest tube drainage include improper positioning of the chest tube, inadequate drainage, bleeding, nerve damage, injury to the diaphragm, infection, surgical emphysema, and problems in the drainage system. Use of the correct technique of insertion and placement, and proper chest tube management while the tube is in place, will go a long way in preventing most of these complications.

Incessant pain may occur after re-expansion of the lung and may evoke a vasovagal response manifesting as bradycardia or hypotension. Intercostal nerve blocks or intrapleural lidocaine may help; parenteral analgesics may be needed, if pain persists. Strong sedatives should however be avoided. Another major complication is re-expansion pulmonary edema following rapid evacuation of a large, long-standing pleural collection. Symptoms usually occur within 6 hours after rapid drainage. This complication can be avoided by slow evacuation of large collections.

After Care of Chest Tube Drainage

- The bottle should never be raised above the chest level, as fluid may drain back into the pleural space and lead to infection, or cause a drowning disaster in the presence of a bronchopleural fistula. However, if the kind of drainage system demonstrated in **Figure 5** is used, this complication can be avoided, because the draining tube never comes in contact with the water in the bottle.
- The fluid level in the tube should oscillate with each breath. Failure to oscillate may be due to blockage or a kink in the chest tube, or may be due to full expansion of the lung.
- The intercostal tube should always be clamped while changing the bottles.
- The original level of water in the bottle should always be marked, so that hourly drainage can be measured.
- Very high negative suction via a suction pump should be avoided. Ideally, a suction control bottle should be added to the drainage system as a safety measure, as described earlier.

Chest Tube Removal

Chest tubes should be removed when there is minimal drainage (less than 100 mL/24 hours), and the chest X-ray shows complete re-expansion of the lung after clamping the outside tube for 24 hours. Check X-rays of the chest should be repeated after removal of the tube. Appearance of a small pneumothorax or minimal surgical emphysema is common and resolves by itself.

■ IMAGING-GUIDED BIOPSIES AND PROCEDURES (FIGS. 6 TO 9)

Imaging is very useful in acting as a guide to obtain material for microbiology as well as histopathology. The main contraindication is the presence of a bleeding diathesis. An international normalized ratio (INR) beyond 1.4 and/or a platelet count less than 50,000 are generally considered contraindications. If the biopsy is necessary for further management, fresh frozen plasma and/or platelet transfusions may be used to minimize the risk of bleeding.

Other relative contraindications are patient's inability to lie still, hold his or her breath, or maintain a prone or decubitus position. Contralateral pneumonectomy, bulla, severe emphysema, or vascular structures anticipated in the path of the biopsy needle are also relative contraindications.

Procedure

The first step is to obtain an informed consent. A detailed explanation of the risks and benefits of the procedure must be explained to the patient and accompanying relatives.

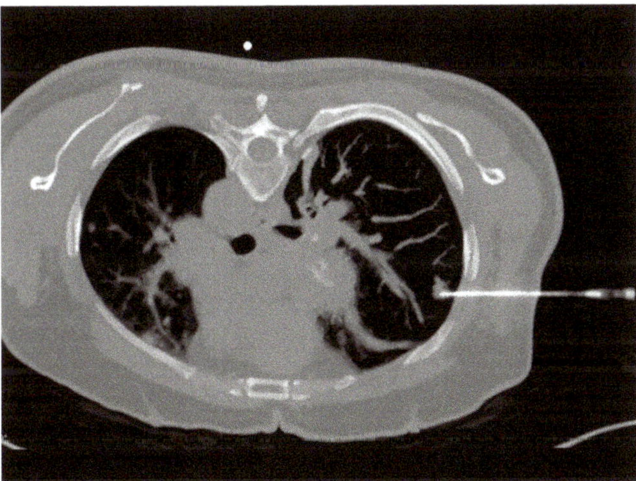

Fig. 6: Computed tomography (CT)-guided fine-needle aspiration cytology (FNAC). CT chest reveals a right lower lobe nodule has been performed with patient in prone position; needle tip is seen in situ in the pulmonary nodule.

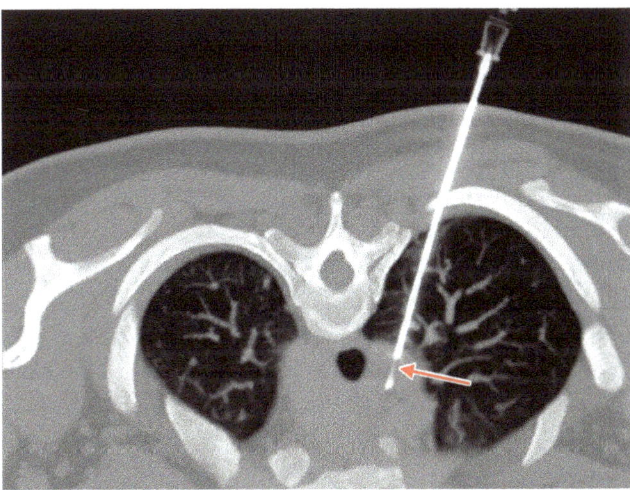

Fig. 8: A Computed tomography (CT)-guided trucut biopsy: CT chest reveals a core biopsy of mediastinal adenopathy with patient in the prone position. Note the open bevel of the tract needle in the adenopathy. This demonstrates the site from where the sample will be obtained.

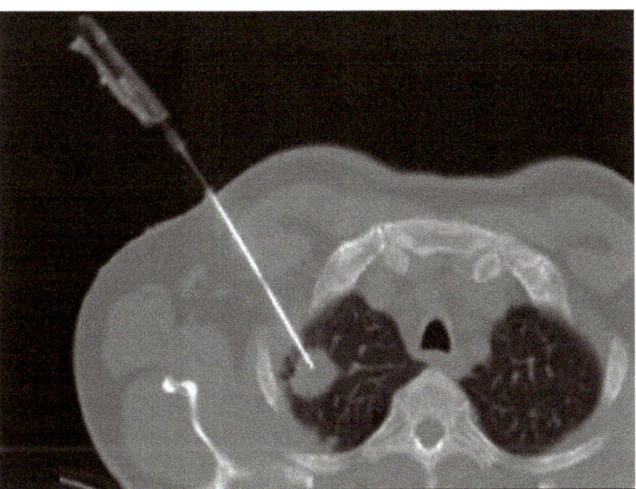

Fig. 7: Computed tomography (CT)-guided biopsy. CT chest reveals a right upper lobe pulmonary nodule. Core biopsy of lesion was performed, note needle within lesion.

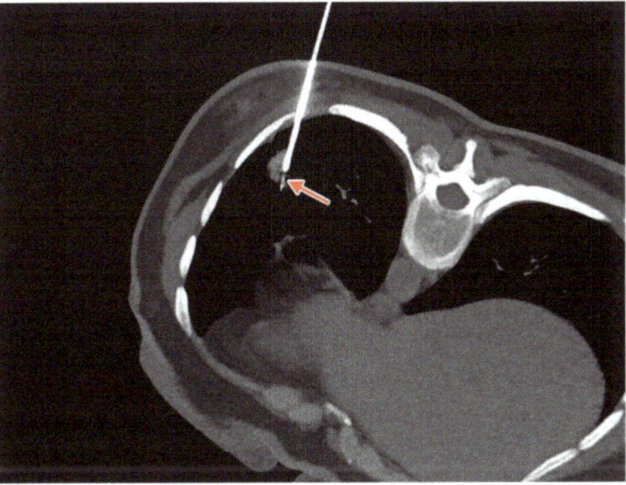

Fig. 9: Computed tomography (CT)-guided trucut biopsy: CT reveals the core biopsy of the left lung nodule with patient in prone position. The open bevel demonstrates the site from where sample was obtained.

The coagulation profile is checked. Patients on aspirin or antiplatelet agents should withdraw these drugs 3–5 days prior to any intervention. Images are obtained of the pathology and a biopsy path is planned. In planning the biopsy path, care should be taken to avoid bullae, emphysematous areas, and vessels. Solid components of necrotic mass lesions should be sampled, as the necrotic component may not yield an adequate result. Once the access path has been decided, the entry point is marked on the skin. This area is thoroughly cleansed with povidone-iodine solution. The entry site is infiltrated with 2% lidocaine solution. Two types of needles may be used—fine-needle aspiration cytology needles or core biopsy needles. It is believed that core biopsy needles have a higher complication rate than fine needles. However, a study of 5,444 biopsies found no difference in the complication rate. The pneumothorax rate after a biopsy procedure is related to the number of passes taken through the pleura. Unless the lesion is less than a centimeter in diameter, core biopsies are preferred vis-a-vis fine needle aspiration biopsies. A coaxial system is used. This consists of a needle with a stylet, which is introduced into the lesion. The stylet is then withdrawn and through this needle a trucut gun is introduced. The advantage of this is that multiple cores can be obtained with only one pass through the pleura. A 20-G coaxial is commonly used; but for mediastinal masses, an 18-G coaxial may be used. It is important that the coaxial needle be placed within the lesion and not in the lung parenchyma. If this is correctly accomplished, the incidence of pneumothorax is very low. After the biopsy is over, the stylet is reinserted and the coaxial assembly removed, as it traverses the lung on its exit. If the lesion is less than 1 cm or fluid filled, an aspiration is performed. A 22-G needle is adequate for fine-needle aspiration cytology. To aspirate infected material, a thicker gauge needle up to 16-G is used. If the lung is to be traversed, the same principle of reinserting the stylet and then removing the assembly should be adhered to; this reduces the incidence of pneumothorax.

Postprocedure, a check scan, preferably in expiration, is obtained for any pneumothorax. The patient is then given oxygen and placed with the biopsy site dependent for an hour. These techniques help to reduce air leak, postbiopsy pneumothorax, and transbronchial spread of biopsy-induced alveolar hemorrhage. A check scan is again obtained at the end of 1 hour; if there is no pneumothorax, the patient is discharged. 98% of all pneumothoraces requiring chest tube insertion develop in the first 1 hour, after a biopsy procedure.

The main complication is a pneumothorax. If the pneumothorax is small, it is treated with nasal oxygen to promote resorption of pleural air. If moderate or large, aspiration of air through a syringe and needle is often tried; if that fails, a chest tube drain is placed ideally anteriorly through the second interspace. In most lung biopsies, alveolar hemorrhage develops within the needle tract. These patients may experience minor hemoptysis. Significant hemoptysis requires observation and further management.

Drainage

Imaging may be used as a guide to drain collection of air, fluid, blood, or pus in the pleural space. Pigtail catheters or intercostal drainage (ICD) may be used. Pigtail catheters are mounted on a needle and stylet. These are introduced into the fluid similar to a biopsy procedure. The stylet is withdrawn, fluid aspirated and sent for examination. The needle is then withdrawn and the pigtail deployed into the fluid collection. The pigtail is fastened to the skin by sutures. Pigtail catheters are available up to 14 Fr in size. They may get blocked by debris, necrotic tissue, or thick pus. Intercostal drains have the advantage of being available from 16 Fr and are excellent for drainage. Intercostal drains are introduced percutaneously under imaging guidance, so that they are appropriately placed **(Figs. 10 to 13)**.

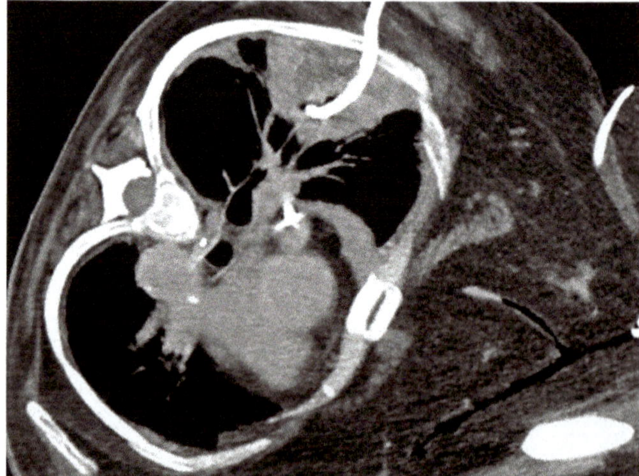

Fig. 10: Computed tomography (CT)-guided pigtail drainage. Under CT guidance a pigtail catheter has been placed into a right upper zone loculated fluid collection. Fluid aspirate revealed pus.

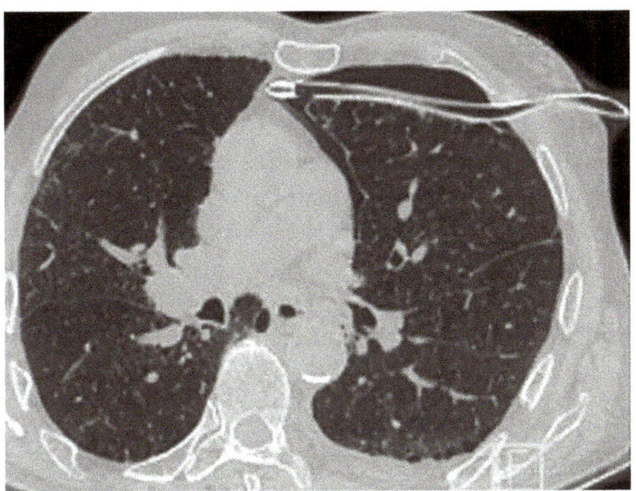

Fig 11: Intercostal drainage (ICD). Computed tomography (CT) chest reveals a left pneumothorax with an ICD *in situ*.

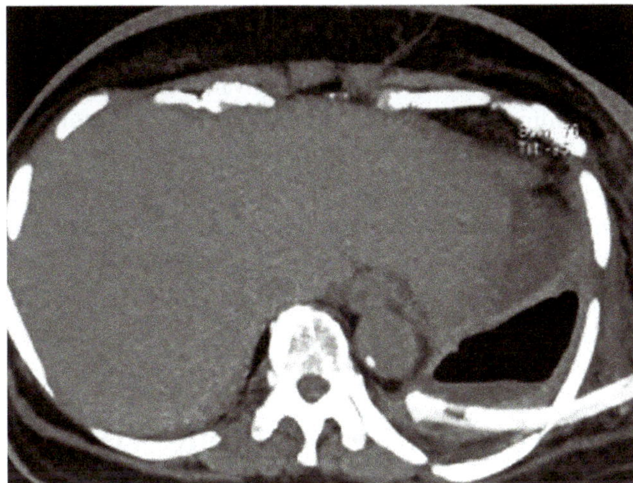

Fig. 13: Computed tomography (CT)-guided intercostal drainage (ICD) insertion. Under CT guidance, an ICD has been inserted into a left basal fluid collection, which has an air/fluid level.

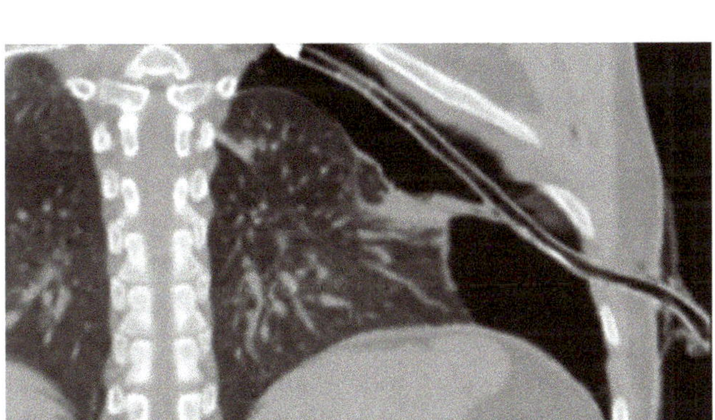

Fig. 12: Intercostal drainage (ICD). Coronal computed tomography (CT) reconstruction reveals a persistent pneumothorax on the left side. An ICD is seen *in situ*. The persistent pneumothorax is due to a pleural adhesion.

Pleural Biopsy

Pleural thickening, pleural-based mass lesions on imaging are investigated by a computed tomography (CT)-guided biopsy. If there is no pleural thickening and the pleural aspirate is nondiagnostic, a pleural biopsy is also warranted. The detection rate of granulomas in tuberculous pleural effusions is close to 50%. Another use of a pleural biopsy is in the detection of a mesothelioma. The most popular needle to perform a pleural biopsy is the Abrams needle. Other needles are the Cope and Raja needle. Pleural biopsies are performed similar to a pleural aspiration. The patient is seated leaning forward, with arms folded resting on a pillow. This helps as the scapula gets rotated forward. After preparation of the skin and instillation of local anesthesia, a stab is made over the skin through a scalpel. The pleural needle is introduced; when the pleura is breached a sudden "give" occurs. Once the needle is in the pleural space, the needle is opened by turning the ferrule, pleural fluid being aspirated and collected for examination. The needle is then withdrawn till the tug of the pleura is felt. When the needle is open, there is an aperture in the outer sheath, which is open and which hooks with the pleura. Once hooked on to the pleura, the ferrule is closed. This closure of the aperture pushes a fragment of the pleura into the aperture. The needle is then pulled sharply out of the pleural cavity. This pulls the bit of pleural tissue in the aperture. The tissue is then put in formalin for histopathology or saline for microbiology. Multiple passes may be taken to obtain multiple bits of tissue. It is important that the aperture is not open between the 10 O'clock and 2 O'clock position, as in this position, there may be danger of damaging the intercostal artery or nerve. A marker on the side of the needle indicates where the aperture is, thereby, helping to avoid the 10–2 O'clock arc. Complications are similar to all pleural procedures, pneumothorax being most common, though this is rare when there is sufficient fluid in the pleural space.

■ RADIOFREQUENCY ABLATION

Inoperable neoplasms, metastases, may be ablated using radiofrequency. In this technique, a radiofrequency probe is inserted into the tumor, the tissues being heated to ablate the tumor. The technique is similar to performing a core biopsy. As the ablation time varies from 5 minutes to 15 minutes depending on the size of the tumor, this procedure is generally performed under sedation or anesthesia. Complications are similar to those of a core biopsy, and include pneumothorax and hemorrhage. The main advantage of radiofrequency ablation is that it is a relatively noninvasive procedure compared to surgery. The procedure may be repeated in the setting of multiple lesions or recurrences **(Fig. 14)**.

■ PERCUTANEOUS TECHNIQUES FOR CENTRAL VENOUS CATHETERIZATION

Presterilized sets of special catheters with associated devices are now available for percutaneous entry into larger veins, e.g. the subclavian, internal jugular, femoral, or brachial veins.

"Catheter-over-needle devices" are most commonly used, and are designed to eliminate the risk of the needle cutting through the catheter; the greatest danger of "catheter-through-needle device" is the shearing of the catheter, if it is accidentally withdrawn through the needle. These devices consist of catheters of variable length, which can be easily passed through the needle lumen, and can be advanced through the peripheral veins into the central veins.

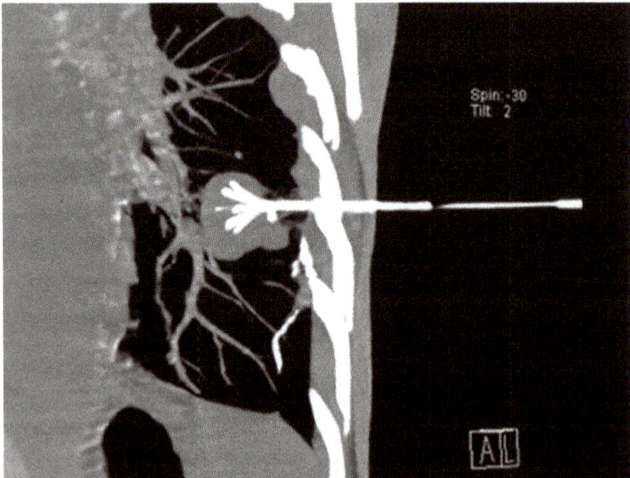

Fig. 14: Radiofrequency ablation: Computed tomography (CT) chest coronal reconstruction reveals a nodular mass lesion with a radiofrequency probe inserted in the mass lesion percutaneously. The prongs are open. Each of these probes will pass an electrical current into the lesion to ablate the lesion.

Both these devices allow placement of a catheter in the central veins by direct puncturing of the vessel. However, if a Swan-Ganz or a pacing catheter needs to be passed through the vein, one may have to use special "Introducer Sets". These are usually expensive units consisting of a needle, guidewire, and a dilator over which a polythene sheath is tightly wrapped. These sets require use of the modified Seldinger technique for introduction of the wide-bore introducer sheath in the vein, through which the catheters can then be passed.

Modified Seldinger Technique (Figs. 15A to D)

The site of the puncture is infiltrated with 1% lidocaine. The vein is cannulated percutaneously with an 18-G thin-walled needle, following the appropriate landmarks and techniques for individual veins as described later. Blood is aspirated from the needle to confirm its entry into the vein, following which the soft end of a J-tip 0.035 inch guidewire is inserted through the needle, and advanced into the superior vena cava (if the subclavian or internal jugular vein is used), or the inferior vena cava (if the femoral vein is used). The guidewire should slide effortlessly through the vein, and should never be forced. After the guidewire is satisfactorily inserted (check that it is not inserted too far in as it may produce ventricular ectopics), the introducer needle is removed, and a small nick is made near the puncture to facilitate the passage of the dilator. The tapered vein dilator carrying an introducer sheath is then advanced over the guidewire with a twisting motion through the skin and subcutaneous tissue into the vessel. Finally, the wire and dilator are removed, leaving the wide-bore introducer sheath in the vein, through which the Swan-Ganz or pacing catheter can be passed. The sheath should be secured well with sutures. Some of the introducer sheaths have a one-way valve at the proximal end to prevent backflow of blood, and a side port to allow continuous infusion of fluid to prevent clotting. Throughout this procedure, care should be taken to ensure that the proximal end of the guidewire always remains outside and does not migrate into the vein. If for any reason during the procedure, the guidewire needs to be removed and reinserted, the whole procedure should be repeated from the beginning; the needle should never be reintroduced over the guidewire, as it can shear the wire.

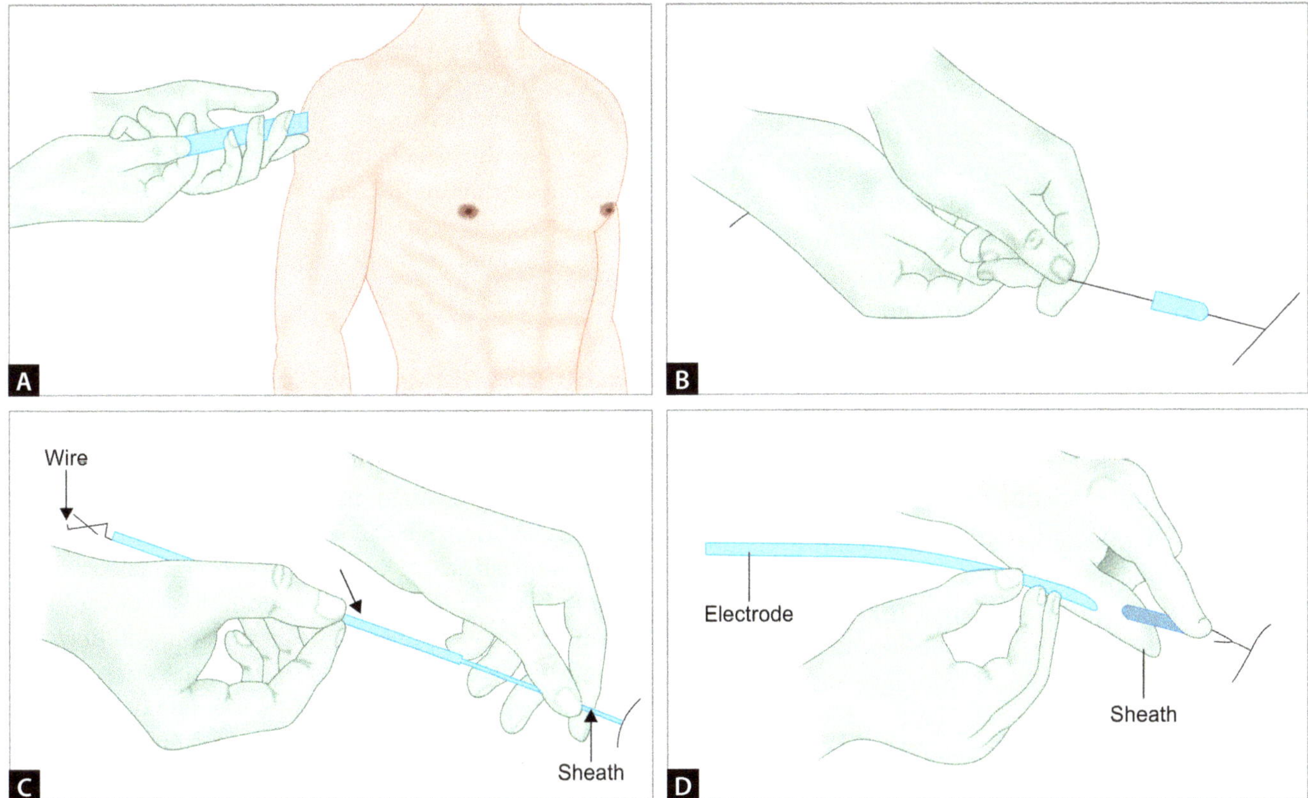

Figs. 15A to D: Modified Seldinger technique of inserting a guidewire and introducer set via subclavian vein puncture. (A) Direction of needle and site of puncture; (B) insertion of guidewire; (C) the introducer sheath (with dilator) is first advanced over the guidewire. Next, with the sheath well in, the guidewire and dilator are removed; (D) an electrode or catheter is inserted through the sheath.
Source: Adapted from Vakil RJ, Udwadia FE. Diagnosis and Management of Medical Emergencies, 3rd edition. Mumbai: Oxford University Press; 198.

Techniques for Specific Veins

Subclavian Vein Catheterization

The patient lies flat or in a slight head-low position. Correct positioning is important; both arms should be stretched straight by the sides, and the patient should be lying on a firm flat surface, so that both the shoulders are in the same plane. The site of puncture is a point just below the junction of the middle and inner thirds of the clavicle.

The skin is now punctured at the selected site with the point of the needle directed toward the suprasternal notch; the plane of the needle should be horizontal to the ground and parallel to the parietal pleura **(Fig. 16)**. The needle is advanced with a gentle suction on the syringe until the subclavian vein is entered, often with a distinct give. It is sometimes necessary to slightly change the angle of the needle, in which case it is always essential that the needle is completely withdrawn before re-entering in a new direction. Once the needle is in the vein, depending

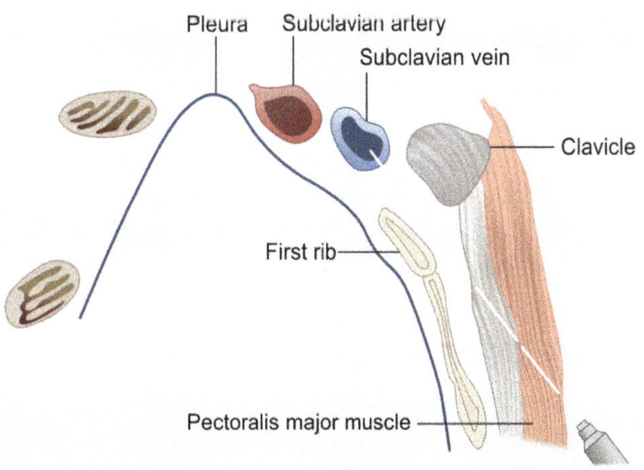

Fig. 16: Percutaneous subclavian venipuncture: anatomical relationship of the subclavian vein.
Source: Adapted from Vakil RJ, Udwadia FE. Diagnosis and Management of Medical Emergencies, 3rd edition. Mumbai: Oxford University Press; 198.

on the catheter design, proceed either with the modified Seldinger technique, or directly introduce the catheter through the needle, or slide it from over the needle.

Complications: Pneumothorax is the most common major complication of this procedure. The incidence of pneumothorax can be reduced by avoiding large-bore needles, multiple punctures, and by disconnecting the ventilator at the time of venepuncture. Other serious complications include air embolism, catheter-induced infection, perforation of the superior vena cava, and hemothorax (due to accidental puncture of the subclavian artery).

Internal Jugular Venepuncture

The patient is placed in the Trendelenburg position, and the skin cleaned and carefully draped. The site of puncture is located two finger breadths above the clavicle at the outer border of the sternomastoid, with the patient's head rotated to the opposite side. The needle with the syringe attached is directed towards the suprasternal notch. Aspiration of blood indicates entry into the vein. Air embolism and thrombophlebitis are the main complications encountered in this procedure. Accidental puncture of the internal carotid artery can also occur. Pneumothorax is rarely observed following this procedure.

Femoral Venepuncture

The femoral vein can also be entered percutaneously. The site of puncture is below the inguinal ligament, just medial to the point where the femoral artery pulse can be palpated. Wound infection is generally more common, and there is an increased risk of thrombophlebitis when the femoral vein is used.

◼ ARTERIAL CATHETERIZATION

Except in unavoidable circumstances, it is wise to choose the radial artery for catheterization, as the risk of occlusion of a proximal artery such as the femoral or brachial could prove disastrous. It is vital to assess the patency of the ulnar artery by Allen's test prior to catheterization, as it is important to be sure that a competent ulnar artery is present. This is done as follows:

- The examiner compresses both arteries, when the patient makes a tight fist to squeeze all the blood out of the hand.
- The patient then extends the fingers, and the examiner observes the blanched hand.
- Compression on the ulnar artery is released, and the examiner observes the hand filling with blood. If filling does not occur, the ulnar artery is presumed to be nonfunctional.

Technique of Radial Artery Catheterization

The wrist is hyperextended and a small area over the radial artery is cleaned and prepared with alcohol and Betadine solution. A small area on both sides of the artery is anesthetized with 1% lidocaine solution. The artery is palpated with the forefinger and middle finger of one hand, and the needle (we prefer a "catheter-over-needle device"), is now inserted percutaneously toward the artery. As the needle touches the vessel wall, the arterial pulsations are "damped"; the needle is now advanced further through the wall into the lumen of the artery. As soon as the blood gushes out, the catheter is advanced slowly over the needle, and the needle is then removed. The catheter hub is attached to a continuous flush system ("Intraflo") via a pressure tubing. The hub of the catheter should be fixed firmly to the skin, and an antibiotic ointment dressing applied over the point of arterial puncture.

Maintaining tight compression over the puncture site, and proper attention to asepsis will go far in avoiding the two most common complications of arterial puncture, viz. local hematoma formation and infection. Clotting of the catheter can be prevented by using a low-dose continuous heparin infusion.

◼ SUGGESTED READING

1. Clark VL, Kruse JA. Arterial catheterization. Critical Care Clin. 1992;8(4):687.
2. Denys BG, Uretsky BF. Anatomical variations of internal jugular vein location: impact on central venous access. Crit Care Med. 1991;19:1516-9.
3. Eapen GA, Shah AM, Lei X, et al. Complications, consequences, and practice patterns of endobronchial ultrasound-guided transbronchial needle aspiration: Results of the AQuIRE registry. Chest. 2013;143(4):1044-53.

4. Frykholm P, Pikwer A, Hammarskjöld F, et al. Clinical guidelines on central venous catheterisation. Swedish Society of Anaesthesiology and Intensive Care Medicine. Acta Anaesthesiol Scand. 2014;58(5):508-24.

5. ED Brewis RAL, Gibson GJ, Geddes DM, et al. Respiratory medicine. Bronchoscopy. New York: Raven Press; 1994.

6. Goumas P, Kokkinis K, Petrocheilos J, et al. Cricothyroidotomy and the anatomy of the cricothyroid space: an autopsy study. J Laryngol Otol. 1997;111:354.

7. Halsted Residents of the John Hopkins Hospital. In: Chen H, Sola J, Lillemoe K (Eds). Manual of Common Bedside Surgical Procedures. Baltimore, USA: Willaims and Wilkins; 1996. p. 20.

8. Isaacs JH Jr, Pederson AD. Emergency cricothyroidotomy. Am Surg. 1999;63:346.

9. Miller KS, Sahn FA. Chest tubes: indications, technique, management and complications. Chest. 1987;91:258.

10. Rosen M, Latto IP, Ng WS. Handbook of Percutaneous Central Venous Catheterization. London: WB Saunders; 1981.

11. Slogoff S, Keats AS, Arlund C. On the safety of radial artery cannulation. Anesthesiology. 1983;59:42.

12. Swanson RS, Uhlig PN, Gross PL, et al. Emergency intravenous access through the femoral vein. Ann Emerg Med. 1984;13:244.

Clinical Approach to Respiratory Disease: Symptoms and Signs

CHAPTER 9

Cough

■ INTRODUCTION

One of the most common symptoms for which a patient seeks advice from the doctor is cough. Cough serves as a protective reflex that protects the lungs against aspiration. It also helps to clear secretions within the respiratory tract. Cough can be voluntary or involuntary. When involuntary it arises from the stimulation of a broad group of rapidly activating irritant receptors (RARs) found in the larynx and tracheobronchial tree. Cough receptors are also present in the pleura, esophagus, stomach and the external auditory canal.

The RARs can be stimulated by diverse stimuli—mechanical, chemical and inflammatory. Inhalation of dust, smoke, or other irritants is an example of mechanical and chemical stimuli causing cough. A tumor in the airway or extrinsic pressure on the airways or distortion of airways due to pulmonary fibrosis causes mechanical stimulation of the RARs and cough. Mucosal inflammation, as for example in tracheobronchitis, is an example of inflammatory stimuli causing cough.

Another cough receptor present in the respiratory tract is the "slowly adapting stretch receptor" (SAR) which terminates inspiration and starts expiration after lung inflation has reached an adequate level. These receptors also influence cough. In addition to the above, there exist thin unmyelinated vagal afferents not only in the mucosa of the respiratory tract but also in the alveolar walls. These receptors have been shown to be exquisitely sensitive to chemicals such as capsaicin sand bradykinin.

■ MECHANISM OF COUGH

Stimulation of cough receptors leads to afferent sensory impulses to the cough center in the medulla via the vagus, glossopharyngeal, trigeminal and phrenic nerves. The vagus carries impulses from the larynx, trachea, bronchi, pleura, esophagus and stomach. The glossopharyngeal nerve carries stimuli from the pharynx; the trigeminal from the nose and paranasal sinuses; the phrenic from the pericardium and diaphragm. The stimulated cough center in the medulla sends impulses through the motor efferents in the cranial nerves, the phrenic nerve and through motor efferents supplying the muscles of the thoracic cage and the accessory muscles of respiration, thereby completing a reflex arc. Cough starts with a rapid inspiration, followed in quick sequence by closure of the glottis, contraction of the muscles of the rib cage and abdominal muscles that leads to a marked rise in pleural and intrapulmonary pressures. There is now a sudden opening of the glottis with a burst of air via the mouth to the outside. The intrathoracic pressure when the glottis is closed can be as high as 100–200 mm Hg so that the velocity of airflow through the airways when the glottis opens is high, propelling secretions upwards to the throat and mouth. The vibrations of the tracheobronchial walls and of secretions present in the airways during the explosive forced expiratory effort are responsible for the sound of a cough.

The effectiveness of cough in propelling secretions depends on the lung volume at which the propulsive expiration is initiated. At high lung volumes (as in healthy individuals) when the "equal pressure points" are located in the large airways, the propulsive force is large. In patients with small lung volumes the "equal pressure points" are closer to the alveoli and the propulsive force "downstream" toward the mouth is feeble. Small lung volumes are particularly observed in critically ill patients or postoperatively after thoracic, cardiovascular or upper abdominal surgery. Retained secretions because of a poor cough in these patients are a cause of atelectasis, which in turn further reduces lung volumes rendering cough even more ineffective.

The cough reflex can be impaired or interrupted at several levels in the reflex pathways. The receptors can be damaged by a lung pathology or their sensitivity diminished by anesthesia or depressant drugs. The reflex may be dampened by a pathology involving the afferent pathways or through depression of the cough center by drugs, disease, or raised intracranial pressure, or following involvement of motor efferents and the muscles supplied by the efferents in neuromuscular disease. At times, the nervous reflex arc is intact, but the effector muscles are weak because of a critical illness, electrolyte imbalance, age, debility or poor nutrition. Tracheostomy eliminates glottic closure, thereby leading to reduced intrapulmonary pressure and a comparatively feebler cough.

■ COMPLICATIONS OF COUGH

Cough when frequent, forceful and prolonged can result in fractures of the ribs, generally the sixth or seventh rib in the mid-axillary line. This can cause severe pain on breathing, more so on coughing. Small hairline fractures of a rib may not be evident on an X-ray of the chest or of the ribs but is always recognized on a computed tomography (CT) of the chest.

Post-tussive syncope is the result of a protracted bout of cough. The syncope ends without sequelae once the cough ceases. It is due to a poor return of blood to the right heart because of marked increase in intrathoracic pressure during the bout of cough. This leads to a sharp fall in cardiac output and syncope. The patients should be instructed to break up the cough into short bouts to prevent post-tussive syncopal attacks.

In older people, particularly in women, severe chronic cough can lead to urinary or even fecal incontinence which can be a source of great social embarrassment.

■ DIAGNOSTIC EVALUATION OF ACUTE COUGH

Diagnostic evaluation is helped by considering cough as acute or chronic. Acute cough starts abruptly and generally resolves within 3–4 weeks. The diagnosis is apparent from other clinical features associated with acute cough. The common causes are acute pharyngitis, laryngitis, and tracheobronchitis either bacterial or viral in origin. Acute allergic rhinitis causing cough is easily recognized by the usual features of rhinitis. More serious causes of acute cough are pneumonia due to bacterial or other microbial infections. Mycoplasmal infection is an important cause of cough. Cough due to mycoplasmal infection is often paroxysmal, either dry or associated with scanty mucoid sputum, and accompanied by flu-like symptoms. Acute asthma may occasionally have cough as the predominant symptom. A careful physical examination will reveal the presence of airways obstruction. An acute exacerbation of chronic obstructive pulmonary disease (COPD) and an acutely evolving pleural effusion are conditions where cough is invariably accompanied by breathlessness and often by tachypnea. Pulmonary infarction is associated with cough. Pleural pain, pleural effusion and dyspnea are often associated features, together with a background of possible deep vein thrombosis **(Table 1)**.

Though acute cough generally ends by 3–4 weeks, occasionally cough caused by an acute viral infection may persist for a couple of months and is probably related to a temporary hyper-reactivity of the airways resulting as a sequel to a viral infection.

■ DIAGNOSTIC EVALUATION OF CHRONIC COUGH

Diagnostic evaluation of a patient with a chronic cough should include a careful history with regard to the nature of cough, whether dry, or productive of mucoid or purulent expectoration, whether there is presence or absence of breathlessness and of associated systemic features. A history of smoking and the number of cigarettes smoked is very important. Though cigarette smoking does often lead to a smoker's cough, a change in the character or intensity of cough always merits further investigation. A history of sinusitis or allergic rhinitis raises the possibility

Table 1: Important common causes of acute cough.
• Acute upper respiratory tract infections
• Acute rhinitis
• Acute sinusitis
• Asthma
• Acute exacerbation of COPD
• Pneumonia; mycoplasmal infection, other acute respiratory infections
• Acutely evolving pleural effusion
• Pulmonary infarction

(COPD: Chronic obstructive pulmonary disease)

of a postnasal drip being responsible for cough. Acid regurgitation, heartburn suggests cough related to gastroesophageal reflux. Chronic bronchial asthma is associated both with cough, wheeze and breathlessness. A history of hemoptysis warrants a thorough investigation. An easily and often forgotten cause of chronic cough is the use of angiotensin-converting enzyme (ACE) inhibitors which disappears when the drug is stopped, though it may take 2–6 weeks for it to disappear completely.

The sudden onset of cough related to aspiration of a foreign body should never be forgotten, particularly in a child. Dyspnea accompanies cough if there is obstruction to the large airways. If the foreign body is small and aspirated deep into the lung, cough is the main symptom. If foreign body aspiration is undiagnosed cough becomes chronic and persistent.

Persistent cough can be the first symptom in tuberculosis and in lung cancer. Cough with purulent expectoration is a feature of suppurative lung diseases such as lung abscess or bronchiectasis. A history of profuse watery or mucoid expectoration is occasionally a feature in some patients with an adenocarcinoma of the lung.

Clinical examination should be meticulous, physical signs pointing to airways obstruction due to asthma, COPD or restrictive lung disease need to be carefully looked out for. The easily recognized dry velcro crackles heard over lung bases are telltale features of interstitial pulmonary fibrosis. A monophonic wheeze suggests obstruction to a large airway. Coarse crackles over the bases in a patient having purulent expectoration suggest bronchiectasis. An examination of the ear, nose, throat and larynx is mandatory.

Investigations should include routine blood tests, an X-ray of the chest and sinuses, sputum examination, including microbiology and cytology, full lung function tests, serial peak flow measurements and if needs be a high-resolution computed tomography (HRCT) chest and bronchoscopy. *It should be remembered that any and every disease involving the lungs, pleura or mediastinum can cause chronic cough.* Almost always, any sinister pathology can ultimately be diagnosed by a careful history, a meticulous physical examination and relevant investigations.

It also needs also to be remembered that *chronic cough is an equally important symptom in diseases of the cardiovascular system. Chronic left ventricular failure or mitral valvular disease may present with cough, often worse in the sleeping posture, relieved when sitting up. It is generally associated with dyspnea, but in some patients cough is the predominant symptom. A meticulous examination and investigation of the cardiovascular system is therefore as important as an assessment of the respiratory system if symptoms and clinical features so warrant.*

The important and frequent causes of chronic cough almost always diagnosed by careful clinical assessment and relevant investigations are given in **Tables 2 to 4**.

The diagnostic problem arises when the history and investigations (which include full imaging studies and bronchoscopy) are noncontributory in discovering the etiology of chronic cough. The patient has generally visited several doctors with no relief. The causes that need special consideration (or reconsideration) are briefly described below. The description is confined to causes of chronic cough due to respiratory disease, or problems involving the respiratory system. The treatment of these diseases or problems has been discussed in different appropriate chapters of this book.

Cough as a Variant of Asthma

Cough and not wheeze or breathlessness is the hallmark of cough-variant asthma. The airway inflammation in cough-variant asthma is similar to that occurring in patients with usual asthma but there is a markedly heightened cough reflex sensitivity in the former. The cough is generally dry or minimally productive; it may be more marked nocturnally, during stress or on exercise. None of these aggravating factors may however be present. Serial peak flow measurement may show variable airflow limitation or obstruction, but this again is not always elicitable. Spirometries with observed bronchodilator response to an aerosolized bronchodilator are routine tests but in most of these patients these tests are noncontributory. Demonstration of bronchial hypersensitivity by an appropriate bronchoprovocation test is both a sensitive and specific pointer to variable airflow obstruction and may be the only positive test in these patients. Eosinophilia and raised immunoglobulin E (IgE) levels are supportive evidence of this variant of asthma. Finally, even if all diagnostic tests are negative, the diagnosis of cough-variant asthma is confirmed by the improvement of cough following the use of aerosolized bronchodilators and inhaled corticosteroids for 2–4 weeks.

Table 2: Causes of chronic cough.
Smoking
Asthma, COPD
Chronic pulmonary infection: • Tuberculosis • Bronchitis • Bronchiectasis • Lung abscess • Fungal infections
Occupational lung diseases: • Pneumoconiosis • Asbestosis • Byssinosis
Interstitial lung disease: • Idiopathic interstitial pneumonia • Interstitial fibrosis from other causes • Infiltrative disorders of the lungs
Granulomatous lung disease: • Sarcoidosis
Foreign body aspiration
Tumors of the lung: • Bronchogenic carcinoma • Alveolar cell carcinoma • Other tumors of the lung
Mediastinal pathology: • Mediastinal tumor • Mediastinal lymphadenopathy
Pleural pathology: • Chronic pleural effusion • Mesothelioma
Cardiovascular causes: • Left ventricular failure • Mitral stenosis • Pulmonary infarction • Aortic aneurysm
Medication-related: • ACE inhibitors
Gastrointestinal causes: • Gastroesophageal reflux • Large diaphragmatic hernia
Unexplained cough

Table 3: Diagnostic evaluation of chronic cough.	
A careful history	• Nature of cough • Expectoration • Breathlessness • Smoking • Sinusitis or allergic rhinitis • Acid regurgitation, heartburn • Chronic bronchial asthma • Hemoptysis • Use of ACE inhibitors
Examination	• Clubbing • ENT examination • Physical signs pointing to airways obstruction (prolonged expiration, wheeze) or restrictive lung disease (like dry 'velcro' crackles) • Careful assessment of CVS
Investigations	• CBC, ESR • Radiographic examination of the chest and sinuses • Sputum examination • Full lung function test • Serial peak expiratory flow rates • *If needed*: HRCT chest and bronchoscopy

(CBC: Complete blood count; ESR: Erythrocyte sedimentation rate; HRCT: High resolution computed tomography)

Table 4: Important common causes of chronic cough.
• Rhinitis with a postnasal drip • Asthma and Cough-variant asthma • Eosinophilic bronchitis • Gastroesophageal reflux • Chronic pulmonary infections, e.g. TB • Postviral due to hyper-reactive airways • ACE inhibitor-related cough • Bronchiectasis (not associated with purulent sputum) • COPD, bronchitis related to smoking, to atmospheric pollution or exposure to biofuels • Interstitial lung disease • Foreign body aspiration • Unexplained cough

Note: Any and almost every pulmonary pathology is capable of causing cough. The above causes need to be considered or reconsidered if history, clinical examination and routine investigations draw a blank.

Nonasthmatic Eosinophilic Bronchitis

Nonasthmatic eosinophilic bronchitis is an increasingly recognized entity characterized by heightened cough reflex, sputum eosinophilia, but with no evidence of either variable airflow obstruction or hyperreactive airways. The cough responds to corticosteroid therapy. The airways inflammation in eosinophilic bronchitis is similar to that in bronchial asthma, the difference being that eosinophilic infiltration in eosinophilic bronchitis is chiefly confined to the bronchial epithelium, whereas in asthma it is more concentrated in the bronchial wall and bronchial muscles. Although eosinophilic infiltration of the airways occurs both in asthma and eosinophilic bronchitis, mast cell infiltration occurs only in asthma which probably explains the difference in airway reactivity. Eosinophils in the sputum (induced if necessary by hypertonic saline) are a pointer to the diagnosis. A definitive diagnosis of eosinophilic bronchitis can only be made by examining bronchial mucosal biopsies; this is however not generally necessary. In the absence of any positive findings, a therapeutic trial with corticosteroids is always worthwhile. *Most patients respond very satisfactorily.* The natural history of eosinophilic bronchitis is variable. A cohort of 367 patients with normal lung functions and eosinophilic infiltration of the bronchial mucosa were followed up for a month. 55% remained symptomatic with normal lung functions; 32% were free of symptoms; 13% developed asthma. Patients with repeated episodes of symptomatic eosinophilic bronchitis seem to have an increased risk for developing asthma.

Rhinitis: Postnasal Drip

Many believe that this is perhaps the most common cause of a chronic innocuous cough in an otherwise healthy individual, where all investigations are negative. Nasal allergy, nonallergic vasomotor rhinitis, nasopharyngitis and sinusitis may cause a postnasal drip resulting in inflammation of the pharynx and larynx stimulating cough receptors which are situated in these areas.

Patients often report nasal congestion or "stuffiness" and examination may reveal secretions dripping or trickling down an inflamed pharyngeal wall. Unfortunately, a drip is not always visible or present at the time of a clinical examination so that the absence of these symptoms or signs does not exclude the diagnosis. Nasal polyps may be present together with tenderness over the sinuses. Investigations for rhinitis include nasal endoscopy, X-ray and CT of the paranasal sinuses which may show mucosal thickening and infected sinuses. An opinion from an ear-nose-throat specialist should always be considered. When an alternative cause of cough is not easily apparent, empiric therapy for a postnasal drip should always be tried before doing extensive investigations.

Gastroesophageal Reflux

There is a bit of dispute as to the frequency of this etiology in patients with chronic cough. Many consider it as a frequent and important cause of chronic cough. The entity exists but perhaps it is often overdiagnosed when no other cause for cough appears plausible.

Gastroesophageal reflux cough is due to relaxation of the esophageal sphincter with reflux of gastric contents into the esophagus. Microaspiration of esophageal contents into the tracheobronchial tree and stimulation of the esophageotracheal-bronchial neural reflex are thought to be responsible for cough. Other factors responsible for cough in patients with gastroesophageal reflux include stimulation of receptors in the upper respiratory tract as in the larynx, and stimulation of receptors in the lower respiratory tract consequent to aspiration of gastric contents.

Gastroesophageal reflux may occur during eating or after a meal, at night during sleep or even in waking hours. Typically, patients complain of heartburn, soreness of the throat or dysphonia, but many patients with gastroesophageal reflux cough may have no such symptoms. Investigations for gastroesophageal reflux include a barium study in the Trendelenburg position which may demonstrate a reflux with or without the presence of a hiatus hernia. An upper GI endoscopy could equally demonstrate a patulous esophageal sphincter with regurgitation of gastric contents, with or without a hiatus hernia. Twenty-four-hour esophageal pH studies have a limited value in the investigation of cough believed to be due to gastroesophageal reflux because they are poor predictors of response to therapy. This test is however considered the optimal diagnostic test with a sensitivity of over 90%, and should be done if surgery is decided upon to relieve cough thought to be due to gastroesophageal reflux.

Laryngopharyngeal Reflux

Laryngopharyngeal reflux is the retrograde flow of gastric contents into the pharynx and larynx causing cough, hoarseness of voice/dysphonia and a constant desire to clear the throat. This is an upper esophageal sphincter disorder that mainly occurs in the upright posture, while bending or exercising. This is in contrast to GERD which is a lower esophageal sphincter problem causing symptoms generally in the recumbent posture.

Pulmonary Tuberculosis

Chronic cough with or without sputum may be the first and for a while the only symptom of pulmonary TB. In areas of the world where TB is endemic, a cough lasting for a month or more always merits an X-ray of the chest and if needs be an HRCT of the chest.

Chronic Bronchitis, COPD

Chronic bronchitis in a patient who is a cigarette smoker is easily recognized. Yet even if there is no history of smoking, chronic bronchitis causing cough with mucoid sputum is not uncommon in large heavily populated and dreadfully polluted cities of the world, including Mumbai, Delhi, Kolkata and Chennai in India. Exposure to combustion products of bio-fuels like wood and coal is an important cause of bronchitis and COPD in North India and should always be asked for in the history. Cough related to an occupational exposure is often missed if a careful occupational history is not taken.

Interstitial Lung Disease

Chronic dry cough, increasing breathlessness on exertion and velcro crackles on auscultation of the bases are features of interstitial lung disease (ILD). Lung functions show a restrictive pattern in contrast to patients with chronic obstructive pulmonary disease who show airways obstruction. Imaging studies generally confirm a diagnosis of ILD.

Bronchiectasis

Some patients with bronchiectasis (generally cylindrical bronchiectasis) have cough but produce little or no sputum. There are generally no physical signs and a radiographic examination of the chest is normal. The diagnosis can be made on an HRCT of the chest.

Aspiration of a Foreign Body

A foreign body aspirated deep into the lung is an important cause of chronic cough. In India, aspiration of a "supari" can lead to persistent cough with varying degree of inflammation generally in the lower lobe of a lung. A history of possible aspiration may only be given on direct questioning. Often the history is noncontributory. A bronchoscopy generally gives the correct diagnosis, but not always so.

Hyper-reactive Airways Following Respiratory Tract Infection

Cough following viral upper respiratory tract infections is common and may last for 4–8 weeks. The most likely cause is hyper-reactivity of airways as well as airways constriction. Inhaled β_2-agonists and corticosteroids help relieve the cough. Another explanation for prolonged post viral cough is that it is the response to exposure of afferent nerves located immediately below the epithelium as a result of viral induced epithelial necrosis.

Cough can also persist after other acute respiratory tract infections, particularly mycoplasma, chlamydial infections. An uncommon cause of persistent chronic cough in adolescents and adults is observed following infection with Bordetella pertussis. Culture of respiratory secretions for these organisms is frequently negative and serological tests need to be performed to help diagnosis.

In persistent cough following nonviral infections, the possible etiology may be a persistent postnasal drip in addition perhaps to bronchial hyper-reactivity.

Angiotensin-Converting-Enzyme (ACE) Inhibitors

Fifteen percent of patients taking ACE inhibitors develop a nonproductive cough. As mentioned earlier, it is believed that the accumulation of bradykinin which is normally degraded by ACE may stimulate C fibers in the airways causing cough. Cough is noticeably an uncommon complication with angiotensin II receptor antagonists which do not increase bradykinin levels. ACE inhibitors causing cough generally do so within the first 2 weeks, though this may extend to 4–6 weeks. The cough generally is relieved within a week of stopping therapy but this may extend at times to 4–6 weeks. It generally does not occur more frequently in asthmatics than in nonasthamatics and is not accompanied by airways obstruction.

Lung Cancer

Bronchogenic carcinoma should be considered in a smoker if there is a recent change in the nature of the "smoker's cough' or a new cough appears. It should also be suspected if cough persists for more than 1 or 2 months after an individual has stopped smoking. Hemoptysis is always a cause of concern and needs prompt investigation as it may be a presenting feature in 5–9% of patients with bronchogenic carcinoma.

Psychogenic Cough

Psychogenic cough is often a diagnosis of desperation or despair. The diagnosis should be entertained when cough is markedly worse during periods of stress, when meticulous examination and investigations have excluded all organic disease, when empiric therapy for some of the important causes of chronic cough discussed above has failed and most importantly, when there is a clear background of emotional instability, or an obvious inability to cope with the ordinary or extraordinary stresses present in a patient's life. One occasionally sees "cough" becoming a "habit"—a respiratory tic, a habit which like any other habit is difficult to break. Even so, it is worth remembering that a patient's attitude and emotional responses may be conditioned by severe chronic persistent cough rather than being responsible for the cough.

Rarer causes of chronic cough are microaspiration in elderly individuals who have difficulty in swallowing, pressure on the trachea due to a superior mediastinal pressure syndrome, impacted foreign body or cerumen in the external auditory canal which causes cough through stimulation of the auricular branch of the vagus nerve. A very rare cause of chronic cough is Holmes-Adie syndrome due to autonomic dysfunction of the vagus nerve.

Undiagnosed Chronic Cough

Chronic cough remains undiagnosed in 10–20% of patients in spite of full investigations. Various diagnostic labels are given to such patients. The cause of very heightened cough reflex is not understood. Symptomatic treatment with codeine or related drugs or the use of nebulized lidocaine for symptomatic relief may be tried. Reassurance that the patient has no grave or dangerous disease often helps. A trial with inhaled steroids and aerosolized bronchodilators should be given to all patients with unexplained cough as cough-variant asthma responds to this therapy. Empiric treatment for a possible gastroesophageal reflux causing unexplained cough may also be tried but more often than not fails **(Table 5)**.

Table 5: Specific treatment for chronic cough.

Causes	Treatment
Rhinitis	Nasal corticosteroids
GERD-related cough	Use of proton pump inhibitors Lifestyle modifications
ACE inhibitor-induced cough	Stop the drug
Asthma	Inhaled bronchodilators and corticosteroids Oral therapy as needed
Chronic bronchitis	Smoking cessation
Bronchiectasis	Antibiotics, postural drainage

■ SUGGESTED READING

1. Bolser DC. Pharmacologic management of cough. Otolaryngol Clin North Am. 2010;43(1):147-55, xi.
2. Holmes RL. Evaluation of the patient with chronic cough. Am Fam Physician. 2004;69(9):2159-66.
3. Irwin RS. Unexplained cough in the adult. Otolaryngol Clin North Am. 2010;43(1):167-80.
4. Iyer VN, Lim KG. Chronic cough: an update. Mayo Clin Proc. 2013;88:1115.
5. McGarvey LP. Future directions in treating cough. Otolaryngol Clin North Am. 2010;43(1):199-211.
6. Rytilä P, Metso T, Heikkinen K, et al. Airway inflammation in patients with symptoms suggesting asthma but with normal lung function. Eur Respir J. 2000;16:824.
7. Silvestri RC, Weinberger SE. Evaluation of subacute and chronic cough in adults. [online] Available from www.uptodate.com [Accessed July, 2018].

CHAPTER 10

Hemoptysis

■ INTRODUCTION

Hemoptysis is the expectoration of blood, the source of bleeding being below the vocal cords, either from the tracheobronchial tree or the lungs. In most cases, hemoptysis though frightening to the patient is mild and self-limiting, requiring no treatment other than rest and sedation. In a few instances it is massive, exsanguinating and life-threatening. There is no generally accepted definition of what constitutes massive hemoptysis. Various reports in the literature use different criteria—hemoptysis varying from a mere 100–600 mL/24 hours to 1,000 mL over a period of several days. From the practical point of view, *hemoptysis should be considered massive when it is life-threatening.*

Hemoptysis should be distinguished from blood originating in the nose or throat at or above the larynx. The patient has an urge to clear the throat and brings up blood when he does so. A careful history suggests the source of bleed and a careful examination of the nose and throat by a specialist will clear the diagnosis. Massive hemoptysis may be difficult to distinguish from severe hematemesis. A carefully taken history is again important. A patient can usually tell even when blood is aspirated and then coughed up, whether it originated in the respiratory tract or the upper gastrointestinal (GI) tract. Blood from the respiratory tract is generally bright red, frothy, mixed with sputum and has an alkaline pH. It may contain macrophages laden with hemosiderin. The bloody material brought up in hematemesis is more often dark rather than bright red; may contain food particles and has an acidic pH. In some cases both a bronchoscopy and an upper GI endoscopy are necessary to ascertain the source of the bleed.

A point worth noting is that the lung has two relatively important sources of blood supply—the pulmonary circulation and the bronchial circulation, so that bleeding with resultant hemoptysis can occur from either of these two vascular beds or from both. Generally speaking, bleeding and hemoptysis due to erosion or rupture of bronchial vessels is brisker and more profuse compared to bleeding from erosion and rupture of pulmonary vessels. This is because the bronchial circulation is part of the systemic vascular bed with a systemic blood pressure which is much higher than the pressure existing in the pulmonary vascular bed.

It is a cardinal principle in medicine that the cause of hemoptysis whether very mild (as with blood-streaked sputum), moderate or severe must be ascertained. At times the cause is evident as, for example, hemoptysis in a patient with acute pneumonia or blood streaking of sputum in acute bronchitis. In other instances the cause is not apparent and deserves not only a good history and clinical examination but also more detailed investigations.

Numerous diseases involving the tracheobronchial tree or the lung can cause hemoptysis. There are, however, some diseases which do so more commonly and which should therefore engage the clinician's attention. In the developing countries of the world, tuberculosis is by far the most common cause of hemoptysis, the next most important common causes being bronchiectasis, lung cancer, pulmonary infarction and mitral stenosis. In the West, lung cancer would head the list if the patient was a smoker over the age of 40–45 years. Bronchiectasis and pulmonary infarction causing hemoptysis are still common in the West but hemoptysis due to mitral stenosis is decidedly rare.

Other pathologies that need to be kept in mind are pneumonia, lung abscess, aspergillomas, Wegener's granulomatosis and intra-alveolar hemorrhage due to vasculitides or autoimmune diseases. It is also important to remember that hemoptysis can occur with acute left ventricular failure as also in coagulopathies or in patients with thrombocytopenia.

We will now briefly discuss the important causes of hemoptysis, followed by an approach to diagnosis and management. The few causes discussed below can be associated with mild, moderate or even life-threatening hemoptysis **(Table 1)**.

■ TUBERCULOSIS

Tuberculosis still remains the most important and most frequent cause of massive hemoptysis in India and other developing countries. Hemoptysis may occur in active tuberculous infection of the lung, or may be a sequel to burnt-out disease. Most patients with active tuberculosis who have severe hemoptysis, have cavitative lung disease with acid-fast bacilli present in the sputum. There are several causes of hemoptysis in tuberculosis. These include:

(a) Bronchiolar ulceration with necrosis and rupture of the underlying bronchial vessels in tuberculous pneumonia. Rupture of pulmonary capillaries due to alveolar necrosis may also be an associated feature.

(b) Rupture of an aneurysmal portion of a branch of the pulmonary artery in cavitative tuberculosis. Rupture of a Rasmussen aneurysm is a well-accepted cause of massive hemoptysis in either active tuberculosis, or in patients with prior infection. Pulmonary arteries traversing thick-walled cavities develop aneurysmal dilatations due to local inflammation of the vessel wall. These aneurysms herniate and project into the cavity lumen. Sudden transient increase in pulmonary artery pressure, or continued inflammation of the vessel wall can cause rupture of the aneurysm with profuse hemorrhage and hemoptysis.

(c) A healed calcified lymph node at or near the hilum can press on a bronchus, and erode through a bronchial vessel into the lumen of the airway, resulting in massive hemoptysis. The patient may cough up this calcified node in the form of a broncholith. This may immediately precede hemoptysis, or occur during a bout of hemoptysis.

(d) Hemoptysis can occur due to bronchiectasis which often occurs as a sequel to tuberculosis. Bleeding occurs due to erosion of tortuous, enlarged bronchial vessels, and a profuse anastomosis between the bronchial and pulmonary circulation.

(e) Chronic tuberculous cavities often predispose to the formation of aspergillomas. The latter can produce profuse bleeding.

■ BRONCHIECTASIS

Bronchiectasis is often associated with bronchial artery hypertrophy, expansion of the peribronchial and submucosal bronchial arterial network, and increased anastomosis between the bronchial and pulmonary circulations. Bleeding can originate from hypertrophied bronchial arteries (under high systemic pressure), or from the submucosal vascular plexus in the bronchiectatic segments.

■ CARDIOVASCULAR DISORDERS

Mitral stenosis is still an important cause of hemoptysis in developing countries, for rheumatic fever though not as frequent as it was four decades ago, still occurs.

Before the era of valvulotomy and mitral valve replacement, hemoptysis occurred in 9–18% of patients with mitral stenosis. Severe hemoptysis is generally due to rupture of engorged, tortuous, dilated varicose bronchial veins that result as a consequence of an elevated left atrial pressure and passive pulmonary hypertension. In these patients, hemoptysis may be precipitated by respiratory infection, by a bout of coughing, or by an increase in intravascular volume, as seen in pregnancy.

Left ventricular failure causes hemoptysis due to pulmonary congestion. Acute pulmonary edema is associated with pink frothy sputum.

Pulmonary thromboembolic disease leading to pulmonary infarction often causes hemoptysis, associated

Table 1: Important causes of life-threatening hemoptysis.

- Tuberculosis
- Bronchiectasis
- Bronchogenic carcinoma, carcinoid tumors
- Lung abscess
- Pulmonary infarction
- Cardiovascular diseases—mitral stenosis, left ventricular failure
- Mycetomas
- Trauma
- Iatrogenic hemoptysis—following bronchoscopy, Swan-Ganz catheterization or transthoracic needle biopsy
- Autoimmune disorders, Wegener's granulomatosis, Goodpasture's syndrome
- Vascular anomalies
- Cryptogenic hemoptysis

with pleuritic pain together with a mild-to-moderate blood-stained effusion.

Rarely, rupture of an aortic aneurysm into the tracheobronchial tree leads to massive hemoptysis and death.

■ BRONCHOGENIC CARCINOMA AND OTHER TUMORS

These very rarely cause massive or life-threatening hemoptysis. Hemoptysis in a smoker beyond 40–45 years should arouse suspicion of a bronchogenic carcinoma. Hemoptysis is rarely massive and is generally characterized by blood-tinged sputum or sputum mixed with blood. Hemoptysis may be the presenting symptom in 10% of patients or it may accompany or be preceded by cough and vague chest discomfort. Hemoptysis in lung cancer can also be due to pneumonia distal to bronchial obstruction. Hemoptysis is an uncommon feature of metastatic carcinoma as these lesions generally do not involve the airways.

Carcinoids in the lung can cause hemoptysis which at times may be life-threatening and difficult to control.

■ LUNG ABSCESS

Bleeding occurs in 20–50% of patients with lung abscess. It is related to necrotizing inflammation of the lung parenchyma eroding bronchial and pulmonary vessels.

■ MYCETOMAS

Mycetomas are fungal balls occurring in patients with preexisting cavitary lung disease. They are most frequently seen in tuberculous cavities, but have been reported in cavitary disease secondary to sarcoidosis, lung abscess, cavitary carcinoma, bronchiectasis, bullous emphysema, and pulmonary infarction. The most frequent mycetoma is an aspergilloma. The cause of massive bleeding in a mycetoma is disputed. Vascular injury by aspergillus-associated endotoxin, aspergillus-related proteolytic activity, and a Type III-related hypersensitivity reaction have all been postulated.

■ TRAUMA

Blunt or penetrating injury to the chest can cause hemoptysis. Steering wheel injuries can cause a rupture of the tracheobronchial tree causing both hemoptysis and pneumothorax.

After a pneumonectomy, a large hemothorax may open into the tracheobronchial tree causing life-threatening hemoptysis. Drainage of the hemothorax with surgical repair of the tear in the bronchus is needed as an emergency measure.

■ AUTOIMMUNE DISEASES

Intra-alveolar hemorrhage can result from Wegener's granulomatosis, other forms of vasculitides, Goodpasture's syndrome and autoimmune connective tissue disorders. The presenting features are hemoptysis, alveolar infiltrates on the X-ray, dyspnea and hypoxemia. The degree of hemoptysis need not always be a guide to the severity of intra-alveolar hemorrhage.

■ IATROGENIC HEMOPTYSIS

This is a potential complication of bronchoscopy, transthoracic needle biopsy, or the use of a Swan-Ganz catheter.

Rupture of the pulmonary artery is the most catastrophic complication following the use of the Swan-Ganz catheter; it carries a mortality of 50% due to massive pulmonary hemorrhage. This complication is more frequently observed in patients with pulmonary hypertension.

■ VASCULAR ANOMALIES

Arteriovenous malformations may rarely cause fatal hemoptysis.

■ CRYPTOGENIC HEMOPTYSIS

About 15% of patients with hemoptysis even after extensive investigation, have no detectable cause of their hemoptysis, and are labeled as cryptogenic hemoptysis. Patients with cryptogenic bleeds generally stop bleeding spontaneously, and require only supportive care. A periodic follow-up is mandatory in these patients.

■ DIAGNOSTIC EVALUATION (TABLES 2 AND 3)

Diagnostic evaluation requires a careful history, a meticulous physical examination, routine blood counts and an X-ray of the chest. Sputum should be sent for microbiological examination and cytology. Culture for acid-fast bacilli should always be done.

When hemoptysis has been severe, blood may well have been aspirated into the opposite lung so that an X-ray of the chest may be misleading.

Brisk hemoptysis also warrants an urgent fiberoptic bronchoscopy to determine the site of the bleed and perhaps also help in management.

A high-resolution computed tomography (HRCT) of the chest is often rewarding though aspirated blood can cast ground-glass shadows in different parts of the same or opposite lung.

The presence of intra-alveolar hemorrhage warrants tests for Goodpasture's syndrome, antineutrophilic cytoplasmic antibodies (ANCA) test for Granulomatosis with polyangiitis (formerly called Wegener's granulomatosis) and for microscopic polyarteritis. A suspicion of connective tissue disorders would dictate tests such as antinuclear antibody test and other relevant tests that may be deemed necessary. A suspicion of a coagulopathy would require a coagulation profile.

The intensity of the search for hemoptysis will depend on the circumstances and clinical probabilities in a given case. An obvious tuberculous lesion on an X-ray of the chest will require no test other than a complete sputum examination.

Hemoptysis due to a lobar pneumonia in a young adult needs no specific test. But if the cause is not determined by basic tests such as X-ray chest, and sputum examination, a thorough investigation is mandatory.

■ MANAGEMENT

Most often hemoptysis ceases on its own and all that is needed is rest and mild sedation. A fall in hemoglobin below 9 g/dL and a fall in the hematocrit below 30%

Table 2: Investigations for hemoptysis.

- CBC, ESR, platelet count
- Sputum examination—microbiological examination including culture for AFB
- X-ray chest, if necessary HRCT chest
- Bronchoscopy
- Other relevant blood tests if there is a suspicion for vasculitides, autoimmune disease, connective tissue disease

Table 3: Investigations for massive hemoptysis.

- X-ray chest
- HRCT chest
- Fiberoptic bronchoscopy
- Angiography of the bronchial and pulmonary circulation to locate site of bleed

particularly in an older individual merits transfusion of packed RBCs. The problem therefore in most patients is not with management but with unravelling the cause when the cause is not apparent.

However, massive life-threatening hemoptysis is a difficult management problem. The first principle is to secure the airway, *with a large bore endotracheal tube* for death in the majority of patients with massive hemoptysis is not due to exsanguination but due to asphyxia produced by blood aspirated in both lungs. These patients invariably need ventilatory support. If the site of the bleeding is known, it is best to posture the patient so that the bleeding site is in the dependent position. This reduces the risk of aspiration. An urgent bronchoscopy is a must. More often than not, the bleeding site cannot be determined because of the blood in the tracheobronchial tree. If however the bleeding is identified as coming from one lung, a single lumen endotracheal tube is inserted into the mainstem bronchus of the nonbleeding lung. The inflated cuff of this tube will prevent spillage into the nonbleeding lung. A potential problem of intubating the right main bronchus is that the origin of the right upper lobe bronchus may become blocked.

Double lumen endotracheal tubes have two separate passageways with differing lengths to the mainstem bronchial and tracheal orifices with two separate cuffs. Usually, a left-sided double lumen tube is preferred over the right as it is technically easier to insert and avoids possible obstruction of the right upper lobe. With the left sided tube the longer lumen terminates within the left main bronchus, while the shorter tube terminates in the distal trachea. Cuffs of both tubes are inflated. The inflated cuff within the left main bronchus prevents spillage of blood from one lung to the other **(Fig. 1)**. The advantage of the double lumen tube is that both lungs can be ventilated. The disadvantage is that it is technically difficult to insert and more importantly the tube is easily and frequently dislodged leading to spillage of blood or even bronchial obstruction. For this reason we have stopped using a double lumen endotracheal tube in the management of massive hemoptysis.

Pari passu with the insertion of the endotracheal tube it is important to provide cardiovascular support through infusion of crystalloids and blood products. Patients receiving heparin or warfarin or who have an elevated prothrombin time should be given fresh frozen plasma infusions; patients who are thrombocytopenic or have been on antiplatelets agents should receive platelet infusions.

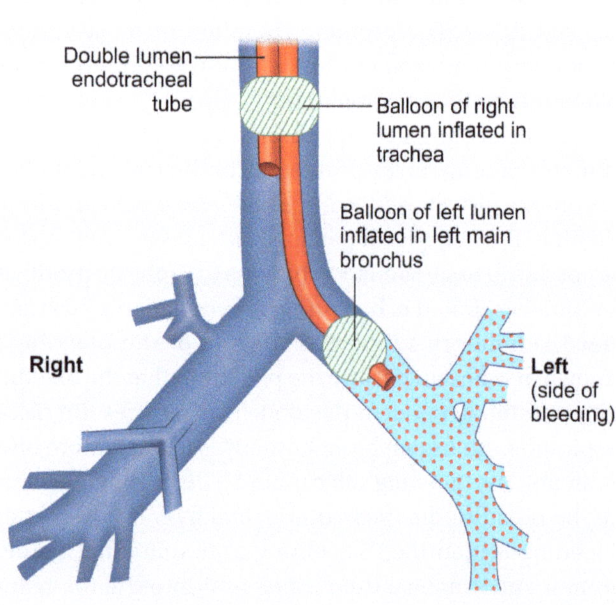

Fig. 1: Schematic representation of proper placement of a left-sided double-lumen endotracheal tube. The inflated balloon in the trachea allows ventilation of the right lung. The inflated balloon in the left main bronchus prevents spill-over of blood from left into right side.

For profuse bleeding which remains uncontrolled, the administration of Factor VIIa should be considered.

Massive hemoptysis often leads to hypoxia or to both hypoxia and hypercapnia. Adequate gas exchange should be maintained with the use of ventilator support after insertion of the endotracheal tube.

Bronchoscopic Techniques to Stop Bleeding

1. *Iced-saline lavage*: The bleeding site identified via bronchoscopy is followed by a lavage with 50 mL aliquots of ice-cold saline. Local vasoconstriction of vessels may lead to hemostasis. On an average 500 mL of cold saline lavage is needed to achieve this effect.
2. *Topical medication*: A vasoconstrictive agent such as epinephrine, or a topical coagulant, such as thrombin or a thrombin-fibrinogen combination can be infused through the bronchoscope into the bleeding site.
3. *Balloon tamponade*: A Fogarty balloon catheter is introduced via the bronchoscope into the segmental bronchus leading to the bleeding site. The balloon is kept inflated for 24–48 hours. It is then deflated and the patient is observed for rebleeding for several hours. The Fogarty catheter is removed if bleeding has stopped.

4. Laser therapy, electrocautery, cryotherapy, argon plasma coagulation may succeed in stopping bleeding from an identified mucosal lesion. Though any of these procedures can be done through a flexible bronchoscope, a rigid bronchoscope is preferred as it allows better visualization of the involved areas and allows more efficient suction.

Arteriography

Arteriography can very often identify the bleeding site, so that the bleeding can be stopped by embolization. Arteriography is indicated in profuse bleeding after bronchoscopy has either failed to identify the source, or when attempts to stop bleeding through the bronchoscope have failed. It should be done only after any existing coagulopathy has been corrected. It can be done on intubated patients on ventilator support. Angiography of the bronchial arteries should be done first, as severe hemoptysis is generally from one or more of these arteries. It should be kept in mind that the anterior spinal artery arises from a bronchial artery in roughly 5% of people. Blockage of the bronchial artery proximal to the origin of the anterior spinal artery could lead to ischemia of the chord with resulting paraplegia.

Pulmonary artery catheterization should only be done if no bleeding site is discovered on angiography of the bronchial arteries. Pulmonary arteries are the source of bleeding in only 10% of patients with massive hemoptysis.

Finally patients in whom the bleeding site is undiscovered should have an angiography of the relevant systemic arteries. The systemic circulation has been reported to be the source of brisk hemoptysis in about 5% patients.

Arteriographic embolization successfully arrests severe hemoptysis in 85% of patients if bronchial, pulmonary and systemic arterial circulations have been well visualized.

Inability to cannulate all bronchial arteries, or failure to identify and/or embolize all of the collateral systemic feeder vessels (which may arise from gastric, intercostal, internal mammary, renal, and hepatic arteries) are reasons for a "failed" arteriographic procedure. Rebleeding after a "successful" arteriographic embolization can occur in a minority of patients after a few months.

Surgery

Uncontrolled bleeding from one or more lobe of the lung in spite of the above-mentioned attempts to arrest hemorrhage may as a last resort require surgery. Prior lung function tests if available may help to judge fitness for surgery. Surgery is contraindicated in the presence of severe underlying pulmonary disease, diffuse bilateral disease and in diffuse alveolar hemorrhage. Both surgical morbidity and mortality are high (20–50%). Empyema and bronchopleural fistula are frequent complications. Postoperative pulmonary hemorrhage, respiratory failure and infection occur frequently.

CONCLUSION

An algorithm for the management of massive hemoptysis is as follows:

a. Infuse crystalloids, colloids, and blood products to maintain circulatory hemodynamic and to correct any coagulopathy if present.

b. Secure airways by intubating patient with a large bore endotracheal tube—use oxygen then "the tube."

c. Urgent bronchoscopy:
   - Bleeding site identified—use methods outlined to stop bleeding via the bronchoscope.
   - Bleeding site identified as coming from one lung—insert endotracheal tube into the mainstem bronchus of the bleeding lung; inflate cuff—this will prevent spillage of blood into the normal lung.
   - Bleeding site undetermined and even after procedure if bleeding actively continues, then go on to—
   - Arteriographic embolization—bronchial, pulmonary and systemic vessels need to be visualized to identify bleeding site or sites for embolization. In a very massive immediately life-threatening hemoptysis, bronchoscopy is unlikely to be of use.

After securing the airway, it is best to proceed with arteriographic embolization.

   - Arteriographic embolization fails and exsanguinating bleeding persists—we have two options:
     – Use Factor VIIa—we have seen this work wonderfully in some patients who were near death.
     – Surgery:
        ◆ If bleeding is from one lobe or one lung, there is no underlying severe diffuse lung disease
        ◆ The procedure carries a high morbidity and mortality.

Note: Maintain as far as possible adequate gas exchange and circulatory hemodynamics.

SUGGESTED READING

1. Bidwell JL. Hemoptysis: diagnosis and management. Am Fam Physician. 2005;72(7):1253-60.

2. Corder R. Hemoptysis. Emerg Med Clin North Am. 2003;21(2):421-35.

3. Dave BR, Sharma A, et al. Nine year single center experience with transcatheter arterial embolization for hemoptysis: medium term outcomes. Vasc Endovasc Surg. 2011; 45:258.

4. Jean-Baptiste E. Clinical assessment and management of massive hemoptysis. Crit Care Med. 2000;28:1642-7.

5. Tang Goh P, Lin M, Teo N, et al. Embolization for hemoptysis: a six-year review. Cardiovasc Intervent Radiol. 2002;25: 17 25.

6. Udwadia FE. Principles of Critical Care, 2nd edition. New Delhi: Oxford University Press; 2005. pp. 301-7.

7. Weinberger SE, Mathur PN, Hollingsworth BS. Etiology and evaluation of hemoptysis in adults. [online] Available from www.uptodate.com. [Accessed July, 2018].

CHAPTER 11

Dyspnea

■ INTRODUCTION

A consensus statement of the American Thoracic Society defines dyspnea in the following way: "Dyspnea is a term used to characterize a subjective experience of breathing discomfort that is comprised of qualitatively distinct sensations that vary in intensity. The experience derives from interactions among multiple physiological, psychological, social, and environmental factors, and may induce secondary physiological and behavioral responses".

This rather cumbersome definition can perhaps be shortened thus—Dyspnea is a term characterized by breathing discomfort or an uncomfortable awareness of breathing, that is comprised of qualitatively different sensations of varying intensity.

Dyspnea is often referred to by the patient as "breathlessness" or "shortness of breath". It is a worrying symptom, prompting the patient to seek medical attention. Dyspnea may be accompanied by tachypnea (faster rate of breathing than normal) but not necessarily so. Being subjective, the sensation of discomfort associated with dyspnea may be interpreted differently by different patients. Some, in particular asthmatics, interpret dyspnea as a feeling of tightness in the chest; others complain of respiratory distress; still others interpret it as a feeling of suffocation. Despite this variability, dyspnea invariably implies discomfort during breathing.

The physiological mechanism underlying dyspnea is complex and not completely understood. The sensation of dyspnea has two components—the first component is the sensory input to the cerebral cortex. The sensory input consists of information derived from several specialized sensory end-receptors. Specialized mechano-receptors are present in the respiratory tract—particularly in the trachea, larynx and large upper airways. Important receptors are also present in the lung parenchyma—the J receptors which are stimulated by stretch and which initiate sensory inputs carried by the vagus nerves to the brain. Sensory inputs are also received from respiratory muscles, the chest wall and from chemoreceptors sensitive to lack of oxygen (a low PaO_2) or to an increase in the $PaCO_2$. Additional sensory inputs not clearly understood may well arise following inadequate oxygen delivery or poor oxygen utilization. These numerous sensory inputs are processed at the spinal level and then at the supraspinal level before they reach the sensorimotor cortex. There is however no specific area in the sensorimotor cortex which is a special locus for dyspnea. The second component is the perception and interpretation of these sensory inputs arriving at the sensorimotor cortex. The interpretation of perceived information in the sensorimotor cortex varies so that the subjective feeling of discomfort during breathing that constitutes dyspnea may be interpreted and expressed in different ways and perhaps more importantly in different degrees by different patients.

In clinical practice one comes across some patients who complain of little or no dyspnea even though they suffer from an underlying disease which if present in others invariably causes significant dyspnea. The reason for this is unclear. Either for some reason they have a blunting or reduction of sensory inputs to the sensorimotor cortex of the brain, or the perception is inadequate so that the interpretation of what is perceived is not enough to produce the expected degree of discomfort on breathing. This is observed in some patients with severe asthma who may complain of little or no discomfort as also in some patients with significant left heart failure who do not (even on direct questioning) complain of dyspnea.

■ PATHOPHYSIOLOGY OF DYSPNEA

Dyspnea is chiefly due to respiratory disease or to cardiovascular disease or to both being present in a patient.

Pathophysiology of Dyspnea in Respiratory Disease

The respiratory system is so designed as to inhale and transport air from the atmosphere into the alveoli of the lungs, where oxygen is exchanged for carbon dioxide by diffusion across the alveolar-capillary membrane. Carbon dioxide is then exhaled and removed from the lungs to the atmosphere. The several components within the respiratory system must function well to enable an appropriate exchange of gases between man and the environment. Derangement or dysfunction at any level can lead to dyspnea. Hence dyspnea due to respiratory disease can be due to disorders involving the respiratory center which controls breathing, to ventilatory pump dysfunction, to disturbance in gas exchange within the lungs, or to a combination of one or more factors, stated above.

Respiratory Center

The respiratory center determines the rate and depth of breathing and stimulation of the respiratory center leads to increased ventilation and breathing discomfort.

Stimulation of the respiratory center can be due to various factors often arising from dysfunction of other components of the respiratory system. For example, hypoxia and hypercapnia that arise from a disturbance in gas exchange due to ventilation-perfusion inequality are strong stimulants of the respiratory center. Hypoxia does so by stimulating the chemoreceptors within the carotid and aortic bodies. Afferents from these bodies reach and stimulate the respiratory center. Carbon dioxide stimulates the respiratory center directly following diffusion of gas into the cerebrospinal fluid. Stimulant sensory inputs may also arise from specialized mechano-receptors present in the trachea, larynx, large upper airways, respiratory and skeletal muscles. J receptors are important stretch receptors present in the interstitium of the lung. They are stimulated by interstitial inflammation as also by interstitial and pulmonary edema. Stimulation of these J receptors is an important cause of dyspnea in both respiratory and cardiovascular disease. Sensory inputs from these receptors reach and stimulate the respiratory center via the vagus nerve. Finally the respiratory center may be stimulated directly by drugs such as aspirin or in metabolic acidosis, as and also by efferents arising from the cerebral cortex.

It is of interest that the breathing pattern in respiratory disease may perhaps reflect attempts by the respiratory control center to reduced breathing discomfort. Hence patients with severe airways obstruction breathe slowly and deeply in order to minimize the pleural pressure needed to overcome airways obstruction. In contrast, patients with restrictive disease as in interstitial pulmonary fibrosis, kyphoscoliosis, or any disease with a lowered lung /chest wall compliance, the breathing pattern is rapid and shallow thereby minimizing the work-load to expand the chest.

Stimulation of the respiratory center in patients with COPD from any cause, e.g. exercise can lead to severe dyspnea and precipitate a crisis leading to respiratory failure. The increase in rate produced by stimulation of the respiratory center in the presence of airways obstruction and airflow limitation leads to increased air trapping within the lungs with every breath. The dynamic hyperinflation that results causes extreme discomfort and dyspnea (*see* chapter on Chronic Obstructive Pulmonary Disease).

In patient with restrictive lung disease, an increase in respiratory rate which results in a tidal volume less than the average resting tidal volume will lead to worsening dyspnea. Increasingly rapid respiratory rate with a shallow breathing pattern lead to an increase in the dead space to tidal volume ratio. This leads to a need for an increase in total ventilation which implies a greater workload and therefore more dyspnea.

The Ventilatory Pump

The ventilatory pump moves air in and out of the respiratory system. It comprises the muscles involved in ventilation, the peripheral nerves which supply the muscles and the skeletal system to which these muscles are attached. It also comprises the pleura which transforms the outward movement of the thoracic cage to negative pressure within the thorax and the conducting airways which are conduits for the flow of air from the outside atmosphere to the alveoli and back. Derangement of the ventilatory pump that results in increased work to move air in and out if the lungs is an important cause of dyspnea. When the work-load to ventilate the lung clearly exceeds the effort available to do so there is not only increasing dyspnea but also hypercapnia. The latter again as mentioned earlier can stimulate the respiratory center. The link between various components of the respiratory system is illustrated in the above situation (*see* chapter on Chronic Obstructive Pulmonary Disease).

Patients with a reduced compliance of the lung (e.g. interstitial lung disease) or of the chest wall (e.g. kyphoscoliosis) perform more work during inspiration and complain of breathlessness.

Neurological problems leading to weakness of the intercostal muscles and the diaphragm (as for example in the Guillum Barré syndrome) require the patient to make a far greater muscular effort to produce a negative intrapleural pressure sufficient to allow air to flow into the lungs. Tachypnea with increasing dyspnea is observed in these patients.

Impaired Gas Exchange

Impaired gas exchange can result in hypoxia and hypoxic respiratory failure, hypercapnia and hypercapnic respiratory failure or a combination of hypoxic and hypercapnic respiratory failure each of which can result in dyspnea. There are two important causes of impaired gas exchange. The first is a ventilation perfusion inequality which results in hypoxia. The hypoxia is relieved by suitably increasing oxygen concentration of inspired air. The second is an intrapulmonary shunt due to perfusion of atelectatic alveoli. This leads to hypoxia which cannot be significantly improved by increasing the oxygen concentration of inspired air. A less important cause is a marked thickness of the alveolar-capillary membrane which reduces the diffusion capacity of oxygen from alveoli into the blood within the capillaries. Almost always, respiratory diseases which reduce the diffusion capacity of oxygen because of thickness of the alveolar-capillary membrane are also associated with well marked ventilation perfusion inequality which remains the main cause of hypoxia. A difficulty in transfer of oxygen through a thick alveolar-capillary membrane may however be significant when the alveolar pressure of oxygen (P_AO_2) is <60 mm Hg.

Pathophysiology of Dyspnea in Cardiovascular Disease

The most important cardiovascular disease causing dyspnea is heart failure whatever its etiology, whether due to left ventricular systolic dysfunction or diastolic dysfunction. Numerous cardiovascular diseases can cause dyspnea. These include ischemic heart disease, cardiomyopathy, valvular heart disease, congenital heart disease, pulmonary hypertension, pulmonary thromboembolus disease, pericardial disease, cardiac tamponade.

Low-output heart disease causes easy fatigability and weakness. Heart failure that results in increased pulmonary venous pressure causes dyspnea which is largely due to stimulation of J receptors present in the interstitium of the lung.

Dyspnea related to anemia and to deconditioning are also customarily included under dyspnea in cardiovascular disease.

Anemia

Oxygen transport to the tissues is equivalent to cardiac output X oxygen content of blood. A fall in the Hb below 7.5 gm% leads to a significant fall in oxygen content and oxygen transport to the tissues. However the exact cause of dyspnea in anemia is not well-understood. Perhaps some degree of anaerobic metabolism may occur in metabolically active tissue cells due to diminished oxygen content of blood perfusing them. A fall in the pH in the microenvironment of these cells is believed to stimulate 'ergo receptors' present in muscles. This as yet remains a hypothesis.

Deconditioning

Cardiovascular fitness is determined by the heart's ability to increase cardiac output to a maximum and the ability of muscles and tissues to utilize oxygen efficiently for metabolism. A lack of exercise and a very sedentary life may lead to a deconditioning of the cardiovascular system so that the patient's limited effort tolerance is not related to cardiovascular disease but to a lack of fitness. A careful history can generally determine that in these patients, effort tolerance is limited more by fatigue than by dyspnea.

Clinical Overview

When patients come with a history of breathlessness on exertion the two most likely causes are a disorder of the cardiovascular system or of the respiratory system. A good history is of immense help. Is the dyspnea on exertion and if so what is the degree of exertion that causes dyspnea? Does it occur at rest? Is there an associated wheeze and/or cough? Is it related to posture? Is it accompanied by substernal or precordial discomfort? Are there any other associated symptoms? These are some of the many questions that need to be asked. A good history should be followed by a meticulous clinical examination—a general examination as also an examination of all systems, in particular, the cardiovascular and respiratory systems. It is important to look out for features of acute or chronic airways obstruction as also for restrictive lung disease. Clinical features characterizing hypoxia and hypercapnia should be carefully sought (*see* the chapter on Acute Respiratory Failure). Clinical examination of the cardiovascular system in particular the size of the heart, the presence of a diastolic gallop at the apex, presence of murmurs suggestive of valvular heart disease and evidence of pulmonary and systemic venous congestion should be noted. The above features are dealt with below in greater detail with regard to the main respiratory and cardiovascular diseases causing dyspnea. A broad differential diagnosis of some important causes of dyspnea is tabled in **Table 1**.

Pulmonary causes of dyspnea broadly fall into three categories:
1. Diseases causing airways obstruction
2. Disease causing a restrictive lung lesion
3. A combination of both obstruction + restriction

Table 1: Broad differential diagnosis of important causes of dyspnea.	
1.	Stimulation of the respiratory center by various factors, e.g. hypoxia, hypercapnia from any cause
2.	*Airways obstruction, airflow limitation* Bronchial asthma, COPD, bronchiolitis, intrinsic or extrinsic obstruction to large airways
3.	*Restrictive lung pathology* Interstitial lung diseases Parenchymal lung diseases; pulmonary edema Diseases involving the pleura, chest wall
4.	Airways obstruction + restrictive lung lesion
5.	Pleural pathologies
6.	*Cardiovascular causes:* Left heart failure, mitral stenosis Pulmonary hypertension Cardiomyopathies Pericardial effusion Congenital heart disease
7.	Pulmonary thromboembolic disease
8.	*Noncardiorespiratory causes:* Anemia, thyrotoxicosis, neuromuscular disease, skeletal thoracic abnormalities, psychogenic, deconditioning

(COPD: Chronic obstructive pulmonary disease)

Diseases Causing Airways Obstruction

The two most frequent diseases causing dyspnea related to airways obstruction are bronchial asthma and chronic obstructive pulmonary disease (COPD). These two diseases have been discussed at length in separate chapters.

The diagnosis both from the history and physical examination is generally easy. Asthma at least in the early part of its natural history is episodic, though in late severe asthma dyspnea may be present not only on exertion but even at rest so that it may resemble COPD. Very occasionally, asthma may present with dyspnea on exertion with no obvious physical findings at rest. Bronchial hypersensitivity can however be demonstrated on appropriate testing. Also, in these patients there is a clear fall in peak flows if measured during the period of breathlessness perceived on exertion.

Chronic obstructive pulmonary disease is a chronic inflammatory progressive disease of the lung chiefly related to cigarette smoking. It is characterized by progressive airflow limitation with incomplete reversibility. Patients with COPD also have a disturbance in the mechanics of breathing, increased lung volumes and a disturbance in gas exchange.

An interesting observation is that some patients with well-marked COPD seem to breathe easily, not complaining of much dyspnea. These patients (termed "blue bloaters") retain carbon dioxide (CO_2) and suffer mainly from chronic bronchitis. Others with the same degree of COPD and with a similar disturbance in lung function are severely dyspneic and manage to keep the $PaCO_2$ within normal limits. These patients suffer chiefly from emphysema and are termed pink puffers. It is now recognized that most patients with COPD have a mixture of bronchitis and emphysema in varying degrees. The pathogenesis of CO_2 retention has been discussed at length in the Chapter on COPD.

One of the important signs of airways obstruction is the presence of a prolonged expiration associated with an expiratory wheeze. The tighter the airways obstruction, the more difficult it is to appreciate a wheeze. The wheeze may indeed be inaudible in patients with COPD obtunded as a result of CO_2 narcosis. It is important to ask the patient to make a forced expiratory maneuver to elicit a tight high-pitched expiratory wheeze. Similarly, the more severe an attack of acute asthma, the poorer the breath sounds with little or no wheeze.

Besides asthma and COPD, airways obstruction causing dyspnea is seen in obstruction to the upper large airways (foreign body, tracheal stenosis, laryngeal stenosis, tumor partially obstructing a large airway, and extrinsic pressure on large airways).

Airways obstruction with dyspnea is also seen in bronchiolitis, bronchiolitis obliterans, cystic fibrosis (*more common in Western countries than in India*), bronchiectasis and some rare infiltrative and granulomatous diseases such as Langerhan's cell histiocytosis and pulmonary lymphangioleimyomatosis. In children airways obstruction causing *acute* dyspnea is more often due to epiglottitis, acute tracheolaryngitis, and foreign body inhalation. Asthma remains an important cause of dyspnea in children and adults.

Disease Causing a Restrictive Lung Disease

Restrictive lung lesions are typically exemplified by interstitial lung disease which indeed has many causes. The most classic is interstitial pneumonia of unknown etiology. Increasing breathlessness with progressive hypoxia, at first on exertion and then even at rest is a feature of this disease. An early sign is the presence of end-inspiratory dry velcro crackles at the bases of both lungs which may precede the complaint of breathlessness on exertion. As the disease progresses and breathlessness increases, velcro crackles gradually extend upward to ultimately involve the whole back and even the front of the chest. The lung functions are characterized by a restrictive defect—small lung volumes, a reduced total lung capacity, normal expiratory flow rates and a reduced diffusion capacity. The latter may be the first lung function defect to be observed in early interstitial lung disease.

Restrictive lung disease with dyspnea can occur with any significant parenchymal pathology such as pneumonia, atelectasis or noncardiogenic pulmonary edema. It can also occur with pleural diseases like pleural effusions, pleural mesothelioma and extensive pleural fibrosis. Diseases of the pleura have been considered in a separate chapter.

Paralysis of both domes of the diaphragm whatever the etiology can lead to marked dyspnea. The patient is unable to lie flat for even a minute, becoming increasingly cyanosed and distressed. Breathing and oxygen saturation both improve when the patient is made to sit up at a right angle. The above complication is occasionally observed after major thoracic or cardiovascular surgery and is related to injury to the phrenic nerves.

A number of patients have a combination of airways obstruction + a restrictive lung lesion. Dyspnea on exertion and in severe disease even at rest is a frequent complaint. Important diseases causing both airways obstruction and a restrictive lung lesion are listed in the accompanying **Table 2**.

Cardiovascular Disease

Cardiovascular disease is an important cause of dyspnea. Acute left ventricular failure causes acute pulmonary edema and acute dyspnea. Chronic left heart failure causes chronic pulmonary congestion and chronic dyspnea.

Dyspnea due to left heart disease can be equated to pulmonary congestion and for clinical understanding is best expressed thus:

Dyspnea on exertion $\cong$ pulmonary congestion $\cong$ LV failure
on exertion on exertion
Dyspnea at rest $\cong$ pulmonary congestion $\cong$ left ventricular
at rest failure at rest
Paroxysmal noctural $\cong$ sudden pulmonary $\cong$ acute LV failure
dyspnea congestion at night at night

A good history and a good clinical examination should make a cardiac cause for dyspnea apparent. A background of heart disease, an enlarged heart, diastolic gallop, relevant auscultatory murmurs and crackles at both bases of the lung are tell-tale features that allow a correct diagnosis. Congestive heart failure is manifested by increased jugular venous pressure, enlarged tender liver, pitting edema of the feet. Pleural effusion (a transudate), generally right-sided may also be present. Relevant investigations may further give the nature of the cardiac ailment.

	Table 2: Examples of obstructive + restrictive lung pathologies.
1.	Bronchiectasis
2.	Extensive or burnt-out tuberculosis
3.	Sarcoidosis
4.	Tropical eosinophilia
5.	Extrinsic allergic alveolitis (some patients)
6.	Inhalation injuries to the lung involving injury to bronchioles and lung parenchyma
7.	Interstitial lung disease associated with small airways obstruction
8.	Langerhan's cell histiocytosis
9.	Lymphangioleimyomatosis

An important clinical observation is that in some patients, acute left ventricular failure presents with paroxysmal dyspnea but instead of the usual crackles there are rhonchi and wheezes all over the chest. This presentation is rightly termed cardiac asthma and needs to be distinguished from bronchial asthma. The presence of background cardiac disease should always arouse suspicion of left ventricular failure. Left heart failure is also the diagnosis in the presence of an enlarged heart or abnormal auscultatory cardiac findings. It is of relevance that when a patient with bronchial asthma or COPD for any reason develops left heart disease and goes into acute left ventricular failure, the presentation is quite often with rhonchi and wheezes over the chest than the usual pulmonary crackles. X-ray of the chest may reveal pulmonary edema but this may not be easily detectable in a patient having large lungs due to longstanding asthma or COPD.

An extremely important cardiovascular condition that can present with breathlessness—generally of acute or subacute onset—is pulmonary thromboembolic disease. The only symptom may be dyspnea and indeed there may be no physical signs whatsoever. A ghastly mistake of dubbing such a patient as functional is often made. A correct diagnosis always rests on an acute awareness of this entity. A background history, such as a long flight or hours of travel in a car or train, or the use of oral contraceptives in a young female, should always arouse suspicion. Even a slight suspicion should prompt the physician to ask for a D-dimmer level, a Doppler of the lower limbs and a high-resolution computed tomography (HRCT) pulmonary angiography. Chronic pulmonary thromboembolic disease presents with dyspnea on exertion, ultimately leading to pulmonary hypertension and right heart failure. It should always be kept in mind where the cause of dyspnea or right heart failure is not apparent (*see* chapter on Pulmonary Embolism). The subject of pulmonary embolism is discussed at length in a separate chapter.

Pulmonary hypertension, in particular idiopathic pulmonary hypertension causing dyspnea, is one other entity where the diagnosis is missed unless physical signs for pulmonary hypertension are sought and confirmed by 2D echocardiographic study.

Diseases other than cardiopulmonary pathologies producing dyspnea should also be kept in mind. These include severe anemia, neuromuscular disease causing weakness of the intercostal and/or diaphragm, myasthenia gravis, thyrotoxicosis, and skeletal abnormalities preventing proper expansion of the rib cage (ankylosing spondylitis, kyphoscoliotic deformity). Dyspnea *on exertion (as has been mentioned earlier)* is also complained by patients who are physically unfit through lack of activity and exercise and by obese individuals.

Dyspnea due to anxiety (psychogenic dyspnea) is typically characterized by sighing breathing, by hyperventilation which may lead to a washout of CO_2 causing carpopedal spasm and even a fainting episode. Tachycardia and inversion of T waves on electrocardiography (ECG) during the episode may lead to a wrong diagnosis of a cardiac disease.

Metabolic acidosis, either diabetic ketoacidosis or metabolic acidosis from any other cause produces deep breaths (Kussmaul's breathing) with or without an increase in the respiratory rate. Usually, the patient does not complain of any discomfort during breathing. Diabetic ketoacidosis has the typical smell of ketones in the breath, while uremic acidosis is associated with an ammonical smell in the breath.

■ CONCLUSION

In conclusion, the differential diagnosis and a final diagnosis of dyspnea can be arrived at by a history, physical examination and relevant investigations **(Table 3)**. Relevant investigations for dyspnea related to respiratory diseases include a blood count, ESR, sputum examination, and X-ray chest. Lung function tests can determine the difference between airways obstruction and restrictive lung disease or point to a combination of both (see chapter on Pulmonary Function Testing). Determining oxygen saturation within an oximeter is important. A study of the arterial PH and blood gases may also be necessary. A fall in the oxygen saturation after a 6-minute walk test is typically observed in interstitial lung disease.

An HRCT of the chest is often necessary to determine the nature and extent of a respiratory disease. Bronchoscopy, a study of the BAL, and if necessary a transbronchial biopsy of a lesion in the lung or mediastinal glands may be necessary in appropriate conditions.

Basic investigations for dyspnea related to cardiovascular disease include basic blood tests, BNP level in the blood, X-ray chest, ESR, echocardiography, ECG, a treadmill stress test or a stress thallium test to determine the presence of myocardial ischemia. A CT coronary angiography or a conventional angiography should be done to determine the presence, degree of ischemic

Table 3: Diagnostic tests in the investigation of dyspnea.

Tests	Abnormalities detected	Possible diagnosis
Basic blood tests	Leukocytosis; low hemoglobin	Infection, anemia
ABG	Low pH; low PaO_2	Acidosis; respiratory alkalosis; hypoxia
BNP	Elevated BNP	Heart failure
X-ray chest	Abnormalities in lung fields, cardiac silhouette, pleura, mediastinum	COPD, interstitial lung disease, infiltrative lung disease; cardiac disease; mediastinal pathology, pleural disease, pneumothorax
Spirometry, lung volumes	Obstructive pattern Restrictive pattern	Airways obstruction; restrictive lung pathology
CO diffusion	Decreased	Interstitial lung disease, pulmonary vascular disease
	Increased	Alveolar hemorrhage
HRCT chest	Various abnormalities, e.g. ground-glass shadows, alveolar shadows, interstitial shadows, centrilobular emphysema, mass lesions, obstruction to central airways	Depends on nature of abnormalities present
HRCT pulmonary angiography	Filling defects or defects in pulmonary arteries	Pulmonary embolism
Fiberoptic bronchoscopy	Obstruction to airways	Tumor, foreign body, extrinsic pressure
Biopsy-fiberoptic CT-guided video-assisted thoracoscopy		Biopsy results may confirm tumor and nature of lung disease

heart disease when strongly suspected on clinical grounds. Further special tests depend on the nature of the cardiovascular disease.

A clinical approach to the symptoms of dyspnea in a patient is to determine whether it is acute or chronic. Acute onset dyspnea has certain important likely etiologies, chronic progressive dyspnea is generally due to another group of causes. Causes of acute and chronic dyspnea are listed in **Table 4**.

The important causes of acute dyspnea in an adult are acute left ventricular failure, bronchial asthma, pneumothorax, acute pneumonia, and acute pulmonary thromboembolism. Atelectasis of a lobe or lung generally from secretions obstructing a bronchus is an important cause of acute dyspnea frequently observed in the critical care unit.

In children acute dyspnea is more often due to upper airways obstruction—acute viral epiglottitis, laryngitis, acute laryngotracheobronchitis, and foreign body obstructing a bronchus. Acute bronchiolitis, pneumonia, bronchopneumonia are other important causes of dyspnea in children.

Chronic progressive dyspnea in adults is most often due to COPD, longstanding severe asthma, cardiac dysfunction leading to chronic left ventricular failure

Table 4: Important causes of acute and chronic dyspnea.

Acute dyspnea in adults	Chronic (often progressive) dyspnea in adults
• Acute episodes of bronchial asthma • Acute left ventricular failure • Acute exacerbation of COPD • Spontaneous pneumothorax • Pneumonia • Pulmonary embolism • Massive atelectasis • Acutely evolving pleural effusion • Foreign body aspiration • A partial obstruction to a large airway • Intra-alveolar hemorrhage • Trauma to the chest wall and intrathoracic structures	• COPD • Chronic left ventricular failure • Asthma • Interstitial pneumonia • Interstitial fibrosis • Slowly evolving pleural effusion • Chronic pulmonary thromboembolic disease • Pulmonary hypertension • Slowly progressive upper airways obstruction (subglottic stenosis, tracheal stenosis, tumor obstructing a large airway, extrinsic pressure on a large airway) • Anemia • Thyrotoxicosis • Neuromuscular disease • Psychogenic dyspnea
In children: Upper airways obstruction due to epiglottitis, laryngitis, tracheobronchitis, foreign body, pneumonia, and bronchiolitis	

and interstitial lung disease. In the elderly there may well be both pulmonary and cardiac components to chronic progressive dyspnea and the degree of contribution to dyspnea by each of these components may be difficult to determine.

Pleural effusion if acute can cause acute dyspnea; a slow accumulation of pleural fluid will cause progressive dyspnea extending over a longer period of time. Progressively worsening anemia is an important cause of gradually increasing dyspnea.

Less common causes of chronic progressive dyspnea are pulmonary hypertension and chronic pulmonary thromboembolic disease. Upper airways obstruction (e.g. tracheal stenosis) or subglottic stenosis or a tumor obstructing a large airway or extrinsic pressure on a large airway causing dyspnea can be misdiagnosed as bronchial asthma.

Psychogenic dyspnea has acute exacerbations but can become chronic if unrecognized and not appropriately managed. Thyrotoxicosis and neuromuscular disease are comparatively uncommon causes that should be kept in mind as they occasionally present with chronic progressive dyspnea.

■ SUGGESTED READING

1. Karnani NG. Evaluation of chronic dyspnea. Am Fam Physician. 2005;71(8):1529-37.
2. Mahler DA. Evaluation of dyspnea in the elderly. Clin Geriatr Med. 2003;19(1):19-33, v.
3. Parshall MB, Schwartzstein RM, Adams L, et al. An official American Thoracic Society statement: update on the mechanisms, assessment, and management of dyspnea. Am J Respire Crit Care Med. 2012;185:435-52.
4. Schwartzstein RM, King TE. Approach to the patient with dyspnoea. [online] Available from www.uptodate.com [Accessed July, 2018].
5. Thomas JR. Clinical management of dyspnoea. Lancet Oncol. 2002;3(4):223-8.

CHAPTER 12

Chest Pain or Discomfort

■ INTRODUCTION

Thoracic pain or discomfort, a common complaint in patients with respiratory problems is equally common or perhaps even more common in several pathologies not involving the lungs, the pleura or the conducting airways. It is therefore vital for the chest physician to be also aware of the important causes of chest pain arising from sources outside the respiratory system. This chapter gives an overall perspective of some important causes of chest discomfort or pain **(Table 1)**.

Table 1: Important causes of chest discomfort/pain.
Cardiovascular causes: • Ischemic cardiac pain   • Pericarditis   • Aortic dissection   • Aneurysms of the ascending arch, descending aorta
Pulmonary embolism
Pleuritic chest pain, pulmonary infarction
Substernal pain associated with acute tracheobronchitis
Pulmonary hypertension
Chest wall pain: • Musculoskeletal pain   • Fracture of ribs, sternum, one or more vertebrae   • Tumor deposits in the ribs or spine   • Myeloma deposits in ribs or spine   • Lung cancer, mediastinal mass lesions   • Pancoast's tumor
Miscellaneous causes: • Peptic esophagitis with esophageal spasm   • Cervical spondylitis   • Tubercle of the spine, metastatic lesions in the spine, spinal chord tumors, transverse myelitis   • Herpes zoster   • Anxiety

■ CARDIOVASCULAR CAUSES

The first principle in the evaluation of chest pain, particularly precordial or substernal pain is to determine whether the pain is related to myocardial ischemia or infarction. Ischemic cardiac pain or the pain of myocardial infarction is often described as substernal heaviness, vice-like, crushing in character. It is the character rather than the severity which is more important for a correct diagnosis. Pricking pain, stabbing pain, pain localized at or below the nipple, pain associated with local tenderness is unlikely to be cardiac pain. Typically, cardiac pain radiates to the left shoulder and arm, sometimes to both shoulders and arms and often to the jaw and to the back. Clinical examination, serial electrocardiography (ECG) tracings and an estimation of cardiac enzymes help in diagnosis.

Pericarditis can cause precordial pain aggravated by breathing. The pain is generally accompanied by a pericardial rub and is often relieved on sitting up. Signs of a pericardial effusion may be evident on clinical examination, or on an X-ray of the chest and on echocardiography.

Aortic dissection is the cause of severe pain generally starting in the back, but is also felt in front of the chest. Unequal pulses, reduced pulsations in the lower limbs, systolic murmur at the base often transmitted to the neck, an audible bruit over the back, are some of the important clinical findings. Patients generally are hypertensive to start with, yet appear to be in shock. The ECG is normal or shows nonspecific changes; the diagnosis is confirmed by computed tomography (CT) or magnetic resonance imaging (MRI) of the chest.

An aneurysm of this ascending aorta, arch of the aorta and the descending aorta may also cause chest pain. This is evident on an X-ray chest and relevant imaging.

PLEURITIC CHEST PAIN

Pleuritic chest pain is due to inflammation and edema of the parietal pleura. It is worse on inspiration, coughing and is described as sharp or knife-like in character. It is generally localized but can be felt across the chest along the distribution of the intercostal nerves that supply the affected area of the pleura. Inflammation of the pleura over the central portion of the diaphragm leads to pain referred to the shoulder, while inflammation of the pleura over the lateral portion of the diaphragm is referred to the abdomen. Pleuritic pain is generally but not always associated with a pleural rub. Systemic features such as fever, malaise are generally present.

Pulmonary infarction can cause localized pleural pain. Systemic features may be absent and a pleural rub is not necessarily present.

SUBSTERNAL PAIN ASSOCIATED WITH ACUTE TRACHEOBRONCHITIS

Acute tracheobronchitis is often associated with a burning or a searing substernal soreness and pain, aggravated by coughing.

PULMONARY HYPERTENSION

Pulmonary hypertension can produce pain indistinguishable from angina on effort. In fact this pain is truly anginal, caused by ischemia to the right ventricle. Anginal pain can also be caused by a fixed very low cardiac output due to the severity of pulmonary hypertension.

Massive pulmonary embolism can cause substernal chest pain indistinguishable from myocardial infarction.

CHEST WALL PAIN

Chest wall pain which is not pleuritic and which does not arise from myocardial ischemia, infarction, or pericarditis, or any other cardiopulmonary problem, may have a musculoskeletal origin. Musculoskeletal pain like pleuritic pain is also aggravated on inspiration. The pain worsens on palpating the painful area.

Acute severe pain localized over one or more ribs in the mid-axillary line is most often seen following cough fractures of these ribs. A crepitus may be felt and imaging studies reveal the fracture.

More serious causes of chest pain are related to tumor or myeloma deposits in the ribs or spine, or local invasion of the thoracic cage from a lung cancer or from soft tissue tumors invading the thoracic cage.

Pancoast's tumor (superior sulcus tumor) described by Pancoast in 1932 causes pain localized to the ipsilateral upper chest, as also pain in the ipsilateral shoulder often radiating along the distribution of the seventh cervical and first thoracic nerves. The condition is often mistaken for shoulder arthritis or cervical spondylitis. The tumor causes Horner's syndrome due to involvement of the sympathetic trunk on the affected side and wasting of the small muscles of the hand if the first thoracic nerve root is infiltrated or compressed by the tumor. An X-ray of chest shows a circumscribed soft tissue shadow at the apex with destruction of C7, T1, T2 vertebrae together with their transverse processes.

Vague chest discomfort or pain is a frequent complaint of patients with lung cancer and of patients with a mediastinal tumor or a mediastinal mass lesion.

MISCELLANEOUS CAUSES

Peptic esophagitis with esophageal spasm can cause substernal pain which may be difficult to distinguish from ischemic myocardial pain.

Cervical spondylitis can also cause pain over the precordium and in one or both upper limbs mimicking myocardial ischemia.

Tubercle of the spine, metastatic lesions in the spine, and spinal cord tumors can cause referred pain to the chest.

Severe unilateral chest pain over a localized area encircling the chest may precede the typical segmental vesicular rash of herpes zoster.

Chest pain is not an uncommon symptom of underlying anxiety. It may be associated with other features of an anxiety state, like hyperventilation, tachycardia, and sweating. The pain often shifts or if fixed is often located at or below the nipple. Clinical examination is normal and basic investigations reveal no abnormality.

SUGGESTED READING

1. Butler KH. Chest pain: a clinical assessment. Radiol Clin North Am. 2006;44(2):165-79, vii.
2. Cayley WE Jr. Diagnosing the cause of chest pain. Am Fam Phys. 2005;72(10):2012-21.
3. Eslick GD. Noncardiac chest pain: evaluation and treatment. Gastroenterol Clin North Am. 2003;32(2):531-52.
4. Hoffmann U, Truong QA, Schoenfeld DA, et al. CT angiography versus standard evaluation in acute chest pain. N Engl J Med. 2012;367(4):299-308.
5. Kelly BS. Evaluation of the elderly patient with acute chest pain. Clin Geriatr Med. 2007;23(2):327-49, vi.

CHAPTER 13

Clinical Examination of the Respiratory System

■ INTRODUCTION

A detailed history and a meticulous physical examination are vital for a thorough assessment of a patient with respiratory disease or for that matter any disease. Unfortunately, with the tremendous advance of science and technology and the advent of sophisticated gadgetry and gleaming machines, the art and science of history-taking and physical examination are sadly neglected. Instead of being in the forefront of a clinical approach, they are increasingly relegated to the background. An evaluation of a patient with symptoms pertaining to the respiratory system can never be complete and correct without a good history and a thorough physical examination. A radiographic examination of the chest is almost an extension of a physical examination in a patient with chest disease. This is because a radiographic examination of the chest can reveal serious disease when physical examination even by an experienced clinician draws a blank. Witness for example, the "uncovering" of a tuberculous infiltrate or cavity, or the presence of a lung cancer, or mediastinal adenopathy by a radiographic examination of the chest in a patient who may essentially have no abnormal physical signs. Yet physical examination may uncover features, which are not evident on a radiographic examination of the chest. For example, the presence of a pleural or pericardial rub heard on auscultation, or the presence of polyphonic wheezes signifying airways obstruction, or a monophonic wheeze signifying obstruction to a large airway are important clinical findings that cannot be detected by a radiographic examination of the chest. The history, physical examination, and chest radiography complement each other to help arrive at a correct diagnosis. Though an X-ray of the chest is mandatory in most patients with persistent respiratory symptoms, its use as a screening procedure to uncover early disease, which is treatable (for example, early cancer) has not been shown to improve mortality and is, therefore, of dubious value. Even so, a routine health check-up in almost all centers of the world includes an X-ray of the chest. The use of high-resolution computed tomography (HRCT) of the chest as a screening procedure is also of unproven benefit.

When the triad of history, physical examination, and radiography of the chest fails to give a diagnosis, further sophisticated tests can be availed of. However, an approach that focuses primarily on these tests is bad medicine.

■ HISTORY

There is no substitute for a good history. Cough and breathlessness or shortness of breath are the two most common symptoms in respiratory diseases. Less frequent complaints are hemoptysis and chest discomfort. A detailed history of each of these symptoms is rewarding. The association of systemic features like fever, weight loss, and joint pains is also of crucial importance and may be elicited only on direct questioning. An occupational history may give the clue to a diagnosis. For example, exposure to asbestos may have occurred several years back, yet the respiratory disease of the present may well be linked to this exposure. Improvement of symptoms over a weekend or on holidays may suggest symptoms related to an occupational exposure. Residence for a short period in India or in other tropical climes may suggest pulmonary problems endemic in these climes. For people living in India, history of temporary residence in a part of the United States where histoplasmosis or coccidioidomycosis is common, may help to clarify the nature of an illness, which resembles tuberculosis (TB) but which has not responded to anti-TB drugs and in which the sputum has no acid-fast bacilli.

A history of smoking cigarettes, bidis, and cigars is important. The duration a patient has smoked and the number of cigarettes smoked (pack years) are of equal importance.

A history of past or associated problems, which produce symptoms outside the respiratory systems, is important. Cough in a patient with scleroderma, for example, may be related to interstitial lung disease which is a pulmonary manifestation of scleroderma, or caused by aspiration pneumonia due to involvement of the esophagus in scleroderma. A pleural effusion in a patient with a history of systemic lupus erythematosus (SLE) may well be due to this disease. A history of cancer of the breast, colon or kidney in the past may relate to respiratory symptoms caused by metastatic disease in the lungs.

It is important to inquire about symptoms unrelated to respiratory disease. Breathlessness and cough may be caused as much by heart disease as by respiratory disease. A history of anginal pains, pedal edema, and a past history of myocardial infarction are all of great relevance. At times, particularly in older people, breathlessness and cough may be related both to respiratory and cardiac disease. Cancer of the lung may occasionally present with symptoms due to paraneoplastic syndromes. The significance of these symptoms in relation to the underlying diagnosis is often lost.

The possibility of human immunodeficiency virus (HIV) infection in relation to opportunistic infections causing pulmonary disease should always be kept in mind, particularly in parts of the world where HIV is highly prevalent. Other conditions where a patient is immunodeficient or immunosuppressed are following chemotherapy or the use of immunosuppressant drugs, hematological malignancies, uncontrolled diabetes, chronic liver or renal disease, transplant patients and patients on corticosteroids.

A careful inquiry into personal habits is important. A history of drug abuse is not easily elicited, but if present, may give the answer to the cause of multiple abscesses in the lungs. The use of methotrexate for rheumatoid disease may be responsible for pneumonia of obscure origin. Bleomycin used as an antimitotic drug can cause crippling interstitial pulmonary fibrosis; Nitrofurantoin used for urinary infection can cause a hypersensitivity response in the lung and pleura with fever, cough and breathlessness.

A family history is also important as in bronchial asthma or cystic fibrosis. To give just one other example—a patient with repeated hemoptysis had visited one hospital after another with no diagnosis as to the cause in spite of full investigations. A careful family history revealed that his brother had recurrent epistaxis and had suffered from malena. The brother was asked to report to the clinic and he was found to have classical telangiectasia on the lip and tongue. The diagnosis rested on the history!

■ PHYSICAL EXAMINATION

A good physical examination of the chest and heart in many hospitals, both here and abroad, unfortunately seems a practice of the past. Yet a meticulous physical examination not just of the respiratory system but also of all systems is crucial for full appraisal of a patient with chest complaints.

General Examination

A general examination even before going to an examination of the chest may present a clue to diagnosis. The presence of prolonged expiration, the use of accessory muscles of respiration, and breathing through pursed lips is a feature of chronic airways obstruction. Flapping tremors or a slightly obtunded mental state point to CO_2 retention. Drowsiness in a patient with cancer lung may well relate to metastasis in the brain. Painful swelling of the ankles and knees together with lesions of erythema nodosum over the skin of the lower extremities is a feature of a number of medical conditions, in particular tuberculosis, sarcoidosis, fungal infection, drug reaction, connective tissue disorders and vasculitides. Painful swelling of the ankles and painful swelling proximal to the wrists, when associated with clubbing is a feature of hypertrophic pulmonary osteoarthropathy.

The presence of iritis may be observed in sarcoidosis and in the vasculitides such as Wegener's granulomatosis. A unilateral miosis is a feature of Horner's syndrome. A puffy face with engorged nonpulsatile jugular veins is seen in the superior vena caval syndrome. In the majority of patients the syndrome is due to a lung cancer.

A firm gland between the two heads of the sternomastoid is always pathological and when biopsied gives the exact diagnosis. Cervical adenopathy when significant occurs in numerous diseases, in particular TB, other infectious diseases, sarcoidosis, lymphoma, and mitotic lesions.

Examination of the skin is of great importance. Erythema nodosum has already been commented upon. Palpable purpura is a classical feature of vasculitides, which could involve the lung as well. Sarcoidosis produces skin lesions some of which are fairly typical so that they provide a clue to the diagnosis of a patient who has cough and breathlessness.

Dilated veins over the skin of the upper chest and shoulders are observed with superior vena caval obstruction.

Raynaud's phenomena in a patient with respiratory symptoms suggest chiefly scleroderma or SLE. Clubbing of the nails occurs in various respiratory disorders—bronchiectasis, lung abscess, interstitial lung disease, lung cancer and in some patients with TB. Central cyanosis in respiratory disease points to well-marked hypoxia, PaO_2 less than 55 mm Hg. It points to severe hypoventilation or ventilation-perfusion inequality, or to a right to left shunt in the lungs. Diffusion defects contribute to hypoxia.

Pitting edema can be due to heart failure—either primary or secondary to lung disease. Deep vein thrombosis is likely in the presence of a swollen painful lower extremity.

These are just a few of the many possible clues that can be unmasked on a general examination.

Examination of the Chest

A careful count of the respiratory rate over a whole minute is of vital importance. A respiratory rate over 20 breaths/min, in particular over 25 breaths/min, is a cause for concern. The pulse: respiratory ratio is often reduced in acute lobar pneumonia. Movements of the chest are best judged from the foot end of the bed. Poor movement of one side of the chest compared to the other is seen with pleural effusion, pneumothorax, pneumonia, TB involving the upper lobe and in atelectasis of a lobe or lung. The pattern of breathing needs to be carefully observed. An indrawing of the upper abdomen during inspiration suggests a diaphragmatic paralysis.

Patients with bilateral diaphragmatic paralysis become breathless, hypoxic and cyanosed on lying flat. They are more comfortable on sitting or standing.

An indrawing of the lower intercostal spaces during inspiration is a sign of respiratory distress. It occurs in the acute respiratory distress syndrome (ARDS) and in severe airflow obstruction due to the high negative intrapleural pressure during inspiration. Paradoxical respiratory

movements are also a sign of respiratory distress and respiratory muscle fatigue. Shallow breathing is seen in hypoventilating patients. Airflow obstruction is associated with prolonged expiration often with an audible wheeze. Restrictive diseases such as interstitial lung disease result in shallow rapid breathing. The same is observed in patients with acute left ventricular failure.

Palpation of the Chest and Neck

One of the most important aspects of palpation is to determine whether the trachea is central or shifted to one side. A shift of the trachea to one side may arise because the trachea is pushed from the opposite side (as in a pleural effusion or pneumothorax) or is pulled toward the same side (as with an atelectasis of a lobe or a lung, or due to upper lobe fibrosis).

Palpation of the neck for lymph glands should never be forgotten if it has not already been done.

The apical impulse should be carefully located. A shift of the impulse is an indication of the shift of the lower mediastinum, either being pushed from the opposite side (as with pleural effusion) or pulled from the same side (as in atelectasis of a lobe or whole lung). The presence of dextrocardia in a patient with chronic cough with expectoration should suggest the possibility of Kartagener's syndrome.

Palpation to test movements of the chest may give the clue to the side of the disease. A lag in the movement of one side of the chest (either the lower, mid-upper or the whole chest) together with a diminished movement of the same side compared to the other is seen with a pleural effusion, pneumothorax, thickened pleura, atelectasis, pneumonia or a large mass lesion in one lung.

Marked local tenderness and swelling over a rib suggests a fracture, a metastatic deposit or a myelomatous deposit at that site. Tuberculosis involving a rib can also cause local swelling, tenderness, and pain.

Tactile fremitus (transmission of sound as a palpable vibration) is best felt with the ulnar border of the hand. It is increased over consolidation and decreased over a pleural effusion or over a pneumothorax.

Localized palpable pulsatile swelling over the chest may be felt in a patient with an empyema necessitans (there is an impulse over the localized swelling on coughing) and in an aneurysm of the arch of the aorta (in the second or third left intercostal space) and of the ascending aorta (second right intercostal space).

Percussion

Auenbrugger discovered percussion when he realized that he could tell how full a beer barrel was by percussing it. The percussion note is normally resonant over an air-filled lung. It is impaired over an area of atelectasis or consolidation and is described as stony dull over a pleural effusion, a markedly thickened pleura or a large mass at the surface of the lung. A hyperresonant note is obtained over large air-filled lungs that characterize emphysema. A localized hyperresonant note is sometimes elicitable over a large-sized bulla. The liver dullness generally observed in the fifth intercostal space in the midclavicular line may be much lower or unelicitable in severe emphysema. The cardiac dullness may be absent in emphysema or in a left-sided pneumothorax.

An impaired note in the first and second left intercostal spaces is occasionally observed with pericardial effusion, aortic aneurysm and in mediastinal tumors.

Auscultation

Even the art of auscultation is falling into disuse or perfunctory use. A resident (ignorant in auscultation) on a ward round in one of the teaching hospitals remarked (rather happily) that soon the stethoscope will be a museum piece allowed to rest on a hook in the wall! Auscultation to the experienced clinician is a guide to the state of the underlying lung.

Breath sounds are normally produced by the vibration of the vocal chords, of the movement of air in the trachea and large bronchi. The quality of these sounds can be determined by listening over the trachea. The breath sounds over the trachea are noted to be hollow with an expiration longer than inspiration and a pause between inspiration and expiration. These breath sounds are transmitted down several orders of bronchi and bronchioles. If one was to hear the sound over these breathing tubes, their character would be the same as over the trachea, only they would be not as loud because of the distance traveled by the sound waves. Once the respiratory bronchioles open into the numerous open air spaces termed the alveoli, the character of the breath sounds changes. No longer do they have the "bronchial" quality. The sound waves are dispersed within the alveoli, so that they now assume the character of normal vesicular breath sounds which are best heard rather than described. These sound vibrations go through the pleura and the chest wall to be heard by the clinician through the diaphragm of the stethoscope. Normal vesicular breath sounds have a rustling quality; the expiration is about one-third the duration of inspiration and there is no pause between inspiration and expiration.

Abnormal Breath Sounds

Bronchial breathing is hollow breathing with prolonged expiration and a pause between inspiration and expiration. One promptly recognizes bronchial breathing most of all by its hollow character. It classically occurs over a consolidated lobe or an atelectic lobe with a patent bronchus. The reason why bronchial breathing is heard over a consolidated lobe is easy to understand. The hollow bronchial sounds produced over the larynx and large airways go down the smaller breathing tubes but are not dispersed within the alveoli because the alveoli are solid and consolidated. These hollow breath sounds go unchanged through the consolidated lobe, through the chest wall to be heard by the listening clinician.

Bronchial breath sounds are termed as tubular, cavernous or amphoric. These all are typically hollow sounds, the difference between them being a difference in the timbre of the sound. Cavernous breath sounds occur over a cavity, the cavity acting as a resonator, which emphasizes some overtones and suppresses others. Amphoric breath sounds may be heard over a pneumothorax or a cavity and are likened to the sound heard when one blows over the top of an open bottle.

Decrease in Breath Sounds

Decrease in breath sounds occurs over a pleural effusion, thickened pleura, pneumothorax, and in atelectasis of a lobe or lung.

Diminished breath sounds are also observed in patients with emphysema, hypoventilating patients, pleural effusion, thickened pleura, pneumothorax, and in patients with paresis of the intercostal muscles or diaphragm. Breath sounds are also diminished when there is a large mass occupying a lobe of the lung. Breath sounds may be absent over a large pleural effusion or over an atelectic lobe with a blocked bronchus.

Prolonged expiration is typically seen in airways obstruction as in chronic obstructive pulmonary disease (COPD) or bronchial asthma. Variation in the intensity of breath sounds over different areas over the lungs is frequent in patients with either COPD or asthma due to uneven distribution of ventilation related to uneven degree of airways obstruction over different parts of the lungs.

Changes in Vocal Fremitus

Vocal fremitus as judged by the transmission of voice sounds when the patients say "one two three" should be carefully elicited. Vocal fremitus is increased over consolidation and over an atelectatic lobe with patent bronchi. It is reduced over a pleural effusion, pleural thickening, pneumothorax, and over a collapsed lobe with closed bronchi. When the vocal fremitus is loud and very clear, it is termed as bronchophony. At times the spoken words take on a nasal quality and this is termed as egophony. This is heard most commonly when consolidated lung and pleural effusion coexist. Clear transmission of a whispered sound is termed as whispering pectoriloquy. It has the same significance as bronchophony.

Adventitious Sounds

Adventitious sounds arising within the lung have been classified in various ways. The earlier classification (first proposed by René Laennec) considered adventitious sounds as:
- Rhonchi (dry sounds), sibilant or high-pitched, and sonorous or low-pitched
- Râles (moist sounds), fine râles (as in consolidation), medium râles (as in a patient with airway secretions), and coarse râles (as in patients with secretions within large airways such as the trachea or major bronchi).

The American Thoracic Society has given a classification based on the acoustic analysis of tape recordings and on the classification introduced by Forgac. This classification is as follows:
- Continuous sounds (wheeze, rhonchi, and stridor)
- Discontinuous sound (crackles).

Wheeze, rhonchi, and *stridor* are continuous musical sounds. Wheezes are high-pitched and originate in airways obstruction caused by spasm, mucosal edema, and secretions. Since airways obstruction is more marked during expiration they are more prominent in that phase of breathing, but they can also occur during inspiration. They are often polyphonic, i.e. vary in pitch and intensity over different areas of the lung in patients with asthma or

COPD. A low-pitched monophonic wheeze is occasionally heard over a partially obstructed main bronchus or lobar bronchus (Chevalier Jackson's sign). Wheezes originate chiefly through vibration of the walls of the bronchi resulting from airflow limitation.

Rhonchi are due to the presence of mucus and secretions within airways. Rhonchi change in location and character on coughing because of movement of these secretions induced by coughing.

Stridor is an inspiratory noise that can be heard at a distance or by auscultation over the neck. It is caused by obstruction to the larynx or trachea or major bronchi.

Crackles (formerly called rales) are due to the explosive snapping opening of numerous small airways that close prematurely during expiration. Crackles are further classified as early inspiratory or late inspiratory. Crackles of interstitial lung disease (as in interstitial pulmonary fibrosis) occur typically in late inspiration. Crackles occurring in early inspiration are noted in patients with COPD. Crackles often heard all through the inspiratory phase are also heard over a consolidated lobe as in pneumonia, atelectasis and in pulmonary edema.

Hypostatic congestion due to prolonged recumbency also gives rise to crackles. These crackles lessen or disappear on making the patient cough.

Crackles have also been classified as wet or dry. Wet crackles, for example, occur in pulmonary edema (typically in left ventricular failure). Dry crackles also called "velcro" crackles are easily recognized with a little practice and are typically heard in interstitial lung disease.

Pleural Rub

Pleural rub is a rough grating friction sound heard during inspiration and early expiration generally in the mid-axillary line and over the lung bases. The sound appears superficial and close to the ear. It signifies pleural inflammation. It is generally easily recognized except when brief in duration and faint; it may then be difficult to distinguish form localized crackles.

An examination of the cardiovascular system is as important as that of the respiratory system as many symptoms of respiratory disease are common to those of cardiovascular disease.

The question (impertinent in our opinion) often asked by students is why should one examine the chest in this detail when we have an X-ray chest at hand and numerous other sophisticated machines to give a diagnosis?

The answer is as follows:
- A doctor who fails to use his eyes, ears and hands is a poor doctor or perhaps no doctor at all. A cultivated power of observation is the hallmark of a good physician.
- If a doctor looks only or almost only at machines and their reports, he has no rapport with his patient. He fails to talk to him, fails to often touch him, and fails to empathize with him. The doctor-patient relationship which lies at the core of medicine stands eroded or broken and medicine is not even a shadow of what it should be.

■ SUGGESTED READING

1. Paul F. Lung Sounds.© London: Bailliere Tindall; 1978.
2. Sarkar M, Madabhavi I, Niranjan N. et al. Auscultation of the respiratory system. Ann Thorac Med. 2015;10(3): 158-68.
3. Sarkar S, Amelung PJ. Evaluation of the dyspnoeic patient in the office. Prim Care. 2006;33(3):643-57.

Section 5

Pulmonary Tuberculosis

CHAPTER 14

Introduction, History, and Epidemiology

■ INTRODUCTION AND IMPACT IN INDIA

Tuberculosis (TB) is a disease that has existed since antiquity. It is a major threat to global health, being the second highest cause of death from an infectious disease after HIV/AIDS. In 2015, there were 10.4 million new cases and 1.4 million deaths from TB globally. Six countries accounted for 60% of the new cases: India, China, Indonesia, Nigeria, Pakistan and South Africa.

Tuberculosis dominates medicine in India, being one of this country's major public health problems. It exists on an epic scale here with India accounting for a third of the world's entire TB burden and a fifth of all the smear-positive cases of the world. 300 million Indians are infected with TB, at least 14 million with active disease. 22% of the world's smear-positive cases reside here giving India the largest concentration of TB cases in the world. The incidence of smear-positive, infectious cases in India is 85 per 100,000. Readily transmitted in impoverished and crowded communities, TB impacts on lives in a manner no other disease can. TB is now the leading infectious cause of adult death in India. At a conservative estimate, each year, at least 500,000 people die of the disease. This works out to one death from TB every minute, a grim statistic that has sadly not changed over the decades. Once considered a disease of slums and ghettos and affecting the socially disadvantaged, TB has widened its reach in India affecting urban and rural communities and people from all walks of life.

Tuberculosis exacts a great price economically as well. The World Economic Forum estimated in 2008 that India loses $3 billion per year from TB annually. Broken down to a personal level, TB causes suffering on an unparalleled scale in India. It devastates entire families by afflicting young bread-earners who lose employment, as a consequence taking on loans that can never be repaid, so that eventually, it causes incalculable human suffering.

■ HISTORY

Skeletal Data

Tuberculosis has probably been a human pathogen for millions of years. Skeletal remains are an important source of TB. The skeletal structure will be affected in about 5% of patients with TB and hence finding a destructive lesion like Pott's disease in the spine is the best evidence of TB for a paleopathologist. The earliest evidence comes from a female skeleton aged 30 years found in the cave of Arma dell' Aquila in Liguria, Italy, dating back to around 5800 BC. TB in mummified remains from Egypt was also noted from around 4500 BC with the most famous being that of the mummy Nesperhan in whom there is clear evidence of both spinal changes and a psoas abscess.

Disease in Asia appears later with the earliest evidence being from around 2700 BC. Skeletal evidence of TB from the Americas is more recent dating back to AD 1000 in North America and AD 700 in South America. In addition to traditional skeletal analysis, biomolecular evidence of TB opened up new insights in the origin and pathogenesis of this disease. Modern molecular and polymerase chain reaction (PCR) began to shed more information and it was now possible to establish the presence of TB even in human remains that had no obvious skeletal remains of TB. This is an exciting field and one that is only a few decades old.

Historical Data

By the 5th century BC, TB was mentioned in the great Hippocrates writings. In India, the ancient *Rig Veda* scriptures make reference to TB as early as 1500 BC. Further elaboration in the Ayurvedas (around 700 BC) makes it clear that the symptoms of TB and its dreaded nature were evident even then—"the physician who wants great fame cures a man attacked by consumption". Ancient Chinese texts (2700 BC) and Egyptian papyrus gave vivid descriptions of glandular TB. TB was mentioned in the writings of nonmedical giants like Homer (800 BC) and Pliny (1st century AD). TB also began to be featured in art sources and engravings; sculpture and paintings began to depict initially kyphotic spines and in the middle ages, emaciated, frail young women in melancholic poses.

By the beginning of the 17th century, TB was becoming exceedingly common and The London Bill of Mortality records that 20% of deaths in England by the mid-1600s were from TB. In the 18th century, John Bunyan famously referred to TB as "Captain of all these men of death". This was merely a reflection of the period, for by the beginning of the 19th century, TB was the main cause of death in most of Europe reaching 800 cases per 100,000 population. The Industrial Revolution in Europe and the poverty and overcrowding seen then, undoubtedly served to fuel the spread of TB in those days. India's current TB epidemic began in the mid-17th century and rates in the community increased to reach their peak in the early years of the 20th century.

A famous catalog of artists, writers, and playwrights died of pulmonary TB adding to its mystique and perpetuating the myth that TB and genius were in some way related. At the height of the romantic era of TB, Alexandre Dumas wrote, "It was the fashion to suffer from the lungs; everybody was consumptive, poets especially; it was good form to spit blood after each emotion that was at all sensational, and to die before reaching the age of thirty years". Indeed Elizabeth Barrett Browning was said to have remarked, "Is it possible that genius is only scrofula?" The list of famous people down the ages who suffered from (and in most cases died of) TB is illuminating, and includes—Alexander Pope, Samuel Johnson, Jean-Jacques Rousseau, Johann Wolfgang von Goethe, Friedrich Schiller, Walter Scott, René Laennec, Niccolo Paganini, Percy Shelley, John Keats, Elizabeth Barrett Browning, Frederic Chopin, Charlotte, Emily and Anne Bronte, Fyodor Dostoyevsky, Anton Chekov, Walt Whitman, Mohammed Ali Jinnah, Franz Kafka, Eleanor Roosevelt, George Orwell, and Nelson Mandela to name a few.

The treatment in those ancient times was largely based on diet, hygiene, rest at high altitudes and sanatoriums, and avoidance of fatigue. In India too, the first sanatoria opened in the temperate hill stations.

The modern era of TB can be said to have begun in 1882 with Robert Koch's epic description of the tubercle bacillus. 3 years later, Conrad Roentgen with his discovery of the X-ray provided a new way to diagnose it. Chemotherapy of TB was only possible after the discovery of streptomycin by Waksman in 1944. Within a few years of the use of streptomycin, it became obvious that resistance was going to emerge rapidly when this drug was used alone. This was perhaps a frightening precursor of the multidrug-resistant TB (MDR-TB) problem that was to leave its full impact only from the 1980s onward. Para-aminosalicylic acid (PAS) was introduced a few years later and added onto streptomycin. It became clear from these early days that combination therapy was the way to prevent resistance developing. The introduction of isoniazid in the 1950s and rifampicin in 1965 paved the way for modern short-course chemotherapy, which was first introduced in the 1970s.

Coming back to India, initial efforts to combat TB only began at the start of the 20th century. These efforts were spearheaded by privately funded voluntary organizations, and though sporadic and inadequate, demonstrated the beginnings of the fight against TB in this country. The earliest sanatoria were set up in the temperate hill stations of India where those afflicted were provided rest and a healthy diet. It was not until India's independence in 1947 that the country took control of its own health and destiny and established two pioneering institutions: (1) the Tuberculosis Chemotherapy Center in Chennai and (2) the National Tuberculosis Institute in Bengaluru. These were under the sponsorship of the Indian Council of Medical Research (ICMR) and the Government of India, respectively. These two centers contributed truly pioneering research that helped shape India's and indeed the world's TB control policies. The famous Madras trials on domiciliary versus sanatorium treatment elegantly and scientifically established the efficacy of domiciliary treatment. Home-treated patients, despite their crowded living conditions and the absence of rest or a diet rich in proteins and vitamins, fared just as well over 5 years of follow-up. The resulting closure of sanatoria across the world that arose as an extension of this study probably saved the developed world millions of dollars.

Several intermittent chemotherapy regimens were also developed by the Madras and Bangalore centers in close collaboration with the British Medical Research Council (BMRC). These served to establish the basis of many of the short-course regimens in use throughout the world. This was indeed the golden age of TB research in this country; an age that has sadly not been equaled by any subsequent generation of researchers.

India's National Tuberculosis Control Program (NTP) was born in 1962, geared at tackling the unique needs of TB control in India. The impact of the NTP will be discussed in the section on epidemiology. Finally, India embraced directly observed treatment, short-course (DOTS) in 1992, and the NTP was reborn as the Revised National Tuberculosis Control Program (RNTCP), which was modeled on the WHO–DOTS strategy.

DOTS in India

No account of the history of TB in India would be complete without discussing the impact of DOTS in this country. Starting with pilot studies in 1993 with coverage of 2.5 million population in just five states to 1996 when coverage of 20 million population was achieved, to 24 March 2006 when 100% DOTS coverage of more than a billion people was achieved, DOTS in India has been the

fastest expanding program in history and is a success story of epic proportions **(Fig. 1)**. The current DOTS program claims 70% case detection rates and 85% success rates; a huge improvement from the earlier program rates **(Fig. 2)**. Mandal et al have estimated that the RNTCP has saved 7.75 million lives from 1997 to 2016 with modelling analysis showing that 40% of its overall impact was due to reduced transmission (*Ref: Mandal S, Chadha VK, Laxminarayan R, et al. Counting the lives saved by DOTS in India: a model-based approach. BMC Medicine. 2017:15;47*).

■ EPIDEMIOLOGY

Global

The natural history of TB epidemics is measured by epidemiologists in secular curves that span centuries. Compared to epidemics of infectious viral disease, TB epidemics progress very slowly through low transmission rates, weak immunity, and a long-generation time. The standard TB epidemic runs over centuries and generates low TB incidence rates. One of the reasons for the slow speed is the immunological fact that only 10% of those infected go on to develop active disease. HIV and other

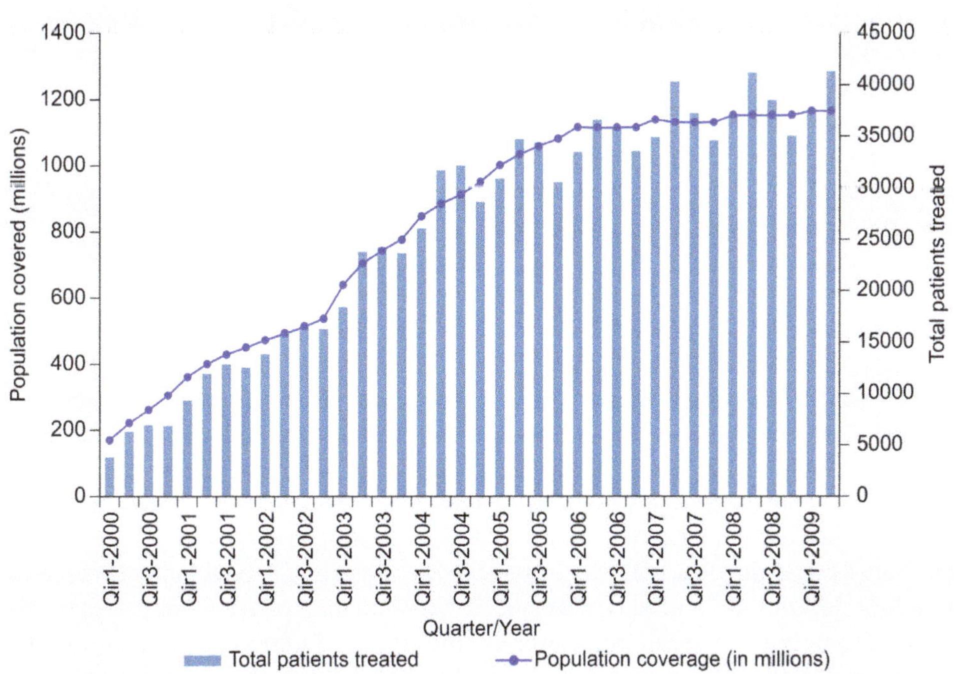

Fig. 1: Population in India covered under directly observed treatment, short-course (DOTS) and total tuberculosis patients put on treatment each quarter.
Source: Ministry of Health and Family Welfare. (2009). Population in India covered under DOTS from 2000–9. (RNTCP performance report, India, 2nd quarter 2009, Central TB division, Ministry of Health and Family Welfare). [online] Available from https://tbcindia.gov.in. [Accessed July, 2018].

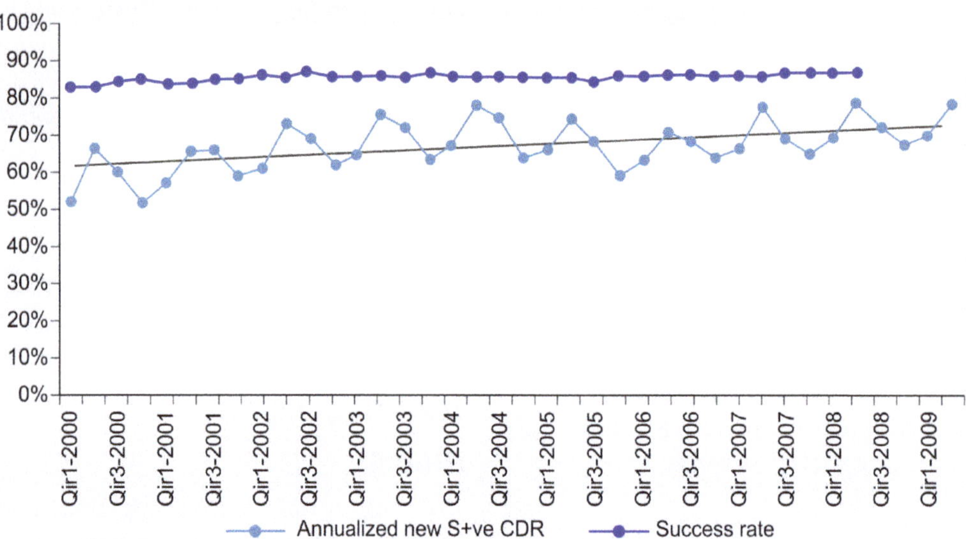

Fig. 2: Annualized new smear-positive case detection rate and treatment success rate in directly observed treatment, short-course (DOTS) areas, 2008–9.
Source: Ministry of Health and Family Welfare. (2009). Annualized new smear case detection rates and treatment success rates. (RNTCP performance report, India, 2nd quarter 2009, Central TB division, Ministry of Health and Family Welfare). [online] Available from https://tbcindia.gov.in. [Accessed July, 2018].

risk factors, of course, dramatically change this equation as will be discussed later. Epidemic modeling shows that in the developed world, TB has been in decline ever since rates per capita peaked in industrialized countries in the early 19th century, interestingly, well before the advent of chemotherapy in the 1950s. The reasons for this 150-year natural decline have been debated by epidemiologists over the years. These include less overcrowding, improved living conditions, caseload shifts to older populations, and most intriguingly the possibility that genetic deletions over the decades have resulted in phenotypes of *Mycobacterium tuberculosis* that are less virulent and less likely to cause cavitary disease. Whatever the factor or combination of factors responsible, it is clear that there was a slow decline in the death rate of TB in Western Europe by 5% per year, starting well before the advent of chemotherapy.

This steady natural decline had ominously leveled off and in some parts of the world actually increased over the last 25 years. In the US, the annual steady 5% per annum decline in TB reduced to just 0.2% in 1985. The next year (1986), in a historic first, cases in the US actually increased for the first time in four decades. In the 1990s, dramatic increases in TB cases began to be reported from several sub-Saharan African countries; in Tanzania cases rose 86%, in Burundi 140% and in Malawi a staggering 180%. It is now clear that both the leveling off and subsequent slight incline in the US and the dramatic incline in Africa were

HIV related. Thus, this disease has had the single most dramatic impact on TB epidemiology since the world's first AIDS cases were described in 1981. An estimated 11% of all new adult TB cases in the year 2015 were HIV related. In the same year, 12% of the 1.84 million TB deaths globally were attributed to HIV. The extent to which HIV is fueling the TB epidemic is difficult to ascertain. Currently, around 15 million people are known to be coinfected with TB and HIV. The clinical features and management of these patients will be discussed in a separate section.

Based on surveys of the prevalence of infection and disease and assessments of surveillance systems and death registrations, there were an estimated 10.4 million new cases of TB in 2015 with an estimated 4.1 million (44%) sputum smear positive. While Africa had the highest estimated incidence rates (around 350 per 100,000 population), the majority of patients with TB live in Asia's most populous countries, with India, Pakistan, Bangladesh, China, and Indonesia between them comprising 60% of all new TB cases in 2015. In 2015, the gap of 4.3 million between notifications of new cases and the estimated number of incident cases reflects the extent of underreporting and underdiagnosis, with India harbouring the majority of these 'missing patients'. **Figure 3** gives the estimated number of new TB cases, by country, throughout the world. As can be readily appreciated, the estimated number of new TB cases in

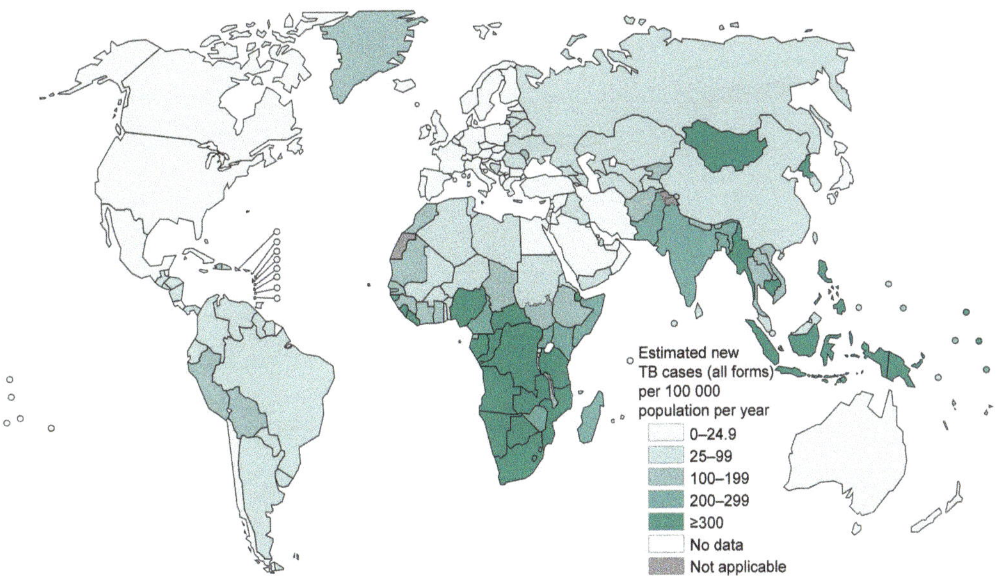

Fig. 3: Estimated tuberculosis (TB) incidence rates, 2015.

India at more than 1,000,000 makes it the country with the highest incident cases. Among the 15 countries with the highest estimated TB incidence rates, 13 are in Africa, almost certainly a reflection of the effect of high rates of HIV coinfection on the natural history of TB. Globally, TB is mainly a disease of adults and affects more men than women. It is a major cause of death amongst young adults, the breadwinners of their families, and the impact both socially and economically is thus devastating. TB is the leading infectious cause of death among people more than 5 years of age in South-East Asia. TB kills 5,000 people a day, 2 million each year. Of these 5,000 daily deaths, over 2,000 occur in South-East Asia. In fact, it is projected that although mortality from many other infectious diseases will continue to decline over the next 20 years, TB will remain one of the 10 leading causes of death unless urgent action is taken. According to the World Health Report, 2015, TB kills more women than all causes of maternal mortality combined. In some areas, women face special problems of access to TB diagnosis and treatment because of stigma and limitations on mobility.

Global Trends over the Last Decade

The fruits of DOTS and increased global attention and funds for TB seem to be finally paying off. From WHO notification data, the global incidence of TB per capita seems to have peaked in 2004 and is now on the decline. According to the latest WHO reports, TB incidence rates have been steady or falling in the South-East Asia and Western Pacific regions, Western and Central Europe, North and Latin America, and the Middle East. They have been increasing until most recently in Eastern Europe (mainly the former Soviet Union), and increasing in sub-Saharan Africa. These encouraging trends are best appreciated in **Figure 4**. While the rise in Africa is being fueled by the HIV epidemic, in Eastern Europe, it is political upheaval, economic decline and failure of TB control and health services that is responsible for the increasing TB incidence. These Eastern European states are also "hotspots" for MDR-TB with more than 10% of new TB cases in Latvia, Estonia, and parts of Russia being MDR-TB. Case reports suggest that over the most recent years, there has been an encouraging trend; a slowing in the rate of increase of TB even in Eastern Europe and Africa. It must not be forgotten, however, that because population growth was faster over the last decades (1.2% per year) than the decline in incidence, the total number of new TB cases arising each year was still increasing.

Epidemiology of TB in India

In India, some epidemiologists have expressed the opinion that the TB epidemic has also entered a phase of slow natural decline. The real situation however belies these theoretical epidemiological models. Indeed, because of India's rapid demographic growth, continuing poverty and malnutrition, and the effects of HIV, the absolute number of cases with TB has actually increased.

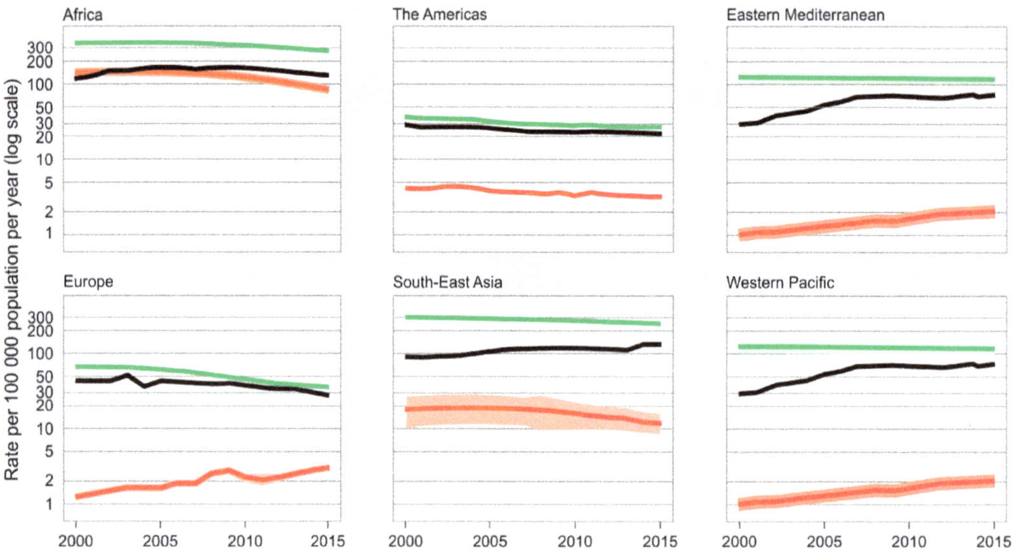

Fig. 4: Regional trends in estimated TB incidence rates (log scale) by WHO region, 2000–2015. Total TB incidence rates are shown in green and incidence rates of HIV-positive TB are shown in red. Shaded areas represent uncertainty intervals. The black lines show notifications of new and relapse cases for comparison with estimates of the total incidence rate.

Although developed countries have reliable notification systems that provide vital epidemiological data, notification for TB (at least from the private sector) is virtually nonexistent in India. Thus, the relevant facts regarding the current epidemiology of TB in India have not been fully elucidated. A number of studies and surveys over the last 50 years have however shed some important light on the subject. These epidemiological studies are of varying degrees of reliability and accuracy. Also, in a country as vast as India with its heterogeneous population, it is difficult to include a group representative of the country as a whole. Despite these limitations, enough data has accrued over the years to enable a reasonable estimate of the magnitude of the TB problem in India. Some of the historically important studies and the broad epidemiological conclusions reached from them shall be presented here.

The National Sample Survey (NSS), conducted between 1955 and 1958 by the ICMR at the behest of the Indian government, remains the main epidemiological source of the TB situation in India. It was on the basis of the findings highlighted by the NSS that the country's TB control programs were structured by the NTP. The country was divided into four broad zones— north, south, east, and west, with urban and rural representative samples being drawn up from each zone.

The total sample size was 3,13,128 people, more or less evenly divided between urban and rural areas. All those over the age of 5 years were screened by miniature mass radiography with two independent radiologists reading each radiograph. Two sputum samples, one spot and one overnight, were collected from all those found to have any type of radiographic abnormality. Individuals were thus divided into bacillary or X-ray cases. The size of this sample has not been exceeded in any subsequent study in the country.

Four important longitudinal surveys done at varying stages between the 1950s and 1980s also deserve individual mention as they greatly added to our understanding of the epidemiological situation in the country. These are the longitudinal surveys from Bengaluru, New Delhi, Madanapalle, and Chingleput. In addition, further epidemiological information came from studies on tuberculin reactivity conducted as a prelude to the Bacillus Calmette-Guerin (BCG) vaccination. From all these studies, a number of epidemiological conclusions can be reached.

Prevalence of Infection

Prevalence of TB infection, as reflected by a positive tuberculin skin test (TST) is a valuable epidemiological index of the burden of TB in a community. In a high-prevalence study like India, most of the population is infected at an early stage with 60–80% of the population being infected by age 25 and having a positive TST. The prevalence rates tended to be higher in males than females in most surveys. No differences were noted between different zones in the country or between urban and rural areas. This realization that rural villagers had similar prevalence rates to those residing in cities helped shape India's subsequent TB control policies. Two confounding factors have long been assumed to limit the diagnostic value of the TST in a country like India; the confounding effect of BCG (which is universally recommended at birth), and the effect of environmental mycobacteria. Hence, interestingly, when we conducted a similar survey using the new interferon-gamma release assays (IGRAs) in healthy urban adult Indians attending a health check at the Hinduja Hospital in Mumbai, rates of around 80% were still seen. This demonstrates that the high rates of positive TSTs noted in earlier surveys were not false positives due to the effect of prior BCG or due to infection with environmental mycobacteria but represented true latent infection.

Incidence of Infection

Incidence of infection is a better indicator of the TB problem than the prevalence. Limited data are available, but it is estimated the overall incidence of infection is around 1.6%.

Annual Risk of Infection

The TB annual risk of infection (ARI) indicates the proportion of the population that will be primarily infected by TB in the course of a year. Indian studies show an ARI of about 1.5% with little decline over 15 years in the Chingleput longitudinal study.

Prevalence of Bacillary Disease

The NSS reported prevalence rates of bacillary disease ranging from 2.3–8 per 1,000. Approximately, half of these were smear positive with males being affected twice as often as females. Subsequent surveys done over three decades have shown essentially similar patterns.

Prevalence of Radiological Disease

Radiological disease is always more prevalent than bacillary disease in all surveys. The NSS and subsequent surveys show rates varying from 14 to 24 radiologically active cases per 1,000 population. Pockets of high prevalence were noted in areas or zones, which were particularly overcrowded. For example, the prevalence rate of 50 per 1,000 in Block number 8 in Kolkata, which is slum-dominated, was more than 20 times higher than the 2.5 per 1,000 prevalence in the more affluent and less densely populated Block 34.

Incidence of Disease

Incidence is a much more sensitive indicator of the TB problem than prevalence. However, because of the expense and manpower involved in maintaining surveillance in even a small area, there are much fewer incidence studies. Available data put the incidence of sputum-positive disease at 1–3 per 1,000, with slightly higher rates in males than females. Incidence figures are on the whole about a third of prevalence figures.

Mortality Rates

A study by Datta showed that case-fatality rates over an 18-month period were about 10% even in those who had completed chemotherapy. The mortality rose to 62% in those who had taken less than half the prescribed medications. Data from death surveys conducted by the Indian government as recently as 1992 showed that the estimated annual current mortality due to TB was around 400,000 deaths of which more than 75% were in the age group 15–45 years. Thus TB remains the single largest contributor to mortality in the productive years of adult life. Indeed, 37% of the world's deaths from TB are estimated to occur in India.

Table 1: Country profile for India from 2015 WHO report.		
Estimates of TB Burden		
	Number (thousands)	**Rate (per 100 000 population)**
Incidence	2840 (1470–4650)	217 (112–355)
Mortality	480 (380–590)	36 (29–45)
TB case notifications, 2015: Total cases notified 1740435 Universal health coverage and social protection 2015: 59%		
Estimated MDR-TB cases 2015: 79000 (72000–87000) MDR-TB cases tested for resistance to 2nd line drugs 2015: 8976 MDR-TB cases started on treatment: 26966 XDR-TB cases started on treatment: 2130		
TB financing, 2016: National TB budget $280 US millions)		

Current Epidemiology in India

In terms of incidence, prevalence, and mortality, the current Indian scenario is best clarified by looking at some data from the 2009 WHO report. Some current Indian data on incidence, mortality and estimated cases from the 2016 WHO Global tuberculosis report is summarized in **Table 1**.

■ SUGGESTED READING

1. Dubovsky H. Tuberculosis and art. S Afr Med J. 1983;64:823-6.
2. Glaziou P. Global burden and epidemiology of tuberculosis. Clin Chest Med. 2009;30(4):621-36.
3. Iademarco MF. Epidemology of tuberculosis. Semin Respir Infect. 2003;18(4):225-40.
4. Toman K. Tuberculosis case-finding and chemotherapy. Geneva: World Health Organization; 1979.

CHAPTER 15

Clinical Features, Diagnosis, and Treatment

■ CLINICAL FEATURES

Primary Pulmonary Tuberculosis

When *Mycobacterium tuberculosis* first infects a nonimmune individual, it results in primary tuberculosis (TB). This involves the combination of a small peripheral focus of infection in the lung parenchyma and affection of the draining regional lymph nodes. The lung lesion can affect any lobe but always affects the periphery of the lung. Pathologically, the lung lesion comprises caseating granulomas. Most often, this remains walled off and heals with or without calcification. It is called the Ghon focus. In a quarter of cases, there may be more than one primary focus.

Within a few days, infection spreads to draining nodes, so peribronchial, hilar, or mediastinal nodes get enlarged either individually or in combination. Whereas right-sided lung lesions only result in right-sided adenopathy, a left-sided lung pulmonary focus may occasionally result in bilateral adenopathy. The combination of the peripheral lung lesion and the associated adenopathy is called a primary complex.

Clinical Features

The majority of patients with primary tuberculous infections are asymptomatic. A strong immune response ensures the infection is overcome without the individual being aware of it. A few patients may have nonspecific symptoms of an upper respiratory tract infection and some may run a short-lived fever. Some children, usually a minority, will be generally unwell, have anorexia, and fail to thrive.

Hypersensitivity Manifestations

Two less common but well-documented hypersensitivity manifestations of primary pulmonary TB are phlyctenular conjunctivitis and erythema nodosum (EN). Phlyctenular conjunctivitis is usually seen within a few weeks of infection but can occur any time within the 1st year. Usually unilateral but occasionally bilateral, it is commoner in children and in African communities. Typically, it appears as a small raised bleb at the limbus with a sheath of dilated vessels radiating outward. The reaction is self-limited and subsides within a week but recurrent lesions can occur over time. The presence of phlyctenular conjunctivitis should always raise the possibility of primary TB and such patients must have a tuberculin skin test (TST) and chest X-ray. Resolution once anti-TB chemotherapy is started is the rule but some patients may need local atropine or steroid drops to dampen the inflammation.

Erythema nodosum is another hypersensitivity manifestation and occurs in 1–15% of primary TB. EN usually occurs within a few days of tuberculin conversion. These lesions may however also occur in postprimary disease. Typically, EN lesions are tender, raised, bruise-like lesions better appreciated in Caucasians than in darker Indians. Joint pains and swelling of the ankle joints may accompany EN and the TST is invariably strongly positive. EN also occurs in sarcoidosis, but here the TST is invariably negative. Apart from TB and sarcoidosis, a host of other infections and noninfectious conditions can be associated with EN.

A primary infection is most often detected when the contacts of an adult infectious case are being screened. A positive TST may be the sole manifestation of primary TB and a chest radiograph may then pick up a primary complex. In children with a primary complex, auscultation is usually normal. On occasion, crackles may be heard over an extensive primary focus. Even less commonly, if the draining glands are markedly enlarged and obstruct a lobar bronchus (usually the middle lobe), a localized wheeze may be heard.

Radiological Features

The primary complex is picked up at the time of tuberculin conversion in no more than a third of all individuals. The pulmonary component appears as a nonspecific and peripheral consolidation. On occasion, there may be a more extensive segmental or lobar consolidation. Atelectasis of a segment or lobe may be seen, if the glands have obstructed a bronchus. The gland group most frequently affected are the hilar nodes. However, hilar and paratracheal gland enlargement on the same side and occasionally bilateral hilar enlargement may occur. Glandular enlargement has been noted to be much more frequent in Asian as opposed to Caucasian children. Mediastinal gland enlargement is also more common in HIV-infected individuals. The natural history of these lesions is that the lung and the glandular component both may calcify over the course of a year. In adults living in endemic areas, small calcific peripheral Ghon foci or calcified hilar glands may be observed on the chest radiographs of entirely asymptomatic individuals. These are the telltale signs of primary infection acquired in childhood and fought off without the patient having any recollection of a childhood infection (**Figs. 1 and 2**).

Diagnosis

In children, the pulmonary component of a primary complex may mimic pneumonia and antibiotics are often first administered. However, if there is history of exposure to an adult with TB and if the TST is positive, the diagnosis of primary pulmonary TB becomes more clear. Since children rarely produce sputum and gastric washings are considered invasive, a trial of anti-TB drugs is often resorted to in a child who is unwell and has the above radiological findings with a positive TST.

Complications

- The enlarged glands can cause subsegmental, segmental, or even lobar atelectasis. This was formerly called epituberculosis. The middle lobe is most commonly affected as mentioned earlier.
- Bronchiectasis occurs due to more permanent damage to the bronchi, most commonly after a lobar collapse.
- *Obstructive emphysema*: Partial compression of a bronchus by a gland can lead to a situation where

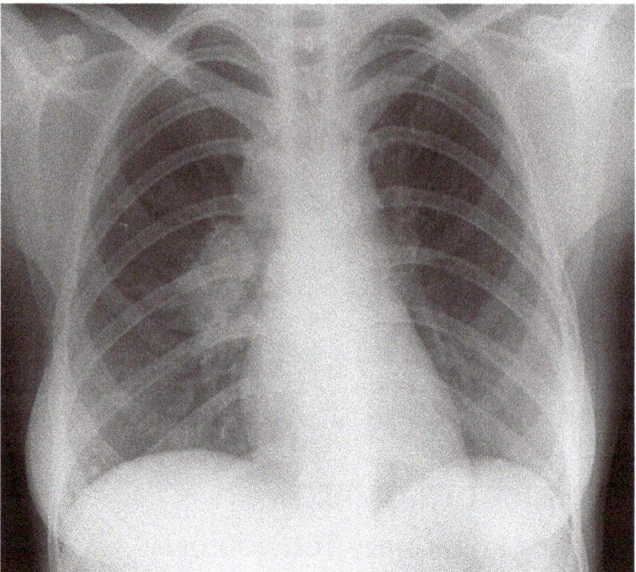

Fig. 1: Primary complex: Chest X-ray demonstrates large mediastinal adenopathy in right paratracheal and hilar regions. Small subtle nodular opacities are seen in the right mid zone representing a primary focus, the combination of both results in a primary complex.

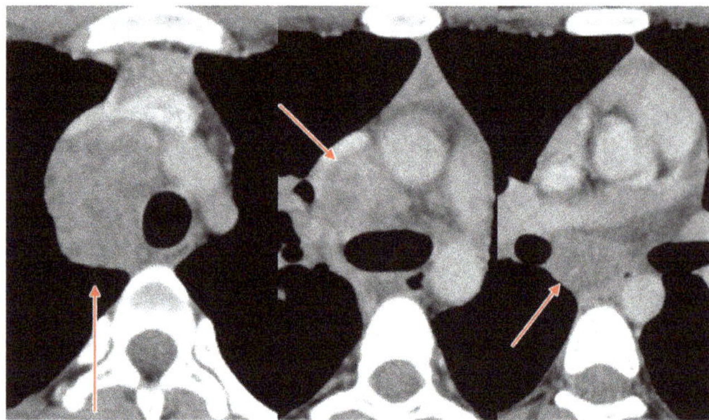

Fig. 2: Primary complex: Axial computed tomography (CT) of the chest demonstrates mediastinal adenopathy in right paratracheal, pretracheal, and subcarinal regions.

air enters a lobe on inspiration but is unable to escape on expiration. This results in an overinflated, "pseudoemphysematous" lobe, often best appreciated on an expiratory chest X-ray. This complication is more often seen in infants below the age of 2 years than in older children or adults.

- *Broncholith*: This is a calcified node, which protrudes into a bronchus and can rarely even be coughed out, often with accompanying hemoptysis.
- *Pleural effusions*: These may sometimes be associated with primary pulmonary TB. They are more common in children and usually resolve even without treatment.

Natural History and Long-term Course of Primary TB

Primary TB is the template from which all future forms of TB develop.

- Primary infection itself is usually asymptomatic and heals with no sequelae apart from TST conversion in 90% of those infected. Such patients are said to have latent TB infection (LTBI). It is believed that a third of the world's population (at least 2 billion) are latently infected.
- The local complications that can complicate primary TB have been discussed above.
- *Postprimary pulmonary TB*: It is the form of TB, which has the most global impact and is the major cause of morbidity and mortality from TB. Only 10% of patients with LTBI will go on to develop postprimary TB; half of these in the 1st year and the rest at any stage in the future, especially as their immune status weakens.
- Pleural effusions
- Miliary TB **(Fig. 3)**
- Meningeal TB
- Disseminated forms of TB affecting almost any and every part of the body but chiefly the skeletal system.

While postprimary pulmonary TB usually develops 1–5 years after the primary infection, pleural effusions and miliary TB usually develop within 6–12 months, while disseminated forms, like skeletal, central nervous system (CNS), and genitourinary TB develop several years after the primary infection.

Postprimary Pulmonary Tuberculosis

Postprimary pulmonary tuberculosis is the form of TB that has the major impact globally. WHO estimated that in 2005, there were 9 million new cases and 1.6 million deaths from this form of TB. This form is also the infectious form and an average case infects about 10 contacts per year. This is, therefore, the form that has the greatest public health impact as well. It will be discussed in detail in this section.

Pathogenesis

Postprimary pulmonary TB may arise in one of three possible ways:

1. Direct progression of the Ghon focus to caseation and cavitation.
2. *Reactivation of primary disease*: Bacteria remain walled off and dormant for decades only to

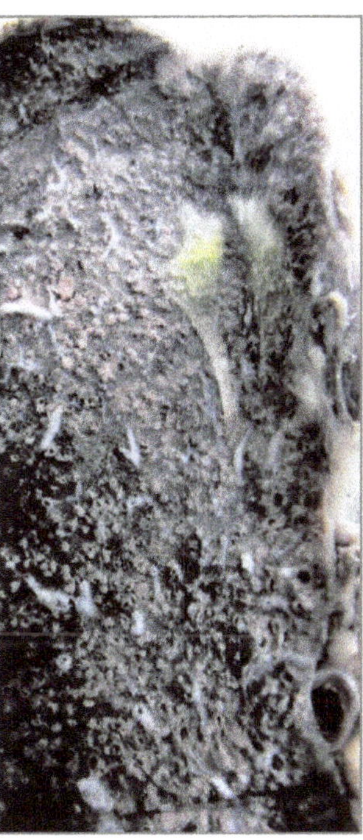

Fig. 3: Miliary tuberculosis (TB): Gross specimen of miliary TB with multiple small miliary lesions disseminated throughout the lungs.

reactivate when host immunity is affected. Diabetes, malnutrition, chronic hemodialysis, steroids, and other immunosuppressive therapies like infliximab, silicosis, and HIV are some of the major risk factors that promote the conversion of latent TB to active disease. The degree of risk is outlined in the **Table 1**.

3. *Exogenous reinfection*: Molecular techniques have shown this to be far more common than previously believed, especially in endemic areas. This route is believed to be very important in the HIV-positive population.

■ CLINICAL PRESENTATION

The common symptoms are:

Fever: Tuberculosis usually causes a temperature, which is of low-to-moderate grade, characteristically has an evening rise and is often accompanied by drenching night sweats. Occasionally, the fever can be high-grade and even accompanied by chills and occasionally rigors. Fever can be the sole symptom of TB and TB (especially extrapulmonary TB), remains one of the leading causes of pyrexia of unknown origin (PUO) in most series throughout the world. TB is especially likely to be the cause of PUO in certain populations like immunocompromised patients,

Table 1: Risk factors for conversion of latent tuberculosis (TB) to active disease.

Risk factor	Relative risk
Past history of TB	1–10
Diabetes	2–4
Malnourished	2–4
Hemodialysis	10
Immunosuppressive Rx	12
Silicosis	30
HIV/AIDS	100–170

(AIDS: Acquired immunodeficiency syndrome; HIV: Human immunodeficiency virus)

diabetics, or the elderly, though it remains an important cause of PUO in any patient. In a recent study, TB was found to be the cause of PUO in 12% of elderly patients compared to 2% of younger patients. In another study of elderly patients from Turkey, TB emerged as the most common cause of PUO prompting the investigators to recommend empiric anti-TB therapy in this population.

The PUO secondary to TB is typically a low-grade fever with an evening rise, accompanied by drenching night sweats. Other temperature patterns associated with TB are intermittent, recurrent, and double quotidian fever (two temperature spikes in the day). The forms of TB most often linked to PUO are miliary TB and glandular TB. These are both paucibacillary forms, hence, the sensitivity of both acid-fast bacilli (AFB) smear and culture is low. The utility of blood and skin tests is also very poor and CT scanning, bone marrow analysis, gland biopsy, or liver biopsy may be needed. Bone marrow biopsy should be strongly considered in patients with PUO with no localizing organ-specific findings, especially if anemia and leukopenia are also present. In this setting, granulomas may be found in 50–80% of cases. Combined histopathology and TB culture seem to be more helpful than histopathology alone. Liver biopsy demonstrates granuloma in 80–90% of patients with miliary TB. About half the number of granulomas shows caseation and half are AFB-positive on smear. Splenic biopsy has also been shown to be useful, especially in patients with PUO and splenomegaly or space-occupying lesions in the spleen. A study from India in 31 patients with PUO, diagnosed TB in 11 patients after splenic fine-needle aspiration. Nearly two-thirds of the samples from

patients diagnosed with TB were AFB-positive, with the highest rate of positivity in samples with inflammatory cells and necrosis without granuloma. The procedure was shown to have a very low rate of complications. Diagnostic laparoscopy may also be a useful procedure in PUO with suspected abdominal TB. Finally, in patients with PUO who are suspected to have TB and whose clinical condition is deteriorating, empiric, anti-TB trials may be considered. In a study by Onal published in 2006, empiric therapy established the diagnosis in 43% of their PUO cases that were caused by TB. A response to empiric therapy with a rifampicin-containing regimen may rarely result from this drug's antibacterial activity, but, as this is the most powerful anti-TB drug, most clinicians would include it in an empiric trial. Fever may abate promptly following initiation of anti-TB treatment or may persist for several weeks.

Cough: Cough is another cardinal symptom. Since the sensitivity of cough as a symptom of TB is very high, any individual with an otherwise unexplained cough of more than 2 weeks duration should be evaluated for TB. The specificity of cough as a symptom of TB is low as cough occurs in a wide range of conditions. The proportion of patients with TB being the underlying cause of chronic cough will depend on the prevalence of TB in the community. These are also the most infectious of all TB patients and inadequate evaluation of a patient with cough results in greater transmission of disease in the community. The cough is accompanied by sputum which is mucoid or purulent and often accompanied by hemoptysis. Sputum of copious quantities is produced when there is accompanying bronchiectasis. Cough may be dry and incessant in glandular TB when cough is secondary to pressure effects of glands on the bronchial tree. Endobronchial TB is characterized by cough with an accompanying wheeze, which is often localized. This is usually misdiagnosed as asthma. Cough may be accompanied by hoarseness of voice in laryngeal TB.

Hemoptysis: Hemoptysis is another key symptom of TB. The presence of hemoptysis should always raise the suspicion of TB, especially when it occurs in a nonsmoker. It may be the presenting symptom of TB and a chest X-ray when done for the first time after a bout of hemoptysis may show extensive TB without any other accompanying symptoms. Hemoptysis is more common in cavitary disease. Hemoptysis may vary from blood streaks in sputum to the sudden coughing up of large quantities of 0.5–1 liter of blood. This degree of massive hemoptysis is not uncommon, may be a presenting symptom, and can be a fatal complication of TB resulting in death by exsanguination. This degree of life-threatening hemoptysis is secondary to erosion of a TB focus into a bronchial artery and can be torrential because bleeding occurs at systemic pressures.

Dyspnea: Parenchymal lung involvement results in dyspnea only if both lungs are extensively affected. Chronic dyspnea may also be the result of the residual scarring and fibrosis that occur after TB is successfully treated. This may, on occasion, be severe enough to lead to respiratory failure.

General symptoms: Symptoms like malaise, fatigue, anorexia, and weight loss are also common in TB. The weight loss can be profound, so that 10–20 kg weight reductions over a few months are not uncommon.

Metabolic and Hematological Manifestations

A broad range of hematological and metabolic manifestations has also been reported in TB. Anemia is not uncommon. This may be the anemia of chronic disease with superimposed nutritional anemia. In some cases, anemia or pancytopenia may result from direct involvement of the bone marrow. Mild leukocytosis occurs in about 10% of patients with TB. On occasion, leukemoid reactions may occur. Leukopenia has also been reported on occasion. Eosinophilia and an increase in monocyte counts may also occur with TB. Hyponatremia is the most common metabolic effect and is reported to occur in about 10% of patients due to inappropriate antidiuretic hormone (ADH) production (SIADH—syndrome of inappropriate antidiuretic hormone secretion).

Evolution of Symptoms

Symptoms are often mild at the onset and evolve gradually in a time course that spans weeks or months. On occasion, however, TB runs a more acute course, and may mimic a bacterial pneumonia clinically and radiologically. Osler's famous dictum of TB being the sole differential diagnosis in a nonresolving pneumonia could equally apply to TB being the main differential diagnosis in what seems to be a lobar pneumonia. In a series of our patients presenting with community-acquired pneumonia (CAP) at the Hinduja Hospital, Mumbai, TB accounted for 7% of all presentations. In a similar study from the University Hospital, Singapore, TB accounted for 21% of all CAPs. In this study, TB was more often an etiological agent than *Streptococcus pneumoniae.*

Physical Findings

Clinical examination is often normal in a patient with pulmonary TB, despite advanced radiological shadowing. General examination may reveal clubbing in advanced suppurative disease and when there is secondary bronchiectasis. A careful general examination is also essential to pick out evidence of TB outside the lung; for example, cervical glands secondary to glandular TB. Scattered crackles are the most common respiratory finding. When there is upper airway stenosis, a localized wheeze may be present. Upper lobe fibrosis may produce tracheal deviation and a flattening of the chest. A large cavity may produce amphoric breathing and this may also be heard over a bronchopleural fistula.

■ DIAGNOSIS

Diagnosis of TB depends on three rather antiquated tests: (1) radiology, (2) sputum and (3) the TST. All these have several limitations, especially in the HIV coinfected population. It is estimated that the world spends a total of 1 billion US dollars on TB diagnostics annually. The cost of seeking a TB diagnosis represents 75% of the annual household income of the poorest socioeconomic classes.

Radiology (Figs. 4 to 25)

Reliance on the chest radiograph alone to diagnose TB results in both underdiagnosis and missed diagnosis. No X-ray pattern is absolutely typical of TB. In fact, 10% or more of the patients found to have TB may have normal-appearing X-rays. Furthermore, as indicated above, 40% or more of the patients who are considered to have TB on the basis of X-ray alone do not have the disease. Therefore, X-ray is an unreliable tool for both diagnosis and monitoring of pulmonary TB.

In an interesting Indian study, which demonstrates the inherent flaws in chest radiography, over 2,000 outpatients had chest radiography and 227 were diagnosed to have

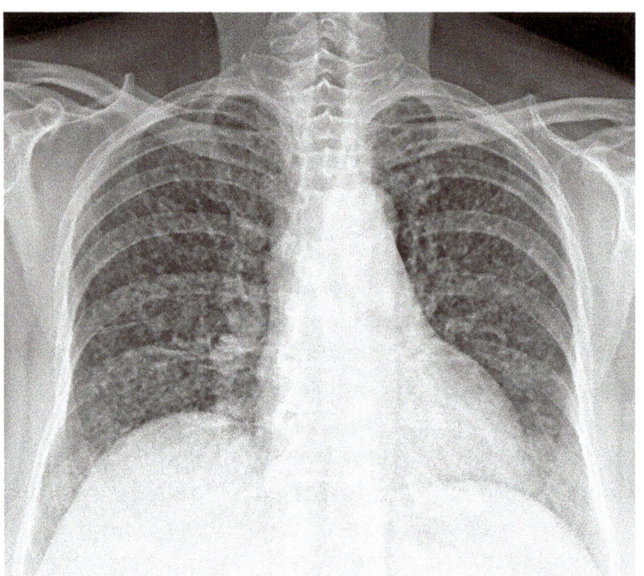

Fig. 4: Miliary tuberculosis (TB): X-ray chest demonstrates multiple miliary nodules in both lung fields.

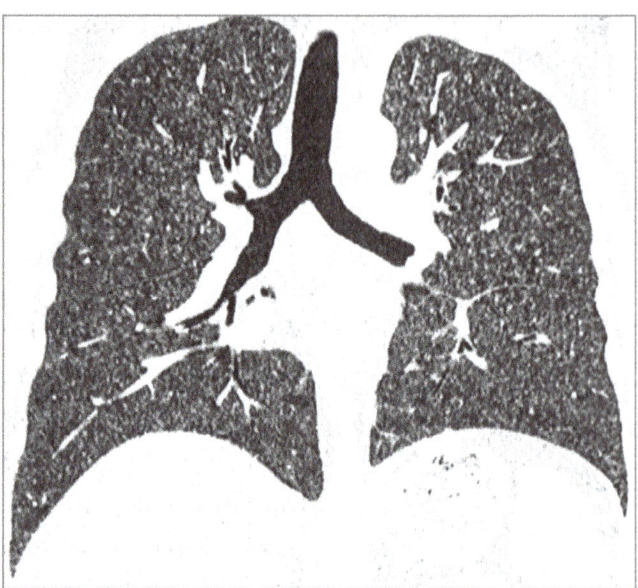

Fig. 6: Miliary tuberculosis (TB): High-resolution computed tomography (HRCT) chest demonstrates multiple small well-defined nodular lesions in both lung fields.

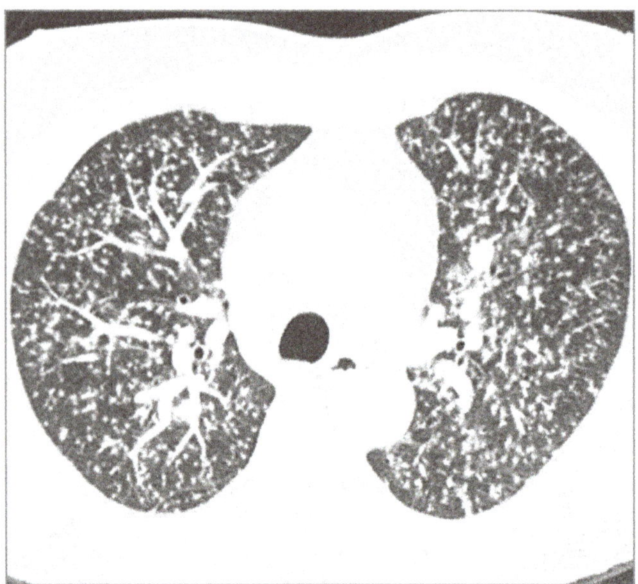

Fig. 5: Miliary tuberculosis (TB): High-resolution computed tomography (HRCT) demonstrates multiple small well-defined nodular lesions in both lung fields.

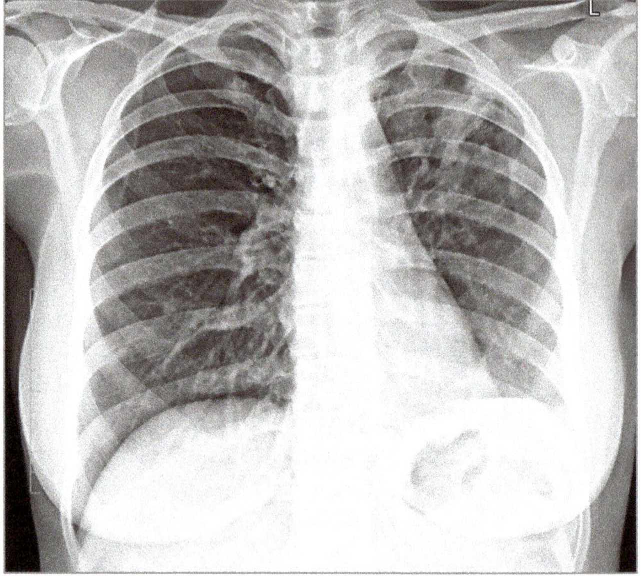

Fig. 7: Pulmonary tuberculosis (TB): Chest X-ray demonstrates ill-defined consolidations in the left upper lobe and mid zone with small cavities interspersed in the consolidation; these consolidations resembling cotton wool, location of the lesions, and cavities are highly indicative of TB, sputum was positive for acid-fast bacilli (AFB).

TB on radiographic grounds. Of the 227, 36% had negative sputum cultures and of the remaining 1,773 patients, 1.5% had positive cultures. From these results, in terms of sensitivity of chest radiographs, 20% of 162 culture-positive cases would have been missed by radiography. Another study by Toman found there is great disagreement between radiologists when asked to read the same X-ray. The disagreement between radiologists on the question: "Is there radiographic evidence of TB in this X-ray?" was as high as 45%. This sounds high but the disagreement index for a question as basic as: "Is this X-ray abnormal?" was 34% and for "Is a cavity present?" was as high as 28%.

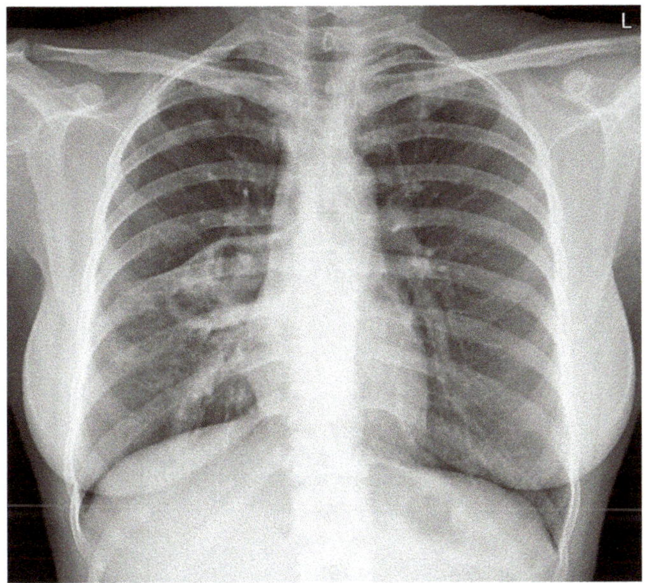

Fig. 8: Pulmonary tuberculosis (TB): Chest X-ray demonstrates a thick walled cavitatory lesion in the right mid zone, however, not obscuring the right cardiac border suggesting its location to be in the apical segment of right lower lobe which is typical of the tuberculosis.

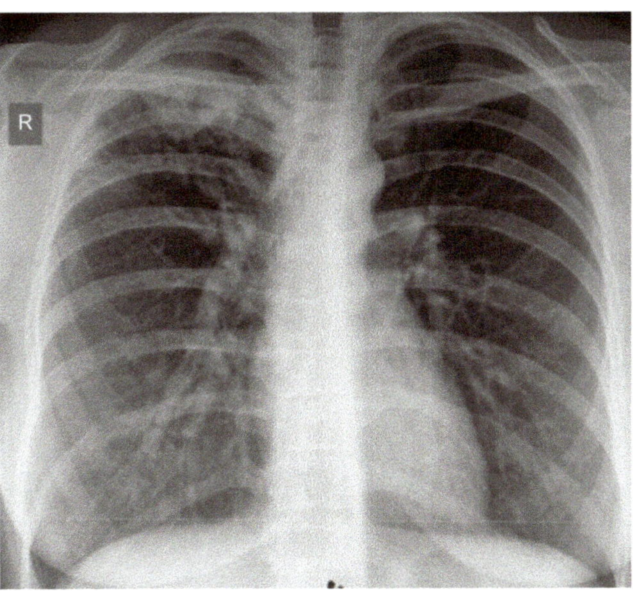

Fig. 10: Pulmonary tuberculosis (TB): Chest X-ray demonstrates a nodular lesion in the right apex with internal cavitation. The location as well as the cavitation is typical for pulmonary TB.

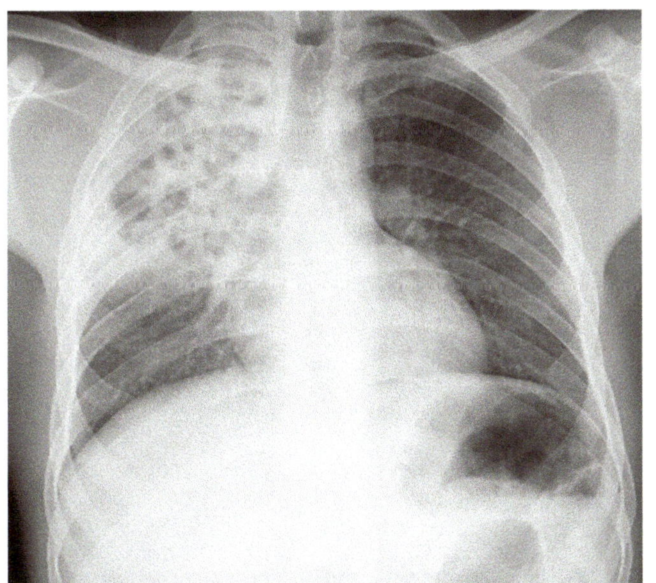

Fig. 9: Pulmonary tuberculosis (TB): PA view of the chest demonstrates ill defined area of consolidations with multiple small interspersed cavities in the right upper and mid zones indicative of active Koch's infection.

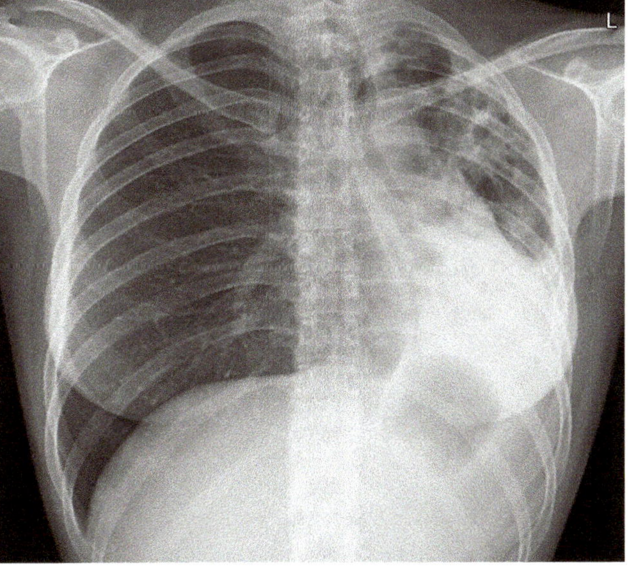

Fig. 11: Pulmonary tuberculosis (TB): PA view of the chest demonstrates multiple areas of ill defined consolidation with internal cavitation in the left upper and mid zones associated with left pleural effusion and mediastinal shift to the left due to volume loss in the involved left lung. Pleural fluid revealed a high adenosine deaminase (ADA) level.

A normal chest radiograph makes pulmonary TB less likely but as almost half the lung volume is obscured on a frontal chest radiograph by the mediastinum and diaphragm and subtle infiltrates at the apex of the lung are obscured by the clavicle and first rib, the X-ray may miss some patients with pulmonary TB and many with

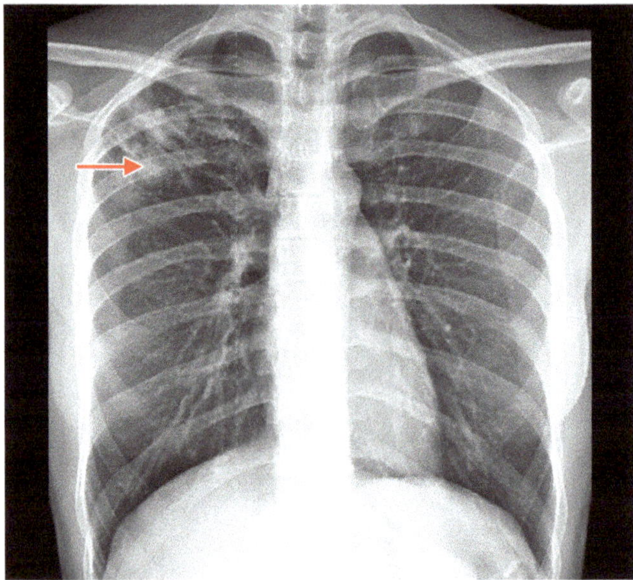

Fig. 12A: Pulmonary tuberculosis (TB): Chest X-ray demonstrates ill-defined fluffy opacities with streaky opacities in the right upper zone. Sputum acid-fast bacilli (AFB) was positive.

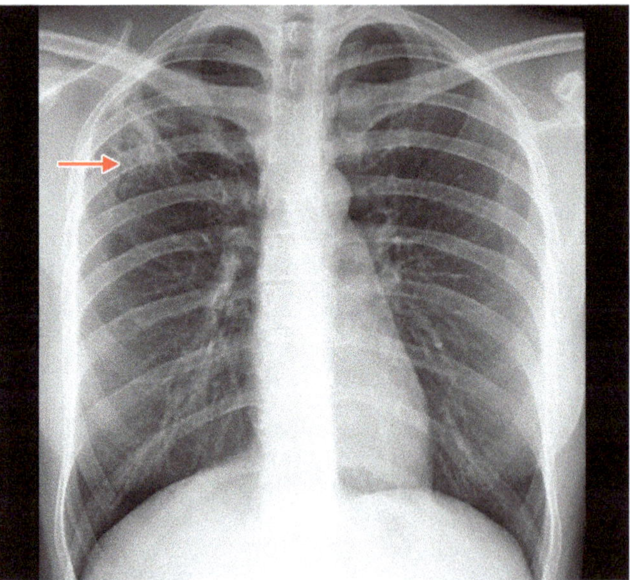

Fig. 12B: Follow-up chest X-ray following eight weeks of anti-Koch's treatment.

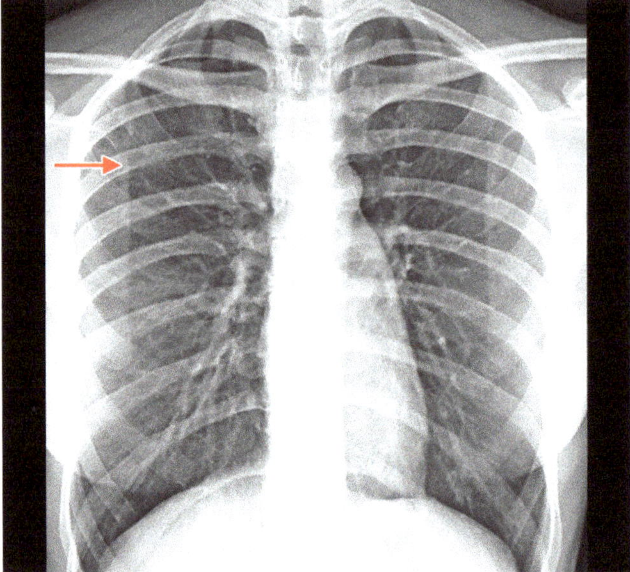

Fig. 12C: Follow-up chest X-ray after six months of treatment demonstrates near total resolution of the previously visualized opacities with minimal associated residual fibrotic lesions.

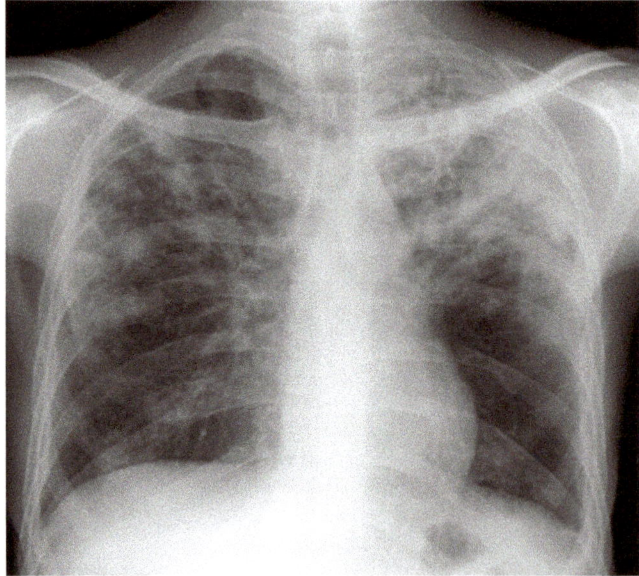

Fig. 13: Pulmonary tuberculosis (TB): Chest X-ray demonstrates ill-defined fluffy consolidations in both upper and mid zones, which tend to conglomerate in the left upper zone. Sputum acid-fast bacilli (AFB) were positive.

glandular TB. A lordotic X-ray may reveal apical TB with far greater clarity than a PA view. A high-resolution computed tomography (HRCT) for lung parenchyma and a contrast CT for the mediastinum may pick up lesions missed on chest radiography. A single X-ray is also often unable to accurately gauge the "activity" of TB. Comparison with old X-rays, if available, is crucial for this distinction. Thus, even more than CT, there is no investigation as important as an old chest X-ray. If an old X-ray is not available, a lesion on an X-ray must not be assumed to be inactive without

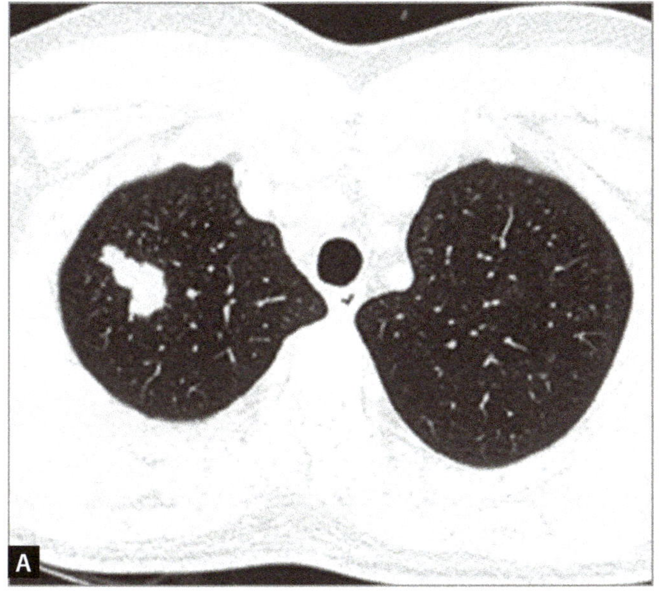

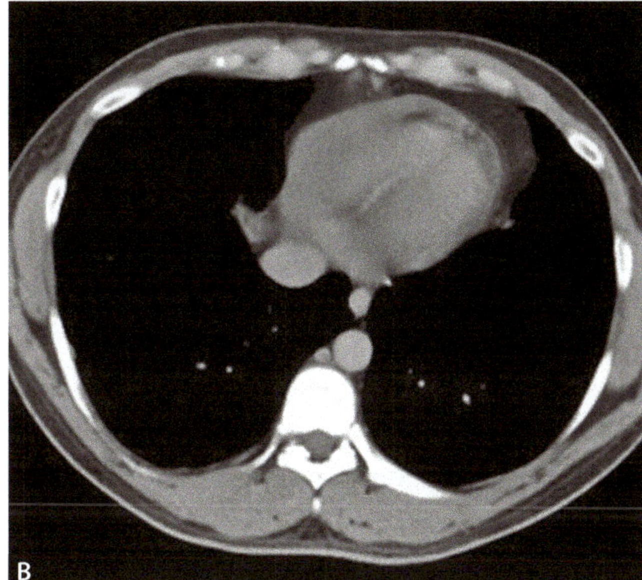

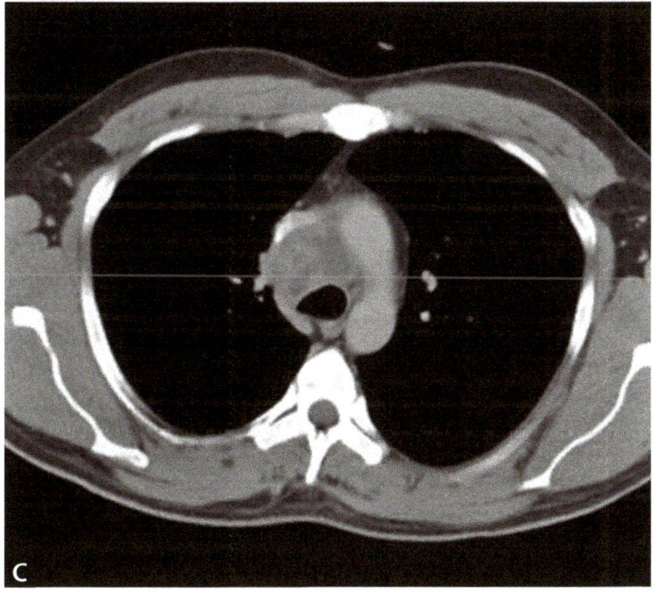

Figs. 14A to C: Pulmonary tuberculosis (TB): Middle-aged male patient presented with fever; weight loss, and a high-erythrocyte sedimentation rate (ESR). Chest X-ray did not reveal any significant abnormality. (A) Chest computed tomography (CT) demonstrates a nodular consolidation in the right apex; (B) additionally there was a small pericardial effusion; and (C) necrotic mediastinal adenopathy. A chest X-ray may miss small nodular consolidations in the apex as they are small in size and may be hidden behind the clavicle and first rib. The mediastinal adenopathy may also not be visualized and hidden by the mediastinal structures, as the adenopathy is retrocaval.

checking the sputum for AFB culture and confirming it is negative. The other classic though rare situation where the X-ray (and indeed CT) may be normal but the patient has a positive sputum smear is endobronchial TB.

The following findings on an X-ray suggest TB: Opacities in the upper lobes or apical segments of the lower lobes, nodular opacities or infiltrates, presence of cavitation, consolidation that persists over several weeks, thus making pneumonia unlikely. Calcification and fibrosis suggest healed disease; but as discussed earlier, this is difficult to confirm on radiographic grounds alone. Other features outside the lung, which may be pointers to TB, include associated pleural or pericardial effusions or the presence of mediastinal adenopathy. CT features of TB include the "tree in bud appearance", which though suggestive is not specific for TB.

Sputum Microscopy

When it comes to the sputum smear, little has changed since Robert Koch's time. Smear microscopy is the most basic and commonly used tool to diagnose TB worldwide. It has the advantage of being inexpensive and simple and operators can be trained easily and rapidly. Results can be provided to the physician within a few hours. A sample of each sputum is smeared on a slide, Ziehl-Neelsen (ZN) stained and then air-dried. The presence of AFB is taken as evidence of TB. While a single smear

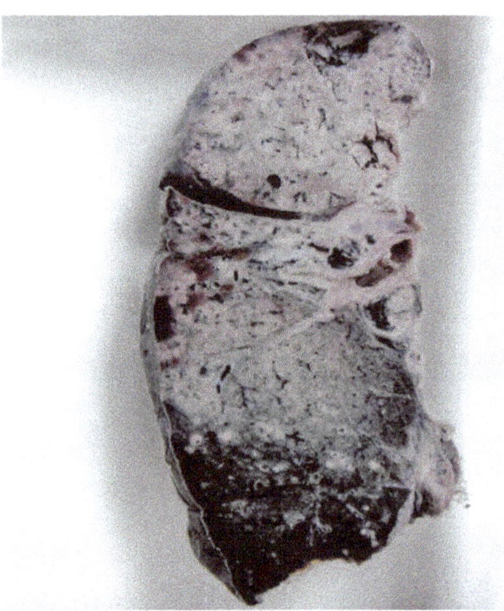

Fig. 15: Cavitating tuberculosis (TB): Gross specimen of cavitating TB, large cavity seen in the apex with tuberculous involvement in right upper lobe, apical segment of lower lobe as well as small tubercles in lower zones.

of a respiratory specimen has a reported sensitivity of between 22% and 43%, when multiple specimens are examined, the detection rate improves considerably. The sensitivity of smears from other specimen sources is even poorer. Overall, sputum microscopy by traditional ZN staining may miss up to 50% of active pulmonary TB. Even the best laboratory will not pick up TB if less than 10,000 bacilli are present per mL of sputum. Add to this the fact that some patients may be unable to produce an adequate sputum sample and that the sputum may not be correctly processed by the laboratory, so that even more cases with TB may be missed. The current WHO recommendation, in their 2007 guidelines, is that the number of sputum sample specimens can be reduced from three to two in countries where workload is high and resources are limited. This was based on the realization that the average incremental yield of the third smear was just 3%. This was confirmed in a recent study we performed at the Hinduja Hospital, which looked at 400 consecutive adult TB suspects and found that the incremental yield of the third sputum sample was 2.8% (seven additional patients). We found that analysis of 57 additional third smears was needed to diagnose one additional case of TB. This minimal additional yield of the third smear does not justify the burden it imposes on both the patient and the Indian healthcare system and the Revised National Tuberculosis Control

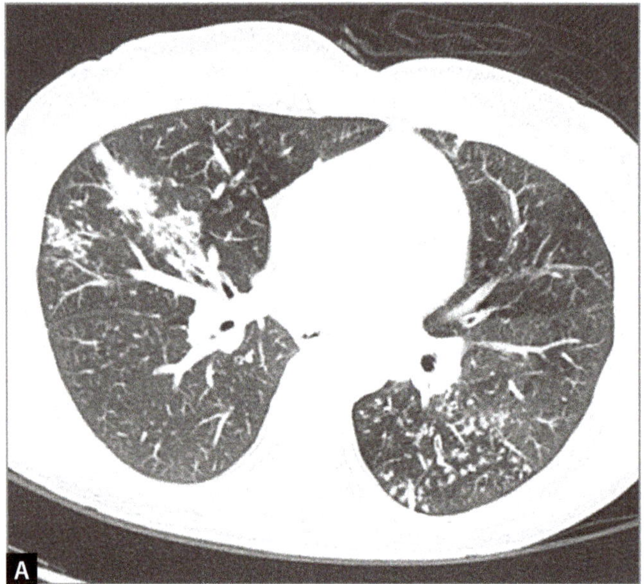
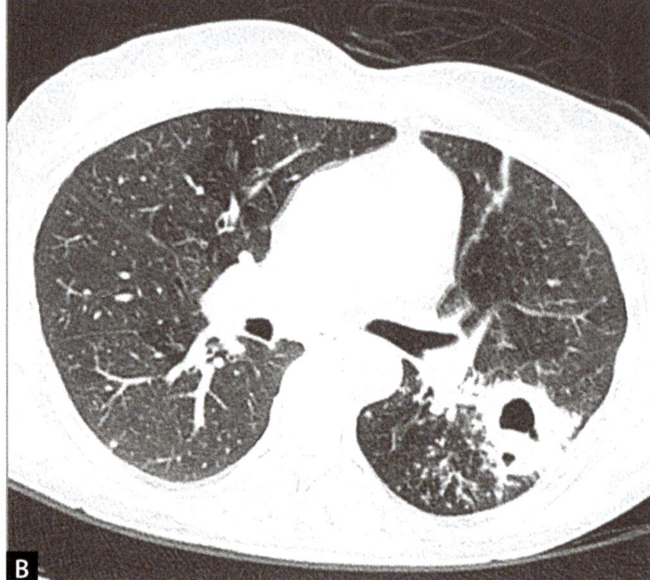

Figs. 16A and B: Pulmonary tuberculosis (TB): Chest computed tomography (CT) demonstrates a thick-walled cavitatory lesion in the apical segment of left lower lobe. Multiple small ill-defined conglomerating pulmonary nodules are seen in left lower lobe and right middle lobe.

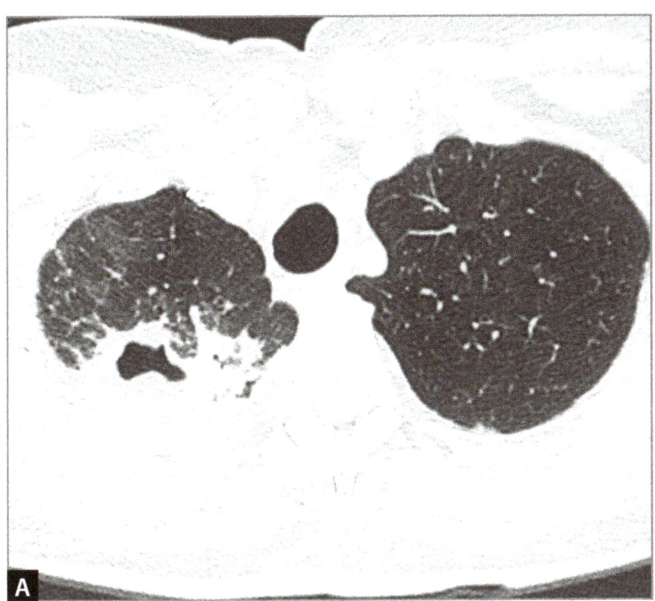
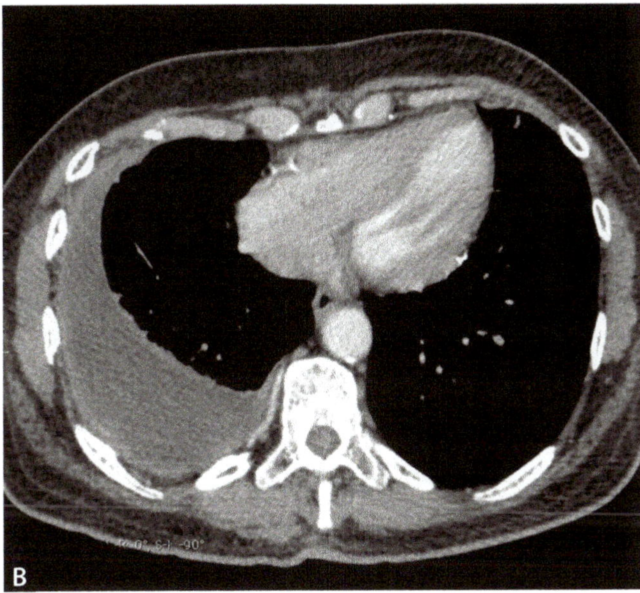

Figs. 17A and B: Pulmonary tuberculosis (TB): High-resolution computed tomography (HRCT) demonstrates ill-defined area of consolidation with cavitation in the right apex. There is pleural effusion on the right side.

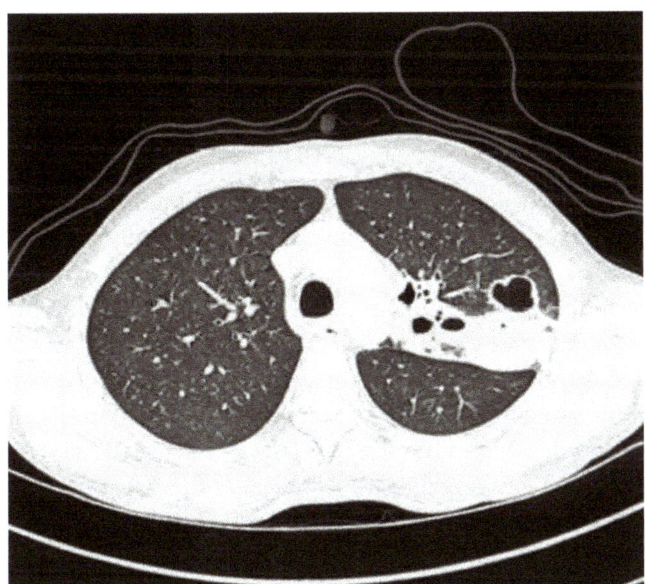

Fig. 18A: Pulmonary tuberculosis (TB): High-resolution computed tomography (HRCT) chest demonstrates left apicoposterior consolidation with internal cavitation.

Program (RNTCP) has rightly revised its guidelines to accept two sputum smears as adequate for diagnosing TB. Samples taken in the early morning are preferred since they are generally acknowledged to be more likely to be positive. For the 50% of patients who are simply unable to produce an adequate sputum sample, hypertonic saline nebulization to induce sputum, or where facilities exist, bronchoscopy with examination of bronchoalveolar lavage (BAL) fluid for AFB is done. In children, nasogastric aspirates may be collected, preferably again in the morning.

Sputum examination, like all other tests, must be considered in the overall clinical context. Operator skill is a crucial variable, and even for experienced microscopists, accuracy has been shown to decline significantly, if the number of slides to be processed is too large due to the physically demanding nature of scrutinizing multiple slides. Laboratory errors and nontuberculous mycobacteria (NTM) are some of the causes of false-positive sputum smears.

Sadly, it is estimated that there are no more than 50,000 microscopy centers in the 22 high-burden countries, which work out to one laboratory for every 75,000 people. Another paradox is that of the global network of 26 supranational reference laboratories (SRNL), only one is housed in India and two in the entire South East Asia region, while 11 are concentrated in Europe.

Sputum Culture

Traditionally, mycobacteria have been cultured on either egg-based solid media or in liquid media and monitored for growth. The main drawback of traditional cultures is

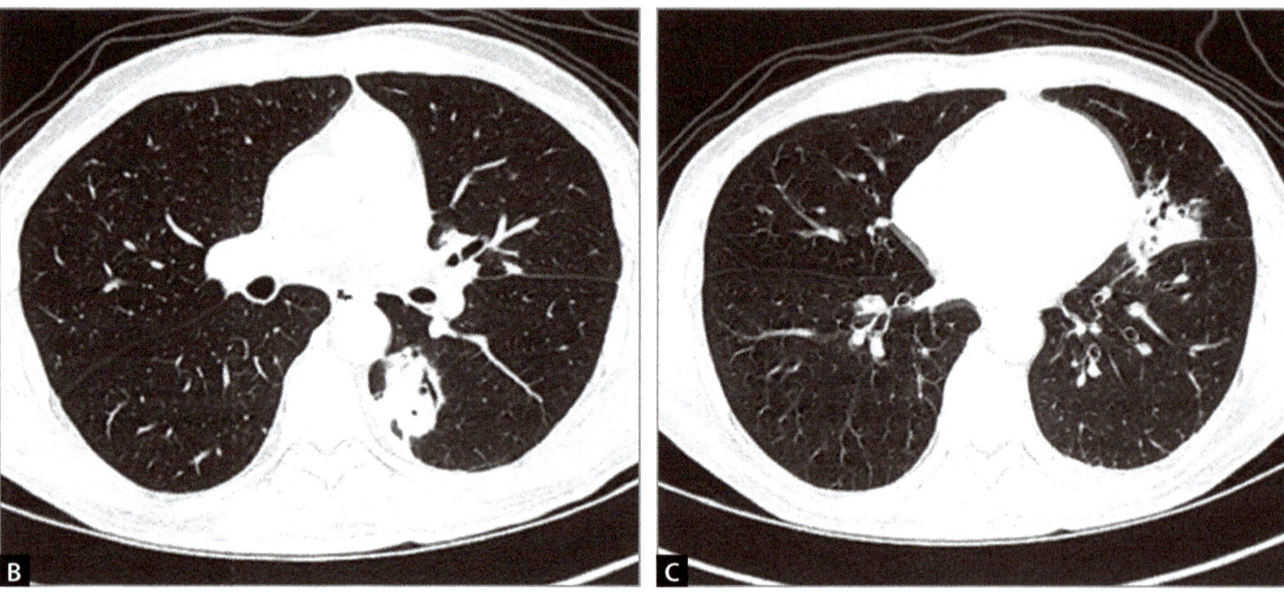

Figs. 18B and C: Nodular consolidations in the apical segment of left lower lobe and the left lingula. These are the typical areas of involvement of tuberculosis (TB).

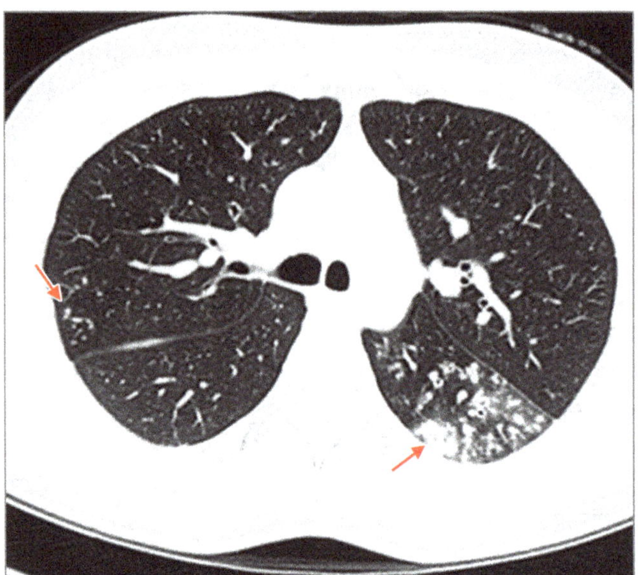

Fig. 19: Endobronchial tuberculosis (TB): High-resolution computed tomography (HRCT) chest demonstrates multiple ill-defined centrilobular nodules in the apical segment of left lower lobe, some of which are conglomerated forming a consolidation as well (arrow). Small centrilobular nodules (arrow) are also noted in the right upper lobe. The presence of centrilobular nodular lesions in 'tree in bud' appearance is highly suggestive of endobronchial TB.

that due to the long division time of *M. tuberculosis,* 16–18 hours under optimal conditions, clinical samples take around 4–6 weeks to turn positive. Lowenstein-Jensen (LJ) medium is the solid culture medium most frequently used throughout the world. It is an egg-based formulation, with glycerol supplement for *M. tuberculosis.* Solid Middlebrook 7H10 and 7H11 containing agar are other culture media that are still in use in laboratories across the world. In the developed world, liquid culture media are more widely used. These have the advantages of faster recovery times and detection rates than conventional solid media. The two liquid systems most frequently used in the developed world are the BACTEC 460 system and the mycobacteria growth index (MGIT) 960 system. Optimal recovery is achieved through a combination of rapid, automated liquid culture systems, and solid LJ slopes. Our experience with both the BACTEC and the MGIT system has been growing and we will discuss the advantages of these systems in the section on advances in diagnosis.

Susceptibility Testing

With the worldwide spread of multidrug-resistant TB (MDR-TB), susceptibility testing assumes great significance. In Mumbai, India, where we practice, an area of high prevalence of isoniazid and multidrug resistance, we would recommend that ideally sputum cultures and sensitivities should be requested in all patients when first seen. This may not be practical on a programmatic level, but it was heartening to note that the new WHO 2009 guidelines have recommended that all patients who

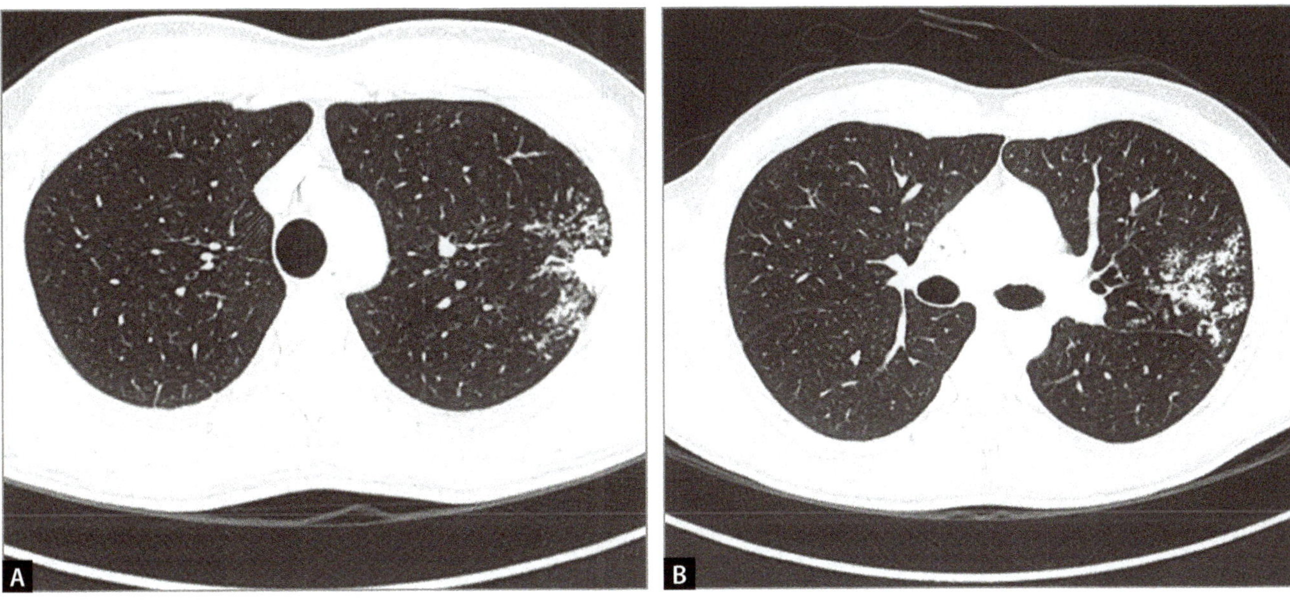

Figs. 20A and B: Endobronchial tuberculosis (TB): High-resolution computed tomography (HRCT) chest demonstrates multiple small nodular lesions in left upper lobe in a branching 'tree in bud' appearance indicative of endobronchial spread of infection. There is also evidence of associated ill-defined subpleural consolidation due to conglomeration.

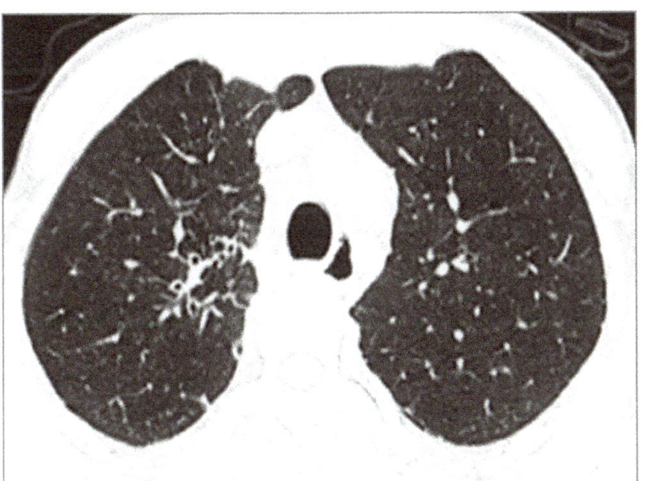

Fig. 21A: Reactivation tuberculosis (TB): High-resolution computed tomography (HRCT) chest demonstrates bronchiectasis and fibrosis in the right apex secondary to old healed TB.

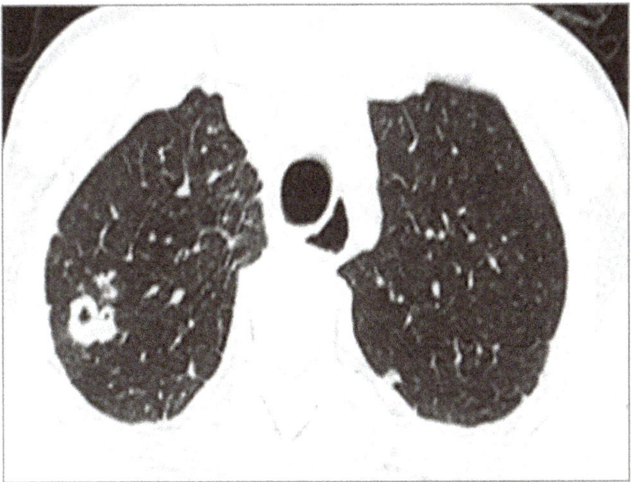

Fig. 21B: Patient presented with low-grade fever, weight loss. High-resolution computed tomography (HRCT) chest revealed a nodular consolidation in the right apex with internal cavitation and small satellite nodular lesions in the apex.

fail directly observed treatment short course (DOTS) Category 1 treatment should have sputum cultures sent off and sensitivity performed on positive cultures instead of wasting a further 8 months of treatment with Category 2 treatment.

The principles of *M. tuberculosis* testing were established by Canetti almost 50 years ago. Generally speaking, direct or indirect tests may be performed by either conventional or rapid methods. The inoculum for the direct tests is the processed clinical specimen in which AFB have been observed (i.e. smear-positive sputum). The advantage of this approach is that the results are obtained sooner and the inoculum is a true representative of bacterial population in situ. The inoculum for the indirect tests on the other hand is the primary isolate culture. This makes preparation of a uniform inoculum easier.

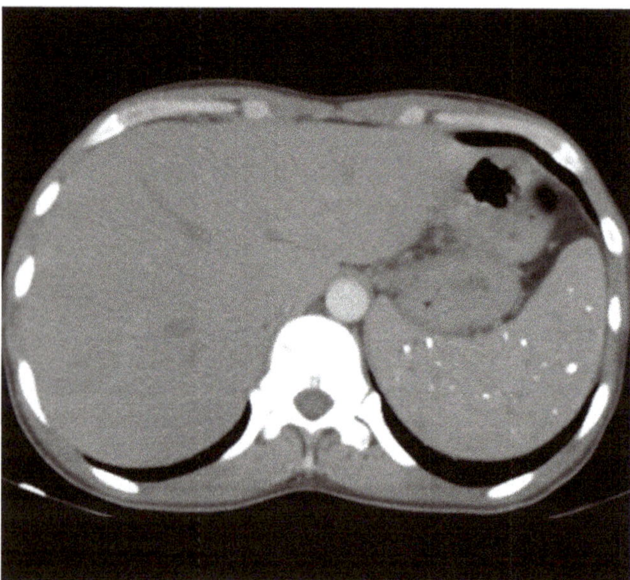

Fig. 21C: Computed tomography (CT) abdomen demonstrates multiple calcified splenic granulomas, a residue from the previous tuberculosis (TB) infection.

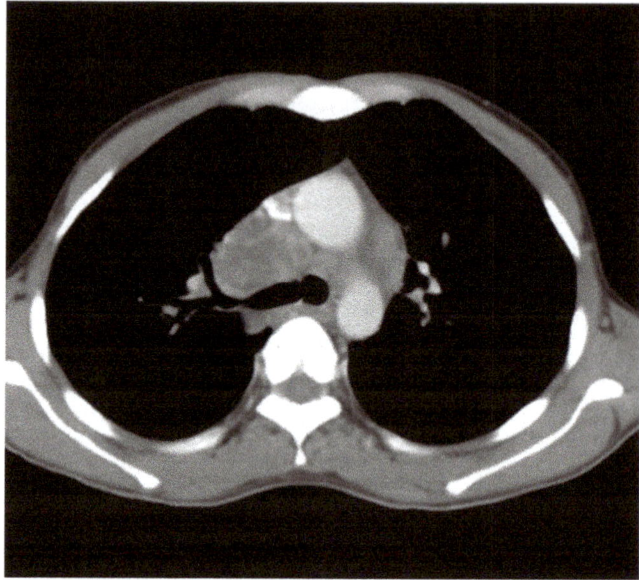

Fig. 21D: Computed tomography (CT) chest with contrast revealed large necrotic mediastinal adenopathy in the right pre-/paratracheal regions. The presence of nodular consolidations with cavitations and large necrotic mediastinal adenopathy is indicative of reactivation of pulmonary tuberculosis (TB) on a background of fibrosis, bronchiectasis, and calcified granulomas.

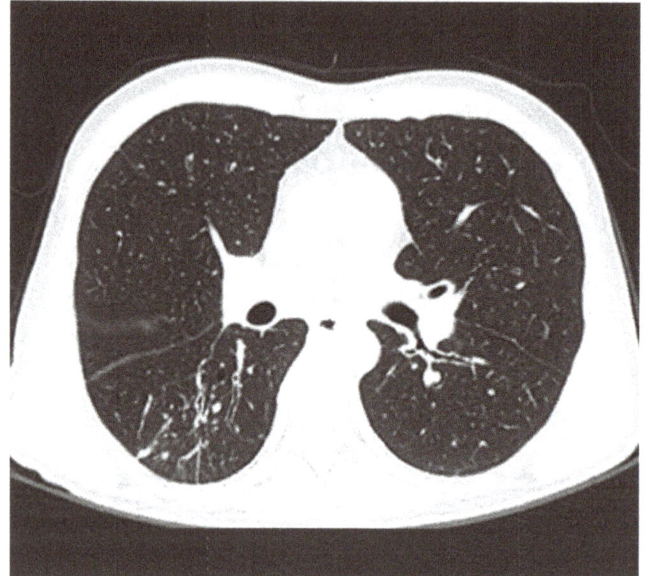

Fig. 22A: Reactivation of pulmonary tuberculosis (TB): Fibrotic lesions with associated bronchiectasis in the apical segment of the right lower lobe. These features are indicative of an old healed inflammatory process. The patient presented with fresh symptoms of fever and cough.

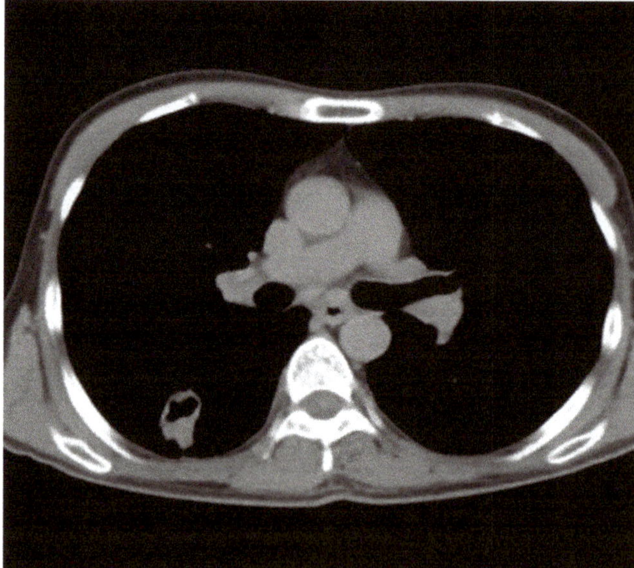

Fig. 22B: Section lower to fibrosis demonstrated thick-walled cavity with air-fluid level confirming reactivation of tuberculosis (TB).

The conventional methods may be performed as direct or indirect tests by inoculating the microorganisms on to a solid medium that has a known concentration of the test drug. For each of the methods described, test concentration of drugs may be prepared in the medium by appropriate dilutions of stock solutions of antimicrobials.

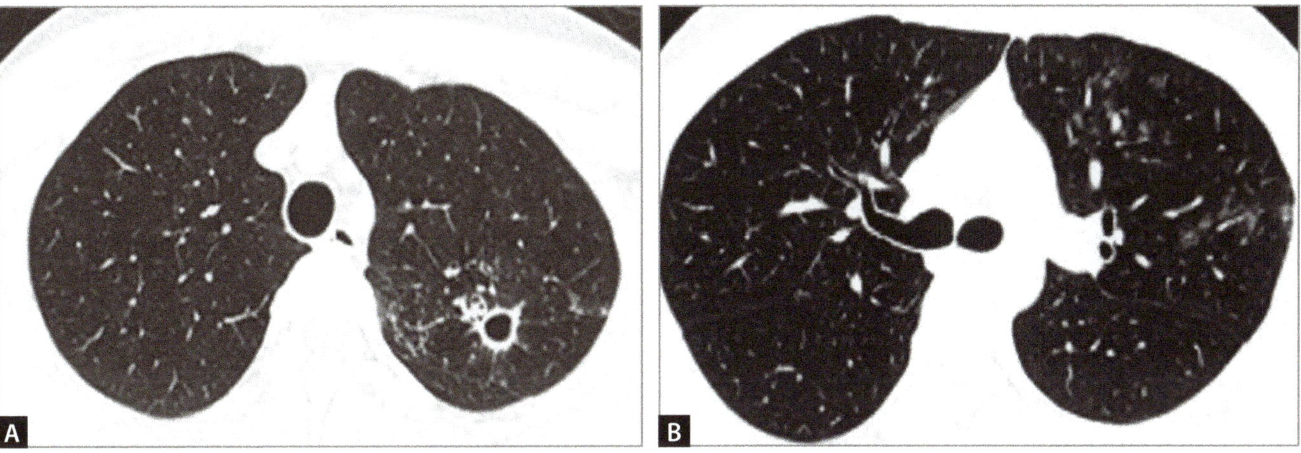

Figs. 23A and B: Cavitary tuberculosis (TB) with hemoptysis: (A) Thick-walled cavity with peripheral small nodular lesions in left apex as a result of pulmonary TB. The patient presented with hemoptysis; (B) sections through lingula demonstrate small ill-defined ground-glass densities in the left lingula.

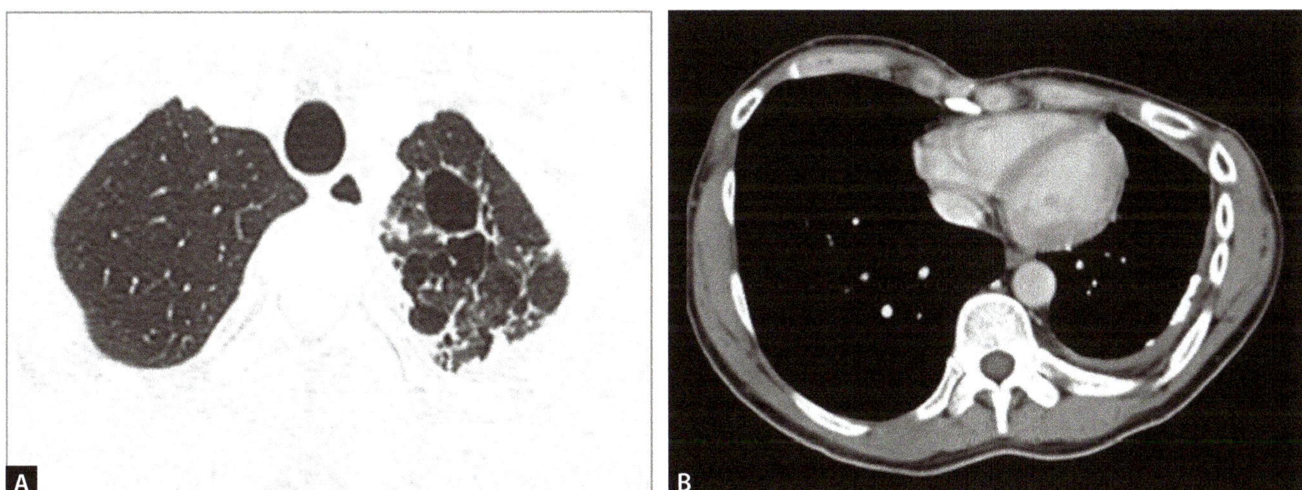

Figs. 24A and B: Old healed tuberculosis (TB): (A) High-resolution computed tomography (HRCT) demonstrates fibrotic lesions with thin-walled air spaces in the left apex. There also appears to be loss of volume as the left apex is smaller in size than the right apex. The walls of the air spaces are not thick, there is no surrounding ill-defined soft tissue or satellite nodules to suggest active infection; (B) lower sections with mediastinal window demonstrate thickened pleura with calcification and loss of volume, small-sized left hemithorax indicative of old healed TB.

This is most easily done in the disk method by incorporating the necessary number of commercially available antimicrobial-containing elution disks in the medium. The three commonly used conventional methods are: (1) the absolute concentration method, (2) the resistance ratio method, and (3) the proportion method. The Centers for Disease Control (CDC) modification of the proportion method is generally considered the standard method in this diverse field. It should be noted that susceptibility tests for pyrazinamide (PZA) can be performed in conventional media only at a reduced pH of about 5.5, a pH at which some strains will not grow. It is, therefore, recommended that PZA be tested by the BACTEC method. Essential to all susceptibility tests, regardless of method, are the critical concentration of drugs to be tested.

During the early 1980s, the BACTEC radiometric system for primary isolation of mycobacteria was developed with a susceptibility test protocol. The use of this system increased the speed with which resistant strains were detected to just 4–6 days after inoculation.

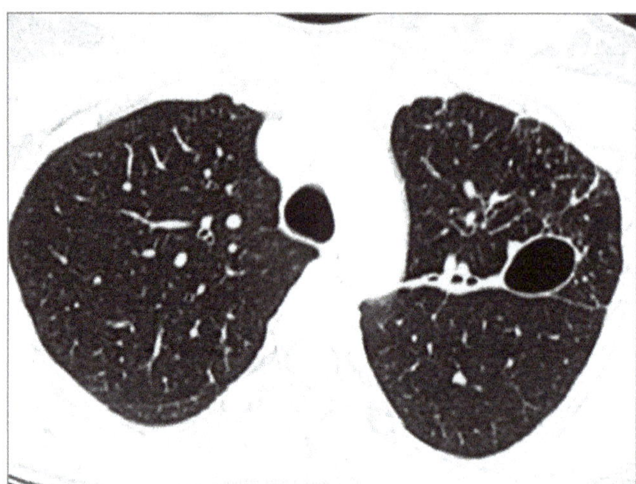

Fig. 25: Old healed tuberculosis (TB): Follow-up computed tomography (CT) in a patient with left apical cavitary TB demonstrates thin-walled cavity in left apex with associated fibrotic lesion and associated bronchiectasis. The thin-walled nature of the cavity, lack of surrounding inflammation, fibrosis, and bronchiectasis are all indicative of old healed quiescent TB.

Another advantage of the BACTEC system is the ability to test for susceptibility to PZA. The MGIT test has also been adapted to susceptibility testing and several studies have found high correlations between the BACTEC, MGIT and proportion methods. The time to detection of resistance with the MGIT system is comparable to that for the BACTEC system. The newer liquid culture methods and molecular methods will be discussed in more detail in the section on advances in diagnosis. The clinician needs to know more about the several available drug-susceptibility testing (DST) methods, both phenotypic and genotypic and these will be discussed in some detail here.

With the emergence of MDR and extensively drug-resistant TB (XDR-TB), the need for new, rapid, and reliable DST is felt globally. Tests can be broadly divided into phenotypic and genotypic methods.

- *Phenotypic methods:* These methods rely on detection of the effects of the drugs on bacterial multiplication or metabolism, compared to controls not exposed to the drugs. The important phenotypic tests are—MGIT, microscopic observation broth-drug susceptibility assay (MODS), slide DST, microcolony method, colorimetric redox indicator methods, nitrate reductase methods (NRA), and mycobacteriophage-based methods.
- *Genotypic methods:* These methods are molecular methods based on identification of resistance

conferring mutations of the bacillary genome. A new generation of genotypic tests is transforming the TB diagnostic horizon. These will be discussed in detail in Chapter 18.

Tuberculin Skin Test

This is one of the oldest tests in medicine to still be widely used in current times. Tuberculin was first prepared by Robert Koch and wrongly assumed to be a cure for TB. The original preparation was purified by Seibert in the 1930s and was standardized a decade later in Denmark where it was labeled PPD-RT23. A final modification came when a small quantity of detergent (Tween 80) was added to the solution. This detergent prevented the absorption of the tuberculin by glass and plastic surfaces that resulted in occasional false-negative reactions. Two techniques may be used to perform the TST—(1) the Mantoux test and (2) the Heaf test. Of these, it is the Mantoux test that is widely used in India and in most of the developing world. This is performed by the intradermal injection of 0.1 mL of PPD containing 5 TU into the volar aspect of the forearm using a 27-G needle with a plastic or glass syringe. The injection must be made just beneath the surface of the skin, so it raises a wheal of 6–10 mm in diameter. The test is read 48–72 hours later when the induration is measured in millimeters and reported. Depending on the size of the induration following a 5 TU Mantoux test, reactions should be considered significant and indicative of TB infection in the following categories of patients:

- *Indurations more than 5 mm:*
  - HIV-infected person.
  - Close recent contact with an infectious case of TB.
  - Persons with chest radiographs consistent with old healed TB.
- *Indurations more than 10 mm:*
  - All other persons with other risk factors for TB apart from those listed above.
- *Indurations more than 15 mm:*
  - Considered positive in all persons (including those with prior BCG vaccine).

Limitations of the TST

The TST has a number of limitations, which have been discussed here. It has a suboptimal sensitivity of only 70–90% in diagnosing active TB. Paradoxically, it is less sensitive in just the high-risk groups where accuracy is most needed like newborns and the immunosuppressed population. Its estimated specificity in healthy people with no known TB disease or exposure is also low at around 50–90%. This is because of its cross-reactivity with BCG and NTM. Another inherent flaw is the practical issue of patients needing to return 48–72 hours later to have the test read again. A study we conducted at the Hinduja Hospital in 2003 showed that a sizeable number of patients (around 40% of the 1,028 tests done) simply do not show up to even have their induration read. No other test has such a high default rate. Technical problems also abound. Batches may be of poor quality, have a relatively short expiry date, and require a cold chain for storage, which is not practical in remote parts of the country. There is also frequent inter-reader variability. Technical issues like the boosting phenomenon and conversion and reversion may make the interpretation of a repeat test difficult. Thus, to state the obvious, the TST is an imperfect test.

The potential confounding effect of BCG on the TST requires special mention. A meta-analysis of the effects of BCG on the TST showed that prior administration of BCG increased the likelihood of a positive TST (relative risk 2.1). This was less likely when BCG was administered in infancy and more likely when given after a year. Tests usually stayed positive up to 15 years of age. After this age, a strongly positive TST should not be attributed to prior BCG.

◼ TREATMENT OF TUBERCULOSIS

The aims of treatment of TB are:
- To cure the patient and restore quality of life and productivity.
- To prevent death from active TB.
- To prevent relapse of TB.
- To reduce transmission of TB to others.
- To prevent the development and transmission of drug resistance.

The first-line drugs are isoniazid, rifampicin, ethambutol, PZA, and streptomycin. The recommended dosing schedule as currently recommended by WHO is tabulated in **Table 2** for daily and intermittent (thrice-weekly) regimens.

Directly observed treatment short course is the accepted standard of care for administration of these first-line drugs. The components of DOTS are discussed here:
- *Uninterrupted, free, and short-course chemotherapy supply*: These days, each registered TB patient has a TB patient kit, which contains the full course of treatment which ensures the treatment will be uninterrupted. The kit provides health workers with a container that has all the required medicines in the right quantities and doses. This helps to limit confusion and wastage and makes it easier to monitor the regularity of treatment. It is hoped that the patient may feel a sense of ownership that helps to ensure he actually keeps returning till he finishes his kit. The standardization that goes into each kit also avoids the chaotic situation that occurs in the private sector where there are a vast and bewildering number of drugs and kits in the market, many of poor quality and questionable bioavailability.
- *Quality microscopy*: It is the next tenet of DOTS. All patients suspected of having pulmonary TB should submit at least two sputum specimens for microscopic examination in a quality-assured laboratory. When

Table 2: Recommended doses of first-line antituberculosis drugs for adults.

| Drug | Recommended dose | | | |
| | Daily | | Three times per week | |
	Dose and range (mg/kg body weight)	Maximum (mg)	Dose and range (mg/kg body weight)	Daily maximum (mg)
Isoniazid	5 (4–6)	300	10 (8–12)	900
Rifampicin	10 (8–12)	600	10 (8–12)	600
Pyrazinamide	25 (20–30)	—	35 (30–40)	—
Ethambutol	15 (15–20)	—	30 (25–35)	—
Streptomycin	15 (12–18)	—	15 (12–18)	1,000

possible, at least one of these should be an early morning sputum specimen as sputum collected at this time has been shown to have the highest yield. A case of pulmonary TB should be considered to be smear-positive, if one or more sputum smear specimens at the start of treatment are positive for AFB.

- *Reporting and monitoring systems in place*: Each patient must be properly registered and the site of TB (pulmonary or extrapulmonary) must be recorded. Record must also be made of whether the patient is a new case (never had treatment for TB or has taken TB treatment for less than a month) or a previously treated patient (one who has received > 1 month of TB drugs in the past). Patient outcomes must also be accurately recorded as—cured, treatment completed, treatment failed, or defaulted. Such accurate data recording lends itself to thorough analysis of the results of the DOTS program. Any deficiencies can be noted and corrective steps can be taken.
- *Direct observation*: This is, perhaps, the most controversial of all the DOTS principles. A healthcare worker must supervise the actual act of swallowing. This is believed to be the most reliable way to ensure compliance. Opponents of direct observation maintain that the act of supervision can be costly and alienating and point to a Cochrane review of four trials that looked at direct observation versus self-treatment and concluded that there was no benefit of direct observation.

Criticisms of DOTS in the Indian Context

Just as we recognized the immense contribution of DOTS to TB control in India, it is equally important to be objective and critical when necessary. A number of criticisms can be raised regarding DOTS in India:

- A verifiable address is mandatory before a patient can be registered in a DOTS center. The homeless, the slum dwellers (50% of Mumbai's population), and the large migrant population are thus automatically excluded. This immediately excludes the most vulnerable members of society, those that would most benefit from being included in a DOTS program.
- Women are even more reluctant to attend a DOTS program as they are even more stigmatized. Thus, there is a skewed male to female ratio of 3:1 in many DOTS centers.

- Indeed, DOTS may be generally too obtrusive for Indians. The disease sadly continues to carry a stigma and seen entering a DOTS clinic leaves no room for doubt that the patient is suffering from TB.
- There is a feeling that the difficult patients are weeded out of many DOTS centers perhaps so that the impressive end of term results is not spoilt. Thus, the marginalized members of society like alcoholics, the homeless and drug addicts, which DOTS programs should be striving to include, are deliberately left out in the cold.
- Private patients are completely outside the purview of DOTS at present. Several studies have shown that as many as 50–80% of new TB patients will choose to go private at the start. Thus, this large TB patient population falls out of the confines of DOTS and falls prey to private practitioners, the majority of whom prescribe drug regimens that are clearly inappropriate. In a landmark study published in Tubercle and Lung Disease by Uplekar in 1993, 143 private doctors practicing in the Dharavi area of Mumbai were asked: "What prescription would you give a sputum-positive patient with no history of prior TB?" The 102 respondents came up with 80 different regimens, the majority inappropriate and more expensive than the standard. Western doctors do not fare much better. In an audit by Iseman of patients eventually referred to his unit in Denver, management errors had been made in 80%. There was an average of 3.93 errors per patient with the single most common error being the addition of a single new drug to a failing regimen.
- DOTS clinic hours are rigid and do not suit daily wage earners who are faced with a choice of either getting their drugs or feeding their family on that day. Travelling the long journey to more distant DOTS centers in more remote parts of the country is especially difficult for the old, the sick, the invalid, and the poor.
- The greatly extra workload imposed on the system by DOTS may eventually overwhelm the system unless far more is allocated in terms of funds and manpower.
- Finally, DOTS alone is clearly inadequate for the MDR-TB and HIV-TB coinfected populations unless DOTS programs include second-line drugs (the so-called DOTS-plus) and antiretroviral drugs.

Despite these critiques, the DOTS-based RNTCP has been remarkably successful in achieving the global targets of detecting 70% of the estimated TB cases and curing 85% of them. Attempts to integrate the private and public sectors and iron out the deficiencies in DOTS outlined above are clearly the way ahead.

Current Treatment Regimens

The current standard regimens for new TB patients is 2 months of isoniazid (H), rifampicin (R), ethambutol (E), and PZA (Z) in the so-called intensive phase followed by 4 months of isoniazid (INH) and rifampicin in the continuation phase. This 6-month regimen is associated with almost 100% bacteriological conversion by the end of treatment in those with drug-susceptible disease and has a relapse rate of roughly 3–5%. The total duration of treatment should be extended from 6–9 months in those patients in whom cavitation is noted on the initial chest radiograph and in those whose sputum is still culture positive despite 2 months of treatment. The standard 6-month regimen can be administered as daily therapy throughout, as intermittent therapy throughout (three times weekly), or as a mixture of approaches with a period of daily administration followed by a period of intermittent administration. In line with increasing evidence of the benefits of daily treatment, India has taken the first steps towards adopting daily fixed dose combination (FDC) for all drug-sensitive patients. The RNTCP's 'recently released new policy standards for TB care in India' endorses this and the switch from intermittent to daily treatment has begun. In the HIV-positive patient coinfected with TB, daily treatment is to be preferred. The latest WHO guidelines permit the use of HR and E in the continuation phase as an alternative to HR in areas where high levels of INH resistance are known to prevent the inadvertent development of MDR-TB while on treatment. Another major and positive change in the latest WHO guidelines is that Category 2 has been phased out. Category 2, previously used in treatment failures, comprised of 2HRZES/1HRZE/5HRE. In our opinion, the majority of people who fail standard treatment have MDR-TB. Subjecting these patients to Category 2, treatment serves only to amplify their resistance and waste an additional 8 months. The current recommendation is that all such treatment failures should undergo DST and be started on an empiric MDR-TB regimen based on knowledge of local resistance patterns. This regimen can be modified and individualized once the DST is available. In countries which lack facilities for DST, the empiric MDR

regimen should be continued throughout the duration of treatment.

First-line Drugs and their Toxicities

Isoniazid

Isoniazid has profound early bactericidal activity against rapidly dividing bacteria. Its major adverse effects are as follows:

- *Asymptomatic elevation in transaminases*: Aminotransferase elevations up to five times the upper limit of normal occur in up to 20% of persons receiving INH alone for treatment of LTBI. The enzyme levels usually return to normal even with continued administration of the drug.
- *Clinical hepatitis*: Data indicate that the incidence of clinical hepatitis is lower than was previously thought. Hepatitis occurred in only 0.1–0.15% of 11,141 persons receiving INH alone as treatment for LTBI in an urban TB control program. Prior studies suggested a higher rate, and a meta-analysis of six studies estimated the rate of clinical hepatitis in patients given isoniazid alone to be 0.6%. In this meta-analysis, the rate of clinical hepatitis was 1.6% when isoniazid was given with other agents, not including rifampicin. The risk was higher when the drug was combined with rifampicin, an average of 2.7% in 19 reports. For INH alone, the risk increases with advancing age; it is uncommon in persons less than 20 years of age but is nearly 2% in persons aged 50–64 years. The risk may also be increased in persons with underlying liver disease, in those with a history of heavy alcohol consumption, and in the postpartum period. Acetylator status may be linked to hepatotoxicity but the link is controversial and screening for acetylator status is not of clinical value. The rate of fatal hepatitis with isoniazid is estimated to be 0.023, but recent studies suggest it may be substantially lower. Death has been associated with continued use of isoniazid despite evidence of hepatitis.
- *Peripheral neuropathy*: It is an adverse effect of isoniazid that is dose related. The risk is increased in patients with other risk factors for peripheral neuropathy like malnutrition, alcohol intake, and diabetes, all common in the Indian context. Pyridoxine supplementation (20 mg/day) is essential to prevent this complication.

- *CNS side-effects*: Seizures and psychosis have been rarely reported but the risk is difficult to quantify.
- *Lupus-like syndrome*: Approximately 20% of patients receiving INH develop antinuclear antibodies. Less than 15% will develop a systemic lupus erythematosus (SLE)-like illness necessitating stoppage of the drug.

Rifampicin

Rifampicin has excellent activity against organisms that are dividing rapidly (early bactericidal activity) and against semidormant bacterial populations, thus accounting for its sterilizing activity.

- *Hepatitis*: Rifampicin interferes with the major bile salt exporter pump and may lead to a conjugated hyperbilirubinemia. This is typically mild, asymptomatic, and of no clinical significance. On its own, rifampicin causes hepatitis (typically of a cholestatic pattern) much less frequently than isoniazid. When given in conjunction with isoniazid, rifampicin may potentiate isoniazid-induced liver injury, and one meta-analysis estimates the rate of hepatitis in patients taking both drugs to be as high as 2.55%.
- *Cutaneous*: Pruritis with or without rash is common, occurring in 6% of patients. It is generally limited and the drug can often be continued, but severe reactions necessitating stopping of the drug can occur in 0.1% of patients.
- *Gastrointestinal (GI) symptoms* like nausea, gastritis, and anorexia are frequent but rarely severe enough to necessitate stopping of the drug. Most can be treated symptomatically.
- *Flu-like syndrome* occurs more frequently in those receiving intermittent rifampicin than in those on daily treatment with the drug.
- *Severe immunological reactions* include thrombocytopenia, hemolytic anemia, acute renal failure, and thrombotic thrombocytopenic purpura. These reactions are rare, occurring in less than 0.1% of patients, and have an immune basis.
- *Drug interactions*: There are a number of drug interactions with potentially serious consequences. Of particular concern are reductions, often to ineffective levels, in the serum concentration of common drugs like warfarin, corticosteroids, and oral contraceptives. Thus, women using this form of birth control should be cautioned that contraceptives will lose efficacy while on rifampicin. In addition, there are important bidirectional interactions between rifamycins and antiretroviral agents, which will be discussed later.

Ethambutol

Ethambutol is a first-line drug for treating all forms of TB. It is included in initial treatment regimens primarily to prevent emergence of rifampicin resistance when primary resistance to isoniazid may be present. It is generally not recommended in children where visual acuity cannot be routinely monitored.

- *Optic nerve toxicity*: Retrobulbar neuritis is the main toxicity associated with ethambutol. This is manifested by decreased visual acuity or decreased red-green color discrimination that may affect one or both eyes. The risk of optic toxicity is dose dependent and is more common at doses of 30 mg/kg body weight or in patients with impaired renal function.
    - *Monitoring for ocular toxicity*: Patients should have baseline visual acuity testing and testing of color discrimination with Snellen chart and Ishihara tests, respectively. At each monthly visit, patients should be asked about blurred vision or scotomas. Monthly testing is recommended in those patients taking doses greater than 15–25 mg/kg for more than 2 months. Ethambutol should be immediately and permanently discontinued, if there are any signs of visual toxicity.
- Cutaneous reactions and pruritis are not uncommon though reactions requiring discontinuation of the drug occur in 0.7% of patients.

Pyrazinamide

Pyrazinamide is most effective against the population of dormant or semidormant bacteria contained within macrophages or in the acidic confines of caseous foci.

- *Hepatotoxicity*: Early studies using higher doses of 40–70 mg/kg per day reported hepatotoxicity at high rates. At the standard dose of 25 mg/kg hepatotoxicity occurs at a rate of 1%.
- *Joint pains*: Nongouty polyarthralgia may occur in up to 40% of patients receiving daily doses of PZA. This rarely requires discontinuation as it responds to nonsteroidal anti-inflammatory drugs (NSAIDs). Asymptomatic hyperuricemia is an expected side

effect of the drug and does not usually require treatment. Acute gout attacks are rare except in patients with pre-existing gout in whom this drug should generally be avoided.

Streptomycin

Streptomycin is equivalent to ethambutol in the intensive phase of a 6-month regimen.

- *Ototoxicity*, which includes hearing and vestibular disturbances, is the most important side effect. The risk increases with age, concomitant use of loop diuretics, increasing single doses and cumulative doses more than 120 g.
- Nephrotoxicity is less common with streptomycin than with amikacin or kanamycin. Renal insufficiency requiring discontinuation occurs in 2% of cases.

- *Symptom-based approach to management of side effects of anti-TB drugs*: The current WHO guidelines give a symptom-based approach to management of common side effects. These side effects may be classified as major and minor. In general, major effects necessitate stopping of treatment while minor effects should be treated symptomatically without discontinuation of drugs. This approach is summarized in **Table 3** below.
- *Managing individual side effects*: Only hepatitis, the most frequently described side effect, will be discussed in detail here.
- *Hepatitis*: Transient elevations of liver function during treatment are relatively common (20% of patients) and may not signify true hepatotoxicity. Drug-induced hepatitis, the most serious common adverse effect, is defined as a serum aspartate aminotransferase

Table 3: Symptom-based approach to management of side effects of tuberculosis (TB) drugs.

Side effects	Drug(s) probably	Management
Major		*Stop responsible drug(s) and refer to clinician urgently*
Skin rash with or without itching	Streptomycin, isoniazid, rifampicin, pyrazinamide	Stop anti-TB drugs
Deafness (no wax on otoscopy)	Streptomycin	Stop streptomycin
Dizziness (vertigo and nystagmus)	Streptomycin	Stop streptomycin
Jaundice (other causes excluded), hepatitis	Isoniazid, pyrazinamide, rifampicin	Stop anti-TB drugs
Confusion (suspect drug-induced acute liver failure if there is jaundice)	Most anti-TB drugs	Stop anti-TB drugs
Visual impairment (other causes excluded)	Ethambutol	Stop ethambutol
Shock, purpura, acute renal failure	Rifampicin	Stop rifampicin
Decreased urine output	Streptomycin	Stop streptomycin
Minor		*Continue anti-TB drugs, check drug doses*
Anorexia, nausea, abdominal pain	Pyrazinamide, rifampicin, isoniazid	Give drugs with small meals or just before bedtime, and advise patient to swallow pills slowly with small sips of water. If symptoms persist or worsen, or there is protracted vomiting or any sign of bleeding, consider the side effect to be major and refer to clinician urgently.
Joint pains	Pyrazinamide	Aspirin or nonsteroidal anti-inflammatory drug or paracetamol
Burning, numbness or tingling sensation in the hands or feet	Isoniazid	Pyridoxine 50–75 mg daily
Drowsiness	Isoniazid	Reassurance: Give drugs before bedtime
Orange/red urine	Rifampicin	Reassurance: Patients should be told when starting treatment that this may happen and is normal
Flu syndrome (fever, chills, malaise, headache, bone pain)	Intermittent dosing of rifampicin	Change from intermittent to daily rifampicin administration

(AST) level more than three times the upper limit of normal in the presence of symptoms, or more than five times the upper limit of normal in the absence of symptoms. Depending on the magnitude of the rise in transaminases, it may be graded as follows: if the AST level is less than five times the upper limit of normal, toxicity can be considered mild, an AST level 5–10 times normal defines moderate toxicity, and an AST level greater than 10 times normal (i.e. greater than 500 IU) is severe. In addition to AST elevation, occasionally there are disproportionate increases in bilirubin and alkaline phosphatase. This pattern is more consistent with rifampicin hepatotoxicity.

If hepatitis occurs, isoniazid, rifampicin, and PZA, all potential causes of hepatic injury, should be stopped immediately. Serologic testing for hepatitis viruses A, B, and C (if not done at baseline) should be performed and the patient questioned carefully regarding exposure to other possible hepatotoxins, especially alcohol.

While waiting for liver function to normalize (generally a few weeks), a decision must be made whether to start a nonhepatotoxic regimen (if the TB is advanced and needs immediate treatment) or to keep the patient off all TB drugs till the liver function normalizes. This latter strategy is acceptable in patients with glandular TB or pleural TB who have a low bacillary load and are not too sick from their TB. On the other hand, if a delay of a few weeks is unacceptable due to the severity of the patient's TB (miliary, meningeal, or cavitary TB), three or more anti-TB medications without hepatotoxicity, such as ethambutol, an aminoglycoside (streptomycin/amikacin/kanamycin/capreomycin), and a fluoroquinolone (levofloxacin or moxifloxacin), may be used until the hepatitis resolves.

Once the AST level decreases to less than two times the upper limit of normal and symptoms have significantly improved, the first-line medications should be restarted in sequential fashion.

The sequence outlined below is based on the current recommendations of the American Thoracic Society, CDC, and Infectious Diseases Society of America. Because rifampicin is much less likely to cause hepatotoxicity than isoniazid or PZA and is the most effective agent, it should be restarted first. If there is no increase in AST after about 1 week, isoniazid may be restarted. PZA can be started 1 week after isoniazid, if AST does not increase. If symptoms recur, or AST increases, the last drug added should be stopped. If

rifampicin and isoniazid are tolerated, and hepatitis was severe, PZA should be assumed to be responsible. In this situation, it may be best to avoid the addition of this drug altogether. In this last circumstance, depending on the number of doses of PZA taken, severity of disease, and bacteriological status, therapy might be extended to 9 months or a fluoroquinolone or aminoglycoside can take its place in the intensive phase.

Close monitoring, with repeat measurements of serum AST and bilirubin and symptom review, is essential in managing these patients.

Treatment of Tuberculosis in Special Situations

- *Pregnancy and lactation*: All the first-line drugs except streptomycin may be safely used during pregnancy and lactation. Pyridoxine supplementation is essential in pregnant women receiving isoniazid. The safety profiles of the second-line drugs have not been ascertained, but they have been used in scattered case studies and small series with good maternal and fetal outcomes. Decisions about which drugs to continue must be individualized after a careful discussion of the possible teratogenic effects with the mother.
- *Renal failure*: In a patient with a creatinine clearance less than 30 mL/min or who is receiving dialysis, isoniazid and rifampicin may be given without any dose adjustment. Ethambutol and PZA must both be given in a three times a week frequency, with the actual dose in mg staying unaltered. All medications should be given postdialysis on the day of the hemodialysis. All the aminoglycosides are best avoided, or, if they must be used, given no more than two or three times a week with serum concentration monitoring. Levofloxacin is also dependent on renal clearance and the frequency of administration must be reduced to three times a week.

■ SUGGESTED READING

1. Blumberg HM, Burman WJ, Chaisson RE, et al. American Thoracic Society/Centers for Disease Control and Prevention/Infectious Diseases Society of America: Treatment of tuberculosis. Am J Resp Crit Care Med. 2003;167:603-62.
2. Dedhia K, Udwadia ZF, Huggett JF, et al. Utility of the antigen-specific interferon-γ assay for the management of tuberculosis. Curr Opin Pulm Med. 2005;11:195-202.

3. Kobashi Y. Transitional change in the clinical features of pulmonary tuberculosis. Respiration. 2008;75(3):304-9.

4. Lalvani A. Diagnosing tuberculosis infection in the 21st century. New tools to tackle an old enemy. Chest. 2007;131:1898-906.

5. Liebeschuetz S, Bamber S, Ewer K, et al. Diagnosis of tuberculosis in South African children with a T-cell-based assay: a prospective cohort study. Lancet. 2004;364:2196-203.

6. Pinto L, Udwadia ZF. The politics of TB: the politics, economics and impact of directly observed treatment in India. Chron Resp Dis. 2007;4(2):101-6.

7. Sharma SK. Miliary tuberculosis: new insights into an old disease. Lancet Infect Dis. 2005;5(7):415-30.

8. Uplekar M, Shepard DS. Treatment of tuberculosis by private general practitioners in India. Tubercle. 1991;72(4):284-90.

CHAPTER 16

Multidrug-resistant and Extensively Drug-resistant Tuberculosis

Drug-resistant (DR) TB has emerged to become a global problem threatening to derail all the progress in TB control made to date.

Terminology

Monoresistant TB is resistance to only one drug. Included here is isoniazid monoresistance which is believed to be widely prevalent in India, and rifampicin monoresistance which is uncommon.

Polydrug-resistant TB is a form of TB resistant to more than one drug but not the combination of isoniazid and rifampicin.

Multidrug-resistant TB (MDR-TB) is TB that is resistant to both isoniazid and rifampicin, the two most powerful anti-TB drugs.

Pre-XDR TB: It is MDR-TB plus resistance to any one fluoroquinolone.

Extensively drug-resistant TB (XDR-TB): It is defined as MDR-TB plus resistance to at least one drug in the fluoroquinolone class and one in the second-line injectable class (kanamycin, amikacin, and capreomycin). These are the two most important classes of medicines in an MDR regimen.

Totally drug-resistant TB (TDR-TB) is defined as resistance to all available first- and second-line drugs (SLD) or resistance to all available drugs. It must be pointed out that the WHO does not recognize the existence of TDR-TB and prefers to use the phrase "resistance beyond XDR".

Types of Multidrug-resistant Tuberculosis

Drug-resistance among new cases (Primary): It is defined as drug-resistance in a patient who has never been treated for TB or who has received less than 1 month of treatment.

Drug-resistance among previously treated cases (secondary or acquired): It is defined as drug-resistance in a patient who has previously received at least 1 month of treatment.

Pathogenesis

Multidrug-resistant tuberculosis is an iatrogenic problem. It is caused by patients not taking the drugs as prescribed to them or by physicians not prescribing the correct drugs in the correct doses and/or for the correct duration. Soon after streptomycin was first introduced as a TB drug in 1947 it became apparent that resistance to individual drugs would develop at a predictable rate if the compounds were used as single agents. Resistance to an anti-TB drug is due to spontaneous chromosomal mutation at a frequency of 10^6 to 10^8 bacterial replications. These rates correspond to the average expected frequency of spontaneous mutation of chromosomes. As mutations resulting in resistance are unlinked, the probability of resistance to all three drugs used simultaneously is in the order of 10^{18} to 10^{20}. Even a large tuberculous cavity would be expected to contain no more than 1 million TB bacteria. Hence the chance of spontaneous drug-resistance is almost impossible when three effective drugs are used in combination. This is the principle of modern short-course chemotherapy. MDR-TB is thus always a manmade or iatrogenic problem occurring when these drugs are prescribed in the wrong doses or taken irregularly.

The genetic basis of resistance to most of the commonly used anti-TB drugs has been recently elucidated **(Table 1)**.

Epidemiology of Multidrug-resistant Tuberculosis and XDR-TB: Global and Indian

Global Epidemiology (Fig. 1)

- *Multidrug-resistant tuberculosis*: Since the launch of the "Global Project on Antituberculosis Drug Resistance Surveillance" in 1994, data on drug-resistance has been systematically compiled and analyzed from 160 countries, which together account for more than 97% of the world's population worldwide, by WHO. Globally, in 2016, an estimated 4.1% of new cases and 19% of previously treated cases were estimated to have MDR-TB. There were estimated to be total of 490,000 MDR-TB cases with 47% of the global total coming from India, China and the Russian Federation. All official reports must be interpreted with the awareness that in many countries the level of underreporting may be high. This is especially the case for those countries where notification is not mandatory. Underdiagnosis can also occur for reasons such as poor geographical and financial access to healthcare, lack or limited symptoms that delay seeking of healthcare, and reliance on diagnostic tests that are not reliable enough to ensure accurate identification of all cases.

- *Extensively drug-resistant TB*: This form of TB was first reported by Gandhi et al. in an important publication in Lancet in 2006 when they reported an outbreak in KwaZulu Natal, South Africa. They detected MDR-TB in 221 patients, of whom 53 had XDR-TB. They reported alarmingly high mortality in these 53 patients with 52 of the 53 dying, with median survival of 16 days from the time of diagnosis. All 44 XDR-TB patients who were tested for HIV were co-infected. Studies have since confirmed the prior existence of XDR-TB in several countries. Since then increasing numbers of XDR-TB have been reported by virtually every country across the globe with 117 countries reporting XDR-TB globally in 2015. A recent study from Emory University and the CDC of over 400 XDR-TB patients in South Africa provided compelling evidence that person to person transmission is the key driver of the spread of XDR-TB. South Africa is experiencing a widespread epidemic of XDR-TB and is reporting a 10-fold increase in cases

Table 1: Mechanisms of drug-resistance in *Mycobacterium tuberculosis*.

Anti-TB drug	Genes involved in resistance	Frequency of mutations
Isoniazid	• *katG* • *inhA*	• 47–58% • 21–34%
Rifampicin	*rpoB*	96–98%
Streptomycin	• *rpsL* • *rrs*	52–59% 8–21%
Ethambutol	*embAB*	50%
Pyrazinamide	*pcnA*	Unknown
Fluoroquinolones	*gyrA*	75–94%

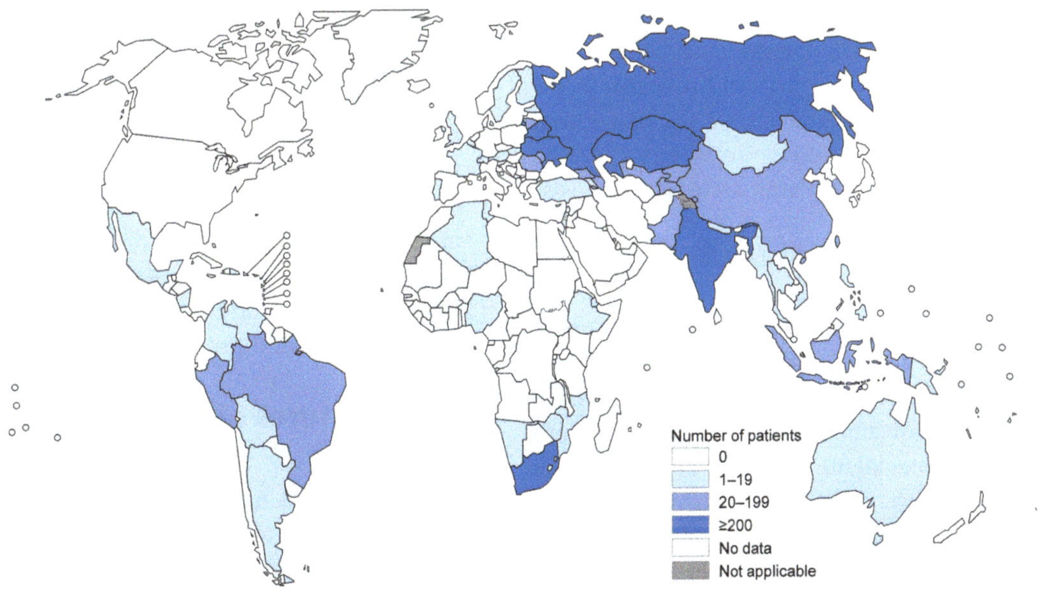

Fig. 1: Number of patients with laboratory-confirmed XDR-TB started on treatment in 2015.

since the initial description. It is estimated that around 9.5% of cases with MDR-TB globally have XDR-TB.

Indian Epidemiology

- *Multidrug-resistant tuberculosis*: The epidemiology of MDR-TB in India is bedeviled by lack of proper notification (only made compulsory in 2012), lack of accurate data recording, sampling of small, nonrepresentative patient groups, and laboratory limitations (few labs capable of performing reliable SLD DST). These limitations must be borne in mind when reflecting on the latest (WHO TB report 2017) estimates that there were 147,000 new cases of MDR-TB in India in 2016. The report goes on to estimate that 2.85 of all new cases and 12% of previously treated TB cases had MDR-TB. For the reasons mentioned above, it is likely that these official figures are probably considerable underestimates. The WHO admits in its global report that in India, multiple surveys in the last few years show considerable underreporting of detected cases, especially in the private sector. Most Indian patients chose to first visit private providers for their TB and large numbers of patients thus slip through the radar. Pai estimated that approximately 1.3 million Indian TB patients (many conceivably with MDR-TB) may either not have been diagnosed or were lost to follow up. There is little doubt that there are hyperendemic urban pockets in densely populated cities where much higher rates of MDR-TB than reported by WHO are routinely encountered. In Mumbai, recent data from Mistry suggests that 24% of new cases and 41%of retreated cases have MDR-TB. Until India completes a truly representative national survey, the true extent of the MDR-TB problem this country faces will be obfuscated by the kind of "statistico-tuberculosis" described above.
- *Extensively drug-resistant TB*: This form of TB has probably existed for years in India because of the cavalier manner in which second-line drugs, particularly fluoroquinolone are abused. India's unsupervised and chaotic private sector provides the perfect template for amplification of MDR-TB into XDR-TB strains. Special mention and condemnation must be made here of the indiscriminate use of fluoroquinolones. An ORG survey of total of 318 million antibiotic prescriptions back in 2004 showed that ciprofloxacin was by far the most commonly prescribed antibiotic across the country. It was cheap, off patent, and dispensed for a variety of nonspecific indications including viral infections and upper respiratory infections. This renders an invaluable group of drugs, the fluoroquinolone, nearly worthless in the Indian MDR-TB context. Fluoroquinolone resistance to M tuberculosis is a global phenomenon after its first description from New York by Sullivan. At the Hinduja hospital clinics, pre-XDR TB (MDR plus fluoroquinolone resistance) is the commonest pattern of resistance encountered and our mycobacterial lab reports resistance rates that have increased from 6% in 1997 to 35% in 2002 to around 74% today in 2017. The first XDR-TB series from India was reported in 2007 from the Mumbai-based Hinduja hospital, a large private hospital, armed with a state of the art mycobacterial laboratory. Here a retrospective analysis of all samples sent for culture and DST to SLDs revealed that as many as 11% of the 329 MDR cases reported in 2007 met the Centers for Disease Control and Prevention definition of XDR-TB. Since this initial report there have been several others from across the country making it apparent that XDR-TB is also firmly entrenched in India. In India too, in keeping with the global average, about 10% of MDR-TB cases have XDR-TB.
- *Totally drug-resistant TB*: In the latter half of 2012, four patients with a more extreme from of drug-resistant TB were encountered and reported by Udwadia et al from the Hinduja hospital. These patients had a DST pattern that made them virtually untreatable, with resistance to all the 12 first and second line drugs that the mycobacterial lab performed DST on. The term "TDR" with its accompanying connotation of untreatable TB, stirred up an unprecedented storm of attention in the lay and medical press both locally and internationally. They did at least serve to put drug-resistant TB on the radar, drawing much needed attention to the large numbers of Indian patients languishing from these extreme forms of TB.

Clinical Features of Multidrug-resistant Tuberculosis

Multidrug-resistant tuberculosis is clinically and radio-logically indistinguishable from drug-sensitive TB **(Figs. 2 to 5)**. It remains essentially a microbiological diagnosis but must be suspected in certain settings.

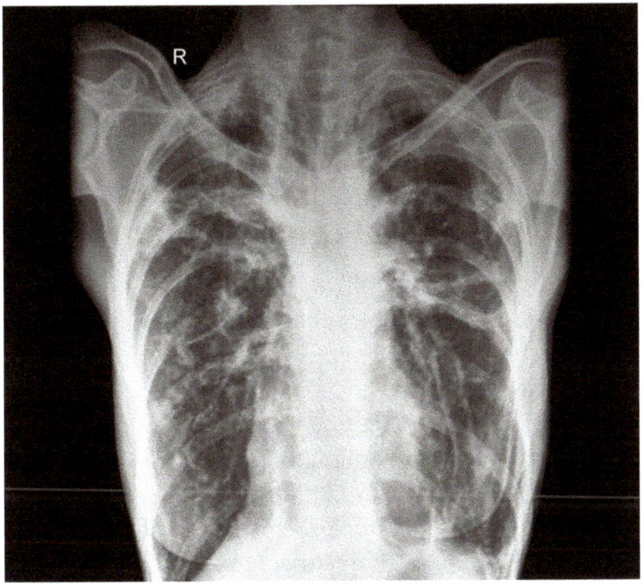

Fig. 2: Multidrug-resistant tuberculosis (MDR-TB). Chest X-ray reveals extensive soft tissue infiltration, cavities in both upper and midzones with calcific and fibrotic lesions.

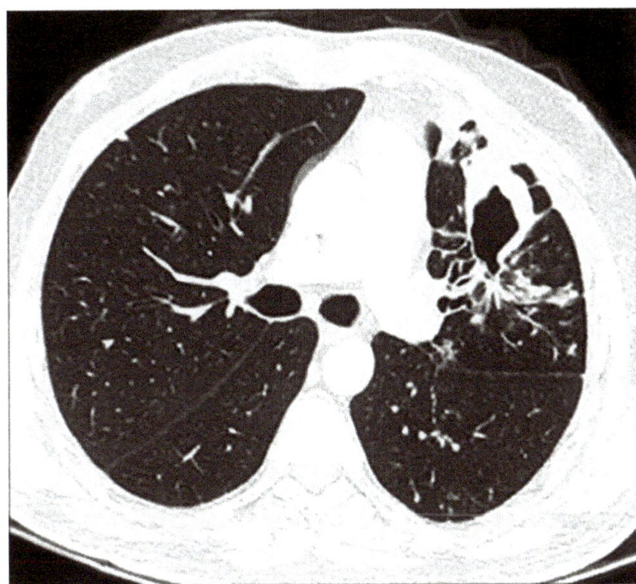

Fig. 4: Multidrug-resistant tuberculosis (MDR-TB). CT chest demonstrates thick-walled cavitating lesions in the left lingula with peripheral fibrotic lesions and dilated bronchi.

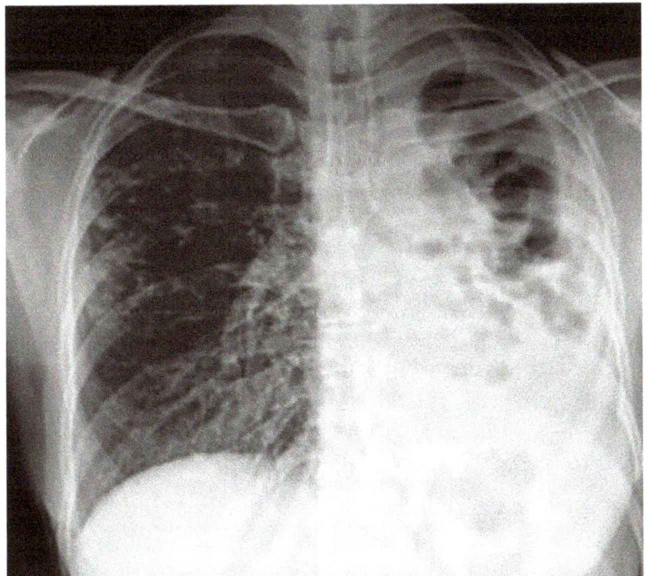

Fig. 3: Multidrug-resistant tuberculosis (MDR-TB). Smear-positive despite directly observed treatments (DOTS) 6 months category 1; DOTS category 2, 8 months; subsequent smears confirm MDR-TB. Chest X-ray reveals destroyed left lower lobe with multiple cavities in left upper lobe, and right lung infiltration.

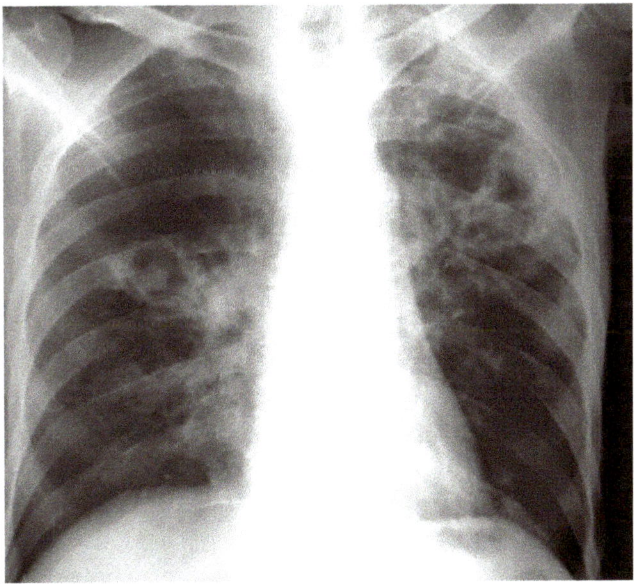

Fig. 5: Multidrug-resistant tuberculosis (MDR-TB). Chest X-ray demonstrates thick-walled cavitating lesions in the right midzone and left upper zone with associated ill-defined soft-tissue opacities.

A cardinal rule is to suspect MDR-TB in any patient with a past history of TB treatment no matter how remote that history. MDR-TB must also be suspected in a patient with TB who gives a history of contact with a patient proven to have MDR-TB. HIV-positive patients are believed by some authorities to have a higher likelihood of developing MDR and XDR-TB but this link has never been proven. In Western countries, MDR-TB is much more common in immigrants from areas of known high prevalence of MDR-TB.

Homelessness, alcohol and substance abuse, and prison populations are also at higher risk of MDR-TB.

Diagnosis of MDR-TB

There is a diagnostic revolution in the manner and the speed with which MDR and XDR TB are now being diagnosed. The Xpert MTB/RIF and the Hain LPA assay are genotypic tests that provide the treating physician with a rapid diagnosis of drug resistant TB in a few days as opposed to the traditional 180–240 days taken by the traditional tests. Sadly, they have not been scaled up in the developing world. Outside South Africa, the number of procured cartridges in 2016 compared with the total number of instrument modules as of 2015 reflects an average rate of only 1.0 test per module per working day globally.

These tests have been discussed in detail in Chapter 18 on Newer Diagnostics.

Problems with diagnosing MDR-TB in India:

- *Too few laboratories*: MDR and XDR remain essentially lab based diagnoses. Despite its population of 1.3 billion India has only 45 laboratories capable of performing DST. This works out to an abysmally low ratio of 0.2 labs per million population. China in contrast with its comparable population has 249 DST capable labs. Without more labs capable of performing quality assured DST, the extent of India's MDR-TB problem will remain submerged from view.
- *Reliance on inappropriate tests*: : Large sums are wasted on inappropriate and misleading diagnostics like serological tests. It is estimated that around 1.5 million TB serological tests are performed annually in India at an estimated cost of $ 15 million a year. Treatment in the private sector is often started or withheld inappropriately based on these tests with disastrous consequences for the patient. The recent decision by the Indian government to pass a directive banning these tests was hailed as a step in the right direction. It remains to be seen if this directive can be rigorously enforced and implemented.
- *Slow to scale out new technologies*: Newer tests like the Xpert MDR/RIF need to be rolled out with greater speed. There are just 54 RNTCP centers across the country offering this test as of 2013. China by contrast had 160 and South Africa which has embraced this new technology with great enthusiasm had 207 Gene Xpert sites. These tests are more costly but far more accurate than traditional sputum tests and if widely rolled out are likely to triple the number of Indian patients diagnosed with MDR-TB.

Impact of Multidrug-resistant Tuberculosis in India

Multidrug-resistant tuberculosis is particularly devastating in India because it is usually suspected and diagnosed late. Very few laboratories reliably perform DSTs in the country. There is no public provision for treating these patients who therefore are compelled to seek out multiple private practitioners of varying quality. Sadly, these patients are still stigmatized, and as second-line drugs are expensive, they end up being partially treated. This results in a huge pool of chronic MDR-TB patients who receive just enough treatment to keep them alive but not enough to cure them. Thus there is exponential spread of this deadly form of TB in crowded communities.

Reasons for the Spread of Multidrug-resistant Tuberculosis in India

- *A failing public program*: India's NTP which originated in 1962 was conceived on sound scientific and social grounds. It was however, poorly implemented and hence made little epidemiological impact over 3 decades. Indeed it begat and bred MDR-TB. Alarm bells were slow to ring and it was only in 1992 that the Indian government finally conceded that the NTP had failed. A joint panel of experts from WHO and the Indian government concluded that it be abandoned in favor of the Revised National Tuberculosis Programme (RNTCP). This was funded by a soft loan of $142 million and based on the five DOTS principles discussed earlier. The RNTCP too, for several decades, sat by, paralyzed, failing to appreciate the scale and severity of the unfolding MDR-TB crisis. There are limits to short course chemotherapy, and even expertly supervised treatment will not help the patient with DR-TB, if he or she is given drugs to which they are resistant. Yet, for years, patients who failed standard treatment and had a high probability of MDR-TB were given a sub-standard regimen of inferior drugs (Cat 2) for 8 months. Category 2 treatment adds a single new first line drug, streptomycin, to the 4 standard drugs. As Engels eloquently argues, the DOTS strategy may have directly contributed to

MDR-TB due to its continuing neglect of socio-cultural factors, the authoritative nature of direct supervision and the lack of co-operation with the private sector.

- *An unregulated private sector*: India has a huge and unregulated private health sector. 70% of hospitals are privately run and 76% of doctors engage in private practice. 50% of practicing doctors are of alternative faiths like homeopathy, Ayurveda, Unani, etc but would not hesitate to take on the initial management of these challenging cases, serving only to amplify resistance with poor prescriptions. A study we conducted in Dharavi, Asia's most densely populated slum in the heart of Mumbai, showed only 3% of the doctors practicing there were able to provide a correct prescription for a patient with MDR-TB. 35% of private practitioners added a single second line drug, usually a fluoroquinolone, to a failing regimen. Without doubt, the poor prescribing practice of Indian private practitioners helped fuel the MDR-TB crisis in this country.
- *Government related factors*: Many of India's health failings have arisen from policy failures, government callousness and bureaucratic myopia with MDR-TB being no exception. Failure of successive governments to grasp the scale and severity of India's MDR crisis have allowed it to escalate to its present desperate situation. Lack of funding and political will have also contributed. The situation is beginning to change and as of 2016, 32,914 MDR and 2475 XDR patients in larger centers had been commenced on treatment with second line drugs in the RNTCP. This is considerable progress and clearly a huge step in the right direction for these desperately ill patients, but the program must find the funds and resources to reach out to, and successfully treat, every MDR-TB patient across the country.
- *Patient related factors*: TB in India is shrouded in secrecy, denial, ignorance and ultimately ostracism. "Doctor shopping" is a peculiar Indian trait with the average urban Indian TB patient visiting 4 doctors before even commencing therapy. Indian TB patients switch doctors and systems of medicine with impunity and there is little continuity of care. These attitudes are borne out of ignorance. Compliance remains poor, with no more than a third of patients completing their treatment.
- *Social factors*: The harsh truth that TB is a social disease is glaringly brought to light in a country like India plagued with seemingly insurmountable social and economic problems. The facts speak for themselves: a population in excess of 1.3 billion, 46% below the poverty line. Childhood malnutrition rates of 47% and the highest infant mortality rates (46%) in the world. Despite this, successive Union budgets have allocated no more than 1% of GDP to health in the public sector over the years.
- *The HIV epidemic*: India now has among the highest absolute number of HIV cases in the world (around 5 million). Though the HIV prevalence in the general population remains steady at 1%, there has been an alarming speed of escalation in high risk populations. TB remains the commonest HIV related co-infection. A large dually infected population of TB-HIV patients is emerging, many with MDR-TB strains. This will pose an enormous added burden on overstretched RNTCP budgets. Whilst antiretroviral therapy is being provided in HIV centers, the government HIV and TB programs work in isolation and are not synchronized as they should be. Ignorance about HIV remains profound with several polls showing that only a small minority of Indian women of reproductive age had even heard of AIDS.
- *Comorbidities*: A number of comorbidities are recently gaining ground. Malnutrition, smoking, indoor and outdoor pollution and diabetes have recently been recognized as drivers of the TB epidemic. All thrive in India making it the perfect incubator for the creation and spread of MDR-TB.

Diabetes mellitus (DM) and TB deserves special mention. India is the diabetes capital of the world with a population of 69.2 million diabetics. There exists a strong epidemiological evidence base demonstrating the coexistence of TB and DM. DM increases the risk of developing TB by 2.5 to 3 fold. The association between a globally prevalent noncommunicable disease such as DM and a serious global infectious disease, TB, has resulted in the creation of a 'syndemic' necessitating urgent synergistic management if it is to be controlled. Globally, 15% of TB cases are associated with diabetes, and India and China account for more than 40% of these. In some states like Tamil Nadu the problem is especially manifest. In a survey by Vishwanathan from five random selected TB units in the state, around 25% of TB patients had DM, of which 9.3% were newly detected diabetics. In the light of these alarming trends, the WHO and the International Union against TB and Lung Disease propose the need for bidirectional screening and efficient comanagement of both diseases. Turning to MDR-TB and diabetes, numerous studies have identified a 2-9 fold increase in the risk of MDR-TB among patients with diabetes compared to normoglycemic individuals. A recent meta-analysis reported significantly higher odds of MDR-TB in patients with DM (OR = 1.71, 95% CI = 1.32; 2.22). The link between DM and TB (both drug sensitive and MDR) will make our efforts to vanquish TB even more difficult and there is real danger of this syndemic careening out of control unless it is tackled on a war footing.

■ TREATING MULTIDRUG-RESISTANT AND EXTENSIVELY DRUG-RESISTANT TUBERCULOSIS

"To tackle TB we need an equity plan that takes seriously the biosocial complexity of a lethal airborne infection that has stalked us for centuries".

—Keshavjee and Paul Farmer

Multidrug-resistant tuberculosis is extremely difficult to treat. It involves prolonged treatment for up to 24 months or longer with combinations of toxic drugs with debilitating side effects. None of the available drugs are backed by any evidence or RCTs, unlike the robust evidence supporting the current short course treatment of drug-sensitive TB. The drugs are expensive and cure rates across the globe, even under optimal conditions are in the vicinity of 60% for MDR-TB and around 405 for XDR-TB (**see Figs. 1 to 5**). High default rates, in the vicinity of 20%, are inevitable when a treatment is so toxic and so prolonged.

Principles of Treatment

The 10 principles outlined here, maximize the chance of successful outcome.

Principle 1: Plan your regimen based on a careful drug history, coupled with the drug susceptibility test (DST) report from a reliable, quality assured laboratory. Make use of the new generation of genetic tests like Xpert and Hain to quickly make an accurate diagnosis and to guide your initial empiric therapy. Treatment can be promptly started based on these tests whilst waiting for the complete DST which is usually available only 4–8 weeks later.

Principle 2: Include the right number of drugs. **Table 2** shows the available new drug grouping by the WHO. At least 4–6 new drugs to which the TB bacteria are sensitive should ideally be used. Too many drugs risks toxicity, while too few increases the risk of treatment failure.

Principle 3: Select drugs from the following groups when composing the regimen:

- Include any first line drug to which the patient is still sensitive, e.g. ethambutol or pyrazinamide. These should be included but not "counted" as one of the 4 new drugs.
- Use a Group A fluoroquinolone (FQ). Moxifloxacin is the preferred FQ. The exact doses are unclear but most experts would recommend 600 mg of moxifloxacin as the ideal dose. If levofloxacin is used, a dose of 750–1000 mg is the ideal dose.
- Use a Group B 2nd line injectable aminoglycoside to which the organism is sensitive. The injectable

Table 2: WHO classification of drugs for multidrug-resistant tuberculosis (MDR-TB).[1]

Group	Drug	Abbrev.
A. Fluoroquinolones[2]	Levofloxacin Moxifloxacin Gatifloxacin	Lfx Mfx Gfx
B. Second-line injectable agents	Amikacin Capreomycin Kanamycin (Streptomycin)[3]	Am Cm Km (S)
C. Other core second-line agents[2]	Ethionamide/Prothionamide Cycloserine/Terizidone Linezolid Clofazimine	Eto/Pto Cs/Trd Lzd Cfz
D. Add-on agents (not part of the core MDR-TB regimen)	D1 Pyrazinamide Ethambutol High-dose isoniazid	Z E Hh
	D2 Bedaquiline Delamanid	Bdq Dlm
	D3 Para-aminosalicylic acid Imipenem-cilastatin[4] Meropenem[4] Amoxicillin-clavulanate[4] (Thioacetazone)[5]	PAS Ipm Mpm Amz-Civ (T)

[1]This regrouping is intended to guide the design of conventional regimens; for shorter regimens lasting 9–12 months the composition is usually standardized (*see* WHO MDR-TB guidelines)
[2]Medicines in Groups A and C are shown by decreasing order of usual preference for use
[3]Refer to the WHO guidelines for the conditions under which streptomycin may substitute other injectable agents. Resistance to streptomycin alone does not qualify for the definition of extensively drug-resistant TB (XDR-TB)
[4]Carbapenems and clavulanate are meant to be used together; clavulanate is only available in formulations combined with amoxicillin
[5]HIV-status must be tested and confirmed to be negative before thioacetazone is started

Source: WHO, Geneva http://www.who.int/tb/MDRTBguidelines2016.pdf

should be used 5 days a week for at least 6–8 months.

- Add Group C and D3 drugs to make up the desired regimen depending on the disease burden and the pattern of resistance. These drugs include older bacteriostatic drugs like (cycloserine, ethionamide clofazamine and PAS) and newer drugs like linezolid. Clofazamine is an old but useful drug and should be part of almost all regimens. The WHO suggests use of ethionamide over PAS but local resistance patterns should be factored in. Linezolid is the most effective but also the most toxic drug in this group and must be used with great caution. Meropenem-clavulanate is the most expensive, and needs an IV port to be inserted for ease of administration. The new 2016 guidelines have dropped clarithromycin and amoxicillin/clavulanate as they are believed to have little or no antimycobacterial activity.
- Try and access the newer D2 drugs for highly resistant strains. Bedaqualine (Sirturo) and Delamanid (Deltyba®) are both difficult to access in India but potentially life saving drugs. Our Indian experience with these drugs will be discussed in a separate section.

Principle 4: Treat for the right duration. The current WHO recommendation for total duration of treatment stands at 22–24 months. Shorter regimens like the 9 month Bangladesh regimen will be discussed in more detail in a separate section.

Principle 5: Use the right doses at the highest end of the range to compensate for the inherent weakness of these drugs. Bear in mind that wrong doses contribute to treatment failure (under dosing) and toxicity and treatment interruption (over dosing). Therapeutic drug monitoring (TDM) is useful but available in no more than a handful of centers worldwide.

Principle 6: Treatment should be administered daily, there is no role for intermittent therapy here. Treatment should ideally be administered under close supervision (i.e. directly observed therapy). Regular cultures are necessary to monitor treatment efficacy.

Principle 7: Monitor closely for toxicity. These are highly toxic drugs and major adverse effects (including life threatening ones) are observed in as many as 40–60% of patients. These side effects must be carefully anticipated and patients carefully monitored.

Principle 8: Early surgery should be considered whenever feasible. Indeed, the more resistant the strain, the lower the threshold for surgery. The most experienced surgeon must be engaged and only patients with localized disease and enough respiratory reserve should be offered this often high-risk procedure.

Principle 9: Empathize, support and motivate your patient. This prolonged and toxic treatment will only succeed with patient-centric support from the treating physician. In the words of Julio Acha who ran the Peruvian program: '*we work with people, not with illnesses or mycobacteria*'.

Principle 10: Address the social determinants and comorbid conditions that accompany TB. Tuberculosis is a social disease and a holistic approach that attempts to improve the general levels of poverty, malnutrition, smoking, bio-mass exposure and diabetes that often co-exist is of vital importance.

Thus treating MDR and XDR Tb are amongst the most challenging problems in medicine but also the most gratifying.

Outcomes and predictors of success: A meta-analysis by Johnston looked at global outcomes from all published studies for MDR-TB. Pooled analysis of 36 studies showed only 62% of patients had successful outcomes. XDR-TB carries even worse outcomes with survival rates around 30%, and mortality even higher in those XDR-TB patients co-infected with HIV. The only 3 predictors of a successful outcome in this meta-analysis included; surgical intervention (OR 1.91), no prior treatment (OR 1.42), and retained fluoroquinolone sensitivity and use (OR 2.20). Other predictors of success or failure in different studies are summarized in **Table 3**.

Treating Multidrug-resistant Tuberculosis in the Private and Public Sectors in India

- *Private sector*: Applying the principles enumerated above to a cohort of Indian patients with MDR-TB in the private sector at the TB clinic of the Hinduja Hospital in Mumbai, we achieved respectable success rates of 64%. These figures are respectable considering these patients were treated under considerable financial constraints. All patients were given individualized treatment, on an ambulatory basis, based on DST where available.

Table 3: Predictors of outcome in MDR and XDR-TB.

Success	Failure
Use of PZA, ethambutol	Previous therapy
Use of quinolones	Number of drugs-resistant
Use of sensitive injectables	Cavitatory disease
Use of more than five drugs	Low BMI
Surgical resection possible	HIV
Noncavitatory disease	Poor adherence
Sputum conversion at 2 months	Positive cultures at 2 months

(BMI: Body mass index; HIV: Human immunodeficiency virus; MDR: Multidrug-resistant; PZA: Pyrazinamide; XDR-TB: Extensively drug-resistant tuberculosis)

- *Public program*: Programatic management of drug-resistant TB is the phrase preferred to DOTS-Plus for treating MDR-TB within the confines of the program. All patients receive a standardized six drug regimen called Category 4 for a period of 24 months. There is real worry in the mind of experts that just as the earlier effete Cat 2 treatment was proven to be worthless and eventually scrapped, the new Cat 4, by attempting the Procrustean crime of giving a standard set of drugs to all MDR-TB patients, irrespective of their resistance pattern, may end up further amplifying resistance. At least 60% of MDR-TB patients in Mumbai are fluoroquinolone resistant and using this, and other drugs to which these patients have been proven to be resistant may not be ideal practice. As Helen Bynum reminds us in her book *Spitting Blood*: "*MDR-TB poignantly illustrates an elementary principle in disease control: only very rarely does a one-size program fit all*". As of 2016, only 32,914 patients had been initiated on therapy. This is a start, but only represents a small drop in the sea of MDR-TB patients in the country. The RNTCP needs to recognize the urgency of getting more patients on appropriate treatment at the earliest. It goes without saying that it makes clinical, economic, epidemiological and moral sense to treat them now, rather than allow the situation to spiral. As Paul Farmer cogently argues: "*It is failure to treat, not treatment failure that is responsible for the vast majority of MDR-TB deaths*".

Drug Toxicities

Shean et al. in a recent publication, sombrely remind us of the major and occasionally life-threatening adverse effects (AE), that complicate the use of second line drugs in drug resistant TB. In their study from South Africa, AE's were encountered in 58% of their cohort of 115 patients. These included hearing loss, psychosis, depression, visual disturbance, renal failure. AEs were often severe, frequently interrupted therapy, and negatively impacted on treatment outcomes. There were 6 deaths directly due to an AE, 5 due to renal failure and 1 due to hypokalemia. All deaths were related to the use of capreomycin.

Drug Costs

There is no little doubt that MDR-TB enacts a tremendous financial burden on its unfortunate victims. These are often poor and marginalized patients anyway, and this is not just a disease of poverty but also results in poverty to the afflicted patient. A recent review of literature showed the cost of treating MDR-TB in high income countries averaged US$83,365. There is limited data from the developing world where the majority of patients are not insured and costs are usually borne out of pocket. In our cohort of patients treated at the Hinduja hospital, the total costs ranged from $1729 to $32,390 with a mean of $5723. The mean cost of XDR-TB was $8401. Drugs comprised the largest proportion of total costs at 37%. Almost 40% of patients incurred catastrophic costs, defined by WHO as more than 40% of the discretionary income.

Newer Drugs

The TB drug pipeline has moved at a glacially slow speed but after almost 40 years of expectant waiting, two new drugs have emerged after rifampicin. These are bedaqualine and delamanid.

Bedaquiline (BDQ): This drug received FDA approval on 31st December 2012. It belongs to a new class of drugs: a diarylquinoline which is a mycobacterial ATP synthase inhibitor. Initial Phase 2 studies showed that addition of BDQ to a standardized regimen led to a dramatic improvement in the proportion of patients who culture converted (48% vs 9%). The Phase 2b study by Diacon in 2014 showed cure rates were 58% in the BDQ group, compared to 32% in the placebo: a striking improvement. The recommended dose of BDQ is 400 mg daily for 2 weeks followed by 200 mg twice a week for 22 weeks. At present WHO only recommends it be used for only 6 months. The drug has a very long half life of 5.5 months. It is well tolerated but can cause QTc prolongation and hence needs meticulous ECG monitoring. The ITC interval must be below 450 ms before starting it and this interval should not exceed 500 ms whilst on treatment. Particular caution must be exercised when it is used with other drugs that increase QT interval like moxifloxacin and clofazamine. At present its use is restricted to adult patients over the age of 18 with pulmonary TB only. This is a moving goal post however and already, it has been safely used in pediatric patients. WHO recommends it be used in patients with MDR or XDR TB where an effective regimen of 4 drugs cannot be designed. However it is important to stress that the best optimal background regimen must also be in place, for even the best new TB drug will not work in isolation and must be part of a regimen. Mycobacteria always seems to inch ahead in the battle of resistance and cases of BDQ resistance are already being reported. In India, as of 2016, a paltry 100 patients had received BDQ on the compassionate use program. 40% of these were from our center at the Hinduja and we reported impressive 65% culture conversion rates even in these highly resistant patients who had run out of most therapeutic options. Apart from the compassionate use program, BDQ has also been made available through the RNTCP. To date only 567 patients have received the drug from the program. Sadly, this represents only a small fraction of all the Indian patients who could benefit from this life-saving drug. The program seems bent on following a restrictive policy, rationing out this precious drug to only a few, the perceived fear of developing resistance being more important in the policy makers minds than the certain death thousands of Indian XDR-TB patients face without it.

Globally, we were part of the large, observational study that was conducted by Borisov et al in 25 centers, and 15 countries in five continents. The results just published in 2017 showed that in the 428 patients who received BDQ as part of their regimen, sputum culture conversion rates were an excellent 91.2% at the end of 6 months. Overall success rates were 71.3% at the end of treatment. The drug was well tolerated, with adverse effects that required interruption of treatment in only 5.8% of patients. Thus global experience suggests that BDQ containing regimens achieve high conversion and success rates.

Recognizing the excellent efficacy and good safety profile of Bedaqualine, the new 2019 MDR-TB guidelines from the WHO have changed to exclude BDQ as a core Group A drug. The problem of course remains of one global access. The new 2019 grouping of medicines for MDR-TB have just been revised and the new recommendations are summarized in **Table 4**.

Delamanid (DLM): Delamanid, a nitro-dihydro-imidazooxazole derivative, is the other new antituberculosis medication currently available. It inhibits mycolic acid synthesis and has shown potent in vitro and in vivo activity against drug-resistant strains of *Mycobacterium tuberculosis*. In a multicenter RCT, 45% of patients who received DLM (100 mg twice daily) plus background drugs had sputum-culture conversion at 2 months, compared to 29% of patients who received a background drug regimen plus placebo (P = 0.008). Based on these results, DLM was approved for use in Europe and Japan in 2014. The recommended doses are 50 mg twice a day for 24 weeks for weight 20 kg to 34 kg; and 100 mg twice a day for 24 weeks for weight over 35 kg. The main side effects are headache, nausea and dizziness. QTc intervals may be prolonged by delaminid as well. WHO recommends that delamanid may be added to a WHO-recommended background regimen in adult patients with pulmonary MDR-TB (conditional recommendation) who have limited drug options. It should be used with caution in patients with HIV, and liver disease, and is contraindicated with QTc > 500 ms. DLM is marketed by Otsuka and is even more difficult to access than BDQ. As of September 2017, only 688 patients globally had received delaminid under programmatic conditions. To date only 51 Indian patients have used delaminid in India, that too on a compassionate use basis.

Table 4: Grouping of medicines recommended for use in longer MDR-TB regimens according to WHO (2019).		
Groups and steps	*Medicine*	
Group A: Include all three medicines	Levofloxacin or Moxifloxacin Bedaquiline Linezolid	Lfx Mfx Bdq Lzd
Group B: Add one or both medicines	Clofazimine Cycloserine or Terizidone	Cfz Cs Trd
Group C: Add to complete the regimen and when medicines from Groups A and B cannot be used	Ethambutol Delamanid Pyrazinamide Imipenem-cilastatin or Meropenem Amikacin (or Streptomycin) Ethionamide or Prothionamide *p*-aminosalicylic acid	E Dlm Z Ipm-Cln Mpm Am (S) Eto Pto PAS

Otsuka has yet to launch Delaminid in India despite getting a patent in 2011. The company has now licensed Mylan to market the drug in India and South Africa. A conditional access program plans to enrol 400 patients on delaminid in India shortly.

Bedaquiline and delamanid in combination: Although the WHO does not currently recommend the combined use of BDQ and DLM, it is possible that these two new potent drugs would be used in tandem as part of future regimens. We have published our results on BDQ and DLM in combination in two Indian patients and reported the combination to be safe and well tolerated.

Bangladesh short-course regimen: It is the only combination regimen that has been through multiple clinical trials. In May 2016, the WHO conditionally recommending this short course regimen for a period of 9–12 months for pulmonary MDR-TB under programmatic conditions, and it is currently already in use in some parts of the world. Although it does not include any new drugs, it's chief advantage is that at 9 months duration, it is shorter than the current standard 2 year regimen. Van Deun laid the groundwork for this regimen with a pivotal initial study in a cohort of 206 patients in Bangladesh. He demonstrated an overall success rate of 87.9%, at a fraction of the cost of traditional regimens (only € 225/course). The regimen was subsequently tested in 507 adult MDR-TB patients in nine African countries with similar, promising outcomes. Currently being used in 23 countries with good success, the Bangladesh regimen comprises of 4–6 months of a later generation fluoroquinolone, kanamycin, prothionamide, high dose isoniazid, clofazamine, pyrazinamide, and ethambutol, followed by 5 months of the fluoroquinolone, clofazamine, pyrazinamide and ethambutol alone. Because of limited global capacity for drug susceptibility testing (DST), WHO does not require that DST for 2nd line drugs be performed prior to starting this short course regimen. Instead it allows the use of treatment history and local surveillance data to guide eligibility for this regimen. Unfortunately, in countries where second line drugs have freely been used outside programmatic conditions, and those with high rates of more extensive patterns of drug resistance, this regimen would not be expected to work and indeed cannot be recommended. There have been several studies from various high prevalence MDR countries suggesting that short course regimen will do limited good in these settings because of the more extreme

Table 5: New drug combinations currently at trial stage.
• STAND: Pretomanid-Moxi-PZA
• STREAM Stage 2: BDQ to replace kanamycin in all oral Bangladesh regimen:
– *NC-005:* Pretomanid-BDQ (Phase 2)
• NIX-TB: Pretomanid-BDQ (Phase 3)
• OPTI-Q: Phase 2
• NEXT: BDQ plus oral OBT (Phase 3)
• ENDTB-Q: BDQ-DLM-OBT (Phase 3):
– *PHOENIX:* DLM versus INH in contacts of MDR patients

(BDQ: Bedaquiline; DLM: Delamanid; INH: Isoniazid; MDR: Multidrug-resistant; OBT: Optimized background therapy; PZA: Pyrazinamide)

patterns of resistance encountered. The available data shows that no more than 4%–50% of patients in some MDR hotspots like Eastern Europe, India, Indonesia, Pakistan and Brazil are likely to be eligible for this regimen. Hence clearly there is need for novel regimens comprising of new and repurposed drugs. Many exciting new trials **(Table 5)** are already underway, with preliminary data expected by 2019. It is not inconceivable that these new, all oral regimens will one day consign the current injectable regimens to the history books.

■ SUGGESTED READING

1. Borisov SE, Dheda K, Enwerem M, et al. Effectiveness and safety of bedaqualine containing regimens in the treatment of MDR and XDR-TB: a multicentre study. Eur Respir J. 2017;49:1700387.
2. Diacon AH, Pym A, Grobusch MP, et al. Multidrug-resistant tuberculosis and culture conversion with bedaquiline. New Engl J Med. 2014;371:723-32.
3. Gler MT, Skripconoca V, Sanchez-Garavito E, et al. Delaminid for multi-drug resistant pulmonary tuberculosis. N Engl J Med. 2012;366:2151-60.
4. Global Tuberculosis Report. 2017 WHO.
5. Johnston JC, Shahidi NC, Sadatsafai M, et al. Treatment outcomes of MDR-TB: a systematic review and meta-analysis. PLOS One Sept 9, 2009.
6. Maryandyshev A, Pontali E, Tiberi S, et al. Bedaquiline and delamanid combination treatment of 5 patients with pulmonary extensively drug-resistant tuberculosis. Emerg Infect Dis. 2017.
7. Shean K, Streicher E, Petersen E, et al. Drug-associated adverse effects and their relationship with outcomes in patients receiving treatment for extensively drug-resistant tuberculosis in South Africa. PLOS One May 7, 2013.
8. Udwadia ZF. Drug-resistant TB: 10 principles of effective management. In Lets Talk TB. Series Editor, Madhu Pai, 3rd edition 2107.

9. Udwadia ZF. MDR, XDR, TDR tuberculosis: ominous progression. Thorax. 2012.

10. Udwadia ZF, Amale RA, Ajbani KK, et al. Totally drug-resistant tuberculosis in India. Clin Infect Dis. 2012;54:579-81.

11. Udwadia ZF, Ganatra SR, Mullerpattan JB. Compassionate use of bedaquiline in highly drug-resistant tuberculosis patients in Mumbai, India. Eur Respir J. 2017;49(3) pii:1601699.

12. Udwadia ZF, Moharil G. Multidrug-resistant tuberculosis treatment in the private sector: results from a tertiary referral private hospital in Mumbai. Lung India. 2014;31:336-41.

13. Udwadia ZF, Pinto LM, Uplekar MW. Tuberculosis management by private practitioners in Mumbai, India: has anything changed in two decades? PLOS One. 2010:5;e12023.

14. Van Deun A, Maug AK, Salim MA, et al. Short, highly effective, and inexpensive standardized treatment of multidrug-resistant tuberculosis. Am J Respir Crit Care Med. 2010;182(5):684-92.

CHAPTER 17

HIV-TB Coinfection

■ INTRODUCTION

One of the reasons for the great increase in the incidence of tuberculosis (TB) over the last 2 decades is because of the impact of human immunodeficiency virus (HIV). Of the world's population of 6 billion, a third (2 billion) people are latently affected by tuberculosis (TB) and around 40 million are HIV-infected. About 15 million, globally, are HIV-TB dually infected; 70% of these reside in Africa and 20% in South East Asia. India which has long housed the world's largest TB population now has the dubious distinction of the largest TB-HIV dually infected population as well. The overlapping epidemics of TB and HIV have had disastrous consequences: about 10% of all TB globally is attributable to HIV and 12% of all the 2 million TB deaths were attributed to HIV.

In 1983, the initial cases of TB in Haitians first came to attention. Then, for the first time, in 1985, the usual annual steady decline (around 5%) in TB incidence in the United States (US) reduced to just 0.2% and then actually increased by 2.6% in 1986, the first time in 35 years that this trend had reversed. This was clear epidemiological evidence of a catastrophe ahead. In the decade that followed dramatic increases in TB incidence were noted in several sub-Saharan countries, especially those with the highest HIV prevalence. In the 1990s, reported TB cases went up by 87% in Tanzania, 140% in Burundi, 154% in Zambia, and an unprecedented 180% in Malawi. This prompted the Centers for Disease Control and Prevention (CDC) to list pulmonary TB as an acquired immunodeficiency syndrome (AIDS)-defining opportunistic infection (OI) in 1993 (extrapulmonary TB had been recognized as AIDS-defining in 1987).

■ IMPORTANCE OF THE LINK

- TB is the earliest HIV-related infection, occurring at CD4 counts averaging around 300/μL.
- TB is also, globally, the most common HIV-related OI.
- TB is the most common cause of mortality in HIV. Globally about a third of all AIDS deaths are due to TB. An autopsy study in Cote d'Ivoire detected TB in 54% of all autopsies.
- TB is the only OI that is transmissible. This has great public health significance in crowded HIV clinics in the developing world.
- HIV patients are more vulnerable to multidrug-resistant (MDR) and extensively drug-resistant (XDR)-TB and have much higher mortality than their counterparts who are seronegative.
- Despite this, with early diagnosis and prompt initiation of treatment, the majority of these patients (especially those with sensitive strains) can be cured.
- TB is preventable in HIV-positive populations and the important role of isoniazid preventive therapy will be discussed later.
- Finally, TB accelerates the course of HIV.

The link between TB and HIV is strong and bidirectional. It is estimated that around 5–10% of HIV patients in the Western world will develop TB at some stage of their illness. In contrast, in Africa, India and South East Asia where large numbers of the population are latently affected, it is estimated that up to 75% of the HIV-positive population will go on to develop TB disease in the course of their HIV.

Looked at from the other side of the coin, the prevalence of HIV in the TB population of a country is also important. It is estimated that 9% and 12% of all TB patients in Mumbai and Manipur, respectively were HIV-positive.

Corresponding estimates for other countries are that 4% of all TB patients in the United Kingdom (UK), 8% in the United States (US), 66% in Uganda, and 81% in Rwanda are HIV-positive.

It would be a missed opportunity not to check the HIV status in all newly diagnosed patients with TB. Sadly, countywide, World Health Organization (WHO) estimates that as recently as 2007, less than 5% of all TB patients in India were being screened for HIV.

Degree of Risk from HIV

Human immunodeficiency virus (HIV) has emerged as the single most important risk factor for converting latent TB to active disease. The relative risk (RR) from HIV is 100–170, thus dwarfing the risk from more traditional factors like diabetes (2–4), hemodialysis (10), immunosuppressive treatment (12) and silicosis (30).

While the risk of latent TB activating in an immunocompetent person is no more than 10% per lifetime, in an HIV-positive individual that risk increases to 10% per year.

Mechanism of the synergy between TB and HIV: CD4-positive T-cells producing gamma interferon play a central role in the defense against TB. Interferon gamma activates macrophages to inhibit intracellular growth of *Mycobacterium tuberculosis (M. tuberculosis)*. HIV causes selective depletion of the very same T-cells, thus decreasing the capacity of these cells to produce gamma interferon. Thus HIV markedly increases TB risk. At the cellular level elegant studies have shown that peripheral lymphocytes from HIV-positive patients with TB produce less gamma interferon compared with lymphocytes from HIV-negative patients with TB. Thus, reduced T1 responses in patients with HIV contribute to their susceptibility to TB. Tuberculosis also has a negative impact on HIV; enhancing local HIV replication in the lung. This may help explain the reduced survival of those dually infected with HIV and TB.

Diagnosis

TB is much more difficult to diagnose in the HIV-positive individual for reasons that will be elaborated: The tuberculin test is often falsely negative in the face of anergy and hence loses its value. Reactivity may be maintained in the early stages but declines as the CD4 count goes down and anergy sets in. The Centers for Disease Control and Prevention (CDC) recommends a 5 mm reaction after 5-TU as a positive reaction in an HIV-positive individual while others have recommended a 2 mm reaction or even a two-stage (boosted) test in these patients. The tuberculin test retains a vital role, and should be routinely done in all HIV-positive individuals, because a recent meta-analysis showed that those with a positive skin test had a 60% reduction in the incidence of TB when given preventive isoniazid therapy while this strategy was of no value in those who were tuberculin-negative. The newer interferon-gamma release assays (IGRAs) may retain their sensitivity in the HIV-positive population but more work is needed to determine their role in these patients. Of the two commercially available IGRAs, the ELISPOT is more accurate than the Quanti Gold in this patient population and is the preferred test.

Sputum microbiology is often negative in HIV-positive patients with TB. A study reported in the Lancet showed that almost 40–70% of all TB is smear-negative in the HIV-positive population. Thus, there is often a considerable diagnostic delay, and, if the clinical suspicion of TB is high, these patients should be commenced on empiric anti-TB therapy. Indeed, because HIV-TB is often paucibacillary and extrapulmonary, cultures from diverse sites like urine, blood, bone marrow, and gland aspirates are more likely to be positive than sputum.

Clinical Features

Early literature was replete with the so-called atypical features in patients with HIV who develop TB. We now know that the spectrum of clinical and radiological findings is no different from seronegative TB patients. The manifestations depend on the level of immuno-suppression, i.e. the CD4 load. Typical manifestations occur when the CD4 count is preserved, but as this drops so-called "atypical" manifestations are noted. Atypical findings in advanced HIV include lower lobe infiltrates, the absence of cavitation and more focal or nodular con-solidation. Normal X-rays may be seen in 7–14% of patients with TB and HIV hence a high index of suspicion is needed. Symptoms and signs cannot on their own distinguish TB from other OIs in the HIV-positive setting but note must be made of two clinical pointers: a prolonged fever [pyrexia of unknown origin (PUO)] and excessive weight loss (>11 kg). While both these are nonspecific and can occur because of other OIs and HIV itself, TB remains the most common cause of PUO in the HIV-infected.

Extrapulmonary TB is more common than pulmonary TB in the HIV-positive setting (odds ratio 2:3). This most frequently takes the form of glandular TB, though pleural effusions and ascites can also occur.

Timing of TB in HIV: Because of the virulence of TB, it can occur at any time in the course of HIV but often occurs early. It precedes other OIs by a few months to years and is often AIDS-defining. It occurs at a higher CD4 count (around 300–350) in most series. In a large Indian cohort of 594 HIV-positive patients followed up over 5 years by Kumarasamy in 2003, pulmonary TB was the most common AIDS-defining illness (50% of all cases). It occurred at a lower median CD4 count of 111/μL and was independently associated with a higher risk of death (OR 3.52).

Treating TB in the HIV-positive Patient

Treating patients who are dually infected is a complicated task. On the positive side, treating these patients with anti-TB therapy results in improvement in symptoms, radiology and sputum clearance, all at the same rate as in the HIV-negative TB patient.

Treatment can be divided into (A) treating the TB and (B) treating the HIV:

(A) *TB treatment*: TB treatment must get precedence over HIV treatment. The drugs and regimen used to treat TB are no different in the HIV-positive from the HIV-negative patient. Standard short-course chemotherapy is used (HREZ) with all drugs being administered daily [ideally, under (directly observed treatment, short course) DOTS], there being no role for intermittent treatment in the context of HIV. The duration of treatment is a controversial issue. Both the American Thoracic Society (ATS) and the CDC recommend the standard duration of treatment (6 months), though the CDC guidelines recommend prolongation of treatment to 9 months in those with slow clinical or bacteriological response. A single study from Zaire showed that relapse rate could be reduced from 9% to 6% if duration of treatment was prolonged from 6 months to a year but even in this study, prolonging the treatment did not translate into improved survival. Hence, at present, 6 months remains the accepted duration of treatment. It must be remembered that significant numbers of patients labeled "relapses", may in reality be "reinfections", and molecular studies will be the way to distinguish these two categories from each other.

Thus, the TB paradox is that despite a number of studies having demonstrated the efficacy of the standard regimen for treating HIV-positive TB patients based on sputum conversion, resolution of radiographic abnormalities and time to clinical improvement, it has been consistently shown that coinfected patients have higher mortality rates. In several studies of TB-HIV coinfected patients from Africa, the risk of dying despite being on anti-TB treatment is 3- to 26-fold higher in the TB-HIV coinfected compared to TB patients who are not HIV-coinfected. A study in South African miners, which was the first to include autopsy data, showed that much of this excess mortality was from nontuberculous AIDS-related conditions. This emphasizes the pivotal role of antiretrovirals (ARVs) in treating TB-HIV coinfected patients and makes a compelling case for their early introduction. Malabsorption of TB drugs must be considered in patients with HIV-related diarrhea and monitoring of drug levels is ideally recommended in this setting. Drug toxicities, drug interactions, and paradoxical reactions will be discussed later.

(B) *HIV treatment*: There is no doubt that antiretroviral therapy (ART) has had a huge impact on survival in the TB-HIV coinfected patient. Controversy has raged on exactly when it should be introduced. Most experts feel that if the patient has a reasonably well preserved CD4 count, ART should be introduced after a delay of a few months of starting the anti-TB drugs. On the other hand, if the patient has a low CD4 count every attempt should be made to introduce ART earlier, even within 2 weeks of starting anti-TB drugs. A study in 2010 from South Africa by Abdool Karim in the *New England Journal of Medicine* attempted to solve this issue. The authors showed that starting ART after completing the intensive phase significantly improved survival compared to commencing ART after completing anti-TB treatment.

Before starting ART, the physician should have a clear knowledge of the drug interactions between rifampicin and most of the PIs (protease inhibitors) and NNRTIs (non-nucleoside reverse transcriptase inhibitors).

Sadly, in India, according to the latest WHO estimates, only 2% of all the HIV-TB cases in the country in 2007 received ART.

(C) *Role of cotrimoxazole prophylaxis therapy (CPT)*: Every HIV-TB patient must be commenced on CPT with a daily trimethoprim-sulfamethoxazole tablet. This simple intervention significantly reduced the risk of death by as much as 46% in an African cohort of HIV-TB patients. This cheap and simple drug is greatly underutilized in the Indian context. Latest WHO estimates are that only 8% of HIV-positive TB cases received CPT in 2007.

(D) Finally, isoniazid retains a vital role as primary prophylaxis in patients who are HIV-positive and have a positive tuberculin skin test. It is crucial to rule out active disease before offering isoniazid prophylaxis. This may be difficult as chest radiographs may be normal and sputum may not be produced. Once active disease has been excluded, isoniazid prophylaxis should be offered as this simple intervention has been shown to reduce the rate of reactivation of tuberculosis by almost 70%. Sadly, implementation is limited in the developing world by logistic deficiencies and poor health infrastructure.

(E) *Antiretroviral therapy (ART) as a means for control of TB in the HIV population*: A number of observational cohort studies (12 in all), from countries across the globe, have demonstrated that the use of triple-drug ART is associated with a 50–92% reduction in TB incidence rates and a halving of the risk of TB recurrence. Most of this benefit occurs in the first 2 years of ART, the benefits being seen across a broad range of immunosuppression although the absolute reduction in TB rates is greatest in those with advanced HIV infection. Mathematical modeling suggests that if ART was implemented with high population coverage, at higher CD4 counts than currently used, it could have a significant impact on TB control at the community level.

Treatment-related Problems

The following problems must be anticipated on treatment:

- *Increased incidence of drug toxicity*: This includes more frequent hepatitis and peripheral neuropathy secondary to rifampicin and isoniazid, respectively and potentially fatal Stevens Johnson syndrome in patients who receive thiacetazone. This drug, which is still commonly used in Africa, though rarely in India, must therefore never be used in the HIV-positive patient. A recent study showed that 34% of patients receiving both TB treatment and ART had to interrupt or discontinue their therapy because of drug-related toxicity.

- *Overlapping toxicity*: The overlapping toxicity of ART and anti-TB drugs makes it difficult to ascertain, which drug has caused the side-effect in question. For example, when hepatitis occurs, it can be caused not just by isoniazid, rifampicin or pyrazinamide but also with nevirapine. Drug rashes can be due to any of the anti-TB drugs but equally secondary to nevirapine, efavirenz, or abacavir.

- *Drug interactions*: Complex drug interactions occur in patients on anti-TB drugs and ART. All the PIs and some of the NNRTIs interact with rifampicin. The mechanism of this interaction is due to rifampicin being a potent inhibitor of the cytochrome P450-3A (CYPA) system. Thus, when rifampicin is coadministered with PIs the consequence of this interaction is high levels of rifampicin (thus increasing the risk of rifampicin toxicity) and low levels of the PIs (thus reducing their efficacy). In fact when coadministered, the levels of all the commonly used PIs drop by almost 80–90% (except for ritonavir), thus compromising the efficacy of the ART regimen. This can be overcome, if a PI must be used, by substituting rifampicin with rifabutin, which is a less potent inhibitor of the CYPA system. Alternatively, it is best to use a non-PI-based regimen. Efavirenz has almost no interaction with rifampicin and hence this drug is to be favored over the PIs when rifampicin is coprescribed.

- *Paradoxical reactions*: These are defined as transient worsening or appearance of new symptoms, signs, or radiographic manifestations of TB occurring after initiation of treatment. They are more correctly referred to as immune reconstitution and inflammation syndrome (IRIS). It is important to distinguish a paradoxical reaction from treatment failure, drug-resistant TB, or a second/new OI. The clinical manifestations of IRIS may be as subtle as a persistent fever or new onset and rapidly expanding adenopathy or brain lesions, which can sometimes prove life-threatening. They occur in about 36% of HIV-positives on anti-TB therapy plus ART as opposed to 7% on anti-TB treatment alone. Most occur within days to weeks of starting ART. The association between a shorter delay between TB treatment initiation and ART initiation is an area of debate. While some investigators have found no difference in time from TB therapy to initiation of ART between IRIS and non-IRIS subjects, others have reported significant differences between the groups, with IRIS generally occurring more often in subjects started on ART within 2 months of TB therapy initiation. In a recent study of 43 cases of *M. tuberculosis-associated* IRIS, the median onset of IRIS was 12–15 days with only four of these cases occurring more than 4 weeks after initiation of ART. They are more common and severe with increasing levels of immunosuppression and are thus more frequently seen when the CD4 count is low and the HIV RNA (ribonucleic acid) viral load is high. Other factors known to predispose HIV-positive patients in general to IRIS include: male sex, younger age, and more rapid fall in viral load on ART. The frequency of IRIS has not been shown to be related to the type of antiviral used. In Gazzard's series of 55 patients with TB-HIV IRIS, patients who developed IRIS were more likely to present with disseminated TB, have a CD4 count less than 100 cells/mm^3 and have a prompt rise in CD4 count in the initial 3 months of highly active antiretroviral therapy (HAART).

Types of Immune Reconstitution and Inflammation Syndrome

Two types of IRIS are recognized in TB-HIV. The first is paradoxical TB-IRIS. This form occurs in patients whose TB has already been diagnosed and is already on anti-TB treatment prior to commencement of ART. In these patients, there is a paradoxical worsening of TB or TB occurring at a different site usually within 3 months of starting ART.

The second type of IRIS is called unmasking TB-IRIS. This form occurs in patients not on TB treatment prior to starting ART **(Fig. 1)**. Active TB develops within 3 months of starting ART. A significant proportion of these cases are those who had preexisting TB, which had not been correctly diagnosed prior to starting ART because of the poor sensitivity of sputum smear and chest radiography in diagnosing TB in these patients.

Mechanism of Immune Reconstitution and Inflammation Syndrome

The mechanism is believed to be restoration of immunity toward mycobacterial antigen. After initiating ART, the CD4+ T lymphocyte count rises rapidly in the 1st month. This represents redistribution of memory cells from sites of immune activation, followed by a more gradual recovery of naive cells. Interestingly, the tuberculin skin test may turn from negative to positive again, evidence of improved CD4 number and function. Subsequent work showed purified protein derivative (PPD)-specific TH1 expansions as the cause of TB-IRIS. Treatment options include careful observation and symptomatic treatment in milder cases to administration of steroids in severe cases.

Interruption of ART is rarely necessary but could be considered in life-threatening cases. Repeated aspiration may be needed for rapidly expanding lymph node masses. **Table 1** gives features suggestive of immune reconstitution inflammatory syndrome in patients infected with *Mycobacterium tuberculosis*.

Table 2 gives the conditions to be considered in the differential diagnosis of IRIS.

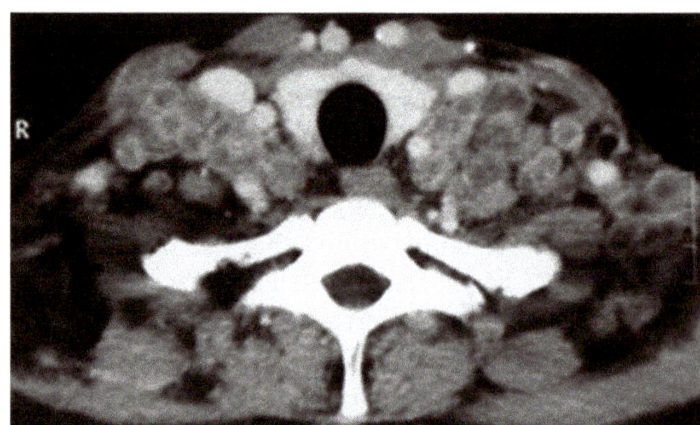

Fig. 1: Immune reconstitution and inflammation syndrome (IRIS). Recently diagnosed seropositive patient started on highly active antiretroviral therapy (HAART) developed large necrotic adenopathy in the neck. This was proven to be due to TB on a fine-needle aspiration cytology (FNAC).

Table 1: Features of immune reconstitution and inflammation syndrome (IRIS).

- Development of new features of the disease or exacerbation of the disease after starting highly active antiretroviral therapy (HAART):
  - New or exacerbation of an already present pulmonary lesion with or without increasing cough, dyspnea
  - New or worsening radiological features of the disease
  - Fresh lymphadenopathy; or worsening of lymphadenopathy already present; cold abscesses
  - New or worsening central nervous system (CNS) disease
  - New or worsening systemic features such as fever, anemia, weight loss, and prostration
- *Immune restoration*: A rise in the CD4 count after HAART
- A fall in the HIV viral load while on HAART

Table 2: Differential diagnosis of IRIS.

- Progression of underlying disease
- Multidrug-resistant (MDR) or extensively drug-resistant (XDR)-TB
- Poor compliance with prescribed anti-TB drugs
- Drug reactions
- Association of TB with another OI (e.g. viral, fungal)
- Association of TB with a malignant disease, e.g. non-Hodgkin's lymphoma
- Association of TB with a nonmalignant, noninfective lung pathology

■ SUGGESTED READING

1. Getahun H, Gunneberg C, Granich R, et al. HIV infection-associated tuberculosis: the epidemiology and the response. Clin Infect Dis. 2010;50(3):201-7.
2. Goldfeld A, Ellner JJ. Pathogenesis and management of HIV/TB coinfection in Asia. Tuberculosis (Edinb). 2007;87(1):26-30.
3. Gunneberg C, Reid A, Williams BG, et al. Global monitoring of collaborative TB-HIV activities. Int J Tuberc Lung Dis. 2008;12(1):2-7.
4. Keshinro B, Diul MY. HIV-TB: epidemiology, clinical features and diagnosis of smear-negative TB. Trop Doct. 2006;36(2):68-71.
5. Michailidis C, Pozniak AL, Mandalia S, et al. Clinical characteristics of IRIS syndrome in patients with HIV and tuberculosis. Antivir Ther. 2005;10(3):417-22.
6. Nunn P, Williams B, Floyd K, et al. Tuberculosis control in the era of HIV. Nat Rev Immunol. 2005;5(10): 819-26.

CHAPTER 18

Novel Technologies for TB Diagnosis

Why does an accurate diagnosis matter?

The average tuberculosis (TB) patient is diagnosed after a delay of 2 months and sees an average of three healthcare providers before he or she commences treatment. For a patient with multidrug resistant-tuberculosis (MDR-TB), the delay is even longer averaging 6 months from the first cough to the time appropriate treatment is actually commenced. Accurate and speedy diagnosis is hugely important, not just for the individual patient, but also to reduce TB transmission and spread in the community.

■ NOVEL TECHNOLOGIES FOR TB DIAGNOSIS

The limitations of our current set of tests are apparent and have been discussed earlier. Indeed, these limitations have been exposed by the HIV epidemic and by the emergence of MDR and extensively drug-resistant tuberculosis (XDR-TB). We continue to rely on three antiquated tests: (1) sputum microscopy, (2) chest radiography and (3) the tuberculin skin test which will collectively miss up to 50% of all cases with tuberculosis.

In the past few years there has been resurgence in interest in developing new and modern tools for the diagnosis of TB. Thus, groups like Foundation for Innovative New Diagnostics (FIND), Global Laboratory Initiative (GLI), and World Health Organization (WHO) have made the development of new diagnostics as their priority. Funds from these ventures have come from the Bill and Melinda Gates Foundation, the Global Fund to Fight AIDS, TB and Malaria (GFATM) and UNITAID. With this influx of funding and political will, it is estimated that the world now spends a total of US$ 1 billion on TB diagnostics annually. No chapter on TB would be complete without a mention of some of these new tests:

1. *Optimized smear microscopy*: Staining is traditionally done using Ziehl-Neelsen stain. This serves as a rapid and inexpensive screen for AFB. The current WHO guidelines recommend performing only two AFB smears instead of three as the incremental yield of the third is low. The overall clinical sensitivity of sputum AFB smear is 22–88% depending on the burden of mycobacteria and the experience of the technician. Besides, AFB smears are not specific for MTB. A preferred alternative is fluorescent staining which consists of a mix of auramine O and rhodamine B dyes. This method is more sensitive and allows more rapid reading of slides and is hence endorsed by WHO with the recommendation that conventional ZN stains be phased out globally. Despite this long standing recommendation, only 7% of labs worldwide had the capability of performing fluorescent staining using light-emitting diode (LED) microscopes. A few points on specimen collection would be appropriate at this stage. Though respiratory specimens (sputum and BAL) are most commonly sent for testing for mycobacteria, virtually any type of specimen can be sent for analysis. Specimens should be collected in sterile, leak-proof containers and do not need special transport media. Tissue should be placed in a small amount of sterile saline to avoid dehydration. Specimens should be ideally be refrigerated during transport to the laboratory to prevent overgrowth of contaminating bacteria. Mycobacteria become more concentrated in the sputum as patients sleep so smear sensitivity increases with the use of early morning sputum. Early morning collection also provides the

best yield for urine samples as organisms collect in the bladder overnight. Normally sterile body fluids such as cerebrospinal fluid, pleural fluid, pericardial and synovial fluid are paucibacillary and may require processing additional volume to achieve adequate sensitivity. Swabs are to be discouraged as they only transfer a minimal volume of specimen onto culture media.

2. *Improved and newer culture methods*: Liquid culture systems such as the BD BACTEC™ MGIT™ (mycobacterial growth indicator tube) system and the fluorescent BACTEC 9000 are currently considered the gold standard for isolating mycobacteria. Both use an O_2-quenched fluorescent dye and measure increasing fluorescence as O_2 is depleted. Both are fully automated systems. Several meta-analyses have shown that these liquid systems are more sensitive for detection of mycobacteria and increase the case yield by at least 10% compared to the traditional media. Another huge advantage is that they reduce the delays in obtaining results to days rather than weeks. Finally, the same samples can be used to monitor drug sensitivity testing (DST) once a positive result is obtained, thus greatly reducing the time required to provide this information to around 10 days compared to 4 weeks for conventional culture. Having said this, it must be remembered that they are more expensive, require greater investment, and are prone to contamination. They require stringent quality assurance systems and training standards. The current WHO policy is to recommend them as a part of a country-specific plan for strengthening laboratory capacity. Sadly, there are less than 40 installations of the BACTEC system throughout the country. The high initial investment (₹20 lakhs) and the higher cost of each culture [₹475 per patient vs ₹40 for Löwenstein-Jensen (LJ) medium] is probably a deterrent. Other concerns about the BACTEC system include the need for syringe and needle for inoculation and the use of radiolabeled products and their eventual safe disposal.

At our Level 2 mycobacterial laboratory at the Hinduja Hospital we have introduced the BACTEC system in 1998 and Rodriguez has recently published her experience with this system in a large and busy reference laboratory. Of the 12,726 specimens sent to the laboratory over 6 years, the overall recovery rate was 39% for the BACTEC system and 29% for the LJ medium. Thus the BACTEC system detected a total of 1,455 (11.4%) additional positive cultures which is statistically highly significant. The average detection time for the BACTEC 460 system was also much faster at 13.3 days versus 31.2 for the LJ medium. The average reporting time for drug susceptibility results was just 6–10 days for the BACTEC system, a huge advantage for the physician keen to begin an individualized treatment regimen in an ill patient with suspected MDR-TB. More recently, our laboratory has begun using the automated MGIT 960 system which has a number of advantages over the BACTEC 460 system. Rodrigues showed that the use of this system also greatly increased the rate of TB cultures. Of 6,413 isolates positive for *M. tuberculosis* (MTB), 41% were positive by MGIT and just 24% by the conventional LJ medium. The mean turnaround time for mycobacterial growth in smear-positive specimens was 9 days for smear-positive and 16 days for smear-negative specimens. The MGIT 960 TB system involves even greater initial investment than the BACTEC 460 (almost ₹3.5 million) but a few sentinel referral centers could clearly use this new technology to great advantage. Higher culture rates and quicker result times are priceless for the individual patient and the physician struggling to treat these patients with resistant TB.

3. *Phage amplification assays*: These have high specificity but lower and variable sensitivity. The prototype is the FAST plaque TB assay which has been field-tested in several parts of the developing world and is attracting great attention as a possible, cheaper alternative to automated systems in the developing world.

4. *Molecular tests*: A new generation of molecular tests have revolutionized TB diagnostics. These can be done from A) Culture growth or B) Directly from patient specimens.

   – *Molecular diagnostics from culture growth*: Confirming the growth of MTB in culture is important for the proper clinical management of tuberculosis cases. There are several molecular techniques currently employed by labs to identify isolates from culture. These will be summarized here:

     • *Nucleic acid hybridization probes*: Food and Drug Administration (FDA) cleared hybridization probes are available from companies for the identification of *M. tuberculosis* complex, *M avium* complex, *M. gordonae* and *M. kansasii*. These culture hybridization probes are highly sensitive and specific and provide results within two hours. The main limitation associated with hybridization probes is that they are only available for four mycobacterial species or complexes.

- *Line probe assays (LPA)*: LPAs are an alternative technique for identification of mycobacteria from culture isolates that make use of hybridization based probes. This technology uses nitrocellulose membrane strips embedded with genus and species specific probes. The most widely used is the GenoType MTBC test from Hain Lifescience. Analytics sensitivity and specificity are generally > 90% for LPAs with results available within 6 hours.
- *MALDI-TOF MS (Matrix Assisted Laser Desorption/Ionization—Time of Flight Mass Spectrometry)*: Maldi-TOF mass spectrometry is a new technology that has recently been applied to identification of mycobacteria. This technique utilizes mass spectrometry to assess the protein content of an isolate for identification. Several studies have documented the accurate identification of mycobacteria species by MALDI-TOF.
- *Whole genome sequencing (WGS)*: Traditional Sanger dideoxy sequencing remains the gold standard for the identification of mycobacteria species. Amplified DNA is sequenced and results compared to established sequence databases. The turn around time is generally 24 hours but this is a labor intensive process that requires a skilled lab and trained technicians. Sequencing is often performed if less expensive and more rapid methods such as hybridization probes and MALDI-TOF fail to produce definitive results. WGS is the gold standard in mapping outbreaks and has tremendous public health utility. Numerous studies confirm that WGS represents a significant advance over previous genotyping methods such as MIRU-VNTR and restriction fragment length polymorphism (RFLP).

– Molecular diagnostics directly from patient specimens:
  - *Xpert MTB/rifampicin (RIF)*: This is a nucleic acid amplification test that has revolutionized the speed and accuracy with which TB and MDR-TB is diagnosed. This is an automated, cartridge based real-time PCR based assay with molecular beacons. It is the most widely validated of the new generation of genotypic tests for TB and hence will be discussed in some detail. The Xpert MTB/RIF does two things concurrently and rapidly: detects TB with high sensitivity and specificity, and detects rifampicin resistance. This test has a number of advantages. It gives a result in about 90 minutes. It is fully automated thus ensuring accuracy and reliability. It is easy for a technician to learn (approximately 2 days training time, opposed to 2 weeks for microscopy), and its sealed disposable cartridge system ensures safety with no special biosafety equipment being needed in the lab. Cross contamination, the Achilles heel of PCR based systems is also therefore not an issue. A single test detects almost all smear positive TB cases and three quarters of all smear negative patients. Following the first landmark study by Boehme et al (NEJM 2005) where it was assessed in centers in India, Peru, South Africa and Azerbaijan, it has been extensively assessed in high burden countries across the globe and identifies 98% of smear positive cases and around 72% of smear negative cases. It also concurrently and rapidly detects rifampicin resistance with 98% sensitivity and 99% specificity compared to a phenotypic DST. It retains its accuracy in the HIV patient population and is also extremely useful in detecting extrapulmonary TB. A systematic review showed respectable sensitivity and specificity in lymph nodes (83% sensitivity, 93% specificity), CSF (80%, 97%), other solid tissue like bone, liver (81%, 98%). The yield from pleural and ascitic fluid remains suboptimal with sensitivity of only 46%. There are some technical limitations which need to be mentioned here: it requires constant electric supply, an operating temperature < 30° Celsius, and humidity control, conditions which may be lacking in tropical countries. The cartridges are expensive (though costs are coming down), and have limited shelf life of 18 months. The machines are also expensive for many parts

of the developing world and need periodic servicing and calibrating. Despite these limitations this test is truly a game changer. In our busy clinics, having a quick diagnosis of TB and even more important, a confirmation of MDR-TB on the same day, the test is a remarkable luxury which has changed the way physicians practice and the speed with which they can commence patients on 2nd line drugs. In recognition of this, the WHO has recommended the Xpert MTB/RIF as the initial diagnostic test in any patient suspected of having MDR-TB or HIV associated TB (strong recommendation). In the Indian context the test needs to be more widely rolled out but modeling analysis has shown that introducing it as the up front test to replace sputum microscopy would result in TB diagnosis increasing 40% and MDR cases increasing almost 5 fold. Whether India really has the resources to treat these large extra numbers of MDR cases, when it is struggling to treat the existing numbers is uncertain. What good is diagnosing MDR-TB if we then don't have the funds to treat it? The cost of the machines and cartridges would also be approximately 40 times the costs of sputum microscopy and providing this test to just 15% of India's huge pool of TB suspects would consume the entire RNTCP budget.

Some limitations of the test need to be pointed out here as well. It detects rifampicin resistance which is a surrogate marker of MDR-TB, but on occasion the patient may still be isoniazid sensitive. Hence this test must ideally be accompanied by a traditional culture and DST. For this reason, in areas where more advanced resistance is common, the lack of information on resistance to isoniazid, ethambutol, fluoroquinolone and aminoglycosides can be frustrating, and a LPA Hain (SLD) is a test that gives all this additional information as well. The test cannot be used for follow up as it remains positive for years after the patient is successfully cured of TB. Finally sometimes discordance occurs between the Xpert MTB/RIF results and the traditional TB culture result with regard to

presence or absence of resistance. This can, understandably, cause great confusion in the mind of physician and patients. Discordant results may be due to low level mutations, or silent mutations, or mutations present outside the rpo beta gene and WGS may be needed to determine the true nature of the resistance.

Thus to conclude, the Xpert MTB/RIF is revolutionizing the diagnosis of TB and MDR-TB across the developed and developing world. It has the potential to transform the TB landscape in India, but whether the program has the capacity to treat the vastly increased numbers of TB and MDR-TB patients that will be thrown up as a result of this test, is unclear at present. Of course it also needs to be stated that even the best new tool inserted into a system that is 'broken' is unlikely to on its own, make an appreciable impact. We need more investment in health systems as well.

Worldwide, as of 2015, international organizations had done a commendable job of rolling out 3553 GeneXpert instruments and 8.8 million Xpert MTB/RIF cartridges to low income, high burden countries.

A new version of the test called the GeneXpert Ultra is available with more advanced TB detection capabilities and increased sensitivity especially in smear negative cases. A recent study showed that this new version might be invaluable in TB meningitis with the Xpert Ultra diagnosing 21/22 microbiologically confirmed cases of TB meningitis.

- *Line-probe assays*: In 2008, LPAs became the first molecular method endorsed by WHO for detection of *M. tuberculosis* and drug resistance from smear-positive patients at risk of MDRTB. Line probe assays may be used for the diagnosis of TB, speciation of nontuberculous mycobacteria (NTM), and drug resistance detection. They are based on the reverse hybridization principle. Specific oligonucleotides are immobilized at known locations on a membrane strip and are hybridized under strictly controlled conditions with the biotin-labelled PCR product. The hybrids formed are detected colorimetrically. Commercially available LPAs include the INNO-LiPA Mycobacteria (Inno-genetics, Belgium) and the GenoType MTBC (Hain Lifesciences, Germany) for mycobacterial species identification and differentiation within the *M. tuberculosis* complex, respectively. The MDRTBplus assay (Hain Lifesciences) allows direct detection of *M. tuberculosis*, isoniazid and rifampicin resistance from smear-positive pulmonary specimens. LPAs are designed for use in reference and intermediate-tier laboratories and can be manual or semi-automated. The manual version is quite laborious with an advertised turnaround time of 6 hours but is usually 1–2 days in most 'real world' settings. Like all open-system PCR assays, there is a risk of cross contamination. Separated laboratories for DNA extraction, amplification and analysis are required, as is exemplary technique. The GenoType MTBDRplus is a new generation of WHO approved assays that can be done directly from samples or cultures and that identifies resistance not just to isoniazid and rifampicin but also to fluoroquinolones and second line injectables. This test can therefore within a day distinguish MDR from XDR TB and help the physician plan an empiric regimen.

- *Other nucleic acid amplification techniques*: In house NAATs use different targets, either DNA or RNA, followed by a detection step performed by various formats. The most commonly used target in these assays is the insertion sequence IS6110. Considerable expertise is needed to run most in-house NAATs and there is risk of contamination if very stringent quality control standards are not met.

5. Serological/Antibody-based tests are mentioned only to be condemned. They are used and abused in this country (TB IgG and IgM antibody tests) despite there being ample evidence that they are nearly worthless with suboptimal accuracy and highly inconsistent results.

6. *Antigen-based tests*: Antigen detection has the potential to overcome some of the well-recognized problems with antibody-based assays. The antigen test showing the most promise is based on the detection of mycobacterial lipoarabinomannan (LAM) antigen in the urine. LAM antigen is a lipopolysaccharide present in mycobacterial cell walls, which is released from metabolically active or degenerating bacterial cells and appears to be present only in patients with active TB disease. Many patients are unable to expectorate a sample of sputum and the urinary LAM assumes great utility in these patients. The overall sensitivity of the test is low but positive LAM results are particularly useful in children and HIV positive patients with low CD4 cell counts.

7. *Interferon-gamma release assays (IGRAs)*: Until recently, the diagnosis of latent TB infection (LTBI) rested solely on the tuberculin skin test (TST). The limitations of this test have been discussed in an earlier section. A recent advance has been the development of the T-cell-based IGRAs. The IGRAs are in vitro tests based on interferon gamma release after T-cell stimulation by antigens that are more specific to *M. tuberculosis* than the purified protein derivative used in the TST. These so-called "Region of Difference" (RD) antigens such as ESAT-6 and CFP10 are encoded by genes deleted in all strains of the Bacillus Calmette-Guérin (BCG) vaccine during its attenuation process. They are also not found in most common nontuberculous mycobacteria (NTM). Thus, no false positives occur in patients who have received BCG in the past or due to NTM. This makes the IGRAs much more specific than the TST. The sensitivity of IGRAs is not consistent across tests and populations but IGRAs seem to be at least as sensitive as the TST (estimated with active TB as the surrogate reference standard). It must be stressed that the IGRAs do not distinguish between latent and active disease hence a positive IGRA must not be construed to necessarily indicate active disease. Equally important, a negative IGRA cannot conclusively rule out active disease in an individual suspected to have TB.

Two IGRAs are currently available as commercial kits that are FDA-approved; the QuantiFERON-TB Gold assay (Celestis) and the T-SPOT. TB assay (Oxford Immunotech). The use of IGRAs is steadily increasing in the developed world and they are especially useful in these countries which have a low TB incidence. In Denmark, Switzerland and Germany the TST has been replaced completely by the IGRA. In the United States, France, Australia and Japan either the TST or IGRA is recommended. In the United Kingdom, Canada, Italy and Spain a two-step approach is currently recommended with the TST being performed first, followed by the IGRA to improve specificity and sensitivity.

Role of the IGRAs in the Developing World

While diagnosing and treating latent TB infection (LTBI) is an essential component of TB control in the developed world, it is clearly a less important strategy in the developing world. There are several reasons for this. Here, the high annual risk of infection and large pediatric burden imply substantial ongoing transmission; the priority of healthcare systems is thus the treatment of large numbers of active cases that promote ongoing spread. A substantial proportion of the population has LTBI and the lifetime risk of these patients developing active disease may be as low as 5–10%. In one of the first studies of its kind from India we showed that as many as 80% of healthy, asymptomatic adults attending the Hinduja Hospital for a health checkup, had a positive IGRA (T-spot TB test). In the face of such a high incidence of latent TB it is easy to understand why the IGRA has less value as a diagnostic test in high-burden countries than it does in the West. Having made these important provisos, the newer IFN-based assays probably do have applications in the developing world, especially since the TST is even less reliable here. BCG at birth, a universal practice in most developing countries, more than doubles the relative risk of a false-positive TST. Furthermore there is a high environmental mycobacterial burden and technical problems like the requirement for a cold chain, improper storage and shortages of syringes and needles are all more acutely felt. Consequently, the utility of the newer tests would be restricted to the following specific situations in the developing world: (i) epidemiological surveillance, (ii) HIV-TB co-infection, (iii) children with TB, and (iv) malnourished TB patients.

8. *Blood gene signatures*: An exciting new area of research is transcriptomic analyses from whole blood specimens to identify patients with latent TB who are likely to go on to develop active disease. Zak in a fascinating study identified a whole blood TB risk signature that predicted with a sensitivity of 66% and specificity of 81% the risk of latent TB progressing to active TB.

■ FUTURE NEEDS: WHAT IS NEEDED TO VANQUISH TB IN INDIA? (TABLE 1)

1. *Social change*: It is stating the obvious, but India will never claw itself out of its present TB crisis until the

Table 1: Future needs to vanquish TB in India.
• Social change
• Demographic control
• Adequate funding
• Global aid
• Efficiency and accountability of District TB Centers
• DOTS, non-DOTS and NGOs
• Education
• Involve and integrate the private sector
• A new TB vaccine
• Need for newer drugs
• Integrate TB and HIV programs
• Legislation

(DOTS: Directly observed treatment, short-course)

entire socioeconomic fabric of the country improves. The standard of living, housing conditions, grinding poverty, level of malnutrition, hygiene and well-being of the community as a whole, and education and literacy rates must improve if any TB program is to make headway. It is sobering to recall that 50% of Indians live on less than US$1 a day and 50% of Indians still do not have access to safe drinking water. The synergy between health and development is clear; investments in health must be accompanied by investments in literacy and infrastructure for health in general to improve in this country.

2. *Demographic control*: India's vast and ever-expanding population is its strength and at the same time its greatest enemy. Unless some attempt is made at population control, the sheer numbers will overwhelm even the best conceived TB program.

3. *Adequate funding*: Funds must be increased to keep pace with India's population explosion. TB control is one of the most cost-effective interventions known but the estimated funds needed to implement the revised TB program alone run at a staggering US$200 million, a sum that exceeds India's entire health budget. If the Indian government is serious about its intentions to eradicate TB, it will have to allocate far more money than it presently does to tackle the problem. That India spends less than 1% of its GDP on health, yet spent US$10 billion on its recent nuclear weapon program, is a sad reflection on the misplaced priorities of its politicians.

4. *Global aid*: External aid from international health organizations and from the developed world is urgently needed. This may make the difference between success and failure of the TB control programs. Sadly, the

containment of TB has, for years, been impeded by a global attitude of silent fatalism. The gross inequalities of wealth and healthcare must be addressed. Direct aid and debt relief are both needed from the developed world. Indeed, at present, just 0.1% of all external aid to developing countries is devoted to TB control. If even 5% of the domestic TB budget of the world's richest countries was diverted to Asia and Africa, the epidemic could be reversed.

5. *Efficiency and accountability of District TB Centers (DTCs)*: It is people who run programs, and unless the apathy and narrow vision of the people who implement the program in each district are replaced by missionary zeal and a sense of purpose, any program is doomed to failure. The activity of each DTC should be marshaled by program managers with vision who can motivate their subordinates. Regular audits should be held to ensure that each DTC keeps its target in terms of case detection, case holding and cure.

6. *DOTS (Directly Observed Treatment, Short-course), non-DOTS and NGOs*: We need to build on the impressive gains of DOTS but strive to make DOTS more adaptive and less disruptive. DOTS should be integrated with the general health services of the country because ultimately the success or failure of DOTS will depend on these. In our quest to expand DOTS, we should not forget the paramount importance of ensuring quality of implementation. Private-public mixes where attempts are made to embrace and include the unwieldy private sector within the ambit of DOTS are essential. Finally, DOTS-plus is essential if our large population of MDR-TB patients is to have any hope of survival.

7. *Educate the people*: As India enters the 21st century, use must be made of every form of media available to educate its teeming masses. Even remote parts of the country have access to television and this would be the ideal medium for transmitting direct, simple and blunt messages educating people in their regional languages. TB must be demystified and destigmatized by bombarding people with messages they can understand on the spread of the disease, treatment options available and the vital importance of regular and prolonged treatment.

8. *Involve and integrate the private sector*: The glaring deficiencies of the private medical sector have already been highlighted in earlier sections of this chapter. No matter how well-structured the RNTCP, a large number of patients will slip through the net by choosing to first consult a private practitioner. There is ample evidence from several pilot projects that Private Public Mixes (PPMs) can be made to work. An applicable model is that private practitioners in these areas hold treatment boxes, undertake DOTS, assist in defaulter tracing and maintain essential records. Such projects have achieved more than 90% cure rates and serve as models of collaboration that can be adopted on a larger scale. The quality of medical education must also improve with doctors being forced to prescribe TB drugs as per standard guidelines. Audits should expose those with substandard prescribing practice. Finally, regular attempts at upgrading the knowledge of all private doctors should be made so that they realize they are crucial partners in the success of TB control programs.

9. *A new TB vaccine*: BCG, the only licensed vaccine against TB was first administered almost a century ago. Since then it has been administered to over 4 billion people, more than 120 million doses annually. Despite this, its efficacy is limited. A recent meta-analysis showed the efficacy of BCG against infant TB was 74% and against TB meningitis was 64%. In spite of this, long-term use of BCG has failed to make a dent in the overall prevalence of TB infection. Research into a new TB vaccine is an intervention that could save millions of lives; a new vaccine offers the potential to change the epidemiology of TB. Sadly, the cost of developing such a vaccine would run at approximately US$1 billion and this has been the main deterrent for researchers. Hence, it is heartening to report recent trials of a new MVA85A vaccine in Oxford. This was administered as a booster to BCG and on its own with encouraging initial results. Another Phase 11b proof-of-concept trial of the MVA85A candidate TB vaccine began in 2009, in 2,800 four-month-old BCG-vaccinated infants in Worcester, Western Cape. Close behind MVA85A, in terms of clinical development, is the AERAS-402/Crucell Ad35 recombinant adenovirus vaccine. This nonreplicating adenovirus expresses three mycobacterial antigens: Ag85A, Ag85B, and Tb10.4. Designed as a boost to BCG or recombinant BCG, it has already been tested in American and African adults and infants, and Phase IIB trials in South Africa are planned. Another trial of an *M. vaccae* vaccine in a cohort of 2000 HIV-positive Tanzanians was also encouraging. These are the first new vaccine trials in 80 years and it is not inconceivable

to hope that a new TB vaccine will finally emerge in the next decade.

10. *The urgent need for new drugs*: A physician struggling to treat a patient with XDR-TB acutely feels the need for new drugs. *M. tuberculosis* has an uncanny ability to mutate and amplify its resistance. This is evident from the Totally Drug Resistant (TDR) strains we first described from India in 2012. Sadly, the drug pipe line does not move with commensurate speed. There is a desperate, unmet need for new drugs and molecules. The primary reason new drugs are not emerging more rapidly is the huge cost of developing a new TB drug. At a conservative estimate it would cost US$ 500 million to develop a new molecule. To be profitable to the drug company, it would then need to be priced high. Yet, TB is overwhelmingly a disease of the developing world where patients and governments would be unable to pay these high prices. Of the 9 million new cases of TB annually, only 1% occurred in the EU or the USA. There are several other reasons why there are so few new TB drugs in the pipeline. TB drug trials are amongst the most difficult and complex to perform. They need a sample size of several thousand in Phase 3 studies. The long duration of trials is also a deterrent. The current gold standard for any drug in Phase 3 trials is 2 years after the study period, during which time the patient must be carefully followed up to ensure there is no relapse. Such trials are difficult to perform, costly, and require great organizational skills and infrastructure, often beyond the capabilities of a developing country where these trials most need to be conducted.

Happily after half a century of waiting, the last few years have seen the emergence of a number of new molecules. The two most important are bedaquiline and delamanid which have been discussed in the section on management. Other new drugs currently undergoing trial are pretomanid and sutezolid. More excitingly trials looking at all new regimens including oral only regimens are already under way (STREAM, NIX-TB). New drugs and trials will be discussed in more detail in Chapter 16.

11. *Integrate TB and HIV programs*: We need to accept that our current approaches to TB control are inadequate in the HIV era. Instead of pretending that these two epidemics exist in isolation, we need to integrate their control programs. This includes more resources, enhanced surveillance, and a minimal package of care (isoniazid and cotrimoxazole prophylaxis) if not DOTS-TB and HAART for all patients.

12. *Legislation*: Finally, strict legislation should be enforced to ensure prescriptions are standardized according to guidelines with only allopathic doctors being allowed to prescribe TB drugs. Second-line drugs should be made available only on the prescription of a specialist. Only a few drugs and fixed drug combinations of proven quality and bioavailability should be allowed in the market.

■ SUGGESTED READING

1. Caulfield AJ, Wengenack NL. Diagnosis of active tuberculosis disease: from microscopy to molecular techniques. J Clin Tubercle Other Mycobacter Dis. 2016;4:33-43.
2. Denkinger CM, Schumacher SG, Boehme CC, et al. Xpert MTB/RIF assay for the diagnosis of extrapulmonary tuberculosis: a systematic review and meta-analysis. Our Respir J. 2014;44:435-66.
3. Dorman SE. New diagnostic tests for tuberculosis: bench, bedside, and beyond. Clin Infect Dis. 2010;50 (Suppl 3): S173-7.
4. Manuel O. QantiFERON-TB Gold assay for the diagnosis of latent tuberculosis infection. Expert Rev Mol Diagn. 2008;8(3):247-56.
5. Mori T. Usefulness of interferon-gamma release assays for diagnosis TB infection and problems with these assays. J Infect Chemother. 2009;15(3):143-55.
6. Pai M, Minion J, Sohn H, et al. Novel and improved technologies for tuberculosis diagnosis: progress and challenges. Clin Chest Med. 2009;30(4):701-16, viii.
7. Piana F. Use of T-SPOT. TB in latent tuberculosis infection diagnosis in general and immunosuppressed populations. New Microbiol. 2007;30(3):286-90.
8. Zak DE, Penn-Nicholson A, Scriba TJ, et al. A blood RNA signature for tuberculosis disease risk: a prospective cohort study. Lancet. 2016:387;2312-22.

Section 6

Infectious Diseases

CHAPTER 19

Community-acquired Pneumonia

■ DEFINITION

Pneumonia is defined as an inflammation and conso-lidation of the lung due to an infectious agent. Pneumonia that develops outside the hospital is considered community-acquired. Pneumonia developing 72 hours after admission to hospital is nosocomial or hospital-acquired. Pneumonitis is occasionally used as a synonym for pneumonia, particularly when inflammation of the lung has resulted from a noninfectious cause, such as a chemical or radiation injury.

■ ETIOLOGY AND EPIDEMIOLOGY

Community-acquired pneumonia (CAP) is a common and often serious illness. In combination with influenza, it is the most frequent cause of infection-related death and is the highest cause of mortality among infectious diseases.

Community-acquired pneumonia can occur at any age but can be particularly lethal at the extremes of age—in children less than 5 years and in adults more than 65 years. Approximately, 120–156 million cases of acute lower respiratory tract infection (ALRI) occur globally every year with roughly 1.4 million resulting in death.

Of these deaths, pneumonia is responsible for an estimated 1 million deaths in children less than 5 years and for 15% of all deaths in children less than 5 years of age. 90–95% of these deaths occur in the developing world. The majority (two-thirds) of pneumonia episodes in children less than 5 years of age occur in just 15 countries, with South Asia and sub-Saharan Africa collectively bearing the largest burden of more than half the total worldwide cases of pneumonia in children. The burden of death has been worsened since the HIV epidemic. Diarrhea and malaria, which are endemic in these areas of the world, are believed to be contributing factors to the high incidence of CAP in these countries.

The estimated average incidence of CAP in children under 5 years in developing countries is 0.29 per child year, in striking contrast to the average incidence in developed countries, which is approximately 0.05 per child year. India bears the maximum morbidity and mortality with regard to childhood pneumonia. It is at the top of the list of 15 countries across the world, which exhibit a high burden of this disease. There are an estimated 43 million new cases of pneumonia in children under 5 years of age every year. Morbidity rates lie between 0.2 episodes and 0.5 episodes per child year and 10–20% of these episodes tend to be severe. Among the high burden countries afflicted with this disease, the estimated mortality in India is 322 per 100,000 in the under 5-year population.

In adults, the incidence of morbidity and mortality of pneumonia increases in individuals beyond 65 years. The predilection of pneumonia for the elderly is not new and led William Osler in 1898 to describe the disease as "the friend of the aged". The overall attack rate of CAP in adults is reported to be approximately 5.16–12 cases for 1,000 persons per year. In the year 2000, severe lower respiratory tract infections were reported to be the cause of death in 120 per million men and 76 per million women in the 15–59 age group worldwide. In more than 60 years age group, the death rate from such infections increased by more than twofold for each further decade of life. Though influenza can strike in any month of the year, there is a seasonal variation in the incidence of influenzal CAP. Both attack rates and mortality rates are higher in winter. However, in tropical countries, there is also an increased incidence in the rainy season.

There are numerous etiological agents known to cause pneumonia. In developing countries and also in a number of other countries in the world **(Table 1)**, *Streptococcus pneumoniae* is the most frequent organism causing CAP. The serotypes of *S. pneumoniae* causing disease in India are Type 1 and Type 3 in adults and Type 6 and Type 1 in children. *Haemophilus influenzae* followed by Mycoplasma are next in frequency as causative agents. In the West, *Legionella* and *Chlamydia* are important causes as well though the lack of facilities in many laboratories in India makes it difficult to estimate the frequency with which these organisms act as causative agents in different regions of our country.

The epidemiology of pneumonia in the West as also in India and other fast developing Asian countries has, however, changed to some extent in recent years and will continue to do so in the future due to: (1) changes in the population at risk; (2) the discovery of new microbes causing pneumonia; (3) changes in the microbial sensitivity to antimicrobial agents; (4) the widespread use of pneumococcal, influenzal, and *H. influenzae* vaccines in the West.

There is a large increase in the number of organ transplant patients all over the world (particularly in the

West) as also a large number in HIV patients, particularly in the poor countries of the world. These individuals form a special subset. Pneumonia in these patients can be caused not only by the usual organisms but also by opportunistic organisms.

Newer pathogens causing CAP have also to an extent altered the epidemiological scene. These newer pathogens (to give some examples) include the Hantavirus, Human metapneumovirus, SARS coronavirus, and *Staphylococcus aureus* carrying the Panton-Valentine leukocidin (PVL) genes.

Viral pneumonias are gaining an increasing prominence. Influenzal pneumonia is the most common and can be lethal when in epidemic form. The frequency of viral pneumonia depends on the degree of sophisticated tests used to identify them. For example in a randomized trial of 107 patients with CAP, real time polymerase chain reaction (PCR) increased the diagnostic yield to 43% compared to the diagnostic yield of 23% by conventional methods. Other viruses (not listed in **Table 1**) causing CAP are adenovirus, coronaviruses, human metapneumovirus. Viral pneumonias are considered in a separate chapter.

An interesting new observation is the finding of complex, diverse microbes within the alveoli (hitherto considered sterile) through culture-independent techniques. It is suggested that these alveolar microbes may have a role in the development of pneumonia either by modulating the host response to infecting organisms or through overgrowth, becoming specific pathogens.

One also needs to consider that in many part of the world, there is an increasing resistance of microbes to the previously effective antimicrobial agents. The incidence of penicillin resistant *S. pneumoniae* is increasing significantly in the West. In the United States, 26% of *S. pneumoniae* are resistant to penicillin and 25% resistant to erythromycin. Multidrug-resistant pneumococci are an alarming problem in the West. Fortunately for India, the resistance of *S. pneumoniae* to penicillin is uncommon. Yet in neighboring Pakistan, it is reported to be as high as 9%. Penicillin resistance is also an important problem in other parts of Asia like Japan. A study from Nagasaki noted that 50% of 49 cases of pneumococcal pneumonia were resistant to penicillin. The importance of such studies cannot be overemphasized. Vigilance and surveillance will go a long way in countering the spread of antibiotic resistance. Finally, in the West, the incidence of CAP due to pneumococci, influenza virus, and *H. influenzae* have registered a fall as vaccination against these organisms is a

Table 1: Common organisms causing community acquired pneumonia.
Aerobic bacteria: • *Group A Streptococci*   • *Streptococcus pneumoniae*   • *Mycoplasma pneumoniae*   • *Haemophilus influenzae*   • *Chlamydia species*   • *Legionella*   • Gram-negative bacteria   • *Moraxella catarrhalis*   • *Staphylococcus aureus*   • *Nocardia species*   • *Mycobacterium tuberculosis*   *Anaerobic bacteria*:   • Oral anaerobes   • Actinomyces   *Viruses*:   • Influenza virus, parainfluenza virus   • Cytomegalovirus   • Respiratory syncytial virus   • Measles virus   • Varicella-zoster virus   *Fungi*:   • Aspergillus   • Histoplasma capsulatum   • *Coccidioides immitis*   • *Blastomyces species*   *Parasites*:   • *E. histolytica*

(*E. histolytica: Entamoeba histolytica*)

standard practice. Unfortunately in India, the importance of this preventive measure is not fully realized by lay people as also by many practicing doctors.

Numerous studies have been reported from the West to determine the frequency of different microorganisms responsible for CAP. However in many large studies, no pathogen could be detected. To give just on example, in the meta-analysis by Fine and Smith [*Ref: Fine MJ, Smith MA, Carson CA, et al. Prognosis and outcomes of patients with community-acquired pneumonia. A meta-analysis. JAMA. 1996;275(2):134-41*] no etiological agent could be identified in the overwhelming majority (11,209) of patients. It is possible that many of these patients with an unidentified etiological agent could be due to the *Pneumococcus*, but they may well have been due to other different organisms.

There is much less data on the etiology of CAP from poor and developing countries. The high cost of routinely performing microbiological, serological, and other relevant sophisticated tests in all patients with CAP is probably the main reason for this. Besides even in rich countries of the West, the ability to exactly determine the microbiological diagnosis of CAP is not encouraging.

Also, the cost-effectiveness of making an exact microbiological diagnosis in every patient has long been debated. At our hospital, a tertiary referral center, a comprehensive pneumonia screen would cost ₹ 10,000 (about $160). In a country, where the per capita income is ₹ 90,000/year, spending this sum of money would be an unjustifiable luxury outside of formal epidemiological studies or in patients with an unusual presentation or in those with serious or life-threatening illness. Empirical antibiotics started promptly as per existing guidelines would be the preferred approach. However, the Asian region is very diverse and existing British or American guidelines cannot and should not be blindly transposed to this region without some idea of the local prevalence of causative organisms and the prevailing antibiotic sensitivity. A relevant review of the available epidemiology from the Asian region is, therefore, given below.

Tuberculosis (TB) presenting as an acute pneumonia should never be forgotten in the Asian continent. Osler used to teach that TB should be the differential diagnosis in any pneumonia that failed to resolve appropriately and this axiom holds true even today in much of Asia, which bears the burden of most of the world's TB. In Tan's series, 16% of patients had TB. Another prospective study of 96 consecutive adults hospitalized with CAP in a University hospital in Singapore found *Mycobacterium*

tuberculosis to be the most common pathogen. In this study, *Mycobacterium tuberculosis* accounted for 21% of all cases of CAP, exceeding those caused by *S. pneumoniae* (12%) and *H. influenzae* (5.2%). A prospective study of CAP from Hong Kong enrolled 90 adults hospitalized at the Prince of Wales Hospital and found that TB presented as CAP in 12% of patients. The authors noted that it could not be differentiated from other causes of pneumonia on clinical or radiological grounds. In this study, pneumococcal infection was diagnosed in only 12% of patients. A Japanese study of 188 cases of CAP found that *Mycobacterium tuberculosis* was the cause of 11% of all cases. These studies emphasize the role of pulmonary TB as an important cause of CAP in the Asian context.

A large study (summarized below) on the etiology of CAP from Mumbai was completed some years ago. Hundred patients with CAP admitted to two hospitals in Mumbai (one private and one public hospital) over a period of 1.5 years were prospectively studied. Despite a thorough search for the etiological agent, no organism could be identified in 44% of the patients. *S. pneumoniae* was the most common organism isolated, accounting for CAP in 22% patients, followed by *Chlamydia* in 14% and *Haemophilus* in 9%. Overall, atypical organisms accounted for 19% of all cases. TB was an important cause of CAP accounting for 7% of the patients. This study demonstrates that when detailed etiological tests are applied to patients with CAP in India, the etiological pattern bears some similarity to that obtained from other Western series, with *S. pneumoniae* heading most series. More such Indian studies from different parts of this vast subcontinent are needed to determine, if there are regional variations in the etiology of CAP. It is only then that rational antibiotic guidelines can be made.

■ RISK FACTORS (TABLE 2)

Age

Age is an important independent risk factor in CAP, the incidence (as already mentioned), being highest in infants

Table 2: Risk factors for community-acquired pneumonia.
• Age (children <5 years and elderly)
• Alcoholism
• Immunodeficiency or immunosuppression
• Poverty
• Poor nutrition
• Smoking
• Aspiration
• Chronic illnesses and comorbid diseases

and the elderly. The frequency of hospitalization due to severe infection increases markedly with age, ranging from 1.6 per 1,000 in adults between 55 years and 64 years to 11.6 per 1,000 after 75 years of age. Mortality in the elderly is significantly higher, 9 per 100,000 rising to 217 per 100,000, if there is one additional risk factor, such as congestive heart failure, diabetes, chronic obstructive pulmonary disease (COPD), and chronic renal failure.

Alcoholism

The defense mechanisms of the respiratory tract are impaired by chronic alcohol consumption. Alcohol facilitates bacterial colonization of the respiratory tract, hinders mucociliary transport, and facilitates aspiration due to impaired swallowing and cough reflexes. Alcoholism is also associated with impaired neutrophil, lymphocyte, monocyte, and alveolar macrophage function contributing thereby to multiplication of bacterial organisms in the lower airways of these patients.

Nutrition

Malnutrition impairs cellular immunity, impairs macrophage function, and decreases the level of immunoglobulin A_2, thereby contributing to an increase in both the incidence and severity of pneumonia. Perhaps, this is one reason for the increased frequency and mortality of pneumonia in children living in poor and developing countries.

Immunodeficiency or Immunosuppression

Immunosuppression or immunodeficiency from any cause is an important risk factor for pneumococcal and other infections.

Smoking

Smoking impairs respiratory mechanisms. Mucociliary transport is adversely affected, as are humoral and cellular immune responses. Smoking is also believed to cause increased adherence of *S. pneumoniae* and *H. influenzae* to the oropharyngeal mucosal surface. Smokers, in particular heavy cigarette smokers, therefore, are at increased risk of pneumonia.

Poverty

Poverty leads not only to poor nutrition but also to poor hygiene, overcrowding, and inhospitable living conditions. These contribute to the risk of pneumococcal and other respiratory infections and the spread of infection from one person to another.

Aspiration

Any background condition, which promotes aspiration of infected oropharyngeal secretions or of gastric contents, is a major risk factor for aspiration pneumonia. Aspiration pneumonia is, therefore, a grave complication in obtunded and comatose patients, in patients who have difficulty in swallowing (either neurogenic or mechanical) and in patients with periodontal disease.

Aspiration of acid gastric contents leads to chemical pneumonitis, the lower the pH of the gastric contents the more intense the inflammation. The chemical inflammation leads to a hemorrhagic bronchitis with well-marked bronchial spasm, alveolar damage, and damage to surfactant with resulting atelectasis.

There is, however, also an increased incidence of aspiration pneumonia in patients whose gastric acid is suppressed, particularly following the use of proton pump inhibitors.

Oropharyngeal secretions often contain anaerobes (anaerobic *Streptococci* and *Bacteroides* species) as also Gram-negative organisms, so that pneumonia resulting from aspiration is often due to these organisms.

Chronic Illness and Comorbid Disease

A study from the Center of Disease Control and Prevention stresses the significant increase in the incidence of invasive pneumococcal disease in patients suffering from chronic diseases. In this study, the overall invasive rate of invasive pneumococcal disease was 8.8 for 100,000 adults. This increased incidence was particularly observed in patients with diabetes, chronic lung disease, asthma, COPD, chronic cardiac failure, and as already pointed out in alcoholism. The rise was highest in adults with solid cancer and HIV. One other study has also noted an increased incidence of pneumococcal pneumonia in patients with dementia, seizures, cerebrovascular disease, and chronic renal failure.

PATHOPHYSIOLOGY (FIG. 1)

The pathogenesis varies with the infecting organism. Aspiration of the organisms residing in the nasopharynx or oropharynx is responsible for pneumococcal pneumonia, as also for pneumonia caused by other Gram-positive, Gram-negative, and anaerobic organisms. Viral infections are due to inhalation of infected droplets from other patients. Inhalation of water droplets contaminated by *Legionella* produces a *Legionella* infection. Inhalation of infected particles from animals can lead to psittacosis and Q fever.

Animal experiments performed several years ago showed that aspirated pneumococci (pneumococci introduced into the trachea) most often produce an initial infection around the hilum (parahilar). This infection then fans outwards toward the periphery. In some instances, when the infection is mild and the body immune response is satisfactory, the infection may remain parahilar; at other times, it extends for a variable distance toward the periphery, so that it may ultimately involve the whole lobe. The inflamed lung goes successively through the process of congestion, red hepatization and finally gray

hepatization before resolution commences. The earliest to be involved parahilar area may be in a stage of red or gray hepatization while the later involved periphery might still be in the stage of congestion. It is easy to understand why pneumonia confined to the parahilar region or extending just beyond it may show no physical signs other than perhaps a few crackles on auscultation, as there is a fair depth of normal lung tissue beyond the pneumonic patch. In fulminant infections, infecting organisms were seen to spread quickly through the lung parenchyma to the pleura and spill into the bloodstream causing a bacteremia.

Pneumonia, in particular staphylococcal infection and also Gram-negative infection may be caused by hematogenous spread. A single lobe may be involved. Multiple areas of consolidation are occasionally observed, often breaking down to form one or more abscesses as, for example, in staphylococcal pneumonia, as also in pneumonia due to *Klebsiella* and *Ps. pyocyaneus*.

CLINICAL APPROACH AND CLINICAL MANIFESTATIONS

The clinical approach to a patient suspected of suffering from CAP consists of a thorough clinical examination, followed by an X-ray of the chest and by microbiological testing of the sputum. A radiographic examination of the chest is an integral feature of the early assessment of a patient suspected to have CAP. A recent study has shown that there is a significant lack of sensitivity in the clinical criteria for the accurate diagnosis of CAP. Even a combination of symptoms and signs (cough, fever, tachycardia, and inspiratory crackles) did not have sensitivity above 50% when using a chest X-ray as a standard (*Ref: Metlay JP, Fine MJ. Testing strategies in the initial management of patients with community-acquired pneumonia. Ann Intern Med. 2003;138:109*). Notwithstanding the above reservation, it is important to be aware of the classic presentation of CAP. CAP has traditionally been thought to present as either of two syndromes—(1) the typical presentation and (2) the atypical presentation. Although recent data suggest that these two syndromes may be less distinct than was once thought, the characteristics of the clinical presentation may nevertheless have some diagnostic value.

The "typical" pneumonia syndrome is characterized by the sudden onset of fever, chills, cough, pleuritic chest pain, and breathlessness. The cough is usually productive; sputum may be rusty in color and sometimes frankly bloody. In case of an anaerobic infection, it may have a foul

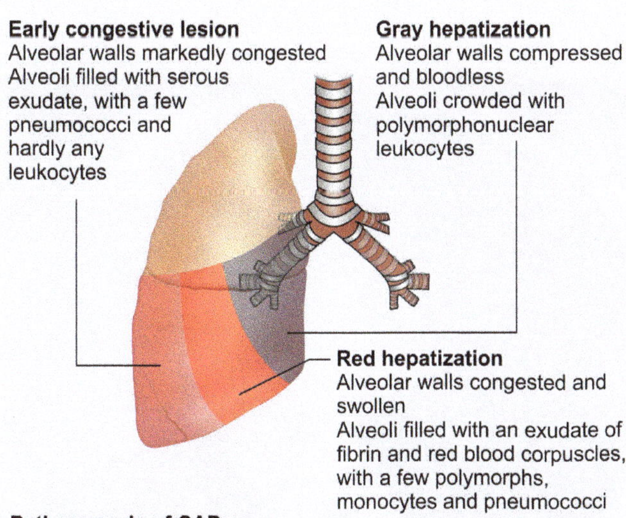

Pathogenesis of CAP:
Parahilar start of pneumonia, fanning outwards. By the time the peripheral portion of the lobe is involved (stage of congestion), the earlier to be involved hilar and parahilar areas may be in a stage of hepatization. The pneumonic patch may stop short just involving the parahilar area, or extend varying distances outwards to ultimately reach the periphery and involve the whole lobe. A small parahilar patch may present with few or no physical signs on examination of the chest and would only be revealed on a radiological examination.

Fig. 1: Pathogenesis of community-acquired pneumonia (CAP).

odor. Fever is usually present, but some patients may be hypothermic (a poor prognostic sign) and some (20%) are afebrile at the time of presentation. General examination reveals a varying degree of tachycardia and tachypnea. In severe infections, there may be central cyanosis and hypotension. On examination of the chest, crackles are heard over the affected area of the lung; physical findings of consolidation (dullness to percussion, increased tactile, vocal fremitus, whispering pectoriloquy, and bronchial breath sounds) are present in about 20% of patients with pneumonia. A pleural friction rub is heard in about 10% of cases.

Leukocytosis, at times marked, is generally present. However, in the elderly, in fulminant infections, and in the immunocompromised, there may be leukopenia. Blood cultures taken before antibiotic therapy are positive in about 10% of cases. Gram stain of a sputum specimen is generally positive for bacteria predominantly of a single type. Radiography shows lobar or segmental consolidation **(Figs. 2 and 3)**. Arterial blood gases show a low partial pressure of oxygen (PaO_2), often low enough in serious infections to result in hypoxemic respiratory failure. In severe cases, there is a combination of hypoxic and hypercapnic respiratory failure.

The typical pneumonia syndrome is usually caused by the most common bacterial pathogen in CAP, *S. pneumoniae,* but can also be due to other bacterial pathogens such as *H. influenzae, S. aureus, Streptococcus pyogenes,* other Gram-positive and Gram-negative aerobes and anaerobes present in the oropharynx. *Most importantly, Mycobacterium tuberculosis infection can also cause a typical pneumonia syndrome.*

Elderly patients usually present with fewer symptoms than younger patients. An interesting study on pneumonia in the elderly by Limthongkul and colleagues in Bangkok, Thailand showed that pneumonia in the elderly might present with no fever, no cough, and no signs of parenchymal infiltration but significant mental changes.

Occasionally, the presentation is with extrapulmonary features. For example, streptococcal pneumonia and staphylococcal pneumonia may present with features of meningitis, cerebral abscess, or endocarditis due to bacteremic spread.

The "atypical" pneumonia syndrome is characterized by a more gradual onset, a dry cough, a prominence of extrapulmonary symptoms (such as headache, myalgias, fatigue, sore throat, nausea, vomiting, and diarrhea) and abnormalities on chest radiographs despite minimal

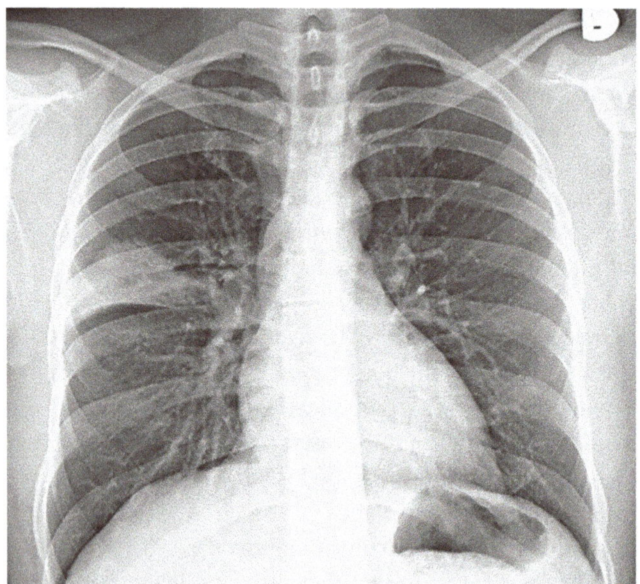

Fig. 2: Pneumococcal pneumonia. Middle-aged female patient with cough and fever of 5 days' duration. Chest X-ray demonstrates an ill-defined consolidation in the right upper lobe limited by the interlobar fissure representing a lobar pneumonia. The offending organism was the *Pneumococcus.*

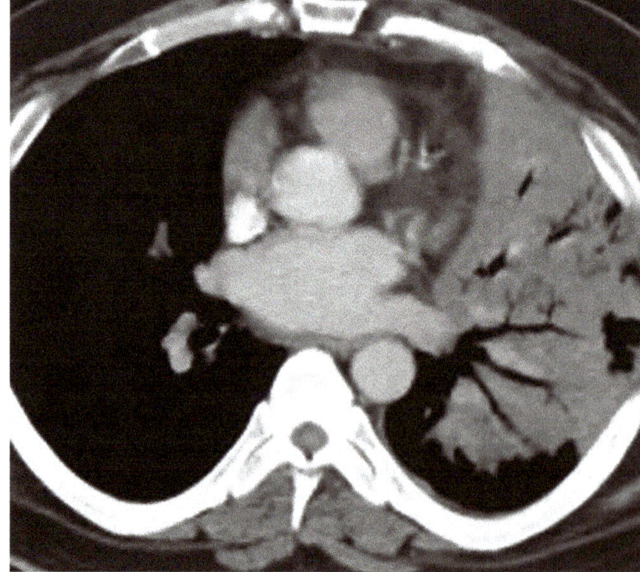

Fig. 3: Middle-aged man presented with high fever, leukocytosis, and hemoptysis. Computed tomography (CT) chest with contrast demonstrated a large ill-defined consolidation in the left upper lobe, and lingula with an air bronchogram.

signs of pulmonary involvement (other than crackles) on physical examination. Atypical pneumonia is classically produced by *Mycoplasma, Legionella,* and *Chlamydia* and the less frequently encountered pathogens *Coxiella burnetii, Francisella tularensis, H. capsulatum,* and *Coccidioides immitis.*

Certain viruses also produce pneumonia that is usually characterized by an atypical presentation, i.e. chills, fever, dry nonproductive cough, and predominance of extrapulmonary symptoms. Primary viral pneumonia can be caused by influenza virus infection (usually as part of a community outbreak in winter), respiratory syncytial virus infection (in children and immunocompromised individuals), measles, and varicella-zoster infection (accompanied by the characteristic rash), and by *Cytomegalovirus* infection (in patients immunocompromised by HIV infection or by immunosuppressive drugs). In addition, influenza, measles, and varicella can predispose to secondary bacterial pneumonia as a result of the destruction of the mucociliary barrier of the airways. Viral infections and fungal infections are considered in the chapter on nonbacterial pneumonias.

■ PNEUMONIA DUE TO SPECIFIC BACTERIAL INFECTIONS

Streptococcus Species

Streptococcus pneumoniae is the most common cause of CAP, presenting generally with the "typical" features described above. However, life-threatening community-acquired pneumococcal pneumonia may present with subtle manifestations. Tachycardia or increased respiratory rate, mental confusion, and rapid deterioration in the clinical state leading to death may be observed, particularly in the elderly and immunocompromised patients.

Streptococcus pyogenes infection also can rarely cause "typical pneumonia". It generally follows viral infections such as measles, varicella in children, and influenza in adults. Pleural effusions and empyema are frequent. Abscess formation with a bronchopleural fistula is more frequently observed.

Staphylococcal Species

Infection occurs by aspiration, inhalation, or by hematogenous spread. Airborne inhalation or aspiration is the route of infection following a viral infection such as measles or influenza or in the presence of a comorbid state such as COPD. Hematogenous spread is from an infective focus, such as within the skin, subcutaneous tissue, or as in endocarditis or following bacteremia secondary to a septic focus anywhere within the body. Direct bloodstream infection can occur following intravenous drug abuse.

The clinical picture may resemble that described under "typical pneumonia" with segmental or lobar consolidation. However, it may be different, because *Staphylococci* frequently cause lysis of lung tissue. This can result (particularly in children) in rapidly expanding thin-walled pneumatoceles or bullae that may push the heart and mediastinum to the opposite side. At times, the greater part of the lung may be occupied by one large pneumatocele or bulla **(Figs. 4 and 5)**. Rupture of the bullae into the pleura can cause a pneumothorax or a pyopneumothorax. In adults, lysis of lung tissue leads to one or more abscess cavities. Nodular infiltrates may coalesce to form areas of consolidation with or without abscess formation. Pleural effusion, empyemas, and bronchopleural fistula are frequent. Metastatic bacteremic spread can lead to meningitis, brain abscess, endocarditis, and rarely to pericarditis. Systemic features may be marked and sepsis with multiple organ dysfunction is observed in fulminant infections. The outcome of staphylococcal CAP depends on the virulence of the organism, the presence

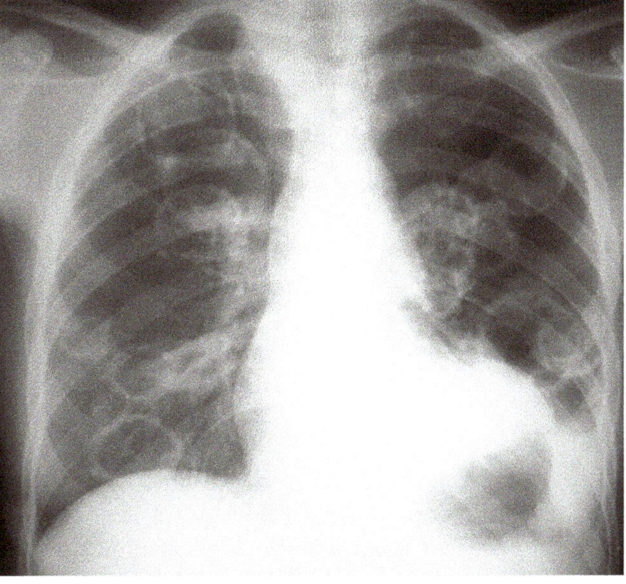

Fig. 4: Staphylococcal pneumonia: Multiple thin air-filled cysts are seen in both lung fields representing pneumatoceles due to staphylococcal infection.

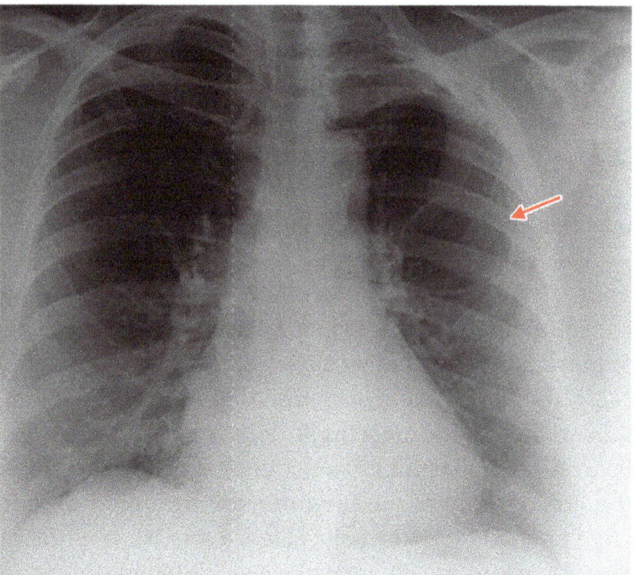

Fig. 5: Staphylococcal pneumonia. Chest X-ray demonstrates a thin-walled pneumatocele, a residue of a healed staphylococcal pneumonia.

or absence of comorbid factors, the age of the patient, presence of sepsis and pleural complications, and the response to antibiotic therapy.

Though most community-acquired staphylococcal infections are methicillin-sensitive, there is an increasing incidence of *methicillin-resistant Staphylococcus aureus (MRSA)* infection in the community, not just in the West but also in India and perhaps also in the other Asian countries. The *MRSA* infections in the community generally affect the skin and subcutaneous tissue but can also cause pneumonia, lung abscess, and empyema. The *MRSA* in the community is a virulent organism usually containing the gene encoding PVL and the SCCmec Type IV element belonging to the USA 200 pulsed field. The PVL contains a toxin that creates lytic pores in the cell membrane of polymorphonuclear leukocytes, thereby causing the release of chemotactic factors that promote inflammation and tissue destruction.

Mycoplasmal Infection

Mycoplasmal pneumonia may occur sporadically but is usually seen in small epidemics. A history of an immediate preceding upper respiratory infection is often present. The clinical features are as described under atypical pneumonia. However, extrapulmonary manifestations are varied and frequent. These commonly include arthralgias,

cervical lymphadenopathy, bullous myringitis, nausea, vomiting, and diarrhea. Immune hemolytic anemia due to the presence of cold agglutinins in the blood is an aid to correct diagnosis. Myocarditis is a rare complication; precordial pain is at times related to pericarditis. Central nervous system (CNS) involvement includes meningitis, meningoencephalopathy, and myelitis. Skin eruptions may be present the most dreaded being erythema multiforme, which may graduate into a full-blown Steven-Johnson syndrome.

A clinical study of mycoplasma pneumonia by Hwang and colleagues in China [*Ref: Hwang JJ, Chen KL. Clinical study of Mycoplasma pneumoniae pneumonia. Gaoxiong Yi Xue Ke Xue Za Zhi. 1993;9(4):204-11*] showed that all patients with *Mycoplasma pneumoniae* complained of fever and cough; 63% had dry cough and 37% had sputum production. Upper respiratory tract complaints such as rhinorrhea, sore throat, or earache were seen in 57% of patients, 55% has gastrointestinal symptoms of anorexia, nausea, vomiting, and diarrhea. Other complaints included myalgia, arthralgia (29%), headache (30%), and general malaise (32%). Dyspnea (17%) and chest pain (20%) were occasionally observed.

Radiological examination reveals diffuse infiltrates in one or both lungs, generally involving the lower lobes; these infiltrates clear slowly over 4–6 weeks **(Figs. 6 and 7)**.

Mycobacterium Tuberculosis (Figs. 8 and 9)

Community-acquired pneumonia due to *Mycobacterium tuberculosis* should always be kept in mind in developing countries. It may present acutely or subacutely, the upper lobe and the apical segment of the lower lobe being most frequently involved. The right middle lobe and the lingular segment of the left lung may also be sites of consolidation. The symptoms and signs may be indistinguishable from CAP due to other organisms. Diagnosis depends on demonstrating acid-fast bacilli in sputum and growing them on culture. It should be a rule that all patients with acute pneumonia in developing countries should have a Ziehl-Neelsen stain of a sputum specimen in addition to other microbiological tests deemed relevant. This would enable the clinician to avoid missing out on the diagnosis of tuberculous pneumonia.

Rarely, acute tuberculous pneumonia presents with bizarre manifestations. An unusual presentation is that of acute respiratory distress, tachycardia, tachypnea,

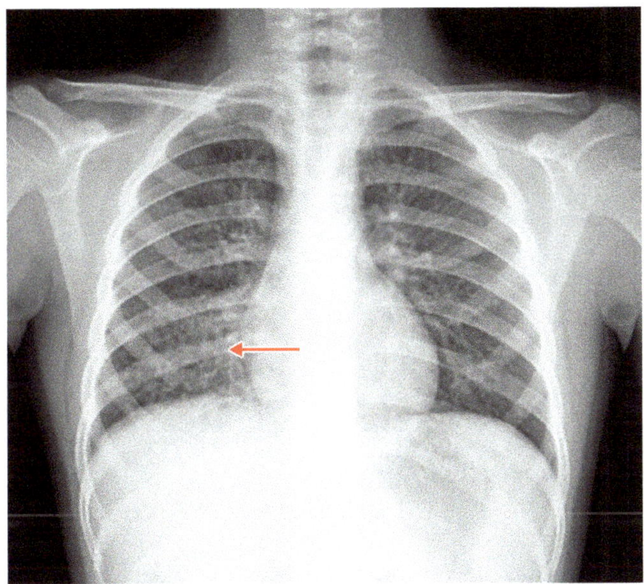

Fig. 6: *Mycoplasma pneumoniae.* A 21-year old male patient presented with fever and cough, total leucocyte count was normal. Antimycoplasma titers were very high. Chest X-ray demonstrated multiple reticular opacities in the right lower zone representing *Mycoplasma pneumonia.*

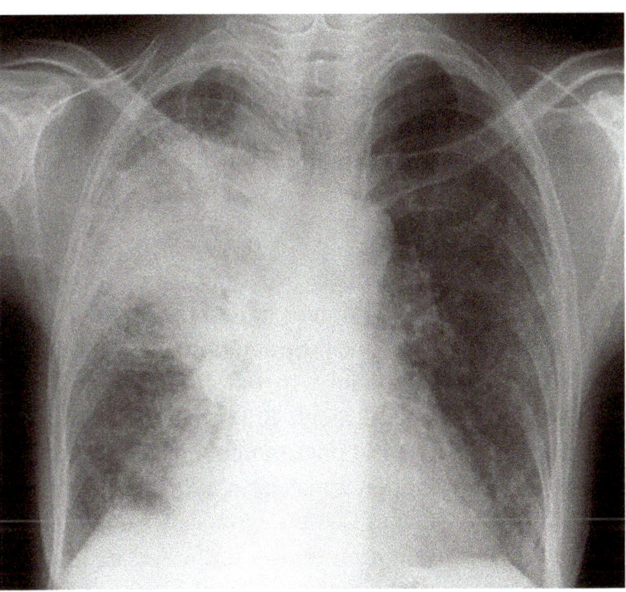

Fig. 8: Acute tuberculous pneumonia. A 33-year-old male patient presented with high fever and chills and mild leukocytosis. Chest X-ray revealed a large lobar consolidation involving the right upper and midzone. Sputum revealed acid-fast bacilli *(Mycobacterium tuberculosis).*

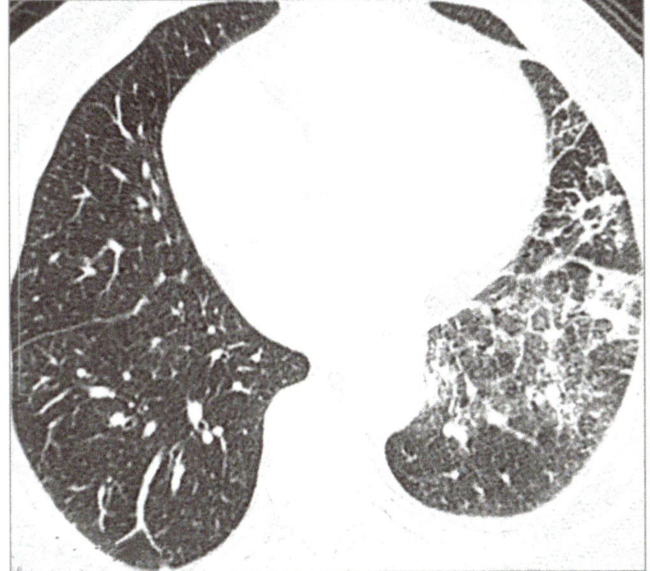

Fig. 7: *Mycoplasma pneumoniae.* Computed tomography (CT) chest of a patient with *Mycoplasma pneumonia* demonstrating ill-defined areas of ground glass densities in the anterior basal segment of left lower lobe with septal and peribronchovascular interstitial thickening.

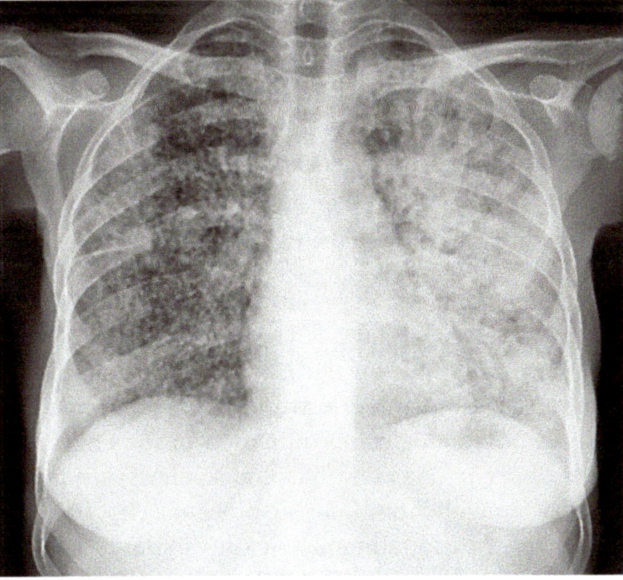

Fig. 9: Tuberculous pneumonia. Chest X-ray reveals diffuse conglomerative consolidations in the entire left lung. Small nodular opacities are seen in the right lung as well. Bronchoalveolar lavage (BAL) revealed acid-fast bacilli.

bilateral shadows in both lung fields, with respiratory crackles on auscultation [acute respiratory distress syndrome (ARDS)]. There is cough but no sputum for examination. The patient can progress to acute respiratory failure with a low PaO_2 (<60 mm Hg) even on supplemental oxygen. Multiorgan failure may be observed. The diagnosis is impossible without an examination of bronchoalveolar lavage (BAL) fluid, which shows acid-fast bacilli. A transbronchial biopsy shows the presence of tubercles (caseating granulomas) on histopathological examination.

Chlamydia Species

The incidence of chlamydia pneumonia is uncertain. A study in Mumbai (mentioned earlier) showed that the organism was responsible for pneumonia in a significant number of patients. Sore throat may antedate the appearance of fever and cough and clinical features are as described under atypical pneumonia. The clinical course is generally mild though it may be severe in patients with comorbid states such as COPD or congestive heart failure. Radiological examination shows unilateral or bilateral infiltrates that may take 4 weeks to resolve.

Legionella Pneumonia

Legionella species are intracellular aerobic organisms. Of the 30 species identified, *Legionella pneumophilia* is the most common. The organism exists in air-conditioning systems and in water. Spread of infection occurs by inhalation of air or droplets contaminated by the organism. Risk factors for Legionnaire's disease include in particular—age, diabetes, smoking, hematological malignancies, cancer, and advanced end-stage renal disease.

Infection may be asymptomatic, mild-to-severe. The incubation period is 2–8 days. Severe infection is characterized by fever with chills, headache, and myalgia followed within 2–3 days by pneumonia. Cough with purulent sputum with or without hemoptysis is often present. Tachycardia and tachypnea are observed. Radiological examination of the chest may show diffuse unilateral or bilateral shadows; segmental or lobar consolidation may also occur **(Fig. 10)**. The presence of extrapulmonary features should suggest the possible diagnosis. These include involvement of many systems. Abdominal pain, diarrhea, and arthralgia are frequent. Headache and mental confusion may be prominent features. Hyponatremia due to syndrome of inappropriate antidiuretic hormone hypersecretion (SIADH) is common and may be a diagnostic clue. Renal involvement may take the form of proteinuria, oliguria, azotemia, and renal failure. Liver functions are often

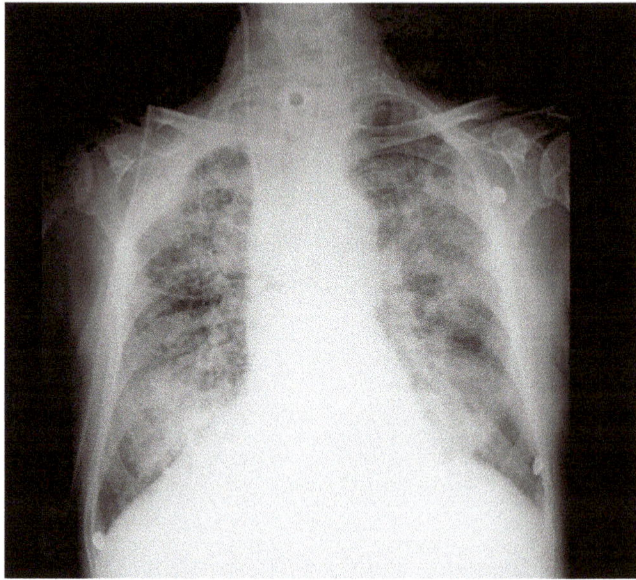

Fig. 10: Legionella pneumonia. An 87-year-old male presented with dyspnea, chest pain, and fever: Chest X-ray demonstrates ill-defined areas of consolidation. Legionella antigen was detected on urine examination.

deranged and hepatosplenomegaly may be present. Pleural effusion, generally mild, may occur, but cavitation is not observed.

The greater and the more severe the extrapulmonary manifestations the more serious the prognosis. The presence of comorbidities as always worsens the outcome. *Legionella* pneumonia is infrequently diagnosed in India, not necessarily because it is very rare, but because it is not carefully looked out for, largely due to lack of laboratory facilities.

Gram-negative Bacilli

Gram-negative bacteria chiefly include *Klebsiella pneumoniae, Escherichia coli, Pseudomonas aeruginosa,* and *Acinetobacter* species. Gram-negative bacteria are most often responsible for nosocomial pneumonia, but CAP attributed to these organisms may occur in old age or in association with comorbid states. Comorbid states include severe COPD, alcoholism, uncontrolled diabetes, neutropenia, immunosuppression, or immunodeficiency states.

Colonization of the oropharynx by Gram-negative bacteria in the above conditions is followed by aspiration into the lungs leading to pneumonia. In some instances, pneumonia results from blood-borne Gram-negative bacterial infection. The clinical presentation is generally that of typical pneumonia. The prognosis, particularly when associated with comorbidities, is poor.

Klebsiella pneumoniae (Friedlander's pneumonia) generally occurs in older patients (>60 years). Acute prostration, purulent sputum with hemoptysis, and extensive involvement generally of one or at times both upper lobes is observed. The extensive consolidation may be associated with breakdown and abscess formation and often causes a downward bulging of the fissure **(Fig. 11)**. This is, however, not pathognomonic of *Klebsiella* infection; it is also occasionally observed in pneumococcal pneumonia caused by *S. pneumoniae* Type III. Hypotension, respiratory failure, and severe sepsis with multiorgan failure characterize severe infection.

Pneumonia due to *P. aeruginosa* usually involves one or both lower lobes and occurs in the elderly and often chronically ill patients. Fever, tachycardia, and quickly evolving acute respiratory failure may follow. Abscess formation and empyema are frequent. The prognosis is poor, death resulting from sepsis, acute respiratory failure, or multiorgan dysfunction.

Pseudomonas aeruginosa is a dangerous organism, which is increasingly resistant to most antibiotics.

Pneumonia due to *Acinetobacter* is often bilateral, quickly progressive, often causes ARDS with severe hypoxemia. Abscess formation and empyema are frequent complications. Death can occur within a few days and is due to respiratory failure or sepsis.

Pneumonia due to *Pseudomonas pseudomallei* has been considered in the chapter on Tropical infections and the lungs.

Nocardia Species

Nocardia are Gram-positive aerobic bacilli chiefly present in soil. The most common *Nocardia* species responsible for pulmonary infection is *Nocardia asteroides.* Most patients with nocardial pneumonia have underlying comorbid states—COPD, malignancy, immunosuppression, and long-term corticosteroid therapy. In 30–50%, there may be no underlying disease. Fulminant nocardial pneumonia is uncommon but when present has a high fatality. In most patients, the onset is subacute with mild-to-moderate fever, cough, increase in breathlessness in COPD patients, and at times pleuritic chest pain. Imaging studies typically show nodules of varying size in one or both lungs, sometimes evident only on a computed tomography (CT) scan **(Fig. 12)**. Infiltrates, lobar consolidation, and abscess formation—either multiple small abscesses or a large abscess cavity may be observed. Metastatic involvement leads to subcutaneous abscesses (presenting as pus discharging from inflamed nodules); metastatic abscesses in the brain lead to varying CNS symptoms depending on the size and location of the abscess. Infection from the

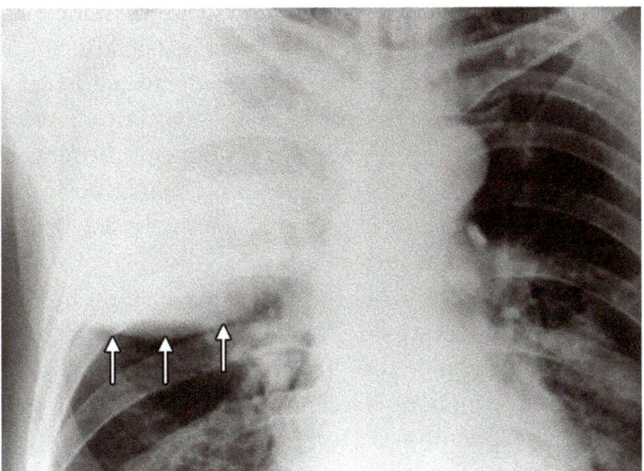

Fig. 11: *Klebsiella pneumoniae*. Chest X-ray demonstrates a large consolidation in the right upper lobe, which is dense and homogeneous; there is downward bulging of the fissure, a common feature of *Klebsiella pneumoniae*.

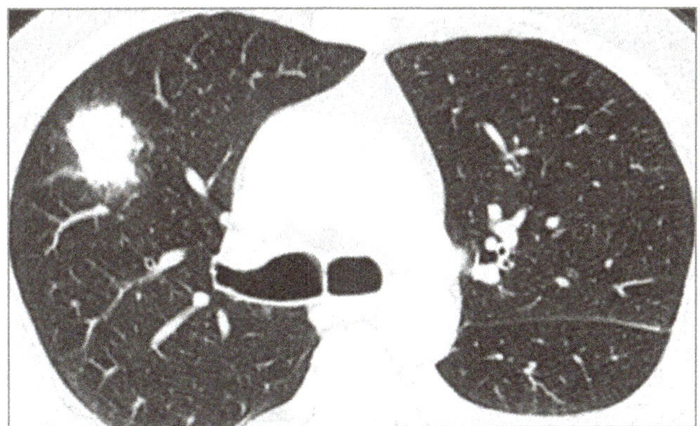

Fig. 12: Nocardiosis: A 57-year-old male patient with history of Churg-Strauss syndrome and with long history of oral steroids developed fever with productive cough. Computed tomography (CT) chest demonstrates nodular mass in right upper lobe and left pleural effusion. CT-guided biopsy was performed and microbiological examination revealed nocardia filaments. Subsequent X-rays revealed progressive reduction and resolution in the nocardiosis.

lung may involve the pleura causing an empyema, and at times, the chest wall causing a fluctuant abscess within the parietes. In the absence of severe associated comorbid states, the prognosis is usually good and provided the diagnosis is made quickly and the patient receives appropriate therapy.

Anaerobic Bacteria

Anaerobic bacterial pneumonia is due to aspiration of anaerobes from the oropharynx into the lungs. Alcoholism, obtunded patients, patients with an inability to protect the airway, prolonged seizures, and bad oral/dental hygiene are background risk factors, which are associated with aspiration pneumonia.

Pneumonia due to anaerobic organisms generally presents as a "typical" pneumonia with fever, cough, dyspnea, and pleuritic pain. Pneumonia generally involves the lower lobe or lobes. Aspiration in the supine posture leads to infiltrates involving the posterior segment of the upper lobe and/or the apical segment of the lower lobe. The sputum is purulent and often has a fetid odor. Necrotizing pneumonia with the formation of multiple abscesses may develop. Empyema is a frequent complication. Prognosis depends on prompt diagnosis and treatment with appropriate antibiotics.

Moraxella Catarrhalis

Moraxella catarrhalis are Gram-negative diplococci commonly found in the oropharynx. On aspiration into the lungs, they may cause pneumonia, particularly in patients with COPD, congestive heart failure, and other comorbid states. The clinical and radiological features are nonspecific. Leukocytosis is common and the outcome generally favorable.

Actinomyces

Actinomyces israelii is a species consisting of Gram-positive filamentous branching bacilli. It was mistaken for a fungus for several years. These organisms are present in the oropharynx and may become pathogenic when aspirated into the lungs. Poor oropharyngeal hygiene, bad dental hygiene, COPD, bronchiectasis are underlying risk factors. The organism produces a subacute to chronic pneumonia (generally involving the lower lobe), which may extend by continuity and contiguity into the pleura and from the pleura to the chest wall, causing one or more sinuses that discharge pus through the chest wall. The clinical features suggest tuberculosis, a fungal infection, or a bronchogenic carcinoma.

The presence of discharging sinuses in the chest wall particularly when they are multiple invariably points to actinomyces infection. The diagnosis is confirmed by examination of the pus, which shows characteristic filamentous branching Gram-positive bacilli. Occasionally, thoracic actinomycosis is associated with cervicofacial actinomycosis. The discharging sinuses in the neck and face are often mistaken for tuberculosis. Actinomycosis can also present as an empyema and the etiology may be missed if proper staining of pus and anaerobic cultures are not done.

Radiological features consist of areas of consolidation with small cavities involving a lobe or a segment. Infection may spread to involve the pleura causing an empyema and may also spread by contiguity to involve the ribs and the chest wall.

Infection due to *Yersinia pestis* and the *Anthrax bacillus* have been dealt within the section on "Tropical Infections Involving the Lung".

Table 3 gives a partial list of clues to the cause of pneumonia that may be obtained from the history and physical examination.

■ RECURRENT PNEUMONIA

Recurrent CAP is always a cause for concern. The most common cause of recurrent pneumonia in the same lobe of a lung is bronchial obstruction. Bronchial obstruction is most often due to carcinoma of the bronchus particularly so in elderly patients. It could also be caused by a foreign body (a "supari" in an adult) or following bronchial stenosis, which is generally a sequel of tuberculosis. An underlying unrecognized bronchiectasis may also be the cause of repeated pneumonia.

Recurrent pneumonia (not necessarily in the same lobe) in young adults may be due to congenital hypogammaglobulinemia. Serum protein estimation and a protein electrophoresis will prove the diagnosis.

Immunoglobulin G (IgG) deficiency in particular may underlie recurrent lower respiratory tract infections. Acquired human immunodeficiency syndrome can also lead to recurrent attacks of pneumonia—to start with, infection is not due to opportunistic organisms. Asplenia, either congenital or following splenectomy predisposes to

Table 3: Clues to the etiology of pneumonia from the history and physical examination.

Environmental:	Organism
• Exposure to contaminated air-conditioning cooling towers, recent travel associated with a stay in hotel, exposure to a grocery store mist machine, visit or recent stay in hospital with contaminated potable water	• *Legionella pneumophila*
• Pneumonia after windstorm in an endemic area	• *Coccidioides immitis*
• Outbreak of pneumonia in shelters for homeless men, jails, military training camps	• *Streptococcus pneumoniae, Mycobacterium tuberculosis, Chlamydia pneumoniae*
• Exposure to contaminated bat caves and excavation in endemic areas	• *Histoplasma capsulatum*
Animal contact:	
• Exposure to infected parturient cats, cattle, sheep, or goats	• *Coxiella burnetii*
• Exposure to turkeys, chickens, ducks, or birds	• *Chlamydia psittaci*
Travel history:	
• Travel to Thailand or other countries in Southeast Asia	• *Burkholderia (Pseudomonas) pseudomallei*
• Pneumonia in immigrants from Asia or India	• *Mycobacterium tuberculosis*
Occupational history:	
• Pneumonia in healthcare workers in a large city with patients infected with HIV	• *Mycobacterium tuberculosis*
Host factors:	
• Diabetic ketoacidosis	• *Streptococcus pneumoniae* and *Staphylococcus aureus*
• Alcoholism	• *Streptococcus pneumoniae, Klebsiella pneumoniae, Staphylococcus aureus*
• COPD	• *Streptococcus pneumoniae, Haemophilus influenzae, Moraxella catarrhalis*
• Solid organ transplant pneumonia (pneumonia occurring 3 months after transplant)	• *Streptococcus pneumoniae, Haemophilus influenzae, Legionella species, Pneumocystis carinii, Cytomegalovirus, Strongyloides stercoralis*
• Sickle cell disease	• *Streptococcus pneumoniae*
• HIV infection CD4 count < 200	• *Pneumocystis carinii*
• CD4 cell count > 200	• *Streptococcus pneumoniae, Haemophilus influenzae, Cryptococcus neoformans, Mycobacterium tuberculosis, Rhodococcus equi*
Physical findings:	
• Periodontal disease with foul-smelling sputum	• Anaerobes
• Bullous myringitis	• *Mycoplasma pneumoniae*
• Absent gag reflex, altered level of consciousness, or recent seizure	• Oral aerobic and anaerobic bacteria due to aspiration
• Encephalitis	• *Mycoplasma pneumoniae, Coxiella burnetii*
• Cerebellar ataxia	• *Legionella pneumophila*
• Erythema multiforme	• *Mycoplasma*
• Erythema nodosum	• *M. tuberculosis, Streptococcus, Mycoplasma*
• Cutaneous nodules (abscesses) and CNS findings	• *Nocardia species*

(CNS: Central nervous system; COPD: Chronic obstructive pulmonary disease; HIV: Human immunodeficiency virus)

fulminant pneumococcal or *H. influenzae* infection, which may recur. Sickle cell disease, neutropenia, or a qualitative defect in neutrophils, T-cell defects or deficiency are other immune-related problems predisposing to recurrent infections.

Aspiration is an important cause of recurrent pneumonia. Achalasia of the cardia when mild or a slowly increasing esophageal stricture is cause which can be easily missed as the patient may not complain of any difficulty in swallowing unless specifically asked. Aspiration following a large hiatus hernia or well-marked gastroesophageal reflux is also occasionally responsible for recurrent episodes of aspiration pneumonia. Aspiration is also probably the underlying cause (together with impaired respiratory defense mechanisms) for recurrent pneumonia in chronic alcoholics. Recurrent pneumonia may occur in patients with pulmonary sequestration. Ciliary dyskinesia with impairment of mucociliary transport also causes frequent lower respiratory tract infections in young adults.

Finally, recurrent pneumonia also occurs in patients with cystic fibrosis—a common entity in the West but less common in the developing countries of the world **(Table 4)**.

■ INVESTIGATIONS

Routine blood count, erythrocyte sedimentation rate (ESR), urine examination, blood culture, and blood biochemistry are necessary. The oxygen saturation should be promptly noted. The diagnostic value of investigations in community acquired pneumonia is given in **Table 5**.

Chest Radiography

According to consensus guidelines from the American Society of Infectious Diseases (ASID) and the American Thoracic Society (ATS), a shadow or an infiltrate on a radiographic examination of the chest, or observed through other imaging techniques is essentially required for the diagnosis of CAP (*Ref: Mandell LA, Wunderink RG, Anzueto A, et al. Infectious Diseases Society of America/ American Thoracic Society consensus guidelines on the management of community-acquired pneumonia in adults. Clin Infect Dis. 2007;44 Suppl 2:S27*).

The radiographic appearance of a CAP includes segmental or lobar consolidation, interstitial infiltrates, or cavitation. Though conventionally segmental and lobar

Table 4: Causes of recurrent pneumonia.
• Bronchial obstruction due to carcinoma bronchus, foreign body, or bronchial stenosis
• Bronchiectasis
• Hypogammaglobulinemia; isolated IgG deficiency
• Acquired human immune deficiency syndrome
• Asplenia either congenital or following splenectomy
• Sickle cell disease, neutropenia, or qualitative defect in neutrophils, T-cell defects or deficiency
• Aspiration:
– Chronic alcoholics
– Achalasia of the cardia
– Esophageal stricture
– Large hiatus hernia
– Well-marked gastroesophageal reflux
• Pulmonary sequestration
• Cystic fibrosis

(Ig: Immunoglobulin)

consolidation are believed to be due to "typical" bacteria and interstitial infiltrates are related to viral infections, to "atypical bacteria" and to pneumocystis infection, it is impossible to distinguish with any degree of surety between bacterial and nonbacterial infection on the basis of radiographic appearances. Also, HRCT of the chest has a greater sensitivity in detecting lesions and defining their extent compared to an X-ray of the chest, though in most instances of suspected CAP a radiographic examination of the chest suffices.

In hospitalized patients with a strong suspicion of CAP and a negative chest X-ray, the IDSA/ATS guidelines suggest starting empiric antibiotics therapy, but repeating an X-ray chest after 48 hours to confirm that CAP really does exist. Alternatively, a CT chest is performed as it is more sensitive than an X-ray chest.

Radiographic response to treatment usually lags behind clinical improvement and pneumococcal pneumonia (especially bacteremic forms) may take 6 weeks to clear on the chest film. *S. aureus* and *Legionella* are amongst the slower resolving pneumonias. Age is the single most important predictor of the speed of resolution. In patients who are elderly, pneumonia resolves at a much slower rate than in younger patients. Persistent, recurrent, and worsening shadowing may indicate either inappropriate treatment or bronchial obstruction by a foreign body, or more commonly, tumor, particularly in patients over the age of 60 years. At times, CT may be especially useful in distinguishing different processes, e.g. pleural effusion versus underlying pulmonary consolidation, hilar adenopathy versus pulmonary mass and pulmonary abscess versus empyema with an air-fluid level.

Laboratory Identification of Infecting Organisms

Laboratory investigation of a case of pneumonia should not delay treatment with antibiotics, the choice of which is based on a knowledge of the likely pathogens and an estimation of the severity of the infection. The lengths to which the clinician is prepared to investigate the microbiological cause of a case of pneumonia is likely to be determined by the severity of the illness at presentation, its response to initial treatment and the laboratory facilities available.

The IDSA and ATS suggest the following testing strategy depending on patient characteristics and severity of illness:

Table 5: Diagnostic value of investigations in community-acquired pneumonia.

Tests	*Remarks*
Routine CBC and biochemistry	There may be leukocytosis, leukopenia, or a normal count
Arterial oxygen saturation and blood gas analysis	Hypoxemia needs prompt correction. The greater the degree of hypoxemia, the more severe the infection
CXR	The etiology of a pneumonia cannot be definitely ascertained by the nature of the radiological shadows
Microbiological	
Sputum—Gram stain/culture	Check, if sample satisfactory Collect sputum prior to starting antibiotics Oropharyngeal contamination may be present Low sensitivity (10%), high specificity (70–80%), if positive Washing/diluting sample helpful
Blood culture	Should be done prior to starting antibiotics; Positive cultures identify organisms
Pleural fluid—Gram stain/culture	If positive, useful in establishing etiological agent
Serological	
Antigen detection	
• Pneumococcal (blood, urine)	Mainly useful for pneumococcal infection
• *Legionella* (urine)	Accurate means of diagnosing *Legionella* infection
• Cold agglutinins	Positive in over 50% of patients with mycoplasmal pneumonia
Serological tests	
• Anti-Mycoplasma	
• Anti-Chlamydia	
• Anti-influenza	Helps in diagnosis of *Mycoplasma*, *Chlamydia*, and viral pneumonias
Invasive tests (only when absolutely necessary)	
Examination of secretions, obtained from protected brush biopsies, bronchoalveolar lavage	Should be done in serious illness not responding to initial empiric antibiotic therapy
Percutaneous transthoracic needle puncture	Diagnostic yield 33–85%. Cannot be used in patients on mechanical ventilation due to the risk of pneumothorax
CT-guided biopsy of lesion	Helps in etiological diagnosis
Transbronchial, thoracoscopic, or open lung biopsy	Helps in diagnosis in the above situation if BAL, protected brush smears and CT-guided biopsies are negative
Newer tests	
PCR assay	Serum of patients with pneumococcal pneumonia: Sensitivity of 100% and specificity of 94%; also useful for other atypical bacteria and many viruses.

(BAL: Bronchoalveolar lavage; CBC: Complete blood count; CT: Computed tomography; CXR: Chest X-ray; PCR: Polymerase chain reaction)

- For outpatients with CAP, routine diagnostic tests are optional.
- Hospitalized patients with special indications should have sputum Gram's stain, sputum culture, and blood culture.
- In India where tuberculosis is endemic, a sputum test should always include smear and culture for acid-fast bacilli.
- Patients with severe CAP in the intensive care unit (ICU) should have sputum Gram's stain and culture, blood culture, pneumococcal and *Legionella* urinary antigen tests.
- Other approved tests include PCR for detecting *Chlamydia pneumoniae, Mycoplasma pneumoniae,* as well as respiratory tract viruses (*see* chapter on Nonbacterial Pneumonia) These tests are rapid with good sensitivity and specificity.

In poorer countries, many consider tests for CAP optional in hospitalized patients without severe CAP. Some microbes are, however, critical to detect because of epidemiological reasons and because treatment differs from standard empiric therapy. These organisms include *Legionella* species, *Chlamydia*, *Mycoplasma pneumoniae*, community-acquired methicillin-resistant *Staphylococci*, and other emerging pathogens. In times of terror that stalks the world today, it may be important to identify agents of bioterrorism.

Sputum Microscopy and Culture

In poorer and developing Asian countries, sputum examination is cheap, easy to perform, and often the mainstay of diagnosis of CAP. Simple Gram staining of sputum, which can be performed even at the bedside, will give an immediate and accurate indication of the pathogen involved, if large numbers of any one pathogen are seen. According to MacFarlane, such positive Gram stains have been shown to have a high specificity in the case of pneumococcal and staphylococcal pneumonia, though the sensitivity is low.

A few practical points about sputum testing need to be labored here as they are particularly relevant in developing countries. First and foremost one must ensure the sample sent to the laboratory is a truly expectorated sample and not saliva. The presence of more than 25 squamous cells per high-power field indicates a sputum sample of poor quality and precious resources may be saved by requesting a repeat sample and not bothering to proceed with sputum culture. The second problem is that lower respiratory secretions are often contaminated by upper respiratory commensals during expectoration and the microbiologist reporting a potential pathogen should be aware that this may not reflect what is actually occurring in the lung. A laboratory trick to counter this is to wash or dilute the sputum, so that only bacteria present in large numbers will grow on culture. The third problem is that even a single dose of an antibiotic can interfere with the culture of common pathogens like *S. pneumoniae* and *H. influenzae.* This is almost certainly the reason why so many hospital-based series of CAP from Asia and the West have no pathogen isolated in the majority of patients despite a careful search. The majority of patients hospitalized for pneumonia have already received one or more courses of antibiotics prior to hospitalization resulting in the sputum yield being very poor. Finally, in as many as a quarter of all patients with pneumonia, sputum is not produced. All these problems conspire to make sputum culture a relatively insensitive method of diagnosing bacterial pneumonia. Less than 50% of patients with bacteremic pneumococcal

pneumonia will have pneumococci isolated from their sputum.

A study from a public hospital in a poor part of India showed that attention to detail with bedside inoculation and dilution of the sputum specimen resulted in a higher yield (34%) of *S. pneumoniae.* If the sputum sample reached the laboratory late or did not undergo dilution the yield of *S. pneumoniae* and Gram-positive cocci was significantly reduced with higher numbers of Gram-negative rods indicating their overgrowth.

Because tuberculosis often mimics pneumonia in Asian countries, it is worth doing acid-fast staining on sputum samples. It is the policy of our microbiology laboratory to perform Ziehl-Neelsen staining on all sputum samples sent to the laboratory for routine culture. This has often helped clinicians make an early diagnosis of tuberculosis even when this has not been initially suspected.

Certain bacteria that can cause CAP are notoriously difficult to culture. *Legionella* is one such example and while occasional isolation on charcoal yeast extract medium may be possible, in the Asian context such a procedure would be expensive and time-consuming and perhaps best performed in only one or two central reference laboratories in poorer countries.

Sputum Immunodetection

The diagnostic rate of pneumococcal pneumonia can be markedly increased by testing for pneumococcal polysaccharide capsular antigen in countercurrent immunoelectrophoresis or latex agglutination. This antigen can also be detected in blood and urine and an advantage of this test is that it is not affected by prior use of antibiotics. The sputum antigen is positive in about 80% of pneumococcal pneumonias, while urine and serum are positive in 36–45% and 9–23% of cases, respectively. A study from Shanghai compared pneumococcal antigen detection by the coagglutination technique with sputum Gram stain and sputum culture. The positive yield was 46% by the coagglutination test, 27% by Gram staining and 17% by culture. Thus, pneumococcal antigen detection by virtue of its speed, sensitivity, convenience, and relative independence of antibiotic therapy provides a new dimension in the etiological diagnosis of pneumococcal pneumonia. The antigen remains detectable for 7–14 days after bacteremic pneumococcal pneumonia.

Other pathogens that may be detected by sputum immunodetection include *Legionella pneumophila, Chlamydia pneumoniae,* and *Pneumocystis carinii.*

It is well-nigh certain that the incidence of *Legionella* pneumonia would rise considerably, if specific tests were done in suspected patients. These include: (1) test for *Legionella* antigen in the urine; (2) positive direct fluorescence antibody test for *Legionella* plus with an antibody titer of more than 1 in 256; (3) isolation of the organism on culture or a fourfold rise in antibody titer.

Blood Culture

In the initial evaluation of a patient with pneumonia, at least two blood samples for culture should be obtained from different venepuncture sites. A positive culture may be obtained in 10–30% of cases, the higher percentage applying to pneumococcal pneumonia. This provides diagnostic proof (i.e. high specificity) of a pathogenic organism, often lacking where sputum culture and other tests are concerned. It is also of prognostic importance because bacteremia is an indicator of more severe infection.

Pleural Fluid

If a pleural effusion is present in a patient suspected of having pneumonia, it should always be examined to exclude an empyema. Gram and acid-fast stains may be useful. The culture of pathogenic organisms is always significant and valuable. The fluid is always an exudate and some biochemical findings (low pH, high lactate dehydrogenase, and low glucose) have been used to predict which parapneumonic effusions may develop into empyemas.

Standard Acute and Convalescent Serological Testing

The usual serological tests involve the measurement of complement-fixing antibody levels in the blood, although the more sensitive enzyme-linked immunosorbent assay (ELISA) and immunofluorescent tests are tending to replace them. Serological tests may be used for infections caused by *Mycoplasma pneumoniae, Chlamydia species, Coxiella burnetii,* and *Legionella species.* By its nature, the complement-fixing test (CFT) is seldom of immediate value and when positive usually provides diagnostic information retrospectively, as two paired sera are required in order to demonstrate a fourfold rise in convalescent-phase antibody titer. It is usual to wait about 14 days between the two samples, although in some infections, such as *Mycoplasma,* a rise may be detected earlier; while in others, notably *Legionella,* the rise may take several weeks.

The problem with paired sampling is that the results are likely to come too late to be of clinical relevance.

Newer Microbiological Techniques

Deoxyribonucleic acid (DNA) probes have been developed for characterizing target organisms and minute amounts of target DNA can be amplified by the PCR to improve the chance of their detection by the DNA probe, so that the sensitivity of the test is increased. A PCR assay has been tested on the serum of patients with bacteremic pneumococcal pneumonia and was found to have a sensitivity of 100% and specificity of 94%. Similar probes have been developed for a wide range of atypical organisms causing CAP including *Legionella pneumophila, Chlamydia, Mycoplasma pneumoniae,* as also for *Blastomyces dermatitidis, Histoplasma capsulatum, Coccidioides immitis, Mycobacterium tuberculosis, Mycobacterium avium, Mycobacterium intracellulare,* and *Mycobacterium scrofulaceum (MAIS group)* and *Mycobacterium kansasii.* Thus, the identification of mycobacterial infection may take hours rather than weeks, although the organism still requires culture in order to allow full antimicrobial sensitivities to be confirmed. Gene expert tests on sputum in suspected tuberculous pneumonia, if positive, will also determine whether the mycobacterium is resistant to or sensitive to rifampicin and isoniazid. These tests are generally outside the reach of all, but a few specialized and referral laboratories in the developing Asian countries.

In a study done by Honda and colleagues in Japan, serologic data was compared with data obtained by capillary PCR to establish the efficacy of capillary PCR for the determination of *Mycoplasma* infection in samples obtained from throat swabs, BAL fluid and sputum of patients with *Mycoplasma* pneumonia. It was found that capillary PCR had a sensitivity of 80.6%.

Invasive Methods for Obtaining Respiratory Secretions

Other methods for obtaining respiratory secretions are more invasive and may be associated with morbidity. Their use is therefore confined to patients who are severely ill and in whom it is considered important to identify the organism rather than relying on an initial empirical antimicrobial approach or in whom such an approach has already been tried and failed.

Fiberoptic Bronchoscopy

Fiberoptic bronchoscopy is usually safe, well tolerated, and has become the standard invasive procedure used to obtain lower respiratory tract secretion from seriously ill or immunocompromised patients with complex or progressive pneumonia and in selected patients with ventilator-associated pneumonia. It picks up oropharyngeal contaminants unless special precautions are taken using a protected specimen brush (PSB). The PSB can be combined with or used separately from BAL to obtain quantitative cultures in order to discriminate between the presence and absence of pneumonia, usually on ventilated patients in an intensive care setting. The diagnostic threshold for pneumonia, rather than airway colonization, has been reported as 10^3 CFU/mL in respiratory secretions obtained by PSB. On the other hand, BAL subtends a wide area of tissue and lung secretions are diluted between 10 and 100-fold, so that when interpreting results, a threshold of 10^4 CFU/mL may be taken. By combining PSB and BAL and by counting intracellular organisms, Chastre and colleagues claimed a sensitivity of 100% (compared with 86% for either technique alone) and a specificity of 96%. Bronchoscopy can therefore provide clues in a difficult case when other methods have failed, even when the picture has been clouded by almost inevitable prior use of antimicrobials. Infection with less usual organisms, such as *Legionalle species, M. tuberculosis, P. carinii,* and other fungi or anaerobes may also be detected in such cases as well as the occasional unsuspected predisposing cause like the mechanical narrowing of a bronchus. On the other hand, negative results have to be treated with caution in patients already treated with antimicrobial therapy, since these may indicate either that the antibiotics are appropriate and that the organisms have been suppressed or that there was no infection there in the first place and the infiltrate was due to a noninfective cause.

In a study in China by Zhong and colleagues, secretions from the lower respiratory tract were taken for bacterial culture using Japanese-made single-sheath catheter (SSC) brush via fiberoptic bronchoscope in 53 cases with CAP. The results showed that bacteria were isolated in 42 out of 53 patients, the organism being pathogenic in 39 out of 53 (73.5%). Among the bacteria isolated from the 42 cases, Gram-negative bacilli accounted for the highest rate of 36% and *Pneumococcus* was next with 31%. There were only three cases yielding contamination. Thus, it showed that SSC has less chances of contamination and is convenient and practical.

Percutaneous Transthoracic Needle Puncture

This procedure employs a small-gauge needle that is advanced into the area of pulmonary consolidation with CT guidance. It requires the patient to cooperate, have good hemostasis, and be able to tolerate a possible associated pulmonary hemorrhage or pneumothorax. Patients on mechanical ventilation cannot undergo lung puncture because of the high incidence of complicating pneumothorax. The diagnostic yield from this procedure ranges from 33% to 85%.

Transtracheal Aspiration

Transtracheal aspiration may be carried out in patients who are unable to produce sputum or in whom the response to the chosen antibiotic is poor. The success of the procedure relies on the assumption that the tracheobronchial tree below the larynx is sterile, but false-positive results occur in patients with chronic lung disease because of tracheobronchial colonization. The technique has also been applied when anaerobic lung infection is suspected. A group from Japan performed this technique on 387 patients over an 8-year period from 1990–98 and isolated anaerobes in 20% of patients with CAP. Popular several decades ago, transtracheal aspiration is rarely carried out today.

Lung Biopsy

Transbronchial, thoracoscopic, or open-lung biopsies tend to be reserved for diffuse pulmonary infiltrates of undetermined cause and in the context of suspected infection are occasionally carried out in sick immuno-compromised hosts in whom the presence of an unusual opportunistic pathogen is likely and in whom less invasive diagnostic approaches like BAL have failed to identify the cause.

Arterial Oxygen Saturation and Blood Gas Analysis

Oxygen saturation performed as a prompt screening procedure and should be followed by arterial blood gas analysis, if desaturation is present. The degree of hypoxemia present is a measure of the severity of the infection and needs prompt correction. The need for inspired oxygen of 40% or more to maintain the oxygen saturation above 90% implies severe pneumonia as does a PaO_2 of 60 mm Hg or less, or a $PaCO_2$ of 50 mm Hg or more. These findings warn that assisted ventilation may become necessary.

Other Laboratory Findings

The white cell count is frequently raised in bacterial pneumonia with a neutrophilia. Elderly patients are not always able to mount such a response. Sometimes when sepsis is overwhelming there may be leukopenia. A lymphocytosis may occur in viral infections or due to "atypical" organisms. The white cell count may be normal in viral pneumonia. The presence of cold agglutinins in a patient's citrated blood is seen in over 50% of cases of *Mycoplasma pneumonia.*

Numerous nonspecific biochemical abnormalities have been noted, such as a raised blood urea, bilirubin, transaminases, and alkaline phosphatase. Hyponatremia due to inappropriate antidiuretic hormone secretion may occur in *Legionella* infection.

Urinalysis may detect small amounts of protein and both red and white blood cells (WBCs) may be seen on microscopy. As mentioned above, pneumococcal antigen may be detected in urine more frequently than in blood but less frequently than in sputum. *Legionella* antigen may also be detected in urine by ELISA, indicating *L. pneumophila* Type 1 infection (thought to account for about 80% of human legionellosis), and this test is well worth doing for a rapid answer in severely ill patients with pneumonia.

■ COMPLICATIONS (TABLE 6)

The most important complication is acute respiratory failure. There is often a large shunt from right to left in pneumonia, particularly when more than one lobe are involved. This leads to a marked fall in the PaO_2 even when the patient is on oxygen at 4–6 L/min. Acute respiratory failure can also occur because of the evolution of the ARDS following a fulminant lobar pneumonia. Multiple shadows in both lungs, with a large right-to-left shunt following a lobar consolidation are now invariably thought to be due to acute lung injury (ARDS), and not due to multilobar pneumonia as was earlier believed.

Acute life-threatening pneumonia is a source of sepsis. All the complications of the sepsis syndrome may be

Table 6: Complications of acute community-acquired pneumonia.

- Acute respiratory failure
- ARDS
- Sepsis syndrome/MODS
- Acute circulatory failure
- Spread of infection to contiguous areas or hematogenous spread, e.g. empyema, acute meningitis, cerebral abscess, endocarditis, acute pericarditis
- Acute left ventricular failure/acute myocarditis
- Acute abdominal distension—acute dilatation of the stomach, ileus
- Femoral vein thrombosis, pulmonary embolism
- Bronchiectasis (as a sequel)

observed. These include hypotension, septic shock, and tissue hypoperfusion with metabolic acidosis culminating in multiple organ failure.

Spread of infection to contiguous areas, or hematogenous spread, add to the gravity of the illness. Empyema is the most common complication of CAP. It may be tucked away posteriorly in the paravertebral gutter and can be missed on a chest X-ray. It is clearly demonstrated on a CT of the chest. It may be responsible for the sepsis syndrome after the consolidation in the lung has resolved. Occasionally, CAP may break down to form a lung abscess; this can occur with infections caused by *S. aureus, Pneumococcus* Type III infection, anaerobic infection or following infections with Gram-negative organisms such as *Klebsiella pneumoniae,* and *P. pyocyaneus.* The abscess may communicate with the pleura causing an empyema and a bronchopleural fistula.

Acute purulent pericarditis is now a very rare complication. It is lethal if undiagnosed and not promptly treated. As little as 300 mL of pus in the pericardium can cause death from cardiac tamponade in a child. The diagnosis should be suspected when there is a sudden clinical deterioration in a patient with acute pneumonia, particularly in the presence of shock with a raised central venous pressure.

Acute pyogenic meningitis may be the presenting feature of an underlying pneumococcal lobar pneumonia. Neck stiffness and a positive Kernig's sign may, however, be present in acute lobar pneumonia even without acute meningitis. Meningism is more frequently observed with upper lobe pneumonia in young adults. A lumbar puncture is always mandatory, as it is the only certain way of distinguishing meningism from meningitis.

A sharp deterioration in the clinical state with confusion, delirium, and severe prostration may also occur when infection from the lungs spreads hematogenously to produce one or more cerebral abscesses. Localizing signs may be present. A CT scan is invaluable in confirming the clinical diagnosis.

In patients with staphylococcal pneumonia with a positive blood culture, it is imperative to test for bacterial endocarditis. The same holds when pneumonia is diagnosed in drug addicts.

Acute left ventricular failure is rare except in patients with pre-existing left ventricular disease. Acute myocarditis can and does however occur in some patients with acute influenza. It is characterized by tachycardia, increase in breathlessness, hypotension, cardiac dilatation, and a diastolic gallop. It may progress to an increasingly severe low output state and death from cardiogenic shock.

In the older age group, we have admitted to the ICU patients severely ill with acute pneumonia presenting with marked abdominal distension. Acute dilatation of the stomach is particularly dangerous, as it compounds respiratory difficulties. Ileus may also occur due to toxemia.

Femoral vein thrombosis is occasionally observed in patients critically ill with pneumonia. Sudden death in acute pneumonia could well be related to pulmonary embolism.

Severe lobar pneumonia may so damage the bronchi within the lobes as to lead to bronchiectasis as a permanent sequel.

Elderly patients with comorbid disease (e.g. ischemic heart disease or cardiovascular disease) may develop arrhythmias, myocardial infarct or a stroke when being treated for a CAP.

■ DIFFERENTIAL DIAGNOSIS

A large pulmonary infarct is an important differential diagnosis of acute lobar pneumonia. The distinction at times is difficult. An important differential diagnosis is pulmonary edema due to left ventricular failure, when the edema is more marked in one lung resulting in a homogenous shadow in the lower lobe of generally the right lung. Atelectasis, aspiration, chemical pneumonitis, pulmonary hemorrhage, connective tissue disorders, drug reactions should also be considered in the differential diagnosis depending on the clinical scenario and associated features. Acute hypersensitivity pneumonitis or acute cryptogenic fibrosing alveolitis may produce bilateral lung shadows with increasing hypoxia. Acute eosinophilic pneumonia should be suspected on the fairly

typical radiological features (peripheral shadows in both lung fields). Acute consolidation due to a vasculitis (e.g. Wegener's) may be indistinguishable from consolidation due to an infection. Pneumonia may occur as a presenting feature of lung cancer or of bronchial obstruction produced by a tumor or a foreign body. Aspiration of betel nut *(supari)* can cause a life-threatening acute necrotizing pneumonia. Cryptogenic organizing pneumonia may, to start with, be an important differential diagnosis of CAP. An infected bulla or cyst may be mistaken for a breaking down staphylococcal pneumonia.

The possibility of an underlying amoebic liver abscess should always be considered in endemic areas in the presence of right lower lobe pathology. A subphrenic abscess may cause a pleural effusion, an empyema, and/or a lower lobe consolidation.

■ MANAGEMENT

When a patient with pneumonia first presents to a general practitioner or a hospital, the cause of pneumonia is generally not known. While sputum and blood culture should be collected at the outset, treatment must start on what are perforce empirical grounds. The first decision the doctor has to make is: "Can this patient with CAP be successfully managed as an outpatient or should the patient be hospitalized?" The second and even more important question is "What should my empirical choice of antibiotic be?"

Estimating Severity of Pneumonia (Table 7)

A number of severity scores have emerged that attempt to determine the severity of a patient's pneumonia. These include:

- *CURB index*: CURB stands for; Confusion, Urea more than 7 mmol/L, Respiratory rate more than 30/min, Blood pressure systolic less than 90 mm Hg, or diastolic

Table 7: Estimating severity of pneumonia.
• CURB index
• CURB-65
• Pneumonia Severity Index (PSI)
• Modified BTS rule
• Revised ATS guidelines

(ATS: American Thoracic Society; BTS: British Thoracic Society)

less than 60 mm Hg. Several elegant British Thoracic Society (BTS) studies have shown that the presence of two of these four denotes severe CAP with such patients having a 24-fold higher risk of death **(Table 8)**.

- *CURB-65*: It includes all four core CURB variables with the addition of age more than 65 years as the fifth variable. Three or more of these five variables are now needed to define severe CAP **(Table 9)**.
- *PSI (Pneumonia Severity Index)*: It uses 20 clinical variables to determine a score. These scores are then used to define five classes of increasing risk of mortality with Class 4 and 5 defining severe CAP.
- *Modified BTS rule*: The BTS rule is based on the presence or absence of three factors on admission: (1) respiratory rate more than 30/min, (2) diastolic blood pressure less than 60 mm Hg, and (3) blood urea more than 7 mmol/L (blood urea done at any time after admission is also applicable). Patients with two or more of these features had a mortality of 19.4% compared with 0.9% in those with none or one of these features. The modified BTS rule included mental confusion as the fourth factor. Those with two or more of the four features had a mortality of 22%.
- *Revised American Thoracic Society (ATS) guidelines*: The presence of at least one major (need for mechanical ventilation or septic shock) or two minor criteria ($PaO_2/FiO_2 < 250$ kPa, multilobar shadowing on chest radiograph, or systolic blood pressure less than 90 mm Hg) is used to define CAP severity **(Table 10)**.

All the scores are more or less comparable in terms of sensitivity, specificity, and predictive value with the CURB score being most strongly recommended because of its simplicity and applicability at the bedside. *When the CURB score was applied to the Indian CAP series in one of our units, it was found to be robust with a PPV (positive predictive value) of 78% and an NPV (negative predictive value) of 94% in predicting who will die or require ICU transfer.*

Would considerations other than the CURB criteria or CURB-65 criteria, the modified BTS criteria or revised ATS guidelines influence the need for hospitalization? In most patients, the CURB or CURB-65 criteria have a high sensitivity and specificity for recognizing patients serious enough to warrant hospitalization—but not always so **(Table 11)**. We would consider hospitalization if just one of the CURB criteria is present and the patient has any one or more of the following:

- Multilobar involvement or cavitation or moderate-sized pleural effusion, or metastatic complications
- PaO_2/FiO_2 less than 250 or a PaO_2 less than 60 mm Hg or an arterial blood pH less than 7.3
- Marked leukopenia or thrombocytopenia or anemia (Hb—8.5 gm%)
- Hypothermia or hyperpyrexia
- Tachycardia more than 120/min
- Presence of significant comorbid disease—moderately severe COPD, cardiac disease, congestive heart failure, immunodeficiency states, or immunosuppression from any cause
- Home management impossible because of poverty, altered mentation, and likelihood of poor compliance.

All patients who have a strongly positive CURB Index, or a PSI, or meet the modified BTS rule, or satisfy the revised ATS guidelines with regard to the severity of the illness, should in our country be preferably admitted to start with in the ICU. The more strongly positive these

---

Table 8: CURB index.

- Confusion
- *Urea* > 7 mmol/L
- *Respiratory rate* > 30/min
- *Blood pressure* systolic < 90 mm Hg, or diastolic < 60 mm Hg. The presence of two of these four denotes severe CAP with such patients having a 24-fold higher risk of death

(CAP: Community-acquired pneumonia)

Table 9: CURB-65.

- Confusion
- *Urea* > 7 mmol/L
- *Respiratory rate* > 30/min
- *Blood pressure* systolic < 90 mm Hg, or diastolic < 60 mm Hg

Group 1: 0 or 1 of the above—mortality low—1.5%—treatment at home

Group 2: 2 of the above, mortality 9.2%—hospitalize

Group 3: 3 or more of the above—mortality 22%—admit in the ICU

(ICU: Intensive care unit)

Table 10: Revised American Thoracic Society (ATS) guidelines.

The presence of any one of the following major or two minor criteria is used to assess the severity of the CAP.

Major criteria:	*Minor criteria*:
• Need for mechanical ventilation • Septic shock	• $PaO_2/FiO_2 < 250$ kPa • Multilobar shadowing on chest radiography • Systolic blood pressure < 90 mm Hg

(CAP: Community-acquired pneumonia; FiO_2: Fraction of inspired oxygen; PaO_2: Partial pressure of oxygen)

Table 11: Criteria for hospitalization.			
Lack of response or further deterioration in condition at home	CURB index (2 or more) CURB-65 (2 or more) Modified BTS rule (2 out of the 3) Revised ATS guidelines (one major or 2 minor criteria)	Multilobar involvement Pleural effusions Metastatic complications Marked leukopenia or thrombocytopenia or anemia Severe hypoxia	Poverty rendering home management impossible
A	B	C	D

(ATS: American Thoracic Society; BTS: British Thoracic Society)
Note: In our setup, all patients who come under category B or C would be cared for in a critical care unit to start with.

guidelines or indices in an individual patient, the greater the need for ICU admission. Presence of one or more of the other clinical features listed separately above also necessitates critical care. While Western countries have clear guidelines on the appropriate initial antibiotics for a patient with CAP, no similar guidelines are available for India or other countries of Asia.

Indeed, because of the vastness and disparity of different parts of the Indian subcontinent, no guidelines could hope to be all-encompassing. Hence, as stressed in the section on "etiology", regional studies, which should be carefully and prospectively performed, must first establish the local epidemiology. Thus, based on the firm knowledge of local epidemiology, patient population profile and economic issues, local guidelines can be individualized for regions of India or other different Asian countries. Blindly transposing Western guidelines to Asian countries would clearly be inappropriate. Worse still however would be empirical treatment given without knowledge or consideration of local epidemiological conditions. Furthermore, a mechanism for regular review at a regional level should ideally be in place to take account of changing patterns of disease such as the reduced susceptibility of common organisms to standard antibiotics and emergence of new or previously unknown pathogens. Such a review by Lim from Singapore noted that there had been a 60-fold increase in the incidence of penicillin resistance in *S. pneumoniae* between 1987 and 1997. The review also made note of the small increase in the number of cases of Legionnaire's disease and the marked increase in the incidence of melioidosis. Similar reviews from Thailand show that melioidosis has become the most common cause of CAP in this region (see Tropical Infections involving the Lungs).

Choice of Antibiotics

The initial treatment is empiric (particularly in hospitalized patients) and should be started promptly once the diagnosis of CAP is considered likely. Sputum or lower respiratory tract secretions (in patients with an artificial airway) should be collected for examination as far as possible, before starting treatment. If for some reason, this necessitates delay, empiric therapy should not be withheld particularly in seriously ill patients. Generally, a limited number of organisms cause CAP, the most common organism the world over being *S. pneumoniae*. Other important pathogens that need to be covered include *H. influenzae* and atypical bacteria in particular *M. pneumoniae*. In contrast to the West, *Legionella* and *Chlamydia pneumoniae* are uncommonly encountered, almost certainly because they are not frequently tested in the laboratory. A cover for oropharyngeal aerobes and anaerobes should be considered in the setting of possible aspiration. Finally, the possibility of a respiratory viral infection needs to be considered under the prevailing epidemiological conditions (*see* chapter on Nonbacterial Pneumonias).

Two important points need to be stressed. First, despite the use of empiric therapy, tests for a microbiological diagnosis are often important, particularly in severe CAP as these tests may suggest infection by organisms that require treatment different from standard empiric therapy. These organisms for example include *Legionella, Mycobacterium tuberculosis, MRSA*, virulent Gram-negative bacteria, and various viruses causing respiratory infection. In appropriate circumstances and situations, it also involves testing for agents of bioterrorism.

Second, though in most parts of our country, the *S. pneumoniae* is sensitive to the penicillin group of drugs, there is an emerging drug resistance to these drugs in different countries of the world, which complicates conventional empiric therapy. Most of these resistant pneumococci respond to higher dose beta lactams other than cefuroxime. Treatment failures have also been demonstrated with the use of macrolides for macrolide-resistant organisms.

Choice of antibiotics in the treatment of CAP is considered separately for patients treated on an outpatient basis and for hospitalized patients.

Outpatient Department Treatment

For patients treated in the community in poorer countries, cost is often an important deciding factor. Cheap but reasonably effective antibiotic choices in India and the developing world would include oral amoxicillin or ampicillin, co-trimoxazole or a tetracycline derivative. A recent trial from one of the poorest areas of the developing world showed that co-trimoxazole was cheap and yet as effective as more expensive antibiotics in 134 Gambian children with pneumonia. It is important that general practitioners and rural healthcare providers are not seduced by the latest (and generally most costly) antibiotics. Responsible prescribing by this group of physicians will go a long way in preventing the emergence of antibiotic resistance. The impact that a rational antibiotic policy can make in reducing pneumonia mortality, even in the poorest part of rural India, can be seen from an inspiring study by Bang et al. This was a community-based intervention trial to reduce childhood mortality from pneumonia in 6,176 children in 58 villages in Gadchiroli, India. These interventions included mass education about childhood pneumonia and case management of pneumonia by trained paramedics and village health workers who were taught to recognize childhood pneumonia and treat it with co-trimoxazole. After a year of intervention, pneumonia-specific childhood mortality was significantly reduced in the intervention area as compared to a control area of 44 villages (8.1 vs 17.5 deaths per 1,000 children under 5 years). The difference in infant mortality (89 vs 121 per 1,000) and total under-five mortality (28.5 vs 40.7 per 1,000) was highly significant. The cost of co-trimoxazole was US $0.025 per child per year. This worked out to a mere $2.64 per child saved.

Another antibiotic, which is a reasonable first choice and relatively inexpensive, is erythromycin. In the many Asian regions, where atypical pathogens are frequently encountered, this would be an appropriate initial choice. A study from Taiwan showed it to be as effective as the more expensive (but better tolerated) clarithromycin.

If cost is not a factor then oral antibiotics with a wider range include a P-lactamase stable antibiotic like co-amoxiclav or a second- or third-generation oral cephalosporin like cefuroxime axetil. Other effective oral choices would be a newer macrolide like azithromycin or clarithromycin. While the newer quinolones are emerging as oral antibiotics for CAP in many parts of the world, it is our opinion that these drugs have a pivotal role as second-line drugs in multidrug-resistant tuberculosis (MDR-TB) and should be reserved for this role in regions where TB is endemic.

Hospitalized Patients

These patients are likely to be more ill at the outset or have associated comorbid conditions and should ideally receive intravenous antibiotics from the start. The initial choice of antibiotics is based on local epidemiology plus an assessment of how severe the pneumonia is.

In the ill-hospitalized patients, all probable pathogens must be covered and an intravenous P-lactamase stable penicillin (e.g. co-amoxiclav) or a cephalosporin (e.g. cefotaxime or ceftriaxone) together with a macrolide provides good initial cover for the majority of typical and atypical pathogens likely to be encountered.

Two situations which deserve separate mention are: (1) infection caused by *Staphylococcus* where flucloxacillin (supported by rifampicin) or vancomycin may be considered and (2) infection caused by Gram-negative enteric bacilli (including *P. aeruginosa*). While the American Thoracic Guidelines recommend cover from the start for these organisms in all severely ill-hospitalized CAPs we do not regard this approach necessary in the initial management of younger previously healthy patients.

In very ill individuals admitted to the ICU with life-threatening pneumonia, particularly in the elderly (in whom community-acquired Gram-negative infections are encountered with increasing frequency), it may be necessary to empirically cover all likely organisms— *S. pneumoniae,* Gram-negative bacteria, staphylococci, and atypical organisms. The antibiotic regime would include amoxicillin or amoxicillin clavulanate to cover pneumococci, piperacillin-tazobactam, or a carbapenem to cover Gram-negative bacteria, vancomycin, if a staphylococcal infection is considered possible and a macrolide for atypical organisms. If an anaerobic infection is suspected one could add either metronidazole or clindamycin, or replace piperacillin-tazobactam with meropenem. This is indeed blunderbuss therapy but is at times unavoidable.

The same empiric regime may need to be followed in younger individuals who fail to respond and appear to worsen after initial therapy with amoxicillin or co-amoxiclav and a macrolide or after initial therapy on a regime consisting of a second-generation cephalosporin and a macrolide.

Once a pathogen causing CAP has been identified through microbiological methods, one should deescalate to target the specific organism. Most clinicians prefer to use two antibiotics for *Pseudomonas* or *Klebsiella pneumoniae* infection.

The appropriate antibiotic therapy for a CAP is listed in **Table 12**.

Patients generally are afebrile or nearly so within 72 hours with appropriate therapy. Cough may be present longer and radiological resolution may take weeks and occasionally even months.

When the patient continues to be hemodynamically stable with marked clinical improvement in his respiratory state and the WBC count, one should switch to oral medication, if this is feasible, provided the patient can swallow comfortably. Elderly patients and those with serious comorbid states [COPD and congestive cardiac failure (CCF)] should receive parenteral therapy for a longer time.

Use of Corticosteroids

In most patients with CAP who are seriously ill and under intensive care, glucocorticoids may be of use. The recommended dose of methylprednisolone is 0.5 mg per kg intravenously 12 hourly or prednisolone 50 mg/day, either one or the other being continued for 5 days. There is some evidence to suggest that infections caused by the influenza virus, or by *Aspergillus* have worse outcomes with the use of steroids as adjunctive therapy. They should, therefore, not be used when these infections are responsible for pneumonia. Corticosteroids should also be avoided in patients believed to be at high risk for side effects, in immunocompromised patients, and in pregnancy.

Duration of Treatment

The antimicrobial treatment for uncomplicated pneumonias due to *S. pneumoniae,* anaerobes, *H. influenzae*, and *M. catarrhalis* should be continued for 7–10 days. The duration of treatment for *Mycoplasma* and *Legionella* infection is 2–3 weeks. However, the presence of *S. aureus* or Gram-negative enteric bacilli or the development of suppurative complications requires a more prolonged course of therapy (e.g. 2 weeks for nonbacteremic staphylococcal pneumonia, 4 weeks for bacteremic staphylococcal pneumonia, and 4–6 weeks in case of an empyema). A study of 186 patients hospitalized for mild-to-moderate pneumonia in nine hospitals from 2000–03 in Netherlands showed 3 days of amoxicillin was as effective as 8 days. Such a strategy, if verified in larger trials, would represent considerable savings in cost and curtail antibiotic resistance.

Assessment of Response to Initial Antimicrobial Therapy

Once antimicrobial treatment is initiated, it is important to monitor the patient for clinical response. Normally no change in antimicrobial treatment should be considered within the first 72 hours unless initial diagnostic studies identify a pathogen not covered by original empirical therapy (e.g. *M. tuberculosis),* a resistant pathogen is

Types of patients	Antibiotic used
Table 12: Antimicrobial therapy in community-acquired pneumonia (CAP).	
Hospitalized patients	β-lactamase penicillin—co-amoxiclav: 1.2 g 8 hourly IV or IV cephalosporin like ceftriaxone: 2 g 12 hourly IV + Oral macrolide like Azithromycin 500 mg 12 hourly
Severely ill patients	Amoxicillin 500 mg QDS + Piperacillin-tazobactam—4.5 g 8 hourly IV or a Carbapenem-meropenem 1 g 8 hourly IV + Vancomycin 500 mg 6 hourly IV (if MRSA suspected) + macrolide Regime to be modified, if infecting organism has been determined. Infection with *Pseudomonas aeruginosa* requires a two-drug combination— meropenem 1 g 8 hourly + aminoglycoside (Amikacin) 1 g IV OD
OPD patients	β-lactamase penicillin-amoxiclav 625 BD orally or cephalosporin-cefuroxime 500 BD orally or macrolide—azithromycin 500 mg BD or levofloxacin 750 mg BD, if atypical organism is suspected

(IV: Intravenous; MRSA: Methicillin-resistant *Staphylococcus aureus*; OPD: Outpatient department)
Note: Quinolones should be used with great discrimination, if at all in countries which have a high prevalence of tuberculosis. In poor rural parts of developing countries, the above drugs are difficult to use. Alternative therapy with amoxicillin 500 QDS or sulfamethoxazole and trimethoprim (Septran DS 1 tablet twice daily) can be effectively used.

isolated from blood or another sterile site (i.e. pleural fluid), or there is clinical deterioration. Even when antimicrobial treatment is appropriate, clinical improvement may be delayed by several factors **(Table 13)**. The presence of coexisting illness and advanced age is associated with delays in improvement. Patients with structural abnormalities of the respiratory tract, particularly COPD, often do not respond as rapidly as previously healthy patients. Unrecognized immunosuppression, e.g. owing to AIDS or prior drug therapy, may also result in delay in clinical improvement. The virulence of the infectious agent may also delay response. Bacteremic patients and patients with Gram-negative or staphylococcal pneumonias are generally slower to respond.

In appropriately treated patients, clinical response is often rapid, especially among patients without prior coexisting disease. In this population, fever usually disappears within two to four days, and the leukocytosis resolves by the 4th or 5th day of therapy. Physical findings remain abnormal in up to 40% of patients at day 7. The chest radiograph may not normalize at 4 weeks even in young (<50-year old), previously healthy individuals and may not reach baseline for up to 6 months in the elderly patients with COPD, or in alcoholic patients. Chest radiographic abnormalities may worsen initially, but significant early (<48 hours) deterioration of chest radiograph, defined as a 50% or greater increase in the size of the infiltrate, progression to significant involvement of multiple lobes, or development of a large pleural effusion should raise concern that therapy is inadequate.

Table 13: Factors involved in poor response to empirical antimicrobial therapy.

- Incorrect microbiological diagnosis
- Inappropriate antimicrobial agent or dosing regimen
- Drug-resistant organism
- Poor drug response (immunocompromised or even otherwise)
- Fulminant infections caused by *MRSA*
- Drug hypersensitivity or drug fever
- Tuberculosis can mimic bacterial pneumonia, also consider unusual organisms such as *Actinomyces* or *Nocardia species*
- Endobronchial obstruction
- Severe aspiration pneumonia, associated renal or liver disease, uncontrolled diabetes, leukopenia
- *Infectious complication*: Empyema, metastatic spread, superinfection
- *Reconsider the diagnosis*: Could it be embolism, malignancy, vasculitis, drug reaction, eosinophilic pneumonia, or cryptogenic organizing pneumonia

Supportive Treatment in Pneumonia

Respiratory Support

Patients who are in obvious respiratory distress with tachypnea are at increased risk of dying and need close monitoring, particularly if they are beginning to show evidence of exhaustion with drowsiness or confusion. The finding of a PaO_2 of less than 60 mm Hg when breathing oxygen at 2–4 L/min indicates a serious situation, as does hypercarbia. Many patients are already receiving supplemental oxygen; a PaO_2/FiO_2 ratio equal to or less than 200 mm Hg is a serious concern. A PaO_2 of 50 mm Hg or less in the presence of rising $PaCO_2$ and acidosis are indications for ventilatory support. Sometimes, improvement in oxygenation can be achieved by postural drainage, so that the "good lung" is dependent. Noninvasive ventilatory support using high-flow oxygen through a continuous positive airway pressure (CPAP) or biphasic positive airway pressure (BiPAP) device may help tide over a crisis and relieve hypoxia provided the patient is sufficiently cooperative, not too tachypneic, hemodynamically stable, and does not have excessive sputum production.

Mechanical ventilation is indicated in hypoxic patients who are hemodynamically unstable, acidotic, have copious respiratory secretions or have a feeble respiratory effort.

Patients who are feeble, are unable to cough and have copious respiratory secretions may need temporary endotracheal intubation to allow proper aspiration of secretions. Ventilatory support may or may not be always necessary.

Inotropic agents such as dopamine or dobutamine and vasopressors such as norepinephrine may be required when severe pneumonia is complicated by hypotension. Pleuritic pain can be relieved by simple nonsedative analgesics. Physiotherapy is of no benefit and should be avoided in acutely ill patients who find cooperation difficult, who may easily become exhausted and even more hypoxic. It may, however, assist expectoration of sputum in less ill patients and in those who are recovering. Elderly or very feeble patients who have a great deal of sputum production, which they cannot expectorate, are aided by a bronchoscopic clearance of chest secretions. **Table 13** gives a list of factors that could be responsible for poor response of pneumonia to treatment.

PROGNOSIS

The outcome of CAP depends on the early diagnosis and effective antimicrobial therapy, along with the age of the patient, the severity of the disease and the underlying associated comorbid conditions. Pneumonia in the elderly is particularly dangerous due to frequent absence of classical symptoms and also due to the higher incidence of adverse effects to antibiotics.

In an interesting study by Chen and colleagues in Taiwan, the following variables were associated with a poor prognosis. They were:

- The presence of septic shock
- The use of ventilatory support
- The presence of radiological spread
- Treatment in an intensive care unit
- Male gender
- Development of ARDS
- *Klebsiella* pneumonia in patients with alcohol habit
- Patients with ultimately fatal underlying disease
- An initial $PaO_2/FiO_2 < 200$
- An arterial pH less than 7.25.

In a study by Dey and colleagues in Delhi, it was found that old age, history of smoking, presence of chronic obstructive airways disease, late presentation to hospital, systolic and diastolic hypotension, high-blood urea, low-serum albumin, and development of septic shock were associated with a poorer prognosis. In their study of 72 patients with CAP, 35% of elderly patients and 14% of young patients succumbed to fulminant sepsis or respiratory failure.

PREVENTION

The prevention of pneumonia aims at strengthening the host's responses, once the pathogen is encountered. This includes the use of chemoprophylaxis or immunization for patients at risk. Chemoprophylaxis can be administered to patients who have encountered or are likely to encounter the pathogen before they become symptomatic (e.g. amantadine during a community outbreak of *Influenza A*, isoniazid for tuberculosis, or trimethoprim-sulfamethoxazole for pneumocystis). Vaccines are available for immunization against *S. pneumoniae, H. influenzae* Type B, *Influenza viruses A* and *B,* and measles virus. Of these, the pneumococcal and influenza vaccines are found to be most effective and are indicated in patients over 65 years of age and in patients with cardiovascular diseases, pulmonary diseases, diabetes mellitus, alcoholism, liver cirrhosis, and immunosuppression (HIV infection, chronic renal failure, organ transplant recipients, sickle cell disease, postsplenectomy state, hematological and lymphatic malignancies). The currently available 23-valent pneumococcal vaccine covers 88% of the serotypes causing systemic disease as well as 8% of related serotypes. The increasing prevalence of multiantibiotic resistance among pneumococci makes the pneumococcal immunization of high-risk individuals of utmost importance. The effect of pneumococcal vaccine lasts for 7–10 years after which it may be repeated. The influenza vaccine should be given yearly to the elderly, and to high-risk individuals.

SUGGESTED READING

1. Apisarnthanarak A, Mundy LM. Etiology of community-acquired pneumonia. Clin Chest Med. 2005;26(1):47-55.
2. Arnold FW, Summersgill TT, Lajoie AS, et al. A worldwide perspective of atypical pathogens in community-acquired pneumonia. Am T Respir Crit Care Med. 2007;175(10):1086-93.
3. Bansal S, Kashyap S, Pal LS, et al. Clinical and bacteriological profile of community acquired pneumonia in Shimla, Himachal Pradesh. Indian J Chest Dis Allied Sci. 2004;46:17-22.
4. Baron ET, Miller TM, Weinstein MP, et al. A guide to utilization of the microbiology laboratory for diagnosis of infectious diseases: 2013 recommendations by the Infectious Diseases Society of America (IDSA) and the American Society for Microbiology (ASM' (a). Clin Infect Dis. 2013;57:e22.
5. Bartlett TG. Diagnostic tests for agents of community-acquired pneumonia. Clin Infect Dis. 2011;52 Suppl 4:S296.
6. Buising KL, Thursky KA, Black JF, et al. A prospective comparison of severity scores for identifying patients with severe community-acquired pneumonia: reconsidering what is meant by severe pneumonia. Thorax. 2006;61(5):419-24.
7. Chen J, Chang S, Liu J, et al. Comparison of clinical characteristics and performance of pneumonia severity score and CURB-65 among younger adults, elderly and very old subjects. Thorax. 2010;65:971-97.
8. Cilloniz C, Ewig S, Polverino E, et al. Microbial aetiology of community-acquired pneumonia and its relation to severity. Thorax. 2011;66:340.
9. Datta Banik ND. Some observations on feeding programmes, nutrition and growth of pre-school children urban community. Indian J Pediatr. 1977;44(353):139-49.
10. Ghimire M, Bhattacharya SK, Narain JP. Pneumonia in South-East Asia Region: public health perspective. Indian T Med Res. 2012;135(4):459-68.

11. Invasive Bacterial Infection Surveillance (IBIS) Group. Prospective multicenter hospital surveillance of *Streptococcus pneumoniae* disease in India. Lancet. 1999;353:1216-20.

12. Ishida T, Hashimoto T, Aria M, et al. Etiology of community acquired pneumonia in hospitalized patients: a three year prospective study in Japan. Chest. 1998;114:1588-93.

13. Mandell LA. Epidemiology and etiology of community-acquired pneumonia. Infect Dis Clin North Am. 2004;18(4):761-76, vii.

14. Musher DM, Thorner AR. Community-acquired pneumonia. N Engl T Med. 2014;371:1619.

15. Niederman MS. Recent advances in community-acquired pneumonia: in patient and outpatient. Chest. 2007;131(4):1205-15.

16. Tarver RD. Radiology of community-acquired pneumonia. Radiol Clin North Am. 2005;43(3):497-512, viii.

17. Woodhead M. Community-acquired pneumonia: severity of illness evaluation. Infect Dis Clin North Am. 2004; 18(4):791-807; viii.

18. Wunderink RG. Community-acquired pneumonia: pathophysiology and host factors with focus on possible new approaches to management of lower respiratory tract infections. Infect Dis Clin North Am. 2004;18(4):743-59, vii.

CHAPTER 20

Nonbacterial Pneumonia

■ VIRAL PNEUMONIA

Epidemiology

Viral upper respiratory tract infections are common at all ages. Viral pneumonia however is uncommon in immunocompetent individuals, except in children and the elderly. The contribution of viral infection to community-acquired pneumonia (CAP) though uncertain is clearly underestimated. This is because reliable tests to confirm viral infections are difficult and outside the scope of the average hospital laboratory and also because of the relative lack of sensitivity of a number of these tests. This is particularly observed in India where there are just a few reference laboratories for virological studies which can claim a standard of excellence. The viral load in CAP in India is unknown though it undoubtedly does exist. In the West, in published series of adults, particularly the elderly, rates of viral pneumonia vary markedly depending on the type of tests, populations and the season in which the study was carried out. Viruses are identified in 0.3–30% of patients who have CAP, in studies using viral culture and serology for diagnosis. In a study on 105 patients with CAP in the West, respiratory viruses were detected in 14% of patients using conventional techniques compared to 56% by the reverse-transcriptase polymerized chain reaction (RT-PCR) technique [*Ref: Templeton KE, Scheltinga SA, van den Eeden WC, et al. Improved diagnosis of the etiology of community-acquired pneumonia with real-time polymerase chain reaction. Clin Infect Dis. 2005;41(3):345-51*]. In all studies, regardless of diagnostic technique, influenza A virus is the most common pathogen, responsible for 4–19% of cases [*Ref: Flamaing J, Engelmann I, Joosten E, et al. Viral lower respiratory tract infection in the elderly: a prospective in-hospital study. Eur J Clin Microbiol Infect Dis. 2003;22(12):720-5*].

The large number of viruses known to cause lower respiratory infection and pneumonia are listed in the accompanying **Table 1**.

The important ones are influenza A, B viruses, parainfluenza virus (PIV), respiratory syncytial virus (RSV), adenovirus, and the *Coronavirus*. The measles virus (which like the parainfluenza and the RSV belongs to the paramyxoviridae family) as also the chickenpox virus can also cause pneumonia. The *Hantavirus*, a rare virus prevalent chiefly in North and South America, can also cause serious pneumonic infection. Pneumonia due to the *Hantavirus* has also been reported from India. [*Ref: Chandy S, Boorugu H, Chrispal A, et al. Hantavirus infection: a case report from India. Indian J Med Microbiol. 2009;27(3):267-70*].

■ SPECIFIC VIRAL PNEUMONIAS

Influenzal Pneumonia

Influenza Virus

Three types of influenza virus have been identified—A, B, and C. Influenza A and B are responsible for close to 50% of all viral pneumonias in immunocompetent adults.

Table 1: Viral causes of pneumonia.	
Common respiratory viruses	***Other viruses***
Influenza viruses A and B	Measles virus
Respiratory syncytial virus (RSV)	Varicella zoster virus
Parainfluenza viruses (PIV)	Cytomegalovirus
Adenovirus	Epstein-Barr virus
Rhinovirus	Hantavirus
Coxsackie virus	

Influenza C virus is a significant cause of respiratory infections in children under-6 years of age. The majority of humans acquire immunity to Influenza C virus early in life so that subsequently clinical disease due to this virus is not generally encountered. The influenza A virus is the only type that can cause influenza to occur in large epidemic and pandemic forms.

Influenza A viruses are endemic gastrointestinal viruses of wild waterfowl, but have evolved elaborate mechanisms to jump species into domestic fowl, farm animals and humans. The major surface glycoprotein antigens on the virus envelope are the hemagglutinin and neuraminidase. The viral hemagglutinin binds to the host cell sialic acid-conjugated glycoprotein, an attachment necessary for viral entry into the cell. Neuraminidase is important for viral release and propagation. The "naming" of the influenza A virus depends on which of these proteins is present in a given virus. Thus, the standard nomenclature is influenza A HxNx (where x is the number corresponding to the specific type of hemagglutinin and neuraminidase).

Periodic gene segment reassertments between human and animal viruses produce important antigenic changes referred to as "shifts". These can lead to explosive deadly pandemics as witnessed in 1888, 1918, 1957 and 1968. The influenza world pandemic of 1918 was responsible for 70 million deaths in the world. In intervening years these "shifted" viruses undergo minor (i.e. less severe) antigenic changes called "drifts" which allows the virus to escape human immune responses raised by previously circulating influenza viruses. The influenza A virus has an amazingly inexhaustible range of mutational possibilities at several epitomes surrounding the viral hemagglutinin site that attaches to human cells. The mechanism as to how zoonotic influenza viruses mix with each other and with human strains to acquire extra properties of human virulence and human to human transmission, thereby causing an explosive outbreak is unknown.

Outbreaks of severe disease occur every 10–40 years. During outbreaks children are usually infected first, before adults, and morbidity and mortality are thus both high. The host immune response is chiefly directed towards the hemagglutinin antigen of the virus and involves both cellular and humoral antibody response. Secretory immunoglobulin A also has a role in host defense. There is marked mucosal inflammation of the respiratory tract, characterized by mucosal edema, hyperemia and in severe cases hemorrhage.

Transmission

Influenza is primarily transmitted from person to person by droplet infection (droplets > 5 μm) when an infected patient coughs or sneezes. Smaller droplets remain airborne longer and thus spread further, being carried by air currents for varying distances (air-borne spread). Contact transmission may also play a role. Infected patients may touch mucous membranes (like nose or nasal secretions) and then touch (e.g. hand shake) other individuals (direct contact). There could also be indirect contact through touching objects or surfaces touched by other noninfected individuals. If either through direct or indirect contact, uninfected patients touch their own mucous membranes, the virus gets deposited and infection ensues.

Seasonal Influenza

Seasonal influenza is generally due to Virus A and occasionally due to Virus B. Epidemics generally occur in winter, anytime between November and April lasting 6–8 weeks and varying in severity. In countries closer to the equator, the influenza season can be prolonged, being a multiphasic or year-round disease and is influenced in particular by the rainy season. Explosive epidemics are common in closed settings such as nursing homes, schools, dormitories. Rates of infection are high in those below 5 years of age, decline in those between 5 years and 49 years of age and rise significantly in those aged 50 years or over. Rates of hospitalization rise significantly with each decade over 60 years rising from 120 per 100,000 for ages 65–69 years to 1,195 per 10,000 for those over 85 years. Mortality rates increase even more dramatically rising from 19 to 358 per 100,000. These figures are from the United States.

The global impact of influenza on morbidity and mortality is considerable, there being 1 million deaths annually worldwide. Recent studies on the burden of influenza in East and South East Asia suggest that 11–20% of outpatient febrile illnesses and 6–14% of hospitalized pneumonia cases had laboratory-confirmed influenza infection.

Epidemiology in South East Asia and India

In temperate climates, influenza shows a marked peak in winter months. In tropical countries, seasonal incidence is less defined there being a high background influenza activity throughout the year in addition to epidemics that occur in intermediate months between the influenza seasons of the temperate countries of the Northern and Southern hemisphere. The reason why the seasonality of influenza varies with latitude is not clearly understood. Environmental factors do not appear to be linked with epidemics, except that the disease appears to be more prevalent in the rainy months of some tropical countries.

The impact of influenza in tropical countries is being increasingly recognized following epidemiological studies on influenza in Hong Kong. Hong Kong is a subtropical rich city located within the likely epicenter of pandemic influenza in South East Asia. It was shown that hospitalization related to influenza varied with age in a U-shaped curve where young infants and elderly patients were at a higher risk of pneumonia and poorer outcomes, a pattern similar to that observed in interpandemic influenza in temperate countries. The results of the epidemiological study of influenza in Hong Kong should not be equated with the likely impact of influenza in poor tropical countries where malnutrition, shortage of antibiotics to treat secondary bacterial infections and poor medical care may well influence the severity and outcome of influenzal infection.

There are two surveillance centers for influenza in India—National Institute of Virology (NIV), Pune and National Institute of Communicable Diseases (NICD), New Delhi. Three surveillance studies have been carried out at the NIV in Pune.

The salient features of the surveillance study extending from 1978 to 1990 showed that the highest number of cases occurred during the rainy months of July, August and September, the viruses isolated being H3N2, H1N1 and influenza-Type B.

The surveillance study in 1980 showed three peaks—in the hot months of March, in the rainy season of July, August, September and a peak in the cool month of November. The viruses isolated were H3N2, H1N1 and influenza-Type B.

The third surveillance study in 2003 showed two peaks—one peak in March-April (H3N2), and another peak in July-August (H3N2). Type B was also prevalent in the rainy months. It was observed that the H3N2 was responsible for severe illness and for the highest hospitalization rate.

More research is needed on the epidemiology of influenza in the tropics. Modeling the influenza burden in tropical countries necessitates reliable surveillance data. Unfortunately, surveillance efforts were initiated very recently in tropical countries so that data on the influenza

burden are of short duration. Laboratory surveillance needs to be strengthened if modeling of disease burden is to be feasible. Also, more studies are needed to determine seasonal influenza patterns across a large range of latitudes, involving tropical countries in both hemispheres. Finally, further research is necessary to determine whether the influenza virus in temperate climes persists in a low-grade activity all through the year with exacerbations in winter or whether the virus is reintroduced from the tropics each year at the beginning of winter. **Figure 1** shows the monthly data of specimens collected for influenza virus detection from 2004 to 2005 at the National Institute of Virology, Pune.

Clinical Features of Uncomplicated Seasonal Influenza

Typical clinical features include an acute onset of fever (ranging up to 100–104°F or even higher), myalgia, cough, usually dry but occasionally productive, sore throat, nasal discharge and congestion and headache. Conjunctival congestion may also be present.

Influenza infection may have other presentations that range from a common cold to systemic features of fever, muscle pains with little indication of respiratory involvement, or fever with general symptoms such as severe weakness, anorexia, malaise.

Physical findings are unremarkable. The pharynx may seem inflamed, cervical glands may be palpable; there are generally few or no respiratory signs. Leucocyte counts are normal or low, high counts suggest a secondary bacterial

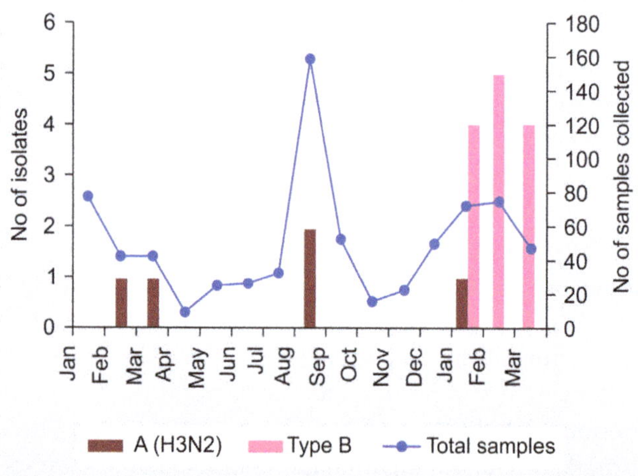

Fig. 1: Monthly data of specimen collection and influenza virus detection during the year 2004–05, NIV Pune.

infection. Uncomplicated influenza lasts for a week; post influenza asthenia and weakness may last much longer, at times several weeks.

Complications of Influenza

Respiratory Complications

- *Pneumonia:* This a major and most common complication, occurring most frequently in those with underlying chronic illness and those considered to be at high risk.
  Influenza pneumonia may take the following forms:
  - Primary pneumonia caused by the virus by itself
  - Influenzal viral pneumonia followed by a secondary bacterial pneumonia—the common organisms being *Staphylococcus aureus, Streptococcus pneumoniae, H. influenza*
  - A combination of primary viral together with a secondary bacterial pneumonia at the same time.
  Primary viral pneumonia though the least common is the most severe. Patients with heart failure, COPD are more prone, but it can also occur in young healthy adults. X-ray of the chest shows a bilateral reticular or reticulonodular shadows or multiple focal areas of consolidation chiefly in both lower lobes. HRCT chest shows multifocal peribronchial or subpleural consolidation and/or ground glass opacities.

  Secondary bacterial pneumonia is an important complication of influenza contributing significantly to morbidity and mortality. It is characterized by the exacerbation of fever and respiratory symptoms after initial improvement in the symptoms of acute influenza. An important complication of secondary bacterial pneumonia is pleural effusion and empyema. The radiological features of secondary bacterial pneumonia consist of segmental or lobar consolidation.

  In fulminant primary influenzal pneumonia both lungs are generally involved, death occurring within 48 to 72 hours.
- *ARDS:* This is a feature of fulminant viral influenza with or without it being complicated by secondary bacterial infection.

Nonrespiratory Complications

- Myositis (exquisite tenderness of the muscles), rhabdomyolysis. Myositis chiefly involves muscles of the lower limbs.
- *CVS complications:* These include ECG changes, myocarditis, pericarditis. Myocarditis is a dreaded but rare complication and is an important cause of sudden death.
- *CNS involvement:* CNS complications include encephalitis, encephalopathy, transverse myelitis, aseptic meningitis, Guillain-Barré syndrome.
  Death when it occurs is generally due to fulminant viral or viral + bacterial pneumonia, ARDS often associated with multiorgan failure, or acute myocarditis.

  It needs *to be mentioned that primary pneumonia due to the influenza virus is rare outside pandemic settings and in nonimmunocompromised patients.* Age *(>65 years)* is an important risk factor as are comorbid conditions such as left heart failure, cardiovascular disease, chronic respiratory disease, diabetes, and well-marked hepatic or renal dysfunction, neurological disorders depressed immune response as in AIDS, cancer, or following the use of antimitotic drugs or glucocorticoids.

  Noninfectious pulmonary complications that can be induced by the influenza virus include bronchiolitis obliterans organizing pneumonia, usual interstitial pneumonia and transient Goodpasture's syndrome. The latter is reported to resolve with the cure of influenza. Perhaps the most important and frequent fatal non-respiratory complication is myocarditis resulting in dilated cardiomyopathy and hypotensive cardiac failure.

Diagnosis

The diagnosis is based on clinical presentation at a time when viral activity causing respiratory infection is high in a community. The clinical features may however be indistinguishable from CAP due to other microorganisms. A specific viral diagnosis can be made by:

- *Culture of respiratory secretions:* Nasal secretions are believed to be better specimens compared to throat swabs to detect the influenza virus. Sputum, endotracheal secretions or bronchoalveolar lavage (BAL) specimens can also be used for culture. Cultures take 2–3 days to become positive and are thus of limited value for making therapeutic or isolation decisions.
- Rapid antigen testing is available for influenza A and B and offers prompt results. These tests have a sensitivity of 50–60% in children and of 90% in adults. False negative tests occur and treatment should not be withheld in these patients if there is a high index of suspicion.

- Immunofluorescent or enzyme-linked immunosorbent assay (ELISA) techniques on nasal or pharyngeal cells obtained by brushing or washing can help in a quick diagnosis (within 15 minutes). This test again requires expertise and is not widely available, at least in developing countries.
- Molecular testing such as RT-PCR offers the best sensitivity and specificity for the diagnosis of influenzal viral infection. It is technically demanding, expensive and available at only a few centers.
- Serological test for antibodies is only useful for epidemiological purposes as it requires two serological assays 14 days apart. There needs to be a fourfold or greater rise in the influenza-specific antibody **(Table 2)**.

Treatment

Antiviral drugs have been approved for the treatment of influenzal infection are amantadine, rimantadine, zanamivir, oseltamivir **(Table 3)**. Amantadine and rimantadine are effective against influenza A, whereas zanamivir and oseltamivir are effective against influenza A and B. These drugs are 70–90% effective for prophylaxis and reduce illness severity, duration of symptoms and virus shedding when given within 48 hours of onset of symptoms.

The Center for Disease Control and Prevention (CDC) recently reported that 92% of influenza A (H3N2) and 25% of influenza A (H1N1) were resistant to the amantadines. The CDC therefore does not recommend the use of this class of drugs at present. Zanamivir and oseltamivir are effective for influenza A and B and are recommended as the current resistant rates are low. These recommendations are based on studies in the US. To what extent they apply to India and other Southeast Asian countries is not known.

It should be noted that each antiviral drug has side-effects that must be considered in treatment selection. Zanamivir can cause bronchospasm and should be avoided in patients with asthma or *chronic obstructive pulmonary disease* (COPD). Oseltamivir is well-tolerated but may cause nausea and vomiting in 10% of patients.

A newer drug Peramivir has been approved by the US Food and Drug Administration in 2014 for treating uncomplicated influenza infection (initiate within 2 days of onset of symptoms of influenza) in adults. The drug is administered as single intravenous injection at a dose of 300 to 600 mg. Peramivir is a neuraminidase inhibitor and its adverse effects are generally few and mild. It is believed to as effective as oseltamivir.

Baloxavir is a new oral selective inhibitor of influenza cap-dependent endonuclease that blocks proliferation of the influenza virus by inhibiting the synthesis of mRNA. It is approved for treatment in healthy adults and in children > 12 years old. A single dose of 40 mg for patients < 80 kg and 80 mg for > 80 kg is shown to be as effective as oseltamivir. However there are reports of emerging

Table 2: Diagnostic tests for influenzal pneumonia.

Test	Time to result	Noteworthy features
Rapid antigen test	<30 minutes	Fast, not technically defective
Immunofluorescent test	1–4 hours	Requires technical expertise
Culture	24 hours to 5 days	Very sensitive—also detects other pathogens
Nucleic acid testing (RT-PCR)	4–24 hours	Very sensitive but requires technical expertise
Antibody testing	Several weeks	High-specific and sensitive

Table 3: Antivirals against influenza.

	Dosage in adult	Dosage in children	Remarks
Oseltamivir	75 mg BD PO for 5 days	≤15 kg; 30 mg twice daily for 5 days ≥15 to 23 kg; 45 mg twice daily for 5 days ≥23 kg; 60 mg twice daily for 5 days >40 kg; 75 mg twice daily for 5 days	Effective; safe Reduced otitis in children Reduced hospitalization rate Side effect—nausea
Zanamivir	10 mg via inhalation BD for 5 days	≥7 years 10 mg inhalation BD <7 years not advised	Equally safe and effective as oseltamivir, no nausea but may cause bronchospasm
Amantadine	Not recommended	Not recommended	High levels of resistance to Influenza A vaccine

resistance to this drug, raising concerns of its long-term use as monotherapy.

The possibility of combined therapy of Oseltamivir + Baloxavir providing greater benefit than oseltamivir alone in hospitalized and immunocompromised patients needs to be explored.

Bacterial pneumonia is a fairly frequent complication (observational studies report 8–36%) of severe influenzal infection. When present or strongly suspected, particularly in elderly patients, an appropriate antibiotic cover should be given. Blood and sputum cultures should help in the choice of antibiotics. Empiric antibiotic therapy may be necessary in critically ill patients and this should cover staphylococcal, pneumococcal and *H. influenzae,* the common bacterial pathogens that cause secondary pneumonias. Vancomycin or linezolid is preferred for staphylococcal infection as *methicillin-resistant Staphylococcus aureus* (MRSA) strains have been reported to cause secondary bacterial pneumonia.

Supportive care is vital. This may necessitate appropriate ventilatory support as also cardiovascular support, since hypotension and dilated cardiomyopathy due to viral myocarditis may be other coexisting complications in patients with influenzal pneumonia. Not uncommonly, influenzal pneumonia precipitates heart failure in patients with a background of heart disease.

It is important to use paracetamol and to avoid aspirin or other salicylates (particularly in children) as symptomatic treatment for headache and fever. This is because salicylates used in this setting are known to be associated with Reye's syndrome. This syndrome is characterized by a noninflammatory encephalopathy, cerebral edema, fatty liver or liver cell dysfunction. This syndrome is associated with influenza A and has a high mortality.

Adjunctive Therapy

Severe adjunctive therapies have been proposed for the management of severely ill patients but none of these have sufficient evidence to support their use. These proposed therapies include the use of glucocorticoids, intravenous immunoglobulins, convalescent plasma and hyperimmune globulin.

Treatment of ARDS

Influenzal infection causing severe ARDS has high mortality. Ventilatory management is on the same lines as with severe ARDS from any other cause. Lung protection strategy with low tidal volumes and adequate PEEP should be employed. In patients who remain severely hypoxemic, rescue strategies is the main include the use of extracorporeal membrane oxygenation.

Prevention

Isolation

A patient diagnosed to be suffering from influenza needs to be isolated as promptly as possible, more so when there is an outbreak of this disease. Delay in isolation could easily result in spread from droplet infection caused by coughing or sneezing. In epidemics, contacts of infected person need to be traced, tested and if needs be isolated.

Influenza Vaccine

Influenza poses both a health and economic burden to the community and is therefore a public health concern. Prevention rests on annual vaccination with trivalent killed virus vaccine. Recommendations are for early vaccinations in all adults over 50 years, children between 6 months to 5 years, patients of any age with chronic medical conditions (particularly those with COPD or chronic respiratory problems), pregnant women, immune suppressed patients, caretakers of high-risk patients and healthcare workers. Unfortunately, the awareness of the need for vaccination is extremely poor not only among patients in the large cities of India (leave aside smaller towns and rural India), but also among practicing doctors.

There is however some conflicting evidence about vaccine efficacy in the elderly and high-risk patients. A Cochrane review of five randomized trials demonstrated a rate of 68% for vaccine effectiveness against influenza, and 43% against influenza-like illnesses. There were few participants beyond 70 years and there seemed to be little efficacy in this group (*Ref: Rivetti D, Jefferson T, Thomas R, et al. Vaccines for preventing influenza in the elderly. Cochrane Database Syst Rev. 2006;3:CD004876*).

Observational cohort studies have also shown conflicting results. In elderly patients vaccination failed to protect against influenza, influenza-like illness or pneumonia, but surprisingly was associated with 26% reduction in hospitalization from influenza and pneumonia, and 42% reduction in all-cause mortality.

Avian Influenza

In 1997 an H5N1 avian influenza virus emerged in Hong Kong, resulting in the death of 6 of the 18 affected patients, mainly young adults. The virus fortunately did not spread from human to human, and was controlled through massive culling of poultry. The H5N1 strain re-emerged in 2003, first in China, Japan, South Korea, then in Thailand, Vietnam, Indonesia, Cambodia, Malaysia leading to massive culling of poultry and attempts to curb the epidemic through vaccination of poultry. More than 60% of patients diagnosed with this viral strain died. In May 2005, a highly pathogenic H5N1 strain emerged in wild birds is Qinghai lake, China, killing not only domestic poultry but wild aquatic birds. This highly pathogenic strain spread to many countries in Asia, Africa, Europe, and was the cause of multiple outbreaks in poultry.

Humans have been affected through close contact with birds and poultry but human to human contact has not been observed except rarely in very close contacts.

In late March 2013, there was a new report of human cases of novel avian influenza A (H7N9) in China. Since then annual epidemics of this virus have occurred, the last fifth wave being in late 2016 and early 2017. Avian influenza A (H7N9) is believed to have resulted from multiple re-assortment events of several (at least four) avian influenza viruses isolated from ducks and poultry.

As of 19 October 2017, a total of 238 cases of human infection with avian influenza A (H5N1) virus were reported from four countries within the Western Pacific Region since January 2003. Of these cases, 134 were fatal, resulting in a case fatality rate (CFR) of 56%. The last case was reported from China and its onset date was 27th December 2015 (1 case, no death) **(Table 4)**.

This "avian flu" differs from the usual seasonal influenza in that it is a serious severe illness with a mortality of 60%. The incubation period is 3–8 days; the disease starts with high fever, cough with severe prostration and myalgia. Tachypnea, dyspnea, respiratory distress and hypoxia

Table 4: Cumulative number of confirmed human cases of avian influenza A (H5N1) reported to WHO, 2003–2017.

Country	2003–2009*		2010–2014**		2015		2016		2017		Total	
	Cases	Deaths	Cases	Deaths	Cases	Deaths	Cases	Deaths	Cases	Deaths	Cases	Deaths
Azerbaijan	8	5	0	0	0	0	0	0	0	0	8	5
Bangladesh	1	0	6	1	1	0	0	0	0	0	8	1
Cambodia	9	7	47	30	0	0	0	0	0	0	56	37
Canada	0	0	1	1	0	0	0	0	0	0	1	1
China	38	25	9	5	6	1	0	0	0	0	53	31
Djibouti	1	0	0	0	0	0	0	0	0	0	1	0
Egypt	90	27	120	50	136	39	10	3	3	1	359	120
Indonesia	162	134	35	31	2	2	0	0	1	1	200	168
Iraq	3	2	0	0	0	0	0	0	0	0	3	2
Lao People's Democratic Republic	2	2	0	0	0	0	0	0	0	0	2	2
Myanmar	1	0	0	0	0	0	0	0	0	0	1	0
Nigeria	1	1	0	0	0	0	0	0	0	0	1	1
Pakistan	3	1	0	0	0	0	0	0	0	0	3	1
Thailand	25	17	0	0	0	0	0	0	0	0	25	17
Turkey	12	4	0	0	0	0	0	0	0	0	12	4
Vietnam	112	57	15	7	0	0	0	0	0	0	127	64
Total	**468**	**282**	**233**	**125**	**145**	**42**	**10**	**3**	**4**	**2**	**860**	**454**

*2003–2009 total figures. Breakdowns by year available on subsequent tables.
**2010–2014 total figures. Breakdowns by year available on subsequent tables.
Total number of cases includes number of deaths.
WHO reports only laboratory cases.
All dates refer to onset of illness.
Source: WHO/GIP, data in HQ as of 27 September 2017.

are noted within a week. The blood shows leukopenia, lymphopenia and thrombocytopenia. The X-ray chest shows patchy interstitial and alveolar infiltrates consistent with primary viral pneumonia rather than secondary bacterial pneumonia. Acute respiratory distress syndrome (ARDS) together with multiorgan failure is seen in patients with severe illness, generally resulting in death. Postmortem studies show diffuse lung injury together with vascular congestion and hyaline membrane formation.

Patients with influenza-like symptoms who have been in contact with poultry afflicted by H5N1 virus should be isolated and tested for H5N1 infection. Diagnostic tests are the rapid antigen test, and direct fluorescent antibody tests which give quick results within 2 hours. Nasal discharge, throat swabs, BAL fluid can be tested by RT-PCR. This test offers the best sensitivity and specificity. Viral cultures are also done for the H5N1 virus. Most of these tests require sophisticated laboratories together with good expertise. Specimens thus need to be sent to accredited laboratories which give reliable results.

Patients with confirmed or suspected H5N1 should be treated with oseltamivir or zanamivir as this viral strain has been shown to be resistant to amantadine and rimantadine. The current recommendation is a 5-day course of oseltamivir in a dose of 75 mg twice daily. Antibacterial agents should be used to target the pneumococcus and *S. aureus,* the two organisms chiefly responsible for secondary bacterial pneumonia.

Critical care is of vital importance. Ventilator support is essential in patients with respiratory failure or with ARDS. Support to all organ systems is crucial as multiple organ dysfunctions are frequently observed.

Many virologists fear that the avian flu due to H5N1 infection has the potential to become an influenza pandemic. Though spread so far has been from infected poultry to man, the possibility of a slight genetic mutation of this virus, or a reassortment of its genetic material may not only enhance its virulence but could give it the property of spreading from human to human, a catastrophe that could well resemble the influenza pandemic of 1916–18. As yet this has not happened but the danger persists.

Swine Flu

The threat of a pandemic of avian influenza still hangs like the sword of Damocles over the world. In the meanwhile in 2009 an H1N1 strain of the influenza virus A was detected in swine-infected humans in Mexico. The H1N1 virus has the property of being transmitted from human to human through droplet infection following coughing or sneezing. There were a number of fatalities in Mexico. In a matter of months this H1N1 virus causing influenza spread to the United States and soon to Europe, Asia and the Far East. The WHO alerted all countries and pronounced this as a world pandemic. A study published in The Lancet Infectious Diseases journal estimates that the death toll from the 2009 pandemic is between 151,700 and 575,400. Maximum deaths have occurred in Mexico; in other countries swine flu is by and large a mild though highly infections illness. This indeed is not so in India where many deaths from H1N1 have been observed. A retrospective study on the epidemiology of influenza A H1N1 infection (Swine Flu) was carried out from May 2009 to April 2010 at the Government Medical College and Hospital (a tertiary center) in Chandigarh. Out of the total of 4,379 patients screened during the period of study, 365 patients were tested, of which 29.8% were found positive. 54 confirmed cases were admitted to the H1N1 isolation ward, of which 54.9% succumbed to the disease. The case fatality ratio was 25.9%. This tertiary center drained patients from Chandigarh, Punjab, Haryana and Himachal Pradesh.

Recurrent episodes of H1N1 infection sometimes in small epidemics continue to be observed in India from 2015 to the present date. Thus, in 2015, out of 42592 infected with H1N1, close to 3000 died. In 2017, of the 38811 infected, 2270 died and in 2019, the first two months have already seen 17366 infected cases, close to 530 have died. It appears that H1N1 continues to pose a serious health hazard to this country (*Source: Integrated Disease Surveillance Programme, Delhi*).

The potential danger of H1N1 is the possibility of a further mutation in the virus or genetic reassortment that could enhance its virulence. If that indeed does transpire, the world may face a catastrophic pandemic.

Strict isolation of patients, tracing of contacts, testing them and if needs be isolating them is crucial for prevention. The pandemic is still active, though perhaps the hot summer months may see a decline in the activity of this virus. However, the rainy season in tropical countries and the winter months to come, hold a serious threat to the whole world.

Clinical Features

The disease starts with usual flu-like symptoms—body ache, fever, prostration, sore throat and a persistent dry cough. A sore throat is invariably present. Running of the nose is not frequently observed. Vomiting and diarrhea are common presentations of pandemic H1N1 influenza A infection both of which are uncommon in seasonal influenza. Patients with underlying co-morbid conditions, extremes of age, pregnant women are at increased risk of severe respiratory complications.

Laboratory Findings

These include leucopenia, a rise in liver enzymes. Anemia and thrombocytopenia may also be observed. A marked rise in CPK is a pointer to ongoing rhabdomyolysis.

Pathology

Autopsy findings in fatal cases of epidemic or pandemic H1N1 infection reveal (a) severe tracheal, bronchial inflammation, edema and even necrosis; (b) diffuse alveolar damage; (c) bacterial coinfection—chiefly with *Staphylococcus aureus* and *Streptococcus pneumoniae*; (d) the primary cells infected by the virus are the alveolar lining cells.

Complications

Risk factors for contacting H1N1 infection in epidemics or pandemic are the same as those mentioned in seasonal influenza.

The following points need to be emphasized:
- Adults hospitalized for H1N1 infection during epidemics are far more likely to have lower respiratory complications, shock/sepsis and organ failure than those with seasonal influenza. Tachypnea and respiratory distress are warning signs of lung involvement **(Figs. 2 to 4)**.
- These H1N1 infected patients are generally more seriously ill, more likely to be admitted to the ICU, require mechanical ventilation or die.
- Bacterial superinfection within the lung is more frequently observed than in seasonal influenza pneumonia. Mortality in these patients is high.
- Neurological complications have been already listed under seasonal influenza. These are far more common in severe pandemic H1N1 influenza A infection. Seizures form an important complication. Confusion, disorientation, encephalitis, encephalopathy, Guillain Barré syndrome, severe acute disseminated encephalitis have been reported in pandemics.
- Other nonrespiratory complications are the same as those in seasonal influenza.

Treatment

Oseltamivir 75 mg twice daily for 5–7 days is the recommended specific therapy. Supportive treatment

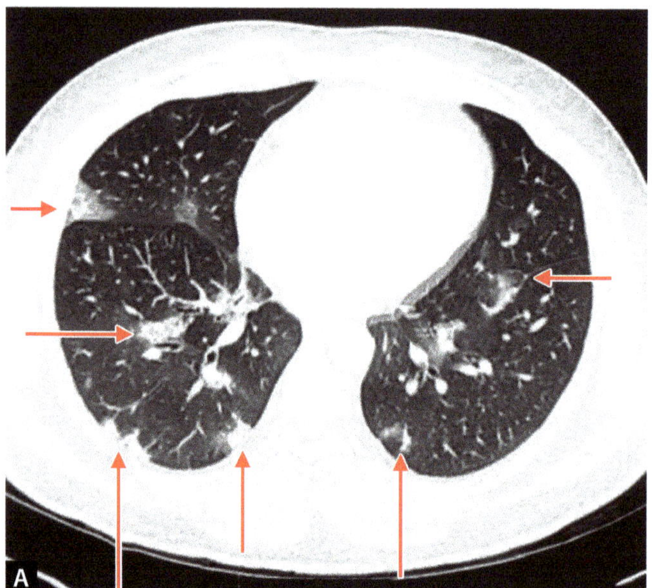

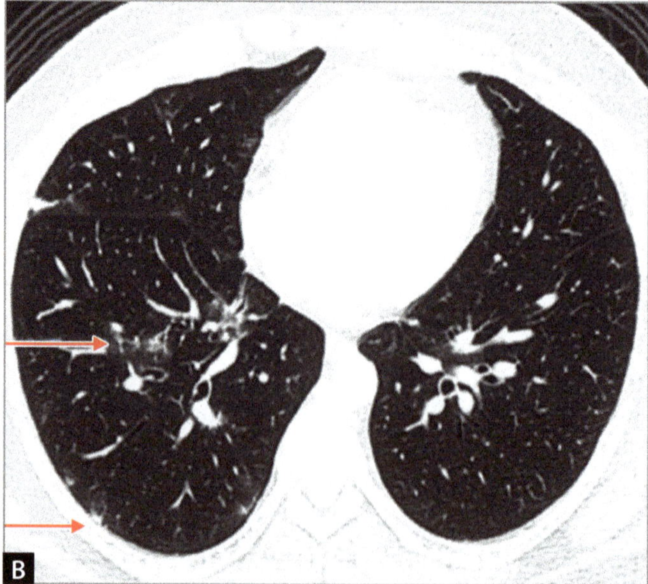

Figs. 2A and B: (A) A 33-year-old male patient presented with high-grade fever cough and dyspnea with ill-defined areas of increased lung attenuation in the subpleural and peribronchovascular regions marked by arrows. This pattern of areas of increased lung attenuation is seen in a number of patients with H1N1. (B) Follow-up CT in patient demonstrates clearing of nearly all areas of increased lung attenuation.

as outlined earlier is imperative in severe infection. Pneumonia, respiratory failure necessitate ventilator support. If conventional ventilator support is unsuccessful to counter hypoxemia, the use of ECMO is indicated, as this rescue procedure has salvaged a number of patients.

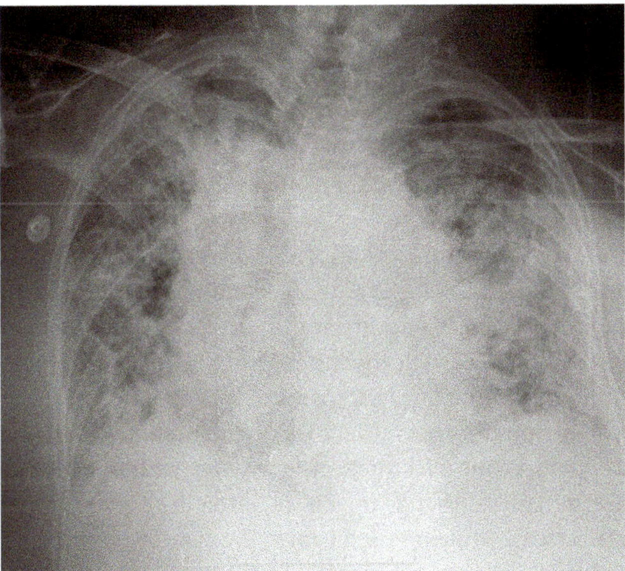

Fig. 3: ARDS in H1N1. Chest X-ray demonstrates diffuse bilateral white out lungs in a case of H1N1 with ARDS.

Prevention consists of the use of the flu vaccine administered once every year.

Dangers of a World Influenza Pandemic

The WHO has predicted that a new influenza pandemic could lead to 1–2 billion cases of flu, 5–12 million cases of severe illness and 1.5–3 million deaths worldwide. It could result in 1–2.3 million hospitalizations and 250,000–650,000 deaths in industrialized countries alone. Its impact on developing countries could be even more devastating. Nevertheless the WHO predicts that the expected pandemic would not be as horrendous as the 1918 pandemic which as stated earlier killed 80 million people, but on par with the 1957 and 1968 pandemics. Whether the present swine flu pandemic will fulfil such ghastly predictions stated above is to be seen. Again, whether avian influenza graduates through a further mutational shift in the future to engulf the world in another dreadful pandemic remains uncertain. Fortunately, so far, the threat of a world pandemic is no longer there, both with regard to H1N1 infection, as also with regard to avian H5N1 infection.

Respiratory Syncytial Virus

Respiratory syncytial virus (RSV) infection is a common and important cause of lower respiratory tract infection in children. For many years it was considered to be a pathogen

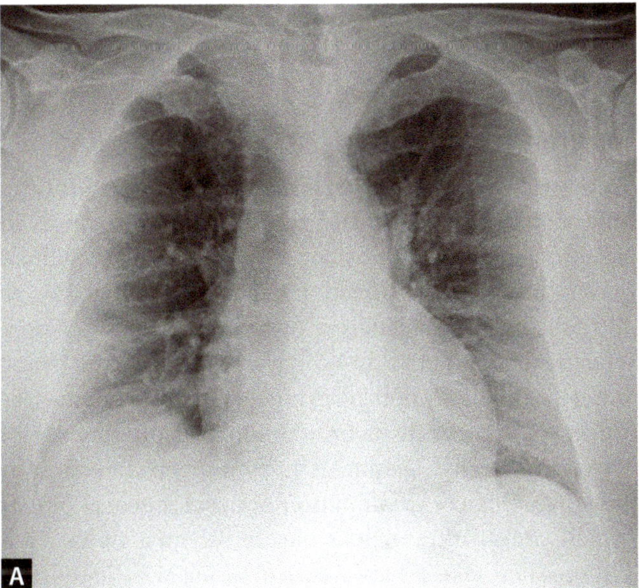

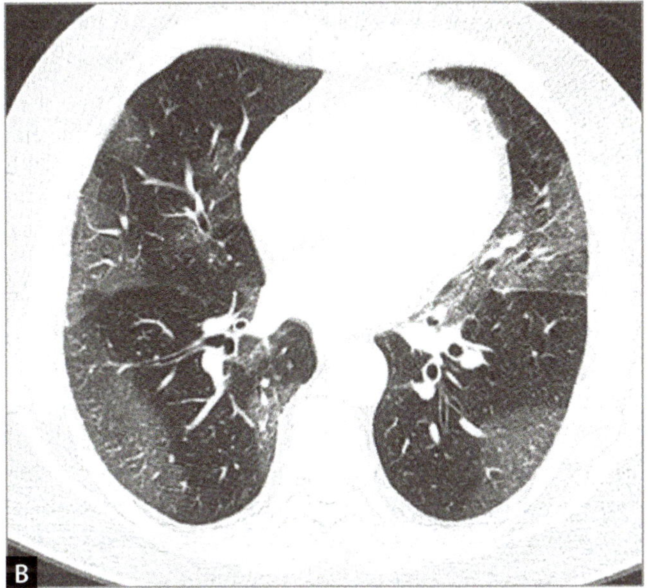

Figs. 4A and B: A 77-year-old presented with high grade fever: (A) Chest X-ray was negative; (B) CT reveals areas of ground glass opacification in subpleural regions of both lung fields suggestive of H1N1.

confined to pediatric practice; however, it is now being increasingly recognized as an important pathogen causing lower respiratory tract infection in adults. The incubation period is 4–6 days and epidemics occur in winter and early spring lasting 1–5 months. Several epidemiological studies in the West indicated that RSV is second to influenza as a cause of serious respiratory disease in adults. Its frequency as a cause of CAP in adults has been estimated at 3–5% over a year. Again there is no reliable epidemiological study to give an estimate of RSV pneumonia in India or for that matter in large metropolitan cities of the country.

Transmission of RSV is by droplet infection produced by coughing or sneezing as also by contaminated skin followed by autoinnoculation in the conjuctiva or nose. Infection leads to increased immunoglobulin E (IgE) production; the degree of rise in IgE predicts the risk of wheezing episodes.

Clinical features include fever, nasal congestion, pharyngitis, cough which is often productive. Lower respiratory tract infection is frequent in 25–30% of infections and takes two forms—(1) bronchiolitis and (2) pneumonia. Clinically, these manifest as dyspnea, tachypnea, increasing cough, wheezing, rhonchi on auscultation and hypoxia. Although difficult to distinguish from influenza there are a few subtle clinical clues that may suggest RSV infection. Patients with RSV infection have more basal congestion with crackles on auscultation, wheezing, a productive cough and a comparatively low-grade fever as compared to patients with influenza. Thus in elderly patients who give a history of a "cold" followed by low-grade fever and wheezing, the diagnosis of RSV infection should be entertained.

The radiological features are characterized by interstitial infiltrates. Patchy segmental shadows and occasionally lobar consolidation have been reported. Bronchiolitis results in patchy atelectasis with areas of hyperinflation.

Diagnosis of RSV infection may be difficult to prove. Cultures of respiratory secretions—sputum, nasopharyngeal washing, and throat swabs may take 2–7 days to show positive results. Immunofluorescent techniques are frequently used on nasal washings; they allow a more reliable and rapid detection of the virus. Rapid antigen tests for RSV have poor sensitivity when compared to influenza. RT-PCR is more sensitive for detection of the virus in adult populations. Serological tests give a retrospective diagnosis if the antibody titer rises to fourfold or more after 2 weeks.

Treatment of RSV pneumonia in adults is supportive—antipyretics, fluids, and oxygen when needed. Corticosteroids are useful in all age groups when there is wheezing, particularly if this is associated with hypoxia. Nebulization with β_2-agonists and budesonide offers symptomatic relief in patients with airways obstruction.

Aerosolized ribavirin improves the clinical course, particularly in severe disease and should be administered (60 mg/mL for 2 hours given by mask, three times a day). RSV-specific immunoglobulin is also approved therapy, particularly in high-risk infants.

Parainfluenza Viruses

Four distinct serotypes are recognized 1, 2, 3, 4A, and 4B. These viruses cause croup, bronchitis and pneumonia in children. PIV-3 is most often associated with pneumonia and is endemic the year around. Pneumonia has also been reported in young adults and in the elderly though the burden of disease in the latter group is unclear. As with influenza, infection is transmitted by droplet infection from respiratory secretions, the incubation period being 2–7 days. Clinical features, even when pneumonia occurs, are nonspecific and are characterized by fever, nasal discharge, hoarseness and cough. Chest radiograph shows diffuse interstitial infiltrates as with any atypical or viral pneumonia.

Viral culture, RT-PCR and serological tests can be used to diagnose PIV infection. Ribavirin has in vitro activity against PIV; its use in patients with PIV infection has not proved curative.

Adenovirus

Adenoviruses are responsible for 5% of respiratory infections in children and less than 2% infections in adults. Epidemics have however been reported in military recruit populations. Infection occurs from inhalation of airborne droplet infection or by feco-oral contamination. The incubation period is 4–7 days. In children and young adults (particularly noticed in military recruits) adenovirus infection can result in bronchiolitis or pneumonia of variable severity. Diagnosis is by antigen detection or histopathological examination of nasal mucosal biopsy which shows intranuclear basophilic inclusions. Viral cultures may take several weeks to be positive. Serological diagnosis depends on a fourfold or more increase in antibodies after an interval of 2 weeks.

NEW CORONAVIRUSES (SEVERE ACUTE RESPIRATORY SYNDROME AND MIDDLE EAST RESPIRATORY SYNDROME)

Coronaviruses are RNA viruses. Two groups of coronaviruses are identified and four strains are known to cause acute respiratory diseases ranging from cold to pneumonia. These include Group 1 (229E and NL63) and Group 2 (OC 43 and HKU 1). A new Coronavirus, SARS-CoV which represents a split from Group 2 was identified as the cause of the severe acute respiratory syndrome (SARS) epidemic which originated in the Guangdong province in China and spread to different parts of the world.

An epidemic associated with a little over 8,000 cases was observed with 774 deaths. The disease then died out perhaps due to effective infection control practices. The human CoV-SARS virus is now believed to be introduced to human population from contact with animal species, likely the civet cats or related animals.

The incubation period of SARS ranges from 2 days to 10 days. It is a serious illness, the older age group being a significant risk factor for death. The clinical features are characterized by fever with chills, cough, and myalgia. Unlike other viral respiratory infections, rhinorrhea and sore throat are uncommon symptoms. About two-thirds of infected patients develop prolonged fever, dyspnea, tachypnea, increasing hypoxia and diarrhea. Chest radiographs show bilateral alveolar shadows which may be quickly progressive **(Figs. 5A and B)**. Age and comorbid medical conditions are independent risk factors and the mortality in those over 60 years is over 50%. Ribavirin, corticosteroids and intravenous gamma globulins have been used as treatment but there is no proof of their efficacy. The disease fortunately is at present quiescent.

In 2012, a similar severe respiratory illness was observed in several Middle Eastern countries due to what is now termed "MERS-CoV". This virus is closely related to *Coronavirus* found in bats but it is believed that a currently undetermined animal host, possibly the camel is involved in transmission to humans. Though MERS-CoV can produce severe respiratory distress just like the human CoV-SARS, sustained person to person contact transmission has not been observed. This in striking contrast to the human CoV-SARS virus which showed a droplet spread, requiring close contact.

Measles Virus

Vaccination against measles has proved of immense benefit, particularly in poor developing countries. Yet there are many in developing countries who have not been vaccinated. In these patients, measles still carries a significant mortality and morbidity.

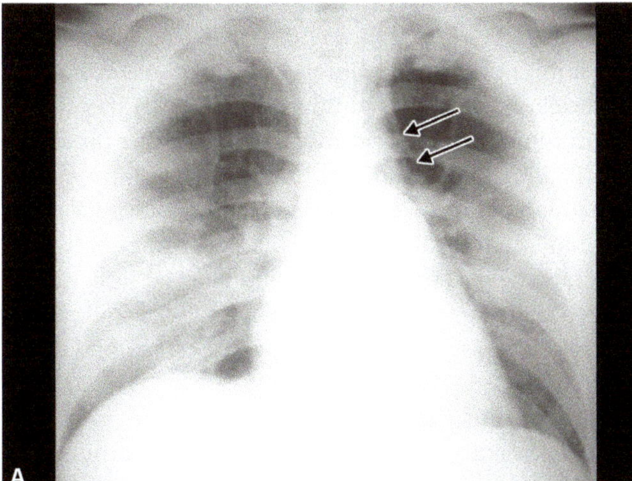
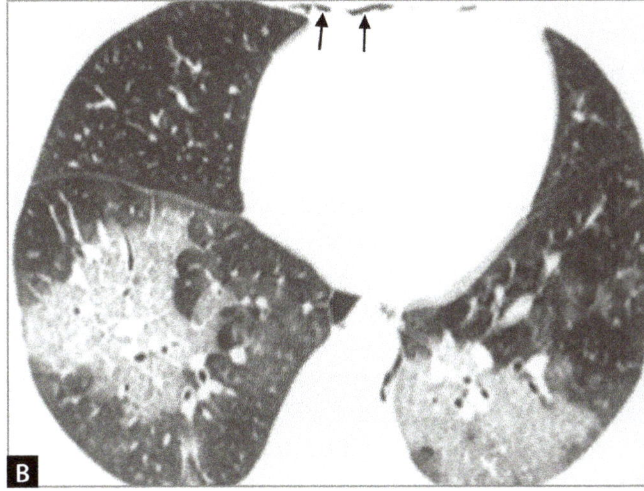

Figs. 5A and B: Severe acute respiratory syndrome (SARS). (A) Chest X-ray demonstrates ill-defined consolidations in both lung fields in the mid- and lower zones. There is a thin paramediastinal air strip on the left side representing mediastinal emphysema; (B) HRCT chest demonstrates ill-defined areas of ground-glass densities in both lower lobes with associated septal thickening noted within.

The measles virus belongs to the paramyxoviridae family like the PIV and RSV. The virus enters chiefly through the respiratory tract. Lower respiratory tract infections occur in close to 50% of patients and take the form of bronchitis, bronchiolitis and viral pneumonia. Measles pneumonia is the main cause of measles-related death in children. Radiographic appearances in measles virus pneumonia are characterized by widespread reticulonodular pulmonary infiltrates. Secondary bacterial pneumonia often occurs. Primary viral pneumonia and secondary bacterial pneumonia may coexist in the same patient.

Treatment is supportive; antibiotics are necessary for secondary bacterial infection. Fortunately, the measles vaccine has reduced the incidence of measles by 98%. If it still does occur, it occurs in the teenage years and is generally mild.

Varicella-Zoster Virus

Varicella hardly ever causes pneumonia in immuno-competent children. But the danger of pneumonia is ever present when varicella occurs in adults. When pneumonia occurs, it generally occurs within 4–5 days of the start of the rash. Cough and pleuritic chest pain are frequently observed. A tell-tale warning sign is tachypnea. Progressive dyspnea, respiratory distress and hypoxia occur in critically ill patients. Radiographic appearances are characterized by nodular infiltrates diffusely spread over both the lungs. At times the X-ray appearance is of military mottling. Hilar adenopathy and small to moderate-sized pleural effusions may occur. The prognosis is grave and death occurs from respiratory failure. If the pneumonia resolves the nodules within the lung calcify; healed calcific nodules may persist for years or even lifelong.

The clinical picture of the characteristic varicella skin and mucosal rash is diagnostic. The virus may be cultured or detected by PCR technique. Serological tests include the fluorescent antibody test, the membrane antigen test and the ELISA test.

Treatment is with early administration of acyclovir (10 mg/kg) intravenously every 8 hours for 10 days in all patients with varicella who develop pneumonia. Preventive administration of oral acyclovir in elderly patients, pregnant women, in patients with COPD or in patients who are immunocompromised is recommended in varicella, even in the absence of pneumonia.

Zoster immune globulin complements the use of acyclovir in patients with varicella pneumonia or in immunocompromised patients even in the absence of pneumonia.

Strict isolation is warranted until all skin lesions have crusted and the crusts have fallen off.

Hantavirus

The *Hantavirus* respiratory syndrome can result from several Hantaviruses. Almost all cases have been reported from North and South America. There have also been reports of proven *Hantavirus* infection from India. Rodents serve as the reservoir and transmission to humans results from aerosolization of the virus contained in their feces. In the first report of evidence of *Hantavirus* in India, a multi-institutional study has confirmed 28 cases of infection among patients with chronic renal disease, warehouse workers and members of the Irula tribe engaged in rodent trapping in the Vellore district of Tamil Nadu (*Ref: Chandy S, Yoshimatsu K, Rainer G, et al. Seroepidemiological study on hantavirus infections in India. T Roy Soc Trop Med H. 2008;102;70-4*).

Clinical features are those of a flu-like syndrome, with fever, myalgia, abdominal pain and diarrhea. Respiratory involvement is characterized by breathlessness, tachypnea and increasing hypoxia. Cough may be absent; if present is not marked. ARDS and shock are observed in severe infection. Hematological examination reveals leukocytosis, thrombocytopenia, hemoconcentration and circulating immunoblasts. In fact the triad of thrombocytopenia, a left shift of the leukocytes with circulating myeloblasts and immunoblasts is strongly suggestive of *Hantavirus* pulmonary syndrome. Multivariate analysis has shown that dizziness, nausea and absence of cough are predictive of HPS. In like fashion, thrombocytopenia, elevated hematocrit and a lowered serum bicarbonate are features that may help to distinguish HPS from other causes of respiratory distress such as pneumococcal infection or influenza. Renal failure may complicate the overall clinical picture. Death is from respiratory failure, shock, and multi-organ dysfunction.

Diagnosis is made by serological and immuno-histochemical techniques. Treatment is supportive. Ventilatory support is essential in severe forms of the disease. Intravenous ribavirin is being used in controlled trials; results are pending.

It should be noted that severe lower respiratory tract infections can occur both from viruses known to cause infections in normal hosts as also from more opportunistic viral pathogens. These opportunistic infections chiefly include those due to cytomegalovirus, herpes simplex viruses, Varicella Zoster virus, adenovirus and RNA viruses. These have been considered in a separate chapter (Pneumonia in the Immunocompromised Patient).

Table 5 lists common respiratory viruses and their associated diseases.

FUNGAL PNEUMONIA

Fungal infections of the lower respiratory tract (causing fungal pneumonia) that occur in normal hosts are histoplasmosis caused by *Histoplasma capsulatum,* blastomycosis caused by *Blastomyces dermatitidis,* and coccidioidomycosis caused by *Coccidioides immitis* and *Paracoccidioides brasiliensis.* These diseases are seen in the north and south American continent. Except for the uncommon presence of histoplasmosis and a few reported cases of blastomycosis, the above mentioned fungal infections are not observed in India and Southeast Asia. They will therefore merit a short description. Cryptococcal infections due to *Cryptococcus neoformans* and certain forms of *Aspergillus* infection due to *Aspergillus fumigatus* can also occur in normal hosts and are observed all over the world including India. Fungal pneumonias that are chiefly restricted to severely immunocompromised patients have been dealt with in the chapter on "Pneumonia in the Non-HIV Immunocompromised Patient".

Aspergillosis

Aspergillus species are ubiquitous fungi. Airway colonization without infection is seen in patients with chronic lung disease such as bronchiectasis, and in burnt-out fibrotic tuberculosis. Invasive *Aspergillus* is almost solely restricted to immunocompromised patients though there are very rare reports of its occurrence in normal hosts as well. Invasive aspergillosis has been described elsewhere (Pneumonia in the Immunocompromised Host).

Table 5: Common respiratory viruses and associated diseases.

Virus	Diseases	Antivirals	Prevention (vacancies)
Influenza	Bronchitis, croup, pneumonia	Oseltamivir Zanamivir	Yes
Para influenza (PIV)	Croup (P1V1) Pneumonia (P1V3)	-	-
Respiratory syncytial virus (RSV)	Bronchiolitis Pneumonia	Ribavirin	-
Rhinovirus	Common cold	-	-
Adenovirus	Croup Pneumonia	-	Yes
Varicella zoster virus	Pneumonia	Acyclovir Famciclovir	-
Herpes simplex virus	Pneumonia	Acyclovir Famciclovir	-
Coronavirus	Common cold (OC43) Pneumonia (HuCoV-SARS)	? Interferon α	-
Measles virus	Croup Pneumonia	-	Yes
Cytomegalo virus	Pharyngitis Pneumonia	Ganciclovir Famciclovir	-
EB virus	Pharyngitis	-	-
Metapneumo virus	Bronchiolitis Pneumonia	-	-
SARS, MERS	Pneumonia	-	-

It is perhaps appropriate to classify the clinical manifestations of *Aspergillus* disease in this chapter **(Table 6)**.

1. Simple colonization without infection.
2. *Hypersensitivity reactions*: Exposure to *A. fumigatus* can lead to allergic asthma, extrinsic allergic alveolitis (hypersensitivity pneumonitis), and allergic bronchopulmonary aspergillosis.

   Spores of *A. fumigatus* when inhaled by atopic individuals can trigger an IgE-mediated inflammatory response in the bronchial mucosa leading to classic features of bronchial asthma.

   In nonatopic individuals, massive or repeated inhalation of *Aspergillus conidia* can lead to persistent airways obstruction and rarely to extrinsic allergic alveolitis (hypersensitivity pneumonitis). This condition is characterized by a flu-like syndrome with fever, malaise, cough, breathlessness and a diffuse neutrophilic interstitial exudate due to a Th1 CD4 response within the lung in the acute phase. The late phase is characterized by reticulonodular opacities within the lung. Nonrecognition of these syndromes can lead to permanent lung damage.

   Allergic bronchopulmonary aspergillosis is a result of sensitization to *A. fumigatus* antigens, in a subset of atopic individuals and in patients with cystic fibrosis. It has been dealt with in a separate chapter.

   Bronchocentric granulomatosis is believed to be a rare hypersensitivity response to *A. fumigatus* and is characterized by replacement of bronchial mucous membrane by granulomas, eosinophilic infiltration and fibrosis. *Aspergillus hyphae* have been recovered from the involved tissue. The condition presents with chest pain, dyspnea, low-grade fever with one or more nodular lesions on a radiographic examination, very similar to the appearance of metastatic lesions. Diagnosis can only be made following a lung biopsy. Multifocal lesions respond to corticosteroids. A single lesion is often surgically removed and generally does not recur.

3. Aspergillomas are fungal balls containing *Aspergillus fumigatus.* These fungal balls exist in preformed cavities—most commonly in tuberculous cavities, but also in bronchiectatic cavities, in Stage IV sarcoid, healed lung abscess and in upper lobe cavities observed in patients with ankylosing spondylitis. Aspergillomas are often silent but occasionally cause hemoptysis which may be mild to moderate and self-limiting, or profuse and exsanguinating, causing death. Radiological appearances are characteristic, showing a solid shadow within a cavity with an airspace above **(Figs. 6A to C)**. Computed tomography (CT) appearances at times allow a diagnosis of an aspergilloma which is missed on routine radiography **(Fig. 7)**.

   Hemoptysis, when severe, is treated with embolization of the culprit bronchial vessel, revealed through angiographies. Both arterial and pulmonary angiographies need to be done so as not to miss out on identification of the culprit vessel. Intracavitatory instillation of Amphotericin B has also been tried. When bleeding persists or recurs, surgical resection if feasible should be undertaken.

4. *Invasive aspergillosis*: Invasive aspergillosis leads to invasion and involvement of the lung parenchyma causing pneumonia. This is dealt with in the chapter on Pneumonia in the Immunocompromised Patient".

   Rarely, chronic necrotizing pneumonia due to aspergillus infection has been recognized in nonneutropenic patients. It may occur on its own or at times appear adjacent to an aspergilloma. Amphotericin B is the treatment of choice in these patients, though voriconazole and caspofungin are new additions to the therapeutic armamentarium. These drugs have been described in detail in the chapter "Pneumonia in the Immunocompromised Patient".

Table 6: Clinical forms of Aspergillus infection.

• Simple colonization without infection
• Hypersensitivity reaction:
  – Allergic bronchial asthma
  – Allergic bronchopulmonary aspergillosis
  – Extrinsic allergic alveolitis
• Aspergilloma
• Invasive aspergillosis (has been considered in a separate chapter)
• Chronic necrotising aspergillus pneumonia

Histoplasmosis

Histoplasma capsulatum is found in soil contaminated by infected bird or bat feces. The disease is chiefly restricted to the central United States, and most of Latin America. This fungus is an important cause of pneumonia in endemic areas. Cases have however also been reported in Africa, India and Southeast Asia. Gopalkrishnan and colleagues have reported 24 cases of proven histoplasmosis from

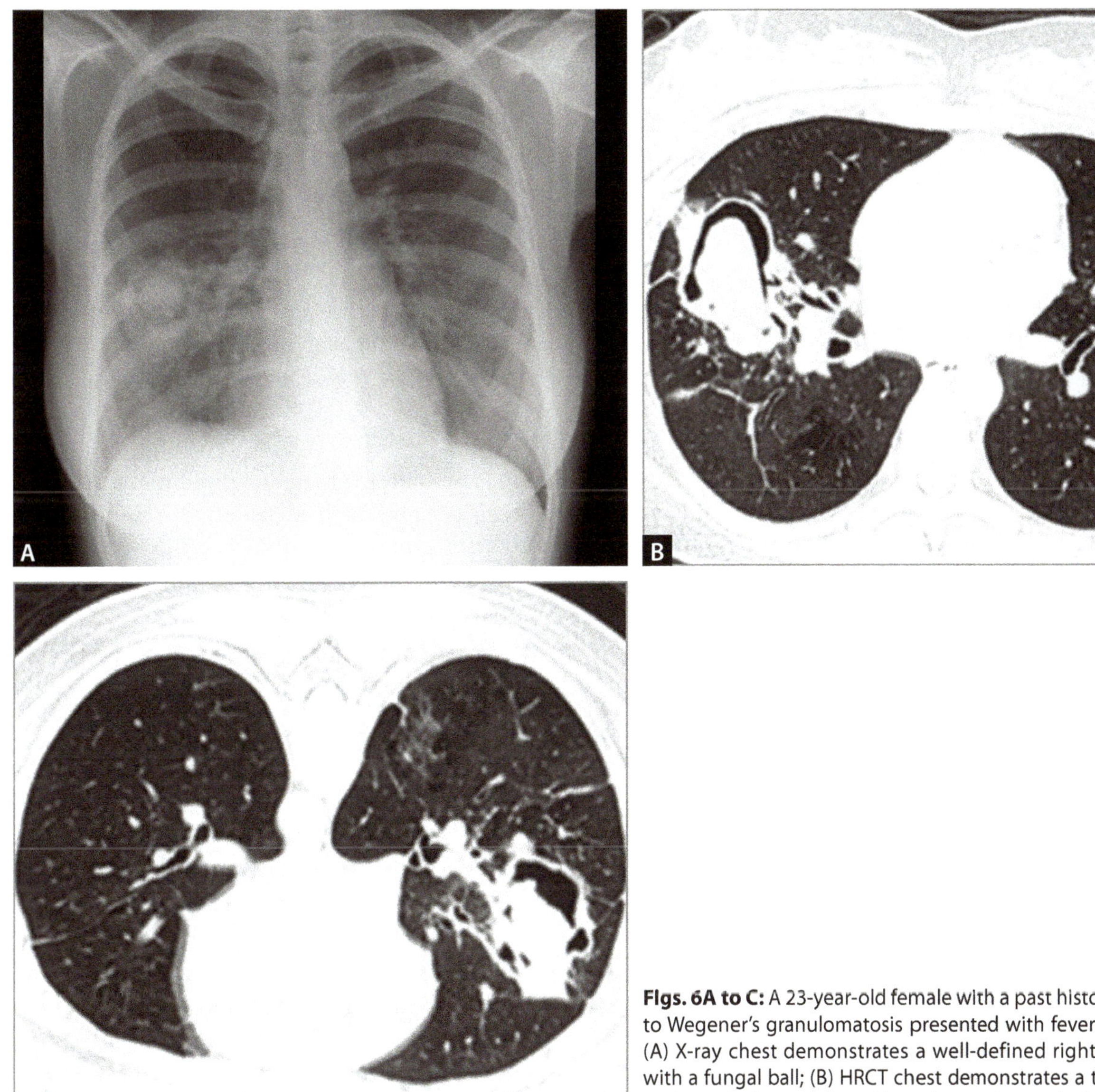

Figs. 6A to C: A 23-year-old female with a past history of cavities due to Wegener's granulomatosis presented with fever and hemoptysis. (A) X-ray chest demonstrates a well-defined right mid-zone cavity with a fungal ball; (B) HRCT chest demonstrates a thin-walled cavity in the right lower lobe with an internal mass lesion representing a fungal ball; and (C) on prone scans the fungal ball is seen to move.

India between 2002 and 2012 showing that the disease is not as rare as is believed.

In India, the majority of histoplasmosis cases were reported from the eastern and north-eastern part of the country, especially from Calcutta (West Bengal) and Assam.

Initially restricted to rural societies it is now also found in urban sites, particularly in association with construction projects involving movement of contaminated soil.

The inhaled spores (2–5 μm in diameter) reach the small airways and alveoli. The spores after inhalation are converted to yeasts which are ingested by macrophages.

The yeast form proliferates in the macrophages and can disseminate to distant metastatic sites.

In the lung the fungus incites a cell-mediated immune response with the formation of a primary granulomatous focus with associated hilar and mediastinal lympha-denopathy very similar to what one observes with a primary complex in tuberculosis. The disease at this stage may be asymptomatic or may present with nonspecific respiratory symptoms with perhaps a low-grade fever. The primary lung lesion may heal and calcify. If it does not heal, the caseous focus may cavitate causing fever, cough with expectoration and occasionally hemoptysis, very similar

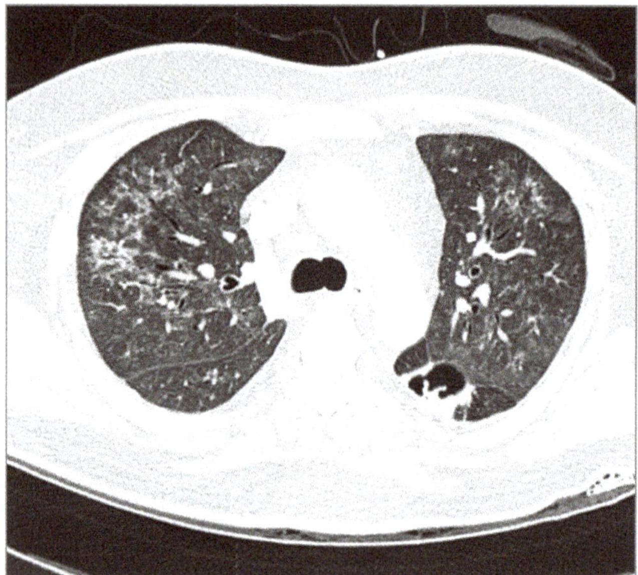

Fig. 7: *Aspergillus* infection: HRCT chest demonstrates ill-defined nodular lesions in the upper lobes as well as a thin cavitating lesion in the apical segment of the left lower lobe representing an aspergilloma. There are multiple thin strands within the lesion representing hyphae.

to the clinical features seen in tuberculosis. Yeast forms of histoplasma may be identified in the sputum on smear or grown on culture. The clinical and radiological picture may be indistinguishable from chronic fibrocaseous cavitative tuberculosis. If the disease is not contained, metastatic lesions may be observed in various organs of the body, particularly the liver and spleen and adrenal glands. Mediastinal fibrosis is a well-known complication of histoplasma infection.

In patients who inhale a large number of spores, an acute syndrome develops generally after an incubation period of 14 days. This syndrome is abrupt in onset and resembles influenza or bacterial pneumonia or an acute form of tuberculosis. Miliary mottling on an X-ray chest indistinguishable from miliary tuberculosis can occur. Rarely, ARDS has been reported as a manifestation of a hyperacute infection.

Diagnosis

In India, histoplasmosis should be considered the differential diagnosis of any patient with an upper respiratory disease resembling tuberculosis where AFB have not been demonstrated on smear or culture and when anti-TB drugs have not proved of use. Hepatosplenomegaly, oral ulcers, pyrexia, adrenal enlargement are other features

of note. When tissue biopsy reveals granulomas and AFB are not observed, fungal stains should be routinely performed.

Direct diagnosis is provided by culture of sputum or BAL specimens, though cultures may take several weeks to become positive. Tissue samples can demonstrate organisms with silver or acid schiff (PAS) staining. Bone-marrow smears may show *Histoplasma capsulatum* in severe metastatic infections.

Indirect diagnosis can be provided by the complement fixation test, immunodiffusion or radioimmunoassay test, all of which take several weeks to become positive.

Treatment

Patients who have chronic progressive pulmonary disease or those with disseminated metastatic disease need to be treated with amphotericin B. The liposomal form of amphotericin B though expensive has less toxicity. Amphotericin B is given intravenously; the drug has many side-effects, notably renal toxicity. Ketoconazole is also effective but has frequent gastrointestinal and anti-testosterone effects. Fluconazole and itraconazole (200–400 mg/day) are as effective as amphotericin B or ketoconazole in patients with mild illness.

Most primary infections are self-limiting, heal on their own and require no treatment. They however need a periodic follow-up to ensure that progressive pulmonary disease or dissemination has not occurred.

Blastomycosis

Blastomycosis is found in North America, Mexico, the Middle East, Africa and India. It is caused by the inhalation of spores of *Blastomyces dermatitidis*. In fact it is endemic in India, though its areas of endemicity, prevalence and natural habitat of the etiological agent remain undetermined. The fungus grows in the soil and the airborne spores are inhaled, reach the alveoli and are converted to the yeast form. Defense mechanisms involve polymorphonuclear leukocytes followed by a cell-mediated immune response that leads to the formation of granulomas. The disease can resemble an acute bacterial infection or mycobacterial infection, again indistinguishable from tuberculosis. Metastatic lesions can occur in the skin, bones, brain and other organs. Extrapulmonary infections can occur years after the primary infection.

Clinical features vary. In North America acute blastomycosis resembles an acute bacterial pneumonia, with fever with chills, cough with purulent sputum and pleuritic pain. In milder cases, the disease resembles tuberculosis with low-grade fever, cough, hemoptysis and weight loss. The radiological findings vary. Lobar consolidation is observed in acute cases. In the milder forms, infiltrates, cavities, rounded densities or even miliary shadowing may be observed **(Fig. 8)**. In the very severe forms of the disease, ARDS can occur even in immunocompetent hosts.

Skin lesions of blastomycosis may occur several years after a self-limiting pulmonary infection.

Diagnosis of blastomycosis is made by examination of respiratory secretions digested by potassium hydroxide. Cultures of respiratory secretions (sputum or BAL fluid) turn positive generally after a week. Silver or PAS staining of infected tissue may reveal the characteristic yeast forms of the fungus.

Treatment

Like histoplasmosis, in many patients blastomycosis is self-limiting and may require no treatment. Patients with acute disease or progressive disease are treated with amphotericin B. Itraconazole or ketoconazole are alternatives for less severe or slowly progressive disease.

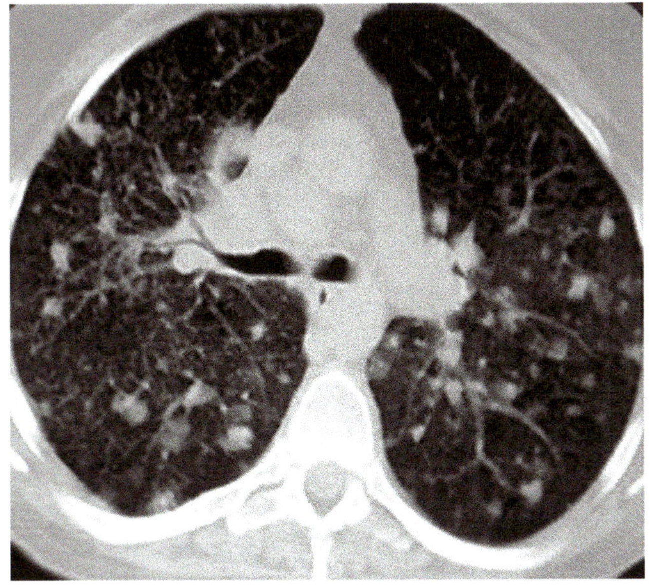

Fig. 8: Intermediate-sized nodules from blastomycosis in a 40-year-old woman with persistent cough, chest pain, and intermittent fevers. The patient had experienced progression of symptoms over several months. CT scan shows multiple bilateral intermediate-sized nodules.

Coccidioidomycosis

Coccidioidomycosis is due to infections with *Coccidioides immitis,* a fungus present in the soil. The disease is endemic in southwestern United States and in Mexico, occurring mainly during hot dry summers. Inhalation of spores leads to both a suppurative lesion and to cell-mediated granulomatous disease within the lungs after an incubation period of about 2 weeks.

Clinical features include fever, chills, arthralgia, pleuritic chest pain, dyspnea and hemoptysis. Physical examination may reveal signs of consolidation and/or cavitation. Pleural effusion may be present. On the other hand, primary infection may be silent, self-limiting and heal on its own.

Chest radiography initially shows one or more areas of consolidation which may cavitate. Hilar adenopathy is often present. The radiographical features as with histoplasmosis and blastomycosis may be indistinguishable from tuberculosis.

The primary lesion may heal as in tuberculosis or may continue to progress with fresh infiltrates, fresh consolidation and cavitation. Persistent fever, cough and weight loss occur. Disseminated coccidioidomycosis may occur several months after the primary infection, involving the skin, bones, joints, meninges and the genitourinary system.

Diagnosis

Diagnosis is made by microscopic examination of sputum after digestion with potassium hydroxide or by silver staining of infected tissues obtained through a tissue biopsy. Cultures of sputum or BAL fluid take almost a week to turn positive. Serological tests and skin tests are of great importance for epidemiological purposes.

Treatment

Many patients with coccidioidomycosis have mild self-limiting disease and require no specific therapy. In progressive disease, fluconazole, itraconazole and ketoconazole are equally effective. In severe disease and in metastatic disease, amphotericin B is the drug of choice.

Cryptococcosis

Cryptococcosis is due to *Cryptococcus neoformans,* a fungus found throughout the world. Cryptococcosis is an uncommon infection and is usually self-limiting and asymptomatic. It may however cause lung infection or meningitis particularly in those with impaired cell-mediated immune responses.

Pulmonary infection can cause pneumonia, presenting with fever, cough, malaise and chest pain. The chest X-ray may show infiltration, consolidation or a mass-like shadow closely resembling a neoplasm. Hilar lymphadenopathy may be present.

Examination of the sputum especially using India ink or sputum culture may show the presence of cryptococci.

However, it must be remembered that *C. neoformans* can colonize the airways of patients with chronic bronchitis or in immunocompromised patients without being responsible for disease. Hence, positive sputum cultures do not necessarily denote disease. Examination of tissue obtained through a transbronchial, CT-guided or thoracoscopic biopsy is often necessary to confirm diagnosis. The presence of *C. neoformans* on staining or on tissue culture confirms the diagnosis with certainty.

Treatment: Patients with progressive disease need treatment with amphotericin B. Ketoconazole, fluconazole and itraconazole are also effective.

■ SUGGESTED READING

1. Cao B, Li XW, Mao Y, et al. Clinical features of the initial cases of 2009 pandemic influenza A (H1N1) virus infection in China. N Engl J Med. 2009;361:2507-17.
2. Chayakulkeeree M. Cryptococcosis. Infect Dis Clin North Am. 2006;20(3):507-44, v-vi.
3. Falsey AR. Community-acquired viral pneumonia. Clin Geriatr Med. 2007;23(3):535-52, vi.
4. Gopalakrishnan R, Nambi PS, Ramasubramanian V, et al. Histoplasmosis in India: truly uncommon or uncommonly recognised? Assoc Physicians India. 2012;60:25-8.
5. Kauffman CA. Histoplasmosis. Clin Chest Med. 2009;30(2):217-25, v.
6. Ksiazek TG, Erdman D, Goldsmith CS, et al. A novel coronavirus associated with severe acute respiratory syndrome. N Engl J Med. 2003;348:1953-66.
7. Lortholary O, Denning OW, Dupont B. Endemic mycosis: a treatment update. J Antimicrob Chemother. 1999;43:321-31.
8. Marr KA. Aspergillosis. Pathogenesis, clinical manifestations, and therapy. Infect Dis Clin North Am. 2002;16(4):875-94, vi.
9. Murthy PR, Ucchil R, Shah U, et al. Hantavirus pulmonary syndrome in a postpartum woman. Indian T Crit Care Med. 2016;20:551-3.
10. Randhawa HS, Chowdhary A, Kathuria S, et al. Blastomycosis in India: report of an imported case and current status. Med Mycol. 2013;51(2):185-9.
11. Riscili BP. Noninvasive pulmonary Aspergillus infections. Clin Chest Med. 2009;30(2):315-35, vii.
12. Rothberg MB. Complications of viral influenza. Am J Med. 2008;121(4):258-64.
13. Scalera NM, Mossad SB. The first pandemic of the 21st century: a review of the 2009 pandemic variant influenza A (H1N1) virus. Postgrad Med. 2009;121(5):43-7.
14. Siddharth V, Goyal V, Kaushal VK. Clinical-epidemiological profile of influenza A H1N1 cases at a Tertiary Care Institute of India. Indian I Community Med. 2012;37(4):232-5.
15. Stamboulian D. Influenza. Infect Dis Clin North Am. 2000;14(1):141-66.
16. Torres AM, Whitney CG. Infectious Diseases Society of America/American Thoracic Society consensus guidelines on the management of community-acquired pneumonia in adults. Clin Infec Dis. 2007;44:S27-72.
17. Zimmer SM, Burke DS. Historical perspective: emergence of influenza A (H1N1) viruses. N Engl J Med. 2009;361(3):279-85.

Pneumonia in the Non-HIV Immunocompromised Patient

■ GENERAL CONSIDERATIONS

Pneumonia in the non-human immunodeficiency virus (HIV) immunocompromised patients carries a significant morbidity and mortality. Thus mortality rates for bone marrow transplant recipients who develop pneumonia and require ventilatory support is close to 90%. The morbidity and mortality are partly related to poor immune response to infection as also to the wide range of potential pathogens that can cause pulmonary infections in these unfortunate patients. Pneumonia can be caused not only by the usual organisms causing community-acquired pneumonia (CAP), but frequently by uncommon organisms and by opportunistic infections, which are very rare in patients with a preserved immune response. Community-acquired Gram-negative pulmonary infections are far more common in the immunocompromised when compared to the immunocompetent. Tuberculosis, particularly in countries like India where the disease has a high-prevalence rate is also an extremely important consideration.

Atypical mycobacteria, *Nocardia*, and chlamydia are also more frequently observed as are fungal infections, in particular *Pneumocystis jirovecii*, *Aspergillus*, *Candida*, and infection with rarer molds. Viral infections, notably due to the *Cytomegalovirus* (CMV) are both frequent and important. Protozoal (toxoplasmal) infection and rarely but importantly hyperinfection with *Strongyloides stercoralis* also are to be considered. The list of potential pathogens is large and the important ones have been tabled below (**Table 1**).

It is obvious that in view of this large range of possible infections, the diagnosis of the cause of pneumonia in the immunocompromised patient is difficult and its management is complex. It is impossible in a given patient to cover such a wide range of possible organisms. An approach that narrows the potential pathogens to a basic minimum is to be aimed at. A specific etiology should be sought and for this bronchoscopy, bronchoalveolar lavage (BAL) studies, and transbronchial biopsies are often early investigational procedures. Bronchoscopy may yield a definite etiological diagnosis in some patients, and even if the procedure is unrevealing, it may enable the physician to exclude infectious agents as the cause of a pulmonary infiltrate or shadow. The early use of computed tomography (CT) scanning is imperative as lesions revealed on a CT may be masked or not evident on routine radiography. In spite of every diagnostic effort, in patients who are critically ill, therapeutic intervention includes the empiric use of broad-spectrum antibiotics together with other

Table 1: Potential pathogens associated with pneumonia in the immunocompromised patients.

Bacteria—pyogenic bacteria:
- Gram-negative—*Pseudomonas aeruginosa*, *Klebsiella pneumoniae*, acinetobacter, *E. coli*, *Proteus*, *Enterobacter*, other Gram-negative organisms
- Gram positive—*Streptococcus pneumoniae*, *Staphylococcus aureus*, *Enterobacter* species
- *Mycobacterium tuberculosis*
- Other bacteria—atypical mycobacteria, *Nocardia*, *Mycoplasma*, *Legionella*, anaerobes

Fungi:
- *Pneumocystis jirovecii*, *Aspergillus* species, *Candida* species, rarer fungi (*Mucor*, *Penicillium*, *Fusarium*), endemic fungi

Viruses:
CMV virus, herpes simplex, *Varicella zoster*, Respiratory viruses—influenza, parainfluenza, Adenovirus, Respiratory syncytial virus

Protozoa

Toxoplasma

Helminths

S. stercoralis

(CMV: *Cytomegalovirus*; E. coli: *Escherichia coli*; S. stercoralis: *Strongyloides stercoralis*)

anti-infective agents covering nonbacterial infections to ensure that the patients receive adequate therapy.

It is certain that with increased use of organ transplants and the associated increased use of immunosuppressants, the increasing incidence of cancer and the use of many new chemotherapeutic drugs in its treatment, the number of immunocompromised patients will increase tremendously in the years to come. This applies not just to the Western world but to developing and poor countries as well. Many of these will be young patients who will have undergone increasingly aggressive treatment in the hope of a cure. Improved outcomes in these patients necessitate better, quicker diagnosis, and organized management protocols.

■ NON-HIV IMMUNOCOMPROMISED PATIENT

The immunocompromised patients considered in this chapter are patients with advanced malignancies, lymphomas, leukemias, aplastic anemia, and severe neutropenia from any cause, and patients receiving organ transplants including bone-marrow transplant recipients **(Table 2)**. Chemotherapy, use of immunosuppressants, corticosteroid therapy, and cytotoxic therapy (use of cyclophosphamide, mycophenolate mofetil) can also compromise immune function, as can the use of monoclonal antibodies against tumor necrosis factor (infliximab).

Lesser degree of immunosuppression is also observed in patients with uncontrolled diabetes, in chronic renal failure, particularly in patients on dialysis, liver cirrhosis,

multiple myeloma, low-dose cytotoxic therapy, and in patients receiving a maintenance dose of corticosteroids for long periods. Many diseases in our country unfold against a background of poor nutrition, which depresses the immune response to infection. Rarely, uncommon infections including opportunistic infections are observed due to poor immune response (in particular cell-mediated response) resulting from extreme old age.

Nature of Immunocompromised Patient

Immune defects can arise from the following causes:
- Severe neutropenia (<1,500/mL)
- A qualitative defect in neutrophil function (rare)
- Cell-mediated immune deficiency (a T-lymphocyte function)
- Deficiency in antibody formation (a B-lymphocyte function)
- From a combination of two or more of these causes.

It needs to be stressed that cell-mediated immune response and humoral defense through antibody production are closely inter-related, interactive, and interdependent.

■ CLINICAL APPROACH TO THE DIFFERENTIAL DIAGNOSIS OF PNEUMONIA IN AN IMMUNOCOMPROMISED PATIENT

It is of great importance to realize that fever, cough, and even hemoptysis in an immunocompromised patient who has a focal or diffuse infiltrate in one or both lungs can be due not only to microorganisms causing a true infective pneumonia, but could equally result from one or more of several noninfective causes. A distinction between the two is at times impossibly difficult. If determined to be of infective etiology, a quick organized attempt should be made to determine the specific or likely microorganism responsible for the pneumonia.

Initial Approach in the Differential Diagnosis is to Elicit a Careful History

The nature of defects in the immune response that can lead to an immunocompromised state has been mentioned earlier. The history should therefore focus on the background disease responsible for the immunocompromised state as also on the current and prior immunosuppressive

Table 2: Immunocompromised patients.
Severely immunocompromised:
• Acute leukemias
• Aplastic anemia
• Severe neutropenia from any cause
• Lymphoma
• Solid organ transplant and hematopoietic stem cell transplant (HSCT) recepients
• Recent chemotherapy, radiation
• Use of immunosuppressant drugs
• Cytotoxic therapy
• High dose of corticosteroid therapy (>30 mg for > 3–4 weeks)
Lesser degree of immunocompromised:
• Uncontrolled diabetes
• Chronic renal failure, particularly patients on dialysis
• Liver cirrhosis
• Multiple myeloma
• Low-dose cytotoxic therapy
• Corticosteroids for long periods
• Malnutrition
• Extreme old age

regimens. This enables the clinician to determine the likely nature of the immune defect as also on the degree of immune dysregulation likely to be present, both of which in turn could point to the likely causes of pneumonia in a particular patient. Thus, patients with neutropenia or those with qualitative defects in neutrophil function are prone to pneumonia due to pyogenic bacteria (in particular *Pseudomonas* and *Klebsiella*), *Aspergillus* infection, and infection with *candida* species. Those with defects in cell-mediated immune response are prone to pneumonia caused by *Mycobacterium tuberculosis, P. jirovecii, Nocardia*, atypical mycobacteria, herpes virus, respiratory viruses, *Legionella*, mycoplasma, toxoplasma, and *S. stercoralis*. Patients who have a defect in antibody formation are prone to infection by *Streptococcus pneumoniae, Haemophilus influenzae*, and herpes viruses. The morbidity and mortality of these infections is forbiddingly high in immunocompromised patients. In one large early study on renal transplant patients, pneumonia occurred in 20% of patients and accounted for 50% of deaths. Though such high figures do not generally apply to current established centers in our country, they are a pointer to the possible morbidity and mortality in poor third world countries caring for renal transplant patients in comparatively less well-established transplant units. **Table 3** gives the nature of the immune defect in relation to the underlying disease/treatment and relates these to the potential pathogens likely to cause infections, including pneumonia in these patients.

As mentioned earlier, fever and pulmonary shadows or infiltrates in an immunocompromised patient are not always related to infection. It is vital to be aware of this fact. Noninfective causes of pulmonary infiltrates or shadows include pulmonary edema, intra-alveolar hemorrhage, pulmonary embolism, drug-induced pulmonary edema, acute respiratory distress syndrome (ARDS), opportunistic neoplasms, and lymphoproliferative disease. Other noninfective lesions include recurrence of underlying tumors, recurrence of lymphoma or of leukemia within the lungs, immune-mediated disorders (acute rejection after lung transplant, obliterative bronchiolitis after lung transplant or after an allogeneic stem cell transplant, or graft versus host reaction after an allogeneic stem cell transplant), engraftment syndrome in hematogenous stem cell transplant and nonspecific focal inflammation. Important noninfective causes of pulmonary infiltrates or shadows in the immunocompromised host are tabled below **(Table 4)**.

The temporal relationship between the initiation of immunosuppression and the onset of pneumonia

Table 3: Nature of immune defects or compromise, causes of defect, related to likely pathogens causing pneumonia.

Immune defect	Cause of defect	Likely pathogens
Cell-mediated	HSCT Lymphoma Leukemia Graft vs host disease Azathioprine Mycophenolate Tacrolimus Corticosteroid therapy	*Mycobacterium tuberculosis,* *Pneumocystis jirovecii,* *Nocardia* Atypical mycobacteria Herpes virus Respiratory viruses *Legionella* *Mycoplasma* Toxoplasma *S. stercoralis*
Neutropenia	Acute leukemia Chemotherapy Aplastic anemia HSCT (early phase) diseases involving or infiltrating the marrow Cytotoxic drugs immunosuppressants	Pyogenic bacteria—in particular Gram-negative infections *Aspergillus Candida*
Functional neutrophil defect	Corticosteroid therapy Azathioprine/ mycophenolate	Same as above
Antibody defect	CLL Lymphoma Myeloma HSCT Splenectomized patients	*Streptococcus pneumoniae* *H. influenzae* Herpes viruses

(CLL: Chronic lymphocytic leukemia; *H. influenzae: Haemophilus influenzae*: HSCT: Hematogenous stem cell transplant; *S. stercoralis: Strongyloides stercoralis*)

or a pulmonary infiltrate plays an important role in the differential diagnosis. In organ transplant and hematological stem cell transplant (HSCT) patients, pneumonia occurring within the first 3 or 4 weeks of the transplant is almost never due to an opportunistic infection but results from usual bacterial pathogens, in particular Gram-negative bacteria such as *Pseudomonas aeruginosa*, and *Klebsiella*. Severe neutropenia may also predispose to invasive fungal infections (IFIs) (*Aspergillus*, other filamentous fungi, and candida) in this time frame.

Cytomegalovirus pneumonia occurs 1–4 months after transplantation. Other opportunistic infections in this time frame include pneumocystis, nocardial, fungal, and viral infections **(Fig. 1)**. After 4 months, patients who have normally functioning grafts and who are on minimal immunosuppressants are more prone to the usual community-acquired infections, though opportunistic infections are possible. Those with poorly functioning

Table 4: Noninfectious causes that mimic infective pneumonia in the immunocompromised host.

- Pulmonary edema
- Intra-alveolar hemorrhage
- Pulmonary infarction
- Pulmonary atelectasis
- Diffuse alveolar hemorrhage (DAH)
- Diffuse alveolar damage
- ARDS
- Drug toxicity, radiation toxicity
- Progression of underlying mitotic disease
- Engraftment syndrome in hematogenous stem cell transplant recipients (HSCT)
- Transfusion-related acute lung injury (TRALI)
- Rejection of graft in graft vs host disease (GVHD)
- Idiopathic pneumonia syndrome
- Bronchiolitis obliterans-organizing pneumonia
- Post-transplantation lymphoproliferative disorders (PTLD)

(ARDS: Acute respiratory distress syndrome)

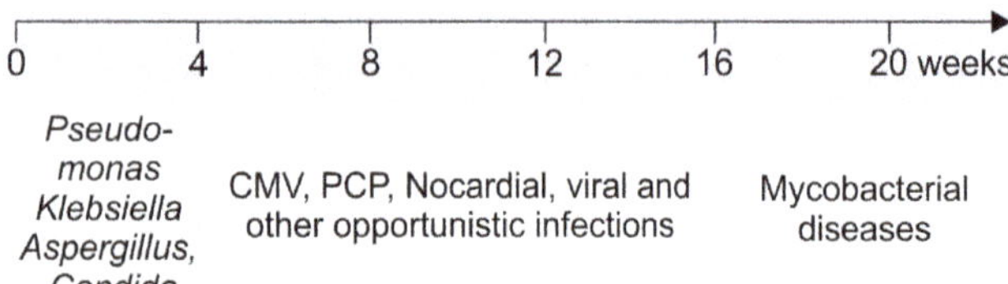

Fig. 1: Various pulmonary infections in transplant recipients in relation to different time frames. (CMV: *Cytomegalovirus*; PCP: *Pneumocystis jirovecii* pneumonia)

grafts who require increased immunosuppressants remain susceptible to opportunistic infections. *Reactivation of latent tuberculous lung infection or a fresh pulmonary infection with M. tuberculosis is of great importance in our country and in countries with a high-prevalence rate of tuberculosis. This is usually a late-onset infection.*

Awareness of the presence of a positive serology for CMV antigen or of a strongly positive Mantoux test prior to immunosuppression may be of diagnostic help. Also, the specific use of prophylactic drugs or antibiotics may make infection with certain organisms unlikely. For example, trimethoprim-sulfamethoxazole has been proved to be very effective in the prevention of *P. carinii* infection. Therefore, a patient on this prophylaxis is unlikely to present with pneumonia due to *P. carinii*. On the other hand, the prophylactic use of fluconazole in single-organ transplant (SOT) and hematopoietic stem cell transplantation (HSCT) in order to prevent candida infections is believed by some authorities to have increased the incidence of invasive aspergillosis. The overuse of fluconazole has also probably created selective pressure promoting the emergence of *Candida tropicalis, Candida glabrata*, and *Candida krusei.*

Epidemiological clues should always be sought. In our country and in other third world countries, depressed cell-mediated immunity is most likely to reactivate or cause fresh infection with *M. tuberculosis*. However exposure to fungi such as *Histoplasma capsulatum* or *Coccidioides immitis* may predispose, particularly in endemic areas, to histoplasmosis or coccidioidomycosis.

Symptoms are generally noncontributory—fever, cough, hemoptysis, and chest pain are common to many infections. In fact symptoms and signs may be absent, the presentation being an asymptomatic "patch" or infiltrate within the lung. Yet at the same time, some patients may present with a fulminant illness that may or may not be marked by high fever but is characterized by increasing tachypnea, spreading pulmonary shadows, increasing hypoxia, cardiorespiratory and multiorgan failure.

Mode of Onset and Tempo of Progression

These often provide critical clues to a diagnosis. Their value is enhanced, if the above features are considered with radiological and CT findings.

An acute onset over 24–48 hours is suggestive of a conventional bacterial infection or certain noninfective causes such as pulmonary edema, pulmonary hemorrhage, pulmonary embolism, or a leukoagglutination reaction. A subacute onset over some days or weeks suggests possible tuberculosis, fungal infection, viral infection, or nocardial infection. The same presentation may, however, also be observed with certain noninfectious causes such as drug-induced pneumonia, radiation pneumonitis, or recurrence of a tumor against the background of a mitotic disease.

Physical Examination

Physical examination may occasionally provide valuable clues. In sophisticated intensive care units (ICUs) with high-technology equipment, physical examination tends to be perfunctory; this should never be so. *Repeated clinical examination might reveal clues, which machines and elaborate investigations fail to detect.* The features enumerated below are merely illustrative of the importance of a careful physical examination.

- Tachypnea in an immunocompromised patient, particularly in the absence of high fever is indicative of sepsis, pneumonia, or acidosis. Physical signs in the chest may or may not be evident; an absence of signs on percussion or auscultation is often observed in these patients.
- Skin lesions are occasionally present in cryptococcal, nocardial, and candidal infections. They take the form of minimally painful or asymptomatic macules, papules, or nodules, which on biopsy provide the correct diagnosis, thereby obviating the need for invasive diagnostic procedures. Erythema gangrenosum is occasionally observed in infections with *Pseudomonas aeruginosa,* and very rarely with other Gram-negative infections.
- A careful search for enlarged lymph glands can be rewarding. Lymphadenopathy strongly suggests a tuberculous infection in our country due to *M. tuberculosis.* An underlying lymphoma, presenting with an obscure pneumonia, has been occasionally diagnosed following the biopsy of a nondescript but clinically palpable lymph node.
- Ocular examination is important, as ocular findings are common with disseminated CMV infection. The retina shows hemorrhages and yellowish-white exudates. Similar ocular findings have been noted in toxoplasmosis, and occasionally in candidiasis and aspergillosis.
- Examination of other systems is of crucial importance. Hepatosplenomegaly with lymphadenopathy may point to an underlying lymphoma or a myeloproliferative disorder. It is also commonly observed in disseminated hematogenous tuberculosis and toxoplasmosis.
- Neurological examination may reveal subtle symptoms and signs suggesting meningitis or a focal neurological lesion. Brain abscess is common in nocardial infection, cryptococcal infection, and in disseminated disease due to *M. tuberculosis.*

Radiological Investigations

Pulmonary infiltrates are never specific enough on a chest X-ray to allow a definitive etiological diagnosis to be made **(Fig. 2)**. Nevertheless, a study of serial chest X-rays when combined with an analysis of the mode of onset and the progress of the disease often help in limiting the diagnostic possibilities. Focal or multifocal consolidation of short

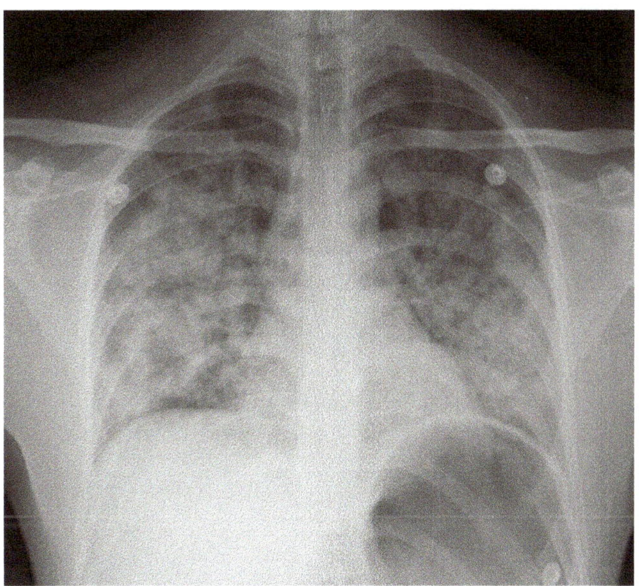

Fig. 2: Chest X-ray reveals ill-defined consolidations in both mid and lower zones more so on the right side.

duration (<48 hours) seen on a chest X-ray is invariably due to an acute bacterial infection. Slowly progressive consolidation with a subacute or chronic history favors tuberculosis, nocardial, or fungal infections. Interstitial infiltrates spreading outwards from the hilar area and evolving in a subacute or chronic manner, suggest pneumocystis, viral or drug-induced infiltration, or may be due to lymphangitis carcinomatosis. Acutely evolving interstitial infiltrates also occur in pulmonary edema or in a leukoagglutination reaction **(Table 5)**.

Acute nodular localized alveolar consolidation or localized nodular infiltrates suggest pulmonary edema or bacterial bronchopneumonia. Nodular infiltrates, which are subacute or chronic and slow in evolving could be tuberculous, fungal, or nocardial in etiology. Such infiltrates could also be due to the recurrence or spread of an original tumor.

These radiological observations are not sacrosanct, and as mentioned at the outset, an exact diagnosis can never be made by the mere description of shadows on a chest radiograph. The overall picture has to be considered.

■ DIAGNOSTIC AND MANAGEMENT PROTOCOLS

Immunocompromised patients who are acutely and severely ill with pulmonary infection need critical care. Diagnostic and management protocols depend on facilities

Table 5: Differential diagnosis of fever and pulmonary infiltrates in the immunocompromised patient, based on radiological signs and onset of symptoms.

Chest X-ray	Acute onset	Subacute/chronic onset
Consolidation	Bacterial Thromboembolic Hemorrhage	Fungal Nocardial Tuberculous
Peribronchovascular	Pulmonary edema Leukoagglutinin reaction	Viral PCP Radiation drug-induced
Nodular infiltrates	Bacterial Pulmonary edema	Tumor Fungal Nocardial Tuberculous

(PCP: *Pneumocystis jirovecii* pneumonia)

available in the ICU and the degree of sophistication of the pathology and microbiology department of the hospital. Routine investigations include a blood count, erythrocyte sedimentation rate (ESR), C-reactive protein estimation, blood culture, sputum examination (if available) for Gram's stain, routine culture sensitivity, acid-fast bacilli (AFB) smear and culture, fungal cultures, and the examination of nasopharyngeal aspirates for viral studies. In some patients, nebulization with hypertonic saline helps to obtain a satisfactory sputum sample.

A radiograph of the chest should be followed by CT of the chest. The latter is far more sensitive in evaluating the site, extent, and nature of lung involvement. Arterial blood gases need to be done to determine the degree of hypoxia, if present, and of hypocapnia or hypercapnia. Severe bacterial pneumonia, pneumocystis infection, and CMV infections are associated with well-marked hypoxia. Invasive tests that may need to be performed are fiberoptic bronchoscopy with a study of BAL fluid for all possible infections, and when necessary a transbronchial biopsy with staining, culture, and histopathological examination of the biopsy material. The purpose is to establish a specific diagnosis that directs specific treatment. In *acutely ill patients empiric therapy should be started without awaiting results of sputum and blood tests* (**Figs. 3 to 5**). Therapy could be changed later, if the results so necessitate.

Diagnostic and management protocols and guidelines depend on the history, the background disease and/or treatment causing immunosuppression (which suggest the nature of organisms likely to cause pneumonia), the acuteness and severity of the illness, the physical signs

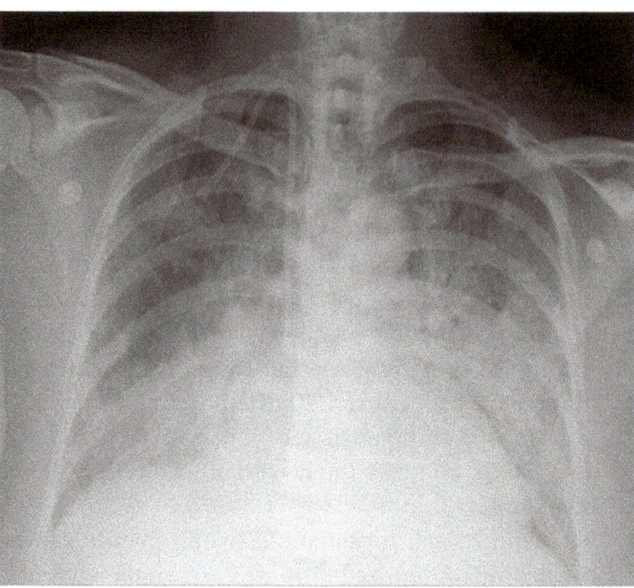

Fig. 3: Chest X-ray reveals ill-defined fluffy opacities in both mid and lower zones. The opacities were secondary to a transfusion-related acute lung injury (TRALI).

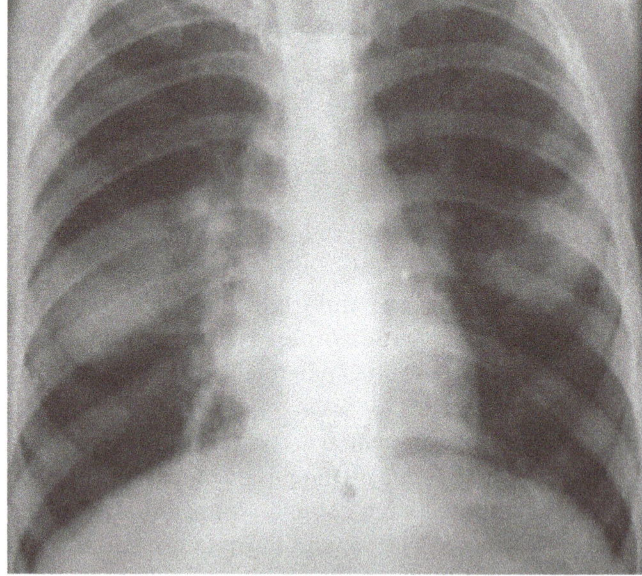

Fig. 4: Chest X-ray reveals bilateral nodular lesions due to staphylococcal pneumonia.

and the nature of imaging findings. *It is unwise to follow protocols rigidly else they can cause more harm than good. They need to be modified for each individual according to prevailing circumstances.*

An overall approach to pneumonia in an immunocompromised patient is given in the algorithm—**Flowchart 1**.

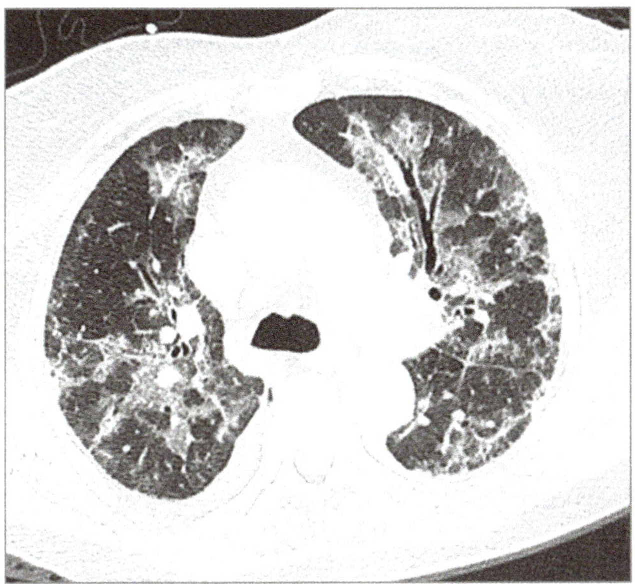

Fig. 5: *Cytomegalovirus* (CMV) infection. High-resolution computed tomography (HRCT) chest demonstrates ill-defined areas of increased lung attenuation in both lung fields representing ground–glass densities. These appearances are very similar to those seen in *Pneumocystis jirovecii* pneumonia. A bronchoalveolar lavage (BAL) is required to differentiate between the two diseases.

Following this, five different clinical scenarios are discussed. It should be noted that a patient may not necessarily fit in any one of these five scenarios. Also, he or she could present with one scenario, which shifts over time to another. Five clinical scenarios are detailed below.

1. *An acutely ill patient with a lobar or one or more areas of focal consolidation or focal alveolar infiltrates*: This is generally due to a bacterial infection and we advocate amoxicillin + piperacillin/tazobactam + a macrolide. This should cover Gram-positive, Gram-negative, and atypical microorganisms. If there is a possibility of a staphylococcal infection, one may need to add flucloxacillin 1 g QDS. In parts of the world or in units where methicillin-resistant staphylococcal infection is prevalent intravenous (IV) vancomycin should be added to the regimen in place of flucloxacillin. Lack of response to the above regime should perhaps lead to a change of antibiotics—meropenem + vancomycin forming a potent effective combination. In pneumonia associated with severe neutropenia, particularly in those who have pleuritic pain, cough, hemoptysis, and whose high-resolution CT (HRCT) is compatible with an *Aspergillus* infection, one should add amphotericin B

or voriconazole to the broad-spectrum antibiotics on an empiric basis. If the patient responds to this regime, the antibiotic course is continued for 10–14 days. A very prompt or dramatic response warrants de-escalation of the antibiotic regime within 7 days of therapy.

If the patient does not respond within 48–72 hours, one should opt to do a BAL with a careful examination of the BAL fluid. A transbronchial biopsy of the lesion, if thought necessary could be done during the same procedure. A specific diagnosis would entail the use of specifically directed drugs toward the etiological agent. If these procedures do not give a specific diagnosis or if the patient is too ill for BAL or transbronchial biopsy or if pathological and microbiological backing is poor as in several developing countries, further management should proceed on an empirical basis. Besides covering Gram-positive and Gram-negative infections, atypical organisms (e.g. *Legionella*, *Mycoplasma*) should be covered with a macrolide given intravenously and a fungal infection (as already mentioned) by the use of amphotericin B.

2. *An acutely ill patient with diffuse bilateral alveolar infiltrates:* Bacterial infections are still possible and the patient needs empiric cover for Gram-positive and Gram-negative infections with IV amoxicillin + a third-generation cephalosporin or piperacillin/tazobactam + an aminoglycoside or a quinolone derivative. The sicker the patient the greater should be the cover for possible invading organisms. If the imaging appearances are compatible with a pneumocystis infection, a trimethoprim and sulfamethoxazole combination should be added to the regime. This is followed by bronchial lavage, and transbronchial biopsy for possible diagnostic help. If this is not possible for reasons stated above or if the diagnostic procedure fails to provide a clue, further treatment remains empiric. Deterioration of the patient should prompt a cover for CMV infection till further tests [in particular a polymerase chain reaction (PCR) for the virus] prove or disprove this. Legionnaire's disease, tuberculosis, and fungal infection may also need appropriate cover depending on the nature of the immune suppression, radiological appearance, and other tests. Algorithm of the management protocol in the first two scenarios is given in **Flowcharts 1 and 2**.

3. *Patient presenting with subacute or chronic focal consolidation on imaging*: If the sputum is unavailable, or is not diagnostic, and if antibiotics used against

Flowchart 1: Algorithm showing an overall approach to pneumonia in an immunocompromised patient. An acutely ill patient with lobar or one or more areas of focal consolidation or alveolar infiltrates.

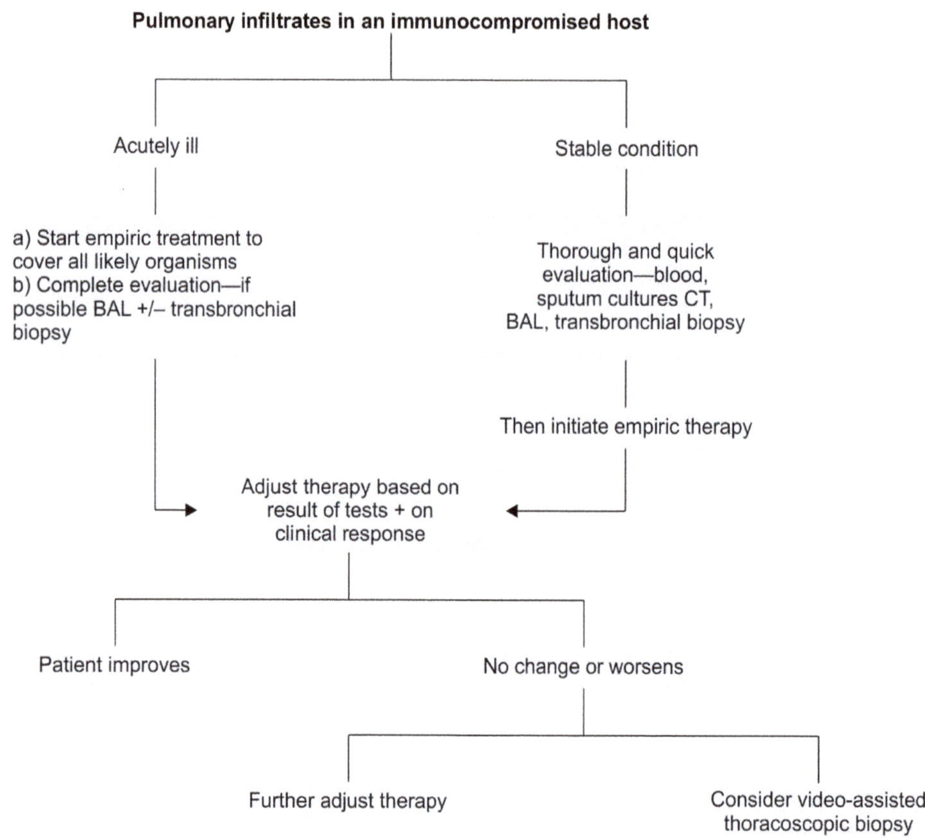

(BAL: Bronchoalveolar lavage; CT: Computed tomography)

Gram-positive and Gram-negative organisms are ineffective, a BAL study and a transbronchial biopsy should help in arriving at a specific diagnosis. If this fails and if the patient's condition allows, a video-assisted thoracoscopic biopsy should be done. This invariably gives the diagnosis. When the consolidated area is peripherally placed a CT-guided biopsy is also of diagnostic help. Among other etiologies, tuberculosis is an important cause of subacute focal areas of consolidation in one or both lungs.

4. *Patients presenting with bilateral perihilar opacities fanning outwards on radiography with diffuse ground–glass opacities in both lungs*: Diffuse ground–glass opacities are met with chiefly in pneumocystis infection, CMV infection, viral pneumonitis, and occasionally with extensive bacterial pneumonias. If the patient is acutely ill or hypoxic as he or she may well be, empiric treatment should be prompt so as to cover organisms

stated above. Investigations should follow. Though BAL may well give a specific diagnosis, it is fraught with risk in severely hypoxic individuals. If done, it is best first to intubate the patient so that the patient if necessary can receive ventilator support with a high fraction of inspired oxygen (FiO_2). A transbronchial biopsy is best avoided particularly if the patient is on ventilator support (for fear of pneumothorax). In stable patients, investigations should include BAL and transbronchial biopsy. Empiric therapy is given or started simultaneously. Treatment is altered depending on the results of investigations and clinical response.

5. *Patients presenting with nodular lesions*: Nodular lesions are often caused by *M. tuberculosis, Aspergillus,* and nocardial infections. Infected central line catheters or indwelling devices can cause metastatic bacterial or fungal nodules in one or both lungs. In the presence of positive blood cultures, these metastatic bacterial

Flowchart 2: Algorithm showing an overall approach to pneumonia in an immunocompromised patient. An acutely ill patient with diffuse bilateral interstitial plus alveolar infiltrates.

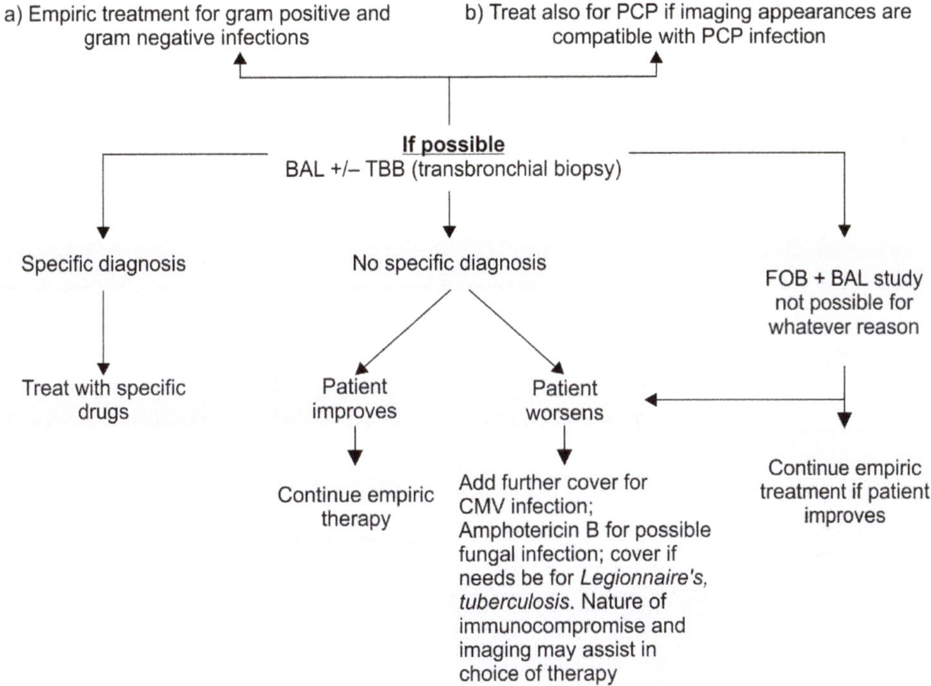

(BAL: Bronchoalveolar lavage; CMV: *Cytomegalovirus*; FOB: Fiberoptic bronchoscopy; PCP: *Pneumocystis jirovecii* pneumonia)

or fungal pulmonary lesions should be treated with appropriate antibiotics without further need for invasive tests.

Nodular lesions caused by viral infections or bacterial infections are generally associated with imaging findings of ground-glass appearance and/or alveolar consolidation. Correct diagnosis necessitates a study of BAL fluid and a transbronchial biopsy. In patients with high-risk factors for *Aspergillus* infection or a CT appearance suggestive of *Aspergillus* infection, empiric antifungal therapy is advisable, if BAL or transbronchial biopsy does not give an appropriate diagnosis. A video-assisted thoracoscopic biopsy, however, invariably enables a firm diagnosis of a fungal pathology.

Bronchoscopy in Immunocompromised Patients

Many immunocompromised hosts with pulmonary infection have either no sputum or a very low positive yield to the sputum they produce. Fiberoptic bronchoscopy with a full study of BAL fluid of the affected area of the lung (for all possible infections) remains a crucial invasive diagnostic procedure.

A study of BAL and if needs be a transbronchial biopsy are almost mandatory in the diagnosis of CMV and in patients with suspected *Pneumocystis jirovecii* pneumonia (PCP) where examination of induced sputum following nebulization with hypertonic saline is not possible or is negative. These tests generally provide a firm diagnosis.

The sensitivity of BAL is, however, dependent on the population studied. In SOT patients, the sensitivity of BAL for CMV infection has been found to be between 20% and 60%. In immunocompromised cancer patients and in HSCT recipients, the yield of BAL for CMV could increase to 95%. BAL remains a sensitive test for the diagnosis of pneumocystis infection in SOT patients, a positive yield being observed in 85–90%. The yield increases even more if transbronchial biopsy material is also studied. In HSCT patients, the diagnostic yield with BAL and transbronchial biopsy for pneumocystis infection is in the range of 80–100%. Therefore unless an immunocompromised host is extremely ill and hypoxic, empiric treatment for CMV or pneumocystis infection based on clinical and radiological criteria alone is rarely justified, given the toxicities of the drugs used for these infections. In our experience, BAL studies supplemented whenever possible by transbronchial biopsy have proved most useful in the diagnosis of tuberculosis (particularly when tuberculosis presents with widespread shadowing in both lungs or as a solid or nodular focal lesion), in nocardial infection and in determining the nature of Gram-negative infections in bacterial pneumonia. On the other hand, BAL with or without transbronchial biopsy is much less sensitive for fungal infections, a positive yield for *Aspergillus* being merely about 60%. We have also been unsuccessful with the diagnosis of Legionnaire's disease and viral infections (other than CMV) through the use of this procedure.

Rano and colleagues studied the use of bronchoscopy in immunocompromised patients with pulmonary infection (causing radiological shadows or infiltrates) and noted that there were three variables that independently predicted mortality—(1) increasing severity of illness, (2) need for mechanical ventilation, and (3) delay in diagnosis. The first two variables are understandable as patients in these categories must be very ill. The third variable is extremely important as in their study it was unrelated to the severity of illness. The risk of death in patients in whom there was a delay of more than 5 days in the identification of pulmonary infection (infiltrate) was more than threefold in this study [*Ref: Rañó A, Agustí C, Jimenez P, et al. Pulmonary infiltrates in non-HIV immunocompromised patients: a diagnostic approach using non-invasive and bronchoscopic procedures. Thorax. 2001;56(5):379-87)].* This study emphasizes the importance of early diagnosis and the early use of a bronchoscopic BAL to achieve a specific diagnosis. Diagnostic delay also has implications with regard to initial therapy. It has been observed several times over that inappropriate selection of antibiotics to initiate therapy adversely affects outcome.

The diagnosis of noninfective infiltrates within the lungs of immunocompromised patients (even after a BAL study) is difficult and almost always is a diagnosis of exclusion. Some noninfective infiltrates, however, can be diagnosed—these include diffuse alveolar damage, alveolar hemorrhage, and presence of tumor cells or lymphoma cells in the BAL fluid pointing to an underlying mitotic disease. The treatment of many noninfective infiltrates in immunocompromised patients is the use of corticosteroids. Corticosteroids may aggravate an underlying infection in the lung. Hence, the need to exclude as far as possible any infective etiology before using steroids.

It must be remembered that BAL through a broncho-scope can aggravate hypoxia and can be dangerous in patients who are already severely hypoxic. Transbronchial biopsies are risky in patients with a coagulopathy or in the presence of thrombocytopenia. Though a number of units in the West perform transbronchial biopsies in patients with a platelet count as low as $10,000/mm^3$, we would avoid transbronchial biopsies in patients with a platelet less than $50,000/mm^3$ unless platelet infusions are given prior to the procedure.

Video-assisted Thoracoscopic (VATS) Biopsy

The advent of VATS biopsy has made open-lung biopsy for diagnostic procedures unnecessary. The VATS biopsy procedure is safe in expert hands, and can be performed under local anesthesia and allows a specific diagnosis in appropriate circumstances.

The question that arises is that if all other tests (including BAL and transbronchial biopsy) are noncontributory, would a VATS yield a diagnosis amenable to treatment? We have found VATS biopsy useful (when other tests were negative) in the specific diagnosis of *Aspergillus* infection, tuberculous infection and infection with atypical mycobacteria. Reports from other units suggest that in fewer than half the patients subjected to VATS biopsy did results warrant a change in treatment. A positive yield was much lower in neutropenic patients and those on ventilator support.

Open-lung surgical biopsy is today hardly ever necessary to establish a diagnosis. Two questions need to be asked before this procedure is undertaken—is the result of the open-lung biopsy likely to alter treatment? Is the patient fit enough to allow this procedure?

◼ IMPORTANT SPECIFIC PNEUMONIA IN THE IMMUNOCOMPROMISED NON-HIV PATIENT

Bacterial Pneumonia

The most common infection in immunocompromised patients is pneumonia caused by bacterial pathogens.

Major risk factors are severe neutropenia and/ or functional defect in neutrophils or phagocytes. Impaired cell-mediated immune response following cytotoxic immunosuppressive therapy is also a risk factor for bacterial pneumonia. Patients with impaired B lymphocyte function as in lymphoproliferative disease, lymphomas, and multiple myeloma are prone to pneumonia caused by *Streptococcus pneumoniae* and *Haemophilus influenzae.*

Immunocompromised patients in hospital and particularly those in the ICU are at grave risk of pneumonia due to organisms such as *Pseudomonas aeruginosa, Klebsiella, Acinetobacter, Escherichia coli,* and other Gram-negative bacteria. *Methicillin-resistant Staphylococcus aureus* (MRSA) infections also cause pneumonia in hospitals or units where this organism is prevalent. Immunocompromised patients treated in hospital and then living in the community are also far more prone to Gram-negative bacterial infection when compared to those who are immunocompetent.

Clinical Features

The clinical features may be the same as in immunocompetent patients, with high fever, cough, rusty sputum, tachypnea, and physical and radiological signs of consolidations.

In patients with severe neutropenia, low-grade pyrexia is more frequent. In fact the patient may be afebrile, presenting with tachypnea and a pulmonary infiltrate. Some patients may have a normal X-ray chest, pulmonary shadowing being revealed only on a *CT* scan of the chest. Some of the other features of bacterial pneumonia in immunocompromised patients have been mentioned earlier in the section.

Diagnosis

Diagnosis is facilitated, if a good sputum sample is available for examination (smear and culture). Blood cultures should always be sent. Patients who do not respond to conventional therapy should have a bronchoscopic BAL study. This often gives a high positive yield. CT scans may reveal focal or dense lobar consolidation and help to distinguish bacterial from fungal or viral pneumonias. Test for *Legionella pneumophila* antigen in the urine should be done, if *Legionella* pneumonia is suspected.

Treatment

The nature of organisms that prevail and cause infection in a hospital or ICU and the antibiogram would help decide therapy in an immunocompromised patient who develops nosocomial pneumonia (NP). In critically ill immunocompromised patients with acute bacterial pneumonia, treatment should never await results of diagnostic tests. To give an example of just one regimen, one could use piperacillin tazobactam + an aminoglycoside as an immediate cover for Gram-negative bacteria. If MRSA is prevalent in a unit, vancomycin should be added. If the patient fails to respond in 48–72 hours, the regime needs to be changed to another combination—for example, a carbapenem + vancomycin. One could add a macrolide, if there is suspicion of *Legionella* or any other atypical organism. Immunocompromised patients admitted to a hospital for a community-acquired bacterial pneumonia need cover for both Gram-positive and Gram-negative organisms.

Severe bacterial pneumonia in immunocompromised patients is often complicated by the *ARDS* and by a pleural exudate that turns into an empyema.

Good oxygenation often with a high-flow oxygen mask is necessary. Ventilator support is frequently necessary in severe pneumonia. All organ systems must be given adequate support.

Pneumocystis Infection

This has been dealt with in the chapter on HIV and the lung. Whereas in AIDS pneumocystis infection is subacute or even insidious in onset, in the immunocompromised non-HIV patient, PCP is more often an acute opportunistic infection producing fever, breathlessness, tachypnea, tachycardia, and progressive hypoxia. Imaging features are those of perihilar shadows fanning out toward the periphery involving the greater part of both lungs. Other possible imaging features have been described in the chapter on HIV and the lung. The yield from BAL in these patients with conventional stains is 80% compared to HIV patients where the yield is over 95%. This is because fewer organisms are recovered in non-HIV patients. The sensitivity of BAL is therefore lowered in non-HIV patients with pneumocystis infection. Similarly, a positive yield (particularly in transplant patients) of induced sputum is low compared to HIV patients.

It is important to bear in mind that PCP can occur in immunocompromised patients besides AIDS. These immunocompromised non-HIV patients prone to PCP have been listed in the chapter on HIV and the lung in the section describing PCP.

Nocardiosis

Nocardia are Gram-positive organisms that grow as branching filaments. Human infection is usually caused by *Nocardia asteroides*. It is an important though a comparatively uncommon cause of pneumonia or pulmonary infiltrates in immunocompromised patients. An important setting for nocardial infection is patients with chronic airways obstruction who have received or continue to receive corticosteroid therapy. Nocardial infection may rarely occur as a CAP even in immunocompetent individuals. This has been briefly described in the chapter on CAP.

Clinical presentation in the immunocompromised patient:
- The initial presentation often seen is that of an asymptomatic pulmonary shadow of uncertain etiology. A radiograph shows one or more shadows often circumscribed, often varying in size and not infrequently cavitating.
- A review of nocardial infection in 260 patients who had undergone heart transplant provides a useful outline of the clinical profile of this disease in the immunocompromised. Fever and dry cough are presenting features and the natural history is subacute, though at times nocardial infection in an immunocompromised host may resemble an acute bacterial pneumonia. Pleural involvement has been reported in a third of these patients. Nocardial infection can disseminate, particularly to the central nervous system (CNS). One or more abscess-like cavities in the lungs and in the brain should always suggest this diagnosis. Skin lesions may present as nodules, which are positive for *Nocardia* on a biopsy.

Diagnosis is difficult, as *Nocardia* are rarely present in sputum samples and sputum cultures are frequently negative. If BAL studies and transbronchial biopsies are noncontributory, a VATS biopsy may help to establish a diagnosis. A CT-guided biopsy of a peripherally placed nodule or abscess has also proved successful in our rather limited experience.

Mycobacterial Infection

Mycobacterial infection chiefly occurs in patients with an impaired cell-mediated immune response. It is a frequent and important cause of focal or nodular shadows on radiography in immunocompromised patients in countries like India where the disease has a high prevalence. The likelihood of tuberculosis also depends on the reason for immunosuppression. Tuberculosis rarely complicates chemotherapy for acute leukemia or HSCT. The incidence is very significant in SOT recipients, being as high as 15–20% in countries where tuberculosis is endemic. Though the risk of tuberculosis is common to heart, lung and liver transplant, it is highest in renal transplant recipients. The disease generally occurs late in the time span after start of immunosuppression, the median time of occurrence being 9 months after transplantation.

Clinical Features and Diagnosis

Clinically, the patients present with pyrexia of unknown origin. Investigations reveal focal, segmental, or lobar consolidation or infiltrates on radiography. CT scans may demonstrate lesions not observed on radiography. The posterior segment of the upper lobe or the dorsal segment of the lower is frequently involved. Miliary shadowing is observed in some cases. In countries where tuberculosis has a high-prevalence rate, the radiological appearances are rarely those of ARDS. Mediastinal and/or hilar adenopathy may be present. Atypical radiographic findings may well be present in immunocompromised patients.

If sputum is not available, a bronchoscopic BAL should be done, combined if possible with a transbronchial biopsy. These procedures are often rewarded by a definite diagnosis. If these tests are negative and there is strong suspicion of tuberculosis, or if there is progressive disease, a video-assisted thoracoscopic biopsy may provide a correct diagnosis.

Treatment is with standard chemotherapy regimen, though it must be kept in mind that infection may well be due to multidrug-resistant strains of the mycobacterium.

The full spectrum of aspergillosis infection has been given in the chapter on NP. This section deals with invasive aspergillosis (IA), which is considered under two heads—(1) invasive pulmonary aspergillosis (IPA) and (2) invasive bronchial aspergillosis (IBA) **(Figs. 6A and B)**.

Invasive Pulmonary Aspergillosis

Invasive pulmonary aspergillosis (IPA) appears to be an increasing cause of pulmonary infection in

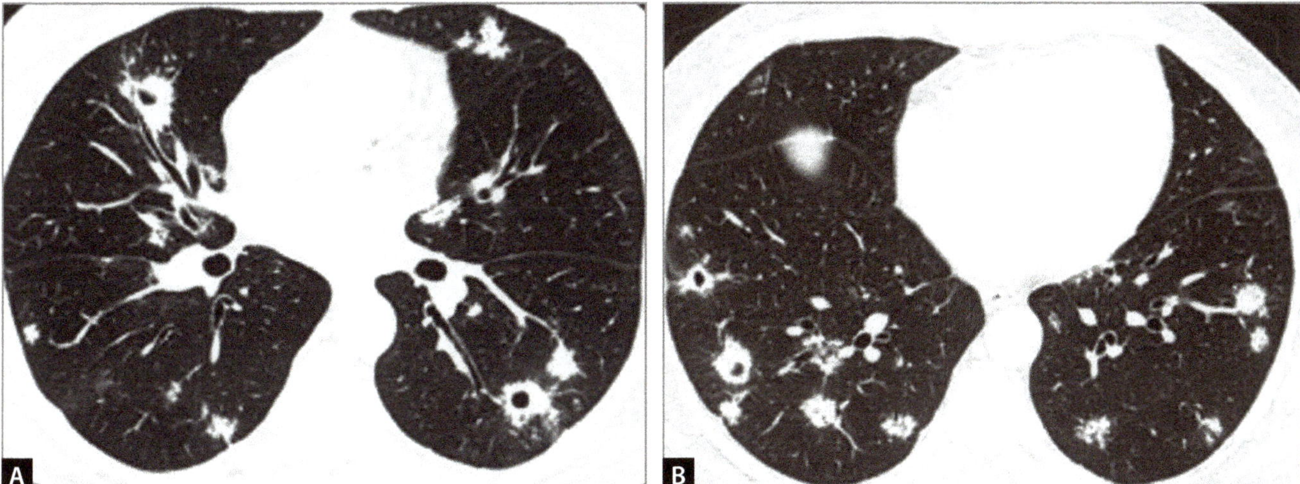

Figs. 6A and B: Invasive aspergillosis: high-resolution computed tomography (HRCT) demonstrates multiple ill-defined nodular lesions in a peribronchial location representing invasive aspergillosis.

immunocompromised patients not only in the West but also in tertiary ICU centers in India. *Aspergillus* species are saprophytic filamentous fungi found in the environment. They propagate by producing spores, which are 2–3 μm in diameter and which on inhalation reach the distal air spaces. Ordinarily, they are innocuous, but in immunocompromised patients with severe neutropenia or with impaired neutrophil or macrophage function these spores germinate into filamentous fungi and invade the lung tissue to cause IPA or invasive involvement of the paranasal sinuses. Metastatic spread to the brain, bones, skin, and other organs may also occur. *Aspergillus* infection is generally due to *Aspergillus fumigatus*. *Aspergillus flavus*, *Aspergillus niger*, and *Aspergillus terreus* may rarely also cause disease.

Risk Factors

The major risk factor is significant neutropenia or poor neutrophil function. The greater the degree of neutropenia and the greater its duration, the greater the risk. IPA is observed in 50% of patients where neutropenia persists more than 4 weeks. Patients most at risk are those with hematological malignancies receiving chemotherapy, patients with aplastic anemia, in stem cell transplant recipients where severe neutropenia is an important complication, in patients with AIDS and in severe immunodeficiency. Patients who develop graft versus host disease are also at risk, as are patients who receive liver, lung, and heart transplants. Patients with acute leukemia develop IPA as a complication 20 times more frequently than patients with lymphoma or organ transplants. Patients on chronic corticosteroid therapy are also at risk of developing this disease. Large prospective multicenter surveillance studies conducted by the Transplant Associate Surveillance Network (TRANSNET) in America have shown that invasive aspergillosis is now the most common fungal infection in HSCT and solid organ transplant recipients, amounting to 43% and 59% of all IFIs, respectively. The overall mortality in these patients was estimated to be approximately 36% and 75% at 12 weeks and 1 year, respectively. In addition to the typical group of patients described above, IPA has been described in other conditions as well—in patients with systemic lupus erythematosus, burns patients, patients with multiple myeloma on high doses of corticosteroids as also in patients with Crohn's disease or rheumatoid arthritis who have received tumor necrosis factor (TNF) inhibitors (e.g. infliximab). Invasive aspergillosis occurring as a nosocomial infection in the ICU is being increasingly realized.

Perhaps the frequency and epidemiology of *Aspergillus* infection to some extent is governed by the presence of airborne *Aspergillus* in a particular eco-environment. Outbreaks of this infection have been related to the increased presence of the organism in the air around construction sites or due to inadequate air-conditioning systems.

Clinical Features

Fever, cough, pleuritic chest pain, and hemoptysis may occur but these symptoms occur with other pulmonary infections as well. Persistent and severe hemoptysis should always raise suspicion of IPA as aspergilli grow into pulmonary vessels producing areas of pulmonary infarction. Massive fatal hemoptysis is known to occur. Chest radiographs may show areas of consolidation or nodules that may cavitate.

About 10% of immunosuppressed patients may present with pyrexia of unknown origin with a radiographic examination of the chest appearing normal. A CT of the chest in these patients may demonstrate nodular infiltrates compatible with IPA.

Invasive pulmonary aspergillosis is sometimes suspected on certain findings in CT studies. These include—(1) a "halo sign"—which is an area of lower attenuation shadowing surrounding a nodule or an area of consolidation; (2) a "crescent sign", which relates to a partially formed cavity due to infarcted lung tissue. The "halo sign" is generally observed within a week of infection; the crescent sign is generally observed after some more weeks. The "halo sign" is neither very sensitive nor specific, for many molds other than *Aspergillus* (e.g. *Fusarium*) can cause a similar pattern on a CT scan. Radiographic appearances are varied. They may vary from nodular infiltrates to dense alveolar consolidation. Because of the angioinvasive nature of the fungus, radiological appearances may resemble wedge-shaped pleural-based infarcts, which may later cavitate. A CT is mandatory as it may reveal lesions not seen on an X-ray chest (**Figs. 7 and 8**).

Invasive Tracheobronchial Aspergillosis

Invasive tracheobronchial aspergillosis (IBA) signifies invasion of the trachea and large bronchi by the Aspergillus. It can be classified as follows:

Tracheobronchitis: This is the least invasive form of *Aspergillus* infection, characterized by inflammation of the tracheobronchial mucosa, without membrane formation or ulceration. It causes a dry cough and pyrexia. A CT may reveal thickening of the mucosa.

Pseudomembranous tracheobronchitis: This condition is characterized by necrosis of the tracheobronchial epithelium and the formation of pseudomembranes. The lesion may progress to extensive invasion of the airways,

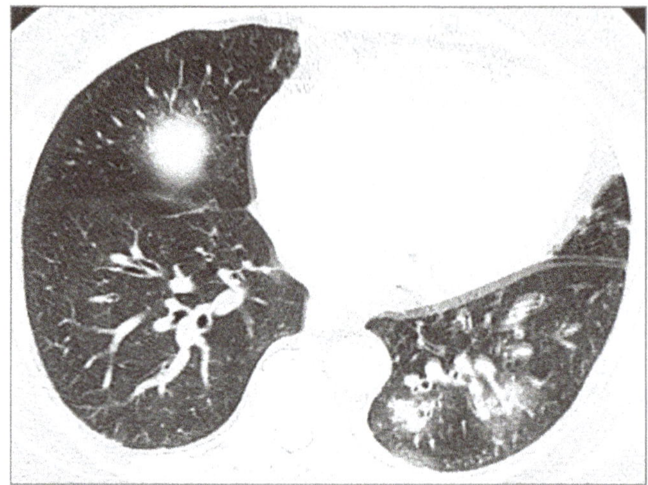

Fig. 7: Halo sign: Computed tomography (CT) chest reveals multiple ill-defined nodular lesions in left lower lobe associated with ground glass halos. This was due to *Aspergillus* infection.

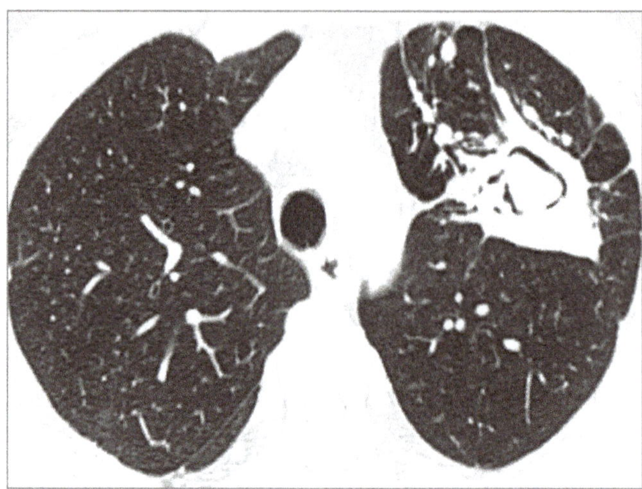

Fig. 8: High-resolution computed tomography (HRCT) chest reveals a nodular lesion with a crescent of air along its superior aspect due to an aspergilloma.

though generally the inflammation does not extend beyond the bronchial cartilage.

Ulcerative tracheobronchitis is the worst and most aggressive form of IBA. It is characterized by necrosis of the epithelium, ulcers, nodules, and plaques. It can extend into and invade the pulmonary parenchyma.

The pseudomembranous form is typically seen in lung transplant recipients. It is occasionally observed in patients with hematological malignancies, HSCT, chronic obstructive pulmonary disease (COPD), AIDS, diabetes, and rarely even in immunocompetent patients. A dry cough is the predominant symptom, the chest X-ray is normal. As the disease progresses, it results in tachypnea, stridor, respiratory failure, and death.

The ulcerative form of IBA occurs almost exclusively at the site of bronchial anastomosis in lung transplant recipients. Bronchoscopy reveals ulcers at the anastomotic site. Symptoms are similar to those of pseudomembranous tracheobronchitis. Complications include anastomotic dehiscence, IPA, and bronchial stenosis.

Bronchial stump aspergillosis is an unusual complication following a pneumonectomy. It generally occurs 6–12 months after surgery causing cough, hemoptysis, and expectoration of putrid brownish sputum in which hyphae of *Aspergillus* can be detected. It is believed to be due to the use of silk sutures (when suturing the bronchial stump) and poor tissue viability. The use of nylon sutures for suturing has reduced the incidence of this complication.

All forms of IBA require systemic antifungal therapy. Systemic voriconazole therapy is often combined with aerosolized amphotericin B deoxycholate (AmBd). Surgical resection with placement of a stent together with systemic antifungal therapy is sometimes advocated.

Chronic Necrotizing Pulmonary Aspergillosis

In milder forms of immunosuppression as in patients on cytotoxic drugs or in patients on a maintenance dose of corticosteroids, *Aspergillus* infection takes the form of an indolent disease characterized by one or more patches of consolidation, which may or may not cavitate. Cough, fever, and weight loss are the presenting features. The course may remain indolent but slowly progressive, or may graduate to a more invasive form of the disease.

Diagnosis

In high-risk patients, the presence of clinical and imaging features compatible with IPA should prompt the use of specific therapy. Even so, a microbiological diagnosis is always to be preferred, because some species of *Aspergillus* infection or infection with other rare filamentous fungi may be resistant to conventional treatment with amphotericin B. Sputum examination including sputum culture is poorly sensitive. Microbiological diagnosis is achieved by BAL study and/or by transbronchial biopsies. The presence

of *Aspergillus* in BAL fluid on smear and/or culture in an immunocompromised patient is highly predictive of IPA **(Table 6)**. However, isolation of *Aspergillus* species by BAL culture can diagnose only 50% of cases of invasive infection. Transbronchial biopsy of affected areas may reveal fungal hyphae infiltrating lung parenchyma. If a transbronchial biopsy is unsuccessful in giving a diagnosis one should attempt a CT-guided biopsy or a video-assisted thoracoscopic biopsy, which usually enables a firm diagnosis.

Noninvasive Tests

Noninvasive tests include—(1) detection of galactomannan or glucan cell wall antigen on BAL specimens obtained through a fiberoptic bronchoscope or in the blood; (2) *PCR* for *Aspergillus* DNA from the blood; (3) β-D-Glucan (β-DG). This is a readily available blood test which detects a cell wall polysaccharide (BDG) found in most fungi with the notable exception of Cryptococcus, zygomycetes and blastomyces. An FDA approved blood assay exists and this test is a useful surrogate marker of invasive fungal infections such as invasive *Aspergillus* or *Candida* or *Pneumocystis jirovecii* infection, though it does not distinguish between them. β-DG levels are also useful in monitoring response to therapy.

Though highly sensitive, the galactomannan antigen test may give false positive results particularly in patients receiving piperacillin-tazobactam. Unfortunately, these tests are not available in many poor developing countries. It is believed that if performed routinely for surveillance in high-risk patients and if found positive, preemptive antifungal treatment could perhaps prevent overt disease.

The diagnosis of *Aspergillus* tracheobronchitis can be made from positive cultures in bronchial washing as also

Table 6: Diagnostic tests for invasive pulmonary aspergillosis (IPA).

- *Microbiological diagnosis*: Culture of sputum, or bronchoalveolar lavage (BAL) fluid
- Transbronchial biopsy
- CT-guided biopsy
- Video-assisted thoracoscopic biopsy
- Detection of galactomannan or glucan cell wall antigen in BAL specimens and in blood
- PCR for *Aspergillus* DNA from the blood

(CT: Computed tomography; DNA: Deoxyribonucleic acid; PCR: Polymerase chain reaction)

from biopsy of tracheobronchial mucosa, which show fungal invasion of bronchial mucosa **(Table 7)**.

The diagnosis of chronic necrotizing pulmonary aspergillosis often requires video-assisted thoracoscopic biopsy or in appropriate circumstances a CT-guided biopsy for confirmation of fungal etiology **(Table 8)**.

Treatment (Table 9)

There is today a better outcome in patients with IPA—even so, the mortality in severely immunocompromised patients is high. Strategies governing treatment include the use of new antifungal agents such as voriconazole, early onset of treatment from suggestive CT appearance or a positive galactomannan antigen test, use of combination antifungal therapy and occasionally surgical excision of localized lesions.

Till the early 1990s, Amphotericin B (AmB) was the only available therapeutic agent. The drug though effective has serious side effects notably on the kidneys. Lipid formulation of AmBd is equally effective and according to some less toxic. However, the introduction of the broad-spectrum triazole, voriconazole, has provided a significant therapeutic advance. In a large prospective randomized in patients with IPA comparing voriconazole with AmB, the response rate was 53% and 32%, respectively and the survival rate of 71% and 58%, respectively. Voriconazole should therefore be the first-line therapy in invasive aspergillosis.

Table 7: Diagnosis of aspergillus tracheobronchitis.
• Positive cultures in bronchial washing • Biopsy of tracheobronchial mucosa

Table 8: Diagnosis of chronic necrotizing pulmonary aspergillosis.
• Video-assisted thoracoscopic biopsy • CT-guided biopsy in appropriate circumstances

Table 9: Treatment of invasive pulmonary aspergillosis (IPA).
• *Amphotericin B*: 0.5–1.5 mg/kg/day IV; lyophilized amphotericin B: 3–5 mg/kg/day IV • *Caspofungin*: 70 mg IV loading dose on day 1, followed by 50 mg/day IV; duration depends on response to therapy • *Voriconazole*: Loading dose: 6 mg/kg IV BD • *Maintenance*: 4 mg/kg IV BD, once patient tolerates the drug, switch to 200 mg PO BD • *Itraconazole*: 200–400 mg daily orally • Surgery in selected circumstances

(IV: Intravenous)

The echinocandins, including caspofungin, micafungin, and anidulafungin are a new class of antifungal agents, which inhibit the synthesis of 1,3-βD glucan, an essential component of the cell wall of many fungi. Caspofungin when used as primary therapy has a response rate of 33–50%; micafungin—a response rate of 50–70%. *Caspofungin used as salvage therapy has a response rate of 50% in invasive aspergillosis.*

Combination therapy: Combination therapy has been tried, since the mechanism of action of echinocandins is different from other antifungals. Echinocandins + voriconazole, voriconazole + anidulafungin are believed to have synergistic effect. The last combination is reported to be associated with a greater survivor benefit when compared to voriconazole alone in patients with hematological malignancies or stem cell transplant recipients.

Surgery: Surgery has been advocated for persistent localized lesions and for aspergillomas which cause recurrent hemoptysis. Surgical intervention may be a lifesaving procedure in patients with IPA who present with or develop exsanguinating hemorrhage provided it is done early, if the disease.

Prophylaxis with voriconazole given orally has been strongly advocated for high risk patients.

Candida Infection

Pneumonia due to candida infection is rare but metastatic lung infection can occur in patients with candidemia or in patients with infected central venous catheters or other infected vascular indwelling devices. Pyrexia, accompanied by nodular lung shadows is observed. Metastatic lesions due to reasons stated above do not need an invasive workup. Fluconazole or amphotericin B should be started promptly and an infected intravascular device should be promptly removed. The frequent use of fluconazole prophylaxis has led to an increased prevalence of strains resistant to usual antifungal drugs. These include *Candida tropicalis, Candida glabrata, Candida parapsilosis,* and *Candida krusei.*

Non-aspergillus Filamentous Fungal Infections

These include infections with Zygomycetes, *Fusarium,* and *Penicillium.* Infection with these filamentous fungi is indistinguishable from IPA. The diagnosis needs to be considered in patients with IPA who do not respond to adequate therapy. Diagnosis can be made from culture of BAL fluid and invasive biopsies. The mortality is extremely high. Infection with *Penicilliosis marneffei* is very rare in India, though a few HIV patients suffering from the infection have been reported from Manipur in Northeast India. It is, however, fairly common in Southeast Asia, particularly in Thailand, and has been reported also in nonimmunocompromised patients. This infection has been briefly dealt with in the section on "Tropical Infections Involving the Lung".

Mucormycosis

Mucormycosis is a rare but important opportunistic infection in immunocompromised patients. The mucorales are saprophytic ubiquitous fungi found in soil. Spores produced by the fungi get air-borne and are inhaled into the respiratory tract but because of their low virulence produce no disease in immunocompetent patients but are pathogenic to immune compromised patients.

Risk Factors

Risk factors are very similar to those observed in invasive *Aspergillus* infection—neutropenia, hematological malignancies, recipients of solid organ transplants, HSCT, and AIDS. In addition, mucormycosis is an important complication of uncontrolled diabetes, renal failure, and particularly in patients with renal failure who are receiving deferoxamine IV therapy.

The usual forms of infection are—(1) rhinocerebral, (2) pneumonia, (3) disseminated, (4) skin and soft tissue.

Clinical Features of the Pneumonic Form

The symptoms are often nonspecific and remain so till late in the disease. Fever not responding to antibiotics, cough, progressive dyspnea, and pleuritic chest pain are often observed. Pneumonia produced by mucormycosis may be indistinguishable from that observed in IPA. The *Mucor* has a propensity to invade vessels causing hemoptysis and cavitative necrotic pulmonary lesions. Infection can also traverse tissue planes of the lung, including bronchi, pleura, diaphragm, and chest wall. Disease can also spread to the contralateral lung.

Death generally occurs from disseminated disease before the advent of respiratory failure.

Radiological Findings

Radiological findings include lobar consolidation, segmental consolidation, nodular infiltrates, and cavitative lesions. They often resemble findings in invasive pulmonary aspergillosis.

Diagnosis

Diagnosis depends on a high index of suspicion and on the histopathological demonstration of tissue invasion by characteristic aseptate hyphae branching at right angles or by the isolation of *Mucorale* species in tissue samples. This generally necessitates invasive procedures like CT-guided biopsy or a VATS biopsy.

Blood cultures are rarely positive; sputum and BAL studies are usually non-contributory. The *Mucor* hyphae pick up fluorescent stains such as calcofluor-white, which in contrast to *Aspergillus* hyphae are nonseptate and branch at right angles.

The PCR testing of selected tissue samples is being recently assessed to help diagnosis.

Differential Diagnosis

The differential diagnosis is from other infections—notably invasive *Aspergillus* infection. If a patient suspected to have IPA has a persistently negative galactomannan test and is not responsive to voriconazole, the possibility of mucormycosis should be entertained.

Treatment

Lyophilized amphotericin B intravenously is the drug of choice. It is given daily till there is significant symptomatic, radiological improvement, and negative tissue biopsies. In a recent study in 24 patients with pneumonia due to mucormycosis the response rate was 71%.

Propiconazole, a broad-spectrum triazole, given in a dose of 800 mg in four divided doses orally is also of use, with a reported response rate of 70%.

The use of hyperbaric oxygen in mucormycosis, which has been tried as adjunctive therapy is unsettled.

Surgery: The angioinvasive property of *Mucor* may prevent antifungals from reaching infected tissue. Surgical debridement of infected tissue is important. A lobectomy or even a pneumonectomy may be necessary to get rid of all visible infection. In a recent review, patients treated with a combination of antifungal agents + surgery had a mortality of 27% compared to a mortality of 55% in those treated with antifungals alone.

Emerging Opportunistic Molds

There is an ever increasing population of immuno-compromised patients in the world and this is one reason we are witness to rare fungal infections not observed before. The two important ones (among others) are filamentous fungi such as *Fusarium*, which cause pulmonary fusariosis and the filamentous fungus such as *Scedosporium*, which can cause pulmonary scedosporiosis. The clinical features resemble IPA; these fungi are resistant to conventional antifungal agents. Infected patients have a poor outcome.

Cryptococcal and Endemic Fungi

Cryptococcal infection is comparatively rare in immunocompromised non-HIV patients. The presentation may be with low-grade pyrexia with focal and multifocal consolidation. In patients with marked suppression of cell-mediated immunity, lobar consolidation may occur. Diagnosis is through staining and culture of sputum and BAL fluid for *Cryptococcus neoformans.* Treatment is with amphotericin B. This may be combined with flucytosine. Oral fluconazole may then need to be continued for prophylaxis.

Infection with histoplasma and coccidioides need not be seriously considered in India, but they remain important considerations in countries where these fungal infections are endemic.

Cytomegalovirus Infection

Cytomegalovirus infection is common in the general population occurring usually in children or adults. The infection is asymptomatic or causes a self-limiting mild disease. Latent infection can be detected by serological testing. In patients with markedly depressed cell-mediated immunity (CD4 counts well below 200) CMV is reactivated and produces CMV disease, infecting the lungs and at times several other organs. Patients with impaired cell-mediated immunity who are serologically CMV-negative are extremely prone to fulminant CMV infection, if given blood products or a transplant organ containing leukocytes from CMV-positive donors. Though most frequently observed in HIV-infected patients with very low CD4 counts, CMV infection can occur occasionally in non-HIV immunocompromised patients.

Clinical Features

The CMV pneumonia is usually insidious in onset presenting with fever, cough, tachypnea, dyspnea, and progressive hypoxia. At the start, chest radiography may be normal; later it shows parahilar shadows fanning out into the periphery, very similar to the radiological appearances in pneumocystis infection.

Computed tomography scans are far more sensitive in detecting infection. They invariably show symmetrical diffuse ground-glass opacities (again similar to pneumocystis infection) with multiple small centrilobular nodules. Rarely, the radiological and CT changes are asymmetrical.

Severe infection is associated with the involvement of other organs. Leukopenia is always present. Liver function can be deranged with a significant rise in liver enzymes and gastrointestinal symptoms can occur from involvement of the colon and the gastrointestinal tract. A telltale feature is the occurrence of CMV chorioretinitis, which is quite distinctive in its appearance.

The differential diagnosis of CMV pneumonia is from other viral infections, from PCP infection, from drug-induced pneumonitis, ARDS, and intra-alveolar hemorrhage.

Diagnosis

- The surest way of proving CMV infection in CMV pneumonia is through a BAL study and a transbronchial biopsy. Intranuclear "owl's eye" inclusion bodies in cytology studies on BAL fluid are confirmatory as are inclusion bodies present in histopathological studies of transbronchial biopsies.
- Cytology on BAL fluid is, however, not a very sensitive test for CMV pneumonia. The main diagnostic techniques in use today are based on probing BAL fluid directly for the presence of CMV antigen or by probing cell cultures inoculated with BAL fluid after 48 hours' incubation.
- Positive viral cultures of BAL fluid or biopsy specimens are the gold standard in diagnosis but the sensitivity of viral cultures is not as good as is desired. Also, cultures take long to give results.

The CMV pneumonia does not occur in the absence of CMV reactivation. CMV reactivation is tested by the presence of CMV antigenemia and by determining the viral load through PCR techniques. A large and increasing viral load substantiates to a great extent the diagnosis of CMV pneumonia **(Table 10)**.

Treatment

The treatment of choice is the use of ganciclovir. Foscarnet and cidofovir are second-line drugs.

Ganciclovir is phosphorylated within infected cells and inhibits viral DNA polymerase. It is given intravenously in a dose of 2.5–5 mg/kg BD or TDS. It has a strong myelosuppressive effect and may prove too toxic in patients who have just received stem cell transplants. An oral formulation of ganciclovir, called valganciclovir has recently been introduced.

The second-line drug foscarnet has a mechanism of action similar to ganciclovir but has renal toxicity, which limits its use. The dosage is 60 mg/kg TDS given intravenously. Cidofovir also has a similar action to ganciclovir, but has both myelosuppressive toxic effects as also renal toxicity. Patients need to be well hydrated and given probenecid before therapy. Treatment with any one of these drugs is for 2–3 weeks.

Patient with CMV disease are also given IV immuno-globulin as a form of passive vaccination against CMV.

Some centers prefer to use one or the other of the three drugs prophylactically in severely immunocompromised patients, whenever there is evidence of increasing CMV reactivation. It is hoped that if such patients do develop CMV infection, the outcome is better, because of the early initiation of therapy.

■ OTHER VIRAL INFECTIONS

Herpes Viruses

Rarely herpes simplex virus (HSV) or herpes zoster virus (HZV) causes pulmonary infection in immuno-compromised patients. Presentation is similar to CMV infection. Skin lesions present in herpetic infections afford the right clue. The virus can be isolated from BAL fluid. Acyclovir is given intravenously in full doses. Severe disease in immunocompromised patients besides causing pneumonia can also involve other organ systems producing multiorgan failure (also *see* Chapter on Nonbacterial Pneumonia).

Respiratory Viruses

Respiratory viruses can cause lower respiratory tract infection in immunocompromised patients. Infection occurs through inhalation of infected droplets. The common responsible viruses are *Influenza A*, parainfluenza virus, respiratory syncytial virus. Infection with adenovirus and rhinovirus has also been reported. There is a woeful lack of appropriate facilities for detecting viral infections in our country and in most countries in the tropical belt.

Respiratory viral infections are generally a late complication of immunosuppressed patients, reflecting persistent poor cell-mediated immune response in transplant patients and in patients on immunosuppressive drug therapy.

Clinical features are those of bronchiolitis—cough, fever, and end-inspiratory high-pitched squeaks. X-ray chest is invariably normal but a CT chest may show evidence of inflammation of small airways with "tree-in-bud" changes. Some degree of alveolar shadowing may also be present. The main differential diagnosis is from mycoplasmal and chlamydia infection. The diagnosis in well-equipped laboratories is confirmed by identifying viral antigen in nasopharyngeal aspirates or in BAL fluid samples by the use of an immunofluorescent test. Viral cultures, if positive, are the gold standard for diagnosis. PCR techniques may perhaps have greater sensitivity. The prognosis of viral infections in the absence of actual pneumonia is good. Obliterative bronchiolitis may, however, occur as a sequel. Treatment with antiviral agents is generally ineffective.

■ SUGGESTED READING

1. Belleza WG. Pulmonary considerations in the immunocompromised patient. Emerg Med Clin North Am. 2003;21(2):499-531, x-xi.
2. Cunha BA. Pneumonias in the compromised host. Infect Dis Clin North Am. 2001;15(2):591-612.
3. Fishman JA. Infection in solid-organ transplant recipients. N Engl J Med. 2007;357:2601.
4. Fishman JA, Kauffman CA, Bond S. (2017). Pulmonary infections in immunocompromised patients. [online]

Table 10: Diagnosis of cytomegalovirus (CMV).
• *BAL study*:
– Intranuclear "owl's eye" inclusion bodies on cytology studies
– Presence of CMV antigen
– Positive viral cultures of BAL fluid
• Transbronchial biopsy
• Positive viral cultures of biopsy specimens
• Serum for PCR and viral load

(BAL: Bronchoalveolar lavage; PCR: Polymerase chain reaction)

Available from https://www.uptodate.com/contents/pulmonary-infections-in-immunocompromised-patients. [Accessed July, 2018].

5. Kotloff RM, Ahya VN, Crawford SW. Pulmonary complications of solid organ and hematopoietic stem cell transplantation. Am J Respir Crit Care Med. 2004; 170:22.

6. Shorr AF. Pulmonary infiltrates in the non-HIV-infected immunocompromised patient: etiologies, diagnostic strategies and outcome. Chest. 2004;125(1):260-71.

7. Tamm M. Pulmonary cytomegalovirus infection in immunocompromised patients. Chest. 2001;119(3): 838-43.

8. Vento S. Lung infections after cancer chemotherapy. Lancet Oncol. 2008;9(10):982-92.

9. Waite S. Acute lung infections in normal and immuno-compromised hosts. Radiol Clin North Am. 2006;44(2): 295-315, ix.

10. Wheat LJ. Approach to the diagnosis of invasive aspergillosis and candidiasis. Clin Chest Med. 2009;30(2):367-77, viii.

CHAPTER 22

Nosocomial Pneumonia

DEFINITIONS

Nosocomial pneumonia (NP) is the most important cause of hospital-acquired infections (HAIs) because it is associated with a significant morbidity and mortality. It consists of three entities: hospital-acquired pneumonia (HAP), ventilator-associated pneumonia (VAP), and healthcare-associated pneumonia (HCAP).

Hospital-acquired pneumonia is defined as pneumonia diagnosed 48 hours or more after hospital admission.

Ventilator-associated pneumonia is defined as pneumonia diagnosed 48 hours or more after endotracheal intubation and ventilator support.

Healthcare-associated pneumonia (HCAP) is defined as pneumonia diagnosed in any patient who was hospitalized in an acute care hospital for 2 or more days within 90 days of the diagnosis; resided in a nursing home or long-term care facility; received recent antibiotic therapy or chemotherapy, or a wound care within 30 days of the current infection; or attended a hospital or hemodialysis clinic. Patient suffering from HCAP are considered to be similar to hospitalized patients in that they are susceptible to colonization with organisms, in particular drug-resistant organisms. There are some workers who consider HCAP to be more akin to community-acquired pneumonia than to nosocomial pneumonia.

Though this chapter centers chiefly on VAP and HAP, the principles can be extrapolated to HCAP.

EPIDEMIOLOGY

Hospital-acquired pneumonia is believed to occur at a rate of 5–10 cases per 1,000 hospital admissions. In 2008, the National Safety Healthcare (NSHC) network, a surveillance branch of the Center of Disease Control and Prevention (CDC) published an annual report to the effect that VAP accounted for 15.9% of all reported HAIs placing third among device-associated HAI The two other device-associated infections being central line-associated blood-stream infection (CLABSI) and catheter-associated urinary tract infections (CAUTI). These figures will vary not only in different countries in South and South East Asia, and in India will also vary in different intensive care units (ICUs) located in a single large city.

Many studies in the West have shown that VAP occurs in 9–27% of all intubated patients. Over 90% of ICU-acquired NPs occur during mechanical ventilation (VAP); close to 50% occur within the first 5 days of ventilator support. In the ICU, VAP comprises one-third or more of the total nosocomial infections. In a 1-day prevalence study involving critically ill patients across Western Europe, pneumonia was the most common ICU-acquired infection occurring in 10% of patients and accounting for 47% of all ICU-acquired infections.

The CDC reports the incidence of NP as 0.9 per 1,000 ventilator days in the medical ICUs and 2 per 1000 ventilator days in the surgical ICUs *[Ref: Dudeck MA, Weiner LM, Allen-Bridson K, et al. National Healthcare Safety Network (NHSN) report, data summary for 2012, Device-associated module. Am J Infect Control. 2013;41(12):1148-66].* Patients who have VAP have worse outcomes and longer hospital and ICU days. There is work to suggest that VAP appears to be an independent risk factor in critically ill patients with a doubling of the mortality rate directly attributed to VAP. This, however, is difficult to determine with reasonable certainty, *as a number of critically ill patients in the ICU may die with pneumonia and not die of pneumonia.* Yet, between 10 and 20% of patients who require ventilation for more than 48 hours will acquire

VAP with a mortality of 15–50%. It has also been shown that early onset VAPs (< 5 days of hospitalization) usually carry better prognosis and are often associated with bacteria sensitive to antibiotics. Late onset VAP (> 5 days) are more likely to be caused by multidrug-resistant (MDR) pathogens and are associated with an increased morbidity and mortality.

Ventilator-associated Pneumonia Rates in India

A recent study published in International Nosocomial Infection Control Consortium (INICC) in 2015 in the American Journal of Infection Control (AJIC) indicates that VAP is the most common healthcare associated infection followed by CLABSI and CAUTI. The pooled VAP rate of 79 ICUs from India between 2004 and 2012 was 9.4/1,000 device days (INICC 2016). The crude mortality rate was 29.6%. The extra length of stay in patients receiving ventilator support was 13.6 days. Another multicentric Indian study also showed VAP to be the leading nosocomial infection with VAP rate of 6.74/1,000 device days.

These rates are significantly greater than what is observed in very good tertiary centers in the West. However, these rates can be reduced to a satisfactory extent in good tertiary ICUs in the large cities of India. To give just one example, in one of the tertiary ICUs in Mumbai (the Breach Candy Hospital and Research Center), VAP rates were brought down to 1.8/1,000 device days in 2015, which have been further reduced to 0.8/1,000 in a 22 bedded ICU (12 medical and 10 surgical beds). This has been possible through strict Infection Control Policies as also an antibiotic policy.

The falling trend over several years in the hospital is illustrated by the **Figure 1**. The rate of VAP in comparison with CLABSI and CAUTI in the above hospital are given below.

◼ PATHOPHYSIOLOGY

Aspiration

Almost always, NP is due to aspiration of infected secretions or particulate matter from the mouth and pharynx into the lower respiratory tract. Retained infected secretions within the large and small airways can also produce NP. In most sick patients in the ICU, the oropharynx is colonized by aerobic Gram-negative bacteria within 5–10 days, whereas in healthy adults the normal organisms

are anaerobic bacteria and harmless commensals like *Neisseria pharyngitis*.

Colonization of patients can occur from exogenous and/or endogenous sources. Exogenous sources include the hands, clothing, equipment of doctors, nurses, healthcare workers, and the unhealthy environment of the ICU. Other exogenous sources include colonized bronchoscopes, stethoscopes, humidifiers, respiratory equipment, and contaminated nebulizers. Endogenous sources include pathogens contaminating and colonizing the oropharynx, the gastrointestinal (GI) tract, the proximal trachea, and the endotracheal or tracheostomy tube **(Flowchart 1)**.

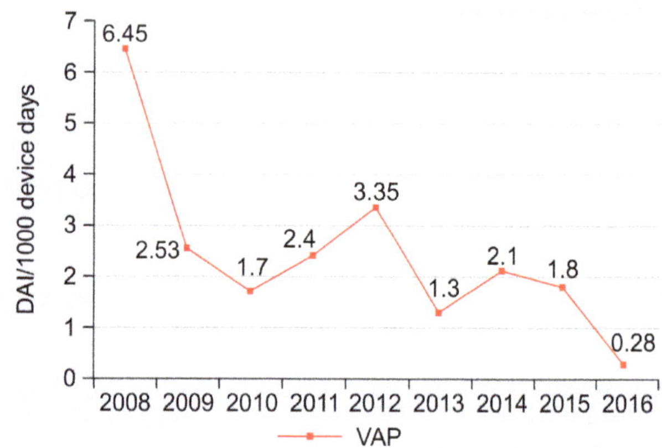

Fig. 1: Temporal trends of VAP at BREACH Candy Hospital Trust (2008–2016).

Flowchart 1: Pathogenesis of nosocomial pneumonia.

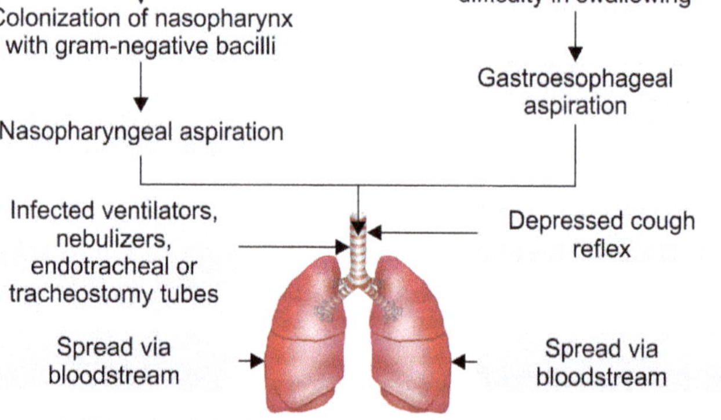

Tracheal intubation is the most important underlying predisposing condition for the development of pneumonia as it aids in aspiration of pathogens and prevents intrinsic respiratory defenses from coming into play. The endotracheal or tracheostomy tube also can further facilitate aspiration, as pathogens often grow on the inner surface and can be aspirated or translocated into the lung. The endotracheal tube is often lined by a biofilm consisting of bacteria embedded in an exopolysaccharide matrix. Embedded bacteria are protected from both antibiotics and the host immune responses and are difficult to eradicate. During tracheal aspiration, mechanical ventilation, and bronchoscopy, particles of this biofilm may be dislodged and pushed into the lung leading to lower respiratory tract infection. The severity of the illness plays an important role in perpetuating this colonization. Invasive diagnostic and therapeutic procedures further promote the aspiration and transfer of infected, colonized oropharyngeal contents into the lower respiratory tract. The upper airway is usually colonized before the lower airway, but organisms such as *Pseudomonas aeruginosa* can colonize the lower airway as a primary event. The reason for colonization of the mouth, oropharynx, and airways by pathogenic bacteria and in particular by Gram-negative organisms, is the subject of research. In healthy individuals, a film of fibronectin covers the epithelium lining the mucosa of the mouth and oropharynx, and prevents the Gram-negative bacteria from adhering to the epithelial cells. This protective coating is lost in very ill individuals, so that pathogenic Gram-negative organisms adhere to receptors present on epithelial cells of the mucosa and soon colonize it. The number of these bacterial receptors on both upper and lower airway epithelial cells is increased in many illnesses. This change is associated with increased colonization at these sites. Risk factors for increased colonization due to enhanced adherence of bacteria to mucosal cells in the airways include serious illnesses, smoking, azotemia, surgery, and malnutrition.

Gastric Colonization

The acid within the stomach serves as a major deterrent to bacteria swallowed in the saliva. If gastric acidity is suppressed by the use of antacids, proton pump inhibitors and H_2 antagonists, the bacteria within the stomach survive, multiply, and soon colonize the upper GI tract. Gastric contents laden with Gram-negative bacteria could easily regurgitate and be aspirated into the lungs, causing aspiration pneumonia. This is particularly frequent in obtunded patients, sedated patients, or following a large vomit. Prophylaxis and treatment of bleeding stress ulcers with sucralfate do not significantly increase gastric pH in most patients, and results in a reduced incidence of NPs.

Hematogenous Pneumonia

Rarely, infected emboli from a septic thrombophlebitis can lead to septic infarcts within the lung. Catheter-related sepsis or any other source of sepsis can cause bacteremia with hematogenous spread of infection into the lungs, causing pneumonia.

Inhalation Pneumonia

Contaminated respiratory equipment (nebulizers, humidifiers, ventilator tubing, etc.) is a source of infected aerosols. Infected particles 3–5 microns in size can be deposited into the terminal bronchioles and alveoli, thereby causing a lower respiratory tract infection.

Iatrogenic Causes

Lack of aseptic precaution during suction of tracheobronchial secretions, either through an endotracheal tube or tracheostomy, is an important cause of lower respiratory tract infection.

■ FACTORS PREDISPOSING TO NOSOCOMIAL PNEUMONIAS

These are given in **Table 1**.

These can be divided into:

- *Host factors*: The factors in which defense mechanisms are suppressed include: (1) overwhelming infections, serious illnesses, e.g. severe sepsis, extrapulmonary infections, prolonged shock, burns or severe trauma, or following major surgery; and (2) background factors which are associated with a greater propensity to infection. These include underlying chronic lung disease (chronic bronchitis), diabetes mellitus, cardiac disease, renal failure, liver cell dysfunction, underlying malignancy, advanced age, malnutrition prior to the onset of a critical illness, or occurring acutely during the course of an illness, and total parenteral nutrition.
- *Therapeutic interventions*: The most important of these are endotracheal intubation, tracheostomy, and mechanical ventilation. Nasogastric tubes encourage gastric colonization with pathogens, and

perhaps provide a scaffolding or conduit for these pathogens to reach the pharynx; aspiration of these pathogens or of infected particulate matter results in pneumonia. Corticosteroids/antimitotic agents are immunosuppressants, and their use both encourages and masks infection. As mentioned earlier, there is evidence that excessive neutralization of acid to treat upper GI bleeds by antacids and H_2-antagonists also facilitates upper GI tract colonization with Gram-negative bacteria, and predispose to pulmonary infection. The use of very high oxygen concentrations in mechanical ventilation over prolonged periods of time may also be detrimental to lung morphology and physiology, and may predispose to infection. Prolonged antibiotic therapy can induce a superinfection by organisms resistant to conventional therapy, and lead to NP resistant to the usual antibiotics.

- *Environmental factors* like overcrowding, an overall unclean environment (which unfortunately is frequently seen in developing countries), increased prevalence of multiple, resistant organisms, and *transmission chiefly through the contaminated hands of ICU personnel,* all predispose to the development of nosocomial infections.

Table 1: Factors predisposing to nosocomial pneumonia (also applicable to other nosocomial infections).

- Host factors:
  - Overwhelming infections or serious illnesses, e.g. severe sepsis, prolonged shock, burns, severe trauma, or following major surgery
  - Background factors, e.g. chronic lung diseases, diabetes mellitus, cardiac, renal, or hepatic dysfunction, advanced age, underlying malignancy, malnutrition
  - Total parenteral nutrition
- Therapeutic interventions:
  - Endotracheal intubation or tracheostomy with mechanical ventilator support
  - Use of invasive procedures (including central lines)
  - Nasogastric tube
  - Use of corticosteroids or chemotherapy
  - Prolonged use of antibiotics
  - Colonization of upper GI tract with Gram-negative bacteria following use of antacids/H_2 antagonists
- Environmental factors:
  - Overcrowding
  - Overall unclean environment (unfortunately so frequently seen in developing countries)
  - Transmission chiefly through contaminated hands of ICU personnel
  - Increased prevalence of multiple, resistant organisms

(GI: Gastrointestinal; ICU: Intensive care unit).

CLINICAL DIAGNOSIS (TABLE 2)

The clinical diagnosis of NP, including VAP, is difficult and often erroneous. This is proven by a postmortem study showing that the clinical diagnosis of pneumonia was incorrect in 60% of cases. The diagnosis of NP requires the presence of the following important features:

- Fever, leukocytosis, purulent sputum or, in the case of VAP, purulent tracheal secretions. At least two of these three clinical criteria should be present.
- A chest X-ray which shows a new or progressive alveolar infiltrate **(Figs. 2 and 3)**. The presence of an abnormal radiographic infiltrate together with at least two out of three clinical criteria stated above has a high degree of

Table 2: Clinical diagnosis of nosocomial pneumonia.

- Chest X-ray which shows a new or progressive alveolar infiltrate
- Fever
- Leukocytosis > 12,000/mm^3 or leucopenia < 4,000/mm^3
- Purulent sputum, or in the case of VAP, purulent tracheal secretions

Note: The presence of an abnormal radiographic infiltrate together with at least two of three clinical criteria stated above has a high degree of sensitivity but a low specificity.
(VAP: Ventilator-associated pneumonia)

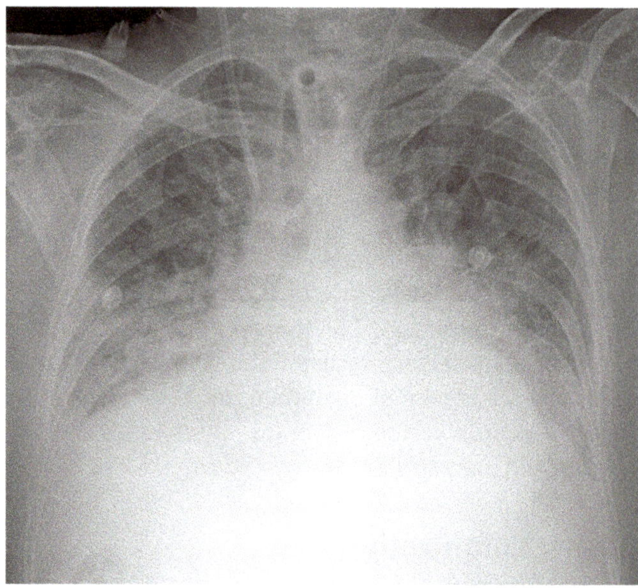

Fig. 2: Nosocomial pneumonia. A 73-year-old man admitted for hernia surgery, developed fever and leukocytosis on day 3 postoperatively. Patient had vomited post-anesthesia and developed aspiration pneumonia. Chest X-ray reveals an ill-defined consolidation in the right lower lobe with evidence of loss of volume; the right hemithorax is slightly smaller in size than the left. These appearances of a consolidation and loss of volume are very suggestive of aspiration pneumonia.

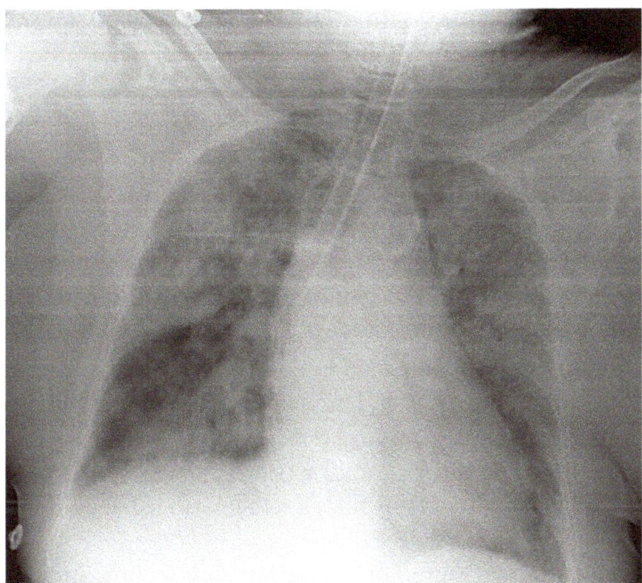

Fig. 3: Ventilator-associated pneumonia. Elderly gentleman was admitted to the intensive care unit and required ventilator support. Within 3 days, he developed fresh and increasing shadows in both lungs suggesting ventilator-associated pneumonia.

Table 3: Other causes of shadows on X-ray chest.
• Atelectasis
• Pulmonary edema
• Pulmonary infarction
• Hemorrhage
• Lung injury (ARDS)
• Drug reaction
• Recurrence or spread of mitotic disease
• Transfusion related acute lung injury (TRALI)

Source: Singh N, Falestiny MN, Rogers P, et al. Pulmonary infiltrates in the surgical ICU: prospective assessment of predictors of etiology and mortality. Chest. 1998;114(4):1129-36.

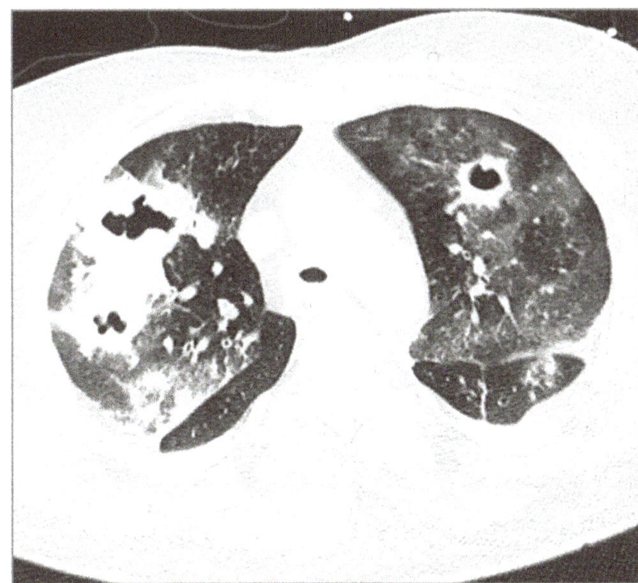

Fig. 4: Nosocomial pneumonia: Computed tomography (CT) chest in a patient admitted for hip replacement surgery. Patient developed fever on fifth postoperative day. CT chest reveals multiple thick-walled cavitatory lesions, ill-defined patchy bronchovascular and subpleural consolidation with ground glass densities. The causative organism was acinetobacter.

sensitivity but a low specificity. When all three clinical criteria are present in a patient with a fresh alveolar infiltrate on an X-ray chest, the specificity improves but the sensitivity falls to an unacceptable level (< 50%).

Diagnostic problems in an individual patient can be formidable for the following reasons:

- A systemic inflammatory response characterized by fever and leukocytosis may be present, but its absence does not exclude the diagnosis of pneumonia. Also, fever and leukocytosis can occur in infections other than pneumonia and in noninfective pathologies in a critically ill patient.
- Absence of sputum or of significant lower respiratory tract secretions in patients with a tracheostomy (with or without ventilator support), does not necessarily exclude pneumonia in the presence of a recent infiltrate on an X-ray chest in a critically ill patient.
- A "shadow" on a chest X-ray is not necessarily inflammatory. Localized shadows in one or both lung fields can be due to pulmonary edema, pulmonary hemorrhage, pulmonary infarction, acute respiratory distress syndrome (ARDS), and other non-inflammatory causes. Atelectasis is often mistaken for pneumonia in a critically ill patient. A clearing of the shadow after vigorous physiotherapy differentiates infiltrates caused by atelectasis from those due to

infection. The other causes of shadows on the X-ray chest are listed in **Table 3**.

It should be remembered that a portable chest X-ray may be difficult to interpret in an intubated critically ill patient. Pneumonia may be difficult to exclude because of the technical quality of the film. Also, the chest X-ray may miss out on subtle features which are quite evident on a computed tomography (CT) of the chest **(Fig. 4)**.

In a study of autopsy-proven VAP, no single radiographic sign had a diagnostic accuracy of more than 68%. The presence of an air bronchogram was the only sign that corresponded best with pneumonia, predicting 64% of pneumonias in this study.

A clinical study showed the presence of lung infection in only 42% of patients diagnosed as VAP, proving that there is a poor correlation between clinical features and bacteriological demonstration of VAP.

- Nosocomial pneumonia in a patient with ARDS may be impossibly difficult to diagnose on a chest X-ray. A number of pathologies can cause asymmetric consolidation in patients with ARDS. An air bronchogram on a chest X-ray in a patient with ARDS is not necessarily predictive of NP.
- In addition to the clinical features mentioned above, it is being increasingly realized that worsening gas exchange is an important consideration in the diagnosis of NP.

Newer Streamlined Surveillance Definitions and Guidelines

With the purpose of improving the efficacy and objectivity of VAP diagnosis, the Centre for Disease Control (CDC) has proposed an approach which focuses on ventilator-associated complications, centered on worsening oxygenation and systemic signs of infection. Remarkably, this new approach includes an algorithm which excludes the use of chest radiography. Instead of merely considering VAP versus non-VAP, the newer guidelines categorizes patients into three groups:

1. Patients with ventilator-associated complications (VAC). These patients are far more sick than those who do not have VAC.
2. Those with infection-related ventilator-associated complications.
3. Patients with probable versus possible VAP. These groups represent patients at various stages in the above spectrum.

The basic features of each of these groups are summarized in **Table 4**.

Certain questions need to be answered with regard to these new definitions and guidelines. Do these guidelines add greater clarity on our concept of VAP? Do they help improve the management of VAP? If chest radiography is excluded, would not one miss a stable VAP which does not significantly alter gas exchange?

Finally, VACs are not always due to infection and the incidence of VAC may not be reduced by measures at VAP prevention. The relation of the quality of patient care to the incidence of VAC is unproven.

We need to wait to see how necessary and useful these new guidelines are, before we set older CDC guidelines of pneumonia and VAP aside.

When considering the older CDC guidelines on NP and VAP, it is apparent from the earlier discussion that though clinical features combined with radiological findings are of help, they lack sufficient specificity in the

Table 4: Newer streamlined surveillance definitions and guidelines.		
Ventilator associated complication (VAC)	*Any one of the following criteria*	
	Minimum daily FiO_2 increased by 0.2 over baseline and persists for >2 days	Minimum daily PEEP increased by >3 cm H_2O over baseline and persists for >2 days
Infection-related ventilator associated complication	*Includes both the features given below*	
	Temperature >38°C or	A new antibiotic started and continued >4 days
	WBC > 12000 or <4000 mm^3	
Possible VAP	*After 3rd day of ventilation and within 2 days of worsening oxygenation, any one of the following criteria is met*	
	Purulent tracheobronchial secretions showing >25 neutrophils and <10 squamous epithelial cells per low power field	Positive culture of sputum/endotracheal aspirate/ BAL/lung tissue or protected specimen brushing (PSB)
Probable VAP	*After 3rd day of ventilation and within 2 days of worsening oxygenation, any one of the following criteria is met*	
	Purulent respiratory secretions from one or more specimen collections and one of the following: • Positive culture of endotracheal aspirate> 10^5 CFU/mL or positive culture of BAL> 10^4 CFU/mL or positive culture of lung tissue > 10^4 CFU/mL or positive culture of PSB> 10^3 CFU/mL	One of the following without the need for purulent respiratory secretions: • Positive pleural fluid culture (specimen obtained following thoracentesis or initial placement of ICD only) or positive lung tissue histopathology or positive serology—common viral Infections like adeno, RSV and influenza

diagnosis of nosocomial and VAP. Bacteriological evidence of pulmonary parenchymal infection is, therefore, also considered necessary to make a firm diagnosis. The cost-effectiveness of different methods used to obtain this bacteriological evidence and the relation of the evidence obtained to ultimate patient management and patient outcome are matters of continued discussion. These methods are briefly discussed below.

CLINICAL FEATURES OF SEVERE NOSOCOMIAL PNEUMONIA

Nosocomial pneumonia can at times be fulminant, particularly when caused by Gram-negative organisms such as *P. aeruginosa* or Acinetobacter. The clinical features are increasing respiratory failure with persistent hypoxia in spite of high FiO_2, PEEP and good ventilator support. There is a rapid progression of radiographic shadowing, severe sepsis, with hypotension and/or multi-organ failure (MOF). The patient soon develops renal failure necessitating dialysis. The mortality is spite of appropriate antibiotics is well over 80%.

Microbiology

Bacteria responsible for nosocomial pneumonia and in particular VAP depend on several factors—ICU population, the gravity of the underlying illness, duration of mechanical ventilation, previous antibiotic therapy and the method used to collect and culture lower respiratory tract secretions. Each ICU will have its own pattern and distribution of bacteria responsible for nosocomial infection, including nosocomial pneumonia. There is no doubt that in recent times aerobic gram negative bacilli (GNB) are the most prevalent pathogens causing nosocomial pneumonia. Organisms typically present in most units in India are Klebsiella, Pseudomonas, Acinetobacter. All these three are often found to be multidrug resistant—resistant even to the carbapenem group of drugs. Occasionally these organisms are also resistant to colistin. Amongst Enterobacteriaceae, one also finds *E. coli*, Enterobacter, Proteus and Serratia species. All these bacteria are ubiquitous in the environment, have minimal nutritional requirement and frequently colonize hospitalized patients.

In some units, methicillin resistant staphylococci (MRSA) have been increasingly reported to cause nosocomial pneumonia. A review of the European Prevalence of Infection revealed *S. aureas* to be responsible for 31% of nosocomial pneumonias.

In a study of device associated infection rates in 40 hospitals from 20 cities of India, the chief causative organisms for VAP were gram negative organisms, all showing significant antibiotic resistance. The three commonest MDR gram-negative organisms in order of frequency were *Acinetobacter baumannii, Pseudomonas species, Klebsiella*. VAP due to *Staphylococcus aureus* was also noted; close to 50% of the isolates tested were resistant strains.

In another Indian study by Rachi Gupta et al. on the epidemiology of multidrug resistant pathogens isolated from VAP in the ICU patients, it was again observed that gram-negative bacteria comprised 88.3% of total isolates among which close to 72% were multidrug resistant. Gram-positive organisms comprised just 5.2% of total isolates and all of these were also multidrug resistant.

In Mumbai, VAP due to *Staphylococcus aureus* infection is for some reason uncommon. In a tertiary hospital in Mumbai (Breach Candy Hospital and Research Center) the gram-negative bacteria profile causing nosocomial pneumonia shows an increasing resistance to beta-lactum/beta-lactamase inhibitor combinations, carbapenams and unfortunately even to colistin. This is indeed a nightmare for both physicians and patients.

Diagnosis

A confirmed diagnosis of NP is difficult as there is no gold standard on which one can rely. Even postmortem histological evidence is not 100% specific. Clinical features described earlier help but fall short in both sensitivity and specificity. A combination of two of the three clinical criteria stated earlier + radiographic infiltrates gave a sensitivity of 69% and specificity of 75% for the diagnosis of VAP in 25 mechanically ventilated patients, using histological and quantitative lung tissue culture on autopsy as the reference. Also in a postmortem analysis of 39 mechanically ventilated patients, clinical criteria did not provide predictive value for histological pneumonia.

This uncertainty in clinical diagnosis leads one to ask whether bacteriological examination of lower respiratory tract secretions could help in diagnosis and thereby allow more specific treatment with improved morbidity and mortality.

Bacteriological examination of lower respiratory tract infections can be obtained by noninvasive and invasive methods.

Noninvasive methods consists of examination of the sputum and in a patient with an artificial airway, examination of the aspirate obtained by suction through this airway. The sputum or the aspirate is stained with Gram's stain and cultured. Qualitative cultures have a high sensitivity (close to 90%) but a low specificity (0–33%) because of contamination of bacteria present in the upper respiratory secretions. A negative culture is however of considerable value, in that it makes the diagnosis of nosocomial pneumonia unlikely. The use of quantitative cultures with a cutoff point at 10^6 CFU/mL increases the specificity of the noninvasive method. Most units in our country use the semiquantitative culture technique as there is no evidence that quantitative cultures (a more technically elaborate procedure) have a decided advantage over semiquantitative cultures.

Invasive Diagnostic Procedures

- Protected specimen brush (PSB) samples of lower respiratory secretions from the area of the abnormal radiological shadow observed on the chest X-ray can be collected by special protected brushes through a fiberoptic bronchoscope. The material is stained with Gram's stain and quantitatively cultured. A culture yielding 10^3 or greater concentration supports the diagnosis of NP and identifies the pathogen.
- *A study of the BAL*: A positive quantitative BAL with a CFU of 10^3–10^5 is considered a positive result.
- *Role of blinded invasive procedures*: These tests include blinded bronchial sampling, mini-BAL, blinded sampling with PSS (BPSB). The sensitivity and specificity are believed to be similar to that of bronchoscopic procedures.

It should be noted that bronchoscopic procedures even when performed expertly can carry a risk to critically ill patients on ventilator support. The main complication is hypoxia during the procedure; this could lead to hypotension, arrhythmia and even death. Hypoxia may persist for several hours after the procedure particularly in patients with ARDS.

Positive Blood Culture, Positive Culture of a Pleural Exudate

In a patient with clinical and radiological features compatible with NP, a positive blood culture is generally a pointer to the nature of the organism causing the infection.

However, a patient could develop NP, for example by aspiration of infected oropharyngeal secretions and also have a separate bloodstream infection from an intravascular device such as the central venous catheter (CVC). On the other hand, cultures of an organism from a tapped pleural exudate are certain specific bacteriological evidence of NP. Unfortunately, pleural effusions or empyemas are infrequent and blood cultures come positive only in a small minority of patients with NP. Summary of a diagnostic strategy for an HAP (including VAP) is given in **Flowchart 2**.

Evaluation of Diagnostic Strategies

Are invasive strategies for culture of lower respiratory tract secretions superior to noninvasive strategies for culture of tracheobronchial secretions?

There have been four randomized controlled trials (RCTs) studying the impact of invasive versus noninvasive strategies on ultimate outcome (mortality), antibiotic use in patients with clinical suspicion of NP. There was no difference in outcome between an invasive strategy (PSB and/or BAL) versus a noninvasive strategy (quantitative endotracheal aspirate culture). One larger trial, however, showed a small reduction in mortality and morbidity using an invasive strategy (PSB or BAL), as also better sequential organ failure assessment (SOFA) scores and lesser use of antibiotics. This study, however, compared invasive strategy with a qualitative culture of tracheal aspirates and could not be strictly compared with the other trials. Most importantly, Shorr et al. reported on a

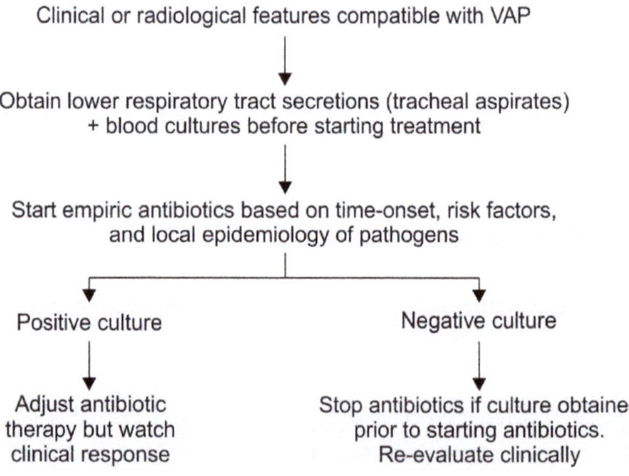

Flowchart 2: Algorithm showing strategy for treatment of ventilator-associated pneumonia.

(VAP: Ventilator-associated pneumonia).

meta-analysis of pooled data from these randomized studies on 628 patients and observed that the invasive approach did not alter mortality. Invasive testing was, however, associated with improved antibiotic utilization, or offered a change of antibiotic therapy after sampling. *It is strongly recommended that cultures within the respiratory tract (either invasive or noninvasive sampling) should be sent before starting a new antibiotic or before changing a previous antibiotic regime. If this is not done, false negative tests are likely to result.* It would appear from the preceding discussion that quantitative cultures of endotracheal aspirates being more specific are to be preferred to qualitative cultures. This concept though sound in theory, is not necessarily true in practice.

Results of a study on qualitative versus quantitative cultures of respiratory secretions for clinical outcomes in patients with VAP are summarized below.

Meta-analysis of five RCTs with 1,367 patients revealed the following:

- Quantitative cultures did not score over qualitative cultures to reduce mortality among patients with VAP.
- There was no evidence to show that the use of quantitative cultures resulted in a higher rate of antibiotic change, reduction in ICU stay, and reduced time on ventilator support, as compared to the use of qualitative cultures.
- Mortality was reduced by the use of prompt appropriate microbial agents from the beginning of the illness.
- The knowledge of local microorganism patterns is important in reducing morbidity and mortality due to VAP.

The evidence present in the above study suggests that (1) invasive modalities for culture of lower respiratory tract secretion are not clearly superior to noninvasive methods for culture of endotracheal secretions; and (2) quantitative cultures have no advantage over qualitative cultures in reducing morbidity and mortality in VAP.

In conclusion, the diagnosis of NP should be based on an overall perspective of clinical, radiological, and bacteriological findings. There is no diagnostic criterion or procedure that serves as a gold standard for the diagnosis of nosocomial (including VAP) pneumonia. There is no definite scientific evidence, or for that matter, expert consensus, to show that antibiotic treatment based on bacteriological examination and cultures of lower respiratory secretions via invasive (special bronchoscopic or other) procedures is superior to empiric treatment

aided by culture sensitivity reports on sputum or on tracheal secretions aspirated through a tracheotomy or endotracheal tube. Currently, it also cannot be maintained that use of quantitative cultures of endotracheal secretions helps to improve ultimate outcome when compared to qualitative cultures of endotracheal secretions.

The only concession in favor of bronchoscopic diagnostic procedures is that specificity in diagnosis is improved, and perhaps the unnecessary use of antibiotics is avoided for clinically insignificant organisms or in situations where smears and cultures are negative. However, patient outcome has not been altered for the better by the use of diagnostic invasive bronchoscopic or BAL procedures. In poor developing countries, where cost is important, expertise limited, and when present, not easily available, it is therefore justifiable to treat NP (suspected on clinical and radiological evidence) empirically with a suitable planned antibiotic regime. Culture sensitivity of endotracheal secretions in VAP prior to the use of antibiotics is advised.

Where expense is not in question and the expertise good and available, bronchoscopic BAL or protected BAL, or protected brush specimens are stained and cultured to guide treatment. This option in our opinion is of use only if performed before starting antibiotics. Its efficacy is reduced, if the patient has already been receiving antibiotics. In any case, empiric therapy with antibiotics should commence promptly after the bronchoscopic procedure. Treatment should never await culture reports. A positive Gram stain could, however, guide initial treatment. Treatment could be later modified, based on culture sensitivity reports.

In our unit, we use empiric antibiotic therapy for NP. Bacteriologic examination of tracheal aspirates by semiquantitative culture is done routinely before starting empiric antibiotic therapy, but it is a moot point as to what extent this helps in management and patient outcome. We use PSB sampling to obtain more specific bacteriological evidence if a patient on empiric therapy fails to improve. The PSB sampling is done before changing the antibiotic regime. Again, it is doubtful if this protocol influences patient outcome. Invasive sampling of lower respiratory secretions in NP (including VAP) is advised in immunocompromised patients where infection due to opportunistic organisms is a strong possibility. Opportunistic infection is often missed if noninvasive sampling is performed.

■ ANTIBIOTIC THERAPY IN NOSOCOMIAL PNEUMONIA

Though antibiotic therapy to start with is empiric, the selection of antibiotic therapy for each patient should depend on:

- A knowledge and awareness of the prevalence of core organisms and their sensitivity to various antibiotics in a particular ICU set-up
- Clinical background, in particular, the presence of risk factors for MDR pathogens
- Time of onset of the VAP
- Whether the patient had received antibiotics prior to the onset of pneumonia.

Awareness of the Prevalence of Core Organisms in a Particular Unit and their Sensitivity to Different Antibiotics

Core organisms responsible for nosocomial infection in units all over the world are predominantly Gram-negative bacteria. It is the exact prevalence of different Gram-negative organisms and their varying sensitivity to antibiotics that is important. This prevalence and sensitivity to antibiotics may vary from unit to unit. Also, prevalence and sensitivity patterns may vary in the same unit from time to time. A bacteriologic surveillance in every ICU is therefore of crucial importance, and the awareness of the nature of organisms generally responsible for VAP in a unit is of help in choosing appropriate antibiotic therapy.

It needs to be repeatedly stressed that there is a marked increase in the incidence of extended spectrum beta lactamase (ESBL) Gram-negative organisms in many ICUs all over India, particularly in the large metropolitan cities of the country. This is largely due to a lack of antibiotic policy in most ICUs all over the country.

Clinical Background

- The feature which is of utmost importance is to determine the presence or absence of risk factors for MDR pathogens. Important risk factors for MDR pathogens are antibiotic therapy within the past 90 days, current hospitalization of 5 days or more, and a high frequency of antibiotic-resistant organisms in a particular ICU or hospital. Other risk factors include immunosuppressed patients, patients with comorbid states, in particular, severe chronic obstructive pulmonary disease (COPD). Risk factors for MDR pathogens are listed in **Table 5**.

- *The severity of the VAP whether mild to moderate or severe*: Severe NP is characterized by one or more of the following features—respiratory failure, rapid radiographic progression, severe sepsis with hypotension and/or multiorgan failure, and acute renal failure requiring dialysis **(Table 6)**.

- In VAP, the time of onset of NP—whether early onset or late onset helps guide the nature of empiric therapy.

Use of Antibiotic Therapy Prior to the Onset of VAP

This factor, if present, further guides the nature of empiric therapy. It is best to choose an antibiotic different from the one used prior to the onset of VAP.

Principles in the Use of Antibiotic in VAP (Tables 7 and 8)

In patients with early onset VAP who have not received antibiotic therapy, the etiological bacteria often found are *Enterobacteriaceae, Haemophilus sp*, or *S. pneumonia*.

Table 5: Important risk factors for multiple drug-resistance (MDR) pathogens.

- Antibiotic therapy within the past 90 days
- Current hospitalization of 5 days or more
- Marked severity of the critical illness
- High frequency of antibiotic resistant organisms
- Immunocompromised patients
- Patients with comorbid states
- Multiple invasive procedures

Table 6: Severe nosocomial pneumonia.

- Respiratory failure, with increasing hypoxia
- Rapid radiographic progression
- Severe sepsis with hypotension and/or MOF
- Acute renal failure requiring dialysis

(MOF: Multiple organs failure)

Table 7: Initial empiric antibiotic therapy in nosocomial and VAP of early onset with no risk factors for MDR organisms.

Probable organisms	Recommended antibiotic (any one of the following may be used)
S. pneumoniae	Ceftriaxone or
Haemophilus influenzae	Amoxicillin-clavulanic acid
Enterobacteriaceae	Piperacillin + Tazobactum

Table 8: Initial empiric therapy for nosocomial or ventilator associated pneumonia of late onset or with risk factors for MDR infection and any degree of severity.

Probable organisms	Recommended antibiotic
Enterobacteriaceae	Cefepime or
Ps. aeruginosa	Piperacillin-tazobactam or
Acinetobacter baumannii Other Gram-negative bacilli	Carbapenem (Imipenem/ Meropenem)

1. The choice of the antibiotic among those listed will depend on the prevalence of the organisms and their sensitivity in a particular unit and also the severity of the disease.
2. Empiric therapy in severe nosocomial pneumonia or when MDR organisms are suspected should include two or more antibiotics, not to prevent resistance for which there is also no convincing evidence, but to provide a wide coverage for all likely infecting organisms.
3. For a wide spectrum coverage of Gram-positive and Gram-negative organisms, a combination like Piperacillin-tazobactam + vancomycin/ teicoplanin OR a carbapenem + vancomycin/teicoplanin is recommended.
4. In case of MDR pseudomonas or acinetobacter, add colistin to any of the above antibiotics, preferably to a carbapenem for maximum synergistic activity.
5. If MRSA is suspected in the unit, add vancomycin to the above antibiotics.

Monotherapy with a third-generation cephalosporin with no antipseudomonal activity (e.g. cefotaxime or ceftriaxone), or the use of clavulanic acid with amoxicillin is appropriate in these patients for about 7 days.

In contrast, VAP occurring in patients after prolonged ventilator support (late onset) and after prolonged use of antibiotics is often caused by multiresistant pathogens such as *P. aeruginosa, Acinetobacter spp., Klebsiella,* or methicillin-resistant *Staphylococcus aureus* (MRSA). The appropriate antibiotic choice should be one which acts against ESBL producing Gram-negative organisms and against Pseudomonas (piperacillin/tazobactam or carbapenems). Vancomycin may be added if a staphylococcal infection is suspected.

In patients with early onset VAP who have received antibiotics, Gram-negative organisms (*P. aeruginosa* and/or other Gram-negative core organisms), as also *Streptococci spp.* and *H. influenzae* are often responsible for the infection.

Finally, in late onset pneumonia occurring without antibiotic use during 15 days prior to infection, *Enterobacteriaceae, Pseudomonas,* or *Acinetobacter* and MRSA are often causative agents.

In both the above groups, i.e. early onset with previous antibiotic therapy and late onset without antibiotic therapy, an appropriate antibiotic choice would be a combination of an antipseudomonal β-lactam with vancomycin to cover MRSA. If NP is thought to result from aspiration of stomach contents, or if there is any other reason to suspect anaerobic infection, metronidazole or clindamycin should be added to the antibiotic regime.

Information obtained from Gram stain of respiratory secretions can guide empiric antibiotic therapy The presence of chiefly Gram-positive bacteria should direct treatment toward *Staphylococcus, Streptococcus,* and *Pneumococcus.* The morphology of stained organisms is also of help in identification. Predominant Gram-negative bacilli direct an appropriate choice of antibiotics. Empiric therapy should start promptly without awaiting culture reports.

Information obtained from culture sensitivity reports though both sensitivity and specificity in identification of the etiological agent in NP leave much to be desired, the culture report may be valuable in patient management, particularly if the empiric therapy decided upon does not prove beneficial.

Follow-up of Nosocomial Pneumonia after Initiating Empiric Therapy

Once culture sensitivity results are obtained, the antibiotic regime should be adjusted as per the microbiological results. If the organism is resistant to one of the two antibiotics in use, it should be omitted. In critically ill patients, another antibiotic which acts against the organism may be substituted for the one omitted. The recommendation to omit aminoglycosides after the first 4 days depends on the gravity of the clinical condition. Monotherapy may be justified in patients who show well marked improvement within 4 days.

Duration of Therapy

A large prospective multicenter trial which compared the efficacy of 8 days to 15 days duration of antibiotic therapy in VAP concluded that an 8-day regimen resulted in reduced antibiotic use, and a decrease in the emergence of multiresistant bacteria when compared to the 15-day regime, without altering the prognosis. It must be remembered that the above is a study on a large group and is not necessarily applicable to an individual patient. Each patient must be considered in relation to several factors which may be applicable to him or her. It is impossible to stop treatment after 7 days or even 15 days in severe

P. aeruginosa or *Acinetobacter spp.* infections. It is often necessary to continue treatment for several weeks, if there is evidence of breakdown of lung tissue with one or more abscesses, or in presence of an empyema, or in the presence of persistent intra-abdominal sepsis. If however a sharp clinical improvement occurs within the first 3 to 4 days of therapy, if PaO_2 and oxygen requirement improve significantly, and inflammatory markers [C-reactive protein (CRP)] sharply decline, antibiotics could be withdrawn safely after 7–10 days.

Lack of Response to Antimicrobial Therapy

There are several reasons for a lack of response to antibiotic therapy. These include a wrong diagnosis of pneumonia, or lack of specific antibiotic coverage against the causative organism. At times though the choice of antibiotic therapy is correct, persistence of the etiological agent leads to a persistent or worsening pneumonia. Persistence of the offending microorganism may be due to several factors; an important cause is inappropriate dosing regimen.

Superinfection pneumonia is a serious problem that often causes death. Superinfection follows prolonged broad-spectrum antibiotic therapy. Organisms causing superinfection are generally drug-resistant and therefore lethal. They include resistant strains of *Pseudomonas* and other Gram-negative bacteria, MRSA, *Enterococci,* fungi and MDR *Enterobacteriaceae.* The possible causes of nonresolution of VAP receiving antibiotic therapy are listed in **Table 9.**

Nosocomial pneumonia when severe can lead to multiorgan dysfunction and/or septic shock, situations where the mortality is high in spite of adequate antibiotic therapy.

Table 9: Possible causes of nonresolution of ventilator-associated pneumonia on antibiotic therapy.

- Wrong diagnosis—a noninfective pathology, rather than an infective one
- Inappropriate antibiotic regime
- Inappropriate dosing of antibiotic
- Persistent respiratory failure; prolonged ventilatory support
- An underlying fatal pathology, e.g. cancer
- Severe gram-negative infection which persists
- Underlying unsuspected immunosuppression
- Acquired resistance to the antibiotic
- Recurrent infection
- Superinfection
- An unexpected pathogen—*Mycobacterium tuberculosis,* fungi, respiratory viruses, *Mycoplasma*

PROGNOSIS AND MORTALITY

Nosocomial pneumonia is the leading cause of death due to HAIs. Mortality rate ranges from 20% to 70%. High-risk organisms that lead to increased mortality include *P. aeruginosa, Acinetobacter spp., Enterobacter spp.,* other Gram-negative organisms, *S. faecalis, S. aureus, Candida* species, *Aspergillus spp.,* and polymicrobial infections. The development of VAP is accompanied by a 1.8–4-fold increase in the risk of death. A French study noted that mortality was inversely related to adequacy of the initial empiric antibiotic therapy. Luna and colleagues found an overall mortality of 52.6% in 76 mechanically ventilated patients with bacteriologically confirmed VAP, if the choice of the initial antibiotic therapy was not appropriate and there was a delay in the start of therapy. Substituting a correct antibiotic cover after culture sensitivity reports are available does not reduce mortality, if the initial empiric therapy has been inadequate.

It must be, however, remembered that nosocomial pneumonia is more common in patients who are critically ill with multiple problems. To what extent death can be attributable to NP per se may be impossible to judge. It is likely that many critically ill patients die with pneumonia rather than die of pneumonia. Death in NP can result from any one or more of the following—septic shock, multiple organ dysfunction, ARDS, cardiovascular instability, and GI bleed. In VAP, it could also be occasionally related to pneumothorax or other forms of barotrauma.

Ventilator-associated Tracheobronchitis

Not all ventilator-associated pulmonary infections constitute pneumonia. They could take the form of a tracheobronchitis characterized by the presence of purulent secretions without any parenchymal involvement. The frequency of ventilator-associated tracheobronchitis (VAT) is less than VAP, but VAT often progresses to VAP. The microbiology of VAT is the same as VAP and can include MDR organisms. Systemic antimicrobial therapy is indicated in VAT. Aerosolized therapy with antibiotics (notably gentamicin) perhaps prevents the occurrence of VAP.

PREVENTION OF NOSOCOMIAL PNEUMONIA (TABLE 10)

Effective measures to prevent NP would reduce the incidence of a disease which is associated with a high

Table 10: Prevention of nosocomial pneumonia.

- Implementation of educational programs for caregivers and frequent performance feedbacks and compliance assessment
- Strict alcohol-based hand hygiene
- Avoidance of tracheal intubation and use of NIV when indicated
- Daily sedation vacation and implementation of weaning protocols
- No ventilator circuit tube changes unless the circuit is soiled or damaged
- Aspiration of subglottic secretions
- Oral care with chlorhexidine
- Avoid stress ulcer prophylaxis in very low-risk patients for gastrointestinal bleed, and consider use of sucralfate when indicated
- Semi-recumbent patient positioning
- Postpyloric feeding in patients who have impaired gastric emptying

morbidity and mortality. The Institute for Healthcare has recommended that infection control measures of proven efficacy should be grouped and implemented as a bundle rather than being implemented individually. This policy has led to better outcome; significant reductions in the incidence of VAP have been reported following the implementation of VAP preventive bundles.

General Prophylactic Measures

General prophylactic measures play an important role. These in brief include:

- Educating all ICU personnel including residents on various aspects of VAP and on the preventive strategies that reduce its incidence. It is important to constantly maintain this high level of education and ensure that there is perfect compliance in relation to execution of preventive strategies.
- *Handwashing*: The World Health Organization (WHO) considers alcohol-based hand disinfection as the single most important strategy to prevent healthcare-associated infection and most studies carried out in ICUs have confirmed the marked reduction of nosocomial infection if alcohol-based hand hygiene is religiously implemented.
- *Daily interruption of sedation*: Daily interruption of sedation avoids constant and continuous impairment of respiratory defense mechanisms. It should be practiced as a general rule with very few exceptions. Avoidance or a sparing use of neuroparalytic agents has also been recommended.
- Both tracheal intubation and mechanical ventilator support predispose to VAP and the longer the period

these interventions are in place the greater the incidence of VAP. As a corollary, the patient should be weaned off support and extubated as soon as it is safe to do so. There are a number of intensivists who opine that protocol-driven weaning procedures help early extubation. Yet, there are some intensivists who opine that early extubation compatible with good patient outcome and safety may also be achieved without following rigid protocols.

- Noninvasive ventilation has the advantage of obviating the use of an endotracheal tube. The risk of NP is thereby reduced. Noninvasive ventilation is particularly useful in acute exacerbations of COPD causing acute respiratory failure, and in respiratory failure due to pulmonary infection in immunocompromised individuals.
- *Improved design of tracheal tube cuff*: Improved design and special material in tracheal tube cuffs have been put into practice with a view to reduce the likelihood of aspiration of infected secretions across the cuff. The new material used for tracheal cuffs include polyurethane, silicone, and latex.
- Before the tracheal tube cuff is deflated, it is important to aspirate secretions in the oropharynx. It is equally important to aspirate tracheal secretions through the tracheostomy tube no sooner than when the cuff is deflated. Coating the internal surface of the endotracheal tube with antimicrobial agents such as silver has been proposed to prevent biofilm formation within the tube. This is a theoretically sound innovation but we have no experience of its use.
- *Aspiration of subglottic secretions*: Subglottic secretions are often colonized and aspiration of colonized secretions through colonized endotracheal tubes reduces hydrostatic pressure above the cuff and prevents leakage of infected supraglottic secretions across the cuff. Aspiration could be through continuous or intermittent suction. Current evidence recommends intermittent suction every 4–6 hours over continuous suction, in order to avoid the potential risk of tracheal injury.
- *Endotracheal tube versus tracheostomy*: Opinions and practices vary in different ICUs. We have always encountered an increased frequency of complications, if an endotracheal tube remains in situ for over 10 days. We replace it with a tracheostomy. In patients with voluminous tracheobronchial secretions, effective suction through an endotracheal tube is often not very effective. In these patients, a tracheostomy is advised

as it allows better suction, less retained secretions, and less chances of areas of infected atelectasis.

- *Management of ventilator circuits*: Ventilator circuit changes should not be made frequently. It is recommended that heated humidifiers be replaced by heat and moisture exchangers as the former are more likely to be contaminated with microorganisms.

  Closed tracheal suction systems have no advantage over open suction. In fact, in patients with excess tracheobronchial secretions, closed system suction is ineffective and is likely to lead to an increased chance of infection.

- *Use of propped up or semirecumbent position*: The patient is best kept with the head of the bed at an angle of 45°. A randomized trial showed a decrease in the incidence of VAP with patients ventilated in a semirecumbent position compared to patients ventilated in the supine position. This is a simple but important preventive measure against VAP.

Stress Ulcer Prophylaxis

The general consensus is that prophylaxis of stress ulcers should be provided by the use of sucralfate as this does not raise the pH of gastric contents. H_2 receptor antagonists and proton pump inhibitors raise the pH of gastric contents and thereby promote increased colonization within the stomach. Aspiration of colonized gastric contents into the respiratory tract can lead to NP.

Enteral feeding has been considered a risk factor for NP because of increased risk of alkalization of gastric contents, and aspiration of gastric contents. Yet, it is unquestionably preferred to intravenous (IV) alimentation which poses a greater risk for bloodstream infection.

Many critically ill patients have delayed gastric emptying. Placing the feeding tube beyond the pylorus reduces but does not obviate the risk of aspiration NP.

Care Over Oropharyngeal Secretions

Oropharyngeal secretions in critically ill patients in the ICU are invariably colonized by pathogenic Gram-negative bacteria which could be aspirated into the lungs. Use of 2% chlorhexidine to clean the oropharynx is a simple but important method to reduce the incidence of aspiration pneumonia. This should be done frequently in all patients and is of particular importance in patients with poor oral and dental hygiene.

Gastric Decontamination

Selective decontamination of the GI tract has been used for many years as a preventive strategy for NP. Antibiotics used are nonabsorbable—tobramycin, polymyxin, and amphotericin B; they are introduced through the nasogastric tube into the stomach in order to prevent gastric colonization with Gram-negative and *Candida spp.,* while preserving the anaerobic flora. Gastric decontamination as a prophylactic measure against NP is often used in the ICUs in Europe. The potential risk of breeding antibiotic-resistant organisms is genuine and results of randomized trials remain controversial.

General Patient Care

Patients should be turned frequently; physiotherapy to the chest, deep breathing, increased mobility in bed, all help to prevent atelectasis and infection. Meticulous asepsis should be observed during suction of tracheal secretions.

■ SUGGESTED READING

1. Berton DC, Kalil AC, Teixeira PJ. Quantitative versus qualitative cultures of respiratory secretions for clinical outcomes in patients with ventilator associated pneumonia. Cochrane Database of Syst Rev. 2008;4:CD006482.
2. Ewig S. Nosocomial pneumonia: de-escalation is what matters. Lancet Infect Dis. 2011;11:155-7.
3. Goff DA, File TM Jr. The evolving role of antimicrobial stewardship in management of multidrug resistant infections. Infect Dis Clin North Am. 2016;30:539-51.
4. Gupta R, Malik A, Rizvi M. Epidemiology of multidrug-resistant Gram-negative pathogens isolated from ventilator-associated pneumonia in ICU patients. J Glob Antimicrob Resist. 2017;9:47-50.
5. Kalil AC, Metersky ML, Klompas M, et al. Management of adults with hospital-acquired and ventilator-associated pneumonia: 2016 Clinical Practice Guidelines by the Infectious Diseases Society of America and the American Thoracic Society. Clin Infect Dis. 2016;63:e61-E111.
6. Kirtland SH, Corley DE, Winterbauer RH, et al. The diagnosis of ventilator-associated pneumonia: comparison of histologic, microbiologic, and clinical criteria. Chest. 1997;112(2):445-57.
7. Swanson JM, Wells DL. Empirical antibiotic therapy for ventilator-associated pneumonia. Antibiotics (Basel). 2013;2:339-51.
8. Udwadia FE. Principles of Critical Care Medicine, 3rd edition. New Delhi: Oxford University Press; 2013.

CHAPTER 23

Nontuberculous Mycobacterial Infections

■ GENERAL CONSIDERATIONS

Pulmonary tuberculosis which is endemic in many countries of the world is caused by the *Mycobacterium tuberculosis* complex, which comprises *Mycobacterium tuberculosis* and its geographical variants, *Mycobacterium bovis, Mycobacterium africanum, Bacillus Calmette-Guerin* (BCG) and *Mycobacterium microti*. This chapter deals with lung disease caused by nontuberculous mycobacteria (NTM). These mycobacteria were previously called by various names, atypical, anonymous, environmental, opportunistic, potentially pathogenic environmental mycobacteria. At present the terminology of non-tuberculous mycobacteria given by the International Working Group on Mycobacterial Taxonomy is universally accepted.

Pulmonary disease due to NTM has become an increasingly recognized and prevalent entity in the last 2–3 decades. Molecular techniques in microbiology and advance imaging techniques have significantly enhanced our understanding of the disease, yet many lacunae and uncertainties remain.

Nontuberculous mycobacteria are ubiquitous in the environment, found primarily in both natural and tap water, in soil, dust, animals and food. Exposure to these organisms is therefore unavoidable. However, unlike *M. tuberculosis* and *M. leprae,* NTM are not obligate pathogens. They do not ordinarily cause disease in humans, nor is there evidence of human to human transmission. They are opportunistic organisms which generally cause disease in immunocompromised individuals or if the skin or mucosal barriers is breached. Infections caused by NTM result in pulmonary disease, skin, soft tissue infections and lymphadenitis.

Disseminated infection may occur in patients with AIDS and in patients with interleukin (IL)-12 and interferon (IFN)-γ receptor abnormalities. The confusing aspect is that NTM can exist as contaminants and also as noninfective colonies in the sputum of a significant number of patients with chronic lung disease, including pulmonary tuberculosis due to the *Mycobacterium tuberculosis* complex. The question that often arises in a particular patient with pulmonary disease is whether these mycobacteria are colonizers or infectious agents producing pulmonary disease. Pulmonary infections caused by NTM are clinically and radiologically indistinguishable from tuberculosis caused by *M. tuberculosis*. Therefore, it is only when the microbiologist has identified the organism on culture and from other characteristics that a clinician becomes aware that he or she may well be dealing with infection due to NTM rather than from classic tuberculosis. It needs to be noted that the identification of acid-fast bacilli in a Ziehl-Neelsen-stained sputum specimen cannot reliably distinguish *Mycobacterium tuberculosis* from NTM which may be contaminants or colonizers rather than agents responsible for actual infection. The question that arises in a patient with pulmonary disease who has NTM isolated on culture is—should one start treatment and when does one do so?

■ EPIDEMIOLOGY

The Developed World and East Asia

The prevalence of classic tuberculosis shows an overall decline in the developed world. Remarkably, the proportion of nontuberculous mycobacterial lung disease has shown an increasing trend.

It is unclear whether this increasing prevalence of NTM lung disease is genuine, or is related to better recognition because of the introduction of molecular and more sensitive laboratory techniques, better imaging techniques and also because of many more sputum specimens being received for culture and exact identification of mycobacterial growth. In the West, the known association of NTM with diseases such as cystic fibrosis, fibronodular bronchiectasis, and pulmonary disease in post-transplant patients and following iatrogenic immunosuppression has led to a greater awareness of the presence of NTM in these situations leading to a reported increase in prevalence. Other reasons offered to explain the increased prevalence of NTM disease in the West in immunocompetent individuals include a reduced immunity to mycobacteria due to the reduced prevalence of tuberculosis, to the well-nigh universal use of BCG vaccine and the use of "showering" during bathing. NTM are frequent in tap water; these organisms are aerosolized and concentrated in shower heads leading to greater concentrated exposure with perhaps greater risk of pulmonary infection.

In spite of what has been written above, available data, especially data derived from population-based studies carried out in North America, Europe and Australia suggest that there is a continuing rise in the prevalence of pulmonary NTM isolates and NTM disease in these continents. Studies from some countries and geographical areas in East Asia such as Japan, South Korea, China, Thailand, Taiwan also corroborate this increase. In Japan, the estimated national prevalence of NTM is recently reported as 33–65 for 100,000 *[Ref: Simons S, van Ingen J, Hsueh PR, et al. Nontuberculous mycobacteria in respiratory tract infections, eastern Asia Emerg Infect Dis. 2011;17(3):343-9]* with most of the cases being due to *M. avium* complex (MAC). The leading role of MAC has also been observed in other countries of East Asia. The other frequently associated species from respiratory secretions include rapidly growing mycobacteria (RGM), *M. kansasii*, *M. scrofulaceum, M. szulgai*, and *M. malmoense, M xenopi*, and *M. fortuitum*.

In some Asian countries and in many countries in Africa, where TB is diagnosed chiefly in the presence of AFB on sputum smear, there are concerns that a number of patients diagnosed as TB, especially drug-resistant TB, may actually have NTM pulmonary disease. A study from China demonstrated that 3.4% of smear positive specimens grew NTM, primarily MAC.

The increasing prevalence of pulmonary disease due to NTM is particularly observed in the elderly. This is of importance considering the aging population in many countries.

A genuine reason for an increase in the prevalence of NTM lung disease is the great AIDS pandemic. The great degree of immune suppression observed in this disease has led to over a million hosts with AIDS rendered susceptible to infections with opportunistic infections, including infection by NTM.

Indian Studies

There is a great paucity of reports of NTM disease from India and the developing world. This is for two reasons—(1) except in well-equipped laboratories of tertiary hospitals in the large cities of India and in a few research centers, mycobacterial specimens positive for AFB on a Ziehl-Neelsen stain are presumed to be related to tuberculosis and are not routinely cultured; (2) there is no paucity of AIDS patients in India and the developing countries and these constitute ready hosts for opportunistic infections. However, tuberculosis is widely prevalent in the developing world and AIDS patients die of tuberculosis or other infections before the CD4 count falls low enough for NTM disease to occur.

There is now increasing evidence to show that NTM are present in our environment. Paramasivan and colleagues from the Tuberculosis Research Centre in Chennai in 1985 reported *M. avium intracellulare* (MAI) to be the most frequent isolated species (22.6% of all NTM), followed by *M. terrae* (12.5%) and *M. scrofulaceum* (10.5%). In 1994, Kamala and colleagues showed that MAI and *M. scrofulaceum* were present in water and dust and could be isolated from sputum samples of individuals.

The data on the pathogenicity of NTM in India is scarce. In 2005, NTM bacteremia was reported by Narang and colleagues in HIV-seropositive patients. This was the first report demonstrating dissemination of NTM infection in India. Similar cases have been reported and many more await recognition in our part of the world.

■ PATHOPHYSIOLOGY

An earlier concept of NTM within the respiratory tract suggested that these organisms were either colonizers or produced invasive disease. In all probability the situation is more complex than the simple dichotomy stated above. NTM can manifest with a graded spectrum of lung involvement, depending on the load and pathogenicity of NTM in question and the susceptibility of the host. The susceptibility of the host is dependent on his general immune status and the state of the local defenses within the respiratory system. Depending on an interaction between the seed (NTM) and the soil (the host), the following outcomes may ensue—colonization, transient colonization, active colonization, indolent infections, overt disease localized to the lung, disseminated NTM infection.

The pathogenicity of important species of NTM in ascending order is as follows: *M. avium, M. xenopi, M. abscessus, M. kansasii, M. szulgai, and M. malmoense,* the last one showing highest pathogenicity.

An overall depressed immune state can understandably predispose to NTM disease as also to other infections. However, impairment of local defenses within the lung can encourage disease due to NTM. Silicosis and cystic fibrosis (CF), for example, are known to be complicated by disease due to NTM. The relationship between non-CF bronchiectasis and NTM is being increasingly elucidated. NTM can cause bronchiectasis by destroying the bronchial wall and bronchiectasis can predispose to NTM colonization/disease. NTM pulmonary disease in bronchiectasis can be further complicated by co-infection with gram-negative organisms and fungi, notably the *Aspergillus* species. Lung damage caused by concurrent or prior *M. tuberculosis* could also be associated with NTM infection. Whether this is due to impaired lung defenses or to a common underlying immunological deficit is unknown.

CLINICAL FEATURES

There is very little or no data from developing countries with regard to pulmonary disease produced by NTM. In the West the four species of NTM most frequently responsible for lung disease are *M. avium-intracellulare-scrofulaceum* (MAIS), *M. kansasii, M. malmoense,* and *M. xenopi.* The clinical and radiological features do not differ among these four species. The following clinical profiles have been reported from the West:

Cavitatory Lung Disease

Over half the patients have preexisting lung disease, chiefly chronic obstructive pulmonary disease (COPD); some have old healed tuberculosis. The clinical features are indistinguishable from pulmonary tuberculosis and include fever, cough, sputum, hemoptysis, weight loss and increasing breathlessness. At least 10% are asymptomatic. There are often added features of chronic obstructive lung disease. The X-ray and CT appearances are indistinguishable from pulmonary tuberculosis and consist of infiltrates with cavitation in either one or both lungs chiefly involving the upper lobes.

Fibronodular Bronchiectasis (Figs. 1 and 2)

In Western studies, 12% of patients with MAC demonstrated a reticular fibrotic radiographic pattern

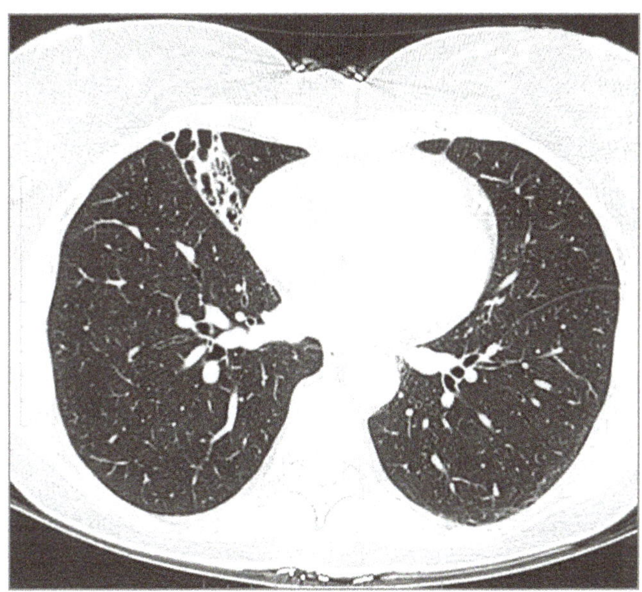

Fig. 1: HRCT chest reveals cystic bronchiectasis in the right middle lobe with atelectasis; BAL revealed atypical mycobacteria. This is an example of Lady Windemere's syndrome.

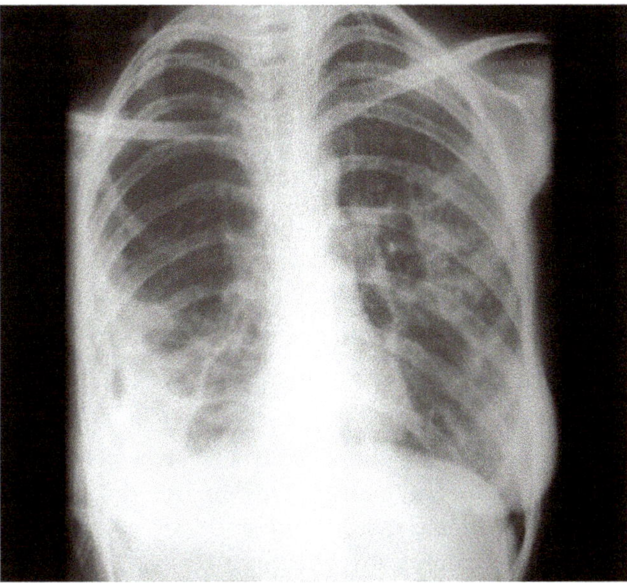

Fig. 2: X-ray chest reveals ill-defined consolidations with associated fibrosis and cavitation in the left mid-zone and right lung bases. BAL revealed MAC.

rather than cavitatory disease. Sputum cultures showed either *M. kansasii* or MAC. Fibronodular bronchiectasis was observed in the absence of cavitation and in patients without preexisting lung disease or immunosuppression. Cough and sputum production are the most common symptoms; hemoptysis may also occur. Fibronodular bronchiectasis has been termed Lady Windemere's syndrome after the play by Oscar Wilde. It is believed to occur in elderly women who suppress their cough so that infected secretions are retained in the middle lobe and lingula. It is suggested that MAC induces peribronchial inflammation and thickening that can progress to severe cystic bronchiectasis.

Hypersensitivity Pneumonitis

A syndrome indistinguishable from hypersensitivity pneumonitis has been described in the West in patients exposed to solutions that contain NTM. Granulomatous disease has thus been reported after exposure to hot tub baths that contain MAC.

■ CONDITIONS ASSOCIATED WITH NONTUBERCULOUS MYCOBACTERIA LUNG DISEASE

It is now increasingly recognized that NTM can perhaps contribute to disease progression and may be present in a number of pulmonary pathologies—COPD, cystic fibrosis, old healed tuberculosis, silicosis, bronchiectasis and pulmonary alveolar proteinosis. Other disorders rarely associated with NTM infections are alpha-1-antitrypsin deficiency and ciliary dyskinesia. It must be accepted that in a given patient it may indeed be difficult to determine whether the presence of NTM constitutes colonization or actually contributes directly to the disease.

Nontuberculous Mycobacteria Pulmonary Disease in the Immunocompromised Patient

Nontuberculous mycobacteria are opportunistic organisms and are more likely to cause disease in immunosuppressed patients as compared to immuno-competent patients.

Nontuberculous mycobacteria disease has been reported after solid organ transplants and in hemopoietic stem cell transplants. NTM pulmonary disease is reported to be relatively uncommon after renal transplants.

The use of tumor necrosis factor antagonists—infliximab and etanercept in rheumatoid disease, Crohn's disease and several other inflammatory conditions has also led to infections with NTM though unquestionably infection due to tuberculosis is more frequent.

Finally, a background of HIV infection with low CD4 counts (<100 cells/uL) is the ideal breeding ground for several opportunistic infections including NTM. Disseminated NTM disease occurs when the CD4 count is less than 50 cells/uL. *M. avium* is the most common cause of disseminated disease in HIV patients. Paradoxically, patients with disseminated disease rarely have pulmonary disease, though the sputum may be positive on culture for *M. avium-intracellulare.*

The other NTM associated with HIV infection is *M. kansasii.* Pulmonary disease due to infection with *M. kansasii* generally occurs without dissemination. This probably reflects the fact that *M. kansasii* is more pathogenic than MAC and that it causes disease in patients who are less immunosuppressed.

■ LABORATORY IDENTIFICATION

The details of microbiological identification of NTM are beyond the scope of this chapter. The species of most clinically relevant NTM can be established by cultural and basic biochemical tests. These involve pigment production, temperature range in which growth occurs, oxygen preference and the ability to hydrolyze Tween 80.

Amplification techniques targeting specific DNA sequences are being used in special reference laboratories for quicker identification. Thus, commercial DNA probes that target ribosomal RNA allows rapid identification of *M. tuberculosis,* MAC, *M. avium,* and *M. intracellulare.* Other methods to identify NTM include genetic techniques directed to 65 kd heat shock protein genes and the 16S ribosomal RNA. These genetic techniques include amplification as in the polymerized chain reaction (PCR), probe hybridization, restriction fragment length polymorphism (RFLP) and DNA sequencing.

■ SUSCEPTIBILITY

The drug sensitivity patterns of clinically relevant NTM are shown below. The *in vitro* sensitivity of *M. kansasii* to rifampicin and ethambutol corresponds to the clinical effectiveness against the *Mycobacterium.* However, with respect to the other NTMs there seems to be a lack of correlation between *in vitro* sensitivity and clinical response to treatment. A prospective trial by the British Thoracic Society has confirmed this *(Ref: BTS research Committee. First randomized trial of treatments for pulmonary disease caused by M. avium intracellulare, M malmoense, and M. xenopi in HIV negative patients: rifampicin, ethambutol and isoniazid versus rifampicin and ethambutol. Thorax. 2001;56:167-72.).* There is also a degree of synergy between rifampicin and ethambutol, in that each drug individually may be ineffective but when combined becomes effective. This is with specific reference to strains of MAIS (*M. scrofulaceum* and *M. avium-intracellulare*), *M. xenopi* and *M. malmoense* (**Table 1**). The significance of *in vitro* sensitivity tests of the newer drugs (quinolones, clarithromycin, azithromycin, and rifabutin) in relation to actual clinical response against NTM infection is not yet known. It is however recommended that in *M. kansasii* infection reported to be resistant to rifampicin, sensitivity tests to all other first-line and newer drugs may help in management.

DIAGNOSIS

Certain principles must be kept in mind if NTM pulmonary infection is to be diagnosed with a fair degree of accuracy once these organisms have been identified by the microbiological laboratory.

- Nontuberculous mycobacteria are ubiquitous, may be present in the water used in the laboratory and contaminate respiratory secretions. Contaminations must be distinguished from infection.
- Nontuberculous mycobacteria may colonize the respiratory tract, particularly in patients with chronic respiratory disease and may not be actually responsible for infection. Colonization should be distinguished from infection. Admittedly, this may at times be impossibly difficult.
- Persistent or progressive symptoms with repeated isolation of the same species of NTM, coupled with progressive radiological changes for which there is

no other explanation suggests infection rather than colonization.

The American Thoracic Society has published the following guidelines as diagnostic criteria before starting long-term therapy:

- Nontuberculous mycobacteria must be cultured a minimum of three times in the preceding years or twice if one of the specimens is positive for mycobacterium in patients presenting with features compatible with NTM pulmonary disease. It is however mandatory by proper testing to exclude infection by *M. tuberculosis.*
- The diagnosis of NTM can also be confirmed if NTM are in greater than 1+ density on stained smear or on culture of bronchoalveolar lavage (BAL).
- The diagnosis of NTM is also confirmed if a lung biopsy shows characteristic features of granulomatous infection together with a sputum or BAL that contain NTM on smear or culture.

Some researchers are of the opinion that recommending repeated positive cultures is too stringent a requirement, in particular for *M. kansasii* infection. Perhaps even a single positive culture when combined with compatible clinical features should warrant start of therapy.

TREATMENT

A diagnosis of NTM lung disease alone does not necessitate immediate treatment against the NTM pathogen. The decision to treat should be based on potential risks of the use of multiple antibiotics for long periods, the age of the patient and the existing comorbid diseases present. Patients with fibrocaseous cavitary lung disease merit immediate treatment because of the higher mortality associated with this form of the disease. On the other hand, nodular bronchiectasis is generally slowly progressive and immediate or early treatment is not incumbent unless the patient is clearly symptomatic and there is no contraindication to the prolonged use of antibiotics. The

Table 1: Sensitivity of opportunistic mycobacteria to individual antituberculosis drugs *in vitro.*

Species	INH	Rifampicin	Ethambutol	Streptomycin	Cipro	Ethio
M. kansasii	R	S	S	B	V	S
MAIS complex	R	R	R	R	R	S
M. malmoense	R	V	V	R	S	S
M. xenopi	R	V	R	S	S	S

(B: Borderline; Cipro: Ciprofloxacin; Ethio: Ethionamide; INH: Isoniazid; R: Resistant; S: Sensitive; V: Variable).

decision to treat may also be aided by molecular analysis, because specific mycobacterial genotypes have been shown to be predictive of disease progression or treatment response in patients with NTM disease **(Table 2)**.

Once the decision to treat has been made, treatment regimens should be formulated according to established guidelines (*Ref: Stout JE. Update on pulmonary disease due to non-tuberculous mycobacteria. Int J Infect Dis. 2016;45:123-34*).

The present recommendation is to use ethambutol and rifampicin or rifampicin, ethambutol, and isoniazid for 2 years. Streptomycin may be added if the response is inadequate. The efficacy of ciprofloxacin and clarithromycin is undetermined.

Table 2: Treatment regimens for different NTM isolates.

Isolate	*Regimen*	
M. kansasii-pulmonary disease	Rifampicin 600 mg daily and Ethambutol 15 mg/kg daily and Isoniazid 300 mg (with pyridoxine 10 mg) daily or azithromycin 250 mg daily or clarithromycin 500 mg twice daily	Antibiotic treatment should continue for a minimum of 12 months after culture conversion
Mycobacterium abscessus-pulmonary disease Clarithromycin-sensitive isolates or inducible macrolide resistant isolates	Initial phase: ≥1month Intravenous amikacin 15 mg/kg daily or 3× per week and intravenous tigecycline 50 mg twice daily and where tolerated intravenous imipenem 1g twice daily and where tolerated oral clarithromycin 500 mg twice daily or oral azithromycin 250–500 mg daily	Continuation phase: Nebulised amikacin and oral clarithromycin 500 mg twice daily or azithromycin 250–500 mg daily and 1–3 of the following antibiotics guided by drug susceptibility results and patient tolerance: oral clofazimine 50–100 mg daily oral linezolid 600 mg daily or twice daily oral minocycline 100 mg twice daily oral moxifloxacin 400 mg daily oral cotrimoxazole 960 mg twice daily
Non-severe M. xenopi-pulmonary disease	Rifampicin 600 mg daily and Ethambutol 15 mg/kg daily and Azithromycin 250 mg daily or Clarithromycin 500 mg twice daily and Moxifloxacin 400 mg daily or Isoniazid 300 mg (+pyridoxine 10 mg) daily	Antibiotic treatment should continue for a minimum of 12 months after culture conversion
Severe M. xenopi-pulmonary disease	Rifampicin 600 mg daily and Ethambutol 15 mg/kg daily and Azithromycin 250 mg daily or Clarithromycin 500 mg twice daily and Moxifloxacin 400 mg daily or Isoniazid 300 mg (+pyridoxine 10 mg) daily and Consider intravenous amikacin for up to 3 months or nebulised amikacin	Antibiotic treatment should continue for a minimum of 12 months after culture conversion
Non-severe M. malmoense-pulmonary disease	Rifampicin 600 mg daily and Ethambutol 15 mg/kg daily and Azithromycin 250 mg daily or Clarithromycin 500 mg twice daily	Antibiotic treatment should continue for a minimum of 12 months after culture conversion

Contd...

Contd...

Isolate	Regimen	
Severe M. malmoense-pulmonary disease	Rifampicin 600 mg daily and Ethambutol 15 mg/kg daily and Azithromycin 250 mg daily or Clarithromycin 500 mg twice daily and Consider intravenous amikacin for up to 3 months or nebulised amikacin	
Non-severe MAC-pulmonary disease	Rifampicin 600 mg 3× per week and Ethambutol 25 mg/kg 3× per week and Azithromycin 500 mg 3× per week or Clarithromycin 1g in two divided doses 3× per week	Antibiotic treatment should continue for a minimum of 12 months after culture conversion
Severe MAC-pulmonary disease	Rifampicin 600 mg daily and Ethambutol 15 mg/kg daily and Azithromycin 250 mg daily or Clarithromycin 500 mg twice daily and Consider intravenous amikacin for up to 3 months or nebulised amikacin	Antibiotic treatment should continue for a minimum of 12 months after culture conversion

■ TREATMENT OF NONTUBERCULOUS MYCOBACTERIA PULMONARY INFECTION IN INDIA AND DEVELOPING COUNTRIES

The identification of the exact species of NTM causing pulmonary infection is a luxury given to very few research laboratories in developing countries. If a diagnosis of NTM infection is made on the basis of clinical features and by laboratory investigations through basic culture and biochemical tests, how does one proceed if species identification is not available. Results of the BTS study show that rifampicin, ethambutol, together with isoniazid are the key drugs in treating these infections. If the response is inadequate, our present state of knowledge dictates that additional drugs should be used empirically. These could include a quinolone or clarithromycin or streptomycin or ethionamide. Two of these may perhaps be added to the basic regime. The simpler the combination of drugs the less toxic the effects and greater the compliance.

Role of Surgery

If a NTM pulmonary infection fails to respond, surgery should be considered if the disease is localized, if the patient is fit for surgery and if lung functions render surgical treatment feasible. Very often, the presence of bilateral disease or crippling background disease in the form of COPD renders surgery impossible. If surgery is performed successfully for localized disease, chemotherapy should be continued for a further period of 18 months to 2 years.

■ TREATMENT OF NONTUBERCULOUS MYCOBACTERIA INFECTION IN AIDS

Response to therapy depends not so much on antimicrobial therapy as on the degree of immunocompromise.

In AIDS, the infection may not be confined to the lungs but may be systemic with persistent bacteremia. In these patients the prognosis is poor. The use of highly active antiretroviral therapy (HAART) has considerably improved prognosis in NTM infection with AIDS. The recommended treatment for MAIS complex, *M. malmoense* or *M. xenopi* is rifampicin, ethambutol and clarithromycin. Therapy should be continued indefinitely as discontinuation leads to either relapse or recurrence. In poor developing countries where species identification is not possible the above regime should be promptly started as it covers the management of all major NTM species causing pulmonary infection including *M. kansasii.*

It should be noted that drug interaction between rifampicin, macrolides and protease inhibitors may render the choice of antimicrobial regimens difficult.

■ SUGGESTED READING

1. BTS Research Committee. First randomised trial of treatments for pulmonary disease caused by *M. avium-intracellulare*, *M. malmoense*, and *M. xenopi* in HIV negative patients: rifampicin, ethambutol and isoniazid versus rifampicin and ethambutol. Thorax. 2001;56:167-72.
2. Field SK. Lung disease due to the more common nontuberculous mycobacteria. Chest. 2006;129(6):1653-72.
3. Glassroth J. Pulmonary disease due to nontuberculous mycobacteria. Chest. 2008;133(1):243-51.
4. Griffith DE. Diagnosing nontuberculous mycobacterial lung disease. A process in evolution. Infect Dis Clin North Am. 2002;16(1):235-49.
5. Kamala T, Paramasivan CN, Herbert D, et al. Evaluation of procedures for isolation of NTM from soil and water samples obtained in Northern India. Appl Environ Microbiol. 2004;70(6):3751-3.
6. Marras TK, Mendelson D, Marchand-Austin A, et al. Pulmonary nontuberculous mycobacterial disease, Ontario, Canada, 1998–2010. Emerg Infect Dis. 2013;19: 1889-91.
7. Martiniano SL, Nick JA. Nontuberculous mycobacterial infections in cystic fibrosis. Clin Chest Med. 2015;36:101-15.
8. Narang P, Narang R, Mendiratta DK, et al. Isolation of *Mycobacterium avium* complex and *M. simiae* from blood of AIDS patients from Sevagram, Maharashtra. Indian I Tuberc. 2005;52:21-6.
9. Piersimoni C. Pulmonary infections associated with non-tuberculous mycobacteria in immunocompetent patients. Lancet Infect Dis. 2008;8(5):323-34.
10. Schluger NW. Tuberculosis and nontuberculous mycobacterial infections in older adults. Clin Chest Med. 2007;28(4):773-81, vi.
11. Stout IE. Update on pulmonary disease due to non-tuberculous mycobacteria. Int J Infect Dis. 2016;45:123-34.
12. van Ingen J, Ferro BE, Hoefsloot W, et al. Drug treatment of pulmonary nontuberculous mycobacterial disease in HIV-negative patients: the evidence. Expert Rev Anti Infect Ther. 2013;11:1065-77.

CHAPTER 24

Bronchiectasis

DEFINITION

Bronchiectasis (bronchus-tube; ectasis-to stretch) is a chronic respiratory disease characterized by a permanent abnormal dilatation of bronchi. This structural abnormality of the bronchi predisposes to retention of respiratory secretions and to bronchial infection. Chronic bronchial suppuration results and is characterized by cough with expectorating of mucopurulent sputum, which in many patients is copious in quantity.

TYPES OF BRONCHIECTASIS

The dilatation of bronchi may take several forms:

- Cystic or saccular bronchiectasis is observed when there is severe damage to the bronchial wall, so that balloon-like dilatation of the bronchial wall is observed. Though this form of bronchiectasis is now uncommon in the developed world because of vaccination against childhood illnesses, improved socioeconomic conditions, and access to good healthcare, it still persists in India and poor countries of the world. Cystic bronchiectasis is generally a result of severe viral (e.g. measles) or bacterial infection in childhood and is characterized by finger clubbing and by the production of large quantities of sputum.
- Cylindrical bronchiectasis results from a lesser degree of damage to the bronchial wall and is characterized by cylindrical dilatation of the bronchi. It is often diffuse, the lower lobes being more frequently involved.
- Varicose bronchiectasis features focal areas of bronchial constrictions, a stenosis in the cylindrically dilated bronchi.
- Traction bronchiectasis occurs in patients with well-marked pulmonary fibrosis, the fibrosis pulling the bronchial walls apart.

EPIDEMIOLOGY

The prevalence of bronchiectasis is difficult to ascertain as published reports even in the West are based mainly on study of chest radiographs, which are not sensitive in diagnosing bronchiectasis. The prevalence is certainly underestimated as the advent of high-resolution computed tomography (HRCT) scans has revealed bronchiectasis in patients who would have otherwise remained undiagnosed. Seitz and his colleagues recently demonstrated that the prevalence of bronchiectasis has increased every year from 2000 to 2007 by an annual percentage of 8.7% *(Ref: Seitz AF, Oliver KN, et al. Trends in bronchiectasis among Medicare beneficiaries in the United States, 2000 to 2007. Chest. 2012;142:432-9).* The prevalence was higher in women, increased with age, peaking at ages 80–84 years. Bronchiectasis is believed to have a higher prevalence in Asian population than in the West, but whether this is a true increase or is due to increased recognition, remains uncertain. Computed tomography (CT) scans have also uncovered milder forms of bronchiectasis as in patients with chronic obstructive pulmonary disease (COPD), chronic asthma, and in smokers with chronic bronchitis. A high incidence of bronchiectasis has been reported in certain ethnic groups, e.g. native Americans in North America, Maoris in New Zealand, and Samoans. It is uncertain whether this increased prevalence is related to genetic factors or to environmental influences. Population surveys to determine the prevalence of bronchiectasis will only be accurate if cheap, widely applicable yet accurate imaging techniques are developed in the future.

ETIOLOGY

There are a number of known causes that are briefly discussed below. Yet in a number of patients (perhaps close to a half), the cause remains unknown.

Postinfective

A lower respiratory tract infection may damage the bronchial walls leading to bronchiectasis. In India, childhood illnesses, in particular measles, other viral infections, and whooping cough are the main culprits. Tuberculosis is another important etiological factor in countries where the prevalence rate of this disease is high. Bronchiectasis related to tuberculosis is generally seen in the upper lobes. However, in lungs severely damaged by extensive tuberculosis, bronchiectasis is often extensive and diffuse. Bacterial infection causing pneumonia could also damage bronchi sufficiently to result in localized bronchiectasis but the cause and effect in many instances remains uncertain. Bronchiectasis is often observed in McLeod's syndrome, a form of obliterative bronchiolitis due to infection occurring in childhood. The insult to the developing lung results in the radiological finding of a unilateral hypovascular, hyperlucent lung with increased air-trapping clearly demonstrated in expiratory film.

Mechanical Obstruction

Mechanical bronchial obstruction, either luminal (foreign body and growth) or due to a bronchial stenosis or due to extrinsic pressure (e.g. from lymphadenopathy) can cause bronchiectasis. Two mechanisms operate: (1) the occurrence of atelectasis causing a pull on the bronchial walls due to negative intrapleural pressure; (2) poor drainage of bronchial secretions with resulting infection and damage to the bronchial wall. The second mechanism is probably the main reason for bronchiectasis in these situations.

Brock syndrome or the middle lobe syndrome is characterized by shrinkage of the middle lobe together with bronchiectasis of this lobe, caused by extrinsic pressure on the middle lobe bronchus, usually due to tuberculous lymphadenopathy. The middle lobe is more prone to atelectasis with subsequent bronchiectasis because it is long, narrow, acutely angulated, and surrounded by a cuff of lymph glands. The narrow acutely angulated middle lobe bronchus may also be predisposed to bronchiectatic changes in conditions associated with poor mucus clearance as in primary ciliary dyskinesia. Nontuberculous adenopathy can also occasionally lead to this syndrome. A stenosis of the middle lobe bronchus, again generally tuberculous in nature, also produces the middle lobe syndrome.

Noninfective Inflammatory Obliterative Bronchiolitis and Pneumonitis

Inhalation of toxic gases like chlorine, ammonia, or smoke can inflame bronchial mucosa and damage bronchial walls leading to bronchiectasis. The basic pathology due to inhalation of toxic gases is an obliterative bronchiolitis; however, damage to walls of the larger bronchi leads to cylindrical bronchiectasis. Acid reflux with aspiration into the lung can cause episodes of airways obstruction. Chronic aspiration may well lead to bronchiectasis.

Immune-mediated Causes

This is classically observed in allergic bronchopulmonary aspergillosis, which results over time to well-marked proximal bronchiectasis chiefly involving the upper lobes. Bronchiectasis is due to two main factors: (1) atelectasis caused by inspissated plugs of mucus, containing fungal hyphae; (2) Type I and III immune-mediated responses to the Aspergillus fumigatus colonizing the airways leading to damage to the bronchial wall. A fuller description of allergic bronchopulmonary aspergillosis is given in a separate chapter.

Conditions causing obliterative bronchiolitis can also damage large airways leading to cylindrical bronchiectasis. This is observed in chronic graft versus host disease, lung transplant rejection, rheumatoid arthritis, other connective tissue disorders, and rarely, following the use of drugs such as penicillamine.

Immunodeficiency

Immunodeficiency should always be suspected in patients with recurrent acute pulmonary infection rather than in those with persistent chronic infection.

Agammaglobulinemia or hypogammaglobulinemia is the most common immunodeficiency detected in these patients. It leads to repeated episodes of lower respiratory tract infections including pneumonia. Bronchiectasis often results. Immunoglobulin G (IgG) subclass deficiency (deficiency in IgG2) is in particular associated with pneumonia due to pneumococcus. Repeated infections can lead to bronchiectasis. IgA deficiency or absence occurs in 0.1–0.2% of the population. In some patients, particularly when associated with IgG2 deficiency, repeated respiratory infections occur resulting in bronchiectasis.

An acquired immunodeficient state exists in patients with multiple myeloma, lymphoma, and lymphatic leukemia. Recurrent respiratory infections can occur, leading to some degree of cylindrical bronchiectasis. Bronchiectasis can also complicate human immunodeficiency virus (HIV) infection following frequent respiratory infections.

Impaired Mucociliary Clearance

Impaired mucociliary clearance results in chronic or recurrent bronchial infection and inflammation leading to damage to bronchial walls and bronchiectasis. The three conditions causing impaired mucociliary clearance are primary ciliary dyskinesia, Young's syndrome, and cystic fibrosis (CF).

Primary ciliary dyskinesia is a rare autosomal recessive condition with incomplete penetration, characterized by ultrastructural abnormalities in the cilia. The abnormalities consist of absence of one or both of the dynein arms, or an abnormality of the microtubules or radial spokes. As a result, the cilia are either immotile, beat slowly or beat in a disorderly fashion or in different directions, thereby impairing mucus clearance.

Cilia line not just the bronchi (right up to the respiratory bronchiole) but the nose, paranasal sinuses, the middle ear and Eustachian tubes and the tail of spermatozoa. Poor ciliary function is present in all these sites, so that bronchiectasis is often associated with chronic sinusitis, middle ear disease, and infertility. Impaired ciliary function may present in the neonatal period with mucus plugging, atelectasis, and pneumonia. More frequently, symptoms of recurrent infection are observed in childhood and adolescence. In 50% of patients with primary ciliary dyskinesia, there is a dextrocardia and some of these patients also have a situs inversus. The triad of bronchiectasis, dextrocardia with or without situs inversus, and chronic sinusitis together with infertility in adult males constitute the Kartagener's syndrome, named after the pediatrician who first described it **(Figs. 1A and B)**. This syndrome is related to a genetic abnormality characterized by the presence of XXY.

Young's syndrome is rare and is characterized by the triad of bronchiectasis, sinusitis, and azoospermia due to functional (i.e. nonobstructive) blockage in the head of the epididymis, which is usually enlarged on palpation. The respiratory secretions are viscid, leading to prolonged,

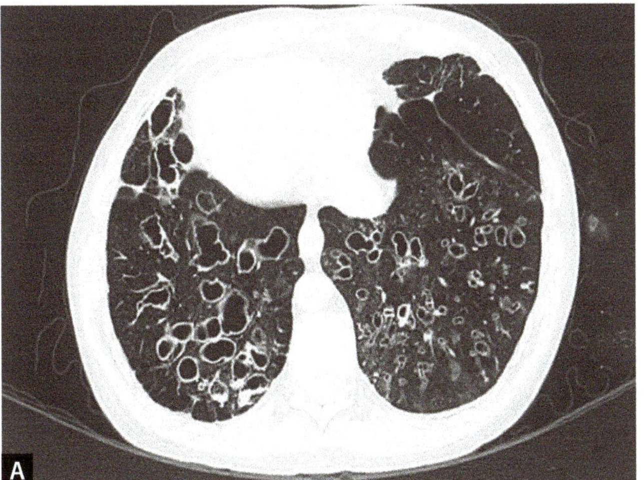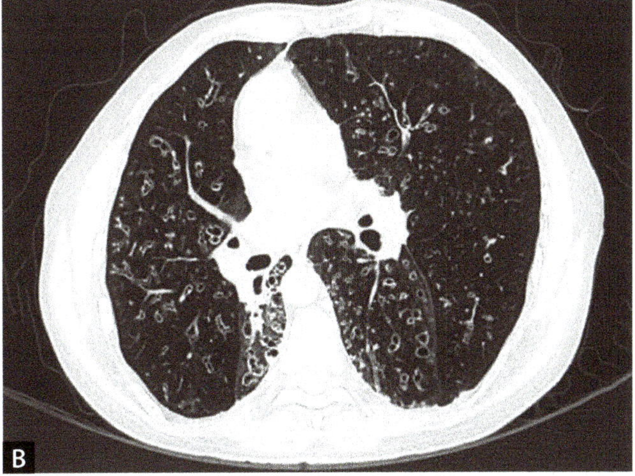

Figs. 1A and B: Kartagener's syndrome. High-resolution computed tomography (HRCT) chest reveals cystic bronchiectasis in both lung fields with dextrocardia.

delayed mucociliary transport. The cause of Young's syndrome is not known though it has been linked to mercury poisoning in childhood.

Cystic fibrosis is the most important cause of impaired mucociliary transport. The disease though common in the West has a comparatively low prevalence in India.

The overall outlook and prognosis is much worse in CF when compared to primary ciliary dyskinesia, despite absent mucociliary clearance in the latter condition. The poor mucociliary clearance in CF is because of reduced hydration and increased viscosity of airway secretions due to abnormal ion transport. Early infection of bronchi is often due to *Staphylococcus aureus* and *Haemophilus influenzae*, but ultimately chronic recurrent infection at a young age is due to *Pseudomonas aeruginosa*. The host–bacteria interaction is probably related to the basic genetic defect in CF. An antimicrobial peptide P deficiency, which normally protects the bronchial epithelium from infection has been shown to be inactivated by the increased salt content of the airway secretion in CF. It has also been shown that *P. aeruginosa* adheres more strongly and in greater numbers to CF epithelial bronchial cells. This again is probably related to the basic genetic mutational defect in the long arm of chromosome 7 in patients with CF, which leads to abnormalities in the CF transmembrane conductance regulator **(Fig. 2)**.

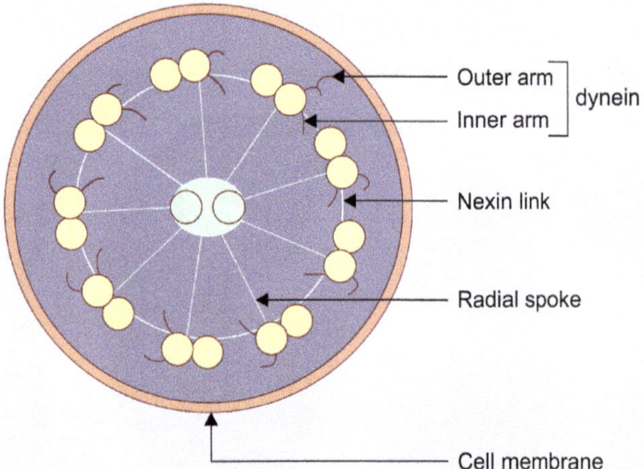

Fig. 2: Normal cilia. Schematic cross-sectional sketch of a normal ciliary shaft is showing the "9–2" arrangement of microtubules, small amount of matrix, and ciliary membrane. In ciliary dyskinesia, there is an absence of one or both dynein arms or an abnormality of the radial spokes. The cilia are therefore immotile, beat slowly or in a disorderly fashion leading to poor mucociliary clearance.

Pulmonary Fibrosis

Fibrosis from any cause (cryptogenic fibrosing alveolitis, sarcoidosis, tuberculosis, and radiation effect) if severe enough, can lead to traction bronchiectasis.

Relation to COPD and Asthma

Large network studies show that a subset of patients who meet the diagnostic criteria of COPD or Asthma have HRCT scans showing bronchiectasis. In a multicenter prospective observational study of 99 patients with moderate to severe COPD by the GOLD (Gold Initiative for Chronic Obstructive Lung Disease) criteria, bronchiectasis was noted on HRCT in 52.7% of patients.

Inflammatory Bowel Disease

Bronchiectasis is a known though uncommon association of ulcerative colitis. To a lesser extent, bronchiectasis is also associated in some patients with Crohn's disease and celiac disease. Two kinds of presentation are observed in ulcerative colitis. The first is after total colectomy in patients with severe ulcerative colitis. Cough and purulent sputum occur soon after, due to bronchiectasis. The second presentation is when patients with one condition develop the other several years later.

Other Causes and Conditions

- Congenital bronchiectasis can result because of absence or diminished amounts of cartilage in the bronchi (William-Campbell syndrome). Bronchial dilatation results because of disruption of the bronchial architecture. Bronchiectasis also occurs in congenital tracheomalacia, in Ehlers-Danlos syndrome and Marfan's syndrome due to atrophy or lack of elastic or muscular elements in the bronchi. Intralobar sequestrations have dead-end bronchi, which retain secretions and can get repeatedly infected leading to bronchiectasis.
- Pulmonary involvement in the form of obliterative bronchiolitis and/or bronchiectasis is an important manifestation of rheumatoid arthritis, Sjogren's syndrome, and other connective tissue disorders. Interestingly, rheumatoid disease, Sjogren's syndrome, Crohn's disease and immunodeficiencies are important causes of bronchiectasis in the West.
- Panbronchiolitis characterized by dyspnea, cough with productive sputum, and inflammation of the bronchial

walls was first described in Japan and then in China and Korea. It is less recognized outside these countries. We have encountered this pathology in a few patients. It can lead to bronchiectasis.

- The yellow nail syndrome is characterized by yellow dystrophic nails, lymphedema, and rhinosinusitis. Pleural effusion may also be associated along with bronchiectasis.
- *Idiopathic bronchiectasis*: A number of patients (perhaps close to 50%) with bronchiectasis have no definite attributable cause. There is at times a history of recurrent colds and cough associated with wheezing in childhood. A latent period of good health is then followed by the development of bronchiectasis between the age of 20 years and 30 years. At times, the features of bronchiectasis seem to be the result of a viral infection, which did not completely resolve. Whether there is any relation between cause and effect in these situations and if so the mechanism of initiation and perpetuation of the disease is unclear.
- *Nontuberculous mycobacteria (NTM) and bronchiectasis*: NTMs known to be associated with bronchiectasis include *Mycobacterium avium-intracellulare* complex (MAC) and *Mycobacterium kansasii*. These cause a progressive bronchiectasis usually restricted to the middle lobe and lingula **(Table 1)**. This affects otherwise healthy, nonsmoking, and middle-aged women of slender build with an ineffective cough; the resulting syndrome is called Lady Windermere syndrome.
- A possible role of vitamin D deficiency as a cause of recurrent exacerbations of bronchiectasis, worse respiratory symptoms and increased colonization of sputum with bacteria was observed in an observational study on 402 patients with bronchiectasis followed for 3 years (*Ref: Chalmers JD, McHugh BJ, Docherty C, et al. Vitamin D deficiency is associated with chronic bacterial colonization and disease severity in bronchiectasis. Thorax. 2013;68:39*). Whether this is an effect of vitamin D induced reduced immunity or reduced outdoor activity due to more severe disease is unclear.

■ PATHOPHYSIOLOGY (FIG. 3)

The development of bronchiectasis depends on an infectious insult leading to mucosal inflammation and tissue damage and/or an impairment of host defenses.

Table 1: Causes of bronchiectasis.

Postinfective	Measles, other viral infection, whooping cough, tuberculosis, bacterial infection
Mechanical obstruction	Intraluminal (foreign body, tumor) and external compression (lymphadenopathy)
Noninfective inflammation	Inhalation of toxic gases
Immune-mediated causes	Allergic bronchopulmonary aspergillosis, chronic graft versus host disease, rejection of lung transplant, connective tissue disorder
Impaired mucociliary clearance	Primary ciliary dyskinesia, Young's syndrome, Cystic fibrosis
Immunodeficiency	Hypogammaglobulinemia, IgG deficiency, IgA deficiency, HIV infection
Pulmonary fibrosis	Tuberculosis, sarcoidosis, cryptogenic fibrosing alveolitis
Congenital	Intralobar pulmonary sequestration; defects in bronchial wall
Miscellaneous	Inflammatory bowel disease, connective tissue disease (Rheumatoid arthritis)

(HIV: Human immunodeficiency virus; Ig: Immunoglobulin)

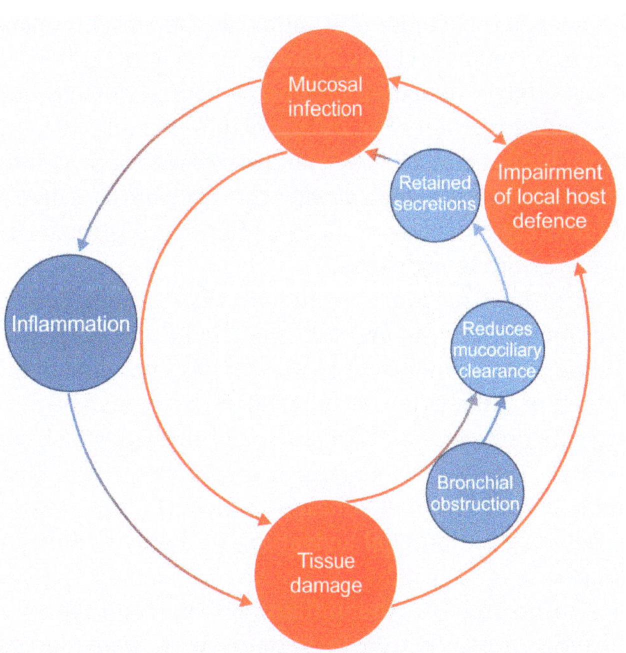

Fig. 3: Pathophysiology of bronchiectasis. Mucosal inflammation and impairment of host defenses result in an interactive self perpetuating vicious cycle leading to bronchiectasis. The initiation of the cycle may predominantly be due to mucosal infection or primarily due to impairment of host defense. Occasionally, bronchial obstruction is the initiating cause; it acts by impairing mucociliary clearance, and thereby promoting mucosal infection. Mucosal infection spreads to involvement of the bronchial walls as well.

These factors interact to form a self-perpetuating vicious cycle. Thus, tissue damage resulting from mucosal inflammation predisposes to recurrent or chronic mucosal infection. Also, tissue damage will impair local host defenses, which in turn predisposes to recurrent or chronic mucosal infection. The initiation of this vicious cycle may be either through an infectious mucosal insult or an impairment of host defense either congenital or acquired, the former being more common than the latter. Bronchial obstruction, whatever the etiology, is one other factor, which could induce bronchiectasis through impairment of mucociliary drainage, which invites infection distal to the obstructed bronchus.

Inflammation results in destruction of the mucosa, the elastin layer of the bronchial wall, as also the muscle and cartilaginous elements of the bronchus, which show varying degrees of destruction. The bronchial architecture is lost and the bronchi permanently dilate. Neutrophils are drawn to the lumen of the bronchi; the bronchial wall shows well-marked lymphocytic infiltration resembling the follicular type of bronchiectasis described several years ago. Copious secretions may block these dilated bronchi as it becomes difficult to clear the viscid mucus through cough or ciliary movement. Bacteria adhere to and multiply within the mucus perpetuating both infection and inflammation. The inflammation extends into the bronchioles and in long-standing cases there results obstruction of the small airways through fibrosis. There is therefore invariably some degree of airways obstruction in patients with bronchiectasis.

The host response to infection is through both B lymphocyte activity and cell-mediated T-cell response. Tissue injury is mediated by neutrophils (attracted to the lumen of inflamed bronchi through chemotaxis) which liberate proteases and oxidants, and through cytokines such as interleukin 8 and other mediators from host cells. Serum levels of adhesion molecules are elevated suggesting endothelial activation, probably within the lungs.

Unfortunately, the inflammatory response fails to eradicate infection in patients with well-marked established bronchiectasis. This is partly due to impaired host defenses, the large bacterial population within the bronchi and perhaps due to certain properties of the infecting bacteria.

Commonly found pathogens in patients with bronchiectasis in our units are Gram-negative organisms like *Klebsiella pneumoniae, H. influenzae, P. aeruginosa,* and Gram-positive organisms like *Staphylococcus aureus* and *Streptococcus pneumoniae.*

A study of 100 patients with bronchiectasis in Hong Kong showed that *P. aeruginosa* was the most frequent pathogen found in the sputum sample with *H. influenzae* being the second most frequent **(Table 2)**.

■ CLINICAL FEATURES

Chronic cough and expectoration of sputum, which is often mucopurulent, are the cardinal features of bronchiectasis. Patients with chronic persistent infection expectorate purulent sputum daily. Those with recurrent episodes of infection bring up large quantities of purulent sputum during periods of exacerbation. In-between acute episodes, some degree of cough with expectoration generally persists. At times, acute exacerbations may be associated with a marked decrease in sputum production because the infected sputum is very viscid and difficult to expectorate. Acute exacerbations are often associated with low-grade fever, pleuritic chest pain, and general malaise. High temperatures are unusual and should suggest the likelihood of a complicating pneumonia. Hemoptysis is often observed. Generally there is just blood-streaking of sputum or the hemoptysis is slight in quantity. Rarely, there is massive hemoptysis (>300 mL), which requires active intervention to avoid a fatal outcome.

Bilateral extensive bronchiectasis or bronchiectasis associated with well-marked airways obstruction leads to dyspnea on exertion or even at rest.

Two unusual presentations of bronchiectasis need to be kept in mind. The first is the patient who comes with

Table 2: Sputum pathogen amongst 100 bronchiectasis patients in Hong Kong.

Pathogen	% of frequency
Pseudomonas aeruginosa	33
Haemophilus influenzae	10
Streptococcus pneumoniae	6
Staphylococcus aureus	5
Other Gram-negative bacilli	5
NTM	3
Moraxella catarrhalis	2
Yeast	1

(NTM: Nontuberculous mycobacteria)

Source: Ho PL, Lam WK, Ip MS, et al. The effects of *Pseudomonas aeruginosa* infection in clinical parameters in steady-state bronchiectasis. Chest. 1998;114(6):1594-8.

recurrent pneumonia. An underlying bronchiectatic lobe is one of the causes of recurrent pneumonia. The second is the patient who has what has been termed "dry bronchiectasis" and who presents with repeated episodes of hemoptysis very often with no abnormality on routine radiography.

Finally, although chronic sputum production is a classic feature of the disease, patients may present with chronic cough, which is nonproductive.

Physical Signs

Clubbing is invariably present in bilateral extensive cystic or saccular bronchiectasis. It is, however, uncommon in the generally observed cylindrical bronchiectasis affecting both lower lobes. Crackles over the bronchiectatic lung are usually heard mostly over one or both bases. Rhonchi are often present as airways obstruction is a very frequent feature in bronchiectasis. A mistaken diagnosis of asthma is therefore occasionally made. During episodes of acute exacerbation, a pleural rub may be heard and there may be signs of a complicating pneumonia.

Lung functions show a normal or more often reduced forced vital capacity (FVC), a reduced forced expiratory volume in one second (FEV1) and a reduced FEV1/FVC. In our experience, at least half the patients show significant improvement in the FVC, FEV1, and FEV1/FVC after the use of an aerosolized bronchodilator or after nebulization with salbutamol. In extensive severe disease, the total lung capacity (TLC) is decreased as is the transfer factor of the lung for carbon monoxide (TLCO).

■ IMAGING STUDIES

A chest X-ray may be normal in close to 50% of patients with bronchiectasis. Peribronchial fibrosis and mucosal hypertrophy lead to thickened bronchial walls, which may be evident as "tramlines" in the lower lobes. Dilated bronchi running perpendicular to the X-ray beam appear as small thick-walled rings. Cystic bronchiectasis is evident as multiple thin-walled ring shadows; when these ring shadows overlap, they may give a honeycombed appearance to the lung. Dilated bronchi filled with secretions give rise to a tubular glove-finger appearance or to opacities that may be mistaken for consolidation. These appearances are particularly observed in bronchiectasis caused by allergic bronchopulmonary aspergillosis.

High-resolution computed tomography of the chest is the diagnostic procedure of choice and has completely replaced bronchography for the definitive diagnosis of bronchiectasis. Occasionally, the CT scan will not only diagnose bronchiectasis but also give the likely diagnosis as in allergic bronchopulmonary aspergillosis, tuberculosis, sarcoidosis, obstruction of a bronchus, and panbronchiolitis. CT findings are related to dilated air-filled bronchi or to dilated fluid-filled bronchi and to crowding of dilated bronchi due to volume loss of the lung in the affected area. Dilated bronchi that are perpendicular to the scanning plane have a circular signet ring appearance because of the smaller pulmonary artery in comparison to the circular dilated bronchus. Dilated bronchi parallel to the scanning plane appear as "tramlines" which do not decrease in diameter as they progress to the periphery. Mucus-filled bronchi appear as branching tubes or nodules; there may be a tree-in-bud appearance. Air trapping due to associated small airways obstruction can be demonstrated by scans taken during expiration; there is increased translucency in areas of air-trapping **(Figs. 4 and 5)**.

Patchy obstruction to the small airways may also give a mosaic appearance in the affected area on the CT scan.

■ DIAGNOSIS

Although the classic features of bronchiectasis have been described above, some patients may present with

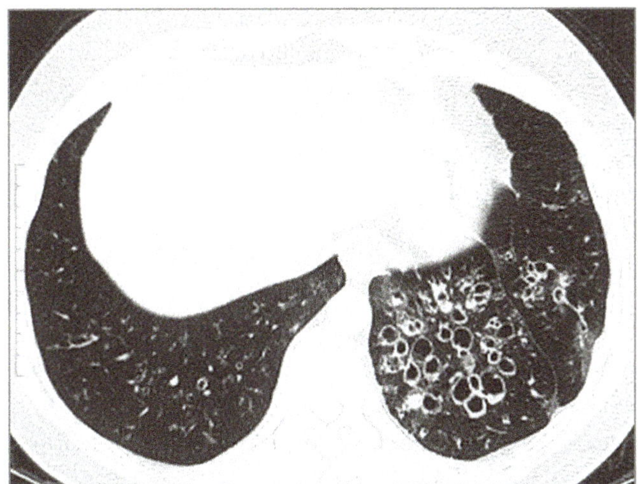

Fig. 4: Bronchiectasis. High-resolution computed tomography (HRCT) reveals dilated bronchi in both lower lobes. The accompanying pulmonary arterial branch is of much smaller diameter as compared to the dilated bronchus. Normally the ratio is 1:1. Also, there is soft tissue in the dilated bronchi in the left lower lobe representing mucoid impaction.

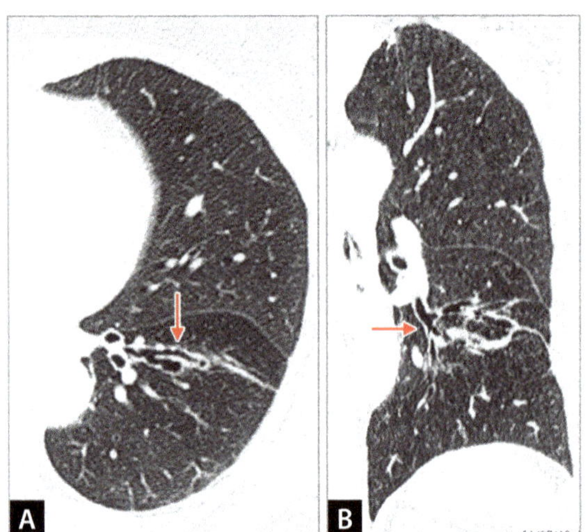

Figs. 5A and B: Traction bronchiectasis. (A) Axial and (B) coronal scans reveal fibrotic lesions in the superior segment of the left lower lobe with dilated bronchi as a result of traction bronchiectasis.

dry cough, low-grade fever, malaise, fatigue, persistent rhinosinusitis, difficult to treat asthma, or as mentioned earlier recurrent hemoptysis.

Investigations

The diagnosis of bronchiectasis is made on the history, clinical examination, and imaging findings, particularly on an HRCT of the chest. Further investigations include a blood count, erythrocyte sedimentation rate (ESR), and C-reactive protein (CRP). Both the ESR and CRP are simple but important markers of the degree of inflammation within the lungs. Serial readings at periodic intervals form a rough guide to the increase or decrease of the inflammatory process within the bronchiectatic lung. A sputum examination for smear, culture, and antibiotic sensitivity is essential as it guides antibiotic selection in treatment. Sputum culture for *Mycobacterium tuberculosis* and atypical mycobacteria should be asked for as well.

Further investigations are directed to determine the cause of bronchiectasis. They are tabled below. In younger patients with associated sinusitis, tests for ciliary dysfunction are important. The saccharin test is a good screening test for ciliary dysfunction. A particle of saccharin is placed 1 cm behind the front edge of the inferior turbinate. The patient is requested to sit quietly with the head looking down and report when a sweet taste is felt. If sweetness is felt in less than 30 seconds, it is normal. Sniffing during the test or looking upwards will give a false quick recording. If the saccharin test is positive, ciliary

integrity and function need to be tested by submitting a sample of the nasal epithelium to light microscopy and electron microscopy. Young patients or even patients between 30 years and 40 years who have recurrent lower respiratory infections or who have recurrent pneumonia should be tested for hypogammaglobulinemia and for deficiency in a subclass of IgG or a deficiency in IgA. It may not be necessary to do all tests tabled below in every patient. Investigations may perhaps be tailored depending on the cause or causes likely to operate in a particular patient **(Table 3)**.

■ COMPLICATIONS

- Extensive bilateral bronchiectasis besides leading to deteriorating health and weight loss can lead to respiratory disability, hypoxia, and chronic hypercapnic respiratory failure, particularly when associated with well-marked airways obstruction. In some instances, cor pulmonale results.
- Pneumonia may complicate bronchiectasis. Occurrence of recurrent attacks of pneumonia is well known. Pleural effusion and empyema may result from contamination of the pleural space.
- In earlier years, when the wide range of antibiotics available today was nonexistent, suppurative bronchial disease was occasionally complicated by the occurrence of a metastatic brain abscess.

Table 3: Protocol for investigation for bronchiectasis.
• CBC, ESR, C-reactive protein (CRP)
• Sputum examination—routine smear, culture, AFB smear, culture
• Pulmonary function tests
• X-ray chest
• HRCT chest
• Skin test for Aspergillus sensitivity
• Saccharin screening test for nasal mucociliary clearance—if positive more detailed test for ciliary function
• Sweat NaCl for suspected cystic fibrosis
• Serum protein electrophoresis for hypogammaglobulinemia particularly in young patients
In selected patients:
• Fiberoptic bronchoscopy
• IgM, IgA, IgG subclass
• Precipitin test for *Aspergillus* infection
• Semen analysis
• Tests for associated conditions
• Test for connective tissue disorder, autoimmune disorders

(AFB: Acid-fast bacilli; CBC: Complete blood count; ESR: Erythrocyte sedimentation rate; HRCT: High-resolution computed tomography; Ig: Immunoglobulin)

- Chronic suppurative bronchiectasis in poor countries where healthcare is unavailable or hopelessly inadequate still remains a cause of amyloid disease.
- Massive life-threatening hemoptysis in an occasional complication.

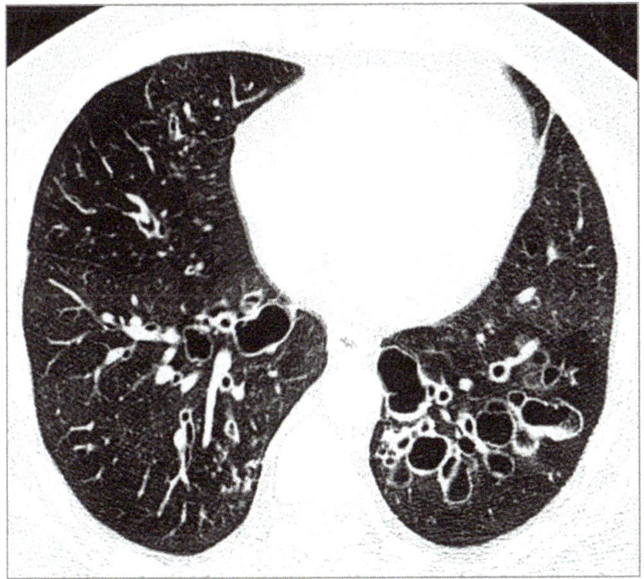

Fig. 6: High-resolution computed tomography (HRCT) reveals cystic bronchiectasis in both lower lobes with few of the dilated bronchi showing mucoid impaction and fluid levels. Multiple peribronchial nodules are seen in both lower lobes. These features are a result of secondary infection.

CLINICAL COURSE

At one time, it was believed that once bronchiectasis occurred in a lobe of the lung it would remain so and was unlikely to involve other lobes and neighboring areas of the lung. This is no longer true. Bronchiectasis may remain localized to one portion of the lung in some patients. In other patients, a follow-up shows involvement of not only the neighboring area of the lung but involvement of the other lung as well. In some patients, the rapidity of involvement is frightening, diffuse bilateral bronchiectasis being observed in a matter of a few years **(Figs. 6 and 7)**.

If causes known to lead to progressive spread of bronchiectasis (such as primary ciliary dyskinesia) have been excluded, rapid spread of bronchiectasis may well be due to abnormalities in the immune response of the host and/or the number and virulence of microorganisms responsible for bronchial inflammation and suppuration.

TREATMENT

Treatment is directed to alleviating symptoms and preventing as far as possible further progression of the disease.

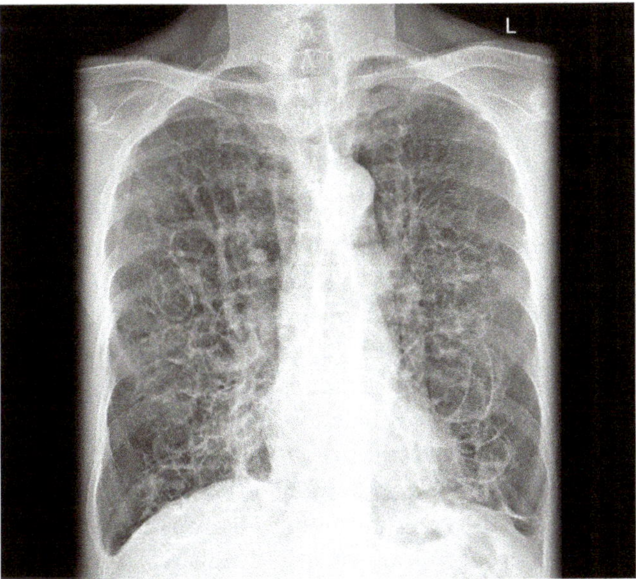

Fig. 7A: PA view of the chest demonstrates multiple thin walled rounded cystic lesions in both mid and lower zones representing cystic bronchiectasis.

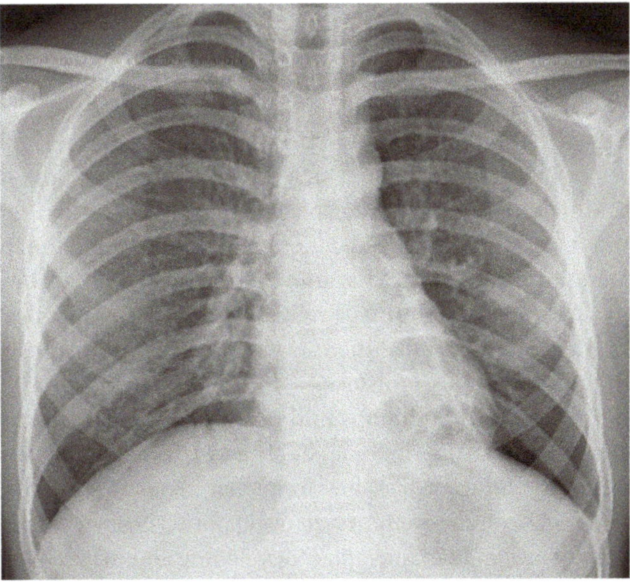

Fig. 7B: PA view of the chest: Multiple thin-walled conglomerative cystic lesions in the left lower lobe in a retrocardiac location.

Medical Treatment

Airway Clearance

The purpose of airway clearance is to mobilize and help expectorate bronchopulmonary secretions, so as to interrupt the vicious cycle of inflammation and infection.

Retained secretions within dilated bronchi lead to bacterial infection. Infection leads to tissue injury as a result of inflammatory mediators and noxious bacterial products. Neutrophils attracted to the bronchial lumen through chemotaxis add to the tissue injury by liberating proteases and oxidants. Retained secretions thus ultimately cause further damage to the bronchial wall with further disruption of bronchial architecture. The cornerstone of treatment is physiotherapy and postural drainage to help keep the dilated bronchi as dry as possible. Postural drainage should be preceded by steam inhalation to help liquefy thick mucopus. Inhaled steam is a far better mucolytic than any other mucolytic agent available today. Nebulized 7% hypertonic saline is equally useful to help improve clearance of secretions by reducing osmolality. Nebulization should be promptly followed by physiotherapy and postural drainage. Mannitol inhaled as a dry powder acts in the same manner as hypertonic saline, but is not used in our part of the world. Postural drainage should be accompanied by percussion and vibration over the affected areas of the lung to help dislodge secretions from the diseased bronchi. Breathing exercises and in particular Yogic breathing exercises also help. Postural drainage should be done at least once daily and during exacerbations at least two to three times in the day. The patient should be told to watch the color of his or her expectoration. Once the bronchiectatic area is drained adequately, the expectoration during and after drainage is often mucoid denoting control of infection. It is important to instill discipline in patients, so that they practice postural drainage religiously. Stopping postural drainage just because there is very little sputum during drainage is always a mistake.

Besides physiotherapy and postural drainage, airway clearance measures include cough-assist devices of various kinds, e.g. flutter valves, low-frequency acoustic vibrators, and high-frequency chest wall oscillators. These of course are not available in most poor developing countries. What is more, they are only of marginal assistance and use when compared to time-tested physiotherapy and postural drainage.

Proper airway clearance through nebulized hypertonic saline or steam inhalation followed by chest physiotherapy (through an assisted device) and postural drainage, improved FEV1, FVC and reduced CRP and sputum neutrophils *(Ref: Kellet F, Robert NM. Nebulised 7% hypertonic saline improves lung function and quality of life in bronchiectasis. Respir Med. 2011;105:1831-5).*

Nebulization with hypertonic saline is also useful to help the patient expectorate extra-viscid sputum as in CF.

Recombinant human deoxyribonuclease (rhDNase) has been used to reduce viscosity and improve transport capacity of purulent respiratory secretions particularly in CF. It is, however, far too expensive and not easily available in poor developing countries. What is more, rhDNase when tried in noncystic fibrosis (NCF) bronchiectasis was found to be harmful. These subjects suffered more frequent exacerbations, hospitalizations, and antibiotic courses than subjects randomized to receive placebo.

Antibiotic Therapy (Table 4)

This is the second cornerstone in the management of bronchiectasis. Antibiotics are tailored as per the organisms grown on culture and their sensitivity tests. It must be remembered that in bronchial infections bacteria are present in the mucus, on the epithelial surface, often invading the mucosa and bronchial wall.

Therefore, the antibiotic used has to reach the site of infection—the bronchial mucosa and bronchial wall. This consideration is important in the choice of an antibiotic. Quinolones and macrolides when administered reach effective concentrations within the lung and the bronchial mucosa, whereas aminoglycosides and beta-lactams do not.

In severe acute exacerbations, antibiotics are given intravenously in appropriate doses and at appropriate intervals for a period of 7–10 days or even longer.

In milder exacerbations, oral antibiotics generally suffice. Infection with *P. aeruginosa* is particularly nasty and difficult to eradicate. An antipseudomonal third-generation cephalosporin like ceftazidime, or piperacillin/tazobactam, or a carbapenem should be given intravenously. Resistant strains of *P. aeruginosa* might require the use of intravenous colistin. When infection is due to other Gram-positive/-negative organisms, the choice of antibiotics is guided by sensitivity tests. Antibiotics often used are cefuroxime, ceftriaxone, and amoxicillin-clavulanic acid in the appropriate doses.

Table 4: Antibiotics in bronchiectasis.

Route	Antibiotics	Dose and duration	P. aeruginosa
Oral	Amoxicillin/clavulanic acid	625 mg BD for 10 days orally	Ciprofloxacin 750 mg for 10–14 days
	Quinolone (ciprofloxacin)	750 mg BD for 7–10 days	
	Azithromycin	500 mg OD for 7–10 days	
	Doxycycline	100 mg BD for 10 days	
Intravenous	Cefuroxime	750 mg TDS for 10 days	
	Ceftriaxone	2 g BD for 7–10 days	
	Amoxicillin/clavulanic acid	1.2 g TDS for 8–10 days	
		4.5 g TDS for 10–14 days	Piperacillin/tazobactam
		2 g BD for 10–14 days	Ceftazidime
		1 g TDS for 10–14 days	Meropenem + an aminoglycoside (dose as per weight)—gentamicin or amikacin given once daily infusion

(*P. aeruginosa: Pseudomonas aeruginosa*)

The problem arises in patients who get recurrent relapses with severe exacerbations in spite of intravenous antibiotics. Many units consider the use of long-term prophylactic antibiotic therapy in these patients. Before embarking on this regime, it is important to ascertain that airway clearance as described above is being correctly and religiously practiced. Prophylactic antibiotic therapy gives rise to many concerns—chiefly the occurrence of resistant organisms that render antibiotics ineffective, as also the side effects and toxicity associated with prolonged use of antibiotics. Three approaches have been recommended:

1. Regular pulsed courses of intravenous antibiotics
2. Prolonged oral antibiotics
3. Inhaled antibiotics given as an isotonic solution via a nebulizer.

Nebulized antibiotics are best administered as prophylaxis to prevent or delay relapses following a course of intravenous antibiotics. Nebulized antibiotics are less effective as treatment for acute exacerbations, perhaps because they do not reach the site of infection due to excessive bronchial secretions and bronchospasm. Antibiotics used via nebulizations include beta-lactams, aminoglycosides (gentamicin, tobramycin) and colistin sulfate. The greatest experience with nebulized antibiotics is in CF for the treatment of *P. aeruginosa* infection. Nebulized gentamicin improved lung functions, reduced airway inflammation and mucous secretion, decreased frequency of exacerbations and hospital admission in these patients. For resistant *P. aeruginosa* strains, nebulization with colistin is to be preferred. Nebulization with antibiotics occasionally causes bronchospasm severe enough to prevent the use of this approach.

Prolonged oral antibiotic therapy has also been shown to be beneficial in the group of patients, which frequently suffer repeated exacerbations of infection. This approach is limited by the side effects of prolonged therapy and by the development of bacterial resistance. Ciprofloxacin or any quinolone therapy is most often used for prolonged oral therapy as quinolones attain satisfactory concentrations in the lung and within bronchi.

Regular pulsed courses of intravenous antibiotics have been advocated, particularly in bronchiectasis associated with CF and benefits have been claimed in 5-year survival. The course is administered before full relapse occurs to keep the bacterial load suppressed and thereby reduce inflammation. The length of time between courses is arbitrarily decided, and varying from 6 to 10 weeks. Regular pulsed therapy with intravenous antibiotics has also been used for bronchiectasis due to causes other than CF, when there are frequently recurring acute infective episodes. The choice of antibiotics is guided by the nature and sensitivity of the infecting organisms. Piperacillin-tazobactam or a carbapenem is often chosen for Gram-negative infections.

Airways Obstruction in Bronchiectasis

Some degree of airways obstruction invariably occurs in bronchiectasis. Aerosolized bronchodilators (salmeterol and fluticasone) often give symptomatic relief when there is a degree of reversibility in the airways obstruction. When bronchospasm is marked during acute exacerbations, nebulization with salbutamol, tiotropium, and budesonide may be of help. Inhaled steroids may reduce inflammation within the bronchi. Oral or even intravenous corticosteroids in a short course of 10–12 days may be of use during acute exacerbations, but prolonged use of oral corticosteroids should be avoided because of side effects and the absence of proven benefit.

Anti-inflammatory Therapy in Bronchiectasis

The goals of therapy in bronchiectasis include not just the control of infection but also suppressing inflammation. Recent work on suppressing inflammation in bronchiectasis has looked at:

1. Macrolides
2. Inhaled corticosteroids.

1. *Macrolides*: Macrolides, besides their antibiotic properties, exert immunomodulatory effects on host inflammatory responses without suppressing the immune system.

These immunomodulatory and anti-inflammatory effects include suppression of inflammatory mediators such as tumor necrosis factor alpha (TNF-α), interleukin-6, interleukin-1, moderating leukocytes recruitment and function, inhibiting biofilm production and reducing mucus production. Clinical benefits of azithromycin have been observed in bronchiectasis due to CF as also in NCF bronchiectasis. Three large published trials have substantiated these benefits. These trials are the Effectiveness of Macrolides in patients with Bronchiectasis using Azithromycin to Control Exacerbation (EMBRACE) trial (*Ref: Wong C, Jayaram L, Karalus N, et al. Azithromycin for prevention of exacerbations in non-cystic fibrosis bronchiectasis (EMBRACE): a randomised, double-blind, placebo-controlled trial. Lancet. 2012;380:660-7*), Bronchiectasis and long-term Azithromycin Treatment (BAT) trial, (*Ref: Altenburg J, de Graaff CS, Stienstra Y, et al. Effect of azithromycin maintenance treatment on infectious exacerbations among patients with non-cystic fibrosis bronchiectasis: the BAT randomized controlled trial. JAMA. 2013;309:1251-9*) and Bronchiectasis and Low-dose Erythromycin Study (BLESS) trial (*Ref: Serisier DJ, Martin ML, McGuckin MA, et al. Effect of long-term, low-dose erythromycin on pulmonary exacerbations among*

patients with non-cystic fibrosis bronchiectasis: the BLESS randomized controlled trial. JAMA. 2013;309:1260-7). Reduced frequency of exacerbation, decreased 24 hours sputum volume, and improved well-being are among the outcomes observed in these studies that used low-dose azithromycin 500 mg twice weekly or 250 mg thrice weekly in NCF bronchiectasis.

Anti-inflammatory treatment with macrolides on a long term 6–9-month basis should therefore be seriously considered in the management of bronchiectasis. Macrolides (azithromycin) are particularly indicated in the following conditions:

- Symptomatic patients
- High-sputum volumes
- Frequent exacerbations
- Pseudomonas colonization.

A potential disadvantage of chronic macrolide use is the potential development of resistant bacterial strains. In the BAT trial, there was observed a greater percentage of resistant pathogens by the end of the treatment period. A greater proportion of resistant oropharyngeal streptococci was observed in the BLESS trial. In the EMBRACE trial, macrolide resistant *S. pneumoniae* developed in 4% of patients in the treatment group.

Long-term use of macrolides can also encourage growth of macrolide-resistant strains of NTM. It could therefore be wise to rule out chronic infection with NTM before starting macrolides in patients with bronchiectasis.

2. *Inhaled corticosteroids in bronchiectasis*: Systemic corticosteroids are not advised in the treatment of NCF bronchiectasis with exception of patients with allergic bronchopulmonary aspergillosis. They do not alter the rate of decline in FEV1 and invariably cause side effects that outweigh benefits.

Inhaled corticosteroids have also been investigated in NCF bronchiectasis. High-dose fluticasone (1,000 µg/day) may reduce sputum volume or inflammatory markers in sputum but have not been shown to reduce exacerbations or improve lung function. Patients receiving medium dose budesonide (640 µg) plus formoterol had less dyspnea, had an increase in cough-free days, and an improved health-related quality of life. However, there was no fall in the exacerbation rate and not any improvement in lung function. Whether the perceived benefits of the medium dose regime are due to a combination of inhaled corticosteroids and long-acting bronchodilators (LABA) or due to LABA alone is uncertain. Perhaps, the use of the medium-dose regime is justified in patients who have airways obstruction showing a fair degree of reversibility *(Ref: Goyal V, Chang AB. Combined inhaled corticosteroids and long acting beta-2-agonists for children and adults with bronchiectasis. Cochrane Database Syst Rev. 2014;6:CD010327).*

Exercise

Pulmonary rehabilitation is of benefit in the management of bronchiectasis. The benefits are related to better mobilization of respiratory secretions, improved exercise tolerance, and an improved health-related quality of life. One retrospective study showed that in addition to the above benefit, there were fewer emergency room visits as well as decreased need for short-acting bronchodilators.

Other Medical Treatment

Bronchiectasis caused by or associated with hypogammaglobulinemia or selective immunoglobulin deficiencies responds well to regular replacement therapy with intravenous immunoglobulin. The interval between infusions depends on the clinical response. A period of 3–4 weeks between infusions is generally chosen at the outset. Selective antibody deficiencies including IgG subclass deficiency can also be treated by replacement. It must be noted that patients with IgG subclass deficiency and complete absence of IgA may develop IgA antibodies after transfusion of blood products or infusion of immunoglobulins containing IgA. This leads to severe anaphylaxis, if immunoglobulins are given. IgA-free infusions should be given to these patients. Massive hemoptysis is a frequent occurrence and complication of bronchiectasis. It is managed by bronchoscopic techniques, bronchial artery embolization, and sometimes by emergency surgery.

Surgical Treatment

Surgical resection of a bronchiectatic lobe is curative. Surgery should only be advised in patients where the bronchiectasis is localized and there is no underlying condition, which predisposes in the future to generalize bronchiectasis, as for example in primary ciliary dyskinesia. Good results are obtained after surgical resection of severe localized bronchiectasis. There is an improvement in general health, and freedom from fever, malaise, and infective episodes. Lung function is not significantly reduced as the diseased lobe contributes very little to lung function.

Every patient with localized bronchiectasis does not require surgery. Patients with mild or even moderately severe bronchiectasis do well with medical therapy—in the main, postural drainage plus the use of appropriate antibiotics during infective episodes. If, however, episodes of recurrent infection are frequent or if bronchiectasis clearly disturbs the patient's lifestyle, surgery is indicated. Surgery is also indicated, if there is repeated hemoptysis as the fear of possible massive hemoptysis in the future always exists. Massive hemoptysis is preferably treated with embolization of the culprit bronchial artery and/or of the pulmonary artery vessel, if that is responsible for the bleed. Surgical resection may be necessary as an emergency procedure, if embolization fails.

Surgery is inadvisable when the disease is not localized and involves both lungs as in cylindrical bronchiectasis, which generally involves both lower lobes. However, in patients where the disease is more generalized, surgery may still be performed as a palliative measure on a grossly diseased local area of the lung, which has not responded to medical treatment and which may act as a source for further spread of the disease.

In our opinion, a contraindication for surgery even in patients with localized bronchiectasis is the presence of significant airways' obstruction unrelieved by aerosolized or nebulized bronchodilators. These patients continue to remain symptomatic after surgery.

Lung transplantation (single lung, double lungs, and heart lung) should be considered in severe bilateral bronchiectasis not responding to medical therapy, particularly if there is chronic respiratory failure. Single-lung transplantation is considered unadvisable for fear of developing bronchiectasis in the transplant lung from the opposite bronchiectatic lung and for fear of dissemination of infection (present in the opposite bronchiectatic lung) following the use of immunosuppressants.

■ OUTCOME

A study by Keistinen et al. in the European Respiratory Journal in 1997 presented the follow-up data from the National Finnish Registry of 842 adult patients with bronchiectasis matched (age and sex) with asthmatics, COPD, and followed up for 8–12 years. There were 1–5 hospitalizations (mean 2.2) and a 28% death rate in the group with bronchiectasis (239 deaths) compared to a 20%

death rate in asthma and 38% death rate for COPD. There is unfortunately no reliable reported follow-up of patients with bronchiectasis in India.

■ SUGGESTED READING

1. Altenburg J, de Graaff CS, Stienstra Y, et al. Effect of azithromycin maintenance treatment on infectious exacerbations among patients with non-cystic fibrosis bronchiectasis: the BAT randomized controlled trial. JAMA. 2013;309:1251-9.
2. Chalmers JD, Aliberti S, Blasi F. Management of bronchiectasis in adults. Eur Respir J. 2015;45:1446.
3. Chalmers JD, Aliberti S, Blasi F. State of the art review: management of bronchiectasis in adults. Eur Respir J. 2015;45(5):1446-62.
4. Chalmers JD, Hill AT. Mechanisms of immune dysfunction and bacterial persistence in non-cystic fibrosis bronchiectasis. Mol Immunol. 2013;55:27.
5. Dimakou K, Triantafillidou C, Toumbis M, et al. Non CF-bronchiectasis: Aetiologic approach, clinical, radiological, microbiological and functional profile in 277 patients. Respir Med. 2016;116:1.
6. Gao YH, Guan WJ, Xu G, et al. The role of viral infection in pulmonary exacerbations of bronchiectasis in adults: a prospective study. Chest. 2015;147:1635.
7. Javidan-Nejad C, Bhalla S. Bronchiectasis. Radiol Clin North Am. 2009;47(2):289-306.
8. King PT, Holdsworth SR, Freezer NJ, et al. Characterization of the onset and presenting clinical features of adult bronchiectasis. Respir Med. 2006;100:2183.
9. Pasteur MC, Helliwell SM, Houghton SJ, et al. An investigation into causative factors in patients with bronchiectasis. Am J Resp Crit Care Med. 2000;162:1277-84.
10. Serisier DJ, Martin ML, McGuckin MA, et al. Effect of long-term, low-dose erythromycin on pulmonary exacerbations among patients with non-cystic fibrosis bronchiectasis: the BLESS randomized controlled trial. JAMA. 2013;309:1260-7.
11. Spencer S, Felix LM, Milan SJ, et al. Oral versus inhaled antibiotics for bronchiectasis. Cochrane Database Syst Rev. 2018;3:CD012579.
12. Wong C, Jayaram L, Karalus N, et al. Azithromycin for prevention of exacerbations in non-cystic fibrosis bronchiectasis (EMBRACE): a randomised, double-blind, placebo-controlled trial. Lancet. 2012;380:660-7.

CHAPTER 25

Lung Abscess

■ INTRODUCTION

A lung abscess is a localized area of infection causing suppurative parenchymal necrosis. A lung abscess is generally single, or may occur as multiple discrete lesions. A tuberculous cavity is excluded from the definition of a lung abscess. However, tuberculosis is an important differential diagnosis particularly in areas where this disease is highly prevalent.

■ ETIOLOGY

- Most lung abscesses are a complication of aspiration pneumonia caused by aspiration of anaerobic organisms colonizing the throat and present in the gingival crevices. Periodontal disease and bad mouth hygiene are often present in these patients. Any condition, which predisposes to aspiration, e.g. obtundation from any cause, inability to protect the airway, difficulty in swallowing, will also predispose to either an aspiration pneumonia or a lung abscess. The more frequent the aspiration and the more infected and greater the volume of the aspirate, the greater the chances of pulmonary complications. Occasionally, the pharynx is colonized by aerobic organisms, chiefly Gram-negative bacteria. This is frequently observed in very sick individuals who have been in the intensive care unit (ICU) for a length of time. Aspiration of these organisms can lead to pneumonia, followed by a lung abscess.

  Rarely, superinfection of a pulmonary infarct, or of damaged lung tissue (as after chemical inhalation injury) by aspirated anaerobes or aerobes can also result in a lung abscess.

- *Suppurative pneumonia*: Progression of pneumonic consolidation to suppurative necrosis is often associated with cavitation. Organisms, which have a potential to cause a suppurative necrosis of a consolidated lobe are *Streptococcus pneumoniae* Type III, *Staphylococcus aureus, Haemophilus influenzae*, and Gram-negative organisms such as *Klebsiella pneumoniae, Pseudomonas pyocyaneus*, and *Escherichia coli*. A lung abscess due to *Entamoeba histolytica* (generally caused by a liver abscess rupturing into the lower lobe of the right or rarely the left lung) is an important cause of a lung abscess in the tropics. In immunosuppressed individuals, *Nocardia asteroides* and fungal infections, in particular infection due to *Aspergillus* species and *Mucor* can cause a lung abscess. Chronic primary pulmonary fungal infection (histoplasmosis, coccidioidomycosis, and blastomycosis) can cause one or more cavitary lesions in patients living in areas where these fungal infections are endemic.
- *Bacteremic spread*: Organisms may reach the lung from a septic focus anywhere within the body. Bloodstream infections from any cause (e.g. an infected central venous catheter) may lead to seeding of the lungs with microorganisms and lead to one or more lung abscesses. Drug addicts who inject heroin or other drugs via the peripheral veins are particularly prone to one or more lung abscesses.
- *Septic pulmonary emboli*: Septic pulmonary emboli originating from septic thrombophlebitis anywhere within the body or septic emboli arising from vegetations on the tricuspid valve (as seen in drug addicts who use drugs through intravenous injections)

in subacute bacterial endocarditis are other causes to be reckoned with.

A unique mechanism in the formation of one or more lung abscesses is observed in Lemierre's syndrome. In this syndrome, infection in the tonsil, peritonsillar area, or pharynx spreads to involve tissue spaces in the neck and the carotid sheath, which contains the internal jugular vein. A septic thrombophlebitis of the internal jugular vein ensues. This leads to a bacteremia generally due to *Fusobacterium necrophorum*, as also to septic emboli to the lungs causing one or more abscesses.

- *Penetrating trauma* to the chest and rarely even blunt trauma to the chest can cause a lung abscess. In the former instance, infection is directly introduced into the lung; in the latter, a contusion caused by the blunt trauma may become secondarily infected.

■ PATHOLOGY

Infection from whatever route causes either a large area of consolidation or causes smaller areas of consolidation, which coalesce to form larger areas. Superadded necrosis of the involved areas is often associated with suppuration. More often than not, this consolidated, necrotic, and suppurative area opens into a draining bronchus. The patient then has purulent expectoration, which may be profuse in quantity. The abscess now communicating with a bronchus has an air-fluid level. The abscess cavity, which contains necrotic pus is lined by inflammatory granulation tissue and is surrounded by a ring of consolidated lung tissue. If it does not heal the abscess becomes chronic. If the abscess is close to the pleura it may cause an empyema or may open into the pleural space causing a pyopneumothorax and a bronchopleural fistula. Metastatic spread of infection to other sites—notably the brain (causing a cerebral abscess) is today a rare complication.

A lung abscess heals with fibrosis, which may obliterate the abscess cavity. Occasionally, a thin-walled sterile cavity remains as a sequel, the inner lining of the cavity being epithelialized or lined by fibrous tissue.

Since aspiration is the most important predisposing factor associated with a lung abscess, the abscess is most frequently situated in the posterior segment of the upper lobe, the apical segment of the lower lobes and occasionally the posterior segment of the lower lobe.

A lung abscess is considered acute, if less than 4 to 6-week-old and chronic, if it persists for a longer period.

■ CLINICAL FEATURES

An acute pyogenic lung abscess in its formative period will cause high fever with chills, severe prostration, and lassitude. A dry cough is generally present. Pleuritic pain may occur, if the abscess is close to the pleura. Once the abscess communicates with the bronchus so that the purulent necrotic secretions are coughed up, the systemic toxicity is reduced. Fever may be low grade or even absent; the patient continuing to cough up dirty, purulent, often fetid sputum. Anaerobic infection is often associated with a fetid smell in the breath and in the sputum that can be perceived from a distance.

Clinical examination reveals tachypnea of varying degree; there may be diminished movement of the chest wall overlying the abscess, and an impaired percussion note because of the surrounding consolidation. Breath sounds could be normal, diminished, or bronchial in character. Bronchial breath sounds when present are related to the surrounding consolidation. At times, the bronchial breath sounds may have a cavernous or amphoteric character. Crepitations may be heard over the involved area of the lung.

The abscess may heal if properly treated, or it may become chronic if diagnosed late or not correctly treated. A chronic lung abscess is often associated with well-marked clubbing and sometimes with pulmonary osteoarthropathy.

A lung abscess may not always be acute in onset. Over half to two-thirds have a subacute or even chronic presentation. Small frequent aspiration of infected material into the lung may lead to small areas of infective necrosis. These may slowly coalesce to form a larger area of infection plus necrosis. The onset in these patients may be insidious with low-grade fever and cough, which to start with is dry and is only later, associated with purulent expectoration. As the areas of involved lung tissue increase, symptoms may become more pronounced. A lung abscess in such patients may be diagnosed late in the natural history of the disease, the diagnosis being established by imaging studies, particularly by high-resolution computed tomography (HRCT) of the chest.

Metastatic seeding of the lung from bacteremia or from septic emboli can cause multiple areas of consolidation, with cavitation. Staphylococcal lung infection of bacteremic or embolic origin often causes multiple abscesses.

Gangrene of the Lung

Gangrene of a segment or lobe of the lung is a rare complication of fulminating necrotizing pneumonia with suppuration. Gangrene is characterized by sloughing of the involved segment or lobe due to thrombosis of both pulmonary and bronchial vessels with resulting infarction. The organisms most commonly involved are *K. pneumoniae;* other organisms implicated include *E. coli,* anaerobes, *Streptococcus pneumoniae, H. influenzae,* and *S. aureus.*

Besides the severity of the illness, the striking feature is the dreadful odor that permeates the whole ward. Though increasingly rare, pulmonary gangrene is still observed in patients with fulminant infection who have not received adequate and timely antibiotic therapy.

■ COMPLICATIONS

Complications include empyema, pyopneumothorax with a bronchopleural fistula; very rarely, there is metastatic spread of infection. Overwhelming sepsis with multiorgan failure can occur in fulminant infection, particularly in immunocompromised patients. In earlier years (five to six decades ago) a chronic lung abscess was an important cause of secondary amyloidosis. This is only rarely observed in present times.

■ IMAGING FEATURES

The chest radiograph to start with shows infiltrates, which coalesce in parts or areas of consolidation most often in segments of the lung mentioned earlier. Cavitation may occur soon or may be observed after a week or even later **(Figs. 1 and 2)**.

A chronic lung abscess appears as an irregular-shaped cavity surrounded by a ring of consolidated lung. The graduation from a "pneumonia" to a "necrotizing pneumonia" and finally to a necrotizing pneumonia communicating with a bronchus so as to produce a cavity (often with an air-fluid level) may take days or weeks.

An empyema may be observed as an associated complication in one-third of the patients. A pyopneumothorax with a bronchopleural fistula may be the presenting radiological appearance in some patients.

An HRCT of the chest may reveal one or more abscesses in a consolidated area well before these become apparent on a radiographic examination of the chest **(Figs. 3 and 4)**.

■ DIAGNOSIS

Clinical features and imaging studies provide the diagnosis. HRCT of the chest is invaluable for a thorough assessment. It may reveal features not evident on a radiographic examination. Bronchoscopy is only useful in

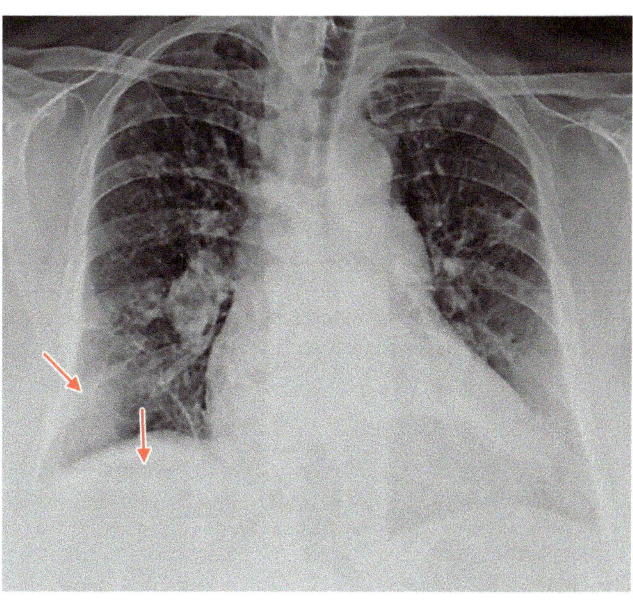

Fig. 1: Chest X-ray reveals an air fluid level in a cavitating lesion with well-defined superior margin and indistinct inferior margin in the right lower zone. This represents an abscess in right lower lobe.

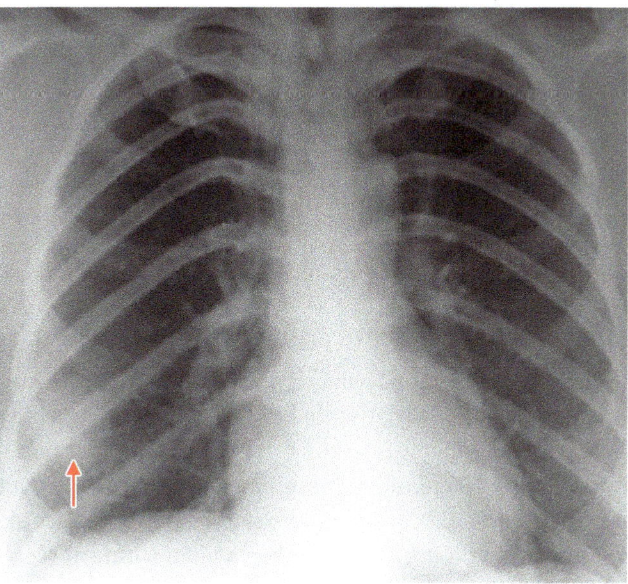

Fig. 2: Chest X-ray reveals a well-defined round nodular lesion in the right lower lobe, high-resolution computed tomography (HRCT) revealed an air-fluid level in the lesion. Computed tomography (CT)-guided aspiration revealed pus indicating a lung abscess.

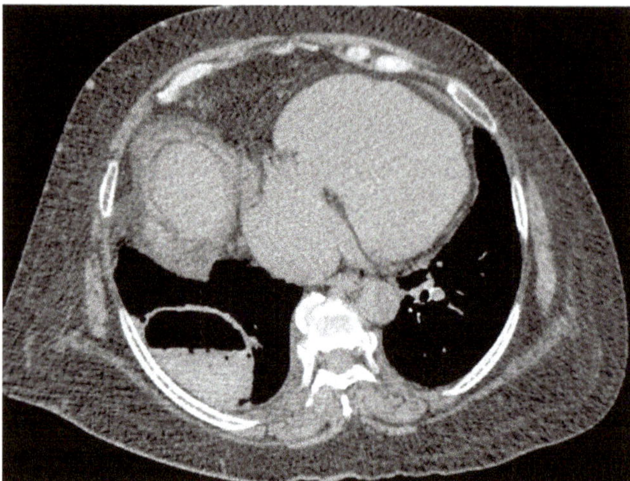

Fig. 3: Computed tomography (CT) chest demonstrates a lesion with an air-fluid level in the right hemithorax. The lesion has acute margins with the chest wall representing an abscess.

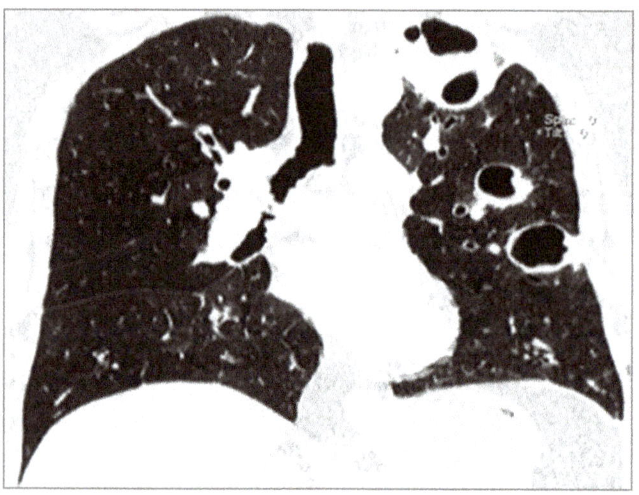

Fig. 4: High-resolution computed tomography (HRCT) chest coronal reconstruction demonstrates multiple well-defined cavities in the left lung representing multiple abscesses. These were staphylococcal in etiology and totally responded to postural drainage and antibiotics.

patients suspected of having an obstruction to a bronchus, or a neoplasm, or to determine the microbiology of a lung abscess, which persists in spite of treatment. A computed tomography (CT)-guided biopsy or a bronchoscopy with a transbronchial biopsy may be necessary to determine whether a cavitating mass is a neoplasm or a lung abscess. Blood cultures are necessary, if a lung abscess is thought to be caused by emboli from a septic thrombophlebitis or from bacterial vegetations on the tricuspid valve as is observed in drug addicts.

Microbiology

Lung abscesses are generally due to polymicrobial infections, chiefly anaerobic and facultative anaerobic bacteria that colonize the oral cavity. The most common organisms are *Peptostreptococcus*, *Prevotella*, *Bacteroides*, and *Fusobacterium* species. These reflect the anaerobic flora of the oral cavity in patients with periodontal disease and poor oral hygiene. Common nonaerobic bacteria that cause lung abscesses are the *Streptococcus anginosus* group and other facultatively anaerobic streptococci.

Other bacteria that can cause a monomicrobial lung abscess include some strains (Type III) of the pneumococcus, *Staphylococcus aureus*, *K. pneumoniae*, *Pseudomonas pyocyaneus*, other Gram-negative bacteria, *H. influenzae*, *Burkholderia pseudomallei*, and *Legionella*. Nocardial infection can also cause lung abscess. *Actinomyces* infection though rare is an easily missed cause. The epidemiology related to causative organisms may vary in different parts of the world. Thus for example *B. pseudomallei* is an important cause of lung abscess in Thailand and Southeast Asia and has also been reported in India, particularly from the Southern states of the country. Nonbacterial pathogens causing lung abscess include fungi, and parasites (*E. histolytica* and *Paragonimus westermani*).

The most common causes of lung abscess in immunocompromised patients are *Pseudomonas aeruginosa*, *K. pneumoniae*, other Gram-negative bacilli, *Nocardia*, fungi (*Aspergillus*, *Mucor*).

It is a cardinal principle that in countries like India where tuberculosis is endemic, the sputum or lower respiratory tract secretions should always be stained and cultured for acid-fast bacilli. A gene expert test on the sputum, if positive, gives an early diagnosis of tuberculosis.

◼ DIFFERENTIAL DIAGNOSIS

In the early phase before cavitation occurs, a formative lung abscess will appear as a pneumonia—either as aspiration pneumonia or a "bronchogenic" lobar or segmental consolidation.

Once a cavity appears, the differential diagnosis is from other cavitating lung pathologies. Pulmonary tuberculosis is an important differential diagnosis particularly in countries where tuberculosis has a high prevalence. Repeated negative sputum for acid-fact bacilli on smear and culture in a patient coughing up frank purulent sputum generally exclude tuberculosis.

An important differential diagnosis of a large lung abscess is a loculated empyema with an air-fluid level (*see* section on Diseases of the Pleura).

A carcinoma of the lung may present as a cavitating lesion indistinguishable from a pyogenic lung abscess. Sputum cytology should always be done particularly in a smoker. Other relevant investigations include CT-guided biopsy or a fiberoptic bronchoscopy only if thought necessary.

A subphrenic pathology, in particular an amoebic abscess should always be considered in the differential diagnosis of a lung abscess in the right lower lobe.

A pyogenic lung abscess due to the usual Gram-positive or Gram-negative infections needs to be differentiated from an abscess due to *Nocardia asteroides, Rhodococcus equi* infections and cavitary lesions caused by fungi such as histoplasma, cryptococcus, mucor or rarely by coccidioidomycosis or blastomycosis in patients living in endemic zones **(Figs. 5A and B)**.

Actinomyces infection of the lung is rare and difficult to diagnose. The appearance of chest wall sinuses discharging "sulfur granules" containing *Actinomyces* in a patient with a chronic lung abscess (often associated with an empyema) allows a definite diagnosis. A bronchoalveolar lavage (BAL) study may help to make a diagnosis when *Actinomyces* presents as a chronic lung abscess or a chronic pneumonia.

Burkholderia pseudomallei should be suspected and looked for even in India. Paragonimiasis as a cause of a cavitary lesion is an important differential diagnosis in Southeast Asia, particularly in Thailand.

Among noninfective lesions (other than lung cancer), the single most important differential diagnosis is Granulomatosis with polyangiitis (GPA) (formerly WG). A cavitary lesion, which spontaneously changes its appearance or disappears to again appear at the same or another site in the lung, is strongly indicative of Granulomatosis with polyangiitis (GPA) (formerly WG) **(Fig. 6)**.

Other causes of noninfectious cavitary disease include lymphomas and intrapulmonary nodules of rheumatoid lung disease and advanced Stage IV sarcoidosis.

■ TREATMENT

Conservative treatment in the management of a lung abscess is based on the appropriate use of antibiotics and on postural drainage to help evacuate the purulent secretions within the abscess plus physiotherapy.

As a principle, empiric antibiotic therapy should not be withheld pending result of microbiological studies on sputum or lower respiratory secretions, particularly in an acute abscess or in patients who are markedly symptomatic. The choice of antibiotic may, however,

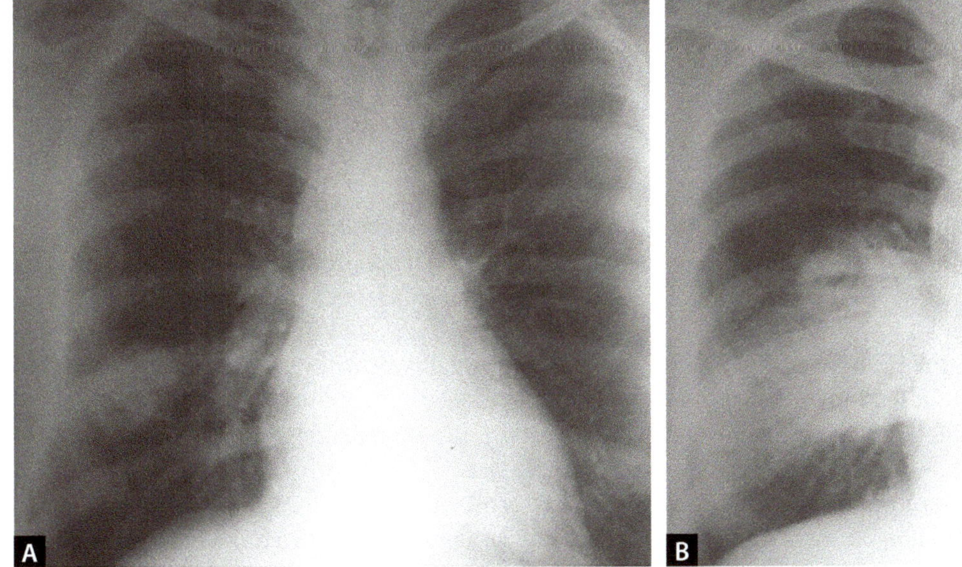

Figs. 5A and B: Cryptococcal lung abscess. (A) Chest X-ray demonstrates a small well-defined nodular lesion in the right lower lobe with internal cavitation; (B) this lesion progressed in a short time to become a large consolidation with a small nodular lesion along its superior aspect with an air-fluid level. At surgery this was a cryptococcal lung abscess.

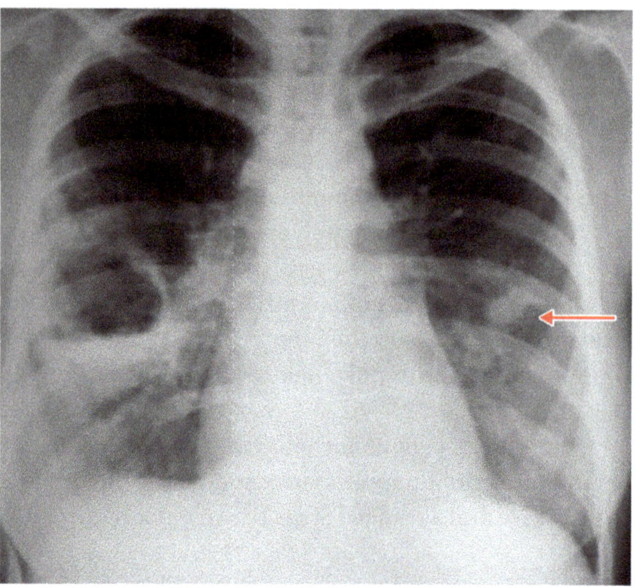

Fig. 6: Chest X-ray reveals a thick-walled cavity with an air-fluid level in the right mid-zone. Nodular lesions are seen in the left mid-zone. The chest X-ray appearances are indicative of an abscess. This patient was febrile, had a very high erythrocyte sedimentation rate (ESR) and was antineutrophil cytoplasmic antibodies (ANCA)-positive. This was due to Granulomatosis with polyangiitis (formerly called Wegener's granulomatosis). Not all air-fluid levels on a chest X-ray are lung abscesses.

need to be altered once culture sensitivity reports are available.

In an acute lung abscess, presenting with severe systemic symptoms, it is important to cover strict anaerobes, facultatively anaerobic streptococci plus important Gram-positive and Gram-negative aerobic bacteria. A reasonable combination is a beta-lactam–beta-lactamase inhibitor (e.g. piperacillin tazobactam 4.5 g IV every 8 hours or a carbapenem (e.g. meropenem 1 g 8 hourly). Either of these two antibiotics would cover most beta-lactamase producing Gram-negative organisms as well.

Clindamycin 600 mg IV every 8 hours followed after 2 weeks by 150–300 mg orally three to four times a day can also be used for anaerobic infections but has the disadvantage of having a greater propensity to cause a *Clostridium difficile* infection.

The use of metronidazole as monotherapy in the treatment of an anaerobic putrid lung abscess has been disappointing with an approximate 50% failure rate. This is probably related to the concurrent presence of facultative anaerobic streptococci that also contribute toward the pathology. If used, it should be combined with an antibiotic, which is a beta-lactam–beta-lactamase inhibitor.

Targeted Therapy

The empiric regimes stated above are appropriate for patients with a mixed anaerobic and streptococcal lung abscess. In a clearly putrid lung abscess, an anaerobic cover must be provided even if an anaerobic organism has not grown on culture. Anaerobes are notoriously difficult to culture.

Once a single organism has been isolated from a culture of the lower respiratory secretions, therapy should be targeted to that organism, choosing the best antibiotic from the sensitivity tests available. This is particularly important for Gram-negative bacilli (e.g. *Klebsiella, Ps. aeruginosa*). Many clinicians would target each of these two organisms with two antibiotics to which these organisms are susceptible.

Duration

Therapy should be continued till such time as symptoms resolve and the chest X-ray shows a small stable residual lesion or is clear. This may take 6–12 weeks of treatment, a good part of which in most cases can be completed by appropriate oral therapy on an outpatient basis.

Response to Therapy

Response to therapy is generally evident within 7–10 days. Fever continuing beyond 10–15 days clearly indicates a lack of response. The patient needs to be reevaluated. Failure to response should suggest the following possibilities:
- Incorrect choice of antibiotics;
- Bronchial obstruction from a foreign body (a supari is an important cause) or a neoplasm;
- A cavitating neoplasm;
- Resistant organisms or unsuspected organisms like fungi;
- Parasites, *Legionella, B. pseudomallei, Nocardia;*
- Tuberculosis;
- Thick loculated pus within the abscess cavity, which has not communicated with a bronchus;
- Poor penetration of antibiotics into the infected lung tissue;
- Presence of a complicating empyema.

Surgical intervention; surgery is indicated:
- If response to conservative management is poor and if the clinical condition worsens;
- In a large abscess, though it is surprising how even very large abscesses can heal on conservative management;
- Severe uncontrolled hemoptysis and bleeding;
- Bronchial obstruction due to tumor or foreign body preventing drainage of abscess contents.

In patients who are very poor surgical risks, percutaneous drainage via catheter with a sufficiently large bore may serve as a temporary measure. Spillage of the abscess content into the pleura during the above procedure may, however, prove disastrous.

Role of Bronchoscopy

If the patient is unable to cough up infected material within the abscess cavity, bronchoscopic drainage, if carefully done may help. This procedure, however, poses the great danger of spillage into healthy areas of the same lung or into the opposite lung leading at times to a serious respiratory crisis. However in critically ill patients who develop a lung abscess distal to a partial bronchial obstruction, bronchoscopic drainage could be life-saving.

■ OUTCOME

Comorbid diseases play an important role in determining the outcome. The patient with no comorbid state who develops a lung abscess has a cure rate of more than 90%, if treated with the appropriate antibiotics. Immunocompromised patients and patients with an obstructed bronchus have mortality rates as high or more than 70%.

■ SUGGESTED READING

1. Bartlett JG. Anaerobic bacterial pleuropulmonary infections. Semin Respir Med. 1992;13:159.
2. Fernandez-Sabe N, Carratala J, Dorca J, et al. Efficacy and safety of sequential amoxicillin-clavulanate in the treatment of anaerobic lung infections. Eur J Clin Microbiol Infect Dis. 2003;22:185.
3. Herth F, Ernst A, Becker HD. Endoscopic drainage of lung abscesses: technique and outcome. Chest. 2005;127: 1378.
4. Hirshberg B, Sklair-Levi M, Nir-Paz R, et al. Factors predicting mortality of patients with lung abscess. Chest. 1999;115:746.
5. Podbielski FJ, Rodriguez HE, Wiesman IM, et al. Pulmonary parenchymal abscess: VATS approach to diagnosis and treatment. Asian Cardiovasc Thorac Ann. 2001;9:339-41.
6. Schweigert M, Dubecz A, Stadlhuber RJ, et al. Modern history of surgical management of lung abscess: from Harold Neuhof to current concepts. Ann Thorac Surg. 2011;92:2293-7.
7. Seo H, Cha SI, Shin KM, et al. Focal necrotizing pneumonia is a distinct entity from lung abscess. Respirology. 2013;18:1095-100.
8. Takayanagi N, Kagiyama N, Ishiguro T, et al. Etiology and outcome of community-acquired lung abscess. Respiration. 2010;80(2):98-105.
9. Yazbeck MF, Dahdel M, Kalra A, et al. Lung abscess: update on microbiology and management. Am J Ther. 2014;21:217-21.

CHAPTER 26

Upper Respiratory Tract Infections

■ SINUSITIS

The paranasal sinuses include the maxillary, frontal, ethmoidal and sphenoidal sinuses. The sinuses are lined by respiratory ciliated epithelium and mucus-producing goblet cells. The ciliated cells move the mucus toward the sinus ostia and from there to the nasopharynx.

■ ACUTE SINUSITIS

The most common cause of an acute sinusitis is a viral infection (e.g. a common cold) which inflames the ciliated epithelium, damages cilia and ciliary movement, obstructs sinus ostia thereby preventing drainage and promoting infection.

Acute allergic rhinitis can also cause sinusitis through mucosal edema with ostial obstruction from edema or from nasal polyps.

Any pathology in the nose or the paranasal sinus or sinuses that blocks ostial drainage can do likewise, e.g. deviated nasal septum, tumor, granulomas, nasogastric or nasotracheal tubes. The organisms causing sinusitis in the above instances are generally bacteria—the *Haemophilus influenzae, Streptococcus pneumoniae* and occasionally gram-negative bacteria. Acute maxillary sinusitis can also occur as a result of spread of infection from infected second bicuspid premolar tooth or infected first, or second molars.

Community-acquired bacterial sinusitis is generally due to *H. influenzae* infection or *S. pneumoniae* and occasionally *Staphylococcus aureus. Moraxella catarrhalis* infection is reported to be more common in children.

Clinical Features

Clinical features consist of nasal congestion, purulent nasal discharge, postnasal drip often causing cough, and sinus pain. The location of pain depends on the sinus involved. Maxillary sinusitis produces pain over the cheek and upper teeth with tenderness on pressure over the maxilla. Frontal sinusitis produces pain over the frontal area and the supraorbital ridges which may be tender on pressure. Infection of the ethmoids causes pain over the bridge of the nose on either side; sphenoidal sinusitis causes retro-orbital pain, occipital pain or pain over the vertex of the head. Purulent sinusitis can produce fever, malaise and leukocytosis.

A differential diagnosis from an acute viral upper respiratory infection is difficult as identical symptoms may occur in the latter.

An X-ray of the paranasal sinuses is helpful only if there is well-nigh complete sinus opacification or mucosal thickening of at least 4 mm. Sinusitis may be present without these findings (**Fig. 1**). A *computed tomography* (CT) of the sinuses is far more sensitive than routine radiography and is essential for diagnosis of sphenoidal or ethmoidal sinusitis (**Fig. 2**).

Nasal endoscopy (done by an otolaryngologist) reveals purulent secretions from the sinus ostia.

Treatment

Amoxicillin-clavulanate or cefuroxime given orally for 8–10 days generally controls infection. Steam inhalation and decongestant nasal drops help sinus drainage. If thick pus is formed within a sinus, surgical drainage is necessary. Surgical attention is also necessary when orbital cellulitis occurs as a complication of sinusitis.

■ CHRONIC BACTERIAL SINUSITIS

Chronic bacterial sinusitis is characterized by pain, fullness and heaviness over the sinuses (at the sites mentioned) for

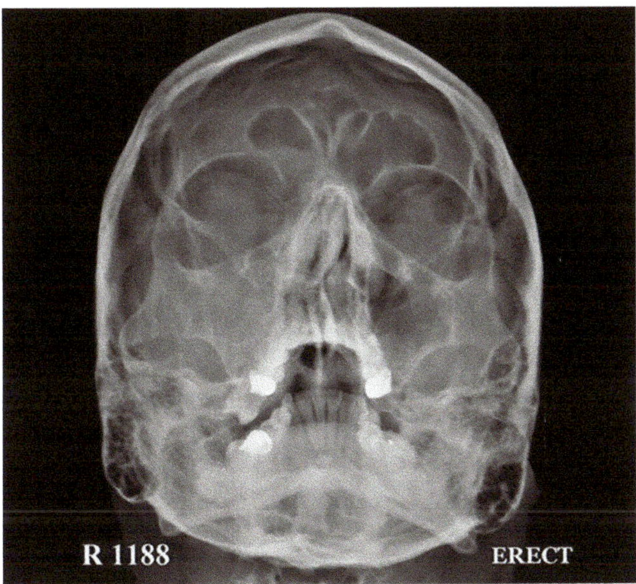

Fig. 1: Sinusitis. Plain X-ray of sinuses; total opacification of the right maxillary sinus due to sinusitis.

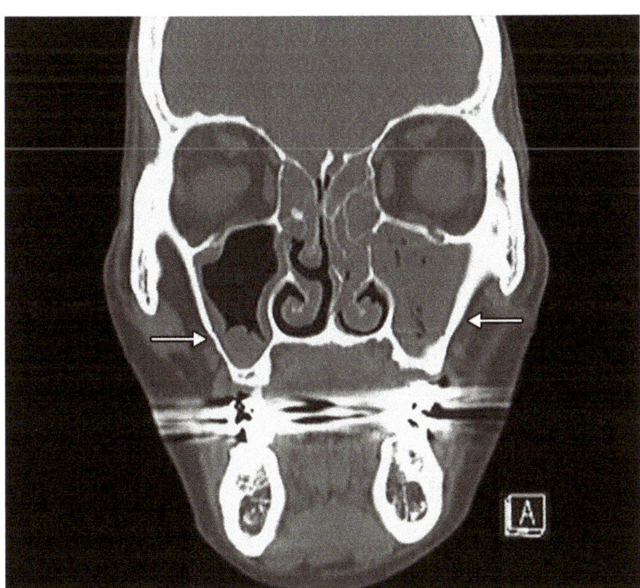

Fig. 2: Coronal CT scan reveals mucosal thickening of the right maxillary sinus, soft tissue opacifying ethmoid, frontal, and left maxillary sinuses. Specks of air are seen in the left maxillary sinus. These changes are due to acute sinusitis.

days, weeks, or months. There is purulent discharge which may occur intermittently from the nose, a postnasal drip causing an inflamed pharynx and larynx, a foul odor and taste and a feeling of malaise and fatigability. A low-grade

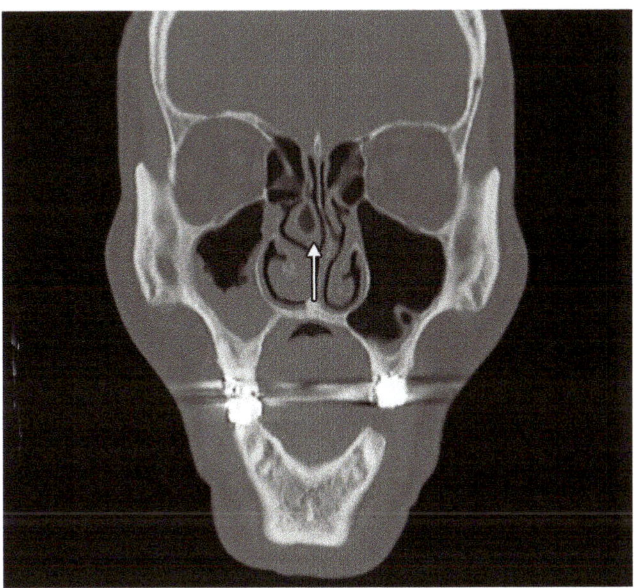

Fig. 3: Chronic sinusitis. Coronal CT reveals pneumatization of the right middle turbinate (arrow) causing narrowing of the right maxillary ostium with resultant right maxillary mucosal thickening in the right maxillary sinus.

evening rise of fever may be present. The above features may occur episodically or persist in a smoldering form with periodic exacerbations.

A CT of the sinuses is important not just to define the sinus or sinuses involved but to define the extent of the disease and to determine if there is any organic pathology blocking the sinus ostia and causing a chronic sinusitis **(Figs. 3 and 4)**. The patient should also be evaluated by an ear-nose-throat (ENT) specialist with the same objectives. Obstruction to the sinus ostia can result from a deviated septum, large nasal polyps, granulomas such as sarcoid or Wegener's granulomatosis and cancers in the region of the nose and sinuses. Impaired mucociliary clearance from whatever cause results in chronic or recurrent sinusitis and recurrent or chronic bronchial infection. Primary ciliary dyskinesia (described under bronchiectasis) is a rare autosomal recessive condition with incomplete penetration which causes both sinusitis and bronchiectasis. Cystic fibrosis is generally associated with chronic sinusitis. Kartagener's syndrome (dextrocardia, sinusitis, bronchiectasis, infertility, with or without situs inversus) has been mentioned under bronchiectasis.

Culture of pus discharged from the nose may identify pathogens. Blind nasal swabs may grow organisms which may be colonizers. Fungal culture, in particular

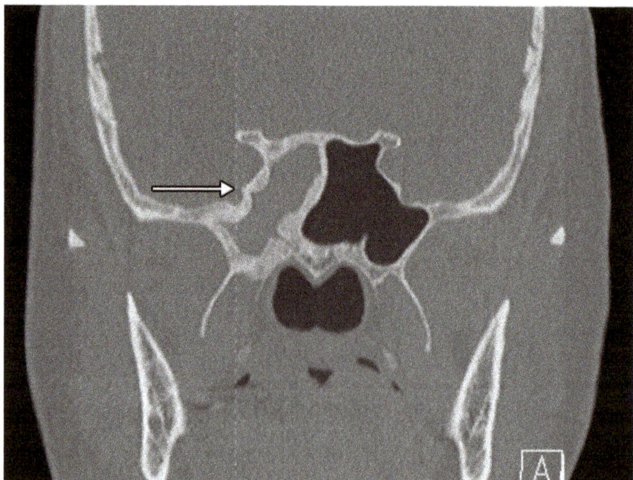

Fig. 4: Coronal computed tomography (CT) demonstrates soft tissue in the right sphenoid sinus with thickening of its walls. The bony thickening is secondary to chronic sinusitis.

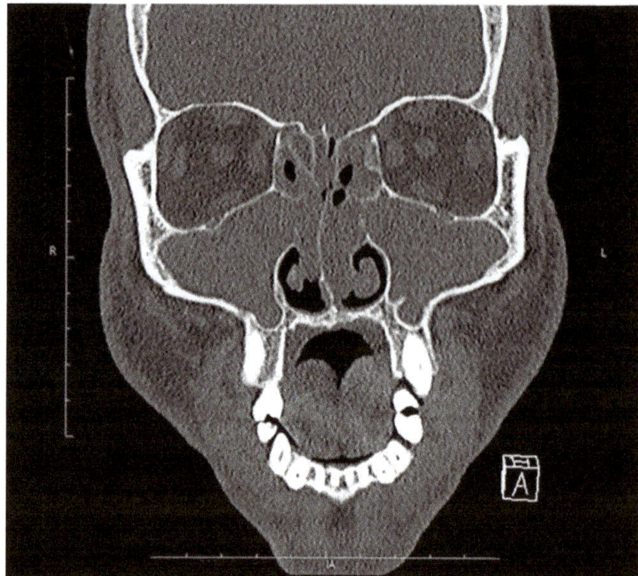

Fig. 5: Extensive soft tissue in the paranasal sinuses, especially ethmoids with extension into nasal cavity, disruption of ethmoidal bones causing obstruction to maxillary ostium and resultant soft tissue in maxillary sinuses. These appearances of soft tissue involving all sinuses, disrupting ethmoidal bones and extending into nasal cavity are typical of *Aspergillus* infection.

for *Aspergillus*, must always be asked for in chronic or recurrent sinusitis. Treatment is the same as for acute sinusitis. Drainage of pus may be necessary. A specialist ENT opinion must be sought.

Complications of Bacterial Sinusitis

The most important complications are preseptal cellulitis and deeper orbital infections both grouped under orbital cellulitis. They both generally occur following ethmoidal sinusitis since the ethmoids are separated from the orbit by just a thin plate of bone. Preseptal cellulitis only involves the eyelids and surrounding structures. The eyelid appears swollen but there is neither restriction of eye movements nor any orbital signs. Orbital cellulitis may go on to graduate into an orbital abscess, causing proptosis, chemosis of the conjunctiva and disturbed vision. When it follows upon an ethmoidal sinusitis, the eye is deviated downward and outward. If treatment is delayed, vision is invariably lost.

Organisms involved are generally *S. pneumoniae*, group A streptococcus and *H. influenzae*. Antibiotics should be given intravenously, providing a broad cover for these organisms.

A CT scan should be done in the presence of even suspicious orbital findings. An orbital abscess necessitates urgent surgical drainage.

Frontal and sphenoidal sinusitis can lead to intracranial complications. These include epidural abscess, subdural abscess, and dural vein thrombosis. Sphenoidal sinusitis can occasionally lead to thrombophlebitis of the cavernous sinus because of the proximity of the latter to the sphenoid sinus.

◼ FUNGAL SINUSITIS

Fungal sinusitis can occur in three forms: (1) sinus aspergilloma, (2) allergic fungal sinusitis, and (3) invasive fungal sinusitis **(Figs. 5 and 6)**.

Sinus Aspergilloma

Sinus aspergilloma is a noninvasive fungal disease occurring as a fungal ball in the maxillary sinus. It causes the usual features of chronic sinusitis often affecting the maxillary sinus. Surgical removal of the aspergilloma ball is curative.

Allergic Fungal Aspergillosis

Allergic fungal aspergillosis is characterized by a hypersensitivity reaction to fungi ubiquitous in the environment and in nasal mucosa where the fungus is trapped following inhalation. The condition is characterized by all the features

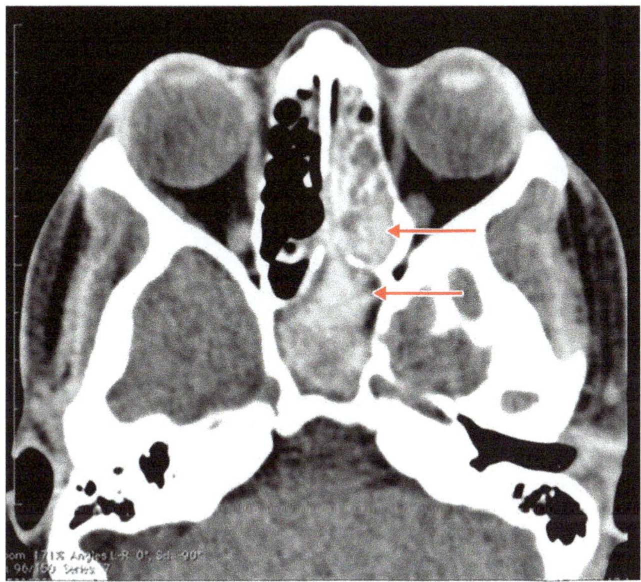

Fig. 6: Axial computed tomography (CT) scan of paranasal sinuses reveals soft tissue in the left anterior and posterior ethmoidal cells as well as in the sphenoid sinuses with internal hyperdensity. The internal hyperdensity is indicative of *Aspergillus* infection.

of chronic sinusitis, nasal discharge, blocked nose and sinus pain. There is often a background history of nasal polyps and bronchial asthma. A CT shows inhomogeneous opacification of one or more sinuses. Bone erosion may be present but this is due to pressure necrosis and not actual invasion. Allergic fungal sinusitis is on par with allergic bronchopulmonary aspergillosis; the former is a hypersensitivity reaction within the sinus and the latter a hypersensitivity reaction in the conducting airways and the lung. The incriminating fungus is invariably *Aspergillus fumigatus.*

The condition is often diagnosed at surgery because sinus secretions are characteristically thick, sticky and brownish (likened to anchovy sauce). Fungal hyphae may be present but there is no evidence of tissue invasion. Fungal cultures most frequently grow *Aspergillus* species. A short course of corticosteroids given over 15 days often serves to clear the allergic fungal sinusitis just as a similar course relieves the clinical features of allergic bronchopulmonary aspergillosis.

Invasive Fungal Sinusitis

Invasive fungal sinusitis carries a high risk of mortality. Mortality is even further increased if the immune state of the patient is impaired and if the ethmoids or sphenoid sinuses are involved because of the proximity of the latter to the orbit, the cavernous sinus and intracranial structures.

■ RHINOCEREBRAL MUCORMYCOSIS

Invasion of the nasal mucosa and of one or more paranasal sinuses by the molds of the order Mucorales (*Mucor, Rhizopus*) is the most devastating invasive fungal infection. Seventy percent of infections occur in diabetics. Other risk factors are immunocompromised patients, the use of immunosuppressants, oral corticosteroids, hematological malignancies and organ transplant patients.

Clinical Features

Early clinical features consist of a swelling around both eyelids of one eye, a purplish discolouration generally of the skin of the lower eyelid, conjunctival injection and pain over the frontal and temporal areas (**Figs. 7A and B**). The clinical features very quickly progress to resemble those of orbital cellulitis. There is proptosis of the eye, limitation of eye movements, diminished vision in the eye that may progress to blindness. Hypoesthesia may be present in the distribution of ophthalmic and maxillary divisions of the trigeminal nerve. Necrotic blisters or eschars may be present over the skin of the eyelid and over the site of the alae nasi, also involving the mucosa of the external nares. Invasion of the neuraxis and spread to the cavernous sinus with cavernous sinus thrombosis can well occur.

Nasal endoscopy shows friable mucosa with black eschars which signifies infarction of the mucosa of the nose and sinuses. Biopsy of the eschars and surrounding friable mucosa shows nonseptal hyphae invading tissue, blood vessels and nerves.

A CT of the paranasal sinuses shows sinusitis with bone erosion and destruction and with varying degree of invasion of the orbit (**Figs. 7C and D**). Absence of eschar does not exclude the diagnosis; biopsy of the mucosa may still reveal the typical nonseptal hyphae of *Mucor.*

Treatment

Treatment consists of extensive surgical debridement of all infected tissue. This may need to be repeated as often as necessary. Amphotericin or lyophilized amphotericin 5–7.5 mg/kg/day over 2 hours intravenously for 10–15 days is the treatment of choice. Voriconazole is of no use against *Mucor.* Posaconazole is a new antifungal that has been used in patients not responding to amphotericin.

Unless diagnosed very early in the natural history of the disease, the prognosis is indeed very grim. Death invariably occurs (with few exceptions), particularly in immunocompromised patients.

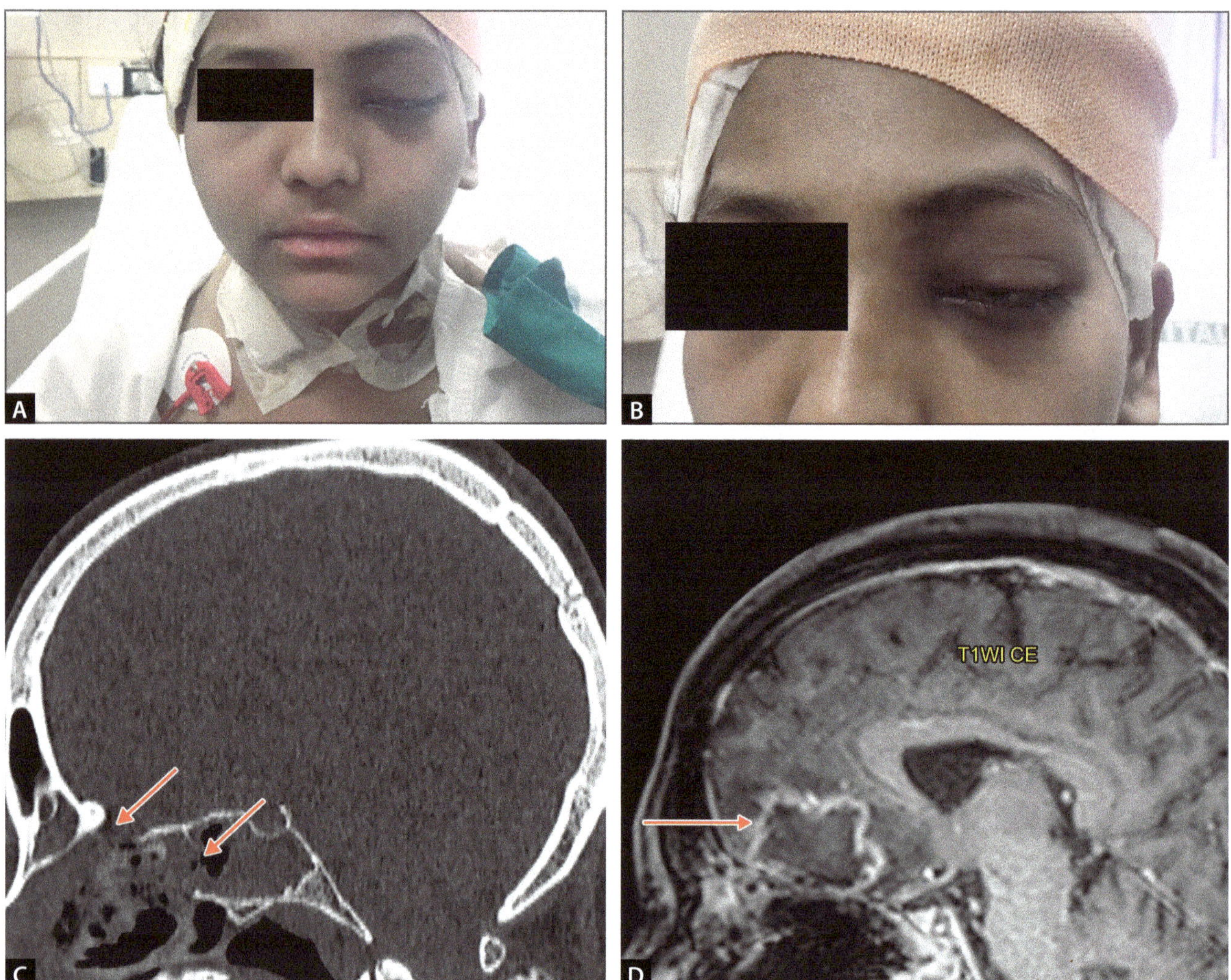

Figs. 7A to D: (A and B) A young girl with uncontrolled diabetes presents with rhinocerebral mucormycosis; (C) Sagittal CT of PNS shows soft tissue in right ethmoidal air cells and right sphenoid sinus with osseous erosions; (D) Sagittal T-1 weighted image reveals altered signal intensity lesion in the right basi-frontal region with peripheral contrast enhancement and destruction of right cribriform plate.

◼ OTHER FUNGI CAUSING INVASIVE SINUSITIS

Other fungi may also cause invasive fungal sinusitis. The most important and the most frequent fungus to do so belongs to the *Aspergillus* species. Again it is the immunocompromised host who is most frequently infected where the onset and course is acute and is as described above. Rarely, invasive *Aspergillus* infection of the nasal mucosa and of the sinuses can occur in normal hosts. Symptoms of orbital cellulitis as described above may evolve subacutely over weeks.

Involvement of the ethmoidal or sphenoidal sinuses by either *Mucor* or *Aspergillus* or other fungi carries the highest mortality. Invasive fungal inflammation spreads quickly to the apex of the orbit with involvement of the second, third, fifth, and sixth nerves. Severe pain, proptosis, and diminished vision quickly leading to blindness is observed. There is ptosis, restricted eye movements and hypoesthesia over the ophthalmic and maxillary divisions of the fifth nerve. Spread to the cavernous sinus is common because of close proximity to the sphenoid and ethmoid sinuses. Fungal invasion of the meninges and the neuraxis is also observed. Death invariably results.

Computed tomography and magnetic resonance imaging show invasion of the sinuses with involvement of the orbit, particularly at the apex. Diagnosis is made by demonstrating fungal invasion of tissue by biopsy.

Treatment

Voriconazole given intravenously is useful for invasive *Aspergillus* infection. It should be given for over 3 weeks and then continued orally. Extensive surgical debridement should be done early in immunocompromised patients. Medical treatment may alone suffice in immunocompetent patients if the disease is diagnosed early.

■ TRACHEOBRONCHITIS

Acute tracheobronchitis is characterized by inflammation of the mucosa of the trachea and bronchi. Mucosal inflammation of the trachea alone is termed tracheitis and of the bronchi is called bronchitis.

Tracheobronchitis is most often due to a viral infection. The viruses most frequently involved being the rhinovirus, coronavirus, influenza virus and adenovirus. Secondary bacterial infection may follow in the wake of a viral infection and is generally due to *H. influenzae* or *S. pneumoniae*. Mycoplasmal infection can be a primary cause of a tracheobronchitis; occasionally, infection is due to *Bordetella pertussis.*

Clinical features consist of fever, cough which may be dry or productive of mucoid sputum. Tracheitis when severe causes substernal tightness and soreness; coughing produces a sharp burning discomfort in the chest. Rhonchi are generally audible on auscultation. Secondary bacterial infection causes the sputum to turn purulent.

Acute viral tracheobronchitis is self-limiting and requires no specific therapy. Symptomatic relief is provided by steam inhalation and oral paracetamol. The presence of secondary bacterial infection may require the use of an antibiotic, particularly in the presence of high fever and other systemic manifestations. Amoxicillin-clavulanate is usually the drug of choice. Severe tracheobronchitis due to a mycoplasmal infection is best treated with a quinolone or a macrolide. Culture of tracheobronchial secretions for *B. pertussis* is necessary if the cough is persistent, paroxysmal or has a clear whoop often followed by vomiting.

■ LARYNGITIS

Laryngitis may be associated with rhinitis or with tracheobronchitis. It is generally due to a viral infection.

Cough which causes pain in the throat and over the pharynx and is accompanied by a hoarse sound points to the diagnosis. Dysphonia or total loss of voice may be present. Systemic features in the form of mild fever may also be noted. A codeine linctus offers symptomatic relief of cough.

Rest to the voice, steam inhalation, lozenges to soothe the throat, warm salt water gargles and symptomatic use of paracetamol offer relief.

Laryngitis that persists needs a careful laryngoscopic examination. Tuberculosis is an important cause. Besides hoarseness of the voice, there is pain over the larynx on swallowing. Tuberculous laryngitis is usually but not always associated with pulmonary tuberculosis. A laryngeal swab is invariably positive for acid-fast bacilli both on staining and culture.

Hoarseness of the voice with discomfort in the throat put down to laryngitis may be the first symptom of a laryngeal cancer involving the vocal cord or the arytenoid region.

Hoarseness of the voice wrongly diagnosed as laryngitis can also result from paralysis of the recurrent laryngeal nerve from various causes. Myxedema may cause a hoarse voice with throat discomfort and may be mistaken as laryngitis. Syphilis as a cause of laryngitis is now very rarely seen.

The dictum should be that a "laryngitis" that persists or is chronic needs an overall review and a laryngoscopic examination.

■ CROUP

"Croup" is the term given to an acute laryngotracheo-bronchitis characterized by subglottic edema. It occurs in children between 3 months and 4 years of age generally in the winter months and in early spring. The disease is most often due to the parainfluenza type 1 virus. Other viruses known to cause croup are the influenza virus, adenovirus, rhinovirus, enterovirus. Rarely, it is due to *Mycoplasma pneumoniae.*

Clinical features include fever, a persistent cough which has the timbre of a "bark" and a stridor due to subglottic edema. The stridor is inspiratory or both inspiratory and expiratory. The course of the illness is often fluctuating with periods of worsening alternating, within hours, with periods of improvement.

The diagnosis is based on clinical grounds. A viral etiology can be proven by using one of the rapid viral antigen detection techniques on nasopharyngeal swabs. The most important differential diagnosis is from acute epiglottitis. The latter is not associated with a "barking" cough. Children with acute epiglottitis are more toxic and ill and worsen rapidly.

Treatment

Treatment consists of nebulizing racemic epinephrine which gives prompt relief. Rebound subglottic edema needs to be carefully watched for. Corticosteroids are also of use. Nebulization of humidified air has also been tried but is of doubtful use.

◼ ACUTE EPIGLOTTITIS

Acute epiglottitis is a life-threatening respiratory emergency as it can cause quick upper airways obstruction and death unless promptly recognized and treated. The condition chiefly seen in children is characterized by a cellulitis at the base of the tongue and the base of the epiglottis. It then involves the epiglottis itself which is swollen, pushed backward so that it quickly obstructs the airways. The disease is rare in children vaccinated against *H. influenzae* type B. In poor developing countries, vaccination against *H. influenzae* is the exception rather than the rule. It therefore still occurs; its prevalence though uncommon is not determined. Epiglottitis can also occur in adults, the most common cause being infection due to *H. influenzae*. Other infectious agents known to cause epiglottitis are *S. pneumoniae*, group A streptococci, *S. aureus*, and *Haemophilus parainfluenzae*.

Clinical Features

Symptoms evolve rapidly within 6–12 hours and in children are characterized by fever, toxemia, sore throat, cough (which lacks the barking character of croup), difficulty in swallowing with drooling of saliva. Upper airways obstruction causes difficulty in breathing so that the child prefers to sit up, is tachypneic with an inspiratory stridor.

Adolescents and adults have a less fulminant course, symptoms being present for 2–4 days. Fever, sore

throat, cough, dysphagia, and difficulty in breathing due to an obstructed airway are the usual symptoms. A flexible fiberoptic nasopharyngoscopy reveals a swollen erythematous epiglottis. A throat swab culture should be obtained to identify the infecting organism.

Treatment

The airway must necessarily be secured and maintained. This is done by immediate insertion of an endotracheal or nasotracheal tube after the child is promptly transported (in a sitting position) to the operation theater of a hospital. If intubation is not possible, a tracheostomy needs to be urgently performed.

Adults who have no impending obstruction should be carefully observed. Broad-spectrum antibiotics (amoxicillin-clavulanate) should be given intravenously for *H. influenzae* infection.

If epiglottitis is due to or is suspected to be caused by *H. influenzae* infection, the patient and all members of the family should be given rifampicin prophylaxis to eradicate carriage of the organism.

◼ SUGGESTED READING

1. Ames WA, Ward VM, Tranter RM, et al. Adult epiglottitis: an under-recognized, life-threatening condition. Br J Anaesth. 2000;85(5):795-7.
2. Brook I. Acute and chronic bacterial sinusitis. Infect Dis Clin North Am. 2007;21(2):427-48, vii.
3. deShazo RD, Chapin K, Swain RE. Fungal sinusitis. N Engl J Med. 1997;337:254-9.
4. Frantz TD, Rasgon BM, Quesenberry CP Jr. Acute epiglottitis in adults. Analysis of 129 cases. JAMA. 1994;272:1358-60.
5. Piccirillo JF. Clinical practice. Acute bacterial sinusitis. N Engl J Med. 2004;351:902-10.
6. Reveiz L, Cardona AF, Ospina EG. Antibiotics for acute laryngitis in adults. Cochrane Database Syst Rev. 2007;2:CD004783.
7. Rosenfeld RM, Piccirillo JF, Chandrasekhar SS, et al. Clinical practice guideline (update): adult sinusitis. Otolaryngol Head Neck Surg. 2015;152(2 Suppl):S1-S39.
8. Spellberg B, Walsh TJ, Kontoyiannis DP, et al. Recent advances in the management of mucormycosis: from bench to bedside. Clin Infe Dis. 2009;48(12):1743-51.

Antibiotic Resistance and its Management

CHAPTER 27

Antibiotic Resistance and its Management

■ INTRODUCTION

Antibiotic resistance is increasing at a dizzying pace today—a remarkable testimony to the ability of bacteria to collect and exchange resistance genes with unimaginable efficiency. The basic mechanisms of bacterial resistance are well-known. These encompass four general mechanisms, namely drug inactivation, altered target, decreased permeability, and multidrug efflux. The earlier challenges that bacterial resistance posed, were well-matched by the discovery of newer molecules by the pharmaceutical industry. Critical new aspects with major implications for emergence, dissemination and maintenance of resistance include hypermutability, integrons and plasmid addiction. Globally, today, the situation has changed and with far fewer therapeutic alternatives for effective treatment, antimicrobial resistance is becoming a major concern. Resistant organisms are associated with greater morbidity and mortality and are certainly impacting the current practice of medicine. Traditionally, infections are different in both hospitals and in the community as they represent different ecosystems and different operational antibiotic selective pressures. This distinction is now becoming blurred. Infections caused by the *ESKAPE* pathogens (*Enterococcus faecium, Staphylococcus aureus, Klebsiella pneumoniae, Acinetobacter baumannii, Pseudomonas aeruginosa, and Enterobacter spps.)* effectively *escape* antibacterial drugs both in hospitals and the community.

From a community perspective, upper respiratory tract infections (URTIs) are probably the most inappropriately treated group of infections. Partly due to the unavailability of cost-effective diagnostic tests to differentiate common viral infections from *Streptococcus pyogenes,* physicians would rather 'cover for bacterial infection' with broad-spectrum antibiotics. Similarly, the leading cause of lower respiratory tract infections (LRTIs) is *Streptococcus pneumoniae* and despite reassuring data that pneumococcal resistance in the Indian subcontinent is not alarming at all, broad-spectrum cephalosporin antibiotics rather than oral amoxicillin are prescribed for a variety of reasons.

■ RESISTANCE IN SPECIFIC RESPIRATORY COMMUNITY PATHOGENS

Streptococcus pneumoniae

Penicillin resistance in *S. pneumoniae* is caused by reduced affinity binding of the β-lactams to the penicillin-binding proteins (PBP). Pneumococcal resistance can occur by homologous recombination of the six PBP genes. PBP2b is the primary resistance determinant for penicillin resistance whereas PBP2x is the primary determinant for cephalosporin resistance. Oral streptococci have been postulated to be the major reservoir for the novel DNA required to create the mosaic genetic sequences demonstrated by the altered pneumococcal PBP genes. Penicillin-resistant strains are resistant to penicillin derivatives, such as ampicillin and the ureidopenicillins, and are generally resistant to first- and second-generation cephalosporins. Cefotaxime and ceftriaxone are often effective because of their high-levels of activity and because of the high tissue levels attained. At present, in India, penicillin, macrolide and fluoroquinolone resistance is reassuringly low, but resistance to co-trimoxazole is alarming. This is in stark contrast to other parts of the world including India's immediate neighbors, where alarming rates of resistance are reported.

A debate is ongoing as to whether infections caused by resistant strains are really associated with poorer outcomes than infections caused by susceptible strains. As a consequence, the Clinical and Laboratory Standards Institute (CLSI) in 2008 revised the parenteral penicillin breakpoints with separate categories for meningeal isolates (S <0.06 µg/mL and raised the breakpoints for nonmeningeal isolates (S < 2 µg/mL and R >8 µg/mL). With this change in interpretive standards, *in vitro* penicillin resistance decreased and does not seem to be a major problem in nonmeningeal isolates. However, penicillin-resistant strains are frequently resistant to non-β-lactam antimicrobial agents and are often multidrug resistant. Resistance to erythromycin, tetracycline, co-trimoxazole, and chloramphenicol are the most common. Macrolide resistance is the most prominent example of pneumococcal resistance with regard to prevalence rate and the level of resistance. A recent surveillance study in the United States shows that prevalence of macrolide resistance in *S. pneumoniae* is approximately 26%. The most common mechanism of macrolide resistance in *S. pneumoniae* is caused by target-site modification encoded by erythromycin ribosome methylation (erm) genes that cause inducible cross-resistance to all macrolides, lincosamides, and streptogramin B. Two other mechanisms of resistance to macrolides include active efflux pump encoded by efflux genes (me/A, *mefE)* that result in resistance to macrolides alone (M phenotype); and ribosomal mutations in the *23S rRNA* gene.

Fluoroquinolone resistance has developed during therapy, especially in patients with prior fluoroquinolone exposures, leading to clinical failure. The older fluoroquinolones (for example, ciprofloxacin) lack reliable activity against pneumococci. Newer fluoroquinolones, such as levofloxacin, moxifloxacin, and gemifloxacin, inhibit most strains at achievable levels. The mechanism of decreased susceptibility to the newer fluoroquinolones is primarily due to mutations in the *parC* gene of topoisomerase IV and the *gyrA* gene of DNA gyrase. However, in the era of MDR/XDR tuberculosis, it is best in poor developing countries to reserve fluoroquinolones for the management of drug-resistant TB.

Haemophilus influenzae

Haemophilus influenzae-related respiratory infections are on the rise the world over. Recognition of nonencapsulated strains as causative agents in acute exacerbations of chronic obstructive pulmonary disease is compelling. In India, *H. influenzae* is not often isolated by microbiology laboratories and thus resistance rates are not clearly defined. In a multicenter study in India, the incidence of β-lactamase production in *Haemophilus* spps. in LRTIs was noted to be 17.2%. Approximately 90% of β-lactamase-producing *H. influenzae* possess the constitutive plasmid TEM-1 enzyme. These isolates are resistant to amoxicillin but remain fully susceptible to the β-lactam or β-lactamase inhibitor combinations. The cephalosporins vary in their activity against the β-lactamase-producing strains. The third-generation cephalosporins are most active and some second-generation cephalosporins such as cefaclor and cefprozil are the least active. Non-β-lactamase-producing strains with altered PBPs are infrequently isolated. *H. influenzae* is usually resistant to erythromycin but susceptible *in vitro* to azithromycin; the 14-OH metabolite of clarithromycin continues to be fairly active.

Moraxella catarrhalis and *Streptococcus pyogenes*

In the US, more than 95% of all *M. catarrhalis* produce a chromosomal, constitutive β-lactamase called the Brovasio enzyme (BRO-1 and BRO-2) which may compromise treatment with amoxicillin. However, most strains are susceptible to cephalosporins, β-lactamase inhibitor combinations and macrolides. In contrast, *S. pyogenes* continues to be susceptible to penicillin but resistance to macrolides and tetracyclines ranges up to 40% in both classes.

Staphylococcus aureus and Community-Acquired Methicillin-Resistant *S. aureus* (CA-MRSA)

Staphylococcus aureus has developed resistance to newer antibiotics over the years. Usually, in complicated post-viral respiratory infections such as influenza, today the world over, more than 90% *S. aureus* produce β-lactamase, rendering penicillin and its derivatives ineffective. Methicillin resistance is also frequent and may exceed 50% in some tertiary care centers. MRSA evolved through the acquisition of the staphylococcus cassette chromosome *mec* (SCCmec). Resistance to methicillin and other β-lactam antibiotics is mediated by the *mecA* gene, which encodes for an additional PBP (PBP2a) that has low affinity for β-lactams. To date, eight types of SCCmec (I-VIII) have been reported. CA-MRSA is both phenotypically and genotypically distinct from Healthcare-associated MRSA (HA-MRSA) and are genotypically SCC*mec* IV and SCC*mec*V types. They are susceptible to multiple classes of antibiotics other than the β-lactams such as clindamycin, co-trimoxazole, tetracyclines, etc. In a recent study in Mumbai, of the SCC*mec* IV strains, 83% were susceptible to many antimicrobial classes and the rest were susceptible to three classes, none being MDR.

The emergence of CA-MRSA especially in skin and soft tissue infections in the community has abolished the belief that resistant organisms bear a fitness cost in the presence of antibiotic stress. These highly-competent clones are capable of spreading locally and internationally. Known to cause severe necrotizing multilobar pneumonia in young healthy adults and children, these strains usually produce the Panton-Valentine Leukocidin (PVL) that enhances their toxigenicity.

■ RESISTANCE IN NOSOCOMIAL ISOLATES

Enterobacteriaceae and Nonfermenters Gram-negative Bacilli

Hospitals today are facing an unprecedented crisis due to the increasingly rapid emergence and dissemination of antibiotic-resistance genes. As hospitals concentrate vulnerable patients, it is an accepted fact that antibiotic resistance is far more prevalent.

Today infections with extended-spectrum β-lactamases (ESBLs) are posing an immense threat to clinical therapeutics. ESBLs are clavulanate-inhibited transferable enzymes that hydrolyze all penicillins, ampicillin, amoxycillin, as also all cephalosporins with an oxyimino side chain (cefotaxime, ceftriaxone, ceftazidime). They are inactive against carbapenems and cephamycins. ESBLs are mainly encountered in organisms like *E. coli, Klebsiella* spps, *Proteus mirabilis, Enterobacter* spps, *Citrobacter* spps, etc. ESBLs are frequently plasmid encoded and may also carry genes encoding resistance to other drug classes like aminoglycosides, quinolones and co-trimoxazole. Nosocomial infections caused by ESBLs as well as by *Amp*C production by Enterobacteriaceae are posing a huge threat to clinical therapeutics. In most Indian city hospitals, the overall prevalence of ESBLs is more than 60%. Though organisms such as *E. coli,*

Proteus spps, *Enterobacter* spps, *Citrobacter* spps, etc. are not traditional respiratory pathogens, *Klebsiella pneumoniae* is known to cause pneumonia in certain risk groups. Risk factors for nosocomial infection with ESBL producers include prolonged hospital stay, use of invasive medical devices, therapy with second or third-generation cephalosporins, penicillins and fluoroquinolones, administration of total parenteral nutrition (TPN), recent surgery, and hemodialysis.

In patients with late-onset ventilator-associated pneumonia (VAP), *P. aeruginosa* and *Acinetobacter baumannii* are established pathogens. In India, with high rates of ESBLs, empiric therapy with carbapenems is the standard of care in seriously ill-patients. Predictably, in patients on carbapenem antibiotics, or in situations with poor infection control practices, the carbapenemases tend to get selected out and easily spread. Carbapenemase-producing gram-negative organisms can hydrolyze all penicillins, cephalosporins, and carbapenems and they have been reported in several large outbreaks in hospitalized patients. *Klebsiella pneumoniae* carbapenemase (KPC) is classically associated with *K. pneumoniae.*

Metallo-β lactamases are β-lactam-hydrolyzing enzymes that contain a zinc moiety and are known to cause several extended outbreaks of nosocomial infections and are commonly found in *Pseudomonas* and *Acinetobacter* species. There are two major groups of metallo-β-lactamases: The IMP-type carbapenemases and the Verona integron-encoded metallo-β-lactamase (VIM) carbapenemases. The emergence of the New Delhi metallo-β-lactamase (NDM)-1 in Enterobacteriaceae that have the potential to spread, is a worrying development. In India carbapenemase producing Klebsiella have become predominant pathogens, leaving behind Pseudomonas and acinetobacter. As a result, we now have to use combinations of polymyxins with other drugs like Carbapenems, Fosfomycin, etc as salvage therapy.

Additional mechanisms augmenting β-lactamase activity involve loss of porin channels in the outer cellular membrane, upregulation of efflux pumps, decreasing antibiotic concentrations in the periplasmic space and facilitating hydrolysis by β-lactamases.

Unfortunately, the emerging threat of pan-resistant gram-negative bacilli with their remarkable resilience and environmental versatility epitomize the opportunistic infections that we will now have to contend with.

■ PREVENTING AND REDUCING RESISTANCE

Antibiotic resistance poses an ever-increasing threat to public health. We propose the following *10 commandments* to reduce overall antibiotic resistance:

1. Establish an etiological diagnosis using rapid diagnostic tests wherever possible.
2. Draw up rational guidelines in the form of an antibiotic policy by the hospital infection control committee core group (infectious disease physician, clinical microbiologist, and clinical pharmacologist) with input from chest physicians for specific lung infections to help curtail unnecessary use. Empiric antibiotic therapy should be based on the knowledge of common causative pathogens for a particular infection **(Table 1)**, known local susceptibility surveillance data, and host factors with special regard to patient comorbidities and specific risk factors. Antibiotic history is also becoming an important consideration in choosing the right drug. From the perspective of the community, knowing the epidemiology of prevalence of organisms with the likely antibiotic-resistance pattern of specific pathogens is vital.
3. Deescalate from broad-spectrum empiric therapy to narrow spectrum as soon as susceptibilities are available. From the perspective of serious infections in the hospital, there is also an urgent requirement to focus on culture and susceptibility before empiric therapy, so that once this has been initiated, streamlining of antibiotics to a narrower spectrum, and to efficacious and more cost-effective options can be quickly instituted.
4. Choosing appropriate dosing for the right duration is an important aspect of antibiotic regimens. Pharmacokinetic (PK) and pharmacodynamic (PD) principles which optimize time above MIC specifically for the β-lactams, area under the Curve (AUC)/MIC ratios for the fluoroquinolones, and peak to MIC ratios (C_{max}/MIC) for aminoglycosides, should be followed. We need to identify antibiotic exposures that prevent amplification of resistant subpopulations of bacteria.
5. Do not treat undrained abscesses or foreign body infections with antibiotics. Abscesses require drainage and infected foreign bodies require to be removed.
6. Distinguish colonization from true infection, especially in the interpretation of positive cultures from nonsterile sites such as sputum or endotracheal aspirates. Within limitations, quantitative cultures may help to delineate true infection.
7. Do not continue to treat only leukocytosis or fever with antibiotics in the intensive care setting, without determining their cause.
8. Methods to detect outbreaks in hospitals, especially those with resistant organisms must be in place.
9. Education and training of doctors helps to ensure appropriate usage. Education alone is the foundation that will enhance and influence prescribing behavior. Strategies that inform rather than dictate work better in curtailing use.
10. Demand compliance with good infection control practices including hand hygiene, barrier precautions and environmental disinfection. Guidelines for infection control certainly serve to stem the tide of dissemination of resistant determinants in the hospital.

■ MANAGING ANTIBIOTIC RESISTANCE

Preserving the effectiveness of the current antibiotics by reducing resistance and improving outcomes is the goal of antimicrobial stewardship. Raising awareness about the escalating problem of antimicrobial resistance with interventional programs is required. Recently, the Infectious Disease Society of America (IDSA) and the Society of Healthcare Epidemiology of America (SHEA) published guidelines for developing an institutional antimicrobial stewardship program. The goals include optimizing clinical outcomes while minimizing the unintended consequences of antimicrobial use by focusing on two evidence-based principles, namely prospective drug use audit with intervention or feedback, and formulary restriction with preauthorization requirements for specific agents. Comprehensive programs are cost-effective with dose optimization, parenteral to oral switches, etc. Indeed, planning and implementing such

Table 1: Percent etiology of community-acquired pneumonia (CAP) in a study in Mumbai.

Streptococcus pneumoniae	30
Chlamydia pneumoniae	13
Haemophilus influenzae	7
Moraxella catarrhalis	6
Mycoplasma pneumoniae	4
Legionella pneumophila	2
Klebsiella pneumoniae	2
Staph aureus	1

stewardship programs in a well-orchestrated and well-designed manner is a huge challenge. Most practicing physicians are not overly concerned about the long-term ecologic effects of antibiotics on microbes. Resistance to antibiotics is unavoidable from an evolutionary perspective, and the simple truth about antibiotics is—the more you use them, the more you will loose them! With the gram-negative antibiotic pipeline practically drying up for the next 10–15 years, it is time to dispel our misplaced optimism that some new drug is bound to arrive.

The 10×20 initiative promises a global commitment to develop ten new antibacterials by 2020. However, we must remember that antibiotic prescribing is the main driver of resistance, and resistance is clearly a function of the volume consumed. No **single** strategy to combat this burgeoning problem of antibiotic resistance seems to be working effectively. Lastly, we must appreciate that we are indeed fortunate to belong to a generation of physicians who have been able to treat and cure infections in this golden era of antibiotics. If we have to pass on this antibiotic legacy to our future generations there is an urgent need for introspection. After all, resistance in bacteria is not a matter of *if but of when*.

■ SUGGESTED READING

1. D'Souza N, Rodrigues C, Mehta A. Molecular characterization of methicillin-resistant Staphylococcus aureus (MRSA) with emergence of epidemic clones of Sequence type (ST) 22 and ST 772 in Mumbai, India. J Clin Microbiol. 2010;48(5):1806-11.
2. Deshpande, Rodrigues, Shetty, et al. New Delhi metallo-β-lactamase (NDM)—1 in Enterobacteriaceae; treatment options with carbapenems compromised. JAPI. 2010:58;147-9.
3. Helen BW, George TH, John BS, et al. Bad bugs, No drugs: No ESKAPE! An update from the Infectious Disease Society of America. Clin Infect Dis. 2009;48:1-12.
4. Jae-Hoon S, Sook-In J, Kwan SK, et al. High prevalence of antimicrobial resistance among clinical Streptococcus pneumoniae isolates in Asia (an ANSORP) study. Antimicrob Agents Chemother. 2004;48:2101-7.
5. Lakshmi V. Need for national/regional guidelines and policies in India to combat antibiotic resistance. Indian J Med Microbiol. 2008;26(2):105-7.
6. Lalitha MK, Thomas K. Antibiotic resistance among Streptococcus pneumonia: In Antibiotic resistance—the modern epidemic: Current status and research issues—proceedings of the 9th Sir Dorabji Tata Symposium. Raghunath D, Nagaraja V, Durga Rao C (Eds). 2009. pp. 147-52.
7. Mehta A, Rodrigues C, Kumar R, et al. A Pilot program of haemophilus surveillance in India. Ind J Clin Pract. 1997;7(10):81-4.
8. Raghunath D. Emerging antibiotic resistance in bacteria with special reference to India. J Biosci. 2008;33(4):593-603.
9. Shanthi M, Sekar U. Multi-drug resistant *Pseudomonas aeruginosa* and *Acinetobacter baumannii* infections among hospitalized patients: risk factors and outcomes. J Assoc Physicians India. 2009;57:636-40.

Section 8

HIV and the Lung

CHAPTER 28

HIV and the Lung

■ INTRODUCTION

The lungs have been at the forefront of the human immunodeficiency virus (HIV) epidemic ever since its first description. The seemingly innocuous first description of what was to become HIV came from the initial historic Morbidity and Mortality Weekly Report (MMWR) report on 5 June, 1981 with the title "Pneumocystis pneumonia—Los Angeles". Not even the most pessimistic reader of that initial account could ever have guessed the scale of the subsequent pandemic less than three decades later with an estimated 78 million people being infected with HIV and 35 million people having died of acquired immunodeficiency syndrome (AIDS)-related illnesses. HIV continues to be a major global public health issue. In 2018, an estimated 33.4 million people were living with HIV (including 1.8 million children)—with a global HIV prevalence of 0.8% among adults. The vast majority of this number lives in low- and middle- income countries. In the same year, 1.1 million people died of AIDS-related illnesses.

An estimated 22.4 million people living with HIV live in sub-Saharan Africa, the vast majority of them (an estimated 19 million) live in east and southern Africa.

Of Thailand's population of more than 60 million, in 2015 it is estimated that 440,000 people were living with HIV and that 15,000 people died of AIDS-related illnesses. After sub-Saharan Africa, Asia and the Pacific are the region with the largest number of people living with HIV, with Thailand accounting for approximately 9%.

The reader is referred to a separate text for a thorough understanding of HIV infection and its natural history.

The table given below **(Table 1)** shows the extent of the HIV pandemic with special reference to Thailand and China **(Tables 2 and 3)**. The Indian data on pulmonary infections in HIV patients is considered separately.

Table 1: Prevalence of HIV or AIDS world wide.

Region	Adults and children living with HIV/AIDS	Adults and children newly infected	Adult prevalence	Deaths of adults and children
Sub-Saharan Africa	22.4 million	1.9 million	5.2%	1.4 million
North Africa and Middle East	310,000	35,000	0.2%	20,000
South and South East Asia	3.8 million	280,000	0.3%	270,000
East Asia	850,000	75,000	<0.1%	59,000
Eastern Europe and Central Asia	1.5 million	110,000	0.7%	87,000
North America	1.4 million	55,000	0.4%	25,000
Western and Central Europe	850,000	30,000	0.3%	13,000
Global Total	33.4 million	2.7 million	0.8%	2.0 million

(AIDS: Acquired immunodeficiency syndrome; HIV: Human immunodeficiency virus)
Source: AVERT.[online] available from: www.AVERT.org [Accessed July, 2018].

Table 2: China AIDS statistics.

Estimated total population, July 2008	1,330,045,000
Estimated number of people living with HIV/AIDS, end 2007	700,000
Proportion of adults with HIV or AIDS who are women, end 2007	29%
Estimated adult prevalence of HIV or AIDS, end 2007	0.1%
Estimated number of AIDS deaths in 2007	39,000

(AIDS: Acquired immunodeficiency syndrome; HIV: Human immunodeficiency virus)
Source: AVERT.[online] available from: www.AVERT.org [Accessed July, 2018].

Table 3: Thailand AIDS statistics.

Estimated total population, July 2008	65,493,000
Estimated number of people living with HIV or AIDS, end 2007	610,000
Proportion of adults with HIV or AIDS who are women, end 2007	42%
Children (0–15) living with HIV or AIDS, end 2007	14,000
Estimated adult prevalence of HIV or AIDS, end 2007	1.4%
Estimated number of AIDS deaths in 2007	31,000

(HIV: Human immunodeficiency virus; AIDS: Acquired immunodeficiency syndrome)
Source: AVERT.[online] available from: www.AVERT.org [Accessed July, 2018].

Table 4: Pulmonary Infections in HIV.

Bacterial Infections:
- *Mycobacterium tuberculosis*
- *Streptococcus pneumoniae*
- *Haemophilus influenzae*
- Nontuberculous mycobacteria (MAC)
- *Staphylococcus aureus*
- *Nocardia and Listeria*
- *Klebsiella* spp and other gram negative organisms
- *Rhodococcus equi*

Parasitic Infections:
- *Toxoplasma gondii*
- *Cryptosporidium spp*
- *Microsporidium spp*
- *Leishmania spp*
- *Strongyloides spp*

Fungal infections:
- *Pneumocystis jirovecii* pneumonia (PCP)
- *Cryptococcus neoformans*
- *Histoplasma capsulatum*
- *Candida albicans*
- *Coccidioides immitis*
- *Aspergillus spp*

Viral Infections:
- *Cytomegalovirus*
- Herpes simplex
- Varicella zoster
- EB virus
- HHV 6
- *JC virus*
- RSV
- HHV-8 (KSAHV) (Kaposi's sarcoma)
- Multiple organisms

(EB: Epstein-Barr; HHV 6: Human herpesvirus 6; KSAHV: *Kaposi's sarcoma-associated herpesvirus*; RSV: Respiratory syncytial virus)

Table 5: Noninfectious pulmonary manifestations.

Malignancy:
- B-cell lymphoma
- Primary effusion lymphoma (body-cavity associated lymphomas)
- Castleman's diseases
- Bronchogenic carcinoma

Idiopathic:
- *ILD*: LIP and NSIP
- *Airway disease*: Bronchiolitis and emphysema
- Diffuse infiltrative CD8 lymphocytosis
- Sarcoidosis
- BOOP
- Primary pulmonary hypertension
- Alveolar hemorrhage

(BOOP: Bronchiolitis obliterans with organizing pneumonia; ILD: Interstitial lung disease; LIP: Lymphoid interstitial pneumonia; NSIP: Nonspecific interstitial pneumonia)

This chapter discusses the pulmonary involvement in AIDS, the lung being the single most common involved organ both on autopsy and clinical studies. According to autopsy findings, the lung was affected with an incidence ranging from 100% in the early part of the epidemic to 70% in the highly active antiretroviral therapy (HAART) era. Even in the current era, pulmonary-related infections not just by AIDS-related opportunistic organisms but also by usual organisms, remain the most important and leading cause of morbidity and mortality in HIV-infected patients worldwide. The spectrum of pulmonary involvement encountered in HIV is given in **Tables 4 and 5**.

■ PULMONARY IMMUNE RESPONSE IN AIDS

The HIV infection besides severely impairing the overall general immune response of the body also impairs the local immune response within the lung. The mechanism underlying the dysregulation of the pulmonary immune response continues to be the subject of research. Immune dysregulation is probably a result of the interaction between the HIV circulating through the lung capillaries, other circulating antigens with a potential to cause disease, airborne inhaled antigens, and local immune cells responsible for local immune responses. This local battle within the lungs takes place under the shadow of an overall generalized depressed immune response (in particular cell-mediated immunity) of the immune system of the body.

Attempts to study the dysregulation of the local pulmonary response to HIV infection includes the use of in vitro cell cultures to mimic the actual pulmonary environment and the study of cells recovered from bronchoalveolar lavage (BAL) fluid through bronchoscopy in infected patients. In the latter form of study, most patients have advanced disease, many are on antiretroviral (ARV) drugs and most have more than one pathogen causing pulmonary disease. Each of these features can influence results of immune studies so performed. An unsettled question is the site or sites of local immune response to HIV infection within the lung and whether the cells within BAL fluid are representative of the immune response arising from one or more of these sites.

■ RISK FACTORS FOR RESPIRATORY DISEASES

Risk factors depend on the following:

Geography

Geography, socioeconomic factors associated with certain geographical areas of the world influence the nature of pulmonary infections, notably with reference to mycobacterial and fungal disease. Pulmonary tuberculosis (TB) is the most common pulmonary infection in HIV patients in India.

Severity of Immunocompromise

The lower the CD4 count and the higher the plasma ribonucleic acid (RNA) viral load, the greater the risk of pulmonary infection. HIV patients with CD4 count below 200 cells/μL are far more prone to recurrent attacks of bacterial pneumonia, and to infection by exotic opportunistic organisms such as *Pneumocystis carinii,* other fungi such as the Aspergillus species and *Penicillium*

marneffei or opportunistic bacteria such as *Nocardia asteroides* and *Rhodococcus equi.* Opportunistic viral infections also make their appearance with very low CD4 counts. These exotic infections are merely a reflection of marked T-cell depletion causing markedly lowered cell-mediated immune response coupled with macrophage dysfunction.

Drug Addiction

Intravenous use of drugs by drug addicts is a great risk factor for the development of pulmonary infection, in particular bacterial pneumonias and mycobacterial infection.

History of Previous Infections

The HIV patients with a previous history of bacterial pneumonia or an episode of *Pneumocystis jirovecii* pneumonia (PCP) in the past are at greater risk of recurrence of these infections. This is perhaps chiefly related to the underlying poor host immune response but may also be influenced by environmental factors. Since HIV-infected smokers seem to have a higher rate of pneumonia than nonsmokers, background structural and functional damage to the lungs (as in smokers) may well be an additional risk factor. Recent studies suggest that chronic obstructive pulmonary disease (COPD) and lung cancer occur more frequently among HIV-infected individuals compared to the general population. This emphasizes the added urgency of stopping smoking in HIV-infected individuals.

Use of *Pneumocystis jirovecii* pneumonia Prophylaxis

Numerous studies have shown that the use of trimethoprim + sulfamethoxazole in all patients with a CD4 below 200 cells/μL has clearly reduced the incidence of PCP. This subject is discussed later in the chapter.

Use of Highly Active Antiretroviral Therapy

The use of specific ARV therapy to combat HIV by controlling and reducing its replication has been shown to clearly reduce the incidence of pulmonary infections and slow the tempo of the natural history of the disease. In the richer countries of the world where HAART is readily available, opportunistic infections (OIs) associated with very low CD4 counts [i.e. cytomegalovirus (CMV) infection and infection by

Mycobacterium Avium-intracellulare] are much less frequent. Malignant diseases such as non-Hodgkin's lymphoma (NHL) are being more frequently observed.

■ EPIDEMIOLOGY

The epidemiology of pulmonary infection in Europe and USA has significantly changed. This is after the use of prophylaxis against pneumocystis; the incidence of PCP has significantly fallen in these countries. Also, following the introduction of HAART, the relative incidence of etiologies causing HIV-related infections has changed, bacterial pneumonia being the most common cause of these infections rather than PCP.

In India, other countries of South Asia and most countries of Southeast Asia and in Africa, pulmonary TB in the most frequent cause of HIV-associated lung infection. Eastern Europe also has a high burden of TB in HIV-infected patients.

Indian Data

Data from India is limited but an early autopsy study by Lanjewar and Duggal in 2001 *(Ref: Lanjewar N, Duggal R. Pulmonary pathology in patients with AIDS: an autopsy study from Mumbai. HIV Med. 2001;2(4):266-71)* showed TB accounted for 61% of all pulmonary disease, with bacterial pneumonias featuring second in terms of frequency at 18%. A more recent study by one of the authors *(Ref: Udwadia ZF, Doshi AV, Bhaduri AS. Pneumocystis carinii pneumonia in HIV-infected patients from Mumbai. J Assoc Physicians India. 2005;53:437-40)* was a prospective study of all hospitalizations for HIV in a tertiary center in Mumbai over 2 years (2002–3). In this study, which looked at 300 consecutive HIV-positive admissions, the lungs were the single most common organ system affected (120 of 300 admissions, 40%). In this study, TB (pulmonary and extrapulmonary) was the most common pulmonary cause of admissions (46/120, 40%). The novel information that emerged from this study was that PCP, previously considered rare in the Indian context, ranked second in importance (34 admissions, 30%). Bacterial infections (pneumonia) ranked third with 30 cases (25%). Malignancies and miscellaneous conditions accounted for 4% each. Another study from Chennai *[Ref: Rajasekaran S, Mahilmaran A. Manifestation of tuberculosis in patients with human immunodeficiency virus: a large Indian study. Ann Thorac Med. 2007;2(2):58-60]* showed that of 12, 750 HIV-confirmed patients visiting the hospital, 4,383 (34.4%) patients had TB. Among them, 2,448 (55.9%) had pulmonary TB, and the remaining 1,935 (44.1%) had either disseminated or extrapulmonary TB. Another recent study from Southern Eastern India showed that amongst 684 patients studied, 18.9% had HIV-TB coinfection; 58.8% amongst these had pulmonary TB *[Ref: Ramachandra K, Vikram S, et al. HIV-TB coinfection: clinicoepidemiological determinants at an antiretroviral therapy center in Southern India. Lung India. 2013;30(4):302-6]*.

■ PULMONARY INFECTIONS IN HIV DISEASE

Coinfection with TB and HIV has been comprehensively covered in the section on "TB". Opportunistic infections (OIs), both bacterial and nonbacterial have been dealt with in an earlier chapter titled "Pneumonia in the Non-HIV Immunocompromised Patient". The clinical features and treatment of different pneumonias including pneumonia caused by OIs in immunocompromised HIV-infected patients and in non-HIV immunocompromised patients are very much the same. The reader is therefore referred to the chapter on "Pneumonia in the Non-HIV Immunocompromised Patient" as also to the chapter on "Nonbacterial Pneumonia". However, the following features in relation to pulmonary infections in HIV-infected patients need to be stressed.

- Tuberculosis is the most common pulmonary infection encountered in HIV patients in India, Africa, and Southeast Asia.
- Severe advanced HIV disease can result in the suppression of cell-mediated immune response with CD4 counts falling to less than 50 cells/μL. As a result, the range of exotic opportunistic pulmonary infections in HIV is generally greater than in non-HIV conditions causing immunosuppression.
- Symptoms and signs of pulmonary infection in HIV-infected patients with very low CD4 counts are meager or even absent rendering diagnosis of various pulmonary infections difficult.
- Multiple infections due to multiple organisms (including opportunistic microorganisms) are to be expected in AIDS patients with very low CD4 counts. As an example pneumocystis pneumonia is often associated with CMV infection and at times with infections caused by *M. Avium intracellulare*.
- Response to therapy, even when this is specific, is perhaps poorest when pulmonary infections occur

in severe HIV disease with very low CD4 counts (<50 cells/μL).

- Specific therapy in relation to both opportunistic and non-OIs in HIV patients needs to be combined with ARV therapy. Specific treatment has been mentioned in the chapter on "Pneumonia in the Non-HIV Immunocompromised Patient". For details on combined ARV therapy, as also complications related to ARV therapy and the interaction between ARV drugs and other medications, the reader should consult another text.
- *Immune reconstitution inflammatory syndrome (IRIS) before the era of ARV therapy for HIV infection.* It was observed that patients with TB on anti-TB drugs who appeared to be responding to therapy, could occasionally develop for a short while, clinical deterioration with exacerbation both in the clinical and radiological features of the disease. Yet the overall patient response to continued medical therapy was good. This "paradoxical reaction" was believed to have an immunological basis.

Following the widespread use of HAART, similar "paradoxical reactions" often of marked severity, have been observed in HIV-infected patients. These "reactions" in the context of HIV-infected individuals have been termed the IRIS. The syndrome has a varied clinical presentation, and has been observed in a wide range of OIs in HIV patients, treated with both ARV drugs as also with therapy directed against the prevailing OI. Typically and most commonly this "reaction" is observed after the initiation of ARV therapy in a patient being treated for pulmonary TB. There is observed a return or exacerbation of TB, together with systemic features such as fever, dyspnea, and a radiological worsening of the lesion. This may be associated with the development of new lesions at different sites. Though IRIS is most commonly observed in infections due to *Mycobacterium tuberculosis,* it is also seen with other OIs due to *Mycobacterium avium* intracellulare, fungi (cryptococcal infection in particular), and viruses (hepatitis and Herpesviridae).

Immune reconstitution inflammatory syndrome has been more fully discussed in the chapter on HIV-TB Coinfection (*see* section on "Pulmonary TB") to which the reader should refer.

The rest of this chapter focuses chiefly on PCP, offers a few pertinent remarks on community-acquired pneumonia (CAP) and briefly discusses malignancies in relation to HIV infection, and idiopathic noninfective nonmalignant disorders associated with HIV infection.

Pneumocystis jirovecii Pneumonia

Introduction and Epidemiology

Globally, PCP accounted for almost two-thirds of the AIDS index diagnoses in the first decade of the HIV pandemic. It remains the most prevalent OI in patients with HIV even today. Considered rare in the Indian, Asian, and African context, our letter in the New England Journal of Medicine in 2004 pointed out that in the developing world it was probably being underdiagnosed due to lack of awareness and lack of special diagnostic facilities such as high-resolution computed tomography (HRCT) scanning, bronchoscopy and BAL studies, and special immunofluorescence stains. Our study not only showed it to be common when diligently searched for but also revealed that almost half of all our cases (49%) would have been missed without access to sophisticated diagnostic techniques. Earlier deaths from TB and more pathogenic organisms may also have been partly responsible for less PCP being reported from Africa and India. In our series, PCP occurred at a mean CD4 count of just 96 cells/μL. Similarly, there is now growing incidence of PCP in other developing countries, notably Africa.

In the developed world while PCP remains one of the most common OIs, there is little doubt that its incidence is declining in the West. There are two reasons for this decline; firstly, effective trimethoprim-sulfamethoxazole (TMP-SMX) is used in almost all patients with CD4 counts less than 200 as such patients are almost nine times more likely to develop PCP. The second reason behind the decline is the widespread availability of ARV therapy. PCP will always retain its importance in HIV and sadly, continue to develop in patients unaware of their HIV status, in those with no access to care, in those unwilling or unable to adhere to therapy and in nonresponders or failures with ARV therapy.

It needs to be pointed out that though the ensuing section is chiefly related to PCP in patients with AIDS, PCP is being increasingly reported in immunocompromised patients not suffering from AIDS **(Table 6)**.

Taxonomy

The long-standing controversy about whether to place PCP in the parasitic or fungal families has finally been settled

Table 6: Important conditions associated with PCP other than AIDS.
• Chemotherapy
• Corticosteroid therapy
• Radiation therapy
• Malignancies
• Leukemia
• Collagen vascular disease
• Hematological disorders
• Nephrotic syndrome
• Congenital immune deficiency disorders

(AIDS: Acquired immunodeficiency syndrome; PCP: *Pneumocystis jirovecii* pneumonia)

by elegant gene sequencing studies by Edman reported in Nature, incontrovertibly linking PCP to the fungal family. *Pneumocystis jirovecii* (PCJ) is the proposed new name after the Czech parasitologist Otto Jirovec. This new name first proposed by Frenkel has now been accepted by Centers for Disease Control and Prevention (CDC) and the National Institutes of Health (NIH) from 2002.

Clinical Features

The PCP infection is characterized by progressive hypoxia, dyspnea, cough coupled with a comparative marked paucity of physical findings. In the AIDS patient with the first episode of infection, the evolution is gradual extending over 2–3 weeks during which constitutional symptoms such as low grade fever and weight loss may be the presenting features. After this period, progressive breathlessness at first on exertion and then even at rest dominates the picture. A dry cough is generally present and there is increasing hypoxia with a marked paucity of physical signs on examination of the chest. Death from hypoxia, respiratory failure results, if the condition is undiagnosed and untreated. To start with in the early part of the natural history, the chest X-ray may be normal. With increasing dyspnea and hypoxia, the typical radiological features described below become evident.

Subsequent infections in AIDS patients may evolve more rapidly. Coinfection with other infections (notably *Cytomegalovirus*, *Legionella*, and mycobacterial species) may accelerate the progression of the disease or even alter its radiological features. These coinfections would also contribute to constitutional symptoms and aggravate hypoxia.

PCP in non-HIV patients: As mentioned earlier, pneumocystis infection is being increasingly recognized in many other immunosuppressed states. In patients on corticosteroid therapy and in transplant recipients, pneumocystis pneumonia is often acute, and far more rapidly progressive than in patients with AIDS. In the organ transplant recipient, PCP occurs generally 2–4 months after the initiation of immune suppression or during periods where immunosuppression is further increased, as for example following the use of pulsed corticosteroids, antilymphocytic serum or following a new CMV infection.

Extrapulmonary pneumocystis—metastatic extra-pulmonary infection is rarely observed in patients with untreated AIDS. Even in these patients, the incidence of extrapulmonary manifestations is less than 1%. Metastatic spread of pneumocystis can involve almost any organ in the body—chiefly the liver, spleen, lymph nodes, and adrenal glands leading to disturbed function of the organ or organs involved. It is noteworthy that respiratory involvement may be minimal or absent in these patients. CT scan may show nonenhancing low attenuation masses. Histopathology may demonstrate granulomas with calcifications. Dual infections of extrapulmonary sites may occur with other opportunistic organisms.

Radiology

In the early stages, bilateral perihilar interstitial shadows are seen. These are often subtle and normal chest radiographs have been reported in 5–34% of series. In our Hinduja Hospital series, 10% of patients had normal radiographs. As the disease progresses, the bilateral perihilar infiltrate spread outwards to the periphery of both lungs in a butterfly pattern, also involving the a apices and/or the bases. This pattern can be succeeded by progressive consolidation with bronchograms, and in severe cases by complete opacification of both lungs fields.

In approximately 10% of cases air-filled cysts or pneumatoceles may be seen in the upper lobes. A variety of atypical radiographic features have been reported. These include—upper lobe infiltrates (especially in patients on nebulized pentamidine prophylaxis), cystic changes, pneumothorax, pleural effusions, focal nodular lesions, cavitation, and adenopathy. It must be pointed out that effusions, upper lobe infiltrates, and adenopathy are all much more likely to be secondary to TB than PCP, especially in the Indian context. Of importance is the fact that while the evolution of the shadows is often rapid, they are slow to resolve. A study by DeLorenzo in Chest in 1987 of 104 PCP patients showed that at 3 weeks only 35% of patients' radiographs had actually improved and at 5 months complete resolution had occurred in only 43%. It should be noted that no radiographic pattern is diagnostic of PCP. For example, CMV infection may produce radiological features indistinguishable from those seen in PCP. In fact both infections may coexist. Also in lung transplant patients, rejection of the allograft or infection can result in perihilar infiltrates also indistinguishable from those seen in PCP (**Figs. 1 to 4**).

Computed Tomography (Figs. 5 to 7)

The HRCT of the chest may demonstrate changes not appreciated on a chest radiograph. The usual pattern observed early in the disease is a ground glass opacity in the perihilar, central region, progressively spreading outwards to the periphery. Resolution of the lesions is better appreciated on a CT scan than on a radiographic study (**Figs. 5A to D**).

Laboratory Findings

A rise in the lactate dehydrogenase (LDH) is often observed; it is a nonspecific marker and is not useful in diagnosis. (1, 3) β-D glucan is a polysaccharide monomer found in many fungal cell walls including pneumocystis. Since (1, 3) β-D glucan also rises in other fungal infections, the specificity of this test in pneumocystis infection is low. False positive tests are also observed in patients receiving immunoglobulin therapy or those on hemodialysis.

Microbiological Diagnosis

Microbiology is crucial to making a diagnosis. Sputum is often not produced, and hence must be induced by nebulization with hypertonic saline for 20 minutes. The yield can be improved by performing a BAL. A transbronchial biopsy is seldom performed but increases diagnostic yield further. In our series, we had four patients with negative BAL but PCP was proven on transbronchial lung

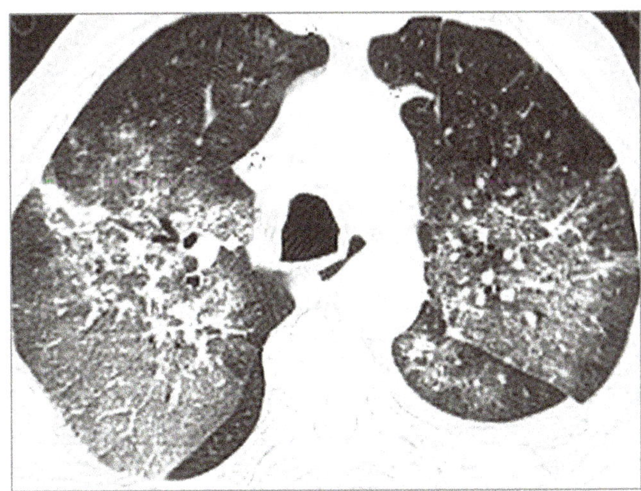

Fig. 2: *Pneumocystis jirovecii* pneumonia. Chest CT demonstrates ill-defined ground-glass densities in both lung fields.

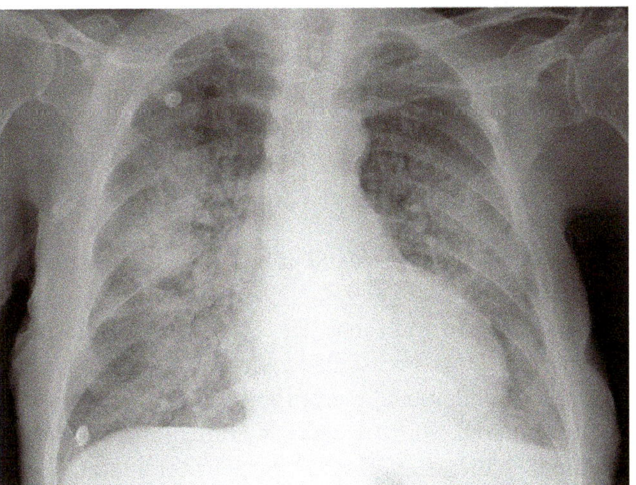

Fig. 3: *Pneumocystis jirovecii* pneumonia. A 43-year-old male patient with a long-standing history of smoking, alcohol abuse, and HIV presented with high-grade fever and low oxygen saturation. Chest X-ray demonstrates ill-defined areas of ground-glass densities in both lung fields, essentially in the parahilar location. Bronchoscopic lavage revealed PCP.
(HIV: Human immunodeficiency virus; PCP: *Pneumocystis jirovecii* pneumonia)

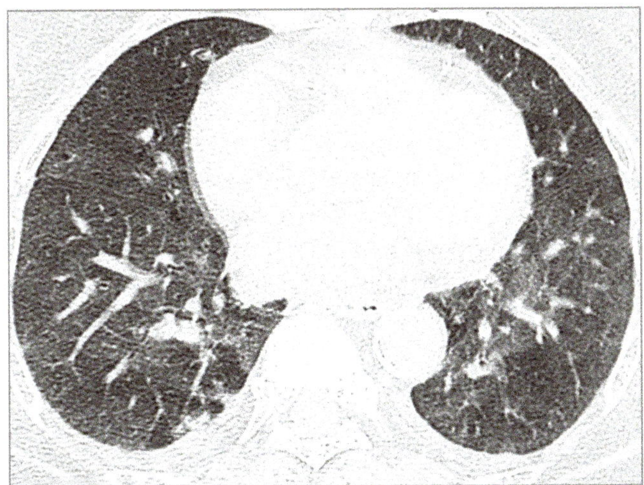

Fig. 1: *Pneumocystis jirovecii* pneumonia. Chest X-ray was normal. High-resolution computed tomography (HRCT) chest was advised for further evaluation and revealed ill-defined ground glass densities in both lung fields.

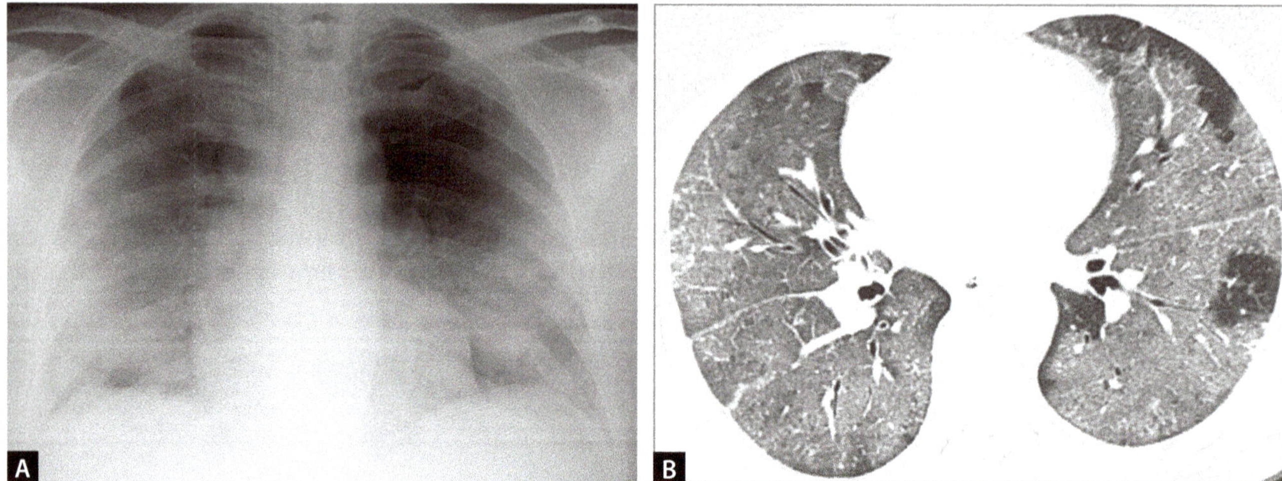

Figs. 4A and B: *Pneumocystis jirovecii* pneumonia in a seropositive male with cough, fever, and dyspnea. Chest X-ray (A) reveals diffuse ground-glass densities in both lung fields. HRCT chest (B) confirms diffuse ground-glass densities in both lung fields.
(HRCT: High-resolution computed tomography)

biopsy only. The stains used are Gomori methenamine, Calcofluor white, Giemsa stain, and Wrights stain. The staining method of choice is the direct immunofluorescent staining with monoclonal antibodies, as it is both very sensitive and specific for identifying trophic and cystic forms of pneumocystis **(Figs. 8A to C)**.

Treatment

The TMP-SMX in a dose of two double-strength tablets thrice daily (TMP-SMX—160 mg trimethoprim and 800 mg sulfamethoxazole constitutes a double-strength tablet) remains the treatment of choice in PCP. Unfortunately, side effects are common at the high doses needed and as many as 50% of patients develop major side effects which demand temporary or permanent discontinuation.

Clindamycin (300 mg TDS/QDS) plus primaquine (15–30 mg OD) is a reasonable alternative and often one that is better tolerated. A large multicenter study by Toma et al. compared clindamycin plus primaquine with TMP-SMX in 87 patients and found it to be better tolerated with similar success rates. Other drugs used include nebulized and intravenous pentamidine (4 mg per kg IV OD), dapsone (100 mg OD), and atovaquone (750 mg orally thrice daily). It is advisable to continue treatment for 2–3 weeks in all patients **(Table 7)**.

- *Role of steroids:* Data from clinical studies has shown that steroids are unequivocally useful in moderate-to-severe PCP. Their use should be reserved for PCP patients who are hypoxic ($PaO_2 < 70$ mm Hg) and have been shown in some series to reduce the rate of worsening respiratory failure and death by as much as 50%. They are most effective when given within 72 hours of onset of the disease. They act by blunting the inflammatory response and are used in a dose of oral prednisolone 40 mg BD × 5 days, 40 mg OD × 5 days, and 20 mg OD × 11 days.
- *Antiretroviral therapy:* The timing of ARV therapy in relation to PCP is controversial. While it was earlier felt best to complete the TMP-SMX therapy before commencing ARV therapy, evidence from the Adult and Adolescent Spectrum of HIV Disease Project showed concurrent prescription of ARV was associated with improved early survival (OR 0.4).
- *Outcome:* There is little doubt that the outcome of PCP has improved. In the Adult and Adolescent Spectrum of HIV Disease Project, which looked at 4,412 patients with 5,222 episodes of PCP, survival at 1 year improved from 40% in 1992 to 63% in 1998 despite emergence of antibiotic-resistant PCP strains. This improvement in survival, although drugs have stayed the same, is due to widespread use of steroids, better intensive care unit (ICU) care of these patients, and earlier introduction of ARVs. Lack of response or inadequate response to specific therapy may be due to one or more of the several factors tabled below **(Table 8)**.

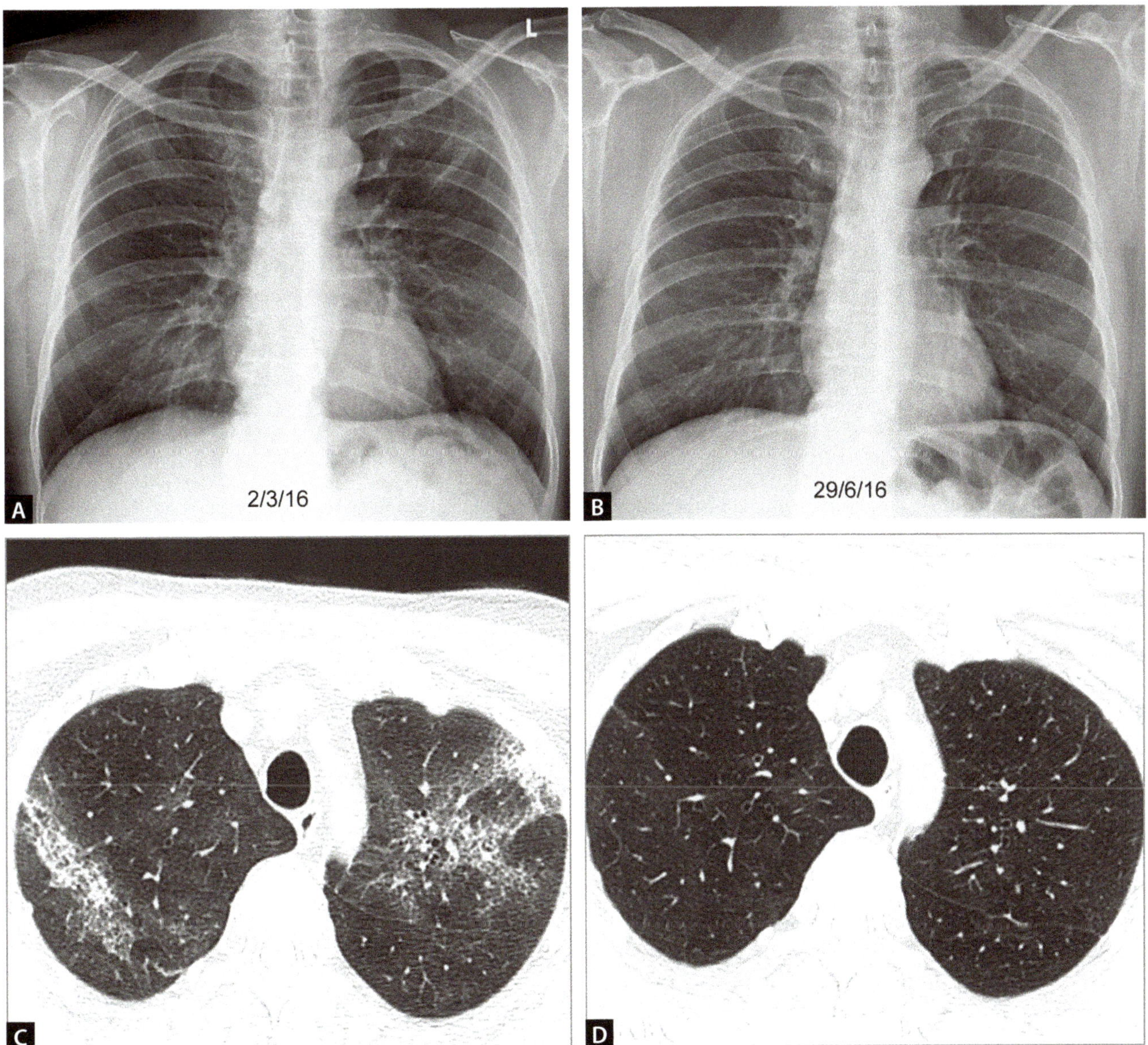

Figs. 5A to D: *Pneumocystis jirovecii* pneumonia: Seropositive middle age man presented with dyspnea, cough and fever. (A) Chest X-ray done on 2/3/2016 revealed ill-defined parenchymal opacities in both upper zones. HRCT (B) revealed ground-glass densities in both upper zones. Sputum revealed PCP. Post-treatment X-ray (C) and HRCT (D) done on 29/6/2016 revealed total clearing of previously visualized opacities.

(HRCT: High-resolution computed tomography; PCP: *Pneumocystis jirovecii* pneumonia)

Prevention

Prophylactic drug therapy should be used in all patients with a CD4 count less than 200. Some prefer to use prophylaxis when the CD4 count less than 400.

The TMP-SMX is the drug of choice for the prevention of pneumocystis infection provided the patient can tolerate the fixed single-strength tablet per day (80 mg TMP + 160 mg SMX). The advantage of using this drug is that it serves as a preventive for a wide range of other opportunistic agents. These include *Toxoplasma gondii*, *Isospora belli*, *Listeria monocytogenes*, and susceptible bacteria such as stains of pneumococci, *H. influenzae*, staphylococci, and some enteric gram-negative organisms. Nocardiosis is also sensitive to TMP-SMX and may to an extent be prevented. TMP-SMX has also been widely used as one tablet thrice a week, than on a daily basis to reduce the toxic effects of the drug. This may, however, reduce its efficacy as a preventive for pneumocystis.

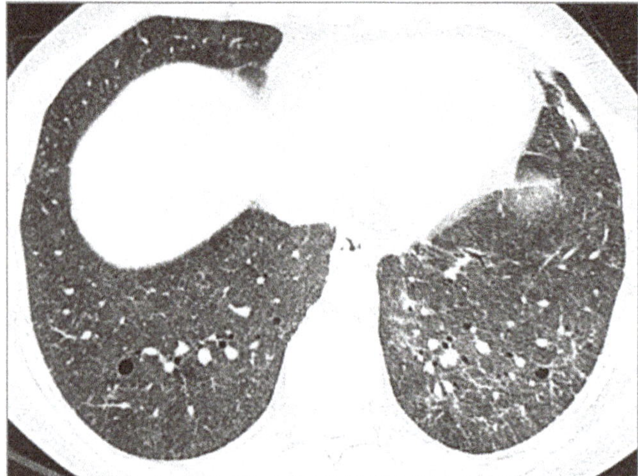

Fig. 6: *Pneumocystis jirovecii* pneumonia. HRCT demonstrates ill-defined ground-glass densities in both lung fields, there are few focal areas of sparing in the lung fields. Multiple pneumatoceles, thin air-walled air space are seen in the both lower lobes. This combination of ground-glass densities and pneumatoceles is important to differentiate PCP from CMV and other conditions presenting with ground-glass densities. The only other condition with ground-glass densities and cysts is lymphocytic interstitial pneumonia (LIP), the cysts in LIP are more numerous and diffuse as compared to the few isolated seen in PCP.

(HRCT: High-resolution computed tomography; PCP: *Pneumocystis jirovecii* pneumonia; CMV: Cytomegalovirus)

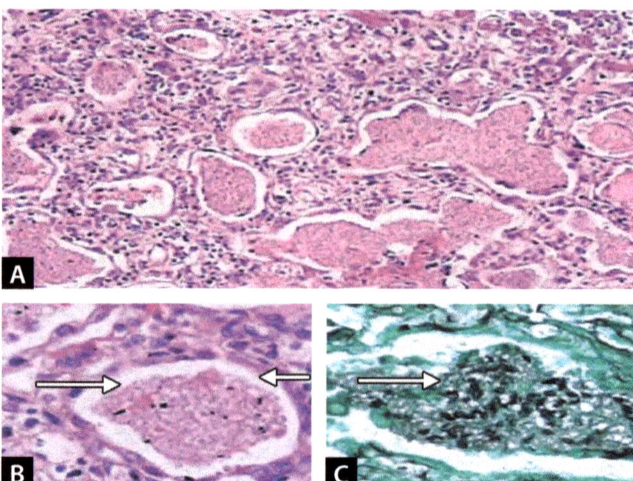

Figs. 8A to C: *Pneumocystis jirovecii* pneumonia (A and B) hematoxylin and eosin stain (H & E) 10X, 100X—the alveolar spaces contain typical granular, foamy honeycombed material showing cysts of *Pneumocystis jirovecii*. The alveolar walls are infiltrated with mononuclear cells. (C) Methenamine silver stain 100X—round and oval, black-colored cysts of *Pneumocystis jirovecii* approximately 4–5 µm in size seen within the alveolar spaces.

Table 7: Prophylactic treatment for PCP infection in HIV.

Drug	
1. TMP-SMX	1 double strength tablet orally/day
2. Dapsone	100 mg orally/day
3. Pentamidine	Nebulized from—300 mg every 4 weeks
4. Atovaquone	750 mg orally BD
5. Azithromycin	1,250 mg orally/weekly

(HIV: Human immunodeficiency virus; PCP: *Pneumocystis jirovecii* pneumonia; TMP-SMX: Trimethoprim-sulfamethoxazole)

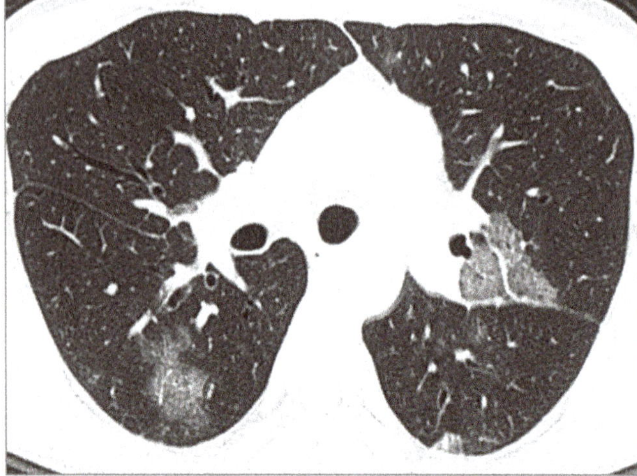

Fig. 7: *Pneumocystis jirovecii* pneumonia. HRCT demonstrates ill-defined ground-glass densities in the left lingula and apical segments of both lower lobes. In a seropositive individual these are highly suggestive of PCP.

(HRCT: High-resolution computed tomography; PCP: *Pneumocystis jirovecii* pneumonia)

Table 8: Possible causes of clinical deterioration in HIV patients with PCP infection.

- Severe PCP pneumonia with persistent hypoxia even on ventilator support
- Iatrogenic
- Drug-induced anemia or methemoglobinemia
- Pneumothorax
- Associated bacterial or viral (cytomegalovirus) infection
- Associated infection with *Mycobacterium avium* intracellulare
- Very low CD4 count (<50 cells/µL)
- Pulmonary embolism
- Inappropriate dosing

(HIV: Human immunodeficiency virus; PCP: *Pneumocystis jirovecii* pneumonia)

Other drugs used for prevention are dapsone, penta-midine, atovaquone, and clarithromycin (*see* **Table 7**).

Community-Acquired Pneumonia

Community-acquired pneumonia (CAP) is 10 times more common in HIV-positive patients. CAPs dominate PCP in Indian, all African, and most Western series. Bacterial infections were the most lung infections in the "Pulmonary Complications of HIV Study". The incidence of CAP increases with declining CD4 counts. Bacteremic pneumococcal pneumonia is commonly seen and in a study by Gilks et al. in the Lancet, accounted for 26% of all CAPs in Nairobi. Gram-negative bacilli and *Staphylococcus aureus* increase in importance as immunosuppression increases. Atypical pathogens are relatively uncommon, but do occur **(Table 9)**.

The mortality of CAP in HIV is also approximately four times higher in HIV-positive than negative patients. Relapses are also more frequent and occurred in 22% of Nairobi prostitutes with CAP. TMP-SMX prophylaxis is useful not just in PCP but also in CAP. It was associated with a 67% reduction in the incidence of bacterial pneumonia in patients receiving this drug. Pneumococcal vaccine is recommended but may be ineffective in preventing disease. A study by French et al. in the Lancet in 2000 showed that the 23 polyvalent vaccines actually increased the risk of developing CAP.

Other Infections

Infections caused by other bacteria, opportunistic infections and endemic fungal infections are also observed. In addition, parasitic infections contribute worldwide to increased morbidity and mortality. Responsible organisms include *Toxoplasma gondii*, *Strongyloides stercoralis*, *Cryptosporidium* and *Microsporidium*.

Table 9: Prevention of other pulmonary infections in HIV-infected.

Drug	Drug used
Bacterial Infections	
Mycobacterium tuberculosis	Isoniazid (6–12 months); often longer
MAC	Clarithromycin daily
Streptococcus pneumoniae	Immunization with 23-valent capsular polysaccharide
Fungal infection	Fluconazole

(MAC: *Mycobacterium avium* complex)

■ MALIGNANCIES AND IDIOPATHIC NONINFECTIVE DISORDERS IN HIV INFECTIONS

Malignancies

Kaposi's Sarcoma

Kaposi's sarcoma (KS) is an angioproliferative tumor now known to be associated with infection with human herpes virus 8 (HHV8). HHV8 has been demonstrated in all forms of KS, the HHV8 RNA and deoxyribonucleic acid (DNA) being present in endothelial cells, mononuclear cells, and spindle cells of the lesion. HHV8 is detectable and shown to replicate in the peripheral blood of patients before symptoms of KS appear. Most patients with AIDS-associated KS have antibodies toward HHV8. HIV is believed to activate this virus, which lies dormant in endothelial cells; this is the trigger for angiogenesis, which results in the development and proliferation of this vascular tumor. The HHV8 genome may exert its oncogenic effect in more than one way. The genome contains genes that are homologs to human genes. Among these is a nuclear antigen that binds to P53 and links viral DNA to human DNA during mitosis. The HHV8 genome also expresses a viral interleukin-8 receptor that induces angiogenesis. Cytokines are required for HHV8 infected endothelial cells to change to a phenotype that leads to the development and growth of KS. The HIV-1 Tat protein regulates cytokines, which promote the oncogenicity of KS cells. Genetic polymorphism of the Fey receptors III A is reported to be associated with an increased risk for developing KS.

Kaposi's sarcoma is more prevalent as the CD4 count declines, but it can occur with comparatively higher CD4 counts as well. In the US, it is 20 times commoner in men who have sex with men. The prevalence has dropped markedly in the West with the introduction of ARV therapy. It is considered rare in India and there are just a few case reports of KS in our country.

Clinical features: KS causes cutaneous, mucocutaneous and visceral lesions, the first two generally preceding visceral lesions by months or years **(Figs. 9A to C)**.

The lesions appear as red or violet papules or nodules, which often fuse to form raised plaques. Any portion of the skin, mucosa, or any visceral organ may be involved.

Pulmonary involvement can cause cough, hemop-tysis, and breathlessness. Though extrapulmonary

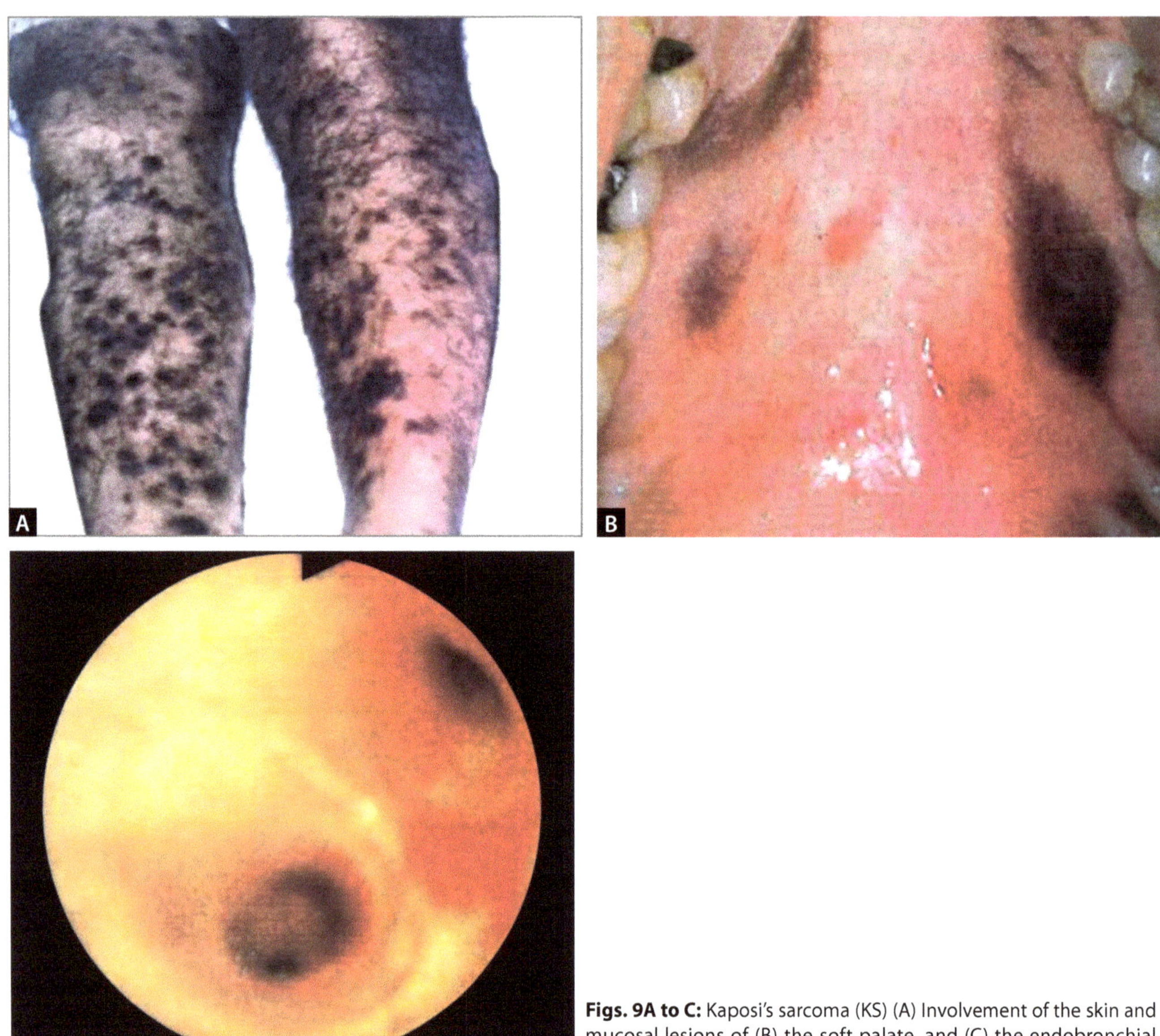

Figs. 9A to C: Kaposi's sarcoma (KS) (A) Involvement of the skin and mucosal lesions of (B) the soft palate, and (C) the endobronchial region in a patient with KS.

involvement is generally evident, 10–15% of KS occur without skin lesions. CD4 counts are generally less than 100/uL. Clinical examination of the respiratory system is usually normal. Typical radiographic features include single or multiple nodules with pleural effusion. HRCT shows peribronchovascular nodules that may be missed on a chest X-ray **(Fig. 10)**. Infiltrates and airspace consolidation may also be present. A fiberoptic bronchoscopy classically reveals purplish raised lesions on the mucosa of the airways. Lesions in the larynx and trachea may rarely cause obstruction. KS lesions are highly vascular and as their appearance is distinctive they are best not biopsied.

Diagnosis: Diagnosis is easy when endobronchial lesions are visible through fiberoptic bronchoscopy. It is difficult if endobronchial lesions are absent, more so if there are also no visible skin or mucosal lesions. Pleural effusions may be serous or serosanguinous; they are exudates with a high LDH. In some patients a CT-guided or a thoracoscopic biopsy of a nodule within the lung or a thoracoscopic visualization (and biopsy if thought necessary) of the pleura is needed for a confirmed diagnosis.

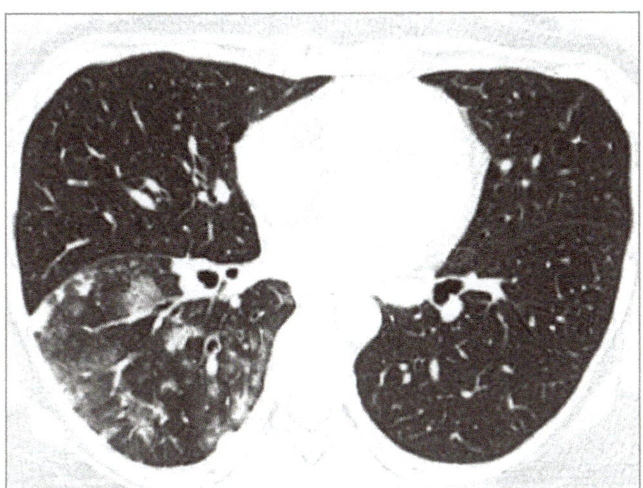

Fig. 10: Kaposi's sarcoma. HRCT demonstrates ill-defined nodular lesions in the right lower lobe in a subpleural and peribronchovascular location. Transbronchial biopsy revealed a Kaposi's sarcoma. (HRCT: High-resolution computed tomography)

Treatment: All patients with KS involving the lung require ARV therapy with concomitant chemotherapy. Prophylaxis against pneumocystis infection should be given to all patients. There are two chemotherapeutic regimes in use:

1. Adriamycin (20 mg/m^2), bleomycin (10 mg/m^2), and vincristine (1.4 mg/m^2)—in four to six cycles. Response rates are about 30–50%.
2. Liposomal doxorubicin (40–60 mg/m^2) or doxorubicin (20 mg/m^2) given every 2 weeks has the same response rate as the first regime with lesser side effects. The risk of drug-to-drug interaction with ARV therapy needs to be kept in mind with both regimes.

Clinical course: The 5-year survival rate of patients with pulmonary KS receiving both ARV therapy and chemotherapy is 50%. Untreated pulmonary KS has a median survival rate of less than 6 months. Very low CD4 counts less than 100/μL, respiratory distress, hypoxia, all worsen prognosis. Early treatment of HIV disease with ARV therapy is the best prevention for KS and other AIDS-related complications.

Non-Hodgkin's Lymphoma

The incidence of NHL in HIV patients has reduced sharply after the introduction of ARV therapy. Even so, it remains an important AIDS-defining illness, particularly in the West. The risk of high-grade lymphoma is increased 600-fold and of primary lymphoma within the brain 3,500-fold in HIV patients. This marked increase is associated with concomitant infections with Epstein-Barr virus (EBV) and/or HHV 8 virus. Other risk factors for NHL are male sex, increased age, and a very low CD4 count less than 100/μL. Most NHLs in AIDS are high grade and belong to either one of the three categories: (1) Burkitt's lymphoma, (2) centroblastic lymphoma, and (3) immunoblastic lymphoma. Burkitt's lymphoma can occur with higher CD4 counts compared to other varieties. Also, the incidence of Burkitt's lymphoma has not appreciably changed following ARV therapy.

Pulmonary NHL can occur as a primary within the lung or may occur secondarily as a spread from a primary elsewhere in the body. The development of NHL in HIV patients is probably influenced by coinfection with EBV and by HHV-8 antigenic stimulation and dysregulation of cytokine response **(Figs. 11A and B)**.

Clinical features: Secondary involvement of the lung from NHL originating outside the lung always means aggressive advanced stage IV disease even at presentation. Fever, weight loss, and presence of disease in lymph nodes or other organ systems is clinically evident.

Primary lymphoma of the lung may present with systemic features of low-grade fever and a high erythrocyte sedimentation rate (ESR). A Pel-Ebstein type of fever may occur though not as frequently as in Hodgkin's disease. Pulmonary symptoms include cough, breathlessness (when there is increased involvement of the lung), and chest pain. The CD4 counts are generally less than 50/μL. Anemia, leucopenia, and thrombocytopenia are frequently present. Imaging studies show single or multiple nodules within the lung parenchyma. Pleural effusion and mediastinal lymphadenopathy may be present.

Diagnosis: A confirmed diagnosis is generally possible through a CT-guided core needle biopsy of a lung nodule. When this is nonconfirmatory, a video-assisted thoracoscopic biopsy may be necessary **(Fig. 12)**.

Treatment: The treatment is as for NHL in general. Two chemotherapeutic regimes are in use:

1. Cyclophosphamide, doxorubicin, vincristine, and prednisolone (CHOP)
2. Etoposide, prednisolone, vincristine, cyclophosphamide, and doxorubicin (EPOCH).

Either one or the other is used in conjunction with ARV therapy.

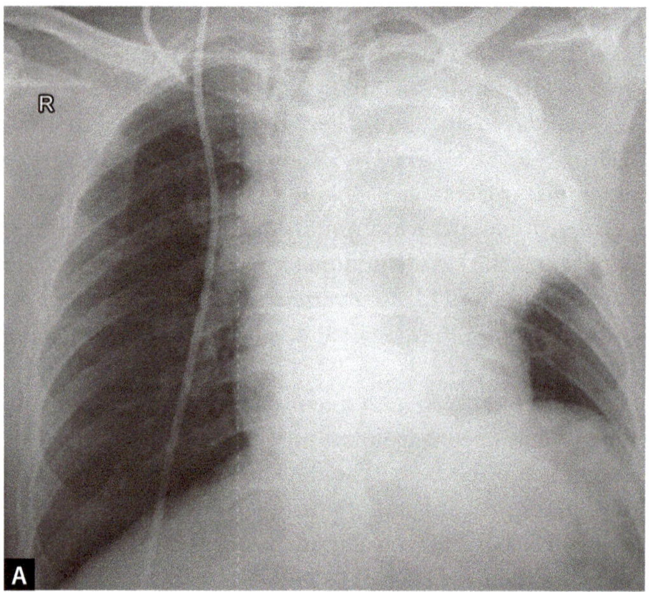 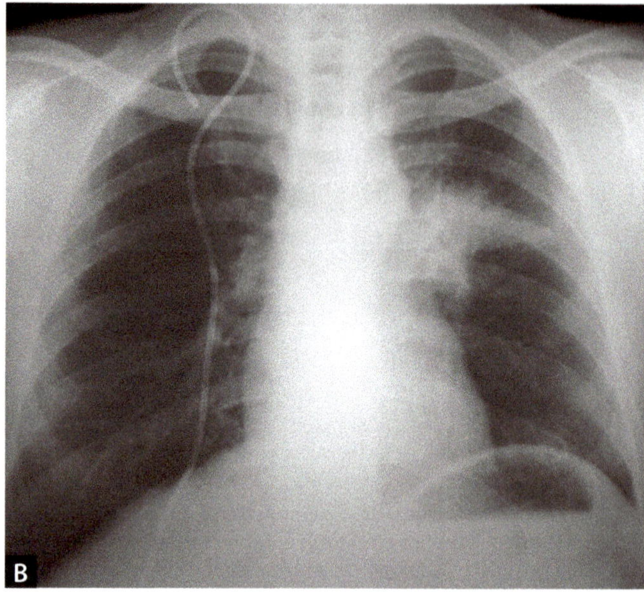

Figs. 11A and B: Non-Hodgkin's Lymphoma. Chest X-ray (A) demonstrates a large mass lesion in the left hemithorax superiorly in a seropositive individual. CT-guided biopsy revealed a non-Hodgkin's lymphoma. Post-treatment chest X-ray (B) reveals marked resolution in the mass lesion.
(CT: Computed tomography)

Primary Effusion Lymphoma (Body Cavity-associated Lymphoma)

Primary Effusion Lymphoma (PEL) is a variant of NHL, which occurs almost exclusively in HIV infections. The pleura, pericardium, and peritoneum may be involved with malignant effusions without identifiable tumor mass in any one of the above. The pleura is more frequently involved. Men are at greater risk, the disease occurring predominantly in men who have sex with men and who are positive for HHV 8. PEL contains HHV 8, EB virus, and expresses CD45.

Clinical features: Fever, weight loss, and fatigue are presenting features. Pleural effusion causes cough, pleuritic pain, and dyspnea. Imaging shows unilateral or bilateral pleural effusions. CT scans may reveal localized masses of NHL in the lung. PEL remains localized to its site of origin—generally the pleura.

Diagnosis: Diagnosis is based on examination of pleural fluid—its immunohistochemistry and molecular characteristics. Demonstration of HHV 8 is considered essential.

Treatment: Treatment is as for NHL and includes chemotherapy with ARV therapy.

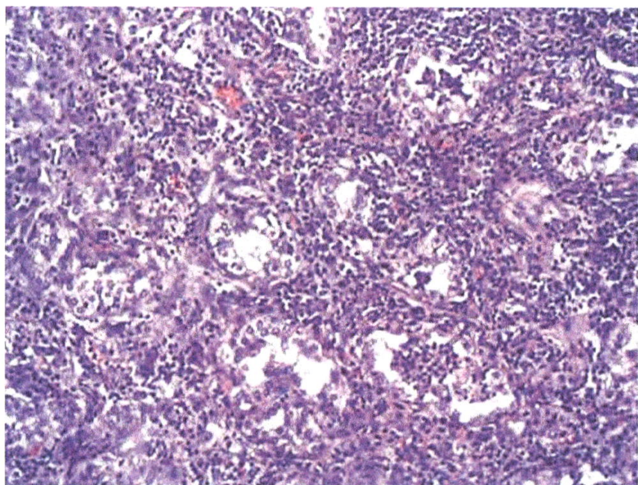

Fig. 12: Non-Hodgkin's lymphoma. Histopathological specimen reveals a dense interstitial infiltrate of small lymphoid cells. IOX magnification shows primary low-grade B-cell non-Hodgkin's lymphoma.

Lung Cancer

Human immunodeficiency virus-positive patients have a two-to-five old increased risk of developing lung cancer. Though this risk extends to all lung cancers, adenocarcinoma accounts for most cases. Men are at greater risk and as in NHLs, lung cancer in the HIV-positive population tends to present in more aggressive and advanced forms. Unlike NHL or KS, the CD4 counts tend to be well-preserved in patients with HIV-associated lung cancer. The risk of lung cancer in HIV-positive patients who smoke is greater than in the normal smoking population. Perhaps smoking added on to HIV infection inflicts greater damage to the lung compared to non-HIV individuals.

Clinical features: Clinical features are the same as lung cancer in general. Patients tend to be younger and the disease is generally more aggressive.

Treatment: Treatment for HIV-associated lung cancer is along the same lines as for lung cancer in non-HIV patients.

Multicentric Castleman's Disease

Castleman's disease is a rare lymphoproliferative disorder showing angioproliferation. There are two clinical variants: (1) localized and (2) multicentric. The multicentric form often transforms to NHL.

There is an increased incidence of Castleman's disease in HIV-infected patients. The disease generally occurs in association with KS with a positive HHV8 infection. Pulmonary involvement in Castleman's disease is exceedingly rare even in the Western world. Neither have we seen one in India and to the best of our knowledge, there is no proven reported case from this country.

Features of the multicentric form of the disease include fever, lymphadenopathy, hepatosplenomegaly, and pancytopenia. Pulmonary involvement often causes cough and breathlessness. Auscultation reveals bilateral basal crackles. CD4 counts vary and need not be very low. There is generally microbiological evidence of HHV8 infection. Imaging studies show mediastinal adenopathy, interstitial infiltrates, and pleural effusion. A lung biopsy is necessary to confirm the diagnosis. Multicentric disease requires chemotherapy with vincristine or etoposide.

With the use of ARV therapy and chemotherapy, the 5-year survival rates reported in the West are close to 50%. NHL is a frequent development.

Idiopathic, Noninfective, and Nonmalignant Disorders

A large number of these disorders have been described in the literature. These disorders should always be considered when microbiological staining and culture together with molecular techniques fail to reveal an infective organism in HIV patients who have pulmonary infiltrates and clinical features compatible with pulmonary infections. A number of these disorders also occur in non-HIV patients; the clinical features and management in HIV patients are similar to that in non-HIV patients.

Only a few of these miscellaneous disorders are considered here.

Lymphocytic Interstitial Pneumonia

Lymphocytic interstitial pneumonia (LIP) is a disease of unknown etiology occurring in patients with HIV infection and in autoimmune disease. It is commoner in children than in adults and generally occurs with advanced disease associated with severe immunosuppression.

Clinical features: Clinical features are nonspecific and include fever, cough, and breathlessness. Generalized lymphadenopathy may be present. Clubbing occasionally occurs in children. Radiography of the chest most commonly shows diffuse interstitial infiltrates. Nodular shadows may also be present. Pleural effusion is a frequent occurrence. Chest CT shows interstitial infiltrates, diffuse ground-glass shadowing, and nodules.

Diagnosis: Diagnosis is one of exclusion. Transbronchial biopsy is necessary for a diagnosis. Biopsy reveals peribronchial, perivascular infiltration of lymphocytes, and plasma cells. Septal infiltration is also present and distinguishes LIP from nonspecific interstitial pneumonia.

Treatment: ARV therapy is believed to cause a regression of this disorder.

HIV-associated Pulmonary Hypertension

Human immunodeficiency virus is an important cause of pulmonary hypertension (PH). It is a rare complication, the reported incidence being less than 0.5% which, however, is significantly greater that the reported incidence of PH in non-HIV patients (0.02%). HIV is assumed to produce vascular changes in the pulmonary arterial tree similar to those observed in primary PH.

The pathogenesis of HIV-associated PH is unclear. HIV is believed to result in increased expression of endothelin-1, a vascular growth factor which may well be responsible for remodeling of the media and adventitia of the pulmonary arterial tree. HIV-related PH can occur at all stages of HIV disease and at any level of the CD4 count.

Clinical features: The main symptom is dyspnea on exertion. Other symptoms include syncope, fatigue, angina, and peripheral edema. The diagnosis is often made late in the natural history of the disease.

The physical signs are similar to those described under primary PH in the section on "Pulmonary Vascular Diseases". Imaging features, echocardiography, and electrocardiography (ECG) findings have been described in the same section. Catheter studies are invariably necessary to measure pulmonary artery pressure, pulmonary occlusion pressure, and the cardiac output.

Diagnosis: It is imperative to exclude all causes of secondary PH described in the section on "Pulmonary Vascular Diseases", before making a diagnosis of HIV-related PH. Also, before a young adult is labeled to have primary PH, care must be taken to exclude HIV disease.

Treatment: Treatment consists of ARV therapy together with drugs helpful in reducing pulmonary artery pressure. These drugs have been discussed in the section on "Pulmonary Vascular Diseases" to which the reader is referred. Interaction between sildenafil and protease inhibitors must be borne in mind.

Prognosis: In spite of newer drugs available for treatment, the disease has a downhill course, leading to heart failure within two years.

■ SUGGESTED READING

1. Benito N, Moreno A, Miro JM, et al. Pulmonary infections in HIV-infected patients: an update in the 21st century. Eur Respir J. 2012;39:730-74.
2. Crothers K, Thompson BW, Burkhardt K, et al. HIV-associated lung infections and complications in the era of combination antiretroviral therapy. Proc Am Thorac Soc. 2011;8(3):275-81.
3. Hull MW, Phillips P, Montaner JSG. Changing global epidemiology of pulmonary manifestations of HIV/AIDS. Chest. 2008;134(6):1287-98.
4. Hussain T, Sinha S, Kulshreshtha KK, et al. Seroprevalence of HIV infection among tuberculosis patients in Agra, India—a hospital-based study. Tuberculosis (Edinb). 2006;86(1):54-9.
5. Lawn SD, Bekker LG, Miller RF. Immune reconstitution disease associated with mycobacterial infections in HIV-infected individuals receiving antiretrovirals. Lancet Infect Dis. 2005;5(6):361-73.
6. Mbulaiteye SM, Parkin DM, Rabkin CS. Epidemiology of AIDS-related malignancies an international perspective. Hematol Oncol Clin North Am. 2003;17(3):673-96, v.
7. Narain JP, Lo YR. Epidemiology of HIV-TB in Asia. Indian J Med Res. 2004;120(4):277-89.
8. Pathni AK, Chauhan LS. HIV/TB in India: a public health challenge. J Indian Medical Association. 2003;101(3):148-9.
9. Sharma SK, Mohan A, Kadhiravan T. HIV-TB co-infection: epidemiology, diagnosis and management. Indian J Med Res. 2005;121(4):550-67.
10. Slotar D, Escalante P, Jones BE. Pulmonary manifestations of HIV/AIDS in the tropics. Clin Chest Med. 2002;23(2):355-67.

Section 9

Tropical Infections Involving the Lung

CHAPTER 29

Helminthic Lung Diseases

■ INTRODUCTION

There are far more people living in the tropical and subtropical areas of the world than in other regions. Besides being exposed to and subject to most diseases and pulmonary infections prevalent in the West and common to the whole world, the billions residing in tropical areas also need to cope with disease and pulmonary infections by and large specific to the tropics.

The battle between "seed" and "soil" is most intensely fought in the tropics. This general geographic term refers to regions of the earth lying between the Tropic of Cancer and the Tropic of Capricorn. Some of the most impoverished countries of the globe lie between these equatorial parallels and include India and Sri Lanka, Thailand, Malaysia, Philippines and Indonesia, most South American countries, Central American and Caribbean islands, all of Africa except its southernmost tip and many South Pacific islands. The climate in these "tropical countries" is characterized by heat and humidity and these climatic conditions coupled with the milieu of poverty and deprivation provide ideal breeding grounds for pathogenic bacteria and parasites and their vectors and intermediate hosts to flourish. Overcrowded, unhygienic living conditions, lack of basic sanitation or access to safe drinking water increase the transmission of these infections. Finally, lack of medical facilities and essential drugs, poorly staffed and funded hospitals and clinics and general lack of infrastructure at all levels of society make practicing medicine in these circumstances a daunting and challenging task. As Maurice King so eloquently pointed out in his monograph, "The main determinant of the pattern of developing care in tropical countries is poverty rather than a warm climate".

The impact of respiratory infections in the tropics is considerable. Pulmonary tuberculosis is an example of one disease, which though prevalent in most parts of the world continues to exert its most devastating effects on the life and economy of poor third world countries. The same is true for pulmonary infections in HIV-infected patients. Both these conditions have been considered elsewhere in this book.

In some tropical and developing countries, childhood mortality may reach 50% in the first 5 years. At least one-third of these deaths are due to respiratory infections. Exotic diseases are also encountered here; the kind the physician practicing in the West may only vaguely remember from his medical-school days. Why are these obscure conditions relevant to all physicians wherever they may practice? The boundaries of countries are shrinking, international travel is becoming common and affordable, and, as the severe acute respiratory syndrome (SARS) epidemic taught us, respiratory pathogens are oblivious to boundaries not even pausing to acquire a visa!

In the last few decades, there have been unparalleled increases in the number of travelers, and populations are now in motion to a degree never before seen in history. Mobile populations include leisure and business travelers, military personnel, long-term expatriates, missionaries, etc. Also included are legal and illegal immigrants and refugees from numerous global conflicts and genocides. Members of these populations travel between countries more frequently and rapidly than ever deemed possible. Back in 1995, it was estimated that 1.5 million tourists crossed international borders every day, an annual total of over 500 million. This number is expected to rise markedly with each passing decade. The huge number of immigrants from the war torn counties of the Middle

East in the last decade, chiefly to Western Europe has magnified this problem immensely. As SARS taught us so compellingly, virtually any destination in the world can be reached from any other in only 36 hours of travel. This 36-hour window is well within the incubation period of most infectious diseases, affording ample opportunity for the unrecognized movement of pathogens from place to place and for rapid global spread of microbes. From the microbe's point of view the global village of the 21st century provides global opportunities for disease emergence and transmission.

■ HELMINTHIC LUNG DISEASES

General Considerations

Parasitic helminths infect billions of people in our world, especially in the tropics, and constitute one of the most important causes of morbidity and mortality. Pulmonary helminthic infections generally manifest with cough, breathlessness and a varying degree of peripheral eosinophilia. An eosinophilic pulmonary infiltrate is often present which may or may not cast a "shadow" on a radiological examination of the chest. In the West, pulmonary helminthiasis is often missed because of its comparative rarity. On the other hand, in the tropics, pulmonary helminthiasis is at times wrongly diagnosed when a radiologically apparent pulmonary infiltrate is associated with peripheral eosinophilia. This is because one fails to take note of the fact that the prevalence of peripheral eosinophilia for several reasons is extremely common in poor tropical countries. A pulmonary infiltrate or shadow may not necessarily be related to either peripheral eosinophilia or proven helminthic infection. It could be due to tuberculosis, other infections or even a noninfective pathology.

In humans, helminths produce a variety of pulmonary diseases, depending chiefly on the nature of the helminthic infection. Also, a pulmonary pathology is observed at a particular phase or stage in the life cycle of the helminth—a phase or stage which involves a transit or a stay within the lungs for a period of time. It is important to be aware of the biological behavior of different helminths in order to arrive at a diagnosis of the pulmonary infections they produce.

Biology and Host-Parasite Relationship

Certain important generalizations need to be kept in mind.

- Helminths are highly evolved human parasites; they have developed elaborate mechanisms that evade the defenses of the host, allowing them to survive in hostile environments.
- The life cycle of these helminthic parasites starts with the egg and then goes on to the larval form and the adult worm. Human infection is by ingestion of the egg or the larvae, penetration of the skin by larvae, transmission of larvae by bites of insects or vectors. Man may constitute a definitive host, an intermediate host, an accidental host or the only host, all depending on the kind of parasite considered.
- Helminths as a rule cannot multiply in the mammalian host. Therefore, the higher the worm load to start with, the greater the pathological consequences. There are two important exceptions to this generalization. The helminth *Strongyloides stercoralis* can autoinfect an immunocompromised patient, causing a hyperinfection syndrome that is often fatal. An echinococcal infection can disseminate and the parasite can multiply following rupture of a hydatid cyst. The released contents seed other sites causing other multiple lesions.
- Helminthic parasites, which at any stage of their life cycle migrate through the lungs, cause generally both a peripheral eosinophilia and a pulmonary eosinophilic infiltrate. This peripheral and tissue eosinophilia is caused by sensitized T-cell lymphocytes, which secrete mediators that induce progenitor cells in the marrow to develop into mature eosinophils. Eosinophilic production and maturation is affected by cytokines, chiefly interleukin 3 (IL3), interleukin 5 (IL5) and granulocyte/macrophage colony stimulating factor (GM-CSF). The eosinophilic response depends on the integrity of the cellular immune response of the host. When the cellular immune response is poor or well-nigh absent as in severe *human immunodeficiency virus* (HIV) infections, the eosinophilic reaction may not occur. Thus, eosinophilia is not observed in Strongyloid infections in HIV patients or in other immunocompromised hosts. Cytokines interact with eosinophils through specific receptors on the cell wall of the eosinophil, stimulating both maturity and metabolic activity.
- Pulmonary manifestations of helminthic disease are due to various factors, again depending on the exact nature of the helminth involved. They could result from the larvae within the lung (as with nematode infection), eggs within the lung (schistosomiasis) or from the

actual worm (paragonimiasis). The pathogenesis of pulmonary manifestation may be due to mechanical obstruction, an inflammatory response to the presence of what the lung considers a foreign body, or as a by-product of the host immune response. In fact, the pulmonary manifestations of many helminthic infections are due to a combination of Type I, Type III, Type IV immune responses of the host.

- It is debatable whether humans develop immunity to a helminthic infection. Unquestionably, ascarial infections are known to recur and filarial infection causing the syndrome of tropical eosinophilia can recur either due to a relapse or re-infection.

■ PULMONARY MANIFESTATIONS OF NEMATODE INFECTIONS

The pulmonary manifestations of nematode infections typically take the form of pulmonary eosinophilia. *Pulmonary eosinophilia* is characterized by pulmonary infiltration with a predominantly eosinophilic exudate, peripheral eosinophilia and the presence of respiratory symptoms, chiefly cough and breathlessness. The nematode parasite infections presenting with pulmonary eosinophilia are *Ascarial infection, Ankylostomal infection, Filarial infection* and *Strongyloides infection.*

Ascariasis

Ascariasis results from the ingestion of embryonated *Ascaris lumbricoides* eggs, which contaminate unwashed vegetables and fruits. The eggs hatch in the gut and the larvae penetrate the gut and reach the lung via the bloodstream. The larvae migrate via the pulmonary capillaries into the alveoli. They then pass up the airways, ascend up the trachea and are swallowed to reach the small intestine where they mature into adult worms.

The presence of larvae in the lungs exerts a hypersensitivity response which is clearly of the Type I kind [immunoglobulin E (IgE) levels are raised], but probably also involves a Type III reaction. The hypersensitivity response in its entirety is characterized pathologically by an eosinophilic pulmonary infiltrate, peripheral eosinophilia, and the presence of a patchy shadow within the lung on a radiographic examination of the chest. The X-ray chest may however appear normal in a number of patients. The peripheral eosinophilia

is not marked and except in rare instances does not exceed a total eosinophil count of 2500/mm^3. The clinical symptoms are cough, often paroxysmal, and breathlessness, which is often associated with a wheeze, so that a mistaken diagnosis of asthma can be easily made. Fever and general malaise may be present. Very rarely, larvae may be expectorated in the sputum. Once the helminths mature in the gut, eggs of *A. lumbricoides* are detected. Lung functions may show a mild obstructive defect with a fair degree of reversibility.

In the more severe cases, the larvae may incite a hypersensitivity pneumonic reaction with a larger shadow occupying part of a lobe. The systemic features are more marked. The larvae are sometimes observed to be fragmented and destroyed, surrounded by a dense cellular exudate chiefly consisting of eosinophils.

The presence of cough, breathlessness, a radiologically observed pulmonary infiltrate or a localized pulmonary shadow (generally in the upper lobe) together with peripheral eosinophilia is often termed Loeffler's syndrome. It denotes a hypersensitivity pulmonary reaction (Type I response) to an antigen and the most common antigenic stimulus is the larvae of either *Ascaris lumbricoides* or the larvae of the ankylostomes. The onset of Loeffler's syndrome caused by intestinal nematodes is generally 2–3 weeks after infection, around the time the larvae migrate from the pulmonary circulation into the alveoli. Other antigens are also known to cause Loeffler's syndrome. Loeffler's syndrome is self-limiting, the pulmonary shadow on the chest X-ray generally clearing within 3–4 weeks. The major mistake frequently made is to consider the pulmonary shadows in Loeffler's syndrome to be due to tuberculosis and to start the patient on 6–9 months of antituberculosis therapy. Nothing is lost in waiting for at least 4 weeks when the possibility of Loeffler's syndrome is suspected. The pulmonary shadows and symptoms disappear by then on their own.

Management is symptomatic. Bronchodilators help and inhaled β_2-agonists give symptomatic relief. No drug acts on the larvae of either Ascarial or ankylostomal infection that cause a hypersensitivity pulmonary response. Albendazole 400 mg once daily or mebendazole 100 mg BD orally daily for 3 days can eradicate both ascarial and ankylostoma infection once the parasite matures into adult worms in the small intestine. Diethylcarbamazine 100 mg thrice daily for a week has the same curative effect on the adult worm.

Ankylostomal Infection (*Ancylostoma duodenale, Necator americanus*)

The parasite found in the tropics is *Ancylostoma duodenale.* It is the infective larvae of this parasite found in soil, which penetrate the skin and through the bloodstream find their way via the pulmonary circulation into the alveoli. Here they excite the same hypersensitivity pulmonary reaction, which often presents clinically as Loeffler's syndrome. The pathogenesis, pathology and clinical features are similar to those described under infection with *A. lumbricoides.* Pulmonary manifestations of ankylostomiasis are not as common as in infections with *A. lumbricoides.* The larvae (as in *A. lumbricoides*) then travel up to the airways, up the trachea and are swallowed into the upper gut where they mature into adult hookworms. These worms attach themselves to the duodenal and jejunal mucosa and suck blood causing well-marked iron deficiency anemia.

Pulmonary Filariasis (Tropical Eosinophilia)

Weingarten in 1943, working at the Breach Candy Hospital in Mumbai, was the first to give the term "tropical eosinophilia" (TE) to a syndrome characterized by severe spasmodic bronchitis, eosinophilic leukocytosis and disseminated mottling of both lungs. The mystery of this exotic tropical syndrome slowly started to unfold, first with the discovery of the clinical efficacy of diethylcarbamazine, then with the unraveling of its histopathology and natural history and finally with studies in etiology and immunology. It is now accepted that *"tropical eosinophilia" as seen in India and other tropical countries is merely an unusual variant of human filariasis, caused by Wuchereria bancrofti and Brugia malayi.*

Epidemiology

Tropical eosinophilia has been reported from filarial endemic regions worldwide. The syndrome is particularly endemic in India, Sri Lanka and Southeast Asia. In India, it is the most endemic along the western coastal strip around Mumbai, Goa, Kerala, the whole of the eastern coast, and in Bengal, Bihar, Orissa, and areas endemic to filarial infection.

Northwest and Central Africa, Tanganyika, West Indies, the coast of China and the Philippines are other countries endemic to this syndrome. Travel from endemic to nonendemic areas also results in the syndrome being occasionally recognized in the West.

Etiology

As mentioned above, the syndrome is a variant of human filarial infection and results from an unusual hypersensitivity reaction to microfilariae liberated by *W. bancrofti* and *Brugia malayi.*

This concept is based on serological, histopathological, therapeutic and immunological studies. The serum of patients with TE shows raised IgE levels and specific antifilarial antibodies. In its early stages, TE responds to diethylcarbamazine both clinically and with regard to a fall in the specific antifilarial antibodies. This drug in vitro has a destructive effect on both microfilariae and the adult filarial worm. Histopathological studies of the lung, liver and lymph nodes in this syndrome often show degenerating fragmented microfilariae in the midst of an intensive eosinophilic exudate.

The role of animal filarial infection in causing TE has been suggested by several workers. Present evidence suggests that animal filarial infection is rare and has little or no role in the overall problem of TE.

Clinical Features

Pulmonary manifestations: Pulmonary manifestations are characterized by paroxysmal cough, breathlessness, wheeze, pulmonary infiltrates on a radiographic examination of the chest and an absolute eosinophil count greater than $3,000–3,500/mm^3$. These symptoms are most marked at night but may also be present in the day. Nonspecific features that accompany pulmonary manifestations include low-grade fever, malaise and weight loss. The absolute eosinophil count in hyperacute cases can be as high as $30,000–50,000/mm^3$. Laboratory features include filarial-specific IgE and IgG antibodies.

Hyperacute manifestations of TE with focal consolidation resembling pneumonia or bronchopneumonia have been described but are now rarely encountered.

Radiological examination: The radiological findings show reticulonodular shadows chiefly in the mid-zones or bases, prominent hila with heavy vascular markings over the bases, and occasionally, miliary mottling indistinguishable from miliary tuberculosis. In about 20% of patients, the X-ray chest may appear normal even though the lung histopathology (on a biopsy) may reveal typical features of TE. The syndrome in the early stages of its natural history invariably responds to diethylcarbamazine. Patients who have not been treated, or have a long history, or who respond inadequately to diethylcarbamazine may progress to chronic respiratory disability due to moderately severe pulmonary fibrosis.

Manifestations involving other systems: Other body systems may be involved. Patients may have lymphadenopathy and hepatosplenomegaly due to involvement of the liver and spleen. Occasionally, the presentation is with a low-grade fever, weight loss, abdominal complaints in the form of abdominal discomfort, diarrhea, the diagnosis being suggested by the very high eosinophil absolute count and the presence of specific antifilarial antibodies. Even here, a lung biopsy may reveal histopathological features of TE.

Lung Functions

About 70% of patients show a dominant restrictive pattern; 30% show airways obstruction + restriction. A lowered single breath transfer factor has also been observed in untreated TE. These findings showed marked improvement following a good clinical response to diethylcarbamazine but do not always return to normal. Some patients continue to progress to interstitial pulmonary fibrosis with permanent impairment of lung function. A study of 162 patients over 5 years by Udwadia revealed an increasing restrictive pattern in patients who had frequent relapses, and in those who responded inadequately to diethylcarbamazine. Patients with a history stretching over 5 years showed lung functions compatible with moderately severe interstitial pulmonary fibrosis. The degree of fibrosis was not as marked as in fibrosing alveolitis and the PaO_2 did not fall below 65 mm Hg. Pulmonary hypertension and cor pulmonale were not evident.

Histopathology and Natural History

This was unraveled for the first time in 1963 when Udwadia and Joshi reported a study of 26 open-lung biopsies in TE. The clinical features of paroxysmal cough, breathlessness, wheeze (resembling spasmodic airways' obstruction), and peripheral eosinophilia are from the very outset characterized by an alveolitis caused by an acute dense eosinophilic exudate. Lung histopathology reveals eosinophilic pneumonia, bronchopneumonia, microabscesses, and granulomas (**Figs. 1A to C**). Lung

functions, even at this stage, show a restrictive pattern on which is superimposed a pattern of airways' obstruction. The latter is due to eosinophilic infiltration of the bronchioles, with edema and disruption of the bronchial mucosa or muscle. Six months to two years after the onset of symptoms, a "mixed-cell" exudate consisting of eosinophils, mononuclear cells and histiocytes is observed in the lungs (**Fig. 1D**). Fibrosis occurs early in the natural history and is slowly progressive. The clinical picture is still readily recognizable because of marked peripheral eosinophilia. Breathlessness on exertion is now the most important symptom. Still later, in patients with a history more than 2 years, the eosinophils in the lung exudate become comparatively sparse, there being an increase in mononuclear cells and histiocytes. Fibrosis is evident and the lung is scarred (**Fig. 1E**). Lung functions show an increasing restrictive pattern. The overall clinical picture is one of mild to moderate interstitial pulmonary fibrosis. This results in respiratory disability due to increasing breathlessness on exertion, increasing restriction on lung function tests and is associated with reticulation of the mid-zones and bases of both lungs on a chest X-ray (**Fig. 2**). The pulmonary fibrosis in TE remains patchy and therefore is never as crippling as that observed in cryptogenic fibrosing alveolitis. The incidence and frequency of pulmonary disability in TE is difficult to estimate. Five out of 19 patients with a history of more than 2 years' duration progressed to a fair degree of pulmonary disability when followed up for 5 years.

The natural history of TE in endemic zones shows frequent recurrences and relapses. In some patients, the peripheral eosinophil count wanes with frequent relapses (the total eosinophil count often being less than $2000/mm^3$), and the predominant symptom is breathlessness on exertion rather than paroxysmal cough and breathlessness. The syndrome if seen at this juncture for the first time is difficult to recognize. It is likely that a number of patients in the tropics who masquerade under the guise of "bronchitis" or "pulmonary fibrosis", are in fact suffering from the end result of TE.

Immunology

In TE, microfilariae from a mature gravid human filarial parasite (*Wuchereria bancrofti, Brugia malayi*) are periodically released but promptly removed from the circulation and "trapped" within the lungs. Microfilaremia in the blood is therefore very rarely

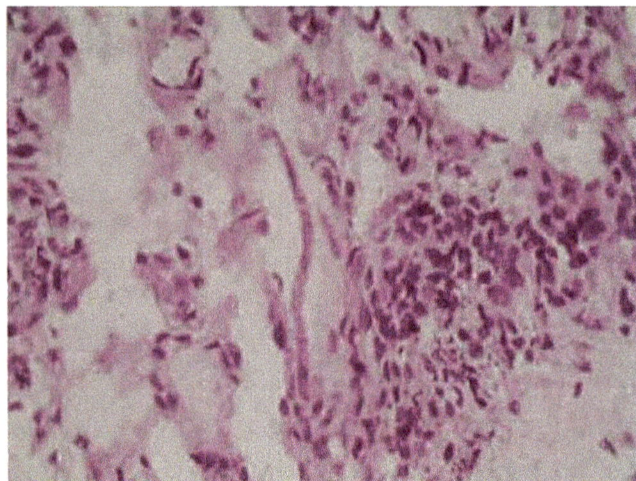

Fig. 1A: Tropical eosinophilia showing the presence of a microfilarial parasite within lung parenchyma.

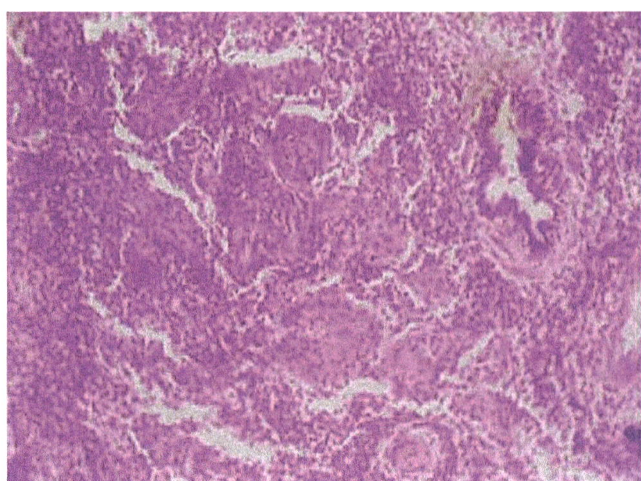

Fig. 1B: Tropical eosinophilia. Histopathological section of eosinophilic pneumonia in a patient with tropical eosinophilia. Note alveoli packed with eosinophils.

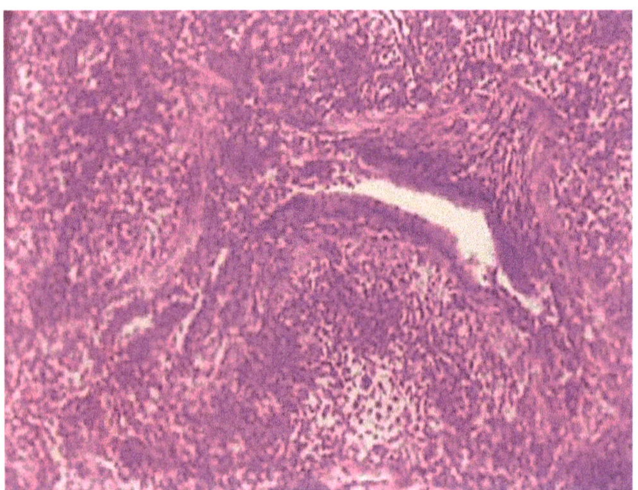

Fig. 1C: Tropical eosinophilia. Histopathological section showing eosinophilic bronchopneumonia. Note infiltration of the bronchial wall with eosinophils with sloughing bronchial mucosa.

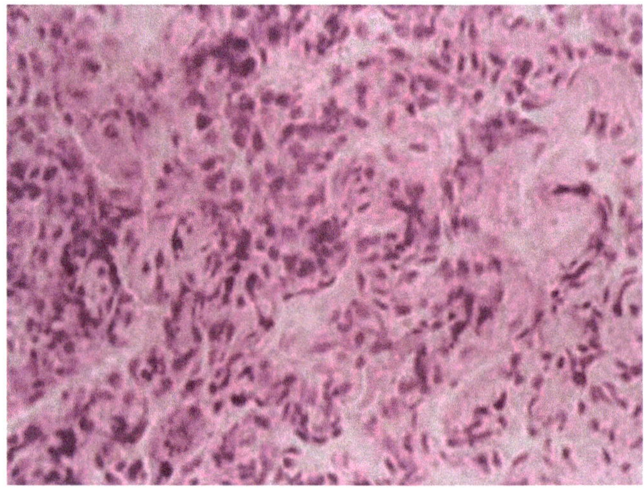

Fig. 1D: Tropical eosinophilia. A mixed-cell exudate consisting of eosinophils, mononuclear cells, histiocytes and lymphocytes. This reaction is observed 6–9 months after the onset of infection.

observed. Within the lungs, the microfilariae excite a severe, immunological response characterized by a marked increase in IgE and high levels of filarial-specific IgG, IgM, and IgE in the epithelial lining fluid. There appears to be an antibody-dependent mechanism of immune-mediated clearance of microfilariae within the lungs. Type I, Type III and Type IV immunological responses are all involved. The role of the eosinophil is crucial in this response. This cell probably has a dual role—a warrior of distinction that helps destroy the microfilariae, and also a role in the destruction of lung tissue due to release of eosinophilic granule components.

Activated eosinophils are capable of releasing major basic proteins, peroxidase and collagenase which injure lung tissue. Eosinophils may also release leukotrienes, which induce bronchoconstriction. The role of the mononuclear cell and macrophages in perpetuating inflammation and in increasing fibrosis is an area of fruitful research. The clinical, physiological and histopathological features characteristic of TE are unquestionably related to the immunological host response to microfilariae. If microfilariae succeed in running the gauntlet of the pulmonary circulation, they can excite an immunological response in the lymph

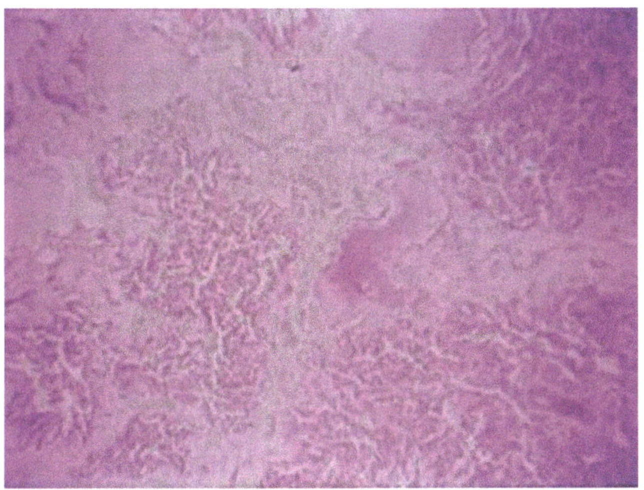

Fig. 1E: Tropical eosinophilia. Histopathological section showing the end-stage of tropical eosinophilia. Note well-marked fibrosis, compartmentalizing the lung. The fibrosis is never marked or as diffuse as in interstitial pulmonary fibrosis. Pockets of eosinophilic infiltration are still recognized, but histiocytes predominate.

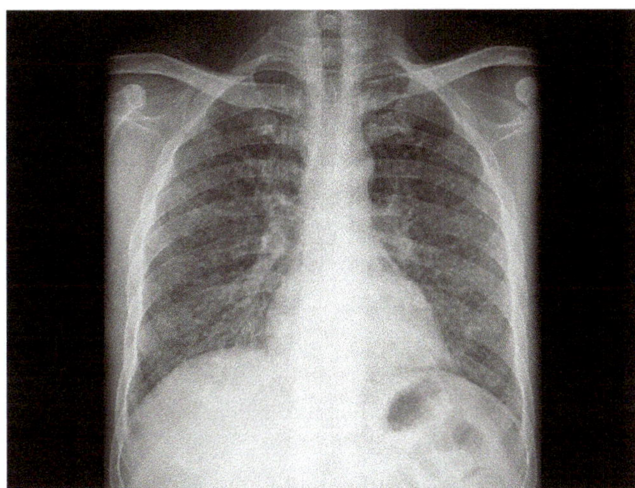

Fig. 2: Tropical eosinophilia: PA view of chest demonstrates predominantly nodular opacities in both lung fields.

glands, liver, spleen and rarely in the muscles and the gastrointestinal tract. Thus, though TE almost always involves the lungs, other organ systems may occasionally also be involved. The reason for the difference between the immunological host response to the same parasite in patients suffering from the usual form of endemic filariasis and in those with TE is an unsolved problem. Racial and genetic factors may play a role, as also the age at which infection occurs and perhaps the frequency of exposure.

The following patterns of human filarial infection can be described:

- Microfilaremia without any clinical features (asymptomatic)
- Microfilaremia with the classic features of endemic filariasis—high fever, severe lymphangitis chiefly involving the lower limbs
- Amicrofilaremia with the clinical features of chronic endemic filariasis
- Amicrofilaremia with the features of TE.

Unfortunately, the term TE is still used by many medical practitioners in the tropics as a "wastepaper basket" for any patient with cough, breathlessness and a rise in the peripheral eosinophil count. Ideally, the term TE should be abandoned and the overall features described above should be considered either as pulmonary manifestations of filarial infection or pulmonary filariasis. This is however easier said than done, because (a) peripheral eosinophilia

is so common in the tropics; (b) a number of conditions in the tropics (including infestation by other helminths) do also produce eosinophilia, cough and breathlessness; (c) The diagnostic confirmation by specific antifilarial antibodies in pulmonary filariasis is a luxury available in very few laboratories in the tropics. A classification of the causes of pulmonary eosinophilia in the tropics is given later in this chapter.

Treatment

Diethylcarbamazine is specific for the treatment of TE. Though a dose of 5 mg/kg/day for 10 days may well be adequate, Udwadia recommends the same dose for a period of 4 weeks. The drug is remarkably free from major side effects. A few patients (<5%) even in the earlier part of the natural history respond inadequately and as many as 20% of patients with a longer duration of symptoms extending from 2–5 years may fail to respond. The lack of response in patients with a long history is understandable as the drug cannot be expected to act on the increasing fibrosis within the lung.

The only 5-year follow-up study of a large series of cases showed that the relapse rate in TE following specific therapy was at least 20%. It was impossible to determine in this study how many were true relapses and how many were due to reinfection. In those living in highly endemic zones, we would recommend repeated monthly courses of diethylcarbamazine at 3-monthly intervals for a period of 1–2 years to help reduce the morbidity in TE. The use of corticosteroids in longstanding cases with evidence of pulmonary fibrosis is worth a trial, though their efficacy has not been studied and is therefore uncertain.

Visceral Larva Migrans

Visceral larva migrans is a disease with pulmonary manifestations caused by the larvae of the dog and cat round worms (*Toxocara canis, Toxocara catis*). These round worms infest the dog and cat respectively and the eggs are passed out via the feces.

These eggs may contaminate food or water and may be ingested by humans. In the intestines, the eggs hatch into larvae which penetrate the gut and reach the liver, lungs and other tissues via the systemic circulation. The larvae excite an immunological plus an inflammatory granulomatous reaction, chiefly in the liver and lungs. The larvae after weeks or months may die and become encapsulated and surrounded by an eosinophilic exudate. The life cycle of these animal parasites is cut short in humans, as the animal larvae cannot mature into adult worms in humans.

Clinical Manifestations

Visceral larva migrans occurs chiefly in children below 5 years, particularly when there is history of pica in the child. Pulmonary manifestations are characterized by cough, breathlessness, eosinophilic pulmonary infiltrates and well-marked peripheral eosinophilia with an absolute eosinophil count more than 3,500/mm^3, as in patients with TE. Breathlessness is often associated with wheezing, the clinical picture being indistinguishable from bronchial asthma. Transient pulmonary infiltrates on chest radiography are observed in over 50% of patients **(Fig. 3)**. Acute eosinophilic pneumonia and respiratory failure have also been observed. The liver is often enlarged; granulomas may be found on histopathological examination of the liver biopsy material. The central nervous system and other body tissues may be rarely involved. Constitutional symptoms in the form of fever, weight loss, malaise, and muscle pains may be present.

Diagnosis

The clinical features of well-marked pulmonary eosinophilia, hepatic enlargement in a young child

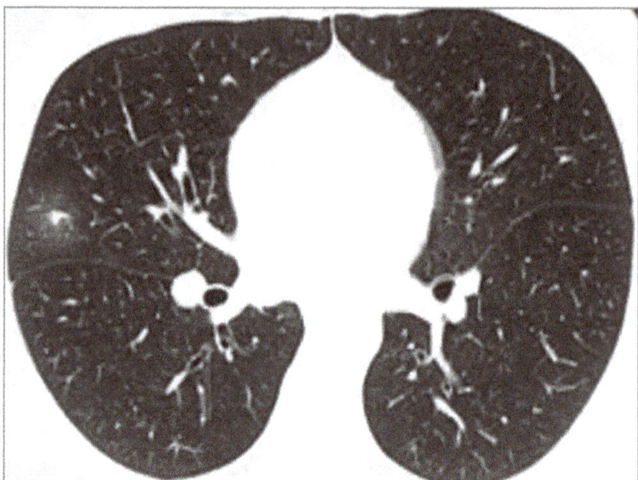

Fig. 3: Visceral larva migrans. High-resolution computed tomography demonstrates a small linear density with a surrounding halo in the right middle lobe.

with no or poor response to diethylcarbamazine should arouse suspicion of visceral larva migrans. A marked elevation of IgE is generally present. An enzyme-linked immunosorbent assay (ELISA) test using larval antigen has a sensitivity of about 70% and a specificity of 90%.

Management

Patients who are symptomatic should be given diethylcarbamazine (6 mg/kg/day) for 21 days or mebendazole (20 mg/kg/day) for 21 days or albendazole (10 mg/kg/day) for 5 days. Treatment could exacerbate an inflammatory reaction following the killing of the larvae. Anti-helminthics may therefore need to be combined with corticosteroids.

Strongyloides stercoralis Infection

Infection with *S. stercoralis* occurs when infective larvae present in the soil penetrate the human skin and travel via the bloodstream into the lungs. The larvae reach the alveoli though the pulmonary capillaries and excite a hypersensitivity lung response that results in the classical clinical features of pulmonary eosinophilia, which have already been described. The larvae ascend up the bronchi and the trachea to be swallowed so as to reach the small gut where they mature into adult worms. These adult worms produce rhabditiform larvae which are noninfective and which are passed out in the stools. In the soil these noninfective larvae turn into infective filariform larvae. It is rare for larvae to be found in the sputum and the correct diagnosis must await the presence of larvae of *S. stercoralis* excreted in the stool.

Hyperinfection Syndrome due to *S. stercoralis* Infection

The most dreaded pulmonary manifestation induced by intestinal nematodes is the hyperinfection syndrome caused by *S. stercoralis.* Invariably, this syndrome occurs only in immunocompromised individuals with a markedly depressed cell-mediated immune response. Very rarely, it has been observed in normal persons. Immunocompromised individuals with depressed cell-mediated immunity include patients with HIV infection, neoplastic diseases such as lymphomas, leukemia, patients on prolonged corticosteroid therapy for whatsoever reason, and patients who have received organ transplants. In these patients there may well occur a change in the reproductive cycle of the parasite. In immunocompetent individuals, the noninfective rhabditiform larvae have to be passed out into stools and only then can develop into the infective filariform larvae. In immunocompromised patients, the change to infective larvae occurs within the host. These numerous infective filariform larvae penetrate the gut, reach the circulation and invade various organ systems, in particular the lungs.

Pulmonary manifestations include severe breathlessness, airways' obstruction with pulmonary opacities on an X-ray and CT chest which may appear as infiltrates, consolidation, cavities or may resemble bronchopneumonia **(Fig. 4)**. Tachycardia, tachypnea and increasing hypoxia are observed. The filariform larvae when they penetrate the gut carry gram-negative gut organisms with them, so that the clinical picture is often combined with that of severe gram-negative sepsis and at times with meningitis due to gram-negative organisms. Interestingly, eosinophilia is absent probably due to poor cell-mediated immunity.

The hyperinfection syndrome caused by *S. stercoralis* is in our experience generally fatal.

Management

Early diagnosis and the stoppage or drastic modification of immunosuppressive therapy (if this is being administered) is imperative. *When an immunosuppressed patient develops pulmonary disease with associated bacteremia and sepsis, the possibility of strongyloidiasis should be seriously entertained* **(Fig. 4)**. Larvae should be carefully searched for in bronchial washings, sputum, duodenal washings and stools. Even reasonable suspicion should warrant the use of specific therapy. Specific therapy consists of albendazole 400 mg orally for 7 days. Two or three courses may be given 10 days apart. Broad-spectrum antibiotics, which cover gram-negative infections, should always be used in adequate dosage for 10–15 days. More often than not diagnosis is made too late to allow survival. Treatment should be initiated in suspect patients.

■ PULMONARY MANIFESTATIONS OF TREMATODE INFECTIONS

Schistosomiasis

Schistosomiasis is the second most common cause of mortality among parasite infections after malaria. It affects 150–200 million people causing 500,000 deaths annually. According to the GeoSentinel database that monitors travelers around the world, schistosomiasis is one of the 10 leading causes of morbidity among travelers, accounting for 6% of all the cases in sub-Saharan Africa. It is reported that 55–100% of travelers on rafting tours in African rivers become infected. The lungs can be affected in both the acute and chronic stages of the illness.

The disease is caused by three important *Schistosoma* species—*S. haematobium, S. mansoni* and *S. japonica.* The disease is endemic in Egypt, Africa, Saudi Arabia, Brazil,

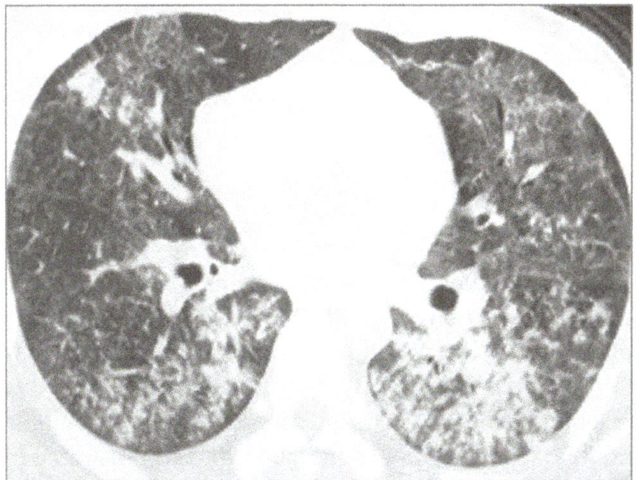

Fig. 4: Strongyloidiasis in an 18-year-old man with hemoptysis. Computed tomography chest clearly delineates the areas of consolidation. Bronchoalveolar lavage (BAL) revealed larvae of *S. stercoralis.*

Philippines and the Yangtze valley of China. It remains a rarity in India.

Pathogenesis

Infection occurs due to exposure to water-contaminated cercariae excreted by snails. These cercariae can penetrate the skin or the intestinal wall and turn within a few hours into schistosomula, which migrate to the lung. Their passage through the lungs often causes an acute hypersensitivity response manifesting clinically as pulmonary eosinophilia. From the lungs they reach the liver where they mature into adult worms. Fecund adult worms then migrate to their final habitat—the vesical plexus around the bladder and uterus *(S. haematobium)* and the mesenteric venous plexus *(S. mansoni* and *S. japonica)*. Eggs of *S. haematobium* besides causing a painful cystitis, enter the systemic venous system and are transported to the lung. Eggs of *S. mansoni* and *S. japonica* are first transported to the liver via the portal circulation where they block the portal radicals causing portal hypertension. These eggs reach the lungs through anastomatic channels between the portal and systemic veins only when portal hypertension is well established.

Eggs reaching the lungs block pulmonary arterioles and excite a granulomatous reaction (eosinophils, lymphocytes, macrophages) within the wall of the arterioles. Granulomatous lesions are also formed around eggs situated within the alveoli. Plexifrom lesions consisting of dilated thin-walled vessels are also observed. There is a progressive blockage of the pulmonary circulation as a result of tissue response (endothelial thickening, fibrin deposition, medial wall hypertrophy) to the eggs within the arterioles. The end result is cor pulmonale and congestive heart failure.

Clinical Features

During the phase of migration from the skin through the lungs to their final habitat, the clinical features are of pulmonary eosinophilia—fever, cough, wheezing, peripheral eosinophilia; the chest radiograph may show mottling due to multiple granulomas caused by ova reaching the lungs via the pulmonary vessels or multiple nodular lesions with ill defined borders as illustrated in **Figure 5**.

During the late phase of the infection when schistosomal ova lead to progressive blockage of the pulmonary circulation, the clinical picture is that of pulmonary

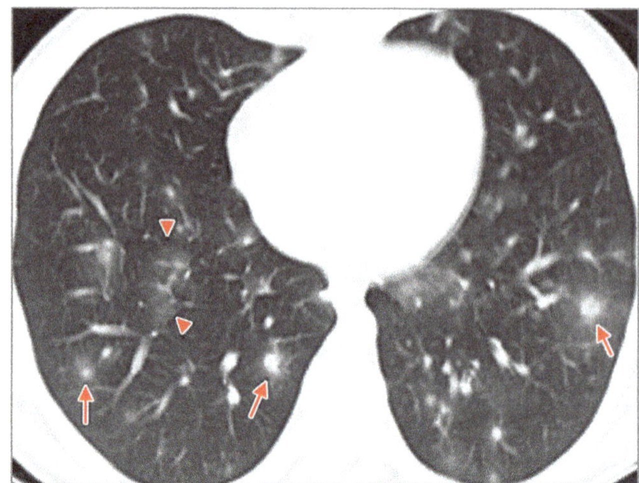

Fig. 5: Computed tomography (CT) chest showing early pulmonary schistosomiasis in a 28-year-old man who had traveled to Mali. Initially, the patient had fever and urticaria, after which he experienced dry cough, predominantly at night. Chest CT scan shows multiple nodular lesions with ill-defined borders in the lower lobes. Histological analysis revealed *S. mansoni*.
Source: Schwartz E, MD, Center for Geographical Medicine and Tropical Diseases, and Rozenman J, MD, Department of Radiology, Sheba Medical Center, Tel Hashomer, Israel.

hypertension and cor pulmonale. Gross aneurysmal dilatation of the pulmonary artery may be observed at this stage. The pulmonary involvement in the chronic phase almost always occurs in those with hepatosplenomegaly and portal hypertension. The opening of portosystemic collaterals allows passage of massive numbers of eggs from the portal vein directly to the lungs. A granulomatous reaction and fibrosis develop, with an acute necrotizing arteriolitis in the pulmonary vasculature leading to pulmonary hypertension and cor pulmonale.

The clinical features of chronic pulmonary schistosomiasis can be categorized into three groups:

1. Asymptomatic patients with eggs within the pulmonary circulation with or without granuloma formation
2. Granulomas with pulmonary hypertension
3. Granuloma formation with cor pulmonale.

The degree of pulmonary hypertension is usually mild to moderate; but may, on occasion, be severe with some patients progressing to cardiac failure or sudden cardiovascular collapse. Pulmonary hypertension and cor pulmonale develop in 5–25% of patients with portal hypertension. Pulmonary arteriovenous fistulae have also been described in this form of schistosomiasis. The exact incidence of schistosomal pulmonary hypertension and cor pulmonale in endemic areas is unclear, but in a study on hospital populations, between 2% and 4% of the total cardiac population were diagnosed as having schistosomal cor pulmonale. Finally, a third form of pulmonary schistosomiasis consists of the reappearance of cough, wheeze, eosinophilia and pulmonary infiltrates during the course of treatment with praziquantel. This is a form of Jarisch-Herxheimer reaction and represents an immunological reaction to newly released antigens from dead worms and eggs in the lungs. Treatment of advanced pulmonary hypertension and cor pulmonale is supportive.

Diagnosis

Urine examination *(S. haematobium);* stool examination (*S. mansoni, S. japonica)* may reveal eggs of the worm. A vesical biopsy may also reveal eggs of *S. haematobium* and *S. japonica*. Serology is also of help.

Treatment

Praziquantel 40 mg/kg in a single dose is the drug of choice. Pulmonary hypertension and cor pulmonale are however irreversible.

Paragonimiasis

Paragonimiasis is a disease endemic in East Asia, Southeast Asia, Africa, and Latin America (particularly in Peru). Human infection is caused by the lung fluke *Paragonimus westermani* and other *Paragonimus* species endemic in the above-mentioned areas. It is believed that 195 million people are at risk and 26.7 million are infected in endemic areas.

Pathogenesis

Human infection occurs from eating raw or insufficiently cooked crustacea such as crabs and crayfish, which contain the encysted infective parasite (metacercariae). These forms excyst in the duodenum, penetrate the wall of the gut, go through the peritoneal cavity, diaphragm and pleural cavity to enter the lungs, where they mature into adult worms roughly measuring $1.2 \times 6 \times 5$ mm. These trematodes (lung flukes) are hermaphrodites and produce brownish eggs coughed up in the sputum or swallowed and voided in feces. Outside the human host, the life cycle goes through a snail intermediate host and then they encyst as metacercariae in freshwater crustacea.

The mature worm tunnels through the lung exciting a granulomatous reaction consisting of eosinophils and neutrophils. The surrounding lung tissue may show consolidation and/or atelectasis. Cystic lesions may enclose the parasite. Secondary infection of these cysts can result in the formation of one or more lung cavities (abscesses) which may communicate with bronchi. The worms as mentioned above lay eggs, which again excite a strong hypersensitivity reaction within the lungs. It needs to be mentioned that though the primary site of infection is in the lungs, the worm may also be found in the brain and very rarely in other tissues.

Clinical Features

Clinical features depend on the worm load present in a given patient. When the worm load is small, the patient may be asymptomatic, and even the chest X-ray may be normal. When moderate or large, clinical features include fever, breathlessness, chest discomfort, cough with expectoration and hemoptysis. The sputum may be rusty or blood-tinged and may contain eggs. Charcot Leyden crystals are frequently present in the sputum.

Chest radiography shows infiltrates, nodular shadows, which may cavitate to resemble one or more abscesses. Fibrosis and areas of atelectasis may be present. Pleural effusion, pneumothorax may also occur, particularly at the time of penetration of the worm into the lung parenchyma. *Computed tomography* (CT) chest often reveals areas of consolidation in one or both the lungs together with associated ground-glass attenuation. The consolidated areas may show cavitation indistinguishable from tuberculosis **(Fig. 6)**. Multilocular radiolucencies, cystic or bronchiectatic, usually without fluid levels, giving a so-called soap bubble appearance have been described. Another characteristic radiographic feature described is a ring shadow with a crescent along one border resembling the corona phase of a solar eclipse. The lesions are predominantly in the bases and peripheries of both lungs. Pleural effusions have been described in 70% of Japanese patients as the *Paragonimus* worms pass through the pleural cavity on their way to the lungs. Pleural thickening and calcification have also been described. Despite this plethora of pulmonary and pleural manifestations, about 20% of paragonimiasis patients are asymptomatic with the lung lesions being detected at routine health checks.

The main differential diagnosis is from tuberculosis or from a bacterial infection. Diagnosis is based on finding eggs in the sputum, in bronchoalveolar lavage (BAL) fluid or feces. Serological tests may also help.

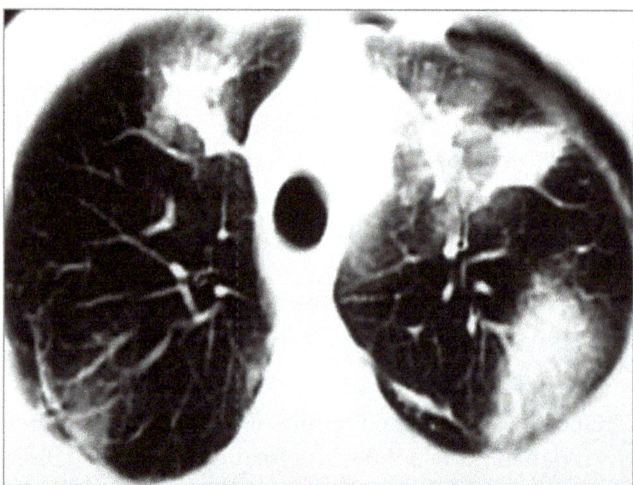

Fig. 6: Pulmonary paragonimiasis in a 35-year-old man. Computed tomography scan demonstrates bilateral ill-defined areas of consolidation and areas of ground-glass attenuation associated with left pneumothorax. Eggs of *P. westermani* were found at bronchoalveolar lavage.

Table 1: Causes of pulmonary eosinophilia.

• *Parasitic diseases*
  – Filaria
  – Ascaris lumbricoides
  – Ankylostomal infection
  – Strongyloidiasis
  – Toxocara canis and catis
  – Paragonimiasis
  – Schistosomiasis

• **Allergic bronchopulmonary aspergillosis**

• **Hypersensitivity response to:**
  – Drugs—penicillin, sulphonamides, trimethoprim-sulphamethoxazole, NSAIDs, carbamazepine, nitrofurantoin, penicillamine
  – Pollen
  – Other fungi
  – Other antigens

• **Asthamatic pulmonary eosinophilia**
• *Pulmonary vasculitis*: **Eosinophilic granulomatosis with polyangiitis (Churg-Strauss syndrome)**
• **Cryptogenic eosinophilic pneumonia**
• **Hypereosinophilic syndrome**

Treatment

The drug of choice is praziquantel given orally 25 mg/kg thrice daily for 2 days. Following treatment the stools within a few days stop containing eggs of the parasite and there is improvement both in the symptoms and in the imaging findings. In patients with pleural effusions, the fluid must be first drained before administering the drug. Triclabendazole, a new benzimidazole derivative has been recently used in small-scale clinical trials and found to be effective and safe in a single dose of 10 mg/kg.

It is seen from the previous descriptions that parasitic nematode and trematode infections often present with pulmonary eosinophilia. Pulmonary eosinophilia can also be due to other causes. **Table 1** lists the causes of pulmonary eosinophilia.

■ PULMONARY MANIFESTATIONS CAUSED BY CYSTODE INFECTIONS

Hydatidosis (Echinococcosis)

Hydatid disease in humans is chiefly caused by the larvae of the cystode *Echinococcus granulosa,* a worm which is found in the intestines of dogs and wolves. These worms release eggs from their gravid segments and the eggs are passed out in the animal's feces. Humans get infected when they ingest these eggs through contamination of food and water. After ingestion, the eggs on reaching the small intestine hatch larvae, which can migrate via the portal vein radicals into the liver where they slowly form hydatid cysts. The larvae could also reach the lungs via hematogenous spread, giving rise to one or more hydatid cysts within the lung. Rarely, hematogenous spread to other organs may also occur. In adults, the liver is the most common site of involvement, followed by the lung. In children, the lung is the most common site of hydatid disease.

Epidemiology

Though worldwide in distribution, particularly involving sheep- and cattle-raising areas (where dogs are also present), the disease is frequent in some tropical countries—particularly parts of Africa, South America and Northern India. It is particularly common in the State of Jammu and Kashmir where hydatid of the lung is one pathology, which most frequently necessitates thoracic surgery. A study from the Postgraduate Institute of Chandigarh in North India has reported an increasing trend in the seroprevalence of human hydatid disease between 1999 and 2003 when compared to the period 1984–98.

Pathology

The larvae reaching the lung slowly give rise to a space-occupying unilocular cyst, which to start with is small but can grow as large as 20 cm in diameter. The cyst is most often solitary (in 60–70% of cases), but multiple cysts also occur. They may be unilateral but in 20% of patients, are bilateral. It is uncommon to observe cysts within the liver and the lungs in the same patient. The cyst wall on histology has three layers:

1. The outer pericyst, which is chiefly composed of fibroblasts and fibrous tissue
2. An acellular middle laminated layer which has a nutrient function
3. An inner germinal layer, which has scoleces and generates daughter cysts. The cyst may lie quiet over years, it may grow to compress neighboring structures, it may rupture into the lung, bronchus, pleura or rarely into the mediastinum or even the pericardium, causing spread of hydatid disease in these areas.

Clinical Features and Complications

A hydatid cyst in the lung is often asymptomatic being discovered on routine chest radiography. Large cyst or cysts may cause cough, breathlessness and vague chest discomfort. An infected cyst behaves as a lung abscess. Rupture of a cyst invariably produces symptoms. The cyst fluid is immunogenic and following rupture can lead to a hypersensitivity reaction or even anaphylaxis. Bronchospasm, hypotension, tachycardia may occur, and anaphylaxis can be fatal. The cyst may rupture into a bronchus, the contents being coughed up in the sputum. Communication with a bronchus also predisposes to infection of the cyst contents and to purulent expectoration. Rupture may also be associated with consolidation of the neighboring lung. If the cyst opens into the pleura, pleural effusion results and pleural dissemination follows with hydatid cysts within the pleura and pleural space. Rarely, rupture into the mediastinum leads to hydatids within the mediastinum and rupture into the pericardium to hydatids within the pericardium.

Imaging Findings

Hydatid cysts appear as round or ovoid cystic, unilocular masses with sharply defined borders which enhance on administration of contrast. The "meniscus sign" is observed when there is air between the outer pericyst and the middle laminated layer. This occurs when a cyst starts to erode an adjacent bronchus or bronchiole. When a cyst ruptures into a bronchus, an air-fluid level is observed within the cyst (**Fig. 7**); the meniscus sign may or may

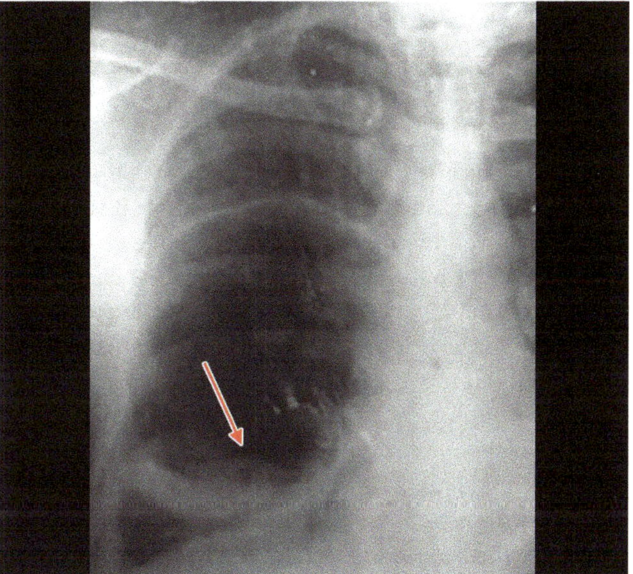

Fig. 7: Pulmonary hydatid cyst. Chest X-ray demonstrates a large air-filled cavity in the right lower zone with a crumpled membrane in the base of the cyst representing a ruptured pulmonary hydatid.

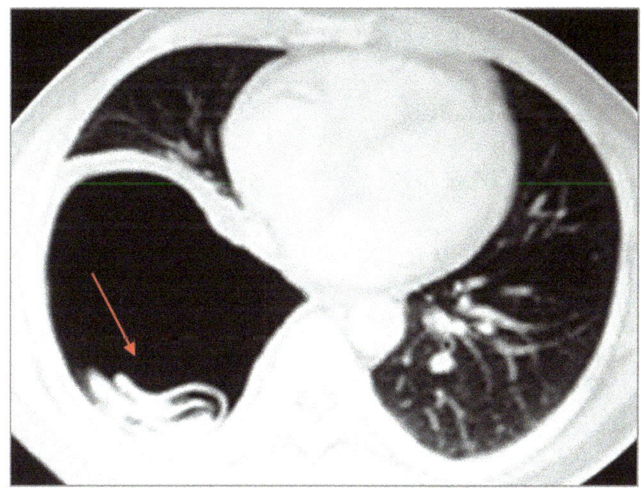

Fig. 8: Hydatid cyst. Computed tomography chest showing the 'water-lily sign', typified by the endocyst floating within the cyst.

not be present at the same time. The "water-lily sign" is typified by the endocyst floating within the cyst (**Fig. 8**).

Diagnosis

The presence of a well-defined cyst, particularly in an endemic area, should arouse suspicion and suggest the correct diagnosis. Indirect hemagglutination tests and the Cansoni skin tests are of doubtful use as they lack sensitivity and specificity. ELISA tests are more useful. Multiple lung cysts may need to be differentiated from metastatic lesions. The liquid nature of the contents of the cyst as judged on CT chest should give a correct diagnosis.

Management

The treatment of choice of a large cyst, which produces compression or is likely to rupture is surgical resection. This is followed by the use of mebendazole (10–15 mg/kg body weight per day) for 8 weeks to take care of any spillage that could have occurred during surgery.

When surgery is not indicated or when there are multiple bilateral cysts or when there is dissemination because of rupture of a cyst, one has to rest content with the use of mebendazole in the dose stated above. The course of mebendazole may be repeated several times. Percutaneous aspiration of a cyst followed by an injection of a cysticidal agent such as hypertonic saline or alcohol, with re-aspiration has also proved successful. It needs to be done under CT guidance. Mebendazole in the dose recommended should be administered.

■ SUGGESTED READING

1. Baharoon SA, Al-Tahdali HH, Bamefleh HS, et al. Acute pulmonary schistosomiasis. J Global Infect Dis. 2011;3(3):293-5.
2. Kim TS, Han J. Pleuropulmonary paragonimiasis: CT findings in 31 patients. AJR Am J Roentgenol. 2005;185(3):616-21.
3. Kunst H, Mack D, Kon OM, et al. Parasitic infections of the lung: a guide for the respiratory physician. Thorax Published Online First: 29 September 2010. doi: 10.1136/thx.2009.132217.
4. Manghani DK, Dastur DK, Udwadia FE. The lung in tropical eosinophilia compared to that in pulmonary hypertension. Fine structural basis of respiratory disability. Zentralbl Pathol. 1992;138:108-18.
5. Martanez S. Thoracic manifestations of tropical parasitic infections: a pictorial review. Radiographics. 2005;25(1):135-55.
6. Ozvaran MK. Pleural complications of pulmonary hydatid disease. Respirology. 2004;9(1):115-9.
7. Ross AG, Bartley PB, Sleigh AC, et al. Schistosomiasis. N Engl J Med. 2002;346:1212-20.
8. Singh TS, Sugiyama H, Rangsiruji A. Paragonimus and paragonimiasis in India. Indian J Med Res. 2012;136(2):192-204.
9. Udwadia FE. Pulmonary eosinophilia. Netaji oration. Part II. J Assoc Physicians India. 1978;26(5):429-37.
10. Udwadia FE. Tropical eosinophilia: a review. Respir Med. 1993;87:17-21.
11. Vijayan VK. Tropical pulmonary eosinophilia: pathogenesis, diagnosis and management. Curr Opin Pulm Med. 2007;13(5):428-33.

CHAPTER 30

Pulmonary Manifestations of Protozoal Infections

■ PULMONARY MANIFESTATIONS OF MALARIAL INFECTION

Malaria is caused by the Plasmodium species—*P. falciparum, P vivax, P. ovale,* and *P. malariae.* The disease is endemic in sub-Saharan Africa, India, Southeast Asia, the Caribbean, and South and Central America. The parasite is transmitted by the female Anopheles mosquito and infects 400–600 million people, causing well over 1 million deaths annually. Some compute deaths close to 2 million annually. Deaths are most common among pregnant women and in children under 5 years living in endemic areas. The majority of deaths are due to *P. falciparum* infection, which can cause a hyperacute fulminant illness that can at times kill the patient within 48 hours. Pulmonary manifestations are almost entirely caused by *P. falciparum* infection.

The infecting mosquito injects sporozoites into the host which then travel to the liver and multiply to form schizonts. These schizonts rupture, liberating numerous merozoites into the blood. The merozoites invade the erythrocytes and develop into mature ring forms (which produce symptoms), and ultimately into erythrocytic schizonts. A few merozoites develop into sexual gametocytes. These do not cause symptoms but when ingested by a mosquito feeding on an infected patient, develop within it to sporozoites thus completing the lifecycle.

Pulmonary Manifestations

Malaria continues to ravage large tracts of the tropics and with the rise in world travel is a disorder that must be considered in any traveller with a recent or remote history of tropical travel. Malaria occurs in 300–500 million individuals annually, affecting 40% of the world's population and an estimated 50–70 million Western travellers are exposed to it annually. It continues to result in 2 million deaths annually. Falciparum malaria is a major cause of death in tropical areas.

A mild degree of "bronchitis" characterized by cough with rhonchi on auscultation is a common feature of all plasmodial infections occurring in 36% of falciparum and 55% of ovale malaria. It is associated with the usual fever with rigors and the disease is mistaken by the unwary as an acute respiratory infection, particularly when the fever is intermittent or continuous as with *P. falciparum* infection.

A study of lung functions in uncomplicated symptomatic malaria showed the presence of increased airways' obstruction, impaired ventilation, decreased gas transfer, and increased pulmonary phagocytic activity in both *P. vivax* and *P. falciparum* infections.

P. falciparum infections can be associated with far more severe pulmonary complications than those mentioned above. These are briefly described:

- Even when radiography of the chest seems apparently normal, some patients with *P. falciparum* infection have a low PaO_2 as low as 60–65 mm Hg. This is due to a ventilator perfusion inequality as the PaO_2 and the oxygen saturation rise with oxygen given at 2–4 L/min. Perhaps interstitial edema and disturbed perfusion to the lungs contribute to this ventilation perfusion inequality.
- *Acute respiratory distress syndrome*: The incidence of acute respiratory distress syndrome (ARDS) is higher in those with more severe malaria. Noncardiogenic pulmonary edema has been reported in 21% of

patients with cerebral malaria and in a third of patients dying of severe malaria. Unlike cerebral malaria which occurs early in the natural history of *P. falciparum* infection, ARDS occurs later, around the same time as renal, hepatic, or coagulation failure. Also, unlike cerebral malaria, there may be little or no evidence of significant parasitemia at the time of its occurrence. The reason for its delayed occurrence, at times several days after antimalarial drugs have been instituted is a mystery. Perhaps the gradual release of cytokines may be responsible for the delayed organ damage. ARDS is more common in pregnant women, in children, and nonimmune adults. In the very severe forms of *P. falciparum*, coexisting cerebral, renal, hematological, and coagulation abnormalities may be seen so that these patients are desperately ill with multiorgan failure.

- Acute respiratory distress syndrome may vary in severity:
    - In mild ARDS, the PaO_2/FiO_2 ratio is between 200 and 300. The increased alveolar arterial gradient in mild ARDS observed with *P. falciparum* infection is largely related to a ventilation perfusion inequality rather than to a right to left shunt within the lung. The prognosis is good and recovery occurs provided there is no serious dysfunction involving other systems.
    - Severe ARDS as has already been mentioned, is a classic feature of fulminant or hyperacute P. *falciparum* infection **(Fig. 1)**. It has, however, also been recently reported with *P. vivax* and *P. ovale* infection. Heavy parasitemia and white blood cells agglutinates are associated with ARDS in patients with *P. vivax* malaria. Dysregulation of cytokine production may be the reason for ARDS in these patients. Increasing tachypnea, respiratory distress, bilateral crackles, fluffy shadows in both lung fields, and severe hypoxia necessitating ventilator support and the use of *positive end-expiratory pressure* (PEEP) are all present. A right to left shunt within the lungs is a prominent feature of severe ARDS, though some degree of ventilation perfusion abnormality correctible by increasing the FiO_2 is also invariably observed.

Acute respiratory distress syndrome rarely occurs as an isolated complication of acute *P. falciparum* infection. It is invariably associated with other organ dysfunction, particularly with cerebral malaria.

Hemodynamic studies of patients with hyperacute *P. falciparum* infection with ARDS and other organ dysfunction reveal hypotension, a low central venous pressure, low pulmonary capillary wedge pressure, with a high cardiac index and a low systemic vascular resistance. The findings are similar to those observed in severe bacterial sepsis and septic shock. In patients who ultimately die, there is marked hypotension, a very low cardiac index, with an increase in the systemic vascular resistance and an increase in pulmonary capillary wedge pressure **(Fig. 2)**.

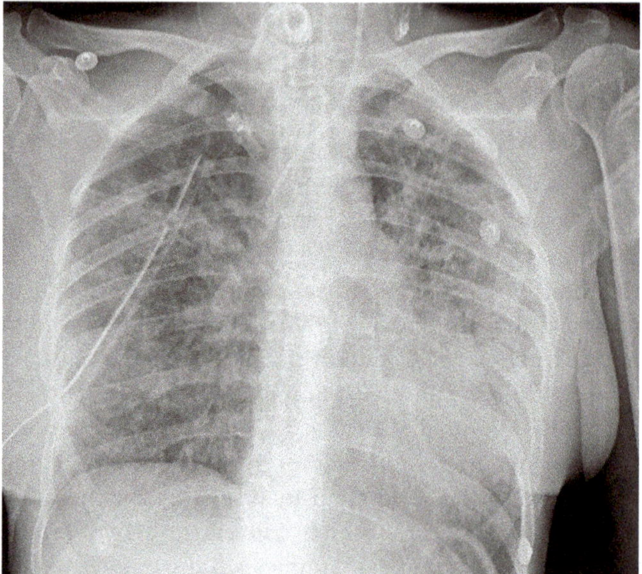

Fig. 1: *P. falciparum* malaria. X-ray chest showing acute respiratory distress syndrome (ARDS) in patient with *P. falciparum* malaria with shadows in both lung fields.

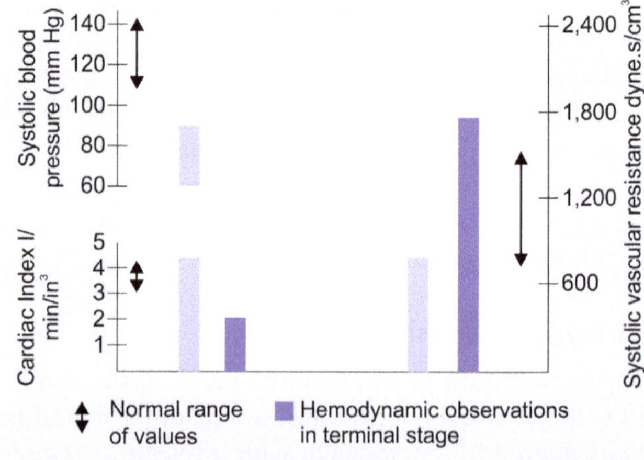

Fig. 2: Hemodynamic observations in fulminant falciparum infections.

- Acute respiratory distress syndrome at times complicates fulminant *P. falciparum* infection associated with disseminated intravascular coagulopathy (DIC). The latter then forms an important pathogenetic factor of ARDS. The features of DIC dominate the clinical picture in these patients.

The pathophysiology of ARDS is characterized by damage to the alveolar capillary membrane causing noncardiogenic increased permeability inflammatory edema. *P. falciparum* infection causes the formation of "sticky knobs" on the surface of infected red blood cells (RBCs). The "knobs" consist of host cells with parasitic antigen and help in binding of infected RBCs to endothelial cells of capillaries and venules. Sequestration and sludging of RBCs blocking capillaries and venules ensues, with hypoxic damage to the alveolar capillary membrane. There is also an increased production and liberation of cytokines, in particular tumor necrosis factor alpha (TNF-α). TNF-α exerts direct cytotoxic effects and also induces the expression in endothelial cells of intercellular adhesion molecule-1 (ICAM-1) and other adhesins which ensure adherence of parasitized RBCs to the alveolar capillary wall. *P. falciparum* merozoite protein could also directly increase pulmonary endothelial permeability.

A study on severe falciparum malaria by Krishnan and Karnad *[Ref: Krishnan A, Karnad DR. Severe falciparum malaria: an important cause of multiple organ failure in Indian intensive care unit patients. Crit Care Med. 2003;31(9):2278-84]* from a busy tertiary referral intensive care unit (ICU) in Mumbai is the largest prospective study to date. Three hundred and one patients with severe falciparum malaria were admitted in the 30-month study period comprising 13% of all ICU admissions in this hospital. ARDS was seen in a relatively higher number (79 patients, 26%) than in any previous study and carried the worst outcome. In this study, ARDS occurred later in the course of the illness (mean 3.1 days, *P* < 0.001) compared with cerebral, renal, or coagulation failure.

- *Pulmonary edema in P. falciparum* infection can be due to *causes other than ARDS.* Pulmonary edema can be due to fluid overload, myocardial dysfunction associated with fulminant *P. falciparum* infection, and rarely due to hyperpyrexia. Rectal temperatures which suddenly shoot up to 108°F or 110°F can cause sudden cardiorespiratory failure with fulminant pulmonary edema. Death can occur within a few minutes to a few hours.

- *Severe P. falciparum infection,* particularly when it occurs in the old, the very young, in pregnant women, or in the malnourished, can cause *marked tachypnea.* The tachypnea in the presence of high fever, electrolyte imbalance, and poor nutrition leads to respiratory muscle fatigue. Respiratory muscle fatigue results in low tidal volumes, a poor cough reflex with inability to clear airway secretions. Areas of atelectasis develop within the lungs with patchy shadows visible on X-ray of the chest. These patients are prone to sudden respiratory arrest. Elective intubation with ventilator support promptly restores normal gas exchange and the pulmonary shadows disappear quickly, distinguishing this condition from ARDS.

- *Aspiration pneumonia* is an important complication, particularly in obtunded patients, more so when injudicious attempts are made to feed them orally.

- *Malarial pneumonia*: While consolidation and pneumonitis on a radiograph in a patient with falciparum or vivax malaria usually represent a superadded bacterial pneumonia, Applebaum and Shrager in 1944 described 4% of their patients with a "malarial pneumonia". The consolidation was lobular in all except 7% who had lobar consolidation. This complication occurred equally in vivax and falciparum malaria. The existence of malarial pneumonia as an entity remains unproven as no convincing demonstration of parasites in sputum has been made nor has there been conclusive exclusion of other pathogens as causative factors. However, the response of the consolidation to antimalarials alone suggests the possibility of malarial pneumonia existing as a distinct but rare entity.

- *Pleural effusion*: Pleural effusions have frequently been found at autopsy in patients dying of pulmonary edema and Applebaum described them in 2.5% of his patients with pneumonia. There is only one report of pleural effusion large enough to require drainage.

- *Secondary bacterial pneumonia*: Secondary bacterial Gram-negative infections are frequent complications of severe complicated malaria and contribute significantly to morbidity and mortality. As early as 1902, Ross alluded to pneumonia being a common cause of death in patients severely debilitated with malaria, and despite the broad-spectrum of antibiotics available today, this statement still holds true. Bacterial sepsis and its associated complications must be avidly sought and excluded or aggressively treated to minimize this high mortality rate. Patients with malaria are prone to bacteremia due to ischemic breakdown of the gastrointestinal mucosal barrier and bacterial translocation. In Krishnan's large series of 301 falciparum patients, secondary bacterial sepsis accounted for 39 patients (35 deaths). Sepsis was the commonest cause of death occurring after the 7th day of hospitalization.

- Patients on ventilator support may develop *nosocomial pneumonia.*
- *Deep vein thrombosis and pulmonary embolism* are important complications to be watched out for.

There are certain points of importance that perhaps need to be stressed.

- Acute respiratory distress syndrome as has been stated earlier is invariably associated with multiple organ dysfunction.
- Once ARDS and organ dysfunction set in, they may continue to evolve even when parasitemia is abolished by specific therapy.
- In hyperacute cases associated with severe hypotension and cardiovascular collapse, ARDS and the full spectrum of multiple organ failure seen with *P. falciparum* infections may occur without detectable parasitemia. This is because most of the parasites remain sequestered within the capillaries of various organs and there are very few circulating in the peripheral blood. Incomplete treatment at home or in another hospital may also be occasionally responsible for inability to detect parasitemia in the peripheral blood. The moral of the story is that in endemic and hyperendemic areas one is justified in treating a patient whose clinical features are compatible with fulminant *P. falciparum* infection with specific antimalarial therapy, even if the diagnosis cannot be confirmed

Pulmonary Complications of Vivax Malaria

The clinical course of vivax malaria is generally benign with lung complications seldom seen. A review of the literature, however, reveals rare cases of ARDS and pulmonary edema secondary to vivax malaria. The possibility of mixed infection with falciparum should always be considered in such cases and it is probably prudent to treat such cases as mixed infections even if falciparum cannot be isolated. Other extremely rare pulmonary complications

of vivax malaria include one reported case of bronchiolitis obliterans with organizing pneumonia (BOOP) and one case of acute interstitial pneumonia.

Pulmonary Toxicity of Malaria Prophylaxis

Antimalarial drug toxicity while rare has been reported. With increasing numbers of travelers on malaria prophylaxis during holidays to endemic areas, this must be borne in mind. Sulfadoxine and pyrimethamine hypersensitivity can cause pulmonary eosinophilia, lung infiltrates, allergic alveolitis, and noncardiogenic pulmonary edema. Methemoglobinemia is well described after use of primaquine and dapsone.

Diagnosis

Diagnosis depends on demonstration of malarial parasites on blood smears. A thick blood smear examined by an experienced pathologist generally allows a definite diagnosis. A thin smear allows identification of the infecting species. Antigen-detecting assays which identify *P. falciparum*-specific histidine-rich protein are of further help in identifying *P. falciparum* infection.

Finally, the need for vigilance even for physicians and patients from the developed world is exemplified by the case of an elderly resident of Germany who developed a sepsis syndrome and respiratory failure. Falciparum was found in the blood on the 6th day of hospitalization. She had never travelled outside the country but lived close to Frankfurt airport and "baggage malaria" from imported anopheles mosquitoes in the luggage or airplane was postulated to be responsible for her illness.

Prognosis

Despite these patients being desperately ill with multiorgan failure, survival rates are better than those with equivalent organ failure from other causes of sepsis. The overall mortality rate in the experienced ICU in Krishnan's study was relatively low at 24% despite severe organ failure. As expected, only 6% of patients with single or no organ failure died whereas mortality rose to 49% in those with multiorgan failure.

Treatment

Artesunate has replaced quinine as the drug of choice in the treatment of *P. falciparum* infection.

The Artesunate-Quinine meta-analysis study group favored artesunate, as it was found to be more active in terms of parasite killing, less toxic, and easier to administer. The dose of artesunate is 2.4 mg/kg initially, 1.2 mg/kg 12 hours later, then 1.2 mg/kg daily for 5 days.

If artesunate is not available (as is indeed so in many areas of poor countries), quinine should be administered intravenously in a dose of 20 mg salt/kg diluted in 10 mg isotonic saline/kg over 4 hours, followed by 8 hours after start of the loading dose with 10 mg/kg over 2 hours every 12 hours, until the patient can swallow, following which the drug is given orally in a dose of 600 mg 8 hourly. The total duration of quinine therapy is 7 days.

Quinine can cause numerous side effects. These include hypoglycemia, tinnitus, impaired hearing, blurred vision, and most importantly ventricular tachycardia particularly when given intravenously. A prolonged QT interval is a warning of the possible occurrence of such arrhythmias. Electrocardiographic (ECG) monitoring is, therefore, very necessary in critically ill patients. Quinine can cause acute hemolysis in patients who are glucose-6-phosphate dehydrogenase (G6PD) deficient.

To counter the threat of resistance of *P. falciparum* to monotherapies, and to improve treatment outcome, combinations of antimalarials are now recommended by World Health Organization (WHO) for the treatment of falciparum malaria. The following antimalarial combination therapies (ACTs) are currently recommended:

- Artemether + lumefantrine
- Artesunate + amodiaquine
- Artesunate + mefloquine
- Artesunate + sulfadoxine-pyrimethamine

Chloroquine should not be used in the treatment of *P. falciparum* infections as the parasite has become resistant to the drug in almost all countries where malaria is endemic. The malarial parasite continues to outwit human ingenuity. There is documentation of in vitro resistance of the *P. falciparum* to artemisinin with delayed clearance of the parasite in Pailin, Cambodia, and possibly in neighboring countries.

The use of ventilator support in ARDS, in severe pulmonary edema from other causes, and in patients who are tachypneic and who show evidence of respiratory muscle fatigue is imperative. Secondary infection, whether iatrogenic or otherwise, requires appropriate antibiotic therapy. Serious pulmonary complications are associated with dysfunction of other organ systems. All systems require support if the patient is to survive. Persistent hypotension in spite of the use of inotropes and vasopressors is of ominous significance. Renal replacement is invaluable in patients with renal shutdown or in overhydrated patients with poor renal function. Patients with a parasitemia of over 25–30% may require exchange transfusion. In our experience, lesser degrees of parasitemia respond to specific treatment with antimalarials and to expert critical care.

Amebic Infections

Amebiasis is caused by the protozoan *Entamoeba histolytica* and is probably the most common cause of mortality among parasitic infections after malaria and schistosomiasis. Amebiasis is responsible for 50–100,000 deaths annually. The disease is endemic in tropical and subtropical regions, having a high prevalence rate in India, Asia, Africa, South America, and Mexico. It spreads by the orofecal route; contamination of food and water, poor hygiene, poor sanitation, and overcrowding help in its dissemination. Globally 10% of the world's population is infected with *E. histolytica* causing significant morbidity and mortality. There are two more points worth noting:

1. Host immunity is negligible in the virginal host. The host antibody response is, however, useful in preventing subsequent invasive episodes.
2. Amebic infection can be fulminant in the very young, in the malnourished, in those on corticosteroids, and in the immunosuppressed. We have observed fulminant amebic infections in some patients with human immunodeficiency virus (HIV) disease.

Pathogenesis

Pulmonary manifestations are invariably secondary to an amebic hepatic abscess. Following the ingestion of cysts, the trophozoites develop in the small gut and are carried with the intestinal contents into the cecum and the large bowel. The trophozoites are motile amebae which attach themselves anywhere along the mucosa of the large gut (particularly in the rectosigmoid and cecum). They produce an ulceration of the mucosa because of the proteolytic enzymes secreted by them. Large flask-shaped ulcers are formed which could bleed or perforate. The trophozoites at the base of these ulcers may enter the portal circulation and reach the liver. Here, the proteolytic enzymes secreted by the trophozoites produce a lytic necrosis of the liver cells resulting in one or more abscesses. A hepatic abscess is most often in the posterio-superior aspect of the right lobe of the liver. Pulmonary manifestations occur as a direct extension of the hepatic abscess through the diaphragm into the pleural space, or into the lung or into both. A left lobe hepatic abscess may extend through the diaphragm into the pericardium and rarely into the left pleural space. Rarely, trophozoites may enter the systemic circulation via the rectal venous plexus so that there is a hematogenous spread of infection to the lung and very occasionally, to other organ systems, particularly the brain. There are some who believe that hematogenous spread could also occur if the trophozoites of a liver abscess gain access to the hepatic veins or the inferior vena cava. Lymphatic spread of amebic infection from the liver through the diaphragm into the thorax remains a theoretical possibility.

In our series, more than 60% of patients with a large liver abscess had serious pulmonary manifestations. It is uncommon to find overt manifestations of amebic ulcerative colitis in patients who have pulmonary manifestations of amebiasis.

Clinical Features and Complications

Pleuropulmonary amebiasis was first described by Simon in 1890 who reported a patient whose liver abscess ruptured into the lung with *E. histolytica* observed in the sputum. Since then, different series from the tropics have reported the incidence of pleuropulmonary involvement to vary from as low as 4% of patients with amebic liver abscesses to as high as 86%. A consistent observation has been that pleuropulmonary complications occur more commonly in developing countries. Like amebic liver abscess, pleuropulmonary amebiasis occurs predominantly in men with a male/female ratio varying from 9:1 to 15:1. While no age is exempt, the age group most likely to develop this complication is young adults in the range of 20–45 years. The onset may be acute, subacute, or chronic. Acute onset is heralded by sudden onset of fever with chills, pain over the right hypochondrium, and pleuritic right-sided chest pain referred to the shoulder and to the back to the right of the midline. There is leukocytosis with a rise in the erythrocyte sedimentation rate. Clinical examination reveals a right-sided pleural rub, dullness to percussion over the right lower chest below the scapula, with diminished breath sounds, or distant bronchial breath sounds. There is invariably an enlarged palpable tender liver; a gentle tap with the fist over the right lower intercostal spaces often produces exquisite tenderness and pain.

Subacute onset is characterized by low-grade fever, weight loss, a milder degree of leukocytosis, pleuritic chest pain and a variable degree of pleural effusion, or the presence of pleuropulmonary complications, the source of which may remain undetected. This is particularly so if the liver is not sufficiently enlarged.

Chronic onset and course are characterized by evening rise of fever, weight loss, pleural effusion which is often wrongly diagnosed as being due to tuberculosis. The presentation could also be that of a chronic lung abscess or pulmonary consolidation, the source of which remains obscure.

Complications (Fig. 3)

- Segmental or total atelectasis of the lower lobe due to upward displacement and fixity of the right dome of the diaphragm are the commonest pulmonary manifestations.
- A sympathetic pleural effusion is equally frequent. It is sterile on culture.
- A hepatic abscess may open through the diaphragm into the pleura leading to a pleural exudate and an empyema. A sudden rupture causes sudden severe

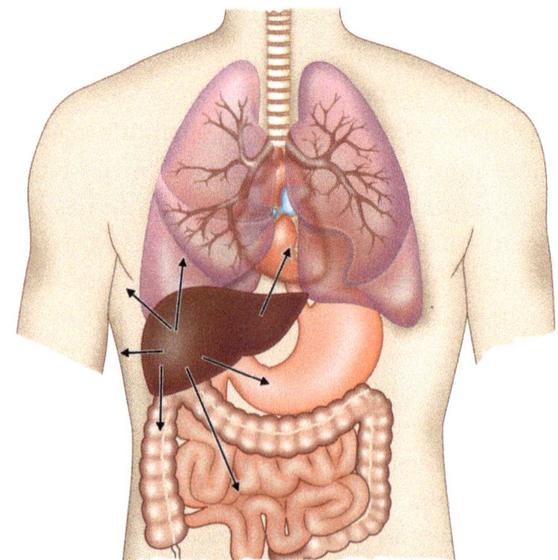

Fig. 3: Possible sites of rupture of an amebic liver abscess.
Source: Vakil RJ, Udwadia FE. 1982. Diagnosis and Management of Medical Emergencies. Mumbai: OUP;1982.

pleural pain, tachycardia, and well-marked dyspnea. The patients can be gravely ill if the hepatic abscess that has ruptured into the pleural space is large; there is danger of death if there is a simultaneous rupture of the hepatic abscess into the peritoneal cavity. A subacute or slow seepage of the hepatic abscess into the pleural space through the diaphragm leads to subacute or chronic clinical features of a right-sided empyema. Pleural paracentesis often reveals dirty brown pus. Trophozoites of *E. histolytica* may be found in the fluid.

- The hepatic abscess may go through the diaphragm into the lower lobe of the lung to cause (1) *consolidation* of part or whole of the right lobe; and (2) a lung abscess; the patient coughing up anchovy sauce material in his sputum. The liver and lung abscess may thereby drain and at times heal. Communication between the liver and lung can lead to a *hepatobronchial fistula* or a *biliary bronchial fistula.*

- Finally, the hepatic abscess may open both into the pleura and the lung causing both an empyema and pulmonary complications stated above.

- A left lobe liver abscess may encroach through the left dome of the diaphragm into the pericardium. Tachycardia of sudden onset with breathlessness is an early sign. It is usually due to a sympathetic pericardial effusion. Actual rupture into the pericardial space of a large left lobe liver abscess is a catastrophe that leads to quick death from cardiac tamponade. A slow leak into the pericardium can, however, be promptly drained and treated. A simultaneous involvement of the left pleura and rarely of the left lower lobe may also be observed.

It should be noted that pulmonary manifestations generally involve the right lower lobe. Occasionally, pulmonary involvement is observed in the middle lobe or at a distance well away from the right dome of the diaphragm. This may well result from a hematogenous spread of trophozoites though the rectal venous plexus into the systemic circulation.

Diagnosis

Pleuropulmonary manifestations involving the right thorax should always arouse suspicion of a possible amebic infection in patients living in endemic areas. Ultrasound of the liver should enable the diagnosis of a possible liver abscess as the source of infection. Radiographic features

include an elevated right hemidiaphragm which is the most common radiographic abnormality being found in well over 50% of amebic liver abscesses. Small sterile right-sided pleural effusions are frequently observed. Basal consolidation is the next most frequent radiographic abnormality; cavitation and abscess formation may occur in the consolidated area. Occasionally, a pulmonary abscess may be seen, distinct from the liver, in any lobe as a result of hematogenous dissemination. Pleural effusions can be small, moderate, or massive. If a hepatobronchial fistula forms, an air-containing cavity may be observed under the diaphragm **(Figs. 4 to 8)**.

Computed tomography of the upper abdomen and chest should further clarify the diagnosis, as it helps to give the exact size, number, and location of the amebic abscess or abscesses. Needle aspiration of a hypoechoic area of the liver draws pus which is reddish brown in color. Trophozoites are only rarely found in the liver aspirate or in the aspirate from an amebic empyema, or in the sputum in patients with a hepatopulmonary or biliopulmonary fistula.

The hemagglutination test for amebiasis is positive and shows a rising titer over the next few weeks. The test may remain positive for several months. Stools very rarely show trophozoites of ameba in patients with pleuropulmonary manifestations. The presence of cysts of *E. histolytica*

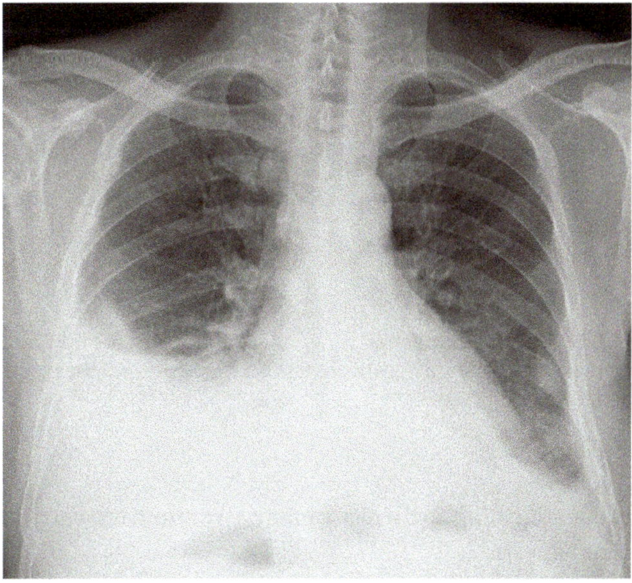

Fig. 4: Pulmonary complications of amebiasis. X-ray chest showing an elevated fixed right dome of the diaphragm, segmental atelectasis of the right lower lobe, and a right-sided pleural effusion.

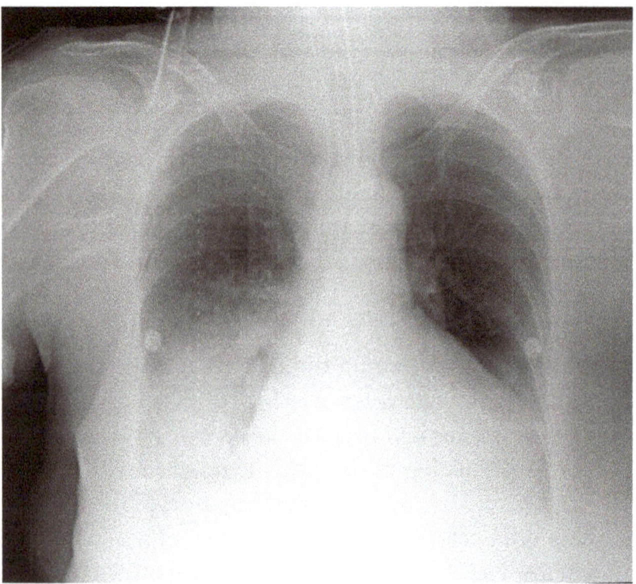

Fig. 5: X-ray chest showing right lower lobe consolidation in a patient with an amebic liver abscess.

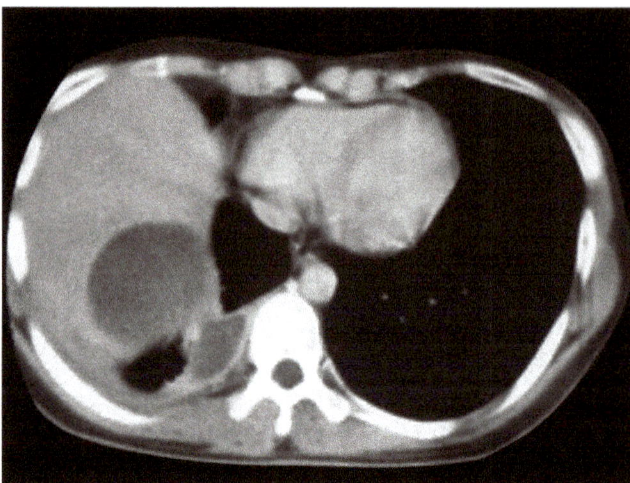

Fig. 7: Amebic liver abscess. Computed tomography (CT) abdomen demonstrates a well-defined hypodense area in the right lobe of the liver, posterior-superior segment. There is extension into the right pleural space; this represents a ruptured amebic liver abscess.

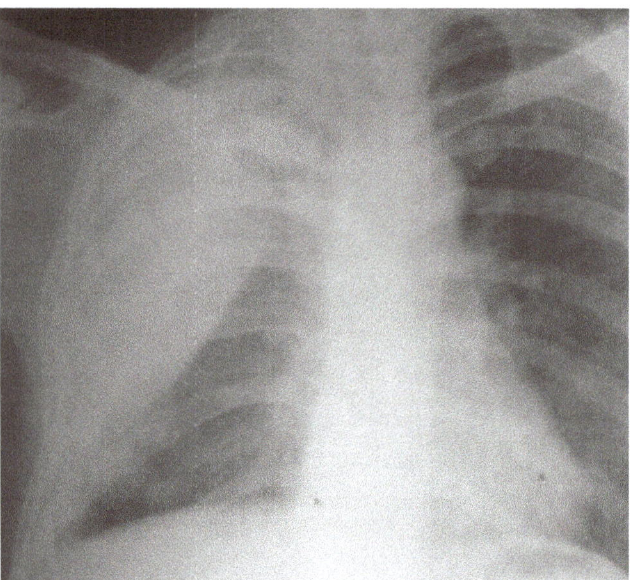

Fig. 6: Amebic empyema. X-ray chest showing a right-sided empyema caused by a hepatic abscess opening both into the pleura and the lung.

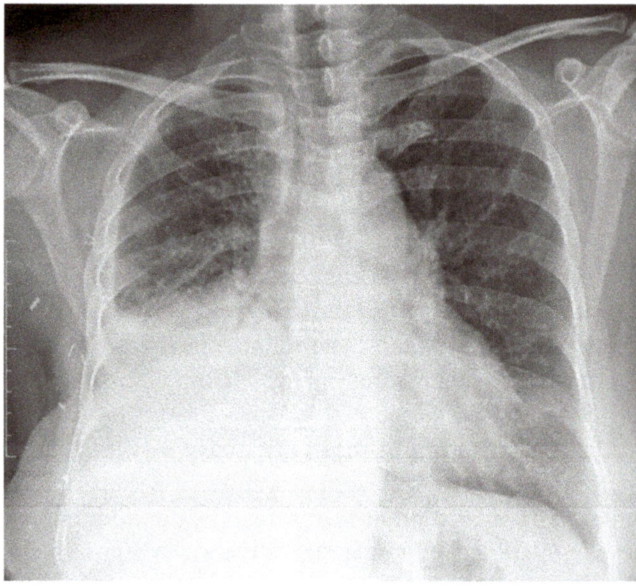

Fig. 8: Large right-sided pleural effusion of amebic etiology. X-ray chest showing right-sided pleural effusion caused by an amebic liver abscess.

has no meaning as there are many asymptomatic carriers of amebiasis.

A combination of serological tests with identification of the parasite by polymerase chain reaction (PCR) or antigen detection is a good diagnostic approach.

Prognosis

If promptly treated, the prognosis is good, except in fulminant infections, in immunocompromised patients, and in children. We have seen one death occur, even though the diagnosis was prompt, treatment adequate, and drainage of the pleural space done as per our protocol. Death when it occurs is due to sepsis, and hypotension with associated myocardial dysfunction. Even with expert critical care, multiple organ failure leading to death can occur. Yet, some patients recover even when they seem on the verge of death. To quote just one example, an elderly diabetic lady was brought into the ICU with a near cardiac arrest. She was resuscitated and was found to have a liver abscess which had ruptured into the peritoneum, pleura, and pericardium. All these spaces were adequately drained as emergency procedures within the ICU and she was given specific antiamebic treatment. The huge liver abscess was also drained a few days later with a large drainage tube. She went into multiorgan failure but after a stormy course ultimately survived.

Treatment

- Metronidazole is the specific treatment for all amebic infections given in a dose of 750 mg thrice daily for 10–15 days. In acutely ill patients, we prefer to give the drug intravenously. Seizures are an important complication of this therapy.
- An empyema or a pleural exudate needs to be drained. Thick pus necessitates tube drainage through an intercostal space. CT studies should help correct positioning of the drainage tube.
- An amebic liver abscess is the source of pleuro-pulmonary manifestations. Ordinarily, after a diagnostic tap, the pus within the abscess need not be aspirated. Specific treatment outlined above leads to healing, though imaging studies may reveal a walled-off space in the liver for weeks or even months. If however the abscess is large, 8–10 cm or more, it should be aspirated dry. Even if it fills up again, repeated aspirations are only occasionally necessary. Repeated aspirations may, however, be necessary if an amebic abscess is complicated by secondary bacterial infection. This is rare, and most often iatrogenic, from improper unsterile aspiration attempts. Very large abscesses which sometimes almost occupy the greater part of the right lobe of the liver may require tube drainage. An important disadvantage of tube drainage is the possibility of introducing secondary bacterial infection **(Table 1)**.
- Secondary bacterial infections of pleuropulmonary lesions are rare; if present, they require appropriate antibiotic therapy.

Table 1: Indications for aspiration of a liver abscess.

- An abscess greater than 10 cm in size—aspiration allows early resolution
- A left lobe abscess greater than 7 cm; a left lobe abscess abutting on the dome of the diaphragm; presence of signs of impending rupture into the pericardium
- Lack of clinical improvement after 4–5 days of specific therapy even if abscess is less than 10 cm in diameter
- Impending rupture into the pleural space
- Seronegative liver abscess (often a pyogenic liver abscess)
- Percutaneous drainage may be necessary when:
  - The abscess is very large
  - Fills repeatedly after tapping
  - Thick pus which is not easily aspirated through a needle, as in patients with a pyogenic liver abscess

- Amebic infection within the gut may be asymptomatic. It is important to use diloxanide 500 mg TDS or iodoquinol 650 mg TDS for 20 days to clear the gut of infection.

■ PULMONARY MANIFESTATIONS OF RARE PROTOZOAL INFECTIONS

Babesiosis

Babesiosis is caused by a tick-borne protozoan parasite *Babesia babesiosis*. The disease is characterized by a malaria-like illness with fever with chills, leukopenia, and thrombocytopenia. The disease is usually mild except in asplenic patients, when it can be severe and even fatal. Pulmonary complications are uncommon but the most frequent manifestation is ARDS.

Giemsa-stained thin blood examination, detection of specific antibodies, and PCR method allow specific diagnosis of pulmonary babesiosis. Treatment consists of a combination therapy with clindamycin 600 mg 8 hourly and quinine 600 mg 8 hourly. Alternatively, one could use atovaquone 750 mg twice daily and azithromycin 500 mg daily for 7 days.

Leishmaniasis

Leishmaniasis (Kala azar) is caused by the protozoan termed *Leishmania donovani*. It is endemic in tropical Africa, South America, and in eastern India, particularly in the states of Bihar, parts of Bengal, and Orissa. The disease is characterized by fever, hepatosplenomegaly, leukopenia, and thrombocytopenia. Bacterial pneumonia may occur as an intercurrent infection.

In endemic zones common to both HIV infection and leishmaniasis, the danger of coinfection of both these diseases is always present and is on the increase. Leishmaniasis in HIV patients can cause serious visceral problems. In these patients, interstitial pneumonia, ARDS, disseminated intravascular coagulation (DIC), and hepatic/renal dysfunction may be the presenting features. Treatment may be ineffective or poorly effective.

Pentamidine, liposomal formulation of amphotericin B, and miltefosine are the drugs for the treatment of this disease.

Pulmonary Toxoplasmosis

Pulmonary toxoplasmosis is caused by a protozoan parasite called *Toxoplasma gondii* which is primarily carried by cats. Humans are infected by parasitic cysts contaminating food or milk products.

Clinical manifestations are an influenza-like syndrome with fever, myalgia, and lymphadenopathy. Pulmonary manifestations are increasingly reported in HIV patients. These include interstitial pneumonia, necrotizing pneumonia, and diffuse alveolar damage.

Diagnosis depends on (1) demonstration of the protozoan parasite in tissue; (2) positive antibodies to the parasite in serological testing; (3) a real time PCR-based assay on bronchoalveolar lavage (BAL) in HIV patients is frequently positive; and (4) histopathological examination of a lymph gland biopsy which is often typical of infection by toxoplasma.

Immunocompetent patients often require no treatment, the disease resolving on its own. When symptoms are severe or fever persists, a combination of pyrimethamine and sulfadiazines is curative.

■ SUGGESTED READING

1. Alvar J, Aparicio P, Aseffa A, et al. The relationship between leishmaniasis and AIDS: the second 10 years. Clin Microbiol Rev. 2008;21(2):334-59.
2. Bora D. Epidemiology of visceral leishmaniasis in India. Natl Med J India. 1999;12(2):62-8.
3. Cheepsattayakorn A, Cheepsattayakorn R. Parasitic pneumonia and lung involvement. Biomed Res Int. 2014;2014:874021.
4. Douglas NM. Artemisinin combination therapy for vivax malaria. Lancet Infect Dis. 2010;10(6):405-16.
5. Krause PJ. Babesiosis. Med Clin North Am. 2002;86(2):361-73.
6. Martanez S. Thoracic manifestations of tropical parasitic infections: a pictorial review. Radiographics. 2005;25(1):135-55.
7. Moonah SN, Tiang NM, Petri Tr WA. Host immune response to intestinal amebiasis. PLoS Pathogens. 2013; 9(8):e1003489.
8. Sarkar S, Saha K, Das CS. Three cases of ARDS: an emerging complication of Plasmodium vivax malaria. Lung India. 2010;27(3):154-7.
9. Shamsuzzaman SM. Thoracic amebiasis. Clin Chest Med. 2002;23(2):479-92.
10. Tan LK. Acute lung injury and other serious complications of Plasmodium vivax malaria. Lancet Infect Dis. 2008;8(7):449-54.
11. Taylor WR. Malaria and the lung. Clin Chest Med. 2002; 23(2):457-68.

CHAPTER 31

Pulmonary Involvement in Fulminant Systemic Tropical Infections

■ INTRODUCTION

Pulmonary involvement is observed in severe tropical infections such as *Plasmodium falciparum* malaria, salmonellosis, leptospirosis, dengue hemorrhagic fever (DHF), other rare hemorrhagic fevers, melioidosis, plague, and anthrax. *P. falciparum* is one infection which when hyperacute often causes pulmonary complications. These have been already described under protozoal infections.

■ TYPHOID AND OTHER SALMONELLA INFECTIONS

Typhoid fever due to *Salmonella typhi (B. typhosus)* is today fortunately detected (at least in metropolitan cities) within the first week and is invariably responsive to ceftriaxone. When diagnosis is delayed pulmonary complications though uncommon may occur.

Respiratory symptoms are common in typhoid infections, being present in about half of all cases at the onset of the disease. Bronchitis causing a dry cough with auscultatory rhonchi is commonly seen. In the tropics, fever lasting a week or more, associated with cough and auscultatory rhonchi is most commonly due to either *S. typhi* or malaria.

In their classic description of 360 cases of typhoid fever, from 1946, Stuart and Roscoe reported cough in 86% of patients, coryza in 60% and chest pain in 60%. In their series, 8% of typhoid cases were initially diagnosed as *chest infection*. Pneumonia is the other pulmonary manifestation being reported in 37 of the 154 patients in this series who had a chest radiograph. The pneumonia usually represents a secondary bacterial pneumonia, often due to *Streptococcus pneumoniae* infection, but lobar pneumonia

occasionally accompanied by pleural effusion secondary to *S. typhi* itself or to *Salmonella choleraesuis*, while rare, is well-recognized. Empyema is occasionally reported, 18 cases being reported in 1929–80 in world literature, *S. typhi* being the causative organism in the majority of cases. Lung abscess is a rare complication and is mostly caused by *S. typhi*. Thailand in Southeast Asia is endemic for salmonella infections. Rare pulmonary manifestations reported from Thailand include interstitial pneumonia, necrotizing pneumonia, and large pneumatoceles of the kind seen in staphylococcal pneumonia. We have never witnessed these complications in India. Rare upper airway complications of typhoid that have been described include laryngeal ulceration and glottic edema.

With increasing international travel to endemic areas, *B. typhosus* and salmonella infections are sporadically seen in the West with the US reporting about 500 cases annually. Nontyphoidal salmonella infection is more common in the US with *S. typimurium* being an important pathogen in the HIV-positive and immunosuppressed populations. The course in the immunodeficient patient is different from that in the immunocompetent. The incidence of bacteremia is high with 75–95% of these patients having positive blood cultures as opposed to 1–4% in the normal host with gastroenteritis. The disease tends not to respond well to antibiotics and often recurs after discontinuation of therapy. Remarkably, *S. typhi* infection is uncommonly reported.

The most dreaded pulmonary complication of *B. typhosus* infection is acute respiratory distress syndrome (ARDS), generally observed in the second week of the fever. ARDS presents with the usual features of breathlessness, tachypnea, auscultatory crackles and radiological features of pulmonary edema **(Fig. 1)**. The patient generally has high fever and there is often evidence of multi-organ dysfunction. Blood cultures for *B. typhosus* are invariably positive in patients with ARDS. The prompt use of ceftriaxone (2 g IV 8-hourly, for 10 days) and appropriate ventilatory support together with support to other organ systems often leads to recovery. Rarely, other salmonella infections (paratyphoid A or B) can also cause ARDS.

Treatment

Ceftriaxone 2 g IV twice daily and in severe cases thrice daily is the drug of choice in India. Azithromycin 500 mg twice daily orally for 5 days is also generally given in addition. Resistance to the quinolone group of drugs is on the rise and unless sensitivity tests permit their use they should be avoided.

Remarkably, *S. typhi* now is sensitive to chloramphenicol, perhaps because the drug was not used for several-years in the treatment of this disease.

◼ LEPTOSPIRAL INFECTION

Leptospirosis is a zoonotic disease. Though worldwide in distribution, it is most common in the tropics and in the developing countries of the world. It is a spirochetal disease, caused by spirochetes belonging to the genus *Leptospira* which comprises a number of serological disease-producing strains. The most common disease-producing strain in India is *Leptospira icterohaemorrhagiae*. Human infection occurs from exposure to rat-infected urine containing the organism present in contaminated water or soil. The organism penetrates the skin and thereby gains entry, following which there is bacteremic spread to various organs of the body, notably the lungs, liver, kidney and the central nervous system.

Leptospirosis is a grave health hazard in tropical and developing countries where rainfall is heavy. It occurs in outbreaks and even larger epidemics during and soon after the monsoon season. In India there are yearly seasonal outbreaks between July and September, particularly where there is heavy flooding from the rains. The disease is endemic in the Indian subcontinent, the whole of Southeast Asia, Andaman Islands, China, Taiwan, South America (particularly in Brazil, Nicaragua) and in Africa. Epidemics in Brazil (1988) and Nicaragua (1995) and periodic yearly epidemics in India have resulted in significant mortality. The disease occurs mainly in farmers exposed to contaminated soil, sewer workers and in city dwellers who have to walk through contaminated water during and following floods caused by heavy rains. People swimming in contaminated swimming pools are also at risk.

Pathophysiology

The leptospirae through bacteremic spread, proliferate in various organs— chiefly the lungs, kidneys, liver, heart and the central nervous system.

Lung pathology reveals congestion; an interstitial inflammatory reaction, intra-alveolar hemorrhage or diffuse alveolar damage causing ARDS. Histopathological examination shows changes in the capillary endothelium with swollen endothelial cells with an increase in pinocytotic vesicles. Inflammatory damage to the alveolar capillary membrane is extensive in severe infection and this is responsible for extensive leak of fluid from the capillaries into the interstitial spaces and the alveoli.

Clinical Features

Leptospiral infections are characterized by high fever, muscle pain and frequent involvement of the liver (causing hepatitis and jaundice), kidneys (causing an acute nephritic picture with acute renal shutdown) and the central nervous system (causing chiefly meningitis).

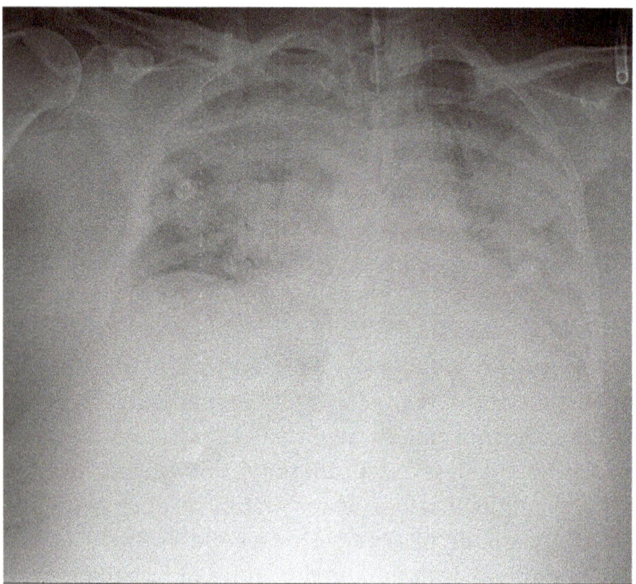

Fig. 1: Acute respiratory distress syndrome X-ray chest in a 30-year-old man who had *B. typhosus* infection.

Pulmonary involvement is common and is usually mild, consisting of a nonproductive cough or cough with blood-tinged sputum.

Severe lung involvement may take the form of ARDS or severe intra-alveolar hemorrhage. Intra-alveolar hemorrhage resembles ARDS. It may occur (and in fact often does) without serious liver, kidney or CNS involvement. The general presentation is high fever of unknown etiology suddenly complicated by acute breathlessness, tachypnea, increasing hypoxia with mottled shadows in both lungs. The shadows may become confluent to resemble pulmonary edema. A wrong diagnosis of pneumonia, aspiration pneumonia or ARDS is often made. The degree of hemoptysis varies. It may be mild, severe and exsanguinating or may not be evident at all. A bronchoalveolar lavage (BAL) study or an endotracheal aspirate if the patient is intubated and put on ventilator support, shows blood-stained fluid with hemosiderin-laden macrophages. The single most important clue to the correct diagnosis of a patient with high fever, sudden onset dyspnea, hypoxia and bilateral alveolar shadows on an X-ray of the chest is the presence of a marked rise in the creatine phosphokinase (CPK) enzyme in the blood. The rise is generally in the thousands. Serological tests for *Leptospira* and in particular a rising titer of antibodies can only be demonstrated after some days or weeks. There is invariably a slight rise in bilirubin and the liver transaminases. A urine examination may show the presence of albumin and red blood cells.

Radiographic Findings

Radiological findings are nonspecific and may be present in the absence of chest symptoms. Common abnormalities include nonsegmental pulmonary opacities, occurring peripherally, particularly in the lower lobes. They are believed to represent a hemorrhagic pneumonitis rather than a bacterial pneumonia. Areas of consolidation may also be observed, not necessarily confined to a segment or lobe. Linear opacities extending upwards from the cardiac border are related to areas of atelectasis. These linear opacities may be unilateral or bilateral in distribution.

Acute respiratory distress syndrome when it occurs has the usual bilateral distribution of opacities, at times causing total *white-out lungs* (*see* chapter on ARDS). Alveolar hemorrhage is characterized by bilateral extensive alveolar opacities. Smaller areas of alveolar hemorrhage produce more localized shadows that could be mistaken for pneumonia **(Fig. 2)**.

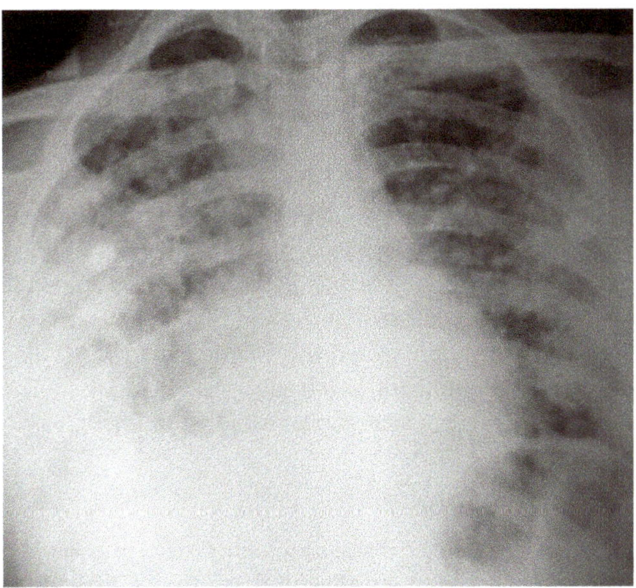

Fig. 2: Leptospirosis. X-ray chest showing bilateral diffuse alveolar shadows in a patient who had intra-alveolar hemorrhage causing severe hypoxia.

Diagnosis

Diagnosis in an endemic area is generally easy. Though lung involvement may occur in isolation, urinary abnormalities, and increase in liver enzymes are generally present. A marked rise in the CPK enzyme is invariably observed. Antibodies to *Leptospira* in the *Leptospira* agglutination test, the ELISA test and the immunofluorescent test may take several weeks to turn positive. A fourfold rise in titer observed between the acute and convalescent sera is diagnostic.

Treatment

It is important to make a prompt diagnosis in fulminant cases of intra-alveolar hemorrhage, else death results. Methylprednisolone 0.5–1 g IV daily for three days followed by prednisolone orally starting with 60 mg daily and tapered off within 2 weeks is lifesaving. Clinical and radiological improvement accompanied by rapid relief of hypoxia within a matter of 8–12 hours is observed following the very first dose of IV methylprednisolone. Ventilatory support is absolutely necessary till recovery occurs. ARDS requires the usual expert ventilatory support with the use of positive end-expiratory pressure (PEEP). The prognosis is especially grave if other organ systems are involved. Specific antibiotics for leptospiral infection also need to be given. Penicillin G, two million unit 4–6-hourly IV for 10 days is the drug of choice. In mild to moderate cases oral medication using amoxycillin, erythromycin, doxycycline or ampicillin can be used.

■ DENGUE HEMORRHAGIC FEVER

Dengue hemorrhagic fever (DHF) is a viral infection caused by the transmission of one of the strains of the dengue virus through the bite of the *Aedes aegypti* mosquito. The disease has a wide distribution in the tropics. It occurs in epidemic form in India, Pakistan and the whole of Southeast Asia, Sri Lanka, Philippines and the Pacific islands. It is also observed in Central and South America and in Africa. The disease in its severe form carries a high mortality.

Pathophysiology

In its severe form, the disease is characterized by a marked increase in capillary permeability leading to leakage of fluid and albumin from the vascular to the extravascular compartment. This leads to a form of severe hypovolemic shock. The disease is characterized by thrombocytopenia and hemorrhages within the skin and also in internal organs, particularly the gastrointestinal (GI) tract. Capillary leak within the lung is responsible for ARDS.

Clinical Features

The usual clinical picture is that of a viral fever with severe aches and pains in the muscles, joints and bones (break-bone fever) which lasts for about a week. Leukopenia and varying degree of thrombocytopenia are invariably present. A skin rash generally macular or maculopapular may or may not be present.

Most patients with dengue recover without complications. Dengue can however take a serious turn and can be fatal. The serious forms of dengue are:

- Dengue hemorrhagic fever, characterized by purpura, ecchymosis, hematemesis, hematuria, bleeding into organ systems. The platelet count is generally below 20000/mm^3 but can be higher. Bleeding can also occur into the pleural and peritoneal spaces. This form of dengue is often associated with a fall in the hematocrit >20% with signs of plasma leakage such as pleural effusion, pulmonary edema, ascites and hypotension.
- Dengue shock syndrome consists of dengue hemorrhagic fever combined with tachycardia, hypotension and shock. Death often occurs.
- Fulminant dengue is characterized by hemorrhage, DIC, shock, ARDS, multiorgan failure, encephalopathy leading to obtundation and deep coma. This has a very high mortality; death invariably occurs.

Pulmonary manifestations are invariably present in the second or toxic phase, though they may also occur in the initial febrile period. These include nonproductive cough, alveolar shadows suggestive of pneumonic consolidation and the rapid evolution of acute lung injury going into ARDS. Tachypnea disproportionate to the degree of fever invariably points to an impending lung injury even when radiographic examination of the chest shows no significant change.

Pleural effusion occurs in the more severe cases. It is a manifestation of a generalized capillary leak syndrome and when marked is often accompanied by severe shock. The pleural fluid does not contain inflammatory cells, is rich in albumin, the albumin concentration being over 60% of that in blood.

Pulmonary manifestations of DHF include hemorrhage, more often into the pleural space and surprisingly much less frequently into the lung parenchyma. Rarely, bleeding into body spaces may precede purpura, epistaxis, GI bleed or hematuria. Of interest is a young lady of 22 years who presented with fever, leukopenia, thrombocytopenia and who developed tachypnea and severe abdominal pain 5 days after the onset of infection. She was strongly positive for the dengue antigen and IgM dengue antibody. Examination and imaging studies revealed bilateral pleural effusion as also fluid within the peritoneal cavity. Examination of the abdomen pointed to an acute abdomen with tenderness, guarding rigidity and ileus. Diagnostic aspiration revealed frank hemorrhage at both these sites. The hemorrhagic fluid accumulated again and again so that she needed drainage tubes in both pleural spaces and in the peritoneal cavity. There was no other bleed at that point in time. The condition was associated with quickly evolving ARDS together with hypovolemic shock. Recovery ensued following replacement of blood loss, measures to counter shock, ventilator support with PEEP for ARDS and support to other organ systems.

High resolution computed tomography (HRCT) of the chest may reveal findings not apparent on a chest radiograph. The commonest finding is bilateral pleural effusions. Lung parenchymal abnormalities that have been reported include ground-glass opacities followed by consolidation, airspace nodules, interlobar septal thickening and peribronchovascular interstitial thickening. The occurrence of ARDS is characterized by alveolar edema and the usual radiological findings observed in this condition. Alveolar hemorrhage is uncommon, but bleeding into the pleural space as already mentioned can occur in severe dengue.

Lung histopathology in fatal cases shows alveolar cum interstitial edema, hemorrhage and thickening of alveolar septa.

Fulminant DHF is associated with a disseminated intravascular coagulopathy (DIC). Massive bleeding from various sites and into organ systems is observed, including massive pulmonary hemorrhage. Death almost always occurs.

Recovery in DHF is characterized by a return to hemodynamic stability, reduction and stoppage of bleeding and a progressive rise in the leukocyte and platelet count.

Diagnosis

Dengue antigen and the IgM antibody to the dengue virus are positive. The IgM antibody test may however take as long as seven days to turn positive.

The differential diagnosis is from other hemorrhagic fevers and other conditions causing ARDS. Secondary bacterial infection in patients suffering from dengue invariably worsens prognosis.

Treatment

The dengue virus is not susceptible to any antibiotic or antiviral agent. Since leukopenia at times is marked ($< 1500/mm^3$), secondary infection is possible and known to occur, particularly in the lungs. Appropriate antibiotics are used to counter such infections. Some clinicians use a prophylactic antibiotic cover in patients with severe leukopenia. It is best not to give an antibiotic except in the presence of secondary infection.

Dengue shock is countered by use of IV crystalloids (normal saline, Ringer's lactate) and if hypotension is severe, by the use of colloids, in particular IV albumin. Shock with ARDS is indeed a difficult management problem. Restoration of hemodynamic stability is of prime importance, but this can aggravate ARDS. Once shock is overcome, fluid intake should be titrated so as not to exceed the urine output. Ventilator support is crucial in the management of respiratory problems causing respiratory failure.

Though severe DIC in dengue is almost always fatal, mild derangement in the form of increased activated prothrombin time is countered by the use of intravenous fresh frozen plasma. Severe bleeding or thrombocytopenia if less than 10,000/mm^3 needs platelet infusions as also packed RBCs to replace blood loss. Appropriate blood products may need to be replaced to counter coagulation defects.

■ TETANUS

Tetanus is an acute often fatal disease caused by the contamination of wounds by *Clostridium tetani*, a gram-positive motile rod shaped obligate anaerobe. Under anaerobic conditions the vegetative form of the organism produces a powerful neurotoxin which on reaching the nervous system causes a marked increase in muscle spasm.

The disease is chiefly prevalent in India, Bangladesh, Pakistan, Southeast Asia, the African continent, and South America. It is indeed a disease of the poorer countries of the world. Spores of *C. tetani* are present in soil, particularly fertile soil, in rural areas where human beings and animals live in close proximity often sharing the same shelter.

The description below first briefly considers the prevalence of tetanus, its pathophysiology, and then discusses the respiratory complications invariably encountered with the disease. Respiratory complications are in fact inherent features of tetanus. They add to its morbidity and mortality and pose problems in management. The management of these respiratory problems involves the basic management of the disease which is therefore finally given brief consideration.

Prevalence

In the very early 1990s it was computed that approximately one million cases of tetanus occurred annually in the world, with a global incidence of 18 per 100,000, with a crude fatality rate at all ages being 40–70%. Around 50% of these patients were neonatal tetanus. The World Bank Development Report states that more than 500,000 reported tetanus fatalities occurred annually in 1993 to 277,000 in 1997. Neonatal tetanus accounted from 20% to 70% of all deaths. For obvious reasons this is an underestimate. WHO reported 12.476 cases in 2017 of which 2266 were neonatal tetanus. The decline is a tribute to the vaccination campaign in mothers and in children. The menace of tetanus with its high fatality remains chiefly in the poorer countries stated above.

Pathophysiology

Tetanus arises from the contamination of a wound by *C. tetani*. It can arise from the most trivial of wounds as after minor needle injuries, or in more serious wounds as in injuries, in accidents, or in war. Unsterile cutting of the umbilical cord and application of various substances by poor ignorant people to the stump of the cord are the common causes of neonatal tetanus. Once the *C. tetani* spores gain entry into a wound, the vegetative form of the organism elaborates a toxin which spreads to adjacent muscles attaching itself to nerve endings in proximity to the wound and in the adjacent muscles. The toxin is internalized and spreads retrogradely along the axons of the peripheral nerves to the anterior horn cells of the related segments of the spinal cord. The toxin also enters the bloodstream from where it reaches the nerve endings of all muscles throughout the body, then along the axonal pathways of all peripheral nerves to reach the motor neuron bodies of the whole spinal cord and brainstem. It also reaches the sympathetic chain, the preganglionic sympathetic neurons in the lateral horns and the parasympathetic center. After reaching the anterior horn cells the toxin passes retrogradely across the presynaptic cleft to bind to receptor nerve terminals of inhibitor interneurons. It then blocks the release of inhibitor neuron transmitters, chiefly glycine and γ-aminobutyric acid (GABA). The motor neurons and the autonomic nerves are now released from all inhibitory control. The unchecked uninhibited motor discharge from motor neurons leads to a marked increase in muscle tone and frequent uncontrolled muscle spasms.

Clinical Features (Figs. 3 and 4)

Tetanus can be mild, moderate, or severe. The severity is often graded in ascending order from grade I to grade IV. Grade III and grade IV correspond to severe and very severe tetanus, respectively. Grade III tetanus is associated with marked rigidity, frequent spasms which also involve the muscles of respiration; spasms occur on the slightest touch or other stimuli (light, noise, for example) or even occur spontaneously. Tachycardia, marked tachypnea (>40 breaths/min), hypoxemia, dysphagia, and a steady increase in autonomic nervous activity is noted. Grade IV (very severe) tetanus consists of all features of grade III tetanus coupled with violent autonomic disturbances amounting to what have been termed *autonomic storms*.

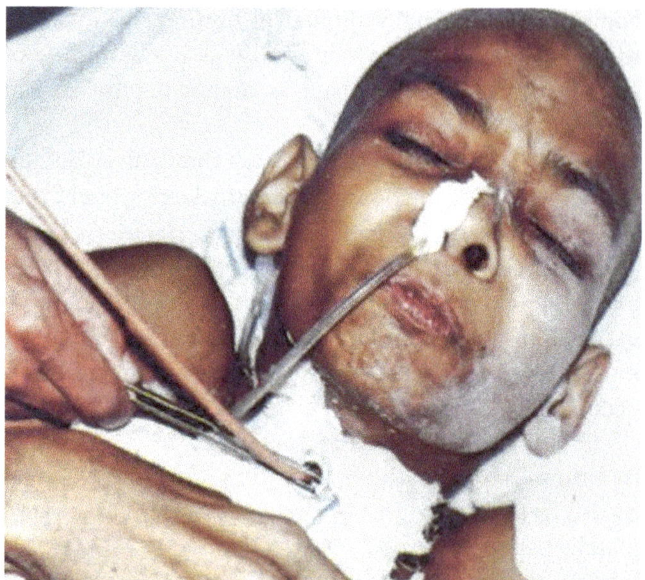

Fig. 3: Tetanus facies with *risus sardonicus.*

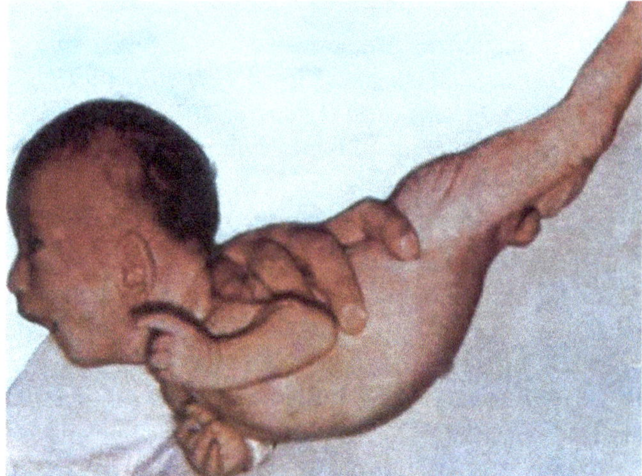

Fig. 4: Opisthotonos in neonatal tetanus.

Complications in tetanus can involve almost any or every system. Only complications involving the respiratory system will now be considered.

■ RESPIRATORY COMPLICATIONS

Respiratory complications are extremely common and contribute significantly to morbidity and mortality. They occur frequently and repeatedly, particularly in severe tetanus and are seen more commonly is those treated conservatively than in those managed with tracheostomy and ventilator support.

Hypoxemic Respiratory Failure

Hypoxemic (type I) respiratory failure occurs frequently in the natural history of even moderately severe tetanus. It is related to ventilation perfusion abnormalities even in lungs which appear normal on clinical and radiological examination and also to some degree of a right to left shunt.

Hypercapnic Respiratory Failure

Patients with severe well-nigh continuous uncontrolled seizures develop hypoventilation with a rise in partial pressure of carbon dioxide ($PaCO_2$) and a fall in partial pressure of oxygen (PaO_2). Excessive sedation (in the absence of ventilator support) worsens the situation. The hypoxemia can be corrected by oxygen given though nasal prongs or a mask, though the hypercapnia remains unchanged.

Further dangerous life-threatening hypoxia often occurs in the presence of other pulmonary complications discussed below. Prolonged or recurrent hypoxia is an important cause of cardiac arrest and death or may produce cerebral damage that can result in coma even when seizures are well controlled.

The use of ventilator support prevents respiratory failure and hypoxia due to pulmonary complications.

Atelectasis, Aspiration Pneumonia, Pneumonia, Bronchopneumonia

These complications are related to the difficulty experienced by patients with tetanus in effectively handling their upper respiratory secretions. The difficulty is related to the following factors:

- Marked increase in oral and pharyngeal secretions.
- The inability to swallow or spit.
- Frequent regurgitation of stomach contents leading to aspiration.
- Rigidity and muscle spasms involving the intercostal and all other respiratory muscles prevent the patients from coughing effectively. Tracheobronchial secretions which are often both infected and excessive gather both in large and small airways leading to infected atelectasis.
- Muscle spasms and marked rigidity of the respiratory muscles markedly reduce chest wall compliance, restricting ventilation and thereby predisposing to atelectasis.

- During the period of prolonged respiratory muscle and laryngeal spasm, there is further accumulation of respiratory secretions within the airways, as well as a fresh reflux of gastric contents. Following prolonged spasms, there often follows a short period of deep breathing resulting in the aspiration of accumulated secretions deep into the lung.
- The aspiration is usually patchy, but can be segmental, lobar or, at times, even involve the whole lung. As expected, atelectasis is more frequent in the apical and basal segments of the lower lobes and in the posterior segment of the upper lobe. Diffuse microatelectasis is frequently observed in patients with severe tetanus. It is characterized by an increase in the alveolar arterial gradient and in the true venous admixture even though the lungs on clinical and radiological examination appear normal. It should therefore be suspected when the PaO_2 is lower in relation to the FiO_2, in the presence of a satisfactory chest X-ray.

In our experience atelectasis occurring in tetanus is more often than not infected in more than 80%, causing aspiration pneumonia, pneumonia and bronchopneumonia. Lung abscess and empyema may also occur. Infecting organisms are usually gram-negative bacteria, the most frequent of which are *Klebsiella* and *P. aeruginosa*. Rarely staphylococci, streptococci, and anaerobes are also found to be responsible for infection in these patients.

Laryngeal Spasm

Laryngeal spasm is a common and a dreaded feature of tetanus. If protracted and unrelieved it causes hypoxia, cyanosis, and sudden death. Laryngeal spasms may accompany or follow a bout of generalized spasms, but may occur alone as an isolated feature. It may occasionally occur as the only spasm in a patient graded as mild tetanus. The very first episode of laryngeal spasm may be sudden and severe enough to cause death. Usually laryngeal spasms occur early in the natural history of severe tetanus or at the height of the disease. Occasionally, an unexpected and even fatal laryngeal spasm may occur, when the patient appears well and is on the way to recovery.

Apneic Attack

Apneic spells, even in the absence of laryngeal spasms, can also occur, leading to severe hypoxemia and cyanosis. They may occur with generalized spasms but more importantly may occur by themselves unrelated to episodes of severe spasms. They always signify severe tetanus. If unrecognized and protracted, the resulting severe hypoxia leads to bradycardia, cardiac arrest, and death.

Episodes of Severe Respiratory Distress

This is a rather unusual respiratory complication observed in both moderate and severe tetanus. It is characterized by episodes of tachypnea, extreme respiratory distress and is not associated with increasing hypoxemia nor with hypercapnia, bronchospasm, or increase in secretions within airways. It is also unrelated to atelectasis. The reason for these attacks is obscure. The explanation perhaps lies in the release of inhibitory control over the respiratory center, or perhaps to the direct action of the tetanus toxin per se on the respiratory center.

Bronchospasm

Tachypnea due to bronchospasm is observed in both moderate and severe tetanus. It is partly related to increased secretions in the tracheobronchial tree producing narrowed airways. In severe tetanus, bronchospasm may be a manifestation of increased parasympathetic activity, many of these patients show evidence of increased vagal tone, in particular bradyrhythm induced by tracheal suction.

Acute Respiratory Distress Syndrome

Acute respiratory distress syndrome can be due to two causes. It is often caused by associated gram-negative sepsis. It then occurs later in the natural history of severe tetanus and the clinical and other features of sepsis are evident. It can also occur early in the natural history of tetanus in the absence of sepsis, and then may well be related to the disease itself.

Diaphragmatic Paralysis

Foccata et al. reported diaphragmatic paralysis in 37% of 115 patients studied both clinically and radiologically. In 97% of patients the paralysis involved the right dome of the diaphragm. We have however been unable to confirm this finding. Whenever the right dome was raised in our patients it was invariably related to a basal atelectasis.

Sudden Death

Sudden death is the most dreaded complication in tetanus. It can result from severe prolonged hypoxia, ventricular arrhythmias, or sudden undetected hyperpyrexia.

■ COMPLICATIONS RELATED TO VENTILATOR SUPPORT

Patients with severe tetanus may need ventilator support for 6 weeks or more. They are critically ill not just with complications involving the respiratory systems, but also complications involving the cardiovascular and often of many other systems. Ventilator support is a challenge to the intensivist and offers him a wealth of experience hardly ever seen with any other disease. Complications include pulmonary infection; significant pulmonary atelectasis (recurrent atelectasis—segmental or subsegmental is an invariable feature of severe tetanus), pneumothorax, pneumomediastinum, accidental disconnection of the ventilator in a paralyzed patient.

Management

In no disease is the dictum that prevention is better than cure more applicable than in tetanus. Tetanus toxoid vaccination at recommended intervals and the use of tetanus toxoid in pregnant mothers who have not been previously immunized could perhaps help to sharply reduce, if not eliminate, the scourge.

Use of Antitoxin

Around 1,000 units of human tetanus immunoglobulin (if available) is given IV. Human tetanus immunoglobulin is free of hypersensitivity reactions. Equine antiserum is unfortunately more easily available in poor countries. A skin test for a hypersensitivity reaction should first be done; fatal anaphylaxis can otherwise occur with use of the equine antiserum.

The details of management of tetanus are beyond the scope of this book. Only management principles are given below.

Use of Sedatives and Muscle Relaxants

The use of sedatives and muscle relaxants is the cornerstone of therapy in grade I and grade II tetanus. The objective is to reduce rigidity and control muscle spasms without depressing respiration. Diazepam, a benzodiazepine and a GABA antagonist is the drug of choice in most units. It should be given in a slow IV infusion over 24 hours and the dose titrated to meet the objective stated above. It is best not to exceed a dose of 120 mg to at most 150 mg over 24 hours in adults even if there is marked rigidity. Higher doses will inevitably depress respiration. Lorazepam with a longer duration of action or midazolam with a shorter duration of action can also be used in place of diazepam. Chlorpromazine and phenobarbital are 2nd line drugs that can be used in combination with diazepam.

Tracheostomy

Tracheostomy is indicated in all patients with grade III and grade IV tetanus. We would also recommend tracheostomy in moderately severe or grade II tetanus as we have seen deaths from sudden uncontrolled laryngeal spasm in these patients.

Induced Paralysis and Ventilator Support

All patients with grades III and IV (severe and very severe) tetanus require both a tracheostomy and ventilator support. Our experience (with many patients) has taught us that mortality in severe tetanus can be markedly reduced if the following principles are followed:

- Ventilator support till such time as spasms cease. Rigidity is markedly reduced and the patients can be successfully weaned. This may take 6–8 weeks in some patients. Efficient ventilator support reduces the risk of respiratory complications.
- The use of neuroparalytic agents to enable effective ventilator support. Pancuronium 2–4 mg IV every 30 min to 2 hours or Vecuronium 0.1 mg/kg is very effective. Alternatively either of these 2 drugs can be given in a slow titrated IV infusion over 24 hours so that ventilation is well-maintained and spasms are well controlled but not necessarily totally abolished.
- During induced paralysis with ventilator support, our experience with the disease dictates that it is best not to give large doses of IV diazepam. We found that 75–100 mg of diazepam is the upper limit of use. Higher doses given over several weeks depress the respiratory and other medullary centers markedly. Sudden death is one of the most important complications of tetanus and resuscitation in these patients is nearly impossible if the medullary centers have been paralyzed through large doses of diazepam.

- Critical care: This is of vital importance. Physiotherapy to the chest given at the time of the maximum effect of the neuroparalytic drug, careful gentle suction to keep the airways open and a constant watch for evidence of atelectasis with prompt efforts to open up an atelectic segment or lobe are of vital importance. Tracheostomy care needs to be meticulous. Prevention and treatment of iatrogenic infection, particularly involving the respiratory system is equally important. There is no complication in or outside a book on critical care medicine that does not occur in some patients with severe tetanus. Looking after and caring for these patients is indeed a great learning experience for the intensivist.

Management of Autonomic Disturbances

Intravenous β-blockers, heavy sedation, IV morphine sulfate, IV labetalol, IV magnesium sulfate and clonidine have all been tried to control autonomic storms. These drugs do not alter the high mortality. Hypotensive spells are best controlled with a volume load or if needs be by a titrated dose of dopamine to maintain a systolic pressure of over 100 mm Hg. Hypertensive spells (BP >200/100 mm Hg) are controlled by a titrated dose of oral propranolol and if needs be by a calcium-channel blocker. IV propranolol should never be used as it can cause sudden death.

Bradyrhythms are treated by a titrated dose of IV atropine; tachyrhythms by a titrated dose of a β-blocker given orally or by the use of verapamil. Meticulous critical care and ventilator support remain the corner stone of therapy in these very ill-patients.

Treatments of complications that arise need expert attention and prompt treatment.

Mortality

The mortality in severe tetanus dropped from 30% to 12% and the mortality of fulminant tetanus from 100% to 23% in the tetanus ward of a large public teaching hospital using basic equipment for critical care and the management principles outlined above. In a well-equipped critical care unit in Mumbai, the mortality of severe tetanus in our unit is as low as 6%. The mortality of severe neonatal tetanus is still between 30% and 70%.

Melioidosis

Melioidosis is an infection caused by the saprophytic bacterium *Burkholderia pseudomallei*. It is endemic in

South and Southeast Asia, the incidence being particularly high in Northeast Thailand. The country with the highest number of recorded cases is Thailand where the average incidence is 4.4 per 100,000 people. The disease is also endemic in South China, Central and South America and parts of Africa. Human infection probably occurs through contaminated scratches and abrasions or occasionally following aspiration of contaminated fresh water. Agricultural workers and rice farmers in close contact with soil and water are at greater risk. It has been reported in India, particularly from Tamil Nadu and Karnataka. Cases have also been reported from Orissa, West Bengal, Assam, Andhra Pradesh, and Maharashtra.

Pulmonary Manifestations

Infection with *B. pseudomallei* causes acute, disseminated, chronic or localized disease. Though melioidosis is a multisystem disease, the lung is a frequent and most important site of involvement.

In the acute form, the lung may be the primary site of involvement or may be part of an acute disseminated disease with multi-organ involvement. Symptoms generally develop within 2 weeks after exposure. There is sudden onset of fever, breathlessness and cough with productive sputum, pleuritic pain and severe prostration. Hemoptysis may occur. The clinical picture is indistinguishable from a severe community-acquired pneumonia or severe gram-negative sepsis. There is well-marked polymorphonuclear leukocytosis. Radiographic examination of the chest reveals lobar consolidation on one or both sides. The consolidated areas may cavitate to form one or more lung abscesses. Pleural effusion and empyema may be associated features.

Though occasionally the lung may appear as the only organ to be involved, most patients with acute disease have evidence of other organ system involvement. There may be cutaneous abscesses, liver abscess, splenic abscess and abscesses within the brain or bones.

Overwhelming sepsis may supervene. ARDS, septic shock and multi-organ failure are observed in fatal cases.

The subacute form is characterized by low-grade fever, weight loss, cough with expectoration and hemoptysis, lasting for weeks or months. These symptoms develop long after exposure to infection or represent reactivation of latent disease.

Radiographic examination reveals consolidation with cavitation generally involving both upper lobes, the X-ray appearances being indistinguishable from pulmonary tuberculosis or a lung abscess **(Figs. 5A and B)**. Pleural effusion and empyema may occur. Even when the lung seems the sole site of involvement, investigations may reveal the presence of one or more abscesses in other organs such as the liver, spleen, bones or the brain. Leukocytosis is generally present.

The chronic form of melioidosis lasts for several months or years with low-grade fever intermingled with apyrexial periods, weight loss, cough and hemoptysis

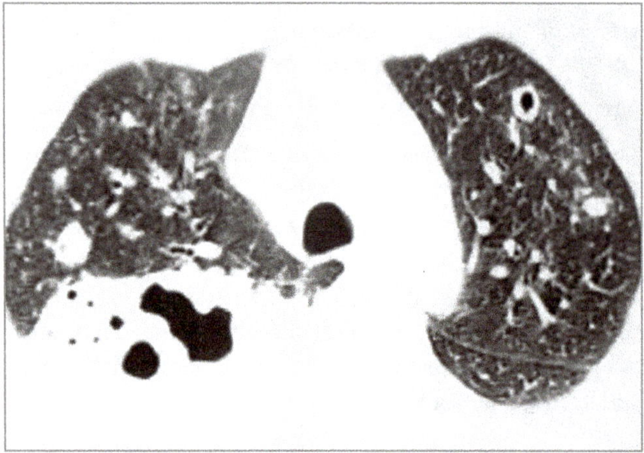

Fig. 5A: CT scan of the chest in an individual whose chest X-ray appearances were highly suggestive of pulmonary tuberculosis. The CT confirms the appearance of a large right upper lobe cavitating lesion. Additionally there are multiple nodular lesions with cavitation seen in both upper lobes.

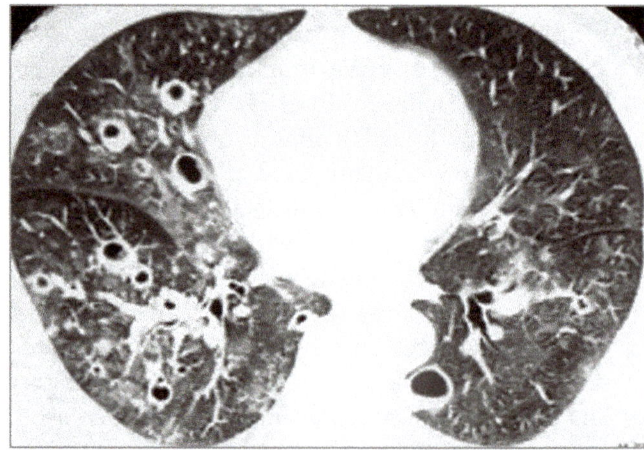

Fig. 5B: Lower CT sections reveal well-defined nodular lesions with cavitations as well as air-fluid levels within the lesions. The location of these lesions in the lung bases as well as the well-defined nature of these lesions is not in favor of tuberculosis. Microbiological evaluation of sputum revealed *B. pseudomallei*.

and pleuritic chest pain. Chest radiographs invariably reveal bilateral upper lobe cavitative disease with fibrosis indistinguishable from tuberculosis. Metastatic spread to other organs may be present or may still occur.

Diagnosis

A clinical diagnosis of melioidosis should always be suspected in upper lobe lesions which resemble tuberculosis when acid-fast bacilli (AFB) smear, culture of sputum or BAL fluid are negative. The diagnosis is confirmed by isolation, identification on culture of *B. pseudomallei* from the sputum. At times isolation of this organism is easier from the discharge of a metastatic cutaneous lesion or from the aspirate of a metastatic liver abscess.

Blood cultures may be positive in septicemic patients. It is important for the clinician to specifically inform the microbiologist if he suspects an infection with *B. pseudomallei*. Identification of the organism in sputum samples which have polymicrobial flora is difficult and often missed.

In patients with little or no sputum, indirect hemagglutination tests and complement fixation tests are performed; they have a high diagnostic sensitivity. People living in highly endemic areas such as Thailand have a high-incidence of seropositivity for this disease. Therefore in these areas the diagnostic titer needs to be high, preferably 1 in 640 or more, to avoid false positive readings.

Treatment

The acute form of the disease or patients with multi-system involvement are best treated with ceftazidime in maximum doses of 2 g IV 8 hourly together with one other antibiotic. This could be doxycycline (4 mg/kg/day) or co-trimoxazole in maximal doses. The antibiotic course should be for 2–4 weeks. Following, this oral antibiotic maintenance thereby is advised for 6 months to a year. Antibiotic for maintenance therapy could either be doxycycline 4 mg/kg/day or co-trimoxazole (trimethoprim 10 mg/kg/day, sulfamethoxazole 50 mg/kg/day) or amoxycillin clavulanate in high doses.

Prolonged courses are necessary because the disease is slow to respond and frequently relapses. Extrapulmonary abscesses may require surgical drainage.

Penicilliosis marneffei

Penicilliosis marneffei is a *Penicillium* that causes disease. Infection with this fungus is rare in India, though a few HIV patients suffering from the infection have been reported from Manipur in Northeast India. It has however been increasingly reported from Southeast Asia—Thailand, Vietnam, South China and Hong Kong. Though more often seen in immunocompromsied HIV patients, it has also been noted in immunocompetent patients. The organism is found in the soil of the countries stated above.

Human infection is through direct skin contact with resulting contamination, or through inhalation of infected aerosols.

Clinical Features

Pulmonary manifestations include cough with or without dyspnea. In HIV patients, the clinical manifestations are those of pneumonia, which may be difficult to distinguish from tuberculous infection, cryptococcal infection, cytomegalovirus (CMV), pneumocystis pneumonia (PCP) or even bacterial infection. A prospective BAL study of HIV patients from Chiang Mai University Hospital, Thailand revealed that *P. marneffei* was found in 40% of patients with fungal infections and in 16% of all cases of pneumonia. Radiological examination of the chest usually showed bilateral involvement with areas of consolidation with or without cavitation or nonspecific reticulonodular or reticular infiltrates. Besides pulmonary manifestations, infection with this fungal species was associated with fever, anemia, lymphadenopathy, hepatosplenomegaly and papular skin eruptions with central umbilication resembling molluscum contagiosum.

Diagnosis

Diagnosis is made by identifying the organism from a Gram stain of sputum or BAL fluid. *P. marneffei* appears as a sausage-shaped gram-negative organism with central septation. Yeast forms of this fungus may also be found. Culture of sputum or BAL fluid is highly specific.

Treatment

Treatment of choice is amphotericin B 0.5 mg/kg intravenously given daily for a total dose of approximately 1 g. Itraconazole 400 mg/day given for 8–12 weeks is also effective. Relapse is frequent in HIV patients; itraconazole 200 mg/day is continued to prevent relapse. Response to treatment is generally observed within 2–3 weeks.

Plague

Plague is caused by the bacterium *Yersinia pestis*. The disease exists as a bacterial zoonosis with rodents being the chief reservoir. The black rat (*Rattus rattus*) and the Oriental flea (Xenopsylla cheopis) are the main reservoir and transmitting agent respectively for human plague in India. Plague is endemic in Africa, Vietnam, India, Myanmar, China, and Peru and has been reported sporadically from the United States. India has seen several outbreaks since 1994, the worst being an outbreak of pneumonic plague in Surat, Gujarat, which caused 52 deaths and resulted in 876 seropositive cases.

Plague generally presents in the bubonic form—painful large buboes (inflamed lymph glands) develop generally in the inguinal region, occasionally in the axillary region and rarely in the cervical region. Bacteremic spread may involve the lungs giving rise to pneumonic plague. This is characterized by pneumonia, often involving both lungs **(Fig. 6)**. Marked toxicity, severe prostration, hypotension and rapidly evolving cardiorespiratory failure can kill the patient in 24–72 hours. Leukocytosis of 10,000–20,000/mm^3 is generally present. Thrombocytopenia and DIC can occur.

In epidemics, the lung may be the primary site of infection. This is due to inhalation of droplets of infected sputum from patients with lung involvement. A rapidly spreading pneumonia often involving both lungs occurs, death occurring within 24–72 hours.

Diagnosis

This is evident in an established epidemic but may be otherwise difficult. Presence of *Y. pestis,* a gram-negative coccobacillus in sputum smear and culture is confirmatory. A passive hemagglutination test or an ELISA test is available in reference laboratories for testing acute and convalescent serum.

Treatment

The drug of choice is streptomycin 30 mg/kg given in two divided doses for 10 days. Patients should be nursed in isolation.

Anthrax

This is a disease caused by *B. anthracis* and is commonly seen in domestic and herbivorous animals. Human anthrax is more prevalent when there is direct contact with infected animals. Anthrax spores are hardy and can remain infectious for months or even years. They are transmitted by contact with infectious carcasses, hides, hairs and bone-meal or from contact with soil contaminated by spores. The disease is endemic in India, Pakistan, Iran, Latin America, and Central Africa. In India, the disease still remains endemic in Tamil Nadu, Karnataka and Andhra Pradesh. The majority of cases are of cutaneous anthrax. However, human cases of pulmonary anthrax, GI anthrax and septicemic anthrax have also been reported.

The pulmonary form is best described as inhalation anthrax (also termed wool sorter's disease).

Pathology

Inhaled anthrax spores are deposited in the alveolar spaces. Macrophages transport these spores to the tracheobronchial and mediastinal lymph glands where they germinate to cause an hemorrhagic mediastinitis with a necrotizing lymphadenitis.

Clinical Features

Initial symptoms are those of a flu-like syndrome with fever, cough, malaise and myalgia. The second stage is characterized by severe respiratory distress, cyanosis and profuse sweating.

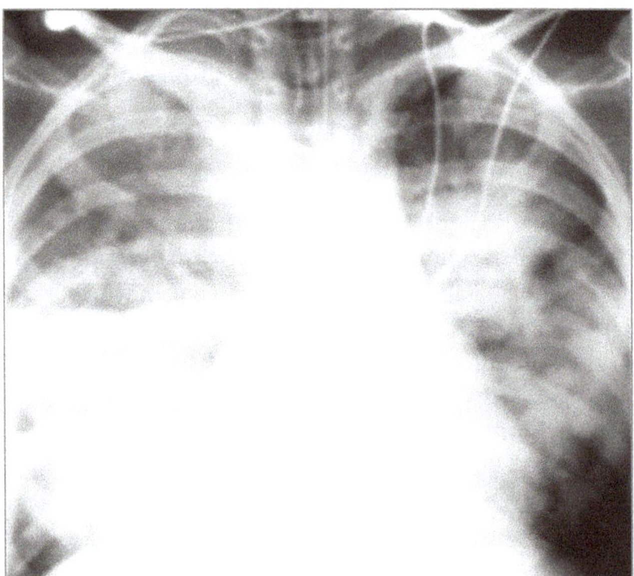

Fig. 6: Plague. X-ray chest showing diffuse bilateral consolidation involving both lungs. There is often subcutaneous edema of the neck; an X-ray of the chest shows symmetrical mediastinal widening with or without a pleural effusion. The mediastinal widening is due to acute mediastinitis and necrotizing lymphadenopathy. Blood culture is often positive for *B. anthracis.* Shock with cardiorespiratory failure occurs within 24–48 hours.

Prognosis

The pulmonary form has a dreadful prognosis. Death occurs from increasing hypotension and cardiorespiratory failure.

Treatment

Penicillin is the drug of choice, four million unit 4 hourly administered for 2 weeks. Intravenous ciprofloxacin (500 mg/day) or IV doxycycline (200 mg/day) may also be used. Intensive support to all organ systems is necessary.

■ SCRUB TYPHUS

Scrub typhus is a zoonotic disease of rural Asia caused by a gram-negative intracellular bacterium Orientia (formerly Rickettsia). This organism is transferred from rats to humans by the bite of a larval mite (chiggers) which has fed on an infected rat. It is believed that more than a billion people are at risk and a million cases are transmitted annually, making it the commonest Rickettsial disease.

Clinical Features

More often than not the disease is mild, short lasting and easily missed. In its typical form it is characterized by fever, myalgia, conjunctival suffusion, generalized lymphadenopathy and the presence of an eschar (which is really an ulcer covered by a thick crust) at the site of the tick bite. Persistent cough is the predominant respiratory feature often associated with bilateral reticular infiltrates at both bases on radiography of the chest. Though most cases are mild, severe cases meriting critical care do occur. These patients develop or present with dyspnea, a progressive increase in the respiratory rate, tachycardia and a fall in O_2 saturation. They may develop a full blown ARDS. High temperature, apathy, confusion may be observed and rarely these may progress to stupor, seizures and deep coma.

Diagnosis

The presence of an eschar is diagnostic but as mentioned earlier it is present only in 50% of cases. Mild leukocytosis and a mild to moderate elevation of liver enzymes are noted.

Treatment

More often than not treatment is based on a clinical assumption of the diagnosis. Tetracycline 500 mg four times a day or doxycycline 100 mg twice daily for 7 days is recommended. In critically ill-patients parenteral doxycycline or parenteral tetracycline or IV chloramphenicol (50–75 mg/kg/day) is administered. Critically-ill patients may require ventilator support as also support to other organ systems. Azithromycin is the drug of choice in pregnant women with scrub typhus or in children who contact the disease, as both tetracycline and doxycycline are contraindicated in the above situation. Azithromycin has also proved successful in patients with drug-resistant scrub typhus.

■ SUGGESTED READING

1. Cunha BA. Osler on typhoid fever: differentiating typhoid from typhus and malaria. Infect Dis Clin North Am. 2004;18(1):111-25.
2. Halstead SB. Dengue. Lancet. 2007;370(9599):1644-52.
3. Martanez S, Restrepo CS, Carrillo JA, et al. Thoracic manifestations of tropical parasitic infections: a pictorial review. Radiographics. 2005;25(1):135-55.
4. Meumann EM1, Cheng AC, Ward L, et al. Clinical features and epidemiology of melioidosis pneumonia: results from a 21-year study and review of the literature. Clin Infect Dis. 2012;54(3):362-9.
5. Pande JN, Kabra SK. Dengue hemorrhagic fever and dengue shock syndrome. Natl Med J India. 1996;9(6):256-8.
6. Peter TV, Sudarsan TI, Prakash JA, et al. Severe scrub typhus infection: clinical features, diagnostic challenges and management. World J Crit Care Med. 2015;4(3):244-50.
7. Udwadia FE. Oxford Textbook of Medicine, 4th edition. New Delhi: Oxford University Press; 2005.
8. Udwadia FE. Tetanus. New Delhi: Oxford University Press; 1994.
9. Udwadia FE, Lall A, Udwadia ZF, et al. Tetanus and its complications: intensive care and management experience in 150 Indian patients. Epidemiol Infect. 1987;99(3): 675-84.
10. Udwadia FE, Sunavala JD, Jain MC, et al. Hemodynamic studies during the management of severe tetanus. Q J Med. 1992;83(302):449-60.
11. Vijayachari P, Sugunan AP, Shriram AN. Leptospirosis: an emerging global public health problem. J Biosci. 2008;33(4):557-69.
12. World Health Organization. Dengue: Guidelines for diagnosis, treatment, prevention, and control. Geneva: World Health Organization; 2009.

Section 10

Airway Diseases

CHAPTER 32

Asthma: Introduction, Epidemiology and Etiopathogenesis

INTRODUCTION

Asthma is a chronic disease characterized by recurrent attacks of cough, wheeze, and breathlessness. It is a public health problem not just for developed countries but across the globe. The World Health Organization (WHO) estimates that 300 million people are afflicted by asthma globally with 250,000 deaths recorded annually. Asthma is the most common chronic disease affecting children and, with the related atopic disorders of eczema and atopic rhinitis, constituted a third of all chronic disorders even 30 years ago. Asthma prevalence is increasing across the globe due to increasing exposure to exacerbating factors like airborne indoor or outdoor pollutants and indoor allergens, and decreasing exposure to protective factors like antioxidants, microbial burden, and physical exercise. It remains an underdiagnosed and undertreated condition creating substantial burden to patients and their families. Despite all the advances in our understanding and treatment of asthma, it continues to kill, with most asthma deaths occurring in the poorer countries. This chapter will focus on the definition, global and Indian epidemiology, types, etiopathogenesis, investigations, treatment, and look at special situations like difficult and fatal asthma, asthma in pregnancy, aspirin-induced and exercise-induced asthma (EIA).

DEFINITION

Asthma is a chronic inflammatory disorder of the airways in which many cells and cellular elements play a role. The chronic inflammation is associated with bronchial hyperresponsiveness (BHR) that leads to recurrent episodes of wheezing, breathlessness, chest tightness, and coughing, especially at night or in the early morning. These episodes are usually associated with widespread but variable airflow obstruction within the lung that is often reversible either spontaneously or with treatment. This definition from GINA (Global Initiative for Asthma) is long but complete, including not just the clinical features but also the key physiological problem (BHR), the inflammation that is the pathological highlight, and the usually but not inevitably reversible nature of the disease.

It encapsulates the huge shift in our understanding of the disease over the last three centuries from the predominantly bronchospastic condition it was postulated to be by Sir John Floyer in his *Treatise of Asthma* in 1698. In fact, it was as early as 1892 that Osler discussed the role of airway inflammation in the pathogenesis of asthma in his *Principles and Practice of Medicine.* Pathological evidence supporting this view appeared as early as 1922. It was only over the last few decades, however, that our view of asthma shifted from that of a disease of airway smooth muscle contraction to one characterized by complex interactions between inflammatory mediators and effector cells. Helping us makes this paradigm shift have been several key clinical studies, postmortem studies, bronchial biopsy studies, and bronchoalveolar lavage (BAL) fluid analysis in asthmatic patients.

EPIDEMIOLOGY OF ASTHMA

Asthma is a complex disease and there are many challenges in studying its epidemiology including the lack of a precise and universal definition and the absence of a single physiological test that is sensitive and specific. Asthma is one of the most common chronic disorders of the developed world. Over the last three decades, there has been an increase in the global incidence of asthma and atopy. There is limited data on the epidemiology of asthma from the Asian continent in general, and the Indian subcontinent in particular, though there is a general impression that the prevalence is lower here than in the Western world. Much of our information on the prevalence of asthma in India comes via the ISAAC study (International Study of Asthma and Allergies in Childhood) in which many Asian countries participated. This and similar studies provided important information on the prevalence and burden of asthma in Asia.

Global Epidemiology

The prevalence of asthma varies from country to country depending upon the definition used to diagnose asthma. Currently, asthma is reported in 1.2–6.3% of the adult population in most countries. On the other hand, diagnosed asthma, (i.e. asthma ever diagnosed by a clinician) runs at 12% in the UK, 7.1% in the US and as high as 15% in Australia. The ECRHS (European Community Respiratory Health Survey) studied the geographic variation in asthma and allergies among the adult population of 22 countries across the globe. Both the ECRHS and the ISAAC surveys demonstrated dramatic variations in the prevalence of asthma symptoms from across the globe. While the ECRHS considered representative samples 20–44 years of age from 22 chiefly Western European countries, ISAAC looked at several (eight participating) Asian countries. In the ECRHS study, the highest prevalence of wheeze was found from Ireland (32%) and the lowest from India (4.1%). In the ISAAC study too, the prevalence of asthma in 13–14-year old varied widely across countries: from a high of 32.2% in the UK, to a low of 1.6% from India. Thus between them, these two major studies showed that asthma prevalence was clearly higher in the Western world than in the Asian region. The wide variation in asthma prevalence seen in the ISAAC study is shown in **Figure 1**. As can be seen India finishes at the lower end of the asthma prevalence league.

Asian Epidemiology

Prior to the 1990s, most of the epidemiological data from Asia was collected in a nonstandardized fashion with different types of written questionnaires. This early data showed there was great variation in the prevalence of "asthma ever" from a low of 1.6% from Guangzhou to a high of 19% from Taiwan. The ISAAC study brought home two important facts. Firstly, that the prevalence of self-reported

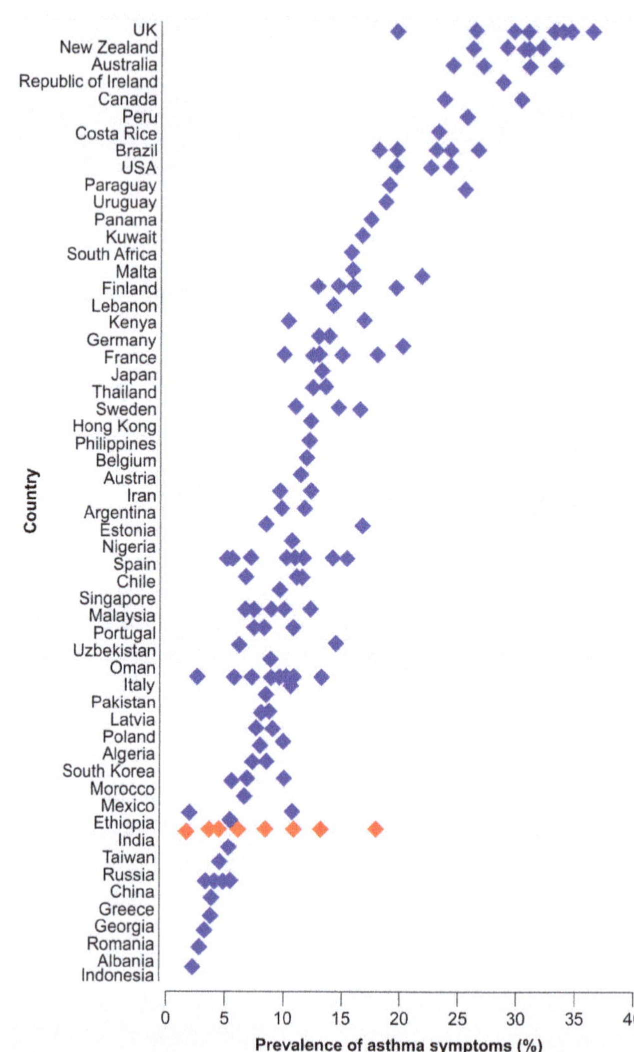

Fig. 1: 12-month prevalence of self-reported asthma symptoms in different countries as reported in International Study of Asthma and Allergies in Childhood (ISAAC).
Source: Richard B. Worldwide variation in prevalence of symptoms of asthma, allergic rhinoconjunctivitis and atopic eczema: ISAAC. Lancet. 1998;351(9111):1225-32.

asthma symptoms in 13–14-year old was much lower in Asian countries than in the West. It also demonstrated tremendous variation even among different countries in the Asian region, with the more affluent Asian countries like Japan and Hong Kong having higher prevalence rates of 10.2% and 10.1%, respectively. However, even these higher prevalence rates lagged considerably behind the prevalence rates reported from New Zealand (18.4%) and Australia (17.6%). Even in younger children aged 6–7 years, the Asian rates mirrored those found in the older children.

Secular Trends in the Asian Region

Several studies from the Asian region confirmed the secular trends of increased prevalence of asthma over the years observed in Western countries. The magnitude of increase was particularly striking in, for example, affluent countries like Singapore, where a study by Leung in 1997 showed the prevalence rates of asthma had increased almost threefold from 5.5% in 1967 to 20.7% three decades later.

Ethnic Differences

Another way to assess the possible changing trend of asthma is to assess the same ethnic group living in a different environment. Such studies demonstrate considerable ethnic differences. A study by Leung and Ho in Chinese children aged 12–18 years from three locations demonstrated that the prevalence of asthma was highest in the children recruited from Hong Kong. In a similar study on almost 3,000 adults from three ethnic groups residing in Singapore, the highest asthma prevalence was found in the Indians (6.6%), while the lowest prevalence was found in the Chinese (3%).

Indian Epidemiology

There is very limited information on the prevalence of asthma among adults in India. The first epidemiological study of asthma prevalence from India emerged from Lucknow in 1966. This study was a questionnaire-based study involving a sample size of 5% of the population of Patna. The prevalence of asthma in the adult population between 30 years and 49 years of age was estimated to be 2.78%. More recent knowledge of the epidemiology of Indian asthma comes from a study by Chowgule et al., which was part of the ECRHS survey in Mumbai residents from 1992–95. In this study a one-in-ten random sample of adults aged 20–44 years was selected from electoral rolls. In Phase 1 of this study, 2,313 adults were interviewed about symptoms, asthma diagnosis and medications in the preceding 12 months. In Phase 2, family and smoking history, serum immunoglobulin E (IgE), skin tests, spirometry, and methacholine challenge were performed on a subset of 20% of patients who had completed the Phase 1 questionnaire. Asthma prevalence in Mumbai was found to be higher than in the Patna study, but still relatively low, at 3.5% (physician diagnosis) and 17% using a very broad definition of asthma. The house dust mite was the most common positive skin test (18%

prevalence) and the only one of the nine applied that was significantly linked to asthma symptoms and physician-diagnosed asthma. In this study, asthma prevalence was strongly associated with positive house dust mite skin test, family history of asthma and total IgE level. When this study cohort was broken down into four age groups, the youngest group aged 20-24 years had the highest prevalence of doctor-diagnosed asthma. Comparison of these results with the prevalence of asthma symptoms overall in all the 48 participating ECRHS centers reveals that the prevalence of asthma and hay fever in Mumbai was significantly lower than the median for most other centers. The highest prevalence rate of wheeze reported in the questionnaire part of the ISAAC survey was 28% in Melbourne, Australia, which was seven times the 4.1% prevalence reported from Mumbai. Thus the ISAAC study established that today, atopic diseases are diseases of privileged countries. The excess in the prevalence of asthma in Western countries is almost totally accounted for by excess in atopic sensitization.

The only other large prevalence study from India comes from the Epidemiology of Asthma Respiratory symptoms and Chronic Bronchitis Study (INSEARCH) conducted by the Indian Council of Medical Research. A total of 169,575 men and women from 12 urban and 11 rural sites in India were studied using a two stage, stratified, sampling strategy using a previously validated questionnaire. The questionnaire used was the IUATLD questionnaire, previously validated in several countries in Europe. The study found the asthma prevalence in India to be 2.05% amongst adults. Female sex, advancing age, residence in urban area, lower socioeconomic status, history of asthma in first degree relative and tobacco smoking were all associated with significantly higher odds of having asthma.

More data exists regarding the prevalence of childhood asthma in India. A literature search identified 15 epidemiological studies on the development of asthma in Indian children from 300 potentially relevant articles. Wide differences in samples, primary outcome variables, lack of consistency in age category, rural-urban variation, criteria for positive diagnosis, and study instruments confounded the outcome variables. The mean prevalence was 7.24% (±SD 5.42). The median prevalence was 4.75% [with interquartile range (IQR) = 2.65–12.35%]. Overall weighted mean prevalence was found to be 2.74. Childhood asthma among children 13–14 years of age was lower than that in younger children 6–7 years of age.

Urban and male predominance with wide inter-regional variation in prevalence was observed. These studies show collectively that the burden of bronchial asthma in Indian children is higher than was previously understood.

■ IMPACT OF ASTHMA IN INDIA

Even figures of 2–3.5% prevalence applied to a country of over a billion translate into large absolute numbers of Indians with asthma. Thus, based on these studies, at least 25–30 million Indians are asthmatic and the economic burden of this disease in India is huge.

India is a vast country of great variation in geographic and climatic conditions, and in socioeconomic and cultural backgrounds. Many large surveys will be needed before a true picture of the prevalence of asthma in this country emerges. More studies from different regions, communities and occupations and from both the rural and urban sectors are needed before a clearer idea of nationwide epidemiology emerges.

■ TYPES OF ASTHMA

Asthma can be classified into several types. These include—childhood asthma, late-onset asthma, chronic asthma, occupational asthma, and difficult asthma. These will all be discussed at appropriate points later.

■ GENETIC FACTORS

In contrast to single-gene disorders like cystic fibrosis, that exhibit classic Mendelian recessive or dominant inheritance, asthma involves multiple genes and expression is influenced by both complex genetic and environmental factors. The multifactorial nature of asthma has confounded genetic studies and despite intensive efforts, no asthma gene has been identified with any certainty.

Asthma is, however, well-known to run in clusters in families. Simply put, the risk that a first-degree family member of a patient with asthma will also develop asthma has been calculated to be two to six times higher than the risk in the general population.

While the search for a specific gene or genes for asthma or atopy remains elusive, the gene that governs airway hyperresponsiveness is located on chromosome 5q near a major locus that regulates serum IgE levels. Marsh first reported this breakthrough announcement of the link between total serum IgE levels and chromosome 5q in

an article in *Science* in 1994. Studies of asthma genetics from the UK, Japan, and the US have also gone on to implicate chromosome 5q as the region that contains one or more susceptibility genes for asthma. Other candidate regions detected by genome-wide searches include chromosome 11q (atopy and positive skin tests and total IgE), chromosome 12q (interferon γ, a mast cell growth factor and the β subunit of nuclear factor-Y), chromosome 6 (eosinophils), and chromosome 16 (total serum IgE).

After determining linkage between asthma and a chromosomal region, the next challenge is to screen this region for candidate genes. A candidate gene has to meet four criteria—(1) the gene product must be functionally relevant to asthma, (2) mutations within the gene must alter the function of the gene, (3) asthma must be linked to the chromosomal region harboring the candidate gene, and (4) finally asthma has to show association with different alleles of this candidate gene. A number of candidate genes have been found that meet these criteria. Chromosome 5q itself has been found to contain numerous candidate genes for asthma and atopy including the cluster of cytokine genes (IL-3, IL-4, IL-5, IL-9, and IL-13) as well as the genes coding for the β_2-adrenergic receptor, the corticosteroid receptor and the granulocyte-macrophage colony-stimulating factor. Other candidate genes include the human leukocyte antigen region at chromosome 6p, tumor necrosis factor-α (TNF-α), and the cytokine gene cluster at chromosome 5q31-33.

Thus, approximately a third of the genetic predisposition to asthma has currently been uncovered. To become relevant to clinical asthma, potential asthma susceptibility genes will now need to be tested in cases and controls with different manifestations of disease and disease severity and in representative population samples with different environmental risk factors. Only then will genotype become a predictor of disease that can be understood in the same terms as other epidemiological risk factors.

Pharmacogenetics—the Role of Genetics in the Treatment of Asthma

Additional genes that are associated with the response to asthma treatment have also been isolated. Thus, it is now clear that different asthmatics respond to β_2-agonists in different ways because of differences in the gene encoding the β-adrenoreceptor. Differences in responses to glucocorticosteroids and leukotriene antagonists are also due to genetic differences in the genes. Thus pharmacogenetics, the genetic variations in individuals that give rise to differing response to drugs, will undoubtedly influence how asthma is managed in the years ahead. A positive association between common arginine-16 variants in the β-adrenergic receptor gene and the responsiveness of asthmatics to β-adrenergic agonists is particularly intriguing. Studies in vitro show that the presence of the Gly16 variant increases downregulation of the β_2-adrenergic receptor following β_2-agonist exposure, while conversely the Glu27 variant protected against agonist-induced downregulation. Intriguingly, studies have shown that the Gly16 variant is more prevalent in asthmatics with nocturnal asthma, while homozygous Gly16 individuals are more prone to bronchodilator desensitization. Already, such genetic information has helped push forward the frontiers of therapy. In a study of 16 moderate asthmatics, albuterol responsiveness was correlated with position in 16 genotypes. The authors found that Arg16 homozygotes gave a higher and more rapid forced expiratory volume in 1 second (FEV1) change compared to Gly16 homozygotes. Similarly, genetic variations may explain the clinical observation that some patients respond well to leukotriene modifiers and some not at all. A series of naturally occurring mutations have been identified within the 5-lipoxygenase gene promoter. In a study of 221 asthmatics, those possessing mutant alleles were relatively resistant to the effects of the leukotriene modifiers.

■ ETIOPATHOGENESIS

In a susceptible host, a number of factors are consistently recognized as triggers of asthma. Some of the important ones will be discussed here.

Allergens

Part of the reason why the prevalence of asthma is so much higher in the West than in the developing world may have to do with the fact that children in the West spend more time indoors and the indoor environment is changing. A number of allergens have been associated with the indoor environment. The most important of these is undoubtedly the house dust mite. Dust mites are arthropods, which grow throughout the world depending on the climate. They thrive in humid environments and some of the highest levels are found in New Zealand, explaining why asthma prevalence is consistently higher in this country. There are different varieties of house dust mite, with *Dermatophagoides pteronyssinus* being the most common temperate species, while *Blomia tropicalis* is the most important type encountered in the tropics. Many different dust mite allergens have been characterized, the most extensively studied are the Group 1 and 2 allergens Der p1 and Der p2, which are 25-kD cysteine protease and 14-kD epididymal proteins, respectively. An elegant longitudinal study by Sears confirmed the relevance of the link between allergy to house dust mite and asthma with sensitivity to house dust mite in childhood (by skin test) being associated with persistent symptoms and relapse of asthma in adult life. A positive skin test for house dust mite allergen at age 13 carried a 3.38 odds ratio (OR) in univariate analysis for predicting wheeze and asthma by the age of 26. Other indoor allergens of note include dog dander, cat dander, and cockroach droppings.

Infections

During infancy, a number of viruses have been associated with the inception of the asthma prototype. Respiratory syncytial virus (RSV) and parainfluenza virus produce a pattern of symptoms, including bronchiolitis that parallel many of the features of childhood asthma. RSV causes significant damage to the respiratory tract epithelium, and epithelial necrosis results in decreased effectiveness of the mucociliary elevator, allowing mucus, inflammatory cells, and plasma exudate to accumulate within the airway lumen. This combination of epithelial damage and resultant airway obstruction can lead to clinical manifestations of asthma. Several long-term prospective studies have shown that as many as 40% of children hospitalized for documented RSV will continue to wheeze or have asthma in later childhood.

In contrast, there is a growing body of literature to suggest that recurrent infections in childhood, especially parasitic, may protect against the development of asthma. This is the basis of the so-called "Hygiene Hypothesis". This was first proposed by Strachan in 1989 when he demonstrated an inverse relationship between birth order in families and prevalence of hay fever and proposed that infections in early infancy, brought home by older siblings, might prevent sensitization. Conversely, lack of early childhood exposure to infectious agents and parasites increases susceptibility to allergic diseases by modulating immune system development. Clearly, there is biological credibility to this hypothesis in that infection will tend to induce a T-lymphocyte helper 1 (Th1) response, promoting the production of interleukin-2 (IL-2) and interferon gamma. These in turn would downregulate the Th2 response associated with allergy, where a different set of mediators (IL-4, IL-5, IL-10, and IL-13) is generated. This hypothesis has been supported by a number of studies. In Germany, the higher pollution levels in East Germany were associated with an increased frequency of respiratory infections and consequently with less allergy. In Japan, an inverse relationship was found between tuberculin responsiveness and allergy. It is intriguing to postulate that this is one reason behind the relatively low asthma prevalence in India. Almost 50–70% of young Indian adults would be tuberculin skin test-positive and this might help to explain the lower asthma prevalence discussed in the section on epidemiology. Similar inverse relationships have been found between allergy and parasitic infections, measles, and hepatitis A infections in childhood. Tuberculosis, measles, and parasitic and viral infections are all more common in the tropics providing an explanation for the global differences in the epidemiology of asthma observed in the ISAAC study. As a corollary to the hygiene hypothesis, so-called helminthic therapy using *Trichuris suis* ova and *Necator americanus* larvae has been tried in a number of immunological disorders including Crohn's disease, ulcerative colitis, multiple sclerosis, and asthma. *Thus, the essence of the hygiene hypothesis is that modern living is associated with too little microbial stimulation early in life. This lack of stimulation of the immune system leads to deficient downregulation of immune responses to the ubiquitous allergens that the individual encounters early in life.*

Pollution

It has become fashionable for the media to blame outdoor pollutants as the cause for increasing asthma and related atopic disorders. While various pollutants can incite asthma, there is no evidence to support the assertion that they induce the disease. Indeed, the study by Von Mutius showed clearly that asthma was less prevalent in polluted East German cities than in cleaner West German cities. Whether this difference was due to pollution or to some other aspect of lifestyle or indoor environment has however not yet been established. A study we conducted in Mumbai tried to correlate the levels of SO_2, NO_2, NH_3, and suspended particulate matter (SPM) with asthma hospitalizations over a period of 3 years in two large private hospitals in different parts of Mumbai. We found no significant correlation between adult asthma hospitalizations and the level of any of these pollutants over the 3 years under study. Thus as this study demonstrates, no simplistic conclusions can be drawn about the exact role of pollution in asthma; the field is a complex one and further, larger, nationwide studies are needed with a prospective birth cohort design to track individual patient exposure to different pollutants more accurately. Such studies would be incredibly expensive and complex to do but would clarify the intriguing link between asthma and outdoor pollution.

Air Pollution and Asthma Epidemics

The relation of ambient air pollution and epidemics of asthma is exemplified by the asthma epidemics of Barcelona in the 1980s. Doctors were struck by clusters of mid-day emergency room (ER) visits for asthma occurring in hospitals located around the docks. Clever epidemiological detective work implicated the unloading of soya beans in the harbor as the cause; affected patients being more likely to be allergic to soya bean. Pollen counts were discounted as a likely cause because levels were not unusually high at these times. NO_2 and SO_2 levels were highest on the days of the epidemics suggesting a possible synergistic role of air pollution. Soya beans have also been implicated in similar epidemics in New Orleans. Discrete asthma epidemics linked to thunderstorms have also been described in London, Birmingham, and Melbourne. Subjects admitted during these epidemics were largely atopic and the levels of air pollution were not exceptional. It is postulated that the dispersal of pollen grains due to aqueous contact after the thunderstorm may release allergens that are small and potent enough to enter the airways and initiate an attack of asthma.

Obesity

Cross-sectional and case-controlled epidemiological studies have shown a modest correlation between obesity and adult asthma prevalence, with relative risk or ORs ranging from 1.0 to 3.0. Some studies show that this effect may be especially pronounced in women. One of the largest studies in the field looked at 86,000 women participating in the Nurses' Health Study, and found that over a 4-year follow-up, the odds of developing asthma were 2.7 times higher in obese (BMI > 30 kg/m^2) than normal weight women. While obesity does not directly cause airway obstruction, it is biologically plausible that it may contribute to airway inflammation. Indeed, obese asthma may be a unique phenotype of asthma, characterized by lack of eosinophilic inflammation, decreased lung volumes, greater symptoms for a given degree of lung function impairment, and poor asthma control. Besides, obesity may induce a state of relative glucocorticoid resistance, which may lead to obese asthmatics responding suboptimally to asthma medications. Weight loss has been shown to improve asthma control and the obese asthmatic should be encouraged and helped to lose weight.

Nutrients

Westernization is characterized by profound changes in dietary habits, so it is conceivable that dietary factors may have caused changes in asthma prevalence. The factors implicated include—increased salt intake, increased consumption of vegetable oil (margarine), decreased consumption of antioxidants, and bottle-feeding practices. None have been confirmed as yet and none explain sibship size and birth order effect, but they remain intriguing hypotheses.

Exercise

Exercise is a potent stimulus to asthma. EIA is particularly common in children and it is estimated that at least 10–12% of school children have EIA. EIA is also commonly seen in professional athletes. A survey of athletes for the 1996 Atlanta Olympics found that 16% of athletes had a history or medication use compatible with EIA. The incidence of EIA varies depending on the sport. The highest rates of EIA are found in winter sports, where 35% of ice skaters, and as many as 40% of cross-country skiers had EIA. Two different hypotheses have been raised regarding the mechanism of EIA. The hyperosmolarity theory states that water loss occurs from the airway surface liquid of the airways during the hyperventilation of exercise. This water loss leads to the release of mediators that cause bronchoconstriction. The other theory is the airway rewarming theory, which states that the hyperventilation of exercise leads to cooling of the airways. After the exercise is complete, there is rewarming of the airway because of dilatation of the small bronchiolar vessels that surround the bronchial tree. This influx of warm blood into these vessels leads to congested vessels, fluid exudation in the submucosa, and mediator

release with consequent bronchospasm. Cross-country skiers have the highest rates of EIA because they exercise over prolonged periods and hyperventilate in cold air. A study of 40 elite cross-country skiers showed that this group of athletes had evidence of a high incidence of airway inflammation and even airway remodeling in bronchial biopsies.

Rhinosinusitis

Several studies dating back to the 1920s have identified rhinosinusitis as a trigger for asthma. A study by Bresciani showed that 100% of severe asthmatics and 88% of patients with mild or moderate asthma will have evidence of sinusitis on computed tomography (CT) scan studies. The verdict is still not out on whether this relationship is causal or an epiphenomenon, i.e. asthma and sinusitis manifestations of the same disease process. Numerous reports do suggest that medical or surgical treatment of rhinosinusitis does undoubtedly improve coexisting asthma. This suggests that rhinosinusitis may have a role as a trigger of asthma. Proposed mechanisms for a causal relationship between the two conditions include nasopharyngiobronchial reflexes, which may be vagal nerve mediated, drip or drainage of inflammatory cells, and mediators from the sinus into the lungs, and local upper respiratory inflammation leading to pulmonary inflammation. Thus the clinician must consider the possible presence of rhinosinusitis in every asthmatic.

Gastroesophageal Reflux

The link between gastroesophageal reflux (GER) and asthma has been known since William Osler first stated that asthma attacks may be due to "reflex influences from the stomach". GER symptoms have since been shown to be extremely common in adults and children with asthma, with as many as 65% of consecutive asthmatics in one study having GER symptoms. More importantly, studies have shown asthma symptoms correlate with esophageal acid events on 24-hour esophageal pH testing. It is important to realize that GER may be clinically silent in asthmatics. Several studies have found abnormal esophageal pH tests in large numbers of "difficult asthmatics", even those without any obvious reflux symptoms. Compared with controls, asthmatics have more frequent reflux episodes and higher esophageal acid contact times. Studies using esophageal manometry conclude that approximately

50–80% of adults and children with asthma have GER. GER has also been linked to increased risk of hospitalizations due to asthma in a few studies. There are several reasons why asthmatics could be more prone to GER than the general population. These include increased pressure gradients between the thorax and abdomen, which tend to overcome the lower esophageal sphincter (LES). Neurogenic reflexes have also been implicated, with autonomic dysregulation and heightened vagal tone releasing more acid in the esophagus, which in turn triggers airway responses. Heightened bronchial reactivity and microaspiration are also postulated mechanisms. Finally, medications like theophylline, albuterol, and oral corticosteroids may all predispose to GER. Studies have shown that GER symptoms increase 170% at night and daytime reflux 24% with theophylline. Nebulized albuterol has been shown to produce a dose-dependent reduction in LES pressure from 17 mm Hg to 8 mm Hg and compromise the amplitude of the esophageal contractions 5 cm and 10 cm above the LES. Oral corticosteroids when given in a dose of 60 mg per day for 7 days have been shown to result in significant increases in esophageal acid contact time at both the proximal and distal esophageal pH probes.

If GER is a potential asthma trigger, then aggressive GER therapy should improve asthma symptoms. Field reviewed the combined results of 12 studies looking at the role of anti-reflux therapy in improving asthma symptoms and found that symptoms improved in 69% and medication could be reduced in 62%. Although pulmonary function did not improve, there was objective improvement in evening peak expiratory flow (PEF) rates in 26%. A more recent Cochrane review however failed to demonstrate an improvement in asthma symptoms. Most of the earlier studies used H_2 receptor antagonists and not the more potent proton-pump inhibitors currently available today. Hence, an important trial from Littner is worth quoting here. This was the only large multicenter, double-blind, placebo-controlled trial in the field and used the highly effective lansoprazole in a dose of 30 mg twice a day or oral placebo and found that treated asthmatics had fewer exacerbations and required significantly fewer oral steroid rescue courses than the controls. Surgical trials have also examined the role of surgery in asthmatics with GER. In a review by Field of 24 trials examining asthma outcomes after antireflux therapy, surgery improved GER variables in 90%, asthma symptoms in 79%, and asthma medication use in 80% of subjects. Pulmonary function improvement occurred in 27% of surgically treated patients.

Food Allergy and Additives

Several studies have shown that food allergy and egg allergy in particular in early infancy increases the risk of asthma developing in later life. Food allergy has also been documented as a risk factor for life-threatening asthma. A case control study found that patients with asthma and food allergy had an OR of 8.58 for life-threatening asthma. The foods known to induce this kind of violent asthmatic reaction include egg, milk, peanut, soy, fish, shellfish, and tree nuts. It must be clarified that food sensitivities causing asthma are rare. Studies where actual food challenge has been used suggest overall rates are no more than 2–5%. Food additives can also be implicated as triggers of asthma. The Food and Drug Administration (FDA) has listed more than 2,500 substances as food additives. Of these, only a few are known to be triggers of asthma. The best known of these are the sulfating agents, which include additives like sulfur dioxide, sodium sulfite, sodium and potassium bisulfite, and metabisulfites. These agents are used as preservatives and antioxidants. About 4% of a random sample of asthmatics will be shown to have sulfite allergy on specific sulfite challenge; however, the risk of reacting to sulfites may be highest in the more severe asthmatics. Tartrazine, a yellow dye, is another food additive known to be implicated in asthma. Other coloring agents are also implicated and it is best to advise asthmatics to avoid exposure to all such agents.

Occupational Triggers

Occupational factors have been implicated in almost 20% of asthmatics. Occupational asthma has been discussed in a separate section (*see* chapter on Common Occupational Lung Diseases).

Psychological Stress

Asthma has long been known to have a psychosomatic basis and is considered by some to be the prototype of a psychosomatic disease. Daily diary studies of patients with asthma have shown that life stressors are associated with lower PEF rates. That stressful life events increase the risk of onset of asthma comes from a large study of over 10,000 Finnish university students where stressful life events like death of a family member were shown to promote development of asthma. Rather than stress directly causing the asthma symptoms, it is thought that stress modulates the immune system to increase the magnitude of the airway inflammatory response to allergens. Difficult asthma has also been linked to stress and depression and several studies have shown the link.

Medications as Triggers of Asthma

A number of commonly used drugs have been implicated as triggers of asthma. Aspirin and other nonsteroidal anti-inflammatory drugs (NSAIDs) are the most commonly implicated agents. Aspirin-induced asthma will be discussed again later. Other important drugs known to worsen asthma include β-blockers, which are contraindicated in asthma and should never be used as they may trigger severe exacerbations. While selective β-blockers have been cleared as safe for use in mild asthmatics, we would recommend that it is wise to avoid these drugs completely. A meta-analysis of randomized, blinded, placebo-controlled trials that studied the effects of cardioselective β-blockers in patients with mild-to-moderate asthma showed that even a single dose of such a drug could reduce FEV1 by 7.5%, though this was not accompanied by a concomitant increase in symptoms. Long-term studies are needed to define the safety profile of cardioselective β-blockers in asthmatics.

Angiotensin-converting enzyme (ACE) inhibitors are well known to cause cough in as many as 10–20% of patients receiving them. Prior asthma is not a risk factor for developing this side effect. ACE inhibitors are thus generally safe in asthmatics though there have been stray reports of bronchoconstriction, asthma worsening, and bronchial hyperreactivity following the use of these drugs in asthmatics. An analysis of the side effects to this group of drugs in the New Zealand Adverse Effects Registry showed that cough accounted for 86% of the 596 adverse respiratory events but bronchospasm and dyspnea occurred in 8% of patients on this drug. Based on this data and case reports, it can be concluded that these drugs are safe but the physician must be aware of their potential to occasionally trigger asthma.

■ PATHOGENESIS OF ASTHMA

Asthma is an inflammatory disorder of the airways, which involves several inflammatory mediators that result in distinct pathophysiological changes. The inflammation, which is a hallmark of asthma, leads to airway hyperre-sponsiveness and asthma symptoms. The major cells and the mediators involved in the asthma process will be discussed here.

Mediators of Asthma and their Cellular Origin

A complex cascade of mediators is involved in the pathogenesis of asthma. These mediators produce their effects by activating specific cell surface mediators resulting in a complex cascade of signaling events. In this section, we will discuss the cells in the bronchial mucosa central to the asthmatic response and the mediators they release.

Cells

Mast cells: Mast cells uniquely populate all vascularized tissue including the upper and lower respiratory tracts. While the role of mast cells in allergic reactions is unequivocal, their precise role in asthma remains controversial. It was believed earlier that mast cells and the mediators they released (histamine, leukotrienes, and prostaglandins) played a central role in the pathogenesis of asthma. Recent evidence argues against the critical involvement of these cells in bronchial hyperreactivity or in the continuing inflammation of asthmatic airways. Mast cell stabilizers like disodium cromoglycate were clinically ineffective and more potent newer mast cell stabilizers have had little or no impact in asthma. β-agonists, which are also potent stabilizers of human mast cells, fail to inhibit late asthmatic responses following allergen challenge or to reduce BHR.

Macrophages: Macrophages are present throughout the respiratory tract and may be activated by IgE-dependent mechanisms. They are characterized by their capacity to synthesize large quantities of a broad array of mediators. These include thromboxane, prostaglandins, leukotriene C, platelet-activating factor (PAF), chemokines, and cytokines, including IL-1, IL-6, TNF, and granulocyte macrophage colony-stimulating factor (GM-CSF), which plays a central role in eosinophil survival and function and regulation of antigen presentation. Macrophages have the capacity to synthesize both pro- and anti-inflammatory cytokines depending on the nature of the stimulus. Inhaled corticosteroids alter the balance of these pro- and anti-inflammatory cytokines in asthma increasing IL-10 production by the alveolar macrophages.

Eosinophils: Eosinophilic infiltration is a prominent feature of asthmatic airways. It is the eosinophil that is found in large numbers in BAL fluid at the time of a late reaction following allergen inhalation. Eosinophils release a variety of membrane-derived mediators including leukotriene C, PAF, and granulocyte-associated proteins such as eosinophilic cationic protein, which are toxic to the airway epithelium. Activated eosinophils in the airway lumen may thus lead to the epithelial damage that characterizes asthma. Eosinophils also synthesize chemokines such as IL-8, MI-1a (macrophage inflammatory problem), and RANTES (regulated upon activation, normal T-cell expressed and secreted) and MCP-1 (monocyte chemoattractant protein), which are inhibited by glucocorticosteroids.

Neutrophils: The role of the neutrophil in human asthma is unclear. In acute severe asthma, high numbers of neutrophils and increased amounts of neutrophil chemoattractant and IL-8 have been described.

T-lymphocytes: T-lymphocytes are also prominent cells in asthmatic airways. They release a variety of lymphokines, which perpetuate allergic inflammatory responses. Thus, for example, IL-3 is important in differentiating mast cells, IL-4 critical for β-cell activation, and IL-5 for maintaining eosinophil survival in tissues.

Inflammatory Mediators

An array of different mediators has been implicated in the pathogenesis of asthma. These account for many of the pathological features of the disease. The important mediators will be discussed in this section.

Histamine: Histamine is released from mast cells and contributes to bronchoconstriction and the inflammatory response.

Chemokines: Chemokines are important in the recruitment of inflammatory cells into the airways and are mainly expressed in airway epithelial cells. Eotaxin is selective for eosinophils; whereas, thymus and activating regulated chemokines (TARC) and macrophage-derived chemokines (MDC) recruit Th2 cells.

Leukotrienes: Leukotrienes are potent bronchoconstrictors and proinflammatory mediators mainly derived from mast cells and eosinophils.

Cytokines: Cytokines orchestrate and amplify the inflammatory response and determine its severity. Keen cytokines include—IL-1β, TNF-α, and GM-CSF. The Th2-derived cytokines include IL-5, IL-4, and IL-13.

Nitric oxide: Nitric oxide (NO) is a potent vasodilator produced from the action of inducible nitric oxide synthase in airway epithelial cells. Exhaled NO is increasingly being used to monitor the effectiveness of asthma treatment as will be discussed in the section on monitoring of asthma.

Prostaglandin D_2: Prostaglandin D_2 is a bronchoconstrictor derived predominantly from mast cells. It is involved in Th2 cell recruitment to the airways.

■ STRUCTURAL CHANGES IN AIRWAYS/ AIRWAY REMODELING

In addition to the inflammatory response, a number of structural changes take place in asthmatic airways over time. These are referred to as airway remodeling. Airway remodeling is defined as an alteration in size, mass, or number of tissue structural components that occur during growth or in response to injury or inflammation. These changes represent repair in response to chronic inflammation and may result in irreversible narrowing of the airways. These structural changes are seen in all asthmatics from an early stage. The remodeling theory is important as it offers crucial insights into the permanent biochemical and pathological alterations of asthmatic patients that have been clinically observed for long. It challenges the assumption that asthma is a reversible disease and explains the accelerated decline in FEV1 seen in some asthmatics.

Pathological Features of Lung Remodeling (Fig. 2)

Airway Thickening

Reticular basement membrane thickening (RBM) is a characteristic feature of asthma not being found in chronic obstructive pulmonary disease (COPD). Collagen Types I, III, V, and fibronectin all contribute to this thickening. The magnitude of deposition has been found to correlate with asthma severity. Thickening of the RBM is an early change being observed in biopsy samples even before the onset of symptoms.

Extracellular Matrix Changes

Deposition of proteoglycans and overexpression of glycosaminoglycan (GAG) hyaluronan have also been

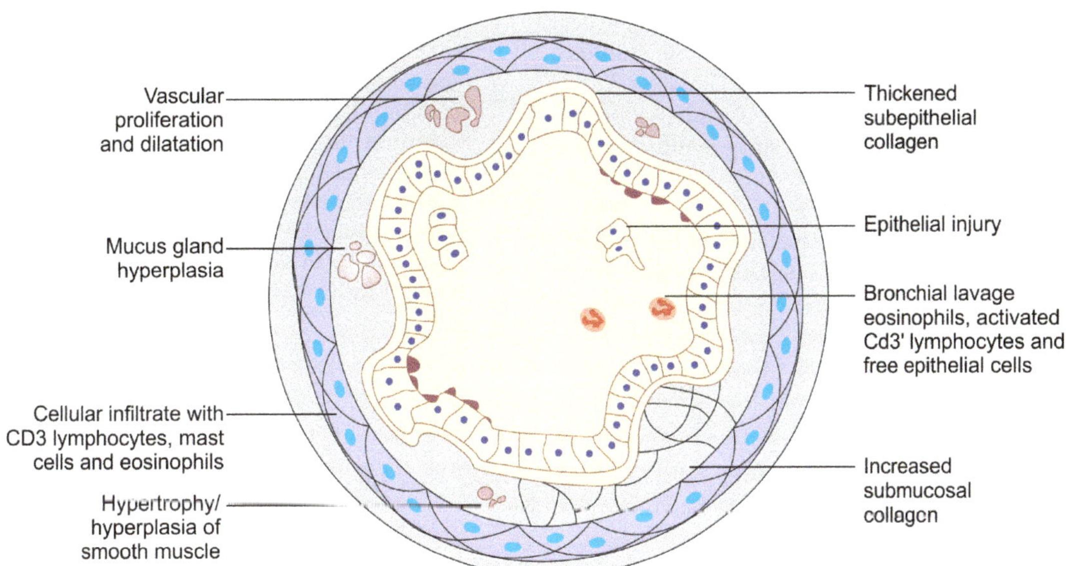

Fig. 2: The features of airway remodeling in asthma.

noted and it is conceivable that airway geometry and subsequently function and dynamics could be affected by this process.

Myocyte Changes

Myocyte hypertrophy and hyperplasia have been linked to asthma remodeling. Several studies show the area of the smooth muscle in the airways increases by as much as 50–230% in fatal cases of asthma and by 25–150% in nonfatal cases. Steroid therapy may have a role in reducing the number of submucosal myofibroblasts.

Mucus Gland Changes

Changes in the subepithelial mucus glands also contribute to airway remodeling. Mucus gland area is increased in subjects with fatal asthma and airway occlusion and plugging secondary to increased mucus production has been a feature noted in several autopsy studies of severe asthma.

Cartilage Changes

Increase in total cartilage area and structural changes like perichondrial degeneration and fibrosis are changes that have been observed in the remodeled airway.

Vascular Changes

Changes in airway vasculature are an important component of remodeling. Vascular congestion, dilatation of vessels and even neovascularization are important components of vascular remodeling. Patients who have fatal asthma also have a marked increase in vessel number and diameter. These changes in vessels contribute to airway wall thickening and increased resistance.

Changes in Enervation

Recent evidence suggests a loss of nerves containing the potent bronchodilator vasoactive intestinal peptide and an increase in nerves containing the bronchospastic agent substance P.

■ SUGGESTED READING

1. Aggarwal AN, Chaudhry K, Chhabra SK, et al. Prevalence and risk factors for bronchial asthma in Indian adults: a multicenter study. Indian J Chest Dis Allied Sci. 2006;48(1):13-22.
2. Chowgule RV, Shetye VM, Parmar JR, et al. Prevalence of respiratory symptoms, bronchial hyperreactivity, and asthma in a megacity. Am J Respir Crit Care Med. 1998;158:547-54.

3. Gibson PG, Henry HL, Coughlan JL. Gastroesophageal reflux treatment for asthma in adults and children. Cochrane Database Syst Rev. 2003;2:CDOO1496.
4. Jindal SK, Aggarwal AN, Gupta D, et al. Indian Study on Epidemiology of Asthma, Respiratory Symptoms and Chronic Bronchitis in adults (INSEARCH). Int J Tuber Lung Dis. 2012;16(9):1270-7.
5. Leung R, Ho P. Asthma, allergy and atopy in three southeast Asian populations. Thorax. 1994;49:1205-10.
6. Singh RB. Asthma in India: applying science to reality. Clin Resp Allergy. 2004;34(5):686-8.
7. The International Study of Asthma and Allergies in Childhood (ISAAC) Steering Committee. Worldwide variations in the prevalence of asthma symptoms: the International Study of Asthma and Allergies in Childhood (ISAAC). Eur Respir J. 1998;12:315-35.
8. Vishwanathan R, Prasad M, Thakur S, et al. Epidemiology of asthma in an urban population; a random morbidity survey. J Indian Med Assoc. 1966;46(9):480-3.

CHAPTER 33

Asthma: Clinical Features and Diagnosis

CLINICAL FEATURES

The classic symptoms of asthma include the triad of cough, dyspnea, and wheeze. These symptoms occur in combination, but on occasion, may occur in isolation. In its classic form, asthma is easy to recognize for both patient and doctor. However, none of these symptoms in isolation or even in combination are specific for asthma, and on occasion the physician may be caught out. Because of the intermittent and nonspecific nature of the symptoms, asthma may remain undiagnosed by both the patient and physician.

Cough

Cough may be the sole manifestation of asthma, in which case it is known as cough-variant asthma. Asthmatic cough is often quite distinctive. It is usually dry, intermittent, has diurnal variation often being significantly worse at night, and may be triggered by talking, laughing or exercise. When accompanied by wheeze, it is easy to diagnose. However, cough is often the sole symptom of asthma and in this setting a high index of suspicion is needed. A history of intermittent seasonal cough or prolonged cough which persists more than a few weeks following a viral upper respiratory tract infection (URTI) (bronchial hyperactivity) is also suggestive of asthma, especially in a young patient with a history of rhinitis or other allergies.

Dyspnea

Dyspnea is another cardinal symptom of asthma but may be absent in milder cases. It may be triggered only after exertion in some younger asthmatics with exercise-induced asthma. It can worsen to extreme levels in asthmatics during acute exacerbations of asthma. In chronic asthma, as in chronic obstructive pulmonary disease (COPD), the breathlessness may be constantly present and worsen with even trivial exertion and activities.

Wheeze

Wheeze is the sine qua non of asthma. The old axiom that all that wheezes is not asthma must of course never be forgotten. Other causes of wheeze are described in **Table 1** and some of these will be discussed in the section on differential diagnosis.

PHYSICAL EXAMINATION

Because of the intermittent nature of asthma, it must be stressed that physical examination may be completely normal at the time the patient is examined, and in this setting, a history based on the symptoms listed earlier is often sufficient to diagnose asthma. Wheeze is the most prominent abnormal physical finding. Wheezes are continuous adventitious lung sounds that can be heard in several diseases including asthma and COPD. The American Thoracic Society (ATS) defines wheezes as high-pitched continuous sounds with a dominant frequency of 400 Hz or more. The mechanism of wheeze production was first compared to a toy trumpet whose sound is produced by a vibrating reed. The pitch of the wheeze is dependent on the mass and elasticity of the airway walls and on the flow velocity. A more current model of wheeze production is based on the mathematical analysis of the stability of airflow through a collapsible tube. According to this model, the fluttering of the airway walls and fluid together, induced by a critical airflow velocity, produces

Table 1: Clinical conditions associated with wheeze.

- Asthma
- Chronic obstructive pulmonary disease
- Pulmonary edema
- Infections such as croup, whooping cough, laryngitis, and acute tracheobronchitis
- Tracheomalacia (laryngeal, tracheal or bronchial)
- Tracheal and large airway stenosis; tumor obstructing large airway
- Interstitial lung diseases especially hypersensitivity pneumonitis and sarcoidosis
- Bronchorreal states: bronchiectasis, cystic fibrosis
- Foreign body aspiration
- Vocal cord dysfunction or laryngeal spasm
- Forced expiration in normal subjects

wheeze. Most wheezes have spectrum peaks with frequencies below 2 kHz, mean frequency between 200 Hz and 800 Hz and probably occur when airflow in large central airways exceeds a critical velocity. Wheezing can appear monophasic, denoting a single note, or polyphonic. Wheezes are often audible at the patient's open mouth or by direct auscultation over the trachea. The clinical value of tracheal auscultation in asthma is well-recognized, and the trachea is superior to the lung for detection of wheeze in most asthmatics.

Paradoxically, of all the variables used to measure the severity of asthma, wheeze is the least sensitive. Occasionally, wheeze may be absent even in the face of severe airflow limitation, as occurs during a severe exacerbation. Godfrey found that only 70% of patients with severe airflow obstruction and the forced expiratory volume in one second (FEV_1) less than 1 L wheeze. The so-called "silent chest" in an asthmatic portends a severe attack that may well end fatally unless promptly recognized and treated.

■ CLINICAL FEATURES OF ACUTE SEVERE ASTHMA

Onset

An acute asthma attack is frightening for patient and physician. The onset is often dramatic, for example, in the atopic patient who is exposed to high concentrations of a provocating allergen, or in the patient markedly sensitive to aspirin. Such a patient may have a catastrophically sudden attack with extreme chest tightness and inability to breathe. More often though, the acute attack may have been building up over several days or even weeks, before

the patient is hospitalized. A study by Bellany revealed that 50% of patients dying of asthma in hospital had been waking up for 5 nights a week in the week prior to their death, and as many as 35% had been waking up that often in the previous month. Clearly an intensification of treatment at that stage, for example, with a short course of steroids, might have prevented the fatal attack.

History

A history of wheeze at night, bad enough to wake the patient from his sleep, must be elicited. Worsening of exertional dyspnea and increasing requirement of inhaled beta-agonists with diminishing relief after each puff are also pointers to a severe attack.

Examination Findings

The patient with an acute severe attack is distressed and able to speak in short sentences only. He gasps for breath, each breath being an audible struggle, often accompanied by a loud wheeze and sometimes by uncontrollable coughing. He is unable to lie flat and always prefers to adopt the sitting position, often bolt upright and leaning forward as he struggles to breathe. A respiratory rate of more than 30/min is a bad prognostic sign. On auscultation of the chest, most patients have loud, widespread, inspiratory and expiratory rhonchi but the occasional patient with severe asthma has a silent chest with hardly any audible breath sounds or rhonchi. A silent chest is another grave prognostic sign and denotes obstruction so severe that there is hardly any airflow. Accessory muscles of respiration are in active use as the patient struggles to overcome the airways' obstruction by sternocleidomastoid contraction and intercostal retraction. Cyanosis may be difficult to detect but when present denotes a severe and dangerous attack. Tachycardia is always present and may be worsened by the medication the patient has taken. A tachycardia more than 110/min denotes a severe attack. The presence of a significant pulsus paradoxus has been shown to reflect lung hyperinflation combined with wide fluctuations in intrathoracic pressure, and when more than 15 mm Hg reflects a severe attack. The features of a severe attack of asthma are given in **Table 2**.

■ DIAGNOSIS OF ASTHMA

The diagnosis of asthma is usually based on the presence of characteristic symptoms. However, because the

Table 2: Features of a severe attack of asthma.

- Inability to complete sentence in one breath
- Obtunded or altered conscious level
- Respiratory rate >30/min
- Silent chest
- Cyanosis
- Respiratory muscle fatigue; apneic spells
- Tachycardia >110/min
- Systolic paradox >15 mm Hg
- Peak expiratory flow <30% of predicted or known best
- PaO_2 <60 mm Hg despite supplemental oxygen at 60% FiO_2
- $PaCO_2$ which is normal or high and rising

symptoms may be nonspecific, and because patients with asthma (especially when the asthma is longstanding) may often have poor recognition of these symptoms, and poor perception of their severity, measurement of lung function abnormalities greatly enhances diagnostic confidence. The following measures of asthma are used in clinical practice.

Peak Expiratory Flow

This is a simple, universally available, and cheap way to diagnose asthma and assess its severity. Just as blood pressure cannot be measured and treated without recourse to sphygmomanometry, it is unwise to attempt to manage asthma without peak flow recordings. Modern peak flow meters, by virtue of their being light and portable, are ideally adapted for use by the patient in home settings for objective recording of the day to day variations that are the hallmark of asthma. Careful instructions must be given to the patient in order to maximize the accuracy of peak expiratory flow (PEF) recordings. PEF is effort-dependent hence the patient must be urged to put maximal effort into the peak flow maneuver. PEF also shows diurnal variation hence the time the peak flow is measured is crucial and must be recorded. Ideally, patients should be instructed to measure their peak flows in the morning soon after waking when the values will be close to the lowest and at night before retiring when they will be higher. Dips in peak flow are the differences between highest and lowest peak flows occurring on a diurnal basis and are a reflection of how well the asthma has been controlled. One method of describing diurnal PEF variability is by noting the amplitude, i.e. the difference in the maximal and minimal peak flows of the day, expressed as a percentage of the mean daily peak flow value and averaged over 1–2 weeks. Another method

of describing PEF variability, and one that is considered the best index lability in clinical practice, is the minimum morning pre-bronchodilator PEF over 1 week, expressed as a percentage of the recent best (min/max). This measure, which involves only a single daily reading and a simple calculation, correlates better than any other index with airway hyperresponsiveness.

Limitations of Peak Expiratory Flow

Apart from the effort-dependent nature of the test, it must be realized that PEF can underestimate the severity of asthma, especially as airflow limitation and gas trapping worsen. It must also be mentioned that PEF is not interchangeable with other measures of airflow limitation like FEV_1. Another inherent problem with PEF is that the values of PEF obtained with different peak flow meters vary considerably. Finally, the range of predicted values is wide and PEF measurements must be correlated with the patient's previously recorded best (when asymptomatic or optimally treated) to more meaningfully assess the severity of his asthma at that point in time.

Utility of Peak Expiratory Flow

In a patient whose history is typical of asthma but who is normal when seen by the physician, the suspicion of asthma can most easily be confirmed by giving the patient a peak flow meter to record PEF at home and demonstrate diurnal variations. In nocturnal asthma, a patient is instructed to record his or her PEF when he wakes up with asthma-like symptoms. PEF readings also have a vital role to play in diagnosing occupational asthma and demonstrating environmental triggers in the patient's workplace. Finally, integral to good asthma management is giving each patient with asthma a written plan with instructions on how to escalate asthma medications based on PEF readings at home.

Spirometry

This is the recommended method of measuring airflow limitation. It involves using a spirometer to perform measurements of FEV_1 and forced vital capacity (FVC). Asthma is characterized by a low FEV_1 and a low $FEV_1/$ FVC ratio. After the baseline measurement has been made, reversibility to two puffs of inhaled beta-2 agonist must be documented. An improvement of more than 12% and more than 200 mL from the pre-bronchodilator value is diagnostic of asthma. The main advantage of spirometric FEV_1 is that it is easy to perform, requires relatively inexpensive equipment, and is reproducible. It must be remembered though that spirometry has many drawbacks as well. It is not as universally available as peak flow meters and is also to some extent effort-dependent. It requires the patient to first take a full inspiration, which some breathless asthmatic patients may be unable to do without coughing. Although most of the flow expired in the first second of the FVC is effort-independent, the initial part of the FVC is effort-dependent and this might slightly affect FEV_1. Hence, detailed instructions need to be given by a trained technician and the highest value of three recordings must be recorded. As with other measurements of airway resistance, the FEV_1 is relatively insensitive to obstruction of the peripheral airways. As ethnic differences in spirometric values have been demonstrated, normal values must have been clearly demonstrated for the population studied. Norms for Indians (in Mumbai) have been established by Udwadia et al. and it is recommended that these be used in our population as they vary considerably from Caucasian values. Normal ranges are also wider and less reliable in younger patients (<20 years) and in the elderly (age >70) *[Ref: Udwadia FE, Sunavala JD, Shetye VM, et al. The maximal expiratory flow-volume curve in normal subjects in India. Chest. 1986;89(6):852-6].*

Measuring Airway Hyperresponsiveness

Airway responsiveness is a term used to describe the ability of the airways to narrow after exposure to constrictor agents. Often a patient with a history consistent with asthma will have normal spirometry when he or she is examined and in this setting, measures of airway responsiveness to direct airway challenges such as inhaled histamine or methacholine or indirect challenges with inhaled mannitol or exercise challenge may help establish the diagnosis of asthma. These tests of bronchial hyperresponsiveness are sensitive for diagnosis of asthma but not specific as they have been reported to be positive in patients with atopic rhinitis, bronchiectasis, cystic fibrosis, and even COPD.

Methods of Measuring Airway Responsiveness

The original method used was inhalation of an aerosolized pharmacological agent in an aerosol generated by a Wright nebulizer inhaled by tidal breathing for 2 minutes. Currently, aerosol is generated by a DeVilbiss 646 nebulizer attached to a Rosenthal French dosimeter and inhaled by five inspiratory capacity breaths.

Factors Affecting the Results

A number of technical factors affect the response including nebulizer output, particle size and speed, and volume of inhalation. If the patient is on medication that controls bronchial hyperreactivity, it will also affect the results and hence beta-agonists and anticholinergic agents must be withdrawn for at least 8 hours and long-acting beta-agonists (LABAs) and anti-histaminics at least 48–72 hours prior to the test. Recent viral infections and ozone may also worsen airway hyperresponsiveness. Therefore in research settings, the test should not be performed within 6 weeks of exposure to these stimuli.

Choice of Bronchoconstrictor Agent

Histamine and methacholine are the two agents used and airway responsiveness to both agents correlates well. Whilst histamine is more easily available, it may result in systemic side-effects like flushing, tachycardia, and headache in high concentration. Another problem with histamine is that tachyphylaxis may be observed following repeated challenges. These side-effects are not noted with methacholine, which is therefore the agent of choice.

Measurement of Response

The response is most commonly measured by assessing the fall in FEV_1 or increase in airway resistance following inhalation of the agent at different concentrations.

Expressing the Results

The usual way of expressing the result is to determine the provocative concentration (PC) of the agent that causes a predetermined drop in FEV_1 from the baseline (usually 20%). This is expressed as PC20 FEV_1.

Measuring Allergic Status

Most patients with asthma have a background of atopy. This can be established by checking the patient's Immunoglobulin E (IgE) levels or performing skin tests to house dust and other allergens. A limitation of these tests is that a positive test does not establish that the disease is allergic in nature or that it is causing asthma, as some individuals have specific IgE antibodies without any symptoms and they may not be causally related.

NONINVASIVE MARKERS OF AIRWAY INFLAMMATION

As asthma is currently considered to be an inflammatory disorder of the airways, it seems logical to include an assessment of this inflammation in the diagnosis and follow-up of this disease. A number of biomarkers in the blood, urine, sputum, exhaled air, and breath condensate have been studied. These are tabulated in **Table 3** and a short account of exhaled nitric oxide (eNO), the most promising biomarker, is given here.

Exhaled Nitric Oxide

Exhaled NO is the most extensively investigated of all the gases present in exhaled air. Over the last decade, measurement of fractional concentration of nitric oxide in exhaled breath (FeNO) has moved from being a research tool to a clinically useful aide to the respiratory physician involved with the management of the asthmatic. It can now be measured easily, quickly, non-invasively and reproducibly in an office setting. The techniques and equipment have evolved and have become simpler and well standardized so estimation of FeNO is now a routine test like spirometry **(Fig. 1)** in most modern PFT laboratories. The cut off points for a significantly raised FeNO in Indian patients remain to be elucidated.

The ways in which FeNO can be useful in different asthma settings are outlined here:

- *FeNO as an inflammatory marker:* Several studies over the years have shown the relationship and correlation between FeNO and other markers of airway inflammation in asthma including sputum, BAL and bronchial biopsy eosinophilia. There is also a strong correlation between FeNO and airway hyperresponsiveness (AHR) to methacholine and an interesting study found that a FeNO above 37 ppb in patients with allergic rhinitis helps identify which of these patients were at risk of developing asthma. A study in infants with recurrent lower respiratory tract "infections" showed that elevated FeNO in infancy predicted which ones go on to develop school-age asthma.
- *FeNO and asthma phenotypes:* Amongst all the inflammatory phenotypes in asthma the eosinophilic phenotype correlates best with elevated FeNO. Even in patients with severe, refractory asthma, FeNO levels were higher in patients with an eosinophilic phenotype. In the EXTRA study looking at which biomarkers predicted response to Omalizumab, FeNO emerged as an important biomarker.
- *FeNO in asthma diagnosis and control:* Whilst reference levels in normal and asthmatic children and adults are still being evaluated, there is little doubt that FeNO can be very useful in differentiating asthma from other diseases, with high sensitivity and specificity. In patients with undiagnosed respiratory symptoms, a FeNO of 26 ppb is the optimum cut-off point for

Table 3: Noninvasive markers of airway inflammation.

- Blood/Serum:
    - Eosinophils
    - Eosinophilic cationic protein (ECP)
    - Eosinophil peroxidase (EPO)
- Urine:
    - Leukotriene E4 (LTE4)
    - 9a, 11p-PGF2
- Induced sputum:
    - Cell differential
    - Soluble mediators (ECP, cysteinyl leukotriene)
- Exhaled air:
    - Nitric oxide
    - Carbon monoxide
    - Hydrocarbons
- Breath condensate:
    - Hydrogen peroxide
    - Leukotriene metabolites
    - 8-isoprostane
    - Nitrotyrosine

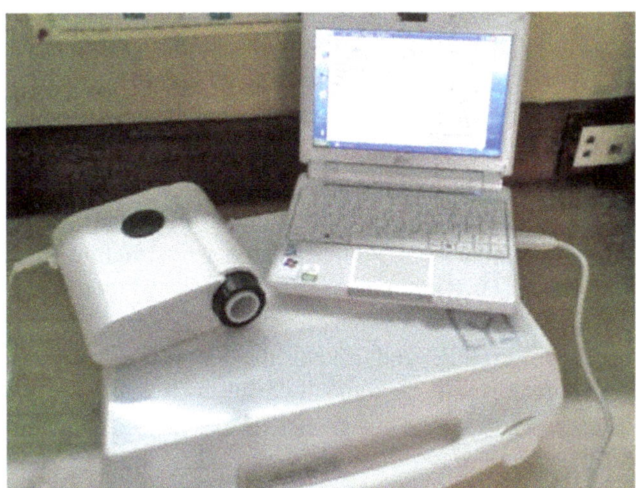

Fig. 1: Exhaled nitric oxide apparatus.

significant (3%) sputum eosinophilia. In addition to initial diagnosis, several studies show that FeNO levels increase further when asthma control worsens or during an acute exacerbation. Conversely FeNO levels improve during inhaled or oral corticosteroid therapy, even before improvements in symptoms or spirometry. Thus, FeNO is a sensitive predictor of asthma control. The ATS guidelines suggest that a FeNO < 25 ppb in adults and < 20 ppb in children is a strong indicator of likely ICS responsiveness.

- *FeNO in asthma management:* Randomized trials designed to assess whether asthma outcomes are improved using regular FeNO measurements as the basis for adjusting the ICS dose have failed to show clinically relevant benefits. Having said that, in the individual difficult asthma patient there is no doubting the clinical utility of making these measurements. Generally speaking, FeNO is highly predictive of ICS response at a cut off point of 33 ppb.

Thus, as this section outlines, FeNO is currently the sole, easily applicable noninvasive biomarker able to help in the diagnosis and management of asthma, more specifically of corticosteroid-sensitive airway inflammation in asthma.

■ DIFFERENTIAL DIAGNOSIS

Whilst the typical asthma attack is easy to diagnose there are a number of asthma mimics that must be mentioned here.

Chronic Obstructive Pulmonary Disease

While the distinction of late-onset asthma from COPD is generally straightforward, on occasion, the difference between these conditions may be difficult. Thus, it is easy to distinguish one from another when the asthmatic is a young atopic subject who has never smoked and has intermittent wheeze and variable reversible airflow limitation. But distinguishing asthma from COPD is much more difficult in a patient whose airway obstruction starts at the age of 60, has smoked in the past for a few years, also has a history of atopy when he was younger, and presents with chronic cough and fixed airflow limitation.

There are many obvious similarities between these two diseases. Both are chronic diseases characterized by airflow obstruction and both are characterized by inflammatory components. In asthma whilst the inflammation is in response to an inhaled allergen and chiefly involves the eosinophil, in COPD the inflammation is secondary to noxious particles in cigarette smoke and is primarily neutrophilic. Despite the obvious differences between these two diseases, including the natural history, the bronchodilator response and the corticosteroid response, actual distinction between the two may be difficult. In a study by Bellia of 128 confirmed asthmatics, 20% were wrongly misdiagnosed as asthma with diagnostic errors especially common in the elderly. Thus, one out of five elderly asthmatics may receive an incorrect label. The distinction is vital when many therapeutic choices exist. Apart from the wrong diagnosis, it is important to realize that there may be genuine overlap between these two diseases. In the NHAHES survey in the US, 17% of participants reported coexisting asthma and COPD and in the UK a study showed that 19% had more than one obstructive lung diagnosis. The coexistence of these two conditions in the same patient is associated not just with increased disease severity but also increased mortality. Finally, a subset of patients can start off as clearly asthmatic and evolve over the years into COPD. The Tucson epidemiological study of airway obstructive disease followed up 3,000 subjects over two decades and established that adult subjects with active asthma had a 12 times higher risk of acquiring COPD than subjects with no asthma even after adjusting for smoking. In another study from Copenhagen which followed up 228 asthmatics over 26 years, 16% had developed nonreversible airway obstruction with a quarter of patients having reduced transfer factor. The factors at initial enrolment that predicted subsequent development of irreversible airflow limitation included initial lower FEV_1 values, less bronchial hyperreactivity, and less reversibility to beta-agonists. Thus, the available literature suggests that around 10–15% of asthmatics will develop fixed airways obstruction. The chances increase if the asthmatic smokes and the asthma is poorly controlled over the initial years. Airway remodeling which has been discussed in an earlier section may help explain why some asthmatics evolve into COPD.

Distinguishing Asthma from COPD
Clinical Features

The important clinical differences between these two conditions are outlined in **Table 4**.

Having said this, the clinical distinction is seldom so cut and dry, and symptoms alone cannot reliably distinguish these two conditions.

Table 4: Clinical differences between asthma and chronic obstructive pulmonary disease (COPD).

	Asthma	*COPD*
Symptoms	Dyspnea episodic, cough dry	Dyspnea persistent and progressive, cough productive
	Wheeze	Breathless on exertion
Onset	Usually childhood	Usually >45 years
Course	Variable, remissions	Progressive
Smoking	Sometimes	Invariably
Bronchodilator response	Good	Poor
Response to steroids	Good	Poor

Spirometry

If the airflow limitation is reversible, this suggests asthma. Having said this, asthmatics may have fixed airflow limitation, especially those with severe or chronic asthma over many years duration and conversely one-third of patients with COPD may show significant (>12%) reversibility after inhaled beta-agonists.

Thus, both asthma and COPD have a spectrum of reversibility and reversibility alone cannot distinguish the two conditions.

Reversibility to Steroids

Reversibility to steroids is a defining feature of asthma but here too there are exceptions. Patients with steroid-resistant asthma will, by definition, be refractory to steroids. On the other hand, significant numbers of COPD patients will show a heartening response to inhaled and oral steroids.

Diffusion Capacity

Diffusion capacity is normal or increased in asthma while it is reduced in patients with COPD. It should be noted that it may also be reduced in smokers without airflow limitation.

Airway Hyperresponsiveness

Even airway hyperresponsiveness, long considered the hallmark of asthma, may be present in COPD and hence cannot reliably distinguish these conditions. A recent study showed that as many as 60% of patients with COPD had evidence of airway hyperresponsiveness with methacholine.

Airway Imaging

Airway imaging is not routinely recommended but high-resolution computed tomography (HRCT) scans can accurately distinguish asthma from emphysema.

Airway Inflammometry

Airway inflammometry is a research tool but can help distinguish these two conditions as well. Induced sputum in the two conditions shows important differences and exhaled NO is also high in asthma and generally normal in COPD.

Asthma-COPD Overlap Syndrome

One of the major changes in the new (2014) GINA Strategy report was the inclusion of a new chapter on the asthma-COPD overlap syndrome (ACOS). Since this report, there has been much published literature and an increased focus on ACOS as a distinct asthma / COPD phenotype. A significant proportion of patients with chronic airway disease are now recognized to have features of both asthma and COPD and meet the definition of ACOS. GINA defined ACOS as persistent airflow limitation with several features usually associated with asthma and several features usually associated with COPD. More recently Louie et al defined ACOS as one of the two clinical phenotypes: asthma with partially reversible airflow obstruction, with or without emphysema or reduced carbon monoxide diffusion capacity (DLCO) to less than 80% predicted, and COPD with emphysema accompanied by reversible or partially reversible airflow obstruction. Clinically, the usual equivalents of ACOS are the asthmatic with a history of smoking who develop non-fully reversible airway obstruction at an older age and/or the COPD patient with increased reversibility. It has been demonstrated that asthma, active smoking, and atopy interact in the development of fixed airflow obstruction. There is a synergy that affects atopic ever smokers with asthmatic patients who go develop COPD with particular inflammatory and clinical characteristics. These individuals share characteristics of both diseases making them difficult to be classified as asthma or COPD in clinical practice.

Epidemiology of ACOS: This condition is more widely prevalent than realized with different studies reporting prevalence rates that vary from 15–55% of patients with airway obstruction. ACOS is reported from countries across the globe: In the Wellington Respiratory Survey the estimated prevalence was 55.2%, in the PLATINO study from South America prevalence rates of 11.6% were reported, whilst in Spain a national consensus study established prevalence rates of 5–21% depending on the population studied. Asian data is limited but a study from Korea using the Korean National Health Insurance database found up to 54.5% of ACOS among COPD patients.

Diagnosing ACOS: In patients with COPD, increased reversibility is one of the pointers to ACOS. Bronchial hyper-responsiveness (BHR) is of course a hallmark of asthma, but BHR can also be demonstrated in up to two-thirds of COPD patients. Consequently some authors recommend the use of provocation tests to diagnose ACOS in patients with COPD. Another diagnostic feature of ACOS in COPD is the presence of sputum eosinophilia. Other potential plasma and sputum biomarkers to diagnose ACOS are being explored.

Importance of identifying ACOS: ACOS patients have more frequent exacerbation than those with COPD. They report more respiratory symptoms and have reduced physical activity and poorer quality of life than those with COPD or asthma alone. They consume, as a consequence, 2–6 fold more healthcare resources than those used by patients with asthma or COPD.

Treatment of ACOS: These patients have to date been systematically excluded from both asthma and COPD pharmacology trials for not being "pure" patients. As a consequence it is difficult to make firm recommendations. A single trial on the role of tiotropium in 472 ACOS patients showed it improved lung function and reduced exacerbations. Of more interest is that patients labeled COPD in the past but actually having ACOS are likely to do better with inhaled corticosteroids than those with COPD alone.

To conclude, the relevance of ACOS is to identify these patients early and commence them on a combination of bronchodilators and inhaled steroids to which they are likely to demonstrate a better response than patients with COPD alone. Clinical trials in this population are needed to evaluate their response to available treatments.

Cardiac Asthma

Cardiac asthma is another close mimic of asthma. Distinguishing one condition from the other may on occasions be difficult on clinical grounds alone. Along with a careful history, chest radiography, electrocardiography (ECG), and echocardiography may be useful in distinguishing cardiac asthma from bronchial asthma. Another useful and new test to help distinguish cardiac asthma from bronchial asthma is the B-type natriuretic peptide (BNP) assay. This helps detect the presence of heart failure, determine its severity, and estimate prognosis. It is a point of care test that is rapid, easy to perform, and relatively inexpensive. Results are available in no longer than 15 minutes from most laboratories. The main advantage of the BNP is its negative predictive value, which stands at around 96%. Thus, heart failure can be confidently ruled out when the BNP is normal (around 100 pg/mL). In a recent emergency room survey, doctors admitted to being unsure of the diagnosis of heart failure in 40% of encounters. The BNP was particularly useful in just these settings with a normal BNP ruling out cardiac failure and suggesting the dyspnea had to be secondary to another cause. The worse the heart failure, the higher the BNP levels and patients admitted with florid congestive cardiac failure (CCF) routinely have levels around 1,000 pg/mL. Serial BNP levels correlate with response to therapy and are thus of some prognostic value. Several studies have shown that patients whose BNP levels reduce in response to treatment in hospital have good outcomes whereas those whose hospital stay ends in death or readmission have rising or only minimal decreases in BNP. It must be noted that BNP levels are higher in older patients, women, patients with renal dysfunction, and those with sepsis. From a management point of view it is worth pointing out that if there is any doubt if the asthma is bronchial or cardiac, it is mandatory to avoid ephedrine and beta-blockers in any form. Other measures like beta-agonists, diuretics, and steroids help both conditions.

Vocal Cord Dysfunction

Vocal cord dysfunction is an important mimic of asthma that is discussed here. It occurs predominantly in women aged 20–40 years and seems more common in those in the medical or nursing profession. Many patients have true asthma coexisting as well, which makes the diagnosis even more difficult. During episodes of vocal cord dysfunction, the "wheeze" is in reality an inspiratory monophasic sound produced at the larynx. The distinction from asthma may be very difficult and some pointers to vocal cord dysfunction are that the sounds resolve with quiet breathing, the patient cannot phonate or cough during the attack, and that there is a normal alveolar arterial gradient during the attack. Other pointers are the absence of hyperinflation on chest radiography and a distinctive inspiratory cut-off on the inspiratory limb of the flow-volume loop. Direct laryngoscopy during an attack is the investigation of choice though this may be difficult to perform. If done, it shows that both vocal cords are in the midline, adducted position during inspiration. On occasion, this finding is only present when provoked after making the patient exercise on a treadmill. Acute attacks can be relieved by breathing an air-helium mixture called heliox. They are all diagnosed late, some even after multiple episodes of ventilator support. As a consequence most develop obesity due to prolonged corticosteroid therapy; iatrogenic Cushing's syndrome is common. These patients have a high incidence of psychiatric problems and hence treatment involves psychiatric help and counseling.

Obstruction to a Large Airway

Intrinsic obstruction produced by a tumor or stenosis or extrinsic obstruction of a large airway (as from a mediastinal mass or an aortic aneurysm) may, at first encounter, be mistaken for asthma. These patients have a monophonic wheeze (instead of the usual polyphonic wheezes heard on asthma). The flow-volume loop shows a clear flattening of the inspiratory limb of the loop. Other relevant investigations also clarify the diagnosis.

Constrictive Bronchiolitis

When idiopathic in origin also presents with cough, breathlessness, and wheeze. The HRCT findings (discussed in a separate chapter) should help to differentiate it from asthma.

■ SUGGESTED READING

1. Barrecheguren M, Esquinas C, Miravitlles M. The asthma-COPD overlap syndrome: opportunities and challenges. Curr Opin Pulm Med. 2015;21:74-9.
2. Berend N. Mechanisms of airway hyperresponsiveness in asthma. Respirology. 2008;13(5):624-31.
3. Ehrlich RI. Wheeze, asthma diagnosis and medication use: a national adult survey in a developing country. Thorax. 2005;60(11):895-901.
4. Field SK, Gelfand GAJ, McFadden SD. The effect of anti-reflux surgery on asthmatics with gastroesophageal reflux. Chest. 1999;116:766-74.
5. Jones SL, Kittelson J, Cowan JO, et al. The predictive value of exhaled nitric oxide measurements in assessing changes in asthma control. Am J Respir Crit Care Med. 2001;164:738-43.
6. King CS. Clinical asthma syndromes and important asthma mimics. Respir Care. 2008;53(5):568-80.
7. Littner MR, Ballard D, Huang B, et al. Twenty four weeks of lansoprazole reduces asthma exacerbations and improves asthma quality of life in subjects with symptoms of acid reflux. Eur Resir J. 2002;20:428.
8. Majid H, Kao C. Utility of exhaled nitric oxide in the diagnosis and management of asthma. Curr Opin Pulm Med. 2010;16(1):42-7.
9. Pollart SM. Overview of changes to asthma guidelines: diagnosis and screening. Am Fam Physician. 2009;79(9):761-7.
10. Ricciardolo F. Revisiting the role of exhaled nitric oxide in asthma. Curr Opin Pulm Med. 2014;20:53-9.
11. Salpeter SR, Ormiston TM, Salpeter EE. Cardioselective beta-blockers in patients with reactive airway disease: a meta-analysis. Ann Intern Med. 2002;137:715-25.
12. Slaughter MC. Not quite asthma: differential diagnosis of dyspnea, cough, and wheezing. Allergy Asthma Proc. 2007;28(3):271-81.
13. Tilles SA. Differential diagnosis of adult asthma. Med Clin North Am. 2006;90(1):61-76.

CHAPTER 34

Asthma: Management

■ ASTHMA MANAGEMENT

Global Initiative for Asthma (GINA) guidelines stress the importance of a six-part management plan. The components are:

1. *Educate patients to develop a partnership*: Education of an asthmatic is an ongoing continual process. It is sobering to note that several studies show that socioeconomic factors like poverty and ignorance are linked to poor asthma control and even asthma deaths. The process of education must include not just the patient but ideally his family as well. Education empowers the asthmatic to understand and manage his disease and helps to build up trust and a relationship between the patient and his healthcare provider. Education not only clarifies the nature of the disease and the medications that must be taken but also serves to teach the patient the correct inhaler technique, the importance of monitoring via a home peak flow meter and allays fears and doubts the patient may have regarding the safety and side effects of the drugs.

2. *Assess and monitor asthma severity*: This is achieved in a number of ways. Symptom reports are the easiest way for the patient to monitor his asthma severity. An asthmatic must be taught that frequent need for reliever medication, nocturnal awakening due to asthma and limitation of activity secondary to worsening asthma are all portends of poor control for which urgent action should be taken. Objective measures of control are based around the peak flow meter at home and every asthmatic must be encouraged to own and monitor his peak flows on an ongoing basis with a written treatment plan geared around changes in peak flow from baseline values. Peak expiratory flow (PEF) monitoring is especially useful in those with poor perception of symptoms. Monitoring in hospital includes spirometry, which is useful for initial assessment, to assess the severity of the airflow limitation and to assess response to therapy.

3. *Avoid exposure to risk factors*: The patient must be urged to avoid exposure to known triggers of asthma including allergens in the environment, food allergens, and additives and medications that can worsen asthma whenever possible. This avoidance should extend to even second-hand or passive tobacco smoke, vehicle emissions in polluted areas, and irritants in the workplace that may be adding an occupational dimension to the patient's asthma.

   It would seem intuitive that establishing a low-allergen environment in the asthmatic patient's home would help in the day-to-day management of his asthma. Although not easy to achieve, substantial reductions in allergen load can be achieved, with gratifying improvements in control, by adopting the measures outlined in **Table 1**.

4. *Establish medication plans for long-term asthma management*: This stepped care approach to asthma management will be dealt with in detail shortly.

5. Management of acute exacerbations.

6. *Provide regular follow-up*: Continual monitoring is essential to ensure that therapeutic goals are met. At each follow-up, an overview of the clinical parameters, a review of home peak flow records and a check of the risk factors and their avoidance, is made.

We will now discuss the following:

- Asthma medications and the long-term, outpatient-based pharmacological management of asthma.
- Management of acute exacerbations of asthma in hospital.

Table 1: Allergen avoidance in the home.

House dust mite reduction measures:
- Cover mattresses, pillows, and blankets in impermeable covers
- Plastic covers (feels uncomfortable)
- Water vapor permeable fabrics (mite guard)
- Wash all bedding at 55°C weekly (hot cycle of washing machine) as this is the temperature that kills mites
- Remove carpets or hoover them frequently
- Acaricides are chemicals that kill mites
- Minimize upholstered furniture, replace with leather
- Keep dust-accumulating objects in cupboards
- Replace curtains with blinds
- Hot wash/freeze stuffed toys
- Reduce humidity

Pet allergen avoidance:
- Get rid of pets
  If this is not possible:
- Keep pet out of bedroom
- Have the pet washed twice a week
- Cleaning the upholstered furniture the pet sits on
- HEPA filters in the main living areas and bedroom

Avoidance of cockroach allergens:
- Remove waste food
- Seal leaks
- Use of chemicals like diazinon, chlorpyrifos, and boric acid

(HEPA: High efficiency particulate air)

ASTHMA MEDICATIONS

Introduction

Medications to treat asthma can be classified into two broad categories—(1) controllers and (2) relievers. Controllers are medications designed to be taken long term to control asthma through their anti-inflammatory effects. Relievers are medicines used on an as needed basis to quickly relieve symptoms, primarily by their bronchodilator properties.

Routes of Administration

Asthma treatment can be administered by a variety of different routes—inhaled, oral, or parenteral (subcutaneous, intramuscular, and intravenous). What is unique about the therapy of asthma is that it is via the inhaled route that medications are primarily delivered to the patient. One of the biggest changes in asthma management in recent times has been the transition from oral to inhaled therapies as the preferred route of administration. The metered dose inhaler (MDI) was first developed in 1955 by Riker Laboratories. Prior to the advent of the MDI, asthma medication was delivered using a squeeze bulb nebulizer, which was fragile and

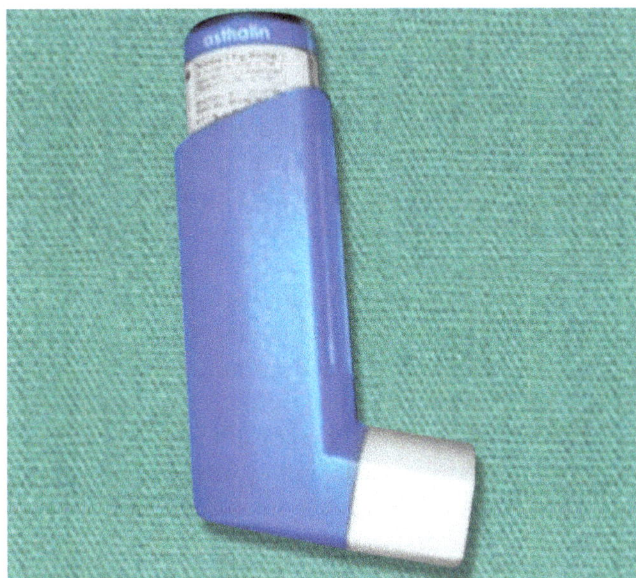

Fig. 1: Metered dose inhaler.

unreliable. The particles this crude device generated were too large for effective lung delivery. Two new technologies converged in the MDI: (1) the chlorofluorocarbon (CFC) propellant and (2) the Meshburg metering valve (originally designed for dispensing perfume). A modern MDI consists of three major components: (1) the canister where the drug formulation resides, (2) the metering valve, which ensures a metered quantity of the drug, is dispensed with each actuation, and (3) the actuator or mouthpiece, which allows the patient to operate the device. The propellant used to carry the active drug contained CFCs. These compounds while safe for the patient were proven to be damaging the earth's ozone layer, hence, CFC-containing inhalers are being phased out the world over and being replaced by CFC-free inhalers as per the Montreal Protocol signed by more than 160 countries including India. The new inhalers, which will use hydrofluoroalkane (HFA) technology, have replaced all CFC-containing inhalers by 2010. Pressurized MDIs are not the only route by which inhaled drugs are delivered to asthmatics **(Figs. 1 and 2)**.

Other inhaler devices include—breath-actuated inhalers (so called accuhalers and turbuhalers), dry powder inhalers (rotacaps and rotahalers), soft mist inhalers, and nebulized or wet aerosols. These different inhaler devices differ in their efficiency of drug delivery to the lower respiratory tract and the ease with which the device can be used by the majority of patients. Individual patient preference, convenience, and ease of use determine which inhaler device is the right one for a particular patient. A good physician is duty-bound to spend part of every consultation teaching and rechecking his patient's inhaler technique as large numbers of patients have very poor inhaler techniques despite using their inhalers (with the same poor technique) for years. The steps to be followed while using an inhaler are outlined in **Table 2**. Several studies worldwide have identified poor patient inhaler technique as a common and persistent problem. Up to 90% of adult patients have been reported to have inadequate inhaler technique with higher rates of errors in children and the elderly asthmatics. The majority of asthmatics using their inhalers do so too poorly to result in reliable drug delivery. Even healthcare professionals themselves are often not familiar with correct inhaler technique and use. In an oft-quoted study from Iran, of 173 healthcare workers (doctors and nurses) who had

their inhaler technique checked, only 7% performed all steps correctly **(Table 3)** *[Ref: Nadi E, Zerrati F. Evaluation of the metered dose inhaler technique among healthcare providers. Acta Medica Iranica. 2005;43(4):268-72].*

Drugs Used in Asthma

- *Controller medications*:
    - Inhaled corticosteroids (ICS)
    - Leukotriene modifiers
    - Long-acting inhaled β_2-agonists
    - Theophylline
    - Long-acting oral β_2-agonists
    - Immunotherapy and biological agents.
- *Reliever medications*:
    - Rapid-acting inhaled β_2-agonists
    - Systemic glucocorticosteroids
    - Anticholinergics
    - Theophylline
    - Short-acting oral β_2-agonists.

Inhaled Corticosteroids

Inhaled corticosteroids are currently the most potent anti-inflammatory drugs for the treatment of asthma. They have a number of positive effects in asthma, which have been outlined in **Table 4**.

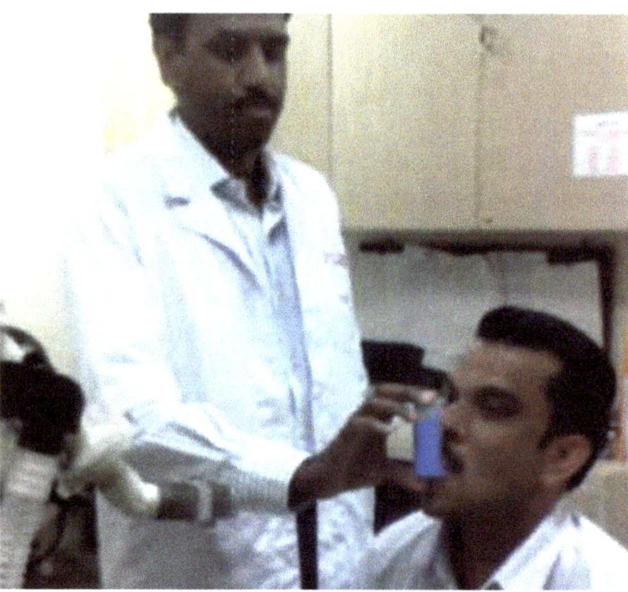

Fig. 2: Pulmonary function test (PFT) technician teaching a patient how to use a metered dose inhaler (MDI).

Table 3: Choice of inhaler device for children with asthma.

Age group	Devices used
Less than 5 years	• MDI + spacer with face mask • Nebulizer with face mask
5–8 years	• MDI + spacer with mouthpiece • Nebulizer with mouthpiece
More than 8 years	• Dry powder inhaler or breath activate inhaler or MDI with spacer and mouthpiece • Nebulizer with mouthpiece

(MDI: Metered dose inhaler)

Table 2: Steps in correct metered dose inhaler (MDI) technique.

1. Take the cap off the inhaler mouthpiece
2. Shake the inhaler
3. Hold the inhaler upright
4. Breathe out
5. Place the inhaler mouthpiece between the lips
6. Activate the inhaler while breathing in deeply and slowly
7. Continue to inhale until the lungs are full
8. Hold the breath for 5–10 seconds
9. Breathe out
10. Gargle immediately after use (while using an inhaled steroid)

Table 4: Effects of inhaled corticosteroid (ICS) in asthma.

- Controls symptoms
- Improves quality of life
- Decreases airway hyperresponsiveness
- Controls inflammation
- Reduces frequency and severity of exacerbations
- Reduces asthma mortality
- Prevents airway remodeling
- Possibly alters the natural history of asthma

What needs to be clarified to patients and their families is that though these drugs have an amazing impact on asthma as outlined in the Box, they do not cure asthma and within a few months of being discontinued, clinical control deteriorates in a significant proportion of patients.

Types of inhaled steroids: There are several generations of inhaled steroids available in the market. Although they differ in potency and bioavailability, because of relatively flat dose-response relationships in asthma, there is not much clinical difference among the different forms.

The different preparations of ICS available in India and their equipotent daily doses are summarized in **Table 5**.

Inhaled corticosteroids are remarkably effective in the vast majority of asthmatics at relatively low doses (equivalent of 400 µg of budesonide per day). However, there is a subset of severe asthmatics where much higher doses of ICS will be needed to achieve optimal control. There does seem to be a close relationship between the dose of ICS and the prevention of acute severe exacerbations. Higher doses of ICS are often required in smokers as cigarette smoke reduces the responsiveness to ICS.

Adverse effects of ICS: The most common side-effects of ICS are oropharyngeal candidiasis, dysphonia, and cough from upper airway irritation. These side effects are reduced, if the patient is instructed to gargle after each dose or advised use of a spacer device. Certain inhaled steroids like ciclesonide, which are activated in the lungs but not in the pharynx are less likely to induce these local side effects. When the dose of ICS crosses 400 µg of budesonide or its equivalent, certain systemic side effects may be noticed. These include—easy bruising, adrenal suppression, decreased bone mineral density (BMD), growth suppression in children, cataracts, and glaucoma. Certain ICS like ciclesonide, budesonide, and fluticasone at equipotent doses have less systemic side effects. It is sometimes difficult in disassociating the effects of high-dose ICS from the effect of the frequent courses of oral corticosteroids taken by patients with severe asthma. ICS do not increase the risk of pulmonary infections including tuberculosis. This is a misconception that is common in India where tuberculosis is endemic. It must be stressed that ICS can be safely used in patients with tuberculosis and are not contraindicated even in patients with active tuberculosis.

There has been ongoing debate on the effect of long-term use of ICS on the bone and on growth and these two important side effects which all asthmatics are concerned about will be put in perspective.

ICS and osteoporosis: There is little doubt that high doses of ICS taken over the years can lead to osteoporosis. In a regression analysis, the lumbar BMD Z-score decreased by 0.5 SD for each 1 mg increment in the daily dose of inhaled steroid, with most patients (71%) taking inhaled budesonide for more than 10 years. An increased risk of hip fracture in patients taking inhaled corticosteroids (dose-dependent) was also noted in a large cross-sectional study in the United Kingdom, with an odds ratio (OR) of 1.19 (after adjusting for use of oral corticosteroids). An almost linear relationship in OR was noted; with the lowest risk at less than 200 µg/day (OR 1.1), to an OR of 1.5 for patients taking 800–1,600 µg/day, to a further exponential risk for those taking more than 1,600 µg/day (OR of 2). In Canada, a similar case-controlled study found that the risk of hip or upper limb fracture increased significantly, by 12%, for each 1,000 µg/day over 1,000 µg dose of inhaled corticosteroid.

Thus, the risk of osteoporosis with high doses of ICS used over prolonged periods of time is real. Recommendations would include keeping the ICS dose to a minimum by using ICS—long-acting β-agonists (LABAs) combinations, and using calcium and bisphosphonate prophylaxis to prevent osteoporosis in vulnerable patients.

ICS and growth: There are three phases of normal childhood growth—(1) nutrition-dependent growth of infancy (the fastest growth phase), (2) the growth hormone-dependent linear second phase from infancy to prepuberty, and (3) the pubertal phase, which ends with epiphyseal growth plate maturation.

When used at the recommended dosages of 100–200 µg/day of beclomethasone dipropionate and HFA or

Table 5: Different inhaled corticosteroid (ICS) preparations available in India.

Drug	Low daily dose (µg)	High daily dose (µg)
Beclomethasone dipropionate	200–500	>1,000–2,000
Budesonide	200–400	>800–1,600
Fluticasone propionate	100–250	>500–1,000
Mometasone furoate	200–400	>800–1,200
Ciclesonide	80–160	>320–1,280

200–400 µg of beclomethasone dipropionate CFC (with volumetric spacer), no significant differences were found in growth velocities (5.27 vs 5.71 cm/year). Fluticasone, when used in doses up to 400 µg/day and ciclesonide up to 160 µg/day also did not seem to have significant effects on growth. Long-term studies with budesonide show a transient slowing of growth in the 1st year of use but no significant effect on final attained adult height. Factors that predisposed to a greater reduction in growth velocity were lower age and lower pretreatment heights. While most studies document slowing of growth in the early stages of long-term inhaled corticosteroid use, it is reassuring to note that when used in the recommended doses, children on inhaled corticosteroids will attain their anticipated height as adults.

Leukotriene Modifiers

The leukotriene modifiers include montelukast, pranlukast, and zafirlukast (which are cysteinyl-leukotriene 1 receptor antagonists) and zileuton (which is a 5-lipoxygenase inhibitor). The only preparation available in the Indian market is montelukast. A mounting body of evidence supports the use of these drugs as an alternative treatment in patients with mild persistent asthma. When used alone, they are weak drugs and as controllers are far less effective than even low doses of ICS. Studies attempting to substitute ICS with these drugs have confirmed that this approach risks a worsening in asthma control. Their optimal role is probably as an "add-on" therapy to ICS, in an attempt to reduce the dose of ICS in patients with moderate-to-severe asthma. Another role for these drugs is in the asthmatic who remains poorly controlled despite high doses of ICS. In this setting, they may help to improve asthma control, though less effectively than the addition of a LABA at this stage.

Side effects: These are well-tolerated drugs and few if any class-related side-effects have been reported. One of the leukotriene modifiers has been associated with liver toxicity. Monitoring of liver function is recommended when this drug is used. As discussed in the section on vasculitis, earlier fears of an association with Churg-Strauss syndrome have proved unfounded.

Long-acting β-agonists

The two drugs in this category are formoterol and salmeterol. Both provide a similar duration of bronchodilatation but formoterol has a more rapid onset of action than salmeterol, which may make it more suitable for symptom relief as well as symptom protection. These drugs must never be used as monotherapy, as they do not influence the inflammation that is the hallmark of poorly controlled asthma. They are most effective when combined with ICS and are the most effective add-on when a medium dose of ICS fails to achieve adequate asthma control. Indeed, in this situation, this is a preferred strategy to increasing the dose of ICS. Several studies have shown that this combination of LABA and ICS in medium doses results in better symptom control, improved lung function, decreased nocturnal attacks, and reduced exacerbations, than ICS alone. Given the synergy between these two groups of drugs, it is only natural that they be combined in fixed dose inhalers that deliver both drugs in standard doses. Several studies have shown that giving this therapy in combination is as effective as giving each drug separately. Thus, salmeterol and fluticasone are combined into inhalers at different concentrations of fluticasone, and formoterol and budesonide are similarly combined with different concentrations of budesonide varying from 100 µg/actuation to 400 µg/actuation. This is not only more convenient and cost-effective than giving each drug separately but also ensures that the LABA is always accompanied by ICS, thus increasing safety. The real concerns of LABAs triggering asthma deaths will be discussed separately. The combination of formoterol and budesonide has an additional advantage. It may be possible to use this single inhaler as both reliever and controller as part of the SMART strategy. This strategy advocates the use of a single inhaler (budesonide and formoterol in combination) for maintenance and reliever therapy in the treatment of asthma and has the advantage of being simple (one inhaler instead of two), and prevents LABA monotherapy. The strategy allows anti-inflammatory therapy to increase in line with disease activity when patients have symptoms. Indeed, some studies have shown that this strategy may provide patients with more sustained control than a fourfold increase in ICS alone.

However, the strategy does have the potential of exposing the patient to high doses of LABAs, albeit with concomitant ICS therapy, and vigilance is warranted in the use of this novel and promising solution to better asthma control. The maximum approved dosage per day with this approach (36 µg/day formoterol in adults and 18 µg/day in children below 12 years of age) needs to be emphasized and made clear to the patients when their asthma control strategy includes this single inhaler approach.

LABAs and the risk of sudden death:
- *An analysis of the controversy*: Inhaled β_2-agonists have been used for almost half a century in the treatment of asthma. Yet their use, especially of the long-acting formulations (LABAs), remains mired in controversy and the verdict on their benefit-to-risk ratio repeatedly questioned. This section attempts to understand the rationale for the debate on their use, and reviews the literature to answer questions raised by both clinicians and patients regarding their use.

Benefits: LABAs, when used with or without ICS, confer beneficial effects to patients with asthma. A Cochrane review that analyzed 85 randomized controlled trials using LABAs found statistically significant improvements in morning PEF rates, asthma symptoms, quality of life, and need for rescue medications when compared to placebo. When used in combination with ICS, there was a significant reduction in asthma exacerbations as well. Guidelines recommend their use in Step 3 or 4 in the management of asthma, i.e. stages associated with a poor level of control despite low-dose ICS.

Controversy: In the 1960s, an epidemic of asthma deaths was noticed in at least six countries including England and New Zealand. This epidemic coincided with the use of an aerosolized formulation of a high-dose β_2-agonist, isoprenaline—called "isoprenaline forte", and was noticed only in countries where this high-dose formulation, containing almost five times the standard dose, was used. In the 1970s, a second epidemic of asthma-related deaths took place in New Zealand, and this temporally coincided with and was attributed to the use of a new short-acting β_2-agonist fenoterol. The termination of this epidemic also coincided with the withdrawal of the drug from the market.

Salmeterol and formoterol, the two LABAs in current use were developed by GlaxoSmithKline (GSK) and Novartis, respectively, in the 1990s. With the apprehension created by the earlier epidemics of asthma mortality associated with β_2-agonists, the Serevent Nationwide Surveillance (SNS) trial was commissioned in the United Kingdom to analyze the safety of salmeterol; 25,189 asthma patients were randomized in a 2:1 ratio to receive either salmeterol 50 µg twice a day or albuterol 200 µg four times a day added to their existing asthma therapy for 16 weeks. The relative risk of death in the salmeterol group was three times that in the albuterol group, although this was not found to be statistically significant.

The largest and the most cited evidence against the use of LABAs comes from the Salmeterol Multicenter Asthma Research Trial (SMART), a study that was conducted as a consequence of the fears raised by the SNS trial. The study was launched in 1996, with the aim of recruiting 60,000 patients. The patients were randomized to receive either salmeterol 42 µg twice a day or placebo in addition to their regular asthma therapy for 28 weeks. In 2003, the study was prematurely terminated because an interim analysis revealed significantly higher rates of secondary outcomes (respiratory-related deaths, asthma-related deaths, and combined asthma-related life-threatening experiences) in those receiving salmeterol. Among the 26,355 subjects studied, adverse outcomes were mainly seen in African Americans, and in this cohort, those patients who were not taking ICS prior to randomization were found to be at greatest risk.

Postulated mechanism of increased mortality due to LABAs: Several hypotheses have been postulated to explain increased mortality due to LABAs.
- *Direct cardiotoxicity*: Direct cardiotoxicity due to overdosing and concurrent hypoxia. Overdosing with LABAs has been postulated to be a consequence of poorly controlled asthma with worsening symptoms. Tolerance to LABAs resulting from a combination of reduced receptor numbers secondary to receptor internalization and reduced production, along with uncoupling of receptors to downstream signaling pathways following repeated activation is also a possible reason why patients overdose on the drugs. Higher doses of LABAs, coupled with hypoxia have been shown in experimental models to be cardiotoxic, causing fatal cardiac depression and asystole. The reduction of peripheral vascular resistance leading to decreased diastolic blood pressure has also been hypothesized as being a contributory factor to death. Hypokalemia caused by these drugs can trigger ventricular tachyarrhythmias as well.
- *Genetic factors*: Genetic polymorphisms of amino acid 16 (arginine or glycine) of the β_2-adrenergic receptor play an important role in clinical response to β-agonists. African-Americans more commonly have the Arg/Arg 16 genotype, a genotype that confers an individual with an increased risk of adverse events with the use of LABAs. Prolonged QTc interval, an

adverse effect of β_2-agonists, has also been postulated to be seen more frequently in certain races.

- *Masking of inflammation*: A likely hypothesis is that the use of these bronchodilators may initially improve symptoms and thus might mask the underlying inflammation, which continues unchecked. It is possibly this worsening inflammation that predisposes these individuals to serious and life-threatening asthma exacerbations.

Current evidence: In a recent meta-analysis that included 215 studies with 106,575 subjects, it was concluded that the OR for risk of asthma mortality was 2.7. However, in the subset of patients not prescribed ICS, the OR was 7.3, while in the 63 studies in which subjects were randomized to receive the combination salmeterol/fluticasone or ICS, no mortality was reported among 22,600 patients. Recent Cochrane reviews analyzing the same question have come to a similar conclusion. A meeting convened by the US Food and Drug Administration to review the risks and benefits of inhaled LABAs for asthma concluded that for adults the benefits of combination inhalers outweighed the risks.

Thus, to conclude, the proven benefits of LABAs in the improvement of subjective and objective parameters of asthma control in patients with moderate-to-severe asthma, and their role in decreasing the need for higher doses of ICS make them valuable drugs in the management of the disease. However, caution needs to be exercised in prescribing them without adequately controlling the inflammation that is the hallmark of the disease. When used along with ICS, they have been found to be safe and effective and can be recommended for use.

Theophylline

Theophylline is traditionally recognized as a bronchodilator, but a growing body of evidence confirms that it also has modest anti-inflammatory properties. While it would not be expected to have any real effect as a first-line controller, it may be beneficial as add-on therapy in patients who are not controlled on ICS alone. Its advantages are that it is a cheap and widely available drug. The main drawback is its toxicity, which has been discussed in the section on acute asthma.

Systemic Glucocorticosteroids

While short bursts of oral steroids lasting for 2 weeks are often required by many asthmatics, a small fraction of asthmatics may only achieve acceptable control by the addition of a low-maintenance dose of oral steroid. If these drugs have to be administered on a long-term basis, attention must be paid to measures that minimize the systemic side effects.

Monoclonal Antibodies in Refractory Asthma (Table 6)

IgE Targeted Antibodies: Omalizumab

The realization that immunoglobulin E (IgE) is an important contributor to the pathogenesis of allergic asthma was the impetus for development of anti-IgE therapy in the form of omalizumab. Omalizumab is a humanized monoclonal antibody to IgE that binds free circulating IgE, thus preventing this molecule from binding to receptors on mast cells, basophils, and dendritic cells. Blocking the attachment of IgE also downregulates the expression of cell-bound IgE receptors. Omalizumab was the first biological agent to be approved for the clinical treatment of asthma and has been in clinical use since 2003. As clinical experience with Omalizumab grows, it is clear that this is an effective drug in some patients with severe asthma.

Table 6: Targeting monoclonal antibodies to individual patients based on Th2-cytokines endotypes.

Target	Biomarkers	Expected clinical benefits	Therapeutic limitations
IgE	+ve skin tests, elevated total IgE, Allergen specific IgE	Reduced exacerbations, decreased asthma symptoms, better QOL, reduced ER visits, improved lung function	Uncertain efficacy in steroid dependent asthma
IL-5	Peripheral blood and sputum eosinophilia, nasal polyposis	Reduced exacerbations, oral steroid reduction, reduced ER visits	Improvement BHR
IL-4/IL-13	Periostin, peripheral blood and sputum eosinophilia, IgE, FeNO	Improvement in FEV1, reduction in ICS dose	Reduction in exacerbations and steroid sparing effect not clearly demonstrated

Source: Modified from Hambly N Monoclonal antibodies for the treatment of refractory asthma. Curr Opin Pulm Med. 2014;20:87-94.

Randomized trials show that Omalizumab reduces not only the rate of exacerbations but also the severity and duration of those that do occur. Patients receiving Omalizumab experience significant improvements in asthma related symptoms, quality of life and lung function. Omalizumab also reduced emergency room visits, hospital admissions and the requirement of both inhaled steroids and rescue bronchodilators. Omalizumab's safety and efficacy in children has also been established, a recent study showing it especially useful in children sensitized to cockroach and dust mite allergen. In the real world setting, Omalizumab is usually reserved as add-on therapy in the treatment of severe refractory allergic asthma. This was specifically evaluated in the EXTRA (Exploring the Effects of Xolair in Allergic Asthma) study. Over 48 weeks, those patients treats with Omalizumab experienced a 25% relative risk reduction in asthma exacerbations, an increase in time to first exacerbation, and improved quality of life. A recent Cochrane review confirmed these results.

The response rate to Omalizumab is variable and difficult to predict. The search is on for biomarkers that will identify responders. A post-hoc analysis of the EXTRA study identified FeNO, peripheral blood eosinophilia, serum periostin as potentially useful biomarkers.

The drug has a good safety profile with a publication reviewing the course of almost 40,000 patients from phase 3 clinical trials and post marketing studies finding anaphylaxis rates of only 0.09%. Earlier reports of small increases in malignancy and lymphoma rates have also proved unfounded, there being no difference in cancer incidence between Omalizumab treated individuals and the general public.

The main disadvantage in the Indian context is the high cost of a course of Omalizumab and the fact that each dose needs to be given under medical supervision.

IL-5 Targeted Antibodies: Mepolizumab

Interleukin-5 (IL-5) is a major cytokines associated with eosinophil recruitment to the airway. Mepolizumab is a humanized monoclonal antibody to IL-5, which provides directed therapy in patients with severe eosinophilic asthma. These patients are characterized by severe exacerbations, progressive corticosteroid hyporesponsiveness, and sputum and blood eosinophilia. Two back to back randomized, double blind, placebo controlled, parallel-group studies published in the same issue of the New England Journal of Medicine established the important role of this drug. The first by Haldar and colleagues in the UK used the drug over 1 year in 61 patients with refractory eosinophilia asthma and recurrent severe exacerbations and demonstrated that its use resulted in significantly fewer exacerbations (by 43%) coupled with reductions in blood and sputum eosinophilia. The second study from Nair and colleagues in Ontario echoed these results. These patients all had severe asthma with persistent sputum eosinophilia despite treatment with oral prednisolone and high dose ICS. Over the 26 weeks of the study, these patients significantly reduced their risk of exacerbations and their dose of oral prednisolone. More recently, the DREAM study evaluated the role of Mepolizumab in 621 patients with severe, exacerbation prone, eosinophilia asthma and found that over 1 year, Mepolizumab significantly reduced the number of exacerbations needing oral corticosteroids by approximately 50%. Mepolizumab was well tolerated in all studies and no neutralizing antibodies were detected.

Reslizumab: An alternative humanized IL-5 inhibitor has also been evaluated, and when given over 15 weeks reduced exacerbations and improved lung function. The benefits of this drug were greatest in those patients with concomitant nasal polyposis.

Interestingly, though serum and sputum eosinophils drop sharply in the presence of monoclonal antibodies to IL-5, bronchial biopsy specimens demonstrate persistent eosinophilic infiltration. This obstacle can be overcome by benralizumab a humanized afucosylated monoclonal antibody that specifically binds the human IL-5 receptor alpha subunit on the target cell. Afucosylation confers enhanced antibody-dependent cellular cytotoxicity that results in highly efficient eosinophil depletion by apoptosis. This drug is better able to penetrate tissues because of its prolonged elimination half life, and it may therefore have better clinical efficacy than Mepolizumab or reslizumab.

Taken as a group, these studies demonstrate that these drugs have a major role in patients with eosinophilia airway inflammation and an eosinophilic phenotype.

IL-4/IL-13 Targeted Antibodies

With the success of anti-IL-5 therapy a large number of drugs targeted at Th2-driven airway inflammation have made their way to clinical trials. One of the more promising is pitrakinra a recombinant monoclonal IL-4 variant that targets both IL-4 and IL-13.

More recently, Wenzel evaluated dupilumab, a fully monoclonal antibody that also inhibited both IL-4 and IL-13 in 104 patients with moderately severe asthma and demonstrated an 87% reduction in asthma exacerbations. Patients receiving dupilumab had both improved lung function and asthma related symptoms differentiating it from anti-IL-5 therapy.

Lebrikizumab a molecule that specifically binds IL-13 may also significantly reduced asthma exacerbations. The Th2 serum biomarker periostin was found to predict a favorable response to lebrikizumab.

Macrolides: Macrolides are antibiotics that have anti-inflammatory and immunomodulatory effects in addition to their antibacterial effects. They have been shown to benefit patients with several neutrophilic airway diseases like cystic fibrosis, and their role in the neutrophilic phenotype of severe asthma is being explored. In the AZISAST study, low dose azithromycin given in a low dose of 250 mg thrice a week for 6 months was associated with a significantly lower rate of exacerbations in patients with severe noneosinophilic asthma. These results need to be confirmed in larger long-term RCTs and biomarkers that will identify the asthmatic with the neutrophilic phenotype need to be elucidated.

Reliever Medications: Rapid-acting Inhaled β_2-agonists

These agents are the drugs most used and abused by asthmatics across the globe. By virtue of the quick relief they provide, they are the preferred medication for relief of bronchospasm during exacerbations and are also used for prevention of exercise-induced asthma. The drugs included in this category are—salbutamol, terbutaline, fenoterol, levalbuterol, reproterol, and pirbuterol. Formoterol, a LABA with a rapid onset of action, is also approved for symptom relief but only when combined with a controller like budesonide as part of the SMART strategy discussed earlier.

It is important to stress that these drugs must only be used on an as-needed basis at the lowest dose and frequency required. Increased requirement and use of these drugs should send a clear signal to the patient and physician that the patient's asthma is suboptimally controlled and that control needs to be intensified.

The side effects encountered when these drugs are used in ever escalating doses include tachycardia, tremors, arrhythmia, and hypokalemia.

Anticholinergics

Anticholinergics include ipratropium bromide and oxitropium bromide. These drugs are less effective relievers in the acute setting than rapidly acting inhaled β_2-agonists but may have some additive effect. They are a viable alternative in the group of asthmatics who cannot tolerate inhaled β_2-agonists because of side effects.

The major side effects reported with these agents include dryness of the mouth and a bitter taste.

Theophylline and Oral β_2-agonists

Short-acting theophylline and oral β_2-agonists (salbutamol and terbutaline tablets and syrups) have some role in relieving asthma symptoms. For millions of Indians who cannot afford or have no access to inhalers, the reality is that these drugs, are often, by default, first-line and sometimes sadly, the sole treatment for their asthma.

■ ALTERNATIVE AND COMPLEMENTARY MEDICINES IN ASTHMA

Like in any other chronic disease for which there is no cure, there are a profusion of alternative therapies available to the asthmatic. Here, we shall only discuss those which have been subjected to the rigors of a clinical trial.

Yoga

Yoga embodies a form of therapy that could conceivably help the asthmatic. It incorporates breathing exercises (pranayama), a cardiovascular component, and relaxation techniques, all of which could be helpful. A recent study from Australia, in 2002, was the first to assess the effect of Sahaja yoga, an Indian system of medication based on ancient Yogic principles, in the setting of a controlled clinical trial. In this parallel-group, double-blind, and randomized controlled study, subjects were randomly allocated to the Sahaja yoga or control intervention groups. The Sahaja yoga group attended a 2-hour yoga session once a week for 4 months with assessments being undertaken at the conclusion of this period and then again 2 months later. The study concluded that the patients in the Sahaja yoga group had limited but definite subjective and objective improvement in some measures of their asthma control with improvement in bronchial hyperreactivity of 1.5 doubling doses and some improvement in aspects of the asthma quality of life score. This benefit was not sustained at the 2-month follow-up period, however. Another older study on the impact of Yoga on asthma showed that it helped lower anxiety and medication use.

Breathing Exercises

The use of breathing exercises in controlling asthma symptoms has been taught and promoted by the American Lung Association in their asthma education series. The type of breathing is "belly breathing" or diaphragmatic breathing. A more specific form of breathing therapy called the Buteyko breathing technique (BBT), which dates back to 1952, has also been found to be beneficial. Four published clinical trials and two abstracts have evaluated BBT and although all reported improvements in one or more outcome measures, results have not been consistent and a recent systematic review concluded that no reliable conclusion could be drawn about the benefit of breathing exercises in asthma.

Homeopathy

There have been six trials with a total of around 500 subjects, but a recent Cochrane review indicated that that there is no evidence that homeopathy is of benefit in asthma.

Hypnosis

Because asthma has a strong psychosomatic component, it would be expected that any form of relaxation therapy would have a positive impact. In keeping with this, a study in the *British Medical Journal* showed that hypnosis was effective in patients with mild asthma and a strong emotional component. In this study by Ewer, hypnosis resulted in an improvement in symptoms coupled with a reduction in medicine requirement and improved bronchial hyperreactivity.

■ USING THE AVAILABLE DRUGS CORRECTLY: THE STEPPED CARE APPROACH

This involves assessing the patient's level of control each time he is seen and then stepping up or down the medications to maintain optimal control.

Assessing Control

Control is assessed from daytime symptoms, limitation of activities, nocturnal symptoms, need for reliever/rescue medication and home PEF and office spirometry. Using all of the above, any asthmatic can be classified into three broad categories of control—(1) well-controlled, (2) partly controlled, and (3) uncontrolled, as can be seen from **Table 7**.

Stepping up or down till Control is Achieved

An asthmatic, who remains uncontrolled on his or her current regimen, should have his treatment stepped up a level till control is achieved. Conversely, if control has been maintained for at least 3 months, treatment can be stepped down to establish the lowest dose that achieves good control.

The five steps listed in **Figure 3** provide options of increasing severity as attempts are made to achieve optimal control. In addition, at each step, GINA guidelines permit use of a short-acting β-agonist as a reliever for quick relief of symptoms. The frequent use of a reliever inhaler is of course one of the components of poor control

Table 7: Levels of asthma control.			
Characteristic	**Well controlled**	**Partly controlled**	**Uncontrolled**
Daytime symptoms	Very occasional; not more than once or at the most twice a week and short-lasting	Two to four times per week	More than four times a week
Full activity	Unrestricted	Slight limitation	Marked limitation
Nocturnal symptoms	None	May have many nocturnal symptoms	May have many nocturnal symptoms
Need for P2 agonist inhaler	Not more than twice a week	Three to five times per week	More than four to five times per week
PEFR	Normal	Normal except during an attack	Reduced, may be markedly so during an attack

(PEFR: Peak expiratory flow rate)

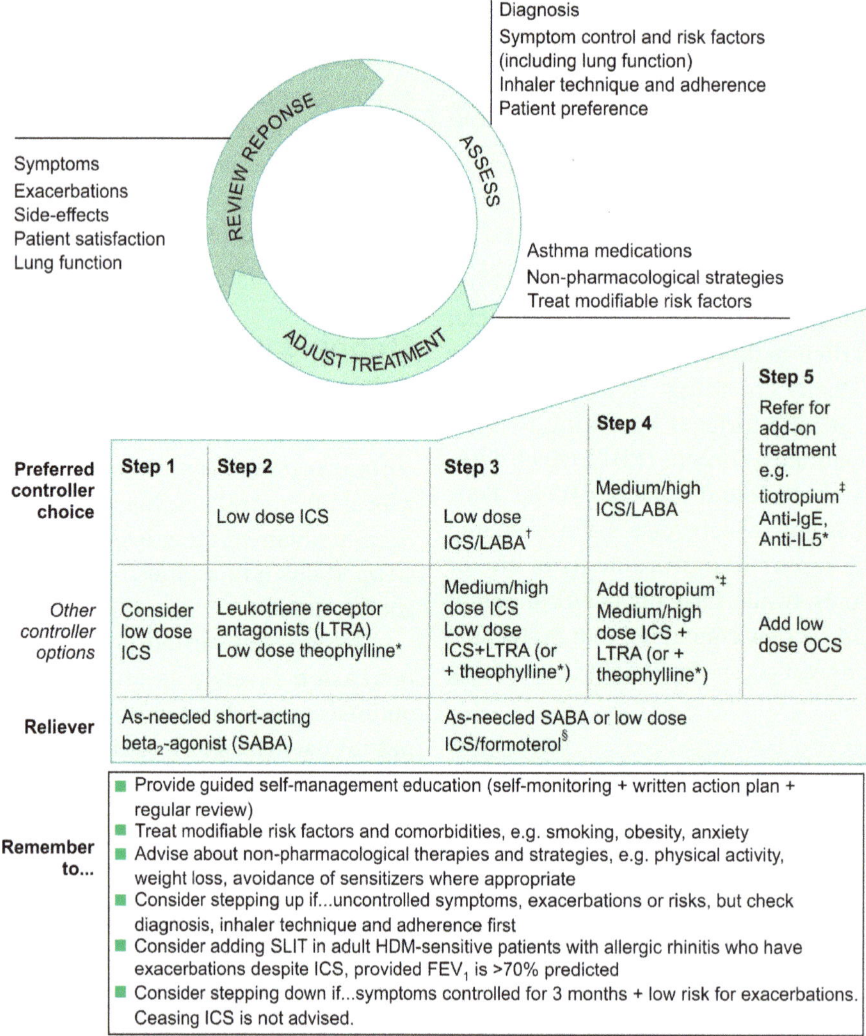

	Step 1	Step 2	Step 3	Step 4	Step 5
Preferred controller choice		Low dose ICS	Low dose ICS/LABA[†]	Medium/high ICS/LABA	Refer for add-on treatment e.g. tiotropium[‡] Anti-IgE, Anti-IL5*
Other controller options	Consider low dose ICS	Leukotriene receptor antagonists (LTRA) Low dose theophylline*	Medium/high dose ICS Low dose ICS+LTRA (or + theophylline*)	Add tiotropium*[‡] Medium/high dose ICS + LTRA (or + theophylline*)	Add low dose OCS
Reliever	As-neecled short-acting beta$_2$-agonist (SABA)		As-neecled SABA or low dose ICS/formoterol[§]		

Remember to...	■ Provide guided self-management education (self-monitoring + written action plan + regular review) ■ Treat modifiable risk factors and comorbidities, e.g. smoking, obesity, anxiety ■ Advise about non-pharmacological therapies and strategies, e.g. physical activity, weight loss, avoidance of sensitizers where appropriate ■ Consider stepping up if...uncontrolled symptoms, exacerbations or risks, but check diagnosis, inhaler technique and adherence first ■ Consider adding SLIT in adult HDM-sensitive patients with allergic rhinitis who have exacerbations despite ICS, provided FEV$_1$ is >70% predicted ■ Consider stepping down if...symptoms controlled for 3 months + low risk for exacerbations. Ceasing ICS is not advised.

* Not for children <12 years of age

† For children 6–11 years, the preferred step 3 treatment is medium dose ICS

‡ Tiotropium by mist inhaler is an add-on option for patients with a history of exacerbations; it is not indicated in childern <12 years

§ Low dose ICS/formoterol is the reliever medication for patients prescribed low dose budosonide/formoterol or low dose beclomethasone/formoterol maintenance and reliever therapy

Fig. 3: Management approach based on control.
(ICS: Inhaled corticosteroids; LABA: Long-acting β2-agonists; IgE: Immunoglobulin E; IL5: Interleukin 5; LTRA: Leukotriene receptor antagonists; SABA: Short-acting β2-agonists; SLIT: Sublingual immunotherapy; HDM: House dust mite).
Source: Reproduced with permission from Global Initiative for Asthma. (2009). Global Strategy for Asthma Management and Prevention, 2009. [online] Available from www.ginaasthma.org. [Accessed July, 2018].

and is clear indication that control needs to be increased a step.

Step 1: As-needed Reliever Medication

Treatment with as-needed short-acting β-agonist inhaler can be recommended only for the patient with mild intermittent asthma who is normal for long periods between episodes. The asthma must be of relatively mild severity and each episode of short duration (no more than a few hours). The patient and even the physician may underestimate the severity and hence if this strategy is to be followed, it is important to document that when the patient is asymptomatic and between episodes, he has normal lung function. In asthmatics intolerant to β-agonists an alternate though inferior approach is an inhaled anticholinergic or oral theophylline though these have a higher incidence of side effects and a slower onset of action. An as-needed β-agonist is also the standard treatment of exercise-induced asthma.

Step 2: Reliever plus Single Controller

This is the initial treatment for the vast majority of asthmatics with persistent symptoms. The controller of choice is low-dose ICS, which is recommended across all age groups as the initial treatment. Alternative but inferior choices are leukotriene modifiers, which are appropriate for patients who are unwilling to use ICS or those asthmatics with severe concomitant atopic rhinitis.

Step 3: Reliever plus One or Two Controllers

At Step 3, the recommended option is to combine a low dose of ICS with an inhaled long-acting β_2-agonist, either in a single combination inhaler or as two separate inhalers. If the combination inhaler chosen is the formoterol–budesonide combination, then this inhaler may double up for both maintenance and rescue because of rapid onset of action of formoterol. Whether this combination can be used with other combinations of inhaler and reliever requires further study.

Other Step 3 options are to increase to medium doses of ICS or add on a leukotriene mediator or oral theophylline.

Step 4: Reliever plus Two or More Controllers

The GINA guidelines recommend that patients at this step should ideally be referred to a specialist who will re-evaluate the reasons for their poor control thoroughly. The preferred treatment at this step is to combine medium or high-dose ICS with a LABA and in addition add on a leukotriene modifier and/or sustained-release oral theophylline. Unfortunately, in the majority of these difficult asthmatics, the change from medium to high doses of ICS provides only little additional benefit but is associated with some systemic side effects.

Step 5: Reliever plus Additional Controller Options

Options at this stage for the difficult-to-treat asthmatic include low maintenance doses of oral steroids, after careful analysis of their risk–benefit balance, or the addition of biologicals like omalizumab.

Scaling Down Treatment

Just as treatment is scaled up a step to improve control, the GINA guidelines also encourage deescalating a step once control is achieved. Such changes should be made by the doctor in conjunction with the patient, with the latter being made fully aware of the potential consequences, including worsening symptoms and an increased risk of exacerbations. Examples of this kind of "step down" include:

- When asthma is controlled with a combination of ICS and LABA, begin by reducing the dose of ICS by approximately 50% while continuing the LABA.
- If control remains, attempt to switch the combination to once daily dosing.
- An attempt could be made to stop the LABA and continue the low dose of ICS alone as monotherapy.
- Controller medicine can be stopped altogether, if the patient's asthma remains controlled on the lowest dose with no recurrence of symptoms for a year.

Asthma Phenotypes and Endotypes; a Personalized Approach to Asthma Management

Although most asthmatics can be managed with the standard conventional approach outlined above, a significant subset of asthmatics suffer from a disease that is more severe and more difficult to control. Such patients may benefit from a more personalized approach, and we are entering a new era in asthma management with the recognition of different and distinct phenotypic clusters with differences in disease onset, clinical features and response to ICS underscoring the clinical heterogeneity of asthma.

Indeed the very definition of asthma as a single disease characterized by chronic airway inflammation and airway remodeling is seen as simplistic and dated. Asthma is now seen as a multidimensional disease involving clinical, physiological and pathologic domains. Wenzel introduced the concept of the "asthma syndrome" indicating that patients with many different characteristics can be grouped under the umbrella term of asthma. The simple and traditional Th2 driven hypothesis, in which allergen combined with genetic susceptibility leads to a heightened Th2-immune response, fails to explain the heterogeneity of asthma. For example, Th-2 targeted treatments do not work in all asthmatics and a deeper understanding reveals that the core physiological abnormality is not always a result of eosinophilic (or Th-2 high) inflammation. The asthma syndrome is now known to be much more complex as would be expected in a disease state driven by over a hundred genes contributing to different asthma manifestations. The asthma syndrome umbrella is now known to include patients with both traditional allergic asthma (Th2 driven) and non-allergic (Th2 low) asthma.

Whilst phenotypes represent the outward manifestations of an individuals' genetics, they do not provide insight into the underlying disease process. Hence, the term "endotype" was proposed to indicate a subtype of the condition defined by a specific biological mechanism. The concept of asthma endotype has been refined further down to a molecular level using gene expression profiling of patient airway samples suggesting "molecular endotypes" of asthma exist as well. Such molecular studies suggest that within the same Th-2 endotype, using bronchial biopsies, different clusters of genes can be demonstrated, suggesting that different molecular endotypes exist.

To conclude this section, it is likely that in the future, stratification of asthma into phenotypes and endotypes will move the field forward in terms of more effective, individualized and personalized therapy for all asthmatics. As newer therapies for asthma become available, recognizing the considerable heterogeneity of this disease will be essential, so that drugs are targeted to the patient population most likely to benefit from them. The one size fit all approach of the last 3 or 4 decades is likely to give way to the personalized approach based on phenotypes and endotypes and driven by biomarkers.

Table 8 represents some of our current knowledge on asthma phenotypes and genotypes, the biomarkers that identify them, and the treatment options available based on this personalized approach.

■ HOSPITAL MANAGEMENT OF ACUTE SEVERE ASTHMA

Acute severe asthma is a medical emergency. Despite asthma being by definition a reversible disease, deaths from asthma continue to occur during severe attacks. Data from India are not available, but in the UK 2,000–4,000 people die of asthma every year with death rates on the incline in every age group, being around 4.5% per annum in the 5–34 year group. Fatal and near-fatal asthma will be discussed in a separate section while management of the hospitalized patient with severe asthma will be discussed here **(Table 9)**.

Oxygen

The majority of patients hospitalized for asthma have hypoxemia of varying degrees of severity at the time of admission. Death when it occurs during an acute asthma attack is almost always a consequence of hypoxemia. Oxygen should therefore be started as promptly as possible. Unlike in chronic obstructive pulmonary disease (COPD), there is little risk of suppression of ventilatory

Table 8: A personalized treatment algorithm for uncontrolled asthma.

Phenotypes	Endotypes	Biomarkers	Therapy
Eosinophilic	Aspirin-sensitive	Eosinophilia, urinary leukotrienes	5-Lipoxygenase inhibitor
Exacerbation prone	Allergic bronchopulmonary mycosis	High IgE, eosinophils, FeNO	Omalizumab, oral steroids, anti-fungal
Exercise induced	Severe late-onset hypereosinophilic	Blood, tissue eosinophilia	Oral steroids, mepolizumab
	Allergic asthma	+ve skin prick tests, high IgE, eosinophils, FeNO, Periostin	Omalizumab, steroids, dupilumab
Poorly steroid responsive			
Adult-onset obesity related	Noneosinophilic (neutrophilic asthma)	Sputum neutrophilia	Macrolides Bronchial thermoplasty
Fixed obstruction			

Source: Modified from Skloot G. Asthma phenotypes and endotypes: a personalized approach to treatment. Curr Opin Pulm Med. 2016;22:3-9.

Table 9: Management of acute asthma.

- *Oxygen*: High flow to maintain $SaO_2 > 95\%$
- *β_2-agonists*: Nebulized initial dose 5 mg salbutamol run continuously in severe attack or every 15 minutes. *MDI*: Initial dose 4–8 puffs. Can be repeated every 15 minutes up to three times
- *Anticholinergics*: Ipratropium bromide nebulized 0.5 mg every 15 minutes or continuously, if necessary. Can be mixed with P2 agonists. *MDI*: Initial dose 4–8 puffs every 15 minutes to be repeated three times
- *Corticosteroids*: Intravenous hydrocortisone 100–200 mg 8 hourly or oral prednisolone 40–60 mg/day
- *Aminophylline*: Loading dose 6 mg/kg in 20 mL of 5% dextrose IV over 20 minutes, subsequent infusion 0.6–0.9 mL/kg/hour via syringe pump
- *Adrenaline*: 0.6 mL of 1:1,000 solution subcutaneously, repeated to a maximum of 2 mL
- *Magnesium*: 2 grams IV
- *Intravenous β_2-agonists*: Salbutamol 4 μg/kg over 2–5 minutes and then as an infusion at 0.1–0.2 μg/kg/min
- *Mechanical ventilation*: When indicated

(IV: Intravenous; MDI: Metered dose inhaler; SaO_2: Oxygen saturation)

drive, hence oxygen should be given at high-flow rates to maintain oxygen saturation (SaO_2) more than 95%. The oxygen should be well-humidified to minimize bronchial irritation and drying of secretions. Since the main cause of hypoxemia in asthma is V/Q mismatch, inspired oxygen concentrations of 35–50% are usually adequate to reverse the hypoxemia. An oximeter is invaluable in detecting the improvement or deterioration in SaO_2 as the attack evolves, though a baseline arterial blood gas on admission is ideally recommended for every patient hospitalized with severe asthma.

Nebulized β-agonists

Nebulized β-agonists are the mainstay of treatment of acute severe asthma. They are the agents of first choice to relieve airflow obstruction in acute asthma. They provide more significant bronchodilatation with the most prompt relief, are cost-effective, and have fewer side effects than other agents. The method of delivery has been the topic of much recent discussion. By the time, a patient with severe asthma is hospitalized, and metered dose inhalers may be less effective because the hyperinflated asthmatic will be too breathless to effectively use his inhaler. These limitations can be overcome by the use of the compressor-driven nebulizer, where drug delivery is less dependent on a coordinated breathing pattern. Also, the more prolonged period of administration permits the delivery of a larger dose. If nebulizer facilities are unavailable, a spacer device may suffice. In a meta-analysis, it has been shown that this was at least equivalent to nebulized therapy. The initial dose of salbutamol or terbutaline is 5 mg diluted with 2–3 mL of normal saline. The dosing frequency can be titrated depending on the response. In severely ill patients, the nebulization can initially run continuously with the dose being topped up as soon as it is finished. Alternatively, it can be given hourly initially and then repeated every 2–4 hours, monitoring for excessive tachycardia. Theoretically, nebulizers driven by air can worsen hypoxemia, if they improve ventilation (by reducing bronchospasm) to a lung unit that is not being perfused. Hence, oxygen mains should ideally drive nebulizers, or, if driven by a compressor, the patient should simultaneously receive supplemental nasal oxygen. If a metered dose inhaler is being used via a spacer, the initial dose is 4–8 puffs of salbutamol, which can be repeated every 15–20 minutes up to three times. In severe disease, the dose can be increased by 1 puff every 30–60 seconds up to 20 puffs as needed. One advantage of the spacer over the nebulizer is that medication given this way can be administered and repeated very quickly (2 minutes versus 10–20 minutes for the wet nebulizer).

Corticosteroids

Corticosteroids have become first-line drugs in the management of asthma, and highlighting the recognition of the increased inflammation associated with such attacks. Every asthmatic sick enough to be hospitalized must promptly receive systemic steroid therapy. The use of steroids has been demonstrated in a large Cochrane meta-analysis to favorably affect the outcome of both admitted and discharged patients. What remains in doubt, however even after decades of use, are the optimum dose, route and frequency of administration, and the type of preparation used. The onset of action of corticosteroids has been historically felt to be slow and a number of recent studies have looked at high doses of inhaled steroids in the setting of an acute asthma attack. In a study by Rodrigo in patients presenting to the emergency department with acute severe asthma, the addition of high-dose inhaled steroid (flunisolide 1 mg every 10 minutes for 3 hours) to salbutamol led to greater bronchodilatation at 120, 150, and 180 minutes than salbutamol alone. In another important study, Harrison showed that orally administered steroids were equally effective even in severe asthma exacerbations, and provided the patient was not vomiting, were a cheaper and simpler option to intravenous therapy.

We would like to offer the following generalizations based on our personal experience when it comes to steroid therapy in acute severe asthma:

- Steroids must be administered early, ideally orally by the patient himself, as soon as his PEF drops less than 50% of his best level.
- In hospital, they should be administered as soon as the patient is first seen as they take around 6 hours to act. Available data suggests that a clear benefit from corticosteroids is unlikely to be noticed in the first 6 hours of administration and becomes evident only 6–12 hours after the initial dose.
- In the hospitalized asthmatic who does not have a very severe attack and who is not vomiting, oral prednisolone in a dose of 40–60 mg/day is as effective as intravenously administered steroids.
- Inhaled steroids may be continued concurrently with systemic steroids though their exact dose and route (spacer versus nebulizer) are unclear. A study by Rowe showed that the addition of inhaled budesonide (800 µg BID) to oral prednisolone in patients discharged from the emergency department led to a reduced relapse rate compared to prednisolone alone, with almost 50% reduction in the relapse rate in those on inhaled and oral steroids compared to those on oral steroids alone.
- In the critically ill asthmatic admitted to the intensive care unit (ICU), we would recommend hydrocortisone in a dose of 200 mg initially then repeated as 100–200 mg every 6–8 hours. Alternatively, methylprednisolone in a dose of 40–80 mg 6–8 hourly can be used.
- There is no evidence that giving much larger doses of steroids significantly speeds up or improves response. The temptation to use heroic doses of steroids must be resisted even when the initial response of the asthmatic seems slow. Indeed, there is a real risk of precipitating an acute steroid myopathy when large doses of steroids are used.
- Complications following a short-duration, moderate-dose course like the one outlined above appear to be minimal, even when continued over 7–14 days.

Anticholinergics

Ipratropium bromide, the anticholinergic agent most commonly used, has a slower onset of action (90–120 minutes vs 5–15 minutes) and produces less bronchodilatation than β_2-agonists. A number of large recent studies have examined the additive effect of the two agents, with one from New Zealand showing a greater improvement in FEV_1 (equivalent to 150 mL) in the combination therapy group. Of even greater impact, the combination of anticholinergics and β-agonists leads to a significant reduction in hospitalization. The initial dose when given by nebulization is 0.5 mg in 2 mL of saline every 15 minutes or even continuously during a severe attack. It may be mixed with the β_2-agonists in the nebulizer chamber. If given via a metered dose inhaler and spacer, the initial dose is 4–8 puffs every 15 minutes, repeated three times.

Intravenous β-agonists

Intravenous β-agonists are less often required with the realization that β-agonists administered via the inhaled route, as discussed earlier, offer at least equal and often superior efficacy with greater safety than parenteral therapy with the same agent. It has been argued that in severe asthma with extensive small airway mucus plugging, nebulized medication may not reach the affected airways. Hence, the addition of intravenous β-agonists may be considered when the severe asthmatic remains refractory despite nebulized β-agonists. Salbutamol is given as an intravenous infusion at 10 µg/min and terbutaline as an infusion at 5 µg/min. When given by this route, β-agonists have a high rate of adverse effects, especially tachycardia and tremors and must be carefully monitored.

Aminophylline

Intravenous aminophylline is a useful bronchodilator that has been used for many years in the treatment of acute asthma. Although a meta-analysis by Littenberg of 13 adequately designed studies could not find conclusive evidence for supporting its use, we have found it to be an extremely effective agent in the asthmatics who remain refractory to nebulized β-agonists and steroids. Aminophylline has a very narrow therapeutic margin and its metabolism is affected by multiple factors, making close monitoring of its levels mandatory if it is used. In patients who are not on oral theophylline preparations at the time of admission, a loading dose of 6 mg/kg body weight diluted in 20 mL of 5% dextrose is given slowly over 25–30 minutes. Following this loading dose, an infusion is set up at a rate of 0.6–0.9 mg/kg/hour via an infusion pump. The plasma concentration must be monitored and maintained within the therapeutic range of 10–20 µg/mL. Although the bronchodilator effect increases when the serum concentration is maintained at the upper end of the therapeutic range, the toxicity increases too, and we would hesitate to cross a serum level of 10 µg/mL. These adverse effects include nausea, vomiting, insomnia, headache, cardiac arrhythmias, convulsions, and death. Unquestionably, some of the deaths from asthma in asthma death audits are linked to theophylline toxicity, hence, it must be stressed again that the drug must be used with caution, monitoring levels where facilities exist. A number of disease states (liver disease, cardiac failure, pneumonia, and hypoxemia) and drugs (macrolides and most fluoroquinolones) affect theophylline clearance and doses need to be adjusted carefully with even more frequent serum level monitoring in these settings.

Adrenaline

Although adrenaline has been used for acute asthma since 1951, with the current availability of more specific β_2-agonists, it is seldom needed. It remains the drug of choice in certain situations like anaphylaxis with prominent bronchoconstriction. It can also be life-saving in a patient with catastrophic asthma who is given preloaded syringes, which they can self-administer, at the start of a sudden attack. The usual dose is 0.5 mL of a 1:1,000 solution given subcutaneously. It may be cautiously repeated, if the patient is being monitored in an ICU to a maximum dose of 2 mL.

Magnesium

A number of studies have evaluated the role of intravenous magnesium sulfate, but not all have shown a positive effect. A recent meta-analysis has shown beneficial effects in patients who fail to respond to standard therapy and those with more severe asthma (FEV_1 < 25% at presentation). A study by Sudlow showed that giving 10–20 g over 1 hour to five ventilated asthmatics resulted in significant falls in P_{plat} (plateau pressure) from 43 cm H_2O to 32 cm H_2O. There may also be a trend toward female responsiveness, as estrogen is believed to augment the bronchodilator effect. There is need for further randomized controlled trials to determine the exact role of magnesium in severe asthma.

Unconventional Therapy

In refractory asthma, there are scattered reports of the use of inhalational anesthetics, extracorporeal oxygenation, or bronchial lavage in patients who are on ventilators. The combination of helium and oxygen (heliox) has also been tried and appears to reduce airway pressure.

Mechanical Ventilation in Asthma

Introduction

Despite all the above measures, a small proportion of patients with acute severe asthma will continue to deteriorate and eventually require mechanical ventilation. Fortunately, only about 10% of asthmatics admitted to hospital will need ICU transfer and no more than 1–2% of them will end up requiring mechanical ventilation.

Rationale

When a patient with severe asthma does not respond to all the medical therapy outlined above, the only way to provide adequate oxygenation may be mechanical ventilation. These patients have a propensity to develop severe airflow limitation, making it difficult to exhale all of their inspired gas, resulting in gas trapping, which leads to dynamic hyperinflation. This is referred to as intrinsic positive end-expiratory pressure (PEEP) or auto-PEEP. One of the most important principles of mechanical ventilation in this setting is to utilize a strategy aimed at reducing the likelihood of this complication occurring.

Noninvasive Ventilation

Unlike COPD where noninvasive ventilation (NIV) has a major role, to date, only two small, prospective, randomized studies have evaluated the role of NIV in severe asthma. Both of these studies suggested that in selected asthmatics NIV could be useful as an initial alternative to intubation and ventilation. Further data is needed and without this, the excellent results of NIV in COPD cannot be transposed to acute asthma **(Table 10)**.

It must be stressed, however, *that arterial blood gas values alone should never dictate when ventilatory support should commence.* Each patient should be evaluated individually; the trends of serial blood gases viewed in conjunction with the patient's clinical status are far more informative than a single blood gas report in isolation.

Table 10: Indications for commencing ventilatory support.

- Cardiac or respiratory arrest with apnea or near apnea
- Deteriorating level of consciousness with inability to protect the airway
- Hypotension
- Increasing respiratory muscle fatigue
- Cyanosis or worsening hypoxemia (PaO_2 < 60 mm Hg despite high-flow oxygen
- Hypercapnia with serial arterial blood gas measurements showing a rising $PaCO_2$

($PaCO_2$: Partial pressure of carbon dioxide in arterial blood; PaO_2: Arterial partial pressure of oxygen)

Intubation

Intubation of the critically ill asthmatic involves considerable risk and hence should be performed deftly and expeditiously by an expert. Many patients have increased bronchospasm and laryngeal spasm during attempted intubation and hence a thorough local anesthetic spray of the pharynx is important. The patient must be preoxygenated and care taken to avoid gastric aspiration. A large-diameter endotracheal tube, ideally more than 8 mm, should be used to minimize airway resistance and facilitate suction. Sedation before intubation is obtained with a small dose of midazolam and, if paralysis is needed, atracurium is preferred.

Ventilatory Strategies

In an attempt to counter the problem posed by traditional ventilation in asthma, Darioli and Perret in a landmark paper in 1984 introduced the concept of controlled hypoventilation. Realizing that high-peak pressures were to be avoided at any cost they set a limit on the peak inspiratory pressure and achieved this by reducing the tidal volume, respiratory rate, minute ventilation, and inspiratory flows. This strategy of deliberate hypoventilation resulted in partial pressure of carbon dioxide in arterial blood ($PaCO_2$) levels around 60–70 mm Hg that were accepted and tolerated by most patients without complication. Arterial pH was maintained with intravenous bicarbonate, if necessary. Adequate oxygenation was maintained by increasing the fraction of inspired oxygen (FiO_2) as necessary. Using this strategy in 34 episodes of mechanical ventilation in 26 asthmatic patients, all survived. Equally important, there was no barotrauma in any of their patients. Hypotension, though it occurred in 45% of cases, was usually transient and fluid responsive.

The fine details of the ventilator settings are not as important as close attention to the basic principles of ventilation in patients with severe asthma—employ low tidal volumes and respiratory rates, prolong expiratory time as much as possible, shorten inspiratory time as much as possible, and monitor for the development of auto-PEEP. Thus, the pressure control mode is used setting the pressure to achieve a tidal volume of 6–8 mL/kg, rate at 11–14 breaths/min. An extrinsic PEEP is only used if there is significant auto-PEEP, the set extrinsic PEEP being clearly lower than the auto-PEEP.

Dynamic Hyperinflation

Dynamic hyperinflation occurs when a machine-preset breath is delivered before the previous expiration is complete, so that elastic equilibrium is not reached before the next inspiration starts. This hyperinflation results in the lungs and chest wall operating on a suboptimal portion of their pressure volume curves. Because gas is trapped in the lungs, there is additional pressure at the end of expiration (auto-PEEP or intrinsic PEEP) above the applied PEEP, which leads to dynamic hyperinflation. Dynamic hyperinflation may thus be defined as the failure of the lung to return to its relaxed volume or functional residual capacity at end-exhalation. Dynamic hyperinflation must be assiduously guarded against when ventilating patients with acute severe asthma. It can be clinically assessed by direct auscultation to make sure expiration is complete before the next breath is delivered. It may also be clinically detected by placing a measuring tape across the patient's chest at the level of the nipples and actually noting the increasing chest girth with each breath, if dynamic hyperinflation is occurring. The most accurate method to detect and quantify dynamic hyperinflation is by measuring the auto-PEEP generated by the end-expiratory occlusion method, where the expiratory limb of the tubing is clamped off at the end of expiration. This method must be routinely used to assess the severity of dynamic hyperinflation while ventilating any asthmatic.

Excessive dynamic hyperinflation has been linked to development of hypotension and barotraumas, the two dreaded complications of ventilation in asthmatics. Hypotension is frequent and is usually fluid-responsive. It also usually responds to briefly disconnecting the patient from mechanical ventilation. A brief trial of apnea (30–45 seconds) is usually diagnostic. When hypotension is due to dynamic hyperinflation, a period of apnea serves to increase venous return and raise the blood pressure. A favorable response to a trial of apnea should lead to a reduction of the respiratory rate and intravenous fluid administration. If on the other hand, a brief trial of apnea and a fluid challenge fail to promptly improve blood pressure, then a mechanism other than dynamic hyperinflation, such as pneumothorax or myocardial depression is likely.

Barotrauma is the other dreaded complication encountered while ventilating patients with severe asthma. It includes not just pneumothorax, but also interstitial emphysema, pneumomediastinum, subcutaneous emphysema, pneumoperitoneum, and tension lung cyst. In older series of mechanical ventilation in asthmatics, barotrauma was a frequently observed complication, with pneumothorax occurring in almost a third of all patients. This was undoubtedly the cause of the high mortality reported when ventilating these patients **(Fig. 4)**.

Weaning

Most patients with asthma do not require prolonged periods of ventilatory support and once bronchospasm has settled and the asthma attack is felt to have resolved on clinical grounds, weaning may be successfully attempted. Difficult weaning may be secondary to respiratory muscle weakness from hypokalemia, hypophosphatemia, acute steroid myopathy, or from prolonged use of neuromuscular blocking agents.

Discharge Planning and Advice

The patient must be discharged when clinically stable. Peak flow monitoring can help to predict when the patient may be safely discharged. A study by Udwadia and Harrison showed that patients discharged from hospital when their peak flows are still fluctuating continue to have major and occasionally catastrophic dips in PEF after discharge. In this study, the authors concluded that it was only safe to discharge patients when the diurnal variation in their PEF falls less than 20%. Discharging them before this target is reached puts them at risk of further severe attacks of asthma requiring rehospitalization and even leading to death.

A hospitalization with severe asthma must be looked at as a failure on the part of the treating physician and his self-management plan. The hospitalized asthmatic offers the physician the ideal opportunity to educate the patient about his disease. Healthcare providers should seize this opportunity to review the patient's understanding of the causes of asthma exacerbations and avoidance of its triggers. He should be taught the correct inhaler technique, taught to use a peak flow meter, and given a written treatment plan. In a study of 150 asthmatics discharged from the emergency department with an action plan which included peak flow monitoring, there was a striking reduction in the risk of relapse in the peak flow action plan group (five readmissions in this group vs 55 in those with no plan). A recent systematic review by the Cochrane airway group looked at 23 studies that compared a written self-treatment plan with usual care and showed that a written plan reduced hospitalization, emergency room visits, and days off work or school.

But we end this section by quoting the words of Thomas Petty, who said—*"the best treatment of status asthmaticus is to treat it three days before it occurs".*

■ HOW IS ASTHMA MANAGED IN INDIA?

In Hospitals

Good guidelines on how to manage asthma exist but are seldom followed. Asthma is a disease that lends itself well to audit, yet there are hardly any audit studies from India. In one such study of acute severe asthma from the Hinduja Hospital, a large private hospital in Mumbai, an audit revealed a number of deficiencies. The authors looked at the hospital records of 80 asthmatics, admitted for an acute exacerbation of asthma over 18 months. A number of deficiencies were identified, chief amongst these being—the respiratory rate was recorded in only 28% of patients, arterial blood gas measurements were made in only 55%, and theophylline levels checked in just 22%. Peak flows were recorded in just 2% of patients and pulmonary function test (PFT) measured in just 43%. More worryingly, errors in management were also highlighted with 20% of hospitalized asthmatics not receiving steroids.

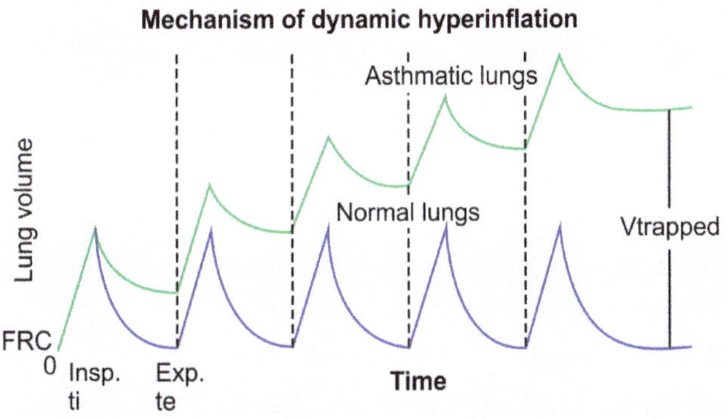

Fig. 4: Mechanism or dynamic hyperinflation in the setting of severe airflow obstruction.
Source: Adapted from Levy BD, Kitch B, Fanta CH. Medical and ventilatory management of status asthmaticus. Intensive Care Med. 1998;24(2):105-17.

Attempts are being made, at local hospital level, to close the audit loop by making recommendations based on this audit and then repeating the audit a few years down the line. It remains to be seen, if such studies actually impact on asthma management or remain academic exercises. We would none the less encourage asthma to be audited in similar fashion at other hospitals in the country, with the audit followed by feedback and implementation of action to close the loop.

In the Community

A study called AIRSA (Asthma Insights and Realities in South Asia), conducted in 2002, contacted 8,000 random households in nine Indian cities (including the big metros like Mumbai, Delhi, Kolkata, and Chennai) to identify 403 asthmatics. These had a face-to-face interview for 45 minutes about their asthma control and treatment. The results highlighted major lacunae in the delivery of treatment and care toward asthmatic patients even in some of India's biggest cities. The survey found that the majority of asthmatics were poorly controlled with 60% of those questioned reporting daytime symptoms and 77% experiencing nocturnal symptoms that disrupted sleep at least once a week in the month prior to the interview. Other reflections of the poor asthma control were that 87% reported limitation in sport and 85% had frequent need for reliever medication in the past month; 27% of adult asthmatics and 53% of children with asthma had missed work or school respectively in the past year due to asthma. Indian doctors seemed to be failing in their duties to their patients; only 58% of patients had actually been taught how to use an inhaler and 10% had a written treatment plan. Only 13% of patients surveyed had even heard of a peak flow meter, only 2% owned one of their own and only 28% of patients had ever had a PFT. The most striking deficiency highlighted by the AIRSA survey was that only 2% of respondents used inhaled corticosteroids for their asthma. Thus, the current level of asthma control in India falls far short of the GINA-set optimal goals for long-term asthma management.

Factors Contributing to Poor Asthma Control in India

- *Asthma is felt to be less of a priority*: Asthma is not felt to be a priority in this country with its huge burden of tuberculosis and other infectious diseases. However, its impact on the health of large numbers of Indians must not be underestimated. The global burden of disease as measured by disability adjusted life years (DALY) lost is 3.4 for tuberculosis and a not inconsiderable 0.9 for asthma.
- *Less healthcare spending on asthma*: Raj Singh from Chennai has estimated that if the prevalence of asthma is 5% and the average cost of asthma medication is about 30 USD per month, 30% of the entire expenditure on health in the country would have to be spent on asthma alone. It is felt that about 10% of patients have access to good quality healthcare, which includes inhalers. However, even less, probably no more than 2% actually use inhalers. If the cost of asthma medication were to be reduced, a greater proportion of those afflicted can be expected to benefit. It is little wonder that the average asthmatic in India still relies on outdated drugs like oral β-agonists instead of inhaled medication. **Table 11** looks at what asthma drugs cost the average Indian as a percentage of his monthly income.
- *Attitudes to health and disease also affect perceptions of asthma in India*: Asthmatics are treated differently by many competing systems of medicine in India. Thus, Ayurveda, which is followed by large numbers of Indians, believes that asthma is caused by an imbalance in one of the three "humors"—Kapha (phlegm), Pitta (bile), and Vata (gas). It is probably these concepts that affect the misconceptions about food many asthmatics in India have. In a survey from Northern India, 88% of parents of children with asthma felt that food was the primary trigger for their children's asthma. A trial we conducted at the Hinduja Hospital of Ayurvedic

Table 11: What do asthma drugs cost the average Indian? Per capita Indian income is equal to ₹ 11,302 Statistical Outline of India, 2000.

Drug	Cost of 1 month tablets/1 MDI	% of monthly income
Oral salbutamol	₹ 12	1.3%
Oral theophylline	₹ 21	2.2%
Salbutamol MDI	₹ 80	8.5%
Budesonide MDI	₹ 214	22%
Nebulizer solution	₹ 1,080	115%
Nebulizer	₹ 4,000	424%
O_2 concentrator	₹ 60,000	6369%

(MDI: Metered dose inhaler; O_2: Oxygen)

drugs in 195 asthmatics in 2001, randomized to receive standard versus Ayurvedic treatment was stopped because only 14% of Ayurvedic patients responded compared to 97% of allopathic patients.

- *Ignorance and superstition*: The Hyderabad fish "treatment" of asthma is another classic example of how superstition and ignorance can combine to hinder the correct medical management of asthma. In this ancient custom, spanning over 150 years, the Murrel fish prepared in a holy well with a herbal cocktail, is forced down the throat of hundreds of thousands of asthmatics desperate for a cure. These gullible and desperate asthmatics throng this venue in Hyderabad on the 7th of June each year for three consecutive years. The family administering the drug claims this treatment will cure asthma, provided it is accompanied by a special diet over 45 days.
- *Poorly trained doctors*: Poorly trained doctors contribute to "difficult asthma" in India. An audit by Bedi of asthma treated by general practitioners, in Punjab, identified an underuse of inhalers and an overuse of ephedrine.
- *Lack of access*: It is estimated that only 10% of asthmatics in India have access to optimal care and less than 2% actually use inhaled medication for their asthma.

Thus clearly the way ahead includes greater public spending on asthma, educating doctors and patients, and improving access to inhalers to large parts of the population.

■ SUGGESTED READING

1. Agertoft L, Pedersen S. Effect of long-term treatment with inhaled budesonide on adult height in children with asthma. N Engl J Med. 2000;343:1064-9.
2. FitzGerald JM. Commentary: intravenous magnesium in severe asthma. Evid Based Med. 1999;4:138.
3. Global Initiative for Asthma. (2009). Global Strategy for Asthma Management and Prevention, 2009. [online] Available from www.ginaasthma.org. [Accessed July, 2018].
4. Hambly N, Nair P. Monoclonal antibodies for the treatment of refractory asthma. Curr Opin Pulm Med. 2014;20:87-94.
5. Harrison BDWH, Stokes TC, Hart GJ, et al. Need for intravenous hydrocortisone in addition to oral prednisolone in patients admitted to hospital with severe asthma without ventilatory failure. Lancet. 1986;8474:181-4.
6. Lazarus SC, Boushey HA, Fahy JV, et al. Long-acting beta2-agonist monotherapy vs continued therapy with inhaled corticosteroids in patients with persistent asthma: a randomized controlled trial. JAMA. 2001;285(20):2583-93.
7. Manocha R, Marks GB, Kenchington P, et al. Sahaja yoga in the management of moderate to severe asthma: a randomised controlled trial. Thorax. 2002;57:110-5.
8. Nelson HS, Weiss ST, Bleecker ER, et al. The Salmeterol Multicenter Asthma Research Trial: a comparison of usual pharmacotherapy for asthma or usual pharmacotherapy plus salmeterol. Chest. 2006;129(1):15-26.
9. Rodrigo G, Rodrigo C. Inhaled flunisolide for acute severe asthma. Am J Respir Crit Care Med. 1998;157(3Pt 1): 698-703.
10. Rodrigo GJ. Comparison of inhaled fluticasone with intravenous hydrocortisone in the treatment of adult acute asthma. Am J Respir Crit Care Med. 2005;171(11):1231-6.
11. Rowe BH, Bota GW, Fabris L, et al. Inhaled budesonide in addition to oral corticosteroids to prevent asthma relapse following discharge from the emergency department: a randomized controlled study. JAMA. 1999;281(22): 2119-26.
12. Rowe BH, Spooner CH, Ducharme FM, et al. The effectiveness of corticosteroids in the treatment of acute exacerbations of asthma: a meta-analysis of their effect on relapse following acute assessment. The Cochrane Library. 1998; Issue 4. Oxford: Update software.
13. Skoner DP, Maspero J, Banerji D. Ciclesonide Pediatric Growth Study Group. Assessment of the long-term safety of inhaled ciclesonide on growth in children with asthma. Pediatrics. 2008;121(1):e1-14.
14. Stather DR, Stewart TE. Clinical review: mechanical ventilation in severe asthma. Critical Care. 2005;9(6):581-7.
15. Udwadia ZF. Acute severe asthma. In: Udwadia FE (Ed). Principles of Critical Care. India: Oxford University Press; 1995. pp. 265-71.
16. Udwadia ZF, Harrison BDWH. An attempt to determine the optimal duration of hospital stay following a severe attack of asthma. JR Coll Physicians Lond. 1990;24(2):112-4.
17. Walters EH, Walters JA, Gibson MD. Inhaled long acting beta agonists for stable chronic asthma. Cochrane Database Syst Rev. 2003;4:CD001385.
18. Walters JA, Wood-Baker R, Walters EH. Long-acting beta2-agonists in asthma: an overview of Cochrane systematic reviews. Respir Med. 2005;99(4):384-95.
19. Weatherall M, Wijesinghe M, Perrin K, et al. Meta-analysis of the risk of mortality with salmeterol and the effect of concomitant inhaled corticosteroid therapy. Thorax. 2010;65(1):39-43.

CHAPTER 35

Asthma: Special Types

■ DIFFICULT ASTHMA

Definition

Difficult asthma may be defined as being present in a patient with a confirmed diagnosis of asthma whose symptoms and/or lung function abnormalities are poorly controlled despite treatment which experience suggests would usually be effective [*Ref: Harrison BD. Difficult asthma. Thorax. 2003;58(7):555-6*].

Pathology

The pathology of severe asthma is distinctive. These patients have persistent airways inflammation and evidence of airway remodeling with structural changes. There is evidence of smooth muscle hypertrophy, thickening of the epithelium and subepithelial fibrosis. Some studies have documented an excess of profibrotic cytokines, like transforming growth factor-beta (TGF-β) in the mucosa of the patient with severe and difficult asthma.

How common is it? Fortunately, most asthma is not difficult, but relatively easy to manage. Difficult asthma constitutes only the tip of the asthma iceberg. Of the more than 200 million estimated asthmatics worldwide, only a small fraction can truly be considered difficult. It is however the difficult asthmatic that consumes most in terms of healthcare resources and time.

In Weiss's study showing that the estimated total annual cost of asthma was a staggering US\$ 4.5 billion in America in 1992, it was noted that 80% of the costs were attributable to 20% of patients with this problem. Studies from Canada and Australia also revealed that patients with severe and difficult asthma though comprising no more than 10% and 6% of the asthma population accounted for 54% and 40% of the annual cost respectively. Thus, the economic burden of asthma is large and derives disproportionately from those with severe disease.

Types of Difficult Asthma

If "difficult" is defined as "a task that demands toil or effort, or a problem that is difficult to solve" then a number of types of asthma can be considered to be difficult. Severe asthma is a heterogeneous disease, in which specific severity phenotypes may respond differently to different therapies. The following clinical phenotypes of asthma can be included under "difficult asthma":

Acute Severe Asthma

Nothing can be more difficult than managing a patient with severe life-threatening asthma in an intensive care unit (ICU).

Brittle Asthma

Brittle asthma is defined as a form of asthma that causes little or no problem on most days but is associated with frequent severe attacks requiring unscheduled hospital or physician visits or frequent courses of oral steroids. A common feature in brittle asthma is the apparent difficulty in controlling the variability in airway function as shown in **Figure 1**.

Fortunately, brittle asthma is not common; it has a prevalence of 0.05% of all asthma. A possible genetic

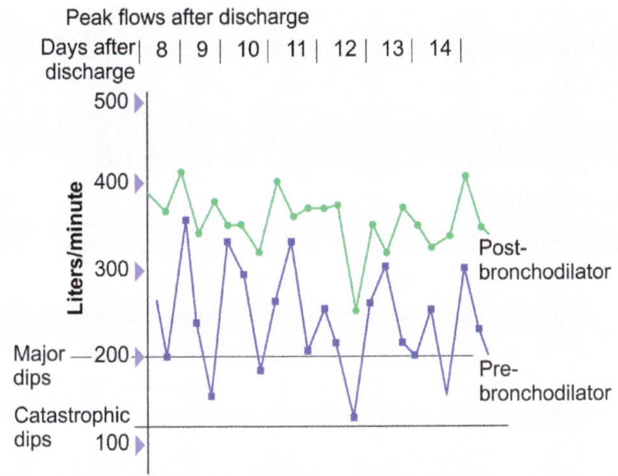

Fig. 1: Peak expiratory flow (PEF) in a patient with brittle asthma. These hectic dips in PEF were even more striking when noted that they began just 8 days following discharge from hospital for an acute attack. This lady was readmitted a few days later.

component is present in brittle asthma; 50% of patients have lost a first-degree relative from asthma.

Two types of brittle asthma are recognized:

Type 1 (brittle asthma): It is characterized by chaotic peak-flow variability for more than 50% of the time for at least 150 days, despite maximal medical treatment. This type is more likely to occur in females. The majority are atopic, with at least one positive skin-prick test. Pet allergies are common and premenstrual factors may contribute in some women with type 1 brittle asthma.

Type 2 (brittle asthma): It is characterized by sudden attacks becoming severe within minutes, against a background of apparently good control. This type has no sex predilection. This form of severe asthma is even more rare. Attacks can occur with catastrophic speed and are believed to be immunoglobulin E (IgE)-mediated.

Both types are difficult to treat and carry a greatly increased risk of death. Multiple hospitalizations and frequent need for mechanical ventilation characterizes both types. Subcutaneous terbutaline, driven by a syringe pump is an intervention that has been found to be of benefit in some patients with brittle asthma. Brittle asthma is really the prototype of difficult asthma and no form of asthma has such a profound impact on the lives, work and psyche of the asthmatic. Psychological disturbance develops in the majority of these patients as shall be discussed later.

Chronic Asthma

Chronic asthma is another clinical phenotype of difficult asthma. This type of asthma rarely causes severe exacerbations but is "difficult" by virtue of it causing symptoms that interfere with the full enjoyment of life despite maximum doses of the best therapies currently available. Every physician can recollect such patients with chronic asthma from his own practice and will agree that they are indeed among the most difficult to treat. This form of asthma usually starts in childhood when it is usually mild and intermittent, but progresses in severity over the years till the patients are disabled almost as severely as patients with advanced emphysema. Indeed, the majority of these patients will need long-term oxygen, just as in patients with severe emphysema, together with a maintenance dose of oral steroids.

Steroid-Resistant Asthma

While asthma is by definition a steroid-responsive disease, there is now increasing awareness that a small fraction of patients with difficult asthma will be truly steroid-unresponsive or resistant. This entity was first described by Schwartz in 1968 in six asthmatic patients who failed to clinically respond to high doses of systemic steroids. He went on to define it as the failure of an asthmatic to improve his forced expiratory volume in 1 second (FEV_1) by 15%, despite an adequate dose of steroid (equivalent of 40 mg prednisolone), with assured compliance, for an adequate duration (2 weeks), despite demonstrating greater than 15% reversibility to an inhaled β_2-agonist. Primary glucocorticosteroid (GCS) resistance is a genetic syndrome, which occurs due to either reduced GCS receptor binding affinity or due to abnormally low numbers of GCS receptors. There is increased activating peptide-1 (API) activity in steroid-resistant asthma. API is a transcription factor complex, which is pertinent to asthmatic inflammation. At a cellular level, steroid-resistant asthma is characterized by impaired in vitro and in vivo responsiveness of monocytes and T-lymphocytes to the suppressive effects of GCSs. Secondary GCS resistance is more common and is due to factors like decreased absorption of steroids or increased metabolism due to interaction with other drugs like rifampicin or carbamazepine.

The importance of recognizing an asthmatic to have steroid resistance is considerable. Early identification can lead to institution of alternative therapies. If on the other hand, steroid resistance remains unrecognized, they continue to be treated with high doses of oral steroid with no clinical benefit but considerable cumulative toxicity. These patients often have a good response to long-acting β-agonists and theophylline and these drugs along with steroid-sparing agents like methotrexate and cyclosporine may be tried.

Approach to the Difficult Asthmatic

A difficult asthmatic requires specialist referral and investigations that encompass the full range of respiratory, imaging, and allergy testing. A multidisciplinary approach is recommended, with close coordination between ear, nose and throat (ENT) colleagues, psychiatrists and counselors offering psychiatric and psychological assessment, and respiratory physicians deciding on therapy. In the West, this is often served by "difficult asthma clinics" where these patients are carefully assessed. In an interesting study by Heaney from one such difficult asthma clinic at a referral hospital in the United Kingdom, of the 80 patients referred with "therapy-resistant" asthma, 95% were found to have an ENT abnormality, 57% had gastroesophageal reflux disease (GERD), 50% had an ICD-10 (The International Statistical Classification of Diseases and Related Health Problems 10th Revision) psychiatric diagnosis, 30% had an additional diagnosis, which was bronchiectasis in nine patients, chronic obstructive pulmonary disease (COPD) in three and vocal cord dysfunction in three. Indeed, one patient did not have asthma at all despite all the referrals to this clinic having come from chest departments from peripheral hospitals with a chest physician confirming the diagnosis of "asthma with persisting refractory symptoms".

Monitoring the Difficult Asthmatic

This is one type of asthma where meticulous monitoring might be rewarded by a reduction in hospitalizations and morbidity. Induced sputum eosinophilia, exhaled nitrogen oxide (NO) levels and other markers of inflammation have all been studied in this group of difficult asthmatics. Exhaled NO has been found to be a reliable, noninvasive and easily measured marker with increasing values serving as a good predictive marker for poor asthma control. Sputum eosinophilia may also be an invaluable marker in further phenotyping severe asthmatics into eosinophilic or neutrophilic categories with the former showing a good

response to biological therapies like mepolizumab, an anti-interleukin-6 (IL-5) agent, which has been discussed earlier.

Approach to Evaluating the Difficult Asthmatic

We would recommend the following 10-point approach when faced with a difficult asthmatic:

1. Question and re-establish the very diagnosis of asthma: spirometry, flow volume loops, methacholine challenge, and tests of airway conductance and resistance may all be used for this purpose.
2. If there is still any doubt, high-resolution computed tomography (HRCT) and fiberoptic bronchoscopy may be needed.
3. Check for coexisting conditions, cardiopulmonary diseases like associated bronchiectasis, COPD, Churg-Strauss syndrome or left ventricular dysfunction.
4. Establish if the asthma is "difficult" because of genuine disease factors, e.g. brittle asthma, steroid resistance, etc.
5. If not, is the asthma difficult because of "doctor"-related factors: being inappropriately treated or undertreated.
6. Are patient-related factors to blame? Is the patient compliant with regard to his therapy? Most often "difficult" asthma boils down to the patient being noncompliant with his inhaled steroid because he is concerned about potential side effects. All that is needed in this situation is to stress the importance and safety of these drugs and spend some time re-educating him. A psychiatric and psychosocial evaluation should be considered in all such patients. Harrison has stressed that underlying depression, denial, personality problems, socioeconomic deprivation, employment problems, marital problems and substance abuse can be found in a significant numbers of these patients and may contribute to the difficulty in controlling their asthma. He has stressed the importance of listening to their problems and concerns and offering sympathy and understanding which may be at least as important as escalating treatment in some of them.
7. Specifically question the contribution of GERD and sinus disease. Both of these have been discussed earlier. Consider 24-hour ambulatory pH monitoring and CT scanning of the sinuses.

8. Check if environmental and occupational factors are worsening the asthma.
9. Are drug-related factors worsening asthma?
10. Finally, are hormonal factors worsening asthma? In significant numbers of women, menstrual factors can contribute to asthma.

Managing the Difficult Asthmatic

The majority of these patients will be on Step 4 treatment, with many requiring in addition oral maintenance doses of steroids. Here too, there are unanswered questions about opting for frequent intermittent high-dose courses each time they exacerbate versus settling for a daily, regular maintenance dose. The risk-benefit comparison of these two strategies in the difficult asthmatic with frequent exacerbations has not been evaluated. What is also unclear is whether there is any clear difference between the different types of oral steroids in terms of long-term side effects. Another unanswered question is whether the route of administration (oral vs injectable) makes a difference. An interesting recent study by Brinke looked at the role of a single intramuscular dose of triamcinolone in 22 patients with severe asthma who had remained uncontrolled despite more than four courses of oral steroids in the preceding year. They found that this strategy not only normalized sputum eosinophilia and improved postbronchodilator FEV_1, but also decreased the use of rescue medicine in the following 6 months. Other studies have looked at high doses of inhaled corticosteroids with fourfold or even much higher than normal doses sometimes re-establishing control. Rodrigo's study showed that repeated and high doses of inhaled fluticasone [3,000 µg/h, administered through a metered-dose inhaler (MDI) and spacer at 10-minute intervals for 3 hours) were more effective than intravenous hydrocortisone in acute severe asthma with more rapid onset of action and a greater response.

This is the group of patients where omalizumab and the other biological therapies discussed earlier may have a real role. A variety of nonsteroidal agents have also been looked at in this patient group, with agents like methotrexate, troleandomycin, telithromycin, macrolides and cyclosporine all being considered. A Cochrane analysis of two of these agents, methotrexate and cyclosporine A has shown a small benefit, but perhaps certain phenotypes would respond better to one or more of these agents.

A novel and exciting new intervention, bronchial thermoplasty has also recently emerged. This involves controlled thermal energy (at 65°C) being applied via the fiberoptic bronchoscope to the bronchial wall in an attempt to reduce smooth muscle mass. Results of a recent trial by Castro of 288 patients where this procedure was compared to a sham procedure showed it improved asthma-specific quality of life with a reduction in severe exacerbations and healthcare utilization in the post-treatment period. The procedure is done with intravenous sedation in three sessions, about a month apart. The bronchi in the lower lobe of one lung, then the lower lobe of the other lung and finally in both upper lobes together are tackled over the three sessions, each lasting about 30–60 minutes. While fears have been raised about the safety of the procedure in patients with severe asthma, the study by Castro found it well-tolerated. Finally, patients with severe asthma increasingly turn to alternative therapies like yoga, acupuncture and behavioral therapy, which prove helpful in the occasional patient.

■ FATAL AND NEAR-FATAL ASTHMA

Historically, asthma was not considered a fatal disease. Osler declared: "the asthmatic pants into old age". Yet, it is now evident that many patients will die of their asthma, some in their youth. No Indian data are available but there are 2,000 deaths in a small country like the United Kingdom from asthma annually. This works out to almost one death from asthma every 4 hours. In the United States, deaths from asthma doubled from 0.6 per 100,000 in 1977 to 1.4 per 100,000 in 1984. Indeed one of the unanswered paradoxes of asthma is why, despite better understanding of the disease and better drugs, asthma mortality is still on the rise when the mortality of all other nonmalignant chronic diseases has declined. Possible explanations for this asthma paradox include increasing incidence of atopy and house dust mite allergen, increasing air pollution, and inappropriate use of inhaled β_2-agonists. None of these on their own are likely to be the real explanation, which is probably that there is a problem in delivering the most crucial disease-modifying agents, inhaled corticosteroids, to the vast majority of asthmatics who need these drugs. A survey by Watson from 24 developing countries in Asia and Africa showed that inhaled steroids were not used by almost 93% of respondents, primarily due to purely economic constraints. As one doctor wrote in his response to Watson's questionnaire: "The poor die, the rich live, matter of cash, really sad." Of course it is not only economics that dictate why asthmatics die, for they also die in significant numbers in the developed world. To understand the causes of death here we have to turn to asthma death audits and confidential inquiries. In a review of seven asthma death audits from the United Kingdom and one from New Zealand, there were a few messages that came through clearly. Harrison succinctly summarized these under the following three headings:

1. DOCTORS fail to assess the severity of asthma because they fail to make objective measurements [peak expiratory flow (PEF), oxygen saturation (SaO_2), arterial blood gas (ABG)].

2. PATIENTS fail to appreciate the severity of their asthma and fail to make the measurements they are meant to (PEF). This is because significant numbers of asthmatics under-perceive their asthma and get accustomed to experiencing severe attacks.

3. As a result of 1 and 2, under-use of the most effective asthma medication, steroids (inhaled and oral) are very common.

Overall, potentially treatable factors occurred in 86% of the patients dying from asthma. An asthma death is always a cause for introspection. Here is a disease, which is by definition meant to be reversible, going on to result in a fatality, that too in a young and productive member of society. What makes it even more poignant is the observation that the vast majority of such deaths could have been prevented.

The factors that come up repeatedly in the asthma audits have been summarized in **Table 1**.

Lessons Arising from the Asthma Death Audits

The studies of asthma deaths from New Zealand and the United States and the results of the confidential inquiry into asthma deaths from East Anglia in the United Kingdom, led to the list in **Table 2** describing the characteristics of a patient at risk of developing a fatal or a near-fatal attack of asthma.

The way ahead lies in education. Education, not just of patients, but also of doctors and family physicians is of crucial importance. The patient who dies of fatal asthma has been getting up for several nights in the week prior to his eventual death. Recognizing the gravity of this and intervening with a short oral course of steroid might save the lives of such patients. Patients at increased risk of developing fatal or near-fatal asthma (NFA) can and should be identified. It is this group that needs extra attention and focus even in a busy outpatient department.

Table 1: Factors contributing to death in asthma death audits.

Patient-related factors:
- Most patients dying of asthma have had previous admissions
- Most give a long history of asthma
- Adverse psychosocial factors found to have been present in significant numbers
- Most are poorly compliant with their medications especially ICS
- Most tend to over rely and use their reliever inhaler (short-acting β_2-agonists like salbutamol and terbutaline)
- Patients become accustomed to a degree of disability
- Not all patients with severe obstruction feel unwell
- The fatal attack of asthma has often persisted for days or even weeks before admission: 50% were waking up 5 nights a week in the week prior to death and 35% were waking up that often for 1 month prior to the eventually fatal admission
- Under use of PEF meters
- Delays in reaching hospital
- The overwhelming majority of deaths occur at home

Doctor-related factors:
- Doctors underestimate the severity of the attack
- Doctors fail to make objective measurements
- Underuse of steroids
- Underuse of agonists
- Overuse of agonists
- Injudicious use of sedation
- Wrong use of drugs like β-blockers and NSAIDs
- Failure to monitor theophylline
- Uncorrected hypokalemia
- Delays instituting mechanical ventilation
- Unrecognized complications of mechanical ventilation

Table 2: Patients at risk of developing fatal or near-fatal asthma (from New Zealand and the United States death audits and the United Kingdom confidential inquiries).

- Previous life-threatening attacks
- Severe disease
- Hospital admission in the previous year
- Unscheduled ER visits in the previous year
- Patient noncompliance
- Psychosocial problems
- Behavioral problems especially denial
- Socioeconomic deprivation
- Three or more categories of asthmatic drugs prescribed
- Requiring frequent courses of oral steroids
- Requiring high-dose inhaled steroids
- Requiring two or more canisters of a bronchodilator monthly
- Discontinuity of medical care

These efforts seem to be paying off and there is now light at the end of the tunnel. Despite the increased prevalence of asthma, deaths from asthma over the last two decades seem to be on the decline in many developed countries. This decline has been noticed in all age groups, but particularly in those under the age of 65 years. Special approaches and management strategies in these, the most difficult and challenging of all asthmatics need to be prioritized.

■ PREGNANT ASTHMATIC

Asthma is a disease that often complicates pregnancy. Recent studies show that 1–4% of pregnancies may be complicated by asthma. Pregnant women have a higher incidence of adverse maternal and fetal outcomes, and are hence a high-risk group that needs to be carefully monitored and optimally treated.

Physiological Changes during Pregnancy

Pregnancy results in enhanced production of progesterone, estradiol and cortisol. Progesterone specifically increases minute ventilation and decreases pulmonary vascular resistance. Changes in lung function noted in pregnancy include reduced functional residual capacity (FRC), reduced residual volume, and reduced total lung capacity. These changes occur even before significant uterine enlargement implying nondirect physiological effects.

FEV_1, and FEV_1/forced vital capacity (FVC) are unaffected by pregnancy hence any change in these parameters can be assumed to be due to respiratory pathology. Minute ventilation can increase by 20–40% and this results in changes in ABGs. The arterial partial pressure of oxygen (PaO_2) rises to 100–105 mm Hg, while arterial partial pressure of carbon dioxide ($PaCO_2$) falls to 32–34 mm Hg. The pH is maintained by renal compensation with increased excretion of bicarbonate. Breathlessness is often present in pregnancy, especially in the last trimester and is due to increased work of breathing or increased respiratory drive. Nasal stuffiness is common in pregnancy, due to a combination of nasal hyperemia and edema and may add to the perceived difficulty in breathing.

Effects of Pregnancy on Asthma

Pregnancy can have varying effects on asthma. A third of all asthmatics will worsen, a third actually improve and a third remain unaffected. The same pattern is usually repeated for the pregnant asthmatic in her subsequent pregnancies. Asthma control is often at its worst at the start of the third trimester with the asthma reassuming its prepregnancy level about 3 months postdelivery. Studies show that the severity and duration of asthma attacks are no different in pregnant asthmatics compared to their nonpregnant counterparts, but due to the reluctance of pregnant patients to commence corticosteroids, they have a threefold increased chance of suffering ongoing exacerbations.

Effects of Asthma on the Mother

Maternal complications associated with uncontrolled asthma include pre-eclampsia, placenta previa, gestational hypertension, hyperemesis gravidarum, vaginal hemorrhage, toxemia, induced and complicated labor, increased cesarean sections and prolonged maternal hospital stay. A study showed that asthmatic females have an odds ratio of 1.6 to 2.2 for each of these complications compared to nonasthmatic females.

Effects of Asthma on the Fetus

Oxygenated fetal blood is normally very low in PaO_2 but because of a remarkable compensatory mechanism this is well tolerated (high fetal hemoglobin concentration, leftward shift in oxygen-hemoglobin disassociation curve, a high fetal cardiac output). Critical respiratory disease in the mother such as an asthma exacerbation results in a fall in maternal PaO_2 and a profound decrease in fetal PaO_2 and tissue oxygenation. As the mother gets hypoxemic during a severe asthma exacerbation, maternal compensatory mechanisms will maintain oxygenation to vital maternal organs at the cost of uterine blood flow. Hence fetal distress can occur even in the absence of obvious maternal hypoxia or hypotension. Fetal complications reported during uncontrolled asthma include increased risk of prenatal mortality, intrauterine growth retardation, low birth weight, preterm birth and neonatal hypoxia.

Management of Asthma during Pregnancy

The treatment of asthma in pregnancy is no different from that in a nonpregnant asthmatic. Of course, the benefit from each medication must be shown to outweigh its possible risk. Having said this, we have seen too many pregnant asthmatics treated suboptimally because of perceived fears of the side effects of asthma medication on the fetus. It must be stressed to the patient apprehensive about taking her drugs that the greatest risk is from uncontrolled asthma and not the drugs. Inhaled and oral steroids may safely be used depending on the situation and inhaled short- and long-acting β_2-agonists are also safe. Oral β-agonists are best avoided near term as they may cause hypoglycemia and palpitation. Epinephrine is also best avoided as it may cause vasoconstriction in the uterus and reduce uteroplacental flow. Theophylline may be used, provided its levels are monitored and it is kept at the lower limit of normal. Not enough is known about the leukotriene modifiers to recommend them safely at present.

ASTHMATIC WITH PREMENSTRUAL WORSENING

A small group of women with asthma may have severe, sometimes catastrophic, worsening in their asthma just prior to their menstrual period. This correlates with falling progesterone levels and increasing estrogen to progesterone ratios. Progesterone is meant to have anti-inflammatory properties, hence its decrease before menstruation could worsen asthma in some patients. Such patients may also demonstrate some degree of steroid resistance. It is vital to recognize this potential link with menstruation in the young asthmatic who has cyclical exacerbations of her asthma. Hormonal treatment with progesterone, usually in depot preparations through the intramuscular route (Depo-Provera) works best in this setting. Recently, goserelin, a gonadotropin-releasing hormone (GnRH) analog has been shown to be effective. On occasion, oophorectomy is the only way to control the catastrophic deterioration in asthma associated with menstruation in some asthmatics.

ASTHMATIC UNDERGOING ANESTHESIA

It is imperative to ensure that the asthmatic goes into surgery with his or her asthma optimally controlled. In a recent study examining almost 18,000 day-care surgeries, asthma was present in 5.7% of all patients and these patients had an approximately fivefold increase in the risk of developing postoperative respiratory adverse effects. Intubation and anesthesia have the potential to induce bronchospasm and worsen pre-existing asthma. Adverse effects included unanticipated admission to ICU, prolonged postoperative stay and unscheduled readmission because of worsening asthma. Poorly controlled and severe asthma, thoracic and upper abdominal surgeries, and general anesthesia involving tracheal intubation were associated with more perioperative problems in asthmatics. Pulmonary function test (PFT) must be checked prior to the surgery and if found to be poor or if bronchospasm is present preoperatively, it is best to delay the surgery (if elective) till the asthma is optimally controlled with bronchodilators and even a short course of oral steroids if necessary. Intravenous hydrocortisone should be given to the asthmatic a few hours prior to surgery if preoperative

FEV_1 is low. Nebulized β_2-agonist should be administered just prior to shifting the patient to the operating theater and continued in the postoperative period. Close monitoring of the patient by the anesthetist perioperatively, and the physician postoperatively, is recommended.

ASPIRIN-INDUCED ASTHMA

Cases of violent bronchospasm following ingestion of aspirin began to be reported shortly after introduction of aspirin into therapy well over a century ago. The association of aspirin sensitivity, asthma and nasal polyposis was first described by Widal in 1922. It was subsequently realized that many other nonsteroidal anti-inflammatory drugs (NSAIDs) shared with aspirin the potential to trigger asthma in sensitive patients.

PATHOGENESIS

Allergic Mechanisms

Since clinical reactions triggered by aspirin are reminiscent of immediate type hypersensitivity reactions, an underlying antigen-antibody mechanism has been suggested. However, skin tests with aspirin are negative and attempts to demonstrate specific antibodies to aspirin have been unsuccessful.

Cyclooxygenase Theory

This theory proposes that precipitation of asthma attacks by aspirin is not based on antigen-antibody reactions, but stems from the pharmacological action of the drug: namely, specific inhibition in the respiratory tract of the enzyme cyclooxygenase (COX). This enzyme is central to the mechanism of aspirin-induced asthma (AIA). This would explain why NSAIDs with anti-COX activity invariably precipitate bronchospasm while those that do not affect COX activity do not provoke bronchospasm. It is now known that the COX enzyme exists in at least two isoforms, COX_1 and COX_2 encoded by distinct genes. Aspirin, indomethacin and piroxicam, which can all trigger AIA in small doses, are all more potent COX_1 inhibitors. Specific COX_2 inhibitors (etoricoxib) and NSAIDs that are more potent COX_2 than COX_1 inhibitors, like nimesulide and meloxicam are generally well-tolerated.

Leukotriene Pathway

Over recent years, the cysteinyl leukotrienes (Cys-LTs) have emerged as major mediators of AIA. In most patients with AIA, basal excretion of Cys-LT in the urine is elevated and increases further upon aspirin administration. In addition, following aspirin challenge there is a release of Cys-LT into both the nasal cavity and bronchial tree. The terminal enzyme for Cys-LT production is LTC4 synthase. In bronchial biopsies from patients with AIA, the expression of this enzyme is fivefold higher than in asthmatics who tolerate aspirin and 19-fold higher than in normal subjects.

Clinical Features

Aspirin-induced asthma is a clear-cut syndrome with a distinct clinical picture. Aspirin intolerance is clearly underdiagnosed in the asthmatic population. Based on history alone, it is estimated that 3–5% of adult asthmatics are aspirin-sensitive. This percentage rises to 6–15% if asthmatics are challenged with aspirin. Many asthmatics who test positive after an aspirin provocation test were unaware of aspirin intolerance prior to the test.

The classic triad of AIA is asthma, nasal polyposis and aspirin sensitivity. Rhinitis is the first symptom to develop. It is perennial, difficult to treat, accompanied by sinusitis and may lead to loss of smell in 50% of patients. In the average patient, asthma starts about 2 years later and intolerance to aspirin and NSAIDs is evident 4 years later. Apart from triggering nasal discharge and acute severe bronchospasm, aspirin can trigger skin manifestations like urticaria and a scarlet flush in 20% of patients, angioedema in 8% of patients and violent anaphylactoid reactions with shock, hypotension and loss of consciousness in about 5% of patients. Females outnumber males by a ratio of 2.3:1 in most series, with symptoms starting earlier in females than males. Asthma runs a protracted course despite the avoidance of aspirin and cross-reactive drugs.

Treatment

Treatment centers around avoidance of aspirin and all NSAIDs as patients with AIA can develop severe and occasionally fatal attacks with not just aspirin but a variety of NSAIDs. The likelihood of an NSAID triggering an asthma attack in these patients correlates with the drug's anti-COX potency and the dosage. If necessary, patients with AIA can tolerate paracetamol in a dose not exceeding 1,000 mg. If an NSAID must be given, a COX_2 inhibitor like rofecoxib is generally felt to be safer.

Several trials have shown that chronic treatment with a leukotriene antagonist may be protective. However, individual AIA cases have been reported who developed bronchospasm after taking NSAID despite being on treatment with montelukast. Inhaled corticosteroids and intranasal fluticasone are also protective. A state of aspirin tolerance can be induced and maintained by aspirin desensitization. Small incremental doses of aspirin are ingested over the course of a few days until 400–650 mg of aspirin is tolerated. Aspirin can then be administered daily, with doses of 80–325 mg used to maintain desensitization. After each dose of aspirin, there is a refractory period during which NSAIDs can be taken. This is important in patients with AIA who have chronic arthritis and rheumatic disease in whom these drugs are regularly needed. Nasal inflammatory disease responds best to this strategy, with a study showing that aspirin desensitization delayed reoccurrence of nasal polyp formation by an average of 6 years in patients who had just completed sinus and polyp surgery.

■ SUGGESTED READING

1. Ayres JG, Miles JF, Barnes PJ. Brittle asthma. Thorax. 1998;53:315-21.
2. Castro M, Rubin AS, Laviolette M, et al. Effectiveness and safety of bronchial thermoplasty in the treatment of severe asthma: a multicenter, randomized, double-blind, sham-controlled clinical trial. Am J Respir Crit Care Med. 2010;181:116-24.
3. Demissie K, Breckenridge MB, Rhoads GG. Infant and maternal outcomes in the pregnancies of asthmatic women. Am J Respir Crit Care Med. 1998;158:1091-5.
4. Harrison BD. Difficult asthma. Thorax. 2003;58:555-6.
5. Heaney LG, Conway E, Kelly C, et al. Predictors of therapy resistant asthma: outcome of a systematic evaluation protocol. Thorax. 2003;58:561-6.
6. Schatz M. Asthma during pregnancy: inter-relationships and management. Ann Allergy. 1992;68:123-33.
7. Watson JP, Lewis RA. Is asthma affordable in developing countries? Thorax. 1997;52:605-7.

CHAPTER 36

Chronic Obstructive Pulmonary Disease: Epidemiology, Etiopathogenesis, Clinical Features, Diagnosis and Imaging

■ INTRODUCTION

Chronic obstructive pulmonary disease (COPD) is a preventable, treatable, yet progressive inflammatory respiratory disease characterized by airflow limitation which is not fully reversible. COPD is a generic term which holds within it separate disease entities, often producing similar overlapping clinical features.

It is important to elaborate upon keywords in the above definition. The disease is considered to be preventable because cigarette smoking (and in India also bidi smoking) is the most important causative risk factor, so that not smoking would sharply reduce its prevalence. Yet COPD does occur in nonsmokers and the importance of other risk factors (some of which are to an extent preventable) are being increasingly recognized.

It is important to stress the word *treatable* with reference to COPD as in the past the disease was considered irreversible and hopeless in its prognosis. This was because patients came for treatment late in the natural history of the disease, at a point in time where treatment was of little or no help. It is now recognized that COPD may be partially reversible and that diagnosis and current treatment at an early stage can and does offer significant relief and benefit to the patient. Yet the disease is not truly curable and in fact is progressive at varying rates in different individuals. The definition given above hinges on the phrase *airflow limitation which is not completely reversible.* This stresses the underlying disturbance in lung function. The hidden clinical message underlying this phrase is that patients with COPD invariably have breathlessness on exertion and in severe cases breathlessness at rest.

According to the Global Initiatives for Obstructive Lung Disease *(Ref: Vestbo J, Hurd SS, Agusti AG, et al. Global strategy for the diagnosis, management, and prevention of chronic obstructive lung disease. GOLD executive summary. Am J Respir Crit Care Med. 2013;187:347-65)* airflow obstruction is present when there is a reduction of the post bronchodilator FEV_1/FVC ratio below 0.70. The severity of this obstruction is then graded or staged by the percentage of the postbronchodilator FEV_1 of the predicted normal FEV_1. The staging as per the GOLD recommendation is as follows in **Table 1**.

■ CHRONIC OBSTRUCTIVE PULMONARY DISEASE AND ASTHMA

A major difficulty is in distinguishing COPD from bronchial asthma, a disease characterized by airways obstruction which is often completely reversible. Yet patients with

Table 1: GOLD guidelines using spirometric findings to stage disease severity.

I	Mild COPD	$FEV_1/FVC < 0.7$; $FEV_1 \geq 80\%$ of predicted
II	Moderate COPD	$FEV_1/FVC < 0.7$; $FEV_1 \geq 50\%$ and $< 80\%$ of predicted
III	Severe COPD	$FEV_1/FVC < 0.7$; $FEV_1 \geq 30\%$ and $< 50\%$ of predicted
IV	Very severe COPD	$FEV_1/FVC < 0.7$; $FEV_1 < 30\%$ of predicted.

Table 2: Differences between asthma and COPD.		
	Asthma	*COPD*
Etiology	Sensitizing allergen	Smoking, other noxious particles or gases
Pathology	An inflammatory disease—chiefly eosinophilic infiltrate + CD4 lymphocytes	An inflammatory disease chiefly macrophages, CD8 lymphocytes, neutrophils in the cellular exudate
Disturbances in function	Significant exacerbations of airways obstruction with good or even complete reversibility	Airflow limitation which may worsen during acute exacerbation Not completely reversible—can be poorly reversible or irreversible
Bronchial hyperactivity	Marked (as judged by bronchial provocation tests)	Poor or absent in most patients
Family history	Often present	Not generally present
Skin allergy	Often present	Not present

difference between the two terms as is explained later) can therefore be considered as a spectrum; at one end is complete reversibility and at the other end is irreversibility. Patients often fall in between these two ends, there being an overlap at times between asthma and COPD.

In recognition of this overlap, GOLD and GINA issued a consensus statement on Asthma, COPD and Asthma-COPD overlap syndrome (ACOS, also referred to as Asthma-COPD overlap (ACO). This overlap is characterized by persistent airflow limitation with several features usually associated with asthma and several features usually associated with COPD. ACOS is therefore defined in clinical practice by the features that it shares with both asthma and COPD [*Ref: Global Initiative for Chronic Obstructive Lung Disease (GOLD). Global Strategy for the Diagnosis, Management and Prevention of Chronic Obstructive Pulmonary Disease: 2018 Report. www.goldcopd.org (Accessed on April 20, 2018)*]. There is on-going study to determine with certainty how treatment algorithms should be constructed for those patients.

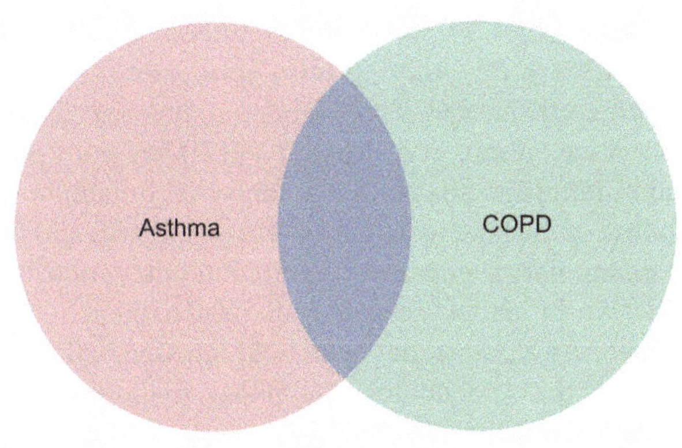

Fig. 1: Overlap seen in some patients with asthma and COPD.

longstanding asthma may show lesser and lesser degree of reversibility and some may ultimately end up showing little or no reversibility whatsoever. Asthmatics, with little or no reversibility may be indistinguishable from patients with COPD. Similarly, patients with COPD who show a fair degree of reversibility in their airways obstruction may be difficult to distinguish from asthmatics. There is also a similarity and overlap in the physiological disturbances underlying chronic asthma and COPD, as also between acute severe asthma and an acute exacerbation of COPD **(Table 2 and Fig. 1)**. Finally, COPD and asthma may coexist; patients with asthma who smoke or are exposed to noxious particles or gases may go on to develop poorly reversible or irreversible airflow limitation. Airflow limitation or airways obstruction (there is a subtle

■ ATOPY AND AIRWAY HYPERRESPONSIVENESS

The Dutch Hypothesis

In 1960 Dutch workers hypothesized that COPD patients with severe, nearly fixed airflow limitation and asthmatics shared a common constitutional predisposition of atopy, airway hyperresponsiveness and eosinophilia. This was contrary to Fletcher's findings that failed to show a relationship between the presence of allergy and an accelerated decline in forced expiratory volume in one second (FEV_1) in smokers. Studies in middle-aged smokers have however shown a relationship between airway hyperresponsiveness (as judged by methacholine or histamine test) and an accelerated decline in FEV_1. COPD patients also have an increase in immunoglobulin E (IgE) and some degree of eosinophilia though this is much less than in asthmatics. There is however, no evidence of atopy (as judged by skin tests) in COPD patients. It is debatable whether airway hyperresponsiveness is a cause or an important contributory factor to COPD as the Dutch maintain, or whether airway hyperresponsiveness is the result of COPD, as is believed by others.

It has been mentioned that COPD is a generic name inclusive of other disease entities. These disease entities are chronic bronchitis, small airways obstruction and emphysema. Whereas the defining feature of COPD is airflow limitation, chronic bronchitis is defined in clinical terms; bronchiolitis (causing small airways obstruction) and emphysema are defined in terms of pathological findings.

■ DEFINITIONS

Chronic bronchitis is clinically (though arbitrarily) defined as chronic cough with sputum on most days for at least 3 months in each of 2 consecutive years, when any other cause of chronic cough has been excluded. Chronic bronchitis need not necessarily cause airflow limitation. It can be classified into simple bronchitis characterized by hypersecretion of mucus; mucopurulent bronchitis characterized by recurrent or chronic mucopurulent sputum and obstructive bronchitis where productive cough is associated with airways obstruction.

Emphysema is defined as abnormal permanent enlargement of airspaces distal to terminal bronchioles accompanied by the disruption of alveolar walls without fibrosis. Emphysema (like chronic bronchitis) need not always cause airflow limitation.

Bronchiolitis causing small airways obstruction is characterized by inflammation and fibrosis in airways is less than 2 mm in diameter. Subtle early inflammatory changes occur in all cigarette smokers; these are undetectable by conventional lung function tests. Yet in susceptible smokers, these subtle changes are progressively amplified, being responsible for the airways obstruction and airflow limitation that characterize COPD.

In an individual case it is difficult to assess the relative contribution of airway disease (large and/or small airways) versus emphysema (air space enlargement with ruptured alveolar walls) to airflow limitation. Most patients have a mixture of both these contributing factors—some more of one and some more of the other. The term COPD was coined in the 1960s to denote airflow limitation from a combination of airway disease and emphysema without assigning the contribution of each of these to the airflow limitation.

The American Thoracic Society and the European Respiratory Society in their statement on the standards for diagnosis and care of patients with COPD have defined the disease as *a preventable and treatable disease characterized by airflow limitation that is not fully reversible. The airflow limitation is usually progressive and is associated with an abnormal inflammatory response in the lungs to noxious particles or gases, primarily to cigarette smoke. Although COPD affects the lungs it also produces significant systemic consequences.* The Global Initiative for Chronic Obstructive Pulmonary Disease (GOLD) has put forth a similar definition stressing the abnormal inflammatory response of the lung to noxious particles or gases and that extrapulmonary events and comorbidities may contribute to the severity of the disease in individual patients.

There are 2 points that need to be stressed before discussion of the epidemiology, pathology, pathophysiology and clinical features of COPD:
- COPD is not just a disease confined to the lungs; it is in a way a systemic disease with a number of comorbidities that influence the severity of the illness. These comorbidities are listed below and include weight loss with significant loss of lean muscle as the disease progresses **(Table 3)**.
- A number of other conditions such as bronchiectasis, bronchiolitis obliterans, cystic fibrosis and sarcoidosis which cause airways obstruction should not be

Table 3: Comorbidities of chronic obstructive pulmonary disease.

- Weight loss
- Loss of lean muscle mass
- Skeletal muscle dysfunction
- Osteoporosis
- Sleep disorder
- Anemia
- Psychosocial problems, in particular anxiety, depression
- Association of ischemic heart disease, diabetes, acid peptic disease

considered under COPD but should be considered in the differential diagnosis. Similarly, burnt out or active tuberculosis with inflammatory damage to the airways, or airway obstruction secondary to or a sequel of any other infective or obstructive pathology is not to be considered under COPD **(Table 4)**.

Yet COPD could well coexist with many of these other diseases which cause airways obstruction. In many developing countries, including India, several Asian and South American countries, tuberculosis and COPD may both be present in many patients, as risk factors for both these diseases are strongly prevalent. In patients with both these diseases each would be expected to contribute to the degree of pulmonary disability. However, there is little recent information on the result of the interaction between these two common diseases. Earlier works suggest that the degree of airways obstruction in patients treated for tuberculosis increases with age, the number of cigarettes smoked and the extent of initial tuberculous disease.

■ EPIDEMIOLOGY

Chronic obstructive pulmonary disease is a significant cause of worldwide morbidity and mortality. Both are clearly on the rise. In 1990, COPD was the 12th leading cause of morbidity and the 6th leading cause of death in the world. In 2002, it was the 6th leading cause of morbidity and the 4th leading cause of death. It is projected that by 2020 COPD will be the 5th leading cause of disability and the 3rd leading cause of death worldwide, the 1st two leading causes being ischemic heart disease and cerebrovascular disease. Its upward climb on the ladder of morbidity and mortality is greater than any of the other chronic diseases.

The prevalence of COPD varies in different countries but is almost certainly more than what is reported. The reasons for this are obvious—for one, in spite of current standard definitions of the disease, there are different concepts of COPD, particularly in Asian countries; also, spirometric studies to confirm the diagnosis of COPD are often lacking. Diagnosis is often made only when the disease is clinically evident, by which time it is already moderately advanced. Patients with early COPD with minimal or no symptoms therefore go undetected.

Global Epidemiology

The global prevalence of physiologically defined chronic obstructive pulmonary disease in patients aged more than 40 years and falling into the category GOLD stage more than 2 is approximately 10%.

The Burden of Obstructive Lung Disease (BOLD) study found that the prevalence of COPD in Gold stage II or higher was 10.1% being 11.8% in men and 8.5% in women. This study revealed marked variance in the prevalence rate between different countries.

The PLATINO study which studied five Latin American countries using post bronchodilator spirometry, reported the prevalence of chronic airways obstruction to be 14.3% and the proportion of those belonging to stage II of the COPD GOLD classification had a prevalence of 5.6%.

The Center for Global Health Research and WHO collaborating Center for Population Health Research and Health training, University of Edinburgh, have published their results on the global and regional estimates of COPD prevalence. These estimates are based on a systematic reviews and meta-analysis of population based studies providing spirometric based prevalence rates of COPD across the world from January 1990 to December 2014. They estimated from the meta-regression epidemiological model, 227.3 million cases of COPD in the year 1990 among people aged ≥ 30 years, corresponding to a global prevalence of 10.7% in this age group. The number of COPD cases increased to 384 million in 2010 with global prevalence of 11.7%. Across WHO regions the highest prevalence was in the Americas (13.3% in 1990 and 15.2% in 2010) and the lowest in Southeast Asia (7.9% in 1990 and 9.7% in 2010). The percentage increase in COPD cases between 1990 and 2010 was highest in the Eastern Mediterranean region (118.7%) followed by the African region (102.1%), while the European region showed the lowest increase (22.5%). The researchers in the above mentioned centers noted a marked paucity of studies in SE Asia, Africa and the Eastern Mediterranean region.

Table 4: Pathologies and clinical entities other than COPD that can present with chronic airways obstruction and which should be distinguished from COPD.

- Bronchiectasis
- Sarcoidosis
- Tuberculosis
- Bronchiolitis obliterans
- Cystic fibrosis
- Other burnt-out infective pathologies
- Tropical eosinophilia
- Langerhans' cell histiocytosis (histiocytosis X)
- Lymphangioleiomyomatosis

The increase in COPD prevalence in many parts of the world is alarming as also the increasing economic burden posed by this increase, particularly in poor countries.

Epidemiological Data in Southeast Asia and India

In the developing world comprising of Southeast Asia, the Asia Pacific region and India, the epidemiological data is scanty, often involving localized areas; also, the data is not easily accessible, as in some Southeast Asian countries it is often published in local languages. Nevertheless there is little doubt that the burden of COPD is significantly underestimated in Asian countries.

Model Estimates of Chronic Obstructive Pulmonary Disease in Asian Countries

Actual scientifically performed studies on the prevalence rate in Asian countries are unavailable. In the absence of such field studies, the Asia-Pacific Round Table Group used a statistical model to project the prevalence of COPD in 12 countries in 2000. The rates varied significantly between 11 Asian countries and Australia from a minimum of 3.5% (Hong Kong, Singapore) to a maximum of 6.7% (Vietnam). The overall prevalence in this study was 6.3% which is higher than the rate of 3.9% extrapolated from the WHO study. The estimated rate for China was 65/1000 which was again 2.5 times greater than that estimated by the WHO study. The considerable variation in the prevalence rate of COPD in the Asia-Pacific region is due to two factors—most importantly the different smoking habits in these countries and also the proportion of the population living in rural areas.

The high-prevalence rates of COPD in many Asian countries projected by the Asia-Pacific Round Table Group in turn reflect the increased prevalence of and exposure to risk factors, chiefly cigarette smoking, but also to occupational factors, indoor pollution from biofuels and environmental outdoor pollution. These projected prevalence rates need to be confirmed by actual field studies. Till then these figures can be used by governmental organizations to allocate resources to mitigate the physical and economic burden caused by the disease.

Field studies in Asia include those from Kim et al., from South Korea in 2005 who reported a prevalence rate as high as 17.2% and of Fukuch et al., from Japan in 2004 who reported a prevalence rate of 10.9%.

The Epidemiology and Impact of COPD (EPIC) Asia population based survey *(Ref: Lim S, Chi-Leung Lam D, et al. Impact of COPD in the Asia-Pacific region: The EPIC Asia population-based survey, Asia Pacific Family Medicine. 2015;14:4)* noted that the overall COPD prevalence was 6.9%, with 19.1 of these subjects having severe COPD, indicating a substantial socioeconomic burden.

Prevalence Studies in India

India is a huge country and there is no study that gives a reliable prevalence rate of COPD for the country as a whole. In fact such a study would pose tremendous logistical difficulties and other problems. In the few studies reported from India in the past 3 decades, the prevalence of COPD was twice as much in men than women with a mean smoking association of 82%. A multicenter study on the epidemiology of COPD and its relationship with tobacco smoking and environmental tobacco exposure was reported by SK Jindal *(Ref: Jindal SK. Emergence of chronic obstructive pulmonary disease as an epidemic in India. Indian J Med Res. 2006;124(6):619-23)* **(Fig. 2)**. They studied urban and rural populations in Bengaluru (South India) and in Chandigarh, New Delhi, Kanpur (all metropolitan cities in North India). COPD was diagnosed in 4.1% of 35, 295 subjects, the male to female ratio being 1.56:1 and the smoker to nonsmoker ratio being 2.65:1.

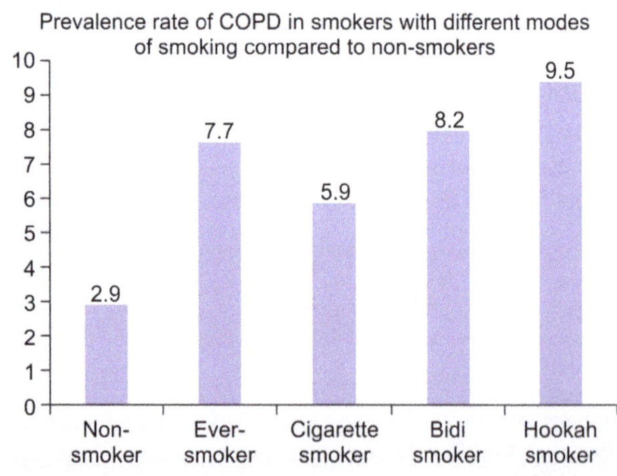

Fig. 2: Indian scenario: Smoking habits.
Source: Adapted from Jindal SK, Agarwal AN, et al. A Multicentric study on epidemiology of chronic obstructive pulmonary disease and its relationship with tobacco smoking and environmental tobacco smoke exposure. Indian J Chest Dis Allied Sci. 2006;48:23-9.

Prevalence of COPD among bidi smokers was 8.2% and among cigarette smokers 5.9%. The odds ratio for COPD was higher for men, elderly individuals and in those from the lower socioeconomic strata. They concluded that both cigarette and bidi smoking had a significant association with COPD. In nonsmokers, especially women, exposure to indoor air pollution due to the use of biofuels (for heating and cooking) was an important risk factor. More significantly, exposure to environmental tobacco smoke was an established cause of COPD. The risk from environmental tobacco smoke exposure in non-smokers was equally significant in children and adults.

A retrospective study (2005) from a chest clinic in Hyderabad showed the prevalence rate of COPD to be 6.85%. The prevalence rate in males was 7.4% and in females 4.64%. A history of 10-pack years of smoking was seen in 87.7% of patients with COPD. Only 12.3% of COPD patients were nonsmokers.

The Indian study on the Epidemiology of Asthma, Respiratory symptoms and Chronic Bronchitis in Adults (INSEARCH), involving a total 85,105 men and 84,470 women from 12 urban and 11 rural centers reported an overall prevalence rate of chronic bronchitis in adults more than 35 years to be 3.4%.

It must be kept in mind that it is impossible to determine how close to or far from the truth are the results reported from Southeast Asia and India. There are hardly if any studies from these regions based on spirometric studies. Mckay and colleagues reported that they could not identify a single high quality study that provided a detailed estimate of COPD prevalence using a relatively standard spirometry based definition , and were therefore unable to perform a meta-analysis *[Ref: McKay AJ, Mahesh PA, Fordham JZ, et al. Prevalence of COPD in India: a systematic review. Prim Care Respir J. 2012;21(3):313-21].*

■ ECONOMIC BURDEN OF CHRONIC OBSTRUCTIVE PULMONARY DISEASE

The economic burden of COPD with regard to cost of healthcare and the indirect drain on economy due to disability caused by the disease is extremely high in Western countries. For example, in the UK, the NHS bears an estimated cost of £ 819 million with 54% of the costs being caused by hospital admissions and 19% caused by drug treatment. Respiratory disease is the 3rd most common cause of disability, COPD accounting for 56% of these lost days in men and 24% in women. Bronchitis,

emphysema, COPD and asthma account for 24.4 million lost working days per year.

Unfortunately, reliable figures for the economic burden in developing countries are unavailable. The World Bank or WHO have introduced a new term called the *Disability Adjusted Life Years* for determining the economic and social burden of a particular disease, which can then be compared with other diseases. This is a composite of years lost by premature death and the number of years lived with disability, adjusted for the severity of the disability. By this yardstick, respiratory diseases account for over 20% of the global economic cum social burden of all diseases. This is likely to increase in the coming years with COPD projected to be the 5th leading cause of disability and the 3rd leading cause of death by 2020. The dramatic projected rise in the global economic and social burden caused by respiratory diseases in general and COPD in particular, will be chiefly related to the increased morbidity and mortality from tobacco smoking and to an ageing population. Both these factors will operate most of all in the developing world, constituted by India, the Asia-Pacific region, the South American continent and perhaps also in Africa. For example the smoking prevalence rate by gender in different countries in Southeast Asia is given in **Figure 3**.

The developing world therefore in the years to come will face a formidable challenge requiring a huge financial outlay on healthcare with regard to COPD and respiratory diseases. The economic burden entailed could well-retard overall prosperity and social welfare in these countries.

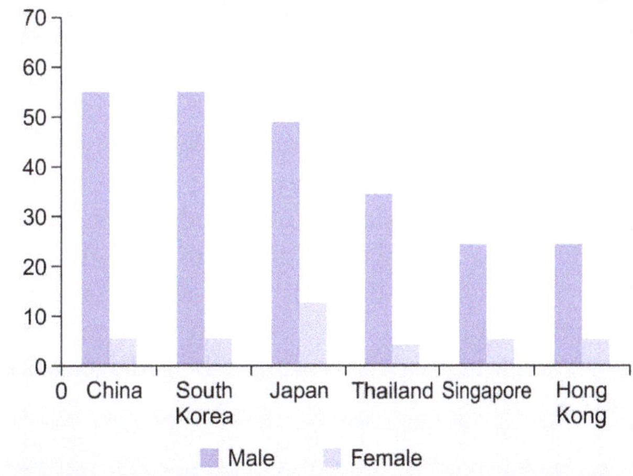

Fig. 3: Smoking prevalence by country-gender in South-east Asia. *Source:* Adapted from Regional COPD Working Group. COPD prevalence in 12 Asia-Pacific countries and regions: projections based on the COPD prevalence estimation model. Respirology. 2003;8(2):192-8.

ETIOLOGY, ENVIRONMENTAL RISK FACTORS

Cigarette Smoking

The evidence pointing to cigarette smoking as the most important cause of COPD is overwhelming. There are certain features in the relation between cigarette smoking, impaired lung function and COPD that need to be stressed:

- All cigarette smokers whose respiratory system is exposed to cigarette smoke on a long-term basis show an inflammatory response within the respiratory system. Also, in general, there is a direct relationship between the degree of smoking and impairment of lung function, those smoking more and for a longer duration having a greater impairment of lung function. Yet a great deal of variability exists, in that some heavy cigarette smokers have near normal lung function. Clinically significant COPD can be said to develop in 10–20% of smokers, though currently this figure is felt to be an underestimate. The evolution of COPD in 20% or more of smokers is related to a marked amplification of the inflammatory response to cigarette smoke. The reason for this is debatable and is the subject of research. *It needs also be noted that 20% or more of patients with COPD have been lifelong nonsmokers, pointing to the role of other etiological or risk factors in the causation of this disease.*

- Fletcher and colleagues in a prospective eight-year study on working men in London showed that while the average decline in FEV_1 in nonsmokers was just 30 mL/year, the average decline in smokers was 60 mL/year. However in the 20% of smokers who developed COPD, the average decline in FEV_1 per year was significantly greater (as high as 100 mL/year) pointing to the increased susceptibility of this group to the effects of cigarette smoke.

Fletcher and colleagues also showed that stopping smoking led to a normal rate of decline of FEV_1. The Lung Health Study confirmed the distinct beneficial effect of quitting smoking on the FEV_1, thereby confirming the important role of cigarette smoking in the pathogenesis of COPD **(Fig. 4)**.

- The work of Doll and Petro in the UK provides strong evidence linking smoking with mortality from bronchitis. The death rate for chronic bronchitis in male doctors between 35 years and 64 years of age fell between 1953–57 and 1961–65 by 24%, compared

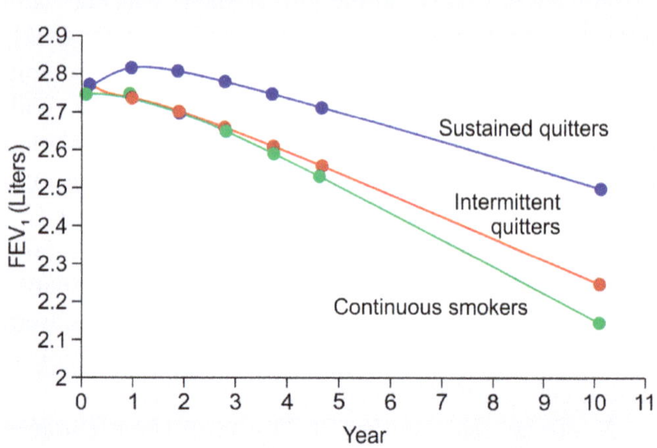

Fig. 4: Decline in FEV_1 over years in sustained quitters, intermittent quitters and continuous smokers.
Source: Reprinted with permission of the American Thoracic Society. Copyright © American Thoracic Society. Anthonisen NR, Connett JE, Murray RP. Smoking and lung function of lung health study participants after 11 years. Am J Respir Crit Care Med. 2002;166(5):675-9. Official Journal of the American Thoracic Society, Diane Gern, Publisher.

to a fall of 4% in other men in the UK of the same age group. These differences in mortality were related to the decrease in smoking habits in doctors in 1961–65.

- There is evidence that in general the risk of developing COPD increases with the increasing degree of cigarette smoking and increasing exposure to cigarette smoke. Work in India suggests that the same holds true for bidi smoking. The bidi is the Indian equivalent of the cigarette, consisting of a rolled up tobacco leaf stuffed with tobacco powder. Pipe and cigar smokers have higher mortality and morbidity rates than nonsmokers, though not as great as cigarette smokers.

The relation of cigarette smoking and the number of cigarettes smoked to the decline in lung function (in particular decline in FEV_1) may perhaps also be influenced by tar, nicotine and other contents within a cigarette, the extent to which the cigarette smoke is inhaled and whether a cigarette is smoked to its bitter end or is discarded midway.

- Studies on exposure to environmental tobacco smoke (passive smoking) suggest a statistically insignificant trend towards an increased relative risk to airflow limitation. Exposure to environmental tobacco smoke all through childhood was associated with significantly low FEV_1 level during adulthood. Maternal smoking is clearly harmful to the fetus, as the newborn child has a low birth weight and presumably reduced lung growth and reduced lung function. To what extent these findings relate to the risk of future development of COPD is difficult to ascertain. Reduced lung function in childhood persisting into adulthood could perhaps accelerate the risk of COPD, particularly in smokers.

Chronic Mucus Hypersecretion

Population studies show that smokers have a greater prevalence of cough and sputum due to hypersecretion of mucus when compared to nonsmokers. Petro and coworkers in an eight-year prospective study in London were unable to show a correlation between the degree of mucus secretion and the accelerated decline in FEV_1 or mortality. They however showed that both mortality and morbidity were strongly related to the development of a low FEV_1. However, another study in a general population in Copenhagen (Copenhagen City Lung Study) in 1976–1994 indicated that mucus hypersecretion is associated with an increased risk of hospitalization for COPD and an increased mortality from COPD. This association between mucus hypersecretion and mortality from COPD is even more marked when the airflow limitation increases and FEV_1 decreases. Mucus hypersecretion in patients with an FEV_1 of 40% of predicted value was then associated with four-fold mortality from COPD compared to a group whose FEV_1 was 80% of predicted.

Bronchopulmonary Infections

Chronic obstructive pulmonary disease patients are prone to recurrent bronchopulmonary infections and one would expect these recurrent infections to accelerate a decline in lung function. However, Fletcher, Petro and colleagues in their prospective eight-year study showed that this was not so. Acute bronchopulmonary infections did cause a temporary decline in lung function which could last for some weeks but which recovered completely. Neither mucus hypersecretion nor bronchopulmonary infections were shown to cause a more rapid decline in FEV_1 after due adjustments were made for age, smoking and the values of FEV_1.

These results have been challenged by the later Lung Health Study which showed an association in smokers between lower respiratory tract infection and an accelerated decline in lung function. Other recent population studies in patients with COPD support this finding.

Differences in the degree of airflow obstruction in the population studied by Fletcher and colleagues from that studied by the Lung Health Study and more recent studies probably explain the different findings.

■ ENVIRONMENTAL RISK FACTORS IN NONSMOKERS

For several years research was chiefly concentrated on smoking as the main risk factor for COPD, so that several prevalence studies in COPD were chiefly done on smokers. However, over the past 10–12 years many studies have suggested that risk factors other than smoking are also strongly associated with COPD. These factors include indoor and outdoor air pollution, bronchopulmonary infection in childhood, occupational exposure to dust and fumes, history of pulmonary tuberculosis, chronic asthma, intrauterine growth retardation, poor nutrition and poor socioeconomic state. Unquestionably smokers whose major risk factor is smoking, could also be exposed to all risk factors experienced by nonsmokers. Some of these risk factors are briefly discussed below.

Prevalence of COPD in Nonsmokers

The United States-based National Health and Nutrition Examination Survey (NHANES III) study reported the prevalence of COPD in nonsmokers to be 6.6%, the diagnosis of COPD being based on a post-bronchodilator spirometric recording of FEV_1/FVC is less than 70%. This study also suggested that a quarter of COPD patients in the US were never-smokers. A similar proportion of COPD never-smokers was reported from the UK (22.9%) and Spain (23.4%).

Figure 5 shows the proportion of nonsmoking COPD patients worldwide. The proportion of non-smoking COPD patient is well over 20% and is reportedly as high as 45% in South Africa. In many studies the diagnosis of COPD was based on the FEV_1/FVC ratio being less than 70%; in some (including the study from South Africa) it was based on the findings observed on a respiratory symptoms questionnaire. A study by Brashier B from the Chest Research Foundation, Pune reported the prevalence of COPD to be 6.7% and the proportion of COPD patients who never smoked as high as 68.6%. This study was on 12,053 subjects over 45 years of age, living in the poorer area of Pune. However, the diagnosis of COPD was based

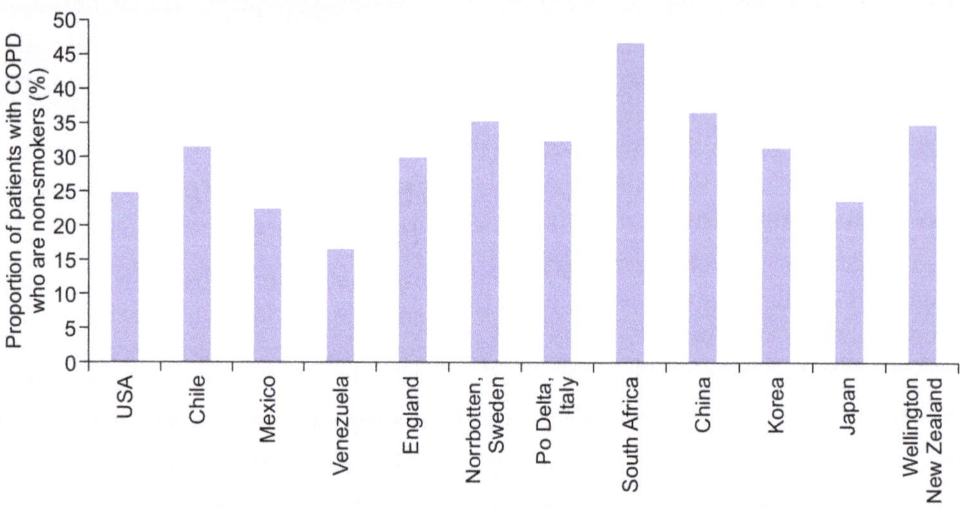

Fig. 5: Proportion of patients with chronic pulmonary disease (COPD) who are nonsmokers worldwide.
Source: Adapted from Salvi SS, Barnes PJ. Chronic obstructive diseases in nonsmokers. Lancet. 2009;374:733-43.

on a respiratory symptoms questionnaire and not on the basis of FEV_1/FVC ratio is less than 70%.

The overall data strongly suggests that the prevalence and burden of COPD in nonsmokers is much higher than what was earlier believed. The risk factors for COPD in nonsmokers are considered below.

Indoor Pollution

Indoor pollution is related to the combustion of biomass fuels which are chiefly derived from the use of wood, grass, vegetable matter, animal dung and charcoal. It is not sufficiently realized that worldwide about 50% of all households and 90% of rural households use biomass fuel as their chief source of domestic energy, chiefly for cooking and heating. By this estimate, about 3 billion people globally are exposed to smoke from incomplete combustion of biomass fuel compared to 1.01 billion who smoke tobacco. More than 80% of households in China, India and Sub-Saharan Africa use this fuel for cooking and 30–75% of homes in South America do likewise. The smoke arising from the burning of biomass fuel is heavily polluted with particulate matter ($< 10\,\mu m$—PM_{10}), nitrogen dioxide, sulfur dioxide, carbon monoxide, formaldehyde, and polycyclic organic compounds, including carcinogens. It therefore appears from the figures stated above that exposure to smoke from these biofuels may be an extremely important global risk factor for COPD. A study suggests that about 50% deaths from COPD in developing countries are due to exposure to smoke from biofuels, of

which about 75% are women. Women are at far greater risk for COPD because they use this fuel for cooking and heating purposes. Studies from India, Pakistan, Nepal, and Turkey have amply confirmed this. In North India, where it is bitterly cold in winter, the use of biofuel for heating and cooking in small rooms with little or no ventilation has led to increasingly severe airways obstruction. Severe COPD with cor pulmonale and right heart failure is observed at a comparatively very young age in these women, in striking contrast to cor pulmonale and right heart failure due to tobacco smoke which generally occurs at a much older age.

Outdoor Air Pollution

The role of outdoor air pollution was recognized following various air pollution episodes, particularly the smog in London in 1952 which led to an excess of deaths from respiratory disease. Though Western countries have cut emission of smoke and sulfur dioxide to an extent, the problem of air pollution in developing countries like India is acute and is likely to increase manifold. The high density of the population in large metropolitan cities (such as Mumbai, New Delhi, Kolkata, Bengaluru, Chennai, Hyderabad) together with the ever increasing number of poorly maintained vehicles careening across narrow congested streets, pose a great risk factor to the development of respiratory symptoms and declining lung function. Current studies show an association between high levels of particulate air pollution that exists in several urban centers and respiratory symptoms and hospital admissions in patients with COPD. Air pollution with particulate matter at more than permissible levels (< 100 $\mu g/m^3$) is the rule rather than the exception in the large cities of India and in many other cities in the world as well. Increased levels of particulate air pollution are associated with deaths from all causes, particularly cardiorespiratory deaths. There is also a clear association between levels of air pollution and exacerbations of COPD. The role of long-term exposure to outdoor air pollution as a risk factor in the development of COPD is perhaps particularly important in the nonsmoking group, though evidence to this effect is not conclusive. There is evidence that air pollution can cause mucus hypersecretion but evidence to show that it causes an accelerated decline in FEV_1 is debatable.

Bronchopulmonary Infections in Childhood

Recurrent bronchopulmonary infections in childhood might adversely affect lung function. It has been suggested that these children grow into adults with unhealthy lungs and have a greater predisposition to COPD as they age.

Children in developing countries are even more prone to recurrent bronchopulmonary infections, particularly when they come from poor homes that use biofuels for cooking and heating. Women who cook and clean in such homes often carry their babies or small children strapped to their back, so that exposure to smoke is as great in the children as in their mothers. Indoor air pollution is therefore a major factor responsible for acute lower respiratory tract infections, which in turn is an important cause of death in developing countries. Around 20% of 12 million deaths in children younger than 5 years of age are due to lower respiratory tract infections. Nearly all these deaths occur in developing countries, the majority in Asia (42%) and Africa (28%). Here again, children who survive these infections may do so with impaired lung function which might predispose them to COPD in later life.

Occupational Exposure

There is a relationship between occupational exposure to organic and inorganic dusts and to the hypersecretion of mucus leading to symptoms of chronic cough and sputum. A longitudinal follow-up of workers exposed to dust over some years has shown a relation between exposure and a decline in FEV_1.

Occupational exposure probably accounts for at least 10–15% of patients who have chronic respiratory symptoms or show a decline in lung function consistent with COPD. In the big cities of India, workers exposed to dust at construction sites, as also those in flour mills grinding grain and those exposed to dust in numerous dusty occupations, are at special risk of developing chronic respiratory symptoms with persistent airways obstruction. Miners exposed to dust in mines besides being at risk for pneumoconiosis are also at risk for developing cough, sputum and increasing airflow limitation. COPD is a hazard faced by welders due to exposure to welding fumes; workers exposed to cadmium are at risk of developing emphysema.

Numerous other factors may interact and perhaps accentuate the effects of occupational exposure. These include smoking and the possible interaction between smoke and dust, as also the effect of air pollution to which many of these poor workers are exposed either at home or in their workplace.

Pulmonary Tuberculosis

There are many who consider that airways obstruction and airflow limitation occurring with active or burnt out pulmonary tuberculosis should not be categorized under COPD. Yet there are many doctors, particularly those working in poor developing countries who question this concept. Pulmonary tuberculosis has been noted to be associated with airflow obstruction during the active phase and also several years after treatment has ended. Airways obstruction is related to the immune response to the mycobacterium that results in airways inflammation and airways fibrosis which is characteristic of COPD. The degree of airways obstruction is correlated with the extent of the disease and the length of time after treatment.

A large population-based study in five Latin American cities showed that the prevalence of COPD (judged by a post-bronchodilator value of $FEV_1/FVC < 70\%$) was 30.7% for patients with a history of tuberculosis and 13.9% in those without this specific history. A history of pulmonary tuberculosis increased the risk of COPD by 4.1 times in men and by 1.7 in women after adjustment for age, sex, ethnicity, smoking habits, exposure to dust, smoke and respiratory morbidity in childhood.

Considering the fact that over 2 billion people in our world are infected with *Mycobacterium tuberculosis* and that there are well over a million new cases of pulmonary tuberculosis every year, the association of COPD with pulmonary tuberculosis is an added burden, especially in developing countries, where the prevalence rate of tuberculosis is very high. The question that needs to be researched is whether this phenotype of COPD is similar to that of COPD caused by smoking; both with regard to natural history and response to pharmacotherapy.

Chronic Asthma

It has already been mentioned that in some severe chronic asthmatics, reversibility of airways obstruction is small or even absent, due to remodeling of the airways from thickening and fibrosis of the bronchial walls. The distinction from COPD in these patients may be impossibly difficult. These asthmatic patients have a pattern of inflammation similar to that of COPD, with increased neutrophils, interleukin-8, proteases, oxidants and a poor response to corticosteroids.

In a retrospective study of more than 300 patients from a rural population in India, it was observed that 75% of patients with poorly-controlled asthma, who had received an oral bronchodilator drug alone, had clinical features characteristic of COPD. Therefore inadequate treatment of severe chronic asthma could well be a risk factor for COPD. This risk is even greater in the developing countries of the world, where for several reasons severe chronic asthma is poorly treated, thereby perhaps contributing to the overall burden of COPD in these countries.

Socioeconomic Conditions

The risk of COPD is greater in those living in poor socioeconomic conditions. This may be related to exposure to indoor and outdoor pollution, poor housing, diet, exposure to repeated infections and other socioeconomic factors.

Gender

Though historically the incidence of COPD is more in men than in women, recent studies in developed countries suggest a near equal distribution between men and women. In North India, where women are markedly exposed to the combustion products of biofuels, the incidence of COPD in women is significantly higher than in other parts of the country.

Growth and Nutrition

Many studies suggest that the incidence of death from COPD varies inversely with the weight at birth and at the age of one year. It seems that impaired growth of the fetus *in utero* is a risk factor in the future development of respiratory disease including COPD. Similarly, impairment of lung growth during gestation is believed to be a potential factor for the future development of COPD.

■ HOST-RELATED FACTORS

Genetic Factors

Genetic factors in COPD are being increasingly researched upon. From the clinical standpoint the possibility that genetic factors may play a role in COPD is suggested by:

- The observation that there is occasionally a clustering of COPD in families.
- Reduction of maximal expiratory air flow rates among nonsmoking relatives of patients with early onset COPD.
- Most importantly, the observation that only about 20% of smokers develop COPD—what is it that prevents 80% of smokers from not developing COPD?

The only proven genetic factor is the one associated with α_1-antitrypsin deficiency. Here again, even in patients with an identified genetic risk factor there is an unexplained variability in the development of COPD.

Polymorphism of genes involved in inflammation, immune response, antioxidant function and protease-antiprotease balance have been implicated in COPD, but none of these has as yet been confirmed. The importance of an interaction between genetic and environmental factors cannot be ignored; it remains a difficult subject for ongoing research.

The reader is referred to the work done by the Genome Wide Associated studies for further details on the subject.

Airway Hyperresponsiveness (AHR)

The Dutch hypothesis stated earlier, believes that an underlying airways hyperresponsiveness is an important contributing factor to the development of COPD. However, smokers do not show AHR until their FEV_1 is already reduced and the experimental induction of emphysema can result in AHR. It is possible and more likely that emphysema may be the cause of AHR rather than AHR contributing significantly to this disease.

■ ALPHA-1 ANTITRYPSIN DEFICIENCY

Alpha-1 antitrypsin deficiency is an inherited disease that can affect the lungs and the liver. In the lung it leads to emphysema and COPD starting in young adulthood. The lung disease progresses, causing crippling respiratory disability and premature death from severe respiratory failure in many patients. In the liver, alpha-1 antitrypsin deficiency may result in the benign neonatal hepatitis syndrome. Some with this deficiency develop hepatic fibrosis progressing to cirrhosis of the liver. Hepatocellular carcinoma can be a complication of cirrhosis related to alpha-1 antitrypsin deficiency. Only the pulmonary manifestations of alpha-1 antitrypsin deficiency are dealt with here.

The alpha-1 antitrypsin deficiency molecule is produced in the liver and its main function in the lung is antiproteolytic, so that it protects the lungs from the proteolytic enzymes which if left unopposed would lead to destruction of lung tissue. The molecule is also believed to regulate immune defense within the lung. A great deal of research has been done on the genetics and the biology of the alpha-1 antitrypsin molecule as also on the pathophysiology of the lung in alpha-1 antitrypsin deficiency. There still remain lacunae on some issues, in particular the reason why only a few patients with this deficiency manifest pulmonary disease.

Features suggestive of alpha-1 antitrypsin deficiency are given in **Table 5**. The genetics, clinical features, diagnosis and treatment have been discussed below.

Genetics

Alpha-1 antitrypsin deficiency is an autosomal recessive disease. The *SERPINA1* gene (formerly known as *PI)*, which encodes the alpha-1 antitrypsin protein, is 12.2 kb, located on the long arm of Chromosome 14 (14q31–32.3) and is markedly pleomorphic. The variants are classified depending on their influence on the alpha-1 antitrypsin level in the blood. The M alleles (M1 to M6) are most commonly found; these are considered to be normal *variants* and are not associated with a fall in alpha-1 antitrypsin levels. Disease occurs as a result of an abnormal mutation of the alpha-1 antitrypsin gene resulting in consequences at several different levels **(Flowchart 1)**. These include deletion of the gene, degradation of unstable m-RNA transcripts, accumulation of alpha-1 antitrypsin in the endoplasmic reticulum, degradation of the antitrypsin protein before its translocation to the golgi complex, and finally difficulty in the effective release of alpha-1 antitrypsin.

The extensive ongoing research on the genetics of this disease is beyond the scope of this book.

The normal serum concentration of alpha-1 antitrypsin is 20–52 μmol/L. It is an acute phase protein whose production is increased during pregnancy, inflammatory diseases and cancer. The released alpha-1 antitrypsin inactivates proteolytic enzymes released in the lungs. Proteolytic enzymes are normally produced in abundance in the lungs as a result of immune responses to air borne pathogens to which the airways and parenchymal lung tissue are constantly exposed. The most important and powerful protease resulting from these immune

Table 5: Features suggestive of alpha-1 antitrypsin deficiency.
• Pulmonary emphysema without risk factors such as smoking, occupational exposure, exposure to dust, exposure to combustion products of biofuels, or heavy environmental pollution
• Pulmonary emphysema at a young age <45 years
• Pulmonary emphysema predominately involving the lower lobes
• Family history of emphysema, or chronic bronchitis or liver cirrhosis in ancestors
• Chronic active hepatitis or cirrhosis of unknown etiology

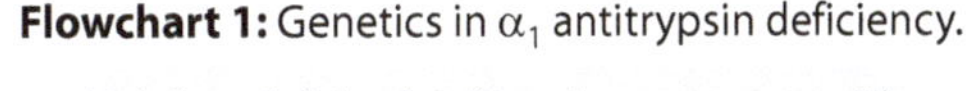

Flowchart 1: Genetics in α_1 antitrypsin deficiency.

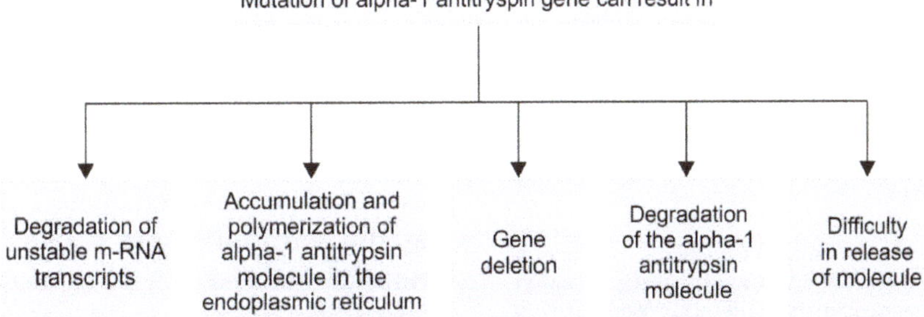

responses is neutrophil elastase, which is effectively inhibited by alpha-1 antitrypsin in a ratio of 1:1. There are other important lung protease inhibitors. These include secretory leucoprotease inhibitor (SLPI) and elafin, both of which are present in a much lower concentration when compared to alpha-1 antitrypsin.

Prevalence

India

The prevalence of alpha-1 antitrypsin deficiency in India is underdetermined as there is no significant reliable data on this subject. Perhaps screening of appropriate patients with COPD or bronchitis may unearth more patients than what is apparent today.

North America, Europe

The highest allele frequencies for alpha-1 antitrypsin deficiency are found in the Caucasians of Europe and America. US African Americans have the lowest. Prevalence estimates for typical deficiency genotypes (SZ, ZZ, SS) of the disease in North America and some of the larger European countries are given in **Table 6**.

Among European countries, Spain and Portugal have the highest prevalence estimate for the deficiency genotypes SZ, ZZ, SS.

Table 6: Estimated percentage of individuals with alpha-1 antitrypsin genotype SZ, ZZ, SS in the total population of North America and some European countries.

Country	SZ	ZZ	SS
France	0.195	0.017	0.578
Germany	0.041	0.010	0.044
Italy	0.075	0.027	0.052
Netherlands	0.044	0.010	0.046
Portugal	0.356	0.019	1.667
Spain	0.360	0.030	1.087
Russia	0.007	0.001	0.009
Sweden	0.113	0.053	0.060
UK	0.065	0.014	0.078
US Caucasian	0.022	0.036	0.052
US African American	0.006	0.002	0.022

Source: Adapted from de Serres FJ, Fernandez-Bustillo E, Lara B, et al. Estimated numbers and prevalence of PI*S and PI*Z alleles of alpha1-antitrypsin deficiency in European countries. Eur Respir J. 2006;27(1):77-84.

Southeast Asia

The database for seven countries in Southeast Asia is given in **Table 7**. The study consisted of twenty cohorts with a total cohort sample of 4,547. The study demonstrated that the PiS and PiZ alleles are found in Malaysia and Thailand, with only the PiS allele found in the Philippines and Singapore, with neither the PiS nor PiZ alleles present in Indonesia, New Guinea or Vietnam. With an estimated total population of 473, 595, 032 for these seven countries, the total population at risk consists of 5, 761, 832 carriers and 93, 062 deficiency allele combinations for PiS and PiZ.

Pathophysiology

It has been shown in all countries that the number of clinically identified patients with lung disease is far less than the anticipated prevalence rate as judged on allele frequencies. However 85% of individuals with the ZZ variants manifest pulmonary disease. The ZZ variants are characterized by the substitution of lysine for glutamic acid at position 342 of the amino acid sequence on the alpha-1 antitrypsin molecule. For this reason, protein synthesis in the endoplasmic cytoplasm of the hepatocytes is delayed, so that 85% of synthesized molecules polymerize into larger concentrates, only a little of the nonpolymerized molecule being released into the blood stream. The antiproteolytic effect exerted by this small release of the alpha-1 antitrypsin molecule is 5 times less than what would accrue with normal levels of alpha-1 antitrypsin. Thus the balance between proteolytic activity within the lung and antiproteolysis is tilted markedly in favor of the former. The released proteases over a few decades destroy the alveolar walls, lung matrix, vessels, giving rise to progressive chronic obstructive lung disease with well-marked emphysema.

The alpha-1 antitrypsin molecule also regulates inflammatory processes in the lung. It exerts an anti-inflammatory effect and perhaps stimulates tissue repair and exerts antibacterial activity.

Current research suggests that polymerized ZZ alpha-1 antitrypsin molecules accumulate not only in hepatocytes but also in peripheral tissue. Bronchoalveolar lavage (BAL) fluid of these patients has revealed the presence of polymerized alpha-1 antitrypsin, suggesting that the antiproteolytic activity within the lung is further diminished. It has also been contended that the polymerized alpha-1 antitrypsin molecule may exert

Table 7: Estimates of the mean gene frequencies in different countries of Southeast Asia.

| Country | Cohorts | | Mean gene frequencies | | | |
	No.	Size	PiM	PiS	PiZ	Total population
Indonesia	5	724	0.9869	0.0000	0.0000	224,784,210
Malaysia	6	1,886	0.9692	0.0241	0.0013	21,793,293
New Guinea	2	182	0.9973	0.0000	0.0000	20,000
Philippines	1	243	0.9918	0.0021	0.0000	82,841,518
Singapore	1	385	0.9792	0.0065	0.0000	4,151,264
Thailand	4	1,064	0.9591	0.0226	0.0132	61,230,874
Vietnam	1	63	0.9921	0.0000	0.0000	78,773,873
Total	20	4,547	0.9732	0.0159	0.0036	473,595,032

Source: Adapted from Worldwide Racial and Ethnic Distribution of alpha-1 antitrypsin deficiency: Summary of an analysis of Published Genetic Epidemiologic Surveys. Chest. 2002;122:1818-29.

a proinflammatory effect in contrast to the monomer form of the molecule which is believed to have an anti-inflammatory effect.

Clinical Features

Pulmonary Manifestations

Cough with expectoration and progressive breathlessness generally occur by the age of 30–40 years. Severe COPD with panacinar emphysema develops over a few decades if the alpha-1 antitrypsin serum concentration is below 35% of the normal mean value (<0.8 g/L or <11 µmol/L). The course of the disease is punctuated by acute exacerbations with worsening of cough and breathlessness. Acute exacerbations are invariably related to airway or pulmonary infections; the additional release of proteolytic enzymes which remain unopposed adds to increasing destruction of alveolar walls, vessels and lung matrix. The end result is progressive crippling respiratory failure similar to advanced COPD unrelated to alpha-1 antitrypsin deficiency.

Physical examination, lung function tests show evidence of airflow limitation with increased lung volumes and reduced CO diffusion capacity. Chest radiography and computed tomography (CT) reveal the classic features of pulmonary emphysema. However, unlike other usual patients with COPD who have predominant emphysematous changes most marked in the upper lobes, patients with ZZ alpha-1 antitrypsin deficiency have emphysematous changes mainly in the lower lobes **(Fig. 6)**. As the disease progresses arterial blood gases

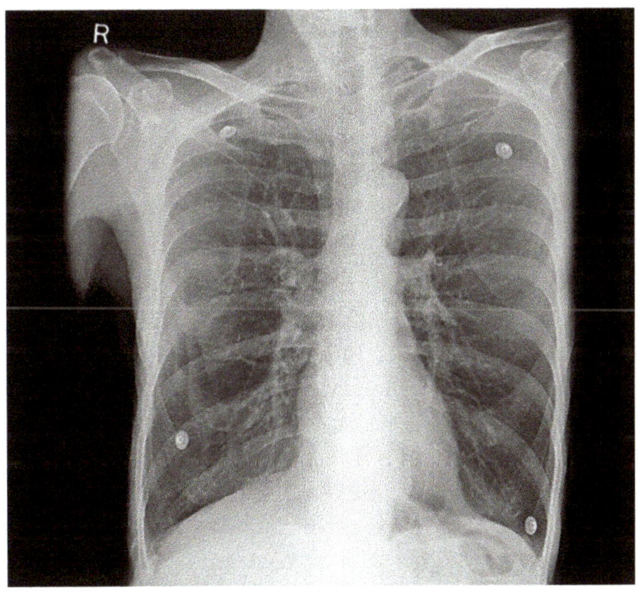

Fig. 6: Alpha-1 antitrypsin deficiency: Chest X-ray PA view demonstrates large areas of hypertranslucency in the lower zones with a tubular heart and compressed lung in the upper zones.

show hypoxemia and ultimately there is increasing hypoxemic plus hypercapnic respiratory failure.

Around 10% of patients with ZZ alpha-1 antitrypsin develop bronchial hyperreactivity. Large bullae may be present and pneumothorax remains a potential dangerous complication.

Other Organ Manifestations

Besides hepatitis and cirrhosis of the liver, alpha-1 antitrypsin deficiency is rarely associated with Wegener's granulomatosis, necrotizing panniculitis and aneurysms that may affect the abdominal aorta and/or cerebral vessels.

Diagnosis

Diagnosis depends on measurement of the concentration of alpha-1 antitrypsin in the serum, the normal range being 1.5–3.0 g/L or 20–52 µmol/L. It needs to be stressed that the alpha-1 antitrypsin molecule is an acute phase protein and the level is upregulated in inflammatory disease. The C-reactive protein should therefore be measured simultaneously, and if found high, the alpha-1 antitrypsin concentration (even if found to be normal) is unreliable, and needs to be repeated when the C-reactive protein is within normal limits.

If the alpha-1 antitrypsin concentration is below normal, a genotyping is performed. This allows genetic counseling of patients and their families and may help predict the severity and course of the disease.

It is unfortunate that screening of alpha-1 antitrypsin is very rarely practiced in hospitals in India. Perhaps screening tests in appropriate patients with COPD would prove that this deficiency is not as rare as is believed.

Treatment

Treatment is similar to that given to any COPD patient. Smoking cessation is imperative, as is exposure to occupational or environmental pollutants. Bacterial infection should be promptly countered with appropriate antibiotics. Lung volume reduction surgery recommended at one time is not generally recommended. Lung transplantation is recommended in severe cases. Replacement therapy with alpha-1 antitrypsin has been used in Europe and America for several years but the evidence for its efficacy is uncertain.

The etiology, risk factors in chronic obstructive pulmonary disease discussed in the earlier sections are summarized in **Table 8**.

■ PATHOLOGY OF CHRONIC OBSTRUCTIVE PULMONARY DISEASE

The pathology of COPD can be summarized as an inflammatory response of the lungs to inhalation of noxious particles or gases.

The overall pathological changes within the lungs in COPD can be summarized as follows:

Table 8: Etiology, risk factors in chronic obstructive pulmonary disease.

- Cigarette smoking, bidi smoking, hookah smoking; cigar, pipe smoking to a lesser extent than cigarette or bidi smoking
- Indoor and outdoor air pollution
- Occupational factors
- Bronchopulmonary infections in childhood
- Pulmonary tuberculosis
- Chronic unrelieved severe asthma
- Genetic factors (alpha-1 antitrypsin deficiency)
- Socioeconomic conditions
- Growth and nutrition (Low birthweight at age of 1-year; impairment of lung growth during gestation)

- Inflammatory changes in the large airways (> 2 mm), but more importantly in the small peripheral airways (< 2 mm), leading to their obstruction, fibrosis, with ultimate distortion.
- Loss of support to the airways because of rupture of alveolar attachments to the airways.
- Loss of elastic recoil of alveoli because of emphysematous changes.
- All three of the above occur in varying degrees in different patients.
- Inflammation of the large airways results in chronic bronchitis which has a clinical definition. Inflammation of the peripheral airways leads to bronchiolitis causing obstruction to the small airways. Inflammation leading to enlarged distal airspaces with rupture of alveolar walls leads to emphysema, a pathological entity.

Chronic Bronchitis

The characteristic pathological features of chronic bronchitis are summarized below:
- Inflammation of the bronchial mucosa and wall. There is in increased mucous secretion due to inflammatory changes in the central airways—trachea, bronchi, bronchioles greater than 2 mm in diameter. Mucous is produced by subepithelial mucous glands in the large airways and by goblet cells in the airway epithelium. There is an increase in the size and number of the mucous glands and of goblet cells. In healthy subjects goblet cells are chiefly present in the proximal airways and decrease peripherally; in chronic bronchitis goblet cells not only increase in number but extend more peripherally. The increase in number and size of mucous-secreting glands and cells leads to an increased volume of mucous secretion not only in the

central airways but also in the peripheral airways, where mucociliary clearance is comparatively inefficient. Inflammation of the bronchial mucosa and submucosa further contributes to excessive mucous secretion. Neutrophilic infiltration is present in the mucosa, submucosa and in mucosal glands; the inflammatory process increases with progress of the disease and during acute exacerbations. Inflammation also involves the bronchial wall. Neutrophils and macrophages are observed in bronchial biopsy specimens together with activated CD8 suppressor cells in contrast to the predominant CD4 cells seen in asthma.

There is in addition metaplasia of the airways epithelium, loss of cilia and disturbed ciliary function resulting in impaired mucociliary clearance. Stagnation of mucous leads not only to obstruction but possible infection. Hypertrophy and hyperplasia of the bronchial muscles with subepithelial fibrosis is also observed.

- Intraluminal inflammation. BAL studies and examination of sputum show evidence of intraluminal inflammation not necessarily associated with airways obstruction. Neutrophils predominate, together with the presence of chemotactic factors which include interleukins and leukotrienes. These inflammatory changes in the central airways induced typically by the noxious influence of cigarette smoke are aggravated during acute exacerbations. The latter are associated with some degree of eosinophilic infiltration of the bronchial mucosa and wall. Neutrophils, macrophages however still predominate in contrast to patients with bronchial asthma where the eosinophil remains the chief inflammatory cell.

Cessation of smoking usually brings symptomatic relief but bronchial biopsy studies indicate that a fair degree of inflammation in the bronchial lumen and wall still persists.

Small Airways Disease

It is believed that silent, often asymptomatic inflammation of the small airways (< 2 mm) is one of the earliest changes to occur in patients with COPD. These inflammatory changes may not be detected by routine spirometry and lung function tests. The nature of inflammation is similar to that described in the large airways, being characterized by an exudate of macrophages, lymphocytes, neutrophils, by goblet cell hyperplasia with excessive mucous production, increase in CD8 lymphocytes and an increase

in the CD8/CD4 ratio. The small peripheral airways (< 2 mm) of the lungs now contribute much more towards airflow resistance. As the inflammatory pathology in the small airways progressively worsens, obstruction increases. There now results a structural remodeling with subepithelial deposition of collagen, increasing fibrosis, scarring and further destruction of the airways.

Resistance to airflow is due to the following factors:

- Physical obstruction to small airways caused by mucous, cell debris, inflammation, narrowing and distortion.
- An airflow limitation caused by loss of alveolar attachments to the peripheral airways. These alveoli through their elasticity normally help to hold the peripheral airways open. The loss of this support leads to premature closing of the airways during expiration.

Emphysema

Emphysema is defined as abnormal permanent enlargement of air spaces distal to the terminal bronchioles and is accompanied by destruction of alveolar walls **(Figs. 7A and B)**. Emphysema is best understood with reference to the acinar unit, which is that unit of the lung being supplied by a single terminal bronchiole. Emphysema is of three main types **(Figs. 8A to C):**

- *Centriacinar or centrilobular emphysema,* in which large airspaces formed by ruptured alveoli cluster around the terminal bronchiole.
- *Panacinar or panlobular emphysema,* in which large airspaces due to ruptured alveolar walls are distributed throughout the acinar unit.
- *Periacinar or paraseptal emphysema,* where enlarged airspaces are found in the periphery of the acinar unit abutting against a fixed structure such as the pleura or septum or a lung fissure.

Centriacinar or centrilobular emphysema has a greater association with cigarette smoking than panacinar emphysema, though both types of emphysema can occur with smoking. Patients with centriacinar emphysema have greater inflammation and pathological involvement of the smaller peripheral airways, the distribution of the emphysema being more marked in the upper lobes. Panacinar emphysema is found in patients with alpha-1 antitrypsin deficiency and alpha-1 proteinase inhibitor deficiency. It is most evident in the lower lobes, but can also occur in patients who have no genetic abnormality.

Paraseptal emphysema occurs peripherally in the acinar unit and is of significance only when it is sufficiently marked in the subpleural region to cause a pneumothorax.

At times emphysematous areas occur irregularly as a sequel to inflammation resulting in scarring and local deforming of lung tissue unrelated to the acinar unit. This does not come under the present definition of emphysema.

Airspace enlargement in emphysema to start with is only visible microscopically. It can be visible macroscopically only when the airspace enlargement exceeds 1 mm **(Figs. 7A and B)**. A bulla is produced by rupture of many adjacent alveolar walls to result in an air space 1 cm or more in diameter. Small bullae may merge with one another to form one or more large bullae which may occupy the greater part of the lobe of a lung. Though the definition of emphysema excludes the presence of fibrosis, some degree of fibrosis is present as a feature of bronchiolitis involving the respiratory bronchioles in smokers.

Vascular Changes

Changes in the vessel walls of the pulmonary arteries occur early in the natural history of COPD. There is thickening of the intima, followed by increase in the smooth muscle of the media with infiltration by inflammatory cells consisting of macrophages and CD8-T-lymphocytes. As the disease progresses, further thickening of the intima and of the muscle within the media, together with deposition of collagen are noted. Hypoxia and hypercapnia so often observed in advanced COPD produce vasoconstriction. Ruptured alveolar walls lead to reduced cross-section of pulmonary capillaries in the lungs and promote further pulmonary hypertension. Pulmonary hypertension is responsible for right ventricular enlargement and right ventricular dysfunction (cor pulmonale).

■ PATHOPHYSIOLOGY OF CHRONIC OBSTRUCTIVE PULMONARY DISEASE

Chronic obstructive pulmonary disease is a heterogeneous disease in its clinical, physiological and pathological aspects. Its pathophysiology is therefore complex as it is dependent on abnormalities in the central conducting airways (> 2 mm), the peripheral airways (< 2 mm), the lung parenchyma, chest wall mechanics, respiratory and skeletal muscle function and structure. The combination of these abnormalities can culminate in crippling respiratory disability, manifest as progressive breathlessness, and disturbed gas exchange leading to respiratory failure and premature death. The function of the heart and lung are interdependent, so that changes in the structure and function of the lungs ultimately result in pulmonary hypertension and right ventricular hypertrophy with or without failure (cor pulmonale).

The starting point of the pathophysiology in COPD is inflammation of the peripheral airways together with destructive inflammatory changes in the periphery of the lung. The physiological disturbances consequent to this inflammation are characterized by obstruction to expiratory airflow and expiratory airflow limitation. There is a subtle but important difference between the terms

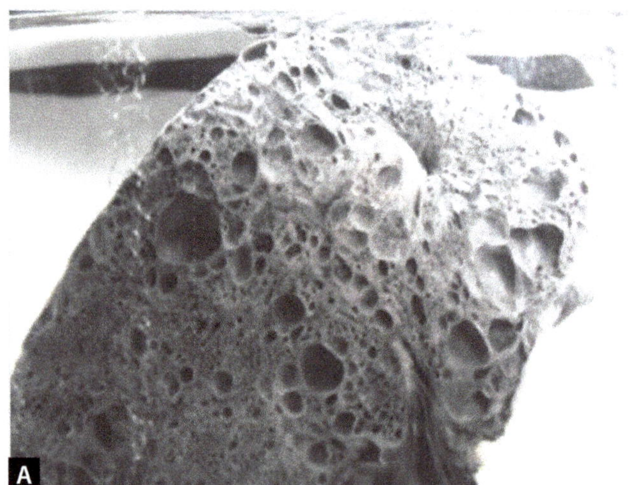

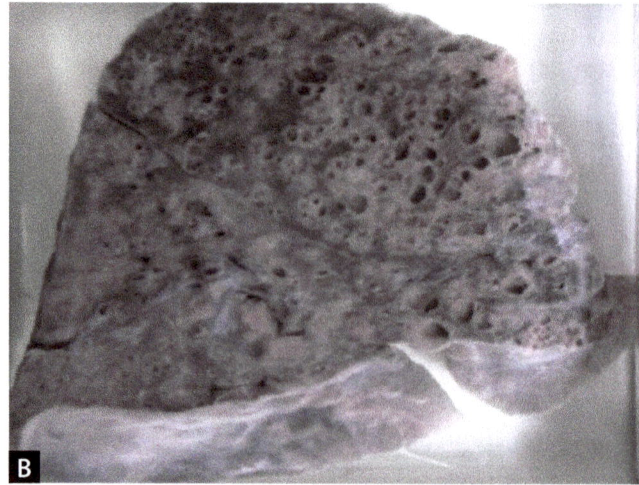

Figs. 7A and B: Cross-section of lung showing emphysematous changes.

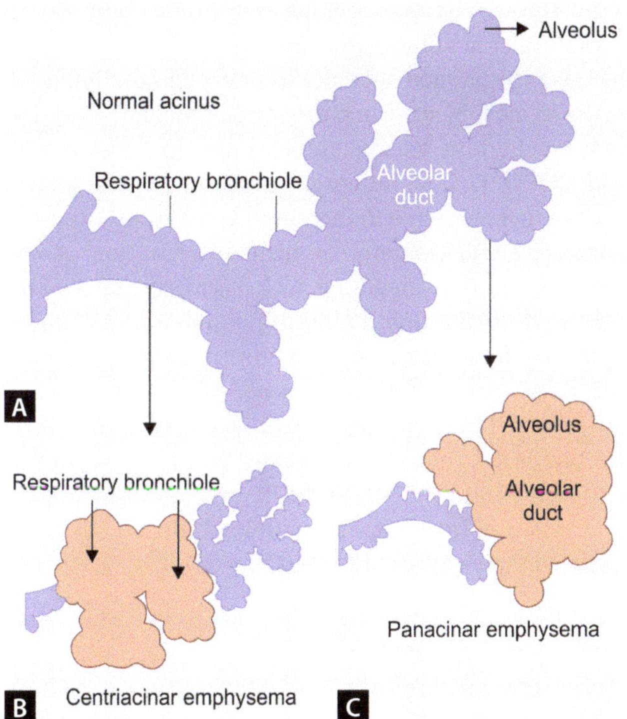

Figs. 8A to C: Major patterns of emphysema. (A) Normal structure within the acinus. (B) Centriacinar emphysema with dilation that initially affects the respiratory bronchioles. (C) Panacinar emphysema in which large airspaces due to ruptured alveolar walls are distributed throughout the acinar unit.
Source: Copyright © 2009 Saunders, An Imprint of Elsevier. This figure was published in, Kumar, Robbins, Cotran. Pathologic Basis of Disease, professional edition, 8th edition.

airways obstruction and expiratory air flow limitation. Expiratory airflow limitation is the expression used in the current definition of COPD. This is as it should be, for expiratory airflow limitation is the key physiological disturbance and the key mechanism that is responsible for progressive dyspnea and disability in patients with COPD.

Peripheral Airways (< 2 mm) in Chronic Obstructive Pulmonary Disease

The pioneering work of Hogg and coworkers *[Ref: Hogg JC, Chu F, Utokaparch S, et al. The nature of small-airways obstruction in chronic obstructive pulmonary disease. N Engl J Med. 2004;350(26):2645-53]* proved that the main site of airways obstruction is in the peripheral airways. As explained under *pathology*, this obstruction results from mucous plugging, inflamed walls, narrowing, fibrosis, distortion and even obliteration of many of these airways. Hogg and coworkers showed that widespread pathological changes in the peripheral airways in COPD

could be demonstrated without detectable abnormalities in routine pulmonary function tests such as spirometry and/or measurement of total pulmonary resistance. This is because of the small contribution of peripheral airways resistance to the total resistance at this early stage of the disease. This prompted Mead to term the small airways in the lungs as the *silent zone*. However, though these peripheral airways lesions were undetected by routine spirometry they can now be detected by special tests for peripheral small airways function. These include measurements of the closing volume (asymptomatic adult smokers have an increase in closing volume compared to nonsmokers), which is volume of isoflow, slope of phase III of the single breath nitrogen washout curve, and frequency dependence of lung compliance (worsening of lung compliance with increased rate of breathing). These are rather esoteric tests performed in special laboratories. Perhaps the only test easily performed and thought to mirror changes in peripheral airways is a reduction in the maximum expiratory flow at lung volume below 50%.

As COPD evolves in its natural history, *in vivo* measurements show a significant increase in total airway resistance, involving both central and peripheral airways. However, central airways resistance is noted to increase by just 50% whereas resistance of the peripheral airways show a fivefold increase.

The inflammation of peripheral airways also involves the periphery of the lung to a varying degree. This inflammation has two effects:

1. Disruption and loss of alveolar attachments to peripheral airways. It is these attachments which normally hold the peripheral airways open during expiration.
2. Disruption of alveolar walls (typical of emphysema) resulting in loss of elastic recoil.

Expiratory Airflow Limitation (Figs. 9 and 10)

Airflow limitation implies that expiratory flow cannot increase at a given lung volume by increasing intrathoracic pressure through forcible contraction of respiratory muscles. COPD is characterized by a reduction in the expiratory flow rates, the lower the flow rate at a given lung volume, the more severe the COPD. This reduction is due to two causes:

- Mechanical obstruction of peripheral airways due to mucus plugging, together with inflammatory changes in the bronchial wall.

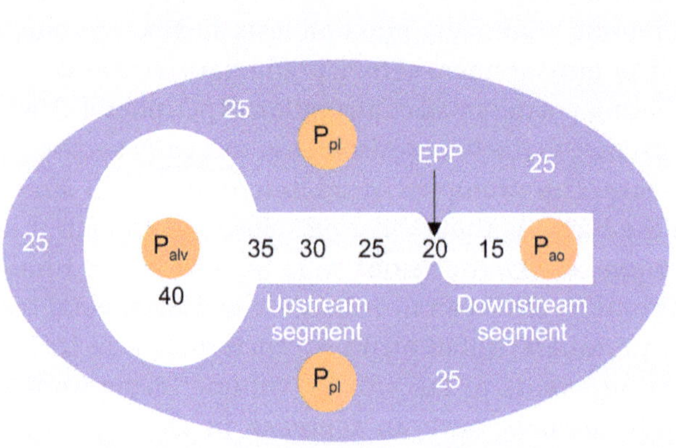

Fig. 9: Airway collapse resulting in an airflow limitation in a normal individual during forced expiration. Just as an example, pressure within the alveolus is equal to the intrapleural pressure of 25 mm Hg + alveolar recoil pressure (say 15 mm Hg), amounting to 40 mm Hg. Once the pressure within the airway falls below the intrapleural pressure, the airway closes thereby limiting expiratory airflow (*see* section on Lung Physiology). (P_{pl}: Intrapleural pressure; P_{alv}: Alveolar pressure; EPP: Equal pressure point).

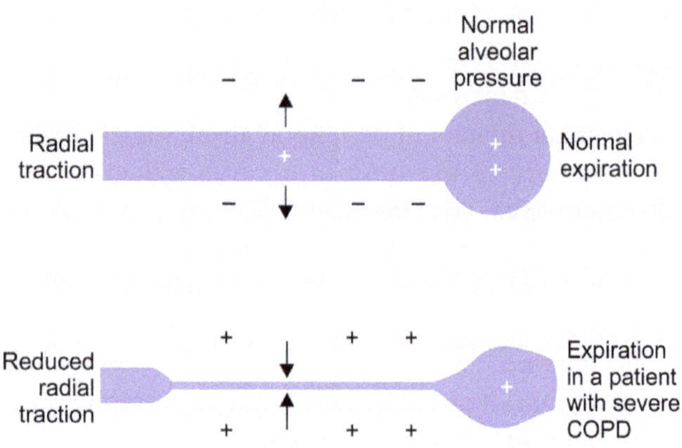

Fig. 10: Expiration in a normal individual and expiratory airflow limitation in a patient with severe COPD. Alveolar attachments to the airway wall keep the airway open during expiration in a normal individual. In severe COPD there is both a loss of elastic recoil and loss of alveolar attachments to the airway walls. The airways collapse even during normal expiration because of dynamic compression leading to a limitation of the expiratory flow rate.

- *Collapse* of the peripheral airways during expiration because of loss of elastic recoil and loss of alveolar attachments to the airways. Expiratory airflow limitation is therefore far more complex than mere

obstruction because it implies dynamic compression of the airways during expiration.

It needs to be pointed out that expiratory air flow limitation occurs in all subjects when the level of maximal flow has been reached. In normal subjects and in patients with mild COPD, airflow limitation occurs as the degree of exercise increases due to increased ventilation. However, in severe COPD, expiratory airflow limitation occurs during resting tidal breathing, which is to say that the flow generated during tidal breathing equals the maximum expiratory flow. These patients are unable to increase their tidal volume to meet increased ventilatory demand necessitated by activity, exercise or increased metabolism. The increased ventilatory demand can only be met by an increase in rate. This results in air-trapping, dynamic hyperinflation (as is explained below), necessitating an increase in the work of breathing.

Pulmonary Hyperinflation

Airways obstruction leads to an increase in the *resistive work* of breathing. The major consequence of expiratory airflow limitation is pulmonary hyperinflation. Pulmonary hyperinflation is characterized by an increase in the functional residual capacity (FRC) above the predicted value. In normal subjects FRC corresponds to the volume at which the inward elastic recoil of the lungs is counterbalanced by the outward elastic recoil of the chest wall. It measures 40% of the total lung capacity.

Static Hyperinflation

In COPD patients the static equilibrium value of the respiratory system is at a higher volume than in normal subjects. This is because of the loss of elastic recoil of the lungs. The outward elastic recoil of the chest raises the resting FRC to the volume of the chest wall.

Dynamic Hyperinflation (Fig. 11)

Dynamic hyperinflation is the mechanism responsible for progressive air-trapping within the alveoli leading to a progressive increase in the intra-alveolar pressure and the FRC. It can occur in severe COPD even when the patient is at rest. In moderately advanced COPD it can occur when the patient exercises or exerts. Most importantly, it can occur with frightening rapidity during an acute severe exacerbation of COPD. The underlying cause is airways obstruction and expiratory airflow limitation. As explained earlier, a dynamic compression and collapse

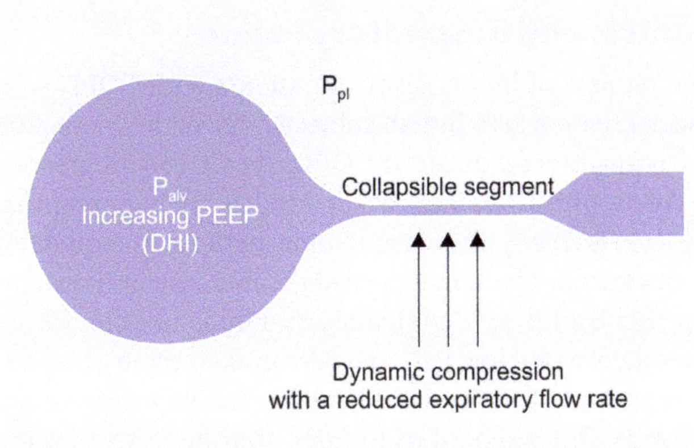

Fig. 11: Dynamic compression of the airways during expiration resulting in dynamic hyperinflation (DHI).

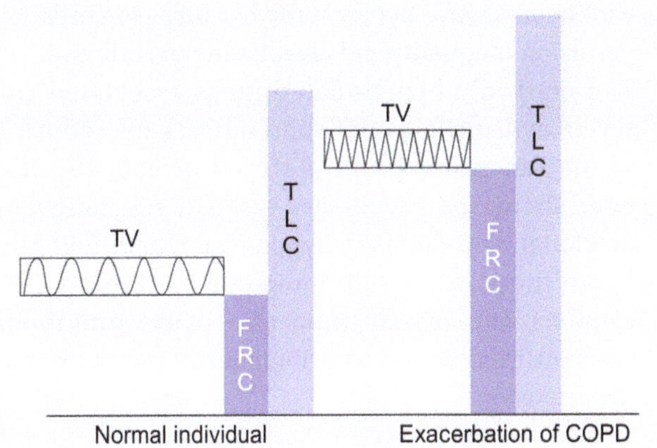

Fig. 12: Increased FRC with the patient breathing at higher lung volumes in severe COPD.

of the peripheral airways during expiration leads to a reduced rate of lung emptying. In these circumstances an inspiratory effort starts before the prolonged expiration is complete. Air is thus trapped in the alveoli causing a rise in the intra-alveolar pressure. The positive end-expiratory alveolar pressure continues to rise every time a prolonged expiration is prematurely cut short or interrupted by an inspiration. This progressive rise in positive end-expiratory alveolar pressure is termed intrinsic PEEP or auto-PEEP; it results in an increase in the FRC and in overinflated lungs.

Dynamic hyperinflation exerts a deleterious effort on the respiratory and circulatory systems:

- Breathing at higher lung volumes is greatly uncomfortable and causes increasing distress **(Fig. 12)**. The work of breathing is significantly increased because of an overinflated chest. An overinflated chest has ribs which are more horizontally placed; also the length tension relationship of the intercostal muscles is far from optimal so that the chest bellows work at a mechanical disadvantage. The low diaphragm and the decreased area of apposition between the diaphragm and the chest wall are further mechanical disadvantages adding to the work of breathing.
- Though it would appear that the expiratory muscles need to work hard because of expiratory obstruction to the airways and expiratory airflow limitation, it is in fact the inspiratory muscles that endure a great workload. This is because with each inspiration the inspiratory muscles need to contract strongly and generate a sufficiently negative intrapleural pressure so that the

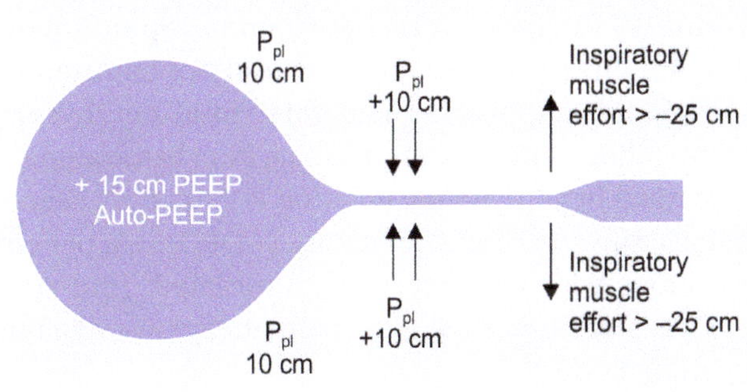

Fig. 13: An increased inspiratory effort is necessary to open collapsed airways and produce a sufficient negative intrapleural pressure to overcome the positive intra-alveolar pressure so as to allow inspiratory air flow. During expiration the intrapleural pressure of + 10 cm H_2O prematurely closes the airways. Total intra-alveolar pressure is 25 cm H_2O. During inspiration the inspiratory muscles must create a negative intrapleural pressure of well over – 25 cm H_2O to allow inspiratory airflow.

collapsed peripheral airways are pulled open and the pressure in the central airways and alveoli is rendered subatmospheric, to enable inspiratory air flow to occur **(Fig. 13)**. This increased work of inspiratory muscles is required when they are for reasons stated above working at a mechanical disadvantage. Therefore when dynamic hyperinflation is marked (as in an acute exacerbation of COPD), inspiratory muscle fatigue occurs, and may lead to a respiratory arrest.

- Increasing dynamic hyperinflation is often associated with hypoxia and hypercapnia because of ventilation-perfusion inequality and alveolar hypoventilation.
- The markedly hyperinflated lungs associated with severe dynamic hyperinflation squeeze the capillaries in the functioning and perfused alveoli, resulting in an increased pulmonary vascular resistance and precipitating pulmonary hypertension and right heart failure in patients with moderate to severe COPD. Hypoxia and hypercapnia also cause pulmonary vasoconstriction and contribute further to pulmonary hypertension.

Severe dynamic hyperinflation is associated with well-marked rise in the positive end-expiratory pressure (auto-PEEP) (*see* **Fig. 13**). This hinders venous return and causes hypotension. When the auto-PEEP is very marked, it exerts an effect similar to that seen in cardiac tamponade (caused by a large pericardial effusion). Severe dynamic hyperinflation with very high auto-PEEP can cause cardiac arrest. Hyperinflated lungs with increase in auto-PEEP can cause barotrauma. Spontaneous pneumothorax is the commonest result of barotrauma. Mediastinal emphysema and interstitial emphysema are two other complications resulting from barotrauma.

Marked hyperdynamic inflation is classically seen in patients with severe exacerbations of COPD, or in patients in a crisis who are incorrectly ventilated. End-stage COPD is also often associated with progressive dynamic hyperinflation.

Respiratory Muscles

The respiratory muscles, as has already been pointed out, work at a mechanical disadvantage. In addition, loss of muscle mass leads to muscle weakness. Malnutrition contributes even further to this muscle weakness. The flattened diaphragm also has a loss of muscle and fails to generate the usual inspiratory force during inspiration. In normal individuals expiration during tidal breathing is generally passive. Patients with COPD need to use their rib cage muscles and accessory muscles of respiration such as the sternomastoids even during quiet breathing. Global function of respiratory muscles has been shown to be impaired in some studies as judged by measurement of maximum inspiratory mouth pressures. Measurement of transdiaphragmatic pressure during inspiration suggests a reduced inspiratory force exerted by the diaphragm in COPD.

Pulmonary Gas Exchange, Ventilatory Control and Respiratory Failure

The pattern of blood gases in patients with COPD with special reference to Indian subjects is given in the section on acute exacerbation of COPD. As COPD progresses, there is often hypoxia associated with hypercapnia. Hypoxia is chiefly due to ventilation-perfusion inequalities or mismatch. There may be a slight increase in the shunt but this is of little significance and does not contribute materially to the low PaO_2. Hypercapnia is often observed in advanced COPD and is due to alveolar hypoventilation. There is still a school of thought that believes that the respiratory center in COPD is insensitive to the rise in $PaCO_2$, compared to normal individuals, so that the ventilatory drive does not increase with increasing $PaCO_2$. All current work, however, suggests that the ventilatory drive in COPD is indeed adequate. In fact Purrel et al., showed that even in very severe end-stage COPD (patients being ventilator-dependent) the ventilatory drive to breathe was not only preserved but was even greater than in stable conditions. Alveolar hypoventilation and CO_2 retention result because of the increase in dead space, and also because the *load* or the ventilatory demands in these patients cannot be matched by the effort the *chest bellows* are capable of.

The reason for mismatch between ventilatory demands (the work of breathing) and the effort required to meet these excessive demands are summarized below:

- Overinflated lungs in COPD can markedly increase the work of breathing.
- The abnormal configuration of the chest puts the *thoracic bellows* including the respiratory muscles and the flattened diaphragm, at a mechanical disadvantage. Wasting of the intercostals and weakness of both the intercostals and the diaphragm adds to the inability of the *effort* to meet the *load* **(Fig. 14)**.
- There is an excessive load on the mechanically disadvantaged inspiratory muscles of breathing because of premature closure of the peripheral airways during expiration with a resultant increase in intra-alveolar pressure (auto-PEEP).

Yet in clinical practice, one occasionally sees COPD patients who do not seem distressed or who do not make any undue effort while breathing. They seem to be breathing *lazily*. Perhaps therefore in some patients a poor respiratory drive in relation to increasing $PaCO_2$ may be at least partially responsible for hypercapnia.

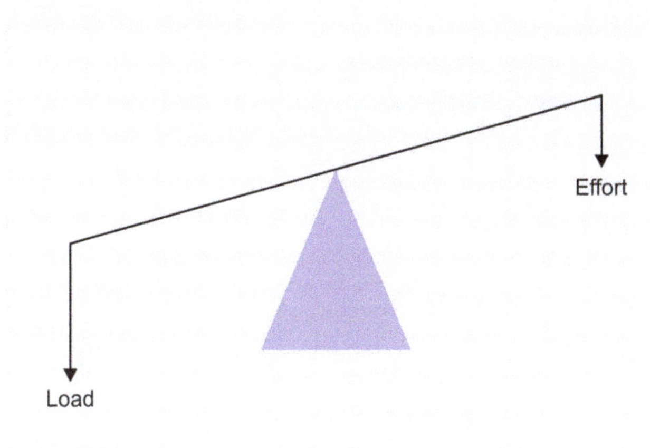

Fig. 14: The above figure shows how effort does not commensurate with the load.

As is pointed out in a subsequent section, though in advanced or severe COPD hypoxia and hypercapnia are present either at rest or during an acute exacerbation, about 10–15% of patients with severe COPD manage to keep their blood gases within reasonably normal limits almost right up to the very end of the natural history of the disease.

Cor Pulmonale

Cor pulmonale is defined as right ventricular hypertrophy with or without right heart failure due to disease of the lungs or the pulmonary circulation or due to chronic alveolar hypoventilation from other causes. The commonest cause of cor pulmonale is COPD. As COPD increases in severity it produces pulmonary hypertension which results in right ventricular hypertrophy and failure. Pulmonary hypertension in COPD is due to several factors:

- Inflammation and narrowing of the walls of pulmonary vessels is an accepted feature of COPD.
- Rupture of alveolar walls in emphysema reduces the total pulmonary vascular bed and contributes to pulmonary hypertension.
- Hypoxia and hypercapnia in advanced COPD lead to pulmonary vasoconstriction and pulmonary hypertension. This is so in stable COPD, but the marked increase in hypoxia and hypercapnia observed in severe exacerbation of COPD can cause an acute rise in pulmonary artery pressure.
- Once pulmonary hypertension is well established, the hypertension itself induces further intimal fibrosis and medial wall hypertrophy.

- Finally, thromboembolic complications are common in COPD and when present add to pulmonary hypertension.

Right ventricular hypertrophy with right heart failure is the end result. Some degree of tricuspid incompetence is also often present. Edema and later, ascites are due to increased systemic venous pressure and hormonal changes leading to salt and water retention.

■ SYSTEMIC EFFECTS OF CHRONIC OBSTRUCTIVE PULMONARY DISEASE

Chronic obstructive pulmonary disease is not just a disease confined to the lungs. It has important systemic effects which influence morbidity and mortality. These systemic effects are marked in patients with severe COPD. They include weight loss, skeletal muscle wasting and dysfunction of the muscles of respiration, including the diaphragm. Weight loss is associated with a poor prognosis. Loss of muscle mass has been shown to be related to systemic inflammation caused by inflammatory mediators, such as tumor necrosis factor, interleukins such as IL-6 and free oxygen radicals leading to oxidative stress. Other systemic effects of COPD include anemia, osteoporosis, nutritional deficiencies, psychological problems, in particular depression and perhaps a higher risk of cardiovascular disease.

■ PATHOGENESIS (TABLE 9)

There are three important factors contributing to the pathogenesis of COPD **(Flowchart 2)**:

- An amplification of the inflammatory response within the peripheral airways and lung parenchyma.
- Increased oxidative stress within the lungs.
- An imbalance between proteases and antiproteases.

Nature of the Amplified Inflammatory Response

The specific pattern of inflammatory response in COPD involves macrophages, neutrophils, T-lymphocytes, B-lymphocytes, and eosinophils. These cells release pro-inflammatory mediators which amplify inflammation and produce both structural and functional damage within the airways and lung parenchyma. Secretion of chemotactic factors attracts macrophages, lymphocytes and neutrophils to the site of inflammation within the respiratory tract.

Table 9: Inflammatory cells and inflammatory mediators in the pathogenesis of COPD.

Inflammatory cells	Inflammatory mediators

• Neutrophils:
  – Present in lumen of airways
  – Increase mucous secretion
  – Release proteinases
  – Increase in number with increasing severity of disease
	• Chemotactic factors:
	  – Lipid mediators, e.g. leukotrienes (LT) B4 which attract neutrophils, T lymphocytes
	  – Chemokines like IL-8

• Macrophages: – Present in lumen and wall of airways, in lung tissue and in BAL fluid	• Proinflammatory cytokines include TNF-alpha, IL-6, IL-8 which amplify the inflammatory process in the lung and are responsible for systemic effects

• T-lymphocytes:
  – Increase in CD8 cells and CD8/CD4 ratio
  – CD8 and Th1 cells secrete interferon γ and express CXCR3
  – CD8 cells cytotoxic to alveolar cells
	• Growth factors, e.g. transforming growth factor (TGF4) which may be responsible for fibrosis
	• Proteases destroying elastin:
	  – Serine proteinases
	  – Cysteine proteinases

• B-lymphocytes—present in peripheral airways and lymphoid follicles as a response to infection and chronic bacterial colonization	
• Eosinophils-increased in sputum and airways during exacerbation of COPD	
• Epithelial cells may be activated to produce inflammatory mediators	

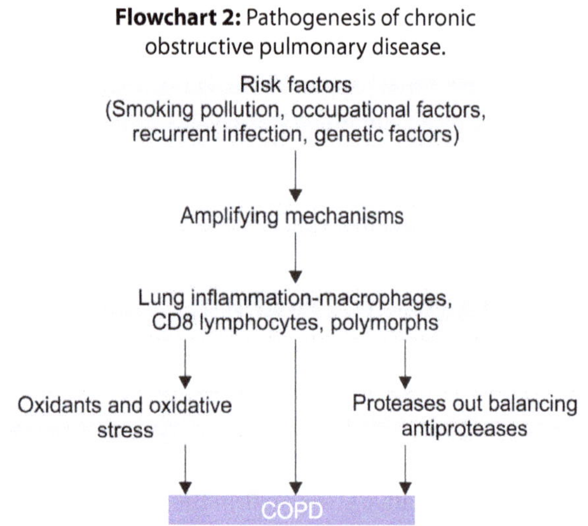

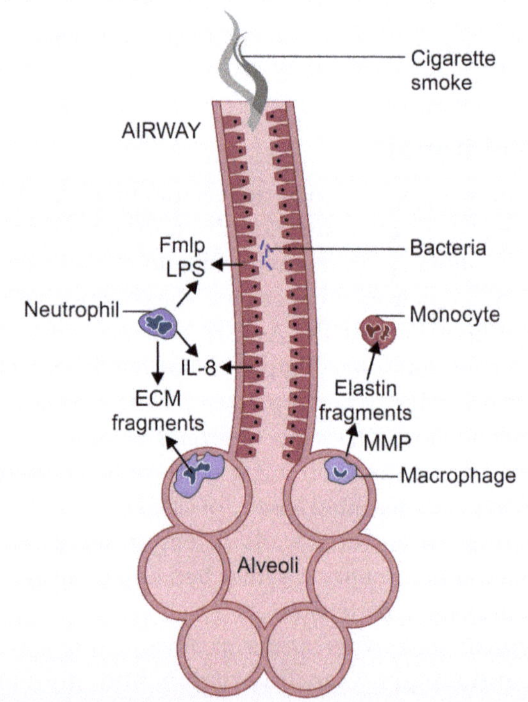

Fig. 15: Mechanism of inflammatory cells accumulation in the lung in COPD— neutrophils are recruited to the airways in response to bacterial products such as lipopolysaccharide (LPS) and IL-8 (from latent viral infections). Inflammatory cell recruitment within the alveolar space is related to activated constitutive macrophages releasing proteinases that produce extracellular matrix fragments (ECM) that are chemotactic for neutrophils and macrophages.

Inflammatory Cells in Chronic Obstructive Pulmonary Disease (Fig. 15)

Macrophages

These are derived from mononuclear cells within the blood but differentiate into macrophages within lung tissue. Macrophages are present in the lumen of the small airways, within the wall and in the lung parenchyma. They produce inflammatory mediators and proteases which amplify the inflammatory response to the irritant effect of cigarette smoke, or other noxious particles or gases.

Neutrophils

They are chiefly present in the lumen of the airways and show a marked increase within the lumen during periods of acute exacerbations. An increase in number is also related to COPD severity. Neutrophils may also be present in the walls and in lung tissue but to a much lesser extent.

T-Lymphocytes

There is a marked increase in CD8 lymphocytes, a lesser increase in CD4 lymphocytes, so that there is an increase in the CD8/CD4 ratio. The CD8+ cells together with the T helper type 1 (Th_1) cells secrete γ-interferon and express the chemokine receptor CXR3. CD8 cells are capable of damaging and destroying alveolar cells through a direct cytotoxic effect.

B-Lymphocytes

There is an increase of B-lymphocytes in lymphoid follicles and in the peripheral airways, perhaps resulting from chronic bacterial colonization and infection within the airways.

Eosinophils

Eosinophils are never as prominent as in bronchial asthma. They are increased within the sputum and within the airways during exacerbations.

Epithelial Cells

Epithelial cells within the airways may also be activated by the irritant effect of cigarette smoke or other noxious particles or gases to produce inflammatory mediators.

Inflammatory Mediators

These can be classified into three classes:
- Chemotactic factors
- Proinflammatory cytokines
- Growth factors.

Chemotactic factors include:
- Lipid mediators such as leukotrienes B4 (LTB4) which are chemotactic to neutrophils and T-lymphocytes.
- Chemokines like interleukin—8 (IL-8), which attract neutrophils and monocytes to the site of inflammation.

Proinflammatory cytokines include tumor necrosis factor (TNF-a), interleukins (IL-8 and IL-6). The interleukins increase inflammatory response and are believed to perhaps contribute to the systemic effects of COPD.

Growth factors include transforming growth factor which helps fibroblasts lay down fibrous tissue. The latter distorts peripheral airways contributing to airways obstruction.

The Role of Oxidative Stress

Oxidative stress plays an important role in amplifying inflammation in COPD. Oxidants are produced by cigarette smoke and other irritant particulate matter; these oxidants are released into the area of inflammation by neutrophils and macrophages. The proof of increased oxidative stress lies in the increase in biomarkers (hydrogen peroxide and B-isoprostane) of oxidative stress in the breath, sputum and systemic circulation of COPD patients. A possible reduction in endogenous antioxidants in COPD may well worsen the effects of oxidative stress.

The adverse effects of oxidative stress in the lungs include increased inflammation, increased mucus secretion, inactivation of antiproteases, and edema due to exudation of plasma from capillaries. The mechanism by which oxidative stress is translated into the adverse effects stated above is explained thus. Nitric oxide is generated by inducible nitric oxide synthase expressed in the peripheral airways and lung parenchyma of COPD patients. The interaction between superoxide anions and nitric oxide leads to the formation of peroxyl nitrite which mediates many of the adverse effects of oxidative stress on the lungs. It is further believed that oxidative stress may lead to an increased expression of inflammatory genes and a marked decrease in the anti-inflammatory action of corticosteroids due to a reduction in the histone deacetylase activity in the lung of COPD patients.

Protease-Antiprotease Imbalance

There is evidence that COPD is characterized by an imbalance between proteases which break down connective tissue and antiproteases which protect against this. Protease-mediated destruction of elastin present within connective tissue is an irreversible, established feature of emphysema. Proteases are derived from both inflammatory and epithelial cells. The 3 important groups of increased proteases in COPD are the serine proteases (represented by neutrophil elastase and proteinase 3), the cysteine proteinases (cathepsins B, K, L, S), and the matrix metalloproteinases (MMP-8, MMP-9, MMP-12).

The antiproteases that counter the serine proteases are alpha-1 antitrypsin, alpha-1 chymotrypsin, and secretory leukoprotease inhibitor. The antiproteases that counter the cathepsins are cystatins, and those countering the MMPs are the tissue inhibitors of MMP (TIMMP 1–4). The proteases outbalance the antiproteases leading to a poorly checked destruction of connective tissue within lung parenchyma, and rupture of the alveolar walls with resultant emphysema.

■ CLINICAL FEATURES

A history of risk exposure is important. Smoking cigarettes, bidis, hookahs, cigars, and pipes is the first and greatest risk. The patient often gives an incorrect assessment of the number of cigarettes or bidis smoked. Smoking history corroborated by a close relative or friend is therefore essential. The duration and intensity of cigarette smoking that should result in COPD varies from one person to another. In the absence of a genetic, environmental or occupational predisposition, smoking less than 10 to 15 pack years (packs of cigarettes per day multiplied by the number of years) is unlikely to result in COPD. The single best variable for predicting which adult will have airflow obstruction on spirometry is a history of more than 40 years of smoking *[Ref: Qaseem A, Wilt TJ, Weinberger SE, Hanania NA, Criner G, van der Molen T, Marciniuk DD, Denberg T, Schünemann H, Wedzicha W, MacDonald R, Shekele P, American College of Physicians, American College of Chest Physicians, American Thoracic Society, European Respiratory Society; Simel D, Rennie D. The rational clinical examination: evidence-based clinical diagnosis, McGraw Hill (Ed), New York 2008].* In most nonsmokers a history of indoor and outdoor urban pollution should be sought as also history of occupational exposure, particularly to dust. Indoor exposure to biofuels might have occurred several years before actual symptoms develop.

Symptoms

The 2 main symptoms of COPD are dyspnea on exertion and cough with expectoration, sometimes accompanied by a wheeze. Breathlessness initially is only on exertion like climbing stairs, walking uphill or walking fast on the level. It gradually worsens so that in the end-stage of the disease the patient is breathless at rest, often sitting up the whole day and night, every breath a struggle. The symptom of breathlessness on exertion in COPD signifies at least moderate airways obstruction and airflow limitation. Yet the perception of the

uncomfortable sensation associated with breathlessness and the increased workload of breathing vary in different individuals, so that a COPD patient with well-marked airflow limitation may clinically be less dyspneic than one with lesser disease.

However, once the FEV_1 is less than 35–40% of its predicted value, patients with COPD are breathless even on minimal exertion. In well-established disease, breathlessness is often worsened in the winter months, or following increased air pollution, or an increased exposure to dust. The degree of breathlessness can be assessed using the Medical Research Council Dyspnea Scale or the Borg Scale **(Table 10)**.

The O_2 cost diagram **(Fig. 16)** is more sensitive to the change in breathlessness with progression of the disease than the MRC scale. The patient marks on a 10 cm line, the point beyond which he or she feels breathless. The distance between *zero* and the marked point enables a score to be obtained.

Cough may be dry but is usually productive, being associated with mucoid sputum. A careful history in smokers generally reveals the presence of cough even before breathlessness appears, the patients ignoring this as a smoker's cough, till such time as breathlessness on exertion ensues either in the natural course of the disease, or is triggered by pulmonary infection. Cough may be severe enough to cause fracture of the ribs, particularly in advanced disease or in osteoporotic patients.

Table 10: Modified MRC dyspnea scale.		
Category	**Degree of dyspnea**	**Effect**
0	None	Not troubled by shortness of breath except with strenuous exercise
1	Slight	Troubled by shortness of breath when hurrying on the level or walking up a slight hill
2	Moderate	Walks slower than people of the same age on the level because of shortness of breath
3	Moderately severe	Has to stop because of shortness of breath when walking at own pace on the level
4	Severe	Stops for breath after about 100 yd or after a few minutes on the level
5	Very severe	Too breathless to leave the house or breathless when dressing or undressing

Based on information to classify the severity of dyspnea according to the categories proposed by the Medical Research Council (MRC).

Source: Mahler DA, Wells CK. Evaluation of clinical methods for rating dyspnea. Chest. 1988;93(3):580-6.

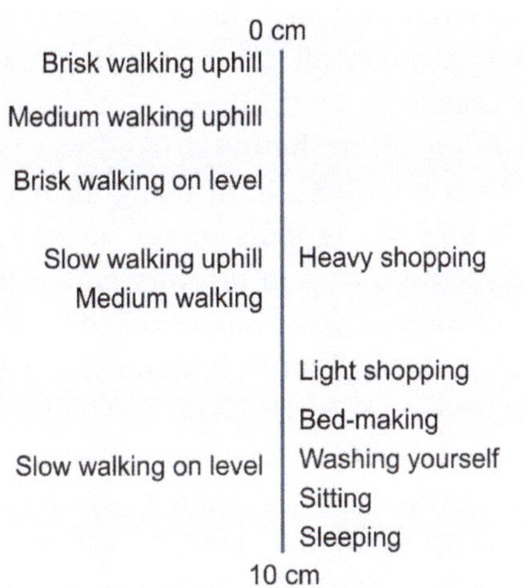

Fig. 16: Oxygen-cost diagram.

Chest discomfort is often complained of, particularly during periods of exacerbation of breathlessness. This discomfort or tightness may resemble ischemic cardiac pain; it is probably related to the increased workload of breathing borne by intercostal muscles working at a mechanical disadvantage.

Pleuritic chest pain should always suggest the possibility of pneumonia, pulmonary infarction or pneumothorax. Hemoptysis may occur with a complicating acute pulmonary infection but should always prompt the search for bronchogenic carcinoma, particularly in smokers. Weight loss with muscle wasting is a frequent feature of advanced COPD, due to poor nutrition and/or increased metabolism. Patients with severe disease are unable to sleep because of breathlessness and cough. Psychiatric disturbances, in particular depression are frequently observed.

Physical Findings

The physical findings may be completely normal early in the natural history of COPD. Physical findings basically ensue from the degree of airflow limitation and the extent of pulmonary hyperinflation that is present.

General Examination

Patients with COPD come for medical attention generally in the fifth or sixth decade. The respiratory rate is often increased, but more importantly the expiration is prolonged, a forced expiratory time greater than 5 sec suggesting airflow limitation. The forced expiratory time can be roughly assessed by auscultation over the trachea during forced expiration. Classically, the prolonged expiration in patients with COPD may be associated with breathing through pursed lips, but this need not be so. The accessory muscles of respiration, in particular the sternomastoids, show active contraction. In severe COPD the nails, lips and tongue may be cyanosed. Clubbing of the nails is absent and when present should suggest underlying bronchiectasis or a bronchogenic carcinoma. The patient may be drowsy or even comatose because of CO_2 retention. Flapping tremors of the hands or of the whole upper limbs (asterixis) may be observed for the same reason. Rarely, CO_2 retention can lead to papilledema and seizures.

Examination of the Respiratory System

In advanced COPD the chest is barrel-shaped with an increase in the anteroposterior chest diameter. This is due to kyphosis, an elevated sternum, elevated and horizontally placed ribs, a prominent sternal angle and a wide subcostal angle. The elevation of the sternum reduces the space (normally 3-finger breadths) between the suprasternal notch and the cricoid cartilage. These peculiarities in the shape of the chest are due to overinflated lungs. Besides the use of the accessory muscles of breathing there is often an indrawing of the intercostal spaces and of the suprasternal notch during inspiration. This is due to the marked increase in the negative intrapleural pressure caused by the strong contraction of the intercostals during inspiration. The flat position of the diaphragm often tugs the lower costal margin inwards during inspiration.

Palpation reveals poor chest expansion. Percussion reveals decreased cardiac and hepatic dullness. In advanced COPD the cardiac dullness may be totally lost. Auscultation typically reveals prolonged expiration with a wheeze more marked during expiration than inspiration. The wheezes are polyphonic though this may be difficult to appreciate. Crackles are also often heard over the bases, chiefly in early inspiration. In many cases with advanced COPD the breath sounds are diminished. An auscultatory wheeze is not always heard. In fact, patients with advanced COPD often have no audible wheeze when breathing normally. It is important to ask the patient to perform a forced expiratory maneuvre when a *tight* wheeze may just be audible.

Cardiovascular System

The heart and lung are closely linked and increasing COPD produces changes in the circulatory system.

Carbon dioxide retention produces a hyperdynamic circulation with tachycardia, a high pulse pressure and a large volume pulse. Pulsus paradoxus though considered an important physical finding, is not often clinically detectable. The marked swings in intrapleural pressure during inspiration (markedly negative intrapleural pressure) and expiration (positive intrapleural pressure) are responsible for the paradoxical pulse. The jugular venous pressure is clinically difficult to gauge because of marked swings during inspiration (the veins collapse sharply) and expiration (the veins fill, mimicking a rise in pressure). The apex is not generally palpable. The heart sounds are often faint but once cor pulmonale occurs, a right ventricular gallop (3rd heart sound) is often heard close to the lower left sternal border. A systolic murmur of tricuspid incompetence (increasing in inspiration) may be present and the pulmonary 2nd sound at the base may be accentuated. The presence of marked pulmonary hypertension leads to a dilated pulmonary artery with pulmonary incompetence, manifested by a blowing diastolic murmur (Graham Steele murmur) best heard in the 2nd, 3rd left intercostal spaces close to the left sternal border. These are the classical findings of cor pulmonale. But there are a number of patients with COPD and cor pulmonale where few or none of these auscultatory findings are elicited. Their absence does not exclude cor pulmonale. The classical ECG findings in cor pulmonale are a peaked p in Lead II, avF, clockwise rotation, tall R in V1 and a RBBB block pattern. They may however not be always present.

When right heart failure occurs, the liver is enlarged and tender. The liver however may be felt well below the costal margin due to the low diaphragm in COPD patients even without heart failure. Pitting edema of the feet is a crucially important physical finding. In the absence of any other obvious cause that explains this finding, it invariably means right heart failure due to cor pulmonale.

It needs to be noted that before the term COPD came into being, patients with this disease were classified into two separate phenotypes—the blue bloater and the pink puffer. The *blue bloater* was puffy in the face, was often cyanosed, *was not unduly tachypneic*, breathing in a lazy and in a not too disturbed fashion. He was both hypoxic and had carbon dioxide retention, and was prone to developing pulmonary hypertension, cor pulmonale and right heart failure with well-marked edema due to fluid retention. The blue bloater was considered to be chiefly bronchitic with regard to his pathology. We know today

that the pathology here is not just in the large airways but is maximum in the small airways leading to increase in airways resistance.

The *pink puffer* on the other hand was tachypneic, could be seen breathing hard using all his accessory muscles. He however kept his arterial blood gases within normal limits almost up to the very end of the natural history of the disease. He was considered to have more of emphysema as the predominant underlying pathology.

It soon came to be realized that such watertight compartments were unsatisfactory, because most patients had varying components of inflammation of the small airways leading to obstruction plus airflow limitation *and* emphysema with airflow limitation. In fact this is the reason why the common generic term COPD was given to the disease.

Assessment of Lung Function

The assessment of lung function is of vital importance for the following reasons:

- The diagnosis of early COPD may be missed on a clinical examination. COPD even today remains grossly under-diagnosed for this very reason.
- An objective diagnosis of COPD needs basic spirometric tests.
- The degree or severity of COPD can be assessed and followed-up objectively through spirometric studies.

Spirometry (Figs. 17 to 20)

In the very early stages, as for example in asymptomatic smokers, the subtle increase in resistance in the peripheral airways can only be made out by special tests (e.g. measurement of closing volume, frequency dependence of compliance) which may be abnormal. These tests are difficult to perform, have a high coefficient of variability and are not advised in routine clinical practice. However, by the time a patient starts to complain of breathlessness, spirometric changes obtained through routine spirometry become evident. The American Thoracic Society (ATS), the European Respiratory Society (ERS) and the Global Initiative for Obstructive Lung Disease (GOLD) have defined COPD to be present in spirometric terms when the post-bronchodilator FEV_1/FVC is less than 70%. This ratio used in spirometric definition holds true irrespective of age, sex and ethnicity. The post-bronchodilator FEV_1 as a percentage of the predicted value is used to assess the

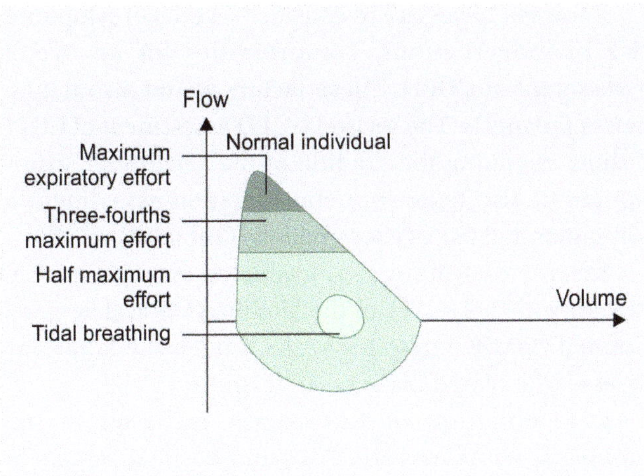

Fig. 17: Flow-volume loop of a normal individual.

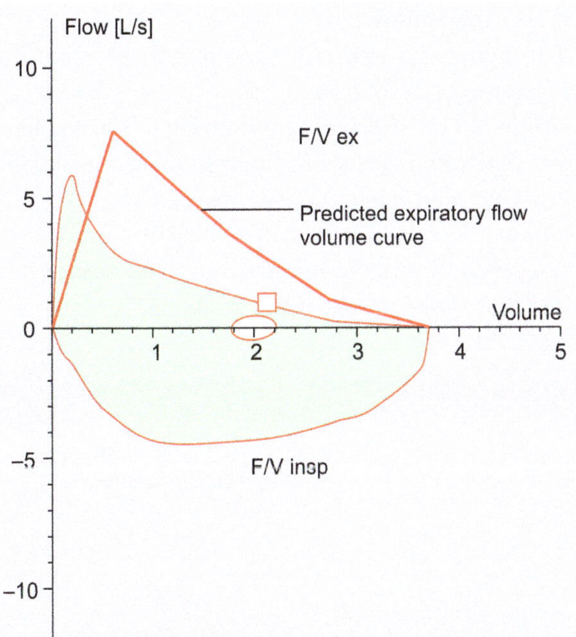

Fig. 18: Flow-volume loop showing mild COPD.

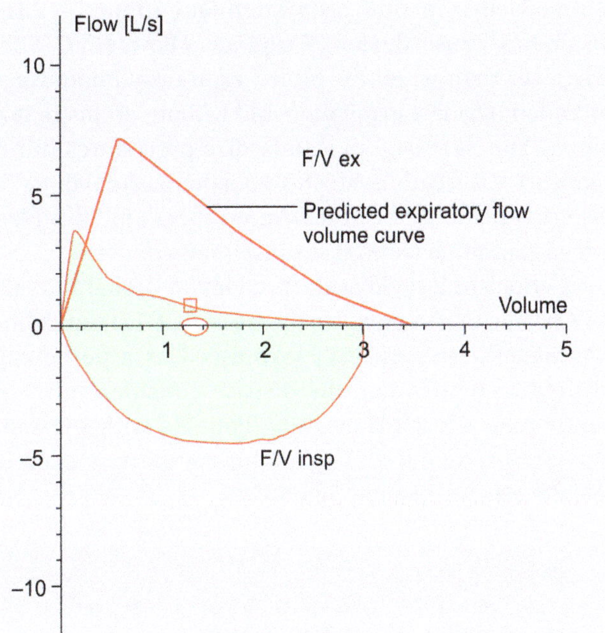

Fig. 19: Flow-volume loop showing moderate COPD.

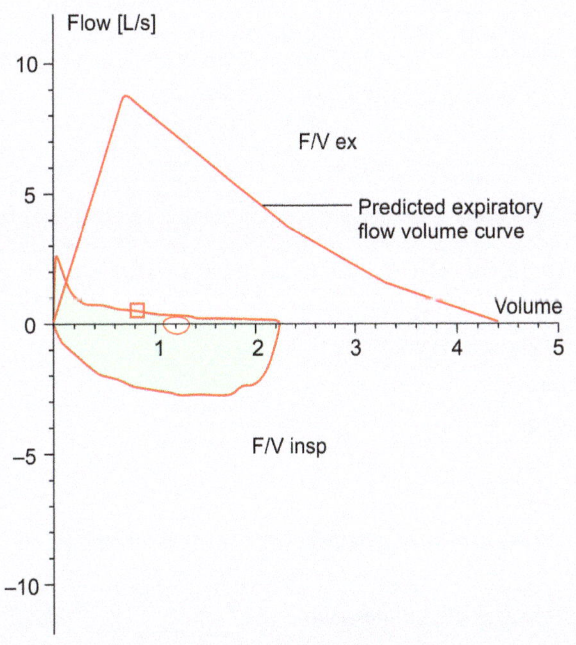

Fig. 20: Flow-volume loop showing severe COPD.
Note: Increasing upward concavity of expiratory curve with increasing
severity of COPD.

degree or severity of COPD. FEV_1 values within ± 20% of the predicted range are considered to be within normal limits.

The GOLD spirometric classification of the degree of COPD severity is given in **Table 11**.

There is indeed an interesting direct relationship between the degree of COPD as judged by the degree of fall in the predicted values of FEV_1 and the degree of inflammatory changes in the small airways as observed in pathological studies.

It is important to note that the speed of inspiration and the presence and duration of the end inspiratory pause before the forced expiration can influence both the FVC and FEV_1 values. If the forced expiratory maneuver is preceded by a slow inspiration and a long (4–5 sec) inspiratory pause, the forced expiratory flows (FVC, FEV_1) are lower than when the forced expiratory maneuver is preceded by a fast inspiration and without an inspiratory pause. The necessity to standardize procedures during spirometry is clearly evident. To obtain maximal flows the inspiration should be at maximum speed, followed by a forced expiration without any inspiratory pause.

A criticism leveled against the initial Global Initiative for Chronic Obstructive Lung Disease (GOLD) guidelines was that the use of FEV_1 (expressed as a percentage of predicted) to stage the disease considers just one component of COPD severity. Patients with the same percent predicted FEV_1 can have different exercise tolerance and different prognosis.

Table 11: GOLD guidelines using spirometric findings to stage disease severity.		
I	Mild COPD	FEV_1/FVC < 70; FEV_1 ≥ 80% of predicted
II	Moderate COPD	FEV_1/FVC < 70; FEV_1 ≥ 50% and < 80% of predicted
III	Severe COPD	FEV_1/FVC < 70; FEV_1 ≥ 30% and < 50% of predicted
IV	Very severe COPD	FEV_1/FVC < 70; FEV_1 < 30% of predicted

It was felt necessary to consider severity of symptoms, risk of exacerbations, comorbidities for an overall assessment of COPD. These factors would also help to assess prognosis. The revised GOLD assessment of COPD besides retaining the grading of the severity of airflow limitation also takes into consideration assessment of symptoms and risk of exacerbations **(Table 12)**.

Severity of symptoms is evaluated through the CAT Assessment Tool (CAT), or the Modified Medical Research Council (mMRC) dyspnea scale, though the latter only assesses the symptoms of breathlessness.

Determination of future risk is based on the number of acute exacerbations and hospitalizations for exacerbations over the past 12 months. A history of zero or one exacerbation in the past 12 months suggests a low risk, two or more exacerbations or a hospitalized exacerbation suggests a high future risk.

The symptoms and risk components are combined into four groups as follows:

- *Group A:* Low risk, less symptoms: 0 to 1 exacerbation per year and no prior hospitalization for exacerbation; and CAT score <10 or mMRC grade 0 to 1.
- *Group B:* Low risk, more symptoms: 0 to 1 exacerbation per year and no prior hospitalization for exacerbation; and CAT score ≥10 or mMRC grade ≥2.

Table 12: Multidimensional assessment of COPD.

GOLD: Severity of airflow limitation (based on postbronchodilator FEV_1).

Stage	*Severity*	*FEV_1 (percent predicted)*
In patients with FEV_1/FVC <0.7:*		
GOLD 1	Mild	≥80
GOLD 2	Moderate	50 to 79
GOLD 3	Severe	30 to 49
GOLD 4	Very severe	<30

GOLD: Assessment of symptoms and risk of exacerbations

	Symptom assessment	
Exacerbations/hospitalizations	*mMRC[¶], 0 to 1; CAT <10[Δ]*	*mMRC ≥2; CAT ≥10*
0 or 1 exacerbations without hospitalization	A	B
≥2 exacerbations or ≥1 hospitalization	C	D

(COPD: Chronic obstructive pulmonary disease; FEV_1: Forced expiratory volume in one second; FVC: Forced vital capacity; CAT: COPD Assessment Test; mMRC: Modified Medical Research Council (mMRC) dyspnea scale)
*The Global Initiative for Chronic Obstructive Lung Disease (GOLD) guidelines (www.goldgopd.org) prefer the threshold of <0.7 to the alternative of the fifth percentile LLN for FEV_1/FVC.
[¶]mMRC dyspnea scale: Refer to UpToDate graphic.
[Δ]http://www.catestonline.org.
Source: From the Global Strategy for the Diagnosis, Management and Prevention of COPD 2017, © Global Initiative for Chronic Obstructive Lung Disease (GOLD), www.goldcopd.org. Adapted with permission.

- *Group C:* High risk, less symptoms: ≥2 exacerbations per year or ≥1 hospitalization for exacerbation; and CAT score <10 or mMRC grade 0 to 1.
- *Group D:* High risk, more symptoms: ≥2 exacerbations per year or ≥1 hospitalization for exacerbation; and CAT score ≥10 or mMRC grade ≥2.

Testing Reversibility of Airways Obstruction and Airflow Limitation

Use of an Aerosolized Bronchodilator: It is important to test for the degree of reversibility to distinguish COPD from asthma. Asthma generally shows good or even complete reversibility, while COPD shows incomplete, poor or no reversibility. There are some who advocate repeating the forced expiratory maneuver after four to five puffs of a β_2-agonist through a metered dose inhaler; others would prefer to nebulize the patient with salbutamol and then repeat the forced expiratory maneuver. In some patients the addition of an anticholinergic drug to a β_2-agonist produces a further increase in FEV_1. Reversibility should be tested at the time of diagnosis. It need not be tested at subsequent follow-ups. A change in FEV_1 greater than 200 mL is considered to be more than random variation, and only then should a change in FEV_1 be taken as significant. In addition to this absolute change in FEV_1, an increase in the FEV_1 by 12% or more is considered significant according to the ERS, ATS and GOLD guidelines. The British Society Guidelines suggest an absolute increase in FEV_1 by 200 mL and an increase of 15% over the baseline value to be significant. Roughly 30% of patients with COPD show significant reversibility.

- *Reversibility to corticosteroids:* Use of corticosteroids to test reversibility in COPD has not been included in the recent guidelines on the assessment and management of the disease. The corticosteroid test does however reveal significant reversibility in some patients with COPD who show no reversibility on using aerosolized or nebulized bronchodilators. Prednisolone in a dose of 30 mg is given for two weeks and standard spirometry is repeated to note the change in FEV_1 as also the degree of change present.

Lung Volumes

The residual volume (RV), functional residual capacity (FRC), total lung capacity (TLC) and ratio of RV/TLC are all increased due to air trapping and hyperinflation of lungs. Using helium techniques to measure static lung volumes might give false low values as the inspired helium may not have sufficient time to equilibrate within the air spaces. Lung volumes measured through body plethysmography are more accurate. This technique measures trapped air in large air spaces, air in poorly ventilated alveoli and gives higher lung volume readings compared to the helium technique.

Flow-volume loops: Flow-volume loops show that the expiratory flow rates at different lung volumes are reduced because of airflow limitation; they also show the degree of airflow limitation in COPD patients (*see* **Figs. 17 to 20**).

Measurement of lung volumes can prove to be of immense use in some patients with severe COPD due to marked airways obstruction and airflow limitation. In these patients the FVC on routine spirometry may be markedly reduced, so that the FEV_1 almost approximates the FVC and the FEV_1/FVC is greater than 70%. A mistaken spirometric interpretation of severe restrictive disease can be made if the lung volumes are not measured. If the lung volumes were to be measured in these patients the RV is found to be markedly increased often with some degree of increase in TLC. The low FVC in these patients is due to a marked increase in the RV. It is of crucial importance to measure lung volumes in these patients to avoid a wrong diagnosis.

Inspiratory Capacity

Greater stress is being placed in noting the inspiratory capacity (a neglected spirometric variable) in COPD. Lung function studies have shown the following:

- The IC reflects the FRC so that any change in the FRC is accompanied by an opposite change in IC, provided the TLC is by and large constant. Millie Emily and Casanova et al., found that a reduced IC correlated both with dyspnea and exercise capacity in COPD. The lower the IC the greater the dyspnea and the poorer the exercise capacity in COPD.
- The IC is a good predictor of maximal tidal volume during exercise and so of maximal exercise ventilation.
- There appears to be a significant inverse correlation between $PaCO_2$ and IC in COPD patients who have significant expiratory airflow limitation.
- The IC is simple to measure and can reflect changes in hyperinflation (either following use of a bronchodilator or an increase in ventilation).
- The IC could help evaluate the status and progress of COPD. A progressive reduction in IC would indicate

reduction in exercise capacity and therefore a progression of the disease. Measurement of IC could perhaps also help assess the efficacy of therapy in COPD. Measurements of FEV_1 and IC should be analyzed to provide better information on lung function in COPD.

CO Transfer

The carbon monoxide transfer factor (TLCO) in advanced COPD is invariably reduced because of a reduction in *ventilated* lung volumes and an inequality in the ventilation-perfusion ratio. However, the diffusion capacity of CO normalized to ventilated alveolar volume (TLCO/VA/KCO) may remain normal, except in the presence of emphysema when it is reduced. A reduced TLCO/VA, KCO excludes bronchial asthma.

The changes in static pressure volume curves of the lungs in COPD in the presence of emphysema consist of an increase in static compliance and a reduction in static transpulmonary pressure at any specific lung volume.

Arterial Blood Gases

Arterial blood gas studies are essential to determine the presence and degree of hypoxemia and hypercapnia in patients with COPD. A lowered PaO_2 and an increased $PaCO_2$ generally occur when the FEV_1 falls well below 50% of predicted values.

But there are many exceptions to this generalization and some patients continue to ventilate well and keep their CO_2 within limits even when the FEV_1 is less than one liter. The pattern of blood gases in Indian subjects and their change during an acute crisis associated with an exacerbation of COPD are considered in the chapter on Acute Exacerbation of COPD **(Fig. 21)**.

Chest Radiography (Figs. 22 to 24)

A chest X-ray is necessary to exclude alternative diagnosis, to diagnose comorbidities or to look out for complications of COPD (pneumonia, pneumothorax). Chest radiography has a sensitivity of about 50% in the diagnosis of COPD of moderate severity.

An X-ray chest of a moderately advanced disease shows increased radiolucency of the lungs, a flat diaphragm, a long narrow heart shadow **(Fig. 22)**. There is increased retrosternal airspace on a lateral radiograph. Bullae defined as radiolucent areas of 1 cm or more in space surrounded by a thin outlining shadow may be observed. Severe COPD

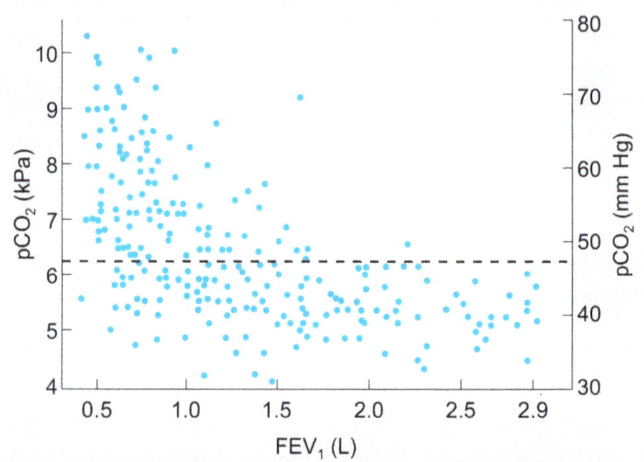

Fig. 21: Relationship between FEV_1 and pCO_2 in COPD during an acute exacerbation of COPD in Indian subjects.

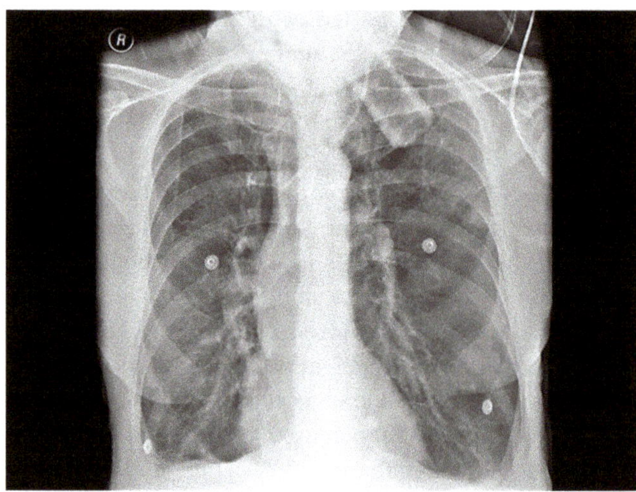

Fig. 22: Chronic obstructive pulmonary disease (COPD): PA view demonstrates a tubular heart, flattened domes of diaphragms and hyperinflated lungs. These are classical features of COPD.

shows an enlarged heart, enlarged vascular hilar shadows and other evidence of pulmonary hypertension.

Computed Tomography (Figs. 25 to 27)

HRCT of the chest has a far greater sensitivity and specificity than chest radiography for the detection of emphysema. Certain features of the CT scan determine whether the emphysema is centrilobular, panacinar or septal.

Complications of COPD

The main complication is pulmonary infection including pneumonia which can precipitate an acute exacerbation of

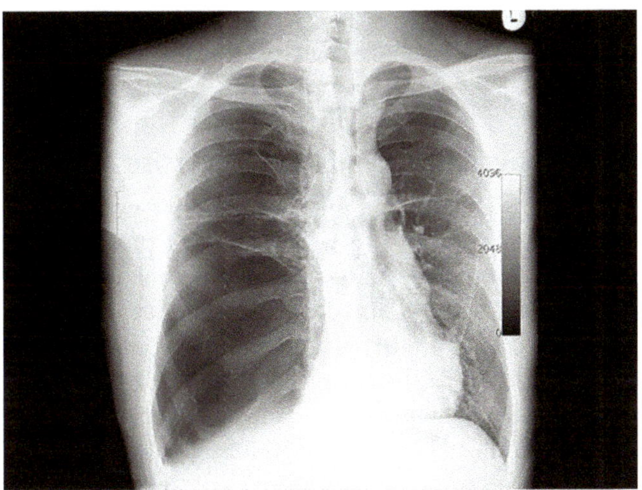

Fig. 23: PA view of the chest demonstrates large emphysematous bullae with intervening septae in the right lung causing compression of the remainder of right lung with marginal mediastinal shift to the left.

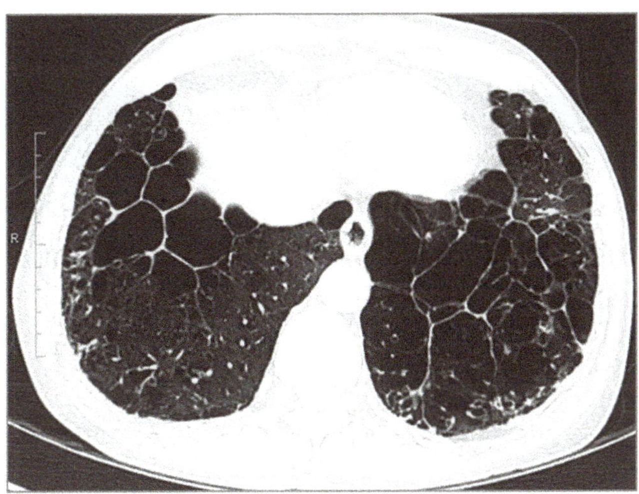

Fig. 25: Emphysema. Extensive thin-walled bullae in both lung fields.

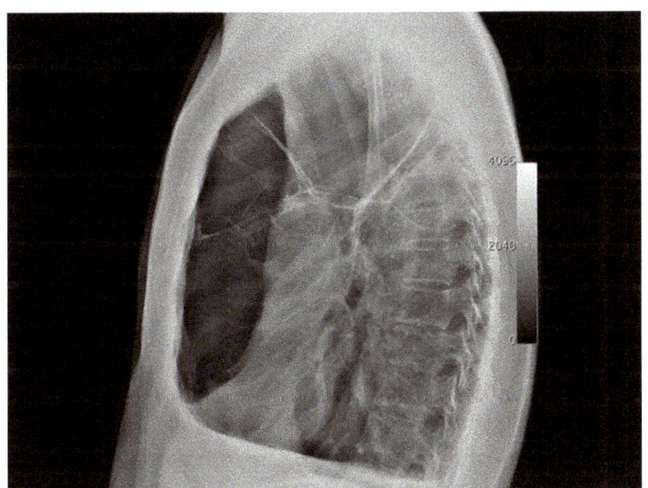

Fig. 24: Chronic obstructive pulmonary disease (COPD): Lateral view of chest demonstrates multiple emphysematous bullae with flattening of domes of diaphragm and markedly widened retrosternal air space and increased anteroposterior thoracic diameter.

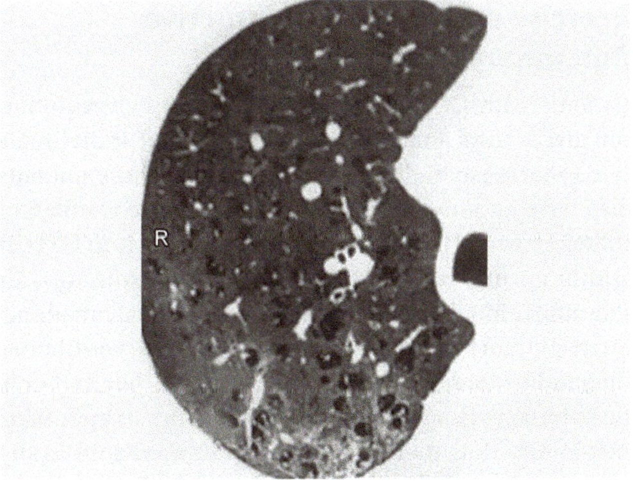

Fig. 26: Centrilobular emphysema-HRCT demonstrates thin-walled well-defined lucencies in the posterior aspect of the right lung. These air spaces demonstrate a vessel in the central portion of the air space representing a centrilobular vessel. This is a classical sign of centrilobular emphysema.

the disease. Other complications include pneumothorax, atelectasis, lung cancer, thromboembolic disease, systemic complications.

Differential Diagnosis

Table 4 lists the main conditions that need to be differentiated from COPD. Each of these conditions has been dealt with at length in separate chapters. Two more conditions need special mention.

1. Obstruction to the central airways caused by benign or malignant tumors, lymph nodes or an aortic aneurysm. These can mimic COPD by causing a progressive dyspnea on exertion. A monophonic wheeze, a flat inspiratory loop on the flow volume curve and imaging studies should give the correct diagnosis.
2. Heart failure can cause dyspnea on exertion and is not uncommonly associated with rhonchi. Clinical examination, imaging and an elevated BNP level in the blood should give the correct diagnosis.

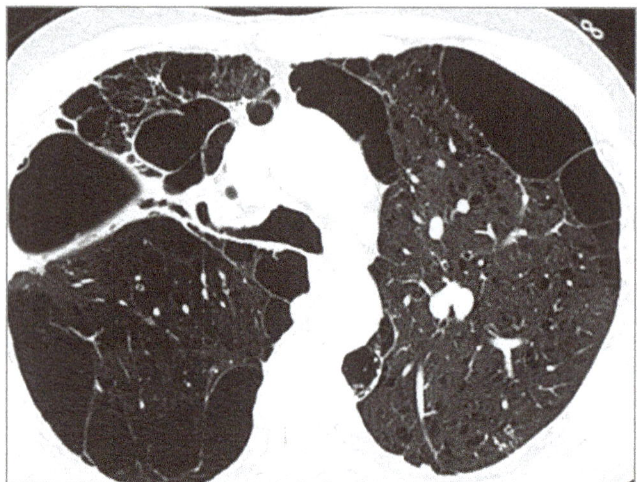

Fig. 27: Emphysema. HRCT demonstrates extensive emphysema in the form of centrilobular emphysema and paraseptal emphysema, compressing lung parenchyma.

Exercise and Chronic Obstructive Pulmonary Disease

Patients with COPD have higher oxygen consumption for given work load compared to normal individuals due to increase in the work of breathing. These patients also have an increase in dead space; minute ventilation therefore needs to be increased if the $PaCO_2$ is to be kept within normal range. As COPD worsens, expiratory air flow limitation occurs even during normal tidal breathing. Such patients cannot meet the increased ventilatory demand by increasing their tidal volume. They can only do so by increasing the respiratory frequency or increasing inspiratory flow thereby causing an upward shift in the end-expiratory volume so that expiratory flow rate can increase. Each of these maneuvers will lead to increased inflation of the lungs and a further increase in the workload of respiratory muscles which are already working at a mechanical disadvantage. Increasing dyspnea would limit their exercise. Exercise is at times also limited by leg muscle fatigue pointing to skeletal muscle dysfunction in COPD.

Exercise increases cardiac output and the increased perfusion of poorly ventilated alveoli lowers V/Q ratios causing hypoxemia and in some instances hypercapnia.

Exercise Test

Exercise testing is quite unnecessary for the diagnosis of COPD. Exercise testing may however offer valuable information on the behavior of the heart-lung combination during the stress of an increased workload. There are three types of tests:

Progressive Symptom Limited Exercise Test

The patient is exercised on a treadmill or cycle with a progressively increasing workload. The patient stops when symptoms prevent further continuation of exercise. A maximum test is defined as one where the heart rate reaches 80% of predicted and the ventilation 90% of predicted. Blood pressure and ECG recordings done simultaneously help assess cardiovascular factors that may contribute to limitation of exercise capacity

Self-Paced Exercise Test

The commonly used test is the 6-minute walk test which is useful only in moderately severe COPD when the FEV_1 is less than 1.5 L. These patients would be expected to have an exercise tolerance of less than 600 m in 6-minute. We would recommend measuring the O_2 saturation at the end of the 6-minute walk. The heart rate, blood pressure and auscultating the heart for a third heart sound in particular may help detect cardiovascular abnormalities. The 6-minute walk test has a coefficient of variation of about 8%.

The Shuttle Walking Test

In this test, the patient performs a paced walk between two points 10 m apart (the shuttle). The pace of the walk is increased at regular intervals until the patient stops the walk because of breathlessness. The number of completed shuttles is noted.

Steady State Exercise Test

The patient is exercised at a sustainable state of maximal activity for 3–6 minutes. Blood gases, V_D/V_T are measured during this test. This test is not necessary for clinical assessment.

Sleep Studies

Nocturnal hypoxemia is often observed in patients with moderate to severe COPD. The association of obstructive sleep apnea with COPD (overlap syndrome) is fairly frequent and these patients can suffer dangerous hypoxic spells during sleep. Sleep studies are indicated in these patients.

Other Investigations

- *Echocardiography:* Echocardiography is often used in suspected or definite cor pulmonale. The tricuspid gradient is used to measure right ventricular systolic pressure and to estimate the pressure gradient across the tricuspid regurgitant jet recorded by the Doppler ultrasound. Right ventricular dimensions, systolic and diastolic function can also be assessed along with the degree of pulmonary hypertension.

- A complete blood count with a determination of the PCV will detect the presence of polycythemia. Polycythemia is always secondary to fairly longstanding hypoxia with a PaO_2 generally less than 55 mm Hg. Polycythemia should be suspected when PCV is greater than 47% in women and greater than 52% in men, the Hb is more than 16 g/dL in women and more than 18 g/dL in men. It is important to recognize polycythemia as it contributes to cerebrovascular accidents, cardiovascular episodes and features of peripheral vascular disease. Other investigations should include a full biochemical study of the blood and ECG, a BNP level in the blood in patients with moderate to severe COPD, and investigations relevant to many systemic features observed in COPD.

- Alph-1 antitrypsin deficiency should be looked out for in all patients is less than 45 years of age with an early onset of emphysema and in all patients with a family history of premature emphysema **(Figs. 23 to 27)**.

■ SUGGESTED READING

1. Adeloye D, Chua S, Lee C, et al. Global and regional estimates of COPD prevalence: systematic review and meta-analysis. J Glob Health. 2015;5(2):020415.
2. Brantly ML, Sandhaus RA, Turino G, et al. The diagnosis and management of alpha-1 antitrypsin deficiency in the adult. Chronic Obstr Pulm Dis (Miami). 2016;3:668.
3. Chan-Yeung M, Ait-Khaled N, White N, et al. The burden and impact of OPD in Asia and Africa. Int J Tuberc Lung Dis. 2004;8(1):2-14.
4. Gershon AS, Warner L, Cascagnette P, et al. Lifetime risk of developing chronic obstructive pulmonary disease: a longitudinal population study. Lancet. 2011;378:991.
5. Global Initiative for Chronic Obstructive Lung Disease (GOLD). Global Strategy for the Diagnosis, Management and Prevention of chronic obstructive pulmonary disease: 2018 Report. www.goldcopd.org
6. Grzetic-Romcevic T, Devcic B, Sonc S. Spirometric testing on World COPD Day. Int J Chron Obstruct Pulmon Dis. 2011;6:141-6
7. Hogg JC, Chu F, Utokaparch S, et al. The nature of small-airway obstruction in chronic obstructive pulmonary disease. N Engl J Med. 2004;350(26):2645-53.
8. Jindal SK. Emergence of chronic obstructive pulmonary disease as an epidemic in India. Indian J Med Res. 2006; 124(6):619-30.
9. Leung JM, Sin DD. Asthma-COPD overlap syndrome: pathogenesis, clinical features, and therapeutic targets. BMJ. 2017;358:j3772.
10. Lopez AD, Shibuya K, Rao C, et al. Chronic obstructive pulmonary disease: current burden and future projections. Eur Respir J. 2006;27(2):397-412.
11. Lopez Varela MV, Montes de Oca M, Halbert RJ, et al. Sex-related differences in COPD in five Latin American cities: the PLATINO study. Eur Respir J. 2010;36(5):1034-41.
12. Mannino DM. COPD: epidemiology, prevalence, morbidity and mortality, and disease heterogeneity. Chest. 2002; 121(5 Suppl):121S-6S.
13. McKay AJ, Mahesh PA, Fordham JZ, et al. Prevalence of COPD in India: a systematic review. Prim Care Respir J. 2012;21(3):313-21.
14. Salvi SS, Barnes PJ. Chronic obstructive pulmonary disease in non-smokers. Lancet. 2009;374(9691):733-43.

Acute Exacerbation of Chronic Obstructive Pulmonary Disease

■ INTRODUCTION

Acute exacerbations of chronic obstructive pulmonary disease (COPD) are in-built features in the natural history of the disease, punctuating its course from time to time. They significantly increase both morbidity and mortality, the in-hospital mortality of COPD exacerbations being as high as 10%. In the UK, COPD exacerbations are the most common cause of medical hospital admissions, amounting to 15.9% of the hospital admissions at a huge cost to the national exchequer. In large metropolitan cities in India, COPD exacerbations are an important and frequent cause of admission to critical care units. Approximately, 1 in 15 patients reporting to the emergency department in a busy Mumbai hospital comes with worsening of symptoms of COPD.

Acute exacerbations are more frequent and often more severe in patients with increasing severity of COPD. The annual frequency of exacerbations in different patients having the same severity of COPD varies for unknown reasons. Predisposition to acute exacerbations may well be related to increasing severity of the disease, greater inflammation of the small airways, greater exposure to and perhaps greater susceptibility to infection and to the presence of lower airways bacterial colonization.

■ DEFINITION

An acute exacerbation of COPD is an acute worsening of symptoms associated with worsening lung functions that could in some patients precipitate acute respiratory failure or the acute worsening of chronic respiratory failure. Respiratory failure (acute or acute on chronic) is often the culminating feature of an acute severe exacerbation of COPD. It is important to stress this fact as it entails awareness for diagnosing this event and necessitates expert critical care in management.

The guidelines of the Global Initiative for Chronic Obstructive Lung Disease (GOLD) define an exacerbation as "an event in the natural course of the disease characterized by a change in the patient's dyspnea, cough and/or sputum that is beyond day to day normal variations, is acute in onset and may warrant a change in medication in a patient with underlying COPD".

■ IMPACT OF CHRONIC OBSTRUCTIVE PULMONARY DISEASE EXACERBATIONS

Besides being a major cause of morbidity, mortality and poor health status, exacerbations of COPD impose a significant burden on healthcare systems all over the world, more so in poor developing countries.

The time course of recovery during an acute exacerbation varies. In one study, 50% of community treated exacerbations recovered to baseline symptoms within 7 days. Yet 14% of exacerbations failed to return to baseline for 35 days.

Recurrent exacerbations lead to accelerated decline in lung function. In one study, recurrent exacerbations led to a fall in FEV_1 of 40.1/mL/year [95% confidence interval (CI) 38–42] verses 32.1 mL/year (95% CI 31–33)] in patients with no or infrequent exacerbations. A 3-year recent longitudinal cohort study observed that exacerbations were associated with a decline in lung function, the FEV_1 showing a mean loss of 2 mL per year per exacerbation. This was associated with a poorer quality of life.

RISK FACTORS

The COPD gene study and the Evaluation of COPD Longitudinally to Identify Predictive Surrogate Endpoints (ECLIPSE) study showed that COPD events do not occur randomly but cluster together in time, so that there is a period characterized by high risk for recurrent exacerbations in the 8-week period after the initial exacerbation. The ECLIPSE study also showed that the more severe the COPD, the more frequent the exacerbations. Thus, 22% of patients in the stage II disease, 33% with stage III disease and 47% with stage IV disease had frequent exacerbations in the first year of follow-up. It was also noted that the single best prediction of exacerbations across all GOLD stages was a past history of exacerbation. Important risk factors for exacerbations in COPD are listed in **Table 1**.

PATHOPHYSIOLOGY

The pathophysiology has been detailed in an earlier section. Acute exacerbations are associated with increased inflammation within the peripheral airways and the lungs. Clinically, this is manifested by worsening dyspnea and sputum production. Pathological features include an even more intense inflammatory exudate and edema of the mucosa of the peripheral airways, an increase in tone of the bronchial muscle and increased mucus production. The acute increase in obstruction to the airways and the further increase in airflow limitation, if sufficiently severe, produce dynamic hyperinflation. As has already been explained in an earlier section, dynamic hyperinflation in acute severe exacerbations can occur with frightening rapidity, the patient becoming increasingly uncomfortable and dyspneic, because he has to breathe at progressively high lung volumes. The work of breathing is substantially increased, well beyond what it was prior to the exacerbation, and there is further impairment of respiratory muscle function. The "effort" expended by the chest bellows and the respiratory muscles is not commensurate with the extra "load" of breathing. This results in alveolar hypoventilation and hypercapnic respiratory failure. Hypoxia is also worsened in severe exacerbations because of increasing ventilation-perfusion inequality (**Flowchart 1**).

Not all acute exacerbations are severe, the degree of exacerbation being probably dependent on the degree of small airways inflammation present in the stable state.

Moderate and severe COPD (Grade III, Grade IV) is associated with a greater degree of inflammation of the small airways, when compared to Grade I and Grade II COPD. This may well be the reason why acute exacerbations are generally more severe in patients with Grade III, Grade IV COPD.

Till a little more than a decade ago COPD was considered a disease confined to the airways. It is now increasingly realized that COPD involves more than the airways, and is frequently associated with a systemic inflammatory response. Exacerbations are thus accompanied by a proinflammatory and a prothrombotic state. A recent study demonstrated elevated levels of interleukin 6, Willebrands factor, D dimer and other surrogate markers for inflammation, endothelial damage and activation of clotting factors during an exacerbation. These returned to baseline with recovery.

Table 1: Risk factors for acute exacerbations in chronic obstructive pulmonary disease (COPD).
Age: • Severity of airway obstruction   • Longer duration of COPD   • Productive cough, wheezing   • Prior history of exacerbations   • Bacterial colonization   • Comorbid conditions such as cardiovascular disease

Flowchart. 1: Pathophysiology of acute respiratory failure (ARF) in exacerbation of chronic obstructive pulmonary disease (COPD).

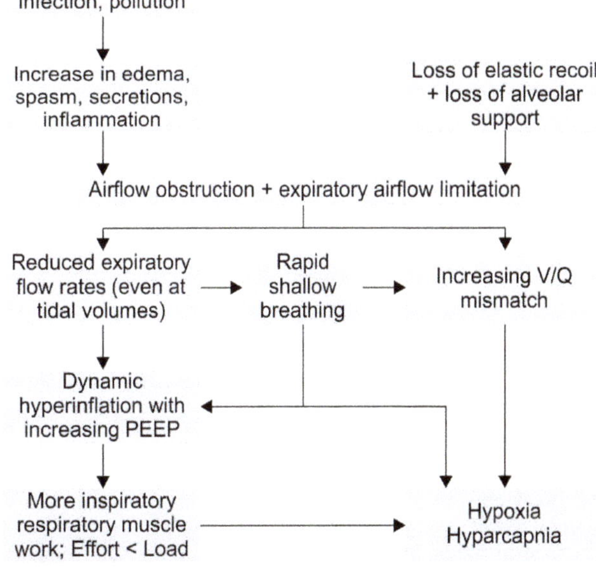

(PEEP: Positive end expiratory pressure)

ETIOLOGY

The most common cause of an acute exacerbation in COPD is infection. The common bacteria causing infective exacerbations are *Streptococcus pneumoniae, Haemophilus influenzae;* in older patients, *Klebsiella pneumoniae* and *Pseudomonas aeruginosa* are often the infecting agents. There is a growing incidence of *Moraxella catarrhalis* as a causative infective agent, both in the West and the developing world. Molecular biology using polymerase chain reaction (PCR) techniques has provided evidence for an increasing role of viruses in the etiology of acute exacerbations. The most common responsible virus is the rhinovirus. Other viruses include the respiratory syncitial virus, coronavirus, influenza virus and the adenovirus. The role of atypical organisms, in particular Mycoplasma and Chlamydia is unclear **(Table 2)**.

Acute exacerbations have also been noted to occur following an acute increase in indoor pollution, exposure to increased outdoor pollution, and due to sudden increase in exposure to an occupational risk factor. One reason for increased incidence of exacerbations during winter is excessive outdoor pollution, which blankets large cities in India at almost ground level. Exposure to pollution from exhausts of cars in traffic jams can lead to acute exacerbations, and is another reason for the emergency visits to hospitals. A sudden and marked spurt in the number of cigarettes smoked has been known to cause an acute exacerbation of COPD.

CLINICAL FEATURES (TABLE 3)

An acute exacerbation of COPD is characterized by a clear worsening of respiratory symptoms, well beyond what the patient is used to experiencing. These symptoms chiefly include increased dyspnea, increased cough with an increase in sputum volume, purulent sputum and an increase in wheeze.

Physical findings include all the features observed with airways obstruction and airflow limitation described earlier. Tachycardia, tachypnea, excessive use of accessory muscles of respiration, in-drawing of intercostal spaces during inspiration with paradoxical breathing are all seen in severe exacerbations. Expiration is clearly prolonged and there is an audible wheeze. Rapidly increasing dynamic hyperinflation will cause an actual measurable increase in the circumference of the chest, increasing tachycardia, hypotension, marked distress and difficulty in breathing, the breath sounds ultimately being reduced to short gasps. Auscultation in the presence of rapidly progressive dynamic hyperinflation may reveal faint or absent breath sounds, the expiratory wheeze often being inaudible. Periods of apnea may interrupt the breathing, which is often irregular. Central cyanosis may be evident because of increasing hypoxia **(Table 4)**. Hypercapnia may progressively worsen, leading often, though not always to flapping tremors and confusion **(Table 5 and Fig. 1)**. Rhythm disturbances may occur in the form of multiple atrial or ventricular extrasystoles, supraventricular tachycardia, chaotic atrial tachycardia, atrial fibrillation and even ventricular tachycardia.

Severe acute exacerbations can precipitate right heart failure, particularly in patients with Grade III and Grade

Table 2: Common organisms and pollutants responsible for acute exacerbation of COPD.
Bacteria: • *Streptococcus pneumoniae* • *Haemophilus influenzae* • *Moraxella catarrhalis* • *Pseudomonas aeruginosa* *Viruses:* • Rhinovirus • Influenza • Parainfluenza • *Coronavirus* • Adenovirus • Respiratory syncytial virus (RSV) *Atypical bacteria:* • *Chlamydia pneumoniae* • *Mycoplasma pneumoniae* *Common pollutants:* • Nitrogen dioxide • Particulates • Sulfur dioxide • Smoke inhalation from fire • Ozone

Table 3: Clinical features of acute severe exacerbation of COPD.
• Increase in dyspnea, cough, sputum • All the clinical features of severe airflow limitation • Features of hypoxia and hypercapnia • Features of right heart failure may be present

Table 4: Causes of hypoxemia.
• V/Q mismatch causing an increased alveolar arterial O_2 gradient • Alveolar hypoventilation • Small shunts amounting to 4–10% of the cardiac output • Low P_vO_2 (observed in some patients with cor pulmonale and severe heart failure)

Table 5: Causes of hypercapnia.
• Alveolar hypoventilation due to increased load and the inability of the respiratory muscles (inspiratory in the main) to meet this load. Inspiratory work of breathing is doubled in acute respiratory failure (ARF); increase in auto or intrinsic PEEP accounts for more than half of this increase in the work of breathing • V/Q mismatch • Change in the pattern of breathing-smaller tidal volume with an increase in respiratory rate. This may be an adaptive mechanism to avoid increasing ventilation and respiratory muscle activation to the point where muscle fatigue ensues

Source: Orozco-Levi M. Structure and function of the respiratory muscles in patients with COPD: impairment or adaptation? Eur Respir J. Suppl. 2003;46:41s-51s.

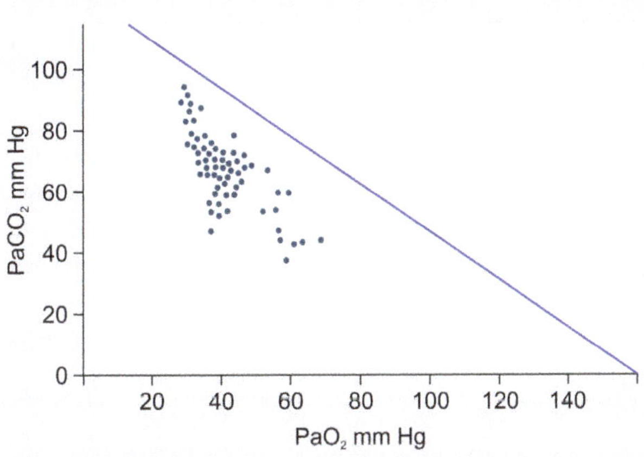

Fig. 1: Arterial blood gas (ABG) in 64 patients with Grade III to Grade IV COPD who developed an acute exacerbation of COPD. Note the severity of hypoxemia and hypercapnia present in most patients with Grade III–IV COPD in an acute severe exacerbation.
Source: Diagnosis and Management of Acute Respiratory Failure, Oxford University Press: Oxford, Delhi, Mumbai; 1979.

IV COPD. This is related to pulmonary vasoconstriction and pulmonary hypertension caused by acute hypoxia and hypercapnia in an individual who often has a baseline increase in pulmonary vascular resistance due to inflammatory changes in the small airways, periphery of the lungs and the pulmonary vessels. The most important and early sign of right heart failure in COPD patients is edema of the feet for which there is no other obvious cause. The edema can worsen and can be so marked as to be generalized. In severe exacerbations in Grade III and Grade IV COPD, electrocardiography (ECG) shows a P-pulmonale often associated with clockwise rotation. There may be evidence of right ventricular enlargement and/or a right bundle branch block pattern. These ECG findings are acute, for they generally regress after recovery and often return to a stable state. Echocardiography may corroborate right ventricular systolic dysfunction, some degree of functional tricuspid incompetence and pulmonary hypertension.

Acute exacerbations of COPD are not necessarily severe; some are indeed mild, easily manageable at home. Apart from a worsening of symptoms more than what is usual for the patient, physical signs are limited to those caused by a modest increase in airways obstruction and airflow limitation.

The duration of acute exacerbations varies. Milder exacerbations often treated at home may be relieved within 4–7 days with adequate treatment, though full recovery with return to baseline symptoms may take as long as 3–4 weeks in some of these patients. Recurrence rate varies in different individuals for unclear reasons. In a cohort of patients with moderate to severe COPD followed up after acute exacerbation, 22% suffered a recurrence within 50 days of the first (index) exacerbation. Perhaps an initial exacerbation may well increase susceptibility to a subsequent one.

Impact of AECOPD on Lung Function

Repeated AECOPD cause an accelerated decline in FEV_1. 25% of those who recover from an AE do not revert to baseline spirometry for 35 days after an AE and 10% do not revert to preadmission baseline for 90 days. At 6 months post AE, 50% of patients, in a large study still required assistance in at least 1 daily activity of living.

■ INVESTIGATIONS

Investigations are done with three objectives in mind:
1. To determine the severity of the exacerbation
2. If infection is the cause, to determine if possible the infective agent responsible for the exacerbation
3. To exclude other complications which can cause an acute respiratory crisis in COPD; a crisis that may be clinically indistinguishable from that caused by exacerbation of COPD.

Investigations include a routine complete blood count (CBC), erythrocyte sedimentation rate (ESR), and C-reactive protein. The latter is believed to be an important marker for the presence and degree of the underlying inflammation in the peripheral airways. X-ray chest and ECG are always done routinely. O_2 saturation, arterial blood gases, and pH are vital tests. The O_2 saturation will serve as a guide to the degree of hypoxia, but it is often impossible to diagnose the presence and degree of CO_2 retention without actually determining the $PaCO_2$. In severe exacerbations causing acute respiratory failure or acute on chronic respiratory failure, arterial pH is of vital importance. *An arterial pH < 7.25 is perhaps the most important single factor associated with high mortality.*

In severe exacerbations, it is important to determine the baseline function of organ systems. Serum creatinine, blood-urea-nitrogen (BUN) levels and serum electrolytes need to be done. Sputum microscopy and culture may help (though not necessarily so) in arriving at the organism responsible for an acute infective exacerbation. It is of particular help if *P. aeruginosa* or *Klebsiella pneumoniae* is grown on culture, as this will dictate the correct choice of antibiotics.

Spirometry is not useful in severe exacerbations as the patient is too ill to allow reliable results. Also, baseline spirometric readings of a patient admitted in an emergency are not generally available.

■ PROBLEMS IN DIAGNOSIS (TABLE 6)

Problems in diagnosis are not infrequent in patients who on clinical examination appear to have an acute exacerbation of COPD. The major difficulty encountered is to distinguish left ventricular dysfunction and failure in a patient with COPD from an acute severe exacerbation of COPD. This difficulty is compounded when acute left ventricular failure is the sole manifestation of ischemic heart disease, without a preceding history of anginal pain and without clear evidence of ischemia on the ECG. Both COPD and ischemic heart disease often manifest in similar age groups. Interestingly, patients with COPD who develop acute left ventricular failure often present with tachypnea and marked wheezing rather than the usual crackles of pulmonary edema. An X-ray chest may be unhelpful and in fact misleading, because occasionally predominantly

Table 6: Problems in diagnosis.
• Association of LV dysfunction and failure in patients with COPD
• Complication of pulmonary embolism in a patient with COPD
• Complication of a pneumothorax in a patient with COPD
• Pneumonia, atelectasis, presenting with acute respiratory failure (ARF) in COPD
• Acute severe asthma
• Nonrespiratory causes triggering ARF in COPD

(COPD: Chronic obstructive pulmonary disease; LV: Left ventricle)

unilateral pulmonary edema may be seen in COPD patients who develop acute left ventricular failure. The unilateral pulmonary edema is often misdiagnosed as pneumonia. Investigations are often noncontributory. We have found echocardiography notoriously unreliable and even misleading in the diagnosis of diastolic dysfunction in acute left ventricular failure.

A case history illustrates this well. Mr S, a heavy cigarette smoker with Grade III to Grade IV COPD was admitted with classic features of an acute exacerbation of COPD due to an acute pulmonary infection. He went into acute respiratory failure with severe hypoxia, hypercapnia and respiratory cum metabolic acidosis. Medical management including noninvasive ventilator support failed to help. He was intubated and put on mechanical ventilator support. He could not be weaned off support for over 10 days. Every night there was a crisis characterized by sudden tachypnea so that he would clash with the machine. There was marked bronchospasm during tachypneic spells, no change in the X-ray chest, with the central venous pressure (CVP) remaining within the normal range. A tracheostomy was done and ventilator support continued. One night he had an exceptionally severe bout of tachypnea with marked wheezing and increased desaturation, requiring a significant step-up in the fraction of inspired oxygen (FiO_2). On this occasion, the tracheal aspirate was frothy and copious, pointing to pulmonary edema. Left ventricular failure due to ischemic heart disease was diagnosed. A coronary angiography showed a tight stenosis in the proximal left anterior descending artery. An angioplasty with stenting was performed. The patient could be weaned off the ventilator support within the next 2 days. He is on continuous oxygen therapy and has a reasonable quality of life.

Pulmonary embolism complicating COPD can also mimic an acute exacerbation. Here again when pulmonary embolism occurs in a patient with COPD, breathlessness is invariably associated with severe wheezing. A negative D-dimer test is a strong point against pulmonary embolism. When in doubt, a pulmonary angiography should be done.

Acute pneumonia, lobar atelectasis due to mucus plugging, are other pulmonary pathologies that can also precipitate severe acute respiratory failure. The clinical diagnosis may be missed as an acute exacerbation of COPD causing acute respiratory failure.

Even a shallow pneumothorax in a patient with moderate to severe COPD can induce acute respiratory failure. This is because an overinflated lung (as occurs in COPD) does not easily collapse even with a good-sized pneumothorax. The pressure within the pneumothorax may be high but it appears quite shallow on the X-ray. This is one reason why any patient with a diagnosis of acute exacerbation of COPD admitted to the hospital, or reporting to the emergency department, should always have an X-ray chest done. It is almost impossible to clinically detect a shallow pneumothorax in a patient with COPD. The only reliable sign is diminished breath sounds over the area of the pneumothorax, but unequal breath sounds over both lungs are not uncommon in COPD, even without pneumothorax.

It is obvious that each of the three complicating conditions listed above can worsen lung function in patients with COPD. This is because each of these conditions will cause tachypnea. Tachypnea in moderate to severe COPD if often characterized by an expiration, which is incomplete, being interrupted by the next inspiration. This will lead to progressive air-trapping, hyperinflated lungs with all the consequent deleterious effects on the work of breathing.

Acute severe asthma may in the absence of a good history be difficult to distinguish from an acute severe exacerbation of COPD when the patient is seen for the first time in an emergency. In fact, some severe asthmatics have very poor reversibility in airways obstruction and airflow limitation, exactly resembling patients with COPD. Fortunately, the management remains exactly the same.

A number of other complications occurring outside the respiratory system may produce an acute respiratory crisis with respiratory failure in patients with well-marked Grade III and IV COPD. For example, narcotic drugs, anesthetics, sedatives, tranquilizers even in small doses can depress the ventilatory drive sufficiently to lead to increasing hypercapnic respiratory failure and a mistaken diagnosis of acute exacerbation of COPD. Trauma causing rib fractures or fractures of the femur, acute systemic infections and sputum retention from any cause are other complications that cause an acute respiratory crisis in COPD patients **(Table 7)**.

It is therefore a cardinal principle in medicine that if a patient with well-marked COPD develops acute respiratory failure or acute on already existing chronic respiratory failure, a careful search for all possible causes must be made. An acute exacerbation of COPD is an important and common cause for the above scenario, but it certainly is not the only cause.

Table 7: Conditions other than acute exacerbation of COPD which are known to precipitate an acute respiratory crisis in COPD patients.

Respiratory conditions
- Pneumonia
- Pulmonary atelectasis
- Pneumothorax
- Pleural effusion
- Pulmonary thromboembolism
- Sputum retention from any cause

Nonrespiratory conditions
- Acute left ventricular failure
- Use of respiratory depressants, drugs, tranquilizers
- Postoperative
- Trauma (fracture ribs, fracture femur)
- Systemic infections
- Severe blood loss

Note: Severe systemic infections increase metabolism thereby increasing ventilatory demands. There is an increase in the "load" on respiratory muscles leading at times to respiratory failure.

Prolonged immobility (as after trauma) can lead to basal atelectasis, sputum retention and worsening lung function.

Blood loss with hypovolemic shock leads to low pulmonary artery pressure with increased V/Q abnormalities, leading to increasing hypoxia.

■ MANAGEMENT

The principles in the management of an acute exacerbation of COPD are:
- Relief of airways obstruction and airflow limitation through a more intensive use of inhaled bronchodilators
- Use of corticosteroids to reduce the increased inflammation within peripheral airways and lung parenchyma
- Use of antibiotics in the presence of bacterial infection
- Use of oxygen to relieve dyspnea and most importantly to relieve hypoxia
- Use of ventilatory support in patients who are in acute respiratory failure or in acute on chronic respiratory failure in spite of conservative treatment mentioned above.

We consider the role of the physiotherapist invaluable in patients who have a great deal of sputum but are unable to expectorate it. *Vigorous percussion to the chest is however harmful and leads to desaturation of oxygen in seriously ill patients.*

Treatment is tailored to the degree of severity of the acute exacerbation. Mild exacerbations may just need intensified bronchodilator therapy. If the sputum is purulent, antibiotics need to be given after collecting sputum for culture/sensitivity but without waiting for the results. If the exacerbation seems more than mild, corticosteroids need to be administered. Controlled oxygen is given for the relief of both hypoxia and dyspnea. It is the first important therapeutic measure in hypoxic patients, and should be started promptly in a patient admitted with acute respiratory failure. Persistence or increasing respiratory failure in spite of conservative management necessitates the use of ventilator support. Noninvasive ventilator support is preferable, but invasive ventilator support should not be delayed if indications so exist.

Inhaled Bronchodilator Therapy

Mild exacerbations of COPD are often controlled merely by increasing the frequency of inhaled bronchodilators. Both short-acting β_2-agonists and an anticholinergic-ipratropium bromide are equally effective bronchodilators and should be inhaled preferably through a spacer device. There is no evidence that the use of both is more effective than the use of either one or the other.

When inhaled the effects of short-acting beta agonists (SABAs) begin within 5 minutes and peak at 15–30 minutes. When ipratropium or an equivalent antimuscarinic agent is inhaled the effects of the drug begins within 10–15 minutes and peak at 30–60 minutes. The effects of these two classes of bronchodilators decline after 2–3 hours but can last 4–6 hours or even longer.

Severe exacerbations necessitate the administration of levosalbutamol (1.25 mg 8-hourly) and an anticholinergic agent like ipratropium (500 µg 8-hourly) through a nebulizer, even though again there is no evidence that this is superior to the use of a metered dose inhaler with a spacer device. Patients in our part of the world who come in with an acute severe exacerbation may have never used a metered dose inhaler and find it impossible to do so effectively at this juncture. Women in particular find it difficult to use the metered dose inhaler even when the COPD is stable. Patients with severe exacerbations are extremely dyspneic, have a poor inspiratory effort and very small tidal volumes. Very little of the drug reaches the airways in spite of using a volume spacer with the metered dose inhaler. The relief in dyspnea due to reduced airways obstruction following a switchover from a metered dose inhaler with a spacer device to the nebulized administration of the drugs, is at times too obvious to be disbelieved.

The frequency of nebulization of salbutamol is generally four times a day, perhaps repeated once in the middle of the night if necessary. Once there is clear relief in airways obstruction, salbutamol can be replaced by nebulization of duolin twice or thrice daily and budesonide 1 mg twice daily.

Use of Corticosteroids

Systemic corticosteroids are indicated in all except the very mild exacerbations that respond well to inhaled bronchodilator therapy alone. A number of randomized trials indicate that the use of steroids relieves airways obstruction producing a rapid improvement in forced expiratory volume in one second (FEV_1). Other outcome effects such as hospitalization, length of hospital stay, and oxygenation are variable. Their effect on mortality has not been determined. Corticosteroids act through their anti-inflammatory effect. The generally accepted dose is 40 mg prednisolone orally for 10–14 days. Critically ill patients, or those in whom absorption of the drug is suspect because of vomiting should be given methyl prednisolone 40 mg 8-hourly intravenously till improvement occurs, following which oral prednisolone is used. Nebulized budesonide also acts through its direct anti-inflammatory effect on the airways. It is however difficult to ascertain to what extent the drug reaches the peripheral airways, where inflammation is most marked.

A randomized controlled trial in inpatients [*Ref: Maltais F, Ostinelli J, Bourbeau J, et al. Comparison of nebulized budesonide and oral prednisolone with placebo in the treatment of acute exacerbations of chronic obstructive pulmonary disease: a randomized controlled trial. Am J Respir Crit Care Med. 2002;165(5):698-703*] compared nebulized budesonide (2 mg TDS for 3 days followed by 2 mg/day for 7 days) with oral prednisolone (30 mg twice daily for 3 days followed by 40 mg once daily for 7 days) and with placebo in patients with COPD who had moderate to severe exacerbation. The inhaled corticosteroid (ICS) group showed the same improvement in FEV_1 as the oral prednisolone group; the duration of hospital stay was similar. *However, in spite of what has been stated above, it would be unwise in COPD patients with severe exacerbations, particularly when associated with hypoxia, to substitute inhaled budesonide in place of the systemic use of corticosteroids.*

Antibiotics

Antibiotics should be used whenever there is an increase in sputum production, particularly when the sputum is purulent—colored yellow or green. These patients should be given antibiotics promptly without awaiting culture sensitivity reports. The choice of antibiotics depends on the organism generally prevailing in patients with acute exacerbation of COPD in a particular locale. The antibiotics used should cover the common organisms generally responsible for acute exacerbations—*Streptococcus pneumoniae, H. influenza* and *Moraxella catarrhalis.* In elderly individuals, gram-negative infections are not uncommon, particularly those due to *P. aeruginosa* and *Klebsiella.* An appropriate cover for gram-negative infections is then necessary. Viral infections (the rhinovirus in particular) are being increasingly recognized as a cause of acute exacerbations of COPD. Antibiotics are of no use when this is so.

The question often arises—does one use empiric antibiotic therapy in patients with severe acute exacerbation, particularly in those with acute respiratory failure, when there is no evidence of bacterial infection? Rightly or wrongly, we do so, as some patients who have infection may have no sputum and the danger of not treating a possible infection in such critically ill patients, particularly when they are old and feeble is great. When such patients need intubation and ventilatory support, suction through the endotracheal tube has often revealed dirty yellow or green tracheobronchial secretions. Interestingly, a meta-analysis of six sufficiently well-designed randomized trials by Sant and colleagues confirmed a statistically significant benefit that favored the use of antibiotics. Also systemic review of placebo-controlled studies showed that the use of appropriate antibiotics in COPD exacerbations reduced the risk of short-term mortality by 77%, treatment failure by 51% and sputum purulence by 44% *(Ref: Ram FS, Rodriquez-Rosin R, et al. Antibiotics for exacerbations of COPD. Cochrane Database Syst. Review 2006. April 19).* Duration of antibiotic therapy is generally not more than 7 days.

Theophylline

Oral theophylline should be given or continued (if the patient is already on the drug) for its bronchodilator effect in the milder forms of acute exacerbation of COPD. In the more severe forms of acute exacerbation, intravenous aminophylline 0.25 g to at the most 0.75 g intravenously over 24 hours through an infusion pump may be given, particularly when there is marked bronchospasm. Great care must be taken particularly in patients who have received oral theophylline during the stable phase of COPD. Theophylline levels in the blood should be carefully monitored and should not exceed 15 mg/dL.

Controlled Oxygen Therapy

Oxygen through nasal prongs or a Venturi mask is used to relieve dyspnea, but most importantly to relieve hypoxia. Patients with Grade III, and Grade IV COPD who develop a severe acute exacerbation, are invariably hypoxic and often hypercapnic. The PaO_2 very often is less than 55–60 mm Hg. These patients always need oxygen and are at risk of death from worsening hypoxia. *It should be a cardinal rule to administer oxygen immediately, and as the very first measure in any acutely ill patient with COPD.* Oxygen should be administered in a controlled manner and should be carefully supervised. Uncontrolled oxygen therapy can be lethal in these patients. Intensive care is crucial for survival. The objective is to increase PaO_2 to a safe level of 60 mm Hg or ensure an oxygen saturation of 90%, without the arterial pH falling below 7.25. Controlled oxygen therapy can be given through a Venturi mask which allows an FiO_2 of 24%; this can be increased through Venturi masks that allow an FiO_2 of 26% or even 28–30%, or more, if dangerous hypoxia is unrelieved. Oxygen given through nasal prongs at a flow rate of 1–2 L/min is a cheap, convenient and effective alternative, as this generally equates to an FiO_2 of 24–27%.

The response to controlled oxygen therapy [starting with an inspired oxygen content of 24%, (and increasing to 26% or even 28–30% if dangerous hypoxia is unrelieved)], falls into the following three patterns:

1. Relief of hypoxemia, with a fall in the $PaCO_2$ and an overall clinical improvement.
2. Relief of hypoxemia, but an initial increase in the $PaCO_2$ with a further fall in arterial pH to not less than 7.25. The $PaCO_2$ then steadies at a higher level, or returns to pretreatment levels. After a couple of days, the $PaCO_2$ generally falls below pretreatment levels. The initial rise in $PaCO_2$ with a fall in arterial pH, is usually observed during the first night after starting oxygen therapy, and is associated with increasing drowsiness, dullness, confusion and apathy. Thereafter, there is a gradual fall in the $PaCO_2$ to pretreatment or even lower levels and a return of pH toward normal, occurring *pari-passu* with clinical improvement.
3. Relief of hypoxemia, but a rapid, progressive, marked increase in the $PaCO_2$ with an increasing respiratory acidosis (pH < 7.25). This response is to be expected if oxygen is administered in an uncontrolled manner, using high oxygen concentrations. It can however also occur with carefully controlled and supervised oxygen

therapy (O_2 concentration between 24% and 28%). The severe respiratory acidosis and the marked rise in the $PaCO_2$ can prove lethal in these patients.

Unfortunately, it is generally the severely hypoxic patient with a fairly high $PaCO_2$ to start with, who is more prone to developing a progressively increasing, dangerously high $PaCO_2$ with a dangerously low arterial pH (< 7.2).

It is important to understand why uncontrolled oxygen therapy (and in some patients even controlled oxygen therapy) can lead to a sharp rise in $PaCO_2$. It used to be believed that the essential drive to breathe in these patients was due to the prevailing hypoxia, because the respiratory center was considered to be relatively insensitive (compared to normal subjects) to the rise in $PaCO_2$. Giving a high FiO_2 (uncontrolled oxygen) would remove the hypoxic stimulus to breathe, so that the patient would have a further rise in $PaCO_2$. This is not true; the ventilatory drive in these patients is even more than normal. Uncontrolled O_2 therapy produces vasodilatation in the pulmonary capillaries due to relief of hypoxia. This leads to a further V/Q mismatch with a low ventilation-perfusion ratio. It is the increasing alveolar hypoventilation due to the above cause that leads to a sharp rise in $PaCO_2$.

Patients who on conservative management (outlined earlier), and on controlled oxygen therapy show poor relief in hypoxia or show a progressive rise in the $PaCO_2$ with a fall in the arterial pH < 7.25, require ventilator support. Ventilator support could be of two types—(1) noninvasive and (2) invasive. It should be noted that many patients with severe Grade IV COPD have a persistent hypercapnia between 50 mm Hg and 60 mm Hg even in a stable state. It is unwise to attempt to reduce very high $PaCO_2$ seen during an acute exacerbation to normal levels. These patients tolerate a $PaCO_2$ between 50 mm Hg and 60 mm Hg fairly well.

Noninvasive Mechanical Ventilation

Noninvasive positive pressure ventilation (NIPPV) has been proven to be useful in several studies of acute respiratory failure caused by an acute exacerbation of COPD. Studies show that the use of NIPPV is associated with a lesser risk of nosocomial infections, less antibiotic use, and a lower mortality when compared to patients who are equally ill but did not receive NIPPV. A Cochrane review by Ram et al of 14 good quality RCT's showed unequivocally that NIV should be used early in the course of respiratory failure before acidosis sets in. It showed that NIV hastens recovery (RR 0.48), reduces hospital deaths (RR 0.52), reduce need for intubation (RR 0.41) and reduces hospital stay (3.2 days).

Noninvasive positive pressure ventilation has the ability to increase alveolar ventilation, rest muscles of respiration, reduce work of breathing and prevent respiratory muscle fatigue. Potential benefits include an increase in tidal volume, a fall in respiratory rate, improved oxygenation, a fall in $PaCO_2$ and greater patient comfort. When these benefits occur, they do so within a few hours of initiating NIPPV. Perhaps the most important advantage of NIPPV in an acute crisis of COPD is that it obviates the need for endotracheal intubation and invasive mechanical ventilation, which is far more inconvenient to the patient, and has more risks—particularly the risk of nosocomial infection.

Having said this, it is our considered opinion that many patients admitted to intensive care units (ICUs) in this country for an acute exacerbation of COPD are offered NIPPV when ventilatory support is not required, i.e. these patients would have recovered on conservative measures outlined above. Also, many such patients are offered NIPPV when they in fact needed prompt intubation and invasive ventilator support.

The indications in our unit for initiating NIPPV in an acute crisis of COPD are **(Table 8)**:

(i) Respiratory rate more than 30 breaths/min

(ii) Respiratory distress due to moderate or severe dyspnea

(iii) pH < 7.30 and/or a $PaCO_2$ > 60 mm Hg, provided these values fail to improve or worsen after a trial of 6–8 hours (or even earlier) of conservative measures.

Indications for NPPV
- Respiratory rate > 30 breaths/min
- Respiratory distress due to moderate or severe dyspnea
- pH < 7.30 and or a $PaCO_2$ > 60 mm Hg, provided these values fail to improve or worsen after a trial of 6–12 hours of conservative treatment

Contraindications to NPPV
- Obtunded patient
- Breathes very poorly, irregularly
- Unable to protect the airway
- Copious respiratory secretions
- Risk of gastric aspiration
- Hypotension; CVS instability
- pH < 7.20 with an acute progressive rise of $PaCO_2$ > 70 mm Hg

Noninvasive mechanical ventilation should not be used as the mode of ventilatory support if the patient is obtunded, breathes poorly or irregularly, is unable to protect the airway, has copious respiratory secretions, and has a risk of aspirating gastric contents. We also prefer to intubate and ventilate those whose $PaO_2 < 45$ mm Hg and who are admitted with a pH < 7.20. Patients who show an acute and progressive rise of $PaCO_2$ of more than 70–80 mm Hg are often obtunded, and in our opinion, are more effectively managed by endotracheal intubation and invasive ventilator support **(Table 9)**. Endotracheal intubation and ventilation should obviously be also resorted to when NIPPV fails to prove of benefit within 6-10 hours of its initiation, or even earlier, if the patient worsens on this mode of support.

Implementation of Noninvasive Positive Pressure Ventilation

Noninvasive positive pressure ventilation can be offered through either a light-fitting face mask or a nasal mask. Each has its own advantages. We prefer the face mask in patients with severe respiratory failure. A wide variety of ventilatory modes can be used in NIPPV. We prefer the biphasic positive airway pressure (BiPAP) mode because it allows for good gas exchange and effectively reduces both the work of breathing and patient distress. Pressure support ventilation (PSV) is perhaps an equally useful mode and is generally better tolerated than the assist-control mode. In a BiPAP mode, to start with, the inspiratory pressure (IP) is kept at 8–10 cm above the end-expiratory pressure (EP), so that if the EP is 5–7 cm H_2O, the IP is 12–15 cm H_2O. The inspiratory pressure can then be slowly (step-wise) adjusted upwards, and the expiratory pressure also suitably adjusted to allow for effective alveolar ventilation and good gas exchange.

If the PSV mode is used for NIPPV, the inspiratory pressure support to start with is kept on 15–20 cm H_2O. A small positive end expiratory pressure (PEEP) of 4–5 cm

H_2O may be of help in patients who have a large auto-PEEP, as it helps reduce inspiratory effort to generate inspiratory airflow in these patients.

Weaning from NIPPV is accomplished by progressively decreasing the level of inspiratory pressure support if the PSV mode is used, or by allowing the patient to be intermittently off NIPPV for increasing lengths of time.

Intubation and Mechanical Ventilation (Table 9)

Patients who show a sharp progressive rise in the $PaCO_2$ with a pH < 7.2 on controlled oxygen therapy, or those whose dangerous hypoxia stand unrelieved on conservative therapy or NIPPV, are best intubated and put on mechanical ventilator support. Selection of cases for this mode of treatment is difficult. It would be disastrous for a patient and his family if after starting mechanical ventilation, it becomes impossible to wean the patient off ventilator support. In our opinion, the best indication whether to opt for invasive ventilator support or not, is the activity and state of health of the patient under basal conditions. If the patient's activity was hopelessly poor under basal conditions to start with (i.e. he was more or less confined to his bed due to poor respiratory reserve), it is unwise to opt for invasive ventilator support, and the family should be advised accordingly. If he was reasonably active prior to the crisis that brought him to the ICU, he should be offered ventilator support.

Endotracheal intubation in patients showing poor response to antibiotics, bronchodilators, corticosteroids and controlled oxygen therapy, offers two advantages. It allows proper access for suctioning of respiratory secretions, and it allows mechanical ventilator support.

Mechanical ventilation is difficult in patients with chronic airways obstruction. We prefer and recommend the assist/control mode in patients with severe acute respiratory failure, so that total support and appropriate choice of ventilator settings can be provided. Sedation and rarely, neuromuscular paralysis may be necessary for effective respiratory support. As recovery proceeds, or in patients who are not very ill, PSV may be used. The principles for successful ventilation are outlined in **Table 10**.

(a) *Small tidal volumes* of 300–400 mL are used with minute ventilation not exceeding 5–6 L/min. Lung protection measures require that peak pressures are not unduly high and that the plateau pressure does

Table 9: Relative indications for endotracheal intubation and ventilator support.
• Respiratory rate > 40 breaths/min
• Respiratory muscle fatigue
• Mental obtundation
• A silent chest—respiratory arrest
• Hypotension
• Falling pH < 7.20
• $PaO_2 < 45$ mm Hg
• Rising $PaCO_2 > 70$ mm close to 100 mm Hg

Table 10: Principles of mechanical ventilation in patients with COPD with acute respiratory crisis.

Ventilator settings	Objectives
• Low tidal volumes of 350 mL (6–7 mL/kg) MV < 5–6 L/min	• Prevents overinflation • Prevents dynamic hyperinflation and progressive increase in auto-PEEP
• Rate: 12–14/min	• Decreases peak inflation pressure
• Flow rate: 40–60 L/min	• Reduces risk of barotraumas
• I:E ratio of 1:3	• Allows good distribution of inspired gas, allows time for expiration
• FiO_2 of 50–70%	• Allows quick correction of hypoxia
• Sedate or use pancuronium	• Allows machine to take over, and prevents clashing with the machine

Notes: (i) Lower $PaCO_2$ very gradually over 24 hours or even longer to 50 mm Hg—a PaO_2 of 60 mm Hg suffices
(ii) If weaning is difficult, use pressure support ventilation.

not exceed 30 cm H_2O. The FiO_2 is increased to 50% or 60% or even more so that dangerous hypoxia is quickly corrected. It is unnecessary to aim for an oxygen saturation more than 90%. The low tidal volumes prevent dynamic hyperinflation, thereby preventing a further increase in auto-PEEP, which is invariably present in these patients (see section on pathophysiology). Low tidal volumes also lead to lower peak inflation pressures. This is a great advantage, as high peak pressures if transmitted to the intrapleural space, cause a sharp reduction in the venous return and the cardiac output, and can produce sudden severe hypotension. In fact, *hypotension should be carefully looked out for, particularly after starting ventilation*. A fall in the arterial pressure should prompt one to further reduce the inflation pressure by further reducing the tidal volume. The blood pressure should also be raised by volume expansion or by using vasopressor support. Once the patient is on mechanical ventilation with the hypoxia corrected by a high FiO_2, an increase in $PaCO_2$ need not be feared. Under these circumstances, death usually does not occur due to a high $PaCO_2$.

Sensitivity: The optimal triggering threshold is difficult in an acute COPD crisis in the presence of dynamic hyperinflation (i.e. auto-PEEP). This is because the patient has to generate a negative pressure at least equal to the level of auto-PEEP before interfacing with the preset sensitivity on the ventilator. If the auto-PEEP is high, the required inspiratory effort (before reaching trigger sensitivity) to initiate airflow is significant and this can lead to patient-ventilator dyssynchrony. Yet if the trigger sensitivity is kept very low, the ventilator could be triggered very frequently and inappropriately. If the auto-PEEP is significantly raised, extrinsic PEEP is applied at a level well below the level of the auto-PEEP. This helps to reduce the effort needed to initiate inspiratory flow.

(b) *Ventilator requirements* are so adjusted so as to bring down the raised $PaCO_2$ level very slowly over 24–48 hours. It is generally unnecessary to reduce the $PaCO_2$ to less than 50 mm Hg unless the basal $PaCO_2$ levels were normal. A sudden drop in the $PaCO_2$ is dangerous as it causes a sudden shift from respiratory acidemia to metabolic alkalosis and alkalemia. This can precipitate dangerous arrhythmias and cause sudden death.

(c) The flow rates used in such patients are usually between 40 L/min and 60 L/min, and the inspiration: expiration ratio is initially set at 1:3.

(d) Patients should not be allowed to clash with the machine; they can be safely given pancuronium, or sedated once they are put on ventilator support.

(e) Mechanical ventilator support is generally necessary for a period of 3–7 days. The maximum period over which we have used ventilator support, and then finally succeeded in weaning the patient, has been 6 weeks. An elective tracheostomy is preferred if ventilator support needs to be extended for more than 7 days, or if the patient has thick copious secretions, which cannot be easily suctioned through the endotracheal tube.

(f) Weaning is generally carried out by the traditional methods. We have used intermittent mandatory ventilation, and PSV, but have never been totally convinced of their absolute necessity. The patient is taken off ventilator support when he can maintain an adequate gas exchange on his own. This generally happens when infection has been controlled, airways obstruction has decreased, and V/Q abnormalities have been significantly rectified. A satisfactory T-tube trial over 2–4 hours invariably allows extubation.

(g) If in a COPD exacerbation weaning fails, NIV should be used. It facilitates weaning, prevents re-intubation and reduces mortality. Early use of NIV in patients who after extubation show a progressive rise in $PaCO_2$ during a spontaneous breathing trial, reduces the risk of respiratory failure and lowers the 90-day mortality in these patients.

(h) Older patients with ischemic heart disease often need careful cardiovascular support. The presence of associated left ventricular failure with pulmonary edema, together with generalized water retention is not uncommon in these patients. *It is indeed remarkable how good ventilator support with improvement in blood gases initiates a diuresis in these patients, even though earlier use of large doses of furosemide might have been ineffective. Correction of severe hypoxia and hypercapnia are probably responsible for the improved cardiac-cum-renal function and diuresis.*

(i) Expert nursing, humidification of inspired oxygen and persistence with the regime outlined earlier, are all essentials of good respiratory care in these patients.

The in-hospital mortality for an AECOPD ranges from 4–30% and averages 12–30% in those with respiratory failure. In survivors 1 year mortality is as high as 43% and 5 year mortality approaches 70%.

Our mortality in patients with acute respiratory failure in COPD who require invasive ventilator support is about 10%.

Treatment of Complications during Acute Respiratory Failure in Exacerbation of COPD

A number of complications may arise in critically ill patients with acute respiratory failure resulting from an acute exacerbation of COPD. These are listed in **Table 11**.

These should be promptly diagnosed and treated. The most dangerous complications outside the respiratory system are cardiac arrhythmias and hemodynamic instability.

Cardiac Arrhythmias: Cardiac arrhythmias are frequently observed in these patients. Supraventricular tachycardia, multifocal atrial tachycardia and atrial fibrillation are common; AV dissociation and multiple ventricular extrasystolies may also occur. The mortality rate is significantly higher in patients having arrhythmias.

Hemodynamic Instability: Patients with COPD often suffer from pulmonary hypertension. An acute exacerbation of COPD worsens pulmonary hypertension due to hypoxic vasoconstriction, dynamic hyperinflation, or the presence of auto-PEEP during mechanical ventilation. A sharp increase in pulmonary artery pressure leads to severe right ventricular dysfunction, right-sided heart failure, with a fall in both systolic and mean arterial blood pressure.

An intravenous fluid challenge expands the intravascular pulmonary bed and improves right ventricular pump function. It should be the initial step in the management of hypotension and hemodynamic instability in an acute crisis of COPD. If the hemodynamic state fails to improve, inotropic and/or vasopressor support become necessary. Ventilator adjustments to reduce dynamic hyperinflation and auto-PEEP are also necessary. The management of acute respiratory crisis in COPD is summarized in **Table 12**.

Hospital Discharge and Follow-up

Patients may be discharged once they are stable, reasonably comfortable with a satisfactory improvement in the FEV_1 and an O_2 saturation of 90% or more breathing room air. Prior to discharge, patients should start optimum therapy for COPD which would include the correct use of inhaled bronchodilators and if necessary inhaled corticosteroids.

Table 11: Complications during acute respiratory failure in COPD.

- Pulmonary infection
- Fluid, electrolyte and acid-base disturbances
- Respiratory acidosis with hypokalemic metabolic alkalosis
- Severe water logging can occur due to salt and water retention
- Cardiac arrhythmias
- Right-sided heart failure
- Hypotension if there is marked auto-PEEP
- Pneumothorax
- Complications due to mechanical ventilation
- Gastrointestinal bleeds
- Pulmonary thromboembolism
- Mental depression

Table 12: Management of acute respiratory crisis in patients with COPD.

- *Improve ventilation, correct ventilation-perfusion mismatch, relieve severe hypoxia and correct low pH:*
  - Controlled oxygen therapy (24–30% oxygen)
  - Treat infection with antibiotics
  - Relieve airways obstruction—nebulize salbutamol 4 hourly, ipratropium bromide 8 hourly
  - Use corticosteroids
  - Theophylline
  - Physiotherapy to help drain copious secretions and prevent sputum retention
  - Ventilator support when so indicated
  - Cardiovascular support when necessary
- *Treat complications encountered during acute respiratory failure:*
  - Correct fluid and electrolyte disturbances
  - Management of cardiac complications, e.g. arrhythmias, hypotension, right-sided heart failure and pulmonary thromboembolism
  - Treat GI bleeds
  - Drain even a shallow pneumothorax

They should be consulted against smoking. Monitoring after discharge should include spirometric readings, clinical examination and the effectiveness of therapy.

Influenza Vaccine

A Cochrane review by Walters et al showed that Influenza vaccine significantly reduced AE compared to placebo (p = 0.006).

Preventing Readmission after Discharge from an AECOPD

About 20% of patients with an AE are readmitted within 30 days of discharge. A post-discharge bundle of smoking cessation, education, inhaler technique assessment and pulmonary rehabilitation reduced readmissions by 6%. Factors associated with readmission included multiple prior admissions, older age, more severe COPD, co-morbidities and lower socioeconomic status.

■ SUGGESTED READING

1. Elliott MW. Noninvasive ventilation in acute exacerbations of COPD. Eur Resp Rev. 2005;14(94):39-42.

2. Holden V, Slack D III, McCurdy MT, et al. Diagnosis and management of acute exacerbation of chronic obstructive pulmonary disease [digest]. Emerg Med Pract. 2017;19(10 Suppl):S1-S2.

3. Jacques R, Man SFP, Sin DD. Prevalence of pulmonary embolism in acute exacerbations of COPD: a systematic review and meta-analysis. Chest March. 2009;135:786-93.

4. Maltais F, Ostinelli J, Bourbeau J, et al. Comparison of nebulized budesonide and oral prednisolone with placebo in the treatment of acute exacerbations of chronic obstructive pulmonary disease: a randomized controlled trial. Am J Respir Crit Care Med. 2002;165(5):698-703.

5. Piquet J, Chavaillon JM, David P, et al. High-risk patients following hospitalisation for an acute exacerbation of COPD. Eur Respir J. 2013;42:946.

6. Singanayagam A, Schembri S, Chalmers JD. Predictors of mortality in hospitalized adults with acute exacerbation of chronic obstructive pulmonary disease. Ann Am Thorac Soc. 2013;10:81.

7. Stevenson NJ, Walker PP, Costell RW, et al. Lung mechanics and dyspnea during exacerbations of chronic obstructive pulmonary disease. Am J Respir Crit Care Med. 2005;172:1510-6.

8. Walters JA, Tan DJ, White CJ, et al. Different durations of corticosteroid therapy for exacerbations of chronic obstructive pulmonary disease. Cochrane Database Syst Rev. 2018;3:CD006897.

CHAPTER 38

Chronic Obstructive Pulmonary Disease: Management

■ INTRODUCTION

By definition, chronic obstructive pulmonary disease (COPD) is incurable yet treatable. Current treatment affords significant symptomatic relief and in particular helps to reduce dyspnea, increases effort tolerance, and improves the quality of life.

Patient compliance with regard to medications prescribed, as also with regard to a disciplined lifestyle and the cessation of smoking (in smokers) is essential for a successful outcome.

Objectives of management are:

- *Prevent progression*: The only way to achieve this objective is to abolish as far as possible all risk factors. Cessation of smoking in smokers is the key to prevent COPD as also to prevent progression of established COPD in smokers.
- *Relieve symptoms*: The main symptoms are breathlessness, poor exercise tolerance, cough often with mucoid or mucopurulent sputum. Symptomatic relief is provided by the appropriate use of aerosolized bronchodilators, the use of inhaled corticosteroids (ICSs), and the use of pulmonary rehabilitation.
- *Prevent and treat exacerbations*: Exacerbations are inbuilt in the natural history of COPD. Their prevention and treatment is of paramount importance and have been considered in a separate chapter.
- *Prolong life*: The use of oxygen in patients who are hypoxic has been clearly shown to prolong life. Oxygen also relieves dyspnea and improves exercise tolerance thereby improving the quality of life.
- *Diagnose and treat any complications* (besides acute exacerbations) that can precipitate acute respiratory failure or can result in acute on chronic respiratory failure in patients with severe COPD. This has been dealt with in the chapter on "Acute Exacerbation of COPD".
- *Improve general nutritional state*: This requires an appropriate diet and graduated exercise under a pulmonary rehabilitation program.
- *Search for and treat comorbidities* like ischemic heart disease, diabetes, liver cell dysfunction, and renal dysfunction, any one of which may have an indirect deleterious bearing on COPD.
- *Symptomatic management of severe hypercapnia* in COPD patients with chronic hypercapnic respiratory failure.
- *Treatment of right heart failure* arising from cor pulmonale in end-stage COPD with appropriate medications.
- *Surgical measures* in a select subset of COPD patients.

■ PREVENT PROGRESSION

Smoking, occupational factors, indoor pollution due to combustion of biofuels and outdoor environmental pollution are the main risk factors. These should be mitigated or abolished. Smoking and indoor pollution can and should be completely abolished. Occupational factors may often be impossible to remove in their entirety but they can and should be appropriately mitigated. Outdoor pollution is impossible for individuals to control, but when feasible, a change of workplace or residence from a very heavily polluted area to an area with little or no pollution may help.

Cessation of smoking is crucial to prevent further progression of COPD and to preserve both lung function and exercise tolerance. Smokers who are susceptible to the adverse effects of cigarette smoke have a sharper decline in lung function, in particular the forced expiratory volume in one second (FEV$_1$) compared to nonsmokers. The Lung Health Study revealed that cessation of smoking in these patients reduces the rate of decline of FEV$_1$ to that of nonsmokers. Cessation of smoking does not cure COPD or reverse the inflammatory damages already present in the small airways and in the lung periphery. Pulmonary function may however show some improvement and not uncommonly the patient feels more comfortable in breathing (**Figs. 1 and 2**).

Smoking Cessation Program

It is important to ascertain the exact habits of patients (both from the patient and for greater accuracy from close relatives or associates), and to assess how motivated they are to quit. An approach to smoking cessation consists of the five "As" detailed in the Gold guidelines.

Ask if the patient is still smoking at every visit.

Advise the patient as to why he should quit, the advantages that would accrue if he did and the dangers inherent in smoking if he did not.

Assess his willingness to quit.

Assist in quitting by educating the patient on nicotine withdrawal and explaining addiction in general and addiction to tobacco in particular. Counseling, support, use of nicotine replacement therapy (NRT) and bupropion are often needed.

Arrange for regular scheduled follow-up; either in person or telephone.

To these five "As" detailed in the Gold guidelines we would add that every time a smoker visits the doctor he should be given a detailed (perhaps even a lurid) expose on the dangers of smoking not just in relation to COPD but also other diseases—notably cancer of the lung, strokes, heart attacks, and dangers of peripheral vascular disease. We have on appropriate occasions directly shown the devastating effects of a massive stroke, cancer of the lung, gangrene of a foot, to help a smoker realize the danger of smoking so that he is further motivated to quit the habit.

It must be admitted that the pressure of work in very busy outpatient departments of large hospitals in metropolitan cities of India and other developing countries leaves little time for a detailed discussion with a smoker on the dangers of smoking. Merely asking him to quit at every visit rarely helps. In fact, in our experience nothing helps (and this includes the use of nicotine replacement patches and bupropion) unless the patient is sufficiently motivated to stop. The aim of the treating doctor is to first arouse this motivation and reinforce it with every visit.

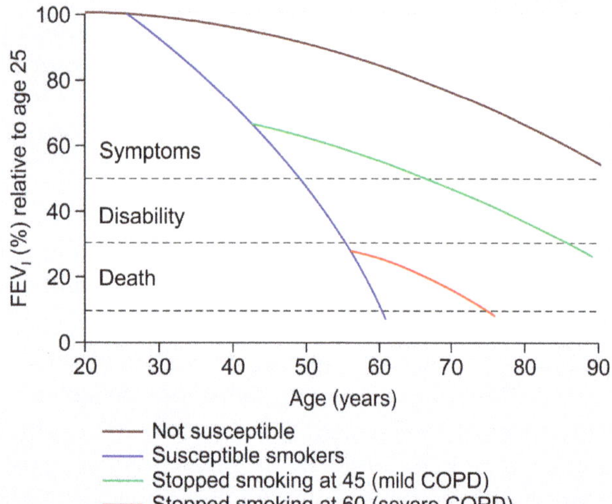

Fig. 1: Decline in lung function in cigarette smokers and the effects of smoking cessation. Lung function declines more rapidly in smokers who are susceptible to the adverse effects of cigarettes compared with nonsmokers. Discontinuing smoking in a 45-year-old with more severe disease reduces the accelerated decline in lung function and delays progression of symptoms.
(COPD: Chronic obstructive pulmonary disease)
Source: Modified from Fletcher C, Petro R. The natural history of chronic airflow obstruction. BMJ. 1977;1:1645-8.

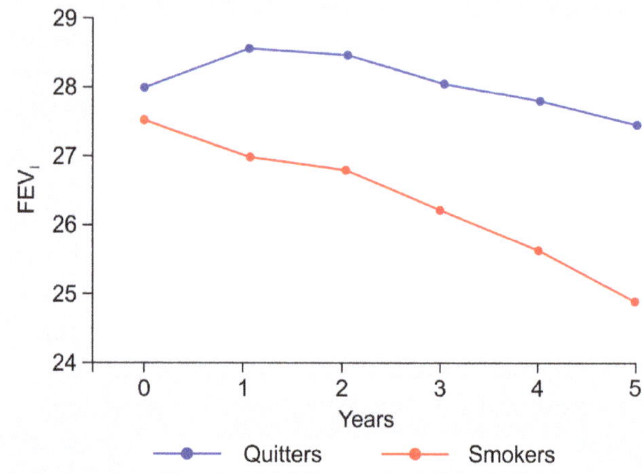

Fig. 2: Effect of smoking cessation on lung function. The forced expired volume in 1 sec (FEV$_1$) improved in the year after smoking cessation.
Source: Adapted from Anthonisen NR, Connett JE, Kiley JP, et al. Effects of smoking intervention and the use of an inhaled anticholinergic bronchodilator on the rate of decline of FEV$_1$. The Lung Health Study. JAMA. 1994;272:1497-505.

The Lung Heart Study showed that patients who were likely to achieve and maintain smoking cessation were married, were accompanied by a relative, friend at counseling sessions, and/or had made previous long-term attempts to quit. Those who were likely to fail had made several short-term attempts to quit, had extra-stressful lives and were still using nicotine patches as replacement therapy 1 year after quitting. Perhaps the main difference underlying those who quit or from those who do not, is the different degree of motivation in these two groups, as also external influences together with personality factors influencing the motivation.

Nicotine Replacement Therapy and the Use of Bupropion

In the West, NRT is reported to result in twice the quit rate compared to placebo. NRT is available as a chewing gum or a skin patch. In the West, it is also available as a nasal spray and an inhaler. The combination of counseling, the use of NRT and bupropion is reported to result in the highest rate for smoking cessation. Bupropion is given in a dose of 150 mg BD for 6–8 weeks. Headache is a frequent side effect, seizures have been occasionally reported, so that it is best avoided in epileptics. Side effects of nicotine are not uncommon with NRT, particularly in patients smoking less than 10 cigarettes per day. In patients with ischemic heart disease (angina, recent myocardial infarction), acid peptic disease, and in pregnant or breast feeding women, NRT is avoided or used with great caution.

Varenicline is a new drug used as an alternative to NRT; it acts as a partial agonist to nicotine acetylcholine receptors and is given as a 12 week course. Randomized trials have shown a better rate of smoking cessation with varenicline than with either placebo or bupropion. Nausea was the main adverse effect observed. Higher suicide rates have been reported in patients on varenicline.

■ PHARMACOTHERAPY

Use of Inhaled Bronchodilators

Bronchodilators in COPD are most often given on a regular basis. They provide symptomatic relief and improve exercise tolerance and capacity. They do so by reducing air-trapping and lung hyperinflation, increasing inspiratory capacity and increasing flow rates during expiration. The FEV_1 may show a significant increase (over

15%), but symptomatic relief may be present even when the FEV_1 is unchanged **(Figs. 3 to 5)**.

The earlier therapeutic strategy of the Global initiative for Chronic Obstructive Lung Disease (GOLD) was

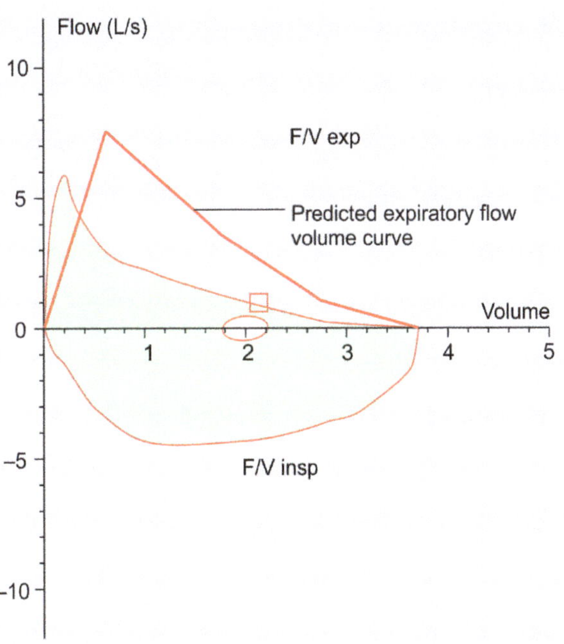

Fig. 3: Flow-volume loop showing mild chronic obstructive pulmonary disease (COPD).

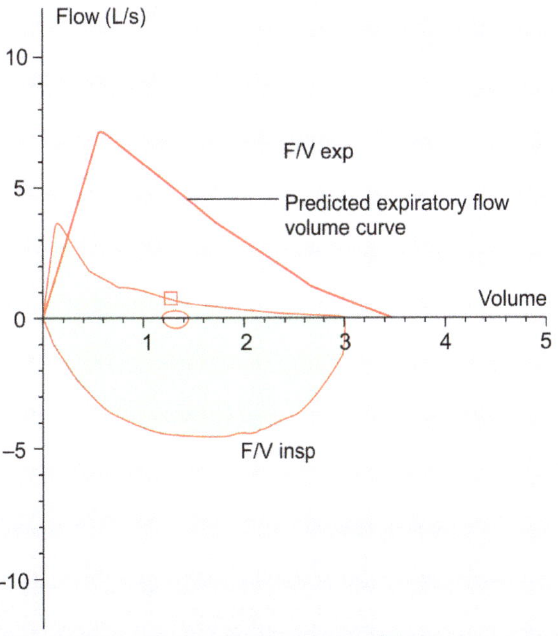

Fig. 4: Flow-volume loop showing moderate chronic obstructive pulmonary disease (COPD).

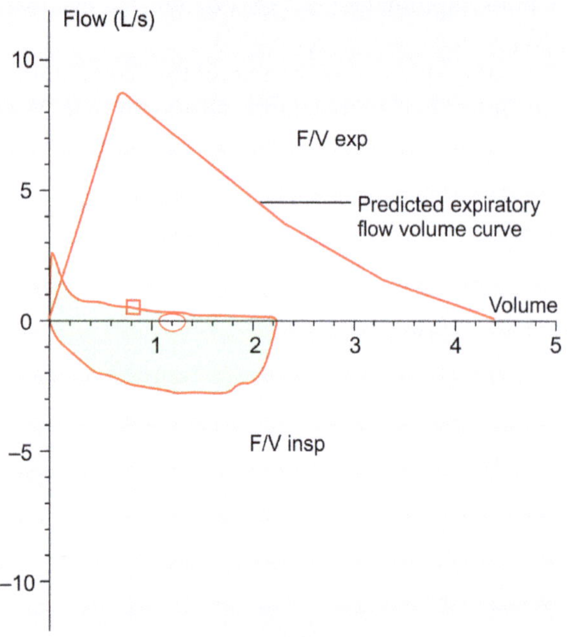

Fig. 5: Flow-volume loop showing severe chronic obstructive pulmonary disease (COPD).

Table 1: Spirometric classification of the degree of COPD severity (based on post-bronchodilator FEV_1).

I	Mild COPD	FEV_1/FVC <70; $FEV_1 \geq 80\%$ of predicted
II	Moderate COPD	FEV_1/FVC < 70; $FEV \geq 50\%$ and < 80% of predicted
III	Severe COPD	FEV_1/FVC < 70; $FEV_1 \geq 30\%$ and < 50% of predicted
IV	Very severe COPD	FEV_1/FVC < 70; FEV_1 < 30% of predicted

based on the degree of severity of disease as judged from spirometric findings **(Table 1)**.

The current therapeutic strategy of GOLD guidelines suggests *using a combined assessment based on severity of individual symptoms and risk of exacerbations to guide therapy*. These guidelines are tabled below **(Table 2)**.

It needs to be stressed that these guidelines are based on studies of large groups of patients with COPD. Therapy should always be tailored to the particular individual under one's care.

Broadly speaking we present a simplified plan for management of COPD, which takes into account the severity of COPD as judged by spirometric findings, the severity of symptoms and the risk of exacerbations.

- Patients who have severe or very severe COPD as judged from spirometric findings, have invariably well-marked symptoms (judged from the mMRC Dyspnea Scale) of breathlessness and most have a high risk of exacerbations of the disease. These are best treated with inhaled LABA + LAMA + ICS .
- Patients who have moderately severe disease as judged from spirometric findings are treated with inhaled LABA + LAMA. If their symptoms increase or are poorly controlled or if they have frequent exacerbations they are best treated with LABA + LAMA + ICS.
- Patients with mild COPD as judged from spirometric findings are advised a short-acting beta agonist (SABA) on an SOS basis to counter a temporary increase in breathlessness. If these episodes of breathlessness are frequent, a LABA daily on a long-term basis is advised.
- Any patient with COPD—even mild or moderate who has frequent exacerbations (>2/year requiring

Table 2: Management of COPD. Therapy based on the GOLD assessment of symptoms and risk of exacerbation.*

Category	Symptoms	Risk	Suggested treatment
ALL			Avoidance of risk factor(s), such as smoking Annual influenza vaccination Pneumococcal vaccination Regular physical activity Regular review/correction of inhaler technique Long-term oxygen therapy if chronic hypoxemia Pulmonary rehabilitation
A	**Less symptomatic** Mild or infrequent symptoms (i.e. breathless with strenuous exercise or when hurrying on level ground or walking up a slight hill)¶ or CAT <10ᐞ	**Low risk** 0 or 1 exacerbations in the past year without associated hospitalization	**Recommendation:** Short-acting bronchodilator or combination of short-acting beta-agonist and anticholinergic, as needed **Alternative:** Long-acting bronchodilator if beneficial

Contd...

Contd...

Category	Symptoms	Risk	Suggested treatment
B	**More symptomatic** Moderate to severe symptoms (i.e. patient has to walk more slowly than others of same age due to breathlessness, has to stop to catch breath when walking on level ground at own pace, or has more severe breathlessness)[¶] or CAT ≥10[Δ]	**Low risk** 0 or 1 exacerbations in the past year without associated hospitalization	**First choice:** Regular treatment with a long-acting bronchodilator, either LAMA or LABA, based on symptom relief. Short-acting bronchodilator available for symptom control as needed **For persistent symptoms:** Regular treatment with a combination of LAMA and LABA
C	**Less symptomatic** Mild or infrequent symptoms (i.e. breathless with strenuous exercise or when hurrying on level ground or walking up a slight hill)[¶] or CAT <10[Δ]	**High risk** ≥2 exacerbations per year with one or more leading to hospitalization	**First choice:** Regular treatment with a LAMA; SABA available for symptom control as needed **For further exacerbations:** Regular treatment with a LAMA plus LABA OR (less preferred) LABA plus ICS
D	**More symptomatic** Moderate to severe symptoms (i.e. patient has to walk slower than others of same age due to breathlessness, has to stop to catch breath when walking on level ground at own pace, or has more severe breathlessness)[¶] or CAT ≥10[Δ]	**High risk** ≥2 exacerbations per year with one or more leading to hospitalization	**First choice:** Regular treatment with combination LABA plus LAMA, LABA plus inhaled glucocorticoid may be preferred, if features of asthma/COPD overlap. SABA available for symptom control as needed. LAMA alone, if LABA contraindicated **For further exacerbations:** Regular treatment with combination of LAMA plus LABA plus ICS OR (less preferred in absence of asthma overlap) switch to LABA plus ICS If exacerbations continue despite triple therapy, additional options for selected patients include roflumilast (if chronic bronchitis and FEV_1 <50% predicted), theophylline, chronic therapy with a macrolide, and stopping inhaled glucocorticoids

Patients must be taught how and when to use their treatments, and treatment choices are adjusted based on patient responses. Medications being prescribed for other conditions should be reviewed.

(COPD: Chronic obstructive pulmonary disease; GOLD: Global Initiative for Chronic Obstructive Lung Disease; LAMA: Long-acting muscarinic (anticholinergic) agent; LABA: Long-acting beta agonist; SABA: Short-acting beta agonist; ICS: Inhaled corticosteroid (glucocorticoid); FEV_1: Forced expiratory volume in one second; FVC: Forced vital capacity)
*All patients with COPD have a reduced FEV_1/FVC ratio that is <0.70% predicted or <5th percentile lower limit of normal. The severity of airflow limitation is determined by the FEV_1.
[¶]Symptom severity based on: Modified Medical Research Council (mMRC) Dyspnea scale.
[Δ]COPD Assessment Test (CAT): http://www.catestonline.org (Accessed on February 10, 2017).
Source: Global Initiative for Chronic Obstructive Pulmonary Disease: Global Strategy for the Diagnosis, Management, and Prevention of COPD, 2017 (Accessed February 10, 2017).
Additional data from:
1. Fletcher CM, Elmes PC, Fairbairn MB, et al. The significance of respiratory symptoms and the diagnosis of chronic bronchitis in a working population. Br Med J. 1959;2:257.
2. Dodd JW, Hogg L, Notan J, et al. The COPD Assessment Test (CAT): response to pulmonary rehabilitation. A multicentre, prospective study. Thorax. 2011;66:425.
3. Dodd JW, Marns PL, Clark AL, et al. The COPD Assessment Test (CAT): short- and medium-term response to pulmonary rehabilitation. COPD. 2012;9:390.
4. Jones PW, Harding G, Berry P, et al. Development and first validation of the COPD Assessment Test. Eur Respir J. 2009;34:648.
5. http://www.catestonline.org

hospitalization) should receive ICS. The latter should not be given alone but with LABA or LAMA.

Exacerbations of breathlessness in any patient with COPD should be countered by the temporary use of an inhaled SABA or an anticholinergic drug, or both.

In moderately severe or severe COPD, once there is significant relief, a de-escalation of therapy may be attempted. The dosage of LABA or LAMA may be reduced, the frequency of use reduced (once daily instead of twice daily), and only if possible the inhaled corticosteroids may be reduced in dosage, frequency, or even stopped.

Theophylline (orally) is a drug introduced very early in the natural history of COPD in our country. A short description of the drug is given later in this chapter.

A relevant discussion on the use of short-acting β_2-agonists (SABAs), LABAs, anticholinergic bronchodilators, theophylline, use of ICSs and the use of the combination of one or more of the above is given below. There is then a brief mention on mucolytic agents and macrolides.

β_2-agonist Bronchodilators

Short-acting β_2-specific Agonists (SABA)

Short-acting β_2-specific agonists bind to and stimulate the β_2-receptors thereby causing smooth muscle relaxation within bronchi and bronchioles. The mechanism of action is through activation of adenylyl cyclase thereby increasing the concentration of intracellular cyclic adenosine monophosphate. SABAs have a rapid onset of action which reaches a peak in 5–15 minutes, the effect lasting for 4–6 hours. Salbutamol (albuterol) is the SABA available for inhalation in most countries of the world. In India, it is available as a metered-dose inhaler (MDI), 100 µg/dose and as a solution for nebulization (2.5 mL = 2.5 mg). It is used in a dose of one to two puffs thrice or at most four times a day. In *mild COPD it is used as and when necessary for symptomatic relief*; it should not be used, as already mentioned earlier, on a regular basis to prevent or reduce symptoms in stable COPD. It can however be used as rescue medication for symptom relief in patients who are using LABAs. Salbutamol can also be nebulized, with the nebulized solution containing 2.5 mg of the drug. Salbutamol is also available as a long-acting oral preparation in the form of a tablet or syrup.

Side effects of inhaled SABA are dose related; they include tachycardia, palpitation, hypertension, electrocardiography (ECG) changes that may occasionally resemble those of subendocardial infarction, and chest discomfort. These effects are due to the binding and stimulation of the β_2-receptors of the heart. Tremor of the hands, nervousness, anxiety, gastrointestinal discomfort, gastroesophageal reflux may also be observed due to systemic absorption of the drug. Hypokalemia is another feature of SABA therapy and is an important effect to be borne in mind, particularly in critically ill patients.

The major disadvantage of SABA is that frequent use as in bronchial asthma leads to a downgrade of the β_2-receptors resulting in tachyphylaxis. They should therefore not be used more than four or at most six times a day. If tachyphylaxis is suspected the drug should be stopped for some days following which it often regains its efficacy.

Levalbuterol tartrate is the R-enantiomer of albuterol. The reason for its development is to reduce the adverse effects believed to be related to the S-enantiomer which is present in the racemic mixture. However, clinical studies show that levalbuterol like other β_2-agonists can produce cardiovascular side effects. Levalbuterol is available as an MDI of 45 µg/dose and as a solution for nebulization.

Long-acting β_2-agonists (LABA)

Salmeterol and formoterol are the LABAs available. LABAs like SABAs, produce bronchodilator effects by direct stimulation of the β_2-receptors. Salmeterol binds preferentially to the lipophilic sites of the β_2-receptors, takes 30–60 minutes to reach its maximum bronchodilator effect which lasts for 12 hours. Formoterol binds equally to hydrophilic and lipophilic sites of the β_2-receptors. It has a rapid onset of action in about 5–15 minutes lasting for 12 hours. Salmeterol is available as 50 µg/dose DPI preparation inhaled twice daily. The regular twice daily use of LABA gives symptom relief to stable COPD patients which may or may not always be reflected in improved lung function.

Though LABAs may significantly improve FEV_1, lung volumes, dyspnea, exacerbation rate and number of hospitalizations, they have no effect on mortality or rate of decline of lung function.

Long-acting β_2-agonists which have a more prolonged action than salmeterol and formoterol, so that they can be administered just once daily, are also in use. They are indacaterol a once daily LABA that improves breathlessness and exacerbation rate, as also olodaterol and vilanterol, once daily LABAs which improve lung function and symptoms.

It should be noted that the regular use of LABA has been implicated in acute exacerbations of severe asthma and in increased asthma deaths. It is possible that tachyphylaxis due to the prolonged regular use of LABA might be responsible for adverse effects. Admittedly these adverse effects have as yet not been reported in patients with COPD.

Anticholinergic Bronchodilators

The commonly used anticholinergic bronchodilator is ipratropium bromide, a short-acting quaternary ammonium derivative of atropine sulfate. It exerts its bronchodilator action by blocking the muscarinic receptors in airway smooth muscles and in cells of the submucous glands.

The drug exerts its blocking effect on muscarinic receptors in a nonselective fashion. It is however the blocking effect on the M_3 receptors in bronchial smooth muscle that is responsible for reduction in bronchomotor tone. There is however no change in mucus secretions following the use of anticholinergic bronchodilators. Ipratropium is available as an MDI containing 20 μg/dose. A combination 20 μg of ipratropium and 50 μg of levosalbutamol is also available. Inhaled ipratropium bromide is not recommended for regular use, but can be used as medication for symptom relief in patients using LABA. Ipratropium is also available as a nebulized solution, the dose being 500 μg nebulized once or twice for symptom relief. Side effects of anticholinergic drugs even when inhaled or nebulized may be observed. The most common is a dry mouth. Other uncommon side effects include skin rashes, headache, constipation, urinary retention, and rarely, hypertension. When nebulized, the drug may affect the eyes (generally through direct contact of the nebulized vapor with the eyes) in patients with glaucoma, causing a further rise in intraocular tension.

The use of ipratropium bromide is not reported to cause tachyphylaxis. Its bronchodilator effect is equal and at times superior to that of inhaled β_2-agonists in COPD. It produces relief of symptoms and improves effort tolerance.

Tiotropium is a long-acting anticholinergic drug (LAMA) which when inhaled has an action lasting 24 hours. Tiotropium binds with equal avidity to M_1, M_2, and M_3 receptors but dissociates quickly from the M_1 receptors. It is available as a 9 μg/dose dry powder inhaler to be given once daily. Its onset of action is between 1 hour and 3 hours and lasts for 24 hours. Clinical studies suggest that tiotropium is more effective than the scheduled doses of ipratropium bromide in improving lung function, relieving symptoms and decreasing the incidence of acute exacerbations. Clinical studies also suggest that tiotropium has a better bronchodilator effect and causes a greater improvement when compared to salmeterol in COPD. The use of tiotropium is not reported to be associated with tachyphylaxis.

The sites of action of β_2-agonists and anticholinergic bronchodilators are given in **Figure 6**.

Other long acting muscarinic agents available abroad but not easily available in India include:

- Aclidinium—a dry powder inhaler, one inhalation twice a day.
- Umeclidinium—once-daily dry powder inhaler.
- Glycopyrrolate—a capsule dry powder inhaler used once daily.

As is emphasized below patients with moderate or severe COPD are best treated by combination of LABA + LAMA inhalational therapy.

Use of Long-acting β_2-agonist Combined with a Long-acting Anticholinergic Bronchodilator

The combination of an inhaled β_2-agonist (LABA) and a long-acting inhaled anticholinergic drug (LAMA) is superior to either one or the other in causing bronchodilation and symptom relief. In COPD patients who remain significantly symptomatic with the use of either one or the other of these bronchodilators, a combination of a LABA plus a long-acting anticholinergic drug should be used, preferably on a regular basis.

Theophylline

Theophylline was the main drug used as a bronchodilator before the advent of inhaled β_2-agonists. It then fell into relative disuse in the West but has now regained its rightful place in the management of COPD. Theophylline is a modest bronchodilator when given orally, but it has additional properties that are being increasingly acknowledged. The drug stimulates the central respiratory drive, is believed to improve diaphragmatic function, reduces diaphragmatic and respiratory muscle fatigue, is a diuretic and in addition has anti-inflammatory effects. This anti-inflammatory action is related to the direct activation of histone deacetylase which takes place even when theophylline blood levels are less than 10 mg/L. A recent review shows that it improves forced vital capacity (FVC), FEV_1, O_2 consumption, PaO_2, and $PaCO_2$ in COPD patients. It is cheap, easily available and is therefore particularly useful to the poor and underprivileged of developing countries such as India, where for several reasons patients in this category are either averse to the use of an inhaled bronchodilator and/or do not manage to use the MDIs in the correct manner.

The mechanisms of action of theophylline are not completely understood. The bronchodilator effect is probably mediated through the inhibition of the two isoenzymes phosphodiesterase III and phosphodiesterase IV. Its nonbronchodilator prophylactic action is probably due to the antagonism of adenosine receptors unrelated to

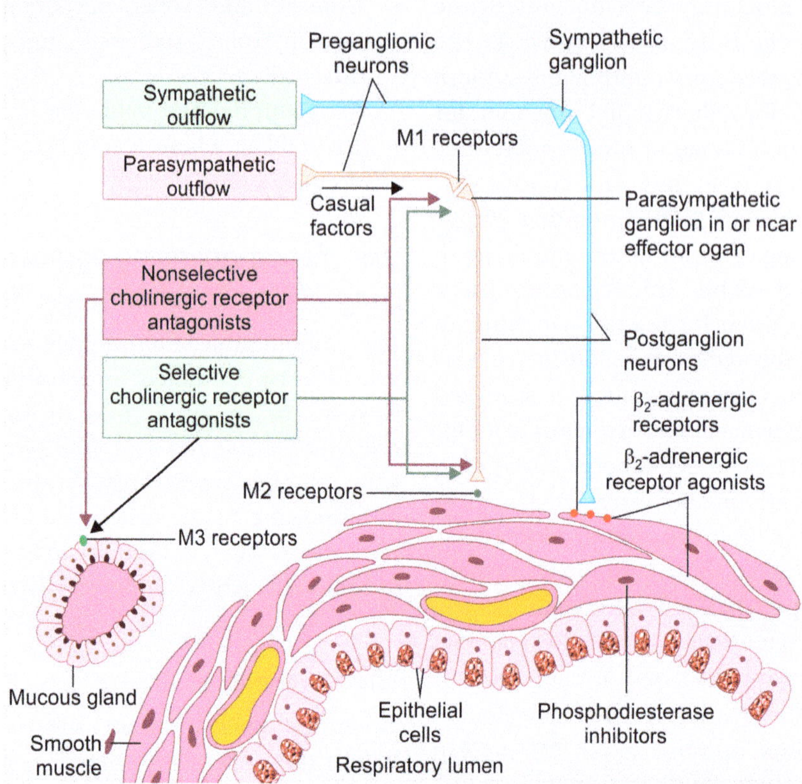

Fig. 6: Sites of action of β₂-agonists and anticholinergic bronchodilators.

inhibition of phosphodiesterase. The drug is metabolized by the cytochrome P450 oxidases. Though the drug unquestionably has side effects, the oral preparation in a dose of 400 mg to at the most 600 mg/day in our experience is well tolerated in Indian subjects. Theophylline levels in the blood should not exceed 20 mg/dL and should preferably range close to 15 mg/dL. Side effects like nausea, vomiting, loss of appetite can occur even when the drug level is in the therapeutic range. Many medications like macrolides and most quinolones interfere with theophylline metabolism. The physician should be aware of the important ones that do so. Besides nausea and vomiting, side effects include abdominal pain, diarrhea, gastroesophageal reflux, anxiety, tremors, nervousness, insomnia and muscle cramps. The two most dangerous toxic effects are arrhythmias, in particular ventricular tachycardia and generalized seizures. Unfortunately, though these dangerous complications are apt to occur when serum concentration of the drug is over 20 mg/dL, and generally over 30 mg/dL, this is not always so. Besides, either of these two dangerous toxic effects may occur suddenly without being preceded by any other minor side

effects mentioned above. Perhaps future studies may prove or disprove the contention that lower serum concentration of the drug may be equally effective in COPD without the danger of adverse side effects.

The GOLD guidelines advocate the use of theophylline in COPD patients who remain symptomatic despite the use of LABA. Theophylline offers greater symptom relief, improves effort tolerance and increases expiratory flow rates when combined with LABA. Stopping the drug reverses this trend. *In developing countries, theophylline is often introduced as a baseline drug, starting in patients with mild COPD and continuing all through to patients with severe COPD.*

Second-generation inhibitors of phosphodiesterase IV are under study. Cilomilast, piclamilast, and roflumilast are some of the newer formulations that have a bronchodilator effect and anti-inflammatory properties with fewer gastrointestinal side effects.

A Cochrane review of 23 randomized trials with selective PDE4 inhibitors concluded that these agents offered benefit over placebo in improving lung function and reducing exacerbations in COPD.

Use of Corticosteroids

It is generally accepted that the long-term use of oral corticosteroids is not indicated and should be strictly avoided in stable COPD patients as their use produces no benefit and results in significant side effects. It is equally accepted, as is discussed in the previous chapter, that the short-term use of systemic or oral corticosteroids for 10–14 days helps recovery in acute exacerbations of COPD.

Role of inhaled corticosteroids in stable COPD: The role of inhaled corticosteroids ICSs has been studied in several large studies of patients with COPD including the Copenhagen study, ISOLDE study, EUROSCOP, and the Lung Health Study. Between them these studies have included almost 5,000 patients with COPD and some generalizations are possible.

Inhaled corticosteroids *do not* slow the inexorable decline in lung function that is a feature of COPD. A recent meta-analysis of 12 trials showed that the change in FEV_1 was an insignificant 51 mL (mean) at 3 years.

Inhaled steroids do have a very important effect on reducing the frequency of exacerbations of COPD. Annual rate of exacerbation in COPD patients getting ICS is 0.99 events/year versus 1.32 events in those on placebo. ICS also provide symptom relief and improve effort tolerance in patients subject to acute "exacerbations. Thus patients on ICS are significantly less likely to be rehospitalized. This may translate into reduced mortality and better quality of life. This protective effect of ICS may take some time to be established. In the ISOLDE study, the effect was apparent only after 3 years.

This effect of ICS on reducing exacerbations may be the main reason behind the improvement in quality of life reported in patients on ICS. It is also certainly the cause of the reduction in mortality observed in patients on ICS. David Sin and colleagues pooled data from seven randomized controlled studies of at least 12 months duration to obtain a database of over 5,000 patients. They showed ICS reduced all-cause mortality by 27%, the effects being more pronounced in women, former smokers, and patients with moderate or severe COPD.

Thus, currently for patients with COPD, it may no longer be relevant to ask whether ICS have a role, but the question that remains is, which COPD patients should be given ICS? The answer based on our present knowledge is that ICS should be reserved for symptomatic COPD patients, probably in GOLD Class III and IV (FEV_1 < 50% of predicted value), who have repeated exacerbations. They are clearly not recommended for all patients with COPD, not only because of the additional cost, but also because COPD patients (unlike asthmatics) tend to be elderly, and are more prone to all the adverse effects of ICS. Another word of caution against the routine use of ICS in COPD came from a meta-analysis of eighteen randomized controlled trials by Sonal Singh which showed conclusively that ICS were associated with a significantly increased risk of pneumonia (RR 1.60) and serious pneumonia (RR 1.71).

Inhaled corticosteroids come in various formulations. Those chiefly used are fluticasone, budesonide, beclomethasone, and triamcinolone. The most frequent side effects are the development of thrush in the oropharynx, bruising of the skin and hoarseness of voice. The possibility of osteoporosis and occurrence of cataracts due to systemic absorption of the steroid need to be considered in older subjects.

Inhaled corticosteroids are not to be used as monotherapy. They are used in combination with LABA. Clinical trials suggest greater improvement in symptoms and in lung function with use of both these agents when compared to either drug used alone. The most common combination used (and approved by FDA) is fluticasone propionate 250 µg and salmeterol 50 µg inhalation powder. One to two puffs twice daily is the regular maintenance dose advocated in patients with moderately severe or severe COPD who are breathless and who have a risk of acute exacerbations.

Mucolytic Agents and Antioxidants

Cough with mucoid or mucopurulent expectoration is an important symptom in COPD. There is no proven effective mucolytic agent available today for COPD patients. DNAse is effective in reducing acute exacerbations of acute infective bronchitis in cystic fibrosis but is ineffective in COPD patients. A recent large randomized controlled trial (RCT) of orally administered acetylcysteine was shown to be ineffective in retarding or arresting deterioration of lung function or preventing exacerbations in COPD.

Steam when inhaled is perhaps the best mucolytic agent and steam inhalation every morning often enables the patient to expectorate sputum; it serves as a bronchial toilet and often results in symptomatic relief.

Macrolides

The use of macrolides has been discussed in the chapter on "Acute Exacerbation of COPD".

■ PULMONARY REHABILITATION

Pulmonary rehabilitation has been defined by a National Heart, Lung and Blood Institute Workshop as:

A multidimensional continuum of services directed to persons with respiratory disease and their families usually by an interdisciplinary team of specialists with a goal of achieving and maintaining the individual's maximum level of independence and functioning in the community *(Ref: Fishman AP. Pulmonary rehabilitation research NIH workshop summary. Am J Respir Care. 994:149;825-33).*

Pulmonary rehabilitation is unfortunately a neglected aspect of therapy even in large centers in India and other developing countries. This is due partly to a lack of appreciation and awareness of its role in producing symptomatic relief in COPD patients and partly because of lack of expertise in implementing and organizing a truly beneficial program.

It is an accepted fact that a carefully implemented rehabilitation program can provide added benefits over and above the benefits due to medication. The most important benefits observed in COPD patients are a relief or reduction of dyspnea and an improved exercise capacity. Studies have also shown a reduction in hospital stay and decrease in health costs. There is a decrease in mental depression so frequently seen in patients with severe COPD, an increased independence in performing daily chores and activities, resulting in an overall improved quality of life. It needs to be stressed that pulmonary rehabilitation program even in the best centers do not improve lung function, airflow limitation or the basic inflammatory pathology that leads to inevitable progression of the disease. This should be explained both to the patient and to those primarily responsible for the patient's health care.

Patient Selection

Candidates selected for pulmonary rehabilitation often have the following features:

- Well-marked dyspnea and poor exercise tolerance or capacity. These patients fall in Grade III-IV severity of COPD. Lung functions are not always an appropriate guide; respiratory symptoms do not always correlate with the degree of reduction in FEV_1. However, patients with an FEV_1 of less than 35% would almost certainly benefit with a rehabilitation program.
- Patients who have frequent hospitalizations or frequent visits to the emergency department.

- Patients in need of psychosocial help and adjustment.

Should patients who insist on smoking be admitted to a rehabilitation program? It is indeed doubtful if any substantial benefit is likely to occur, particularly in heavy smokers. Their commitment to the program is always suspect. Yet a rehabilitation program if regularly attended, may be an ideal ground for motivating such patients to stop smoking, and giving them social and emotional support to help them to do so.

It is important to ensure a thorough examination and investigation of a patient before selection for a rehabilitation program, so as to exclude comorbidities such as significant ischemic heart disease, hypertension, or arthritis that may preclude exercise **(Table 3)**.

Though this section deals with pulmonary rehabilitation in COPD, the rehabilitation program is also applicable to other respiratory diseases like bronchial asthma and interstitial lung disease.

Finally, rehabilitation is a multidisciplinary approach carried out by a team headed by a coordinator. It should include a physician, an experienced exercise trainer, nurses, physiotherapists, respiratory therapists, psychiatrists, and dieticians. The team should provide a coordinated plan of rehabilitation, a plan which most importantly is individualized for each patient's disability and needs, and also a plan which is set to achieve realistic goals and does not promise impossible results. Only then is patient participation good and effective.

Features of Rehabilitation

Realistic patient-centered long-term and short-term goals should be set and aimed at after a thorough overall assessment. Many centers prefer to put the patient through an exercise test to unearth significant ischemic heart disease or development of arrhythmias **(Table 4)**.

Table 3: Patient selection for pulmonary rehabilitation.
Thorough assessment to exclude significant ischemic heart disease, valvular heart disease, arrhythmias, arthritides is done. Following this, selection of patients with: • Well-marked dyspnea and poor exercise tolerance—Grade III/IV severity of chronic obstructive pulmonary disease (COPD) • Dyspnea and reduced effort tolerance in patients with Grade II COPD • Patients who have frequent hospitalizations or frequent visits to the emergency department • Patients in need of psychosocial help and adjustment

Note: Respiratory symptoms (dyspnea, poor exercise tolerance) do not always correlate with degree of reduction in FEV_1).

Table 4: Features of pulmonary rehabilitation.

- Realistic patient-centered long-term and short-term goals and objectives
- *Exercise training*: Graduated exercise under close supervision. Walking or cycling as exercises for the lower limbs. Use of oxygen when necessary during exercise training
- *Breathing exercises and training*: Pursed lip breathing with slow complete expiration followed by a slow inspiration. Diaphragmatic breathing, rhythmic breathing during activity, allowing for full expiration. Yogic breathing exercises. Proper use of body mechanics to conserve energy and reduce energy requirements in conjunction with rhythmic breathing
- Psychological counseling to counter in particular anxiety, depression
- *Education:*
  - A healthy, disciplined and if needs be a suitably modified life style
  - Education on the technique and timing of medications
  - Individual and group instructions
  - Reinforce motivation to quit smoking in smokers
- Nutritional guidance
- Outcome evaluation
- Exercise as an inbuilt program in daily life even after rehabilitation program is complete (6–12 weeks)

- *Exercise training*: Exercise training, starting at a low level with a slow increase (if that is possible) improves exercise capacity and reduces dyspnea. The only type of exercise to the lower extremities is in the form of walking or cycling. Training programs to gradually increase exercise capacity follow the same regime as in healthy individuals. An exercise trainer and physiotherapist supervised by a physician help to provide this graded exercise.

- *Breathing exercises*: Breathing exercises help in reducing dyspnea—the uncomfortable feeling associated with breathing. Pursed lip breathing, diaphragmatic breathing, controlled rhythmic breathing improve tidal volume, reduce airtrapping and hyperinflation and thereby reduce the work of breathing. Yogic breathing exercises are truly beneficial, provided they do not involve holding the breath or using forced expiratory maneuvers. Coordinating breathing with special activities, learning not to hold the breath, breathing rhythmically and ensuring a full expiration during any activity help to reduce dyspnea. Training to use proper body mechanics to conserve energy and to reduce energy requirements is particularly useful in those with poor respiratory reserve. When necessary, oxygen inhalation during training sessions helps the patient increase his workload during exercise sessions, adding to the benefits of rehabilitation.

PSYCHOLOGICAL COUNSELING

Chronic obstructive pulmonary disease particularly when marked often causes psychological stress in the form of anxiety and depression. Psychiatric help and counseling can prove of significant benefit.

EDUCATION

Education is centered on:
- A healthy, disciplined, and if needs be a suitably modified lifestyle.
- A behavioral approach requires education on the technique and timing of medications which are carefully incorporated into the patient's daily activities.
- Individual and group instructions are important features of this program.

NUTRITIONAL GUIDANCE

Chronic obstructive pulmonary disease patients lose muscle mass and body weight. In fact a loss of body weight (<90% ideal) is a marker for increased mortality in this disease. Nutritional guidance to improve muscle mass is of help in these patients. On the other hand, patients who are overweight clearly benefit with nutritional guidance that allows them to lose weight. In those patients where body weight is not a problem, a balanced diet with enough calories to meet caloric expenditure during exercise is provided.

The optimal duration of a rehabilitation program has not been established. Most programs have two to three sessions a week, for a 6–12-week period. Patients with severe symptoms benefit with longer programs. Ideally, an exercise rehabilitation program should be inbuilt in the daily life of every COPD patient.

OXYGEN THERAPY

Patients with severe COPD often have marked chronic hypoxemia. Long-term oxygen therapy (LTOT) should always be prescribed for patients with COPD who have a PaO_2 < 55 mm Hg or a pulse oxygen saturation < 88%. LTOT in these patients has been shown to improve quality of life as also improve survival **(Table 5)**.

The objective of oxygen therapy is to increase the PaO_2 to more than 60 mm Hg (O_2 saturation of 90%). A pulse oximeter is useful to ensure that oxygen flow is adequate to permit oxygen saturation of not less than 90% at all

Table 5: Indications for continuous oxygen therapy in patients with chronic obstructive pulmonary disease (COPD).	
Stable obstructive pulmonary disease on optimal medical therapy + $PaO_2 < 55$ mm Hg with O_2 saturation < 90%	$PaCO_2 > 55$ mm Hg together with a PCV > 55%; Right heart dysfunction—P pulmonale, peripheral edema.

times—during rest and activity. Oxygen flow at night may need to be increased to allow a saturation of 90%. Besides clearly improving survival, oxygen relieves dyspnea at rest and during activity, reduces pulmonary hypertension, improves cognition and significantly improves the quality of life.

Some patients with COPD may not meet the requirements for use of oxygen at rest in the day. They may however desaturate well below 90% during activity or exercise, or may show significant desaturation during sleep at night, even in the proven absence of obstructive sleep apnea. These patients require to be given oxygen during exercise as also during sleep to enable the oxygen saturation to be more than 90%. Nocturnal hypoxemia is particularly dangerous as it can induce dangerous arrhythmia, pulmonary hypertension, poor cognition during the day, associated with hypersomnolence. Oxygen is often used intermittently to relieve breathlessness after exertion or activity even in the absence of hypoxemia or right heart failure. Though of no proven benefit, there should be no objection to its use if the patient feels quicker relief.

In patients who have significant hypercapnia, oxygen administration should be controlled, as uncontrolled therapy using high oxygen flow rates may relieve hypoxia but worsen hypercapnia, rendering the patients increasingly drowsy or even comatose. Controlled oxygen is best delivered by a Venturi mask, or through nasal prongs at a flow rate of 1–2 L/min.

The role of oxygen in COPD should be carefully explained to COPD patients who require it. This educational aspect can be reinforced during the pulmonary rehabilitation program.

The 5-year survival rate of COPD patients who require continuous oxygen therapy is poor with a life expectancy of 50% at the end of 5 years.

Control of Hypercapnia

The end-stage of advanced COPD is often characterized by mounting hypercapnia, with its added feature of drowsiness, which could progress to a comatose state. Hypercapnia often worsens during the night, so that the patient is difficult to arouse in the mornings. The excessive drowsy state leads to a poor cough reflex, sputum retention, which in turn causes pulmonary infection with an exacerbation of COPD. Noninvasive ventilatory support at night using a BiPAP or CPAP machine often helps to prevent an undue rise of $PaCO_2$. This leads to greater alertness in the morning and a better quality of life. If needs be, a BiPAP machine may need to be used during some hours in the day as well, again to prevent an undue rise in $PaCO_2$.

Treatment of Right Heart Failure due to Cor Pulmonale

Symptomatic treatment consists of salt restriction, restriction of fluid intake and the use of loop diuretics such as frusemide.

Digoxin may be used, but is of doubtful benefit. Aldactone 50-100 mg/day may help in salt and water excretion, but care must be taken to avoid hyperkalemia. Relief of hypoxia and hypercapnia is important, as this reduces to an extent the vasoconstrictive aspect of pulmonary hypertension and thereby helps right ventricular function. Measures to reduce hyperinflation of the lungs also help to reduce pulmonary hypertension. It is of practical importance to note that markedly hypercapnic patients who are severely waterlogged because of right heart failure due to cor pulmonale often do not respond to even large doses of diuretics. The response is however often dramatic (with regard to sharp reduction of generalized edema) when these patients are ventilated so that $PaCO_2$ is brought down to reasonable levels (45–55 mm Hg) **(Table 6)**.

Table 6: Treatment of right heart failure in chronic obstructive pulmonary disease (COPD).
• Continuous oxygen • Salt and water restriction • Loop diuretics • Aldactone (check for hyperkalemia) • Noninvasive ventilation (NIV) or if necessary temporary invasive ventilatory support to patients with marked hypercapnia who are severely waterlogged—diuresis often ensues • Digoxin (doubtful value) • Measures to reduce hyperinflation of lungs • Treatment of complicating arrhythmias • Prophylaxis and treatment of pulmonary thromboembolism • Treatment of complications as of when they arise

Treatment of arrhythmias, recognition and treatment of complicating pulmonary infections and of pulmonary thromboembolism are important aspects of management.

INTERVENTIONAL THERAPY IN STABLE CHRONIC OBSTRUCTIVE PULMONARY DISEASE

Interventional therapy is the only available option in patients who in spite of full supervised medical therapy continue to remain very dyspneic, have very poor exercise tolerance and continue to be hypoxic and hypercapnic.

Interventional therapy may take the following forms:

- *Bullectomy*: In patients with one or more large bullae, surgical removal of bullae relieves dyspnea and improves effort tolerance.
- *Lung volume reduction surgery*: In selected patients with a predominant severe upper lobe emphysema, lung volume reduction surgery (LVRS) improves survival and exercise tolerance.
- *Bronchoscopic interventions*: In selected patients with severe asthma bronchoscopic intervention through the appropriate placement of valves and/or coils helps to reduce end-expiratory volume and improves exercise tolerance 6–12 months after the procedure.
- *Lung transplantation*: In carefully chosen patients lung transplantation if successful, prolongs survival, improves quality of life, and effort tolerance.

Details of interventional therapy are outside the scope of this book; however relevant information, useful to the physicians with regard to LVRS and lung transplantation is given below.

Lung Volume Reduction Surgery (LVRS)

Lung volume reduction surgery is useful in a subset of patients with emphysema who have localized bullae, chiefly in the upper lobes. The bullae serve no purpose; in fact they contribute to an increased dead space and thus to alveolar hypoventilation. The National Emphysema Treatment Trial (NETT) has shown that when lung volume reduction was undertaken in a select subset of patients with emphysema there was an overall survival advantage when compared to medical therapy with a 5-year risk ratio of death of 0.86 (p = 0.02). Survival, exercise capacity improved in the subset of patients with upper lobe predominant disease and low exercise capacity. Patients with upper lobe predominant disease with good exercise capacity had further improvement in exercise capacity together with an improvement in quality of life, but not in survival. The NETT also identified a high-risk group characterized by FEV_1 less than 20% of predicted, and either a homogeneous distribution of emphysema or a CO-diffusing capacity (DLCO) less than 20% of predicted. These patients had a significant operative mortality and surgery was not recommended.

The NETT study was the largest RCT with 1,218 patients. This study showed a 6.6% lower absolute mortality rate in the bilateral LVRS group compared to the medical arm. The indications and contraindications to lung volume reduction are given in **Table 7**.

The inclusion criteria for LVRS included:

- High-resolution computed tomography (HRCT) evidence of bilateral emphysema, upper lobe predominance
- $FEV_1 \leq 45\%$, TLC $\geq 100\%$, RV ≥ 150, 6MWD ≥ 140 m
- $PaO_2 \geq 45$ mm Hg, $PaCO_2 \leq 60$ mm Hg
- Nonsmoking ≥ 4 months, BMI ≤ 31.1 kg/m^2
- Prednisolone ≤ 20 mg/day.

Note: 6MWD: 6-minute walk distance.

Lung Transplantation

Chronic obstructive pulmonary disease is the most common indication for lung transplantation. Transplantation can be done for single or both lungs depending on the severity of the disease and the patient's age. Indications for lung transplantation are:

- Advanced COPD patients who are severely symptomatic in spite of optimal medical therapy
- One or more of the following:
  - $FEV_1 < 25\%$ of the predicted value
  - $PaCO_2 > 55$ mm Hg; pulmonary hypertension; right heart failure
- A life expectancy < 2 years

Table 7: Indication and contraindications for lung volume reduction surgery.

- *Indications*:
  - Severe emphysema confined to upper lobes and low exercise capacity inspite of optimal medical treatment
  - Low exercise capacity with no lower lobe disease
  - Upper lobe disease and fair to good exercise capacity
- *Contraindications*:
  - $FEV_1 < 20\%$ of predicted, and either a homogeneous distribution of emphysema or a CO diffusing capacity (DLCO) < 20% predicted
  - Low exercise capacity with no upper lobe disease

- Age < 55 years for heart lung transplant; <60 years for a bilateral lung transplant; <65 years for a single lung transplant.

Lung transplantation is contraindicated if there is a history of malignancy within the past 2 years, persistence of substance addiction within 6 months of surgery, presence of hepatitis B, C or HIV infection and dysfunction of any other organ system.

The survival rate after transplantation varies in different centers but averages as follows:
- 90% at the end of 1 year
- 65–90% at the end of 2 years
- 41–50% at the end of 5 years.

A successful lung transplant leads to an improved quality of life and significant improvement in both lung function and exercise capacity. Patients remain on immunosuppressive drugs and are thus prone to infection. Rejection is another complication that can occur soon after transplantation or may occur months or years later.

Lung Transplantation in India

Lung transplantation is slowly but steadily establishing itself in India—chiefly at the All India Institute of Medical Sciences, Delhi and at the Apollo Hospitals, Chennai. At Apollo Hospitals, Chennai, the first isolated single lung transplant was performed in 2011. The transplant unit has then progressed to performing double lung transplants and preferentially performs double lung transplants whenever possible.

The results of this transplant team at the Apollo Hospitals in Chennai are comparable to other good transplant centers in the rest of the world, the survival rate being 80% at 1 year, 65% at 3 years and 54% at 5 years.

The indications for lung transplantation laid down by the center at the Apollo Hospital, Chennai are given in **Table 8**.

Table 8: Indications for lung transplantation.
1. Timing of listing
2. BODE index ≥7
3. FEV_1 ≤15 to 20% predicted
4. Three or more severe exacerbations during the preceding year
5. One severe exacerbation with acute hypercapnic respiratory failure
6. Moderate-to-severe pulmonary hypertension

(BODE: Body mass index, degree of airflow obstruction and dyspnea, and exercise capacity; FEV_1: Forced expiratory volume in 1 s)
The BODE index is calculated using these factors and arriving at a Total Criteria Point Count.

Perhaps Point 4, 5 are debatable as good medical management and follow-up when available may be associated with lesser mortality vis-a-vis the mortality during or soon after a lung transplant.

Future Hopes

Several new approaches to the management of COPD are being investigated. Invasive techniques using the bronchoscope for lung volume reduction, placement of one-way valves, endobronchial instillation of biological sealants, thermal airway ablation and airway stents to decompress bullae are being practiced in specialized centers.

Mepolizumab is a monoclonal antibody against interleukin (IL)-5 now being used in eosinophilic asthma. There are ongoing studies to determine the role of eosinophils in COPD. Research on drugs directed against eosinophils may perhaps be of use in some patients.

■ MORTALITY

Chronic obstructive pulmonary disease is the only important chronic disease where the death rate continues to increase steadily. As already mentioned, it has been projected to be the third leading cause of death by 2020. In 2002, the WHO estimated the global mortality from COPD as 44.2/100,000. Mortality was highest in the Western Pacific region (79.8/100,000) and lowest in Africa (18.1/100,000). In all regions, mortality was higher in men than in women except in the West Pacific region.

Chronic obstructive pulmonary disease accounted for 140,000 deaths in the United States; the mortality increased with age and for patients more than 45 years. The current trend shows a slight decrease in mortality in men, and a slight increase in mortality in women. In the United Kingdom in 2003, there were 26,000 deaths from COPD which represents 4.9% of all deaths. Mortality rates were higher in urban compared to rural areas.

Mortality figures from Southeast Asian countries are similar or even higher than in the West. It is believed that just as there is an underestimation of prevalence figures of COPD, there is an equal underestimation of mortality figures. This is because COPD is often given as a contributory cause of death rather than a primary cause. Also, terms such as chronic bronchitis and emphysema are often given as the cause of death instead of COPD; this lowers the reported mortality rates for COPD. The epidemiological data gathered from mortality rates given

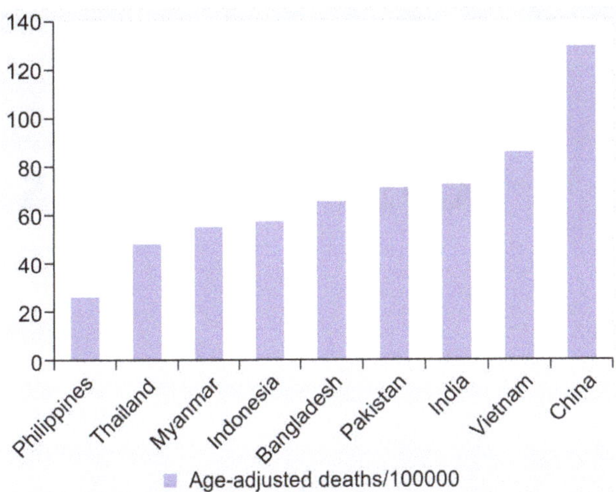

Fig. 7: Age-adjusted deaths/100,000 due to chronic obstructive pulmonary disease (COPD) in Southeast Asia.
Source: Adapted from Lopez AD, Mathers CD, Ezzati M, et al. Global burden of disease and risk factors. New York: Oxford University Press; 2006.

in national statistics of developing countries may therefore be unreliable. Even so, the mortality rates are forbiddingly high **(Fig. 7)**.

In China, death from chronic respiratory disease ranks as the first cause of death. In 1994, the mortality rate for the whole population was 161.57/100,000 in the rural areas and 94.4/100,000 in urban areas. In Thailand, the mortality rate ranged from 500 to 4,400/100,000 in men aged 51 years and older and 600 to 3,400/100,000 in women. In Singapore between 1991 and 1998, COPD deaths were reported to be 16.3/100,000 in individuals more than 55 years, being four times higher than in women. In Hong Kong, the death rate from COPD in 1997 was 31.1/100,000 of the population and in Japan COPD mortality in 1999 was 10.4/100,000.

■ SUGGESTED READING

1. Almagro P. Recent improvement in long-term survival after a COPD hospitalisation. Thorax. 2010;65:298-302.
2. Barnes PJ. Emerging pharmacotherapies for COPD. Chest. 2008;134:1278-86.
3. Burge PS, Calverley P. Inhaled steroids in obstructive lung disease in Europe, the ISOLDE trial: protocol, and progress. Am J Respir Crit Care Med. 1994;149:A312.
4. Global Initiative for Chronic Obstructive Lung Disease (GOLD). Global Strategy for the Diagnosis, Management and Prevention of Chronic Obstructive Pulmonary Disease: 2018 Report. www.goldcopd.org
5. Grimes GC. Medications for COPD: a review of effectiveness. Am Fam Physician. 2007;76:1141-8.
6. Karner C, Cates CJ. The effect of adding inhaled corticosteroids to tiotropium and long-acting beta2-agonists for chronic obstructive pulmonary disease. Cochrane Database Syst Rev. 2011;CD009039.
7. Kew KM, Mavergames C, Walters JA. Long-acting beta2-agonists for chronic obstructive pulmonary disease. Cochrane Database Syst Rev. 2013;CD010177.
8. Pauwels RA, Lofdahl CG, Pride NB, et al. European Respiratory Society study on chronic obstructive pulmonary disease (EUROSCOP): hypothesis and design. Eur Respir J. 1992;5:1254-61.
9. Pavord ID, Chanez P, Criner GJ, et al. Mepolizumab for eosinophilic chronic obstructive pulmonary disease. N Engl J Med. 2017;377:1613.
10. Rabe KF, Hurd S, Anzueto A, et al. Global strategy for the diagnosis, management, and prevention of chronic obstructive pulmonary disease: GOLD executive summary. Am J Respir Crit Care Med. 2007;176:532-55.
11. Reardon J. Pulmonary rehabilitation for COPD. Respir Med. 2005;99:S19-27.
12. Singh S, Amin AV, Loke YK. Long-term use of inhaled corticosteroids and the risk of pneumonia in chronic obstructive pulmonary disease: a meta-analysis. Arch Intern Med. 2009;169(3):219-29.
13. Suissa S, Drazen JM. Making sense of triple inhaled therapy for COPD. N Engl J Med. 2018;378:1723.
14. Vestbo J, Lange P, Sorensen T, et al. The Copenhagen City Lung Study—a clinical trial of inhaled corticosteroids in COPD: design and progress. Am J Respir Crit Care Med. 1995;151:A466.
15. Vestbo J. TORCH Study Group. The TORCH (towards a revolution in COPD health) survival study protocol. Eur Respir J. 2004;24:206-10.
16. Welsh EJ, Cates CJ, Poole P. Combination inhaled steroid and long-acting beta2-agonist versus tiotropium for chronic obstructive pulmonary disease. Cochrane Database Syst Rev. 2010;12:CD007891.

CHAPTER 39

Cystic Fibrosis

■ INTRODUCTION

Cystic fibrosis is a fatal or life-limiting autosomal recessive genetic disease. In its epidemiology it has an ethnic distribution, being most common in the Caucasian race with a frequency of 1 in 3,300 live births. It is less common in the black population, the incidence being 1 in 17,000. The incidence in African-Americans is believed to be in 1 in 15,000 and in Asian-Americans 1 in 31,000. The disease is believed to be comparatively rare in India and Southeast Asia. This may or may not be factual. Its apparent rarity at least in India may well be related to a lack of awareness of the problem, so that diagnostic tests for the disease, particularly in adolescents and young adults presenting solely with respiratory features, are not performed. The Indian scenario with regard to cystic fibrosis is briefly discussed later in the chapter.

Cystic fibrosis involves many organ systems giving rise to a variety of clinical features. Involvement of the respiratory system is however generally most pronounced so that the clinical presentation of cystic fibrosis is often dominated by progressive respiratory disease.

The underlying abnormality in cystic fibrosis is defective chloride transport in sweat glands and respiratory epithelium and other epithelial cells. An increase in sweat sodium and chloride in cystic fibrosis provides an early available diagnostic marker for the disease. The genetic defect responsible for the disease was discovered as late as 1989. The cause of cystic fibrosis was then proven to be due to a mutated gene encoding a defective chloride channel in epithelial cells. This has unquestionably improved our understanding of cystic fibrosis and given us at least some insight into the different manifestations involving different organ systems encountered in this disease.

■ GENETICS

Cystic fibrosis is caused by a mutation on a gene on chromosome 7 which encodes a protein responsible for ion transport across epithelial cells. This protein is named the cystic fibrosis transmembrane conductance regulator or (CFTR). Numerous genetic mutations have been described with regard to this gene; most of these mutations are rare. The CFTR mutations are grouped into five classes:

Class I —CFTR is not synthesized
Class II—CFTR is inadequately processed
Class III—CFTR is unregulated
Class IV—CFTR shows abnormal conductance
Class V—CFTR is partially defective in its production or processing.

Over 60% of patients with cystic fibrosis in the West have a class II mutation caused by deletion of phenylalanine in Portion 508 (F508) of CFTR. F508 A CFTR is incorrectly folded and trapped in the endoplasm and is then proteolytically degraded, thereby losing its function. The little CFTR that escapes this degradation reaches the membrane of the epithelial cells and shows functional activity.

It has been shown that patients who carry 2 severe mutations causing a loss of function of CFTR (class I, II, III) have the typical features of cystic fibrosis characterized by pancreatic insufficiency, elevated sweat chloride and early age of diagnosis. On the other hand patients who have just one mild mutation with partial function of CFTR do not have pancreatic insufficiency, have sweat chloride values close to upper limits of normal and are diagnosed at a later age. Class IV and V mutations have been shown to be linked with pancreatic insufficiency. Attempts to correlate specific mutations with lung disease have shown significant variations with regard to severity of lung involvement. Because of this wide variation, it has been suggested that environmental factors and/or genes other than the one related to CFTR may perhaps play a role in the evaluation, progression and severity of the disease.

PATHOPHYSIOLOGY

The pathophysiology of cystic fibrosis is best understood by contrasting the normal ionic transport within the airways mucosa with that of the deranged ionic transport in cystic fibrosis.

In normal subjects, airway epithelial cells secrete chloride and absorb sodium chloride and water. This is regulated through *channels* by the CFTR. The balance between *secretion* and *absorption* determines water transport and allows an adequate layer of airway surface liquid which supports the thin mucous layer present over epithelial cells. This mucous layer is constantly escalated upwards and out of the airways through regulated ciliary movement.

In patients with cystic fibrosis, absence or dysfunction of the CFTR leads to reduced chloride secretion and increased absorption of sodium chloride. This is detrimental for water transport so that the airway surface liquid which supports the mucous layer present over epithelial cells is lacking. In the absence of the airway surface liquid, respiratory cilia are dysfunctional and there is a breakdown of mucociliary transport. Mucous which becomes increasingly viscous accumulates and plugs the smaller airways. This is the basic and primary pathological event in cystic fibrosis.

Sequentially, there is now trapping of inhaled bacteria in the poorly moving viscous mucous. These microorganisms produce an ongoing inflammation in the small airways. Airways inflammation, obstruction, distortion, with progressive lung damage leads ultimately to hypoxic or hypoxic cum hypercapnic respiratory failure.

INFECTING ORGANISMS IN CYSTIC FIBROSIS

There is generally a small spectrum of infecting organisms that perpetuate inflammation in cystic fibrosis. The commonest isolate is *Pseudomonas aeruginosa,* followed by *Staphylococcus aureus* and *Haemophilus influenzae.* Initially these organisms form nonmucoid colonies.

However, the mucous in cystic fibrosis lacks oxygen, leading to anaerobic growth of bacteria and a switch of the above organisms from the nonmucoid form to the mucoid form. The mucoid forms produce a fine biofilm which hinders the action of antibiotics on these bacteria and also enables them to resist killing by the immunological responses of the host.

As the disease progresses and worsens, other multiresistant bacteria may come on the scene. These are *Stenotrophomonas maltophilia, Alcaligenes xylosoxidans,* and the *Burkholderia cepacia* complex. These organisms are isolated in 10% of patients with cystic fibrosis. Occasionally, nontuberculous mycobacteria *(Mycobacterium avium-intracellulare)* are isolated. It is a matter of dispute whether these organisms are colonizers or are responsible for infection, inflammation and progress of the disease. Perhaps they may be playing a dual role. The *B. cepacia* complex is recognized to be an unusual but dangerous organism. This organism, normally present in soil and water, causes chronic infection only in cystic fibrosis and chronic granulomatous disease. It is a multiresistant organism with poor or no response to antibiotic therapy and worsens the progress in patients with cystic fibrosis. There is evidence that in patients with cystic fibrosis, the *B. cepacia* complex can cause cross-infection by spreading from one patient to the other. What is more, 10–15% of patients with cystic fibrosis who are infected by the *B. cepacia* complex develop the *cepacia syndrome* characterized by a necrotizing pneumonia, marked leukocytosis, bacteremia and an almost 100% mortality.

There are a few important features in relation to inflammation of the airways in cystic fibrosis. Firstly and importantly, inflammation of the airways starts very early in the first months of life in a patient with typical cystic fibrosis. It antedates symptoms of respiratory disease by a long period of time stretching from months to years. Secondly, the inflammatory process is neutrophilic and sustained. There is an exaggerated inflammatory response to both bacterial and viral pathogens. Whether the absence or defect of the cystic fibrosis membrane regulator plays a direct role in inducing this inflammatory response or whether it only plays an indirect role by causing mucous plugging is a matter of dispute. Unquestionably, it is persistent, exaggerated sustained inflammation within the airways which determines the downhill course of cystic fibrosis.

CLINICAL FEATURES

Cystic fibrosis has a wide spectrum of symptoms which involve the respiratory system, gastrointestinal system and in adults the reproductive system.

The classic triad in cystic fibrosis consists of cough with sputum, steatorrhea and failure to thrive. Pulmonary symptoms may not be present at birth but may occur later in childhood, adolescence or even later. At times clinical features of the disease may only involve the lungs, evidence of steatorrhea due to pancreatic insufficiency not being clinically manifest in 10–15% of patients. As the child matures into an adult, infertility due to azoospermia caused by obstructed or absent vas deferens is almost always present.

Cystic fibrosis is generally not evident at birth except in 10–15% of patients who present with meconium ileus. Meconium ileus is actually a manifestation of pancreatic insufficiency though it is not associated with more severe manifestations of pancreatic disease. The respiratory and nonrespiratory features of cystic fibrosis are tabled separately **(Table 1)**.

This section chiefly deal with the respiratory manifestations of cystic fibrosis **(Table 2)**. The chief symptom of respiratory involvement is cough, which to start with occurs during exacerbations, but later becomes chronic and is associated with productive sputum. The sputum is mucoid but during periods of infection it becomes purulent and colored yellow or green. Persistent untreated infection results in persistent cough with purulent expectoration. Minor hemoptysis may occur during exacerbations. As the disease progresses there is increasing breathlessness on exertion. Pansinusitis is often present.

Some patients have hyperactive airways and so have wheezing, paroxysmal bouts of cough and a fair degree of reversibility of airways obstruction. They are often diagnosed and treated as *asthma*; the underlying disease remaining undetected.

As the disease progresses there is worsening dyspnea, bouts of fever due to recurrent or persistent infection. Bronchiectasis chiefly involving the upper lobes is observed. Weight loss or failure to increase weight (in childhood and adolescence) is invariably present. The nails are often clubbed.

The end-result is hypoxemic respiratory failure and still later hypoxemic plus hypercapnic respiratory failure. This generally occurs when the FEV_1 is less than 30% of predicted value. Cor pulmonale occurs late in the illness.

Patients with cystic fibrosis invariably have a sinusitis involving almost all paranasal sinuses. The sinusitis may be clinically manifest or may be silent being diagnosed on imaging studies.

IMAGING

Although the disease is present at birth, radiographic abnormalities may not become apparent for years. The earliest findings are recurrent pneumonia, mucoid impaction, bronchiectasis and focal atelectasis. The involvement is predominantly in the upper lobes. With time there is advancement in the disease process with progressive worsening of radiographic abnormalities. The hila may be enlarged due to adenopathy or pulmonary hypertension **(Figs. 1A and B)**.

Computed Tomography of the Chest

The findings vary with duration and severity of disease. The predominant findings are of bronchiectasis with or without mucoid impaction mainly in the upper lobes. Due to chronic inflammatory changes, there is bronchial wall thickening with peribronchiolar inflammation. There may be mosaic perfusion due to bronchial wall thickening involving the smaller airways **(Fig. 2)**. Focal areas of consolidation and atelectasis are often seen. Pulmonary hypertension develops late in the course of the disease. There may also be hypertrophy of the bronchial arteries contributing to episodes of hemoptysis.

Table 1: Nonrespiratory features of cystic fibrosis.

- Gastrointestinal disease:
  - Meconium ileus, distal intestinal obstruction syndrome
  - Steatorrhea due to pancreatic insufficiency
  - Pancreatitis
  - Failure to thrive, hypoalbuminemia
  - Deficiency of fat-soluble vitamins
  - Biliary cirrhosis
- Infertility due to azoospermia caused by obstruction to the vas deferens

Table 2: Respiratory features of cystic fibrosis.

- Chronic productive cough with increasing periods of purulent expectoration
- Colonization and infection with *S. aureus*, *P. aeruginosa*
- Airways obstruction with progressive reduction in FEV_1
- Radiological abnormalities with bronchiectasis involving chiefly the upper lobes
- Clubbing
- Pansinusitis
- Hypoxemia or hypoxemic + hypercapnic respiratory failure

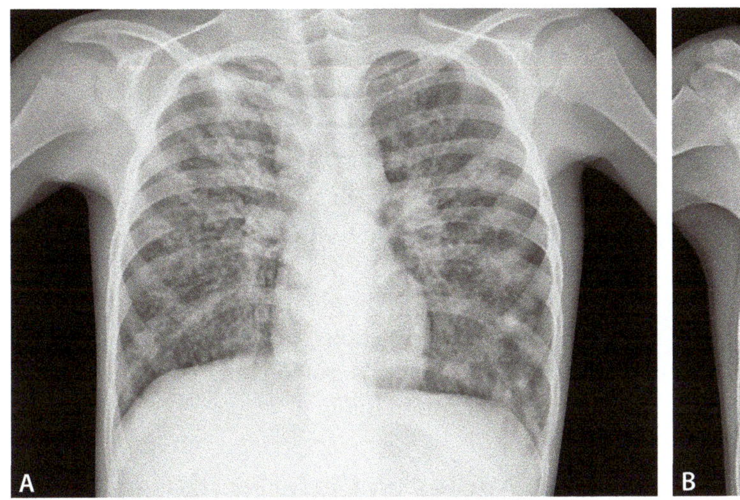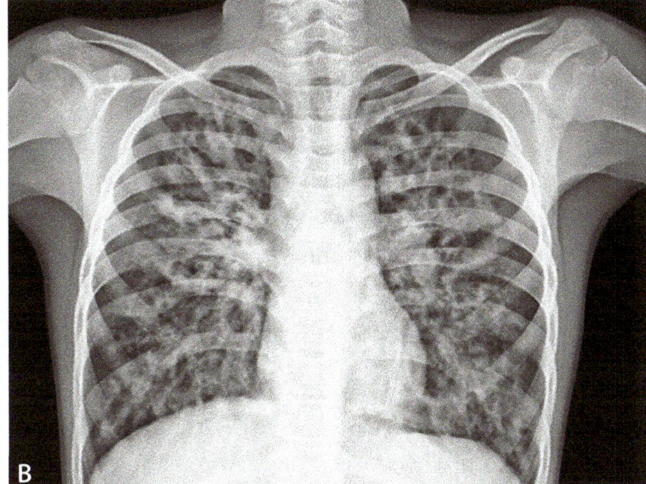

Figs. 1A and B: Cystic fibrosis: In a young boy with cystic fibrosis. (A) The X-ray done in 2010 reveals an ill-defined consolidation in the right apical region with multiple small nodular lesions in both lung fields; (B) Subsequent X-ray done in 2014 demonstrate ill-defined reticular opacities in both lung fields associated with multiple cystic lesions indicative of bronchiectasis. This is an example of extensive bronchiectasis in cystic fibrosis.

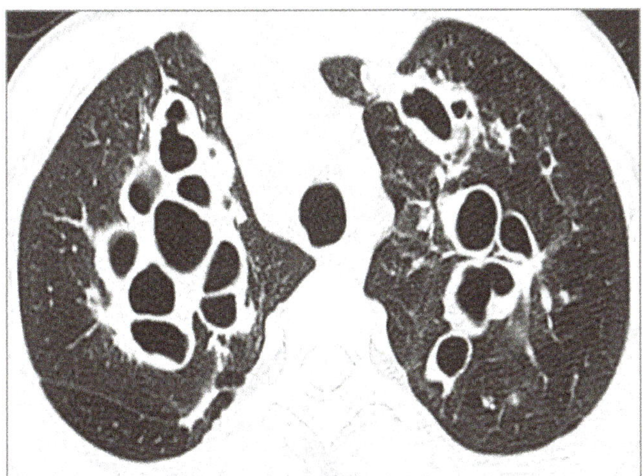

Fig. 2: Cystic fibrosis: High-resolution computed tomography (HRCT) chest demonstrates extensive cystic bronchiectasis in both upper lobes.

◼ DIAGNOSTIC TESTS (TABLE 3)

- *The sweat sodium chloride test:* A suspicion of cystic fibrosis should prompt the measurement of sweat sodium and chloride. Abnormal ion transport in this disease is reflected in the high sodium and chloride levels in sweat. Chloride content of sweat is greater than 60 mmol/L on repeated testing is diagnostic of the disease. Sweat chloride content between 30–60 mmol/L is a borderline result which may be observed in patients with cystic fibrosis.

Table 3: Diagnostic tests for cystic fibrosis.
• The sweat sodium chloride test; sweat chloride > 60 mmol/L
• Genotyping of the most common CFTR mutations
• Assessing CFTR function by measurement of the nasal potential difference
• Fat estimation of stools over 48–72 hours, determining concentration of chymotrypsin or pancreatic specific elastase in feces
• Imaging studies (X-ray, CT) of the paranasal sinuses and of the chest
• Sputum culture
• Seminal fluid test for azoospermia

- *Genotyping of the most common CFTR mutations.*
- *Assessing CFTR function by measurement of the nasal potential difference:* These tests need to be done only if the sweat test and the CFTR genotyping are not diagnostic. The transport of sodium and chloride across the nasal mucosa produces an electrical potential difference. Changes in potential difference as a result of stimulation or inhibition of ion channels by nasal perfusion can be measured. The normal nasal mucosa gives a different response when compared to cystic fibrous mucosa. This test is difficult, highly technical and requires special expertise.
- *Most patients with cystic fibrosis have pancreatic insufficiency.* This can be tested by fat estimation of stools over 48–72 hours, to prove the presence of steatorrhea and by decreased concentration of

chymotrypsin or pancreatic-specific elastase in feces.

- *Imaging studies (X-ray, CT) of the chest and of paranasal sinuses.*
- *Sputum cultures* typically show the presence of *S. aureus* or *P. aeruginosa* or *H. influenzae,* particularly during infection exacerbation.

Western studies suggest that in 5–10% of patients the diagnosis of cystic fibrosis is not made until adulthood. These patients do not have the classic features of cystic fibrosis and may present with involvement of just one system—sterility due to azoospermia from obstructed vas deferens, recurrent acute pancreatitis or chronic airways disease with bronchiectasis. Pancreatic insufficiency is not present in these patients and the sweat chloride test is not clearly diagnostic. Mutations of the CFTR gene test through commercial genetic screening panels in these adults are also not those classically associated with cystic fibrosis. Perhaps, mutations of the CFTR gene in adult patients are mild and therefore escape the genetic screening panels conventionally used for this disease. The nasal potential difference may prove of diagnostic use in these patients, only the test is highly technical requiring special expertise.

The presence of obstructive azoospermia should always prompt genetic testing for cystic fibrosis. However, a diagnosis of cystic fibrosis should only be made in these adults if proper diagnostic criteria are met—sweat chloride is greater than 60 mmol/L, two CFTR causing mutations and nasal potential difference observed with cystic fibrosis.

Western studies claim that despite sophisticated diagnostic tests a definite diagnosis of cystic fibrosis cannot be made in a number of adults who have clinical features suggestive of the disease including typical cystic fibrosis bronchiectasis.

Indian Scenario

Though the precise incidence of cystic fibrosis among Indians is unknown, current evidence suggests that the disease is more common in people of Indian origin than is thought. Of the 3,500 new cases registered in the Pediatric Chest Clinic from 1995–2002 at the All India Institute of Medical Science, Kobra and his colleagues diagnosed cystic fibrosis in 120 (3.5%) children. The diagnosis was based on a sweat chloride greater than 60 mEq/L and a positive genetic test for DF 508 mutation.

There are no reliable studies to document even the approximate incidence or prevalence of cystic fibrosis in India. A study of cord blood samples investigating carrier state of ΔF508 mutation in India calculated the incidence of cystic fibrosis as 1 in 40,000 newborns. There is evidence to suggest that prevalence of cystic fibrosis and the ΔF508 mutation is far more common in North India than in the South of the country. In Pakistan ΔF508 mutation is observed chiefly in the province of Baluchistan. It is hypothesized that population migration from this province was responsible for introducing this specific genetic mutation into Northern India.

Genetic Studies on Cystic Fibrosis in India

There are very few studies that describe the genotype of Indian children in cystic fibrosis. Ashavaid TF, Raghavan R, et al., report that the frequency of ΔF508 mutation in Indian children with cystic fibrosis is between 19% and 56%. Likewise in other Asian countries the incidence of of ΔF508 mutation is less than in Caucasians. The spectrum of mutations in Indian children (apart from ΔF508) is reported to be heterogeneous and variable; rare and new mutations have also been described. *Mandal A, Kabra S, Lodha R [Ref: Kabra SK, Kabra M, Lodha R, et al. Cystic fibrosis in India. Pediatr Pulmonol. 2007;42(12):1087-94]* believe that the heterogeneity of the mutation profile could well be related to variations in ethnic background.

Clinical Manifestations

Clinical manifestations of cystic fibrosis is India are similar to those observed in the West.

Respiratory features included repeated attacks or persistent pneumonia in almost all patients, airways obstruction with hyperinflated lungs in 83%, crepitations on auscultation in 92% and wheezing in 25%. Organisms cultured from sputum in order of frequency were *P. aeruginosa, S. aureus, Klebsiella* spp.

Failure to thrive, malabsorption and malnutrition were prominent clinical features outside the respiratory system. Mandal A, Kabra S, Lodha R report that clinical manifestations of cystic fibrosis which to an extent were different from the West included—a late and advanced stage of the illness at diagnosis, hypochloremic acidosis, vitamin A and D deficiencies, higher colonization rate of the lungs with *P. aeruginosa* and lower rates of common mutations. Cystic fibrosis patients in India were noted to have a higher prevalence of peripheral neuropathy and allergic bronchopulmonary aspergillosis when compared to the West.

Almost certainly, the disease in India and perhaps in Southeast Asia is not as uncommon as is believed. The apparent rarity is due to the lack of awareness of the problem and the lack of diagnostic facilities even if the awareness is present. The disease, presenting with airways obstruction, chronic respiratory systems or bronchiectasis in adolescents or young adults is missed for the above-mentioned reasons. The question also arises whether in India and other Asian countries a *forme fruste* of cystic fibrosis exists, with borderline sweat chloride tests and with lesser degree of CFTR mutation, or mutations not considered typical for the disease. A greater in-depth study of patients presenting with chronic airways obstruction, recurrent respiratory infections or bronchiectasis of the type and distribution seen in cystic fibrosis or of patients with obstructive azoospermia may perhaps prove rewarding.

Natural History of Lung Disease in Cystic Fibrosis

Pathological abnormalities in the small airways precede clinical symptoms. These abnormalities take the form of mucous plugging with dilatation distal to the obstructed small airways. Chronic productive cough is associated with a steady decline in lung function. Acute exacerbations are triggered by infection and as the disease progresses a well-nigh permanent colonization with *S. aureus* and *P. aeruginosa* is observed. Exacerbations cause a worsening of symptoms, a decline of FEV_1 and if unrecognized and untreated may cause a permanent further decline in lung function. A greater awareness of this fact has led to more vigorous treatment of pulmonary manifestations of this disease. Evaluation of clinical features, periodic FEV_1 measurements and imaging studies are important in assessing the outcome of these patients. Some patients progress to hypoxemic cum hypercapnic respiratory failure with cor pulmonale in spite of assiduous care.

■ MANAGEMENT OF PULMONARY FEATURES OF CYSTIC FIBROSIS

There is no cure for cystic fibrosis. Treatment is symptomatic. Principles of treatment are:

- Early initiation of treatment.
- Use of CFTR modulators after genotyping.
- Combating the cycle of mucus retention, infection and inflammation.
- Recognition and treatment of acute exacerbations.

CFTR Modulators

CFTR Modulators are a new class of drugs that act by either improving production, intracellular processing, or function of the CFTR protein. Wherever facilities are available all patients with cystic fibrosis should have their CFTR genotyped to determine if they carry a genotype which can be modulated by CFTR modulator therapy. The CFTR mutation would determine the selection of the CFTR modulator (*Ref: Simon R. Cystic fibrosis: overview of the treatment of lung disease.www.uptodate.com. Nov 2018*).

Ensuring Patency of Airways

Patency of airways and airway clearance is maintained by physiotherapy and by a combination of drugs-inhalation of a beta agonist like albuterol as also by a combination of inhaled drugs that loose and liquefy the viscid mucus. These inhaled drugs in the main are hypertonic saline and DNase.

Physiotherapy to the chest and regular supervised exercise are of critical importance. Physiotherapy helps to dislodge viscid secretions and enables the patient to expectorate and thereby keep the airways patent.

Physiotherapy includes percussion, vibration, postural drainage. It also includes breathing, coughing maneuvers as also the use of oscillating positive expiratory pressure devices.

Hypertonic saline: Hypertonic saline 4 mL of 5–7% should be nebulized twice daily for several weeks. An aerosolized bronchodilator is preferably given before each dose. Patients treated with hypertonic saline are reported to have fewer pulmonary exacerbations requiring antibiotics.

DNase: Recombinant DNase nebulized daily and on a long term bases reduces sputum viscosity, improves lung function and reduces the number of exacerbations in mild and moderately severe disease (*Ref: Yang C, Montgomery M. Dornase alfa for cystic fibrosis. Cochrane Database Syst Rev. 2018;9:CD001127*). DNase is however very expensive, not easily available; few in poor countries can manage to use it. Moreover the efficacy of nebulized hypertonic saline is almost as good as that of nebulized DNase.

DNase and hypertonic saline have different modes of action. DNase decreases viscosity of purulent sputum by cleaving the DNA released by degenerating neutrophils thereby liquefying the sputum. Hypertonic saline hydrates the viscid mucus, thereby liquefying it so that it is more easily expectorated. Both these agents can be used one after the other but should not be mixed.

Treatment of Airway Infection

Treatment of airways infection is of crucial importance. The organisms most frequently responsible for infection are *S. aureus, H. influenzae* and most of all, particularly in advanced disease, *P. aeruginosa.* The following points are noteworthy **(Table 4)**:

- Acute exacerbations of the disease are related to infection and need immediate antibiotic treatment.
- Threshold for administering antibiotics should be low; else each exacerbation can cause further permanent damage.
- Antistaphylococcal antibiotics should be given for 3–4 weeks. There is insufficient evidence to use antistaphylococcal antibiotics as prophylaxis. In fact prophylactic therapy may perhaps promote the emergence of *P. aeruginosa.*
- *P. aeruginosa* is the prominent colonizer and infective agent in cystic fibrosis in adult patients. Patients generally become chronically infected with mucoid strains of this organism and this has a significant negative impact on the disease.

Table 4: Drugs in cystic fibrosis.

Pathogen	Antibiotic used	Dosage
1. S. aureus		
MSSA	Amoxicillin/clavulanate	625 mg BD orally 1.2 g 8 hourly IV
MRSA	Linezolid	600 mg BD
2. H. influenzae	Cefuroxime	500 mg BD orally
	Ceftriaxone	1–2 g 12 hourly IV
3. P. aeruginosa	Ciprofloxacin	500 mg BD orally
	Piperacillin/tazobactam	45 g 8 hourly IV
	Nebulized tobramycin	300 mg BD
	Nebulized colistin	150 mg BD

- It is impossible to eradicate chronic infection caused by *P. aeruginosa,* but early antibiotic therapy against this organism is an important advance in management. Inhaled antibiotic therapy with tobramycin together with oral therapy with ciprofloxacin has been used successfully to reduce the incidence of chronic *P. aeruginosa* infection.
- Inhaled antibiotic therapy with tobramycin or colistin or one alternating with the other is the treatment of choice for maintenance therapy in patients infected with *P. aeruginosa.* In addition to inhaled antibiotics, azithromycin 500 mg once or twice daily is reported to reduce exacerbations of *P. aeruginosa* infection in this disease and improve lung function. The reason for this is unclear. It may be related to the anti-inflammatory effect of the macrolide or the drug may have an effect on the organisms growing in biofilms, even though the drug has no efficacy against *P. aeruginosa* when tested in routine cultures. There is concern that long term use of azithromycin in patients with active or occult nontuberculous mycobacteria (NTM) could lead to resistance of NTM to this drug. Patients should therefore be screened for NTM before initiating therapy and reassessed periodically.
- Acute exacerbations of severe infection are treated with an intravenous combination of piperacillin + tazobactam with an aminoglycoside. Less severe exacerbations are treated with oral ciprofloxacin. Some centers treat chronically infected patients with IV antibiotics for 2–3 weeks every three months on a continuous basis. There is insufficient evidence to advocate use of this protocol.
- Occasionally, patients with cystic fibrosis are infected by other gram-negative organisms. These include *B. cepacia* complex, and *S. maltophilia.* Their relation to progression of disease in patients with cystic fibrosis is undetermined. Patients chronically infected with *B. cepacia* respond to doxycycline or trimethoprim-sulfamethoxazole during minor exacerbations. More severe exacerbations may require IV meropenem, inhaled tobramycin in *combination* with ceftazidime or chloramphenicol. Prolonged antibiotic therapy extending for several weeks may be necessary before clinical response occurs. The occurrence of the cepacia syndrome in 10–15% of patients of cystic fibrosis infected by the *B. cepacia* complex has already been commented upon.

S. maltophilia is best treated with trimethoprim-sulfamethoxazole combined with ticarcillin-clavulanate or levofloxacin.

Treatment of Inflammation

Cystic fibrosis is characterized by an intense neutrophilic inflammation of the airways. Prednisolone in a dose of 1 mg/kg given on alternate days was found to reduce decline in lung function in patients infected with *P. aeruginosa.* However, serious side-effects which included hyperglycemia, growth retardation in children and cataract were observed. The current recommendation in cystic fibrosis is not to use systemic corticosteroids on a chronic bases except in the presence of asthma and allergic bronchopulmonary aspergillosis because of associated side-effects.

Inhaled corticosteroids are widely used but have not been shown to improve lung function in cystic fibrosis. Short-term use of inhaled β_2-agonists may benefit patients with increased airway hyperresponsiveness, commonly observed in CF. Inhaled β_2-agonists are also advocated in patients with allergic bronchopulmonary aspergillosis immediately or prior to sessions of physiotherapy and exercise and immediately prior to nebulized hypertonic saline, DNase or nebulized antibiotics to limit nonspecific bronchial hyper-reactivity and improve penetration of these drugs.

Use of Nonsteroidal Anti-inflammatory Drugs

A Cochrane review on the use of ibuprofen concluded that high-dose ibuprofen can slow the progression of cystic fibrosis, especially in children, provided the serum ibuprofen concentrations were maintained at as high as 50–100 µg/mL. This is impractical in many countries of the world; the drug is therefore best avoided in India.

The possible anti-inflammatory effects of macrolides in particular azithromycin has already been mentioned.

New Drugs

Ivacaftor: Ivacaftor is a potentiator that activates the defective CF transmembrane conductance regulator (CFTR) at the cell surface. The basic target for this therapy is the mutated CFTR in which glycine has been replaced by aspartic acid at position 551, interfering with the gating of the channel. It was observed in studies extending close to 1 year that ivacaftor in a dose of 150 mg twice daily led to fewer pulmonary exacerbations compared to placebo. There was also a decrease in sweat chloride concentration in treated patients compared to placebo.

Aerosolized Aztreonam for Moderate to Severe Disease

P. aeruginosa infection of the airways in cystic fibrosis leads to a more rapid decline in lung function and reduced survival. Studies have shown that aerosolized aztreonam was effective in reducing exacerbations and improving lung function. This therapy was not associated with increased resistance of *P. aeruginosa* to the drug. There are not enough studies to determine the use of aerosolized aztreonam in patients with mild cystic fibrosis.

Vaccinations: Patients with CF should be vaccinated against pneumococcal disease using the protocol for "high risk"patients. Annual influenza vaccination is also important.

Gene Replacement Therapy

Cystic fibrosis is caused by gene mutation leading to deficient or absent CFTR. Therefore gene replacement therapy if successful would be both appropriate and specific. Gene therapy trials have targeted the respiratory system using adenovirus and cationic lipids as vectors. A transient effect on CFTR expression and function has been observed in human trials but there is no long-lasting effect. Gene therapy therefore cannot be recommended as a specific treatment for cystic fibrosis as yet.

Lung Transplantation

Lung transplantation is the only treatment available for end-stage cystic fibrosis. A patient should be ill enough so that there is a survival benefit if given a lung transplant, yet he or she should not die while on the waiting list. An FEV_1 is less than 30% of predicted value in a patient receiving maximum medical treatment for the disease is accepted as an indicator for a double-lung or heart-lung transplant. The above value of FEV_1 is associated with a median survival rate of two years. Generally, survival is better for adults than for children. Survival is particularly poor in patients infected with *B. cepacia* so that some centers considered the presence of this infection as a contraindication to surgery. Current data from the International Society for

Heart and Lung Transplantation (ISHLT data) has shown a one-year survival rate of 80%, 5-year survival rate of 55% and 10-year survival rate of 35% after lung transplantation.

Indications for transplant surgery advised by the Transplant Unit of the Apollo Hospitals, Chennai include:

- Hypoxia (PaO_2 < 60 mm Hg); hypercapnia ($PaCO_2$ > 50 mm Hg)
- Long-term noninvasive ventilation therapy
- Pulmonary hypertension
- Frequent hospitalization
- Rapid lung function decline
- World Health Organization Functional Class IV.

(*Ref: Sunder T, Ramesh TP, Kumar KM, et al. Lung transplant: the Indian experience and suggested guidelines—Part 1 selection of the donor and recipient. J Pract Cardiovasc Sci. 2018;4:88-95*).

TREATMENT OF RESPIRATORY COMPLICATIONS IN CYSTIC FIBROSIS

Pneumothorax

Pneumothorax is a complication in patients with more severe disease and is related to rupture of an emphysematous area in the lung. A chest tube drain is invariably necessary. The lung may not expand readily because of the underlying fibrosis.

Pneumothorax may be recurrent and pleurodesis may be necessary with talc or tetracycline. If pneumothorax with air leak still persists, a video-assisted thoracoscopic surgical procedure needs to be done to close the leak.

Hemoptysis

Hemoptysis is usually a symptom of infection but can also occur from the dilated bronchial circulation in bronchiectatic areas of the lung. Use of antibiotics to counter infection and of vitamin K is advisable. Massive hemoptysis which is life-threatening is best treated with bronchial embolization once the site of bleeding is localized through angiographic studies. It is important to secure the airway in a patient with severe hemoptysis.

Allergic Bronchopulmonary Aspergillosis

Aspergillus is frequently present in sputum cultures of patients with cystic fibrosis without being responsible for any symptoms. However, some patients with cystic fibrosis have hyperreactive airways; an exacerbation of this hyperreactivity is at times related to allergic bronchopulmonary aspergillosis. The diagnosis may be difficult, as cough, wheezing, bronchiectasis, presence of *Aspergillus* in the sputum are common in patients with cystic fibrosis. The presence of fleeting pulmonary shadows, markedly elevated immunoglobulin E (IgE) specific to *Aspergillus*, positive skin test and precipitins against *Aspergillus* support the diagnosis of allergic bronchopulmonary aspergillosis.

Corticosteroids in a dose of 30–40 mg daily tapered over 2-weeks improve both symptoms and the FEV_1. Itraconazole can be used as adjunctive therapy, though its efficacy has not been proven in cystic fibrosis.

Bronchiectasis

Bronchiectasis is not a complication but a feature of progressive cystic fibrosis.

Treatment of Other Features of Cystic Fibrosis

Cystic fibrosis in its full form causes pancreatic insufficiency, malabsorption, with malnutrition and infertility due to obstructive azoospermia. These need attention and treatment for overall success in the management of the disease.

SUGGESTED READING

1. Kabra SK, Kabra M, Lodha R, et al. Cystic fibrosis in India. Pediatr Pulmonol. 2007;42(12):1087-94.
2. Michel SH, Maqbool A, Hanna MD, et al Nutrition management of pediatric patients who have cystic fibrosis. Pediatr Clin North Am. 2009;56(5):1123-41
3. Mogayzel PJ Jr, Naureckas ET, Robinson KA, et al. Cystic fibrosis pulmonary guidelines. Chronic medications for maintenance of lung health. Am J Respir Crit Care Med. 2013;187(7):680-9.
4. Robinson TE. Imaging of the chest in cystic fibrosis. Clin Chest Med. 2007;28(2):405-21.
5. Sueblinvong V, Suratt BT, Weiss DJ. Novel therapies for the treatment of cystic fibrosis: new developments in gene and stem cell therapy. Clin Chest Med. 2007;28(2):361-79.
6. VanDevanter DR, Kahle JS, O'Sullivan AK, et al. Cystic fibrosis in young children: a review of disease manifestation, progression, and response to early treatment. Cyst Fibros. 2016;15(2):147-57.

Allergic Bronchopulmonary Aspergillosis

■ ALLERGIC BRONCHOPULMONARY ASPERGILLOSIS

Allergic bronchopulmonary aspergillosis (ABPA) was first described by Hanson and colleagues from the Brompton Hospital, London in 1952 and again in 1967 by Scadding who noticed an association between this disease and central bronchiectasis. It is a potentially progressive disease characterized by a hypersensitivity host response to intermittent or continuous colonization of the bronchi by hyphae of *Aspergillus fumigatus*. This hypersensitivity response leads to eosinophilic infiltration of the periphery of the lung (eosinophilic pneumonia), plugging of bronchi with mucus plugs often containing hyphae of the fungus, and an inflammation of the bronchial walls which in time to come can lead to bronchiectasis. In the vast majority of cases, ABPA is associated with bronchial asthma; the incidence of ABPA is higher in patients with cystic fibrosis, in pre-existing idiopathic bronchiectasis, and in individuals with atopic disorders.

Epidemiology

There are a number of asthmatics who show an immediate type cutaneous hypersensitivity to the *Aspergillus fumigatus (A. fumigatus)* antigen but just a few of these develop ABPA. The reason for this is not known. The prevalence of ABPA in an asthmatic population is probably between 1 and 2%; it is as high as 7–14% in corticosteroid-dependent asthma. Cystic fibrosis is an uncommon disease in India, but in the West, ABPA complicates 7–15% of patients with cystic fibrosis. Very occasionally, ABPA is diagnosed in nonasthmatics. This is either due to the fact that these patients have a mild asthma of which they are unaware, or even if they do not have asthma they are atopic individuals.

Allergic bronchopulmonary aspergillosis can occur at any age, but is most frequently diagnosed in the third to sixth decade. Familial cases have been reported in the West suggesting that genetic factors may have a role in its development.

Pathogenesis

Aspergillus spores are 2–3 mm in diameter and when inhaled are principally deposited in the proximal large bronchi where humidity and temperature (37°C) provide optimal growth conditions for *A. fumigatus*. The fungal spores within the bronchi turn into hyphae and colonize the bronchial wall. Epithelial damage within the bronchi with impaired ciliary function observed in both bronchial asthma and in cystic fibrosis probably encourage colonization and therefore predispose to ABPA. The fungal hyphae are believed to further impair ciliary function thereby helping even more in colonization. This effect is mediated by gliotoxin, produced by *Aspergillus* as also perhaps by other toxins. Adhesion of *A. fumigatus* to the bronchial wall may be also important for colonization and the development of ABPA in susceptible individuals. Adhesion of *A. fumigatus* to extracellular matrix has been observed, in particular to fibronectin and other subepithelial components exposed after tissue damage within the bronchial wall.

Though fungal metabolites may enhance inflammation, they are not central to the pathogenesis of ABPA. The pathogenesis is almost completely based on the immunological response of the host to the antigen-colonizing fungus within the airways of the patient. The immunological response is a Type I response, a Type III response, and a Type IV T-cell-mediated response.

Allergic bronchopulmonary aspergillosis is almost always associated with a markedly elevated level of both nonspecific and *Aspergillus*-specific Immunoglobulin E (IgE). A Type I reaction is proposed with degranulation of mast cells and release of histamine, leukotrienes, and other cytokines.

There is not just an increase in IgE levels, but also a polyclonal antibody response to the *Aspergillus* antigen, resulting in high levels of both total and specific IgG and IgA as well. The local high concentration of antigen and specific antibody leads to local immune-complex deposition—a Type III immune response results, causing an inflammatory exudate that damages the bronchial wall.

A Type IV immune response is also believed to underlie the pathogenesis of ABPA. The *Aspergillus* antigen is processed and presented to T-cells with activation of TH2 CD4—T-cell response. The TH2 cytokines [interleukin-4 (IL-4), IL-5)] lead to submucosal inflammation featuring both the abundant prevalence of eosinophils together with granuloma formation.

In addition to lymphocytes, eosinophils and basophils also contribute to airways inflammation and injury. Neutrophils also cause tissue injury, there being a correlation between the rise in IL-8 levels and the degree of neutrophilia observed in the sputum in patients with ABPA.

It is probable that the fungus itself plays a significant role in the pathogenesis. Proteases derived from the hyphae of *A. fumigatus* can cause epithelial injury and trigger hypersensitivity by allowing penetration of fungal antigens into bronchial walls. Proteases derived from the *Aspergillus* may also release proinflammatory cytokines which cause tissue damage and contribute to the development of bronchiectasis.

The question that arises is why do only some individuals with asthma develop ABPA while the majority do not. One reason may be genetic predisposition in those asthmatics who develop ABPA. T-cell antigen responsiveness has been observed only with specific human leukocyte antigen (HLA)-DR subtypes. Six HLA-DR subtypes have been identified accounting for most cases of ABPA. The pathogenesis of ABPA is illustrated in **Flowchart 1**.

Pathology

Three features are of note:

1. Eosinophilic infiltration of the lung parenchyma which is responsible for fleeting radiological shadows. The eosinophilic infiltration is compatible with an eosinophilic pneumonia.
2. Occlusion of bronchi, by mucus plugs containing Charcot Leyden crystal (eosinophilic degradation products), Curschmann spirals, and fungal hyphae. Mucus plugging can lead to atelectasis of a lung segment, a lobe or rarely, the whole lung.
3. The bronchial walls show infiltration with eosinophils, granuloma formation, leading to thickening of the walls, fibrosis, and bronchiectasis, typically proximal, and chiefly involving the upper lobes.

Clinical Features

Allergic bronchopulmonary aspergillosis occurs chiefly in patients with asthma. It is more frequent in adults with pre-existing asthma but also occurs in asthmatic children and has been reported in infants as well. It is an important complication of cystic fibrosis, a disease which fortunately is uncommon in our part of the world. Rarely, it may occur in nonasthmatic but atopic individuals. ABPA has the following presentations:

- The classic presentation is that of an exacerbation of asthma with fever, malaise, and cough with expectoration of brownish- or brownish-black viscid pellets of sputum containing hyphae of *Aspergillus*. Imaging findings are compatible with ABPA.
- Acute exacerbation of bronchial asthma or an acute severe asthma: A diagnostic search for ABPA is at times rewarding in this setting.
- Asymptomatic presentation: Asthmatic symptoms are no worse and may even appear better to the patient, the diagnosis of ABPA being suggested by findings on an incidental radiological examination of the chest.
- Repeated episodes of ABPA in an asthmatic patient may lead to proximal bronchiectasis. The symptoms and signs of bronchiectasis may predominate over those of asthma, and the clinical features of repeated episodes of bacterial bronchopulmonary infection may be difficult to distinguish from episodes of allergic bronchopulmonary aspergillosis.

In the hope of aiding diagnosis and management, ABPA has been classified into five stages: stage I—acute; stage II—remission; stage III—exacerbation; stage IV—corticosteroid-dependent asthma; and stage V—fibrotic end-stage chiefly involving the upper lobes.

Individuals with features consistent with ABPA but with no radiological evidence of bronchiectasis are termed

Flowchart 1: Pathogenesis of allergic bronchopulmonary aspergillosis.

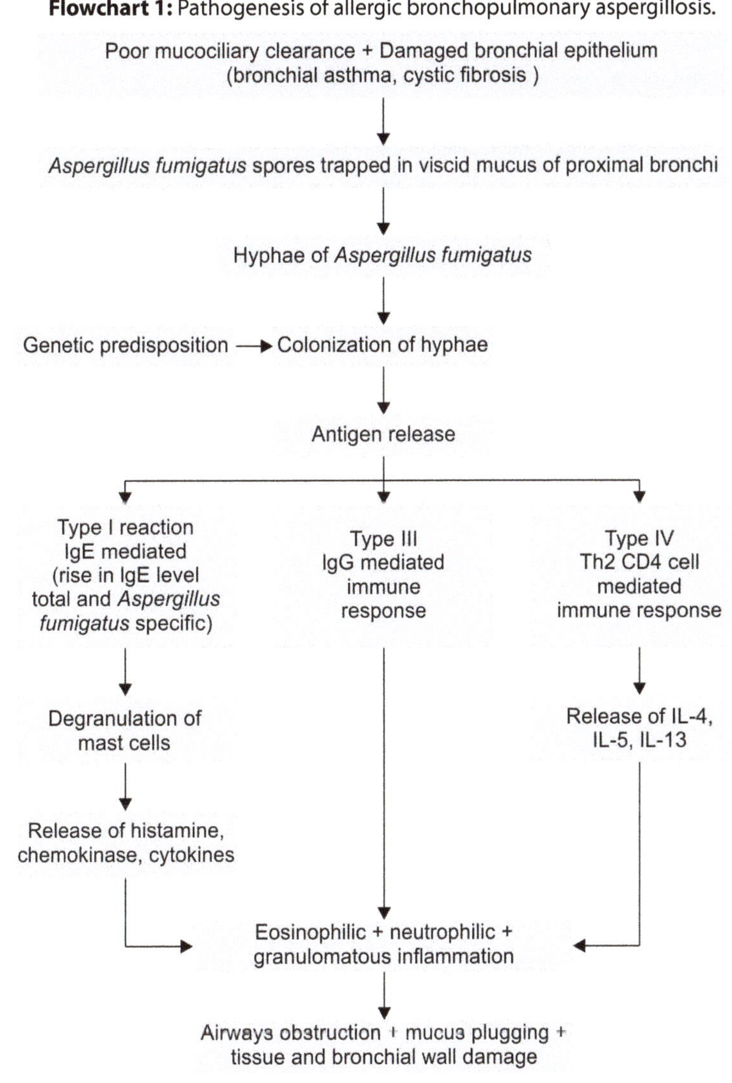

seropositive ABPA (ABPA-S). Those with radiological evidence of bronchiectasis are termed ABPA-B. It is difficult to ascertain whether ABPA-B is the natural sequel or the end result of ABPA-S followed over a varying period of time, or whether the ABPA-S and ABPA-B are two different clinical patterns of the disease.

Diagnosis (Table 1)

The diagnosis of ABPA is often made on clinical grounds but needs to be confirmed by serological and radiological findings. There are no absolute diagnostic criteria, but over several years guidelines for diagnosis have continued to evolve and have recently been updated. These guidelines are given in **Flowchart 2**.

Table 1: Criteria for diagnosis of ABPA.

Seropositive ABPA
- History of asthma
- Immediate cutaneous reactivity to Aspergillus species or A. fumigatus
- Total serum IgE concentration greater than 1000 IU/mL
- Elevated serum IgE or IgG to A. fumigatus or presence of serum precipitins

ABPA-Central Bronchiectasis (ABPA-CB)
- Above criteria present
- Central bronchiectasis on CT chest or CXR

Other supportive clinical findings
- Peripheral blood eosinophilia
- Patchy fleeting infiltrates
- Expectoration of brown mucus plugs
- Sputum culture positive for A. fumigatus
- Mucoid impacted bronchi evident on radiographic studies

Flowchart 2: Approach to diagnosis of allergic bronchopulmonary aspergillosis (ABPA).

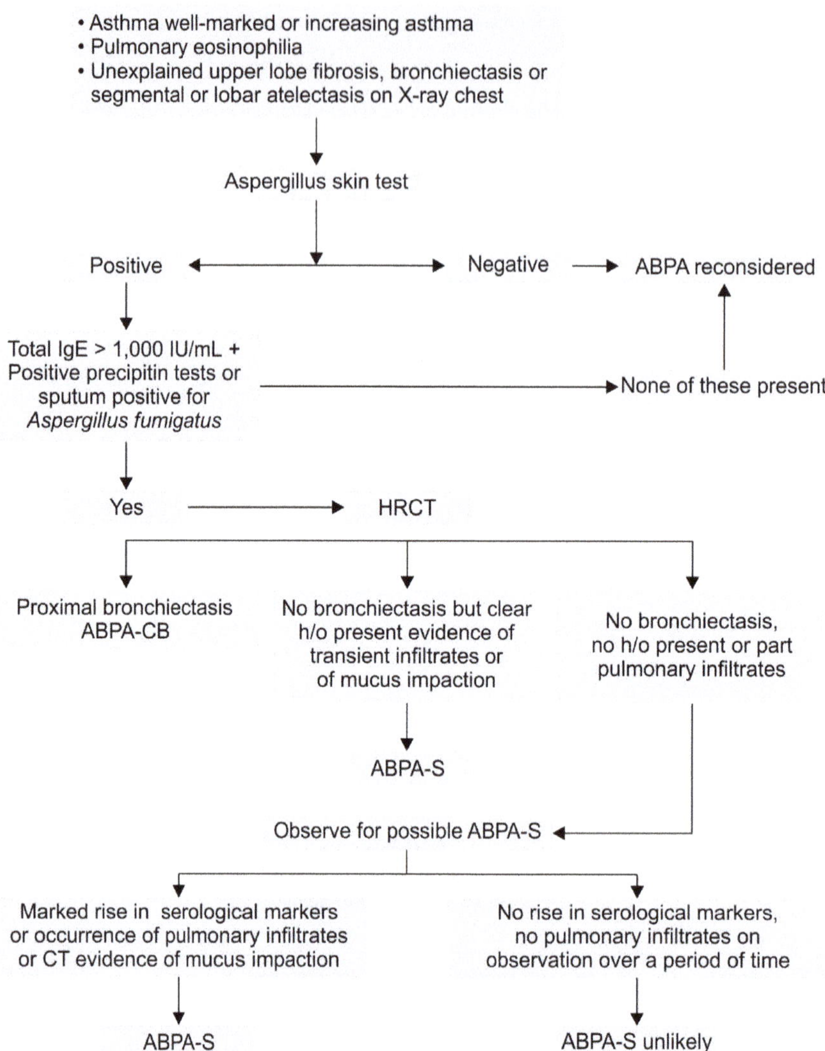

(ABPA-CB: ABPA-central bronchiectasis; ABPA-S: ABPA-seropositive; CT: Computed tomography; h/o: History of; HRCT: High-resolution CT; Ig: Immunoglobulin)

The reason why these guidelines are not sacrosanct is that when the disease is in remission the serological evidence may be markedly attenuated. Also if serological studies are done on patients with ABPA who have been receiving corticosteroids, the serological evidence given in **Flowchart 2** again may not be quite forthcoming. The importance of not being bound by guidelines but considering clinical, serological, and radiological findings during different stages in the natural history of ABPA is self-evident.

It has been earlier mentioned that allergic bronchopulmonary aspergillosis exists in two forms—ABPA seropositive (S) and ABPA—central bronchiectasis (CB).

The ABPA-S includes patients in whom the skin test and serological findings noted in **Table 1** are all positive. These patients show the following features: a history of asthma, IgE levels more than 1,000 IU/mL, elevated IgE and IgG specific antibodies against *A. fumigatus,* immediate positive skin test to *A. fumigatus,* and/or serum IgG antibodies against *A. fumigatus.* These patients have normal chest radiographs (except for occasional fleeting shadows) and show no evidence of central bronchiectasis [on computed tomography (CT) studies].

Clinically, these patients are less symptomatic, have fewer exacerbations of asthma, and less severe degree of airways obstruction.

In contrast, patients with ABPA-CB have severe advanced disease, often expectorate mucus plugs containing hyphae of *A. fumigatus,* and have central bronchiectasis on CT chest or on a chest X-ray. In addition, they are positive for all the criteria of ABPA-S listed above.

It is debatable whether ABPA-S is a milder form of the disease due to a milder and a different form of host response or an earlier stage of the disease which over time progresses to ABPA-CB.

Although it has been mentioned earlier that the serological features of the disease may depend on the natural history of the disease, it is important to stress that a normal IgE level in symptomatic untreated patients with asthma virtually excludes ABPA.

Relevant details with regards to skin prick tests, IgE, IgG levels, precipitin antibodies, and sputum cultures with reference to the diagnosis of ABPA are given below.

Skin Prick Test

The skin prick test using standardized extracts of *A. fumigatus* antigen is positive in all patients with ABPA. A positive test detects specific IgE and is characterized by a positive wheal and flare of 3 mm or more (when compared to the negative control) within 15 minutes. The skin prick test is extremely sensitive but is not specific for ABPA as 25% of patients with uncomplicated asthma also have a positive test.

Serum IgE and IgG Levels

There is a marked rise in total IgE level—far more than in uncomplicated asthma. The rise is due chiefly to a nonspecific increase in IgE. IgE specific to *A. fumigatus* is also raised and the absence of rise in this specific IgE makes the diagnosis of ABPA unlikely. The total IgE is generally more than 1,000 IU/mL, though during remission lesser values may be obtained. In the latter group of patients, a follow-up during exacerbation is often associated with a rise of IgE more than 1,100 IU/mL. There is also a rise in specific IgG in ABPA. It needs to be stressed that although *A. fumigatus*-specific IgE and IgG are generally higher in ABPA than in uncomplicated asthma, there is a considerable overlap between these two groups.

Serum Precipitin Antibodies

Immunoglobulin G precipitin antibody to *A. fumigatus* is found to be positive in 70% of patients with ABPA. It is less sensitive compared to the *Aspergillus* prick test, but is more specific. Even so, the precipitin test is also positive in a very small proportion of healthy individuals, in 10–12% of asthmatics and in 27% of patients with farmer's lung.

Presence of A. fumigatus in Sputum

The detection of hyphae of *A. fumigatus* in patients with asthma (on smear and/or culture) is confirmatory of ABPA, as it clearly points to a colonization of the bronchial wall with the fungus. Unfortunately, hyphae are not always found in the sputum of patients with ABPA. They are more likely to be seen on culture during exacerbations. Even then, sputum containing hyphae of *A. fumigatus* is produced intermittently in patients with ABPA so that a negative sputum examination does not exclude the diagnosis.

The diagnosis and management of ABPA is considerably helped by being aware of the natural history of the disease **(Table 2)**.

Radiographic Changes

Abnormalities in the chest X-ray may be transient or permanent **(Figs. 1 to 3)**.

Table 2: Natural history of allergic bronchopulmonary aspergillosis.
Stage I: Acute   • Symptoms of acute asthma   • Peripheral eosinophilia   • All immunological features observed in ABPA-S will be positive in this stage   • Fleeting pulmonary infiltrates   • Response to steroids and antifungal therapy   *Note:* 2, 3, and 4 may be markedly attenuated in patients receiving corticosteroids.
Stage II: Remission   • Resolution of symptoms and pulmonary infiltrates   • Lessening of peripheral eosinophilia and significant attenuation of all immunological response
Stage III: Exacerbation of the disease   • Recurrence or worsening of clinical symptoms   • Recurrence of peripheral eosinophilia and other immunological features   • Recurrent pulmonary infiltrates
Stage IV: Steroid dependent asthma   • Persistent elevation in immunological features
Stage V: • Refractory steroid dependent asthma   • Fibrotic lung disease   • Lung function shows always obstruction and restriction   • Bronchiectasis-recurrent infection

Transient Changes

These are of two kinds:

1. *Transient pulmonary infiltrates of eosinophilic pneumonia*: These are typically not segmental in distribution, fleeting in character, changing positions spontaneously, and invariably accompanied by well-marked peripheral eosinophilia. At times, the infiltrates are perihilar and when large simulate a tumor mass or marked hilar adenopathy.

2. *Areas of atelectasis due to mucus plugging of bronchi*: These areas of atelectasis may be segmental, lobar or rarely, whole lung atelectasis. The atelectatic area opens up on coughing up a mucus plug or after bronchoscopic removal of the mucus plug. Persisting occlusion of one

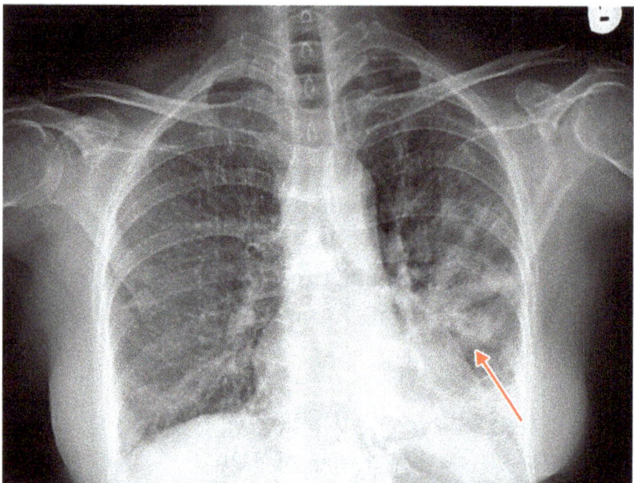

Fig. 1: Allergic bronchopulmonary aspergillosis (ABPA). Chest X-ray demonstrates well-defined tubular densities in left hilar and paracardiac regions, finger-in-glove appearance, typical of central bronchiectasis with mucoid impaction in ABPA.

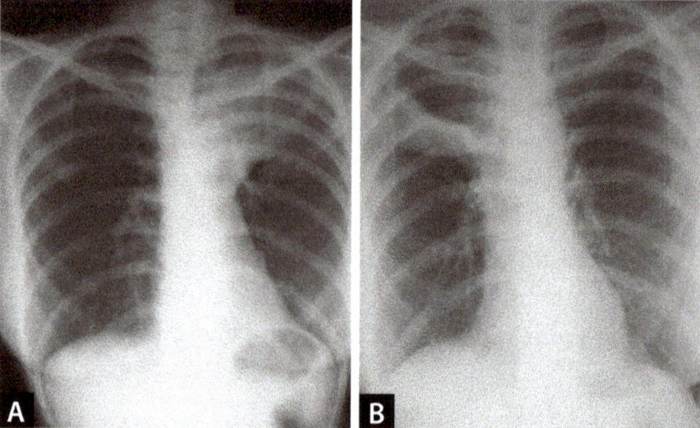

Figs. 2A and B: Allergic bronchopulmonary aspergillosis (ABPA). (A) Elderly asthmatic lady presented with left upper lobe collapse as evidenced by an ill-defined opacity in the left upper zone. (B) One and half years later she presented with right upper lobe partial collapse. Fleeting collapse consolidations are typical of ABPA.

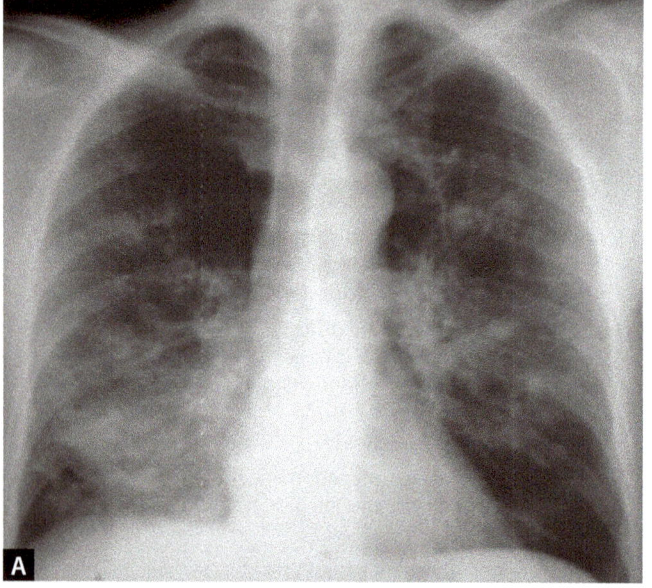

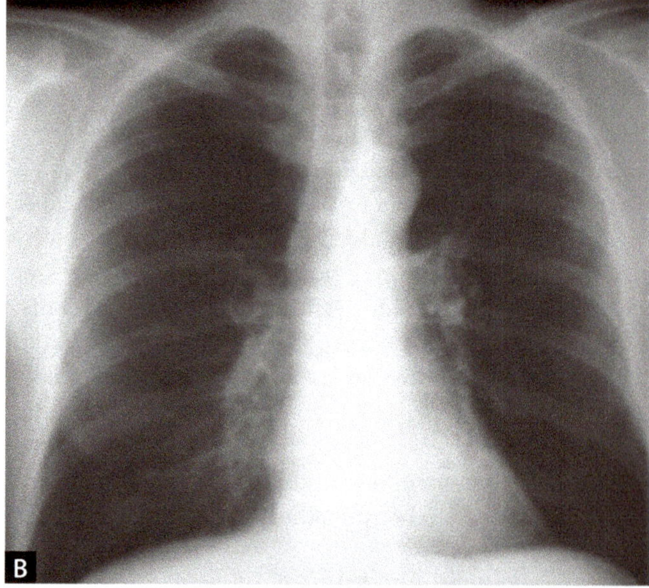

Figs. 3A and B: Allergic bronchopulmonary aspergillosis (ABPA). (A) Chest X-ray reveals ill-defined areas of consolidation in the right lower lobe as well as patchy areas of consolidation in the left lung. Serum IgE levels were very high. Patient was treated for ABPA. (B) Chest X-ray subsequently demonstrated complete resolution.

or more bronchi is likely to lead to bronchopulmonary damage—bronchiectasis + fibrosis.

Permanent Changes

These include the following:

- Parallel line (tram-line) shadows extending from the hilum outward represent dilated bronchi with thickened walls. In cross-section, dilated bronchi may appear as ring shadows or as cysts of proximal saccular bronchiectasis. Presence of associated fibrosis may cause volume contraction, chiefly of the upper lobes.
- When large dilated bronchi are filled with mucus, they cast a shadow similar to a gloved finger or gloved fingers (if there is more than one bronchus so impacted) appearance. Mucus may be expectorated from these bronchi but there remains a permanent distortion and thickening of the bronchial walls.

It is important to realize that changes on a radiological examination of the chest in some patients of ABPA may be inconspicuous, even in the presence of well-marked bronchiectasis that is brought out only on a CT of the chest. Again, upper lobe changes with fibrosis and bronchiectasis can also occur in asthmatics who develop tuberculosis or sarcoidosis, or in patients who have cystic fibrosis not complicated by ABPA.

Computed Tomography Findings

High-resolution CT (HRCT) of the chest is imperative for the diagnosis of ABPA **(Figs. 4 and 5)**.

- HRCT is vastly more sensitive than the chest X-ray in detecting bronchiectasis. Bronchiectasis chiefly involves the upper lobes and is classically central in character. In our experience exclusively, central bronchiectasis seldom occurs in any pathology other than in ABPA, though admittedly there is some disagreement with others on this statement. In advanced cases, the bronchiectasis can be more widespread.
- Pulmonary infiltrates (transient) are observed on a CT chest when none appear on an X-ray chest. Areas of eosinophilic consolidation may at times resemble tumor masses, particularly when situated in the parahilar region.
- Areas of distal atelectasis and mucus plugging of bronchi may be observed on an HRCT of the chest but may not be evident on an X-ray chest. Mucus

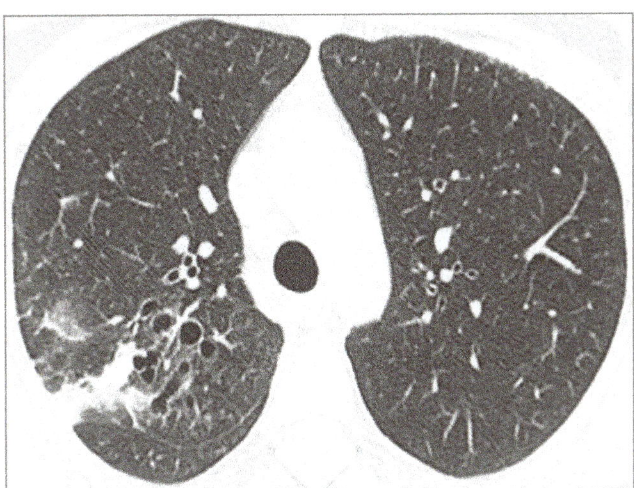

Fig. 4: Allergic bronchopulmonary aspergillosis. Computed tomography chest reveals tubular branching consolidation in the right middle lobe with dilated bronchi in the right middle lobe and left lingula. The tubular branching structures represent dilated bronchi with mucoid impaction.

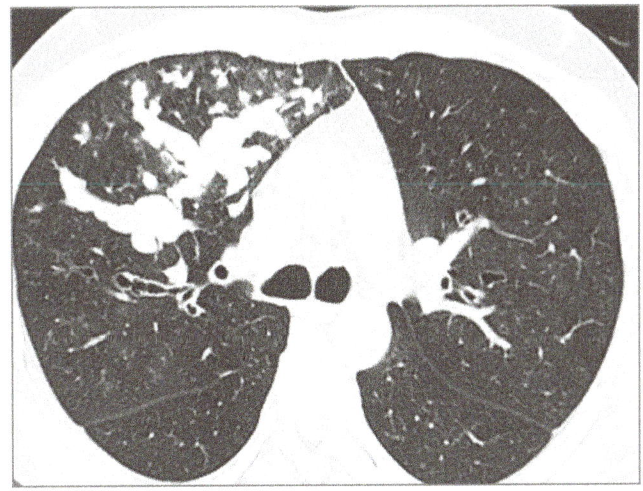

Fig. 5: Allergic bronchopulmonary aspergillosis (ABPA). High-resolution computed tomography (HRCT) chest demonstrates dilated bronchi in the right upper lobe with tubular consolidation along the periphery. Dilated central bronchi with mucoid impaction is typical of ABPA.

impaction may manifest in cross-section as centrilobular nodules.

The distinction between skin test-positive uncomplicated asthma and ABPA may be difficult on clinical grounds. HRCT studies may help. It is suggested that dilated bronchi in more than three lobes, the presence of mucus impaction, and centrilobular nodules favor the diagnosis of ABPA.

Pulmonary Function Tests

Lung function tests show airways obstruction, worse during exacerbation with improvement during remission. The occurrence of fibrosis and bronchiectasis may lead to a superadded restrictive defect. Worsening airways obstruction in chronic asthma, particularly when there is little or no reversibility, should warrant a search for complicating ABPA.

Treatment

Corticosteroids are the mainstay in the treatment of ABPA, and should be used early in the natural history of the disease as their use may prevent increasing damage to the lung. Though there is no convincing evidence that the early and rational use of corticosteroids will prevent bronchiectasis, retrospective studies suggest that corticosteroids may prevent or reduce increasing pulmonary fibrosis.

- Treatment for stage I and stage II disease warrants the use of prednisolone 0.5 mg/kg given for 2–3 weeks. The dose is then tapered by 5–10 mg every 2–3 weeks to a maintenance dose of 5–7.5 mg daily.

  Some patients require a maintenance dose on a long-term basis to control the disease and prevent recurrence. Systemic corticosteroids relieve symptoms, reduce airways obstruction, and reduce serum IgE levels and peripheral eosinophilia. Pulmonary infiltrates, if present, resolve satisfactorily.

- IgE levels should be monitored within a few months of an acute episode and followed up subsequently at periodic intervals. A significant rise in IgE points to increased disease activity and may herald an acute exacerbation or may even occur in the absence of clinical symptoms. A doubling or more of IgE levels should warrant a reintroduction of a course of steroid therapy or an escalation of steroid dosage, if the patient is already on a maintenance dose.

- Patients who are stable with very occasional exacerbations should receive steroids only during exacerbations. Long-term maintenance corticosteroids therapy should be considered only in those who have frequent exacerbations of ABPA or who show progressive bronchopulmonary damage.

- Monitoring of IgE levels, chest X-ray, and pulmonary functions is important. This may throw light on advancing disease even in the absence of symptoms.

- Inhaled β_2-agonists (e.g. salmeterol) together with inhaled corticosteroid do not constitute primary treatment for ABPA but help to relieve airways obstruction and may offer some steroid sparing effect.

- Itraconazole, an antifungal, has now been proven to be of use for ABPA. It probably acts by reducing colonization of the bronchial wall and is given in a dose of 200 mg twice daily for 16 weeks. The drug also allows a reduction in corticosteroid dosage, reduces IgE levels, helps to resolve pulmonary infiltrates, and improves exercise tolerance and lung function. It should be noted that itraconazole has a number of drug interactions. It may also cause adrenal insufficiency by directly depressing the adrenal glands or may do so by reduced steroids clearance in patients on steroid inhalers. Liver functions need to be monitored as the drug can be hepatotoxic. The drug has been found to be useful even during exacerbations of ABPA.

- Omalizumab, a biologically engineered antibody against IgE has been used in ABPA. Most patients with difficult to treat ABPA will not meet the criteria laid down for use of this drug. Even so, multiple case reports and a study of small series suggest that in a dose of 375 mg subcutaneously every 2 weeks, the drug helps to control disease activity and has a steroid sparing effect. More trials on this drug need to be done to determine its use in patients with advanced ABPA.

- Patients of ABPA with bronchiectasis should receive standard airways clearance treatment and other measures as discussed in the chapter on "Bronchiectasis".

- Secondary bacterial infection particularly in patients with bronchiectasis should be treated with appropriate antibiotics.

■ CONTROL OF UNDERLYING DISEASE

Underlying asthma needs to be optimally controlled. Mucus plugging with the formation of bronchial casts is far more likely to occur in narrow airways than when the airways have a normal or near normal caliber. Hence, the need to control asthmatic symptoms and improve expiratory airflow rates as far as is possible. This necessitates the use of inhaled corticosteroids and β_2-agonists, preferably a combination of salmeterol and fluticasone. In some patients, adequate control of asthma necessitates the use of a maintenance dose of oral corticosteroids.

Similarly, good control over cystic fibrosis is important when ABPA complicates this disease. It is indeed difficult to diagnose ABPA in patients with cystic fibrosis. Symptoms of ABPA and symptoms caused by an infective exacerbation of cystic fibrosis bronchiectasis are similar. CT findings of ABPA may also be present in cystic fibrosis. *Aspergillus* skin test and the precipitin test are positive in some patients with cystic fibrosis. However, pulmonary infiltrates do not usually occur with infective exacerbations of cystic fibrosis bronchiectasis. If these infiltrates do occur and if they clear with steroids, they lend support to the diagnosis of ABPA.

The complication of ABPA in a patient with cystic fibrosis may present difficulties for a possible future lung transplant. Even colonization of the airways with *Aspergillus* without ABPA may present difficulties. If sputum cultures are positive for *Aspergillus* in the pretransplant period, the patient is treated with oral itraconazole and nebulized amphotericin. This is continued for a month after transplant surgery.

LONG-TERM SEQUELAE AND COMPLICATIONS OF ABPA

Severe airways obstruction, bronchiectasis, and pulmonary fibrosis are the sequel of advanced unchecked ABPA. Other complications include the development of an aspergilloma, lobar and rarely whole lung atelectasis, and allergic *Aspergillus* sinusitis. Very rarely, there may be *Aspergillus* tissue invasion and a mildly invasive *Aspergillosis*.

Patients crippled with advanced ABPA have successfully received lung transplants. Recurrence of ABPA in the transplants has been reported.

Severe Asthma with Fungal Sensitivity

Some patients with severe asthma have well marked fungal allergy. These allergic fungal states have some of the features of ABPA-S, but do not meet all the requirements observed in the latter. The criteria for the diagnosis of severe asthma with fungal sensitivity (SAFS) include:

- Poorly controlled asthma in spite of more than 500 µg of inhaled fluticasone and the near continuous use of oral corticosteroids
- Serum IgE levels less than 1,000 IU/mL
- Positive prick test to *A. fumigatus* or elevated specific IgE level to *A. fumigatus*

- Absence of serum precipitins and elevated specific levels of IgG
- Absence of bronchiectasis or lung infiltrates.

It is possible that there is a continuum starting with severe asthma, progressing to severe asthma with fungal allergy and still further progressing to ABPA.

Besides the use of oral corticosteroids, antifungal therapy with itraconazole improves asthma control and has a steroid sparing effect.

ALLERGIC ASPERGILLUS SINUSITIS

Allergic *Aspergillus* sinusitis has the same histological features as ABPA. Clinically, patients present with a sinusitis not responding to antibiotic therapy. X-ray of the paranasal sinus shows opaque sinuses and CT of the sinuses shows soft tissue densities filling the sinuses without any bone destruction. Nasal polyps are often present. The *Aspergillus* skin test is positive; the precipitin test is also positive in the majority of patients. Treatment with oral steroids is very effective and obviates the need for surgical intervention.

SUGGESTED READING

1. Agarwal R. Allergic bronchopulmonary aspergillosis. Chest. 2009;135(3):805-26.
2. Bedi RS. Allergic bronchopulmonary aspergillosis: Indian perspective. Indian J Chest Dis Allied Sci. 2009;51(2): 73-4.
3. Denning DW, Pleuvry A, Cole DC. Global burden of allergic bronchopulmonary aspergillosis with asthma and its complication chronic pulmonary aspergillosis in adults. Med Mycol. 2013;51(4):361-70.
4. Muldoon EG, Strek ME, Patterson KC. Allergic and noninvasive infectious pulmonary aspergillosis syndromes. Clin Chest Med. 2017;38(3):521-34.
5. Patterson K, Strek ME. Allergic bronchopulmonary aspergillosis. Proc Am Thorac Soc. 2010;7:237-44.
6. Rosenberg M, Patterson R, Mintzer R, et al. Clinical and immunologic criteria for the diagnosis of allergic bronchopulmonary aspergillosis. Ann Intern Med. 1977;86:405-14.
7. Shah A. Allergic bronchopulmonary aspergillosis: a review of a disease with a worldwide distribution. J Asthma. 2002;39(4):273-89.
8. Stevens DA, Schwartz HJ, Lee JY, et al. A randomized trial of itraconazole in allergic bronchopulmonary aspergillosis. N Engl J Med. 2000;342:756-62.

CHAPTER 41

Bronchiolitis

■ GENERAL CONSIDERATIONS

Bronchioles are small conducting airways less than 2 mm in diameter. They constitute a transition area between the tertiary bronchi (which have cartilage in their walls) and the lung parenchyma. They lack cartilage, have a very thin fibromuscular wall lined by epithelium and have fundamentally a centrilobular location. Because of their large number, their easily collapsibility (lack of cartilage and small diameter) and because they form the immediate conduits that transport gases to and from the alveoli, they are particularly vulnerable to "injury" from infectious and noninfectious causes. Bronchiolitis is an inflammatory narrowing and obstruction of these small (<2 mm in diameter) conducting airways. The inflammation is the result of an "insult" or "damage" to the bronchiolar epithelium, the fibromuscular wall and/or the peribronchiolar tissue due to an infective, noninfective or undetermined cause. Inflammatory cells and granulation tissue may be present in the lumen, within the bronchiolar walls as also peribronchially. The sequel to this inflammation is often a narrowing, a distortion and, in some cases, a total obliteration of the involved small conducting airways. In most instances, involvement of the small airways is chiefly proximal to the respiratory bronchioles. Among notable exceptions are patients with diffuse panbronchiolitis (DPB) and the entity termed respiratory bronchiolitis in smokers, where the brunt of the inflammatory pathology is borne by the respiratory bronchioles and the adjacent alveoli. Involvement of the respiratory bronchioles together with an alveolar infiltrate is also noted in bronchiolitis obliterans with organizing pneumonia (BOOP), also termed cryptogenic organizing pneumonia (COP).

■ SEMANTICS

The semantics in relation to bronchiolar disorders is confusing as different descriptive terms are either synonymous or perhaps overlap, or represent different stages of the same disease. For example, terms which are synonymous and in use are constrictive bronchiolitis, obstructive bronchiolitis, obliterative bronchiolitis and bronchiolitis obliterans. Again, the term bronchiolitis obliterans has been applied to two different histological patterns of bronchiolar fibrosis as also to different clinical syndromes ranging from progressive airway obstruction (constrictive or obliterative bronchiolitis), to a predominant infiltrative process involving the alveoli and producing a restrictive lesion (BOOP) or COP.

Bronchiolar abnormalities may also exist as a feature of parenchymal lung involvement as in bronchopneumonia, or as an associated feature of involvement of the more proximal airways as in bronchiectasis. Secondary bronchiolar involvement is also observed in interstitial lung disease, such as sarcoidosis, extrinsic allergic alveolitis, and Langerhans cell histiocytosis. Finally, inflammation involving the small airways in chronic obstructive pulmonary disease (COPD) is the major factor responsible for airflow limitation in this disease.

Table 1 gives an overall perspective of disorders or diseases involving the bronchioles. *The subsequent discussion centers solely on primary bronchiolitis.*

■ PRIMARY BRONCHIOLITIS

Primary bronchiolitis constitutes a group of bronchiolar wall disorders in which the pathology is anatomically limited to the bronchioles. This is in striking contrast to secondary bronchiolitis, where bronchiolar wall

Table 1: Bronchiolar wall disorders.

- Primary bronchiolitis—disorder or disease confined anatomically to the bronchiolar wall
- Secondary bronchiolitis in which interstitial lung disease is associated with significant bronchiolar involvement:
  - Cryptogenic organizing pneumonia
  - Extrinsic allergic alveolitis
  - Respiratory bronchiolitis with interstitial lung disease
  - Other interstitial lung diseases, e.g. sarcoidosis, Langerhans cell histiocytosis

abnormalities are secondarily associated features of different interstitial lung diseases or are prominent components of obstructive airways' diseases such as COPD and asthma.

Primary bronchiolitis can be further classified into: (1) *Constrictive bronchiolitis* (also termed obstructive bronchiolitis or bronchiolitis obliterans); and (2) *Other forms of primary bronchiolitis*. These include DPB, mineral dust bronchiolitis, respiratory bronchiolitis, follicular bronchiolitis, and other rare forms of primary bronchiolitis.

Constrictive Bronchiolitis (Obstructive Bronchiolitis or Bronchiolitis Obliterans)

Constrictive bronchiolitis is characterized histologically by constriction followed by obliteration of the small airways. This histological end result can occur in different clinical settings with different etiological factors. When no obvious cause is evident, the disease is termed cryptogenic constrictive bronchiolitis or cryptogenic bronchiolitis obliterans. Known etiological factors are connective tissue disorders (rheumatoid disease, systemic lupus erythematosus in particular), acute viral infections, inhalational injury, as a complication in recipients of heart-lung and bone marrow transplants and as a toxic effect of certain drugs. Rarely, obliterative bronchiolitis is observed in association with inflammatory bowel disease, neuroendocrine cell hyperplasia, multiple carcinoid tumors and paraneoplastic pemphigus.

Histopathology

Histopathology of constrictive bronchiolitis is characterized by a distinctive pattern of peribronchiolar fibrosis which first constricts bronchioles and then obliterates their lumen. This histological feature is common to all etiological factors. The fibrotic process surrounds the bronchioles, strangling the small airways

through external compression and constriction. Even in advanced severe cases, the disease is patchy in its distribution and can therefore be missed if the appropriate areas of the lung have not been sampled. Transbronchial biopsy often does not allow a correct diagnosis which can only be made by a video-assisted thoracoscopic biopsy.

Acute Infective Bronchiolitis

Acute infective bronchiolitis is seen mostly in infants and children as a feature of acute viral infection. In fact, it is the commonest respiratory disease in infancy occurring in epidemic form in the winter months. It is also observed in India and other developing countries, but its prevalence remains undetermined because of the general difficulty in performing reliable virological studies. The respiratory syncytial virus is the commonest cause of acute bronchiolitis in infants and children. Other viruses such as the adenovirus, measles, influenza and parainfluenza virus can also do so. Acute bronchiolitis has also been reported following mycoplasmal and chlamydial infection.

Acute bronchiolitis in adults is uncommon, though it can occasionally be caused by the viruses stated above. Symptoms in adults are generally not severe when compared to infants and children, perhaps because the small airways in adults contribute less to total pulmonary resistance. Acute bronchiolitis may also be seen in adults following aspiration (particularly of gastric acid as in Mendelson's syndrome), inhalational injuries and bone marrow transplant and Stevens-Johnson syndrome.

Pathology: The mucus membrane of the bronchioles in acute infective bronchiolitis is acutely inflamed, with edema and necrosis of the epithelial cells. In viral bronchiolitis (in particular respiratory syncytial viral infection), the respiratory epithelial cells produce several chemokines such as macrophage inflammatory protein 1a, several proinflammatory interleukins and RANTES (regulated upon activation, normal T-cell expressed and secreted). These cytokines recruit and activate eosinophils, lymphocytes, macrophages, neutrophils and natural killer cells at the site of inflammation. Inflammatory edema of the bronchiolar wall, increased mucus secretion and hyper-reactivity of the small airways form the end result.

Clinical features: Clinical features are characterized by tachypnea, tachycardia and breathlessness with prolonged expiration. Wheeze may be audible at a distance and there may be, in some infants and children, severe respiratory distress with indrawing of the intercostal spaces during inspiration, flaring of the alae nasi and use of accessory muscles of respiration. Rhonchi, together with crackles, are the usual auscultatory signs. Radiography of the chest typically reveals hyperinflated lungs. High-resolution computed tomography (HRCT) of the chest in acute infective bronchiolitis reveals ill-defined centrilobular nodules. These nodules relate to inflamed bronchioles impacted with secretions, coupled with peribronchial inflammation. The inflamed bronchioles cause linear branching lines on imaging study. Focal areas of consolidation may be present.

Treatment: In most instances, the disease is mild. Treatment is then supportive. When severe and in the presence of respiratory distress, the patient needs to be hospitalized and given supplemental oxygen. Bronchodilators, corticosteroids and antiviral agents need to be used. The overall mortality is generally not more than 1%.

In a few patients, acute infective bronchiolitis may result over a period of time in progressive constrictive bronchiolitis. This is observed in particular with adenovirus infection as also after measles and influenza A infection. Occasionally, MacLeod's syndrome may evolve as a sequel of acute infective bronchiolitis.

Other Causes of Constrictive Bronchiolitis (Table 2)

Inhalational injury: Constrictive bronchiolitis is a frequent complication of inhalation of toxic gases. In the Bhopal gas tragedy, necrotizing bronchiolitis following inhalation of methyl isocyanate gas (MIC) led to a crippling obliterative bronchiolitis in a number of patients. Other toxic gases that cause inhalational injury (characterized by constrictive bronchiolitis) include NO_2, chlorine, inhalation of smoke emanating from fires, ammonia and SO_2. Constrictive bronchiolitis presenting as increasing airway obstruction may be observed several weeks after the initial insult.

Transplant recipients: Patients with allogenic bone marrow transplant, heart-lung transplant or lung transplant may develop constrictive bronchiolitis as a chronic rejection phenomenon. Constrictive bronchiolitis is a major cause of death in lung transplant patients. It occurs in over 50% of lung transplant patients over 5 years. Confirmation of the diagnosis of this complication is often not possible, as transbronchial biopsy in constrictive bronchiolitis generally yields negative results. Diagnosis is based on the clinical and objective evidence of airway obstruction; a fall in FEV1 below 20% of its previous stable value being considered significant.

Connective tissue disorders: Rheumatoid disease is the commonest connective tissue disorder causing constrictive bronchiolitis. The course of the disease varies. In some patients, it is rapidly progressive; in others, the progress is slow. Constrictive bronchiolitis generally occurs in patients with longstanding disease. It is possible that subclinical forms of obliterative bronchiolitis may be present in a larger number of patients than what is suspected. Penicillamine and gold (both uncommonly used today) used as therapy for rheumatoid disease have been known to cause obliterative bronchiolitis.

Association with other diseases: The association of constrictive bronchiolitis with inflammatory bowel disease, neuroendocrine cell hyperplasia, carcinoid tumorlets and paraneoplastic pemphigus is rare and though reported, has not been witnessed by us as yet.

Finally, when no etiological factor can be implicated one is left with the diagnosis of *cryptogenic constrictive bronchiolitis* or *cryptogenic bronchiolitis obliterans.* It is a rare disease occurring mostly in women. In some patients, there is a history of a mild flu-like infection in the recent past, but a confirmed etiological diagnosis generally cannot be substantiated.

Pathogenesis

As mentioned earlier, different etiological factors causing constrictive bronchiolitis ultimately lead to the same histopatholgical end result. The pathogenetic mechanisms may however vary. For example, inhalational

Table 2: Etiology of constrictive bronchiolitis.

- Cryptogenic
- Connective tissue disorders (perhaps the most common cause in clinical practice):
  - Rheumatoid arthritis, systemic lupus erythematosus, polymyositis, systemic sclerosis
- Acute viral infection:
  - Respiratory syncytial virus, adenovirus, influenza, parainfluenza virus, other viruses
- Inhalational injury:
  - Toxic gases (e.g. oxides of nitrogen, ammonia, SO_2, chlorine, phosgene, etc.)
- Allograft recipients:
  - Heart-lung transplants, lung transplant, bone marrow transplant
- Drugs:
  - Gold, penicillamine, busulfan, cocaine
- Associated with other diseases:
  - Inflammatory bowel disease, neuroendocrine cell hyperplasia, carcinoid tumors, paraneoplastic pemphigus

injury has a direct chemical toxic effect on mucosal cells and also on the bronchiolar wall structure. Viral infections cause an inflammatory reaction, cytokine production, leading to eventual fibrosis. In constrictive bronchiolitis following lung transplants, the pathogenesis is based on alloreactivity to human leukocyte antigens (HLA), airways inflammation, viral infections and airway ischemia. Constrictive bronchiolitis occurring in patients with pemphigus, a paraneoplastic syndrome is characterized by deposition of IgE on epithelial cells and acantholytic changes. Multiple pathogenetic mechanisms, some of which are known and some not yet evident, may ultimately lead to the same end result.

Clinical Features

Patients with constrictive bronchiolitis present with progressive breathlessness and cough. There may be few or no physical signs; few crackles may be heard over the bases. If lung function tests are not done, the diagnosis may well be missed in early cases. Lung functions show airway obstruction with air trapping. There is well-marked reduction in the mid and late expiratory flow rates. Residual volume and total lung capacity are both increased. Diffusing capacity is reduced. Aerosolized bronchodilators cause no improvement in the airway obstruction.

Imaging

In the early part of the natural history, the chest X-ray may be passed off as normal. As the disease progresses, there is hyperinflation with peripheral attenuation of vascular markings. Serial radiographs of the chest show increasing lung volumes. Thickening of the bronchial walls may occasionally be observed.

High-resolution computed tomography of the chest shows a mosaic pattern due to areas of decreased attenuation and vascularity. Images during expiration show evidence of air trapping. Thickened bronchiolar walls with distal bronchiectasis may occur. The mosaic appearance is due to decreased perfusion in areas of bronchiolar obstruction and redistribution of blood to normal areas. Mosaic appearance of the lung described above though a classic feature of constrictive bronchiolitis, is also observed in pulmonary vascular disease, and airway disease. HRCT imaging with contrast enhancement of pulmonary vasculature helps in the differential diagnosis **(Figs. 1 and 2)**.

Natural History

In most patients, the disease is progressive and ultimately leads to respiratory failure and death.

Treatment

Bronchodilators are generally ineffective and response to corticosteroids, both oral and inhaled is poor.

Management of posttransplant obliterative bronchiolitis consists of increasing the dose of immuno-suppressants in the hope of slowing or countering the rejection phenomenon. The use of statins has been

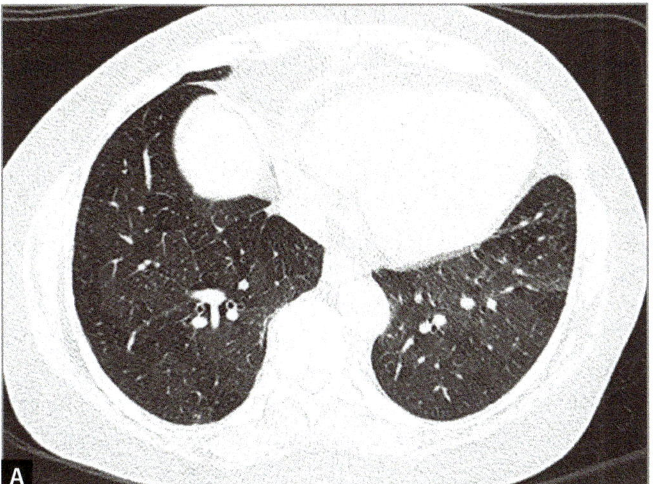
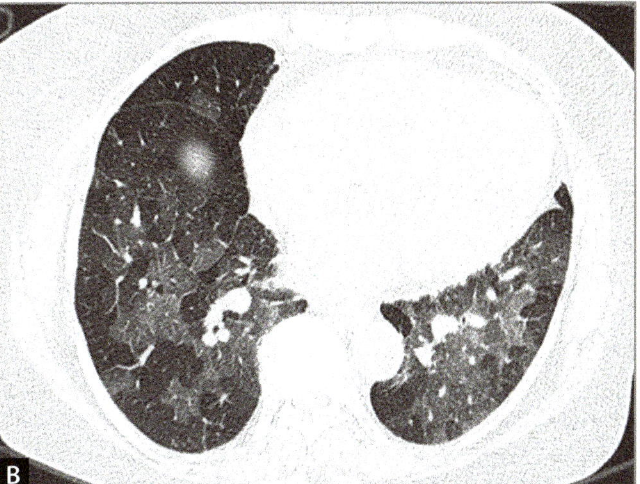

Figs. 1A and B: Bronchiolitis obliterans (A) Inspiratory high-resolution computed tomography (HRCT) demonstrates subtle areas of decreased lung attenuation in the lung periphery bilaterally; (B) Expiratory CT demonstrates marked air trapping in the subtle areas seen on the inspiratory CT scan.

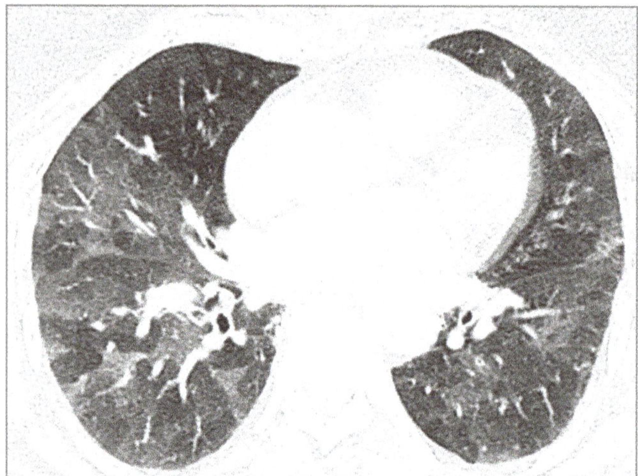

Fig. 2: Bronchiolitis obliterans. Focal areas of air trapping on an expiratory high-resolution computed tomography (HRCT). Note small-sized vessels in lucent areas.

reported to reduce the risk of rejection in lung transplant patients.

Other Forms of Primary Bronchiolitis

Bronchiolitis due to Mineral Dust Exposure

Inhalation of mineral dusts generally results in pneumoconiosis (a restrictive lung pathology). However, mineral dust can sometimes be deposited in the bronchioles, particularly in respiratory bronchioles and in alveolar ducts, inciting a chronic inflammatory response with fibrosis at the site of deposition, thereby causing a well-marked airway obstruction. A number of inorganic dusts can result in this form of bronchiolitis. These dusts include iron, talc, mica, aluminum, silica and coal. The degree of fibrosis depends generally on the local dust burden the patient experiences.

Respiratory Bronchiolitis

Respiratory bronchiolitis is a specific disease of the small airways related to smoking. The distinguishing features of this smoking-related disease is the presence of pigmented macrophages within the lumen of respiratory bronchioles and adjacent alveoli. The disease is invariably asymptomatic except when it is associated with interstitial lung disease—respiratory bronchiolitis-associated interstitial lung disease. It may then cause cough and breathlessness.

Radiographic examination of the chest is normal in respiratory bronchiolitis. An HRCT of the chest shows centrilobular nodules. No treatment is required other than cessation of smoking.

Follicular Bronchiolitis

Follicular bronchiolitis is characterized by the presence of hyperplastic lymphoid follicles with reactive germinal centers along bronchiolar walls. It is a frequent accompaniment of bronchiectasis involving the large airways. Follicular bronchiolitis may also occur as a part of lymphoproliferative disorders within the lung. Lymphoproliferative disorders may be (a) reactive non-neoplastic lesions; (b) lymphoproliferative malignant lesions; (c) lymphoproliferative disorders and lymphomas related to AIDS. In some patients, peribronchial lymphoid hyperplasia and infiltration may extend into the adjacent interstitium so that there is an overlap with lymphoid interstitial pneumonia.

Follicular bronchiolitis may be idiopathic in origin or is secondary, occurring with rheumatoid arthritis, Sjogren's syndrome, mixed connective tissue disease, immunodeficiency states including AIDS, and in poorly defined hypersensitivity reactions.

Clinical features: Breathlessness on exertion is the usual symptom. Physical signs may be absent or may reveal scattered crackles over both lungs.

Radiography of the chest may appear normal or may reveal bilateral small nodular or reticulonodular infiltrates. HRCT of the chest may reveal centrilobular nodules—1–10 mm in size, together with peribronchial nodules and ground-glass opacities. The nodules and ground-glass opacities are diffuse and bilateral in distribution. Bronchial walls may show thickening. A distinctive pattern which has been associated with bronchiolar disease is a "tree-in-bud" appearance due to impaction of the bronchiolar lumen with mucus or an inflammation exudate. The presence of peribronchiolar inflammation and peribronchiolar lymphoid follicles may appear as tree-in-bud on HRCT chest.

Treatment: Treatment is directed to the underlying cause. If no cause is evident, corticosteroids and immunomodulation have been tried with varying success. Recently, erythromycin has been reported to be of use.

Rarer Form of Bronchiolitis

Three rarer forms of primary bronchiolitis have been reported.

The first is aspiration bronchiolitis due to repeated aspiration of foreign particles causing chronic inflammatory bronchiolitis. Most patients are elderly or bedridden.

The second is a distinctive form of lymphocytic bronchiolitis observed in lung biopsies of nylon flocking industry workers. It is probably caused by an immunological response to inhaled antigenic material.

The third is a form of chronic bronchiolitis obliterans recently described in workers at a microwave popcorn factory. Patients present with progressive dyspnea, increasing obstructive airway disease with a normal chest radiograph. It is believed that this form of bronchiolitis is caused by exposure to diacetyl, an organic compound used to add a buttery flavor to popcorn.

Diffuse Panbronchiolitis (DPB)

Diffuse panbronchiolitis is a distinct clinical entity that was fist described in Japan over 40 years ago. It is an inflammatory disease of the small airways diffusely involving both lungs, the inflammation extending to all layers of the respiratory bronchioles. DPB is both a suppurative and obstructive airway disease which if untreated leads to bronchiectasis, respiratory failure and death.

Epidemiology: Though most frequent in Japan (prevalence 11 per 100, 000), it has also been reported from other Southeast Asian countries, including Korea, China, Thailand, Malaysia and Singapore.

In Mumbai, we have encountered a few patients whose clinical and radiological features are indistinguishable from those described in DPB. Though confined almost entirely to East Asians, recently the disease has been occasionally encountered and reported in Caucasians, Hispanics and African-American populations in Europe and America.

There is no remarkable sex predominance; the disease occurs chiefly between the second and fifth decades, the average age of onset being around 40 years. Studies from Japan state that two-thirds of patients are nonsmokers.

Etiology: The etiology is unknown but the fact that the distribution of this disease is chiefly in East Asians suggests an ethnic and genetic predisposition. This view is strengthened by the observation that many patients with DPB possessed the HLA-BW54 antigen. The HLA-BW54 antigen is primarily confined to the Japanese, Chinese and Korean races and perhaps can be used as a marker for DPB as this antigen has a very low frequency in the general population. The association of HLA-A11 has been noticed in Koreans suffering from panbronchiolitis.

Pathology: The lesions are diffuse and widespread, though the lower lobes are more involved. The pathology is centered around the respiratory bronchioles with transmural and peribronchial infiltration with lymphocytes, plasma cells, distinctive lipid-laden foamy macrophages and histiocytes; most of the alveoli are however unaffected. There is widespread narrowing of respiratory bronchioles, dilatation of the proximal membranous bronchioles with ultimate widespread bronchiectasis as the disease progresses. The functional abnormality that ensues is essentially obstructive.

Clinical features: Chronic cough with expectoration of purulent sputum, dyspnea on exertion and wheezing are the predominant clinical manifestations. Chronic paranasal sinusitis is present in over 75% of patients and may precede symptoms of chest disease by months or a few years. As the disease progresses, the volume of sputum increases because of widespread bronchiectasis. An important clinical feature is the frequent isolation of *Haemophilus influenzae, Streptococcus pneumoniae* and in advanced cases, *Pseudomonas aeruginosa* from the sputum.

Physical findings reveal crackles all over, though more marked in the lower lobes. Airway obstruction causes scattered wheezes on both sides. When airway obstruction is marked, wheezes may not be apparent unless the patient is asked to perform a forced expiratory mano euver. Clubbing is uncommon, hypoxic and still later hypoxic and hypercapnic respiratory failure occurs as the end result of the disease.

Radiological features: A radiographic examination of the chest reveals 2 mm nodular opacities scattered diffusely through both lungs often accompanied by hyperinflation. HRCT of the chest reveals that these nodular opacities are centrilobular in distribution with branching linear densities (tree-in-bud appearance). The opacities correspond to thickened dilated bronchial walls with intraluminal mucopurulent plugs. Areas of air trapping within the lungs are often present. Bronchiectasis is observed as the disease progresses in the form of ring-shaped or tram-line shadows.

Lung function studies: Lung functions are characterized by severe small airways obstruction with little or no reversibility following the use of an aerosolized bronchodilator. Lung volumes are often increased. Occasionally, a combined obstructive plus restrictive pattern is observed. The CO diffusion capacity may be reduced. As the disease progresses, chronic hypoxic or hypoxic plus hypercapnic respiratory failure ensues.

Differential diagnosis: Differential diagnosis from other forms of chronic bronchitis or obliterative bronchiolitis may be difficult. DPB is both an obstructive and persistent suppurative disease of the small airways. The pathological distinction lies in the involvement of the respiratory bronchioles, whereas most other forms of bronchiolitis involve bronchioles proximal to the respiratory bronchioles. The frequent association of chronic sinusitis in DPB, the strongly suggestive appearances on the HRCT of the chest and the frequent isolation of *H. influenzae, S. pneumoniae* and in advanced stages, *P. aeruginosa* from the sputum help in diagnosis.

Management

- *Use of erythromycin:* Many studies in Japan have shown that 600 mg erythromycin given daily for more than 2 years has a curative effect. There followed an improvement in symptoms, lung functions, CT appearance and survival rates.

Macrolides besides countering acute infection in the airways have other modes of action:

- They have an anti-inflammatory and immunoregulatory action. They do so by inhibiting the production of many proinflammatory cytokines such as interleukin (IL)-1, IL-6, IL-8. They also inhibit the formation of leukotrienes which attract neutrophils and inhibit release of superoxides.
- Macrolides block the release of adhesin molecules necessary for neutrophil migration. The bronchoalveolar lavage (BAL) fluid after use of erythromycin shows marked reduction in neutrophils.
- Macrolides cause a significant decrease in sputum volume.

The above anti-inflammatory effects lead to reduced airways infection and increased survival.

Beside erythromycin, the newer macrolides like clarithromycin have also been successfully used in the treatment of DPB.

- *Use of β₂-agonist and ipratropium or tiotropium:* Use of β_2-agonist and ipratropium or tiotropium through inhalation may help mucociliary clearance and bronchodilation, when there is some degree of reversibility in airway obstruction.
- *Use of corticosteroids:* Though commonly used, the evidence supporting their use is lacking.
- *Use of nonsteroid anti-inflammatory drugs:* These may exert nonspecific, anti-inflammatory effects and reduce sputum production but here again their efficacy is unproven.
- *Use of antibiotics:* Acute bacterial infection should be promptly treated with appropriate antibiotics, the choice of antibiotic being governed by sputum culture sensitivity reports.

■ BRONCHIOLITIS AND ASTHMA

Early onset of severe bronchiolitis is associated with onset of bronchial asthma, especially if the bronchiolitis is due to respiratory syncytial virus. An increased risk of asthma may persist into early childhood. A genetic predisposition to severe early bronchiolitis in life and the subsequent development of asthma is suggested by reports of an association between polymorphism in genes in the innate immune response, allergic response and inflammatory cytokines.

Differential Diagnosis of Bronchiolitis

The differential diagnosis is chiefly from bronchial asthma. Most patients with asthma show fair degree of reversibility though the more severe ones may show little or no reversibility. A reduction in CO diffusion is rare in asthma but often observed in bronchiolitis. The perfusion mosaic pattern observed on an HRCT of the chest is rare in asthma and observed in more than 50% of cases in bronchiolitis.

Sarcoidosis has been reported to occasionally produce strictures within the bronchi leading to airflow limitation. The bronchioles are however not involved.

Bronchocentric granulomatosis again involves the bronchi. The HRCT appearance is different—parahilar rounded shadows which on biopsy may reveal hyphae of *Aspergillus fumigatus.*

A very rare entity termed diffuse idiopathic neuroendocrine cell hyperplasia is a neuroendocrine proliferation of cells confined to bronchial and bronchiolar epithelium. It is associated with a carcinoid tumor, occurs predominately in women and presents with dyspnea, cough, airflow limitation and multiple small nodules on HRCT chest. Serum levels of chromogranin A may be elevated. Diagnosis can be made only on a transbronchial or a video-assisted thoracoscopic biopsy.

■ SUGGESTED READING

1. Alvarado A, Arce I. Bronchiolitis in adult: a review. Clin Res Trials. 2017;3:1-7.
2. Barker AF, Bergeron A, Rom WN, et al. Obliterative bronchiolitis. N Engl J Med. 2014;370:1820.
3. Carr LL, Chung JH, Achcar DR, et al. The clinical course of diffuse idiopathic pulmonary neuroendocrine cell hyperplasia. Chest. 2015;147:415.
4. Devakonda A, Raoof S, Sung A, et al. Bronchiolar disorders: a clinical-radiological diagnostic algorithm. Chest. 2010;137:938-51.
5. King TE Jr. Bronchiolitis. In: Interstitial Lung Disease, 5th ed, Schwarz MI, King TE Jr (Eds). People's Medical Publishing House, Shelton, CT, USA 2011, p.1003.
6. Laohaburanakit P, Chan A, Allen RP. Bronchiolitis obliterans. Clin Rev Allergy Immunol. 2003;25(3):259-74.
7. Poleth V, Casoni G, Chilose M, et al. Diffuse panbronchiolitis. Eur Resp J. 2006;28(4):862-71.
8. Scott AI, Sharples LD, Stewart S. Bronchiolitis obliterans syndrome: risk factors and therapeutic strategies. Drugs. 2005;65(6):761-71.
9. Tsang HWT. Diffuse panbronchiolitis: diagnosis and treatment. Clin Pulmonary Med. 2000;7:245-52.

CHAPTER 42

Oxygen Therapy

■ GENERAL CONSIDERATIONS

Cells require oxygen for their metabolic activity. Cellular hypoxia results when oxygen supply and oxygen stores within the cells do not meet the oxygen demand.

Oxygen stores are limited so that in acute respiratory failure or in cardiovascular catastrophes when oxygen supply is acutely reduced, tissue hypoxia can cause death. It is both the severity and the acuteness of hypoxia which determine the issue. However, in chronic respiratory failure [as in chronic obstructive pulmonary disease (COPD)], hypoxia evolves slowly over years, inducing metabolic changes that enable the cells to survive.

Hypoxia can be considered to be hypoxemic when associated with a fall in the oxygen saturation of arterial blood (SaO_2). Anemic hypoxia is due to a lowered hemoglobin content which lowers the oxygen content of the arterial blood ($CaCO_2$). Hypoxia can also be due to poor supply of oxygen to the tissues vis-à-vis their demands, as occurs in low cardiac output syndromes or in shock from any cause. Histotoxic hypoxia is due to the inability of tissue cells to utilize oxygen because of an abnormality in mitochondrial cell respiration (*see* chapter on Acute Respiratory Failure in Adults).

Hypoxemia, defined as a fall in SaO_2, is nearly always associated with a fall in the arterial pressure of oxygen (PaO_2). However, the PaO_2 may remain normal even though the SaO_2 is reduced when carboxyhemoglobin (HbCO or COHb) or methemoglobin is increased, because there is a decrease in the available functional hemoglobin. Conversely, the PaO_2 may be low in the presence of a normal SaO_2 when there is an increased affinity of hemoglobin for oxygen. This occurs when there is an intrinsic change in the structure of the hemoglobin molecule (as with variants of normal adult hemoglobin) or when there is an altered response to 2,3-biphosphoglycerate. Oxygen is used as therapy in most critically ill patients. It can be lifesaving in acute respiratory failure yet can be lethal if incorrectly used. Oxygen administration aims at increasing the P_AO_2, and thereby the PaO_2 and the SaO_2. Except in some instances, it is enough to aim at a saturation of 90%; an oxygen saturation less than 90% generally corresponds to a PaO_2 less than 60 mm Hg, and denotes the presence of moderate hypoxia. A moderate degree of hypoxia disturbs normal cell metabolism and function; marked hypoxia results in cellular death. A PaO_2 less than 20 mm Hg for a significant length of time generally produces brain death; yet a PaO_2 a little above 30 mm Hg probably maintains adequate cell function if the blood flow is adequate.

We have no means of accurately assessing cell function, and there is no doubt that the sensitivity of certain tissues (such as the brain and the heart) to lack of oxygen is far greater as compared to other tissues (e.g. skin and muscle). It is possible that even minor degrees of hypoxia which are easily tolerated in a young healthy individual, might pose problems in critically ill individuals, or in those with a poor coronary circulation, or with impaired cerebral blood flow due to diffuse cerebrovascular disease. It is important to relieve hypoxia of even mild intensity in all such critically ill patients, and preferably aim at an oxygen saturation of at least 90%, preferably even greater than 90%.

■ INDICATIONS FOR OXYGEN THERAPY (TABLE 1)

Hypoxia is the prime indication for oxygen administration. Dramatic relief with oxygen therapy is chiefly observed

Table 1: Indications for oxygen therapy.

- Hypoxemia:
  - Cardiopulmonary or respiratory arrest
  - Anesthetic error or accident
  - Hypoventilation from any cause
  - Respiratory diseases characterized by ventilation-perfusion mismatch, with or without impaired diffusion across the alveolar capillary membrane; a right to left shunt within the lungs or the heart
  - Respiratory distress with a respiratory rate more than 24/minute
- Pneumothorax
- Myocardial infarction and unstable angina
- Decreased oxygen content of arterial blood:
  - Severe anemia
  - Carbon monoxide poisoning
  - Methemoglobinemia, sulfhemoglobinemia
- Decreased transport of oxygen with impaired perfusion of tissues:
  - Shock from any cause
  - Left ventricular failure
  - Cardiac arrhythmias causing hemodynamic instability
  - Cardiac arrest
- Poor uptake or utilization of oxygen in tissues
- Postoperative states

when arterial hypoxemia (i.e. a low PaO_2) is due to a low PAO_2 or ventilation-perfusion (V/Q) mismatch within the lungs. Relief of hypoxia in such patients often brings in its wake three other effects:

1. Decrease in the work of breathing. Hypoxia often causes increased ventilatory work and relief of hypoxia is often followed by a decrease in the work of breathing.
2. Decrease in myocardial work. The heart and circulatory systems are frequently involved in compensatory responses to hypoxia; once the hypoxia is reversed, these compensatory responses abate and the work of the myocardium is reduced.
3. Improvement in cell function involving various organ systems of the body is a welcome aspect of adequate oxygenation to the tissues.

   Indications for oxygen therapy are stated here.

Hypoxemia

In an acute setting, hypoxemia (low SaO_2 with a low PaO_2) is the most important and most frequent indication for administering oxygen. These patients (particularly when hypoxemia is due to a respiratory problem) benefit the most with oxygen therapy. The following situations are included in this group.

- Cardiopulmonary or respiratory arrest. Administration of oxygen is of vital importance, but is of no avail unless the patient is simultaneously ventilated and cardiac resuscitation (in a cardiac arrest) is successfully performed.
- Anesthetic error or accident.
- Hypoventilation from any cause.
- Respiratory diseases characterized by V/Q mismatch, with or without impaired diffusion across the alveolar capillary membrane. These include severe COPD, acute severe asthma, as also interstitial lung disease. The most common cause of hypoxemia in clinical medicine is a V/Q mismatch. Patients who have this underlying abnormality benefit the most with oxygen therapy. In fact, if in a hypoxemic patient administration of oxygen leads to a sharp rise in the PaO_2 and SaO_2, the underlying cause of hypoxemia can be confidently attributed to a V/Q mismatch or to hypoventilation.
- Respiratory diseases associated with an increase in the right to left shunt within the lungs as in acute respiratory distress syndrome (ARDS), atelectasis, and pneumonia. When there is a true right to left shunt in the lungs (desaturated blood pumped by the right ventricle perfusing totally atelectatic alveoli), there can be no relief of hypoxemia following use of oxygen. However, even in well-marked ARDS there also exists some degree of V/Q abnormality with V/Q ratios less than 1. Some degree of relief may therefore be expected. The larger the right to left shunt the lesser the relief. Patients with shunts more than 20–25% may show little or no relief from administered oxygen.
- Respiratory distress with a respiratory rate more than 24/minute is an indication for oxygen therapy as per American College of Chest Physicians—National Heart, Lung, and Blood Institute (NHLBI) Conference on oxygen therapy *[Ref: Fulmer JD, Snider GL. American College of Chest Physicians (ACCP)—National Heart, Lung and Blood Institute (NHLBI) Conference on oxygen therapy. Arch Intern Med. 1984;144:1645-55].*

Pneumothorax

High concentration of pure oxygen [fraction of inspired oxygen (FiO_2) 60%] has been shown to quicken resolution of a pneumothorax. This is related to an increase of pressure in the gases within the pleural space following use of pure oxygen at a high FiO_2, so that the increased pressure gradient between the air in the pleural space and the surrounding tissues accelerates the absorption of nitrogen from the pleural space.

Myocardial Infarction and Unstable Angina

The American Heart Association guidelines for Advanced Cardiac Life Support recommend the use of supplemental oxygen in all patients with the acute coronary syndrome regardless of the presence or absence of hypoxemia. Though undoubtedly useful in hypoxemia (as may be present in the acute stage of a myocardial infarct), the administration of oxygen in patients who are normoxic is not based on convincing data.

Decreased Oxygen Content of Arterial Blood (Other than that Caused by a Decrease in PaO₂)

- Severe anemia.
- Carbon monoxide poisoning.
- Methemoglobinemia, sulfhemoglobinemia.

The use of high concentration of oxygen is useful but limited in scope as the PaO_2 is generally normal in this group; it is the oxygen content which is low.

Chronic anemia is generally well-tolerated. In acute severe anemia, use of high-flow oxygen through a nonrebreathing mask is of help, in addition to blood transfusions.

In carbon monoxide poisoning, carbon monoxide combines avidly with hemoglobin to form a stable compound COHb, thereby sharply reducing the oxygen-carrying capacity of the blood. Management consists of administering oxygen at 10 L/minute through a tight-fitting reservoir mask. The use of close to 100% oxygen provides one-third of the body requirement of oxygen through the extra oxygen dissolved in plasma. It also reduces the half-life of COHb from 4 hours to 1.5 hours. Hyperbaric oxygen can further reduce the half-life to 20 minutes and can provide enough oxygen in solution to fully take care of the oxygen requirements of the body.

In acute severe methemoglobinemia, inhalation of a high concentration of oxygen is a useful temporary measure (for reasons stated above) till the methemoglobinemia is reversed.

Decreased Transport of Oxygen with Impaired Perfusion of Tissues

- Shock from any cause.
- Left ventricular failure.
- Cardiac arrhythmias causing hemodynamic instability.
- Cardiac arrest.

A fall in systolic blood pressure to less than 100 mm Hg, a low cardiac output with metabolic acidosis (bicarbonate <18 mmol/L), severe shock from any cause are indications for oxygen therapy.

A marked fall in the venous partial pressure of oxygen (PvO_2) due to a fall in the cardiac output leads to a significant fall in the PaO_2. Also, many of these conditions produce an increase in the physiological dead space and/or a V/Q mismatch. It is important to maximize both the PaO_2 and the oxygen content, as also increase oxygen transport through an increase in the cardiac output in these patients.

Poor Uptake or Utilization of Oxygen in Tissues

Poor uptake and/or utilization of oxygen in tissues is seen in septic shock, ARDS; here again the PaO_2, oxygen content and oxygen transport or delivery to the tissue cells must be adequate if cellular and organ functions are to be well-maintained.

Oxygen is not utilized by tissues in cyanide poisoning as cyanide inactivates the enzyme cytochrome oxidase within the cells. A high FiO_2 is only of marginal help; reversal of cyanide toxicity by suitable antidotes is of prime importance.

Postoperative States

General anesthesia usually induces a decrease in the functional residual capacity, an increase in venous admixture and a slight to moderate V/Q mismatch. This is particularly observed following thoracic surgery, coronary artery bypass graft surgery, open-heart surgery, upper abdominal surgery and any protracted surgical procedure. A mild to moderate hypoxemia results, easily relieved by administering oxygen for an appropriate period of time.

It is important to remember that even though oxygen helps in the relief of hypoxia, it does not eradicate the root cause of hypoxia. It is therefore no substitute for adequate alveolar ventilation, neither does it solve the problem of

V/Q abnormalities, nor does it abolish a right to left shunt within the lungs. Again, the oxygen content of blood is not only dependent on the PaO_2 but also on the hemoglobin concentration of the blood. The importance of an adequate cardiac output to ensure good oxygen transport cannot be overstressed. Finally, the proper uptake and utilization of oxygen by the tissue cells is necessary if tissue hypoxia is to be countered or prevented.

Important Considerations in Oxygen Administration

When uncontrolled oxygen (at high flow rates) is given to relieve hypoxia in patients with severe COPD or in patients who suffer an acute exacerbation of COPD, relief of hypoxemia may be accompanied by a sharp rise in the arterial partial pressure of carbon dioxide ($PaCO_2$). Marked hypercapnia is undesirable and can cause a sharp fall in the pH of the arterial blood increasing both morbidity and mortality in these patients. The hypercapnia that results in the above circumstances is largely related to alveolar hypoventilation rather than to the inability of the respiratory center to respond to an increasing $PaCO_2$. This has been dealt with in the chapter "Chronic Obstructive Pulmonary Disease".

Therefore, an important consideration is to use controlled oxygen therapy to relieve hypoxemia in patients with an acute exacerbation of COPD. This is achieved by administering oxygen through a Venturi mask (24.5% or 28%) or using low-flow oxygen at 2 L/minute via nasal prongs. Arterial blood gas analysis should be done prior to starting oxygen and 30–45 minutes after starting oxygen therapy. The incidence of sharply increasing hypercapnia with controlled oxygen therapy is observed only in a small percentage (13% in a recent study) of patients. If the PaO_2 during controlled oxygen therapy rises close to 60 mm Hg and the arterial pH is not lower than 7.25, controlled oxygen therapy should be continued. If however even with controlled oxygen therapy, the $PaCO_2$ continues to rise so that the arterial pH falls below 7.25, or it is impossible to relieve hypoxemia (PaO_2 <55 mm Hg) without increasing hypercapnia and a falling arterial pH, other measures such as ventilator support become necessary. The ventilator support may be noninvasive or invasive depending upon prevailing circumstances (*see* chapter on Chronic Obstructive Pulmonary Disease).

One other consideration to be remembered is that in patients who hypoventilate due to neurogenic diseases, respiratory muscle weakness, poisonings (and in other conditions where to start with the lungs are essentially normal), administering oxygen will relieve hypoxemia but will have no effects on the hypercapnia observed in these patients. Finally, it should be remembered that oxygen is a dry gas and should always be humidified before administration, particularly so when the upper airway is bypassed by the use of an endotracheal tube or a tracheostomy. Ventilation of the lungs with dry gases produces heat loss, and moisture loss from the respiratory passages, and also alters pulmonary function. Heat loss causes a fall in body temperature and increases oxygen consumption. Moisture loss leads to drying or dehydration of the respiratory mucosa. The most important effect consequent to this drying is a reduced activity of the mucociliary escalator with sputum retention. Blocked airways from inspissated respiratory secretions result in V/Q inequalities, and may lead to or accentuate hypoxia. Thus, the importance of humidifying oxygen in inspired gas cannot be overemphasized.

■ METHODS OF OXYGEN ADMINISTRATION

Routine Oxygen Therapy using Low-flow Oxygen Administration Devices

A moderate rise of oxygen concentration in the alveoli suffices to relieve moderate hypoxia. An oxygen concentration of approximately 40% may be achieved by using nasal catheters, nasal prongs, or simple orofacial masks, if the flow rate is maintained between 6 L/minute and 8 L/minute. Patients cannot ordinarily tolerate flow rates higher than 6–8 L/minute through the above-mentioned devices.

Nasal Catheters and Nasal Prongs

These are the simplest and most commonly used techniques of oxygen administration. If a nasal catheter is used, its tip should be advanced to the fold of the soft palate, and then pulled back very slightly. If it is introduced too far, it can produce gaseous distention of the stomach, as oxygen finds its way into the stomach rather than into the lungs. Irritation of the nasal mucosa can be minimized by lubricating the catheter with Xylocaine jelly. The catheter can be changed from one nostril to the other every 6–8 hours.

Most units prefer nasal prongs to nasal catheters. Nasal prongs (two short plastic prongs that fit into the external nares) **(Fig. 1)** offer the advantage of simplicity and comfort. An added advantage over an orofacial mask is that the administered oxygen does not have to be discontinued during eating, speaking or coughing.

When oxygen is administered through nasal prongs or a nasal catheter, at a flow rate of 1–2 L/minute, the oxygen concentration is approximately 24%. At flow rates of 6–8 L/minute, the oxygen concentration approximates 40%. Further increase in flow rates is poorly tolerated and produces very little additional increase in oxygen concentration.

The effect of a given flow of oxygen through a nasal catheter or prongs is dependent not only on the flow rate, but the tidal volume and minute ventilation of the patient. If the tidal volume and minute ventilation decrease, i.e. the patient hypoventilates, then the inspired oxygen concentration will rise. Precise regulation or control over inspired oxygen concentration is thus not possible with nasal prongs or catheter. Other methods of administering supplemental oxygen include the use of reservoir cannula, transtracheal oxygen delivery, pulsed oxygen delivery, as also oxygen delivery through a face mask, face mask with reservoir bag, face mask with reservoir bag and directional valves.

Transtracheal oxygen delivery is effected via a small catheter inserted into the trachea at the base of the neck. It is totally unnecessary for intensive care unit (ICU) use though it has some benefits for patients on domiciliary oxygen therapy. Pulsed oxygen devices deliver oxygen only during inspiration. This conserves oxygen, yet provides a PaO_2 equivalent to that obtained with a continuous flow system through prongs or a face mask. Pulse type devices deliver fixed oxygen volume and flow each time a pulse is triggered. Demand devices vary the volume of oxygen delivered from breath to breath depending on the depth of inspiration.

Face Mask

A simple oronasal plastic mask **(Fig. 2)** fed with oxygen at a flow rate of 6–10 L/minute, is a frequently used method for administering oxygen. The oxygen fed directly into the mask (after humidification), displaces air and creates a small oxygen reservoir. During inspiration, oxygen in the mask is inhaled; room air is also entrained through the ports and through the space between the face and the mask. The oxygen concentration of inspired gas is thus much less than 100%. The extent to which inspired oxygen concentration can increase depends on the size of the mask (and therefore of the oxygen reservoir), and the flow rate of oxygen. Higher flow rates are generally better tolerated through the use of a mask as compared to nasal prongs or catheters. At a flow rate of 6–10 L/minute, an oxygen concentration of approximately 35–55% can be achieved.

The face mask is less easy and less comfortable to wear than nasal prongs. The major disadvantage is that it has to be removed when the patient speaks, eats, drinks, coughs, or expectorates.

Face Mask with Reservoir Bag

The addition of a reservoir bag to the face mask **(Fig. 3)** increases the potential reservoir of oxygen,

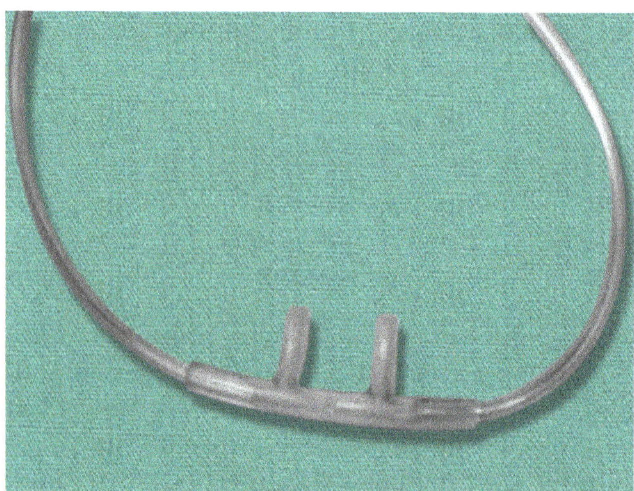

Fig. 1: Nasal prongs.

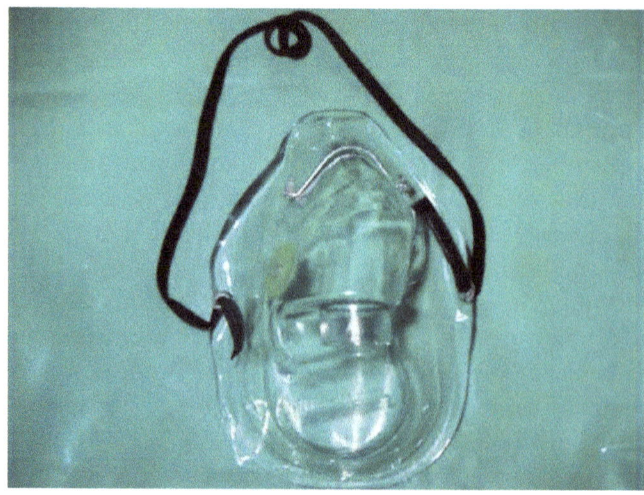

Fig. 2: Simple face mask.

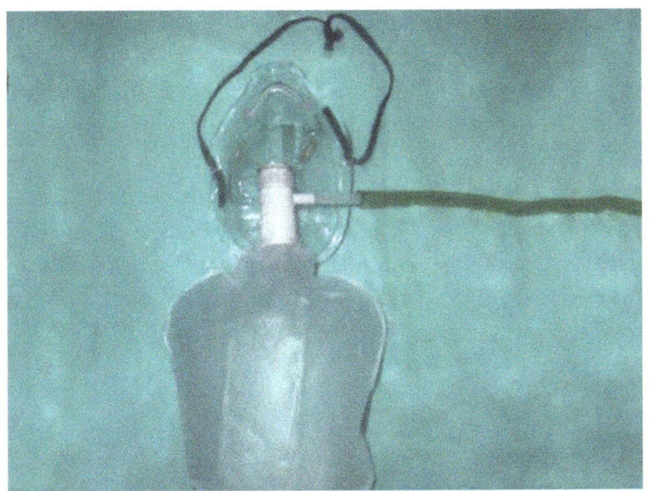

Fig. 3: Face mask with reservoir bag.

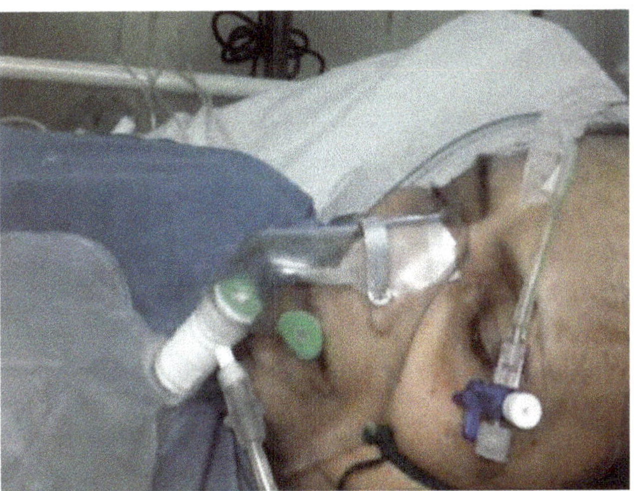

Fig. 4: A patient breathing through a face mask with reservoir bag and directional valves.

and allows a further increase in the concentration of inspired oxygen.

Inspired oxygen consists of oxygen from the reservoir bag of the face mask, together with some air entrained through the side ports and the small space between the mask and the skin of the face. During expiration, most of the exhaled gas passes out through the side ports, but some expired gas may return to the reservoir bag. This could lead to a fall in partial pressure of oxygen (pO_2) and a rise in the partial pressure of carbon dioxide (pCO_2) in the reservoir bag, and should be avoided by a sufficiently high rate of oxygen flow to keep the bag washed out. Oxygen flow rates of 8–12 L/minute are commonly used with this device, and can provide an inspired oxygen concentration between 50% and 80%. The flow rate of oxygen must be so adjusted that the reservoir bag is not emptied by more than half during inspiration.

Face Mask with Reservoir Bag and Directional Valves

The entrainment of room air during inspiration can be almost completely prevented by covering the side ports with directional valves (**Fig. 4**). Except for some air passing between the mask and the face, the entire volume of inspired gas consists of oxygen from the reservoir bag and the face mask. During exhalation, the side port directional valves open and air passes out from the mask into the atmosphere. The passage of expired air back into the reservoir bag can be prevented by a directional valve.

Table 2: Clinical differences between asthma and chronic obstructive pulmonary disease (COPD).

Device	O_2 flow (L/min)	O_2 concentration
Nasal cannula	Approx. 6	Approx. 40–45%
Facial mask	Approx. 8	Approx. 35–55%
Mask with reservoir	Approx. 10	Approx. 50–80%
Mask with reservoir and directional valves	Approx. 12	Approx. 90–95%

It is important that the flow rate of oxygen fed into the mask and reservoir bag with directional valves is in the range of 10–15 L/minute. The inspired oxygen concentrations can thereby be raised in such instances to as high as 90–95%. It is also extremely important to ensure that there is no failure in oxygen supply nor a sharp fall in the flow rate, as breathing is dependent on oxygen fed into the mask-reservoir device. If the reservoir bag is inadvertently empty, asphyxia results. **Table 2** compares the oxygen flow (L/minute) and oxygen concentrations (%) obtained by using low-flow oxygen administration devices.

Oxygen Therapy using a High Flow Administration Device

High flow nasal cannula (HFNC): Traditionally, nasal oxygen has been delivered at low flows (1–8 L/min) through nasal cannula or prongs. Recently, heated, humidified oxygen at flows of up to 60 L/min has been delivered in patients with hypoxemic respiratory failure via specially designed nasal cannulas. A number of commercially available devices are already available. The components of one such prototype are seen in **Figure 5**. The potential clinical applications of high flow nasal oxygen are hypoxemic respiratory failure caused by severe pneumonia, ARDS of any etiology, ILD with respiratory failure, and cardiogenic pulmonary edema. HFNC has also been used postoperatively in operation theatres and ICU's. Patients in respiratory distress have high inspiratory flow rates that greatly exceed the flow rates of traditional oxygen delivery. Entrained room air then dilutes the supplemental O_2 often substantially reducing the delivered FiO_2. HFNC generates much higher flow rates than the patients peak inspiratory flow rates, as a consequence less mixing with room air occurs and the desired oxygen is more reliably delivered. When a patient in respiratory distress breathes rapidly, considerable metabolic cost is extended by the patient in warming and humidifying the air. Reducing this metabolic cost by delivering warm and humidified air may explain why HFNC is so well-tolerated. Warming inspired air to core temperature (37° C) and humidifying it to saturation maintains mucosal function. We have seen patients who cannot tolerate CPAP or NIV comfortably tolerating HFNC for several days, thus avoiding in some cases the need for intubation and ventilation. There is much less nasal trauma and none of the facial pressure ulcers that make long-term treatment with NIV so difficult.

HFNC elevates nasopharyngeal pressure, thus resulting in the generation of PEEP (approximately 0.7

for each 10 L flow). This results in an improved breathing pattern with increased tidal volume, reduced respiratory rate and less work of breathing. Much data on the use of HFNC is being generated and a recent metaanalysis of 6 RCTs showed that compared to conventional oxygen therapy, HFNC, was associated with a lower intubation risk. Overall, as HFNC is being increasingly used in ICUs across the globe it would be no exaggeration to say it is an innovative and powerful technique that has the potential to change the management of respiratory failure.

Controlled Oxygen Therapy

Principles

The purpose of controlled oxygen therapy is to relieve dangerous hypoxia by producing an adequate increase in the P_AO_2 and the PaO_2, and yet control and limit the associated rise of $PaCO_2$. This would also limit the fall in arterial pH due to respiratory acidosis.

Technique

The concentration of inspired oxygen is controlled by using high air flows with known oxygen enrichment. The principle underlying this technique is entrainment of air with constant-pressure jet mixing. High air flows allow the immediate space or environment around the patient's face to be so thoroughly flushed, that there is no rebreathing and no contamination with room air. In this manner, the concentration of inspired oxygen can be controlled to within 2%.

Ventimask

The Ventimask works on the Venturi principle and allows perfectly controlled oxygen administration. Oxygen is delivered to the mask through a nozzle, and the aperture of the nozzle is of set size so that as the oxygen is released through the aperture, it entrains a fixed portion of air through the side holes of the mask. Thus if an oxygen concentration of 24% is desired, the aperture of the delivery nozzle is such that 1 L of oxygen/minute will entrain 20 L of air, and 2 L of oxygen/minute will entrain 40 L of air. The entrainment ratio is 1:20, and is independent of the flow rate; the oxygen concentration of the inspired gas is thus independent of the flow rate.

Different Ventimasks have different aperture size nozzles, and provide different but fixed oxygen concentrations. For example, a mask that is designed to provide an

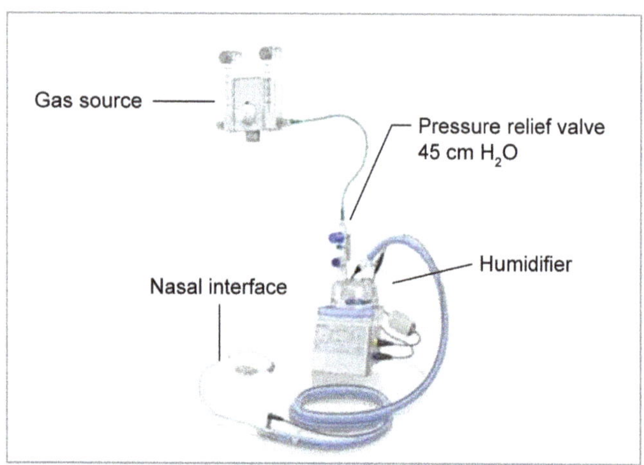

Fig. 5: High flow nasal cannula (HFNC).

oxygen concentration of 28% will have a nozzle aperture that allows 1 L of oxygen delivered through the nozzle to entrain 10 L of air through the side holes, i.e. a 1:10 entrainment ratio, which is again independent of the flow rate of oxygen.

As mentioned at the outset, the Ventimask works on the Venturi principle, and the Venturi is fairly accurate at the recommended total flow of 40 L/minute (i.e. 2 L of oxygen/minute for a 24% mask, and 4 L of oxygen/minute for a 28% mask). The gas flow around the patient's nose and mouth flushes the mask continuously, washing out the expired carbon dioxide, and ensuring that the patient only breathes the oxygen-air mixture provided to him.

The greatest advantage of the Ventimask is that the oxygen concentration it provides is independent of the flow rate, and also independent of the patient's tidal volume and minute ventilation. It can be easily used by all nurses, and requires no special adjustment. Also, the concentration of oxygen delivered is not at the mercy of faulty flow meters or reducing valves. The disadvantage as with all oronasal masks is that it has to be removed during coughing, eating, speaking, or drinking. In a seriously ill patient, removing the mask during feeds can cause a dangerous deterioration due to a sharp fall in the PaO_2 and worsening hypoxia. In severely hypoxic patients, the administration of oxygen should be continued, even when the patient is being fed, via nasal prongs at a flow rate of 1–2 L/minute; this prevents the temporary but dangerous hypoxia.

Currently, other commercially available high-airflow systems have been designed to deliver oxygen concentrations varying from 24% to 50%, using the same principle as the Venturi mask. A jet of oxygen from a wall or tank source is passed through a precisely designed (exact size) orifice, and this results in the entrainment of room air through the ports in the surrounding cylinder.

Nasal Prongs

Many ICUs in Mumbai and other large cities (leave aside smaller towns all over the country) do not use Ventimasks or other high-airflow oxygen-enriched delivery systems to provide controlled oxygen therapy. It is recommended that in the absence of these devices, nasal catheters or nasal prongs be used in an attempt to give controlled oxygen therapy. Oxygen at a flow rate of 1–2 L/minute through nasal prongs or catheters is generally effective in providing controlled oxygen concentrations of 24–28% in inspired gas. The flow rate should be initially kept at 1 L/minute;

if this is well-tolerated, it is increased to 2 L/minute. Measurements of the PaO_2 and the $PaCO_2$ are of help, and the patient is kept under a close watch, especially as regards his ventilation. If the patient has marked hypoventilation, administration of oxygen even at 1–2 L/minute can lead to an uncontrolled or higher than desired concentration of oxygen. In such patients, the flow rate should be reduced to less than 1 L/minute. Oxygen delivered through nasal prongs or catheters at low flow rates as stated above, is generally effective in relieving hypoxia without producing a dangerous rise in the pCO_2 **(Table 3)**.

Hyperbaric Oxygen

Hyperbaric oxygen is not administered in the ICU. Yet some critically ill patients under intensive care have to be transported to hyperbaric oxygen chambers in the same or distant hospitals to avail of this therapy. The administration of oxygen at higher than atmospheric pressure has certain advantages. When breathing air at atmospheric pressure, the oxygen in solution in plasma is 0.3 mL/dL; when breathing oxygen at a pressure of 2 atmospheres, it is 4.5 mL/dL. This is just a little less than the amount of oxygen taken up by tissues in unit time, and goes a long way in aiding jeopardized tissue perfusion, and relieving tissue hypoxia. The main use of hyperbaric oxygen is in the treatment of carbon monoxide poisoning. The dissolved oxygen relieves hypoxia, and the markedly increased oxygen tension helps the quick dissociation of carbon monoxide from HbCO. Hyperbaric oxygen therapy is also

Table 3: Effect of oxygen (administered through a nasal catheter at flow rate of 2 L/min) in relieving hypoxia without causing dangerous hypercapnia in 7 patients with obstructive airways disease.

Patients	Before O_2 therapy		After O_2 therapy			
			4 hours		24–36 hours	
	pO_2	pCO_2	pO_2	pCO_2	pO_2	pCO_2
	(mm Hg)		(mm Hg)		(mm Hg)	
1	50	56	75	60	80	55
2	48	52	66	60	75	46
3	45	50	60	54	70	56
4	55	48	70	48	86	46
5	42	48	65	54	68	50
6	40	68	60	76	66	58
7	38	72	60	86	60	65

Source: Adapted with permission from Udwadia FE. Acute Respiratory Failure. Bombay, India: Oxford University Press; 1979.

useful in the management of sepsis secondary to wounds contaminated by anaerobic gas-forming organisms, and in the treatment of wounds with a poor blood supply.

■ COMPLICATIONS OF OXYGEN THERAPY

Progressive Hypercapnia

The danger of progressive hypercapnia, particularly after uncontrolled oxygen therapy in a number of patients with hypoxia due to COPD, has already been discussed (also *see* chapter on Chronic Obstructive Pulmonary Disease).

Circulatory Depression

This is very rare, but has been occasionally observed in patients who have been acutely, severely hypoxic, and whose circulation is maintained by excessive sympathetic activity and excessive catecholamine discharge, induced by the severe hypoxia. Sudden relief of hypoxia abolishes this sympathetic overactivity, causing temporary hypotension, and occasionally circulatory collapse. We have observed this phenomenon following sudden relief of acute severe hypoxia in glottic or subglottic obstruction, after establishing an open airway (through a tracheotomy) and administering a high concentration of oxygen. Circulatory depression is temporary, and can be corrected by a volume load, or by an infusion containing a sympathomimetic agent.

Drying and Crusting of Secretions in the Respiratory Tract

Oxygen should always be humidified prior to administration. This is particularly imperative in patients with artificial airways. Unhumidified oxygen causes drying of secretions, and this can result in blockage of the bronchi by inspissated mucus. Partial or complete blockage of artificial airways (endotracheal or tracheostomy tube) by crusted secretions can have disastrous consequences.

Danger of Oxygen Withdrawal

Moderate or severe hypoxia warrants continuous oxygen therapy till such time as the hypoxia is relieved. Some hypoxic COPD patients may become drowsy or disoriented even on controlled oxygen therapy. To discontinue oxygen in such a situation is dangerous and wrong. If oxygen administration is stopped with the $PaCO_2$ markedly elevated, the P_ACO_2 (and consequently the PaO_2) falls to an even lower level than that prior to starting oxygen therapy.

This is because the P_ACO_2 has risen to a higher level than that prevailing at the start of oxygen therapy. Such patients therefore have a worsening of their already severe hypoxic state. Intermittent oxygen therapy can be dangerous in a hypoxic patient, and is wrong on principle. It only serves to give periods of relief from hypoxia, followed by periods of worsening and often extreme hypoxia. Oxygen, if indicated, needs to be *given continuously* till hypoxia is relieved.

Oxygen Toxicity

Lung Toxicity

High concentrations of oxygen over a prolonged period of time can produce changes in the lungs characterized by atelectasis, damage to the surfactant, interalveolar edema, and interstitial thickening and fibrosis. It is generally accepted that oxygen concentrations up to 50% are safe for long periods. We have used 60% oxygen for weeks, and have observed that the patients have recovered without residual effects. We have also been forced to use 100% oxygen in two patients (who would otherwise have died of hypoxia) for as long as 24 hours, followed by 80–90% oxygen for the next 4–7 days, and then 60–70% oxygen for another week. Both patients survived without any significant residual damage to the lungs. *This does not mean that very high oxygen concentrations should be used with abandon.* It does however signify that in our experience, the use of 100% oxygen is not as lethal as is often made out to be.

The practical applications to be derived from experimental and clinical studies on oxygen toxicity are summarized here.

- For patients with chronic hypoxemia (as in severe chronic airways obstruction), it is sufficient to use a concentration of oxygen that will correct dangerously low PaO_2 levels. A PaO_2 between 55 mm Hg and 60 mm Hg (O_2 saturation—90%) is generally adequate in these patients.
- Positive end-expiratory pressure (PEEP) should be used during mechanical ventilation if an inspired oxygen concentration greater than 50% fails to relieve dangerous hypoxia.
- In acute pulmonary problems with severe hypoxia, the oxygen concentration must be sufficient to allow an oxygen saturation of about 90%. If in spite of the use of PEEP, very high oxygen concentration (>80%) is needed over a prolonged period of time to maintain an oxygen saturation of 90%, it may be permissible to allow mild to moderate hypoxemia (O_2 saturation around 85%) so as to enable a reduction in the FiO_2. The degree

of hypoxia one allows will depend on the patient's tolerance to hypoxia, the age of the patient, and the ability or otherwise to increase oxygen transport to the tissues.

- *Life-threatening hypoxia must always be relieved, even if this requires the use of 100% oxygen for prolonged periods of time.* The fear and danger of possible oxygen toxicity is never an argument to allow a patient to irreversibly deteriorate and die of hypoxia.
- It is difficult, if not impossible, to detect signs of lung toxicity due to high oxygen concentrations in critically ill individuals with serious pulmonary problems. A fall in the compliance and the PaO_2 can occur due to very high oxygen concentrations, but we have found it impossible to ascertain in clinical practice, whether this is related to the disease, or is iatrogenic due to oxygen toxicity.

Retrolental Fibroplasia

This complication occurs in the neonatal period, and is related to high P_AO_2 levels. If the inspired oxygen concentration is high enough to raise the P_AO_2 to about 160 mm Hg even for a few hours, retrolental fibroplasia can occur. Therefore, in neonates, PaO_2 levels should never exceed 100 mm Hg.

Cerebral Oxygen Toxicity

This is occasionally observed when oxygen is breathed at hyperbaric pressures above 1 atmosphere. The syndrome is chiefly characterized by epileptic fits and is termed the Paul Bert effect, after the individual who first described it.

◼ LONG-TERM OXYGEN THERAPY

Long-term oxygen therapy (LTOT) finds its greatest and proven use in patients who have COPD and suffer from well-marked hypoxemia. The objectives of LTOT are:

- To relieve hypoxemia so that the PaO_2 is greater than 60 mm Hg (with an O_2 saturation >90%), without inducing or increasing hypercapnia.
- Reduction of polycythemia
- Prevention of right heart failure
- Improvement of quality of sleep
- Improvement in cognition and neuropsychiatric function
- *Most importantly, improve survival.*

Accepted Indications for LTOT in COPD

The first prerequisite is that the patient should have received optimal treatment and should have stopped smoking. LTOT is then indicated in patients with COPD who have a stable PaO_2 of less than 55 mm Hg breathing air. This cutoff point is chosen because it lies on the steepest part of the O_2 dissociation curve, so that any further fall would lead to severe hypoxemia.

Long-term oxygen therapy in COPD patients is also indicated if the PaO_2 is between 55 mm Hg and 59 mm Hg (between 7.3 kPa and 7.8 kPa) with PCV greater than 55% (erythrocytosis) and right heart dysfunction— P pulmonale, pulmonary hypertension or clinical evidence of cor pulmonale, such as peripheral edema for which there is no other cause.

The use of LTOT in COPD under the right indications has been clearly shown to improve survival rates compared to controls not on LTOT in quite a few studies. The Medical Research Council (MRC) Working Party Trial showed that mortality was less when COPD patients with severe hypoxemia and CO_2 retention were treated with long-term domiciliary oxygen for 15 hours daily when compared to those who were not given oxygen.

The Nocturnal Oxygen Therapy Trial (NOTT) group in the United States studied 203 patients with hypoxemic COPD being treated randomly either with nocturnal oxygen only for 12 hours daily or with continuous oxygen therapy. Results at the end of 3 years showed increased mortality in those being treated with nocturnal oxygen as compared to those receiving continuous oxygen **(Fig. 6)**.

The recommendation therefore is that hypoxemic COPD patients who satisfy the indications stated earlier should as far as possible be advised LTOT continuously through 24 hours. It is not as if nocturnal oxygen therapy is of no use. It helps survival but not to the extent of continuously administered oxygen. As a corollary, it could be stated that the greater the number of hours that oxygen is administered during LTOT, the greater the survival benefit.

Possible Indications for LTOT in COPD

Oxygen is often prescribed by a number of physicians in COPD patients whose PaO_2 is less than 60 mm Hg but more than 55 mm Hg even in the absence of hypercapnia, pulmonary hypertension, polycythemia or clinical evidence of cor pulmonale. In a French study of 7,770 COPD patients prescribed LTOT via the French ANTADIR network, 18.5%

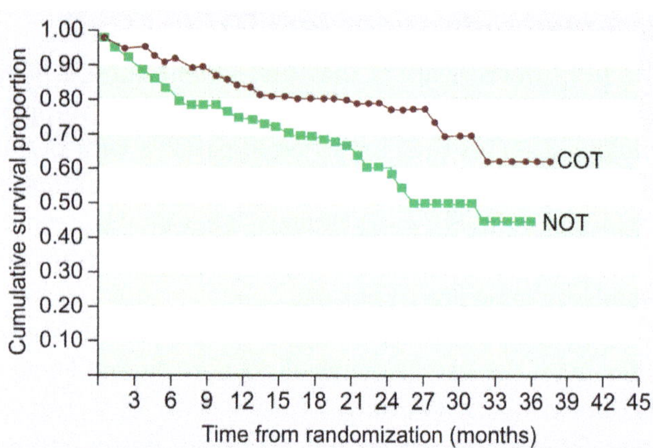

Fig. 6: The Nocturnal Oxygen Therapy Trial (NOTT) survival data. (NOT: Nocturnal oxygen therapy; COT: Continuous oxygen therapy)

had a PaO_2 of 60 mm Hg or more at the start of the trial. Over an 11-year period (1984–1995), the patients with a PaO_2 of 60 mm Hg who were prescribed LTOT were shown to have severe COPD and their survival was similar to that of more hypoxemic patients. However, another study by Górecka and colleagues *(Ref: Górecka D, Gorzelak K, Sliwiński P, et al. Effect of long-term oxygen therapy on survival in patients with chronic obstructive pulmonary disease with moderate hypoxemia. Thorax. 1997;52:674-9)* gave different results. A randomized study over 3 years on 135 COPD patients with a stable PaO_2 between 55 mm Hg and 65 mm Hg, comparing air and LTOT showed no difference in survival rate. This study casts doubt on the need to use LTOT in patients with moderate hypoxemia. Many practicing physicians would prefer to be on the safer side and give the benefit of doubt to the patient by prescribing LTOT when the PaO_2 is less than 60 mm Hg (yet >55 mm Hg) or the O_2 saturation is less than 90% provided the patient can afford the therapy.

Long-term Oxygen Therapy and Noninvasive Ventilator Support in COPD with Severe Chronic Hypoxemic plus Hypercapnic Respiratory Failure

In patients with COPD who are in chronic respiratory failure with well-marked hypoxemia plus hypercapnia, the use of noninvasive positive pressure ventilatory support in combination with LTOT controls nocturnal hypoventilation, improves quality of sleep, may lead to improved PaO_2 and $PaCO_2$ levels in the day and thereby improves the quality of life. It is impossible to give noninvasive ventilator support all through 24 hours every day. It should therefore be given all through the night and for some 4–6 hours during the day. Yet noninvasive ventilator support by itself is generally of little use in the above circumstances. It needs to be combined with LTOT.

Nocturnal Oxygen Only in COPD

The use of nocturnal oxygen should benefit patients with COPD (daytime PaO_2 >60 mm Hg) who desaturate sharply at night during sleep. Severe nocturnal desaturation in these patients could (1) disturb sleep; (2) trigger cardiac arrhythmias, particularly in older patients with ischemic heart disease, (3) perhaps cause episodes of pulmonary hypertension during periods of desaturation. The suggestion that these episodes could accelerate the evolution of permanent pulmonary hypertension and cor pulmonale though not proven, cannot be ignored.

Long-term Oxygen Therapy in Chronic Respiratory Failure due to Causes other than COPD

Chronic hypercapnic respiratory failure is also observed in patients with severe kyphoscoliosis, neuromuscular disease and other diseases extensively involving the lungs. If hypercapnia is not marked and if hypoxemia (PaO_2 <55 mm Hg) can be countered by oxygen at 1–2 L/minute without significant increase in the hypercapnia, then the patient can be kept comfortable on LTOT at a low flow rate. If however the hypercapnia is marked (>60–65 mm Hg) or is sharply increased following oxygen therapy, LTOT needs to be combined with noninvasive ventilator support for as many hours in the day and night as possible. More often than not these patients receive noninvasive support at night and for a few hours in the day.

Patients with severe restrictive disease may become increasingly hypoxic as the disease progresses. LTOT or nocturnal oxygen therapy may become necessary if the PaO_2 falls less than 55 mm Hg. The same holds for severe hypoxemia caused by bilateral destructive lung disease. In end-stage disease of the nature described above, the flow rate of oxygen may need to be increased to 4 L or more per minute to counter worsening hypoxemia.

Dosage of Oxygen

Hypoxemic COPD patients satisfying the criteria stated above generally need a flow rate of 1–2 L/minute. Even then, they may desaturate during sleep. Arbitrarily an increase in the flow rate by 1 L/minute is administered during the night. Uncontrolled oxygen therapy can however precipitate increasing hypercapnia. Oxygen given to counter severe hypoxemia due to end-stage restrictive lung pathologies (such as interstitial lung disease) often requires a higher rate of greater than 2 L/min, often as high as 6 to 10 L/min.

Nocturnal Oxygen Therapy in Central Sleep Apnea in Patients with Congestive Heart Failure

Sleep disordered breathing in the form of Cheyne-Stokes respiration (CSR) and spells of central sleep apnea (CSA) have been frequently reported (30–100%) in patients with congestive heart failure, contributing to increasing deterioration in the cardiac condition.

The pathogenesis of CSR-CSA is believed to be related to:

- Heightened responses of the respiratory center to hypoxia and hypercapnia leading to an unstable respiratory center
- Hypocapnia
- Prolonged circulation time.

Cheyne-Stokes respiration with CSA is associated with increase in sympathetic tone, which is generally deleterious to patients in congestive heart failure. Nocturnal oxygen when administered to these patients improves CSR-CSA. This improvement was noted to correlate with increase in peak oxygen consumption during exercise, perhaps due to reduction in the sympathetic tone following the use of nocturnal oxygen.

Long-term Oxygen Delivery System

The most common source of oxygen for LTOT is the oxygen concentrator. Other systems include compressed gas or liquid oxygen. Oxygen concentrators are heavy (about 35 lbs), require a wall current and therefore can only provide a stationary source of supplemental oxygen. Unless patients are immobilized, confined to their room or bed, mobile oxygen delivery system should also be used. Both compressed gas and liquid portable oxygen systems are available for use. Liquid oxygen containers are easier to refill when compared to high-pressure cylinders. However, liquid oxygen is not used in our country chiefly because of its expense and difficult availability. The devices for oxygen administration chiefly include nasal prongs and cannulae. Devices to "conserve" home oxygen include nasal reservoir nasal cannulae, electronic conserving devices and transtracheal catheter. These have already been briefly discussed earlier. Transtracheal catheter, though convenient to the patient, carries the risk of infection and is perhaps the least frequently used mode of domiciliary long-term oxygen delivery.

■ SUGGESTED READING

1. Carpagnano GE, Kharitonov SA, Foschino-Barbaro MP, et al. Supplementary oxygen in healthy subjects and those with COPD increases oxidative stress and airway inflammation. Thorax. 2004;59(12):1016-9.
2. Continuous or nocturnal oxygen therapy in hypoxemic chronic obstructive lung disease: a clinical trial. Nocturnal Oxygen Therapy Trial Group. Ann Intern Med. 1980;93:391-8.
3. Croxton TL, Bailey WC. Long-term oxygen treatment in chronic obstructive pulmonary disease: recommendations for future research: an NHLBI workshop report. Am J Respir Crit Care Med. 2006;174(4):373-8.
4. Eastwood GM, O'Connell B, Gardner A, et al. Evaluation of nasopharyngeal oxygen, nasal prongs and facemask oxygen therapy devices in adult patients: a randomised crossover trial. Anaesth Intensive Care. 2008;36(5):691-4.
5. Long-term domiciliary oxygen therapy in chronic hypoxic cor pulmonale complicating chronic bronchitis and emphysema. Report of the Medical Research Council Working Party. Lancet. 1981;1(8222):681-6.
6. Veale D, Chailleux E, Taytard A, et al. Characteristics and survival of patients prescribed long-term oxygen therapy outside prescription guidelines. Eur Respir J. 1998;12:780-4.
7. Zielinski J. Long-term oxygen therapy in COPD patients with moderate hypoxaemia: does it add years to life? Eur Respir J. 1998;12:756-8.

Lung Tumors

CHAPTER 43

Lung Cancer and Other Lung Tumors

■ INTRODUCTION

At the turn of the 20th century lung cancer was considered a rare malignancy. Since then, the incidence has progressively increased and for several past decades, lung cancer has become the most common cancer in the world. According to Globocan 2018 there are estimated to be 1.8 million new cases in 2018, (12.9% of the total). The incidence of lung cancer varies widely in different countries and geographical areas of the world and this will be discussed shortly.

The overall mortality from lung cancer is horrendous. It is the most common cause of death from cancer worldwide and is estimated to be responsible for 1 in 5 deaths (1.5 million deaths, 18.4% of the total). Though mortality figures in special world class centers continue to improve, the overall fatality from this disease remains high (the overall ratio of mortality to incidence is 0.87). There is a relative lack of significant variability in survival in different regions of the world. Hence, the mortality observed in different geographical regions of the world is closely related to the incidence of the disease in each of these geographical regions. The 5-year survival in the more developed regions according to Globocan 2018 is about 15%, and the 5-year survival in the less developed region is less than 10%. In the very poor countries of the world where statistical figures are scanty and unreliable, the survival rate is probably well below 5%.

The reason for this horrific mortality is twofold. Firstly, many patients with lung cancer, even advanced lung cancer, are either asymptomatic or have few symptoms, so that by the time they are diagnosed it is too late for curative therapy. Secondly, the natural history of most lung cancers is characterized by rapid intrathoracic spread and frequent metastatic spread to distant organ systems.

The chief cause of lung cancer in 85–90% of cases is smoking, a fact brilliantly proven by the excellent epidemiological studies by Doll and Hill in the early 1950s. Not smoking and cessation of cigarette smoking is undoubtedly the best and the most certain method to reduce the risk of lung cancer. It is indeed a sad commentary on human affairs that a disease currently preventable is allowed to flourish and cause so many deaths in the world.

The term lung cancer is used for cancers arising in the airways or lung parenchyma, and these are classified into two main subtypes—small cell lung cancer (SCLC) and nonsmall cell lung cancer (NSCLC). About 95% of all cancers are SCLC or NSCLC. The remaining 5% of cancers are other tumors of comparative rarer cell type originating in the lung. The thrust of this chapter is chiefly on SCLC and NSCLC. A few of the rarer cancers, as also metastatic lesions from primary sites outside the lungs are dealt with briefly at the end of the chapter.

■ EPIDEMIOLOGY

In 2018, lung cancer was the most frequently diagnosed cancer worldwide and was the leading cause of cancer death among males. Among females lung cancer was the third leading cause of death in the more developed countries. The Lung Cancer Incidence and mortality rates (age standardized rate per 100,000) for 2018 in different countries and geographical areas of the world are given in **Figure 1**.

A few comments on the incidence rates in various geographical areas of the world are given below. The first point to notice is that the incidence of lung cancer in all geographical regions in 2018 was more in males than in females. The highest age standardized rate incidence rates in men were observed in Central and Eastern Europe (49.3

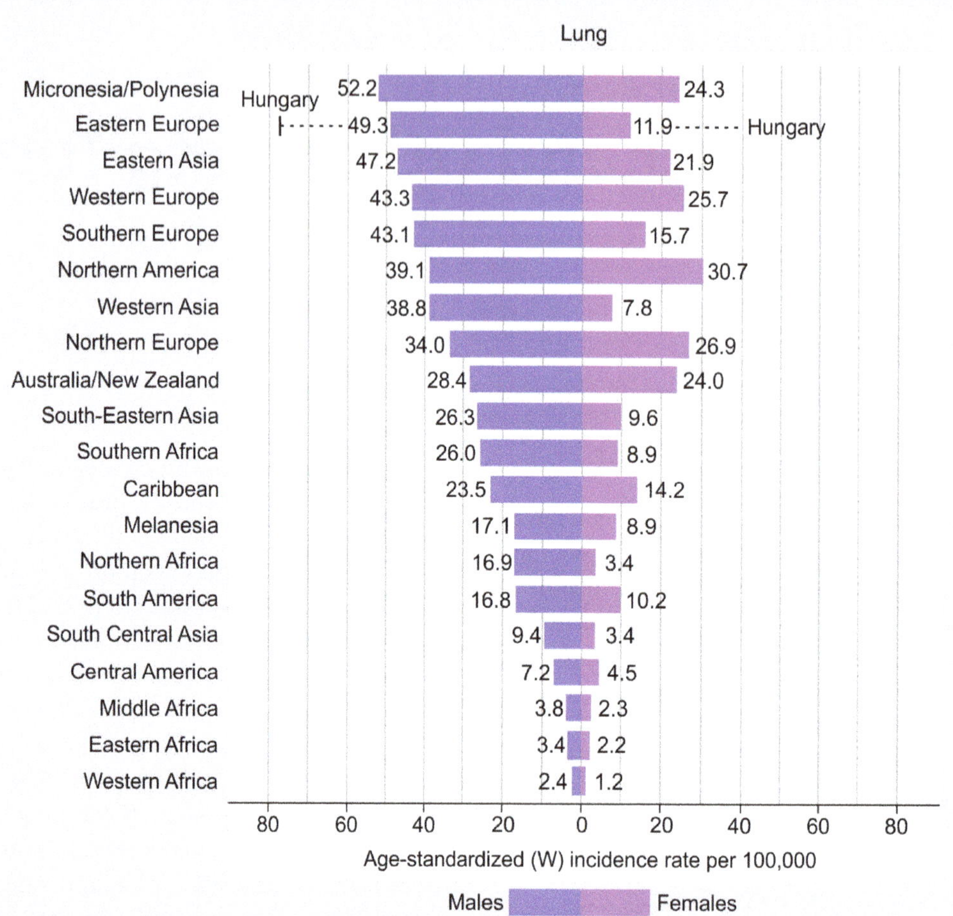

Fig. 1: Worldwide estimated incidence and mortality of lung cancer—GLOBOCAN, 2018.

per 100,000) and Eastern Asia (47.2 per 100,000). Closely following the high incidence rates stated were Southern Europe (43.1 per 100,000) and Northern America (39.1 per 100,000). Notably low rates were observed in western and Middle African 2.4 and 3.8 per 100,000, respectively.

Among women the highest lung cancer rates were in Northern America, Northern and Western Europe, Australia or New Zealand and East Asia. Lung cancer rates in Chinese women were as high as 20.4 per 100,000, despite the fact that the prevalence of smoking in Chinese women was less than that observed in women in the European countries. This is believed to be due to increased indoor pollution resulting from cooking on coal stoves which prevails in many parts of China.

Incidence of lung cancer rates in different regions of the world reflects the stages and degree of tobacco smoking in these regions. In the United States, the United Kingdom and Denmark, the tobacco epidemic began earliest and peaked around the middle of the last century. Lung cancer rates in these countries have been decreasing in men and plateauing in women. In countries like Spain where the tobacco epidemic peaked later, lung cancer rates are observed to be decreasing in men but continue to increase in women. In contrast in countries where the tobacco epidemic has been established more recently and smoking tobacco has perhaps yet to peak, as in China, Indonesia, and some countries in Africa, lung cancer rates are likely to increase for at least a few more decades.

The trends in the incidence of lung cancer in men and women (in a few countries) are given in **Figure 2**.

The high incidence of cancer of the lung in Asia (in particular East Asia) is cause for worry. 51% of the world's lung cancer cases occur in China. The "tobacco epidemic" in China shows no sign of abating. China continues to be the largest consumer of tobacco in the world, with about 301 million current smokers. More than two-thirds of

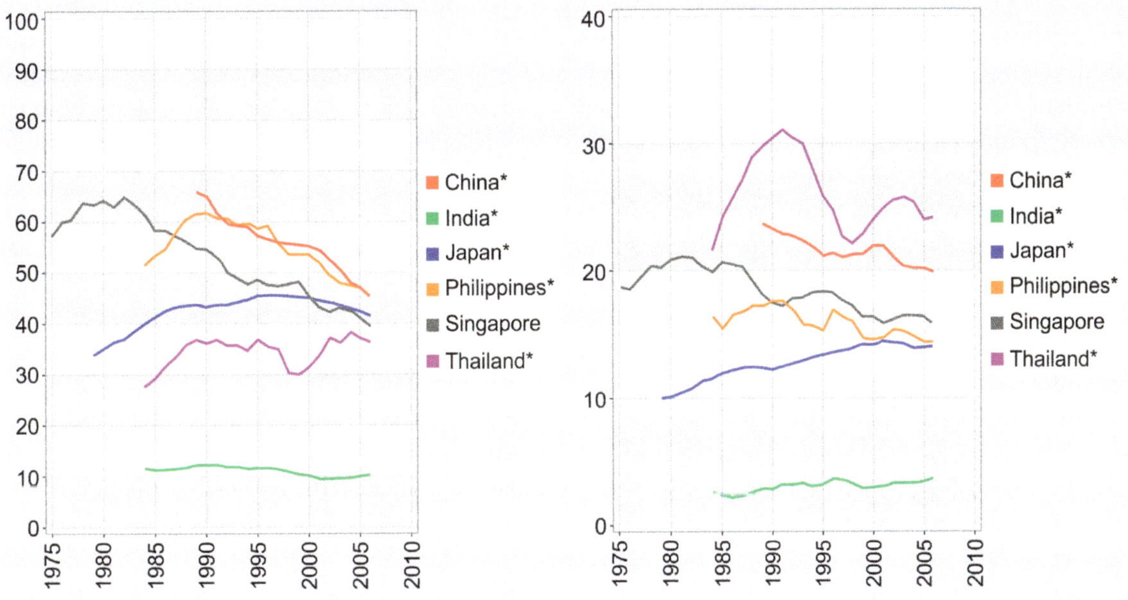

Fig. 2: Trends in incidence of lung cancer in selected countries: age-standardized rate (W) per 100,000, men and women, GLOBOCAN 2012.

Chinese men smoke and it is estimated that half of them will die of smoking unless they quit. Deaths from smoking in China are estimated to be about 2 million in 2030 and are expected to be close to 3 million people in 2050.

United States: In the United States, there has been a precipitous rise in the incidence and death rate from decade to decade starting from 1930 onward. In 1930, the age-adjusted lung cancer deaths in males were 5/100,00 per year and in females 3/100,000 per year. In 1987, in males they rose to 74.9/100,000 and in females to 28.5/100,000. As mentioned in the introductory remarks, today lung cancer would account for 31% of all cancer deaths in males and 27% of all cancer deaths in females.

United Kingdom: The lung cancer rates in the UK are approximately 100 per 100,00 per year. The UK incidence rates in men peaked in the 1970s when it ranked highest in the world. Since then they have fallen by 10% every 5 years. In contrast the incidence of lung cancer increased by 5% every 10 years in women until the 1980s, following which the rise has slowed. The fall in the incidence in males and the rise in the incidence in females mirror the changing smoking trends in the country.

Europe: The incidence of lung cancer in Europe standardized to the population of Europe is about 43–57 per 100,000 in men and 11–15 per 100,000 in women. Increased cigarette smoking in females between 1985 and 1995 in France led to an increase in the incidence rate by 56% in women and 5% in men under the age of 65 years. As expected, female mortality more than doubled, while male deaths increased by just under 50%.

Asia and Africa: Within Asia the standardized mortality rates were highest in China and lowest in the South Pacific Islands—29.1 and 13.8 per 100,000, respectively. In all developing countries lung cancer in males accounts for close to three quarters of patients. The rates in females are low, except among Chinese women who have a comparatively higher rate.

In the last decade there has been a progressive increase in lung cancer in China and South Korea, mostly in men. In South Korea, the age-adjusted mortality increased from 3.7/100,00 in 1980 to 17.8/100,000 in 1994 in males and from 1.4 to 7/100,000 in women. The projected average annual age-adjusted mortality in 2000–2004 was 65.5 and 15.1/100,000 for males and females, respectively.

Age-standardized mortalities in both North and South African regions were low—7.9 and 11.5 /100,000, respectively in males and 3.2 and 5.3 per 100,000 in females.

The lung cancer incidence in Australia is higher compared to the UK and Canada but lower than the US. However, the mortality rate for lung cancer is lower in Australia compared to the US—32% lower than the US in males and 48% lower in women.

The increasing trend of 1–5% in age-related mortality rates in lung cancer is universal involving most countries of the world. Overall mortality is less in females. There is however evidence to show that in countries where women show increasing smoking habits, the rate of rise in female mortality per year is more than in males.

The Indian Scenario: Several epidemiological studies performed across various and different demographic cohorts confirm the significant morbidity and mortality due to lung cancer in India **(Fig. 3)**. According to the Globocan 2012 report, the estimated incidence of lung cancer in India was 70.25 in all ages and both sexes; the crude incidence rate was 5.6 per 100,000, the age standardized rate (world), i.e. ASR (w) was 6.9 and the cumulative risk was 0.85.

In terms of incidence rates, lung cancer ranked fourth overall among all cancers, after breast, cervical, and oral cancer. In males, lung cancer ranked second whilst in females it was sixth in terms of cancer incidence.

Among Indian males, lung cancer was the most common cause of cancer mortality. Among Indian females it was the seventh cause in relation to cancer mortality behind breast, cervix, colorectal, ovary, stomach, lip or oral cavity cancer. It is almost certain that this is an underestimation of the overall burden of lung cancer in India because of incomplete registration in different states of India.

As per the GLOBOCAN 2008 report, male:female ratio for lung cancer in India was 4.5:1, this ratio varies with age and smoking status. The ratio increased progressively from 51–60 years and then remained steady.

Smoking is the greatest risk factor (80–90%); 10–20% of cancers could perhaps be attributed to occupational exposure to various carcinogens. The percentage of tobacco-related products smoked in India are *beedis* (28.4–79%), cigarettes (9.0–53.7), *hookah* (3.477.3), and mixed (7.5–13.6). The relative risk of developing lung cancer is 2.64 for *beedi* smokers and 2.23 for cigarette smokers, and 2.45 as the overall risk for smoking tobacco. Passive smoking and environmental tobacco smoke (ETS) are known risk factors, environmental tobacco exposure carrying a relative risk of developing lung cancer of 1.48 in males and 1.2 in females. The risk increases with an increase in exposure.

The epidemiological description of lung cancer varies in different regions as collected from different cancer registries across the country.

Lung cancer is the first and leading cause of cancer in males in metropolitan cities of Mumbai, Delhi, Kolkata, Bhopal, and Ahmedabad. The three urban registries of Bhopal, Delhi, and Mumbai have registered lung cancer as the most frequent site of cancer, constituting around 10% of cancers at all sites. It is the second leading site of cancer in Chennai and Thiruvananthapuram and the third leading site in Bengaluru, Nagpur, and Pune.

The National Cancer Registry Programme has adjudged that Aizwal in Mizoram state and Imphal in Manipur state had one and a half times the mean age-adjusted rate (MAAR) of the highest urban population-based cancer registry—Delhi (11.5 per 1000,00). In fact nine other districts were judged to have MAAR higher than that of the MAAR of Delhi.

The disease though more common in urban areas also has a grip over rural areas as evinced by rural registries from Karunagappally in Kerala where lung cancer is the most frequent of all cancers.

Population-based cancer registries show that cancer of the lung in Indian women is not as frequent a site for cancer when compared to men. Among cities the highest

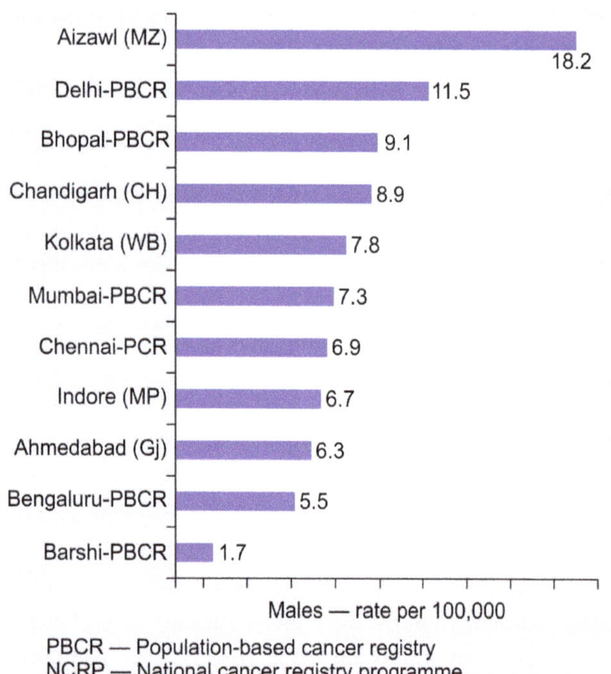

Fig. 3: Lung cancer in India—district-wise comparisons of age-adjusted incidence rates with that of population-based cancer registries (PBCRs) under National Cancer Registry Program (NCRP) (2001–4). We have been unable to access data subsequent to 2004. *Source:* Modified from National Cancer Registry Program (2001–4).

incidence of lung cancer in women is observed in Mumbai with age-adjusted rate of 4.2/100,000. Even this age-adjusted rate for females in Mumbai is lower than that of Indian women in Singapore and other women in areas of high incidence in the world.

The influence of ethnic and genetic factors is suggested by the very low incidence of lung cancer in Parsee males living in the rural areas of Maharashtra and Gujarat. The age-adjusted incidence rate in non-Parsee males (12.6) is almost thrice the rate in Parsee males (4.2) while the rates are similar in Parsee and non-Parsee females (3.7). In Mumbai the same difference in incidence of lung cancer in the Parsee and non-Parsee population is only apparent after the age of 54 years and not before. The role of cigarette smoking and air pollution in Mumbai, in addition to ethnic and genetic factors may all be important reasons for the above findings.

The average age at the time of diagnosis of cancer is 56 years for males and 52 years for females as per the hospital-based cancer registry at Tata Memorial Hospital, Mumbai. Data from Kerala, North India, and Rajasthan suggest the same average age.

Risk factors influencing the incidence of lung cancer have been dealt with in the section on "Etiology" in this chapter.

■ ETIOLOGY AND PATHOGENESIS OF LUNG CANCER

Etiology

Cigarette smoking is unquestionably the most important cause of lung cancer. This fact is chiefly based on epidemiological studies, supplemented by pathological findings related to the effect of cigarette smoke on bronchial mucosa.

Smoking

The relation of cigarette smoking to lung cancer was established in the 1950s through the elegant and sound epidemiological studies of Doll and Hill in the UK. These studies convincingly proved that the majority of patients with cancer of the lung were heavy smokers and that the incidence of cancer of the lung in nonsmokers was low. Prospective studies again carried out by Doll and Hill, were equally conclusive. The best of these was a study on 40,000 doctors in the UK. In 1951, each of these gave details of their smoking habits. By 1964 the link between death from lung cancer in this group and smoking habits was incontrovertible. Similar results were noted in the US. The US Surgeon General's Report on Smoking and Health in 1964 concluded that cigarette smoking was causally related to lung cancer. It has been estimated that close to 20% of all cancer deaths worldwide could be prevented if tobacco smoking was stopped. The cumulative lung cancer risk can be as high as 30% in lifelong heavy smokers as compared to a lifelong risk of 1% in nonsmokers. These and other epidemiological studies established the following facts in relation to smoking and lung cancer **(Table 1)**.

- The risk of lung cancer is increased in smokers compared to nonsmokers by a factor of 10. Pipe smokers and cigar smokers have a comparatively lower incidence than cigarette smokers probably because the smoke is not inhaled into the lungs to the same degree.
- The risk of cancer increases with the number of cigarettes smoked and increases proportionally with the time a person has smoked. The greater the number of years a patient has smoked and the larger the number of cigarettes smoked, the greater the risk of lung cancer. Current smokers smoking one pack a day for 20 years have a risk of lung cancer 10–15 times that of those who have never smoked. This risk increases to 25 times if two or more packs are smoked for 20 years. Lung cancer risk is also proportional to the age at which smoking started, the degree of inhalation during tobacco smoking, and the tar and nicotine content of cigarettes.
- A British study showed that in those who stopped smoking, the risk begins to decline almost immediately; it however takes 15 years for the risk to decline to a level which is still approximately twice that of those who never smoked. The Multiple Risk Factor Intervention Trial showed similar results. It is apparent that even if cigarette smoking were to cease today the current spate of lung cancer would continue for long.

Table 1: Relation of smoking to lung cancer.
• Risk of lung cancer is increased in smokers compared to nonsmokers by a factor of 10
• The risk of cancer increases with the number of cigarettes smoked and increases proportionally with the time a person has smoked
• Risk of developing lung cancer decreases with cessation of smoking
• Passive smoking is an associated risk for lung cancer

- Passive smoking by which is meant inhalation of cigarette smoke exhaled by others or smoke inhaled from smoldering cigarettes, i.e. environmental tobacco smoke (ETS) also carries a small but clear increase in risk for lung cancer. Studies showed 1.2 times risk for lung cancer in women who lived with husbands who smoked compared to women who lived in smoke-free homes. Passive smoking is estimated to give rise to 300 new cases of cancer every year in the US. The ban on cigarette smoking in many public places in many countries of the world is indeed a welcome step.

Smoking and Lung Cancer in India

Smoking is the main causative factor in India just as in the rest of the world. A history of active tobacco smoking is present in 87% of males and 85% of females. A history of passive exposure to tobacco smoke was found in only 3%. The relative risk of developing lung cancer in *bidi* smokers was noted to be 2.64 whereas in cigarette smokers it was 2.23, the overall relative risk being 2.45. Studies in India further suggest that *beedis* are more carcinogenic than cigarettes *[Ref: Jussawalla DJ, Jain DK. Lung cancer in Greater Bombay: correlations with religion and smoking habits. Br J Cancer. 1979;40(3):437-48].*

Hookah smoking has also been associated with lung cancer.

In a study by Gupta D, Boffetta P, et al. *(Ref: Gupta D, Boffetta P, Gaborieau V, et al. Risk factors of lung cancer in Chandigarh, India. Indian J Med Res. 2001;113:142-50)* 80% of men and 33% of women among the patients were ever-smokers compared to 60% of men and 20% of women among controls. The odds ratio (OR) for ever-smoking was 5.0 (95% class interval CI = 3.11–8.04) among the men and 2.47 (95% CI = 0.79–0.75) among women.

What is the cause of the "tobacco epidemic" that has led to lung cancer? The cause of the tobacco epidemic is the addiction to nicotine contained within tobacco, an addiction perhaps as bad as addiction to alcohol, and nearly if not quite as bad as addiction to heroin or morphine. How does cigarette smoke cause lung cancer? Cigarette smoke is an aerosol composed of numerous gaseous and particulate compounds. Mainstream smoke (MS) results from inhalation of air through the cigarette and is the main source of smoke exposure to the smoker. Side-stream smoke is that which arises from the cigarette between puffs and is a main source of ETS.

The tar present in the mainstream smoke is a risk factor for lung cancer, while the pleasurable effect of the inhaled nicotine perpetuates the addiction.

The International Agency for Cancer Research has identified numerous chemical compounds in the mainstream cigarette smoke which act as carcinogens **(Tables 2 and 3)**. Of the 81 constituents found in mainstream smoke, 48 carcinogens are present in the particulate form, the rest are present in the vapor form or both in the vapor and the particulate form.

The major carcinogens of great concern are the tobacco specific N-nitrosamines (TSNAs) formed by the nitrosation of nicotine during smoking. Some are important inducers of lung cancer. Other potential carcinogens include polycyclic aromatic hydrocarbons, aromatic amines, benzene, arsenic, chromium, and vinyl chloride. The above carcinogens can be destroyed and the cancer risk in an individual patient perhaps lies in the balance between activation and destruction of the above carcinogens. How do these carcinogens act? Carcinogens in particular N-nitrosamines can bind to the DNA (deoxyribonucleic acid) and form DNA adducts. If repair mechanisms of DNA are poor or absent, DNA deformities can lead to adverse permanent

Table 2: Important carcinogens in cigarette smoke.

Carcinogenic to humans:
- N-nitrosamines (TSNAs)
- Benzene
- Chromium
- Polycyclic aromatic hydrocarbons
- Arsenic
- Aromatic amines
- Vinyl chloride
- Benzo[a]pyrene

Table 3: Important carcinogens in cigarette smoke.

Probably carcinogenic to humans:
- Acrylonitrile
- 1,3-Butadiene
- Formaldehyde
- N-Nitrosodiethylamine
- N-Nitrosodimethylamine
- Lead
- 5-Methylchrysene
- NNK
- 2-Nitropropane
- Ortho-toluidine
- Urethane (ethyl carbamate)

mutations. TSNA through signaling pathway activation can modulate oncogenes and tumor suppressor genes leading to cellular proliferation and tumor formation. DNA mutations caused by nitrosamines can result in the activation of K-ras oncogenes. Activation of K-ras oncogenes has been detected in a number of adenocarcinomas of the lung in ex-smokers, suggesting that such mutations persist even after cessation of smoking. This perhaps explains the persistent risk of lung cancer even after the stoppage of smoking. Another carcinogen present in tobacco smoke—benzo[a]pyrene can damage *p53* tumor suppressing loci that have been found to be abnormal in 60% of lung cancer patients. There is probably a genetic susceptibility to the carcinogenic effects of poisonous chemicals in tobacco smoke in those who develop lung cancer. How this genetic susceptibility is translated into the occurrence of actual disease is a subject of research.

Pathological evidence for the dangers of cigarette smoking on the bronchial epithelium is evidenced by the close association between metaplasia and atypia of mucosal cells in relation to the number of cigarettes smoked. Animal experiments lend further proof of the link between lung cancer and tobacco smoke.

Cigarette smoking can cause all histopathological types of lung cancers. The strongest association is with squamous cell carcinoma and small cell cancer which generally arise in the central airways; a weaker association exists with adenocarcinoma of the lung which generally arises in the periphery of the lung.

Smoking Habits in the World

Smoking habits in the world are a matter of considerable alarm. Smoking habits in the US have fortunately declined over the last four decades from 52% in men and 34% in women to 25% for men and 19% for women. The World Health Organization Report of 2002 mentions that about one-third of all men worldwide smoke and that approximately 15 billion cigarettes are sold daily.

Smoking habits in Europe and Asia though varying from country to country are even higher in Europe; on an overall estimate 30—40% of men and 15–30% of women smoke. Smoking rates in men in China are horrendous—close to 67% though in women it is much lower—4%.

It is obvious that the worldwide epidemic of lung cancer due to cigarette smoking will continue to rise for decades.

Cancer of the Lung in the "Never Smokers"

Though smoking tobacco is the most common cause of lung cancer, the latter also occurs in nonsmokers. Ideally, never smokers should be defined as those who have never smoked, but included in this term are also individuals who have never smoked more than hundred cigarettes in their whole lifetime. 15% of lung cancers in men and approximately 53% in women worldwide occur in never smokers. This accounts for 25% of all lung cancer cases. However, there is a significant variation in the proportion of lung cancer in never smokers ranging from approximately 10–11% in males in the Western world up to 40% in females in Asia. If lung cancer in never smokers is considered a separate entity then it becomes the seventh cause of cancer-related deaths in the world.

The age-adjusted rate for lung cancer in never smokers (age 40–79 years) ranges from 4.4–13.7 per 100,000 person year for men and 14.4–20.81 per 100,000 person years for women. In current smokers of the same age group the rates are 12–20 times higher *[Ref: Pallis AG, Syrigos KN. Lung cancer in never smokers: disease characteristics and risk factors. Crit Rev Oncol Hematol. 2013;88(3):494-503]*.

Adenocarcinoma of the lung is the main cancer observed in never smokers. Risk factors for nonsmokers include environmental exposure to carcinogens, outdoor and indoor air pollution, exposure to asbestos, arsenic, and perhaps importantly exposure to ETS. Genetic factors have also been considered to be important; the genes implicated being the epidermal growth factor receptor (EGFR), the human repair gene, cytochrome *p50*, and glutathione S transferase.

Interestingly, a multivariate analysis of adenocarcinoma of the lung showed that the survival rate in never smokers was significantly better (23%—5 year survival) than in smokers (16%—5 year survival). This finding suggests that adenocarcinoma in nonsmokers may have a distinct biology and natural history which is different from those observed in smokers.

In 2010, the first genome-wide associated study reported genetic variations in never smoking females which may perhaps be responsible for a distinct biological profile. It was noted that a large percentage of these patients had driver aberrations [EGFR and human epidermal growth factor receptor (HER-2) mutations, anaplastic lymphoma kinase (ALK) and ROS-1 rearrangements). These alterations could perhaps in the future be targeted through agents already in clinical use, or which are under development.

Good results have been observed with erlotinib and gefitinib in EGFR mutated patients. *Therefore, understanding the biology of lung cancer in never smokers, in particular the distinct clinical, pathological, and genetic features, as also risk factors, is crucial for better management.*

Other Risk Factors

Exposure to ionizing radiation: Radon exposure due to ionizing radiation is perhaps the most important cancer risk for nonsmokers not exposed to asbestos. Radon is a decay product arising from radium which in turn is a breakdown product of uranium. Exposure to radon through ionic radiation is present in miners mining rock faces for various metals and most importantly miners mining for uranium. These miners are therefore prone to lung cancer. This has been observed for several decades in miners mining various metals in the mountains between Saxony and the Czech Republic.

Radon is also present in indoor and outdoor air and the greater the exposure, the greater the risk of lung cancer. In the US, radon in the general environment has been held responsible for 10% of all lung cancers, so that it forms the second most important cause of cancer. To what extent this risk applies to other countries is not known.

Asbestos exposure and other occupation hazards: There exists a clear link between asbestos exposure and lung cancer. The increased risk is translated into actual disease 20 or more years after initial exposure. Asbestos is chiefly used in the construction industry and for its fire-resistant properties. There are many types of asbestos fibers, some being more carcinogenic than others. The subject has been dealt with at length under Occupational Lung Disorders.

Occupational factors reported to be associated with increased risk of lung cancer have been listed in **Table 4**. Unfortunately, information on occupational risk for lung cancer in India is sadly lacking.

Air pollution: Atmospheric pollution is also considered a risk for lung cancer. In Western countries, even allowing for smoking habits, the risk of cancer is higher in the polluted urban areas compared to the less polluted rural areas. Atmospheric pollutants are mainly polycyclic hydrocarbons from the combustion of fossil fuels—wood and coal fires. These have now been given up in almost all cities of the world. The main sources of pollutants today

Table 4: Occupational risk factors associated with lung cancer.

Chemicals	*Occupation involved*
Arsenic	Smelter workers and vineyard workers
Asbestos	Insulation workers and shipyard workers
Nickel	Refinery workers
Radiation	Uranium mining
Chromium	Ore miners and pigment manufacturers
Chloromethyl	Industrial workers
Radon	Hematite miners
Soot, tars	Coke oven workers
Oils and coke	Gas houseworkers, rubber workers

Note: Other probable carcinogens are beryllium, cadmium, formaldehyde, and silica.

in most countries of the world are exhausts from motor vehicles, particularly diesel smoke, and emissions from factories within or close to cities.

Environmental tobacco smoke: It is estimated that at least 17% of lung cancers in nonsmokers are related to high levels of ETS during childhood and adolescence. In an analysis of 37 epidemiological studies on nonsmokers who lived or did not live with smokers, it was estimated that a nonsmoker living with a smoker had a 27% increased risk of developing lung cancer. However, the risk of a nonsmoker developing cancer of the lung is quite low so that an increase in this background low risk by 27% may not significantly increase this risk. Evidence suggests that there is an overall OR of 1.34 in the risk for lung cancer associated with exposure to ETS.

Race and ethnicity: The incidence of lung cancer is higher among blacks, Polynesians, and lower in Japanese Americans, Hispanics than among Whites in the United States. The reason for this difference is not apparent though it could be related partly to differences in smoking habits and partly perhaps to genetic causes.

Dietary factors: The role of dietary factors in increasing or decreasing risk for lung cancer remains unproven. Retrospective case-controlled studies suggest a protective role for fruit consumption. Vegetable consumption is reported to be associated with decreased lung cancer risk, and there are studies that support a protective role for beta carotene and vitamin C. Three randomized controlled studies have however shown that supplementation with beta carotene failed to exert a protective effect against lung cancer.

Genetics: There is a great deal of ongoing research on the role of genetics in lung cancer. A genetic component could influence lung cancer in three ways: (1) it could influence the overall susceptibility to lung cancer; (2) it could influence the susceptibility to a certain type of lung cancer; (3) it could influence the patient's responsiveness or unresponsiveness to different therapies available against lung cancer. The last factor is indeed of crucial importance as it envisages a day when optimal therapy could be tailored for each patient with lung cancer.

The work of Spitz and his colleagues shows the influence of family history of cancer as an important risk factor for lung cancer in never smokers, former smokers, and current smokers. The risk of cancer lung seems also to be significantly increased in persons with a family history of an early onset (<60 years) lung cancer. There is a twofold increase in the risk for lung cancer in individuals with a family history of lung cancer. This applies both to smokers and nonsmokers.

Current research is focused on genetic markers of host susceptibility to lung carcinogens—notably those present in tobacco smoke. The susceptibility genetic factors include high penetration low-frequency genes and low penetration high-frequency genes. The objective is to target genes which encode enzymes that influence absorption, metabolism, conjugation, removal or neutralization of carcinogens present in tobacco smoke, as also other lung carcinogens.

Numerous enzymes have been studied, the details of which are beyond the scope of this book. Genes encoding for the interleukins (IL)-1, IL-6, IL-8 or the cyclooxygenase enzymes or the metalloproteinases (MMP 1-2-3-12) have been shown to be associated with an increased cancer risk. Acquired changes in the DNA chromosome are also a cause of increased cancer risk. The details of these genetic studies are best left to the research geneticist, but the awareness of the possible increasing role of genes in lung carcinomas is important. However, it must be emphasized that in spite of ongoing extensive research in this field, the genes responsible for conferring an increased risk of lung cancer have not yet been identified.

Chronic obstructive pulmonary disease: Recent studies suggest that chronic obstructive pulmonary disease is a risk factor for lung cancer over and above that caused by cigarette smoking.

The Lung Health Study has supported this view based on a study of 580 patients who had mild airways obstruction and a history of smoking. These were followed up and assessed for the effectiveness of stopping smoking and use of anticholinergic therapy. Lung cancer was the leading cause of death over a 5-year follow-up. Perhaps it may well be that instead of airways obstruction predisposing to lung cancer both airways obstruction and lung cancer were related to the common factor—smoking.

The incidence of lung cancer is also increased in patients with pulmonary fibrosis (even after adjustment for smoking habits), the OR for lung cancer being 8.25, compared to control subjects.

Etiology and important risk factors associated with lung cancer are given in **Table 5.**

Pathogenesis

The pathogenesis of bronchogenic carcinoma can be summarized as a step-by-step process altering normal bronchial mucosal cells into malignant cells under the influence of a carcinogenic agent. The most common carcinogenic agents responsible for this are one or more of the many carcinogens present in cigarette smoke. Carcinogens act by inducing a genetic damage to mucosal cells so that a step-by-step progression to malignancy occurs.

The multistep gradual evolution from normal epithelium to hyperplasia—metaplasia –dysplasia—carcinoma in situ—invasive carcinoma has been studied by cytopathologists in uranium miners in the United States. Similar evidence demonstrating the presence of dysplasia preceding carcinoma was observed in a large autopsy study in which the whole bronchial tree was examined in several patients dying of lung cancer.

Squamous metaplasia has therefore been regarded by many as a premalignant change. This is supported by the presence of metaplasia and dysplasia frequently observed adjacent to invasive carcinoma as also by the presence of genetic abnormalities which are similar to those prevailing in adjacent invasive cancerous cells.

These premalignant changes are quite extensive and explain the high incidence of a second primary lung cancer

Table 5: Etiology and important risk factors associated with lung cancer.

- Smoking, exposure to environmental cigarette smoke
- Exposure to ionizing radiation
- Asbestos exposure and other occupational hazards
- Air pollution, indoor and outdoor
- Genetic factors
- Chronic obstructive pulmonary disease; pulmonary fibrosis

in the same individual. It has been shown that 4% of lung cancer patients have more than one lung tumor and that a further 4–6% develop a second lung tumor later.

Atypical alveolar hyperplasia has also been noted as a focal premalignant change accompanying bronchogenic carcinoma, chiefly an adenocarcinoma of the lung. It is possible though not proven that alveolar cell carcinoma (a variant of adenocarcinoma) may perhaps evolve from these atypical hyperplastic premalignant cells.

The mechanism by which carcinogens in the smoke of cigarette smokers induce a multistep change in the bronchial epithelial cells resulting in malignancy is poorly understood. Carcinogens in cigarette smoke probably induce a genetic change in the bronchial epithelium. Early cancers have shown a number of genetic and molecular alterations. These include mutations in the *p53* tumor suppressor gene and K-ras proto oncogene as also diminished expression of *p16* tumor suppressor gene because of hypermethylation.

Both NSCLC and SCLC have been known to have chromosomal abnormalities. Mutations of *p53* tumor suppressor gene are present in 50% of NSCLC and 70% of SCLC. An increased expression of epidermal growth factor together with its receptor is present in about 60% of NSCLC. Identification of critical early molecular alterations may perhaps help in the early detection of cancer.

Finally, it is an accepted fact that there is a survival discrepancy between patients suffering from the same stage of cancer. This means that the biology of tumors may vary even though the disease stage is identical. The reason for this biological variation is a subject of research. Differences in outcome for tumors classified as belonging to the same stage could be related to oncogene amplification, mutations in tumors, suppressor genes, nature and level of tumor antigens, and other biological factors.

The unravelling of the genetic profile of lung cancer may in the future serve two purposes—(1) a better prediction of patient survival; (2) tailoring patient-specific treatment (chemotherapeutic agents) to enhance survival rates.

■ PATHOLOGY OF BRONCHOPULMONARY CARCINOMA

According to the WHO classification, although there are many types of lung cancer, just four of these account for over 95% of the total. These are squamous cell carcinoma, adenocarcinoma, small cell carcinoma, and large cell carcinoma. For clinical purposes, cancer is best divided into NSCLC, which in the main includes adenocarcinoma and squamous cell carcinoma, and SCLC. It is important to distinguish between these two main types **(Table 6)**. A histopathological diagnosis is not always easy as there is a significant interobserver variation among pathologists in identifying various subtypes of NSCLC. Though this may not be of clinical significance with regard to therapy at present, it may prove relevant in the future if the treatment of NSCLC becomes specifically related to the subtypes.

Squamous Cell Carcinoma (Fig. 4)

The main histopathological features of squamous cell carcinoma are the presence of keratinization and/or

Table 6: Classification of lung cancer used in clinical practice.

Types:
 • Nonsmall cell lung cancer:
  – Adenocarcinoma:
   - Adenocarcinoma in situ (AIS)
   - Minimally invasive adenocarcinoma (MIA)
   - Invasive carcinoma and its variants
  – Squamous cell carcinoma
 • Small cell lung cancer:
  – Large cell undifferentiated carcinoma
  – Others:
   - Carcinoid tumors
   - Mucoepidermoid carcinoma
   - Carcinoma of the sarcomatoid and sarcomatous type
   - Carcinoma of the salivary gland type

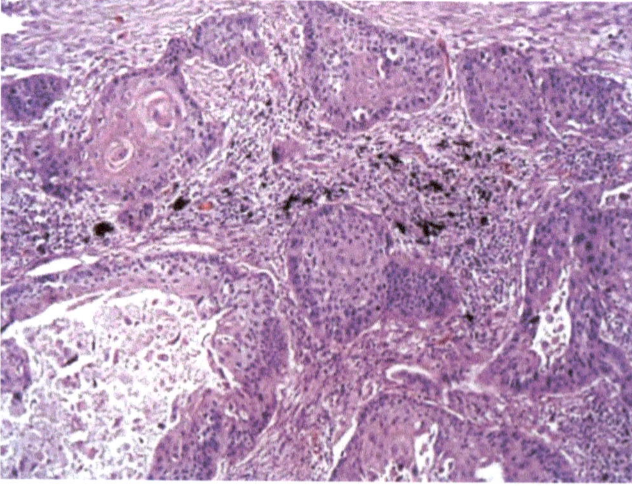

Fig. 4: Squamous cell carcinoma of the lung. H&E (hematoxylin and eosin) microscopy image at 20x magnification demonstrates nests of tumor cells with central keratinization indicating a squamous cell carcinoma of the lung.

the presence of intercellular junctions or bridges often termed "prickles" or desmosomes. Squamous cell carcinomas generally arise centrally in association with central airways—trachea, main stem, lobar, and also with segmental bronchi. They are the least malignant of the four main types and have a high correlation with smoking history. As these cancers are usually centrally placed, they cause clinical and radiological features of obstruction to the large airways. In the very early stages, the tumor may be radiologically occult even on a computed tomography (CT) examination of the chest.

Squamous cell carcinoma may also originate peripherally presenting as a mass lesion which may cavitate and be mistaken for a lung abscess. Cavitation is more often seen in squamous cell carcinoma than in other cell types. There are four histological variants described in squamous cell carcinoma. These are papillary, clear cell, small cell, and basaloid pattern.

Adenocarcinoma (Figs. 5 to 8)

Adenocarcinoma is the most frequent form of lung cancer in most countries. There is an increasing incidence of

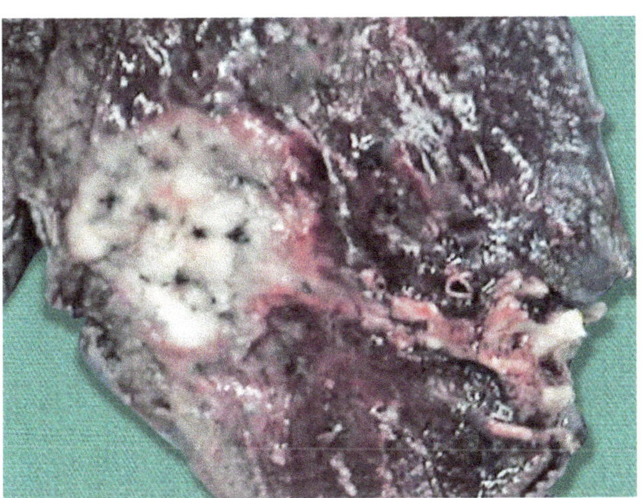

Fig. 5: Adenocarcinoma of the lung. Gross lobectomy specimen demonstrates a peripherally placed solid mass lesion, fairly distant from the lobar bronchus.

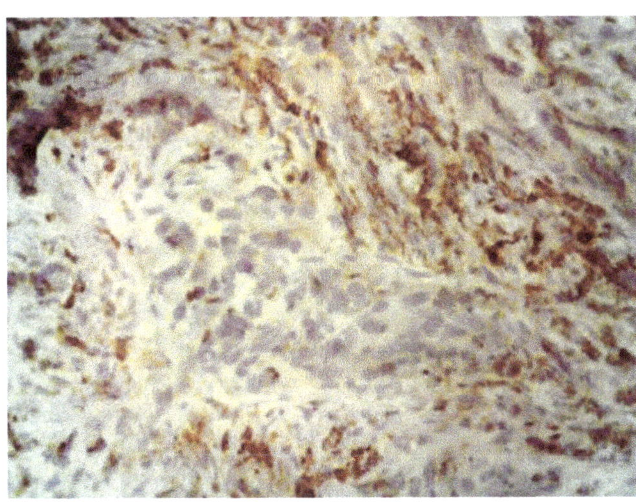

Fig. 7: Adenocarcinoma in situ. Histopathology shows alveoli lined by malignant cells. The framework of the lung is preserved indicating that this is an adenocarcinoma in situ.

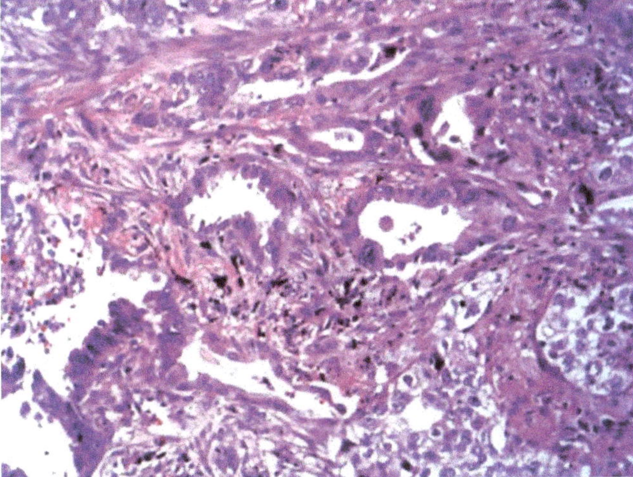

Fig. 6: Adenocarcinoma of the lung. H&E (hematoxylin and eosin) microscopy at 20x magnification reveals tumor cells disposed in glandular pattern, separated by desmoplastic stroma indicative of an adenocarcinoma of the lung.

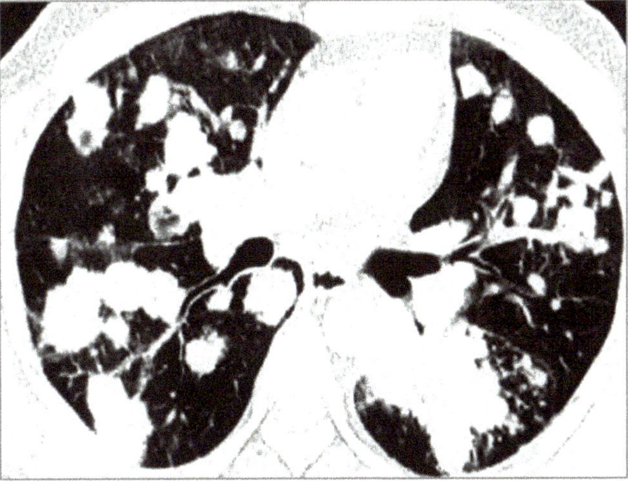

Fig. 8: Adenocarcinoma (previously termed as bronchoalveolar carcinoma). CT of chest demonstrates multiple well-defined lesions in both lung fields with ill-defined lesions in the right upper lobe posteriorly. CT-guided biopsy revealed an invasive adenocarcinoma.

adenocarcinoma in India as well, as will be discussed in the next section of this chapter.

Adenocarcinoma of the lung is characterized by diverse histological features; it has a variable natural history, a wide range of radiological findings and molecular characteristics. The 2004 WHO classification of adenocarcinoma included the following subtypes—acinar, papillary, bronchoalveolar, solid, and mixed. The definition of the bronchoalveolar subtype required that the tumor had a pure lepidic growth pattern without evidence of stromal vascular or pleural invasion. The term lepidic implies that the proliferating tumor cells should uniformly line the alveolar walls, using the latter as a scaffolding.

The new 2011 comprehensive classification of adenocarcinoma of the lung as agreed upon by IASLC/ATS/ERS does away with the term bronchoalveolar carcinoma altogether in favor of adenocarcinoma in situ (AIS). For small (<3 cm) solitary adenocarcinomas with predominant lepidic growth and minimal or small foci of invasion, the term minimally invasive adenocarcinoma (MIA) is recommended. By definition the term MIA is only applicable to a solitary discrete lesion except in the rare instance of multiple tumors that are synchronous primaries. Both AIS and MIA show good 5-year survival statistics and typically are characterized by ground glass opacities on a high-resolution computed tomography (HRCT) of the chest, without a solid component. The majority are nonmucinous though some show a mixed mucinous and nonmucinous pattern.

The IASLC/ATS/ERS consensus further proposed the following subtypes for invasive carcinomas—lepidic predominant adenocarcinoma with tumor cells mainly growing and spreading along alveolar walls, papillary predominant adenocarcinoma, acinar predominant adenocarcinoma, micropapillary adenocarcinoma, and solid predominant adenocarcinoma with mucin.

The *variants* of invasive adenocarcinomas as proposed in the 2011 update are invasive, colloid, fetal, and enteric adenocarcinoma. The details of these variants in terms of both recognition and significance lie in the domain of the pathologist.

The majority of adenocarcinomas arise in the periphery of the lung. Some specific subtypes are associated with for example EGFR mutations or the ALK fusion genes, but one cannot predict the mutations from the histology. Molecular tests are therefore necessary to determine if a particular cell type would respond to targeted therapy.

The main histological differential diagnosis of a primary adenocarcinoma of the lung is from a metastatic lesion arising from a primary outside the lung—for example ovarian, or pancreatic cancer. It may also be difficult to distinguish a peripheral adenocarcinoma of the lung with extensive pleural involvement, from diffuse pleural involvement by a metastatic tumor, or from a pleural mesothelioma.

Small Cell Lung Cancer (Figs. 9 to 11)

Small cell lung cancers are believed to arise from neuroendocrine cells and account for about 20% of lung cancers in most series. SCLCs are strongly associated with

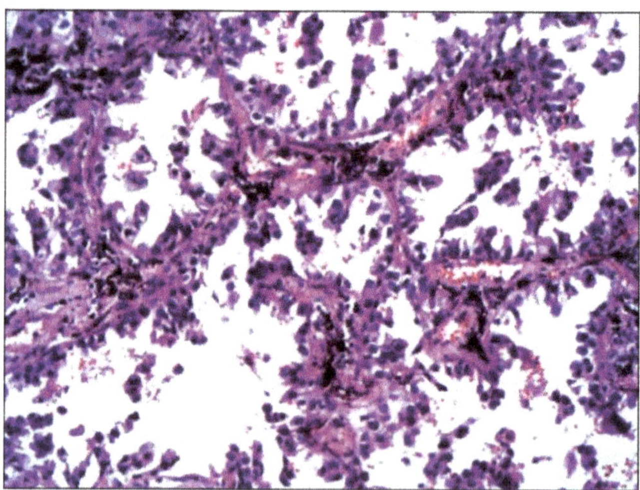

Fig. 9: 20x. Small cell carcinoma lung. Immunohistochemistry with leukocyte common antigen. It is important to differentiate a lymphoma from small cell carcinoma. This marker helps to differentiate, as lymphoma will be positive and small cell cancer will be negative.

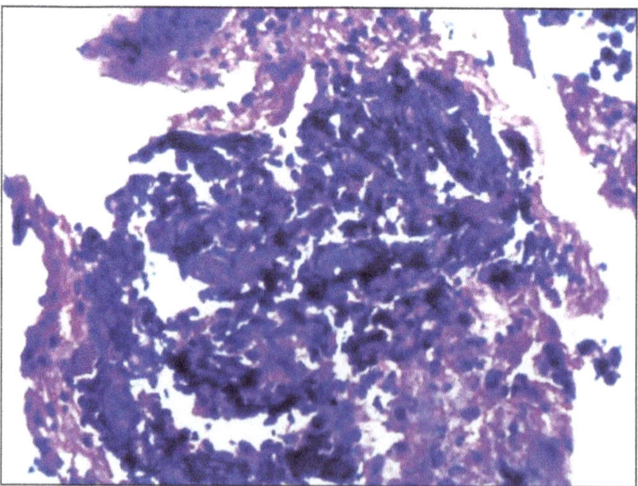

Fig. 10: Small cell carcinoma of the lung. Nests of darkly stained small to medium-sized cells with scant indiscernible cytoplasm. Crush artifact is noted which is an important diagnostic feature.

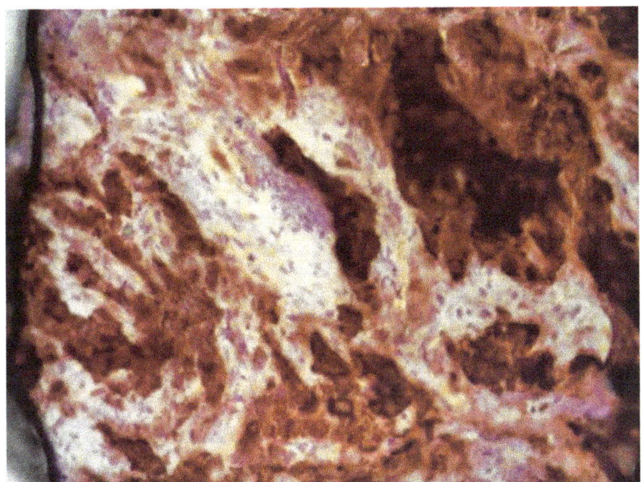

Fig. 11: Small cell carcinoma of the lung. Immunohistochemistry using cytokeratin shows strong positivity in tumor cells.

smoking, generally occur centrally, invariably causing early metastatic mediastinal adenopathy. Imaging features usually show a large mediastinal adenopathy, the primary site of origin being unclear. SCLC is the lung cancer most frequently associated with distant metastatic spread and most frequently associated with one or more of the paraneoplastic syndrome. The latter may precede the clinical or even the imaging presence of SCLC by several months.

Small cell lung cancer is considered a systemic disease, even in the limited stage, the only exception being SCLC presenting as a localized peripheral nodule without any hilar or mediastinal adenopathy.

Histologically, SCLC consists of small oval cells with little cytoplasm closely packed together, the tumor cells appearing to press on one another to produce what has been termed nuclear molding. The cell nuclei are pyknotic with a distinct nucleolus and a dispersed granular chromatin pattern.

Large Cell Undifferentiated Carcinoma

These tumors lack either squamous or glandular differentiation, the tumor cells being arranged in sheets. The cells have a fair amount of cytoplasm, vesicular nuclei with prominent nucleoli. Large cell undifferentiated carcinomas generally present as a peripheral mass; necrosis is often present within the mass.

Some of the other rarer pathological forms of lung cancers are adenosquamous carcinomas which partake of features of both adenocarcinoma and squamous cell carcinoma, carcinoid tumors, carcinoma of the salivary gland type, mucoepidermoid carcinoma, carcinoma of the sarcomatoid and sarcomatous type, lymphomas, and metastatic tumors from primaries situated outside the lungs.

Scar Cancer

Peripheral lung cancers, usually adenocarcinoma, sometimes exhibit a central area of sclerosis resembling a scar. The question has been debated whether this scar tissue is a product of the tumor or whether the tumor has arisen from the scar. Perhaps both are possible. The diffuse scarring in usual interstitial pneumonia and in some other conditions causing interstitial lung disease has a well-recognized association with the development of lung cancer. Though there are reports of this association and occurrence in the West, we have very rarely encountered a bronchogenic carcinoma arising from scar tissue in our centers.

■ PREVALENCE OF HISTOLOGICAL CELL TYPES OF LUNG CANCER

The prevalence of different histological cell types is affected by the geographic areas and the population under study as also by the method in which the pathological material is obtained. There are differences in the prevalence of different cell types identified from biopsy specimens, from surgically resected specimens and from autopsy studies.

The World Scenario

Earlier in the Western world, squamous cell carcinoma was by far the most common subtype of lung cancer. Close to 1980, there were twice as many squamous cell carcinomas as adenocarcinomas in men, whereas adenocarcinomas were slightly more frequent in women. By 1990, adenocarcinomas (29–37%) in the United States were as frequent as squamous cell carcinomas (27–34%) and today the most common subtype of lung cancer in the United States, both in men and women, is adenocarcinoma.

It thus appears that to start with, the surge of lung cancer in men was related to a marked increase in squamous cell carcinomas while that in women was mainly due to adenocarcinomas, there being an overall preponderance of squamous cell carcinoma. Then how does one now explain the present increase in the overall prevalence of adenocarcinoma? Wynder and Higgins believe that the change is related to the change in smoking habits.

Following the introduction of filter-tipped cigarettes in the 1960s, smokers needed to take more frequent and deeper puffs to fulfill their need for nicotine. Cigarette smoke therefore reached more distally into the smaller bronchioles where adenocarcinoma occurs.

To summarize, the surge of squamous cell cancer in men before 1980 was due to smoking habits before the introduction of filter cigarettes. The surge in cancer among females after 1970 is related to smoking filter cigarettes and the change in the increased incidence from squamous to adenocarcinoma is also related (according to Wynder and Higgins) to the changeover in men to smoking filter cigarettes.

The Indian Scenario

Most of the older and even some recent Indian studies have reported that squamous cell carcinoma is the most common histological type in India. In a review article of 2004 by Behera D, Balamugesh T, the biological cell type which had a predominant prevalence in India was squamous cell carcinoma (45%). Small cell carcinoma had a reported prevalence of 20% and adenocarcinoma of 25% *(Ref: Behera D, Balamugesh T. Lung cancer in India. Indian J Chest Dis Allied Sci. 2004;46:269-81).* Other studies from northern India came to the same conclusion. In western countries and many Asian countries, adenocarcinoma is the most frequent cell type. Current studies from two large hospitals in India suggest that even in this country, adenocarcinoma is the leading histological cell type of lung cancer, pushing squamous cell carcinoma into second place. A research article on the Clinicopathological Profile of Lung Cancer at AIIMS—A Changing Paradigm

in India *[Ref: Malik PS, Sharma MC, Mohanti BK, et al. Clinicopathological profile of lung cancer at AIIMS: a changing paradigm in India. Asian Pac J Cancer Prev. 2013;14(1):489-94]* reported that of the 435 pathological proved lung cancers by an independent expert, there were 85% NSCLC and 14.7 SCLC.

Among the NSCLC, adenocarcinoma was the most common histological type (37.3%), followed by squamous cell carcinoma (32.1%), large cell carcinoma (2.8%), and other rare lung cancers.

The histological cell types studied in 2006 by the Tata Memorial Hospital, Mumbai which drains cancer patients of all classes from all over India reported adenocarcinoma as the most common cell type. The current data (2012–2014) comes to the same conclusion. The histological cell types reported by this hospital in males and females in the year 2004 and 2012–14 have been shown in **Table 7**. The increasing incidence of adenocarcinomas in males (48.5% of all lung cancers) and especially in females (55.2% of all lung cancers) is noteworthy.

Lung Cancer in Chinese Women

There has been a dramatic increase in lung cancer deaths in Chinese women *[Ref: Zou XN, Lin D, et al. Histological subtypes of lung cancer in Chinese women from 2000 to 2012. Thoracic Cancer. 2014;5:447-54)* in recent decades]. The predominant histological cell type again is adenocarcinoma. The study by Xia Zou and colleagues has shown that incidence of adenocarcinoma increased with relative frequency from 72% in lung cancer cases identified in 2000–2002 to 76.49% in 2011–2012. This significant increase of adenocarcinoma in Chinese women

Table 7: Prevalence of histological cell types of lung cancer at the Tata Memorial Hospital.

Annual Report, Mumbai Cancer Registry, 2006			Annual Report, Mumbai Cancer Registry, 2012–14		
Histology	**Male (%)**	**Female (%)**	**Histology**	**Male**	**Female**
Small cell carcinoma	10.4	6.1	Neoplasm malignant	20.5	31.3
Large cell carcinoma	1.6	1.1	Large cell carcinoma	–	0.6
Squamous cell carcinoma	14.6	9.4	Undiff/Anaplastic carcinoma	0.2	
Adenocarcinoma	17.3	31.1	Small cell carcinoma	7.8	1.8
Others	25.2	22.8	Squamous cell carcinoma	19	4.3
No histology	31.0	29.4	Other carcinomas	2.2	4.3
	100	100	Adenocarcinoma	48.5	55.2
			Others	1.9	2.5

suggests the likelihood of persistent and strong exposure to potential carcinogens in the Chinese population.

■ CLINICAL FEATURES

The clinical presentation and clinical features of lung cancer vary enormously. 10–20% of cases are asymptomatic, being discovered fortuitously following a radiographic examination of the chest performed for a routine health check. Symptoms when they occur may be related to a gradual obstruction of one of the larger airways, or due to local spread within the lungs or the thorax. The very first clinical presentation may take the form of a distant metastatic lesion, or of multiple metastatic lesions so that the interval between the time of presentation and death is indeed very short. Finally, at times the clinical presentation and features are dominated by symptoms caused by nonmetastatic (paraneoplastic) syndromes. More often than not, a combination of clinical features described above is observed. It is unfortunately a truism to state that in most patients, by the time the diagnosis of cancer of the lung has been made, treatment to alter the natural history of the disease is of little or no avail.

Local Symptoms

The cell-type of lung cancer may determine the pattern of dissemination as also the nature of problems for which the patient seeks advice. An adenocarcinoma generally arises within the lung parenchyma and is often peripherally situated. Local intrathoracic symptoms may be delayed, the disease announcing itself through one or more metastatic lesions or by a pleural effusion. On the other hand, squamous cell carcinomas tend to be confined to the thorax for a longer time so that symptoms related to the lungs and to intrathoracic spread are more common. SCLCs are rapidly-growing tumors, usually arising in the central airways, spreading locally and metastasizing quickly so that symptoms at the time of presentation are often related both to the chest and the distant metastasis.

Cough

This is the most common presenting clinical feature of lung cancer and is invariably present when a tumor arises in one of the central airways and tends to narrow or obstruct it. Cough is caused by ulceration of the bronchial mucosa and/or because of obstruction to the lumen of the airway. Close to 70% of lung cancers involve the major central airways—the carina, main and lobar bronchi. A tumor in any one of these situations, besides causing ulceration of the mucosa and obstruction, impairs mucus clearance, thereby promoting further cough. Pneumonia—a single attack or recurrent episodes distal to a partially obstructed bronchus is a feature of bronchogenic carcinoma. Increasing bronchial obstruction can lead to atelectasis of a lobe or even a lung, causing both cough and breathlessness.

Since lung cancer occurs most frequently in cigarette smokers, cough caused by the lung cancer is often mistakenly looked upon as a smoker's cough, or attributed to chronic bronchitis, or to an upper respiratory tract infection. Persistent cough or increasing cough in a smoker merits a chest radiograph, particularly in a patient over 40 years of age. A change in the character of cough (particularly in a smoker's cough) also necessitates investigation. An ulcerating or obstructing cancerous lesion in a large bronchus often causes paroxysms of a dry brassy cough (with a metallic sound) which may be accompanied by a wheeze, noisy breathing or even stridor.

Cough is generally dry, or in a smoker may be associated with mucoid sputum; the sputum may be yellow in the presence of infection. Excessive sputum production, amounting to a bronchorrhea is occasionally seen in an invasive adenocarcinoma that starts by lining the alveoli of one lung but often also involves the other.

Hemoptysis

Hemoptysis is the sole presenting feature in 5–10% of patients with bronchogenic carcinoma. It occurs as one among other presenting features in 30%. When it is the sole presenting feature, it prompts immediate concern and investigation. Hemoptysis is rarely profuse; more often it takes the form of streaking of sputum with blood, or sputum mixed with blood, particularly in the mornings. An X-ray of the chest is imperative; an abnormal chest X-ray necessitates further investigation. Even if the chest radiography is normal, hemoptysis, particularly in a smoker warrants a fiberoptic bronchoscopy. It needs to be noted however that the yield of endobronchial tumors following bronchoscopy in patients with hemoptysis who have a normal chest X-ray is not more than 5%. Occasionally, a bronchogenic carcinoma is diagnosed on a CT of the chest with a normal bronchoscopic study. The diagnosis of a bronchogenic carcinoma can be excluded in a patient presenting with hemoptysis, if the chest X-ray, sputum cytology, fiberoptic bronchoscopy, and a CT thorax are normal.

Dyspnea

Dyspnea may be a presenting symptom together with cough and sputum in 25% of patients with lung cancer. It occurs early in the natural history of this disease in over 50% of patients. Most importantly, dyspnea occasionally may be complained of as the presenting symptom (or in association with other symptoms), even though the chest X-ray is normal. Dyspnea in the above situation is related to progressive obstruction of a major bronchus, together with increasing obstructive emphysema of a lobe (if the lobar bronchus is involved) or the whole lung (if the main bronchus is involved). Dyspnea may then be associated with a fixed monophonic inspiratory wheeze (Chevalier Jackson's sign) and is often mistaken for bronchial asthma. Ventilation perfusion scans have shown well-marked abnormalities disproportionate to any radiological abnormalities. A flow volume loop shows flattening of the inspiratory portion of the loop followed later by a flattened expiratory portion of the loop as well.

As the disease progresses, dyspnea may be due to several other causes. It may be due to pneumonia distal to the obstructive lesion, due to lobar atelectasis, or due to a pleural effusion. It can also result from extensive involvement of the lung parenchyma, from left vocal cord paralysis due to pressure on the left recurrent laryngeal nerve and occasionally from extrinsic pressure on large airways due to extensive involvement of the mediastinum by the disease. More than one factor may be responsible for this symptom. Dyspnea is also a prominent and distressing symptom in lymphangitis carcinomatosis and in pericardial effusion caused by malignant invasion of the parietal pericardium.

Chest Pain

Chest pain occurs in 25–50% of patients at the time of diagnosis. It is on the side of the tumor, is dull aching in character, often ill-defined and may be either intermittent or continuous. It can be related to extension of the tumor to the mediastinum, chest wall, vertebrae or pleura. Pleural involvement may cause pleuritic chest pain but not always so **(Fig. 12)**. Most importantly, pain due to chest wall involvement does not exclude operability as these

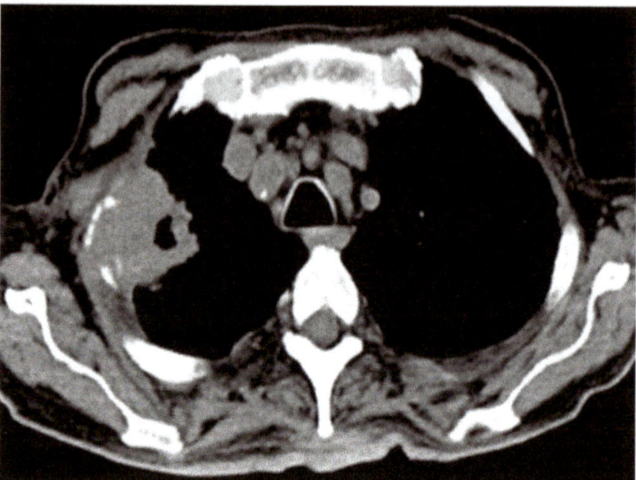

Fig. 12: Computed tomography of chest demonstrates cavitating mass lesion in apical segment of the right upper lobe destroying underlying rib with chest wall involvement.

patients, in the absence of lymph node involvement, have T3 lesions (as discussed later under Staging) and have fairly good survival rates after surgery.

Bronchogenic carcinoma arising at the apex of the lung or the superior sulcus (Pancoast tumor) causes shoulder pain often radiating down the arm. These patients are often diagnosed as cervical spondylitis or "arthritis", with a delay in the correct diagnosis.

Wheezing

Wheezing as a symptom of central airways obstruction together with cough and dyspnea has already been mentioned earlier. It may be the presenting symptom in a few patients. The fixed monophonic wheeze should be distinguished from the polyphonic wheezes present in asthma or chronic bronchitis. Significant localized airways obstruction (involving the main bronchus or proximal lobar bronchus) may give rise to "noisy breathing" or even a stridor indistinguishable from that observed with an obstructed glottis. Breathlessness and a wheeze due to central airways obstruction necessitate urgent planned treatment.

Systemic Features

Low-grade fever, lassitude, weight loss, loss of appetite may occasionally be the presenting features of lung cancer with or without respiratory symptoms.

Intrathoracic Spread

Bronchogenic carcinoma involving a central airway may involve the bronchial wall and extend outward into the surrounding lung tissue, producing an increasing "mass" lesion. A lesion starting within the lung parenchyma may do likewise. Spread of the tumor may extend into the mediastinum and mediastinal structures, the pleura, the pericardium, the thoracic cage, and the vertebrae **(Figs. 13 to 15)**. The clinical presentation and clinical features may be directly related to the intrathoracic spread.

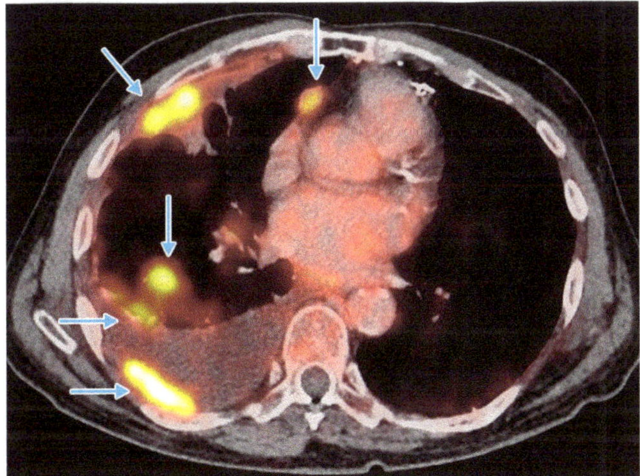

Fig. 13: Carcinoma of the lung spread to pleura, pericardium. Axial PET-CT image demonstrates primary lung neoplasm, metastatic right pleural effusion and multiple pleural deposits as evidenced by increased FDG uptake. Cytology of the pleural fluid confirmed metastatic adenocarcinoma cells.

Hoarseness of the voice together with a rasping soundless cough due to left recurrent laryngeal nerve involvement as it loops round the aortic arch is a presenting symptom in close to 10% of patients. Involvement of the sympathetic trunk leads to a Horner's syndrome on the affected side, manifested by slight ptosis, a small pupil and absence of sweating on the ipsilateral affected half of the face.

The superior vena caval (SVC) syndrome is characterized by obstruction and occlusion of the superior vena cava by pressure of the tumor, or by thrombosis due to slowing of blood flow through the vein due to extrinsic pressure or infiltration of the wall of the vein by tumor cells **(Figs. 16A and B)**. It is invariably associated with metastatic involvement of the paratracheal glands from a tumor within the right lung. The SVC syndrome occurs most commonly with a small cell carcinoma of the lung, being a presenting feature in 10%. Patients complain of fullness of the face and neck, particularly on bending forward. The face is puffy, plethoric with congested conjunctivae. These clinical features may take time to evolve. The presence of engorged jugular veins with absent or poorly perceptible pulsations is the first sign of this syndrome occurring well before other symptoms or signs appear. A blocked superior vena cava is associated with opening of collateral veins visible in the upper chest; these maintain adequate venous return to the heart.

Malignant mediastinal adenopathy is due to spread of tumor along lymphatics to mediastinal nodes. Malignant

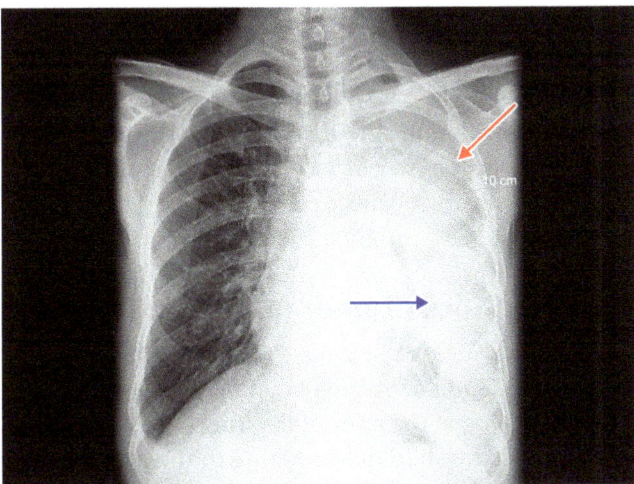

Fig. 14: Bronchogenic carcinoma. Chest X-ray reveals ill-defined mass lesion in left upper zone (red arrow) with loculated pleural effusion on the left side (blue arrow). No midline shift is noted. Small pleural effusion is seen on the right side.

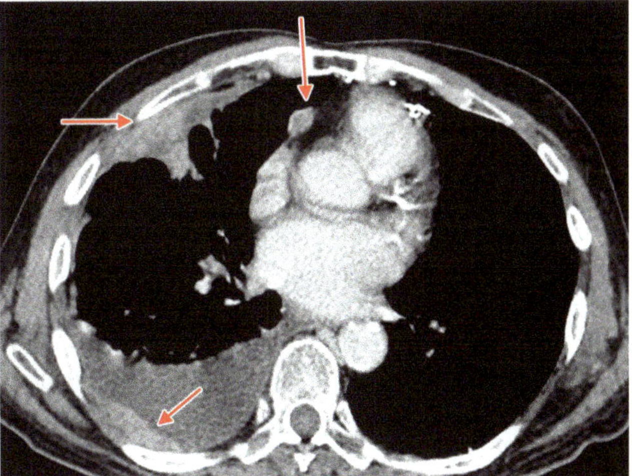

Fig. 15: Pleural metastasis from carcinoma lung. CT chest reveals moderate right pleural effusion with multiple nodular pleural lesions. Pleural fluid cytology revealed adenocarcinoma cells representing metastatic spread from primary lung carcinoma.

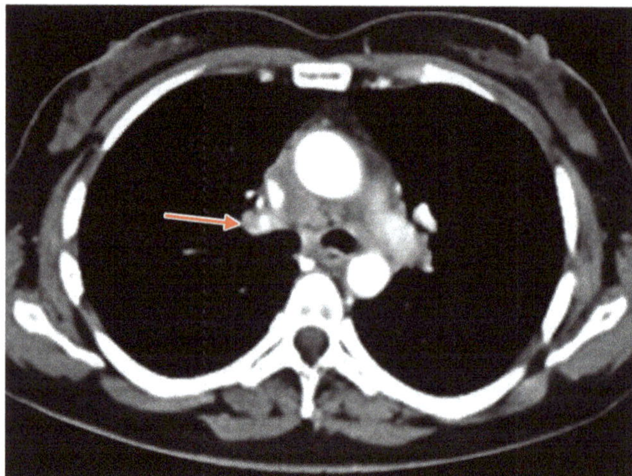

Fig. 16A: Superior vena caval (SVC) syndrome. Computed tomography of chest demonstrates an ill-defined mass lesion in the mediastinum encasing the SVC. Biopsy revealed a small cell carcinoma.

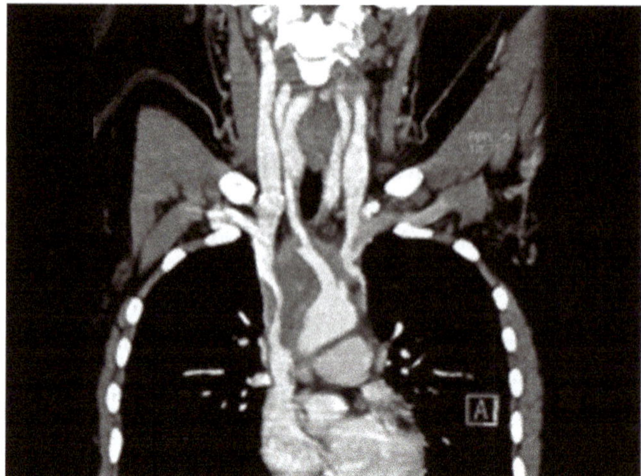

Fig. 16B: SVC syndrome. Coronal computed tomography reveals mass lesion encasing and narrowing the SVC.

infiltration of the mediastinum can also occur through contiguity. Dysphagia can result from pressure of malignant nodes on the esophagus, and rarely through direct tumor invasion and compression.

Pericardial involvement causes pericardial effusion and occasionally cardiac tamponade. Mitotic cells are not invariably recovered from the pericardial fluid.

Invasion of the chest wall by contiguity or of the vertebrae may result in chest pain, discomfort or back pain. Ribs and vertebrae are however more often involved by blood-borne metastasis.

Spread of malignant disease to the pleura by continuity or of contiguity leads to pleural effusion. Malignant pleural effusions are exudates, which may be serous, serosanguinous or frankly bloody. The presence of malignant cells in the pleural fluid points to unresectability of the tumor. Symptoms of pleural involvement are pleuritic chest pain, cough, and dyspnea.

Yet close to 20% of patients with bronchogenic carcinoma with pleural effusions due to direct or metastatic spread are asymptomatic.

It is important to note that not all pleural effusions in lung cancer are malignant in etiology. Pleural effusions could also be due to pneumonia distal to an obstructive lesion within the bronchus, due to pulmonary embolism, lymphatic obstruction, atelectasis, or coexistent heart failure. Therefore, the mere presence of a pleural effusion in a patient with bronchogenic carcinoma does not always point to unresectability in the presence of an otherwise resectable tumor. Proof of a malignant pleural effusion rests in the demonstration of mitotic cells in the pleural aspirate. Unfortunately, the yield of a positive fluid cytology in malignant pleural effusions is about 65%. In retrospective studies, it has been shown that this yield remains the same whether the fluid accumulation within the pleura is small or large. Blind pleural biopsy increases the yield only to a small extent. Therefore, if the initial cytology is negative, a repeat study should be done. If still negative, a video-assisted thoracoscopy allows a good look into the pleural space as also a biopsy, enabling one to make a firm diagnosis. It is important that the diagnosis of pleural metastasis is confirmed or excluded, so that the chance of a successful surgical resection of the tumor is not missed.

Involvement of the pleura can also occur from blood-borne metastasis from a bronchogenic carcinoma, or from retrograde spread of cancer cells along the lymphatics to the pleura.

Superior Sulcus Tumor (Pancoast Tumor)

The superior sulcus is a groove made by the subclavian artery on the vault of the pleura and the apex of the lung. A tumor arising at the apex of the lung presents typically with pain in the shoulder radiating to the arm down to the fingers. It is associated with erosion of the posterior portion of the first two ribs and often the seventh cervical and first, second dorsal vertebrae (**Fig. 17**). Involvement of the sympathetic trunk causes Horner's syndrome

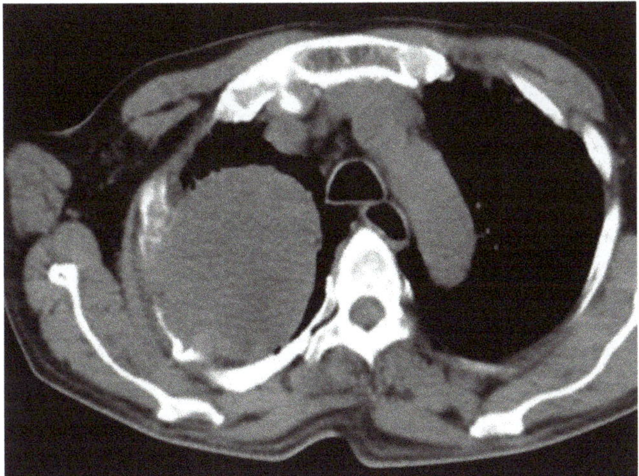

Fig. 17: Pancoast tumor: Computed tomography scan demonstrates large mass in the right upper lobe destroying chest wall and adjacent ribs.

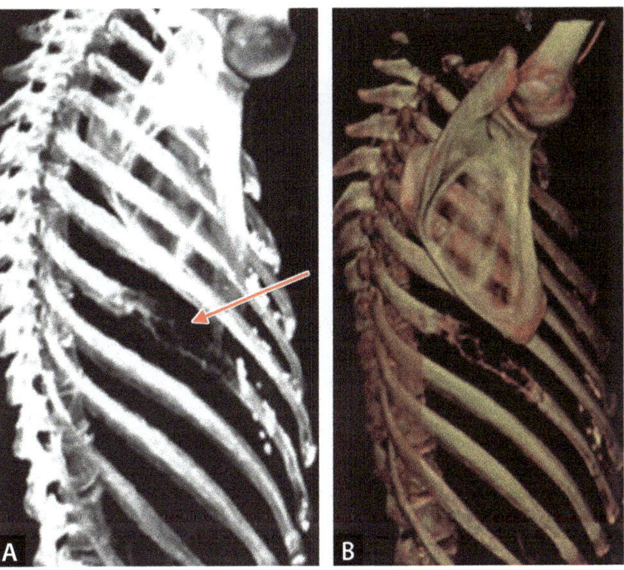

Figs. 18A and B: Computed tomography scan of ribs demonstrates destructive lesion of 8th rib representing a metastatic deposit.

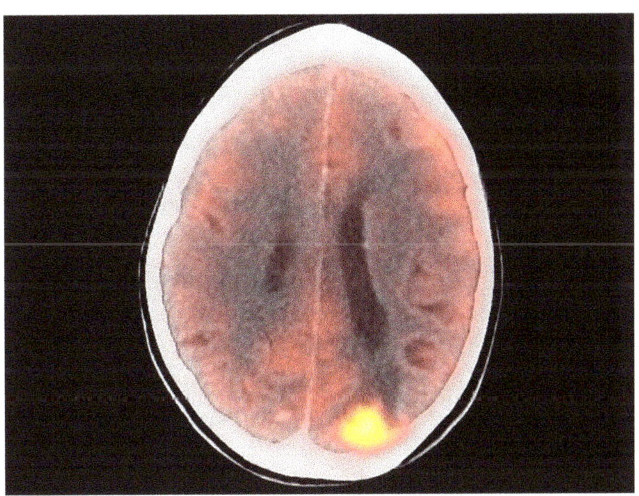

Fig. 19: PET-CT scan demonstrates mass lesion in the left occipital region showing increased uptake representing metastatic deposit.

and involvement of the first thoracic nerve root is often associated with wasting of the small muscles of the hand.

An X-ray of the chest in the early stages may show a faint opacity over the apex often missed as a soft tissue shadow. An HRCT however clears the diagnosis by not only revealing the tumor mass but also showing bony erosions of the ribs and vertebrae.

Distant Extrathoracic Metastatic Manifestations

Distant metastatic blood-borne spread is the presenting feature in about one-third patients. Distant metastasis can involve any organ or organ system. Bone metastases are particularly frequent—the ribs, vertebrae, the long bones such as the humerus and femur often being involved **(Figs. 18A and B)**. Bone pains are present in over 20% of patients at presentation and should arouse suspicion of bony metastasis. Spontaneous fracture of the femur or a fracture after trivial injury is often due to a metastatic lesion.

Metastases to the brain are frequent and may be single or multiple. Secondary metastatic tumor generally arising from the lung is the most common cerebral tumor occurring in adults after 40 years of age **(Fig. 19)**.

Small cell lung cancer has the greatest tendency to metastasize while squamous cell carcinoma has the least tendency to do so. Cranial metastasis may be asymptomatic or may produce symptoms of increased intracranial tension such as headache, vomiting, blurred vision, diplopia and/or focal signs depending on the situation of the metastatic lesion. Intracranial metastases have been reported in 30–50% of patients with lung cancer at autopsy. Spinal cord metastases are uncommon and when present are usually associated with cerebral metastasis.

Liver metastases are frequent; they are generally silent except when large or multiple when they may produce an enlarged tender liver **(Figs. 20A and B)**. Liver functions are not significantly disturbed, except again when the metastases are numerous and large. Jaundice is rare except when metastatic glands at the porta hepatis press upon the bile duct.

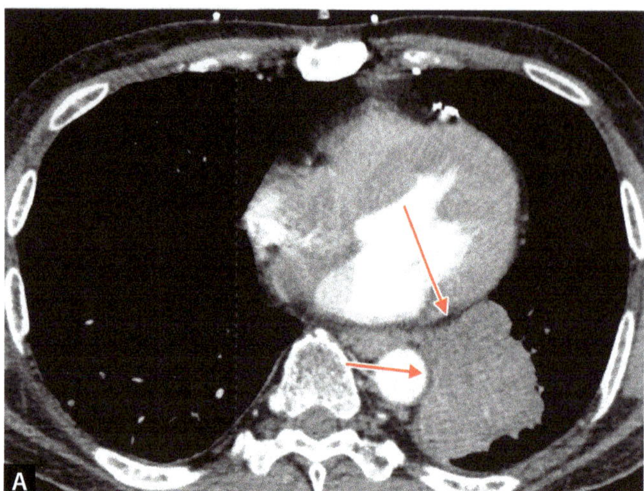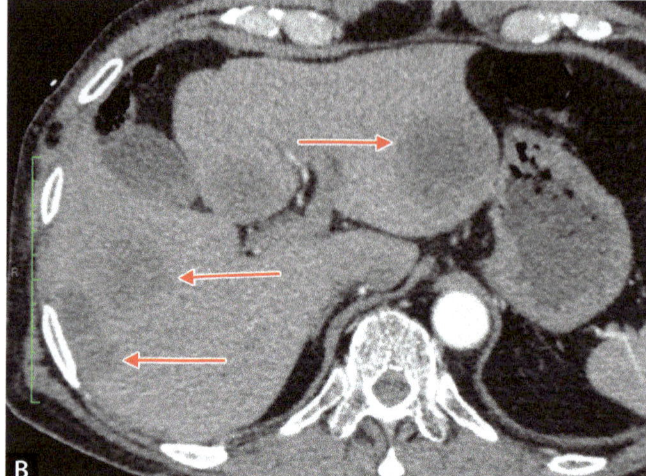

Figs. 20A and B: (A) CT scan of the chest demonstrates nodular left lower lobe mass with multiple lesions in the liver (B). Lung lesion on biopsy was the primary neoplasm, liver lesions were the metastatic deposits.

Metastatic deposits in the suprarenal glands and in the intra-abdominal lymph nodes are common, particularly in small cell carcinomas. Adrenal metastatic lesions are the presenting features in close to 10% of patients with small cell carcinoma of the lung; they are less commonly observed in squamous cell carcinoma and adenocarcinoma. Destruction of the adrenal glands can lead to adrenocortical deficiency **(Fig. 21)**.

Spread of disease to the supraclavicular and anterior cervical lymph glands has been noted to occur in 15–30% of patients during the course of the illness.

There is no organ or organ symptom that is exempt from possible metastatic spread arising from lung cancer.

Nonmetastatic Paraneoplastic Manifestations (Table 8)

Paraneoplastic syndromes are related to those remote effects of lung cancer that are not caused by direct invasion or spread or metastasis. They occur in about 10–20% of patients with bronchogenic carcinoma. Paraneoplastic syndromes are most commonly (though not solely) associated with SCLC and are caused by the production of polypeptide hormones by the tumor cells. 70% of patients with SCLC and 15% of NSCLC show an elevation of one or more of these polypeptide hormones at the time of diagnosis. However, only a small minority of these presents with clinical manifestations of a paraneoplastic syndrome.

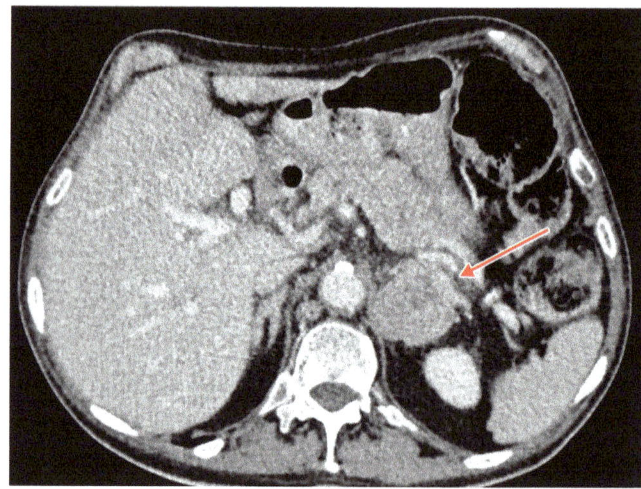

Fig. 21: Computed tomography scan of the abdomen reveals a well-defined mass lesion in the left adrenal gland representing a metastatic deposit.

Small cell lung cancers show neuroendocrine characteristics. These include cytoplasmic and membrane-bound neurosecretory granules containing amines and polypeptide products. However, 15% of nonsmall cell tumors also have elevated serum polypeptide levels at the time of diagnosis. Hormonal peptides are also produced by other solid tumors, lymphomas, and some leukemias. It has been postulated that all lung cancers originate from a common stem cell and that hormone production occurs at an early stage of cell development.

Ectopic hormone production is most frequently observed in SCLC, the most frequently elevated hormone

Table 8: Nonmetastatic paraneoplastic manifestations of lung cancer.
Endocrine system: • Hypercalcemia • Syndrome of inappropriate antidiuretic hormone secretion Ectopic corticotropin hormone syndrome • Hyperthyroidism (usually with squamous cell tumor) • Gynecomastia • Pigmentation associated with α and β melanocyte stimulation • Somatostatin release mimicking a pancreatic tumor • Hyperglycemia • Hypoglycemia • Galactorrhea • Growth hormone excess
Musculoskeletal system: • Finger clubbing • Hypertrophic pulmonary osteoarthropathy • Dermatomyositis • Polymyositis
Neurological features: • Peripheral neuropathy • Lambert-Eaton myasthenic syndrome • Encephalomyelopathy • Cerebellar degeneration • Autonomic neuropathy • Impaired vision

being calcitonin. The adrenocorticotrophic hormone, melanocyte-producing hormone, lipotropin, and the antidiuretic hormone (ADH) are also frequently raised in patients with SCLC.

Polypeptides, in particular neuropeptides, have been investigated in the hope that they may serve as tumor markers of disease. The neuropeptide bombesin is often present within cells of SCLCs but the serum levels are low. However, the neuron-specific enolase present in the brain, in neuroendocrine tissue and in SCLCs, shows a high serum level in patients with clinical manifestations of SCLC. The levels of elevated polypeptides fall following tumor response to chemotherapy but are not sensitive enough to predict relapse. All said and done, the hope that polypeptides may serve as tumor markers in the diagnosis of lung cancer or in predicting relapse of lung cancers has so far not been fulfilled.

The paraneoplastic manifestations of lung cancer caused by the production of polypeptide hormones are briefly described below.

Hypercalcemia

Hypercalcemia is most frequently due to multiple bony metastases. Less commonly it is due to a parathyroid hormone-related protein (PTHP), calcitriol or other cytokines that have an osteoclastic effect. Serum parathyroid hormone levels are normal but an elevated PTHP is detected in 50% of patients. PTHP not only has an osteoclastic effect but also prevents renal reabsorption of sodium and water thereby causing polyuria. Hypercalcemia is most often associated with squamous cell carcinomas of the lung. Generally, patients with hypercalcemia have inoperable disease, the median survival rate after symptomatic hypercalcemia being 1 month.

Clinical features of hypercalcemia include anorexia, nausea, vomiting, lethargy, constipation, polyuria, and dehydration. Confusion, drowsiness, coma, and renal failure occur later. Cardiovascular effects include shortened QT interval, heart block, ventricular arrhythmias, and cardiac arrest. Various combinations of the above clinical features may be observed.

Patients with a serum Ca above 12 mg/dL require treatment. The principles of treatment are:

- Correction of dehydration with intravenous normal saline—three or more liters of fluid need to be given.
- Use of IV frusemide to promote diuresis, taking care that intake of fluid at least equals the increased output.
- Inhibiting bone resorption and osteoclastic activity by the use of calcitonin and bisphosphonates. Zoledronate is the most effective of the bisphosphonates and is given in a dose of 4–8 mg intravenously over 15 minutes. Normal calcium levels are generally achieved within 4–10 days and are maintained for 30–40 days. Calcitonin decreases bone resorption, reduces the serum Ca level by 2 mg/dL. It is a weak agent and is given in a dose of 4 IU/kg intravenously or subcutaneously every 12 hours. It is useful to urgently bring down a high serum calcium level while waiting for the more slow acting but more effective zoledronate to take effect. Tachyphylaxis to calcitonin generally sets in after 48 hours. Combined treatment of zoledronate with calcitonin has an additive effect in lowering serum calcium.
- *Treatment of the underlying cancer*: Successful treatment (either chemotherapy or resection) is associated with a return of serum calcium levels to normal levels.

Patients with hypercalcemia who have widespread metastatic lesions die generally within a month and are best given supportive treatment.

Syndrome of Inappropriate Antidiuretic Hormone Secretion

Syndrome of inappropriate antidiuretic hormone secretion (SIADH) is due to increased secretion of the antidiuretic hormone and is observed in about 10% of patients who have SCLC. SCLC is by far the most common cause of SIADH accounting for over 75% of cases of this syndrome. Diagnostic criteria of SIADH are:

- Hyponatremia (serum sodium <135 mEq/L)
- Hypotonicity (plasma osmolality <280 mOsm/kg)
- Inappropriately concentrated urine (>100 mOsm/kg water)
- Elevated urine sodium concentration (>20 mEq/L), except during sodium restriction
- Clinical euvolemia
- Normal renal, adrenal, and thyroid function.

Symptoms of SIADH depend on the degree of hyponatremia and the rapidity of fall in serum sodium. A slow fall of serum sodium to below 120 mEq/L may be tolerated without untoward symptoms. Symptoms of hyponatremia include vomiting, drowsiness, confusion, coma, and seizures; these are caused by increased water content within nerve cells of the brain.

Treatment in mild to moderate cases consists of fluid restriction to below 1,000 mL/day. Further treatment consists of using Tolvaptan, a vasopressin receptor antagonist which works by regulating the sodium and water levels in the body. It is given in a dose of 15 mg OD initially and can be given 12 hourly if required.

When central nervous system (CNS) symptoms due to marked hyponatremia (Na <115 mEq/L) are severe, it is best to use a titrated solution of 3% hypertonic saline 100–150 mL given intravenously over 4–6 hours. Hypertonic saline can be dangerous in patients with poor pump function or diastolic dysfunction and can precipitate pulmonary edema. The serum sodium should be carefully monitored and should be increased slowly by a maximum of 8 mEq/day and not more than 16–18 mEq in 48 hours. A sharp rise in serum sodium can precipitate central pontine myelinosis which may manifest with drowsiness, coma, quadriparesis, and even death.

Patients with SCLC who have an associated SIADH should be promptly treated with chemotherapy. Successful chemotherapy leads to improvement in SIADH within a few weeks. Relapse of the disease is invariably associated with the return of SIADH.

Ectopic Corticotropin Hormone Syndrome

This syndrome is chiefly confined to SCLC, but is occasionally observed in carcinoid tumors of the lung, thymic tumors, neuroblastoma, and medullary carcinoma of the thyroid. The syndrome is due to ectopic production of corticotropin or corticotropin-releasing hormone. Though plasma corticotropin levels may be elevated in close to a quarter to a third of patients of SCLC, the short natural history of SCLC generally does not allow the evolution of a full-fledged Cushing's syndrome. Occasionally, one encounters a partial evolution of Cushing's syndrome characterized by proximal muscle myopathy, pigmentation, hypokalemic alkalosis, and increased plasma cortisol levels which are not suppressed with dexamethasone. Marked elevation of free cortisol in the urine (>500 µg/24 hrs) and of plasma corticotropin levels (>200 pg/mL) are strongly suggestive of ectopic corticotropin as the cause of the partial Cushing's syndrome described above.

Ketoconazole is the drug of choice for the treatment of Cushing's syndrome in the above setting. It is given in a dose of 200 mg thrice daily, slowly increasing (in the absence of toxic effects) to 400 mg thrice daily. Liver functions should be carefully monitored. If ketoconazole does not reduce cortisol secretion effectively, metyrapone is added at 250 mg 2–3 times a day, increased slowly to a maximum of 4 g/day. Hypoadrenalism occasionally results with this treatment and may require the use of dexamethasone 0.25–0.5 mg/day.

Appropriate treatment of SCLC with chemotherapy may help to reduce cortisol secretion and improve symptoms. Cushing's syndrome related to tumors other than SCLC is treated if possible by resection of the tumor.

Dermatomyositis and Polymyositis

Dermatomyositis and polymyositis have been reported as paraneoplastic features of an underlying malignancy, chiefly a bronchogenic carcinoma. The incidence is debatable, perhaps about 10%, though population-based studies in Australia and Sweden suggest a higher frequency of 15–25%. The risk of developing an overt malignancy is most within the first 2 years of the diagnosis and is more with dermatomyositis than pure polymyositis. Cancer surveillance is therefore important and should consist of a careful clinical examination together with appropriate screening, in particular mammography, chest X-ray, and colonoscopy.

Finger Clubbing, Hypertrophic Pulmonary Osteoarthropathy

Clubbing of the fingers and toes is characterized by loss of the angle between the nail bed and the cuticle. The angle is first straightened and then becomes convex. Rounded nails and bulbous fingertips develop due to enlargement of the connective tissue in the distal phalanges. Clubbed nails occur in 10–30% of patients with lung cancer.

Hypertrophic pulmonary osteopathy may be preceded by clubbing and is characterized by periosteitis, painful arthropathy and often marked finger clubbing. Besides lung cancer, it has been reported in thymic carcinoma, thyroid carcinoma, chronic myeloid leukemia, Hodgkin's disease, adenocarcinoma of the esophagus, bronchial carcinoid tumors, and pleural fibroma. It also has been observed in a number of nonmalignant conditions.

Among lung cancers, both clubbing and hypertrophic pulmonary osteopathy are most commonly associated with squamous cell carcinoma and occasionally with adenocarcinoma and large cell carcinoma. It may precede the diagnosis of lung cancer in 30% of patients. The painful periosteitis chiefly affects the distal ends of the radius, ulna, tibia, and the fibula. Besides the usual painful wrists and ankles, a painful arthropathy of the knees and elbows may also occur. Radiological changes may be observed in the femur and humerus even in the absence of pain in knees and elbows. Pain may prevent walking and may restrict movements at the wrists.

The cause of hypertrophic pulmonary osteoarthropathy is unknown but it may be caused by a humoral agent. The diagnosis should be considered in a cigarette smoker when there is a short history of arthralgia or an arthropathy chiefly involving the ankles and wrists. An X-ray of the long bones in suspected hypertrophic pulmonary osteoarthropathy reveals periosteitis with periosteal new bone formation. A bone scan reveals diffuse uptake in the long bones at the site of periosteitis. Amazingly, hypertrophic pulmonary osteoarthropathy has been reported to resolve after a thoracotomy even if the cancer has not been resected. Treatment is with anti-inflammatory drugs. The use of bisphosphate pamidronate has been reported to give good relief. Successful resection of the tumor leads to a regression of hypertrophic pulmonary osteoarthropathy.

Other rare paraneoplastic syndromes include hyperthyroidism (usually with squamous cell tumor), gynecomastia, and pigmentation associated with α- and β-melanocyte stimulation. Somatostatin release mimicking a pancreatic tumor has also been described. Hyperglycemia, hypoglycemia, galactorrhea, and growth hormone excess are some of the other rarer endocrine manifestations of the paraneoplastic syndrome.

Fever, weight loss, and anemia may be observed as the presenting features in some patients with an underlying cancer of the lung. They are considered by many as paramalignant.

Neurological Syndromes

Paraneoplastic syndromes with neurological features are most often met with in small cell cancer of the lung. The frequency of their occurrence varies; some workers estimate the frequency of any of these neurological syndromes at close to 5%. Neurological symptoms may precede the diagnosis of SCLC by months and at times as much as 2 years, the mean interval being about 8 months.

The most common neurological paraneoplastic feature is a peripheral neuropathy. It is most often a sensory neuropathy that could be painful; occasionally, a sensory motor neuropathy may occur. Other neurological syndromes include the Lambert-Eaton myasthenic syndrome, encephalomyelopathy, cerebellar degeneration, autonomic neuropathy, and impaired vision due to autoantibodies in the serum against a specific subset of retinal neurons.

Paraneoplastic syndromes are thought to be immune-mediated because a number of autoantibodies have been identified. Two important autoantibodies that have been shown to be associated with SCLC are antinuclear neuronal antibody I (ANNA I) and ANNA II. Another recently described autoantibody termed CRMP-5 has also been found to be associated with SCLC and thymomas. An anti-Purkinje antibody (anti-Yo) has been recently identified; it is found to be associated in patients with ovarian cancer and breast cancer. These autoantibodies may predict the nature of the neoplasm but do not identify the nature of the paraneoplastic syndrome. More than one autoantibody may be present in a patient with SCLC.

In a review of 162 sequential patients with a positive ANNA I, 88% were found to develop lung cancer most of which were SCLCs. In the vast majority of these cases, the diagnosis of SCLC was made within 6 months of the manifestation of the neurological syndrome; in a small minority it occurred later. Most of these patients (90%) had limited-stage disease confined to the lung and mediastinum. In another study, ANNA antibodies were again associated with limited-stage disease, good response to therapy, and longer survival than patients who had SCLC without ANNA I autoantibodies.

It is important to note that in patients who present with a paraneoplastic neurological syndrome due to an underlying SCLC, the mitotic lesion may not be identified by the initial investigational workup. A careful high-resolution computed tomography (HRCT) of the chest is therefore imperative, particularly in smokers when neurological features compatible with a paraneoplastic syndrome are present. A search for autoantibodies described above should be made if the required facilities are available. Positron emission tomography (PET) scan is also advised; a positive PET scan may help to locate and identify the lesion, facilitating biopsy and allowing confirmation.

The Lambert-Eaton myasthenic syndrome is most commonly observed in association with SCLC. About 50% of patients with the Lambert-Eaton myasthenic syndrome have an underlying malignancy, the majority of these malignancies being SCLCs. The overall incidence of this syndrome in SCLC is reported to be about 2–4%.

The syndrome is characterized by proximal muscle weakness, depressed tendon reflexes, and autonomic disturbances and is related to an impaired release of acetylcholine at the motor nerve endings. This syndrome is associated with allotypes Gm2 and HLA-B8 and precedes the diagnosis of lung cancer by 8 months to 2 years.

The Lambert-Eaton myasthenic syndrome has been strongly associated with antibodies against P/Q type presynaptic voltage-gated calcium channels of peripheral cholinergic nerve endings. These autoantibodies block the release of acetylcholine at nerve endings and are present in over 90% of patients with the Lambert-Eaton syndrome. The same antibodies have also been identified in 25% of patients with SCLC who do not have Lambert-Eaton myasthenic syndrome. Diagnosis of Lambert-Eaton syndrome is based on the clinical features together with characteristic electromyography (EMG) findings.

Treatment of the cancer often induces remission of this syndrome. The use of acetylcholine esterase inhibitors has very limited value, the response to the drug often being absent or poor.

■ THE ASSOCIATION OF VENOUS THROMBOSIS WITH LUNG CANCER

Venous thrombosis and thrombophlebitis migrans can antedate the appearance of an adenocarcinoma of the lung. If these occur in a middle-aged or elderly smoker without obvious cause, a careful physical examination and basic screening tests for an underlying lung cancer are advisable.

Venous thrombosis also often complicates the natural history of an established lung cancer. The reason for the hypercoagulable state responsible for venous thrombosis in underlying malignancies (including lung cancer) is not known. Venous thrombosis associated with an underlying malignancy is difficult to control and may extend in spite of anticoagulants. The American College of Chest Physicians has opined that low molecular weight heparin is superior to the use of oral anticoagulants in treatment of venous thrombosis occurring in patients with malignant disease. Two recent studies showed that apixaban and rivaroxaban were effective in preventing venous thrombosis in patients with cancer at high risk for thrombosis.

■ DIAGNOSTIC ASSESSMENT AND STAGING

Diagnostic assessment and staging are essential prerequisites for the management of lung cancers **(Table 9)**. There are three objectives that must be kept in mind. First, to establish a definite diagnosis of lung cancer, second to determine the histological cell type of lung cancer, and third to determine the degree of dissemination, both with regard to local and metastatic spread. Unnecessary investigations should be avoided in patients with obvious advanced disseminated disease unsuitable for either surgery or chemotherapy. Investigations should also be kept to a minimum in elderly people or in patients with advanced disease caused by a cell-type unlikely to respond to systemic therapy. A balanced assessment is necessary before planning management.

A careful history and a meticulous physical examination is the first requisite. No routine investigation

Table 9: Diagnostic assessment of lung cancer.
• A careful history and a meticulous physical examination
• Radiography of chest
• Sputum cytology
• HRCT of the chest
• PET study
• Bronchoscopy
• Biopsy:
– Transbronchial via fiberoptic bronchoscope
– Endobronchial ultrasound-guided biopsy
– CT-guided biopsy
– Mediastinoscopic biopsy (rare)
– Video-assisted thoracoscopic biopsy (rare)

will, for example, pick up a firm gland palpable between the two heads of the sternomastoid muscle or in the supraclavicular fossa, or diagnose a slight ptosis with a smaller pupil on the affected side due to an early Horner's syndrome from involvement of the sympathetic trunk. Again, no investigation will detect a monophonic wheeze due to partial obstruction of a large airway, or detect a pleural rub, or detect clubbing with early pulmonary osteoarthropathy, or diagnose some of the neurological paraneoplastic syndromes associated with lung cancer. The importance of a thorough physical examination cannot be overemphasized.

Radiology

The chest X-ray is usually abnormal by the time symptoms appear. Radiographic abnormalities on chest X-ray that are likely to be missed are briefly mentioned below.

Obstruction to a Large Airway (Fig. 22)

Lung cancers most often occur in the central airways. The earliest sign of large airways obstruction is obstructive emphysema of the involved lobe or lung best picked up on an expiratory film. Subsequent to this there will be shrinkage of a lobe or lung as judged by a loss of lung volume with a displaced fissure or an elevated dome of the diaphragm. Complete endobronchial obstruction will

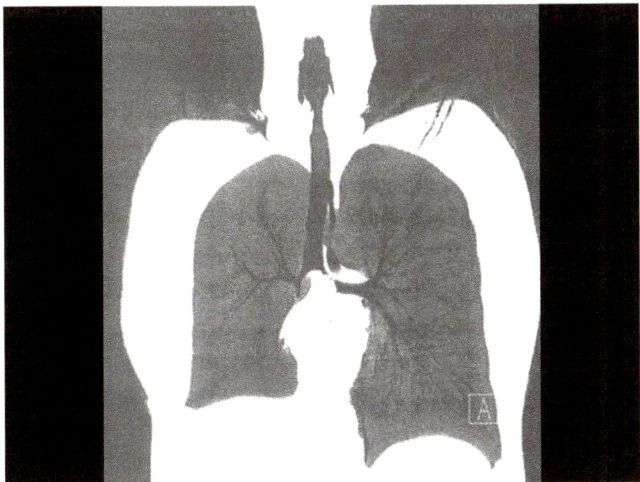

Fig. 22: Coronal computed tomography reconstruction reveals a subcarinal mass lesion causing encasement of the right lower lobe bronchus with resultant right lower lobe collapse and consolidation. There is extension of the lesion to involve the left lower lobe bronchus which is significantly narrowed by the mass lesion.

manifest as a collapse of a lobe. A left lower lobe collapse can easily be missed on an X-ray because it lies behind the heart. An abnormal hilum (an absent lower leash of vessels when the left lower lobe is collapsed or an upward shift of the hilum when an upper lobe collapses) should suggest the diagnosis.

A Hilar Pathology

A mass in the hilar region may be difficult to detect when it is small because of the superimposition of the hilar vessels. An asymmetry in size between the two hilar shadows or a difference in the densities of the two shadows should arouse suspicion.

Small Peripheral Nodule

About 30–35% of lung cancers present as a peripheral lesion. A nodule must be at least 1 cm in size before it is visualized on chest X-ray. Even then it may be difficult or impossible to recognize if it is situated behind a rib, behind the heart or in the costophrenic space.

Lung Cancer against a Background of Other Lung Diseases

Lung cancer developing in a patient with asbestosis, or in interstitial pulmonary fibrosis or in systemic sclerosis (all of which have a greater incidence of lung cancer) may be difficult to detect on a radiological examination of the chest.

Sputum Cytology

Sputum cytology is a simple, inexpensive useful test in the diagnosis of lung cancer. It should always be availed of in the presence of cough with sputum. If a bronchoscopy is done the bronchoalveolar lavage (BAL) fluid should also always be sent for cytological study. Sputum cytology is generally not positive when the disease presents as an isolated peripheral nodule. Further discussion on sputum cytology is given later in this section.

High-resolution Computed Tomography of Chest

Any suspicion of bronchogenic carcinoma on radiography of the chest necessitates an HRCT of the chest. HRCT chest provides fuller detailed information not only in relation to the tumor but also about the presence or absence of obvious local spread.

Bronchoscopy

Bronchoscopy provides direct visualization of the tumor arising in the central airways. It allows a biopsy that will help determine cell type. Bronchoscopy is also important to help evaluate the patient for surgery. A tumor arising within a lobar bronchus is fit to be removed by a lobectomy. However, if the tumor extends into the main bronchus, a pneumonectomy is the answer provided the tumor is more than 1 cm away from the carina. A spread of the tumor to mediastinal structures is at times evident by the widening and fixity of the carina due to involvement of the subcarinal lymph glands, or by the presence of inward pressure on the lateral wall of the bronchus or trachea by enlarged paratracheal glands. These bronchoscopic findings often denote unresectability.

Positron Emission Tomography Study

Positron emission tomography study when available is becoming a part of the protocol for both the diagnostic assessment and staging of lung cancers. Its usefulness is discussed later in this chapter.

Biopsy

A confirmed diagnosis of lung cancer (except in obvious advanced disease where any specific therapy is of no use) requires histopathological proof and cytological examination.

Biopsy of a tumor in the central airways is through a fiberoptic bronchoscope. A peripherally situated "nodule" within the lung is best approached through a CT-guided biopsy. A percutaneous aspiration needle biopsy gives a poor yield and may give misleading results. A core biopsy of a peripheral nodule has a diagnostic yield of 80–90% for a single sample and a yield of 95% for two or three samples.

Rarely, a mediastinoscopic biopsy or video-assisted thoracoscopic biopsy may be needed to confirm a diagnosis or to establish the presence and degree of dissemination.

■ SOLITARY PULMONARY NODULE

The presence of a solitary pulmonary nodule (SPN) on a plain X-ray of the chest often poses a problem in management **(Fig. 23)**. Is the nodule benign or malignant? That is the question!

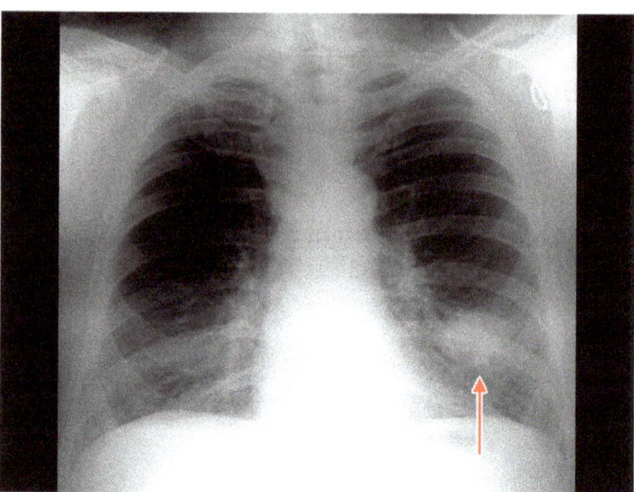

Fig. 23: Solitary pulmonary nodule. Plain X-ray of the chest reveals a pulmonary nodule in the left lower lobe. The whiskered outline is highly suggestive of a malignancy.

An SPN is defined as a single small (<30 mm) fairly well circumscribed lesion that is completely surrounded by lung parenchyma. Patients are usually asymptomatic and typically there are no other abnormal imaging features, i.e. no evidence of mediastinal or hilar adenopathy, no pleural effusion or atelectasis. More often than not, an SPN is discovered fortuitously on chest X-ray done as a routine health check. An HRCT of the chest may reveal an SPN not evident on X-ray of the chest.

Radiologically, a solitary lesion less than 30 mm is considered a nodule and a lesion more than 30 mm is considered a mass lesion. The distinction is important. When patients present with a SPN, the evaluation is geared to assess the probability of malignancy. This involves a planned CT scan surveillance and as and when necessary a nonsurgical or surgical biopsy.

In contrast, when a nodule or a mass lesion causes symptoms or is associated with other imaging abnormalities (e.g. mediastinal or hilar adenopathy) the work-up is for a suspected cancer. An isolated mass lesion (>30 mm) without any other imaging abnormality warrants a biopsy or surgical excision.

Differential Diagnosis

An SPN may be due to several causes. **Table 10** lists the causes of an SPN more commonly met with in clinical practice. **Table 11** illustrates the vast differential diagnosis.

Table 10: Common causes of solitary nodule detected by chest radiography.
• Metastasis • Primary bronchial carcinoma • Tuberculosis • Abscess • Pneumonia (localized) • Bronchial carcinoid • Hamartoma

Table 11: Uncommon causes of solitary nodule detected by chest radiography.

• Lymphoma
• Bronchogenic cyst
• Pulmonary infarct
• Nocardial infection
• Wegener's granulomatosis
• Rheumatoid nodule
• Hydatid cyst
• Arteriovenous aneurysm
• Cryptogenic organising pneumonia
• Sarcoid
• Foreign body
• Rarer tumors:
  – Fibroma
  – Leiomyoma
  – Papilloma
  – Chondroma

The prevalence of different etiologies in different studies varies, depending on the age, ethnicity, geography, and the smoking habits of the patient group under study. Surprisingly, contrary to expectations, screening studies of smokers who are at high risk of malignancy suggest that the vast majority of SPNs identified on an HRCT of the chest are benign. In the Pan-Canadian Early Detection of Lung Cancer and the British Columbia Cancer Agency Studies, among the 12,029 nodules found, only 144 (1%) were malignant.

An SPN may be malignant or benign.

Malignant

Common causes of a malignant SPN are a primary lung cancer, a metastatic lesion, and a carcinoid.

- *Primary lung cancer*: The most common primary lung cancer presenting as an SPN is histologically an adenocarcinoma followed by a squamous cell carcinoma and large cell carcinoma. An adenocarcinoma and large cell carcinoma more often present as a peripheral nodule; a squamous cell carcinoma is more often a central lesion rather than a peripheral one. Rarely, a small cell carcinoma as also a primary extranodal lymphoma may present as a SPN.
- *Metastatic cancer*: Most metastatic lesions are multiple; occasionally a metastatic lesion may present as an SPN. This is particularly observed in patients with a carcinoma of the breast, colon, kidney testicle as also in patients with a malignant melanoma; a metastatic pulmonary lesion may however be secondary to other primary sites.
- *Carcinoid tumors*: Carcinoid tumors are generally endobronchial but may present as an SPN in about 20% of cases. Rarer tumors listed in **Table 11** may occasionally present as a SPN.

Benign Causes

- *Infections*: Infectious granulomas cause the majority of isolated circumscribed pulmonary nodules. In countries where tuberculosis is endemic, it is unquestionably the most common cause. Histoplasmosis and other specific fungal causes are important in parts of the world where these infections are endemic. Granulomas may or may not show calcification.

  Occasionally, a localized pneumonia or abscess or a single hydatid cyst may present as an SPN. Rarely, a fully calcified SPN may be due to dirofilariasis, because of the granulomatous response to the larvae of the dirofilaria within the lung.
- *Benign tumors*: The most common benign tumor presenting as an SPN is a hamartoma, which constitutes about 10% of benign nodules in the lung. They generally present in middle age and are histologically heterogeneous containing cartilage, fat, muscle myxomatous tissues, and fibroblastic tissue. The characteristic CT appearance (thin slices <2 mm) shows areas of fat attenuation with areas of calcification which is diagnostic of a hamartoma.

  The classic popcorn calcification described in hamartomas occurs only in 10% of patients. Hamartomas grow very slowly over years and for all practical purposes do not turn malignant.

  Less common benign neoplasms are fibromas, leiomyomas, hemangiomas, amyloidoma, and plasmacytoma.
- *Vascular causes*: The most common vascular cause is an arteriovenous malformation, which is common in hereditary hemorrhagic telangiectasia but which

can also be idiopathic. A contrast enhanced CT scan usually demonstrates a feeding artery and vein. A biopsy should not be attempted for the risk of severe bleeding.

- *Uncommon causes*: There are a number of uncommon causes; these include benign granulomatosis with polyangiitis (formerly Wegener's granulomatosis), sarcoidosis, rheumatoid disease, rounded atelectasis, cryptogenic organizing pneumonia, and pulmonary infarction.

An Approach to the Assessment of a Solitary Pulmonary Nodule

History and Clinical Examination

It is always best to start with a carefully taken history and a detailed physical examination, an art and a science increasingly being relegated to the background in modern medicine.

A history of past tuberculosis, a recent chest infection or a history of past malignancy is important. Malignancy can recur after several years; this is particularly so for example, with breast cancer, a seminoma, and a hypernephroma. It is important to ask for symptoms of systemic illness in the form of fever, or weight loss, or other systemic features associated with some of the etiological factors listed in the **Tables 10 and 11**. History of recent travel to parts of the world where fungal infection is endemic may point to an underlying coccidioidomycosis as the cause of SPN. On clinical examination, one should specifically look out for peripheral lymphadenopathy, hepatosplenomegaly or physical signs of infection or underlying vasculitides. A significant polymorphonuclear leukocytosis or an erythrocyte sedimentation rate more than 50 mm in the first hour suggests an infective or nonmalignant etiology. A strongly positive Mantoux test is in favor of a tuberculous granuloma though it does not exclude malignancy, particularly in an older man or woman who is a smoker.

Review of Previous Radiographs of the Chest

Review of previous radiographs or radiograph is perhaps the single most important investigation to obtain. A lesion that is unchanged in size over 2 years is almost certainly not malignant and a nodule unchanged for over 1 year has a higher chance of being benign. The most common cause of a nodule that remains unchanged over 2 years is a

healed granuloma. In parts of the world where tuberculosis has a high prevalence rate, the etiology of the granuloma is invariably tuberculosis.

HRCT of the Chest with Contrast (Figs. 24 to 26)

An HRCT of the chest gives information often not attainable on radiography. It is therefore an absolutely necessary investigation both for initial diagnostic purpose and for a future follow-up. An HRCT chest defines the nodule more accurately, whether solid with a homogenous density, or part-solid, or nonsolid. The latter is a ground glass density which may have a solid component. It defines its exact size, its margins whether smooth and well-defined or irregular. An HRCT may reveal the presence of other nodules within the lung not visible on radiography, or the presence of undetected mediastinal or hilar adenopathy.

An SPN may be calcified; an HRCT defines the nature, pattern, and extent of calcification, which is often different in benign and malignant lesions.

If the presence of multiple nodules on the CT with or without mediastinal adenopathy suggests metastatic disease, a search for a primary through appropriate investigation and imaging studies is warranted.

Positron Emission Tomography Study (Figs. 27A and B)

The use of PET to help diagnose malignancy in an SPN has a further advantage that it provides a diagnostic accuracy

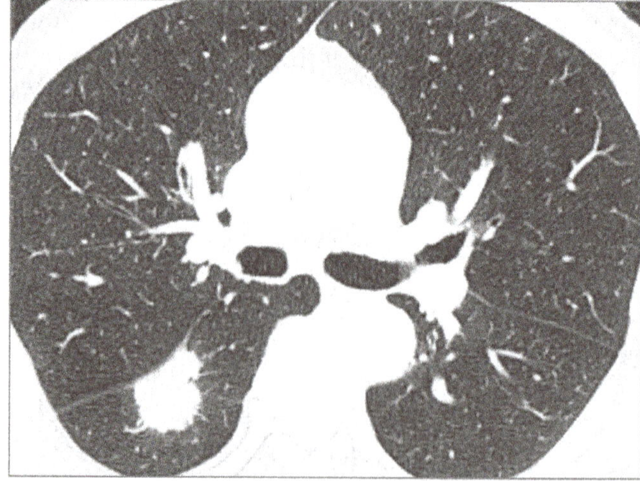

Fig. 24: Computed tomography scan in a middle aged smoker revealed a mass lesion in the right lower lobe with a whiskered margin. Fine-needle aspiration cytology (FNAC) revealed it to be a squamous cell carcinoma.

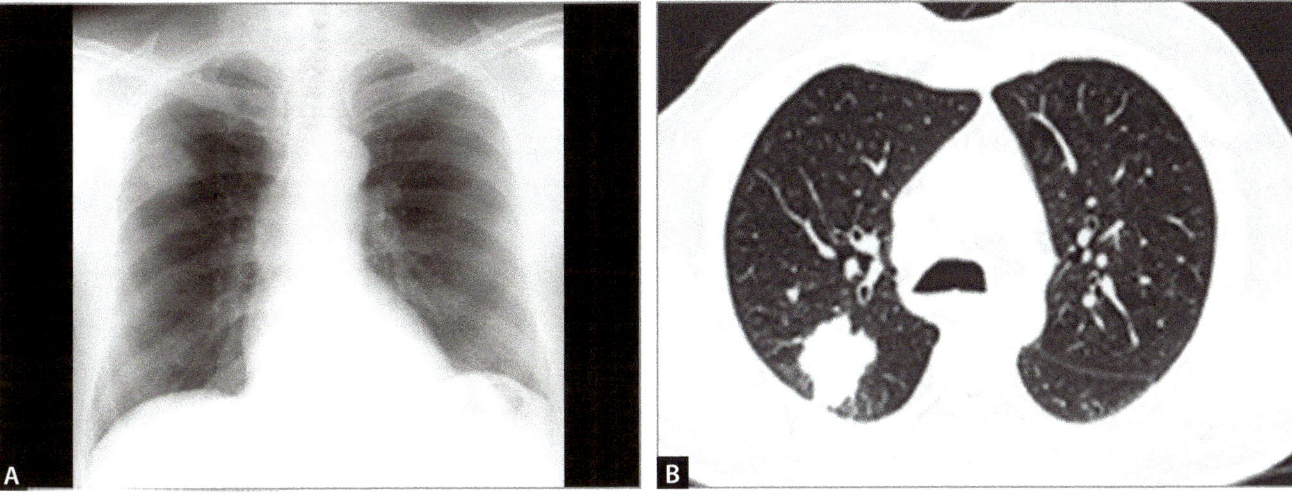

Figs. 25A and B: Solitary pulmonary nodule: (A) Chest X-ray demonstrates a lobulated mass lesion in the right upper lobe; (B) CT of chest demonstrates the mass lesion to have a mildly whiskered outline raising the possibility of a neoplasm. CT-guided biopsy revealed an adenocarcinoma.

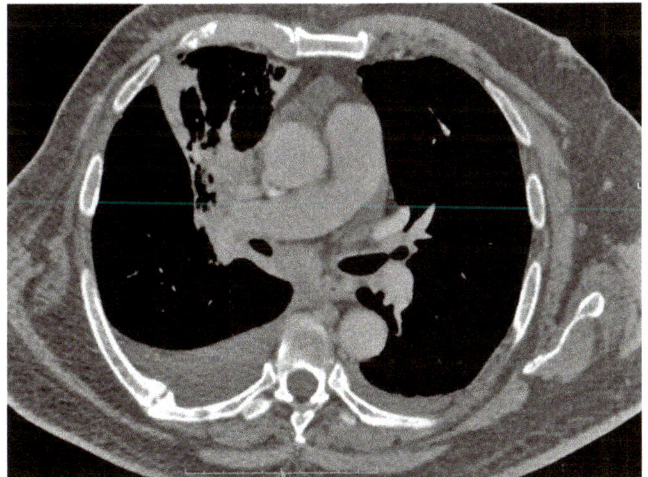

Fig. 26: Mass lesion in right parahilar region causing segmental atelectasis of middle lobe. Bilateral pleural effusions are seen.

of about 90% (sensitivity 90%, specificity 95%) in lesions more than 1 cm in size. The resolution limit of a nodule that can be evaluated through PET is 7–8 mm. An added advantage of the PET scan is its ability to detect occult metastatic disease, thereby changing the approach to management.

In most PET studies that assess sensitivity, standardized uptake value (SUV) more than 2.5 is typically used to distinguish SPNs that have a high probability of malignancy. In spite of the unquestionable value of PET studies, it must be noted that PET can give false-positive and false-negative findings.

False-positive findings occur with inflammatory and infectious conditions—tuberculous granulomas, sarcoidosis, pneumonia, and rheumatoid nodules. False-negative may occasionally occur with less metabolically active tumors—AIS, MIA, and mucinous adenocarcinoma. False-positives may also occur in patients with uncontrolled hyperglycemia. Very small lesions less than 8 mm, may occasionally not be picked up by PET because there needs to be a critical mass of metabolically active malignant cells for detection by PET.

Assessment of Risk of Malignancy in SPN

Assessment of risk is a vital important as management strategies are dependent on the assessment. The probability of malignancy should be assessed clinically or by qualitative predictive models. We prefer to do so clinically. There seems to be a good agreement between the probability of malignancy arrived at clinically or by the use of prediction models. Assessment should determine:

- Is there a low probability of malignancy? (<5%)
- Is there an intermediate probability of malignancy? (5–65%)
- Is there a high probability of malignancy? (>65 %).

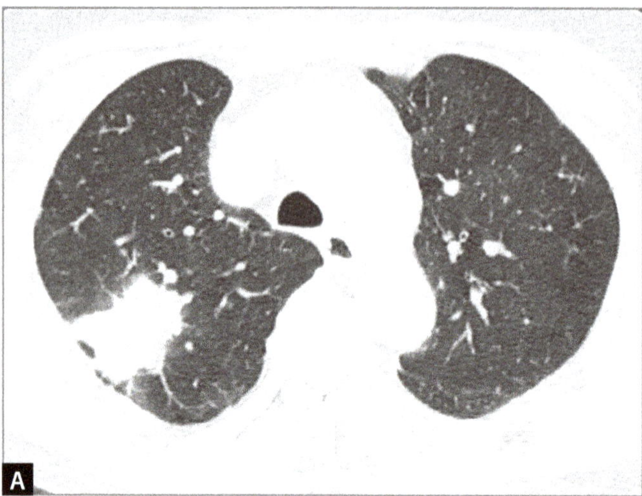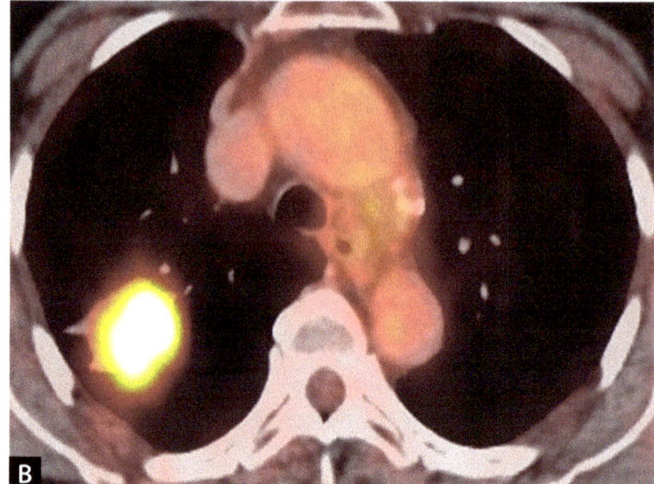

Figs. 27A and B: (A) Computed tomography of chest demonstrates a solitary pulmonary mass in the right upper lobe, fine-needle aspiration cytology revealed an adenocarcinoma; (B) PET-CT done for staging revealed markedly increased uptake. No other lesions demonstrated uptake indicating a Stage 1 lesion.

Clinical Assessment

- *Age*: The probability of malignancy increases with the patient's age. A study showed that the percentage of malignant SPN increased with age: 35–39 years—3%; 40-49 years—15%; 50-59 years—43%; more than 60 years—50%.
- The probability of malignancy is higher in current smokers and to a slightly lesser extent in those with a history of smoking.
- Other risk factors include family history of cancer, prior malignancy, asbestos exposure, and emphysema.
- *Size of the SPN*: Studies have consistently shown that the size of the SPN measured at its maximum diameter is an independent predictor for malignancy. The larger is the size, the greater is the risk.

  The increasing risk as per the increasing size of the tumor is given below:
  - Nodules less than 5 mm: less than 1%
  - Nodules 5–9 mm: 2-6%
  - Nodules 8–20 mm: 18%
  - Nodules >20 mm: >50%.
- *Attenuation*: Solid SPNs are dense and homogeneous on imaging. Subcentimeter nodules (<8 mm) are unlikely to be malignant. Subsolid nodules should be further assessed for the presence or absence of a solid component. The risk of malignancy is greater in subsolid lesions that have a large and newly developed solid component.
- *Growth*: HRCT is the method of choice to assess the growth. An SPN which has grown on serial imaging is at high risk for malignancy, necessitating biopsy or excision. A solid nodule which has been stable for 2 years and a subsolid nodule which has been stable for 5 years is likely to be benign and tissue biopsy can be avoided. It is obvious that every attempt should be made to obtain older imaging studies.
- *Border*: The risk of malignancy is lower when the border is smooth and higher in SPN with a scalloped border, an irregular border or a spiculated border.
- *Calcification*: Asymmetric or eccentric classification is suspicious of malignancy. Laminated (concentric), central or homogenous calcification suggests that the SPN is benign.
- *Location*: Although malignant nodules can occur in any lobe of the lung, in a study of over 7,000 nodules, two-thirds of the malignant nodules were located in the upper lobes.
- A positive PET scan with an SUV more than 2.5 has a high sensitivity for malignancy, though false-positives and false-negative scans can occur.

The risk for malignancy (low, intermediate, and high) can be assessed from the clinical and imaging features described above. The risk can also be assessed by quantitative predictive models. A full and simplified version of one model was derived using data collected from the Pan-Canadian Early Detection of Lung Cancer screening study and validated using data from the British Columbia Cancer Agency study. Predictors of cancer were identified in 2,961 patients with nodules found on first screening study. These included older age, female sex, family history of lung cancer, emphysema, larger nodule size, location of the nodule in the upper lobe, part-solid nodule type, and spiculation. The negative predictive value of this model was consistently high (99%), the sensitivity ranged from 60% to 86% when different cut-off thresholds were used. The probability of malignancy was calculated using the calculator.

Management Strategies

Once the risk for malignancy of an SPN in an individual patient has been properly stratified, management decisions can be taken with a fair degree of confidence.

- *Patients with adequate prior imaging*: This includes patients with prior imaging done and therefore allows proper assessment of growth or stability of the SPN.
    - *Growing nodule*: A nodule that has grown on serial imaging carries a high risk of malignancy. It should be evaluated pathologically with excision or biopsy.
    - *Stable nodule*: An SPN which is unchanged over 2 years or a subsolid nodule which is unchanged over 5 years is likely to be benign and does not need further revaluation. CT surveillance may be necessary in individual cases suspected of a low-grade adenocarcinoma.
- *Patients with no previous imaging available*:
    - *Solid nodules more than 8 mm*: When growth or stability cannot be determined, a consensus of opinion is given below.
        - A nodule that has a low probability (less than 5%) can be followed up by serial CT scans at 3 to 6 months, 9 to 12 months, 18 to 24 months provided the nodule remains unchanged.
        - A nodule with intermediate probability should be biopsied or excised if PET is positive. If PET is unavailable or indeterminate, the decision is individualized for each patient. Most clinicians would opt for a biopsy or surgical excision.
        - A nodule which has a high probability (> 65%) of being malignant is preferably excised. A PET is advisable but not absolutely necessary.
    - *Solid nodule less than 8 mm*: A solid nodule less than 8 mm should be followed by serial CT scans. If unchanged over 2 years, it is benign; if it grows it should be excised.
    - *For nodules less than 6 mm*: Routine CT follow-up is not required. A CT after 12 months is advisable in patients with a suspicious nodule morphology located in the upper lobe.
    - *For nodules more than 6 and less than 8 mm*: A CT follow-up at 6–12 months is advised. A CT at 18–24 months may also be done if the stability of the nodule is in question.
    - *Pure ground glass nodules*: Most ground glass nodules (also called nonsolid), SPNs more than 6 mm, should be followed up by serial CT scans. Many of these nodules resolve spontaneously. However, some grow and develop a solid component. This is suspicious of malignancy and necessitates biopsy or excision. Ground glass nodules which remain stable over a period of 5 years follow-up require no further observation.
    - *Part-solid nodules*: These nodules have a greater likelihood of malignancy. In patients with part-solid SPNs more than 6 mm, CT surveillance should be carried out at 3–6 months and then annually for 5 years. Nodules that are growing and have a growing solid component, or a solid component more than 8 mm are highly suspicious of malignancy and should be biopsied or excised.
- *Multiple nodules*: At times CT studies show multiple nodules. Prospective studies of patients during staging and evaluation of lung cancer have shown that most of these nodules are benign. However, benign and malignant nodules may coexist in the same patient. The risk of malignancy should be based on assessing the largest nodule.

The strategies outlined meet general consensus but are not sacrosanct.

There are some centers who to play safe would excise SPN more than 8 mm even if the probability of malignancy as judged by risk stratification is low. It is likely that this approach may result in excision of malignant lesions; it is equally likely that a number of unnecessary surgeries are performed to remove lesions which are benign and did not merit surgery.

■ STAGING OF LUNG CANCER

The Tumor Node Metastasis (TNM) Staging System for lung cancer is an internationally accepted system used to determine and characterize the extent of disease. The TNM system combines features of the tumor and its spread if present into disease stage groups that correlate with survival and optimize treatment. As yet treatment that best influences survival is surgery, and for this staging is vitally essential. One must make a distinction between clinical staging and pathological staging. The former is based solely on clinical examination and noninvasive imaging techniques. The latter depends on the study of histological material obtained either by invasive imaging studies or at the time of surgical resection. The invasive histological studies combined with clinical evaluation and staging allows a physician to stage the disease in its entirety. Also awareness of the histological cell type of lung cancer may enable the treating doctor to better understand the natural history of the disease. Despite the evolution of the staging system over several years that has helped optimize management, "the links between disease-stage and treatment have become weaker, because studies of stage-specific treatments were done at a time which predated the most sophisticated staging methods and clinical practice of the present".

Two facts need to be further borne in mind:

1. Two-thirds of patients with bronchogenic carcinoma at the time of diagnosis are inoperable. This may primarily be due to extrathoracic spread but could also be determined by age, very poor lung function or presence of serious comorbid conditions.
2. Staging investigations detailed below are applicable only to NSCLCs, because almost all SCLCs at the time of presentation have intrathoracic spread, chiefly to the mediastinal nodes or extrathoracic metastatic lesions or both.

Guidelines for staging have been published by the American College of Physicians, the American Thoracic Society and European Respiratory Society. These clinical guidelines, as expected, recommend that all patients have a careful history, detailed physical examination, basic blood chemistry, and a CT of the chest extending through the liver and adrenal glands.

Determining presence of tumor markers is not recommended. Pulmonary function tests are absolutely necessary when the tumor is deemed resectable. Ventilation perfusion scans may help in deciding for or against surgery in patients with impaired pulmonary functions.

TNM Staging Classification on Nonsmall Cell Lung Cancers

The TNM classification is based on the size, situation and local extension of the lung tumor, the presence or absence of regional lymph node involvement and if present the extent of nodal involvement, the presence or absence of distant metastasis. The classification first devised in 1975 and subsequently reviewed and upgraded in 1997 (from a database of 5319 patients assessed for surgery) remained unaltered in the sixth edition published in 2002. The classification is applicable to NSCLCs.

The sixth edition of the staging system was upgraded and the seventh edition was published in 2009. The seventh edition was based on the collected data on 68,463 patients with NSCLC registered or diagnosed from 1990 to 2000, whose records had adequate information for analyzing the tumor, node, metastasis classification. The T, N, and M descriptors were analyzed, and recommendations for changes in the seventh edition of the TNM classification were proposed based on observed differences in survival.

We now have the eighth edition of the staging system (2017). The revision is planned to incorporate new survival data accruing from advances in imaging techniques, clinical testing, and current treatment.

The database was from 90,041 patients and cases from an electronic data capture system developed by Cancer Research and Biostatistics (CRAB, 4,667 patients). Data from 70,967 patients with NSCLC were used to validate the prognostic value of this new TNM system.

The eighth edition is effective as of January 1, 2018 in the United States. However, outside of the United States, the Union for International Cancer Control (UICC) has implemented the eighth edition changes as of January 1, 2017 **(Table 12)**.

Results of Clinical Staging

The survival results are indeed dismal and have shown very little improvement in the last decade. Of the 100 patients diagnosed as NSCLC, close to 65% will be deemed inoperable. Inoperability will be based on the extent of disease and its spread based on clinical examination and on radiography of the chest and to a lesser extent on age, serious comorbid disease, and poor lung function. A further 10–15% who have a normal mediastinum on the chest X-ray will have mediastinal nodes on an HRCT of the chest or on a PET scan. In the majority, these nodes will be positive for malignancy. Finally, of the 25% operated upon, 20% will have a resectable tumor; in 5% the tumor will be inoperable on the table. Finally, of the 20% patients in whom the tumor is resected only 5% will survive for 5 years. A more dismal story in medicine or surgery is difficult to

Table 12: Descriptors and T and M categories of the eighth edition with seventh edition for comparison*.

Descriptor in 8th edition	N categories: 8th edition (7th edition)			
	Overall stage			
	N0	N1	N2	N3
T1a (≤ 1 cm)	**IA1** (IA)	**IIB** (IIA)	IIIA	IIIB
T1b (>1 to ≤ 2 cm)	**IA2** (IA)	**IIB** (IIA)	IIIA	IIIB
T1c (>2 to ≤ 3 cm)	**IA3** (IA)	**IIB** (IIA)	IIIA	IIIB
T2a (>3 to 4 cm)	IB	**IIB** (IIA)	IIIA	IIIB
T2b (>4 to 5 cm)	**IIA** (1B)	**IIB** (IIA)	IIIA	IIIB
T3 (>5 to 7 cm)	**IIB** (IIA)	**IIIA** (IIB)	**IIIB** (IIIA)	**IIIC** (IIIB)
T3 (>5 to 7 cm)	IIB	IIIA	**IIIB** (IIIA)	**IIIC** (IIIB)
T4 (>7 cm)	**IIIA** (IIB)	IIIA	**IIIB** (IIIA)	**IIIC** (IIIB)
T4 (> 7 cm)	**IIIA** (IIB)	IIIA	**IIIB** (IIIA)	**IIIC** (IIIB)
T2a (>3 to 4 cm)	**IB** (IIB)	**IIB** (IIIA)	IIIA	IIIB
T2b (>4 to 5 cm)	**IIA** (IIB)	**IIB** (IIIA)	IIIA	IIIB
T4 (>7 cm)	IIIA	IIIA	IIIB	**IIIC** (IIIB)
M1a (Intrathoracic)	**IVA** (IV)	**IVA** (IV)	**IVA** (IV)	**IVA** (IV)
M1b (Single extrathoracic)	**IVA** (IV)	**IVA** (IV)	**IVA** (IV)	**IVA** (IV)
M1c (Multiple metastatic)	**IVB** (IV)	**IVB** (IV)	**IVB** (IV)	**IVB** (IV)

* Where there is a change, the resultant stage groupings for the eighth edition are in bold, and the stage in the seventh edition is given in parenthesis. M1b is single extrathoracic lesion; M1c is multiple metastatic lesions; N1 is ipsilateral peribronchial and/or hilar lymph nodes; N2 is ipsilateral mediastinal and/or subcarinal lymph nodes; N3 is contralateral mediastinal and/or hilar, as well as any supraclavicular lymph nodes.

Source: Goldstraw P, Chansky K, Crowley J, et al. The IASLC Lung Cancer Staging. J Thorac Oncol. 2016;11:39. Table used with the permission of Elsevier Inc. All rights reserved.

recount. The above scenario prevails in most centers of developing countries. In highly specialized centers the 5-year survival rate has now improved to 12–15%.

Staging for Small Cell Lung Tumors

The TNM staging described earlier when applied to SCLC makes no difference to the prognosis. The Veterans Administration Staging System categorized SCLC into "limited disease" and "extensive disease". Limited disease is limited to one hemithorax and ipsilateral cervical nodes. Extensive disease is one that has spread beyond the hemithorax—to the contralateral hilar mediastinal, cervical nodes, or to a malignant pleural effusion or to distant extrathoracic metastatic sites.

Extrathoracic Staging of Nonsmall Cell Lung Cancers (Table 13)

Examination may help detection of obvious disease, as with the presence of palpable nodes, bony tenderness,

Table 13: Steps for extrathoracic staging of nonsmall cell lung cancer.

1	Clinical examination
2	Biochemical examination
3	Relevant blood tests for paraneoplastic syndromes if clinically suspected
4	CT of the chest which includes the upper abdomen (with contrast)
5	Isotope bone scan only in the presence of musculoskeletal symptoms
6	CT brain
7	PET scan of the whole body

and the presence of a firm or even nodular enlarged liver. Neurological symptoms may point to metastatic spread to the nervous system or to paraneoplastic neurological syndromes. Biochemical examination of blood may show important findings such as hypercalcemia and hyponatremia. Hyponatremia occurs almost exclusively in SCLCs. Hypercalcemia may indicate bone metastasis or may be due to a paraneoplastic syndrome caused by a parathyroid hormone like peptide.

Organ screening of the liver and the adrenals is important and is provided by a CT of the chest which includes the upper abdomen. HRCT studies may reveal the presence of asymptomatic metastasis in the liver, adrenal, bone, abdominal lymph glands, and the brain in some patients. It must, however, be stated that the result of CT scans of the brain and liver are usually normal in patients who have neither organ-specific features nor any nonspecific features such as fever, weight loss, altered liver functions, suggesting metastatic spread to these organs.

Isotope bone scans are important to detect bony involvement in the presence of bone pains but many clinicians do not advise bone scans in the absence of musculoskeletal symptoms. This is because as many as 40% of bone scans may prove falsely positive, showing thereby the poor specificity of the test.

The role of PET in the evaluation of patients with known or suspected cancer is assuming increasing importance. Several studies have shown that PET may reveal unsuspected mediastinal or extrathoracic spread, so that thoracotomy is avoided in about 1 in 5 patients. Cancer cells have a high rate of glycolysis and an increased uptake of glucose by the cells because of the increased number of transport proteins compared to normal cells. The PET tracer 18-fluorodeoxyglucose (18-FDG) is therefore selectively taken up by the neoplastic cells and accumulates within them. PET has been shown to detect distant metastatic lesions in 10–15% of patients who are thought to be operable and alter management in 40% of cases. A study that compared whole body PET scan to CT chest, CT brain, bone scan or magnetic resonance imaging (MRI) in staging lung cancer showed that PET correctly and accurately staged 83% of patients with NSCLC compared to pathological findings. Not only did PET scan pick up distant metastasis, not picked up by other techniques, but it also showed that lesions which were considered suspicious by other techniques but which were not PET-positive, were benign. It must however be remembered that PET scan may show false-positive reports in 10–15% of patients. It is therefore absolutely essential that a biopsy of a distant metastasis (positive on a PET scan) is obtained to decide whether the patient has truly inoperable disease.

To summarize, extrathoracic staging for metastatic lesions to start with requires a careful history, physical examination, and a study of biochemical and other basic parameters. An HRCT of the chest which is essential for intrathoracic staging should include the upper abdomen so as to view possible metastasis in the liver and adrenals. PET scan of the whole body is the best investigation to detect occult metastasis. Since false-positive results are found in 10–15% of patients, biopsy of a metastatic site deemed positive by a PET study should be done for confirmation. A brain CT is not recommended as a routine screening test. However, 1–2% of asymptomatic patients have brain metastasis who would otherwise be operable. For this reason many specialized oncology centers insist on a head scan as a necessary staging investigation. Bone scanning is advised only in patients with musculoskeletal pains or in patients with nonspecific symptoms such as weight loss and fever. Bone scans have a high false-positive rate; a single focal abnormality on a bone scan necessitates confirmation by CT or by a biopsy of the area concerned.

Intrathoracic Staging (Tables 14 and 15)

Clinical history and examination will identify mediastinal spread from the presence of pressure symptoms such as the SVC syndrome, Horner's syndrome, presence of dysphagia, and hoarseness of the voice caused by recurrent laryngeal nerve palsy. An HRCT of the chest is indispensable for intrathoracic staging (**Figs. 28 to 31**). The diagnosis of the primary malignant tumor and

Table 14: Approach to biopsy procedures to establish both staging and cell type in lung cancer.

Types of lesion	Investigation of choice
Peripheral nodule	CT-guided core biopsy
Large central mass	Bronchoscopy
Endobronchial malignant tumor	Biopsy through fiberoptic bronchoscope
Mediastinal adenopathy	CT-guided or endobronchial ultrasound-guided transbronchial biopsy
Paratracheal, subcarinal, hilar nodes	Transbronchial needle aspiration

Table 15: Steps for intrathoracic staging.

1	Clinical history and examination; sputum cytology
2	Evaluation of a pleural effusion
3	HRCT of the chest with contrast
4	Biopsy of the tumor and/or mediastinal adenopathy
5	PET scan

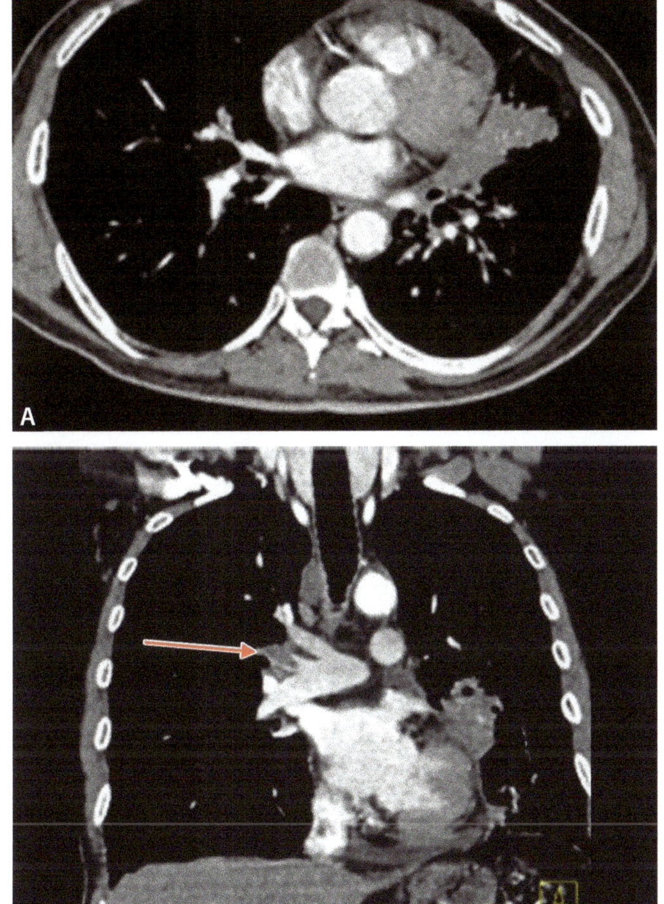

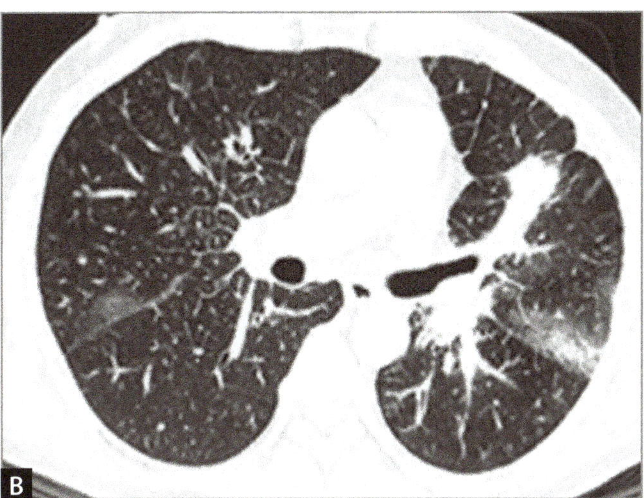

Figs. 28A to C: (A) Computed tomography scan demonstrates a mass lesion in the left lingula flush with the pericardium; (B) Lung window demonstrates irregular mass lesion with adjacent lymphatic thickening as well as lymphatic thickening in opposite lung. This appearance of smooth lymphatic thickening without distortion of lung parenchyma is classical for lymphangitis carcinomatosis; (C) Contrast CT demonstrates a thrombus in the right upper lobe pulmonary vessels representing thrombi.

its histopathology can be made by a biopsy through a fiberoptic bronchoscope for an endobronchial tumor within the larger bronchi or by a CT-guided biopsy of a more peripherally placed lesion. A centrally arising tumor may however be inaccessible for a biopsy. The presence of mediastinal pressure symptoms or just the presence of large mediastinal lymphadenopathy on a posteroanterior and lateral radiograph of the chest points to inoperability. Further evaluation is then unnecessary.

Mediastinal adenopathy in a suspected lung cancer should be sampled for malignancy through a CT-guided biopsy. With the increasing availability of endobronchial ultrasound (EBUS) sampling of mediastinal nodes and CT imaging, the need for mediastinoscopy for patients with lung cancer has lessened markedly. However, many centers still consider mediastinoscopy a useful diagnostic staging technique. It needs to be

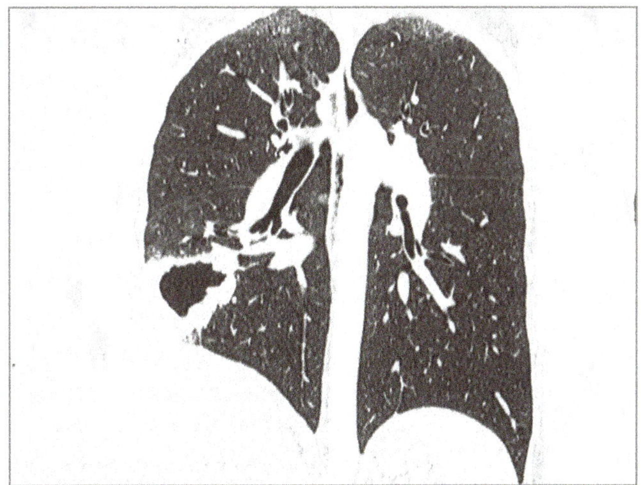

Fig. 29: Coronal CT image of the chest demonstrates cavitating right lower lobe neoplasm and mild elevation of the right hemidiaphragm.

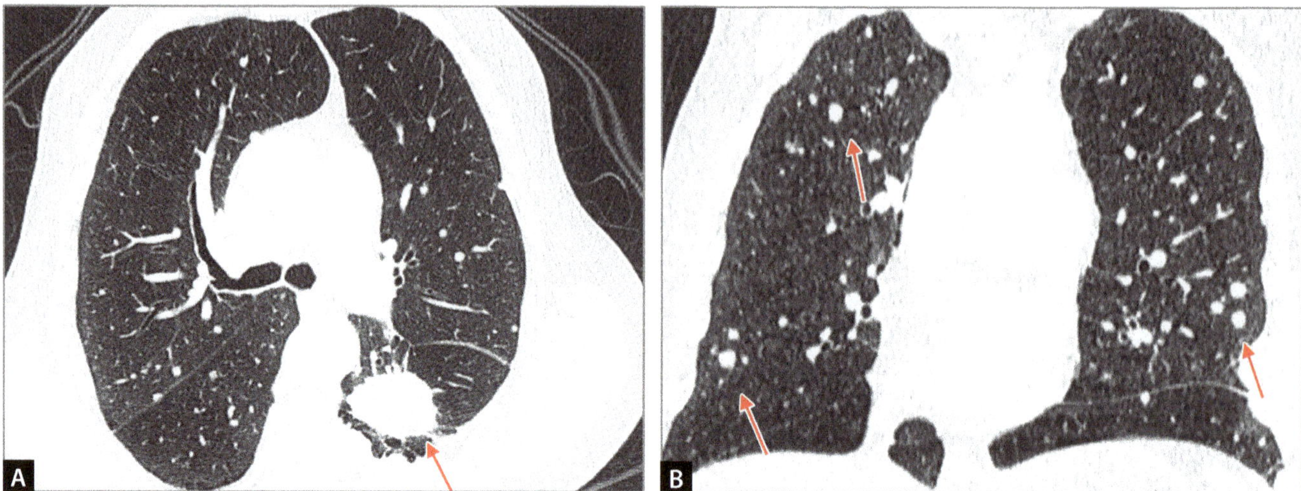

Figs. 30A and B: (A) Non small-cell carcinoma. Chest CT demonstrates a large irregular mass in the left lower lobe with irregular margins representing primary lung neoplasm; (B) Chest CT demonstrates multiple pulmonary nodules representing metastatic deposits.

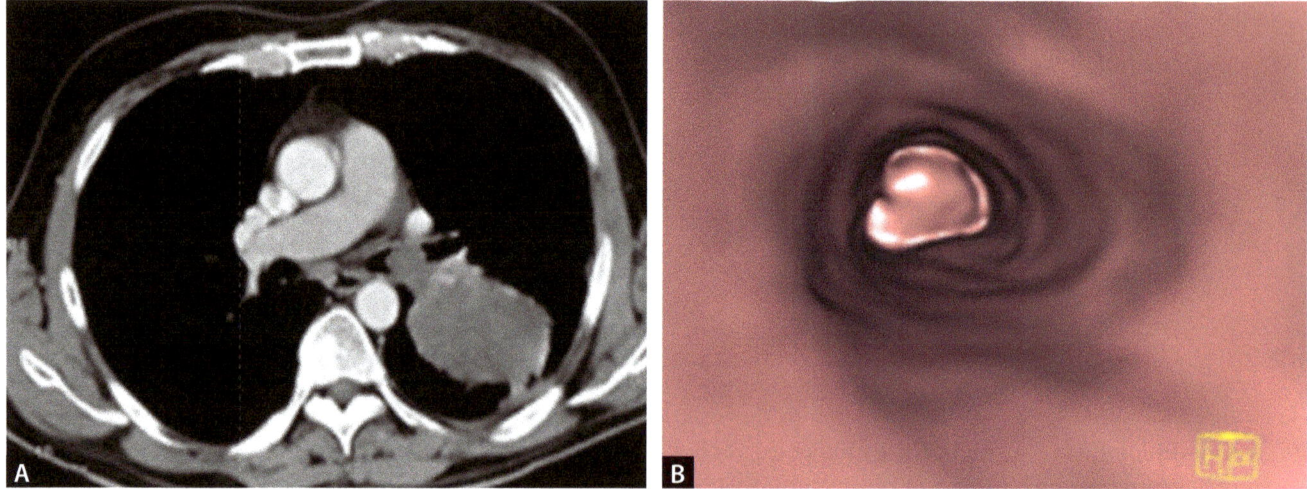

Figs. 31A and B: (A) Large left upper lobe mass lesion with left intrabronchial extension; (B) Intrabronchial extension demonstrated on virtual bronchoscopy.

pointed out that the subaortic nodes (level 5) and para-aortic nodes (level 6), both of which are situated in the aortopulmonary window, cannot be assessed by standard cervical mediastinoscopy.

A pleural effusion in a proven lung cancer is due to metastatic spread, lymphatic obstruction, lymphangitis carcinomatosis, and rarely due to medical causes unrelated to cancer. Pleural aspiration, repeated if necessary, reveals mitotic cells within the pleural fluid in only 75% of cases. Direct proof of malignancy can only be obtained in these instances by a video-assisted thoracoscopy which enables the thoracoscopist to view the pleura and take multiple biopsies. It is perhaps important to do so, as a nonmalignant etiology of a pleural effusion should allow surgery to proceed in an otherwise operable patient.

High-resolution CT contrast study is essential in evaluating the extent of pulmonary disease, identifying small pulmonary nodules, detection of pleural involvement, and detecting mediastinal lymphadenopathy. HRCT chest should include the upper abdomen to view possible metastasis to the liver and adrenal glands.

An MRI can occasionally be more accurate in detecting invasion of mediastinal structures and involvement of the diaphragm, spine, and spinal cord. On the whole it does not have significant advantage over HRCT contrast study of the chest.

Rarely a video-assisted thoracoscopic biopsy may be necessary to confirm or refute the presence of malignant disease.

Positron Emission Tomography (Figs. 32A and B)

The value of PET in detecting distant metastasis for extrathoracic staging has already been commented upon. It is equally valuable for intrathoracic staging. PET scans detect focal pulmonary lesions with a sensitivity of 96% and specificity of 88% and has an accuracy of 94% in lesions 10 mm in size or more. It however allows for a much poorer spatial resolution so that the anatomic assessment compared to a CT is inadequate. It should be remembered that false-positive results are observed in 10–15% of patients. False-positive results have been reported in tuberculosis, fungal infection, sarcoidosis, inflammatory disorders such as cryptogenic organizing pneumonia and rheumatoid nodules. False-negative reports can occur in alveolar cell carcinoma, carcinoids, and in tumors less than 1 cm in size. Hyperglycemia from whatever cause can interfere with 18-FDG uptake and can result in a false-negative scan.

A meta-analysis of the literature reveals that PET scans can identify mediastinal lymph node metastasis with an appropriate sensitivity of 90% and specificity of 85%. CT scan staging of the mediastinal lymph nodes has shown false-positive and false-negative results of about 30–40%, PET scans compare more favorably to CT scans in this regard. PET scans have also been shown to decrease nodal staging as initially determined by CT scan. The value of PET scan in both intrathoracic and extrathoracic lung cancer cannot be denied. PET study is therefore today an integral investigation in the diagnosis and staging of NSCLC.

In the final analysis, the investigation or the test chosen to diagnose and stage lung cancer depends on the site of the tumor in the lung and the degree and nature of spread. The test chosen should be one that gives the most information with the least risk.

A tumor presenting as a peripheral nodule is best diagnosed and staged through a CT-guided core biopsy as has been mentioned earlier. A biopsy through a fiberoptic bronchoscope has a very poor yield except when the CT shows a bronchus leading into the peripheral nodule (*see* **Table 14**).

A tumor presenting as a large central mass is often easily diagnosed by bronchoscopy. An endobronchial malignant tumor is diagnosed with 100% accuracy by a biopsy through a fiberoptic bronchoscope. The visual extent of the tumor, its relation to the carina, the fixity or otherwise of the carina also help to judge the operability or inoperability of the tumor (*see* **Table 14**).

When the primary tumor is not evident and the suspicion of a malignancy is aroused by the presence of a mediastinal adenopathy (identified by either CT or PET)

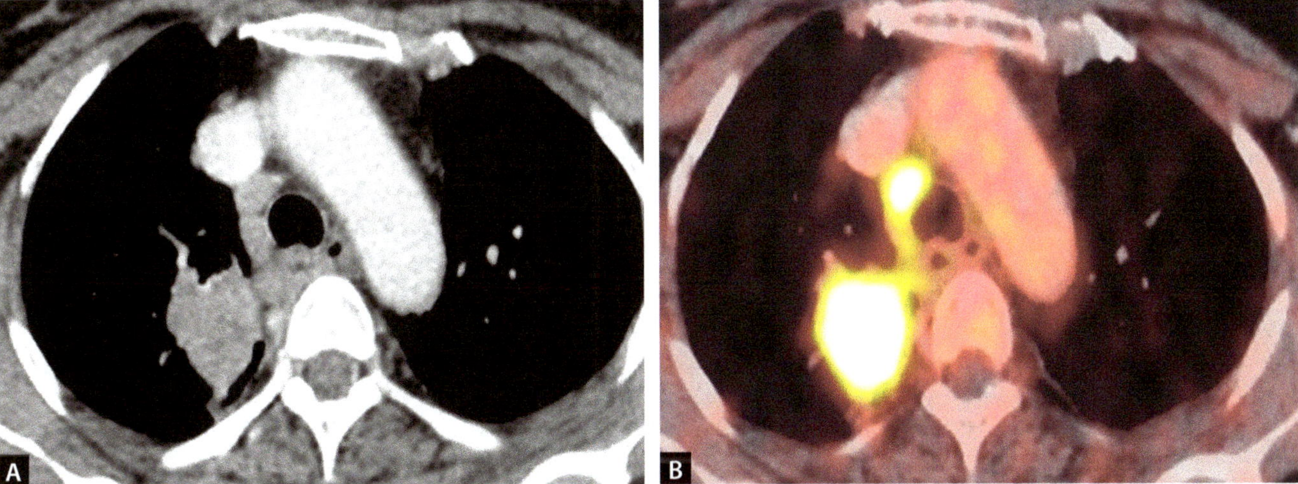

Figs. 32A and B: PET-CT demonstrates marked uptake by a large irregular central mass lesion in the right hilar region. There is another focus of uptake in the anterior mediastinum representing a metastatic adenopathy.

biopsy of mediastinal lymph nodes is necessary. Biopsy of mediastinal nodes is also necessary for proper staging even when a tumor in the lung is visible on imaging. If a CT-guided lymph node biopsy is deemed difficult or risky, transbronchial needle aspiration through a fiberoptic bronchoscope may be used to sample lymph nodes in the paratracheal, subcarinal, and hilar regions. This method may then allow both diagnosis and staging of the disease. Several studies have shown a significant improvement in the positive yield using EBUS compared to blind bronchoscopic needle aspiration. EBUS allows real-time imaging of mediastinal nodes so that the bronchoscopist can see the needle in the mediastinal node at the time of sampling. The use of EBUS obviates the need for mediastinoscopy to stage ipsilateral (N2) and contralateral nodes in lung cancer. Mediastinoscopy to sample mediastinal lymph nodes is today an increasingly uncommonly used procedure (*see* **Table 14**).

In advanced stage disease, the test which establishes a diagnosis in the simplest and preferably noninvasive way is to be chosen. For example, rather than biopsy a mass lesion in the lung, biopsy of a fair-sized lymph node in the neck may establish the diagnosis and also prove metastasis.

When lung cancer presents as a pleural effusion, both diagnosis and staging can be accomplished by cytological examination of the pleural fluid. If positive for malignancy, it establishes T4 (Stage IIB) disease.

Role of Sputum Cytology

Though mentioned last in this discussion, sputum cytology is among the first modalities that should be availed of in the diagnosis of lung cancer. Sputum cytological examination is cheap and when positive has a high specificity. In countries where the prevalence of tuberculosis is high, all sputum specimens sent for cytological examination should also be stained and cultured for acid-fast bacilli. The latter when present on smear or culture point to tuberculosis as the cause of a lung or mediastinal pathology. Sputum cytology is less likely to be positive when lung cancer presents as a peripheral nodule and much more likely to be positive with central tumors or large tumors, particularly large cavitating tumors. Sensitivity of a single sputum specimen for the diagnosis of cancer is approximately 50%. Repeated examination of the sputum increases sensitivity. Occasionally, a radiographically occult squamous cell carcinoma may be diagnosed by a sputum examination which shows mitotic squamous cells on cytology.

Management and Prognosis of Nonsmall Cell Lung Cancer (Flowchart 1)

Only 15–25% of patients with NSCLC present when the disease is in early stage, so that they can be offered potentially curative surgical intervention. About 30–35% have locally advanced stage disease and need management

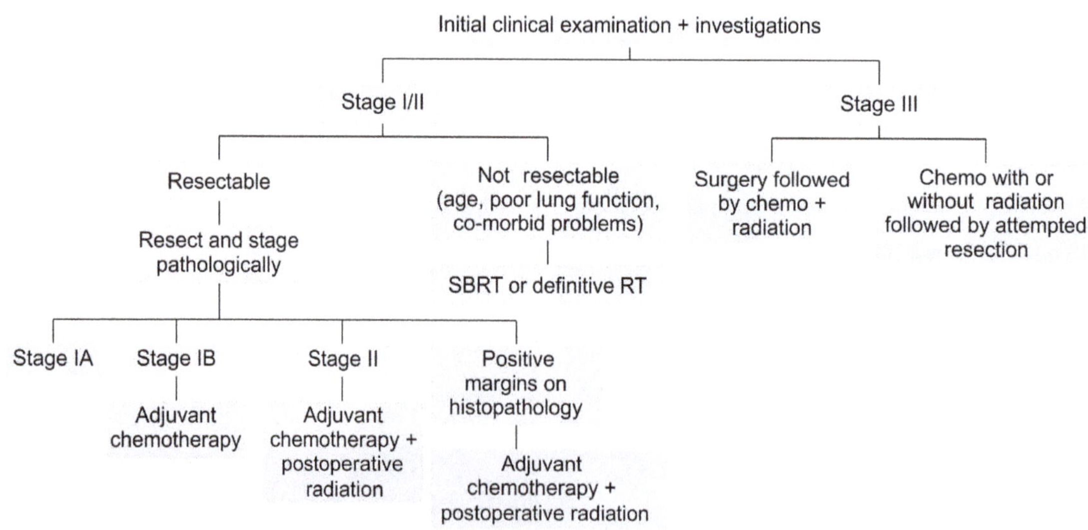

Flowchart 1: Algorithm for NSCLC in patients who on clinical examination and investigations (listed in text) are felt to be potential resectable.

SBRT: Stereotoxic body radiation therapy—preferred for tumors < 5 cm.
Definitive radiation therapy for tumors > 5 cm . See text for discussion on surgery in Stage III NSCLC.

through combined modality protocols. Close to 50% have advanced metastatic disease and can only be offered palliative treatment.

Complete staging on NSCLC is of utmost importance because the presence or absence of mediastinal lymph node involvement is the key prognostic marker in this disease. Also, the mere presence of mediastinal adenopathy in a patient with NSCLC does not always imply that the nodes are malignant. The majority of patients with NSCLC should therefore have mediastinal lymph node biopsies, either transbronchial biopsies thorough a fiberoptic bronchoscope or CT-guided biopsies or biopsies obtained thorough mediastinoscopy.

All large metropolitan cities in India are now making increasing use of the PET scan in the staging of NSCLC. As mentioned earlier it is more accurate in the detection of mediastinal node involvement compared to the CT. It is however an expensive test and is unavailable in many developing countries of the world. Moreover, the sensitivity of PET in poor developing countries is not as good compared to the West because of the high incidence of infections, notably tuberculosis in our part of the world.

Stage 0, I, II (Table 16)

The treatment of choice for Stage 0 (carcinoma in situ), IA/B or IIA/B NSCLC is surgical resection provided there is no strong medical contraindication against surgery.

Lobectomy, the surgical resection of the involved lobe, is the treatment of choice for early NSCLC, provided the patient has adequate pulmonary function to withstand the procedure. In most surgical centers this involves a formal thoracotomy. However in specialized centers lobectomy together with a dissection of mediastinal nodes through video-assisted thoracoscopic surgery is gaining increasing acceptance.

Proximal tumors are not easy to resect by lobectomy. In this situation sleeve resection is preferred over pneumonectomy as it allows better preservation of lung function and prevents complications associated with pneumonectomy.

Surgery for early NSCLC should always be accompanied by sampling of mediastinal nodes from four or five sites or a dissection and removal of mediastinal nodes. Most surgeons today are in favor of radical dissection of mediastinal nodes.

Limited resection: A sublobar resection which constitutes either a segmental resection of one or more anatomical segment (segmentectomy) or a nonanatomical wedge resection may be the considered approach in some patients who because of old age, poor pulmonary reserve, or other comorbid conditions are unfit for lobectomy. A study by the Lung Cancer Study Group that randomly assigned patients with a peripheral T1N0 (stage 1A) NSCLC to either lobectomy or a more limited resection (segmentectomy or wedge resection) concluded that there was a threefold increase in the rate of local recurrence and a lower survival rate with local resection compared to lobectomy. Even so, limited resection may well be an alternative in a selected subgroup of patients with a small early peripheral NSCLC.

Chest wall disease: For patients with chest wall involvement Stage IIB (T3 N0 M0) an en bloc resection may be indicated. A 40% survival rate for 5 years has been observed in a series constituting 212 patients.

Adjuvant chemotherapy is indicated for patients with pathological stage II disease. It may also well be indicated for patients with stage 1B disease. It is also indicated for patients who after postresection are noted to have stage III disease; sequential postoperative radiation therapy is generally administered for those with mediastinal node involvement.

Adjuvant therapy is not indicated for patients with resected stage Ia tumors.

Radiation therapy is indicated only in patients where surgical margins of the tumor after resection show cancerous infiltration. It is not indicated for the patients with stage I, II disease, with negative resection margins.

Table 16: Management of nonsmall cell lung cancer (NSCLC).
Stage 0, IA/B, IIA/B: • Surgery for NSCLC with mediastinal lymph node dissection • Adjuvant chemotherapy for IIA, IIB, IIIA disease; can be given in IB as well; radiotherapy for patients who are unfit and have a tumor <5 cm
Stage IIIA: • Surgery is followed by adjuvant chemotherapy
Stage IIIB: • Generally considered inoperable but in a small subset of patients, surgery may be offered • Pancoast tumor without involvement of mediastinal nodes— chemoradiotherapy followed by surgery
Inoperable stage IIIA, IIIB: • Concurrent chemotherapy plus radiotherapy without surgery
Stage IV: • Palliative treatment plus possible control of the disease • Chemotherapeutic agents like cisplatin plus etoposide or carboplatin plus paclitaxel (combined with radiotherapy)

Radiation therapy is an alternative for those unfit for surgery or those who refuse surgery. For those patients who have a tumor size less than 5 cm, stereotactic body radiation therapy (SBRT) is the treatment of choice, provided the equipment and expertise are available. Full-dose fractional radiotherapy is advised for a large lesion and for lesions less than 5 cm if SBRT is unavailable.

Operative Mortality

Thirty days' operative mortality is 1–3% for a lobectomy and 5–7% for a pneumonectomy. Morbidity and mortality are chiefly due to respiratory failure, particularly in patients with borderline respiratory reserve, nosocomial pneumonia, empyema, and bronchopleural fistula. Occasionally, death can result in the postoperative period from acute myocardial infarction or pulmonary embolism.

Prognosis after Surgery (Table 17)

Prognosis is always better in specialized oncology centers or when performed by experienced oncology surgeons in hospitals with good facilities and staff.

The 5-year survival for Stage IA lung cancer is close to 70% and for IB between 50% and 60%. For patients with Stage IIA disease, the 5-year survival is 40–55% and survival for IIB is close to 40%.

When long-term survival rates are analyzed in a large patient population subject to complete resection at thoracotomy, the overall results leave much to be desired. Thus, 40–60% of patients who have been operated upon successfully for IB, IIA/B NSCLC have a recurrence within the first 5 years. It is believed that this is due to a dissemination of micrometastasis to distant sites early in the natural history of the disease and/or to cancer cells left behind at the local site at the time of surgery. Modern immunohistochemical techniques on mediastinal nodes and bone marrow biopsies have demonstrated the presence of disseminated cytokeratin-positive cells.

Table 17: Prognosis of nonsmall cell lung cancer (with appropriate management).

The 5-year survival for stage	IA—73%; IB—58% IIA—46%; IIB—36%
Pancoast tumor	25–35%
Inoperable stage IIIA, IIIB	10–20%
Inoperable stage IV	1–3%

It is for this reason that adjuvant therapy is invariably recommended for Stage II and Stage 1B NSCLC. The role of postoperative radiotherapy as mentioned earlier, be reserved in only selected situations.

A number of studies from North America, Europe, other countries and even India have shown increased survival rates in patients who have undergone lobar resection for IIA/IIB disease and have received four cycles of adjuvant cisplatin-based chemotherapy compared to those who received no adjuvant chemotherapy after resection. When both adjuvant chemotherapy and radiotherapy are planned, adjuvant chemotherapy is given first and is followed by radiation as concurrent therapy may because of toxic effects, prevent the delivery of the recommended doses and cycles of chemotherapy.

Management of Stage III NSCLC (*see* Table 16)

Stage III NSCLC are a heterogeneous group varying both with regard to the extent of the tumor within the lung and its nodal spread. Different surgical centers have different approaches to management, suggesting that treatment of stage III NSCLC is controversial.

In the early TNM classification (7th edition) Stage III NSCLC was defined as the primary tumor extension into extrapulmonary structures (T3 or T4) or involvement of the mediastinal nodes (N2 or N3). The current TNM classification (8th edition) includes also under Stage III tumors greater than 5 cm in size with hilar, intrapulmonary or peribronchial spread (T3 N1) or tumors more than 7 cm regardless of lymph node involvement.

The description given below really outlines the general principles in the management of stage III NSCLC.

- *T3 N1 disease (Stage IIIA)*: For T3 N1 tumors or for multiple tumor nodules with no mediastinal node involvement, surgical resection is advised subject to technical feasibility. Surgery is followed by adjuvant chemotherapy. If surgical resection is incomplete, concurrent chemoradiotherapy is indicated. Radiotherapy is not indicated in a complete resection of T3 N1 disease, but is advised in patients with positive surgical margins or in strongly suspected or proven mediastinal node involvement at the time of surgery (N2 disease). It should be pointed out that some units do not advise radiotherapy in patients with single station N2 disease, particularly if they are old, feeble, or poorly nourished, so as to avoid radiation-induced toxicity.

The management of a superior sulcus (Pancoast tumor) tumor is different. Pancoast tumor with or without hilar involvement is generally treated first with concurrent chemoradiotherapy followed by surgery.

- *T4 N0-N1 disease (Group IIIB)*: T4 lesions are generally unresectable and most of these lesions are treated with chemoradiation therapy, as in patients with mediastinal involvement. There is however a small subset of patients that can be offered surgery. Surgery for T4 disease is contraindicated in the presence of N2 involvement or if the disease is unlikely to be completely resectable.

- *Adjuvant-based chemotherapy*: Adjuvant cisplatin-based chemotherapy is always recommended in all completely resected stage II and stage III NSCLC. There are numerous clinical trials proving that adjuvant therapy following surgery prolongs survival in these patients.

- *Adjuvant radiation therapy*: As mentioned earlier, adjuvant radiation therapy is included in Stage III NSCLC in the following circumstances:
  - When the margins of the surgically resected tumor are infiltrated with cancer, overall survival is greater in patients who have received adjuvant radiotherapy than in those who did not—five-year survival rates been 32.4% vs. 23.7%.
  - In patients staged as IIIA but who at or after surgery are found to have N2 involvement. Survival was greater in patients with N2 disease who received radiation therapy compared to those who did not. Survival was also greater in patients with N2 disease who received adjuvant chemotherapy as against those who did not. Remarkably, in striking contrast, in patients with N1 disease, radiation therapy had a negative effect on survival in those given adjuvant chemotherapy.

- *N2 disease (mediastinal involvement)*:
  - If mediastinal node involvement (N2 disease) is substantiated before contemplated surgery, in most patients concurrent chemotherapy is standard treatment, using platinum-based chemotherapy and full-dose radiation.
  - Surgery is also offered in a subject of these patients after induction chemotherapy or chemoradiation. The role of surgery however remains controversial and debatable. Some centers use the surgical approach sparingly while others do so more freely.

Some points need to be taken into consideration with regard to a surgical option in patients with N2 disease.

- There are no prospective randomized trials to advise on or define the subset of patients that would benefit from surgery. Perhaps those with single station N2 disease—less than 3 cm to start with, those that respond to induction therapy, and those in whom the disease can be resected via lobectomy rather than a pneumonectomy are suitable candidates.
- Surgery is avoided in those who have not benefited by induction therapy in multistation N2 disease, in T4 disease, and in those with poor cardiorespiratory reserve.
- For those undergoing surgery, prior induction therapy could be chemoradiation or chemotherapy, though this subject remains controversial.

In conclusion, surgery performed routinely and unselectively in N2 disease is not likely to improve survival. However in a selected subset of patients, surgery after induction therapy may help local control and may perhaps improve survival, though this latter hope has not been definitely substantiated.

- *N3 disease—advanced NSCLC*: Patients with NSCLC with N3 disease are not surgically resectable. They are treated with concurrent chemotherapy plus radiotherapy without surgery. Initially, sequential chemotherapy plus radiotherapy was used to reduce overall toxicity, but the superiority of chemo-radiotherapy has been demonstrated in two large phase III trials. The difference in the median survival (between concurrent and sequential therapies) is however indeed negligible, making one wonder whether the side effects of the above treatment in many ways could well be worse than the disease itself.

Choice of Chemotherapy in Advanced NSCLC

The details of chemotherapy are beyond the scope of this book. Two chemotherapeutic regimes are in common use:

1. *Cisplatin + Etoposide (combined with radiotherapy)*: In a multiphase trial of 50 patients with pathologically confirmed Stage IIIB disease and a follow-up of 52 months, the 3- and 5-year survival rates were 15% and 13%, respectively.

2. Carboplatin + Paclitaxel (combined with radiotherapy) used in a specific protocol resulted in a median survival of 16.3 months.

Target Drugs for Stage IV NSCLC

There is now an increasing emphasis on the use of targeted drugs for lung cancer. The first class of these neoagents is the EGFR tyrosine kinase inhibitor. It has shown a survival benefit when used in Stage IV NSCLC. The drug in use belonging to this class is erlotinib; it has been approved as second and third-line treatment of Stage IV NSCLC. The EGFR tyrosine kinase inhibitors are of no benefit when added to standard chemotherapy.

The second class of new drugs involving targeted therapy is the antiangiogenesis drug bevacizumab. This drug is an antivascular endothelial growth factor monoclonal antibody shown to increase survival in Stage IV nonsquamous NSCLC. Severe bleeding at times with fatal results is a known complication following use of this drug.

In conclusion, though chemotherapeutic regimens may prolong survival to a small extent, do they improve quality of life during the small extended period to any significant extent? Assessment of quality of life is difficult; it is conditioned not only by physical discomfort but by mental attitudes to bodily discomfort and to impending dissolution. Measurements of quality of life by various questionnaires such as the Quality of Life Index or the Functional Living Index Cancer Instrument are to our mind of very dubious value.

Palliative therapy in the treatment of NSLC is given in **Table 18**.

Bronchoscopy in the Management of Lung Cancer

The main use of bronchoscopy is to help stage lung cancer. Bronchoscopy also had limited use in the treatment of lung cancer through photodynamic therapy (PDT), laser therapy, brachytherapy, and through the use of airway stents in patients where an endobronchial growth is obstructing a large airway. PDT can only be used in NSCLC (in particular squamous cell carcinoma) if the tumor is within the reach of a flexible fiberoptic bronchoscope, if the lesion is smaller than 3 cm in surface area and does not extend more than just a few mm into the bronchial wall. Superficial squamous cell carcinoma or carcinoma in situ not evident on radiographic examination can be successfully treated by this method. 70–80% have a good response; there is a recurrence rate of 15–20%. Even so, in the above situation surgical resection is the treatment of choice if the patient is operable, PDT being reserved for patients who are unfit for surgery because of poor lung function or comorbid states.

Laser Therapy

Laser therapy is for palliative use in lung cancers obstructing central airways. The maximum clinical experience is with the neodymium:yttrium aluminum garnet (Nd:YAG) laser. Laser produces its effects by causing tissue necrosis + photocoagulation. Indications for use are: (a) lesions obstructing the central airways, particularly the trachea or main stem bronchi; (b) presence of a visible bronchial lumen and of functioning lung tissue beyond the obstructing cancerous lesions; (c) patients unresponsive to other modalities of treatment.

Relief of symptoms follows promptly on successful laser resection but median survival after this palliative treatment is generally not more than 6 months.

Brachytherapy

Brachytherapy is again a form of palliative therapy used to relieve both luminal obstruction of large airways and obstruction of large airways from extrinsic pressure. It is most often used in patients who have already received external beam radiation. Brachytherapy consists of an application of a titrated radiation dose applied through a nylon catheter placed into the lesion endoscopically. Successful and significant relief of an obstructed airway is observed in about 50% of patients, but median survival rate after brachytherapy does not extend beyond a few months.

Use of Prosthetic Stents

Bronchoscopic placement of airway stents is again a palliative treatment to relieve airways obstruction involving large airways or lobar bronchi. The largest experience is with silastic stents and metal stents. Combination of metal plus silastic and other materials in the stent have also been used. Stent insertion is done through either a

Table 18: Palliative treatment for nonsmall cell lung cancer.

- Photodynamic therapy
- Laser therapy
- Brachytherapy
- Use of prosthetic stents

flexible or rigid bronchoscope. Prompt relief of obstructive symptoms is observed after successful placement of the stent. Complications of the use of a stent are: (a) migration of the stent; (b) obstruction of the stent by secretions; and (c) granulation tissue formation.

An advantage of the silastic stent over the metal stent is that the former can be removed; while the latter can became incorporated within the bronchial wall and is then not removable. Even when a stent is appropriately placed, in time to come the growth can extend proximal or distal to the stent, again leading to airway obstruction.

■ SMALL CELL LUNG CANCER

Small cell lung cancer is a rapidly growing lung cancer characterized by a high growth fraction and the early development of widespread metastasis. It is initially highly responsive to chemotherapy and radiotherapy but almost all patients relapse generally within a few months with resistant disease that kills the patient.

Epidemiology

Small cell lung cancer occurs almost exclusively in smokers, particularly in heavy smokers. It is very rare in nonsmokers. A case-control series study revealed that it represented just 2.9% of cases in women and none in men who never smoked. In countries like the United States where the smoking habit is on the decline, the proportion of patients diagnosed as SCLC has reduced. The increased prevalence of smoking habit in women may be reflected in the next few decades with an increasing incidence of SCLC in women.

Classification and Pathology

Initially, the WHO classified SCLC into three histological subtypes—the oat cell, intermediate cell type, and combined. The combined SCLC had a NSCLC component, usually squamous cell or adenocarcinoma. The classification has changed so that histological changes could correlate better with clinical behavior. The present WHO classification (2004) of lung tumors does away with the intermediate cell type substage and introduces a new variant of large cell carcinoma, termed large cell neuroendocrine carcinoma (LCNEC), as this subtype is similar in clinical features, cell biology, and natural history to SCLC.

Small cell lung cancer, combined SCLC, LCNEC and carcinoids, typical and atypical are malignancies that have a neuroendocrine origin. The first three are highly malignant; atypical carcinoids are intermediate grade tumors and typical carcinoids are low-grade tumors.

Histology

The diagnosis of SCLC is based on the histological findings characterized by the presence of small "blue" cells, the size of lymphocytes. The cytoplasm is sparse and the nuclei do not show distinct nucleoli.

Tumor markers: SCLC has immunohistochemical markers which establish that the origin of the tumor is from within the lung. However, there are no molecular markers that can be targeted for treatment selection in SCLC. This is in striking contrast to NSCLC where biomarkers such as EGFR mutations can be targeted by therapeutic agents, and programed death ligand 1 (PDL-1) which can be targeted by immunotherapy.

Genetics: Multiple genetic defects have been detected in SCLC but even a brief description is outside the scope of this book. We mention just four genetic mutations out of the several that have been observed:
- *p53* mutations are detected in nearly all SCLC tumors.
- Haploinsufficiency due to loss of material on chromosome *3p* at multiple sites leads to loss or poor expression of many tumor-suppressor genes in SCLC.
- Loss of the retinoblastoma gene function at 13q14, either through absence or the presence of an abnormal gene product is observed in almost all patients with SCLC.
- A large number of alterations are observed in DNA samples of patients with SCLC.

Clinical Findings

Patients may present with any one or a combination of features described below:
- Approximately 70% of patients present with overt metastatic disease. The frequent sites of metastasis are the liver, adrenals, bone, bone marrow, and brain. Though often symptomatic (depending on the metastatic site) metastatic disease in organ symptoms may be silent and produce no symptoms to start with.
- Symptoms referred to the chest in SCLC chiefly include cough and dyspnea. Hemoptysis and atelectasis or pneumonia are not as frequently observed as in NSCLC due to the diffuse submucosal involvement in SCLC

in contrast to intraluminal growth pattern in NSCLC which leads to obstructive features.

- The most common presentation is the presence of a well-marked mediastinal adenopathy causing a big mediastinal mass and the presence of hilar adenopathy. The natural history of SCLC is to start in the central airways, infiltrating the submucosa of the bronchus, and quickly spreading to the mediastinal glands. Over time there could be narrowing of the bronchial lumen because of endobronchial spread or extrinsic pressure from the mediastinal adenopathy.
- One or more neuroendocrine paraneoplastic complications may occasionally be the presenting feature underlying the presence of a SCLC.
- Weight loss, debility, low-grade fever may occasionally be presenting symptoms. A SCLC is discovered on investigation.

Very occasionally, a SCLC can present as an isolated peripheral nodule without mediastinal or hilar adenopathy. This finding often leads to a CT-guided fine needle biopsy. Findings of a fine needle biopsy cannot be relied upon to distinguish SCLC from other neuroendocrine tumors; for example, typical or atypical carcinoids. In this situation, mediastinal staging followed by resection of the tumor should be done.

Staging

A modification of the two-stage staging of SCLC introduced by the Veterans Affairs Lung Study Group (VALSG) continues to be used in staging SCLC. This modified staging system is both simple and clinically useful in assessing prognosis in these patients. SCLC has two stages:

1. *Limited disease*: The tumor is confined to the ipsilateral hemothorax, so that the tumor and the involved nodes can be in a simple tolerable radiotherapy port.
2. *Extensive disease*: The tumor spreads outside the boundaries of limited disease (stated above). Extensive disease includes distant metastatic spread, spread to the pleura or pericardium, spread to the contralateral hilar or cervical lymph glands. Extensive disease implies spread to any one or more of these sites.

The TNM Staging System

The TNM Staging system for NSCLC proposed by the International Association of the Study of the Lung Cancer in 2017 (8th edition) recommends the same staging system for SCLC as well. The improved prognostic ability with

regard to survival in SCLC using the currently proposed staging system was confirmed in a separate Cohort of 4,884 patients in the Surveillance, Epidemiology and End Results (SEER) data base. The results showed a decreasing trend in survival with increase of T, N and increase in stage groupings.

The application of the TNM Staging system to SCLC has unfortunately not significantly impacted management of patients with SCLC because most patients present with advanced stage extensive disease. It however helps to identify patients who after a thorough evaluation and investigation are found to have T1 N0 disease. These patients need surgical resection of the tumor followed by chemotherapy. Unfortunately this applies to less than 5% of patients with SCLC. Hence, the major therapeutic impact of staging is to guide chemoradiation in these patients. All patients with a histological diagnosis of SCLC (even the few successfully resected) need systemic therapy with chemotherapy and more often with chemoradiation.

Workup of a Patient with SCLC

The objective is to quickly stage the disease in order to guide chemoradiation therapy and in rare cases resection of the tumor. However, SCLC has a very short doubling time and patients may deteriorate or even die without effective treatment. Staging should therefore be quick and not delay treatment for more than a few days.

A workup for a patient with SCLC includes a thorough clinical examination, a complete hematological and biochemical profile. Imaging is of crucial importance. It includes an X-ray of the chest, HRCT of the chest and abdomen, MRI of the brain, and a PET scan to detect metastatic lesions. A bone marrow biopsy is a necessary feature of a workup protocol. 15–30% of patients present with bone marrow involvement. Rarely, the bone marrow may be the sole site of metastatic involvement. Pleural and/or pericardial paracentesis may need to be done when necessary.

Importance of PET screening:

- The use of PET scan has already been elaborated upon in patients with NSCLC. A few points with reference to SCLC need to be stressed.
- Positron emission tomography has 100% sensitivity for SCLC and its use in the initial workup gives a more complete picture of the staging of the disease.
- Metastatic lesions may be silent. A PET scan reveals the silent lesions **(Fig. 33)**.

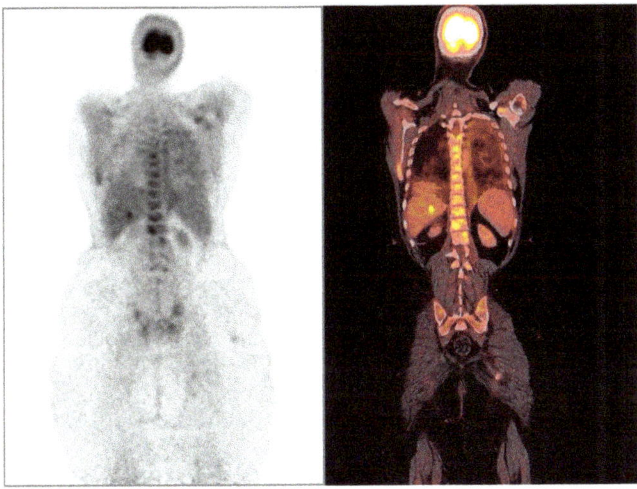

Fig. 33: PET-CT demonstrates multiple focal lesions in the vertebrae as well as the liver representing metastatic deposits from a left parahilar primary neoplasm.

- Positron emission tomography may alter treatment either through change in disease stage or by refining thoracic radiation fields and doses.
- Positron emission tomography in combination with CT of the chest is of help in restaging post-thoracic radiation by distinguishing effects of radiation reaction in normal tissue from progressive malignant disease.

Initial Management of Limited SCLC

The management of limited SCLC is summarized below.

Patients with stage 1 (T1 to T2 N0) with limited stage (LS) SCLC who have no evidence of mediastinal node involvement and who have no metastasis should be offered resection (lobectomy) which is then followed up by four cycles of cisplatin-based adjuvant chemotherapy **(Table 19)**. It is important that these patients have had a thorough workup before surgery is contemplated. This includes invasive staging of mediastinal lymph nodes to ensure as far as possible that there is no mediastinal involvement as also a workup to ensure the absence of metastatic disease. SCLC presenting as a localized solitary peripheral nodule when surgically resected has a survival rate 25–35% provided surgery has been followed up by adjunct chemotherapy.

For patients with LS-SCLC who have pathological involvement of mediastinal and/or hilar lymph nodes, surgery is contraindicated. Chemotherapy is the initial treatment. The preferred chemotherapy in LS-SCLC is a two-drug combination of four cycles of cisplatin and etoposide. Carboplatin may be substituted for cisplatin

Table 19: Management of small cell lung cancer (SCLC).
Patient with stage 1 (T1 to T2 N0) with limited stage (LS):   • Surgical resection followed by four cycles of cisplatin-based adjuvant chemotherapy
LS-SCLC who have pathological involvement of mediastinal and/or hilar lymph nodes: • Chemotherapy with the use of concurrent radiation therapy
Extensive stage SCLC: • Combination therapy with cisplatin or carboplatin plus etoposide

in patients with contraindications to the use of cisplatin. The chemotherapy should be combined with the use of concurrent radiation therapy, the latter being administered with the first or second cycle of chemotherapy. Baseline PET scans at diagnosis should help plan the dose, schedule, and field of radiotherapy. The details of radiotherapy are outside the scope of this book. Recently etoposide was compared with another alkylator-based regimen, cyclophosphamide, epirubicin, and vincristine. Studies confirmed that etoposide combined with cisplatin is the standard preferred regime for treatment of LS-SCLC.

Prophylactic cranial irradiation is indicated for patients with complete or very good to partial remission.

The combination modality therapy, (chemotherapy + radiation) should be given concurrently without interruption.

Supportive care with regard to pain relief, nutrition, and hydration is important.

For most patients with SCLC who develop the superior vena cava obstruction syndrome, initial therapy should be chemotherapy rather than radiation. Most patients respond dramatically to chemotherapy. Radiation may however be required in those who are in extreme distress or who do not respond to chemotherapy.

Benefits of Treatment

Patients with SCLC do not generally survive for more than few months without treatment. In patients with LS-SCLC who have been treated with chemoradiotherapy and prophylactic cranial irradiation, the response rate is 80–90% with 50–60% complete response rates. The disease however recurs, so that the median survival rate is about 17 months and the 5-year survival rate is about 20%.

Initial Management of Extensive SCLC

- Over 70–75% of patients with SCLC present with extensive disease. These patients should receive combination therapy with cisplatin or carboplatin plus etoposide. Reasonable alternative regimes that are offered substitute irinotecan, topotecan or epirubicin for etoposide. Initial chemotherapy is usually limited to four to six cycles of induction chemotherapy.

- Maintenance therapy of three or four drug combinations and alternating or using sequential non-cross-resistant regimens have shown no advantage when compared to two-drug regimens.
- Patients who show a good improvement following chemotherapy but who have residual thoracic disease should be given appropriate radiation therapy. Prophylactic cranial irradiation is also indicated in these patients.
- Finally as discussed in the management of very advanced NSCLC, perhaps discretion is the better part of valour so that treatment of these patients should be tempered with common sense. Many patients in our part of the world who are poor and unaffording should perhaps be cared for with humaneness and palliation without recourse to drugs, which at most give a few more months of painful existence.

It should be kept in mind that from time of diagnosis, the median survival rate of extended SCLC is 8–13 months. Less than 5% of those with extended SCLC survive beyond 2 years.

If response to initial first-line therapy (cisplatin or etoposide and carboplatin) has been good so that there has been a remission for over 6 months then a subsequent relapse is best treated with the same chemotherapeutic regime used initially.

◼ CLINICAL COURSE OF LUNG CANCER

Many aspects of the clinical course have been covered in the earlier discussion on lung cancer. The following points are however briefly summarized and are worthy of note **(Table 20)**:

- The overall 5-year survival in patients who have lung cancer even today is just 15% in good experienced oncology centers. In the average surgical centers and in most centers in developing countries, the 5-year survival is even more dismal—around 5–7%.
- The most important prognostic determinant is the tumor stage. As mentioned earlier, NSCLC Stage IA after successful surgical resection has a 5-year survival rate of 70% compared to 10% survival rate in patients with NSCLC-Stage-IA cancer who are

Table 20: Clinical course of lung cancer.

- Overall 5-year survival in patients—15%
- The most important prognostic determinant is the tumor stage
- Asymptomatic patients diagnosed with lung cancer have a better long-term survival rate compared to symptomatic patients
- Squamous cell cancer of the lung in younger patients has a better prognosis. Surgically unresectable nonsmall cell lung cancer and small cell lung cancer have a poor prognosis
- Squamous cell cancer of the lung has a greater incidence of local recurrence and lower rate of metastatic lesions
- Small cell lung carcinoma has the highest rate of metastatic spread
- Genes may influence survival
- Functional state has been shown to be an important predictor of survival
- After surgical resection of lung cancer, second primary lung cancer may develop in 2–3% per year

not operated upon either because they are unfit or refusing surgery.

- Patients detected with lung cancer (at various stages) who are asymptomatic have a 35% long-term survival vs. 10% survival in those detected with the presence of symptoms.
- Squamous cell cancer of the lung in younger patients has a better prognosis. Surgically unresectable NSCLC and SCLC have a poor prognosis.
- Squamous cell cancer of the lung has a greater incidence of local recurrence and lower rate of metastatic lesions compared to adenocarcinoma and large cell carcinoma.
- Patients with SCLC have the highest rate of metastatic spread.
- Genes may influence survival. A meta-analysis has shown that KRAS mutations were associated with poorer survival, especially in adenocarcinoma.
- Functional state has been shown to be an important predictor of survival. A number of performance status scales have been devised to assess functional state. A patient who is unable to carry out normal activities but is confined to his home and manages to care for himself is an example of an independent predictor of poor survival. Significant weight loss of more than 10% and the male gender are also independent predictors of shortened survival in unresectable disease.
- After successful surgical resection of lung cancer at any stage of the disease, Western literature has reported a second primary lung cancer developing in 2–3% per year. This suggests that patients successfully treated for

lung cancer should be closely followed up for at least 5 years and preferably 10 years. Follow-up, however, has not been shown to improve overall survival. No reliable and comprehensive Indian data with regard to the incidence of second primary lung cancers is available.

OTHER LUNG TUMORS

Pulmonary Metastasis

A pulmonary metastatic lesion from a primary cancer arising outside the thorax may present as a single solitary nodule or multiple nodular lesions. These are generally evident on chest X-ray and are often asymptomatic. Occasionally, an HRCT of the chest may reveal single or multiple pulmonary metastatic lesions not picked up by routine radiography.

The lung is a common site of metastatic deposits **(Fig. 34)**. Sources of primary cancer causing frequent blood-borne metastasis to the lungs include the breast, kidney, thyroid, colon, stomach, and head and neck cancers. Melanomas also metastasize frequently to the lung as do sarcomas. Besides metastatic pulmonary nodules, metastasis may involve the pleura and result in

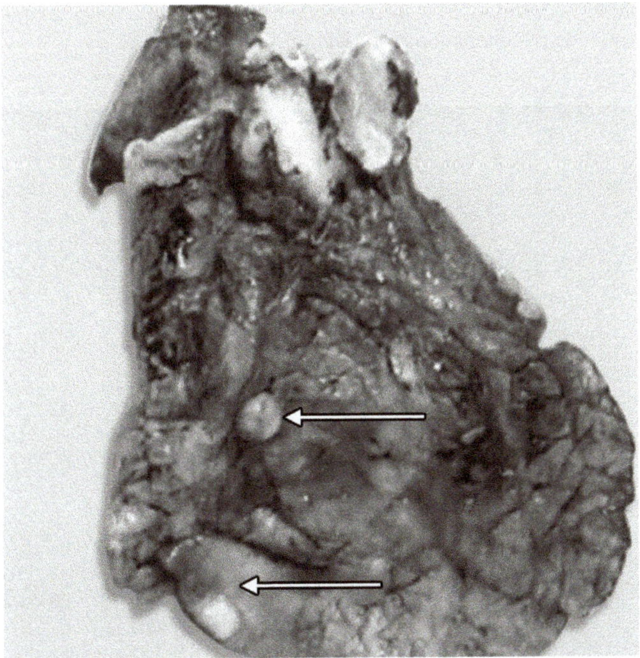

Fig. 34: Gross lobectomy specimen which demonstrates multiple subpleural well-defined homogenous rounded nodules. These represented metastatic deposits from a chondrosarcoma of the rib (arrows).

lymphangitis carcinomatosis. The latter is particularly frequently observed with breast and stomach cancers. Endobronchial secondary deposits may also occur.

The diagnosis of a pulmonary metastasis depending on the size and situation of the lesion can be made by a CT-guided biopsy or a transbronchial biopsy through a fiberoptic bronchoscope. A video-assisted thoracoscopic biopsy may occasionally be necessary to establish a definite diagnosis. A video-assisted thoracoscopy may also be necessary to confirm or refute the diagnosis of a metastatic pleural effusion. Multiple metastases need requisite systemic chemotherapy depending on the source or site of the primary cancer.

Role of Surgery in Pulmonary Metastasis

Metastasectomy has gained acceptance among oncosurgeons for patients who present only with metastasis to the lung, from a primary elsewhere. There are however no randomized studies to compare patients who have had metastasectomy to those receiving medical therapy or observation.

The International Registry of Lung Metastasis assessed the long-term results of pulmonary metastasectomy through a retrospective review of several thousand patients who had undergone this procedure. Patients with a solitary pulmonary metastasis had a survival period of 43% at 5 years after metastasectomy; those with two or three metastasis had a survival of 34% at 5 years, and patients who had 4 or more metastasis had a survival of 27% at 5 years. The ability to achieve complete resectability was the main determinant of survival. The 5-year survival of patients whose metastatic lesions were completely resectable was 36% with a median survival of 33%. Patients whose lesions were not completely resected had a 5-year survival of 15% with a median survival of 13 months. Pulmonary metastasectomy should be considered if:

- There are no other distant metastatic lesions in any other organ system
- Complete resectability of the lung lesion is achievable without crippling respiratory reserve
- The primary mitotic lesion has been taken care or is controllable and the site of the resected primary tumor shows no evidence of recurrence.

The two parameters that should be considered as a prognostic index for surgical metastasectomy are—a disease-free period more than 36 months and the number of pulmonary metastasis. The prognosis and survival over

5 years is best when the disease-free interval is more than 36 months and there is a solitary metastasis. It is worst if disease-free period is less than 36 months and there are multiple metastases. Surgery is inadvisable in the latter group. The prognosis lies in-between, if either the disease-free period is less than 36 months or there are multiple metastases.

Staging for distant metastatic disease is an absolute prerequisite, before surgery on even a single pulmonary metastatic lesion is considered.

Neuroendocrine Tumors (Carcinoids)

Carcinoid tumors are now termed neuroendocrine tumors, because they originate from neuroendocrine cells. These are malignant tumors—many with a low-grade malignancy, some with an intermediate grade malignancy and some with a high-grade malignancy (cells showing marked mitosis). Even the low grade malignancy neuroendocrine tumors have a potential to metastatize.

Neuroendocrine tumors (carcinoids) constitute 1 to 2% of lung tumors. They generally present between 50 years and 60 years of age.

Patients with carcinoid tumors may be asymptomatic, the tumor being discovered as a solitary nodule on chest radiography. 70% or more of carcinoid tumors are centrally situated and are often endobronchial; the presentation then is with cough, hemoptysis, and features of partial or complete bronchial obstruction. These include clinical features of pneumonia distal to the tumor or of atelectasis of a lobe or lung when the obstruction to the airway is complete.

Though a neuroendocrine tumor is composed of neuroendocrine cells, the carcinoid syndrome characterized by episodes of flushing, urticaria, diarrhea, and hypotension is rare and generally occurs in carcinoids that have metastasized to the liver. This syndrome is due to excessive production of serotonin and bioactive amines. An uncommon but important manifestation of the carcinoid syndrome is severe tricuspid regurgitation with resulting congestive heart failure due to fibrosis of the tricuspid valves.

Radiologically, as mentioned earlier, a neuroendocrine tumor presents as a well-defined nodule which may show calcification. An HRCT of the chest typically shows a localized central tumor deforming an airway **(Figs. 35 and 36)**. Punctate calcification may or may not be present. Homogenous contrast enhancement with or without hilar

adenopathy is observed. An MRI demonstrates high-signal intensity on T2-weighted images. Carcinoids are hypometabolic on FDG-PET scan. Somatostatin receptor scintigraphy can detect occult primary tumors and localization of metastatic disease.

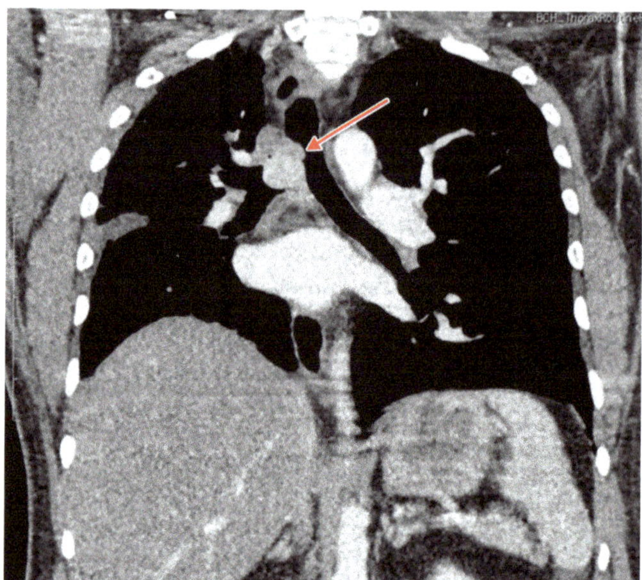

Fig. 35: Carcinoid tumor. Coronal image demonstrates lobulated nodular lesion in the distal trachea and carina extending into the right main bronchus with consequent reduced right lung volume and mild hyperinflation of the left lung.

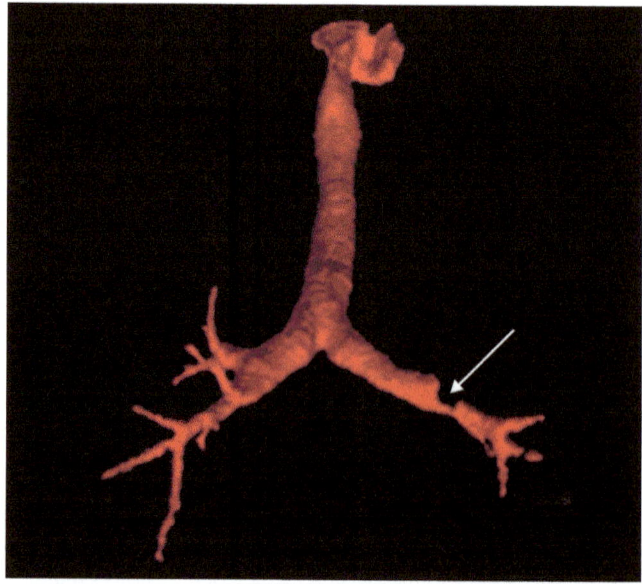

Fig. 36: Neuroendocrine tumor: CT volume-rendered image of the tracheobronchial tree reveals the intrabronchial extension of the neuroendocrine tumor.

Diagnosis is made by bronchoscopy as these tumors are often endobronchial. A carcinoid within the lung parenchyma can be diagnosed through a CT-guided biopsy. These tumors are often vascular and biopsy at times leads to significant bleeding.

Uncommonly neuroendocrine tumors may present with a paraneoplastic syndrome, such as Cushing's syndrome due to ectopic adrenocorticotropic hormone secretion.

Surgical resection of the tumor, lobectomy with lymph node resection, is curative in the absence of any nodal or extrathoracic spread (chiefly to the liver). The 10-year survival rate in such patients is well over 90%. Survival rates are reduced if the tumors is more than 3 cm in size, or in the presence of nodal metastasis; it is even further reduced with liver metastasis.

Neuroendocrine tumors with high grade malignancy as judged by degree of mitosis, necrosis, atypia **(Figs. 37 to 39)**, tend to recur, have a higher rate of metastasis to regional lymph nodes and the liver, and are usually larger at the time of diagnosis. Surgery if possible is still the optimal line of treatment, the 5-year survival rate being 60%. Neuroendocrine tumors respond poorly to radiotherapy or chemotherapy compared to NSCLC.

Pulmonary Lymphoma

Pulmonary lymphomas are invariably of the non-Hodgkin's variety and form less than 1% of all tumors. The diagnosis is generally made on a CT-guided biopsy. It is uncommon to come across a non-Hodgkin's lymphoma solely involving

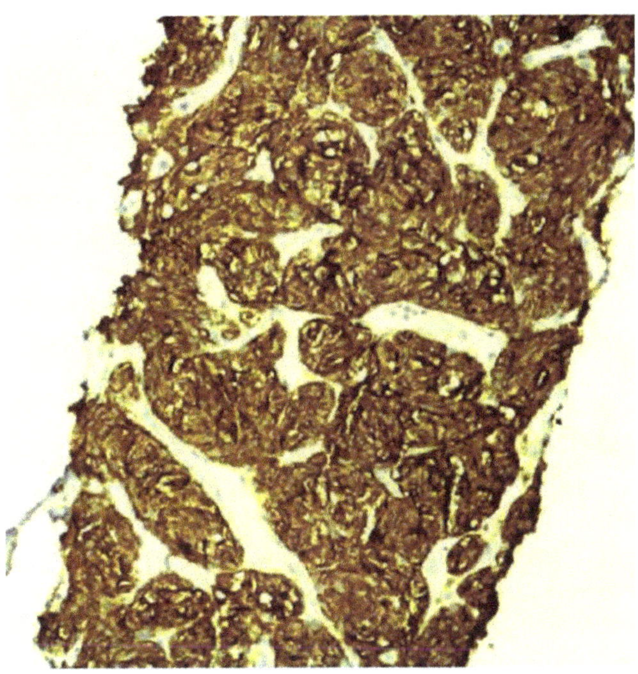

Fig. 38: Neuroendocrine tumor of the lung. H&E (hematoxylin and eosin) 20x magnification microscopy demonstrates discrete nests of tumor cells with uniform oval nuclei in a neuroendocrine tumor of the lung.

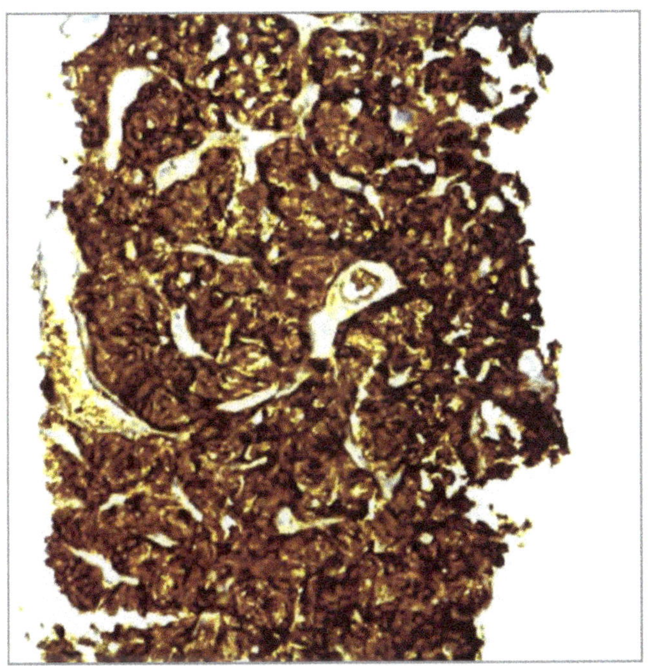

Fig. 37: 10x. Neuroendocrine tumor—immunohistochemistry for neuroendocrine marker synaptophysin. Strong cytoplasmic positivity is noted.

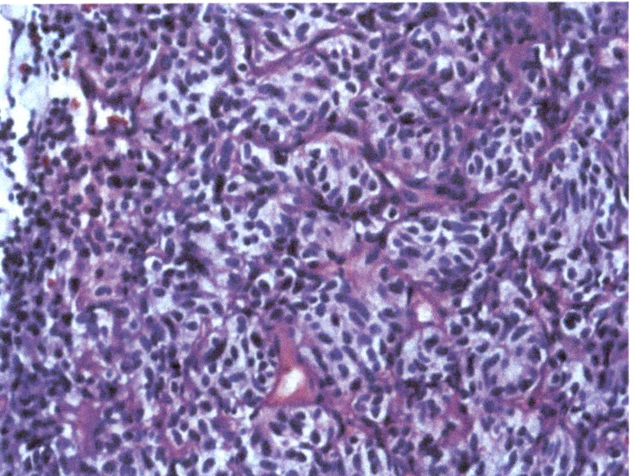

Fig. 39: 10x. Neuroendocrine tumor—immunohistochemistry for neuroendocrine marker chromogranin. Strong cytoplasmic positivity is noted.

the lung. A clinical plus other investigational search for involvement of lymph glands and other organ systems should be made. Surgical resection for a single, isolated non-Hodgkin's lymphoma may be curative. Chemotherapy is indicated in patients with more extensive pulmonary or disseminated disease.

Microepidermoid Carcinoma

Microepidermoid carcinomas are rare tumors involving the large airways—the trachea or the proximal bronchi. They arise from salivary gland tissue within the large airways. Being endotracheal or endobronchial, they present with cough, hemoptysis, dyspnea, stridor, and obstructive symptoms. They are low-malignancy tumors but may metastasize to lymph nodes.

Treatment is by surgical resection if this is feasible—complete resection is rewarded with an excellent prognosis.

Adenoid Cystic Carcinoma

Adenoid cystic carcinoma is a salivary gland tumor arising from the trachea, main stem or lobar bronchi, constituting less than 1% of all lung tumors. Rarely, it arises peripherally. Presenting symptoms, because of its endobronchial situation, are cough, hemoptysis, dyspnea, and obstructive clinical features distal to the obstruction.

The treatment of choice is surgical resection though this is often incomplete. Local recurrence as well as metastasis is observed.

Hamartoma

Hamartoma is the most common benign neoplasm of the lung with the highest frequency of occurrence in the fifth or sixth decade. A hamartoma is invariably asymptomatic and is detected as a well-defined nodule either on chest radiography or CT of the chest **(Fig. 40)**. Histologically, a hamartoma consists of mixed tissue, a combination of cartilage, muscle, fat, connective tissue, and respiratory epithelium. Calcification is often noted; it may take the form of popcorn calcification in about 25% of patients. The radiographic appearance is generally typical and no treatment is advised other than periodic observation. A radiographically doubtful or indeterminate nodule however warrants surgical resection.

■ PREVENTION

Avoidance of smoking (never-smoking) and stopping smoking are the prime preventive measure considering

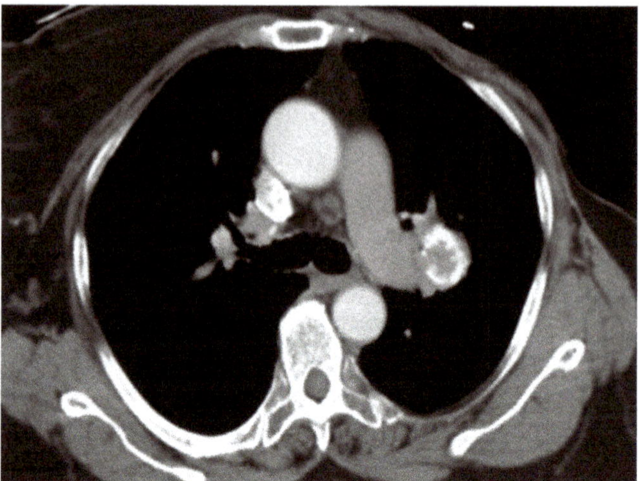

Fig. 40: Computed tomography of chest confirms the irregular internal calcification indicative of a hamartoma.

the fact that 85% of lung cancers occur in smokers or former smokers. Tobacco is addictive and smoking cessation proves difficult. Motivation through repeated meetings with the physician often helps—but only to a small extent. Use of supplemental nicotine patches, hypnosis, group therapy, and acupuncture has at various times led to one year abstinence rates of 20% or more. The drug varenicline, a nicotine agonist, has been shown to be superior to bupropion in stopping cigarette smoking in randomized trials. The cessation rate for smoking at 12 weeks is 44% with varenicline, 29.5% with bupropion, and 17.7% with placebo. A recent study suggests that electronic cigarettes (e-cigarettes) may have a role as a smoking cessation aid. In our opinion, in addition to what is mentioned above, patients addicted to cigarette smoking can give up cigarettes only if they are sufficiently motivated from within to do so. The incidence of lung cancer would indeed fall precipitously if smoking of tobacco is declared a dreadful poison and is banned all over the world.

■ SUGGESTED READING

1. Behera D, Balamugesh T. Lung cancer in India. Indian J Chest Dis Allied Sci. 2004;46(4):269-81.
2. Bryant A. Differences in epidemiology, histology, and survival between cigarette smokers and never-smokers who develop non-small cell lung cancer. Chest. 2007;132(1):185-92.
3. Dela Cruz CS, Tanoue LT, Matthay RA. Lung cancer: epidemiology, etiology, and prevention. Clin Chest Med. 2011;32(4):605-44.
4. Erasmus JJ. CT, positron emission tomography, and MRI in staging lung cancer. Clin Chest Med. 2008;29(1):39-57.

5. Ginsberg MS. Lung cancer. Radiol Clin North Am. 2007;45(1):21-43.

6. Glisson BS, Byers LA. Pathobiology and staging of small cell carcinoma of the lung. [online] Available from https://www.uptodate.com/contents/search?search=Pathobiology%20and%20staging%20of%20small%20cell%20carcinoma%20of%20the%20lung&sp=0&source=USER_INPUT&searchOffset=1&autoComplete=false&language=en&max=10&index=&autoCompleteTerm=[Accessed July 2018].

7. Globocan 2012: Estimated Cancer Incidence, Mortality and Prevalence Worldwide in 2012. [online] Available from http://globocan.iarc.fr/Default.aspx [Accessed July 2018].

8. Gould MK, Tang T, Liu IL, et al. Recent trends in the identification of incidental pulmonary nodules. Am J Respir Crit Care Med. 2015;192:1208.

9. Kelley MJ. Prevention of lung cancer: summary of published evidence. Chest. 2003;123(1 Suppl):50S-9S.

10. Kelly K. Extensive stage small cell lung cancer: Initial management. [online] Available from https://www.uptodate.com/contents/search?search=Extensive%20stage%20small%20cell%20lung%20cancer:%20Initial%20management&sp=0&source=USER_INPUT&searchOffset=1&autoComplete=false&language=en&max=10&index=&autoCompleteTerm= [Accessed July 2018].

11. Ost D, Fein AM, Feinsilver SH. Clinical practice. The solitary pulmonary nodule. N Engl J Med. 2003;348(25):2535-42.

12. Planchard D, Besse B. Lung cancer in never-smokers. Euro Respir J. 2015;45:1214-7.

13. Schild SE, Ramalingam SS, Vallieres E. Management of stage III non-small cell lung cancer. [online] Available from https://www.uptodate.com/contents/search?search=Management%20of%20stage%20I%20and%20stage%20II%20non-small%20cell%20lung%20cancer&x=0&y=0 [Accessed July 2018].

14. Subramanian J. Molecular genetics of lung cancer in people who have never smoked. Lancet Oncol. 2008;9(7):676-82.

15. Tanoue LT, Gettinger S. Treatment of lung cancer in older patients. Clin Chest Med. 2007;28(4):735-49, vi.

16. Thomas KW, Gould MK. Tumor, Node, Metastasis (TNM) staging system for lung cancer. [online] Available from https://www.uptodate.com/contents/search?search=Tumor,%20Node,%20Metastasis%20(TNM)%20staging%20system%20for%20lung%20cancer&sp=0&source=USER_INPUT&searchOffset=1&autoComplete=false&language=en&max=10& index=&autoCompleteTerm= [Accessed July 2018].

17. Travis WD, Brambilla E, Nicholson AG, et al. The 2015 World Health Organization Classification of Lung Tumors: Impact of Genetic, Clinical and Radiologic Advances Since the 2004. J Thorac Oncol. 2015;10(9):1243-60.

18. Travis WD. Pathology of lung cancer. Clin Chest Med. 2002;23(1):65-81, viii.

19. West HJ, Vallieres E, Schild SE. Management of stage I and stage II non-small cell lung cancer. [online] Available from https://www.uptodate.com/contents/search?search=Management%20of%20stage%20I%20and%20stage%20II%20non-small%20cell%20lung%20cancer&x=0&y=0 [Accessed July 2018].

20. Zou XN, Lin D, Chao A, et al. Histological subtypes of lung cancer in Chinese women from 2000 to 2012. Thoracic Cancer. 2014;5:447-54.

Section 12

Interstitial Lung Diseases and Other Diffuse Lung Diseases

CHAPTER 44

Interstitial Lung Disease: Idiopathic Interstitial Pneumonia

■ INTRODUCTION

Interstitial lung diseases (ILDs) are a group of diffuse lung diseases that affect not just the interstitium of the lung but also the airspaces, peripheral airways and vessels along with their respective epithelial and endothelial linings. Diffuse parenchymal lung diseases (DPLD) may hence be a more accurate description of these disorders.

The ILDs may be classified as those secondary to a known cause or disease state like drugs or collagen vascular disease or granulomatous conditions like sarcoidosis or rarer diseases like Langerhans cell or pulmonary alveolar proteinosis. At last count there were at least 150 diseases which were known to present with ILD. Many of these have been discussed in different parts of this text. More often than not, the cause of the ILD remains unknown despite a detailed history, physical examination and investigation. Osler first described the generic *chronic interstitial pneumonia* over a century ago but these idiopathic forms of ILD are currently called idiopathic interstitial pneumonias (IIPs).

The first modern classification schema was proposed in 1969 by Liebow and Carrington who described 5 distinct histopathological patterns in patients with IIP: Usual interstitial pneumonia (UIP), desquamative interstitial pneumonia (DIP), lymphocytic interstitial pneumonia (LIP), bronchiolitis obliterans organizing pneumonia (BOOP) and giant cell interstitial pneumonia. Each of these patients had a distinct clinical profile suggesting that they represented separate diseases.

Katzenstein and Myers revised Liebow and Carrington's classification in 1998, excluding BOOP (felt to represent an intraluminal rather than an interstitial process), LIP (as it was a lymphoproliferative disorder) and giant cell interstitial pneumonia (felt to be a hard-metal pneumoconiosis). They instead divided IIPs into 5 groups, maintaining UIP and DIP, but adding 3 newly recognized entities: Respiratory bronchiolitis-associated interstitial lung disease (RB-ILD), acute interstitial pneumonia (AIP), formerly Hamman-Rich syndrome) and nonspecific interstitial pneumonia (NSIP).

Most recently, the American Thoracic Society (ATS) and European Respiratory Society (ERS) convened a consensus panel of clinicians, radiologists and pathologists to establish a uniform set of criteria for diagnosis of IIPs. They combined the two earlier classifications into the current schema with seven distinct disease entities now falling under the umbrella of IIP. This classification is outlined in **Table 1** which describes the clinical entity and its corresponding histopathological pattern.

Table 1: The American Thoracic Society/European Respiratory Society consensus classification of idiopathic interstitial pneumonias.

Histopathological pattern	*Corresponding clinical diagnosis*
Usual interstitial pneumonia	Idiopathic pulmonary fibrosis
Nonspecific interstitial pneumonia	Nonspecific interstitial pneumonia
Organizing pneumonia	Cryptogenic organizing pneumonia
Diffuse alveolar damage	Acute interstitial pneumonia
Respiratory bronchiolitis	Respiratory bronchiolitis—associated ILD
Desquamative interstitial pneumonia	Desquamative interstitial pneumonia
Lymphocytic interstitial pneumonia	Lymphocytic interstitial pneumonia

■ EPIDEMIOLOGICAL SPECTRUM AND DISTRIBUTION OF INTERSTITIAL LUNG DISEASES IN INDIA

In India, the ILDs remain significantly under-diagnosed and under-reported. This is probably due to the lack of awareness and lack of easy availability of computed tomography (CT) scanning and surgical centers offering open and video-assisted lung biopsy. The considerable expenses involved in these special investigations are also a deterrent for the Indian patient with ILD. Finally, the overwhelming burden of tuberculosis (TB) in India tends to dominate respiratory medicine in this country. TB can mimic some of the ILDs, especially sarcoidosis, and leads to diagnostic errors and delays. Nevertheless, in the last few decades, ILDs and DPLDs have been increasingly recognized in India. The surge in the recognition of ILD in India corresponds to the turn of the century when high-resolution computed tomography (HRCT) scanning became more readily available as a primary diagnostic aid. Most of the earlier reports on ILDs in the 1980s and 1990s generally referred to the diffuse interstitial involvement that occurred in systemic diseases like connective tissue disorders. In that era there were very few reports on idiopathic pulmonary fibrosis (IPF) in the Indian literature. At one of our hospitals, a tertiary referral center in Mumbai, we analyzed 274 biopsy-proven cases of DPLD over a 7-year period. In this series, IPF constituted the single largest disease group, accounting for 43% of all patients encountered. The spectrum of secondary causes was no different from that seen in Western countries. Drug-induced DPLD, pneumoconiosis, sarcoidosis, extrinsic allergic alveolitis, histiocytosis X, Wegener's granulomatosis, pulmonary alveolar proteinosis and lymphomatoid granulomatosis were all encountered (*Ref: Sen T, Udwadia ZF. Retrospective study of ILD in a tertiary care center in India. Indian J Chest Dis Allied Sci. In Press*). Another retrospective study from the same center looked into the clinical features, radiology, pulmonary function test (PFT) and follow-up of 117 biopsy-proven cases of IPF over 7 years. We found that 6% of these cases had familial IPF. Another comprehensive retrospective review revealed 34 cases of biopsy-proven cryptogenic organizing pneumonia (COP) encountered from 2000–05, establishing that COP was not uncommon in India although the majority of cases were initially mislabeled as TB before the final diagnosis was made. There are several smaller Indian case series of ILDs secondary to different

connective tissue diseases with recent Indian studies pointing out the presence of ILD in 65% of patients with systemic sclerosis and 25% of patients with rheumatoid arthritis. A step in the right direction is Singh et al's efforts to maintain a prospective national registry between 2012 and 2015 involving 27 investigators in 19 cities in India. Including clinical and radiological data on 1,084 patients with ILD, the authors claimed that the commonest type of ILD encountered in the country was hypersensitivity pneumonitis (HP), (encountered in almost 50% of all their patents), with ILD secondary to connective tissue disease and IPF both accounting for around 14% of cases.

Their contentious claim that the majority of cases of HP were linked to mold growth in air coolers has been disputed however as it was backed up with serological testing in very few patients. Despite the criticisms, studies like these that can give a panoramic view of the ILD spectrum across the country are useful and needed. The fact that the registry is active and prospective will hopefully result in a more comprehensive representation of the subcontinent in the future (*Ref: Singh S, Collins B, Sharma B, et al. Interstitial lung disease in India, results of a prospective registry. Am J Respir Crit Care Med. 2017:195;801-13*).

Thus to conclude the results of nationwide and other smaller studies suggest that ILD is widely prevalent in India with a spectrum and distribution not substantially different from that encountered in the West.

■ DIAGNOSIS OF INTERSTITIAL LUNG DISEASES

History

The patient's age, gender and smoking status often provide the initial clues in the history. Patients with IPF are usually more than 60 years old. Indeed, it is essential to rule out a secondary cause before labeling a young patient as having IPF. Patients with IIP of the NSIP variety are usually less than 60 years old. Sarcoidosis usually occurs at a younger age. Lymphangioleiomyomatosis (LAM) is exclusively a disease of women, while pulmonary Langerhans cell granulomatosis (also called histiocytosis X or eosinophilic granuloma) occurs in young cigarette-smoking males. A family history of ILD in parents, siblings or children raises the possibility of familial IPF. A detailed environmental and occupational history is essential and may provide vital clues to the etiology of the ILD. At-risk occupations include farmers (extrinsic allergic alveolitis), miners (pneumoconiosis), workers in nuclear, aerospace, computer or electronics industries (berylliosis), and shipyard workers, mechanics and electricians (asbestosis). Hobbies such as bird breeding or pigeon feeding as is common in this country and exposure to pets like budgerigars or parakeets may also be relevant and must be specifically inquired for. Several drugs are known to cause ILD; the use of amiodarone, methotrexate, penicillamine and chemotherapeutic agents must be checked for.

Symptoms

The two cardinal symptoms of ILD are cough and dyspnea. Though these are nonspecific symptoms, a careful teasing out of these symptoms can often provide clues to ILD being the underlying cause. The cough is always dry and nonproductive. Unlike the dry cough caused by asthma which is intermittent and often nocturnal, the cough of patients with IPF shows no diurnal variation. It does not wax and wane and can be incessant. It may worsen (as the dyspnea does) with exertion. It is a disabling and distressing symptom for the patient and one which is often mislabeled asthma or bronchitis by the physician, especially in the early stages. It is often refractory to all therapies. The other cardinal symptom is dyspnea. In the early stages this may be present only on undue exertion like climbing stairs and absent at rest or with routine activity. It is relentlessly progressive however and there is no more crippling symptom than the dyspnea of advanced IPF. As the disease progresses it occurs with trivial activity and eventually at rest. It is relieved to some extent by oxygen, but eventually persists despite high-flow oxygen. Other respiratory symptoms are rare and if present may provide important clues to the etiology or complications. Thus, for example, hemoptysis points to underlying alveolar hemorrhage which may complicate the ILD of collagen vascular disorders like systemic lupus erythematosus (SLE) or raise suspicions of pulmonary embolism or malignancy, both known complications of ILD. Pleuritic pain should raise the possibility of the occurrence of a pneumothorax. Wheeze may occur in ILD related to sarcoidosis or extrinsic allergic alveolitis (both being ILDs with frequent airway involvement). Symptoms outside the lungs like fever and joint pains raise the possibility of sarcoidosis or collagen vascular disorder.

Signs

Crackles are the distinctive physical finding. The crackles are typically dry or Velcro-like and heard in the very bases of the lung during end-inspiration. In the early stages they are very subtle and must be carefully auscultated for with the patient instructed to lean forward and breathe very deeply. They are different in character from those heard in bronchiectasis and do not change with coughing. Once heard they are almost pathognomonic and must never be ignored even if the patient has few symptoms and a normal chest radiograph at the time. The only condition which produces similar crackles is interstitial pulmonary edema. While crackles are heard in all the ILDs they are relatively less common in granulomatous ILDs like sarcoidosis. Squawks and wheeze may be heard in extrinsic allergic alveolitis (EAA) and occasionally in sarcoidosis with airway involvement. Finger clubbing is another common sign. It is more commonly seen in IPF and is rare in sarcoidosis, collagen vascular disease-associated ILD and BOOP. Signs of pulmonary hypertension must be carefully assessed and are not uncommon in advanced ILD, often portending a grave prognosis. Finally, extrapulmonary signs like erythema nodosum (sarcoidosis), Raynaud's phenomenon and sclerodactyly (systemic sclerosis), subcutaneous nodules (rheumatoid arthritis) and café au lait spots (underlying tuberous sclerosis and associated LAM) must be carefully checked for **(Table 2)**.

Chest Radiography (Figs. 1 to 5)

The chest radiograph remains an integral part of the workup of a patient with suspected ILD. However, the chest radiograph has shortcomings with regard to sensitivity and specificity which must be borne in mind. Various limitations of the chest radiograph can be listed:

Table 2: Clinical features of idiopathic interstitial pneumonia.

Symptoms:
- Cough
- Dyspnea
- Wheeze in case of sarcoidosis or extrinsic allergic alveolitis
- Extrapulmonary features suggest association of collagen vascular disease or sarcoidosis

Signs:
- Crackles-dry or *Velcro* crackles
- Wheeze in sarcoidosis or EAA
- Finger clubbing
- Signs of pulmonary hypertension
- Extrapulmonary signs like erythema nodosum (sarcoidosis), Raynaud's phenomenon and sclerodactyly (systemic sclerosis), subcutaneous nodules (rheumatoid arthritis) and café-au-lait spots (underlying tuberous sclerosis and associated LAM)

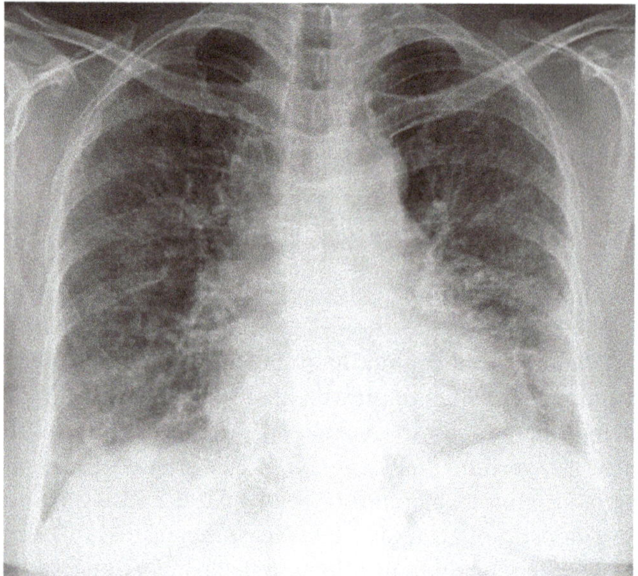

Fig. 1: Idiopathic pulmonary fibrosis. X-ray chest demonstrates reticular opacities in both lung fields, particularly the right lung base. HRCT chest confirmed presence of reticular opacity in a case with a UIP pattern.

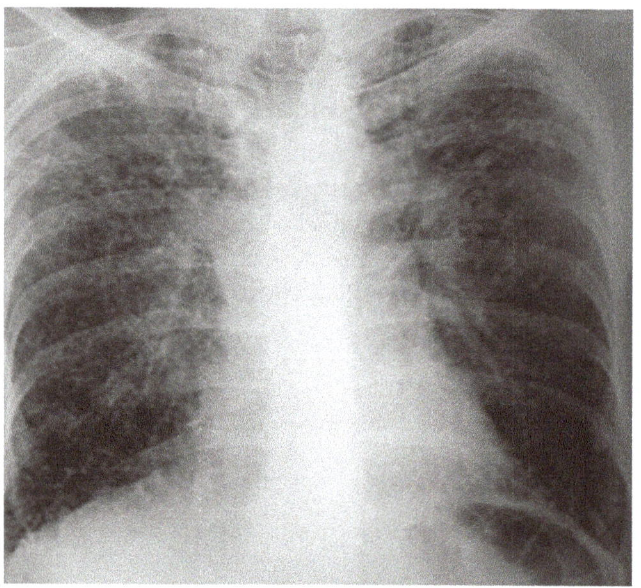

Fig. 2: Interstitial lung disease (ILD): Chest X-ray reveals reticulonodular opacities in the upper and mid-zones. The reticulonodular opacities indicate ILD. In view of the upper and mid-zone involvement, the possibility of an IPF is less likely. High-resolution computed tomography (HRCT) chest revealed peribronchial interstitial thickening as a result of chronic hypersensitivity pneumonitis.

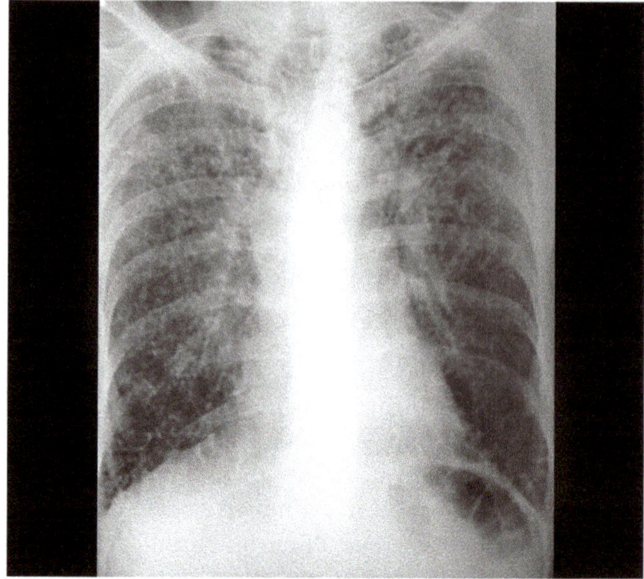

Fig. 3: Idiopathic pulmonary fibrosis. X-ray chest demonstrates reticulonodular opacities in the upper and mid-zones. The reticulonodular opacities indicate ILD. In view of the upper and mid-zone involvement, the possibility of an IPF is less likely HRCT chest revealed peribronchial interstitial thickening as a result of chronic hypersensitivity pneumonitis.

- The range of patterns on a chest radiograph is obviously limited even when the ILD is obvious.

  About half the lung volume is obscured on a frontal chest radiograph by the mediastinum and diaphragm making early ILD often impossible to pick. The sensitivity of chest radiography is difficult to gauge but one historical series showed that at least 10% of cases with biopsy-proven ILD had an apparently normal radiograph.

- A diagnosis made on chest radiograph is seldom confident. In a large series by Mathieson (*Ref: Mathieson JR, Mayo JR, Staples CA, et al. Chronic diffuse infiltrative lung disease: comparison of diagnostic accuracy of CT and chest radiography. Radiology. 1989;171;111-6*). a confident diagnosis could be made in less than a quarter of the cases by experienced radiologists and this diagnosis correctly matched the histological diagnosis in only 77%.

- The chest radiograph cannot determine disease activity or whether the disease is likely to be reversible or not.

  Having pointed out these limitations, the chest radiograph has a number of advantages:

- It is useful for pattern recognition; for example, the bilateral hilar adenopathy and upper lobe preponderance of sarcoidosis or the lower lobe honeycombing of IPF.

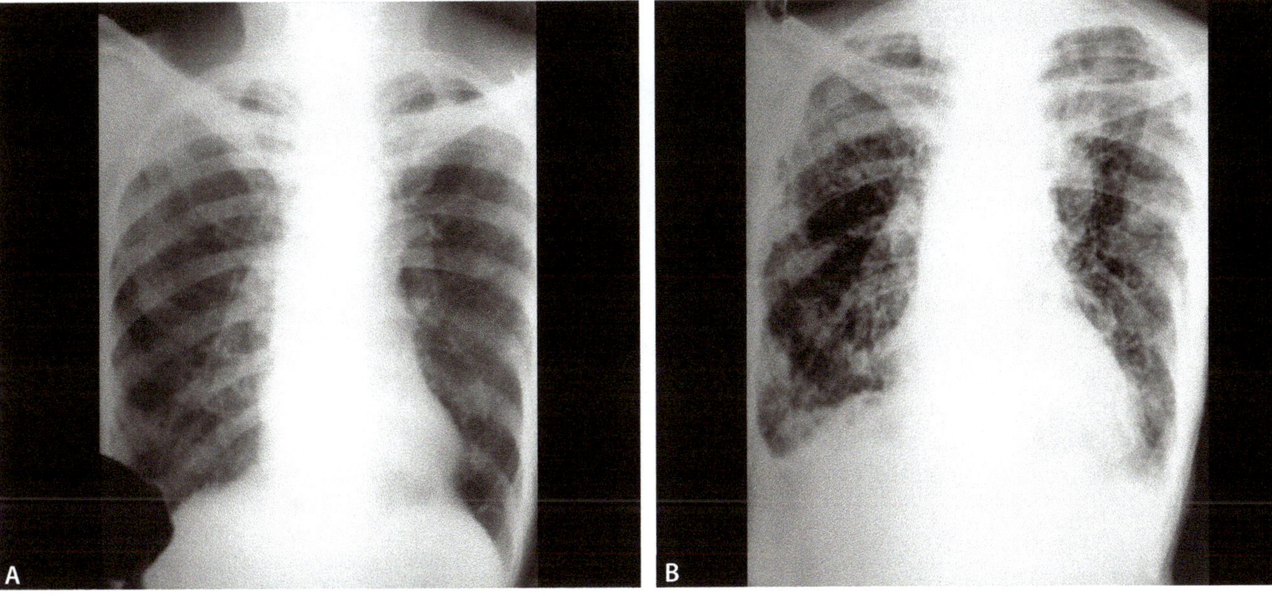

Figs. 4A and B: (A) Chest X-ray reveals reticular opacities in a patient with IPF. (B) Follow-up X-ray after 6 years demonstrates progression of disease process. The chest X-ray has a low specificity and sensitivity in diffuse lung diseases but is an easy and cheap modality to assess progression of the disease.

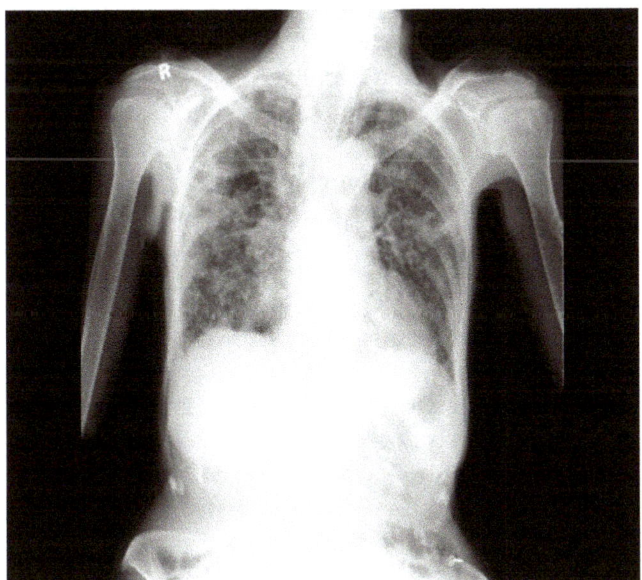

Fig. 5: IPF with opportunistic infection. Chest X-ray reveals reticular opacities in both lung fields as a result of IPF, ill-defined areas of consolidation with cavitation in right upper lobe. Patient was on long-term treatment with immunosuppressants for IPF, developed cough with expectoration and fever. The right upper lobe consolidation with cavitation was due to an opportunistic infection. Sputum was positive for acid-fast bacilli (AFB).

- It is widely used for serial monitoring of progress (along with PFT) as it is impractical to use HRCTs too frequently in this role.

- It is more than adequate to detect complications such as pneumothorax or superadded infection.

Thus, in summary, chest radiography though inferior to the HRCT scan remains a pivotal screening tool. Because of its ready availability it is often the first and only tool in parts of the developing world.

High-resolution Computed Tomography

High-resolution computed tomography provides cross-sectional images of the lungs that possess spatial and contrast resolution such that submillimeter structures in the lung are clearly visible.

Sensitivity of High-resolution Computed Tomography

The sensitivity of HRCT for ILD is believed to be in the vicinity of 95%. This is much higher than that of chest radiography but is not yet 100%. Thus, it is possible on rare occasions to have biopsy proof of ILD with a normal HRCT. In one series of biopsy-proven IPF by Orens et al., CT appearances were considered normal in 3 of 25 cases (i.e. 12%). The clinical significance of such subtle and early ILD is unclear.

Specificity of High-resolution Computed Tomography

Many reports have shown that HRCT is significantly more accurate than chest radiography in diagnosing individual ILDs. In the study by Mathieson referred to earlier, a confident diagnosis was reached more than twice as often with CT than with chest radiography. This diagnosis was correct in 93% of cases compared with 77% of cases of first-choice radiographic diagnosis. If clinical features, chest radiography and HRCT are combined there is an exponential increase in diagnostic accuracy to 66–80% of patients with ILD. It must be noted that the diagnostic accuracy of HRCT is highly disease-dependent. Thus, when the HRCT appearance is typical of UIP, the diagnosis is correct more than 90% of times. On the other hand, the wide range of HRCT patterns of NSIP makes this a difficult diagnosis to accurately make on CT.

Observer Variations

Observer variations among thoracic radiologists when making a histospecific diagnosis are not uncommon and interobserver variation is especially divergent in NSIP.

High-resolution Computed Tomography and Biopsy

High-resolution computed tomography may make a biopsy unnecessary. A typical HRCT pattern of UIP in an elderly male with the classic history is diagnostic of IPF so often that a biopsy is not indicated in this situation. More and more centers are relying on typical CT features to help them decide which patients need not undergo biopsy, thus sparing these elderly patients from undergoing an invasive procedure. Conversely, if the CT findings are atypical in any way then a biopsy should be ideally performed. An HRCT may also provide invaluable information to the surgeon on which lobes or segments of the lung he should sample for biopsy. The HRCT features of UIP, desquamative interstitial pneumonia, NSIP and acute interstitial pneumonia are illustrated in **Figures 6 to 11**. A brief description of the histopathology of various IIPs is given in **Table 3**.

High-resolution Computed Tomography and Biopsy and Disease Reversibility

A ground-glass pattern on HRCT predicts the response to treatment and increased survival compared to patients

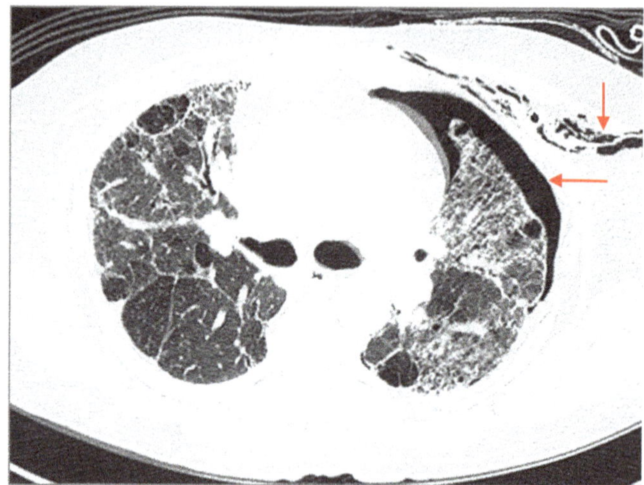

Fig. 6: Usual interstitial pneumonia: High-resolution computed tomography (HRCT) chest demonstrates thin-walled honeycomb cysts in a subpleural location, especially with adjacent septal thickening. Note patchy areas of intervening normal lung. There is associated mild pneumothorax and subcutaneous emphysema on the left side.

in whom the predominant CT type is reticulation. The HRCT pattern of honeycombing is highly predictive of an irreversible pattern that is unlikely to respond even with high doses of immunosuppressive therapy.

High-resolution Computed Tomography and Detecting Complications

High-resolution computed tomography is an accurate way of picking up complications of an ILD in a patient faring poorly. TB is an important opportunistic infection and may be impossible to pick up on traditional chest radiography in a patient with preexisting fibrosis. An HRCT may, on the other hand, pick up a cavity or infiltrate that can be a useful pointer to TB. A septal carcinoma is another complication that can be picked up more accurately on CT scanning compared to chest radiography.

Pivotal Role of CT in diagnosing IPF: Thus, the CT scan has a pivotal role in making a diagnosis of IPF as emphasized in the 2011 ERS, ATS guidelines.

These guidelines describe the key radiological findings in patients with IPF. For a confident diagnosis of Usual Interstitial Pneumonia (UIP) pattern to be made, the four key radiological features mentioned in **Table 3** must all be met:

- Subpleural, basal predominance
- Reticular abnormalities
- Honeycombing
- None of the 7 features listed as inconsistent with UIP.

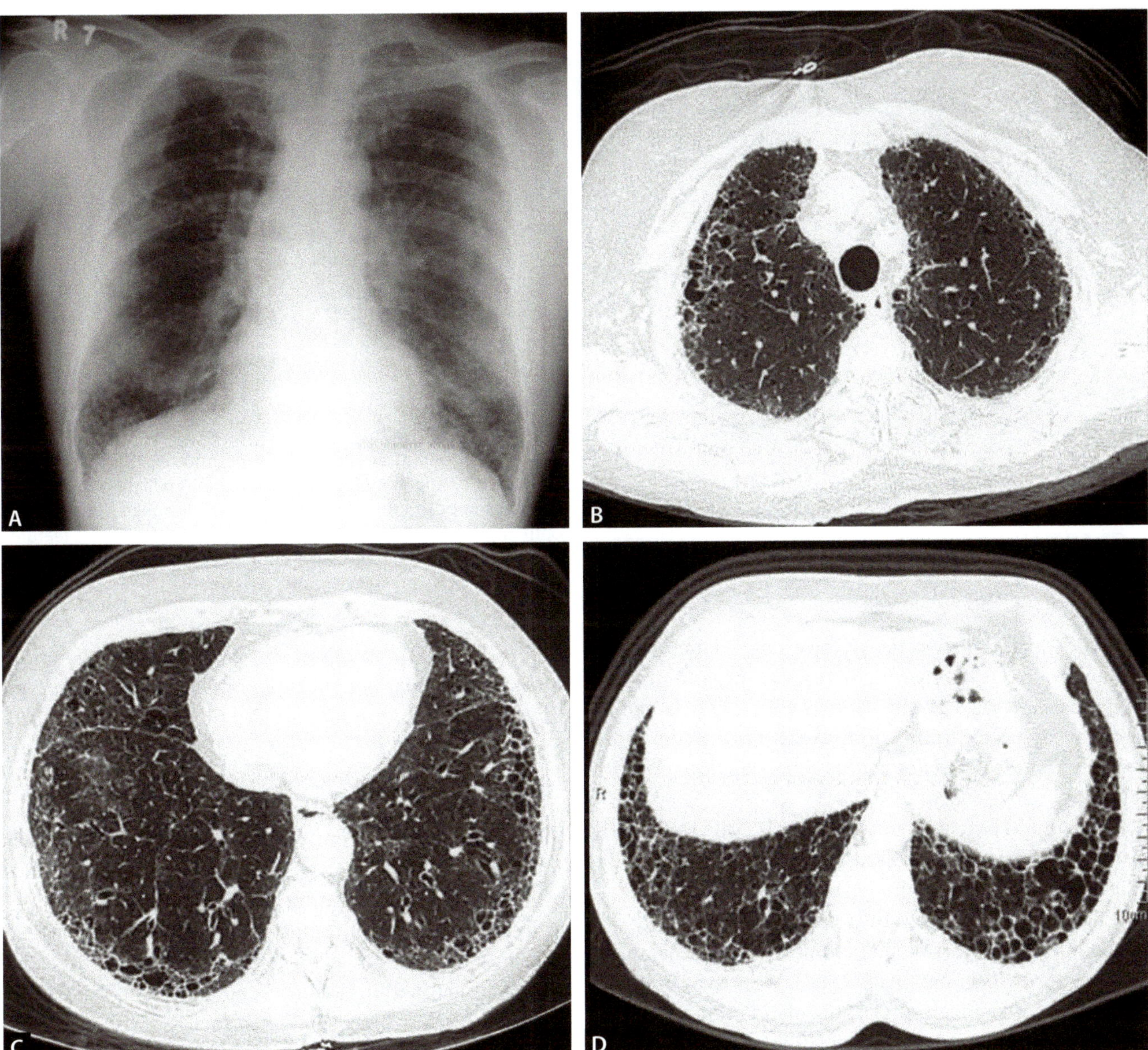

Figs. 7A to D: Usual interstitial pneumonia: (A) Chest X-ray demonstrates reticular and honeycomb changes in both lung fields, especially lung bases. HRCT chest (B to D) demonstrates similar appearances of honeycomb cysts with septal thickening in subpleural regions. No ground-glass densities are seen indicating UIP pattern of interstitial pneumonia.

It must be stressed that the presence of a UIP pattern on HRCT alone is not sufficient to label a patient IPF. History and context are all important as a UIP CT pattern can be encountered in other conditions like hypersensitivity pneumonia, secondary to collagen vascular disease and asbestosis. The guidelines stress that a confident diagnosis of IPF (without need for a biopsy) can only be made in a patient with a UIP pattern on CT scan if the patient also has clinical and demographic features of IPF, and all other known causes of ILD can be excluded

(Table 4) (*Ref: An official ATS/ERS/JRS/ATLT statement: idiopathic pulmonary fibrosis, evidence-based guidelines for diagnosis and management. Am J Respir Crit Care Med. 2011:183;788-824*).

Pulmonary Function Testing

A restrictive defect is the most frequent ventilatory abnormality in patients with ILDs. A drop in the transfer factor may be the only abnormality in patients with ILD; spirometry may be normal in early stages. Some ILDs

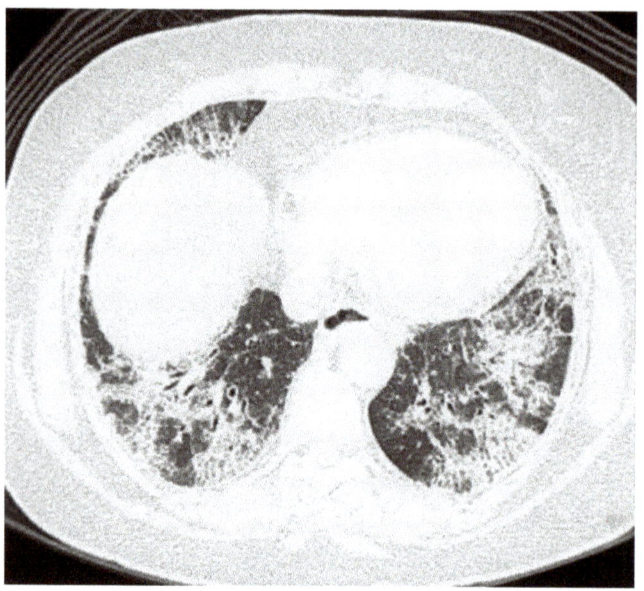

Fig. 8: Usual interstitial pneumonia, late stage. Marked fibrotic thickened interstitial septae with collapse of alveoli.

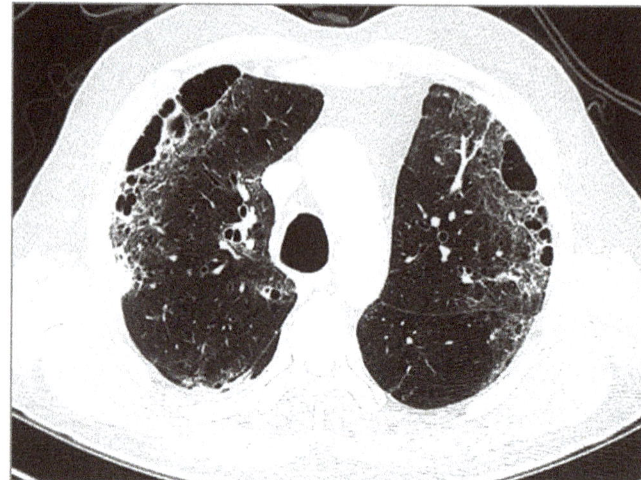

Fig. 9: Desquamative interstitial pneumonia. High-resolution computed tomography (HRCT) demonstrates diffuse ground-glass densities in both lung fields. There are thin-walled cysts seen in both upper lobes. The patient was a chronic smoker. These features of ground-glass densities with lung cysts are typical in smokers, representing desquamative interstitial pneumonia.

such as LAM and histiocytosis X have a mixed picture with evidence of gas trapping with increased lung volumes and an increased RV/TLC ratio. Patients with ILD who smoke and have concomitant emphysema have even more severely reduced transfer factors than nonsmokers with ILD.

The aims of lung function testing in ILD are to quantify disease severity, monitor disease progression and, ideally, to identify variables that predict mortality.

Several studies have shown that the worse the PFT at presentation the worse the outcome. A transfer factor of the lung for carbon monoxide (TLCO) less than 35% was associated with a mean survival of only 24 months with no difference in the outcome between IPF and NSIP. Thus, the severity of IPF is best staged by TLCO estimation.

Serial lung function is a simple, noninvasive and easily reproducible way to monitor disease progression. Change in forced vital capacity (FVC) and TLCO have emerged as the serial PFT measurements most consistently predictive of mortality. A decline in FVC of 10% and a decline in TLCO of 20% from their baseline values are predictive of a 2.4-fold increase in mortality. A study by Latsi et al., showed that serial FVC trends are even more reliable than serial TLCO trends in predicting poor survival. Even more interestingly, his study showed that the histological diagnosis is irrelevant once lung function changes over 12 months have been taken into account *[Ref: Latsi*

PL, du Bois RM, Nicholson AG, et al. Fibrotic idiopathic interstitial pneumonia: the prognostic value of longitudinal functional trends. Am J Respir Crit Care Med. 2003;168(5): 531-7].

Desaturation during exercise is a sensitive but not specific test for diagnosing ILD. The 6-minute walk test (6MWT) has only recently been applied to ILD but has provided powerful prognostic information in 4 studies of IPF. Indeed, desaturation to 88% in a baseline 6MWT either during or at the end of the walk has emerged as a much more powerful predictor of mortality than resting lung function tests. A recent study concluded that desaturation less than 88% was associated with a survival of 3.2 years compared to median survival of 6.6 years in those patients who maintained saturation greater than 88%. Two recent studies have also confirmed the prognostic significance of distance walked in the 6MWT in IPF patients. Those walking less than 212 m had a significantly lower survival than those walking further distances. The distance walked may also be of prognostic value. Attempts to formulate a combined measure of desaturation and distance covered may represent a novel and useful marker of disease severity and prognosis. Serial 6MWT is also useful in following up disease progression. Thus, 6MWT is a cheap, simple, reproducible but underutilized monitoring tool in patients with ILD. It requires no equipment apart from an oximeter and a

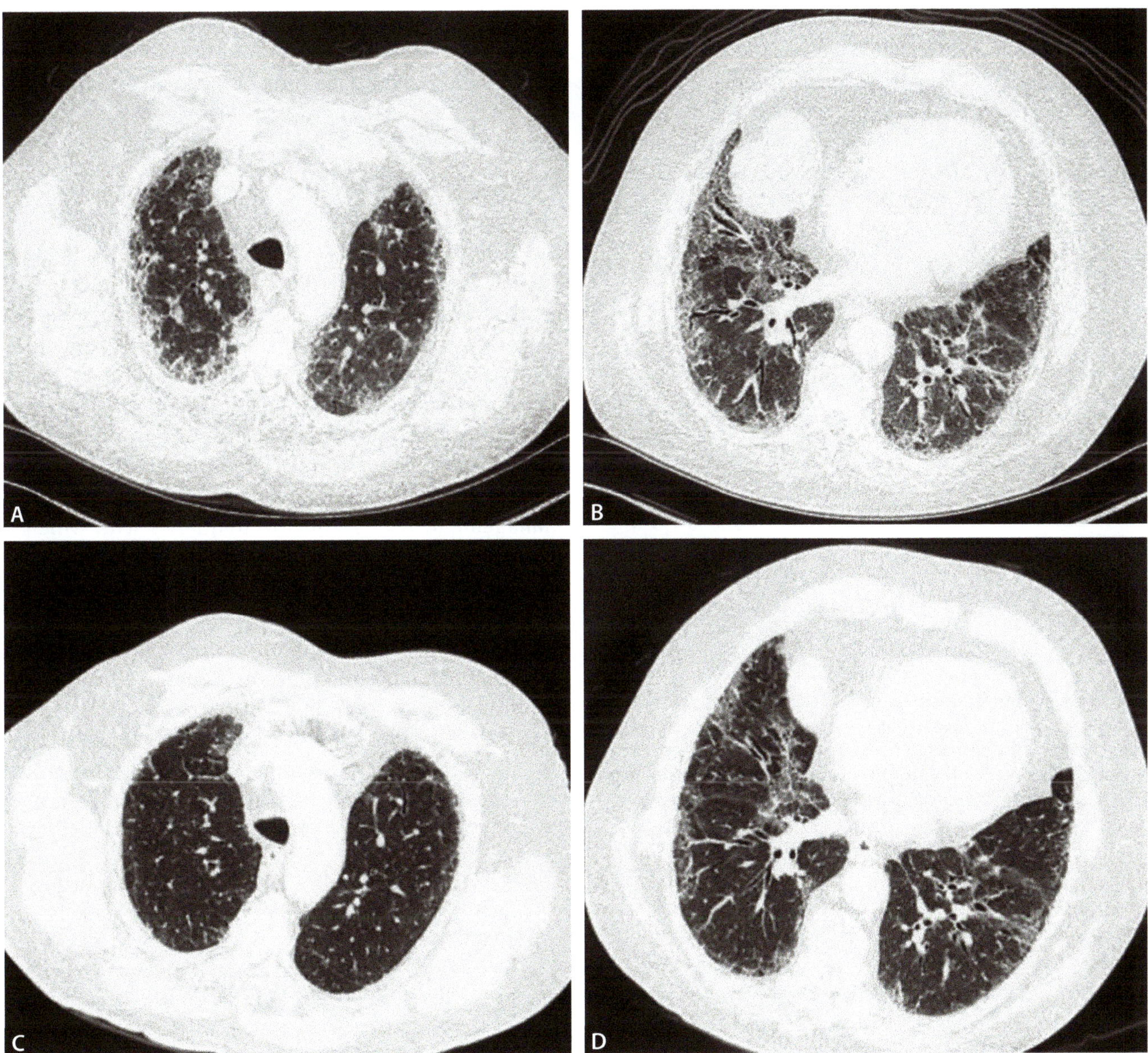

Figs. 10A to D: Nonspecific interstitial pneumonia (NSIP): (A and B) High-resolution computed tomography (HRCT) demonstrates ill-defined ground-glass densities in a peribronchovascular and subpleural location with associated traction bronchiectasis. No significant honeycomb changes are visualized. These features are of NSIP; follow-up CT (C and D) studies after treatment reveal resolution in ground-glass densities with residual traction bronchiectasis.

clock and can be done even in smaller centers without facilities for measuring transfer factor.

Bronchoscopy, Bronchoalveolar Lavage, and Transbronchial Lung Biopsy

Bronchoscopy and BAL are likely to add diagnostic value in only a few situations. BAL is useful if a secondary infection like TB is suspected in a patient with ILD. BAL may also be of value in rarer ILDs with eosinophilia or in pulmonary alveolar proteinosis when proteinaceous PAS positive material may be of diagnostic value. Outside these settings, BAL remains a research tool. BAL lymphocyte ratios (CD4/CD8) are raised in sarcoidosis but lowered in EAA. Other BAL cell fractions have been studied as well: BAL neutrophilia is believed to be linked to the extent and severity of disease, while BAL eosinophilia is linked to disease progression. However, these generalizations are not discriminatory enough for us to recommend BAL in the routine workup of a patient with ILD.

Transbronchial lung biopsy cannot replace a surgical biopsy. It cannot determine the type of IIP encountered. Having said this, it may be of great diagnostic value in sarcoidosis, EAA, BOOP and occasionally in PAP. We

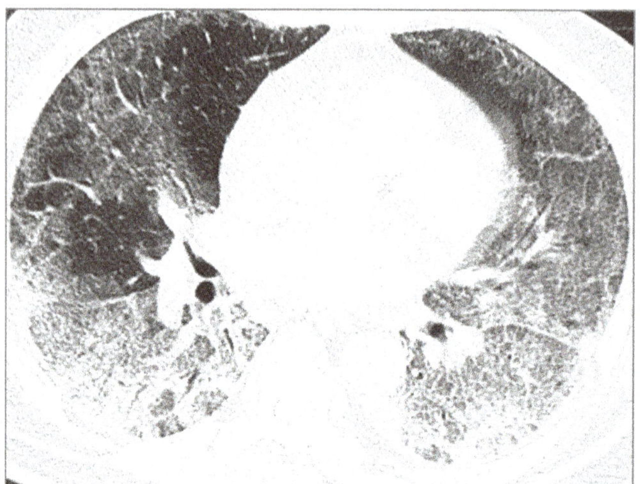

Fig. 11: Acute interstitial pneumonia. HRCT demonstrates diffuse ill-defined ground-glass densities or consolidation with air bronchograms in both lung fields. Patient presented with acute onset of respiratory failure. This represents acute interstitial pneumonia, patient responded well to corticosteroid therapy.

recently reported a series of over 30 cases of BOOP all of whom had been diagnosed on transbronchial lung biopsy (TBLBx) thus sparing the patient the need for open lung biopsy.

Open Lung Biopsy

An open biopsy is the only way to accurately determine which of the seven types of IIP a patient has. It is also often the only way to make a definitive diagnosis in patients with many of the rarer DPLDs. There is a natural reluctance in the minds of many physicians to subject their patients to an invasive procedure like an open lung biopsy. These patients are often elderly, have impaired lung function and multiple comorbidities. Furthermore, it is often argued that since there are limited effective therapies for IPF, pathological diagnosis does little to change overall management. As a result the frequency with which a surgical lung biopsy is performed is very low.

A number of questions need to be asked:

a. *With advances in HRCT, is a biopsy still needed?*
   High-resolution computed tomography is a critical element in the diagnosis of IIP but unfortunately often cannot be relied on to make an accurate diagnosis. When the classic findings of reticulonodular opacities at the bases and peripheries of the lung, with associated traction bronchiectasis and honeycombing

Type of pneumonia	Radiology	Histopathology
UIP	Reticular abnormality, honeycombing, basal peripheral predominance, often patchy with intervening normal lung	Heterogeneous areas of young connective tissue, scarring, honeycomb changes, normal lung
NSIP	Ground-glass abnormality. Reticular shadows, traction bronchiectasis, basal predominance with or without subpleural sparing	Alveolar septal thickening by inflammation/fibrosis Spatially and temporarily homogenous
DIP	Ground glass, basal peripheral predominance with or without cysts	Diffuse macrophage accumulation within alveolar spaces, mild interstitial thickening. Homogenous involvement
RBILD	Centrilobular nodules Ground-glass attenuation Diffuse or upper lobe predominance	Bronchogenic accumulation of alveolar macrophages. Mild bronchiolar fibrosis
AIP	Ground glass consolidation, organizing architectural distortion, traction bronchiectasis	Acute edema, hyaline membrane, interstitial inflammation, airspace organization
LIP	Ground glass, septal thickening, cysts, diffuse or lower lung distribution	Diffuse alveolar Infiltration by lymphocytes Infrequent lymphoid Hyperplasia
OP	Consolidation in peribronchial or subpleural distribution	Intraluminal organizing fibrosis in bronchioles, alveolar ducts and alveoli. Temporarily homogenous patchy distribution.

Table 3: Radiology and histopathological features of various interstitial pneumonias.

Table 4: The American Thoracic Society/European Respiratory Society criteria for diagnosing idiopathic pulmonary fibrosis.

Major criteria (mandatory):
- Exclusion of other causes of ILD
- Abnormal PFT
- Bi-basal reticular abnormalities with minimal ground glass opacities on HRCT
- BAL or transbronchial biopsy excluding all other alternative diagnosis

Minor criteria (3 of 4 mandatory):
- Age > 50 years
- Insidious onset of otherwise unexplained dyspnea on exertion
- Duration of illness of > 3 months
- Bi-basal, inspiratory, dry crackles

are present, the diagnostic accuracy of CT approaches 90–100% and can then obviate the need for a biopsy. Unfortunately these features are found in only 50% or less of patients with IPF. For the non-UIP subtypes, radiographic specificity drops even further. An elegant study asked how frequently combined clinical and HRCT data can confidently diagnose IPF making open lung biopsy unnecessary *[Ref: Hunning-Hake GW, Zimmerman MB, Schwartz DA, et al. Utility of a lung biopsy for the diagnosis of idiopathic pulmonary fibrosis. Am J Respir Crit Care Med. 2001;164(2):193-6].*

When expert pulmonologists and radiologists agreed on a core diagnosis of IPF **(Table 4)** with high clinical confidence, the positive predictive value approached 90%. Unfortunately a confident clinical diagnosis can be achieved in only 50% of these patients. The accuracy decreased even more when the diagnosis was less certain and especially in non-UIP subtypes. Thus often an open lung biopsy remains the only way to obtain a definite diagnosis.

b. *Is it safe?*
In experienced hands a surgical biopsy is safe. Advances in anesthesia and surgical techniques have made the procedure much safer. A study for risk factors showed that advanced age, low diffusion capacity, need for oxygen therapy and pulmonary hypertension are all independent risk factors for complications and mortality after a surgical biopsy. Video-assisted thoracoscopic surgery (VATS) has revolutionized the procedure and the 30-day mortality is no more than 1–3% when these high-risk patients are excluded.

c. *Technical considerations?*
Biopsies should be ideally taken early in the disease not only because this is safer but because when end-stage fibrosis has developed little further histological information can be gleaned.

Biopsy should be taken after careful discussion with the radiologist, from more than one lobe (preferably both upper and lower) to improve the overall yield. When discordant findings are obtained in samples from different sites (e.g. UIP in one lobe and NSIP in another), these patients must be presumed to have UIP for their prognosis is comparable to concordant UIP.

d. *What advantages are there from obtaining a surgical biopsy?*
A definite label of UIP on biopsy allows a patient to be labeled a definite case of IPF. This has great prognostic value and such information is useful for patients and their families. Novel therapies are constantly being developed and such patients can ideally be enrolled in trials with these new agents armed with the knowledge that their survival with routine immunosuppressives alone is likely to be dismal.

e. *So who should it be done on?*
Even the most aggressive-minded physician would agree that there is little to be gained in subjecting an 80-year-old male with gross clubbing and distinctive crackles who has an HRCT showing classical basal and peripheral honeycombing to an open lung biopsy. However, in younger patients or those with atypical features on HRCT a surgical biopsy would be ideal and might provide useful insights into the patients' further course and outcome.

The histopathological features of usual interstitial pneumonia and nonspecific interstitial pneumonia are illustrated in **Figures 12 to 14**.

Putting it all Together

In no other branch of respiratory medicine is close coordination between clinician, radiologist, and pathologist more important than in the ILDs. Thus, pathology on open lung biopsy is not the gold standard here, as even an expert pathologist will be lost without the input provided by clinician and radiologist.

From this arose the concept of MDD or multidisciplinary-discussion where a final diagnosis should ideally only be reached when these three specialists sit together and discuss each case, coming to a final, unifying diagnosis. It has been convincingly shown that the accuracy of diagnosis shows an incremental increase and improvement with this approach. Thus, the κ value which

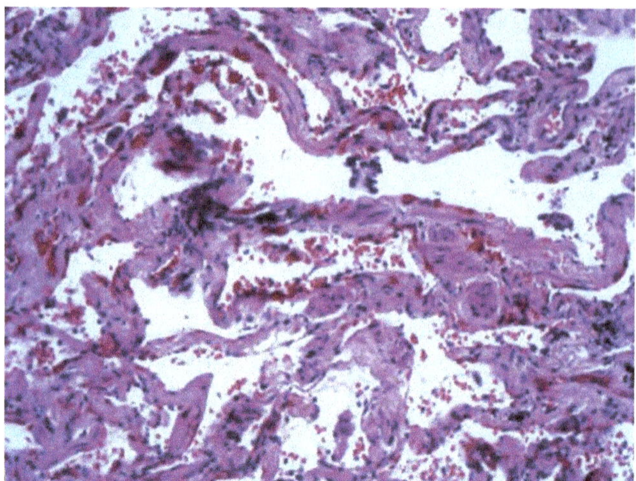

Fig. 12: Usual interstitial pneumonia, markedly thickened, widened fibrotic interstitial septae.

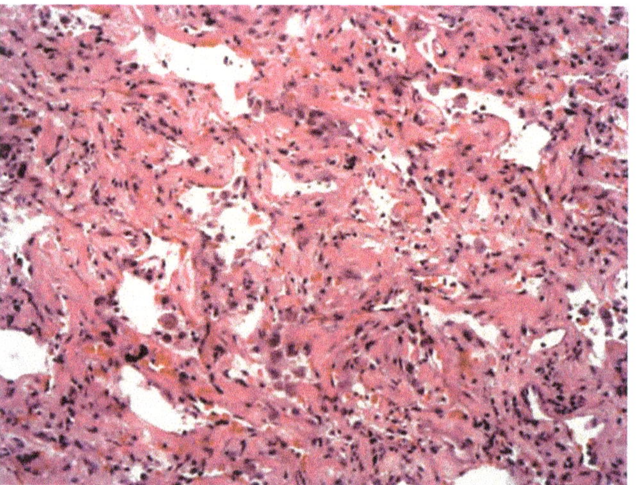

Fig. 13: Nonspecific interstitial pneumonia HRCT chest demonstrates ill-defined ground-glass densities in both lung bases in a peribronchovascular and subpleural location, there are no honeycomb changes. These features are indicative of NSIP pattern of interstitial pneumonia.

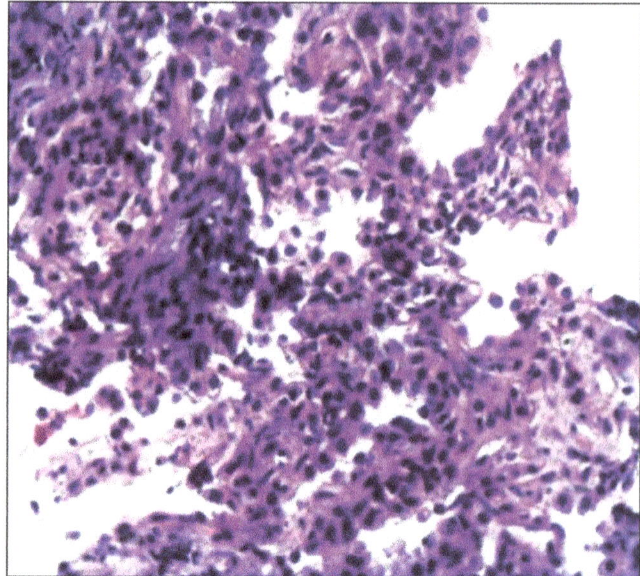

Fig. 14: Nonspecific interstitial pneumonia (H&E, 40x). NSIP cellular phase. Diffuse uniform interstitial inflammatory infiltrate is present in the interstitium, composed predominantly of lymphocytes. The alveoli show hyperplasia of Type II pneumocytes. Temporal uniformity is noted. Fibrosis is indiscernible.

reflects diagnostic agreement increases from 0.42 (fair) when the CT is looked at in isolation by the radiologist to 0.67 (substantial) when clinician and radiologist meet and discuss, to 0.84 (excellent) when clinician, radiologist and pathologist meet and have a multidisciplinary discussion. **Table 5** lists the key features in the diagnosis of ILD.

■ TREATMENT

Patients with newly diagnosed IPF currently have a median survival of 3–4 years. No current drug can reverse or even halt the relentless decline in lung function in IPF. However, while most of the earlier drugs have been shown to be ineffective and sometimes even harmful, there have emerged novel antifibrotic agents in the last few years that have changed the landscape.

Earlier Treatment

Most of the earlier drugs used for the treatment of IPF have fallen by the wayside to be replaced by newer antifibrotic agents. Agents that were in use and have been shown to be ineffective are summarized here:

- Steroids: We have clear evidence that the high doses of steroids that were the mainstay of earlier decades do more harm than good. Earlier studies have been subject to scrutiny and a recent Cochrane review by Richeldi concluded that there was no role for steroids alone in the management of this condition (*Ref: Richeldi L, Davies H, Spagnolo P, et al. Cochran Database of Systematic Reviews; 2009, Issue 2. Art No:CD002880*).
- Triple therapy: of low dose steroid, azathioprine, and N-acetylcystine (NAC) used by most chest physicians over many years has also been recently shown in the recent PANTHER-IPF trial, to be worse than placebo [*Ref: Raghu G, Idiopathic Pulmonary Fibrosis Clinical*

Table 5: Diagnosis of interstitial lung disease.

- *History*: Dry cough, dyspnea
- *Clinical examination*: Dry *Velcro* crackles, specific features related to ILD secondary to a known cause (e.g. connective tissue disease)
- *Chest radiography*: Useful for diagnosis, pattern recognition and for serial monitoring
- *High-resolution computed tomography chest*: Sensitivity of 95% for diagnosis, ground-glass pattern predicts reversibility, detects complications
- *Pulmonary function test*: Restrictive pattern. Reduced transfer factor; reduced FVC; reduced lung volumes. Some ILDs have a mixture of obstructive + restrictive pattern. Helps monitor disease
- *Bronchoscopy, bronchoalveolar lavage (BAL)*: Adds diagnostic value in just a few situations
- *Video-assisted thoracoscopic surgery/Open lung biopsy*: Only way for a definitive diagnosis in the rarer forms. Not required in the typical UIP

Research Network, Anstrom KJ, et al. Prednisolone, azathioprine, and N-acetylcysteine for pulmonary fibrosis. N Engl J Med. 2012;366(21):1968-77].

- In fact, the NIH stopped the trial prematurely when only 50% of the data had been collected when a planned interim analysis showed increased death and hospitalization rates in the patients receiving triple therapy over placebo. This coupled with no evidence of clinical or physiological benefit prompted the safety board to recommend trial termination.
- N-acetylcysteine (NAC): As mono therapy was also put to the test against placebo and found to be ineffective [*Ref: Martinez FJ, IPF Clinical Research Network, de Andrade JA, et al. Randomized trial of acetylcysteine in idiopathic pulmonary fibrosis. N Engl J Med. 2014;370(22):2093-3101].*
- Other agents shown in recent trials to be of no value in IPF include: Interferon gamma (IFN-γ), anticoagulants, bosentan, cyclosporine A, colchicine, etanercept, sildenafil, and ambrisentan. All these agents have recommendations against their use in current ATS-ERS guidelines.
- In contrast to these consistently negative studies the silver lining has been the remarkable, proven efficacy of two novels antifibrotic agents: Pirfenidone and nintedanib. The pivotal studies for both these drugs was published in the same issue of the New England Journal of Medicine in 2014 and they both received rapid FDA approval for IPF within a few months of this publication. With the advent of these two new agents

we have truly entered a new era in the management of IPF.

- *Pirfenidone*: It is a novel antifibrotic agent that inhibits TGF-β_1 stimulated collagen synthesis and blocks fibroblast proliferation. Overall, data from four RCTs provides evidence of its effect on preserving lung function. In the CAPACITY and ASCEND trials the drug was shown to slow the annual decline of FVC by about 50% compared to placebo. When the data from these two trials was pooled, for the first time in any IPF study, a significant benefit in all-cause mortality was observed. The drug is given in a dose of 1,800 mg a day but because of the high rates of nausea and gastric distress reported (32%), at this dose, it is best to escalate the dose gradually and always administer the tablets after food. Apart from the gastric side effects, other important side effects worth mentioning include photosensitivity reactions (12%), and deranged liver function (3%).
- *Nintedanib*: Nintedanib is a potent inhibitor of several tyrosine kinase receptors—Platelet-derived growth factor (PDGF), fibroblast growth factor (FGF) and vascular endothelial growth factor (VEGF). These receptors mediate signaling pathways known to be involved in the development of fibrosis. Nintedanib acts by binding to the intracellular receptors blocking substrate binding. After an earlier phase II study TOMORROW in 2011, the INPULSIS trial, two replicate, parallel, 52-week, randomized, double-blind Phase III studies showed that a dose of 150 mg twice a day of nintedanib slowed the speed of decline in FVC by around 50% compared to placebo. The most frequent adverse effect reported with this drug is diarrhea reported with a frequency of around 60% in the INPULSIS study.

The availability of two new drugs, and with them, for the first time a real choice, begs the interesting question of which agent is to be preferred. On the basis of available data, the superiority of one drug over the other has not been established. Both drugs do the same: Slow the decline in FVC in mild to moderate IPF to the same extent (about 50%) with acceptable side effects. Head to head comparisons in a single trial will never be made it and is ill-advised to compare data from one trial with the other as each trial had nuanced differences in inclusion and exclusion criteria and the way the primary outcome FVC was analyzed.

We would recommend choosing the initial drug, based on patient preference, physician familiarity, availability, cost, side effect profile and tolerability. If the patient cannot tolerate the initial agent chosen, or his FVC and TLCO continue to decline at a rate signifying treatment failure (decline in FVC is more than 10% at 6 months, and in TLCO, then a switch can be made from one agent to the other. At present, a case cannot be made for combining agents as the potential toxicity may outweigh benefit. However, as our knowledge and experience with these agents grows, it is likely that combination therapy will be used in the future to treat IPF.

General Measures

- Oxygen should be provided to all patients with IPF who are hypoxic or who desaturate with exercise. Unlike in COPD, there is no evidence that oxygen therapy impacts on long-term survival in IPF. However, breathlessness is one of the most distressing symptoms for any patient with IPF and oxygen undoubtedly provides some relief. Nebulized morphine has been tried without effect, but oral opiates, in small and carefully titrated doses may provide some relief from the crippling breathlessness experienced in end stage patients.
- *Cough*: It is another disabling and distressing symptom in these patients and one that does not respond to standard antitussives. A small study showed thalidomide may have an effect and may be considered in carefully selected patients.
- *Gastroesophageal reflux disease*: Patients with IPF have been shown to have a higher incidence of GERD than the general population. After confirming its presence (24 hour pH studies and manometry), treatment with proton-pump inhibitors is recommended as there is a hypothesis that reflux of acid, bile salts, and pepsin can accelerate the progression of fibrosis.
- *Sleep apnea*: It is another common association and patients of IPF found to have coexisting obstructive sleep apnea (OSA) may benefit from continuous positive airway pressure (CPAP).
- *Pulmonary rehabilitation*: All patients with IPF should ideally be referred for pulmonary rehabilitation. Recent studies show it improves quality of life and effort capacity.

Lung Transplantation

Lung transplantation is often the only option for the younger patient with advanced IPF. It is one of the commonest indications for lung transplantation at most centers. The actuarial survival after lung transplant for IPF approaches 75% at 1 year and 50% at 5 years. The optimal timing for transplant varies from center to center. Our center at the Hinduja hospital was among the first to perform a single lung transplant for a patient with advanced lung fibrosis in 2012. Unfortunately the patient survived for a little more than 3 months. The current lung transplant scenario in India is discussed later in this chapter.

■ COMPLICATIONS OF INTERSTITIAL LUNG DISEASE (TABLE 6)

Acute Exacerbation of Interstitial Lung Disease

Acute exacerbation of IPF (AE-IPF): It is defined as an acute worsening of dyspnea and lung function without an obvious identifiable cause. This phenomenon has been recognized to occur in other fibrotic lung diseases as well, including HP and collagen vascular disease associated ILD. The following diagnostic criteria have been proposed for AE-IPF:

- A previous or concurrent diagnosis of IPF.
- Unexplained worsening of dyspnea within the past 30 days.
- High-resolution computed tomography with new bilateral ground-glass opacities and exclusion of alternative causes including pulmonary infection.

This is a common event occurring with an annual incidence varying between 1–20% of IPF patients depending on the population studied. A consistently higher rate has been reported in Korean and Japanese populations. AE-IPF is a major cause of morbidity and mortality in patients with IPF, accounting for over half of all hospital admissions. AE-IPF is also the

Table 6: Complications of interstitial lung disease.

- Acute exacerbations of IPF
- Opportunistic infections
- Bronchial carcinomas
- Heart failure and ischemic heart disease
- Pulmonary embolism
- Pneumothorax

commonest cause of death in patients with IPF. The short-term mortality is around 50%, but the mortality approaches 90% in patients admitted in the ICU. Autopsy findings in these patients reveal a background of usual interstitial pneumonia and a pattern of diffuse alveolar damage (DAD), with or without concurrent organizing pneumonia.

Management involves hospitalization and supplemental oxygen. Mechanical ventilation is avoided in most centers because of the almost uniformly bleak survival at this stage. The patient and his or her family must have this eventuality discussed in advance and ideally have an advance directive in place.

Noninvasive ventilation may eliminate the need for intubation and should be offered to all patients. Antibiotics in a broad empiric spectrum should be given to all patients with inclusion of co-trimoxazole to cover possible PCP. Large pulses of steroids (typically 500 mg of methylprednisone) are given daily for 3 days without any good evidence that this approach really works. Other agents like cyclophosphamide pulses, tacrolimus, cyclosporine, polymyxin B-immobilized fiber cartridge, and thrombomodulin have all been looked at in scattered case reports and small, uncontrolled trials. The new antifibrotics, pirfenidone and nintedanib may have a role in preventing acute exacerbations in IPF patients already receiving them on a regular basis. They should be continued in the patient who is admitted with an AE-IPF.

Opportunistic Infections

Opportunistic infections are frequent in these immunosuppressed patients. TB is the most frequent in the Indian setting. It is difficult to diagnose and the clinician must have a high index of suspicion if he is not to miss it completely.

Bronchial Carcinomas

These are not uncommon. In a review of the causes of death in 550 patients with IPF, 10% of all deaths were due to bronchial carcinoma. These are usually scar carcinomas arising from diffuse areas of scarring. They are most often localized adenocarcinoma or alveolar cell carcinomas. They are again difficult to diagnose and can only be treated palliatively as these patients are generally not candidates for resection or chemotherapy.

Heart Failure and Ischemic Heart Disease

Pulmonary hypertension and right heart failure are almost inevitable in advanced ILD and may contribute to mortality. These patients are usually elderly hence coexisting ischemic heart disease and LV dysfunction is also common.

Pulmonary Embolism

It has been reported to cause 3–7% of deaths in IPF. The real incidence may be higher because most of these patients are bedridden in the late stages of this disease.

Pneumothorax

It can complicate fibrotic lungs. If it occurs it is often difficult to treat since the lung is stiff and difficult to expand. Prolonged intercostal tube drainage may be required as these patients are usually too unwell to undergo thoracoscopic intervention.

A study by Panos looked at the causes of death in 550 patients with IPF. Mean survival ranged from 3.2 years to 5 years. Respiratory failure (39%), heart failure (14%), bronchogenic carcinoma (10%) and ischemic heart disease (10%) were the four commonest causes of death in this series [*Ref: Panos RJ, Mortenson R, Niccoli SA, et al. Clinical deterioration in patients with idiopathic pulmonary fibrosis: causes and assessment. Am J Med. 1990;88(4):396-404*].

■ FEATURES OF INTERSTITIAL LUNG DISEASE SPECIFIC TO INDIA (TABLE 7)

Overlap with Tuberculosis

Because of the very high burden of TB in India, most patients with pulmonary symptoms and diffuse radiological opacities are invariably initially labeled TB.

Table 7: Features of interstitial lung disease specific to India.

- Overlap with tuberculosis
- Chest radiography is the main diagnostic tool but has significant limitations
- Scarcity of HRCT machines (1 scanner per million populations)
- Lung function tests—only a few tertiary centers can perform CO diffusion studies
- Surgical biopsy using VATS is underutilized
- TB reactivation on treatment, increase in or precipitation of diabetes with treatment of the disease
- No lung transplant facilities in India

In our series of 134 patients of biopsy-proven sarcoidosis at the Hinduja hospital, Mumbai, over a third (37%) were initially labeled TB and received several months of inappropriate anti-TB therapy before the correct diagnosis was confirmed. Another series of biopsy-confirmed BOOP from the same institution revealed that 10% were mislabeled TB and received inappropriate anti-TB therapy. Additionally, pulmonary infections like TB continue to remain frequent causes of pulmonary fibrosis. In a follow-up study of patients with newly diagnosed TB, residual fibrosis was seen in 40% of patients at 3 months and in 25% at 12 months. In all these patients follow-up HRCT scans showed evidence of fibrosis with irregular linear opacities. There is a tendency to over-diagnose such post-tubercular fibrosis as ILD. Post-tubercular fibrosis is neither progressive nor active. It usually affects the upper lobes and is limited to the site where the active TB originally occurred. A careful review of old chest radiographs should make the diagnosis of post-TB scarring obvious.

Limitations of Chest Radiography

In a resource-limited setting like India, the chest radiograph is per force given undue weightage for the diagnosis or exclusion of any condition. In a series of 117 biopsy-proven cases of IPF from the Hinduja hospital in Mumbai, the chest radiograph was reported normal in as many as 27% of patients though subsequent CT scans showed them to have fairly advanced disease. Thus, overdependence on chest radiographs for the diagnosis of DPLD may result in delays in diagnosis with large numbers of patients remaining undiagnosed or misdiagnosed till advanced fibrosis sets in.

High-resolution Computed Tomography Scanning in India

The first attempts at HRCT scanning of the chest began in 1991, in centers in Mumbai and New Delhi. Currently, India has a CT scanner base of 3,000 machines which works out to 1 scanner per million populations. This penetrance is considered very low when compared to other countries in the region: Korea and Japan have 31 and 92 per million populations respectively. Besides the numbers it would not be unfair to claim that no more than a handful of radiologists countrywide would have an interest in chest imaging and in using the correct end-inspiratory breath-holding techniques needed to obtain good-quality images.

Lung Function Testing in India

Only a few tertiary referral hospitals in the country have the equipment to perform diffusion capacity studies. 6MWTs although not requiring any specialized equipment are underutilized.

Surgical Biopsy

Video-assisted thoracoscopy (VATS) is underutilized. Countrywide there are no more than 15 thoracic surgeons capable of performing this procedure. This results in delays in making a definitive diagnosis.

Treatment Issues in India

Tuberculosis Reactivation

Interstitial lung disease patients on steroids and immuno-suppressants are prone to develop opportunistic infections of which TB is the most common. In a country where the rates of latent tuberculosis infection (LTBI) are as high as 50–70%, reactivation of TB is a constant worry in patients on immunosuppressants. In a study from the Hinduja hospital, of 146 patients with systemic lupus erythematosus (SLE) who received steroids in a median cumulative dose of 7.5 mg for a median duration of 12 months, 17 patients went on to develop active TB. Ideally a tuberculin skin test or one of the IGRAs (IFN-γ release assays) should be done prior to starting immunosuppressives, and isoniazid prophylaxis offered to those with a positive result. However, there is no consensus on the protective effect of isoniazid in this setting and care must be taken to rule out active disease prior to starting a single drug.

Diabetes Flare-up

India has the largest diabetic population in the world (30 million) and many patients with ILD will have preexisting diabetes prior to starting steroids, while several will go on to develop it after commencement. It is vital to aim for tight control of diabetes in these patients on steroids.

Lung Transplantation in India

Lung transplantation is slowly but steadily establishing itself in India—chiefly at the Apollo and Global Hospitals, Chennai and PSG Hospital, Coimbatore. At the Apollo Hospital, Chennai, the first isolated single lung transplant was performed in 2011. The transplant unit has then progressed to performing double lung transplants and preferentially performs double lung transplants whenever possible.

The indications for lung transplant in ILD according to this team are:

- Decline in FVC > 10% during 6 month follow-up
- Desaturation < 88% or distance < 250 m on 6 min walk test or 50 m decline in 6 min walk test over 6 months
- Pulmonary hypertension on catheterization or ECHO with clinical deterioration
- Hospitalizations due to respiratory decline, pneumothorax, or acute exacerbations.

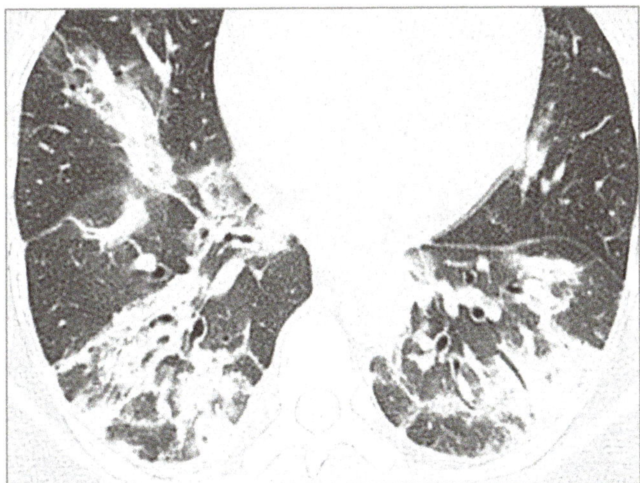

Fig. 15: COP HRCT chest demonstrates ill-defined subpleural and peribronchovascular consolidations in the right lung. Patient had a high ESR, biopsy of subpleural consolidation revealed COP. Patient had an excellent response to oral corticosteroid therapy.

BRONCHIOLITIS OBLITERANS ORGANIZING PNEUMONIA (FIGS. 15 TO 18)

In 1983, Davidson described a clinicopathological entity which he called cryptogenic organizing pneumonia (COP). Two years later Epler reported the same condition but labeled it bronchiolitis obliterans organizing pneumonia (BOOP). These two terms for the same disease, from different sides of the Atlantic have stood the test of time. COP probably is a better descriptor as it captures the clinical and radiological profile which is that of an alveolar rather than an airway disease. This is the term that will be used in the rest of this discussion. BOOP is the more commonly used term however, but care must be taken not to confuse it with *bronchiolitis obliterans* which is a completely different and unrelated entity or from respiratory bronchiolitis observed in chronic smokers **(Fig. 19)**.

Etiology

Organizing pneumonia can occur secondary to a number of diseases including infection, drug toxicity and connective tissue disorders. When it occurs in the absence of any of these known etiologies it is termed cryptogenic. It can, on occasion, be found accompanying other histological patterns seen in patients with IIPs, such as UIP and NSIP in which case it is considered to be a secondary phenomenon.

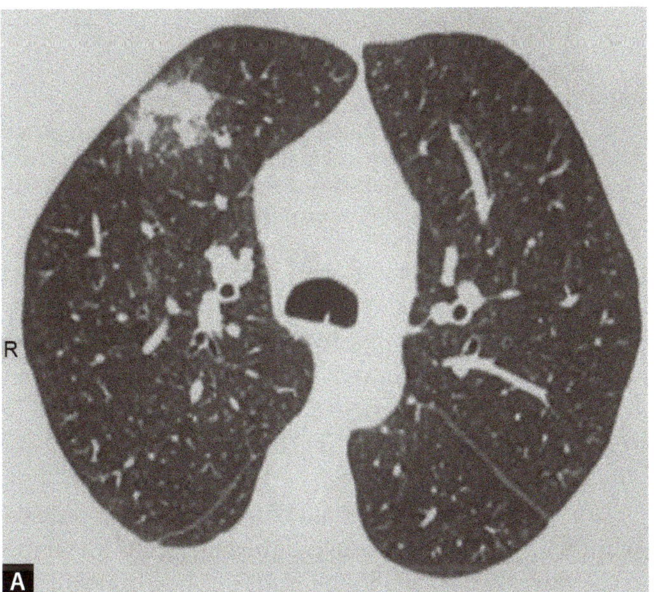
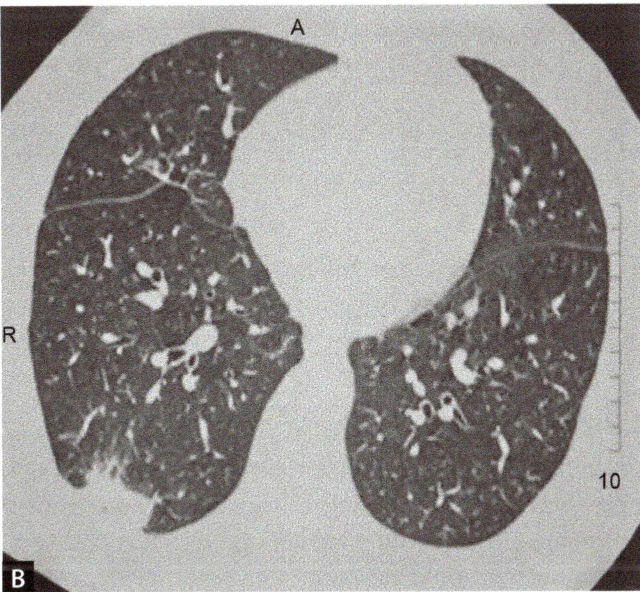

Figs. 16A and B: Middle-aged man with a right upper zone opacity treated with antibiotics and antitubercular drugs. (A) Opacity in right lung upper zone persisted. HRCT chest revealed ill-defined peribronchial and subpleural consolidation (B) right lower zone lesion. Biopsy revealed COP.

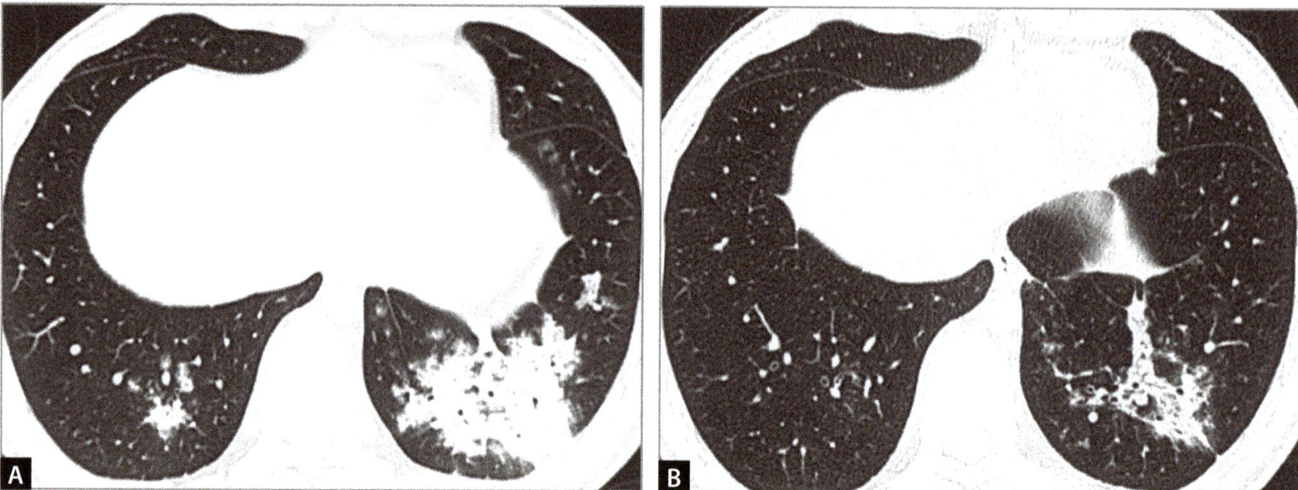

Figs. 17A and B: Middle-aged man presented with cough and breathlessness with opacity noted in left lower zone on the chest X-ray. HRCT demonstrates (A) ill-defined peribronchovascular consolidation in both lung bases. Patient has high ESR, biopsy revealed COP; (B) Treatment with corticosteroid showed good response.

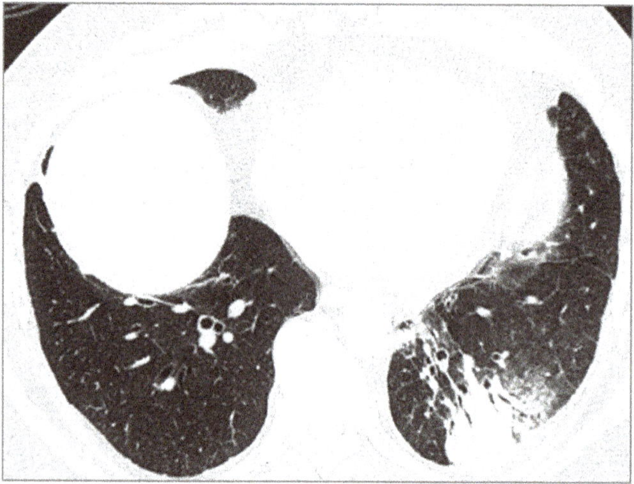

Fig. 18: High-resolution computed tomography (HRCT) chest performed on 17/08/2012 demonstrates subpleural consolidation in the left lung base, biopsy revealed COP.

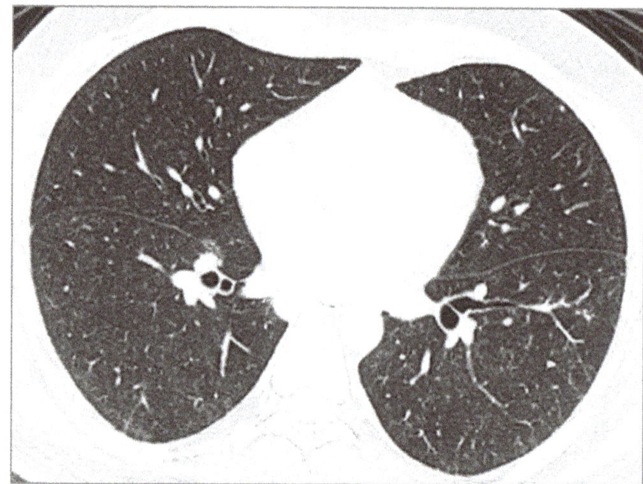

Fig. 19: Respiratory bronchiolitis. High-resolution computed tomography (HRCT) chest in a chronic smoker demonstrates small centrilobular nodules in both lung fields. These are small with ill-defined margins representing respiratory bronchiolitis.

Thus when organizing pneumonia is found on lung biopsy, a careful search for other underlying pathology patterns and clinical conditions should be performed.

Clinical Features

Cryptogenic organizing pneumonia often has a mean age of presentation of 50–60 years but has been reported at an age range of 20–80 with no gender predilection. Patients present acutely or subacutely with fever, malaise, cough and dyspnea. It mimics a viral infection or a community-acquired pneumonia and most patients are labeled as such and receive multiple courses of antibiotics.

Spontaneous remissions can occur in up to 50% of patients and in correctly treated patients the outcome is usually good with prompt resolution of symptoms and a slower improvement in radiology. Relapses are common but unpredictable and occur as the steroid dose is reduced with a 58% relapse rate being reported in a recent European Cohort.

An acute fulminant variant of COP is also recognized without pulmonary fibrosis, presenting as an acute respiratory distress syndrome (ARDS). These patients are extremely ill and require mechanical ventilation but have an excellent and rapid response to steroids even at this stage. Fibrosing COP is another variant with this subtype having extensive fibrosis which can progress to a fatal outcome despite treatment. Finally, a unifocal form of COP occurs in about 10% of patients. Such forms present as a solitary pulmonary nodule (SPN) and undergo resection with the correct diagnosis being made only after histopathology is available.

High-resolution Computed Tomography

High-resolution computed tomography in COP shows a number of distinctive features. There are bilateral, patchy, air space consolidations with a subpleural or peribronchial distribution often with ground-glass opacities. Shadows sometimes resolve spontaneously on serial radiographs only to reappear in another area. Honeycombing is rare.

Other Tests

These patients often have a leukocytosis making the distinction from community-acquired pneumonia even more difficult. The ESR is almost always markedly elevated. BAL shows increased lymphocytes and foamy macrophages.

Pathology

Cryptogenic organizing pneumonia can be definitively diagnosed only after a tissue biopsy. While earlier authors stressed the need for an open lung biopsy, our experience and that of others suggests that this is one IIP that can often be diagnosed by transbronchial lung biopsy. The characteristic lesion of COP is granulation tissue which proliferates within the distal air spaces, occluding the terminal bronchioles and alveolar ducts and spaces. These buds are called Masson's buds and are the pathological hallmark of BOOP.

■ MANAGEMENT AND OUTCOME

Cryptogenic organizing pneumonia responds very well to steroids. It is, in fact, the most steroid-responsive of all the IIPs with a favorable response in more than 80% of cases. Rarely, especially if COP is diagnosed late, it can continue to progress despite steroids. These patients then behave like an NSIP. Treatment with steroids in COP needs to continue for at least 6–12 months and relapses are not uncommon, especially as the steroid dose is tapered. Second-line immunosuppressives are sometimes needed. Recent case reports have shown a beneficial effect of macrolides in COP probably due to their anti-inflammatory effect.

Indian Data on Cryptogenic Organizing Pneumonia

The first Indian case of COP was described from our institution. We recently published the only large case series from this country where we reported on 34 cases of biopsy-proven COP from a single center from 2000–05. This study provides the first detailed analysis of the clinical and radiological presentation of COP from India. This is a good-sized cohort from a single center and shows that COP is not uncommon in India but underrecognized. Our patients had almost all received multiple courses of antibiotics and often prolonged anti-TB chemotherapy before the correct diagnosis was eventually made. Because of these long delays, as many as 21% of our patients responded suboptimally to steroids. Other distinctive features in our patients were female preponderance with females being affected 3 times as frequently as males. Transbronchial lung biopsy yielded the correct diagnosis in all our patients thus making surgical biopsy unnecessary *(Ref: Sen T, Udwadia ZF. Cryptogenic organizing pneumonia: clinical profile in a series of 34 admitted patients in a hospital in India. J Assoc Physicians India. 2008;56:229-32).*

■ SUGGESTED READING

1. Cordier JF. Cryptogenic organizing pneumonia. Clin Chest Med. 2004;25(4):727-38.
2. Davies G, Wells AU, du Bois RM. Respiratory bronchiolitis associated with interstitial lung disease and desquamative interstitial pneumonia. Clin Chest Med. 2004;25(4):717-26.
3. du Bois RM. Evolving concepts in the early and accurate diagnosis of idiopathic pulmonary fibrosis. Clin Chest Med. 2006;27(1 Suppl 1):S17-25.
4. Leslie KO. Pathology of interstitial lung disease. Clin Chest Med. 2004;25(4):657-703.
5. Lu BS, Bhorade SM. Lung transplantation for interstitial lung disease. Clin Chest Med. 2004;25(4):773-82.
6. Noth I, Martinez FJ. Recent advances in idiopathic pulmonary fibrosis. Chest. 2007;132(2):637-50.
7. Patel NM, Lederer DJ, Borczuk AC, et al. Pulmonary hypertension in idiopathic pulmonary fibrosis. Chest. 2007;132(3):998-1006.
8. Pipavath S, Godwin JD. Imaging of interstitial lung disease. Clin Chest Med. 2004;25(3):455-65.
9. Vourlekis JS. Acute interstitial pneumonia. Clin Chest Med. 2004;25(4):739-47.

CHAPTER 45

Sarcoidosis

■ GENERAL CONSIDERATIONS

Sarcoidosis is a disease of worldwide distribution characterized by the presence of noncaseating epitheloid granulomas in affected organs or organ systems; it is caused by an immune response to an unknown antigen in genetically susceptible individuals.

Sarcoidosis is a multisystem disease that can involve any organ in the body. The lungs and intrathoracic nodes are, however, most frequently involved. The mere presence of noncaseating granulomas is not proof of the disease. Preferably, there should be granulomatous lesions in more than one organ system and it is important that other causes of noncaseating epitheloid granulomas have been excluded. Unfortunately, as yet there is no test of sufficient sensitivity and specificity to help in the diagnosis, which therefore is based not just on histological evidence but on clinical and imaging features compatible with the disease.

Clinical, epidemiological, and familial studies have stressed the role of genetic susceptibility in the occurrence of the disease. Sarcoidosis has a variable clinical presentation and clinical course, and though corticosteroids form the cornerstone of treatment, there is as yet no specific cure for the disease.

■ EPIDEMIOLOGY

Sarcoidosis has a worldwide distribution though it is commoner in some parts of the world compared to others. Prevalence rates are underestimated even in the West and the US because a large number of people have asymptomatic disease and are therefore unaware of it. The highest prevalence rates are in Sweden, Denmark and in African Americans. African-Americans (particularly African-American women), are three and a half times more commonly affected, with a reported age-adjusted incidence of 35.5/100,000 compared with 10.9/100,000 in whites. The overall prevalence rates in the US, Southern Europe and Japan are reported as 10–40 per 100,000.

In the West, the disease occurs most frequently in the age group of 20–40 years with a second peak in women after the age of 50 years. The disease is more common in women than in men.

In the ACCESS study, one-third of the patients were between 50 years and 65 years. Sarcoidosis is known to recur after years or even decades of remission. It presents with recurrent involvement of the original organ involvement, or a new onset neurological or a different organ system involvement.

Geography and ethnicity often determine clinical presentation and severity of the disease. Erythema nodosum and Lofgren's syndrome are frequent clinical presentations in Scandinavian countries. They are comparatively less frequent in the US and Europe and infrequent in blacks and Japanese. However, cardiac involvement with sarcoidosis is more commonly observed in the Japanese than in any other race or country. More than 50% of Japanese with sarcoidosis have cardiac involvement.

African-Americans and Africans are more likely to have severe disease, carrying a higher morbidity and mortality compared to Europeans or the white population in US. In South Africa, skin lesions such as lupus pernio, nodules, plaques, and psoriasis like lesions are more common, often leading to a misdiagnosis of leprosy. In the United Kingdom, Southern Europe, US and in most other countries of the world, mortality is most often due to progressive pulmonary sarcoidosis. However, in Sweden and Japan, cardiac involvement is the leading cause of death in sarcoidosis. The overall mortality of sarcoidosis as judged from Western figures is 1–5%.

India and Southeast Asia

In the fifties and sixties sarcoidosis was considered a rare disease in India. It is now accepted that the disease is not uncommon, there being reports of fairly large series from western India, eastern India and northern India. The disease appears to be more frequent over the age of 40 years, partly because of lack of awareness of the problem among physicians and partly because the disease is often wrongly diagnosed and treated for a long time as tuberculosis. SK Gupta, working on sarcoidosis in Kolkata was able to trace 640 proven cases of sarcoidosis in India, published in 11 series up to December 2001. This number will probably have more than doubled now. The disease seems to be commoner in Kolkata and Bengal than in any other part of India. Interestingly, in Kolkata and Bengal the disease is commoner in the ethnic Rajasthani patients (Rajasthani migrants who have migrated from Rajasthan in northwest India to Kolkata and Bengal) than in the local Bengali population. Many patients seeking advice in our units in Mumbai are also Rajasthanis living in Bengal and Rajasthanis from Rajasthan. Ethnicity and perhaps geography are responsible for this case selection. The true prevalence rate of sarcoidosis in any part of India (leave aside the whole country) is however undetermined. The differences in clinical phenotypes of sarcoidosis as reported in the West and in studies from India are probably determined by geography and ethnicity. These are discussed later in the chapter.

Sarcoidosis is an uncommon disease in Southeast Asia, with the exception of Japan. Luo Wei and colleagues have reported just 223 patients (59% women) with histological evidence of sarcoidosis from the many different provinces of China.

The disease is barely seen in Hong Kong; in Korea sarcoidosis is believed to be very rare. However, a nationwide survey in Korea between 1992 and 1999 reported 309 biopsy-proven cases from 58 hospitals, the incidence of sarcoidosis being 0.125/100,000.

The incidence of sarcoidosis is significantly more in Japan than in all other Southeast Asian countries. In 2004, a large study of 1,027 patients enrolled from a cluster encompassing 79.4% of the entire Japanese population was designed using the National Epidemiological Survey, with the objectives of determining clinical phenotypes in sarcoidosis and the incidence of the disease. The study revealed an average incidence rate of 1.01 per 100,000 inhabitants (0.73 for males and 1.28 for females). The female to male ratio was shown to have increased from 1.12 in 1973–77 to 1.82 in 2004 (*Ref: Morimota T, Azuma A, Abe S, et al. Epidemiology of sarcoidosis in Japan. Eur Resp J. 2008;31:372-9*).

The increased incidence of cardiac sarcoidosis in the Japanese has already been commented upon. In a comparative study of cardiac sarcoidosis in the Japanese, African-Americans, and US Caucasians, by Iwai and coworkers, the incidence of cardiac sarcoid granulomas was 67.8%, 21.2% and 13.7% respectively (*Ref: Iwai K, Sekigutti M, Hosoda Y, et al. Racial difference in cardiac sarcoidosis incidence observed at autopsy. Sarcoidosis. 1994;11:26-31*).

■ ETIOLOGY

The etiology of sarcoidosis, in spite of a great deal of research, is still unknown. It is probably the interaction between an unknown antigen in the environment, the host response and genetic factors that results in disease. One hypothesis states that there may well be multiple causes of sarcoidosis, and different patterns observed may at least partly be related to different causes.

Noncaseating granulomas are the essential and characteristic features of sarcoidosis. Granulomas can be caused by mycobacteria, fungi, viruses, other micro-organisms and by inorganic agents. None of these have been consistently or convincingly demonstrated in sarcoid tissue. The occasional demonstration of one or the other does not prove causality. Also, a microorganism may trigger the disease and then could be destroyed by the host immune response. The immune response may, however, continue to be directed against undegradable antigenic protein products of the microorganism. Alternatively, an autoimmune response may be induced by the host-antigen reaction thereby perpetuating the inflammatory disease. In either case it could be impossibly difficult to identify the antigen triggering the disease.

Recently several potential autoantigens, such as vimentin, ATP synthetase and Lysil tRNA have been identified. Derived peptides from these antibodies stimulated Th_1 lymphocytes in the blood or lung of sarcoidosis patients, suggesting that they may support and sustain granuloma formation.

The link between environmental exposure and sarcoidosis is suggested by the seasonal clustering of the disease in winter and early spring months, both in the

Northern and Southern hemispheres. The ACCESS (A Case Control Etiological Study of Sarcoidosis) is a multicentered US-based study of over 700 newly diagnosed biopsy-proven patients with sarcoidosis compared to age-sex-race-matched controls. The results of this study showed an absence of environmental or occupational exposure positively linked to sarcoidosis (Odds ratio > 2 and exposure prevalence > 5%). Weak positive associations (Odds ratio 1.5) were found for insecticide use at work, mold/mildew exposure at work and musty odors, suggesting a possible role of microbial-rich environment. The ACCESS study found a negative association between smoking and risk for sarcoidosis. The study demonstrated that there was no single dominant environmental exposure responsible for the disease, again suggesting the importance of the interaction between the gene, the environment and the host response in initiation of the disease.

The possibility of an infectious agent causing sarcoidosis has been considered and researched upon for several years. There are reports of systemic sarcoidosis developing in transplant recipients following transplant of donor organs of patients with active sarcoidosis. This clearly suggests a transmissible agent as the likely cause of sarcoidosis.

American, European and Japanese researchers have demonstrated mycobacterial DNA in a number of biopsy specimens. A meta-analysis of numerous studies revealed a 10–20 fold likelihood of detecting mycobacterial DNA RNA in sarcoid tissue compared to control tissues. Researchers using homogenized sarcoid tissue extracts, mass spectrometry and protein immunoblotting were able to identify the mycobacterial catalase protein (mKatG), a potential pathogenic antigen. Several studies have shown that a majority of sarcoidosis patients (70%) have lung and blood T cell responses to mycobacterial antigens, including mKatG. Perhaps mKatG antigen may be responsible for a subset of patients with sarcoidosis. There is always the possibility that more than one antigen (perhaps multiple different antigens) can trigger the disease. Other similar mycobacterial antigens may well be identified in the future.

Other organisms implicated in the etiology of sarcoidosis, include chlamydia, rickettsia, lymphotropic DNA viruses (EB virus, cytomegalovirus, human herpes virus) and the human lymphocytic T cell virus (HTLV1). This is mere conjecture, as there is no definite evidence to support their role in the etiology of the disease. Japanese workers identified *Propionibacterium acnes* DNA in 80–90% sarcoid tissue in Japan and Europe, but also in 0–60% of controls.

Although there is no definite evidence to prove an infectious etiology in sarcoidosis, many investigators believe that certain organisms may trigger the disease against the background of genetic susceptibility.

In clinical practice there does seem to be some relation between *Mycobacterium tuberculosis* and sarcoidosis. Besides clinical similarities, patients with sarcoidosis may occasionally develop proven tuberculosis (TB) and very occasionally patients with proven TB may in later years develop biopsy-proven sarcoidosis. In the last situation there is no response to anti-TB drugs but a good response to corticosteroids. Yet it needs to be stated that though different mycobacterial proteins may perhaps cause sarcoidosis, *Mycobacterium tuberculosis* does not cause this disease. The fact that anti-TB drugs are ineffective in sarcoidosis is sufficient proof of this.

■ GENETIC FACTORS

Familial clustering and racial differences in incidence and in clinical presentation point to the importance of genetics in the etiology of sarcoidosis. Studies in the West have shown that familial clustering of the disease occurs in 3–14% of patients, more in the blacks than in the whites. The US ACCESS study found siblings of patients with sarcoidosis having a higher relative risk (Odds ratio approximately 5.8) compared to parents (Odds ratio approximately 3.8). The US ACCESS study also suggests that genetic factors have a greater influence in susceptibility to sarcoidosis in whites than in blacks.

Genetic studies have examined the role of human leukocyte antigen (HLA) alleles (both Class I and Class II) and non-HLA genes in relation to sarcoidosis.

Role of Genetics in Sarcoidosis

The differences in the incidence of sarcoidosis in various ethnic groups as also disease clustering in families suggests that genetics may well play an important role in the etiology of sarcoidosis. The importance of ethnicity has already been mentioned, specifically with African-Americans who are three-and-a-half times more commonly affected than the rest of the population in the United States. Worldwide, familial sarcoidosis occurs in 3–14% patients. The ACCESS study (A Case-Control Etiological Sarcoidosis Study) showed that cases were five times more likely than control subjects to report an affected sibling or parent.

The current advances in genetic marker maps and genotyping technology make present-day investigations and exploration of genes linked to sarcoidosis both exciting and challenging.

Human Leukocyte Antigens

Human leukocyte antigens (HLAs) play an important role in antigen presentation. The search for a link between HLAs and sarcoidosis began several years ago. Early reports revealed an association of acute sarcoidosis with HLA Class I antigen HLA-B8, and noted that HLA-B8/DR3 genes were inherited as a sarcoidosis risk haplotype, a haplotype which is also associated with autoimmune disease in whites. Studies in HLA Class I antigens were followed by studies on HLA Class II antigens. The current belief is that both HLA Class I and II genes work together in the evolution of the pathophysiology of sarcoidosis.

Though current work on the genetics of sarcoidosis is in a state of flux, some important observations from genetic research on this subject are worth noting.

- The HLA-DRB1 is associated with sarcoidosis, with variations of the HLA-DRB1 gene affecting both susceptibility and prognosis of sarcoidosis.
- HLA-DR3 has been shown to be associated with susceptibility to sarcoid; HLA-DR1 and DR4 offer disease protection in Scandinavian and European populations.
- Other studies have shown that class II HLA-DR17 (DR3) halotype and specifically HLA DRB1 0301 or the closely linked DQB1 0201 allele to be associated with mild disease, which is —stage I X-ray chest, Lofgren's syndrome, acute arthritis, remission within 2 years in European and Japanese population.
- One study identified four *DR* and nine *DQ gene* polymorphisms associated with increased susceptibility to sarcoidosis. On the other hand, HLA DPBI and the closely linked DQB1 alleles have been shown to be associated with decreased disease susceptibility in some studies.
- Several different HLA class II genes acting in concert or independently predispose to sarcoidosis.
- The linkage disequilibrium (LD) within the major histocompatibility complex (MHC region) limits the ability to exactly identify the HLA genes.

An important negative finding is the lack of association of sarcoidosis with HLA-DPB1*0201, the allele that carries glutamate in amino-acid position 69 (Glu69). This allele has been consistently associated with berylliosis, a disease very similar to sarcoidosis.

Non-HLA Candidate Genes

Genes that influence antigen processing, antigen presentation, macrophage and T-cell activation, and cell recruitment are considered sarcoidosis candidate genes. Numerous such genes have been investigated in relation to sarcoidosis. Some of the candidate genes investigated in relation to sarcoidosis include the following:

Angiotensin-converting enzyme (ACE), CC chemokine receptor + a receptor for monocyte chemoattractant protein; CCR5 which serves as a receptor for macrophage inflammatory proteins and for monocyte chemotactic protein 2. Other candidate genes investigated include Clara cell 10-kD protein, Heat Shock Protein A1L, interleukins IL-1, IL-4R, IL-18, IFN-α and Vascular Endothelial Growth Factor. Not one of these or several others that have been investigated show a significant or consistent association with sarcoidosis. For a fuller review on this subject, the reader is referred to the article (*Ref: Iannuzzi MC, Rybicki BA. Genetics of sarcoidosis. Am Thorac Soc. 2007;4:108-16*).

In conclusion, sarcoidosis probably results from an interaction of environmental factors and alleles of many genes. A genetic association has been extensively researched upon in the hope that identifying alleles and candidate genes influencing risk and phenotype will increase our understanding of the disease. A few HLA genes have been shown to be associated with sarcoidosis. No convincing association has been found with candidate genes. Unfortunately many of the reported associations have not been corroborated by different groups of researchers.

Future research in this field holds promise. Profiling gene expression in BAL fluid and blood at the time of presentation may perhaps help to predict disease progression, resolution, and response to treatment. Functional analysis of candidate genes identified by linkage analysis in conjunction with genome association studies may throw greater light upon the pathogenesis of this disease.

■ IMMUNOPATHOGENESIS

Noncaseating granulomas within affected tissue is the characteristic feature of sarcoidosis. These granulomas are a result of a cell-mediated immunological response of the host to an unidentified antigen. Though the immunological mechanisms and the molecular biology of the immune response are now better elucidated, the interaction between antigen, host response and genetic factors that ultimately causes sarcoidosis is poorly understood.

The initial or primary event in the immunopathogenesis is an alveolitis due to the accumulation of activated CD4$^+$ T helper cell lymphocytes within the alveoli. Bronchoalveolar lavage (BAL) studies show a marked increase in the CD4:CD8 ratio. An increase beyond 3.5–4 is considered to be highly specific for sarcoidosis. In fact, in acutely presenting sarcoid the CD4:CD8 ratio may exceed 10 and may be as high as 30.

The activated CD4$^+$ T helper cells seem to be derived from the blood, the lymphocytes from the blood being trapped and then compartmentalized within the lung. The T4 lymphocyte count in the blood is thereby reduced. The migration of T4 lymphocytes from the blood into the lungs is due to increased production of cytokines and chemokines. Two active chemokines that attract peripheral lymphocytes into the lungs are IP-10 and RANTFS. These are present in a high concentration in patients with active sarcoidosis. The increased number of CD4 cells within the lungs is also due to the local proliferation of lymphocytes within the lung, probably a response to an antigen.

The depletion of CD4 cell lymphocytes within the blood is responsible for the depressed cell-mediated immunity present in patients with sarcoidosis. This is evinced by a negative tuberculin test as also by a depressed immune response to viral and fungal antigens.

Alveolar macrophages also proliferate (in addition to CD4$^+$ helper lymphocytes) within the lungs. These are derived from mononuclear cells within the blood as also from local proliferation. Alveolar macrophages are activated, are monocytic in appearance and have two functions. They are antigen-processing and antigen-presenting cells and produce proinflammatory cytokines that induce further proliferation and activation of T4 cells and alveolar macrophages. The characteristic inflammatory response in sarcoidosis is of the Th1 type with the production of Th1-associated cytokines, IL-2, interferon (IFN)-γ and TNF-α. The production of IL-12 by activated alveolar macrophages intensifies Th1 response as it induces production of TNF-α by T cells and natural killer (NK) cells. Another cytokine produced by activated macrophages and lymphocytes is IL-18, which acts in synergy with IL-12 to increase the production of IFN-γ by T cells and NK cells. Both IL-12 and IL-18 are present in increased concentrations in patients with sarcoidosis.

The earlier described T cell-mediated immune response directed against an unknown but perhaps persistent antigen is responsible for the characteristic sarcoid granulomas. TNF-α, IFN-γ, interleukins, in particular IL-1 are necessary for the formation and persistence of these granulomas. Under the influence of chronic cytokine influence and stimulation, alveolar macrophages differentiate into epitheloid cells. Some of these epitheloid cells fuse to form giant cells. The cluster of lymphocytes and mononuclear cells forming the granuloma may be encased by fibrous tissue laid down by fibroblasts.

The upregulated cytokine expression described earlier is associated with increased activation of the transcription factor NF-kβ and a downregulation of the inflammation suppressive transcription factor peroxisome proliferation activated receptor-γ.

Role of Immunoregulatory Cells

Immunoregulatory T cells maintain immune homeostasis by controlling the immune response. It is hypothesized that in sarcoidosis the immune regulatory function of these cells is suppressed so that there is little or no suppression of proinflammatory cytokine expression or of granuloma formation. There is a diminished number of immune regulatory natural killer T (NKT) cells and this may contribute to the chronicity of the lesions in sarcoidosis.

Role of Host Protein Amyloid A

Chen ES and colleagues noted that there is a high concentration of host protein serum amyloid AA (SAA) in the granulomas observed in sarcoid, but not so in granulomatous inflammation observed in other diseases. They hypothesized that the pathobiology of sarcoidosis was due to the accumulation of SAA within the granulomas. SAA and its released peptides amplify the proinflammatory Th1 response to pathogenic antigens at the sites of granulomatous inflammation.

Pulmonary Fibrosis

Research is directed toward the identification of markers associated with an increased risk of fibrosis. It is possible that a switch from a Th inflammatory profile to a Th2 inflammatory profile may contribute to fibroblasts and fibrosis. IL-4 production is a feature of the Th2 inflammatory profile and IL-4 is chemotactic for fibroblasts stimulating them to lay down fibrous tissue. Other fibrogenic factors are insulin-like growth factor binding protein (IGFBP), platelet-derived growth factor, IGF1 and granulocyte-macrophage colony stimulating factor (GM-CSF).

Though the immunopathogensis of sarcoidosis is chiefly T-cell-mediated, there is also a polyclonal activation of B cells in this disease. This leads to presence of antibodies to numerous viral antigens and to the formation of immune complexes which are associated with and which may be responsible for erythema nodosum. It has been postulated that increased B cell activity may contribute to arthralgia, uveitis and erythema nodosum seen in sarcoidosis.

■ PATHOLOGY

The classic feature of sarcoidosis is the well-defined noncaseating granulomas without the presence of microorganisms on staining or even on tissue culture. The granuloma consists of epitheloid cells, T-lymphocytes of the CD4 kind, and a few macrophages, and multinucleated Langhan's giant cells **(Figs. 1 to 3)**. The giant cells may contain inclusion bodies of calcium carbonate or form asteroid bodies. There is an outer peripheral layer of CD8 T cells, monocytes and B lymphocytes. Both CD4$^+$ and CD8$^+$ T cells carry the aP form of the T cell receptor (TCR). T cells carrying y8-TCR are rarely observed within or at the periphery of the granulomas.

Fibroblasts with collagen and fibrous tissue are often present surrounding the granuloma. In the lungs the

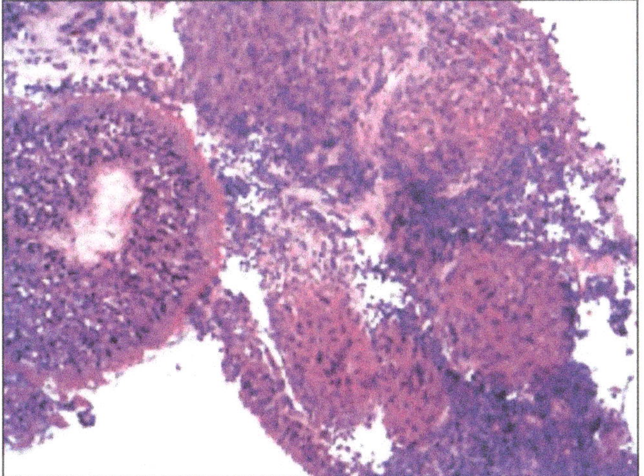

Fig. 1: Transbronchial biopsy of the lung. Presence of noncaseating granulomas consistent with sarcoidosis is noted (Hematoxylin and eosin stain).

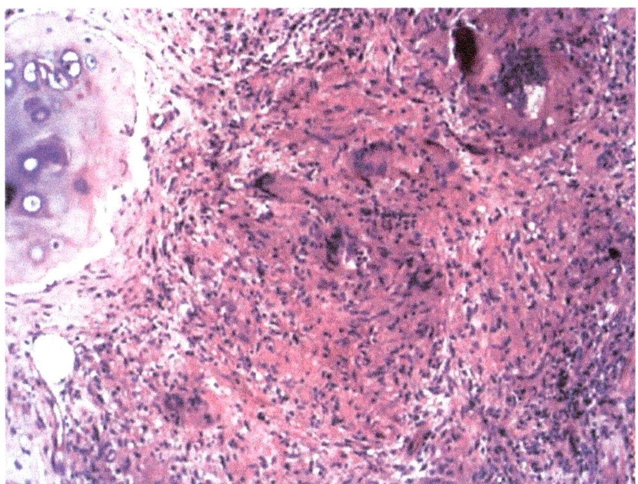

Fig. 2: Sarcoidosis—transbronchial biopsy of the lung. Presence of noncaseating granulomas, replete with Langhan's and foreign body type giant cells (20× H&E).

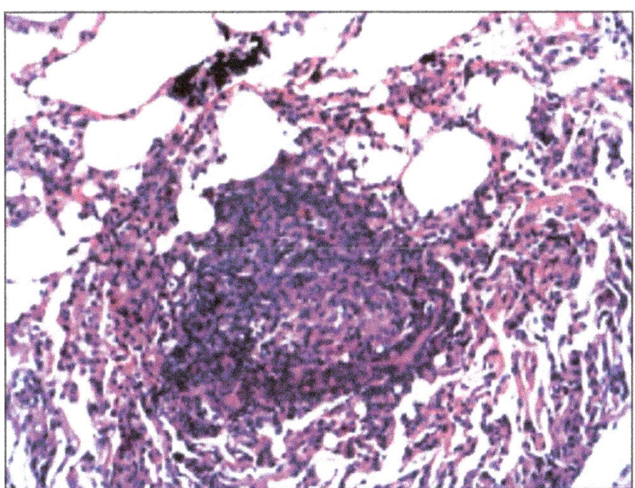

Fig. 3: Sarcoidosis—transbronchial biopsy of the lung (20× H&E). Presence of noncaseating granulomas in the interstitium is noted.

granulomas are distributed peribronchially, perivascularly and are noted to "dot" the fissures. The granulomas may resolve, persist, or coalesce to destroy lung tissue and ultimately lead to progressive fibrosis, which chiefly involves the upper lobes.

It is to be noted that noncaseating granulomas are not specific for sarcoidosis. They may occur in tuberculosis, berylliosis and hypersensitivity pneumonitis and can be caused by a number of other microorganisms.

The epitheloid cells in the granuloma secrete ACE so that serum levels of ACE are often though not always elevated in sarcoidosis. The ACE level in the serum is used as a nonspecific marker of the total granuloma burden and of sarcoid activity. Another product secreted by the sarcoid granuloma is vitamin D_3 which when secreted in excess leads to increase in serum calcium levels. The vitamin D receptor gene has two allele variants; the B allele of the vitamin D receptor gene is believed to be associated with sarcoidosis.

■ CLINICAL PRESENTATION

Sarcoidosis is a multiorgan disease; any one or more organs or organ systems can be involved. The clinical presentation, the clinical features and the course of the disease therefore vary considerably. Patients with symptomatic disease may seek advice from an internist or from any one of the different medical specialties depending on which organ or organ system is clinically involved.

The following section first deals with the overall clinical presentation, clinical features of pulmonary sarcoidosis and extrapulmonary sarcoidosis. It then gives a brief description of sarcoidosis in the Indian scenario.

Close to two-thirds of patients are asymptomatic and have sarcoidosis diagnosed accidentally following a routine chest radiograph on the basis of a bilateral hilar adenopathy. When symptoms do occur, the most frequent presentation is that of a dry cough and exertional dyspnea. This is because the lungs and/or intrathoracic lymph nodes are involved in over 90% of patients with sarcoidosis. Exertional dyspnea when present suggests that the disease has probably been in existence for some months. In the ACCESS study more than half the patients were initially seen with pulmonary symptoms.

Constitutional symptoms in the form of fever, malaise, lassitude, weight loss and arthralgias occur in 20% of patients in most Western reports. These can occur in association with clinical features of any organ involvement or may occur as the sole presenting feature. Pyrexia of unknown origin is not an uncommon presentation of sarcoidosis.

Ethnicity plays an important role in the clinical presentation of the disease. African-Americans are noted to develop more severe constitutional and respiratory symptoms compared to Caucasians. Uveitis is commoner in the Japanese. Lupus pernio characterized by disfiguring lesions of the cheek and nose is more commonly observed in elderly women of the Afro-Caribbean race.

The disease may present acutely or may be subacute or insidious in onset and progress. The two well-recognized acute forms of the disease are Lofgren's syndrome and Heerfordt's syndrome. Lofgren's syndrome is described later under "Clinical Features". Heerfordt's syndrome is characterized by fever, parotid gland enlargement, uveitis, xerostomia and unilateral or bilateral facial nerve palsy.

A classification scheme given by Fishman (*Systemic Sarcoidosis; Fishman's Pulmonary Diseases and Disorders*) based on the initial presentation of patients with sarcoidosis is as follows: asymptomatic, acute sarcoidosis with or without erythema nodosum, intermediate sarcoidosis with symptoms or signs of pulmonary disease for less than 2 years, chronic pulmonary sarcoidosis of more than 2 years and predominately extrapulmonary sarcoidosis. Patients who have persistent disease for more than 2 years, usually, though not always have persistent long-term disease.

■ CLINICAL FEATURES

The clinical features are best described under the following heads—asymptomatic sarcoidosis, acute sarcoidosis with or without erythema nodosum, pulmonary sarcoidosis, extrapulmonary sarcoidosis.

Asymptomatic Sarcoidosis

As mentioned under "Clinical Presentation", up to two-thirds of patients are asymptomatic, the diagnosis being made on the basis of a radiographic examination of the chest which shows bilateral hilar adenopathy. Pulmonary infiltrates may be occasionally present in some patients; these are more evident on a high-resolution computed tomography (HRCT) of the chest.

Acute Sarcoidosis with or without Erythema Nodosum (Lofgren's Syndrome)

Lofgren's syndrome is manifested by acute onset of high fever, bilateral hilar adenopathy, erythema nodosum, polyarthritis often associated with uveitis. Erythema nodosum is characterized by painful reddish nodules, several centimeters in diameter, chiefly involving the lower limbs. The nodules change color to a dull brown with time, may disappear, but often return in crops. Biopsy of the nodules reveals a panniculitis. Occasionally, the nodules also involve the thighs and the upper limbs. The polyarthritis is very painful, chiefly involving the ankles and knees, and occasionally the wrists and elbows as well. Variants of this syndrome are important to recognize. The chest radiograph is normal in 10% of patients; an HRCT of the chest may reveal a hilar adenopathy in these patients. Some patients manifest fever, constitutional symptoms, bilateral hilar adenopathy, polyarthritis, but have no erythema nodosum. This syndrome either in its full form or its variants has a good prognosis. 80% of patients enjoy a remission in weeks or months. Recurrence generally does not occur.

In Scandinavia one-third of patients with sarcoidosis may present with Lofgren's syndrome; the incidence is lower in the Caucasian race, and still lower in African-Americans, Africans, and in India and South-East Asia.

Pulmonary Sarcoidosis

Dry cough is an early symptom. Dyspnea on exertion is observed as the disease progresses. Dyspnea progressively worsens and in late stages of the disease is present even at rest. Dyspnea is due to airways' obstruction or due to restrictive lung disease or more often due to both airways' obstruction plus restrictive lung disease. Occasionally, enlarged mediastinal lymph glands pressing on large airways may contribute to or be chiefly responsible for dyspnea. With advanced pulmonary disease leading to pulmonary fibrosis and bronchiectasis, cough is associated with expectoration. Hemoptysis may also then occur. Wheezing is common in patients with endobronchial disease causing airways' obstruction or in patients with late fibrocystic disease. Bronchodilators may offer relief only to patients with increased bronchial hyper-reactivity. Vague chest pain, the cause of which is uncertain, is a frequent complaint. Though diffuse endobronchial involvement may be present, segmental atelectasis or localized bronchial or tracheal stenosis is rare. In the late stage of pulmonary sarcoid characterized by fibrocystic disease and bronchiectasis, an aspergilloma may form in a cystic space or in a bronchiectatic cavity. This may remain silent or may at times cause profuse hemoptysis.

Physical Findings

Physical findings are sparse. Rhonchi may be heard in patients with airways' obstruction only on forced expiration. Crackles are infrequent being present in less than 20% of patients. Clubbing is rare; it is generally absent.

Imaging Studies

An X-ray chest is abnormal in over 90% of patients with sarcoidosis and to an extent has prognostic implications **(Table 1)**. The chest radiograph should be used as the basis for a grading or staging system **(Figs. 4 to 7)**. The stages range progressively from Stage 0 to Stage IV.

- *Stage 0:* Stage 0 is characterized by a normal chest radiograph. A normal chest radiograph is found in 5–10% of patients with sarcoidosis, invariably in those with extrapulmonary sarcoidosis.
- *Stage I:* Stage I is characterized by bilateral hilar adenopathy and is present in about 40% of patients. This may be associated with a right paratracheal adenopathy, and in some patients there may also be a subcarinal, and pretracheal adenopathy.
- *Stage II:* Stage II is characterized by hilar adenopathy with or without mediastinal adenopathy and with the presence of pulmonary infiltrates. This is seen initially in 30–50% of patients. Pulmonary infiltrates take the form of perivascular or peribronchial reticulonodules in the upper and mid-zones of the lungs. Discrete nodules may also be seen along the fissures of the lungs. Radiographic findings may also take the form of fluffy alveolar shadows resembling small areas of consolidation. Rarely, a miliary pattern resembling miliary TB is observed. Calcification of lymph nodes may be observed in longstanding cases.
- *Stage III:* Stage III is characterized by the presence of pulmonary infiltrates without hilar or mediastinal adenopathy. Pulmonary infiltration takes the form of reticulonodular shadows or alveolar shadows chiefly involving the upper and mid-zones of both lungs.
- *Stage IV:* The radiograph of the chest in Stage IV shows extensive fibrosis. The hila are pulled up; there is extensive fibrocystic disease, bronchiectasis, together with small and large bullae and honeycombing of the lungs chiefly involving the upper lobes, the lingula and the right middle lobes. There is also a significant loss of lung volume. The radiological features are akin

Table 1: Approximate frequency of different stages in radiological examination of the chest on presentation as reported in the West and in western India.

	Western figures	Mumbai
Stage I	40%	43%
Stage II	30–50	36%
Stage III	15%	21%

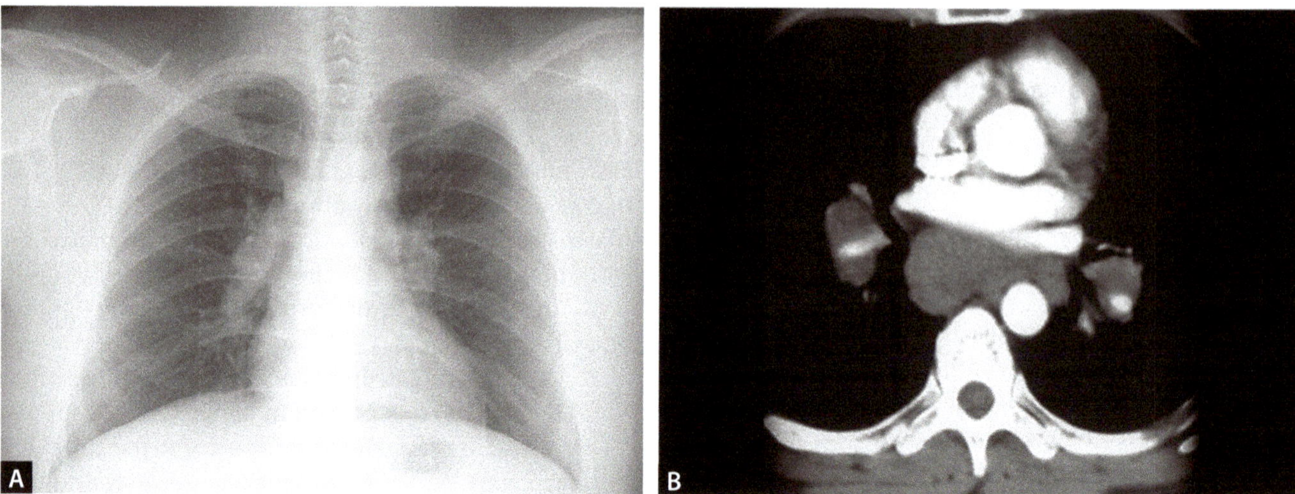

Figs. 4A and B: (A) A 33-year-old man at a routine pre-employment health check. Chest X-ray demonstrates bilateral hilar adenopathy due to Stage I sarcoidosis. (B) Stage I sarcoidosis—contrast-enhanced CT scan demonstrates large bilateral hilar adenopathy and large subcarinal adenopathy. No necrosis is seen in the adenopathy.

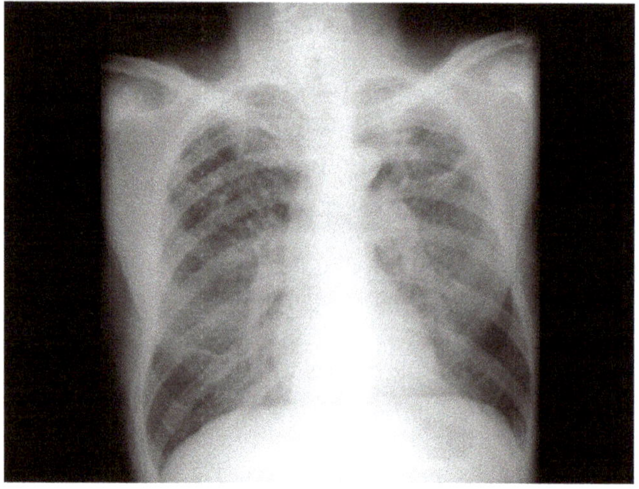

Fig. 5: Stage II sarcoidosis: Chest X-ray demonstrates enlarged hilar adenopathy as well as extensive bilateral interstitial lesions.

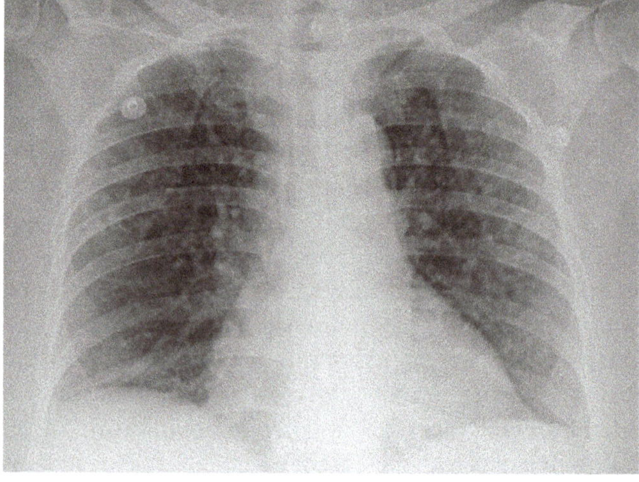

Fig. 6: Stage III sarcoidosis. Chest X-ray demonstrates extensive interstitial nodules in both lung fields. No significant mediastinal adenopathy.

to longstanding bilateral burnt-out TB involving the upper lobes of both lungs.

Unusual radiographic findings in sarcoidosis include the presence of a mycetoma in one of the cystic spaces or in a bronchiectatic cavity, an isolated nodule, or nodules, pleural involvement in the form of a pleural effusion or rarely, a pneumothorax.

HRCT Scan

HRCT scan of the chest may reveal details, particularly in relation to an adenopathy or to pulmonary infiltrates not visible on plain X-ray. HRCT of the chest also reveals the exact nature and distribution of pulmonary infiltrates; these are generally centrally distributed, peribronchially, perivascularly and along lung fissures. Ground glass opacities and honeycombing not present on an X-ray chest may be seen on an HRCT examination **(Figs. 8 and 9)**. CT of the chest is often useful—(1) in the evaluation of suspected sarcoidosis presenting with extrapulmonary manifestations but with a normal chest X-ray; (2) prior to planned biopsy of enlarged mediastinal nodes; (3) to evaluate uncommon X-ray appearances in sarcoidosis; (4) to evaluate the degree of fibrocystic disease or bronchiectasis, or detect the presence of a mycetoma in a patient with sarcoidosis who has well-marked hemoptysis.

FDG-PET Scan

The FDG-PET scan has a small role in the evaluation of sarcoidosis. It may help to identify occult lesions more accessible to biopsy than lung lesions. It does not differentiate sarcoidosis from malignancy as the FDG-PET may be positive in both these conditions. The FDG-PET together with MRI may be useful in the evaluation of cardiac sarcoidosis.

Lung Functions

Lung functions may show a restrictive pattern, an obstructive pattern and more often, as the disease progresses, features of both airways' obstruction and a restrictive ventilatory pattern. It needs to be remembered that lung functions may be normal even when there are pulmonary infiltrates on an X-ray chest.

The earliest features of a restrictive ventilatory defect are a fall in CO diffusion with a decrease in the total lung capacity. Later, there is a fall in the forced vital capacity, the residual volume and the functional residual capacity. Obstructive lung disease is typically characterized by decreased forced expiratory volume in the first second, forced vital capacity, FEV_1/FVC ratio and by reduced expiratory flow rates. Typical features of combined obstructive + restrictive patterns are a reduced CO diffusion, reduced FVC, reduced lung volumes, with a significant reduction in the expiratory flow rates and in the FEV_1/FVC ratio. Extensive fibrosis in end-stage sarcoid is often associated with a fall in oxygen saturation after a 6 minute walk test.

Bronchial hyper-reactivity may contribute to airways' obstruction in a small subgroup of patients. These patients may respond to aerosolized bronchodilators.

Resting hypoxemia is observed in some patients with Stage IV disease in the presence of well-marked airways'

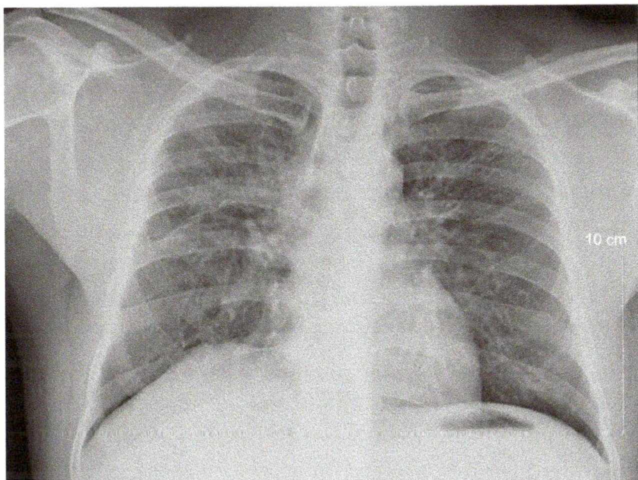

Fig. 7: Stage IV sarcoidosis. Chest X-ray demonstrates extensive fibrotic and interstitial opacities in the upper zones due to burnt-out sarcoidosis.

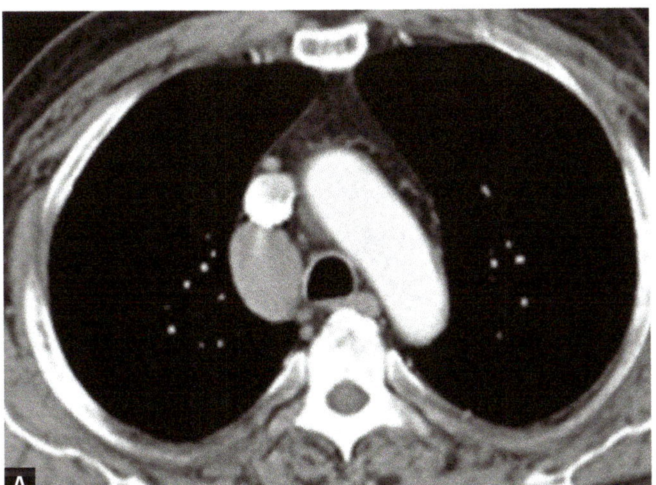

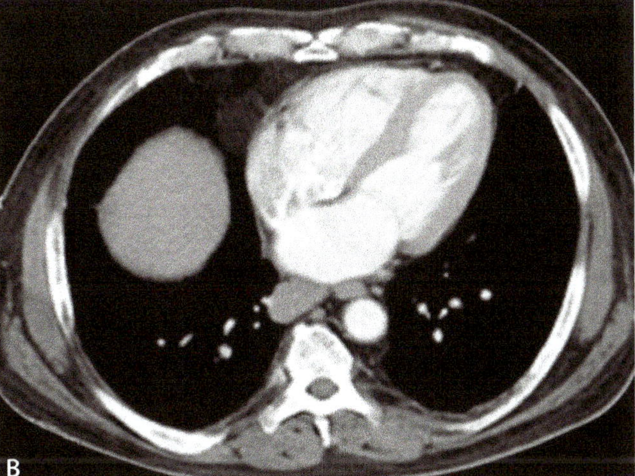

Figs. 8A and B: Chest CT reveals large right paratracheal adenopathy as well as moderate-sized subcarinal adenopathy, no necrosis is seen in the adenopathy.

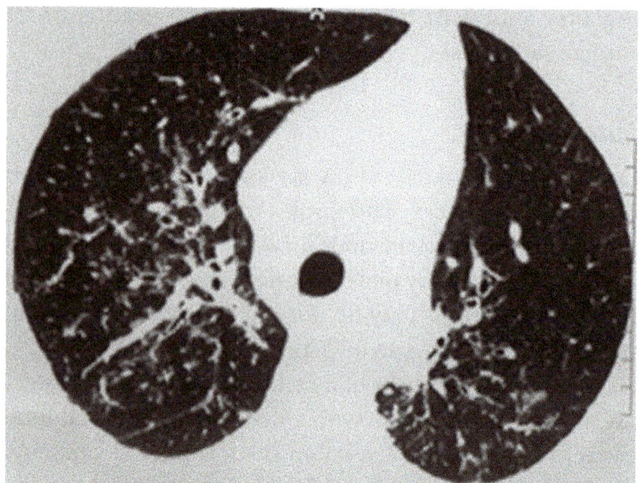

Fig. 8C: HRCT reveals multiple small interstitial nodules as well as peribronchial interstitial thickening due to sarcoidosis.

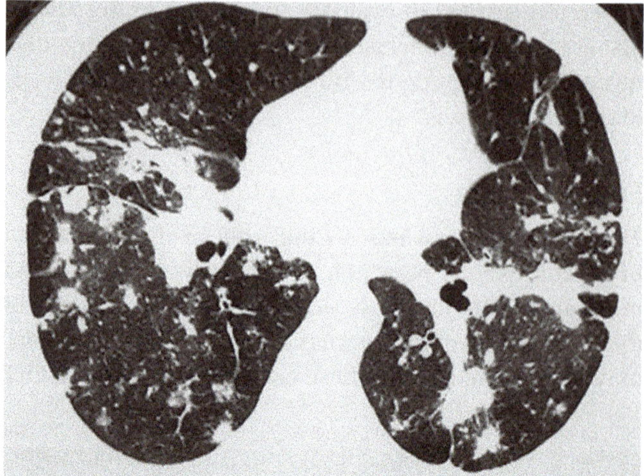

Fig. 10: Necrotizing sarcoidosis—HRCT demonstrates large nodules in both lung fields in a peribronchovascular location bilaterally. Transbronchial biopsy revealed necrotizing granulomas.

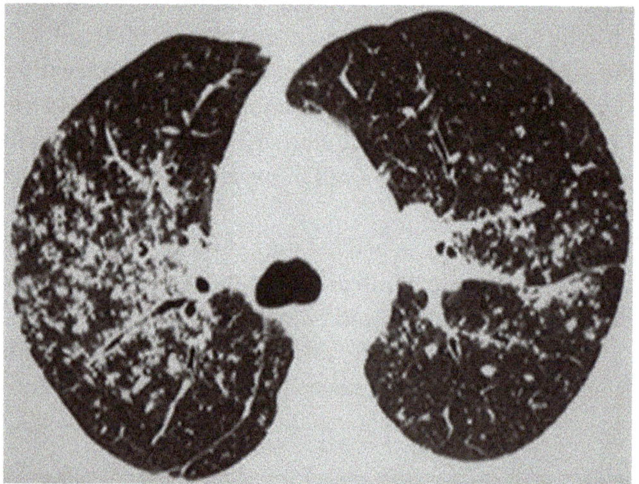

Fig. 9: Extensive sarcoid granulomas on an HRCT chest demonstrating multiple nodules along the fissures, subpleurally as well as along bronchovascular structures, typical location for interstitial nodules.

obstruction and restriction. Further oxygen desaturation occurs with exercise. We have seen two patients of sarcoidosis with miliary mottling of both lungs developing respiratory failure with well-marked hypoxemia. There was dramatic response to corticosteroid therapy. CO_2 retention does not occur except in the presence of advanced pulmonary disease.

Necrotizing Sarcoid Granulomatosis (Fig. 10)

Necrotizing sarcoid granulomatosis is a rare disorder characterized by the presence of one or more solid noncaseating granulomas involving pulmonary arteries and veins without evidence of systemic vasculitis. The condition has similarities to *granulomatosis with polyangiitis* but is considered to be a variant of sarcoidosis. The patient may be asymptomatic or may present with constitutional symptoms, chest pain and dyspnea. Chest radiography demonstrates solid, generally multiple, noncavitatory nodules resembling metastatic lesions. Pleural effusion has been reported in a majority of these patients and should lend suspicion to a possible correct diagnosis. A thoracoscopic biopsy is imperative to confirm the diagnosis of this rare variant of sarcoidosis. The lesions have been reported to improve spontaneously; there is also a rapid response to corticosteroid therapy.

Pulmonary Hypertension

Pulmonary hypertension is observed generally with advanced pulmonary sarcoidosis and is associated with an increased mortality. The overall incidence of pulmonary hypertension is less than or equal to 6% but it occurs in as many as 70% of patients with advanced disease. Pulmonary hypertension should always be suspected when the degree of dyspnea is disproportionate to pulmonary function impairment. Patients generally present with increasing dyspnea. The cause of pulmonary hypertension is extensive interstitial lung disease, severe fibrosis causing a marked decrease in the pulmonary vascular bed. In patients with sarcoid involvement of the heart, left ventricular dysfunction contributes to pulmonary hypertension. Echocardiography is useful in the diagnosis of pulmonary hypertension. Right heart catheterization is however generally necessary to confirm the diagnosis and note its severity.

Extrapulmonary Manifestations of Sarcoidosis

Some patients have sarcoid involvement of one or more organ systems either in addition to pulmonary involvement or without evidence of pulmonary disease. The incidence of involvement of different organs or organ systems in extrapulmonary sarcoidosis depends on the geography as also the ethnicity of the population studied; it clearly varies in different parts of the world. The incidence of the involvement of different organ systems, as reported in the West and as reported in studies from the Indian subcontinent is given later in this section. *Extra pulmonary manifestations of sarcoidosis should always be sought in patient with pulmonary sarcoidosis.* Hence investigations in a patient with pulmonary sarcoidosis should include a CBC, urine examination, blood biochemistry, an ophthalmic examination, a tuberculin test, ECG, USG of the abdomen for adenopathy and/ or hepatosplenomegaly. Further investigations may be necessary in patients with suspected neurosarcoid or in those with cardiac involvement. A brief description of possible extrapulmonary manifestations of sarcoidosis that may well occur in conjunction with pulmonary manifestations is given below.

Cutaneous Sarcoid

In Indians, the skin is the most frequently involved organ system outside the lungs and intrathoracic lymph nodes. The incidence would perhaps be greater than that reported if a meticulous search for skin sarcoid is made on every patient with pulmonary sarcoid. Skin involvement takes the form of small yellowish papules, plaques, subcutaneous nodules and erythema nodosum **(Fig. 11)**. Typically, the lesions are noted along the hairline, nose, ears, extensor surfaces of the arms and legs and the back. Lupus pernio is a disfiguring skin lesion of the face characterized by dull red or reddish-brown plaques on the nose (the tip and the alae nasi in particular), the cheeks and the skin below the eyes **(Fig. 12)**. The lesions disfigure the nose and the face.

Sarcoid nodules have a propensity to form in scar tissue (an operation scar, for example). The diagnosis of sarcoid is at times made when a tumor removed from within and below an operation scar is noted on histology to be a noncaseating granulomatous mass.

Ocular Sarcoid

Ocular sarcoid typically takes the form of an anterior uveitis affecting one or both eyes. It is often associated with a hilar adenopathy but may occur in isolation. Though uveitis is known to occur as a manifestation of TB, it is far more frequently observed with sarcoid. Rarely, optic neuritis or chorioretinitis may occur causing a dramatic loss of vision. Conjunctivitis can also result from sarcoid involvement of the conjunctiva.

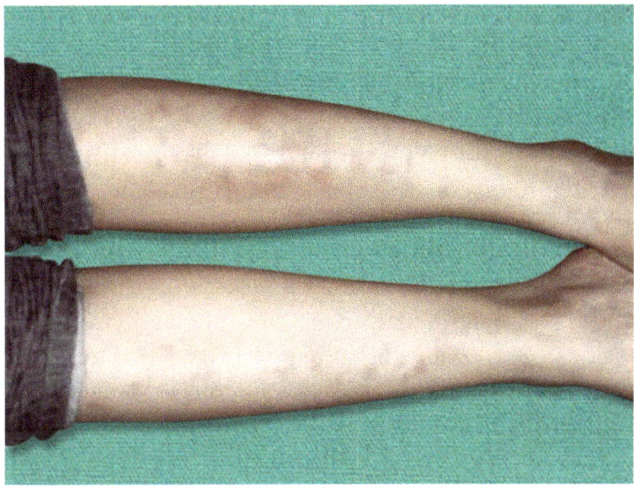

Fig. 11: Erythema nodosum. Reddish nodules on the skin of both lower limbs, more marked on the extensor surface. This was associated with severe pain in the ankles and knees.

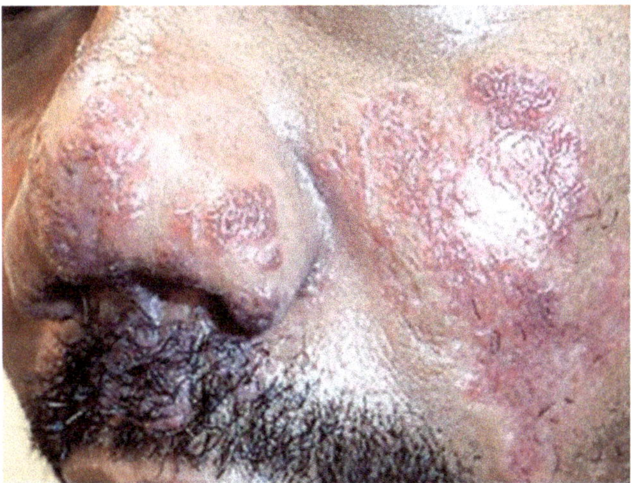

Fig. 12: Lupus pernio. Sarcoid involvement of nose, alae nasi, cheek, nasolabial folds characterized by destructive lesions.

Lymph Glands

Sarcoid involvement of the lymph glands outside the thorax is often mistakenly diagnosed as TB. The lymph glands generally show mild to moderate enlargement, are mobile and nontender. Any group of lymph glands including those within the abdomen may be involved.

Liver and Spleen Involvement

The incidence of hepatosplenomegaly varies in different geographic areas. Splenic involvement is being increasingly observed with the advent of HRCT studies of the abdomen. Though generally asymptomatic, involvement of the spleen on CT studies is manifest in the form of one or multiple hypoechoic lesions. The spleen may be palpable in a few of these patients.

Granulomatous hepatitis may cause an asymptomatic rise in liver enzymes, chronic cholestasis and very rarely has been reported to result in cirrhosis with portal hypertension.

An important presentation of sarcoid is pyrexia of unknown origin with hepatomegaly or hepatospleno-megaly. A liver biopsy shows noncaseating granulomas and the splenomegaly if present shows hypoechoic lesions on a CT of the abdomen **(Fig. 13)**. There is a dramatic response to corticosteroids. It is to be noted that similar clinical findings and CT appearances may also occur with TB.

Neurosarcoid

Neurosarcoid is not as rare as is believed and we have dealt with a number of patients either in association with pulmonary involvement or occurring without pulmonary disease. The most important and frequent symptom is persistent headache. Change in the mental state, confusion and seizures may also occur as presenting symptoms. Cranial neuropathy chiefly involving one or both facial nerves is an important feature of neurosarcoid.

Other cranial nerves may be involved; optic neuritis can cause blurred vision, field defects and blindness. Sarcoid deposits in the hypothalamus and/or in the pituitary gland can cause hypothalamic and/or pituitary dysfunction. Aseptic meningitis and spinal cord sarcoid deposits causing transverse myelitis are also a feature of neurosarcoid. The imaging findings on an MRI are fairly characteristic showing dural thickening over the convexity of the cerebral hemispheres and dural

thickening in the tentorial area **(Figs. 14A and B)**. Lesions obstructing the third ventricle can cause obstructive hydrocephalus.

Sarcoid Involvement of the Heart

This disorder is again not as uncommon as supposed and probably occurs in about 5% of patients. The classical presentation is that of a dilated or congestive cardiomyopathy with a fall in systolic ejection fraction to at times as low as 15–20%. Left ventricular failure followed

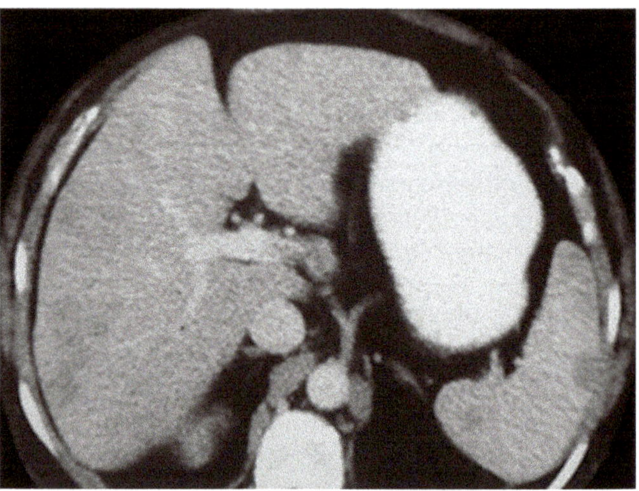

Fig. 13: Abdominal CT reveals multiple focal hepatic and splenic lesions. Biopsy revealed noncaseating granulomas.

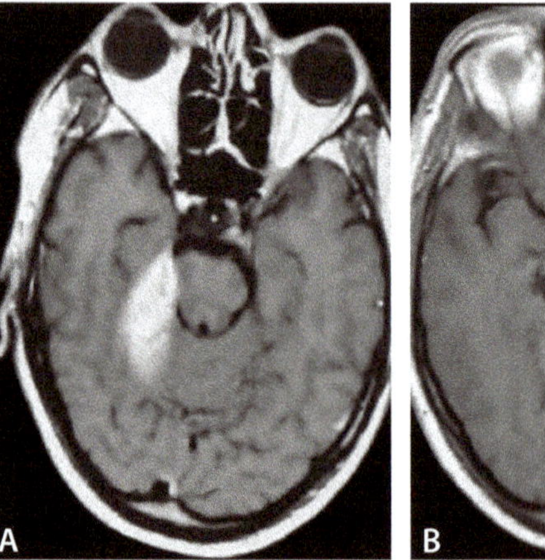
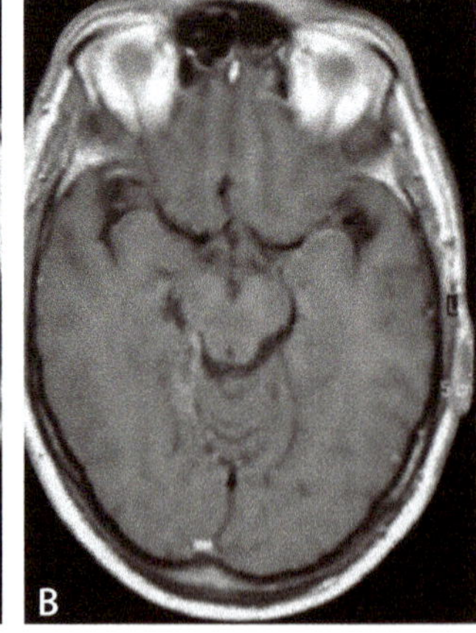

Figs. 14A and B: A 43-year-old man with biopsy-proven pulmonary sarcoid presented with blurring of vision and headaches. On examination, the only positive finding was papilloedema. (A) Contrast-enhanced MRI demonstrates plaque-like enhancement along the dura. Intracranial sarcoid often manifests as dural mass lesions. (B) After treatment MRI demonstrates nearly total disappearance of dural mass lesion.

by congestive heart failure occurs. Echocardiographic findings often show focal hypokinesia. Gallium studies show a positive pickup of gallium by sarcoid tissue within the heart muscle. Another classic presentation is the presence of heart block—either a bundle branch block or complete heart block, or the presence of arrhythmias. An important etiology of dangerous ventricular arrhythmias in young individuals between 20 years and 40 years of age, for which there is no obvious cause, is sarcoidosis. An HRCT of the chest showing hilar or mediastinal adenopathy in such a patient should strongly suggest this diagnosis. A therapeutic trial with high-dose corticosteroids is often rewarding. Electrophysiological studies with high-frequency ablation of ectopic foci and the use of an implantable defibrillator is the treatment of choice today. Death has occurred during such procedures even in excellent specialized clinics.

Hypercalcemia

Hypercalcemia is an infrequent observation in our units. Sarcoid granulomas result in increased conversion of 1-hydroxy-vitamin D3 to 1,25 dihydroxyvitamin D3. Increased absorption of calcium from the gut occurs, leading to hypercalcemia. Renal stones and nephrocalcinosis may result. Noncaseating granulomatous lesions may occur in the kidneys. They may occasionally cause serious renal dysfunction. Significant renal dysfunction in the presence of granulomatous lesions (as seen on renal biopsy) is more likely to be related to *granulomatosis with polyangiitis* than to sarcoidosis.

Other Organs and Organ Systems

Any organ or organ system may be involved. Sarcoid involvement of the upper respiratory tract may cause epistaxis, nasal congestion, sinusitis; involvement and destruction of the nasal septum can cause a saddle deformity of the nose. Laryngeal sarcoid can cause stridor, hoarseness and marked upper airways obstruction.

Granulomatosis involvement of the parotid, submandibular or lachrymal glands can lead to xerostomia and dry eyes. The association of bilateral parotid enlargement, facial palsy, fever and uveitis has been mentioned earlier.

Muscle pains and muscle weakness may be observed, the clinical picture resembling polymyositis. Muscle biopsy often shows the presence of sarcoid granulomas. Punched out bony lesions with cystic changes and loss of trabeculae may be observed, particularly in the metacarpophalangeal and interphalangeal joints. Lytic bony lesions involving the spine or long bones have been reported but in our experience these lesions in patients with proven sarcoid involving the lungs are invariably related to separate metastatic disease than to sarcoid.

Hematogenous involvement may consist of granulomatous lesions in the bone marrow, peripheral lymphopenia and hypersplenism.

■ THE INDIAN SCENARIO

It is worth briefly highlighting the clinical features of sarcoidosis in India, so as to enable comparison with observations on the disease in the West.

A study of 135 patients with biopsy-proven sarcoidosis over a 7-year period (1994–2001) from one of our units in Mumbai showed that the disease presented at a mean age of 48.5 years with a male to female ratio of 1:1.4. The most common presenting symptoms were cough (64%), exertional dyspnea (43%), fever (36%), weight loss (35%), and arthralgia (25%). There appears to be an increase in the incidence of constitutional symptoms compared to Western figures. Skin involvement (17%) and ocular symptoms (13%) were commonly seen. On the other hand hepatosplenomegaly, peripheral lymphadenopathy, and parotid enlargement were infrequent clinical manifestations. Contrary to the above, studies from eastern India (Kolkata, West Bengal) show an increased incidence of hepatomegaly (43.5%) and splenomegaly (32.5%) and peripheral lymphadenopathy (22%). Hypercalcemia, uncommon in the study from Mumbai, was much more frequent in eastern India. These differences between eastern and western India are probably related to geography and difference in ethnicity. Other clinical features as observed in the subcontinent of India are worthy of comment. The acute form of sarcoidosis, characterized either by Lofgren's syndrome or Heerfordt's syndrome is rarely observed. Sarcoid involvement of the heart and neurosarcoid though not common, do occur. In fact, any and every organ has been seen to be involved just as in the West. **Table 2** gives the frequency of organ involvement as reported in the West and as observed in India.

The multisystem involvement in sarcoidosis is illustrated by the brief case report given here.

Table 2: Approximate frequency of commonly occurring organ involvement in the west as compared to western India (Mumbai).

Organ involved	Western studies	Western India (Mumbai)
Lung	> 90% (on conventional X-ray)	> 90% (on conventional X-ray)
Respiratory symptoms (cough, dyspnea)	40–60%	64% cough; 43% dyspnea
Constitutional symptoms	20–25%	> 35%
Cutaneous	25%	17%
Ocular	20–30%	13%
Peripheral lymphadenopathy	35%	<10%
Hepatic sarcoid	65% (on biopsy) much less frequent with regard to clinical manifestation	<5% frequency on liver biopsy undetermined
Musculoskeletal system (including arthralgia)	25%	25%
Neurosarcoid	5–10%	5–7%
Cardiac sarcoid	5–10%	5%
Exocrine gland sarcoid	10%	<2%
Hematogenous sarcoid	<5%	<2%

Note: Studies from eastern India (Kolkata) showed a greater frequency of hepatomegaly (43.5%), splenomegaly (31.5%), peripheral lymphadenopathy (12%) and hypercalcemia compared to a study in western India (Mumbai).

Case Study

A 40-year-old man had a bladder neck obstruction requiring transurethral resection of the prostrate. Histological study of the prostate showed noncaseating granulomas compatible with sarcoid. A CT and MRI study of the abdomen and pelvis and chest done subsequent to this procedure showed enlarged seminal vesicles which also showed granulomatous lesions on a CT-guided biopsy. Abdominal lymphadenopathy, hypoechoic lesions in the liver and spleen and Stage II sarcoid on imaging of the chest were also present. The serum ACE (SACE) level was markedly elevated. The patient refused treatment, preferring Ayurveda to Allopathy. He returned 6 months later, very ill, with increased sarcoid involvement of all systems mentioned earlier, together with sarcoid epididymitis and sarcoid of the skin, muscles and joints. He also had hypersplenism manifested as an enlarged spleen, anemia, leukopenia, and thrombocytopenia. Bone marrow biopsy showed the presence of multiple sarcoid granulomas. After admission to hospital he developed an acute cholecystitis necessitating emergency surgery. The wall of the gallbladder on histology showed noncaseating sarcoid granulomas. His response to corticosteroids given in a dose of 40 mg/day was excellent except for a persistent severe hypersplenism. A splenectomy brought relief with the blood count and platelet count returning to normal. It is now many years since the onset of his disease and he now has a persistent low-grade sarcoid activity in many of his organ systems; he is on a maintenance dose of 10 mg prednisolone/day + azathioprine 100 mg/day.

■ CONDITIONS ASSOCIATED WITH SARCOIDOSIS

Common Variable Immunodeficiency

Common variable immunodeficiency (CVID) is a rare disorder and the association of sarcoidosis with this disorder must indeed be doubly rare. Recurrent sarcoidosis (biopsy proven) has been recorded in a subset of patients with CVID. CVID should therefore be suspected in patients with recurrent sarcoidosis, or in children with sarcoidosis, given the low frequency of the disease in this age group.

Autoimmune Disease

Sarcoidosis has been known to be associated with a number of autoimmune disorders such as ulcerative colitis, Crohn's disease, scleroderma, Sjogren's syndrome, biliary cirrhosis, autoimmune hemolytic anemia. It is probable that these associations are related to a common immune disturbance characterized by altered Th1 immunity.

Recently immune-mediated disorders have been described in patients with elevated level of IgG4. The disorder is characterized by constitutional symptoms adenopathy and tumor-like masses. Granulomatous inflammation is observed in a subset of these tumors that mimic sarcoidosis.

Cancer

Noncaseating granulomas can be observed in 3–10% of tumors, and in appropriately 4–10% of draining lymph glands. Uncommonly, lymphadenopathy at more than one site may be observed in patents with recent or past diagnosis of cancer or after chemotherapy. Diagnosis is established by biopsy of a lymph node which shows sarcoidosis and not a recurrence of the earlier cancer.

■ DIAGNOSIS AND DIAGNOSTIC APPROACH

Diagnosis of sarcoid needs to fulfill three requisites—(1) a compatible clinical picture, (2) presence of noncaseating granulomas on biopsy, and (3) the exclusion of other causes of noncaseating granulomas. The importance of pulmonary function tests and imaging studies in the diagnosis of pulmonary sarcoidosis has already been discussed in a previous section. Two important causes of noncaseating granulomas are *TB and fungal infections*. Other causes of noncaseating granulomas include brucellosis, *granulomatosis with polyangiitis*, and *eosinophilic granulomatosis with polyangiitis*. *Occupational diseases* or *work-related diseases* such as *berylliosis, hypersensitivity pneumonitis* and *drug-related lung diseases* should also be considered. It is therefore imperative that noncaseating granulomas in biopsy material should be stained for all relevant organisms, particularly for TB and fungal infection. Culture of biopsy material, in particular for *Mycobacterium tuberculosis* is also advisable. Negative staining for acid-fast bacilli, negative culture and a negative polymerase chain reaction (PCR) for acid-fast bacilli strengthens the diagnosis of sarcoidosis in a patient with a clinical picture compatible with the disease. *In poor, developing countries TB remains the main differential diagnosis as noncaseating granulomas can occur in TB and acid-fast bacilli are not necessarily always present on staining.* A negative Mantoux

skin test in the above circumstances favors the diagnosis of sarcoidosis.

Chronic berylliosis, an occupational hypersensitivity disorder due to exposure to beryllium is indistinguishable from sarcoidosis. Exposure to beryllium occurs in nuclear, aerospace, computer and electronic industries. The disease is characterized by noncaseating granulomas in the affected organs, chiefly the lungs and the skin. The diagnosis is made by a careful occupational history and demonstrating sensitivity to beryllium by a positive beryllium lymphocyte proliferation test. Chronic berylliosis is generally resistant to corticosteroid treatment. If undiagnosed, in the presence of continued exposure the mortality is as high as 25%. Resolution of the disease has been reported after cessation of exposure to beryllium.

As a rule, biopsy to confirm the clinical suspicion of sarcoidosis should be performed from a site which is most easily accessible and which is least traumatic. Thus if pulmonary sarcoidosis is also associated with skin involvement or peripheral lymphadenopathy or enlargement of the parotid or lachrymal glands, a biopsy of the skin lesion or an excision biopsy of a lymph gland or lachrymal gland biopsy may give the diagnosis with the least trauma.

Isolated pulmonary sarcoidosis needs a *fiberoptic bronchoscopy with a transbronchial biopsy*. The diagnostic yield in a patient with hilar or mediastinal adenopathy varies from 60% to 90%, if at least four to six biopsies are taken, depending on the experience and expertise of the bronchoscopist. It is even higher if hilar or mediastinal adenopathy is associated with pulmonary infiltrates on radiography or a chest CT. Intrathoracic lymph nodes can be sampled when technically feasible through a transbronchoscopic needle aspiration biopsy or through a CT-guided biopsy. An *endoscopic bronchial ultrasound guided transneedle bronchial* biopsy gives a better yield, reduces injury to mediastinal vessels and other structures and is superior to the standard transbronchial needle aspiration. These procedures in combination with a transbronchial lung biopsy increase the diagnostic yield to over 90%. Bronchial mucosal biopsies may yield positive results in over 50% of patients even in the absence of endobronchial involvement as judged by the naked eye. It *needs to be remembered that transbronchial biopsy in Stage IV of pulmonary sarcoidosis has a low yield.*

BAL studies show a CD4:CD8 ratio greater than 3.5 in sarcoidosis; this test has a high specificity but a low sensitivity and is not recommended for diagnostic purposes.

Mediastinoscopy with **mediastinoscopic** biopsy may have to be resorted to when fiberoptic transbronchial biopsy or a CT-guided biopsy fails to give definite results, provided the intrathoracic lymphadenopathy is accessible through a mediastinoscope **(Figs. 15A and B)**.

Rarely, a **video-assisted thoracoscopic biopsy** becomes necessary to establish a diagnosis, particularly in rare manifestations of pulmonary sarcoidosis—as with solid lesions due to necrotizing sarcoid granulomatosis.

It is to be noted that though bilateral hilar adenopathy, fever, polyarthritis and erythema nodosum occurring in Lofgren's syndrome are typically due to sarcoidosis, they also occur with TB in countries where TB is strongly endemic and in histoplasmosis and other fungal infections in areas of the world endemic to these infections. A diagnostic hilar or mediastinal gland biopsy may not be necessary in Lofgren's syndrome in Western countries but is on occasion advisable in poor developing countries of the world, particularly if use of corticosteroids is contemplated. A strongly positive Mantoux test in a patient with erythema nodosum, arthralgia and hilar plus mediastinal adenopathy is invariably due to TB; a biopsy is generally neither indicated nor necessary.

Asymptomatic bilateral hilar adenopathy with a negative Mantoux skin test, in our opinion, does not need a diagnostic biopsy. It invariably points to sarcoidosis, though TB and a lymphoma may enter into the differential diagnosis. A close follow-up is, however, warranted.

Sarcoidosis presenting as a mediastinal adenopathy needs to be differentiated from all other causes of such adenopathy—notably TB, Hodgkin's and non-Hodgkin's lymphoma, and metastatic involvement of mediastinal lymph nodes. The presence of well-marked necrosis of lymph glands on an HRCT of the chest invariably points to TB. Lymphadenopathy due to sarcoid involvement does not show necrosis. Lymphomas and metastatic lymphadenopathy though generally non-necrotic may occasionally show necrosis. A CT-guided biopsy, *an* ultrasound-guided transbronchial biopsy through a fiberoptic bronchoscope or if necessary a biopsy obtained through a mediastinoscopy should give the correct diagnosis.

A histopathological study of mediastinal adenopathy in 100 Indian patients (using EBUS transbronchial aspiration biopsy) revealed tuberculosis and sarcoidosis as the most common causes, followed by malignancy. An uncommon cause in this study was adenopathy due to anthracosis (in 5% cases).

Diagnosis of sarcoidosis involving other organ systems without pulmonary involvement may be difficult. Fortunately, more often than not, one or more of the organ systems involved are accessible to a biopsy procedure. Neurosarcoid has fairly characteristic though not absolutely specific imaging findings. Very rarely, a brain biopsy becomes necessary to exclude malignant or infectious disease.

Sarcoidosis involving the heart is suggested by clinical features stated earlier, by suggestive echocardiographic

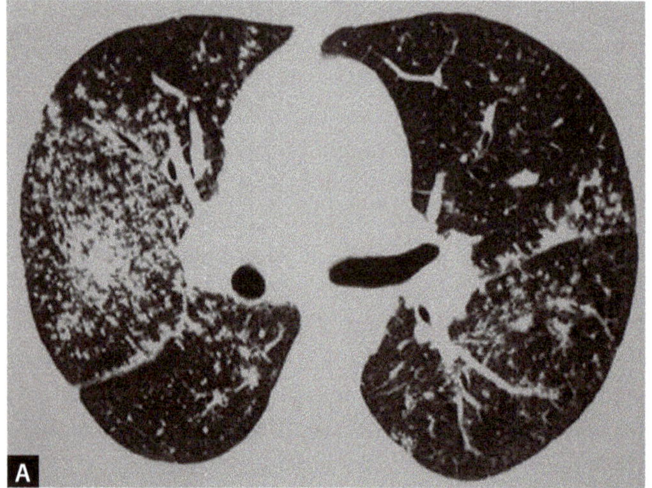
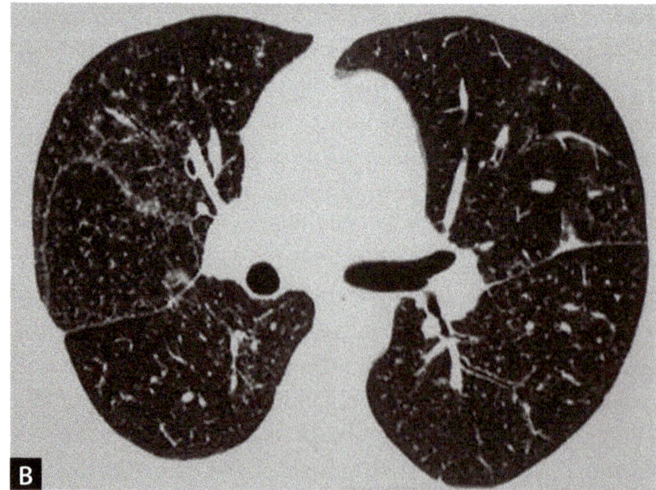

Figs. 15A and B: Extensive interstitial nodules. (A) Interstitial nodules seen. (B) After 6 months of treatment nearly all nodules have disappeared.

findings and by a positive gallium scan. Endomyocardial biopsy is not advised as the diagnostic yield is less than 10-20%.

For organ involvement which is difficult to biopsy, imaging techniques such as gallium 67 scan or ^{18}F-fluorodeoxyglucose positron emission tomography (FDG-PET) may help to pick up areas of occult inflammation that could then allow easy biopsy for confirming the diagnosis. It has been suggested that a gallium 67 scan showing an uptake in bilateral hilar and right paratracheal glands (lambda sign) together with an uptake in the parotids, submandibular, and lachrymal glands' regions (panda sign) is pathognomonic of sarcoidosis. PET scanning is associated with much less radiation exposure, provides excellent resolution, and will probably replace gallium scan to help locate sites of inflammation which are not clinically evident.

Other laboratory tests may be necessary to exclude other diseases. There is no laboratory test that is specific for sarcoidosis. Serum angiotensin converting enzyme (SACE) levels are elevated in 40-80% of cases with clinically active disease. Elevated SACE levels are, however, also seen in TB, other granulomatous disease, lymphoma, hepatitis, thyroid disorders, Hansen's disease and a few others. In our experience we have found the SACE level elevated in close to 80% of active sarcoidosis. The test, however, lacks the specificity to allow a diagnosis on this basis alone, more so as the test is not infrequently positive in TB and lymphoma—two conditions that need to be especially considered in the differential diagnosis of sarcoidosis. In a histologically proven case of sarcoid an elevated SACE level is a fairly good marker of the activity of sarcoidosis. A fall is consistently though not always observed in clinical remission. A subsequent rise often heralds a recurrence of the disease. The test is however variable and has no prognostic value.

■ PROGNOSIS

The ACCESS study has given valuable information with regards to the natural history of sarcoidosis in patients living in the West. The following features are of note:

- Organ involvement is defined early in the natural history of the disease. Only 23% of patients in the ACCESS study were noted to have a new organ involvement during a 2-year follow-up.
- Patients who undergo remission generally do so within two to three years. Sarcoidosis rarely recurs after a prolonged period of remission. Notable exceptions are neurosarcoidosis and sarcoid uveitis.
- Patients who do not show remission continue with chronic sarcoidosis and these patients constitute 30-50% of all known patients with sarcoidosis. These patients have progressive organ involvement, the rate of progression varying from patient to patient.
- Acute presentation of sarcoidosis as in the Lofgren's syndrome is associated with a good prognosis, the remission rate being 70–80%.
- Patients presenting with Stage I chest radiograph have a spontaneous remission rate of 60–90%. Those presenting with a Stage II chest radiograph have a poorer outcome with a spontaneous remission rate of 40–70%. Patients presenting with a Stage III chest X-ray have a remission rate of 10–20% and those with Stage IV chest radiographs showing extensive pulmonary fibrosis do not undergo remission.

Death when it occurs is generally due to progressive pulmonary fibrosis causing chronic hypoxemic or hypoxemic plus hypercapnic respiratory failure. Pulmonary hypertension and cor pulmonale are end-stage phenomena.

Occasionally, TB occurs as a complication, particularly in countries where the prevalence rate of TB is high. Pneumothorax can complicate sarcoidosis in rare instances, particularly when the radiograph of the chest is at Stage IV level.

Secondary infection with gram-positive or gram-negative organisms in the fibrocystic stage of the disease is also observed. An aspergilloma is not an uncommon complication in patients with severe fibrocystic disease and bronchiectasis. Aspergillomas can cause exsanguinating bleeds.

■ TREATMENT

Many patients with sarcoidosis have a good prognosis; some indeed have an excellent prognosis. For example, asymptomatic or mildly symptomatic patients presenting with Stage I disease (with reference to radiological examination of the chest) may show remission rates as high as 90%. These patients require a follow-up but no specific therapy, even if the glands are large. Patients with Stage II radiographic findings who have minimal or no symptoms, very little pulmonary infiltrates on an X-ray chest and who have normal lung functions may also be closely observed to determine if there is evidence of remission or progression. Clear evidence of progressive pulmonary infiltration or the presence of impaired lung function or of disturbing symptoms warrants systemic therapy. The mild form of Lofgren's syndrome either in its full form or a variant form responds to rest and nonsteroidal anti-inflammatory drugs. The severe form of this syndrome characterized by high fever, painful arthropathy and painful erythema nodosum warrants systemic corticosteroid therapy. The presence of uveitis, even in mild Lofgren's syndrome, is an indication for corticosteroid therapy.

As a general principle, systemic corticosteroids are indicated:

- When there is significant disturbance of organ function in the organ or organs affected by sarcoidosis;
- When there are constitutional symptoms in the form of persistent fever, weight loss, lassitude, arthralgias or painful arthropathy.

Systemic Therapy

Use of Corticosteroids (Table 3)

Corticosteroids form the mainstay of therapy for sarcoidosis. They provide prompt symptomatic relief and reverse organ dysfunction. The extent to which organ dysfunction is reversed depends on the degree of damage to organ structure already present and in particular to the degree of fibrosis before starting therapy. Most clinical trials conclude that the use of corticosteroids favorably influences the outcome in chronic pulmonary sarcoidosis.

There is however some controversy as to whether steroids significantly influence the long-term natural history of the disease. Many authorities are of the view that they neither influence the natural history nor improve the ultimate survival. Comparative studies of patients receiving corticosteroid treatment for 18 months and those not receiving corticosteroids suggest that though steroid therapy improved symptoms and suppressed granulomas, there was no evidence of improvement in long-term prognosis.

The British Thoracic Society Sarcoidosis Study was conducted on a multicenter basis to determine the long-term effects of corticosteroids in pulmonary sarcoidosis. A group of 58 patients was treated for one and a half years starting with 30 mg/day for a month; 20 mg daily for the next month; 10 mg daily to complete a year, following which the drug was very slowly tapered and stopped after a further 6 months. Another group of 31 patients was offered selective treatment; in these, treatment was offered only if there was a development of symptoms or there was deteriorating lung function. The initial dose of prednisolone was 30 mg/day and this was tapered and stopped after 6–9 months. The average follow-up of the two groups was 5 years. The group on prolonged one and a half years' treatment with the arm of optimizing radiographic appearance of the chest showed significantly better long-term functional outcome, though in the final analysis the difference between the two groups though significant, was not very large.

Regardless of the controversy, corticosteroids should be given in pulmonary sarcoidosis in presence of significant or worsening symptoms or if there is deteriorating lung function.

Dosage of corticosteroids: The optimal dose and duration of therapy has not been determined by prospective randomized controlled trials. Treatment is therefore individualized depending on the organ or organs involved, the severity of symptoms, the degree of organ dysfunction and the patient's response to therapy.

Initial treatment is generally started with 30–40 mg prednisolone per day in an average-sized adult. Sarcoid involving the heart, neurosarcoid, involvement of the kidneys or the presence of hypersplenism may warrant a dose of 60 mg/day to start with. The dose is slowly tapered every 3–4 weeks to a maintenance dose of 5–10 mg/day. Treatment should preferably be continued for at least 12 months since tapering the dose completely before this period generally leads to a relapse. Some patients require a maintenance dose of prednisolone for 2–3 years or even indefinitely to keep the disease under control. Inhaled steroids may offer symptomatic relief in patients

Table 3: Indications for systemic corticosteroids.

- Chronic pulmonary sarcoid which is invariably associated with symptoms and deteriorating lung function
- Severe form of Löfgren's syndrome
- Neurosarcoidosis or sarcoidosis involving the heart
- Persistent hypercalcemia
- Renal or hepatic dysfunction
- Uveitis not responding to topical corticosteroids or showing frequent relapse while on topical corticosteroids
- Palpable spleen with multiple hypoechoic areas on imaging studies—hypersplenism
- Sarcoid myopathy
- Disfiguring skin sarcoids
- Persistent disabling constitutional symptoms in the form of fever, weight loss, tiredness, arthralgias

who have airways' obstruction and hyper-reactive airways. They do not replace oral steroids in the management of pulmonary sarcoidosis.

Corticosteroid dosage in patients presenting with severe life-threatening neurosarcoidosis or with severe ocular involvement with impending blindness (as with acute optic neuritis or chorioretinitis) needs to be larger than that stated above. Pulse therapy of IV methylprednisolone 0.5–1 g daily for 3–4 days is followed by 60 mg prednisolone daily. Immunosuppressive therapy (discussed later) is often used for its steroid-sparing effect, as therapy may need to be continued for years.

Disease Refractory to Glucocorticoid Therapy

Though most patients respond to glucocorticoid therapy, about 10% are unresponsive and progress to increasing organ failure involving one or more organs. These patients need immunosuppressive agents as drugs may also allow a sharp reduction in steroid dosage in patients who have severe untoward side-effects related to steroids. It is important to ensure that " refractoriness" is not because of end stage pulmonary fibrosis, non-compliance, infection or co-morbid disease **(Table 4)**.

Before starting alternative therapy, one needs to check the blood count, liver function and creatinine as therapy can cause myelosuppression as well as hepatic and renal dysfunction. These tests should be repeated at periodic intervals to ensure that the blood count, liver and renal function are normal. The immunosuppressive drugs mainly used are methotrexate, azathioprine, leflunomide, mycophenolate. Methotrexate is generally the first choice as studies suggest that the drug benefits 50–70% of patients though a response may only be observed after 6 months. The dose is 5 to 7.5 mg weekly increased by 2.5 mg every 2 weeks to a total dose of 10–15 mg/week given orally or preferably intramuscularly. Folic acid is routinely given daily to reduce the incidence of myelosuppression. A low dose of prednisolone preferably not more than 10 mg may be continued with methotrexate therapy.

If methotrexate is ineffective or not tolerated, another immunosuppressive drug is tried—either azathioprine, leflunomide, or mycophenolate.

Anti TNF Therapy

If patients do not respond to one or other of the immunosuppressive agents stated above given alone or in

Table 4: Drugs used in the treatment of sarcoidosis.		
Systemic therapy		
Corticosteroids	Start with 30–40 mg prednisolone/day. Cardiac sarcoid, neurosarcoid, involvement of the kidneys or the presence of hypersplenism–60 mg/day	Taper till maintenance dose of 5–10 mg/day is reached in 12 months
	Pulse doses with intravenous methyl prednisolone 0.5–1 g/day for 4 days are needed in severe neurosarcoidosis or with severe ocular involvement with impending blindness	Switch to oral prednisolone 60 mg/day and taper slowly
Systemic side-effects of corticosteroids should be periodically monitored and prophylactically treated, if possible		
Systemic therapy		
Hydroxychloroquine	Skin sarcoidosis and in neurosarcoidosis	
Doxycycline, minocycline	Skin sarcoid—200 mg/day	
Azathioprine	Severe corticosteroid resistant sarcoidosis 50 mg/day for 2 weeks, increase up to 100 mg/day	
Methotrexate	Steroid resistant sarcoidosis 10–20 mg/week	
Leflunomide	Steroid resistant sarcoidosis—20 mg/day	
Mycophenolate mofetil	Neurosarcoid, ocular, hepatitis and corticosteroid resistant pulmonary sarcoidosis	
Cyclophosphamide	Rarely tried in neurosarcoidosis	
Anti-TNF therapy—Infliximab	Experimental	

combination with glucocorticoids, the next step would be to add TNF-α antagonist—infliximab or adalimumab or etanercept. These drugs can precipitate serious infections, notably tuberculosis, hepatitis B and C. Prior to their use, a tuberculin test, a peripheral blood interferon release assay, as also serology for HBsAg, anti-HBc and anti-HCV should be done.

The dose of infliximab is 3 to 5 mg/kg at 0, 2, 6, 12 weeks and adalimumab 40 mg every week or other week.

The optimal dose of adalimumab in pulmonary sarcoidosis is not known. The recommended dose is 40–80 mg subcutaneously every week or every other week.

A randomized trial of infliximab in chronic pulmonary sarcoid found the drug effective in several endpoints including improvement in FVC after 6 months of therapy.

Other Investigational Drugs

Several medications have been proposed for the use in sarcoidosis but are not too commonly used in pulmonary sarcoidosis as there is no data to support their efficacy.

Of these the one which still continues to be used is hydroxychloroquine. Though chiefly used for cutaneous sarcoid, it is often used in difficult cases of pulmonary sarcoidosis as a supplement to steroid therapy.

Other drugs which have been used without data for any significant benefit include cyclophosphamide, golimumab (a humanised TNF-α antibody), ustekinumab (monoclonal antibody to interleukin), colchicine, cyclosporine, non-steroidal anti-inflammatory agents, tetracycline, thalidomide, pentoxifylline. There drugs are best avoided.

Symptomatic Therapy

- Profuse hemoptysis from an aspergilloma in advanced fibrotic pulmonary sarcoidosis may need embolization of culprit bronchial or pulmonary vessels. Surgery is usually contraindicated in view of very poor lung function in these patients.
- Hypoxemic respiratory failure in advanced cases requires continues oxygen at 1–2 L/min if PaO_2 at rest is less than 55 mm Hg.
- Pulmonary hypertension and cor pulmonale require symptomatic treatment. There have been several reports of treatment of sarcoid associated pulmonary hypertension. The prostacyclin epoprostenol has been successfully used in the long-term management of patients. In an open label trial half of the number of patients had hemodynamic improvement or improvement in exercise tolerance. The oral agents sildenafil and bosentan have also been reported to benefit close to 50% of patients of sarcoid associated pulmonary hypertension.
- Sarcoidosis involving the heart and manifesting with arrhythmias necessitates the use of appropriate anti-arrhythmic drugs and if needs be the insertion of an automatic implantable cardioverter + defibrillator. Congestive cardiomyopathy needs conventional treatment in the form of diuretics, afterload reducing agents, digoxin, aldactone and the judicious use of a β-blocker. These patients require larger doses of corticosteroids initially and may also need higher maintenance dose of 15–20 mg/day for many months.

Lung Transplant

In specialized centers in the West, lung transplantation is an important option in patients with advanced pulmonary sarcoidosis who show severe impairment of pulmonary function refractory to medical therapy. Timing of transplantation is both difficult and challenging. Mortality rates in Western countries for patients with sarcoidosis awaiting transplants are high (27–53%). There are as yet no clear guidelines even in the West for candidate selection as there are, for example, in patients with idiopathic pulmonary fibrosis. For the present, it has been suggested that selection of patients with sarcoidosis for lung transplantation should be based on an extrapolation of prevalent guidelines for lung transplantation in patients with severe idiopathic pulmonary fibrosis. These guidelines are:

- Forced Vital Capacity (FVC) of less than 50% of predicted;
- Diffusion Capacity (DLCO) less than 50% of predicted;
- Hypoxemia at rest or hypoxemia induced by exercise;
- Deteriorating lung function on optimal medical therapy.

Special risk factors associated with mortality in patients on *Lung Transplant Waiting List* as observed in the West are:

- Elevated right atrial pressure (>15 mm Hg)
- Pulmonary hypertension
- Increased quantity of supplemental oxygen used
- The African-American race.

It is to be noted that after lung transplantation, recurrent sarcoidosis in the lung allografts can occur though this does not affect survival or the risk of complications.

In India where (except at the All India Institute of Medical Science and the Apollo Hospitals, Chennai) lung transplantation is not frequently performed, advanced sarcoidosis will continue to be treated on medical lines. It would be of relevance to study the life expectancy of advanced pulmonary sarcoidosis in Indian and other Asian patients who are hypoxemic at rest or on a standard 6-minute walk, and whose FVC and CO diffusion capacity are less than 50% of predicted, while continuing optimal medical therapy which includes supplemental oxygen.

■ SUGGESTED READING

1. Badgwell C. Cutaneous sarcoidosis therapy updated. J Am Acad Dermatol. 2007;56(1):69-83.
2. Baughman RP, Culver DA, Judson MA. A concise review of pulmonary sarcoidosis. Am J Respir Crit Care Med. 2011;183(5):573-81.
3. Baughman RP. Treatment of sarcoidosis. Clin Chest Med. 2008;29(3):533-48.
4. Chen ES. Etiology of sarcoidosis. Clin Chest Med. 2008;29(3):365-77.
5. Gupta SK. Sarcoidosis: a journey through 50 years. Indian J Chest Dis Allied Sci. 2002;44(4):247-53.
6. Gupta SK, Gupta S. Sarcoidosis in India: a review of 125 biopsy proven cases from eastern India. Sarcoidosis. 1990;7(1):43-9.
7. Iwai K, Sekigutti M, Hosoda Y, et al. Racial difference in cardiac sarcoidosis incidence observed at autopsy. Sarcoidosis. 1994;11:26-31.
8. Judson MA. The diagnosis of sarcoidosis. Clin Chest Med. 2008;29:415-27.
9. Kim JS. Cardiac sarcoidosis. Am Heart J. 2009;157(1):9-21.
10. Mihailovic-Vucinic V. Pulmonary sarcoidosis. Clin Chest Med. 2008;29(3):459-73.
11. Morimota T, Azuma A, Abe S, et al. Epidemiology of sarcoidosis in Japan. Eur Resp J. 2008;31:372-9.
12. Nagai S. Outcome of sarcoidosis. Clin Chest Med. 2008;29(3):565-74.
13. O'Regan A, Berman JS. Sarcoidosis. Ann Intern Med. 2012;156:ITC5.
14. Rizzato G, Tinelli C. Unusual presentation of sarcoidosis. Respiration. 2005;72:3.
15. Rose AS. Hepatic, ocular, and cutaneous sarcoidosis. Clin Chest Med. 2008;29(3):509-24.
16. Sharma OP. Sarcoidosis around the world. Clin Chest Med. 2008;29:357-63.
17. Sharma SK. Uncommon manifestations of sarcoidosis. J Assoc Physicians India. 2004;52:210-4.
18. Stern BJ. Neurologic presentations of sarcoidosis. Neurol Clin. 2010;28(1):185-98.
19. Valeyre D, Prasse A, Nunes H, et al. Sarcoidosis. The Lancet. 2014;383(9923):1155-67.
20. Wijsenbeek MS, Culver DA. Treatment of sarcoidosis. Clin Chest Med. 2015;36:751.

CHAPTER 46

Pulmonary Langerhans Cell Histiocytosis

■ GENERAL CONSIDERATIONS

Pulmonary Langerhans cell histiocytosis (LCH) is characterized by the monoclonal proliferation and infiltration of Langerhans cells in the small bronchioles and interstitium of the lungs. The earlier designation was histiocytosis X and eosinophilic granuloma. The term histiocytosis X was coined in 1953 by Lichtenstein for a group of three clinical entities, each with a differing clinical spectrum, but having as a common feature, the proliferation of a histiocytic-appearing cell. The three clinical entities considered by Lichtenstein under histiocytosis X were:

1. Letterer-Siwe disease—an aggressive, lethal disorder of young children, characterized by multisystem involvement.
2. Hand-Schüller-Christian syndrome—generally occurring in children and young adults, characterized by multiple focal bone lesions (invariably involving the skull bones), exophthalmos and diabetes insipidus.
3. Eosinophilic granuloma of the bone or the lungs—focal lesions involving one or more bones or lesions involving both lungs.

The underlying offending proliferating histiocytic-appearing cell present in all these three clinical entities was later identified as the "Langerhans cell". Therefore, LCH is now preferred to the term histiocytosis X and pulmonary involvement in histiocytosis X is termed pulmonary LCH. A simplified current classification of LCH is given in **Table 1**.

Pulmonary LCH is a rare smoking-related interstitial disease affecting young adults. Lung involvement usually occurs in isolation; uncommonly involvement of other organ systems is also observed, notably of the bones, pituitary gland and the skin.

Table 1: Simplified system of classification of Langerhans cell histiocytosis in adults.

Single-organ involvement:
- Lung (occurs in isolation in >85% of cases with lung involvement)
- Bone
- Skin
- Pituitary
- Lymph nodes
- Other sites: thyroid, liver, spleen, brain

Multisystem disease:
- Multiorgan disease with lung involvement (5–15% of cases with lung involvement)
- Multiorgan disease without lung involvement
- Multiorgan histiocytic disorder

■ EPIDEMIOLOGY AND ETIOLOGY

The incidence and prevalence of pulmonary LCH is unknown. It is a rare disease, but the incidence and prevalence may well be underestimated, because some patients are asymptomatic, some show spontaneous remission and the exact diagnosis of an interstitial disease like pulmonary LCH may be missed if a lung biopsy has not been performed.

Pulmonary LCH is a smoker's disease occurring in young adults generally between 20 years and 40 years of age. Tobacco smoke is the causative factor; no other environmental or occupational factor has been incriminated. Though previously thought to have a male preponderance in the West, current literature suggests equal distribution between males and females or even predominance in females, perhaps related to the increasing smoking habit of women in the West. A smoking history is obtained in more than 90% of patients. We have seen a patient in his early teens who was a nonsmoker, but passive smoking may have played a role in this patient as the father was a heavy smoker. There is no evidence of a genetic predisposition though familial clustering in children has been reported in Western literature. The disease is believed to be more common in Whites than in Blacks or Asians.

An interesting feature is an association of this disease with other malignancies, prompting the belief that it may possibly be a premalignant condition. Lymphomas, hematological malignancies, solid cancers have been reported with pulmonary LCH. This association however may well be related to the role that tobacco smoke plays both in the pathogenesis of cancers and pulmonary LCH.

PATHOGENESIS

Though the disease is characterized by several disturbances in immune function, its pathogenesis is unknown. Abnormalities in immune function include:

- A non-specific increase in IgG in bronchoalveolar BAL fluid.
- Immune complexes both in the blood as also bound to tissues.
- Abnormalities in T cell function.

Whether these changes represent a nonspecific activation of the immune system or play a significant role in the pathogenesis of LCH is unclear.

Cigarette smoking unquestionably plays an important role in PLH as it is present in nearly all patients. Remarkably enough, cigarette smoking does not seem to be associated with extrapulmonary LCH.

A prevailing hypothesis is that the production of a Bombesin like peptide plays an important role. Bombesin is a neuropeptide produced by neuroendocrine cells which are increased in the lungs of smokers. These peptides are chemotactic to monocytes, stimulate multiplication of epithelial cells and fibroblasts and also stimulate the cytokine production by macrophages, which in turn activate and stimulate Langerhans cells within the lung.

Tobacco contains glycoproteins which are immuno-stimulant. These glycoproteins together with other regulatory glycoprotein peptides may contribute to the pathogenesis.

In conclusion PLH is a reactive polyclonal proliferation of Langerhans cells induced by antigens in cigarette smoke, though the exact pathogenesis remains unclear.

In contrast, other systemic forms of LCH are unrelated to cigarette smoke and are the result of a monoclonal proliferation of Langerhans cells.

RELATIONSHIP TO MALIGNANCY

Though PLCH is regarded as a non-neoplastic process associated with smoking, a subset of PLCH patients may be due to a clonal process associated with BRAF V600 mutation. These mutations play an important role in the development of cancer. Lymphomas, bronchogenic carcinoma, pulmonary carcinoid tumor, mediastinal ganglioneuroma have been reported with pulmonary LCH. Malignancy may precede, accompany or follow the diagnosis of Pulmonary LCH. The above association may, however, well be related to the role that tobacco smoke plays in the pathogenesis of some malignant tumors.

PATHOLOGY

The characteristic infiltrate and granulomas consist typically of Langerhans cells. On light microscopy, these cells are usually mononuclear with abundant acidophilic cytoplasm and highly characteristic nuclei. The nuclei are irregular, elongated with prominent grooves and folds traversing in all directions. Eosinophils are also frequently present as are a few lymphocytes and plasma cells. As the lesions heal, fibrosis occurs; Langerhans cells and eosinophils are scarce or even absent in fibrotic lesions, being replaced by lymphocytes, macrophages and plasma cells. Fibrosis may lead to marked honeycombing of the lungs, most marked in the upper lobes where the disease is more marked from the very beginning.

On electron microscopy, the Langerhans cell has a characteristic appearance. Within its cytoplasm can be found typical granules termed the Birbeck granules. Birbeck granulas are rod-shaped, with zipper-like striations and sometimes have a bulbous racket-shaped end **(Fig. 1)**. Immunostaining shows CD1 antigen on the cell surface and S100 protein in the cytoplasm.

CLINICAL FEATURES

The clinical presentation varies. A history of cigarette smoking is important.

- The patient may be asymptomatic (10–25% of patients), the disease being discovered on a routine X-ray chest which shows small nodular lesions chiefly in the upper- and mid-zones of both lungs. At times the X-ray

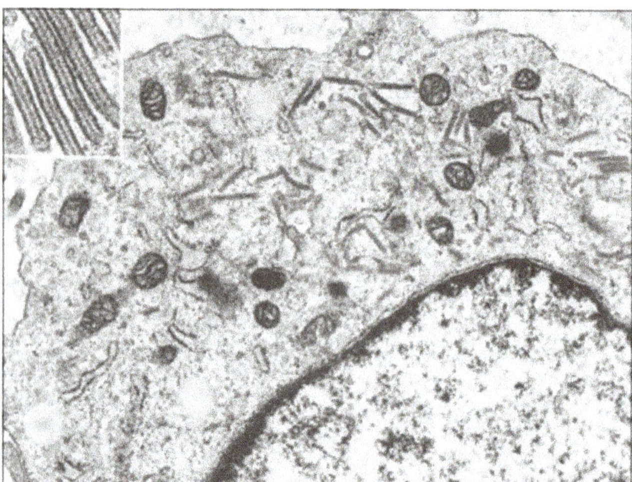

Fig. 1: Ultrastructurally the Langerhans cells contain Birbeck granules, which are seen in the cytoplasm of the cell and in the inset.

appears indistinguishable from miliary tuberculosis (TB) and is treated for a time as such. The absence of any change in the miliary lesions after treatment prompts an open lung biopsy which reveals the true nature of the pathology.

- The two important respiratory symptoms are cough and dyspnea on exertion. Increasing dyspnea is observed when there is progression of the disease.
- The first manifestation of the disease may be a spontaneous pneumothorax which may recur on the same side or may occur after a varying interval on the other. We have observed a patient with spontaneous pneumothorax occurring simultaneously on both sides causing acute respiratory distress and failure.
- Constitutional symptoms include low-grade fever, weight loss, and fatigue occurring in 20% of patients. A mistaken diagnosis of miliary TB is frequent when these patients also have small nodular shadows in the lungs.
- Rarely (5–10% of patients) extrapulmonary manifestation may occur.

Bone lesions may cause pain or pathological fractures if the skeletal bone or bones are involved. More often the disease involves the flat bones. Bone lesions may be the sole manifestation of the disease or may precede pulmonary involvement.

Central nervous system involvement generally takes the form of diabetes insipidus; the prognosis in these patients is poor.

Skin lesions may be observed in the form of erythematous, maculopapular lesions; the scalp may show crusted seborrheic lesions.

Pulmonary arteriopathy and veno-occlusive disease may occur independently from the bronchoalveolar lesions. These may impair diffusion capacity and exercise tolerance to a degree disproportionate to radiological findings.

Hemoptysis is an uncommon complication and should prompt a search for infection or a tumor.

■ PHYSICAL FINDINGS

There may be no physical finding on examination of the chest. Clubbing of the nails is uncommon. Some patients have rhonchi on auscultation, others may have fine crackles, particularly in the upper lobes and a few have both rhonchi and crackles.

In patients who show progression of the disease, increasing pulmonary fibrosis produces hypoxic respiratory failure, pulmonary hypertension, cor pulmonale and congestive heart failure.

■ NATURAL HISTORY

The natural history is variable. In 25% of patients, there is complete spontaneous remission. In 50% of patients, the disease stabilizes after mild to moderate progression. There is however always the possibility of the disease resuming activity after a varying period of stabilization. In 25% of patients, there is progressive deterioration. In the last group, the end result is chronic hypoxic cum hypercapnic respiratory failure and increasing pulmonary hypertension with cor pulmonale and congestive heart failure; the median survival is reported to be 13 years. The natural history can be punctuated at any point in time by pneumothorax. Pulmonary infection or systemic sepsis from any other cause is an important complication, particularly in those on corticosteroids and/or cytotoxic drugs.

■ INVESTIGATIONS

Chest Radiography (Figs. 2A to J)

An X-ray of the chest shows micronodular lesions, at times miliary lesions, chiefly involving the upper- and mid-zones of both lungs, with a sparing of the costophrenic angles. The lesions on a careful examination are often

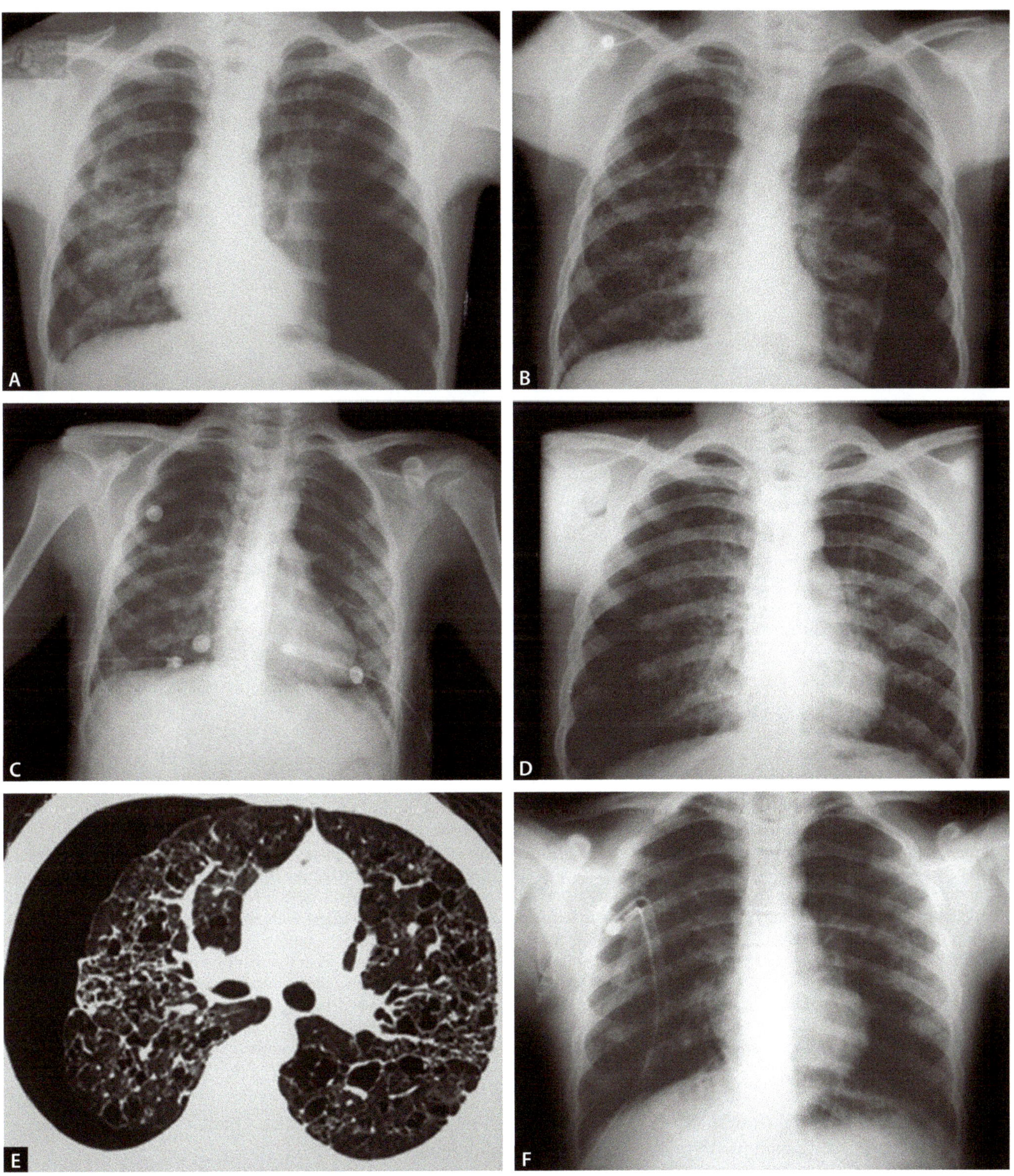

Figs. 2A to F

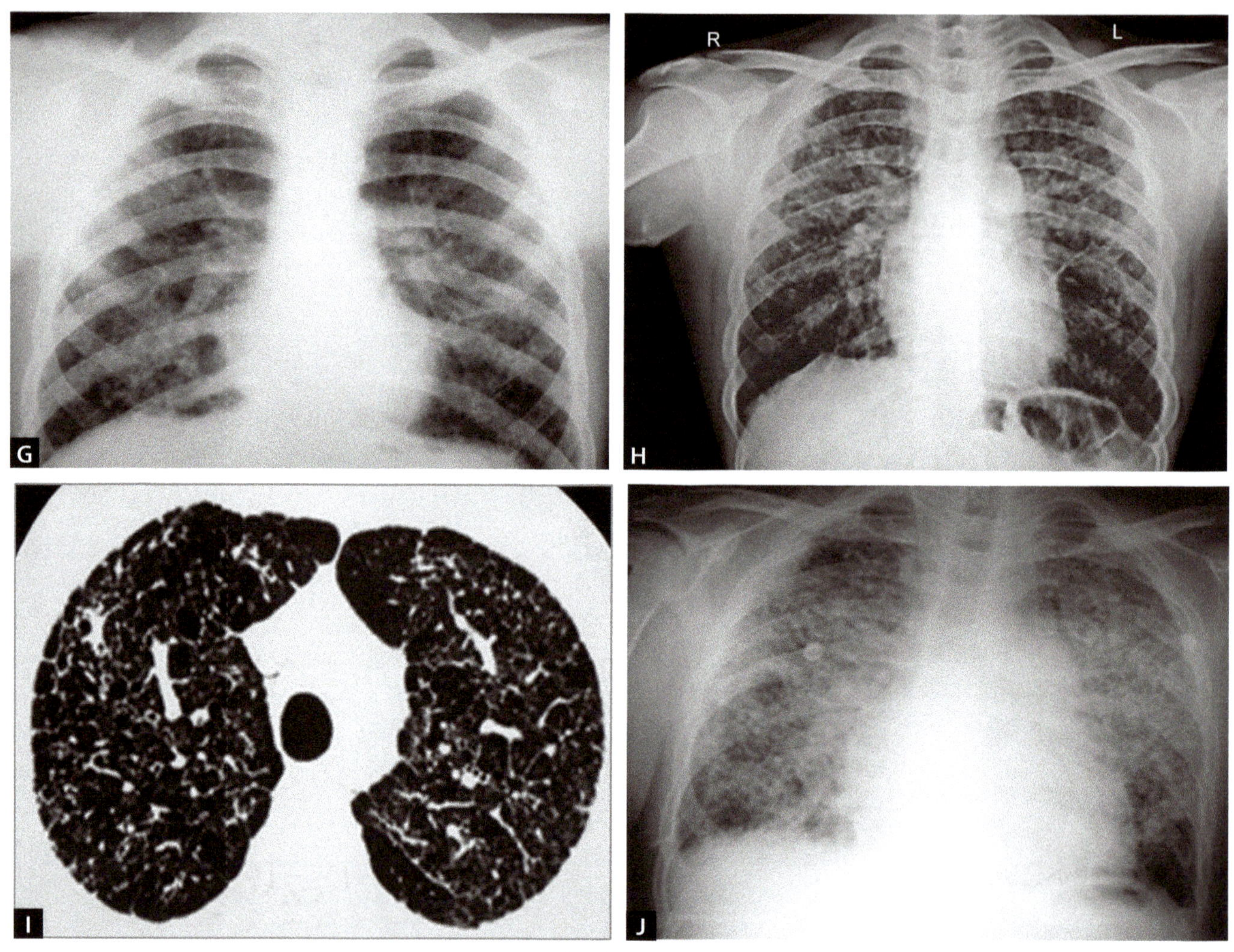

Figs. 2G to J

Figs. 2A to J: Pulmonary Langerhans cell histiocytosis. An 11-year-old boy presented with sudden onset chest pain, breathlessness. (A) Chest X-ray revealed bilateral pneumothorax, larger on the left side. Pneumothorax resolved with intercostal drainage (ICD) tube insertion; (B) Four months later; he developed bilateral pneumothorax again; (C) Treated with bilateral ICD and subsequently left pleurodesis done; (D) Three years later developed recurrence of right pneumothorax. Visualized lung parenchyma reveals reticulonodular lesions in both lung fields; (E) High-resolution computed tomography (HRCT) chest reveals cysts which are bizarre in shape with abnormal intervening parenchyma, a typical finding of Langerhans cell histiocytosis; (F) Subsequently right pleurodesis done; (G) Postpleurodesis X-ray reveals extensive reticulonodular lesions in both lung fields; (H and I) Follow-up X-ray and CT chest, 10 years after the first pneumothorax reveals bilateral reticulonodular opacities which have considerably increased, CT chest at this point reveals progression in size, shape and extent of the cysts. Note presence of nodules indicating that the disease is still active; (J) Chest X-ray a short while later demonstrates extensive bilateral pulmonary opacities denoting acute respiratory distress syndrome (ARDS) related to overwhelming bacterial sepsis. Note enlarged cardiac silhouette with dilated pulmonary artery denoting chronic cor pulmonale at the end stage of the disease.

superimposed on cystic ring shadows 5–10 mm in diameter; the cystic ring shadows represent cavitation of the nodular lung lesions. As the disease progresses there is increasing fibrosis; the smaller cyst lesions merging to form larger thin-walled cysts and bullae. Well-marked honeycombing of the lungs is evident with progression of the disease. Very importantly the lung volumes on a chest X-ray remain normal, unlike what is observed in interstitial pulmonary fibrosis.

High-Resolution Computed Tomography of the Chest (Figs. 2E and 2J)

High-resolution computed tomography (HRCT) of the chest in the early stages shows nodules in the upper- and mid-zones of both lungs. Serial CTs over time show a progression from nodular lesions to cavitation and cystic lesions. Increasing fibrosis leads to honeycombing of the lung, most marked in the upper and middle lobes.

The above typical pattern is not always present. Ground-glass attenuation may accompany the typical changes noted above. Also, at times, large cysts and bullae may be formed all over, including the lower lobes.

It has been shown that nodular lesions on an HRCT chest are an indication of active disease. Cystic lesions cannot however be considered inactive, as it is impossible to distinguish inactive cysts from cavitating granulomas.

PET Scan

FDG-PET scan often shows an increased uptake in the early stage of the disease associated with a nodular radiological pattern. Negative PET scans are generally observed in later stages if the disease is associated with fibrosis and honeycombed cysts.

Lung Function Tests

Lung function tests show typically a mixture of an obstructive plus restrictive pattern. At times one pattern predominates over the other. A fall in the diffusing capacity of carbon monoxide may be an early finding. A standard 6-minute walk may show a fall in oxygen saturation. In the presence of increasing airways obstruction, the forced expiratory volume in 1 second/forced vital capacity (FEV_1/FVC) is progressively reduced and there is an increased ratio of residual volume to total lung capacity.

Bronchoalveolar Lavage

The presence of more than 5% Langerhans cells in the bronchoalveolar lavage (BAL) fluid is considered to be diagnostic of the disease. However, the BAL may be negative with regard to Langerhans cells in more than 50% of patients. A lower proportion of Langerhans cells (<4%) can be seen in interstitial lung disease, bronchiolitis, and bronchoalveolar carcinoma.

Lung Biopsy

Transbronchial lung biopsy generally affords a poor yield of 10–40%. A thoracoscopic or open lung biopsy is the diagnostic procedure of choice. Even here the diagnosis may not be proven because of sampling errors since the lesions are focal and sampling of a cystic area may show no evidence of active disease.

■ DIAGNOSIS

The diagnosis should be suspected in young adults who are smokers and who have nodular lesions in the upper- and mid-zones of both lungs. The HRCT chest appearances should be compatible with those described earlier. In the typical patient with the expected clinical features and typical imaging findings, a BAL study and/or a lung biopsy may not be necessary. A BAL study, failing which a lung biopsy, is indicated when the imaging findings are atypical; as for example in symptomatic patients where the shadows are purely nodular or to distinguish lymphangiomyomatosis from LCH. A differential diagnosis of TB, extrinsic allergic alveolitis and sarcoidosis may need to be entertained in some patients with LCH.

■ TREATMENT

The patient should be instructed to stop smoking. The disease has been then known to regress or at least stabilize in some but not all patients.

If a period of observation shows that the lung disease is progressive, corticosteroids are indicated. Prednisolone in a dose of 40 mg/day is given for 4 weeks; reduced by 5 mg every 3–4 weeks to a maintenance dose (preferably not >10 mg/day) that controls the disease.

In rapidly progressive disease uncontrolled by corticosteroids, cytotoxic drugs such as cyclophospha-mide, methotrexate, chlorambucil have been tried. Their effect on the natural history of progressive disease is undetermined. In disseminated disease, a combination of corticosteroids and cytotoxic drugs is advocated from the very beginning.

The role of corticosteroids or cytotoxic drugs in this disease remains unproven.

Cladribine (2-chlorodeoxyadenosine), a cytotoxic agent that is toxic for lymphocytes and monocytes has been effectively used in patients with progressive LCH. This drug has also been used successfully in combination with cytotoxic alkylating agents plus corticosteroids for the aggressive multisystem form of the disease. Cladribine needs to be tried on a large number of patients before its therapeutic role can be correctly evaluated.

The BRAF V600E mutation is observed in 35 to 50% of patients with PLCH. Identification of these patients allows targeted therapy with BRAF inhibitor, Vemurafenib. This results in non-progression and stabilization of the disease. However, relapse invariably occurs on stopping treatment.

Pulmonary hypertension when present may partially respond to conventional therapy.

Radiotherapy has proved useful as a palliative treatment for painful bone lesions.

Pneumothorax invariably necessitates chest tube drainage. Pleurodesis may be necessary in patients with recurrent pneumothorax.

In rapidly progressive systemic disease, bone marrow transplantation has been successfully performed. Advanced pulmonary disease with respiratory failure or pulmonary hypertension has been treated with lung transplantation. The disease may however recur in the transplanted lung.

Complications such as pulmonary or any other systemic infections need requisite treatment.

■ SUGGESTED READING

1. Aricò M, Girschikofsky M, Généreau T, et al. Langerhans cell histiocytosis in adults. Report from the International Registry of the Histiocyte Society. Eur J Cancer. 2003;39:2341-8.

2. Brown RE. Pulmonary Langerhans'-cell histiocytosis. N Engl J Med. 2000;343(22):1654-5; author reply 1656.

3. Fukuda Y, Miura S, Fujimi K, et al. Effects of treatment with a combination of cardiac rehabilitation and bosentan in patients with pulmonary Langerhans cell histiocytosis associated with pulmonary hypertension. Eur J Prev Cardiol. 2014;21:1481-3.

4. Lorillon G, Tazi A. How I manage pulmonary Langerhans cell histiocytosis. Eur Respir Rev. 2017;26.

5. Mendez JL, Nadrous HF, Vassallo R, et al. Pneumothorax in pulmonary Langerhans cell histiocytosis. Chest. 2004;125:1028-32.

6. Roden AC, Hu X, Kip S, et al. BRAF V600E expression in Langerhans cell histiocytosis: clinical and immunohistochemical study on 25 pulmonary and 54 extrapulmonary cases. Am J Surg Pathol. 2014;38:548.

7. Sundar KM, Gosselin MV, Chung HL, et al. Pulmonary Langerhans cell histiocytosis: emerging concepts in pathobiology, radiology, and clinical evolution of disease. Chest. 2003;123:1673-83.

8. Tazi A. Adult pulmonary Langerhans' cell histiocytosis. Eur Respir J. 2006;27:1272-85.

9. Wei P, Lu HW, Jiang S, et al. Pulmonary langerhans cell histiocytosis: case series and literature review. Medicine (Baltimore). 2014;93:e141.

CHAPTER 47

Pulmonary Lymphangioleiomyomatosis and Other Rare Diffuse Lung Diseases

■ GENERAL CONSIDERATIONS

Pulmonary lymphangioleiomyomatosis (LAM) is a rare, generally progressive disease affecting women in the childbearing age, characterized by infiltration of the lung by an unusual form of smooth muscle cell (termed LAM cells) causing extensive cyst formation and destruction of lung tissue. It is characterized clinically by dyspnea, cough, recurrent pneumothorax, chylous pleural effusion, and in most patients, progression to respiratory failure. Some patients with pulmonary LAM show the presence of benign angiomyolipomas (AML) in the kidneys and/or enlargement of the axial retrocrural and retroperitoneal lymphatics.

The pulmonary manifestations of LAM predominate, but rarely, the disease may present exclusively within the abdomen, or the extrapulmonary abdominal presentation may precede involvement of the lungs.

Therapy for this disease is unsatisfactory but advances in molecular biology have identified several potential targets for future clinical trials with appropriate drugs.

■ EPIDEMIOLOGY

The prevalence in the UK, France, and USA is about 1 per million of the population. It is also met with as a rare disease in India and other countries but the prevalence is unknown. The mean age of onset as judged from several studies is 35 years. Though almost exclusively occurring in females of childbearing age, there are reports of this disease in post-menopausal women receiving hormonal therapy.

There are two forms of LAM—sporadic LAM (S-LAM) and LAM occurring in association with tuberous sclerosis (TSC-LAM). Both are associated with mutations of tuberous sclerosis genes which regulate pathways that control energy supply and nutrients to cells. Global estimates indicate that the prevalence of TSC-LAM is probably five times more than S-LAM. However, women with S-LAM form more than 85% of the 1,300 patients registered by the LAM foundation, suggesting that TSC-LAM may perhaps be a milder disease than S-LAM. It has been estimated that 30–40% of women with TSC may have high-resolution computed tomography (HRCT) findings consistent with LAM.

■ GENETICS—MOLECULAR PATHOGENESIS OF LAM

Lymphangioleiomyomatosis and TSC both are caused by mutations of either the hamartin (TSC-1) gene on chromosome 9 or the tuberin (TSC-2) gene on chromosome 16. These are tumor suppressor genes which form a complex that has a negative regulatory effect on the cell cycle. These genes control cell growth and survival through the rapamycin signaling pathway. Deficiency or dysfunction of the encoded proteins hamartin or tuberin results in a loss of regulatory cell control. The consequent activation of the mTOR kinase and S-6 kinase leads to increased protein synthesis, cellular proliferation, migration, and invasion.

It is believed that mutation and loss of heterogeneity in the *TSC-2* gene, or less commonly in the *TSC-1* gene, is responsible for sporadic pulmonary LAM. Pulmonary LAM cells and cells of AML in the kidney in sporadic LAM have been shown to possess the same *TSC-2* gene mutation, not present in normal cells. There is evidence to suggest that LAM cells can metastasize. When a lung transplant performed for this disease shows a recurrence of pulmonary LAM in the transplant, the same TSC-2 mutation is observed in LAM cells of the recurrent disease as is present in the LAM cells of the original disease.

The mechanism whereby the mutations described above are translated into the clinical features of pulmonary LAM is uncertain. It is possible that factors in addition to mutations in the *TSC-2* gene may be necessary for the development of LAM. The disease is limited to women, is exacerbated by the administration of estrogen and may regress after menopause. Also LAM cells have estrogen and progesterone receptors. These findings suggest that female sex hormones, in particular estrogens, may have a role in the evolution of the disease.

■ PATHOLOGY

The macroscopic appearance is of numerous cysts distributed all through the lungs. Microscopically, there is a proliferation of LAM cells. Proliferation within the wall of the airways leads to airways obstruction and airflow limitation; proliferation within the lymphatic walls leads to lymphatic obstruction; and proliferation within vessel walls leads to obstruction and rupture of vessels with intra-alveolar hemorrhage.

Lymphangioleiomyomatosis cells appear to be a type of smooth muscle cells as they express actin, desmin, and vimentin. The cells are however, not typical of smooth muscle cells as they contain electron-dense membrane-bound vesicles. The cells stain with HMB-45, a feature useful for diagnosis in biopsy specimens of patients suspected to have this disease. LAM cells express receptors for estrogens and progesterone. The estrogen receptors are associated with anti-apoptotic protein Bcl-2. It is likely that suppression of apoptosis by estrogen may be the mechanism underlying hormonal dependence in this disease.

■ CLINICAL FEATURES

Pulmonary LAM presents most frequently with cough and progressive breathlessness on exertion. The breathlessness may be associated with a wheeze. Hemoptysis though less common may also occur. An important presentation is with pleural chest pain caused by a pneumothorax. Pneumothorax may occur in either or both sides, may be recurrent, and can occur at any time in the natural history of the disease. An important and often classical clinical feature is the presence of a unilateral or bilateral chylous pleural effusion, which recurs promptly

on tapping and which may be occasionally associated with chyloptysis. A chylous pleural effusion may be the presenting clinical feature or may occur later in the course of the disease.

Rarely, extrapulmonary symptoms may be the presenting features. Extrapulmonary features include angiomyolipoma, abdominal lymphadenopathy, abdominal LAM, and chylous ascites. Angiomyolipomas are within the kidneys (very rarely outside, within the abdomen); they are generally small and asymptomatic, but occasionally are large and may bleed. Mediastinal and abdominal lymphadenopathy is a frequent feature. LAMs within the abdomen are large, lobulated, generally retroperitoneal masses containing chylous fluid. They can cause abdominal pain and chylous ascites **(Figs. 1A to E)**.

The clinical features of tuberous sclerosis should always be sought because of the clear association between LAM and this disease. Pulmonary and extrapulmonary features of LAM are listed in **Table 1**.

■ NATURAL HISTORY

In most, but not all cases, pulmonary LAM is a progressive disease chiefly producing airways obstruction but often a combination of obstruction plus restriction. It leads to progressive hypoxic or hypoxic + hypercapnic respiratory failure. The natural history is punctuated by pneumothorax which is often recurrent and by chylous pleural effusion. Life expectancy from the onset of symptoms is reported at 4 to 16 years. Currently, the median survival is around 10 years though patients with milder disease and slower progression may live longer. The disease may regress after menopause.

■ DIAGNOSIS

The major differential diagnosis is Langerhans cell histiocytosis occurring in a female. Langerhans cell histiocytosis invariably has a smoking history, chiefly involves the upper and mid-zones, and spares the costophrenic region. The cysts occur against the background of small nodules in the lung, are thicker walled, more irregularly shaped, and often not as symmetrical as in pulmonary LAM.

Airflow limitation due to emphysema with lucent cysts on imaging studies is another important differential diagnosis. More often it is pulmonary LAM which is mistaken for emphysema than vice versa. Cystic spaces

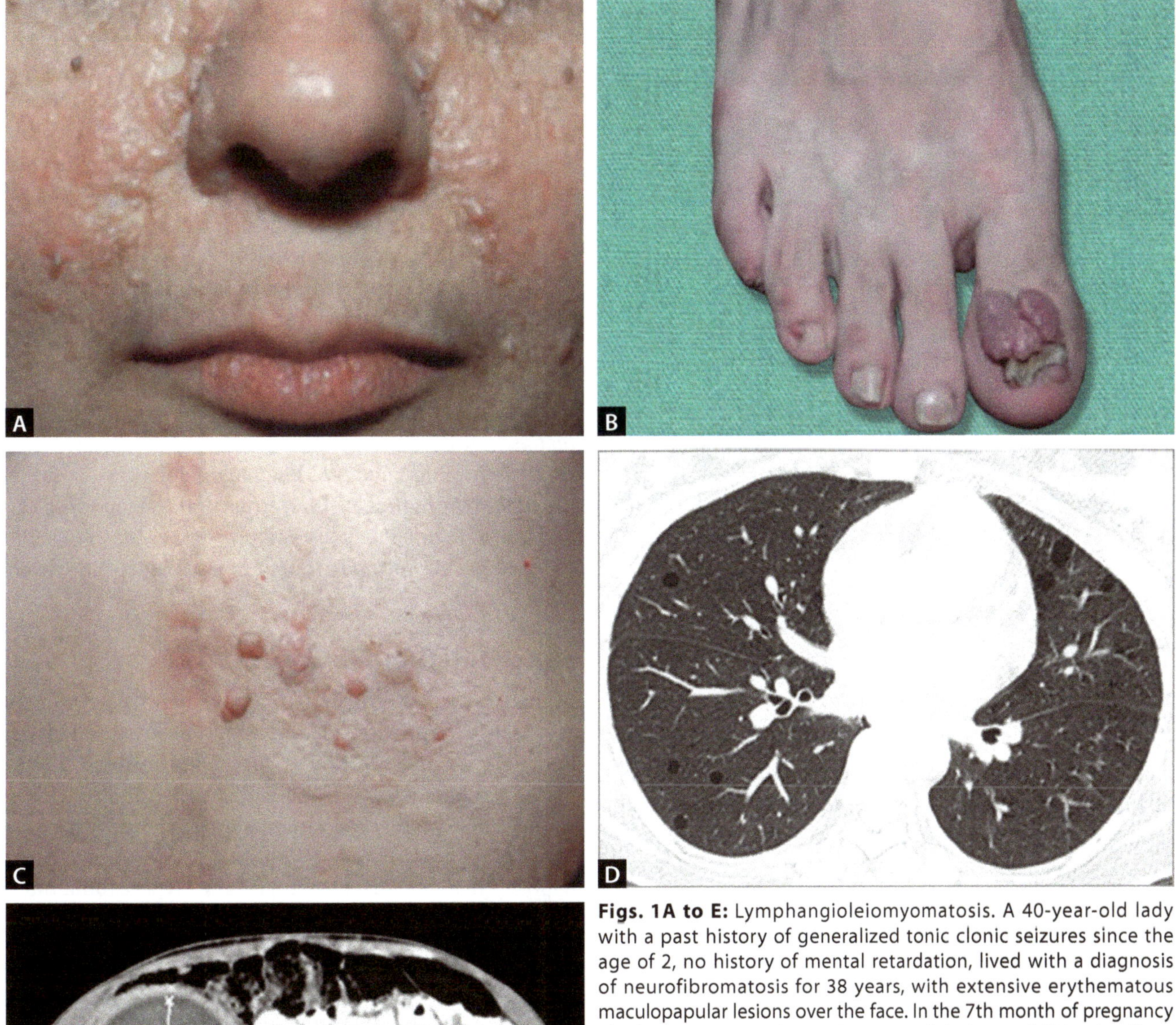

Figs. 1A to E: Lymphangioleiomyomatosis. A 40-year-old lady with a past history of generalized tonic clonic seizures since the age of 2, no history of mental retardation, lived with a diagnosis of neurofibromatosis for 38 years, with extensive erythematous maculopapular lesions over the face. In the 7th month of pregnancy she had a pneumothorax, intercostal drainage (ICD) tube. Note (A) facial angiofibroma; (B) ungual fibroma; (C) shagreen patch. (D) Post-pleurodesis high-resolution computed tomography chest reveals multiple thin-walled cysts in both lung fields. The intervening lung parenchyma is normal. These are not as a result of centrilobular emphysema as they are in the lower zones, the centrilobular vessels are on the periphery of the cyst and patient denied a history of smoking. The cysts are thin-walled and rounded as compared to pulmonary Langerhans cell histiocytosis cysts which are thick-walled and irregular in shape. (E) CT of the abdomen reveals a well-defined mass lesion which is relatively homogenous in consistency with internal hyperdensities representing hemorrhage. Surgical excision revealed an angiomyolipoma.

in emphysema have no clear defining walls in contrast to LAM. Other diseases that can mimic LAM are cavitating metastatic lesions, extrinsic allergic alveolitis, bronchiolitis, bronchopulmonary dysplasia, and the Birt-Hogg-Dubé (BHD) syndrome. The latter is a very rare tumor suppressor syndrome characterized by spontaneous pneumothorax, skin lesions, pulmonary cysts, and inherited renal cell cancer.

Table 1: Pulmonary and extrapulmonary features of lymphangioleiomyomatosis (LAM).

Pulmonary	Extrapulmonary (during course of the disease)
Dyspnea	Angiomyolipoma (generally renal, rarely extrarenal)
Cough	Lymphadenopathy
Chest pain	Lymphangioleiomyomas
Hemoptysis	Chylous ascites
Pneumothorax	
Chylous effusion	

A definite diagnosis of LAM can be made from the characteristic HRCT-coupled with a lung biopsy showing the typical features of LAM.

A lung biopsy may not be possible in all patients. The diagnosis is however *very probable* in the presence of a characteristic HRCT, the presence of an angiomyolipoma, chylous pleural effusion, lymphangiomyoma, and tuberous sclerosis. A *likely* diagnosis can be made in the presence of appropriate clinical features and a characteristic HRCT.

A contributing blood test in the diagnosis is the estimation of vascular endothelial growth factor D (VEGF-D) level in blood. VEGF-D is a lymphangiogenic factor which is a measure of lymphatic involvement in LAM. In the presence of an appropriate clinical and imaging feature, a VEGF-D serum level more than or equal to 800 pg/mL is diagnostic of LAM. This test to the best of our knowledge is not available in India.

■ INVESTIGATIONS

Chest Radiography

As the disease progresses, radiography of the chest shows reticular shadowing with thin-walled cysts distributed all over. Septal Kerley-B lines are visible. Cysts may merge to form larger cysts. Pneumothorax or chylous pleural effusion may be present. The cystic changes in the lung may become more evident and discernible when a pneumothorax produces a partial collapse of the lung. An important feature is that the lungs are normal-sized or often hyperexpanded, and not small in volume as is observed in the honeycombed lungs of interstitial pulmonary fibrosis.

High-Resolution Computed Tomography

An HRCT of the chest very often strongly suggests the correct diagnosis. The following features are noted:

- The presence of evenly distributed thin-walled cysts in both lung fields with normal intervening parenchyma. The cysts vary in size, generally from 2 mm to 20 mm but may merge to form much larger cysts of 5–10 cm. The cysts even when large invariably have discernible thin walls unlike in emphysema where they do not have discernible walls.
- Ground-glass densities may be present and represent recent pulmonary hemorrhage.
- Hilar and retrocrural lymphadenopathy may be present.

High-resolution computed tomography of the abdomen often reveals extrapulmonary features which may be silent and asymptomatic. These include AML recognized by the presence of areas of fat density (<10 Hounsfield units); lymphadenopathy along the course of the axial lymphatics in the retrocrural, retroperitoneal, and pelvic regions may also be present. LAMs are visible as large cystic, retroperitoneal masses with thick well-defined walls.

Lung Function Tests

In the early stages, the lung functions may be normal. As the disease progresses, an increasingly obstructive pattern is observed on spirometry. Very often the ventilatory pattern is characterized by both obstructive and restrictive changes. Reduced carbon monoxide (CO) transfer occurs early in the disease. Arterial blood gases show increasing hypoxemia as the disease progresses. Hypercapnia often occurs later in the course of the disease.

■ PROGNOSIS

Chylous effusion, lymphangioleiomyomas are generally associated with a more severe form of disease. Patients presenting with exertional dyspnea or hemoptysis have a worse prognosis than those presenting with pneumothorax. Marked elevation of VEGF-D levels generally point to progressive disease and a poorer prognosis.

Angiomyolipomas

Angiomyolipomas occur in the kidney. The main complication of a large angiolipoma is bleeding. This should be treated by embolization rather than resection. Severe pain is also another indication for selective embolization. Here again, sirolimus reduces tumor size in 50% of patients and so may prevent bleeding and the need for embolization. The drug should be used in all patients with large angiolipomas. Discontinuation of the drug leads to a return of the tumor to its previous size. *Pregnancy leads to a sharp deterioration of patients with LAM who are symptomatic. Patients should be advised against pregnancy.*

■ MANAGEMENT

Hormonal Therapy

Treatment for this disease is unsatisfactory. Since the disease was thought to be hormone-dependent, attempts at treatment were directed toward estrogen depletion or blockade. Though earlier reports on the use of progesterone (orally or intramuscular depot preparation) suggested that the drug may be of some benefit, a retrospective meta-analysis by Taveria Da Silva et al., showed that progesterone did not prevent a decline in forced expiratory volume in one second (FEV_1) and appeared to accelerate the decline in diffusion lung capacity for carbon monoxide (DLCO) compared to untreated patients. The early enthusiasm for progesterone treatment has therefore waned.

Oophorectomy was earlier recommended as a method of causing estrogen depletion. There is however no evidence that oophorectomy is of any use and currently this treatment has also fallen out of favor.

Sirolimus in the Treatment of LAM

Ever since the discovery that *TSC gene I* and *TSC gene II* are involved in the pathogenesis, important advances in the treatment of LAM have been achieved. *TSC I and TSC II* are suppressor genes that encode hamartin and tuberin, respectively. These proteins form a complex that regulates the intracellular mTOR, thereby regulating cell growth and proliferation. Two different complexes involving mTOR, mTOR 1 and mTOR 2 have been identified. Sirolimus is an immunosuppressive drug that provides partial inhibition of mTOR 1 and has some degree of inhibitory on mTOR 2. Sirolimus has been found to be of some efficacy in a number of trials in patients with tuberous sclerosis or LAM who had AML. Tumors were reduced by 50% in a year's therapy. Withdrawal of the drug led to a partial increase in size of the tumors. The effect of sirolimus on pulmonary functions (MILES trail) resulted in an improvement of forced vital capacity (FVC), FEV_1, in the quality of life and in functional performance. Withdrawal of the drug led to decline of lung functions. In a new study, sirolimus was tried on 19 patients with chylous effusion and lymphangioleiomyomas for 2-and-half years, nine of these

19 patients had complete remission of chylous effusion and abdominal lymphangioleiomyomas.

The current recommendation is to use sirolimus in patients with LAM who are symptomatic, or who have chylous effusion or ascites. The dose of sirolimus is 2 mg/day, trough serum levels being maintained at 5–15 ng/mL. Many prefer to start with 1 mg/day except in patients who show sharp decline, who should receive 2 mg/day, the dose being titrated back to 1 mg/day, once stability in lung functions is achieved. Current recommendation supports targeting a trough level ≤10 ng/mL in the blood. Sirolimus is a suppressive drug rather than a curative drug and since the omission of the drug leads to regression of lung function to pretreatment levels, the current recommendation is to continue the drug indefinitely or as long as the drug is tolerated. Adverse effects of the drug include mucosal ulcers, renal impairment, hyperlipidemia, infection, amenorrhea, and sirolimus-related interstitial pneumonia, anemia, thrombocytopenia, hypertension, allergies, susceptibility to latent neoplasms. It is not yet known how long the drug should be continued and whether ultimately the disease develops a resistance to the drug.

Everolimus

Patients who do not tolerate or respond to sirolimus may respond to the second line drug everolimus. The drug is not approved for sporadic LAM, the dose used in clinical studies being 2.5 mg/day increasing to 10 mg/day. A multicenter study in patients with pulmonary LAM suggests that this drug has the same efficacy and side-effects as sirolimus *(Ref: Goldberg HJ, Harari S, Cottin V, et al. Everolimus for the treatment of lymphangioleiomyomatosis: a phase II study. Eur Respir J. 2015;46:783).*

Inhibitors of Autophagy

Autophagy is the mechanism whereby cells maintain energy hemostasis and recycle proteins. Hydroxychloroquine is known to induce cell death by blocking autophagy. On the other hand, blockage of mTOR signaling by sirolimus could result in an increased survival of LAM cells. Inhibition of autophagy by chloroquine could potentially enhance the effect of sirolimus on LAM. A current study (SAIL trial) is ongoing to test the effects of sirolimus and hydroxychloroquine on LAM. Results of Phase I show that a combination of sirolimus and hydroxychloroquine is well-tolerated in these patients.

Symptomatic Treatment of Airways Obstruction in LAM

The use of bronchodilators in the form of inhaled or nebulized β_2-agonists may afford some relief to patients with some degree of reversibility to their airflow limitation.

Oxygen affords a degree of relief to those who are increasingly dyspneic and in those who have hypoxic respiratory failure.

Pneumothorax

Pneumothorax is associated with a fair degree of morbidity, more so as it recurs in over 50% or more of patients. Pleurodesis may be necessary but this may increase complications for future lung transplantation. Lung transplantations with current techniques have however been successful even in patients with pleurodesis.

Chylous Effusions

Chylous effusions are due to rupture of subpleural lymphatics or blockage of the thoracic duct. Management consists of:

- Use of octreotide which reduces the production of lymph through reduction of splanchnic blood flow
- A low-fat diet which reduces production of lymph
- Aspiration of fluid when the chylous effusion is symptomatic. Repeated aspirations may however lead to significant loss of fat and protein
- Surgical measures when conservative methods fail. These include pleurodesis, pleurectomy, thoracic duct ligation, and pleuroperitoneal shunt
- The current finding that sirolimus is effective in reducing and stopping recurrent chylous pleural effusions and lymphangioleiomyomas suggests that the drug should be tried in place of invasive surgical procedures such as pleurodesis.

Angiomyolipomas

Angiomyolipomas in the kidney, if large, can cause bleeding, which may be severe. This is preferably treated by embolization of involved vessels. Surgical treatment if decided upon, should be aimed at conserving as much renal tissue as possible. A close follow-up of angiomyolipomas by frequent 3 to 6-monthly ultrasound examinations is important. Here again sirolimus has been shown to significantly reduce the size of the tumors over a period of a year.

Lung Transplantation

Lung transplantation is the only available and effective treatment for advanced disease. The presence of marked dyspnea, hypoxemia, and a significantly reduced DLCO is an indication for considering lung transplantation even when airflow obstruction is not critical. Dyspnea with severe airflow obstruction as judged by FEV_1 near 30% of its predicted value is in itself an indication for lung transplantation. The cumulative survival rate for patients with pulmonary LAM who had lung transplantation in the United States is 65% at 5 years which is better than the survival rate for other lung diseases requiring transplant surgery. Many centers prefer double-lung transplants to single-lung transplants even though survival rates are similar, because double-lung transplants are associated with lower rates of bronchiolitis obliterans and greater improvement in the FEV_1.

■ PULMONARY AMYLOIDOSIS (FIGS. 2A AND B)

Amyloidosis is characterized by the homogenous extracellular deposition of material that stains with Congo-red and that has an apple-green birefringence under polarized light. Amyloid is laid down in the form of fibrils 7–10 mm in diameter and these can be generated from a number of precursor proteins in the blood. The two major amyloid proteins are AL and AA proteins. The AL protein is derived from the light chains of immunoglobulins and is associated with primary amyloidosis, amyloidosis complicating multiple myeloma, and in isolated tracheobronchial and nodular pulmonary amyloidosis. The AA is derived from a protein normally found in serum and is present in secondary amyloidosis, occurring in patients with chronic inflammatory disorders and rheumatoid arthritis.

Amyloid involvement of the lung takes three forms:

1. Pulmonary involvement in primary systemic amyloidosis. The pulmonary parenchyma or the alveolar septa or both show amyloid infiltrates. The frequency of pulmonary involvement in primary systemic amyloidosis is 36–60%. The mean age is around 60 years, both sexes being equally affected. It is often discovered on imaging studies and generally produces few or no symptoms. X-ray of the chest shows a diffuse reticular infiltrate or reticulonodular infiltrates. The prognosis is poor being related to the

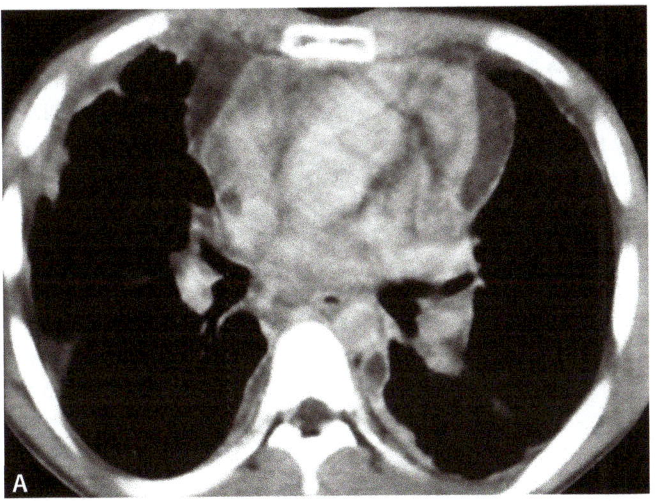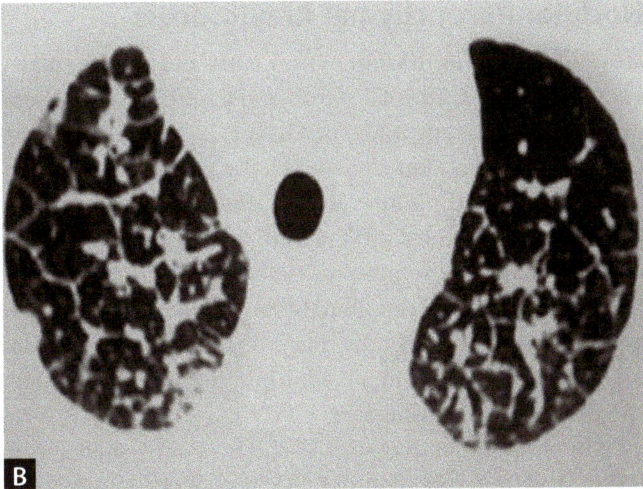

Figs. 2A and B: Amyloidosis. CT chest reveals a small pericardial effusion with bilateral pleural thickening. High-resolution computed tomography chest reveals septal thickening with nodules along the septa. The lung architecture is preserved; such an appearance may be seen in lymphangitic carcinomatosis. Transbronchial biopsy revealed amyloidosis.

primary systemic amyloidosis of which pulmonary amyloidosis is just a part. The median survival rate is generally not more than 1.5 years.

2. Pulmonary involvement in secondary amyloidosis. Amyloid deposition in the lung is rare in secondary amyloidosis. It is generally limited and clinically silent.

3. Isolated pulmonary amyloidosis. This is a rare disease and can present in three forms—tracheobronchial amyloidosis, nodular amyloidosis, and diffuse parenchymal amyloidosis.

Tracheobronchial Amyloidosis

Tracheobronchial amyloidosis is characterized by the deposition and infiltration of amyloid deposits in the tracheobronchial tree. The presentation may be in the form of one or more strictures in the trachea or the large airways due to local and focal deposits of amyloid.

Clinical presentation could also be related to a more diffuse deposition of amyloid involving the entire or greater part of the tracheobronchial tree causing bronchial constriction.

Rarely, amyloid deposits may take the form of endobronchial or tracheal polypoid or tumor-like lesions.

The amyloid deposits in tracheobronchial amyloidosis are of the AL type and are generally deposited in the submucosa. Calcification and even ossification within deposits may be observed.

Clinical Features

Cough, wheezing, and breathlessness on exertion are the most frequent symptoms; these may be indistinguishable from the clinical features observed in chronic obstructive pulmonary disease (COPD). If strictures form in the trachea or large bronchi, noisy breathing or stridor is observed. Hemoptysis is not frequent. Bronchial strictures could cause atelectasis, repeated episodes of pneumonia, and ultimately bronchiectasis of the affected segment or lobe. Hilar and mediastinal adenopathy due to amyloid deposits may occur.

The differential diagnosis is from COPD and asthma. Atelectasis or lobar collapse due to a bronchial stricture may raise the possibility of lung cancer, particularly in the presence of hilar and mediastinal adenopathy.

Diagnosis and Treatment

Diagnosis is by bronchial biopsy through a fiberoptic bronchoscope. Bronchoscopic appearance is that of shiny pale plaques with areas of focal narrowing. The biopsy material stains positive with Congo-red. Focal strictures or lesions can be generally resected by laser therapy. Solitary polypoid masses can be resected with excellent results. Diffuse amyloid tracheobronchitis has a poor prognosis. Breathlessness and airways obstruction progress, leading to death from respiratory failure. In one series, 30% patients died within 4–6 years. Hemoptysis is frequent in diffuse tracheobronchial disease and can be fatal.

Nodular Parenchymal Amyloidosis

Isolated nodular parenchymal amyloidosis is rare, occurs generally after 60 years of age with an equal sex distribution. The amyloid is of AL type.

The disease is characterized by the presence of one or multiple amyloid nodules within the lung parenchyma, the size of the nodules varying from 0.5 cm to 5 cm. Larger nodules may also be present. Calcification or cavitation has been reported in one-third of the nodules. Mediastinal and/or hilar adenopathy may occur when there is multinodular involvement. Multiple nodules can cause cough and breathlessness.

The differential diagnosis is chiefly from a metastatic lesion, and from tuberculosis (TB) or other granulomatous diseases.

Diagnosis is generally made on examination of a solitary nodule removed at surgery. A thoracoscopic biopsy of a nodule gives the diagnosis when there is multinodular involvement of the lung. The multinodular form of the disease cannot be cured surgically; even so the prognosis is good, far better than for the tracheobronchial form of the disease.

Diffuse Parenchymal Amyloidosis

Isolated diffuse parenchymal amyloidosis is extremely rare, amyloid being deposited in the alveolar septa and in the media of the blood vessels.

In contrast to parenchymal lung involvement occurring as a feature of primary systemic amyloidosis, patients with isolated diffuse lung involvement with amyloid are always symptomatic, with cough, progressive dyspnea leading to progressive hypoxemia, and respiratory failure. End-inspiratory crackles are generally present as with other interstitial lung diseases. Death generally occurs within 2 years of the diagnosis.

Imaging studies, involving both chest X-ray and high-resolution computed tomography (HRCT), show progressively increasing reticulonodular infiltrates; hilar and mediastinal nodes may be enlarged in some cases. The imaging features are indistinguishable from other pathologies causing interstitial lung disease.

Corticosteroids and/or immunosuppressive drugs have not been shown to be of any use. A number of novel approaches and treatment of amyloidosis are under investigation and perhaps in time to come may be of use.

■ PULMONARY ALVEOLAR PROTEINOSIS (FIGS. 3 TO 5)

Pulmonary Alveolar Proteinosis (PAP) is characterized by the accumulation of surfactant within the alveoli and terminal bronchioles. When alveolar filling with surfactant is extensive, gas exchange is affected resulting in hypoxemic respiratory failure. PAP occurs in many different clinical conditions. Research has identified its molecular basis

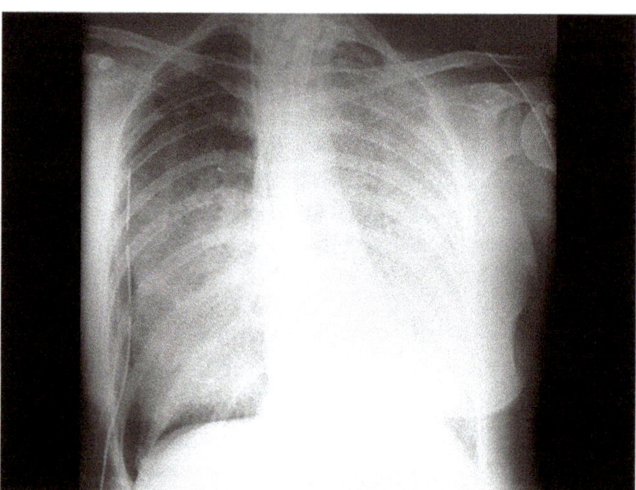

Fig. 3: Pulmonary alveolar proteinosis. Chest X-ray demonstrates diffuse ground-glass densities in both lung fields. Thoracoscopic biopsy revealed pulmonary alveolar proteinosis. Intercostal drainage (ICD) tube in situ, right side following the thoracoscopic biopsy.

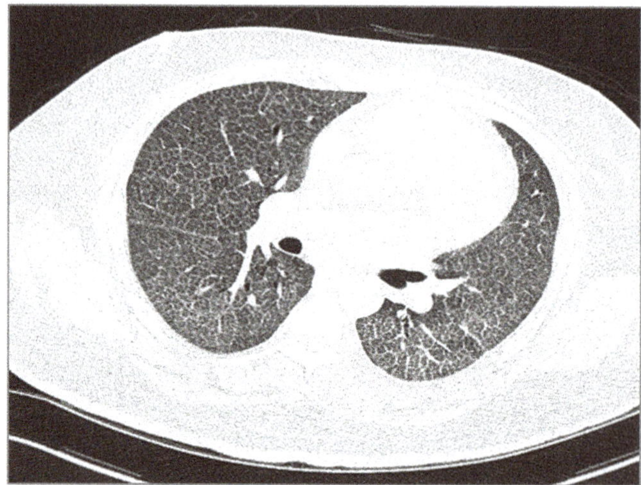

Fig. 4: Pulmonary alveolar proteinosis. High-resolution computed tomography chest demonstrates diffuse ground-glass densities with septal thickening indicative of a crazy pavement appearance. These features are fairly diagnostic of pulmonary alveolar proteinosis.

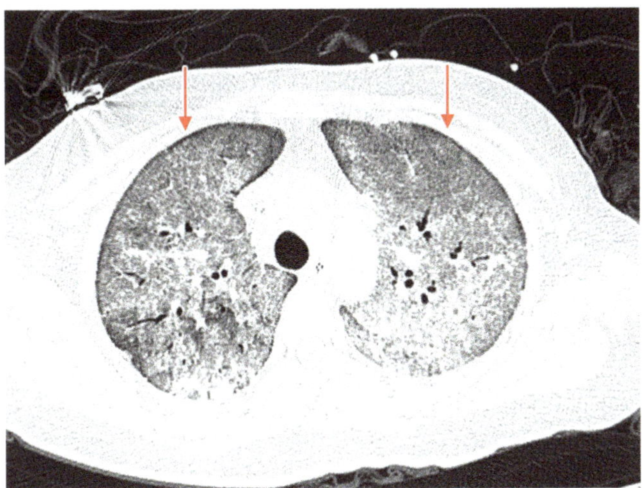

Fig. 5: Pulmonary alveolar proteinosis. High-resolution computed tomography chest demonstrates diffuse ground-glass densities in both lung fields with a thin dark subpleural line; this is due to the proteinaceous material being compressed away from the chest wall.

in over 90% of cases. In particular, the molecular basis underlying the role of the granulocyte-macrophage colony stimulating factor (GM-CSF) in surfactant homeostasis is well-understood.

Epidemiology

Alveolar proteinosis is a rare disease occurring predominately in men (male-female ratio 3:1). We have encountered five proven patients as yet. There is an increased incidence in smokers. The peak age of onset as judged by reviews is between 30 years and 50 years. However, it has also been reported in neonates, infants, and children. Familial incidence is rare but reported.

Pathophysiology

PAP can be primary, hereditary, congenital or acquired. Primary PAP accounts for 90% of cases of PAP. Hereditary, secondary and congenital PAP account for the remainder.

In primary PAP the fault lies in the functioning of the GM-CSF, a 23-kDa cytokine produced by respiratory epithelium and other cells. Besides stimulating granulocyte and macrophage colonies from hematological progenitors, GM-CSF has effects on the alveolar epithelium (Type II alveolar cells) which are not well-understood, as also on alveolar macrophages, the effects on which are very well defined. In primary PAP there is a break or disruption of

the GM-CSF signaling to alveolar macrophages because of neutralizing autoantibodies against GM-CSF.

- *Hereditary PAP* is due to recessive variants of the GM-CSF receptor genes (CSF2RA, CSF2RB); these genetic variants impair signaling by the intact GM-CSF.
- *Congenital PAP* is due to disorders of surfactant production.
- *Secondary PAP* develops in adults and is due to high level dust exposures (silica, aluminium, titanium, indium-tin oxide), myelodysplastic syndrome, hematological malignancies and other allogeneic hematopoietic cell transplantation for myeloid malignancies. In most cases, secondary PAP is due to a relative deficiency in the GM-CSF and related macrophage dysfunction.

This chapter is chiefly focused on primary PAP.

The disturbance in surfactant homeostasis which is the basic cause of primary PAP needs further elaboration. Surfactant within the alveoli plays a vital role in preventing alveolar wall collapse by reducing surface wall tension. It consists of 90% phospholipid and 10% protein (surfactant protein A, B, C, D). Surfactant proteins B and C through their surface active properties keep the alveoli open; surfactant proteins A and D help in host defence. Surfactant lipids and proteins are synthesized, stored and secreted into the alveoli by Type II alveolar cells. The surfactant secreted into the alveoli by type II alveolar cells is released in the form of lamella bodies which are converted into tubular myelin. After use, the surfactant is internalized by Type II alveolar cells and macrophages in roughly equal amounts. Type II alveolar cells recycle and catabolize the internalized surfactant via poorly defined mechanisms which do not involve GM-CSF. In striking contrast, alveolar macrophages can only catabolize the internalized surfactant in the presence of an appropriately delivered 'signal' from the GM-CSF. In the absence of control and 'signaling' by the GM-CSF, alveolar macrophages fail to catabolize surfactant, leading to its accumulation within the alveoli.

It has been shown for several years that primary or idiopathic PAP is associated with a high level of GS-CSF autoantibodies which neutralize GM-CSF, thereby eliminating or reducing its controlling activity and directives to alveolar macrophages. Surfactant instead of being catabolized by the latter accumulates within alveolar spaces-alveolar proteinosis results. These GS-CSF autoantibodies are of the IgG class-chiefly IgG_1 and IgG_2.

Further studies have provided convincing evidence of the pathogenicity of these antibodies in primary or idiopathic PAP, leading to the recommendation that the name be changed from 'Primary' or 'Idiopathic ' PAP to autoimmune PAP.

Clinical Features

The disease to start with is often silent and is then only discovered by imaging studies. Presenting features chiefly include increasing breathlessness on exertion and cough. Low-grade fever, hemoptysis, and vague chest discomfort may also be present.

Physical examination in some patients is essentially normal. Crackles on end inspiration may be heard in 50% of patients. Mild to moderate clubbing is observed in one-third of patients. Extensive or advanced pulmonary alveolar proteinosis may present with cyanosis, hypoxic respiratory failure, and cor pulmonale.

Though the disease is invariably insidious in onset and has a fair degree of chronicity before it is diagnosed, very rarely, a subacute onset presenting with low-grade fever, increasing shadows in both the lungs (resembling ARDS), increasing hypoxemia, and respiratory failure necessitating ventilator support may occur. The clinical picture is often mistaken to start with for ARDS. We have encountered one such patient, but this presentation must indeed be very rare.

An important complication of alveolar proteinosis is a complicating infection, in particular by *Nocardia*, Mycobacteria, and fungi. These complications are rare if therapeutic lavage is offered appropriately. In rare instances interstitial pulmonary fibrosis results as a sequel to longstanding alveolar proteinosis.

Investigations

Chest X-ray shows diffuse bilateral alveolar shadows, generally more marked centrally and less marked peripherally. This distribution gives rise to "bat-wing" shadows resembling pulmonary edema. Air bronchograms are clearly visible through these shadows.

Occasionally, atypical findings are present, consisting of focal or diffuse asymmetrical shadows, consolidation or reticulonodular shadows.

HRCT of the chest is often diagnostic and shows the following features:
- Ground-glass opacification with a sharp differentiation from the normal lung
- Marked septal thickening with the formation of polygonal shapes—crazy pavement pattern
- Areas of consolidation with air bronchograms. These may be surrounded by ground-glass densities.

Lung Functions

Lung function shows a restrictive pattern with well-marked reduction in the diffusion capacity. With progressive disease there is increasing hypoxemia which increases with exercise.

There are no specific laboratory markers for this disease. The lactate dehydrogenase (LDH) is raised; it declines after therapeutic lavage. The levels of surfactant protein A and D may be increased but this again is not specific to this disease.

Diagnosis

The diagnosis of alveolar proteinosis should be suspected in patients with varying degree of dyspnea who on an X-ray of the chest show alveolar shadows resembling the bat—wing appearance of pulmonary edema. The HRCT findings are often typical in this disease though rarely atypical features may be present. The chief diagnostic tool is a BAL study; the BAL fluid having a characteristic milky appearance. Examination of BAL fluid on light microscopy shows:
- Acellular globules that stain positive with periodic acid-Schiff (PAS) and are basophilic with the May-Giemsa stain
- Presence of few macrophages
- Cell debris which also shows a positive though weak PAS stain. Electron microscopy of BAL fluid is unnecessary for diagnosis. An examination of the BAL sediment through electron microscopy shows myelin-like multilamellated structures and lamellated bodies.

Besides a study of BAL, transbronchial or surgical lung biopsy can identify the syndrome but cannot determine the cause. The GM-CSF autoantibody has now been defined and evaluated in a multinational validation study. The presence of this autoantibody in the serum demonstrates a 100% sensitivity and 100% specificity for autoimmune PAP. Similarly a rise in GM-CSF in the serum is sensitive and specific for hereditary PAP, which has a genetic basis.

Differential Diagnosis (Table 2)

Alveolar shadows on imaging may occur in the following situations—pulmonary edema, intra-alveolar hemorrhage, bronchoalveolar carcinoma, chronic eosinophilic pneumonia, exogenous lipid pneumonia, AIP, COP, drug induced pneumonitis.

An overall assessment of the clinical features and imaging studies, in particular the HRCT of the chest, allows a definite diagnosis in most instances. The appearance of the BAL fluid is pathognomic in alveolar proteinosis.

Complications

Secondary infections are the main complications of primary or autoimmune PAP. These contribute to increased morbidity and mortality. Opportunistic infections are often observed, including aspergillus, nocardia, pneumocystis, mycobacterial infection. Infection can also occur at extra-pulmonary sites, suggesting an overall defect in the host defence due to poor antimicrobial function of macrophages and neutrophils.

Management

The disease does not continue to progress in all patients. In fact, spontaneous remission occurs in one-third of patients. Patients should be offered treatment if symptoms are bothersome enough to interfere with the quality of life or when pulmonary functions deteriorate.

The only effective treatment is lung lavage with normal saline. This should only be done by an experienced team with constant monitoring of O_2 saturation, electrocardiography (ECG) and blood pressure. The lung more severely affected is lavaged first. If both are equally affected then the left lung is first lavaged as the right has a larger volume and greater ventilatory capacity compared to the left.

Whole lung lavage is done under general anesthesia after intubating the patient with a double-lumen, endotracheal tube (Carlen's tube). Both lungs are first oxygenated with 100% oxygen for 15 minutes, to wash out nitrogen. This is then followed by a single-lung lavage. The volume used for each filling is 500–1,000 mL. The lavage fluid is then allowed to drain out by gravity, helped by mechanical chest percussion. Filling of the lung with isotonic saline followed by drainage of the lavage fluid is done repeatedly till the effluent loses its milky appearance and is virtually clear. This may require 10–30 L of isotonic saline lavage.

At each cycle there should be a careful record of the inflow fluid into the lung and the outflow fluid out of the lung. The inflow and outflow should match. If fluid retention exceeds 1.5–2 L, the procedure should be stopped and leakage into the pleural space or contralateral lung should be suspected. The procedure is generally well-tolerated. Complications include pneumonia, hydropneumothorax, and bronchoconstriction.

Whole lung lavage of the other lung should be done 3 to 7 days after the first. If the patients are too ill for whole lung lavage, partial lavage of segments or a lobe through a fiberoptic bronchoscope may provide a degree of relief. In very ill patients whole lung lavage has been performed with the help of extracorporeal membrane oxygenation.

Whole lung lavage produces a permanent remission in 25–50% of patients with marked clearing of radiological shadows, relief of symptoms, and marked improvement in lung function. In the others, the disease returns and the lavage procedure may have to be repeated as and when necessary, often at intervals of 3–6 months.

Currently, recombinant GM-CSF has been used subcutaneously, the response rate being slightly lower than 50%. The dosage is 250 µg/day for a month increasing to 5 mcg/kg/day for the second month, and 9 mcg/kg/day for the third month. Recombinant GM-CSF has also been reported to improve lung function tests in these patients. Finally in refractory disease, a few studies have investigated the role of rituximab, although more work needs to be done on its use. Small number of reports have also shown the use of therapeutic plasma exchange in patients who have failed to respond to whole lung lavage. However, the data is insufficient to recommend its use.

Table 2: Differential diagnosis of alveolar shadows on imaging.

- Pulmonary edema
- Intra-alveolar hemorrhage
- Pulmonary infections (e.g. mycoplasma)
- Bronchoalveolar carcinoma
- Chronic eosinophilic pneumonia
- Exogenous lipid pneumonia
- Acute interstitial pneumonia (AIP)
- Cryptogenic organizing pneumonia (COP)
- Drug induced pneumonitis

■ NEUROFIBROMATOSIS AND PULMONARY ALVEOLAR MICROLITHIASIS

Neurofibromatosis

Neurofibromatosis (NF) is an autosomal disorder with various clinical presentations. NF Type 1 is related to the *NF1* gene on chromosome 17 which codes for neurofibromin. NF Type 2 is related to the *NF2* gene which codes for merlin.

Pulmonary involvement takes the form of intrathoracic neurofibroma, meningocele, and parenchymal lung disease with fibrosis. Kyphoscoliosis is also a feature observed with NF. A large earlier series suggested that 7–23% of patients with NF had parenchymal lung involvement. A more recent study of 156 patients of NF at the Mayo Clinic revealed parenchymal involvement in only 1.9% of patients. All the rest with parenchymal disease had other causes for pulmonary infiltrates such as smoking-related lung disease, rheumatoid disease, and recurrent pneumonia. The true incidence of parenchymal involvement in NF is perhaps therefore much less than what was reported earlier.

Pulmonary Alveolar Microlithiasis

Pulmonary alveolar microlithiasis is characterized by the diffuse deposition of concentrically laminated calcium phosphate particles in the form of microliths within the alveoli of both lungs.

The diffuse deposition of microliths within the alveoli produces distinctive calcific micronodular shadows in both lung fields, likened to a "sand-storm" appearance. The mean age at diagnosis reported in studies is in the mid-thirties. The disease however can occur at any age. The disease is an autosomal recessive disorder with a familial presence in about one-third of patients. It is due to a mutation on the gene (SCL34A2) present on chromosome 4. This gene is strongly expressed in type II alveolar cells and its function is to encode a sodium phosphate co-transporter thereby preventing its accumulation within the alveoli. A mutation of this gene prevents this function—hence the accumulation of microliths within the alveoli.

A large review revealed that more than 50% of patients were asymptomatic in spite of the frightening appearance of the lung on radiographic examination. The others had cough, dyspnea, and chest pain. Progress of the disease was slow; death from progression was due to cardiorespiratory failure.

Diagnosis can be confirmed by transbronchial lung biopsy and by the increased uptake during ^{99m}technetium scanning of the lungs. There is no therapy, though attempts at lung transplantation have been made. Calcific microliths have been reported to regress in pediatric patients treated with bisphosphonate.

■ IDIOPATHIC PULMONARY HEMOSIDEROSIS (FIGS. 6A TO D)

Idiopathic pulmonary hemosiderosis is a very rare disease of unknown etiology characterized by a single or by recurrent episodes of diffuse alveolar hemorrhage; each episode typically presenting with dyspnea, hemoptysis, anemia, and bilateral acinar infiltrates, generally in the parahilar and lower zones of the lungs. The disease occurs chiefly in children and adolescents with an equal male–female ratio. It is also observed in adults generally under 30 years of age, but has been reported in older individuals as well.

Pathogenesis

The etiology is unknown. The current belief is that idiopathic pulmonary hemosiderosis has an immunological basis. This assumption is based on the following:

- Its association with other autoimmune diseases, such as hemolytic anemia, thyrotoxicosis, celiac disease.
- Idiopathic pulmonary hemosiderosis is known to occur in children who show hypersensitivity to cow's milk. The disease improves when cow's milk is struck off the diet.
- Treatment with immunosuppressive drugs has been successful in several cases.

Pathology

There is intra-alveolar hemorrhage together with an accumulation of hemosiderin-laden macrophages within the alveoli. The alveolar capillaries are often dilated; various other structural abnormalities of the alveolar capillaries have been reported. As a consequence of repeated hemorrhage, the alveolar walls are thickened with increased interstitial connective tissue. In patients with a longstanding history, there is well-marked interstitial pulmonary fibrosis.

Immunological studies do not show the presence of either immunoglobulin or complement deposition. Microscopic examination may reveal various abnormalities in the basement membrane of the capillaries. These are nonspecific in nature and are more severe in children than in adults.

Clinical Features

Intra-alveolar hemorrhage occurs episodically and each episode is characterized by dyspnea, cough, and hemoptysis. Low-grade fever is often present. A single

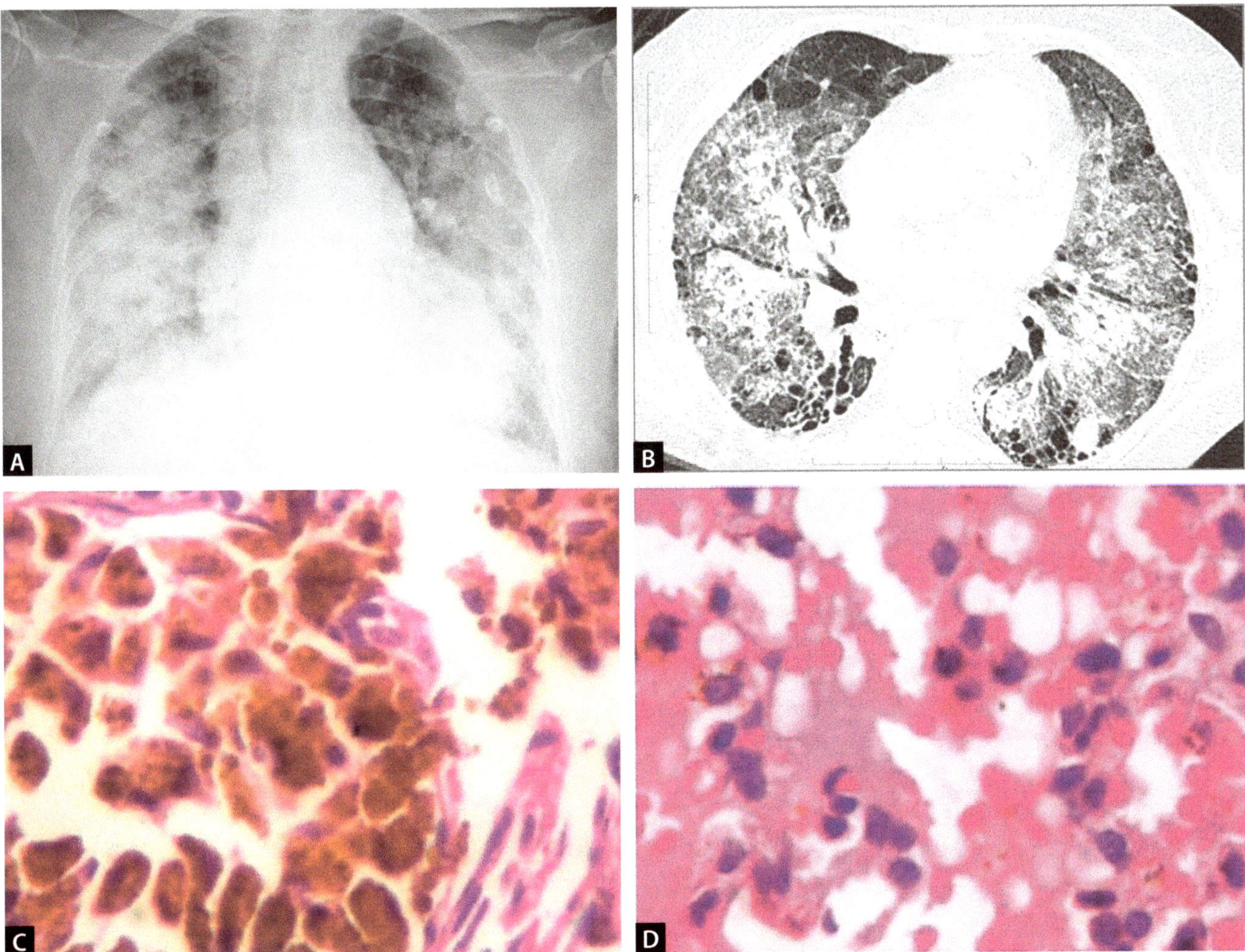

Figs. 6A to D: Idiopathic pulmonary hemosiderosis. A 13-year-old boy presented with history of repeated episodes of hemoptysis over the last 9 months. (A) Chest X-ray reveals diffuse alveolar opacities in both lower zones as well as the left mid-zone (B) High-resolution computed tomography revealed ill-defined ground-glass densities in the subpleural regions of both lung fields. Thoracoscopic biopsy was performed. (C and D) Histopathology revealed mild bronchiolitis with fresh and old intra-alveolar hemorrhage, and clusters of hemosiderin pigment-laden macrophages in many of the alveolar spaces. No evidence of granulomas, capillaritis or vasculitis.

severe episode or frequent episodes cause iron deficiency anemia. Icterus with an increase in unconjugated bilirubin may be present following the release of bile pigments from the blood in the alveoli. Physical findings during an episode of intra-alveolar bleed include tachycardia, tachypnea, pallor, and fine crackles generally over the mid-zones and bases. Severe episodes cause arterial hypoxemia, the degree of hypoxemia being directly related to the severity of the intra-alveolar hemorrhage. Hepatosplenomegaly and generalized lymphadenopathy have been observed in chronic cases.

When intra-alveolar hemorrhage is mild but fairly frequent, the presenting feature is that of an iron deficiency anemia of obscure origin. The chief complaints are fatigability, weakness, and breathlessness on exertion.

Repeated intra-alveolar hemorrhage leads to interstitial pulmonary fibrosis, characterized by increasing breathlessness on exertion, end-inspiratory crackles over the bases and arterial hypoxemia. Mild to moderate clubbing may occur. Progressive fibrosis can lead to hypoxemic respiratory failure.

Imaging Findings

An episode of intra-alveolar hemorrhage leads to bilateral basal and parahilar alveolar shadows. Rarely, the shadows may be unilateral or may involve just one lobe. Once the alveolar bleed subsides, the shadows clear over a week or two. Repeated bleeds produce interstitial fibrosis with characteristic reticulation chiefly involving the lung bases. HRCT of the chest is more sensitive in picking up intra-alveolar bleeds and later the presence of interstitial pulmonary fibrosis.

Lung Function Tests

Lung function tests show a restrictive ventilatory defect which becomes more pronounced with increasing fibrosis. During an active bleed, particularly in the early part of the natural history of the disease, CO diffusion may be more than normal, the CO being picked up by the hemoglobin within the alveoli.

Blood Examination

The peripheral blood shows all the features of iron deficiency anemia—a low serum iron, high iron-binding capacity, and low-iron saturation. Mild peripheral eosinophilia may be present; cold agglutinins have been reported in half the patients.

Differential Diagnosis

The diagnosis of idiopathic pulmonary hemosiderosis can only be made if all other causes of intra-alveolar hemorrhage have been excluded. These causes have been listed in the section on pulmonary vasculitis.

In longstanding cases, the condition is often mistaken for interstitial pulmonary fibrosis of undetermined origin or related to one of the interstitial pneumonias.

When iron deficiency anemia together with hepatosplenomegaly is a presenting feature, the diagnosis is often missed.

Bronchoalveolar Lavage

Bronchoalveolar lavage shows bloody or pink-tinged BAL fluid during an acute episode. Microscopic examination during a fresh bleed shows free RBCs and phagocytosed erythrocytes within macrophages; a few days later hemosiderin-laden macrophages are observed.

Lung Biopsy

Transbronchial biopsy may show hemosiderin-laden macrophages within the alveoli with thickened alveolar walls and an increase in interstitial connective tissue.

A thoracoscopic lung biopsy may be necessary in longstanding cases who present with interstitial lung fibrosis or when it is important to exclude with certainty other causes of intra-alveolar hemorrhage.

Natural History

The disease may take the following courses:

- Spontaneous remission even after many years
- Recurrent episodes over many years of typical intra-alveolar bleeds, leading to chronic interstitial pulmonary fibrosis
- Hypoxemic respiratory failure and chronic cor pulmonale may result
- Mild disease with occasional hemoptysis, iron deficiency anemia, and a varying degree of interstitial pulmonary fibrosis
- Rapid progression, with death from massive diffuse intra-alveolar hemorrhage.

Treatment

For adults without impending respiratory failure due to acute alveolar hemorrhage, methylprednisolone 500 mg daily for five days is recommended. After resolution of the acute episode, the patient is shifted to oral steroids. Azathioprine is also used in this disease. Also a gluten free diet would prevent recurrent episodes of alveolar hemorrhage in coexistent celiac disease.

Massive intra-alveolar bleeds need packed RBC transfusions and hemodynamic support. Endotracheal intubation accompanied by ventilatory support is often necessary.

■ SUGGESTED READING

1. Berk JL. Persistent pleural effusions in primary systemic amyloidosis: etiology and prognosis. Chest. 2003;124(3):969-77.
2. Bonella F, Bauer PC, Griese M, et al. Pulmonary alveolar proteinosis: new insights from a single-center cohort of 70 patients. Respir Med. 2011;105:1908.
3. Collard HR. Diffuse alveolar hemorrhage. Clin Chest Med. 2004;25(3):583-92.
4. Engel PJ. Pulmonary hypertension in neurofibromatosis. Am J Cardiol. 2007;99(8):1177-8.
5. Glodstein LS, Kavier MS, Curtis-McCarthy, et al. Pulmonary alveolar proteinosis clinical features and outcomes. Chest. 1998;114:1357-62.
6. Harari S, Elia D, Torre O, et al. Sirolimus therapy for patients with lymphangioleiomyomatosis leads to loss of

chylous ascites and circulating LAM cells. Chest. 2016;150: e29.

7. Ioachimescu OC, Sieber S, Kotch A. Idiopathic pulmonary haemosiderosis revisited. Eur Respir J. 2004;24:162.

8. Johnson S, Tattersfield A. Clinical experience of lymphangioleiomyomatosis in the UK. Thorax. 2000;55: 1052-7.

9. Johnson SR, Cordier JF, Lazor R, et al. European Respiratory Society guidelines for the diagnosis and management of lymphangioleiomyomatosis. Eur Respir J. 2010;35: 14-26.

10. Kavuru MS, Sullivan EJ, Piccin R, et al. Exogenous granulocyte-macrophage colony stimulating factor administration for pulmonary alveolar proteinosis. Am J Respir Crit Care Med. 2000;161:1143-8.

11. Lachmann HJ, Hawkins PN. Amyloidosis and the lung. Chron Respir Dis. 2006;3:203-14.

12. Lauta VM. Pulmonary alveolar microlithiasis: an overview of clinical and pathological features together with possible therapies. Respir Med. 2003;97(10):1081-5.

13. McCormack FX, Gupta N, Finlay GR, et al. Official American Thoracic Society/Japanese Respiratory Society Clinical Practice Guidelines: Lymphangioleiomyomatosis Diagnosis and Management. Am J Respir Crit Care Med. 2016;194:748.

14. McCormack FX, Gupta N. Sporadic lymphangioleiomyomatosis: clinical presentation and diagnostic evaluation. UpToDate. 2018.

15. McCormack FX. Lymphangioleiomyomatosis: a clinical update. Chest. 2008;133:507-16.

16. Michaud G. Whole-lung lavage for pulmonary alveolar proteinosis. Chest. 2009;136(6):1678-81.

17. Presneill JJ. Pulmonary alveolar proteinosis. Clin Chest Med. 2004;25(3):593-613.

18. Ryu JH, Moss J, Beck GJ, et al. The NHLBI lymphangioleiomyomatosis registry characteristics of 250 patients at enrollment. Am J Respir Crit Care Med. 2006;173:105-11.

19. Seymour JF, Presneill JJ. Pulmonary alveolar proteinosis: progress in the first 44 years. Am J Respiratory Crit Care Med. 2002;160:215-35.

20. Stewart DR. Is pulmonary arterial hypertension in neurofibromatosis type 1 secondary to a plexogenic arteriopathy? Chest. 2007;132(3):798-808.

21. Suzuki T, Trapnell BC. Pulmonary alveolar proteinosis syndrome. Clin Chest Med. 2016;37:431.

22. Tachibana T. Pulmonary alveolar microlithiasis: review and management. Curr Opin Pulm Med. 2009;15(5):486-90.

23. Takada T, Mikami A, Kitamura N, et al. Efficacy and safety of long-term sirolimus therapy for Asian patients with lymphangioleiomyomatosis. Ann Am Thorac Soc. 2016; 13:1912.

CHAPTER 48

Hypersensitivity Pneumonitis

■ INTRODUCTION

Hypersensitivity pneumonitis (HP) constitutes a group of immunologically mediated diseases characterized by an inflammatory response of the alveoli, bronchioles and the interstitium of the lung to the repeated inhalation of a wide variety of antigen-containing organic dusts.

Hypersensitivity pneumonitis is often an occupational, work-related disease though it can occur from exposure to specific antigenic dust in the home or in the outside environment. Only a minority of the many people exposed to environmental or work-related antigens develop HP. Risk factors are governed to an extent by the antigen concentration, duration, frequency and intermittency of exposure, as also by the local seasons, climate and the use of respiratory protective devices. Farmer's lung for example is most frequently seen in the monsoon when damp harvested hay is stocked in poorly ventilated enclosures. Bird fancier's lung occurs with greater frequency in the hot summer months, when exposure to avian antigen is increased. In Japan, HP is most frequently seen in the hot, wet summer months and is associated with microbial contamination of damp indoor furnishings. Host factors which increase susceptibility must also play an important role. The nature of these factors is poorly understood.

■ ETIOLOGY

Numerous antigenic dusts when inhaled have been shown to cause HP. The list has grown over the years and presumably will continue to grow. An important common feature of all antigenic dusts causing HP is that the particle size of the antigenic dust must be less than 3 μm so that it reaches the periphery of the lungs.

Antigenic dust or particles causing HP can be broadly divided into microorganisms (which serve as antigen) in dust, animal proteins, chemicals and drugs. In a number of instances, the antigen responsible for HP remains undetected or is unknown. A list of important causes of HP is shown in **Table 1**.

Perhaps the most common antigens responsible for HP are the thermophilic actinomycetes, which are ubiquitous, found in soil, decaying vegetable matter and compost. A survey of clinically important thermophilic actinomycetes covering numerous soil samples from different sites in Delhi, Punjab, Uttar Pradesh, and Jammu and Kashmir (North India) revealed that *Thermoactinomyces vulgaris* was the most common species occurring in 56% of the samples. This was followed by *Saccharomonospora viridis* (29%), *Thermoactinomyces thalpophilus* (27%), *Saccharopolyspora rectivirgula* (21%) and *Thermoactinomyces sacchari* (40%). The most common substrate for *S. rectivirgula* was hay, yielding 44% of its isolates. This survey carried out by the Vallabhbhai Patel Chest Institute, Delhi, showed the widespread environmental presence of thermophilic actinomycetes suggesting the propensity for frequent exposure of humans to these antigenic microorganisms *(Ref: Randhawa HS, Chowdhary A. Medical mycology in India (1957-2007): contributions by the VPCI Mycoses Group. Indian J Chest Dis Allied Sci. 2008;50:19-32).*

Antigens present in fungi such as the *Aspergillus* species or animal proteins (e.g. from birds) or in certain chemicals have also been shown to cause HP.

All over the world, the most common form of HP is farmer's lung caused chiefly by exposure to moldy hay. The antigen was initially named *Micropolyspora polyspora*, classified as a mold. It was then termed *Micropolyspora*

Table 1: Causes of hypersensitivity pneumonitis (HP).	
Plant proteins	*Exposure*
• Farmer's lung	Moldy hay
• Bagassosis	Moldy pressed sugarcane
• Mushroom-worker's lung	Moldy compost and mushroom
• Malt-worker's lung	Contaminated barley
• Compost lung	Compost
• Tobacco-worker's lung	Mold on tobacco
• Wood pulp worker's lung	Contaminated wood pulp or dust
• Summer-type HP	Contaminated house furnishings
Animal proteins	
• Bird-fancier's disease exposure to pigeon dust	Pigeons, parrots, chickens, parakeets, geese, ducks
Insect proteins	
• Miller's lung	Contaminated grain
Chemicals	
• Chemical worker's lung	Polyurethane foams, spray paint, glues
• Epoxy resin lung	Heated epoxy resin
• Thatched roof lung	Dried grasses and leaves
• Humidifier lung; air conditioner lung	Contaminated humidifiers and air conditioners
Others	
• Coffee-worker's lung	Coffee bean dust
• Tea-grower's lung	Tea plants

faeni. The current classification is *S. rectivirgula. T. vulgaris* and *Aspergillus* species are also contributory antigens.

An exploratory prevalence study of farmer's lung carried out by the Vallabhbhai Patel Chest Institute in Delhi showed that 30% of 197 farmers (who formed the test subjects) with respiratory complaints related their symptoms to exposure to wheat straw, thresher's dust or other vegetable matter in their environment. There was an overall prevalence of 13.2% precipitating antibodies against clinically important thermophilic actinomycetes. Of these *S. rectivirgula* accounted for 55% of the positive reactors. Based on clinical history, imaging studies, lung functions and serum precipitation antibodies to *S. rectivirgula,* farmer's lung was diagnosed in flour workers *(Ref: Randhawa HS, Chowdhary A. Medical mycology in India (1957-2007): contributions by the VPCI Mycoses Group. Indian J Chest Dis Allied Sci. 2008;50:19-32).* The results of a large prospective registry of TLD in India

have recently been published. Singh et al enrolled 1084 adults with ILD from 27 centers across India and found that HP was the commonest diagnosis being found is as many as 47% of all patients. They postulated that contaminated air coolers were probably the source, though this conclusion is debatable as actual tests for bio-allergens were seldom done.

A variety of fungi, *Aspergillus* species and *Penicillium* species are implicated in causing HP in a variety of occupations such as farming. They are also responsible for disease acquired in home environments (summer-type HP in Japan).

Obviously, a large epidemiological study is warranted in view of the huge farming population in our country.

Another important cause of HP is exposure to avian antigen. The antigens are glycoproteins with immunoglobulin A (IgA) activity and are present in bird droppings, serum and bloom from the feathers of several birds. These include pigeons, parrots, chicken, ducks, geese and turkeys.

In large metropolitan cities of India, exposure to pigeon droppings and bloom from feathers is an important cause of HP. This is because pigeons abound and feeding pigeons (which gather en masse at certain places in the city) with grain is a semireligious custom. Pigeons also frequently dirty the window sills and terraces of buildings. Heavy exposure to avian antigen is to be anticipated in these circumstances.

Exposure to moldy pressed sugarcane can lead to a form of HP termed bagassosis. This is common in the sugarcane belt in the province of Maharashtra, the offending antigens being *T. sacchari* and *T. vulgaris.*

Inhalation of antigen-contaminated grain and grain dust is another important cause of the both allergic asthma and HP in many cities of India where the grinding of grain in poorly ventilated shops leads to exposure to a great deal of grain dust.

Occasionally, low-molecular-weight chemicals can react with protein in the airways to form antigens causing HP. These chemicals include trimellitic anhydride and phthalic anhydride used in plastic, and causing plastic worker's lung. Diisocyanates such as toluene diisocyanate have also been reported to cause HP.

Free-living amoeba and nematodes contaminating hot water and ventilation system were thought in the past to cause HP. It has now been shown that the real culprit is the colonization of the above by nontuberculous mycobacteria (NTM) which are resistant to heat and disinfection.

Drugs such as amiodarone, gold, procarbazine have also been reported to cause HP.

■ PATHOGENESIS

Hypersensitivity pneumonitis is a disease resulting from repeated exposure to a variety of antigens. The question that needs to be answered is that considering the increasing number and wider distribution of offending antigens, why should only few individuals develop the disease. It has been hypothesized that *pre-existing genetic susceptibility* and/or *environmental factors* form the background which increase the chances of developing HP. In essence, genetic and environmental factors act as *risk factors* and antigenic risk exposure constitutes the initiating factor responsible for HP. The list of frequently observed antigens has been given in **Table 2**. The most common and important antigens responsible for HP have been discussed under etiology.

The following section in relation to promoting and protecting factors, genetic susceptibility and immunopathology has been almost entirely based on the concise clinical review, "Hypersensitivity pneumonitis—insights in diagnosis and pathobiology" by Selman et al. in 2012 [*Ref: Selman M, Pardo A, King TE. Hypersensitivity pneumonitis—insights in diagnosis and pathobiology. Am J Respir Crit Care Med. 2012;186(4):314-24*].

■ GENETIC SUSCEPTIBILITY

The major histocompatibility complex (MHC) plays an important role in regulating the immune response system of the body. The polymorphism and the heterogeneity within the MHC genome allow the immune system to fight disease pathogens and yet at the same time add to the risk of inducing different immunopathological disorders. Class II MHC molecules are believed to be the primary susceptibility locus in HP—DR and DQ have been associated with increased risk for HP in different people with different genetic backgrounds.

It has also been observed that polymorphisms of the transporter associated with antigen processing (TAP) genes increase the susceptibility to HP.

Just as there are genetic factors which predispose to HP following repeated antigenic challenge, there are genetic factors which resist the antigenic challenge thereby preventing the disease. Two studies performed in patients with different ethnic backgrounds demonstrated that promoter variants in tissue inhibitor of metalloproteinase-3 have a protective effect. The mechanism by which TMP-3 may decrease the risk for HP is not clear.

Environmental Promoting Factors

Many patients with acute HP to start with have initial symptoms suggestive of viral infection. Also, in a large heterogeneous farming population, exposure to pesticides was strongly associated with farmer's lung. Pesticide exposure should be considered an important factor in this disease.

Paradoxical Effect of Cigarette Smoking

Hypersensitivity pneumonitis is less frequent in smokers than in nonsmokers. It has been observed that when smokers are exposed to many environmental antigens they produce lower levels of specific antigens when compared to nonsmokers. Interestingly, when smokers do develop HP, the disease runs a chronic course, has frequent

Table 2: Probable antigens associated with various conditions.

• Farmer's lung	*Saccharopolyspora rectivirgula, Thermoactinomyces vulgaris*
• Bagassosis	*Thermoactinomyces sacchari, T. vulgaris*
• Mushroom-worker's lung	*S. rectivirgula, T. vulgaris*
• Malt-worker's lung	*Aspergillus clavatus*
• Compost lung	*Aspergillus* spp., *T. vulgaris*
• Tobacco-worker's lung	*Aspergillus* spp.
• Humidifier lung; air conditioner lung	Nontuberculous mycobacteria
• Wood pulp worker's lung	*Alternaria* spp.
• Thatched roof lung	*Saccharomonospora viridis*
• Summer-type HP	*Trichosporon cutaneum*
Animal proteins	
• Bird-fancier's disease	Avian droppings, serum, feathers
Insect proteins	
• Miller's lung	*Sitophilus granarius*
Chemicals	
• Chemical worker's lung	Diisocyanates, trimellitic anhydride
• Epoxy resin lung	Phthalic anhydride

exacerbations and has a poor survival rate compared to nonsmokers.

Tolerance as Protective Factor

Many individuals exposed to an environmental antigenic challenge develop a mild lymphocytic alveolitis but are asymptomatic pointing to a tolerance to antigen-inducing HP. This tolerance may well be mediated by regulatory T cells, a special subset of CD4+ T cells that play an important role in maintaining a balance between tissue damaging and tissue protective effects of immune response. Regulatory T cells probably play an important anti-inflammatory role.

■ IMMUNOPATHOLOGY

Hypersensitivity pneumonitis is a hypersensitivity response to an inhaled antigen. It is believed that both type III and type IV hypersensitivity responses as defined by Coombs and Gell are involved.

Type III response is characterized by the formation of antigen-antibody immune complexes which excite a hypersensitivity response in the lung through activation of the complement system. Though IgG antibodies predominate, IgM and IgA antibodies are also found. There is an elevation of C1q, C3, C5a levels in the bronchoalveolar lavage (BAL) fluid of affected patients. Immune complexes release proinflammatory cytokines, notably tumor necrosis factor-alpha (TNF-α) and interleukins (ILs) which can induce inflammatory changes within the lungs.

Type IV reaction plays an equally important role in the pathogenesis of HP. BAL fluid in the initial stages shows the presence of neutrophils; this is soon followed by activated lymphocytes, there being an increase in CD8 lymphocytes so that the CD4:CD8 ratio is reduced. Histological studies show the presence of granulomas, a feature observed in type IV response, as also the presence of activated lymphocytes and macrophages in the alveolar and interstitial cellular infiltrates in the lungs.

Details of immunopathogenesis are beyond the scope of this book and readers are referred to specialized works on the subject. Very briefly, immune complexes mediate the acute form of HP. Subacute and chronic forms of HP are provoked through T lymphocytes through a Th1 immune response. Interaction between the HP antigen and CD4+ T cells leads to differentiation of CD4+ T cells into a variety of effector subsets. The induction of granulomatous inflammation requires the expression of the Th1 cytokines, including TNF-α, IL-12, interferon-α as well as a toll-like receptor 9-mediated dendritic cell response. The coexistence of the above with genetic or environmental promoting factors leads to an exaggerated immune response resulting in marked granulomatous lung inflammation.

Further, in the presence of repeated antigenic exposure coupled with a genetic predisposition, changes occur within the lungs inducing expansion and activation of fibroblasts which lay down fibrosis.

Though HP is chiefly an antigen-dependent and antigen-driven disease, there is a suggestion that nonantigenic factors may also perhaps play a role. Inhaled dust particles themselves can cause a degree of inflammation. Also, organic dust may contain toxins such as mycotoxins or endotoxins and histamine-releasing substances that are directly or indirectly toxic to alveolar cells. There are also a number of protein antigens that have immunological adjuvant effects which can activate macrophages and the complement system. The above view has been based on animal experiments. To what extent these nonantigen challenges to the lung play a role in HP in conjectural.

■ HISTOPATHOLOGY (FIGS. 1 AND 2)

The main histopathological features of HP are: (1) the presence of small scattered granulomas which may be poorly defined; (2) a mononuclear and lymphocytic alveolar cum interstitial infiltrate; (3) a bronchiolitis. Granulomas are a distinguishing feature, which help to differentiate HP from interstitial pneumonia.

However, granulomas are not evident in 30% of surgical lung biopsies from patients with HP.

It has been shown that the detection of granulomas may be helped by staining with cathepsin K, a cysteine protease markedly expressed in activated macrophages and epithelioid cells. Intense expression of cathepsin K is observed in epithelioid cells and macrophages present in all diseases with granulomas. In contrast, diseases characterized by a mere collection of alveolar macrophages as in desquamative interstitial pneumonia or in respiratory bronchiolitis with interstitial lung disease (ILD) were negative.

Chronic HP is characterized by architectural distortion of lung tissue with progressive fibrosis, chiefly involving the upper lobes, but also involving other lobes of both

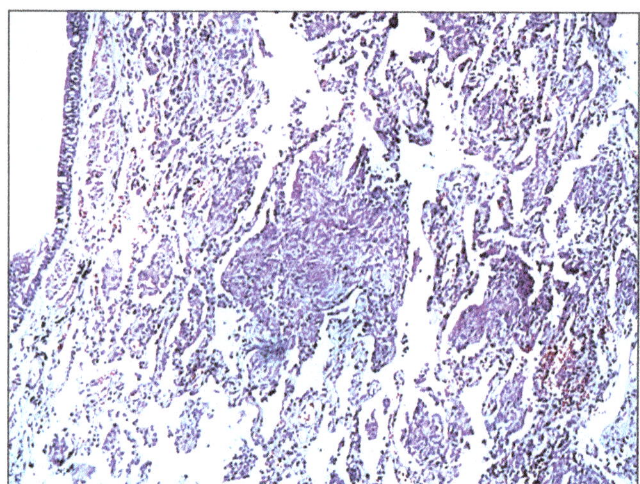

Fig. 1: Hypersensitivity pneumonitis (H&E 100x): Interstitium shows a poorly formed non-necrotizing granuloma. The surrounding lung shows widespread lymphocyte rich interstitial inflammation.

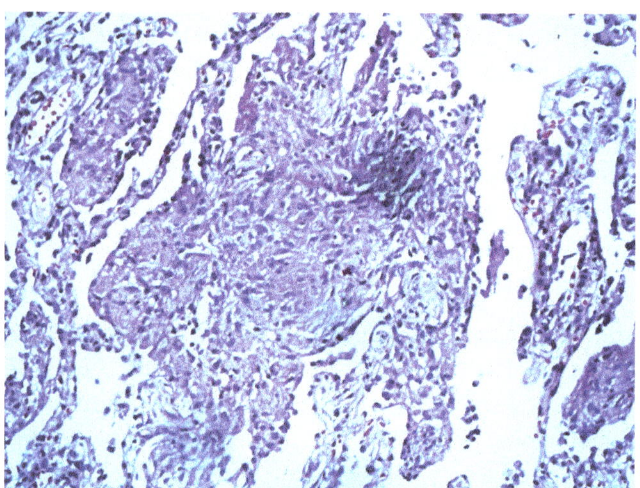

Fig. 2: Hypersensitivity pneumonitis (H&E 200x): Interstitium shows a poorly formed non-necrotizing granuloma comprising loose aggregate of epithelioid histiocytes.

lungs. The histopathological pattern may be difficult to distinguish from nonspecific interstitial pneumonia (NSIP) and usual interstitial pneumonia (UIP).

Although the histopathological features in HP are generally uniform in distribution, it is a well-accepted fact that occasionally discordant findings may be observed—in one specimen typical findings of HP may be seen, and in another, findings resemble those observed in UIP or NSIP.

A complication of chronic HP is lung cancer, particularly observed in cigarette smokers. A recent study reported the coexistence of HP with alveolar proteinosis.

CLINICAL FEATURES

Hypersensitivity pneumonitis may present in an acute, subacute or chronic form. In the classic acute form, symptoms are observed 4–12 hours after antigenic dust exposure. Constitutional symptoms observed are fever, chills, myalgia, and prostration. Respiratory features include cough, breathlessness, tachypnea, basal crackles and in rare instances hypoxemia severe enough to cause cyanosis. The symptoms generally peak within 6–24 hours and subside even without treatment within 2–4 days if antigenic exposure has ceased. In many patients, antigenic exposure remains unsuspected and the condition is often diagnosed as an acute infection, particularly when peripheral blood examination reveals polymorphonuclear leukocytosis with a raised erythrocyte sedimentation rate.

In farmers, the differential diagnosis should include the organic dust toxic syndrome (ODTS) usually related to unloading silos.

Occasionally, symptoms in acute HP may be mild and the disease is diagnosed as a nonspecific febrile illness. Both acute and subacute HP may be associated with wheezing, bronchial hyper-responsiveness and a normal chest X-ray. The differential diagnosis in these patients includes bronchial asthma, related to some occupational exposure. Generally acute HP is nonprogressive, remits spontaneously but can recur on repeated exposure to the antigen. However, some patients with repeated acute episodes of farmer's lung may develop chronic airways obstruction with centrilobular emphysema.

In the subacute and particularly in the chronic form, the relation between antigenic dust exposure and clinical presentation is not often apparent. Dyspnea which is gradually progressive, cough with or without expectoration, fatigability, and malaise are present. Digital clubbing may occur in the chronic form. Progressive fibrosis occurs in the chronic form if antigenic exposure continues, the clinical picture being that of interstitial pulmonary fibrosis. An important distinguishing feature from some of the other forms of ILD is predominant involvement of the upper and middle lobes of the both lungs. The interstitial pulmonary fibrosis consequent to the chronic form of HP may progress to result in chronic hypoxemic respiratory failure and cor pulmonale. It is likely that after a certain stage is reached the disease not only fails to regress but may continue to progress even after exposure to the offending antigen ceases.

The differential diagnosis in the subacute form includes tuberculosis, sarcoidosis, NSIP, lymphocytic interstitial pneumonia, drug-induced lung toxicity. Sarcoidosis is generally associated with lymphadenopathy and the granulomas on histopathology are far better defined than in HP. The differential diagnosis in the chronic form associated well-marked progressive fibrosis is from NSIP or even UIP.

Some patients with chronic HP develop acute exacerbations with increasing dyspnea and hypoxemia with fresh ground-glass shadows on high-resolution computed tomography (HRCT) chest. These exacerbations are reported to be more frequent in smokers, who at the time of initial diagnosis had well-marked fibrosis with poor lung function tests. Histopathology reveals organizing diffuse alveolar damage against the background of marked fibrosis.

Lung Functions

Acute HP is characterized by a restrictive ventilatory defect—a low forced vital capacity (FVC) with a low carbon monoxide (CO) transfer factor.

Some degree of small airways obstruction as evinced by reduced expiratory flow rates may be observed.

Subacute and chronic forms show a restrictive pattern with a loss of lung volume. Arterial hypoxemia on exercise, later even at rest, may be present. Mixed ventilatory defects may also be observed, there being a combination of obstruction to small airways (reduced mid-expiratory flow rates) and restriction [reduction in FVC, total lung capacity (TLC) and CO diffusion]. Some patients, particularly patients with farmer's lung, show well-marked airways obstruction with hyper-reactive airways.

Imaging Studies

Chest X-ray

A normal X-ray does not exclude acute or even subacute HP. Abnormalities if present take the form of diffuse ground-glass shadowing and reticulonodular infiltrate. Radiographic examination of the chest in chronic HP shows bilateral upper lobe fibrosis with upward retraction of the hila, volume loss chiefly affecting the upper and middle lobes. Reticular opacities may be present.

High-resolution computed tomography is often far more revealing than a chest X-ray. The following features are observed **(Figs. 3 to 5)**:

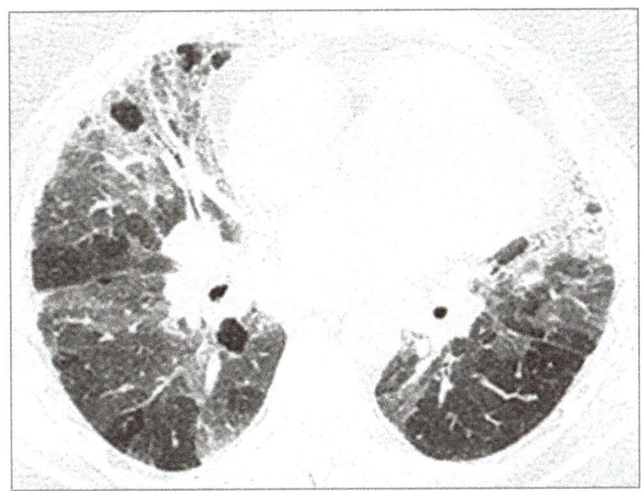

Fig. 3: High-resolution computed tomography (HRCT) chest reveals diffuse ground-glass densities in both lung fields in a geographical pattern with small nodules within the areas of ground-glass density. There is presence of mosaic perfusion as evidenced by areas of reduced lung attenuation interspersed in these areas of ground-glass density.

- *Centrilobular nodules*: Centrilobular nodules which are small in size (between 2 mm and 4 mm) are frequent, chiefly occurring in the middle and lower lobes. Their close relation to bronchioles (bronchocentric) probably corresponds to an underlying bronchiolitis.
- *Ground-glass opacities*: These are hazy confluent opacities which may dominate the imaging findings in acute HP. But they also occur in varying degrees in the subacute and chronic forms. They probably indicate an alveolitis related to ongoing antigenic exposure. Rarely, consolidation may be observed in the acute form of the disease, resolving spontaneously or with treatment.
- *Expiratory air-trapping*: Expiratory air-trapping leads to a mosaic appearance of portions of the lung fields. The portion of the lung where air is trapped during and following expiration appears dark and lucent compared to its surrounding areas. This imaging feature is best viewed on HRCT cuts taken at end-expiration; it represents small airways obstruction caused by bronchiolitis.
- *Fibrosis*: Chronic HP leads to fibrosis characterized by linear reticular opacities, volume loss, traction bronchiectasis and ultimately in honeycombing of the lung. Fibrosis chiefly involves the upper and middle lobes but the lower lobes may also be involved. Computed tomography (CT) features may at times be

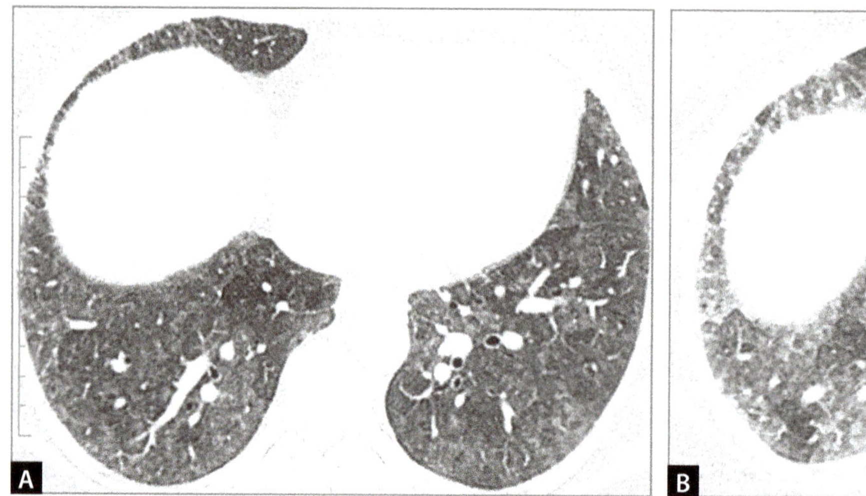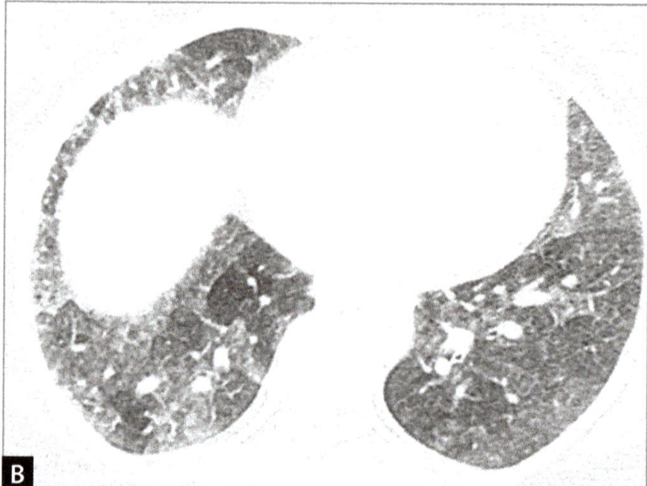

Figs. 4A and B: (A) HRCT chest demonstrates diffuse ground-glass densities in both lung fields with presence of mosaic perfusion as evidenced by areas of reduced attenuation interspersed in the areas of ground-glass density. The vasculature in these areas of reduced attenuation has small-sized vessels; (B) On the expiratory image, there is evidence of air trapping as the areas of mosaic attenuation are further accentuated.

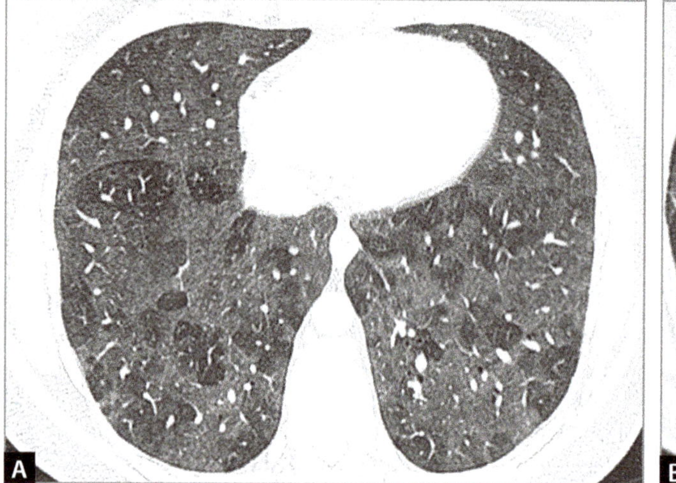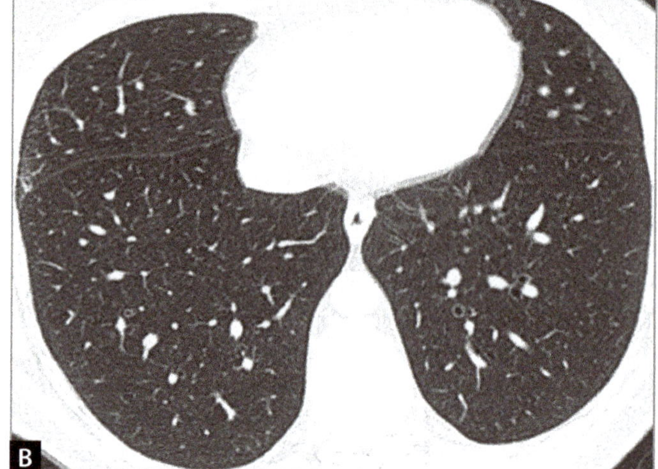

Figs. 5A and B: (A) HRCT chest reveals diffuse ground-glass densities in a middle-aged female with a history of hypersensitivity to cat hair representing hypersensitivity pneumonitis; (B) Follow-up HRCT after the cat was given away and a short course of steroids reveals clearing up of all lesions.

indistinguishable from those observed in NSIP. Greater involvement of the upper lobes and the presence of discernible centrilobular nodules help in correct differentiation.

- *Emphysema*: Recent studies in chronic farmer's lung suggest that emphysema is more frequent than fibrosis. The distribution of emphysema is more in the upper lobes, similar to that observed in smoking-related emphysema. Emphysema probably results from obstruction to the small airways due to ongoing bronchiolitis.

Bronchoalveolar Lavage Studies

Bronchoalveolar lavage fluid shows a marked increase in the T lymphocytes (50%) with CD8 predominance. This marked increase is unusual in UIP, NSIP, sarcoidosis, entities generally considered in the differential diagnosis of HP. The determination of CD4 and CD8 subsets or the CD4/CD8 ratio does not help in clinical practice as these diverge according to a number of situations, type of inhaled antigens, smoking habits and chronicity of HP. Abnormalities in BAL fluid may persist after clinical symptoms abate and have no correlation with clinical features, or lung function abnormalities.

DIAGNOSIS

There is no single diagnostic test (including lung biopsy) which clinches the definite diagnosis of HP. Diagnosis should be made taking several factors into consideration—history, exposure to an antigenic dust known to cause HP, pulmonary function tests, imaging features, particularly an HRCT of the chest and the demonstration of antigens contained in the dust, together with precipitating antibodies within the blood to these antigens.

Diagnostic criteria proposed by the Hypersensitivity Pneumonia Study Group include the following:

1. Exposure to a known antigen
2. Precipitating antibodies
3. Recurrent respiratory symptoms
4. Inspiratory crackles
5. Symptoms 4–8 hours after exposure
6. Weight loss.

The diagnostic sensitivity is believed to be 80%, with specificity also of 80%, if all six variables are present. In clinical practice one rarely encounters patients who satisfy all the above criteria. A clinical diagnosis is often necessary on lesser evidence. Imaging studies are of significant help in an overall assessment.

The two important differential diagnoses for acute HP are: (1) an acute chest infection and (2) the ODTS. The latter is a toxic syndrome related to exposure to organic dust; it is characterized by high fever, chills, but little or no dyspnea. Lung functions and chest X-ray are normal.

The differential diagnoses of chronic HP include sarcoidosis, tuberculosis, and other pathologies causing interstitial pulmonary fibrosis, notably idiopathic interstitial pneumonia.

In patients who have some degree of airways obstruction, the differential diagnosis includes chronic bronchitis and asthma. It needs to be remembered that allergies known to cause HP can also cause allergic asthma.

MANAGEMENT

The mainstay of treatment is to avoid exposure to the offending antigen. At times, particularly in poor developing countries, this may be impossibly difficult. Avoidance of exposure to the offending antigen in farmer's lung requires precautionary measures such as dust masks with filters, improved ventilation, adequately improved storage facilities, mechanization of farming processes, all of which are often beyond the reach of most farmers in poor developing countries.

As mentioned earlier, HP due to exposure to pigeon dust and pigeon droppings is largely preventable. There are religious groups in India (notably Jains) who feed large flocks of pigeons which gather at certain sites in the large cities of India. Antigen exposure in this setting can be overwhelming and if avoided completely can prevent HP and afford relief to those patients in whom HP is due to such exposure.

Removing pet birds from the home is of vital importance if an inmate is found to have HP even if precipitins of avian antigen are absent, provided there is no evidence of any other antigenic exposure. This should be followed by a thorough cleaning of the apartment as dust containing avian antigen may persist in the environment long after the birds have been removed.

A detailed occupational history and a history of a specific environmental exposure are of help in identifying possible antigens. Not uncommonly, at least in our experience no such incriminating antigen can be identified.

Corticosteroids are often used in the treatment of acute HP, though the acute episodes are known to resolve spontaneously without treatment. A placebo-controlled therapeutic trial by Kokkarinen et al. on farmer's lung showed that those treated with steroids showed significant improvement in physiological parameters, particularly in the diffusion capacity at the end of 2 months, compared to placebo-treated patients. There is however no documented improvement in long-term prognosis.

In patients with subacute disease, if antigen exposure is avoided, prednisolone is given in a dose of 0.5 mg/kg over 3–4 weeks and then gradually tapered and stopped after 4–6 months. Remission usually occurs. However, in patients with subacute progressive or chronic disease, prednisolone is given in the above dose for 4–6 weeks followed by a gradual tapering of the dose over 4–6 months till a maintenance dose of 10 mg/day is reached. In a number of cases, withdrawal of the drug can lead to relapse, particularly if the nature of the antigenic challenge remains unknown. However, once symptoms abate and lung functions are close to normal, an attempt should be made to withdraw the steroid completely.

Patients who show evidence of airways obstruction should be given the benefit of inhaled β_2-agonist and steroids. Patients with HP need a careful follow-up, both clinical and with regards to lung function tests.

Chronic HP may continue to progress to pulmonary fibrosis even if antigen exposure is absent. These patients should also be given the benefit of corticosteroid therapy. Cytotoxic therapy using azathioprine or cyclophosphamide has been added to corticosteroids in poorly controlled patients with chronic HP. Their efficacy with regard to outcome has not been proven.

■ SUGGESTED READING

1. Cormier Y, Brown M, Worthy S, et al. High-resolution computed tomographic characteristics in acute farmer's lung and in its follow-up. Eur Respir J. 2000;16:56-60.
2. Glazer CS, Rose CS, Lynch DA. Clinical and radiologic manifestations of hypersensitivity pneumonitis. J Thorac Imaging. 2002;17:261-72.
3. Hariri LP, Mino-Kenudson M, Shea B, et al. Distinct histopathology of acute onset or abrupt exacerbation of hypersensitivity pneumonitis. Hum Pathol. 2012;43: 660-8.
4. Lacasse Y, Selman M, Costabel U, et al. Clinical diagnosis of hypersensitivity pneumonitis. Am J Respir Crit Care Med. 2003;168:952-8.
5. Randhawa HS, Chowdhary A. Medical mycology in India (1957-2007): contributions by the VPCI Mycoses Group. Indian J Chest Dis Allied Sci. 2008;50:19-32.
6. Selman M. Hypersensitivity pneumonitis: a multifaceted deceiving disorder. Clin Chest Med. 2004;25(3):531-47, vi.
7. Selman M, Pardo A, King TE. Hypersensitivity pneumonitis—insights in diagnosis and pathobiology. Am J Respir Crit Care Med. 2012;186(4):314-24.
8. Singh S, Collins B, Sharma B, et al. Interstitial lung disease in India. Results of a prospective registry. Am J Respir Crit Care Med. 2017;195:801-13.
9. Solaymani-Dodaran M, West J, Smith C, et al. Extrinsic allergic alveolitis: incidence and mortality in the general population. QJM. 2007;100:233-7.
10. Spurzem JR, Romberger DJ, Von Essen SG. Agricultural lung disease. Clin Chest Med. 2002;23(4):795-810.
11. Tillie-Leblond I, Grenouillet F, Reboux G, et al. Hypersensitivity pneumonitis and metalworking fluids contaminated by mycobacteria. Eur Respir J. 2011;37: 640-7.

CHAPTER 49

Eosinophilic Pneumonia

■ INTRODUCTION

Eosinophilic pneumonia is a consolidation of a portion of the lung due to the filling of alveoli with inflammatory cells, which are predominately eosinophils. This is usually but not always accompanied by peripheral eosinophilia. In clinical practice, a diagnosis of eosinophilic pneumonia is often made in the presence of a pulmonary shadow accompanied by peripheral eosinophilia, without a tissue diagnosis. This may be incorrect for several reasons—(a) peripheral eosinophilia is very common in the tropics, chiefly due to past parasitic infection. The lung pathology may be unrelated to the peripheral eosinophilia; (b) peripheral eosinophilia has been very occasionally noted to occur in pulmonary tuberculosis, Hodgkin's disease and lung cancer.

Eosinophilic pneumonia has also been variously termed Loeffler's syndrome or pulmonary infiltration with eosinophilia (PIE) syndrome) or pulmonary eosinophilia.

■ PATHOLOGY

Gross pathologic features of the lung are similar in spite of different etiologies. The lung tissue involved appears solid, airless and grey. Microscopic examination reveals alveoli filled with eosinophils; mononuclear cells, chiefly macrophages are also present. The eosinophilic infiltration often extends to the interstitial tissue and may involve the bronchial walls. There is a perivascular inflammation noted around the vessels but no actual infiltration of the vessel wall.

■ CLASSIFICATION OF EOSINOPHILIC PNEUMONIA

A classification of eosinophilic pneumonia is given below. There is a certain degree of overlap in the conditions described in an individual patient. For example, the prevasculitic phase of eosinophilic granulomatosis with polyangiitis (EGPA) (previously called Churg-Strauss syndrome) may be difficult to distinguish from cryptogenic eosinophilic pneumonia (CEP) or from asthmatic pulmonary eosinophilia.

- *Parasitic causes* (particularly in the tropics) (*see* section on Tropical Infections Involving the Lungs)
- *Other known and unknown antigens:* These include drugs, in particular nonsteroidal inflammatory drugs, pollen, and other agents. Pulmonary infiltrates with peripheral eosinophilia have been described in patients in contact with nickel, following sensitization to ivy, rarely in brucella infections and in the early stages of the Spanish toxic oil syndrome. These conditions may or may not be associated with airways obstruction.
- Allergic bronchopulmonary aspergillosis
- Pulmonary vasculitis—Eosinophilic granulomatosis with polyangiitis (EGPA)
- Unknown causes:
    - Associated with asthma (intrinsic, extrinsic)
    - Acute eosinophilic pneumonia (AEP)
    - Cryptogenic chronic eosinophilic pneumonia or CEP.
- Hypereosinophilic syndrome.

Eosinophilic pneumonia (also called pulmonary eosinophilia) due to parasitic causes has been dealt with in the section on *Tropical Infections Involving the Lung*. Allergic bronchopulmonary aspergillosis has been considered in the section on *Airways Diseases* while EGPA has been considered in the section on *Pulmonary Vasculitis*.

This chapter will deal mainly with just five and six of the classifications described above.

ASTHMATIC PULMONARY EOSINOPHILIA

Asthmatic pulmonary eosinophilia is a rare condition and in large series in the West was found in just 0.4% of patients with asthma. It is probably related to more than one cause; there are two groups of patients—one with extrinsic asthma and the other with intrinsic asthma.

Pulmonary Eosinophilia in Extrinsic Asthma

These patients are generally atopic children often less than 10 years of age. The immunoglobulin E (IgE) levels are significantly raised and there is a close resemblance to allergic bronchopulmonary aspergillosis. However, the skin test to *Aspergillus* antigen is negative and precipitins to *Aspergillus* are absent in the peripheral blood. The condition probably arises from unidentified inhaled antigens in atopic children.

Segmental atelectasis due to mucus plugging in children with extrinsic asthma is often mistaken for eosinophilic pneumonia.

Pulmonary Eosinophilia in Intrinsic Asthma

The onset of intrinsic asthma in these patients is rapidly followed by diffuse bilateral mottling. The condition is generally observed in the third and fourth decade. There is no history of atopy and the IgE levels are normal. The peripheral eosinophilia is generally mild to moderate.

A radiological examination shows bilateral shadows more often peripherally distributed. The response to corticosteroids is dramatic. It is impossible in a given patient to distinguish the above entities from the prevasculitic phase of EGPA. The histopathology shows eosinophils filling alveoli and involving the interstitial tissue, which again is indistinguishable from the prevasculitic phase of EGPA. Upper lobe

involvement needs to be distinguished from allergic bronchopulmonary aspergillosis, in which the skin-prick test to *Aspergillus* antigen is positive.

A follow-up of these rare patients after steroids have been stopped may clarify the diagnosis.

ACUTE EOSINOPHILIC PNEUMONIA (AEP)

Acute noninfectious pneumonia characterized by alveoli filled predominantly with eosinophils and with a few macrophages has been described since 1989. The patient generally presents with a 10–30-day illness, which is characterized by fever, progressive dyspnea, mottled lung fields, again chiefly involving the peripheries. Hypoxic respiratory failure requiring ventilatory support is often present. The response to corticosteroids is excellent, the mottled shadows clearing within 1–2 weeks. Generally, there is no recurrence on withdrawal of the corticosteroids. Bronchoalveolar lavage (BAL) fluid with eosinophilia more than 25% in the absence of identifiable infectious causes is the criterion used for diagnosis.

The etiology of AEP is unknown and the pathogenesis is unclear. Both in AEP and CEP, there is the presence of significant inflammatory cytokines in the BAL fluid. For example, chemokine CCI 17 has been detected in high concentrations in BAL fluid both in AEP and CEP. This is consistent with the role of T cells in the pathogenesis of AEP. There are also an array of Th2 and Th1 cytokines in the BAL, in particular many interleukins, reflecting the secretary potential of eosinophils. Elevated levels in particular of the cytokine IL-5 in BAL fluid is the key factor responsible for differentiation, migration, and survival of eosinophils in AEP. Vascular endothelial growth factor is present in BAL fluid; it promotes vascular permeability and perhaps contributes to the pathophysiology of the disease. Eosinophils are known to produce cationic proteins and inflammatory lipid mediators both of which can be detected in the blood of patients with AEP.

Though no fungal infection has been shown to cause AEP, it is of interest that high concentrations of beta glucan have been found in the BAL fluid.

Finally, there is a strong association between cigarette smoking, in particular cigarette smoking of recent onset and AEP. Secondhand smoke exposure and smoking of flavored cigars have also been associated with AEP.

CRYPTOGENIC CHRONIC EOSINOPHILIC PNEUMONIA (CEP)

This entity was first described by Carrington and his associates. It is characterized by eosinophilic pulmonary infiltrates generally involving both lungs, with peripheral eosinophilia. Asthma may be associated but not always so. Subsequently, the same entity was described by Turner-Warwick (who used the term cryptogenic eosinophilic pneumonia) as also by Pearson and Rosenov.

Cryptogenic eosinophilic pneumonia is more common in women, generally occurring in the third decade. The clinical picture has the features of a systemic illness with fever, weight loss, night sweats, and anemia together with respiratory symptoms of cough and breathlessness. In addition to peripheral eosinophilia, there is often a polymorphonuclear leukoytosis, an erythrocyte sedimentation rate (ESR) which is often as high as 100 mm/hour and a raised C-reactive protein. The IgE may be just slightly raised, quite disproportionate to the degree of peripheral eosinophilia present. Rarely, pulmonary eosinophilia may not be associated with peripheral eosinophilia. This renders diagnosis doubly difficult.

The radiograph of the chest shows bilateral shadows generally peripherally placed and this distribution should arouse suspicion as to the nature of the lesion. This is termed the photographic negative of pulmonary edema. Lack of this pattern does not however exclude CEP. CT of the chest shows patchy airspace consolidation generally with a peripheral distribution. Pleural effusions are a rare manifestation. Lung functions show a restrictive pattern or features of both obstruction and restriction (**Figs. 1A and B**).

The etiology and pathogenesis are unknown. As in AEP, numerous inflammatory cytokines have been identified in the BAL fluid of CEP. Eosinophils in CEP secrete increased eosinophilic cationic protein and major basic protein. Eosinophil-derived neurotoxin has been observed in the urine of patients with CEP. T-cells probably play an active role in the pathogenesis, there being an increase in the number of activated T4 cells in the alveoli. How all these factors interact in the pathophysiology of this condition is not known.

Diagnosis is best proven by a video-assisted thoracoscopic biopsy which reveals typical eosinophilic consolidation of alveoli.

Examination of BAL fluid obtained through a bronchoscope shows numerous eosinophils, the eosinophil count in the BAL fluid exceeding 40% in more than 80% of patients. Video-assisted thoracoscopic biopsy is not necessary for diagnosis if the BAL fluid has eosinophilia more than 40%. The main differential diagnosis is from EGPA (Churg-Strauss syndrome).

Treatment is with corticosteroids 0.5–1 mg/kg. There is dramatic improvement starting within a few days and being complete with regard to symptoms, pulmonary infiltrates, and peripheral eosinophilia within about

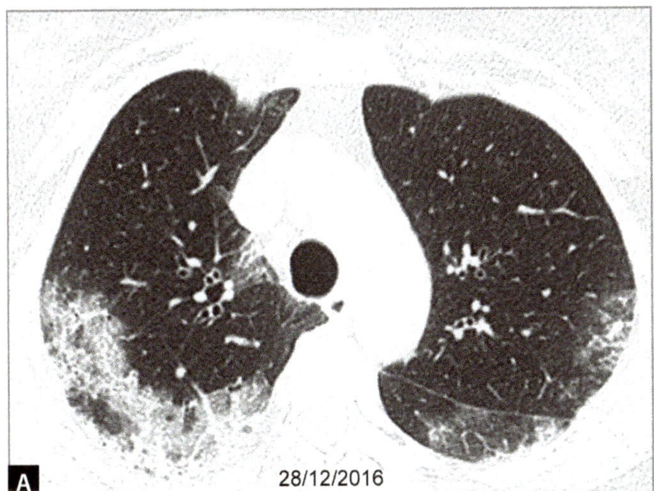

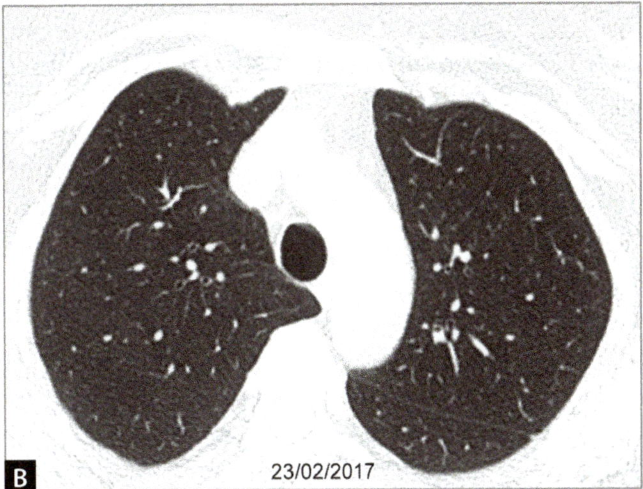

Figs. 1A and B: High-resolution computed tomography (HRCT) chest demonstrates ill-defi ned peripheral subpleural groundglass densities. Patient presented with low-grade fever, cough and well-marked peripheral eosinophilia. A video-assisted thoracoscopic biopsy revealed eosinophlic pneumonia. Good response to corticosteroid theapy.

2 weeks. However, after steroid withdrawal, there is a tendency for the eosinophilic pulmonary infiltrates to return, often at the same sites within the lungs as where they first appeared. A maintenance dose of corticosteroids is preferably given for a year. Even then, the disease may recur several months after stoppage of corticosteroids.

THE ROLE OF THE EOSINOPHILS IN EOSINOPHILIC PNEUMONIA

The role of eosinophils in eosinophilic pneumonia continues to be a subject of research. Type I IgE-mediated responses probably initiate the eosinophilic syndrome. Mast cells release an eosinophilic chemotactic factor which attracts eosinophils to the site of reaction. IgE levels in blood generally mirror the degree of disease activity though IgE levels in chronic CEP are not significantly elevated.

Eosinophils have a protective function and yet can also cause tissue damage. Their protective function is conceivably related to the presence of lysosomal enzymes which include sulfatase, arylsulfatase, glucoronidase, and histamine. These enzymes help to neutralize products secreted by the mast cells. Their protective action extends to attenuating type I regain-mediated hypersensitivity reactions. Eosinophils can phagocytose immune complexes, and mast cell granules. In pulmonary eosinophilia due to parasitic infection, the eosinophil is a warrior of distinction, particularly in pulmonary eosinophilia associated with filarial infection. The microfilaria trapped in the lungs are destroyed chiefly through the action of eosinophils which secrete certain proteins such as major basic protein, eosinophilic cationic protein, each of which is toxic to parasites within the lung. Yet these very secretory products are also toxic to normal lung tissue—to alveolar cells, bronchial epithelium and to the vascular endothelium. Tissue damage, therefore results.

HYPEREOSINOPHILIC SYNDROME

This is a multisystem disorder involving the heart, the lungs, the central and peripheral nervous system, other organs and is associated with a very high peripheral eosinophilia. Eosinophilia is marked, with mean eosinophil levels of 20×10^9/L going as high as $160–200 \times 10^9$/L. The eosinophils in the peripheral smear show increased vacuolation and degradation.

Clinically, this syndrome is characterized by systemic features of fever, weight loss, anorexia, and hepatosplenomegaly. The cardiovascular system is involved in the majority of patients. Involvement takes the form of arrhythmias, heart failure, thrombosis within the cardiac chambers with thromboembolic episodes, and finally to gross subendocardial fibrosis which causes mitral cum tricuspid incompetence and resultant recalcitrant congestive heart failure.

Respiratory involvement is characterized by cough, focal infiltrate or diffuse lung consolidation and eosinophilic pleural effusions. Generally, asthma is not a feature of the disease.

Central nervous system (CNS) involvement takes the form of focal lesions in the brain, either caused by focal arteritis or thromboembolic episodes. Peripheral neuropathy, in particular mononeuritis multiplex, may be observed.

Other features include skin rashes, abdominal pain, proteinuria, hypertension, muscle weakness and polyarthropathy.

Thromboembolic episodes punctuate the natural history of the disease. Bone marrow examination shows massive eosinophilic infiltration, with masses of eosinophils in all stages of maturity. The serum IgE level may be raised but not unduly so.

Diagnosis

Diagnosis is based on the clinical features of multisystem involvement, together with marked peripheral eosinophilia for which there is no obvious cause. When the main brunt of the disease is on the lungs causing well-marked eosinophilic pneumonia, the differential diagnosis is from EGPA. The latter is hardly ever associated with the degree of peripheral eosinophilia seen in the hypereosinophilic syndrome. Also, EGPA in its fully evolved form is characterized by a significant degree of vasculitis.

Treatment

Prednisolone often produces a remission, especially in the presence of pulmonary eosinophilia, heart failure and raised serum IgE level. Hydroxyurea and vincristine have been reported to be of help. Plasmapheresis has been used but with indeterminate results. Immunomodulatory drugs such as imatinib are often used. A recent placebo-controlled trial has shown that specifically targeting eosinophils with a monoclonal antibody against IL-5 is useful as adjunct therapy for the hypereosinophilic syndrome. The presence of marked mitral and tricuspid incompetence causing heart failure may prompt valve replacement surgery.

Remissions are associated with relief of symptoms and with a fall in the peripheral eosinophilia. Nevertheless, the disease has a high morbidity and mortality.

■ SUGGESTED READING

1. Akuthotaa P, Weller PF. Eosinophilic pneumonias. Clin Microbiol Rev. 2012;25:649-60.
2. Guillevin L, Cohen P, Gayraud M, et al. Churg-Strauss syndrome. Clinical study and long-term follow-up of 96 patients. Medicine (Baltimore). 1999;78:26-37.
3. Janz DR. Acute eosinophilic pneumonia: a case report and review of the literature. Crit Care Med. 2009;37(4): 1470-4.
4. Keogh KA, Specks U. Churg-Strauss syndrome. Semin Respir Crit Care Med. 2006;27:148-57.
5. Roufosse F, Goldman M, Cogan E. Hypereosinophilic syndrome: lymphoproliferative and myeloproliferative variants. Semin Respir Crit Care Med. 2006;27:158-70.
6. Savani DM. Eosinophilic lung disease in the tropics. Clin Chest Med. 2002;23(2):377-96.
7. Udwadia FE. Eosinophilic lung disease and tropical pulmonary eosinophilia. In: Munjal YP (Ed). API Textbook of Medicine, 8th edition. New Delhi: Jaypee Brothers Medical Publishers; 2008. pp. 390-3.
8. Udwadia FE. Tropical eosinophilia: a review? Respir Med. 1993;87:17-21.
9. Uptodate. (2017). Chronic eosinophilic pneumonia. [online] Available from https://www.uptodate.com/contents/ chronic-eosinophilic-pneumonia/print [Accessed July 2018].
10. Wechsler ME. Pulmonary eosinophilic syndromes. Immunol Allergy Clin North Am. 2007;27(3):477-92.

Pulmonary Vascular Disorders

CHAPTER 50

Pulmonary Vasculitis

■ INTRODUCTION

Pulmonary vasculitis is characterized pathologically by destruction of the blood vessel wall, cellular inflammation and tissue necrosis. The pulmonary vessels may be involved as part of a systemic vasculitis or primarily affected as the sole site of involvement. Thus, vasculitis may be classified as primary idiopathic, primary immune complex-mediated, and secondary vasculitis. Primary vasculitides are of unknown etiology. They form a heterogeneous group with overlapping features; they, however, share one important feature, in that all respond to immunosuppressive agents. Primary vasculitides are further classified by the size of the vessels involved, the nature of the inflammatory infiltrate and the predominant location of the affected vessels.

The classification and terminology of primary vasculitides was recently updated at the 2012 Chapel Hill International Consensus Conference. This classification is given in **Table 1**. We have also included in this Box the term secondary vasculitides. These vasculitides are secondary to an underlying systemic disorder—for example, systemic lupus erythematosus (SLE). Secondary vasculitides may also be a histopathological feature of severe infection of the lungs or the side effects of some drugs.

The small-vessel vasculitides, which present most commonly with respiratory symptoms, are granulomatosis with polyangiitis (GPA)—formerly termed Wegener's granulomatosis (WG), eosinophilic granulomatosis with polyangiitis (EGPA)—formerly termed Churg-Strauss syndrome (CSS), and microscopic polyangiitis (MPA). This group of small vasculitides include patients who most often have antineutrophilic cytoplasmic antibodies (ANCA) are therefore often referred to as ANCA-associated

Table 1: Classification of vasculitis.

Classification:
- *Primary idiopathic vasculitis*:
  - *Small vessel*:
    - Granulomatosis with polyangiitis
    - Eosinophilic granulomatosis with polyangiitis
    - Microscopic polyarteritis
    - Idiopathic pauci-immune rapidly progressive glomerulo-nephritis
    - Isolated pauci-immune pulmonary capillaritis
  - *Medium vessel*:
    - Polyarteritis nodosa
    - Kawasaki disease
  - *Large vessel*:
    - Giant cell arteritis
    - Takayasu's arteritis
- *Primary immune complex-mediated vasculitis*:
  - Goodpasture's syndrome
  - Henoch-Schonlein purpura
  - Behcet's disease
  - IgA nephropathy
- *Secondary vasculitis*:
  - *Autoimmune disease*: SLE, RA, polymyositis, scleroderma
  - *Miscellaneous*: Infections in the lung, drugs (propylthiouracil, diphenylhydantoin)

(Ig: Immunoglobulin; RA: Rheumatoid arthritis; SLE: Systemic lupus erythematosus)

vasculitides. ANCA are of two kinds—(1) c-ANCA and (2) p-ANCA. c-ANCA are antibodies directed to the cytoplasm of the neutrophils; they react with neutrophil granule enzyme proteinase 3 (PR-3 ANCA). They cause a cytoplasmic immunofluorescence on ethanol fixed neutrophils. In contrast, p-ANCA cause a perinuclear immunofluorescence on ethanol fixed neutrophils and react with myeloperoxidase (MPO-ANCA). Most patients with GPA are positive for the c-ANCA, while many patients with EGPA and MPA are positive for the p-ANCA, i.e.

MPO-ANCA. Interestingly none of these three primary small vasculitides have immunoglobulin deposits in tissue lesions, in striking contrast to the group of vasculitides classified as immune–complex small-vessels vasculitides.

The pathophysiology, clinical features, diagnosis and the management of the three ANCA-associated vasculitides is given below.

ANCA-ASSOCIATED VASCULITIDES

Granulomatosis with Polyangiitis (formerly Wegener's Granulomatosis)

GPA is the prototype of an ANCA-positive vasculitis. It was first described by Friedrich Wegener, a young German pathologist in 1936. It was not till 1985 that the link between GPA and ANCA was established and only in 1990 that the antigen responsible was identified as PR3, a 29 kd serine proteinase called proteinase 3. GPA was considered a uniformly progressive fatal disease in 1955 when Churg reviewed the available data. It was only in 1973 when Fauci treated 18 GPA patients with steroids and cyclophosphamide that it was realized that sustained remissions could be achieved in this disease once thought uniformly fatal.

GPA is characterized by a triad of findings; necrotizing granulomatous inflammation of the upper and/or lower respiratory tract, generalized focal necrotizing vasculitis of the lungs and other organs, and focal necrotizing glomerulonephritis. All findings may not be apparent at the time of diagnosis although up to 90% of patients will ultimately manifest renal disease.

The initial clinical features vary from the mild and nonspecific (fever, arthralgia, myalgia, and malaise) to the dramatic (massive hemoptysis) depending on the site of involvement. The American College of Rheumatology (ACR) criteria for diagnosis of GPA include—nasal or oral inflammation, abnormal chest radiographs, abnormal urine sediment, and granulomatous inflammation on biopsy. If biopsy is not available, hemoptysis can be substituted as the fourth criterion. This definition has a diagnostic sensitivity of 88% and specificity of 92%. Before discussing important organ-specific manifestations of GPA, the pathophysiology of all ANCA-associated vasculitides is given below.

Pathophysiology of ANCA-associated Vasculitis

The etiology of ANCA-associated vasculitides is unknown and various views have been put forth with regard to the pathophysiology. This pathophysiology is common to all three ANCA associated vasculitides—GPA, EGPA, and MPA. A brief and basic description of what little that is known is given below:

- It is believed that genetic predisposition to autoimmunity coupled with environmental triggers, in particular infection, play a role in the development of ANCA vasculitis in predisposed patients.
- A study of genetic factors suggests that GPA and MPA are genetically distinct. PR3-ANCA-positive patients, for example, show a strong association with HLA-DP, the serpin A gene (SERPENAI), which codes for the α-1 antitrypsin, the major inhibitor of PR3 and with the PRTN3 gene, which encodes PR3. In patients who are positive for MPO-ANCA only an association with HLA-DQ has been found. Whether these genes influence the disease process, how and to what extent they do so is a subject for research.
- Clinical observations suggest that the presence or absence of ANCA and the specific type of ANCA (PR3 or MPO) determine the disease phenotype. To give just a few examples, patients with "limited" or "less severe" disease and a negative ANCA do not generally develop systemic vasculitis and patients who are PR3-ANCA-positive have more relapses than those who are MPO-ANCA positive.
- Most importantly, ANCA is not just a diagnostic test or tool. Both PR3 and MPO-ANCA have strong proinflammatory effects chiefly on neutrophils but also on monocytes and endothelial cells, initiating, enhancing, and perpetuating endothelial cell and tissue damage.

Many *in vitro* studies suggest that ANCA increases the adhesion of neutrophils to the endothelial cells. ANCA then activates primed neutrophils resulting in release of oxygen radicals and proteolytic enzymes, which damage endothelial cells. It is likely that ANCA may also directly exert a cytotoxic effect on endothelial cells.

- Finally the crucial question: What are the factors responsible not only for ANCA production but also its perpetuation? We do not know with any degree of certainty. It is hypothesized that infection may be responsible for ANCA in genetically predisposed individuals. It is a fact that many patients with ANCA-associated vasculitis relate a relapse or recurrence of their disease to a preceding infection.

The ANCA directed against a variety of infections—viral, fungal, bacterial, and protozoal has been observed. The

ANCA are shown to disappear when these infections are successfully treated. It is suggested that the persistence of ANCA in patients with vasculitis is related to molecular mimicry in susceptible hosts. This supports the theory that *Staphylococcus aureus* infection is a contributory factor to the development of vasculitis. Antigens produced by *S. aureus* induce potent B- and T-cell activity, initiating and maintaining ANCA production and cytokine release, thereby causing a cascading effect that results in granulomatous inflammation and vasculitis.

Clinical Features

The important specific manifestations of GPA are now discussed.

Upper airway and lung: The lung is the most commonly affected organ. There is evidence of lung involvement in more than 80% of patients with GPA at some stage of their disease. Indeed, 90% of patients with GPA will first seek medical attention for pulmonary or upper airway involvement. While lung involvement is part of multisystem involvement in most patients, the lung may be the only organ affected in 10% of patients.

Limited GPA: The current concept of limited GPA needs to be mentioned. It signifies that (1) granulomatosis is the main pathological feature, the vasculitis being of much lesser significance; (2) there is no immediate risk to life nor irreversible damage to an affected organ. In this context the term "limited" should be changed to "nonsevere", in contrast to "severe" GPA, which poses a risk to life and significant damage to an affected organ. For example, GPA may be limited to the CNS or limited to the kidneys and yet can be "severe" enough to be a danger to life and cause significant damage to the organ concerned.

Spectrum of respiratory system involvement in GPA: Every part of the respiratory system may be affected:

- *Involvement of the nose, sinuses, ear, and throat*: Nasal involvement is characterized by congestion, crusting, epistaxis due to mucosal friability and ulceration. Chronic recurrent sinusitis and otitis media leading to deafness are other presenting features. A saddle nose deformity and perforation of the septum can occur from ischemia to the nasal cartilage. Oral manifestations include oropharyngeal ulceration and gingival hyperplasia.
- *Tracheobronchial*: Subglottic stenosis may be the presenting symptom of GPA and the patient may present with dyspnea and stridor, which may initially be misdiagnosed as asthma. The subglottic area is the most common site of tracheobronchial involvement as it is a watershed area of the microcirculation. Bronchial stenosis and endobronchial granulomatous occluding lesions are also described. Subglottic stenosis is reported to occur in 16–23% of patients with GPA. It has been reported to occur more commonly in females than males and the median age at diagnosis is 26 years. Patients with GPA who develop subglottic stenosis tend to have more sinus involvement and saddle-nose deformity and less pulmonary involvement than other GPA patients. Subglottic stenosis can present and progress in the absence of any other systemic involvement. Thus in any patient with subglottic stenosis an ANCA test should be mandatory. In a series of patients with GPA and subglottic stenosis, only 57% initially showed a positive ANCA. Interestingly, 85% of the cohort became positive at a later date emphasizing the need to perform serial ANCAs, if there is diagnostic uncertainty. A spirometry will show characteristic, box-like flattening of the flow–volume loop in the inspiratory and expiratory portions, and dynamic computed tomography (CT) with tracheal reconstruction may outline the extent of the stenosis. A laryngoscopic examination is the definitive procedure needed to document the subglottic stenosis and grade the severity of circumferential narrowing by the Cotton-Myer classification. Biopsies of the subglottic stenosis are usually not sensitive for the diagnosis of GPA with only 10% of subglottic biopsies revealing changes consistent with GPA. In contrast, nasal biopsies on a similar cohort of patients yield a positive biopsy in 80% of patients.
- *Pulmonary involvement*: Symptoms from pulmonary involvement include cough, dyspnea, chest pain, and hemoptysis. A variety of radiological abnormalities have been described including infiltrates, nodules, infiltrates with cavitation, and nodules with cavitation. The nodules are rounded, range in size from a few millimeters to several centimeters and are commonly bilateral. Overall, 50% of nodules will cavitate. Solitary nodules may be the presenting feature in some patients. The most common form of pulmonary involvement in GPA is the radiological presence of nodules, which may vary from a small to large "mass lesions" that often cavitate. These cavitating lesions may have an air-fluid level. The pathological basis of these lesions is a necrotizing granulomatosis. They

may be well-nigh silent, or cause symptoms when they are in large numbers. The most common symptoms are persistent cough and breathlessness on exertion. Fleeting shadows appearing and disappearing within short periods of time are another important feature of this disease.

Another important radiographic pattern is alveolar filling shadows secondary to alveolar hemorrhage. Unusual appearances include lymphadenopathy, consolidation, and large pleural effusions. Chest CT may pick up more than radiography and frequently reveals nodules and ground-glass opacification not apparent on chest radiography.

Diffuse alveolar hemorrhage (DAH) is another distinctive, potentially life-threatening manifestation of GPA and can on occasions (10%) be a presenting feature. It occurs with an incidence of 7–45% in GPA and 10–30% in MPA. It is rare in EGPA, though it has been reported. It is a major cause of morbidity and mortality in vasculitis with the acute mortality from vasculitis and DAH being six times that of vasculitis alone. DAH is recognized by the diagnostic triad of anemia, hemoptysis, and pulmonary infiltrates. The hemoptysis may be massive and exsanguinating. On the other hand, one-third of patients with DAH may not report significant hemoptysis but may have alveolar hemorrhage. This group is more difficult to diagnose and a sudden drop in hemoglobin accompanied by alveolar filling shadows should alert the physician to possible DAH even in the absence of overt hemoptysis. An increase in the corrected transfer factor (KCO), due to increased Hb-CO binding, to more than 30% above baseline may be another clue. Diagnosis of DAH is often made by fiberoptic bronchoscopy, which demonstrates diffuse bleeding throughout the bronchial tree. Hemosiderin-laden macrophages can be stained by Prussian blue stain and are often of diagnostic value. Transbronchial or open lung biopsy is rarely required and often not possible in these very sick and hypoxic patients. If performed they reveal pauci-immune hemorrhagic necrotizing alveolar capillaritis without evidence of granulomatous inflammation.

- *Pleural*: Pleural effusions are not common but have been reported in GPA. They are more common in EGPA when they may be rich in eosinophils.
- *Pulmonary artery*: Pulmonary vessel involvement in GPA chiefly involves the small and medium-sized vessels but pulmonary hypertension has been reported

in scattered case reports, presumably secondary to larger vessel involvement.

Renal: Renal involvement takes the form of glomerulonephritis. It may be silent and become only evident when it culminates in severe renal failure. Clinical manifestations include—(1) asymptomatic hematuria, which may remit and relapse with normal renal functions. The diagnosis of ANCA-related vasculitis may be delayed in favor of IgA nephropathy in these patients; (2) a progressive rise in serum creatinine over days or weeks with urine showing albumin, red blood cells (RBCs), casts; (3) very rapidly rising creatinine, hematuria, hypertension, edema—a result of necrotizing vasculitis—a medical emergency; (4) proteinuria, which is generally subnephrotic less than 3 g/day, but rarely exceeds 3 g/day; (5) rapidly progressive glomerulonephritis. It is noteworthy that some patients with GPA may present with glomerulonephritis as the sole feature of the disease.

Other systems:

- *Skin involvement* is frequent and takes the form of vasculitic necrotic ulcers, nodules, and palpable purpura.
- *Ocular involvement* is observed in one or more parts of the eye and may threaten vision. They include conjunctivitis, keratitis, episcleritis, scleritis, retinal vasculitis, and retro-orbital inflammatory pseudotumors affecting one or both eyes. The pseudotumor causes proptosis, double vision, field defects, and can sharply impair visual acuity.
- *Neurological involvement* may occur as mononeuritis multiplex due to inflammation of the vasa vasorum. Central nervous system (CNS) involvement takes the form of vasculitis and pachymeningitis and may lead to irreversible damage and impaired function.
- Other systems that can be involved include the heart (regional wall motion abnormalities on Echo) and the gastrointestinal (GI) tract. *Almost any and every organ has been reported to be involved in GPA.*

Occasionally, GPA may present with a pyrexia of unknown origin (PUO). The erythrocyte sedimentation rate (ESR) is invariably raised in these patients.

Diagnosis of GPA (Figs. 1 to 6)

- Routine tests include complete blood count (CBC), ESR, urine analysis (proper microscopy, not dipstick), creatinine, other antibodies like ANA and

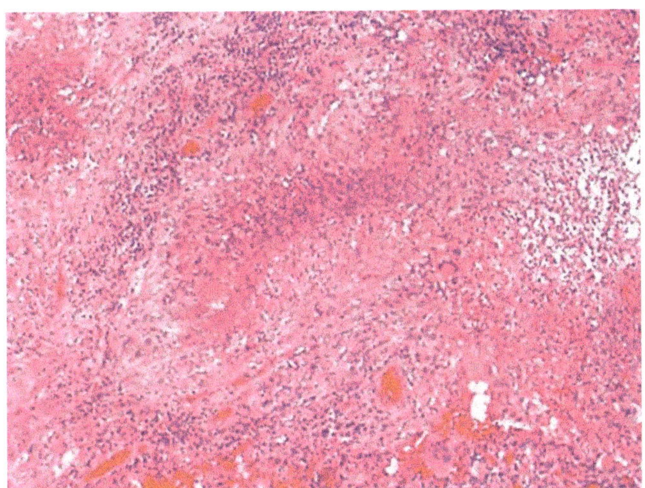

Fig. 1: Granulomatosis with polyangiitis involving the lungs. Necrotizing granulomas, the central necrosis contains amorphous pink material, nuclear debris and inflammatory cells and is surrounded by palisaded histiocytes and giant cells. Cytoplasmic antineutrophil cytoplasmic antibodies (c-ANCA) done prior to the biopsy was strongly positive.

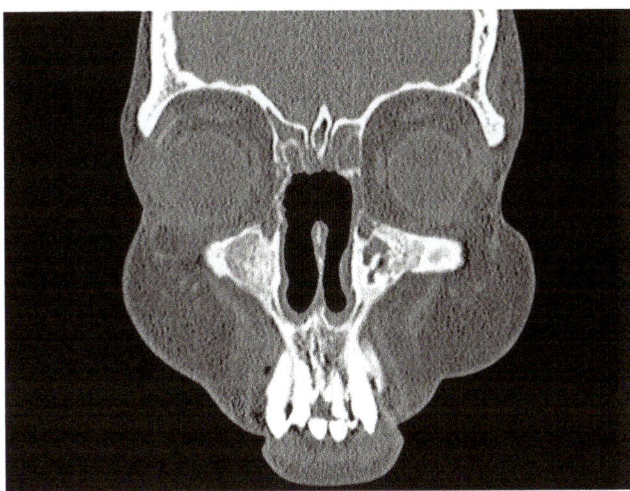

Fig. 3: Wegener's granulomatosis. Paranasal sinuses (PNS) CT demonstrates considerable thickening of the wall of paranasal sinuses with marked sclerosis and irregularity. Note the destruction of the nasal septum, medial walls of the maxillary sinuses and the turbinates.

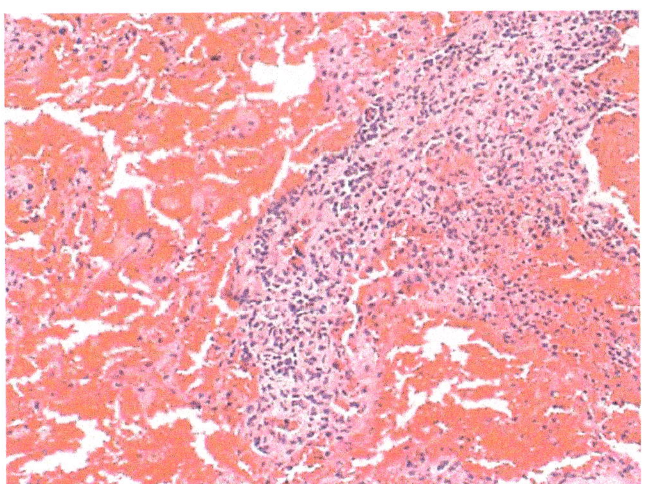

Fig. 2: Granulomatosis with polyangiitis. Intra-alveolar hemorrhage with marked perivascular inflammatory infiltrate.

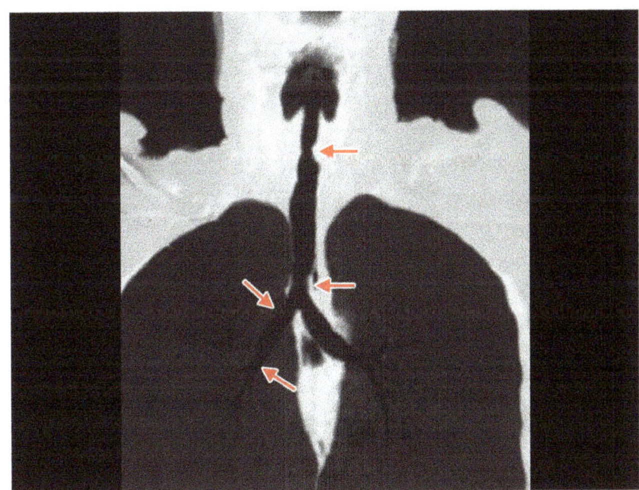

Fig. 4: Subglottic stenosis. 3D computed tomography (CT) using maximum intensity projection (MIP) of tracheobronchial tree demonstrates multifocal strictures in trachea—subglottic region, distal trachea, proximal right bronchus, and distal right bronchus.

anti-glomerular basement membrane (GBM) antibody **(Table 2)**.

- *ANCA*: A positive ANCA is highly sensitive and specific for GPA. c-ANCA is positive in about 90% of patients with active generalized GPA and in 40–60% of those with "limited" or "less severe" GPA. A p-ANCA is positive in less than 10% of patients with GPA but in the majority of patients with MPA and EGPA.

Specificity is, however, not absolute and a weakly positive c-ANCA may be found in tuberculosis (TB), HIV, infective endocarditis, and monoclonal gammopathy of unknown significance (MGUS). Hence, a positive ANCA supports the diagnosis of GPA, but is not a replacement for tissue diagnosis. We have seen inappropriate administration of powerful cytotoxics to patients with suspected GPA based on a positive ANCA with disastrous

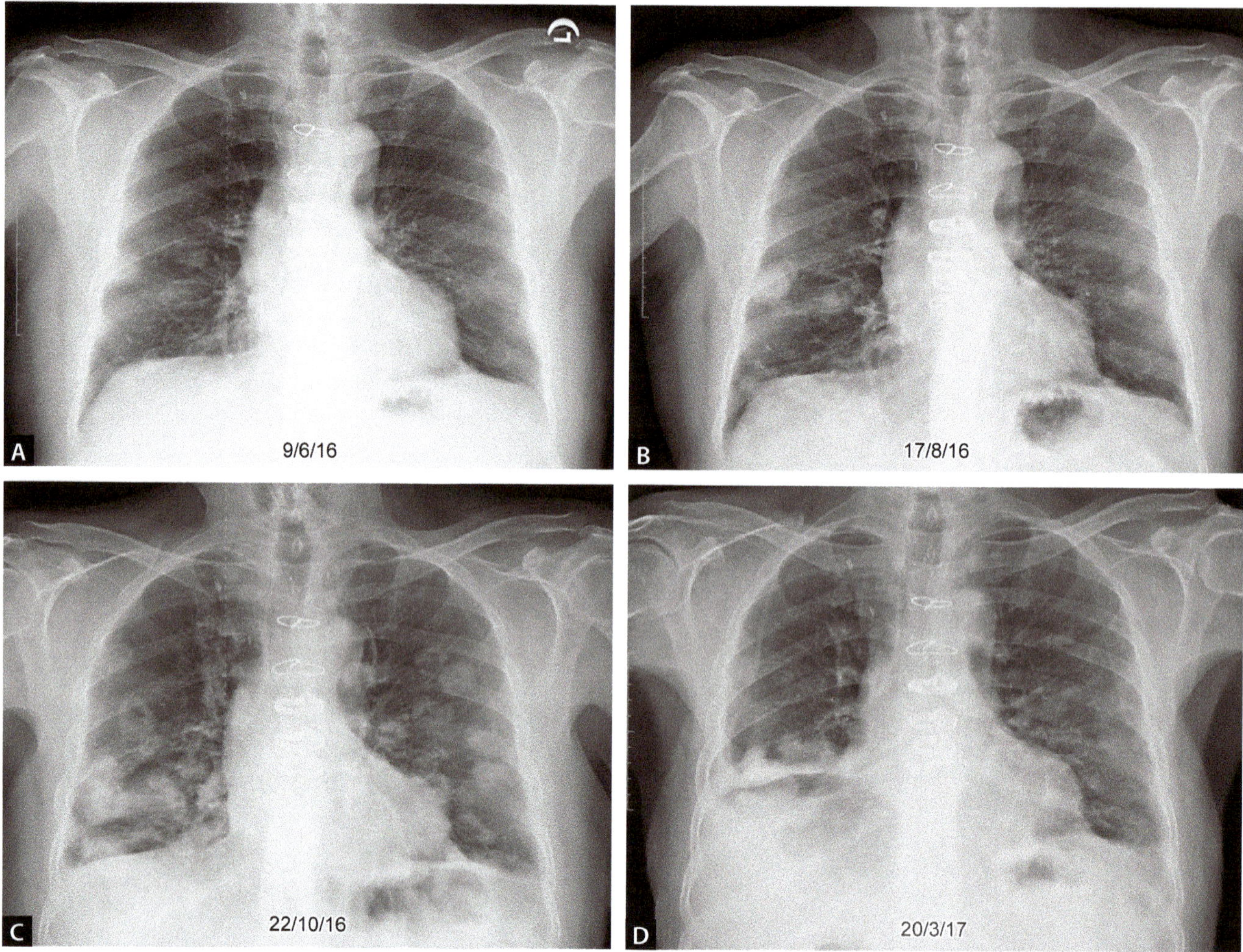

Figs. 5A to D: Wegener's granulomatosis in a 66-year-old male patient who presented with hemoptysis and systemic features of weight loss, fever and anemia. Serial chest X-rays showed cavitation and consolidation, more importantly, changing area of consolidation and changing cavities (A) done on 9/06/2016 revealed pleural based nodular opacity in the right mid zone; (B) done on 17/08/2016 revealed multiple thick walled cavitating lesions in both mid and lower zones; (C) done on 22/10/2016 revealed multiple circular opacities in both mid and lower zones, few of them showed necrotic centers; (D) done on 20/3/2017 revealed almost complete resolution of the previously seen lesions and a pleural effusion on the right side. This is typical feature of Wegener's granulomatosis where the lesions appear and disappear or change in size spontaneously.

consequences, as the ANCA was falsely positive due to TB.

Much interest has also focused in recent years on the role of ANCA in diagnosing relapses of GPA. This disease remits with appropriate treatment but relapses are common. There is evidence that changing ANCA titers can mirror these relapses. A meta-analysis by Cohen showed that 81 of 157 relapses were preceded by a rise in ANCA titer. Overall, this meta-analysis showed that a rising ANCA titer had a sensitivity of 85% and specificity of 52% in diagnosing relapses. The pragmatic conclusion that can be reached from this is that while a rising ANCA titer may herald a flare and justify heightened vigilance, it cannot be the sole basis for acceleration of therapy.

- *Biopsy*: A biopsy is usually needed to confirm the clinical suspicion of vasculitis. Tissue must be obtained from an involved but accessible organ or site. Lung, upper-airway lesions, skin, and kidney are all potential biopsy sites. Biopsy yield is best from the lung (>90%). A firm diagnosis can rarely be made from a transbronchial biopsy or a CT-guided biopsy of a lung lesion. An open lung or video-assisted thoracoscopic surgery (VATS) biopsy is usually needed to make a definitive diagnosis. Biopsy should show the distinctive

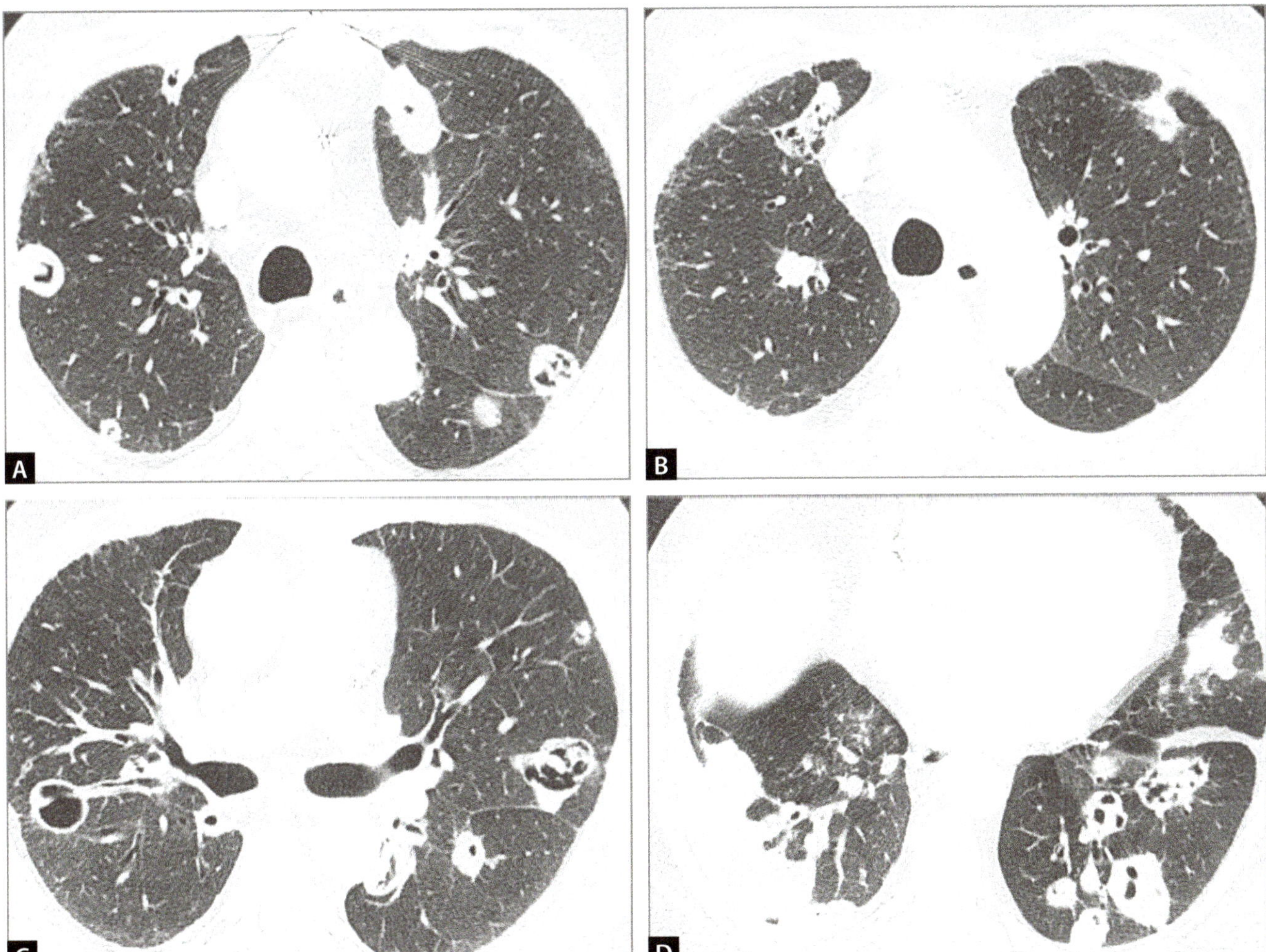

Figs. 6A to D: Wegener's granulomatosis: High-resolution computed tomography (HRCT) chest done for the same patient on 28/12/16 reveals multiple, variably sized, cavitating lesions with associated thick, irregular walls seen widely distributed in both lung fields. There are ill-defined conglomerating consolidations seen in right lung base.

Table 2: Diagnosis of GPA.
• CBC, urine analysis, creatinine
• ANA and anti-GBM antibody
• ANCA—p-ANCA and c-ANCA
• Biopsy—tissue biopsy from skin, lung, kidney, upper airway open lung or VATS biopsy for a definitive diagnosis

(ANA: Antinuclear antibodies; ANCA: Antineutrophil cytoplasmic antibodies; c: Cytoplasmic; CBC: Complete blood count; GBM: Glomerular basement membrane; VATS: Video-assisted thoracoscopic surgery)

triad of—necrotizing granulomatous inflammation, necrotizing vasculitis, and microabscesses. This is not always realized. Depending on the site of disease that is biopsied, some biopsies may show only granulomatous inflammation, or only a vasculitis. Biopsy findings should be considered in relation to the overall clinical picture and results of the ANCA test. Biopsy specimens are always stained and at times cultured to exclude infective etiologies.

Subglottic stenosis, airway lesions, and skin have a low yield, while sinus and nasal mucosa have a higher yield. Percutaneous renal biopsy may be indicated, if glomerulonephritis is suspected, though kidney biopsy is seldom diagnostic.

• A bronchoalveolar lavage (BAL) study is important when there is a suspicion of intra-alveolar hemorrhage in the absence of hemoptysis. Bronchoscopy reveals diffuse bleeding within the lung and BAL reveals the presence of macrophages, staining positive for iron.

Treatment (Table 3)

Treatment consists of:
- Induction of remission
- Maintenance of remission
- Prevention of relapse
  - All of which should be undertaken with:
    - Minimal morbidity and mortality either from the disease itself or the therapy.

Modern treatment has transformed GPA from a near uniformly fatal rapidly progressive disease to a chronic relapsing one with a 5-year survival of around 80%. This has, however, come at the cost of significant treatment-related morbidity.

The principles of therapy are:
- Induction phase to achieve remission
- Maintenance phase, where treatment is carefully deescalated
- Assessment of disease activity with dose titration
- Careful monitoring for drug toxicity
- Monitoring for opportunistic infections
- Add-on therapies in failures.

Induction phase: For active, severe, generalized disease, steroid and cyclophosphamide remain the gold standard.

Table 3: Management of GPA.

Induction of remission:
- Oral prednisolone can be used in a dose of 1 mg/kg + cyclophosphamide in a dose of 2 mg/kg daily
- IV cyclophosphamide
- IV rituximab (see text)

Maintenance therapy:
- Azathioprine, methotrexate, mycophenolate mofetil, cyclosporine and trimethoprim/sulfamethoxazole

Monitor for toxicity:
- Monitor for opportunistic infections like tuberculosis or PCP

Treatment of patients refractory to treatment:
- Rituximab

Management of special situations:
- Mild indolent disease localized to the upper and or lower airways, trimethoprim/sulfamethoxazole—150/180 mg twice daily

Limited GPA or patients with early generalized disease:
- Methotrexate 20–25 mg/week

Rapidly progressive fulminant disease—methylprednisolone in doses up to 1 g/day for 3 days

Subglottic stenosis—intralesional steroids plus endoscopic dilatation or cold knife lysis. Laser therapy, airway stents, and surgical procedures like laryngotracheal reconstruction and tracheostomy

(PCP: *Pneumocystis jirovecii* pneumonia GPA: Granulomatosis with polyangiitis)

Oral prednisolone can be used in a dose of 1 mg/kg not exceeding 80 mg/day and cyclophosphamide in a dose of 2 mg/kg daily. Intravenous (IV) pulse therapy with cyclophosphamide consisting of three pulses of 15 mg/kg given 2 weeks apart, followed by 15 mg/kg pulses every 3 weeks for 6 months is equally effective in inducing remission. A steroid plus cyclophosphamide regimen will achieve remission in 90% of patients. In recent years, rituximab has also been used to induce remission in severe ANCA-associated vasculitis. It is administered as an IV infusion in four weekly doses of 375 mg/m^2 of body surface. Studies have shown that the above course of rituximab has the same efficacy as cyclophosphamide, and is equivalent to the daily oral therapy with cyclophosphamide followed by azathioprine for 18 months.

Special situations:
- In patients with mild indolent disease localized to the upper and or lower airways, trimethoprim/sulfamethoxazole in a dose of 160/180 mg twice daily may be tried. Such patients must be carefully monitored and if there is any evidence of other organ involvement stronger immunosuppressants must be started.
- Limited or nonsevere GPA or patients with early generalized disease without renal involvement can receive oral prednisolone at 0.5–1 mg/kg not exceeding 80 mg/day in combination with methotrexate 15–25 mg once weekly, either orally or subcutaneously. This dose should be supplemented by folic acid 5 mg/day for 6 days (omitted on the day of methotrexate therapy) and standard *Pneumocystis jirovecii* pneumonia (PCP) prophylaxis. This milder immunosuppression avoids the more serious toxicity of cyclophosphamide and is equally effective in this group of patients.
- Rapidly progressive fulminant disease, DAH, and rapidly progressive renal failure are best treated with pulses of methylprednisolone in doses up to 1 g/day for 3 days. A large recent study, the MEPEX trial (methylprednisolone versus plasma exchange) showed that 2 weeks of plasma exchange was clearly superior to pulses alone in terms of renal recovery. Recombinant factor VIIa and desmopressin have also been tried to control torrential hemorrhage in patients with DAH.
- *Subglottic stenosis*: Subglottic lesions are generally unresponsive to systemic therapy. Success rates of medical therapy in relieving the obstruction run at 20–25%. Intralesional steroids have been used with

some success, methylprednisolone being injected in a four-quadrant and submucosal pattern. The steroid injections are best combined with endoscopic dilatation or cold knife lysis. Lasers have been used but may result in extensive scarring making such patients more difficult to manage later. The use of airway stents to maintain airway patency is also controversial. Most experts feel that the long-term safety of these stents has not been well established; stent fracture, migration, excess granulation tissue, and even death have been reported. A number of surgical techniques involving laryngotracheal reconstruction have been described and involvement of a skilled ear, nose, and throat (ENT) surgeon is mandatory in all such cases. Tracheostomy is of course the procedure of choice when the airway is critically compromised or in an emergency setting.

Maintenance therapy: Once remission is achieved, prednisolone is tapered off and stopped over 3–6 months. Patients with limited or nonsevere disease are maintained on methotrexate. Patients who had received cyclophosphamide as induction therapy should preferably be maintained on azathioprine. Mycophenolate mofetil is an alternative to azathioprine but is less effective. The objective is to maintain remission therapy for a minimum of 12 months after remission has been achieved. In a number of patients who to start with were seriously ill, or who experienced relapses, the duration of remission therapy may extend for a much longer period. Long-term maintenance therapy with trimethoprim-sulfamethoxazole (Tmp/Smx) in a dose of 160/180 mg has also been found to be beneficial in preventing relapses.

Monitor for toxicity: Cyclophosphamide is a very toxic agent and careful monitoring of blood counts is essential. The optimal dose is one that reduces the lymphocyte count but maintains the total white blood cell (WBC) count over $3,500/mm^3$. To avoid bladder toxicity, the patient must be advised to take the entire dose in the morning and drink plenty of water. Regular checks of urine are also advised. Steroid-related side effects must also be monitored and every attempt made to get down to alternate day maintenance doses to minimize toxicity. Concomitant calcium, vitamin D, and bisphosphonates are also recommended in most patients on steroids to prevent osteoporosis.

Monitor for opportunistic infections (OIs): OIs like TB or PCP are common after immunosuppression and must be carefully monitored for. In our setting, TB is of special importance and is difficult to diagnose as the clinical and radiological features may mimic flare-up of GPA. The role of isoniazid prophylaxis in patients of GPA with positive tuberculin skin tests (latent TB) has not been established. Tmp/Smx prophylaxis against pneumocystis infection is recommended in all patients receiving cyclophosphamide or methotrexate for remission induction or maintenance.

Treatment of patients refractory to treatment: About 10% of patients do not respond to therapy. Patients who have not responded to cytotoxic agents, high-dose steroids, or plasma exchange are deemed to have refractory disease. Novel therapies considered in this small but critically ill group of patients include tumor necrosis factor (TNF) blockers (etanercept, infliximab) and rituximab. A large study showed no efficacy of etanercept when added to standard therapy. In fact, such patients had a higher incidence of malignancy. On the other hand, rituximab in the dose mentioned earlier has proved very effective in inducing remission in refractory cases. It is the standard drug for treatment of refractory cases. Relapse following rituximab therapy has been treated with a second course of the drug with very satisfactory results.

Two further points are worth stressing:

1. *Some patients are wrongly dubbed "refractory":* Their so called refractoriness may be due to noncompliance with therapy, inadequate initial immunosuppression or to infection related to the use of immunosuppressive drugs.
2. Two manifestations of ANCA-related vasculitis in GPA are largely unresponsive to treatment rather than being termed resistant. These are orbital pseudotumor and subglottic stenosis.

Eosinophilic Granulomatosis with Polyangiitis (formerly Churg-Strauss Syndrome)

Definition

The Chapel Hill Consensus Conference defines EGPA as an eosinophil-rich and granulomatous inflammation involving the respiratory tract, and a necrotizing vasculitis involving the small to medium vessels, with associated asthma and eosinophilia.

Background

The syndrome was first described in 1951, in an article in the American Journal of Pathology, by Churg and Strauss in 13 patients with asthma, eosinophilia, granulomatous inflammation, necrotizing systemic vasculitis, and necrotizing glomerulonephritis.

Diagnosis

The ACR has proposed six criteria for the diagnosis of EGPA. These include:

1. Asthma
2. Eosinophilia (>10% in the peripheral blood)
3. Paranasal sinusitis
4. Pulmonary infiltrates (often transient)
5. Histological evidence of vasculitis with extravascular eosinophils
6. Mononeuritis multiplex or polyneuropathy.

The presence of four or more criteria helps to diagnose EGPA with a sensitivity of 85% and a specificity of 99.7%.

Epidemiology

The incidence of EGPA in the US is one to three cases per 100,000 adults per year. Globally, the incidence is similar at 2.5 cases per 100,000 adults per year. There is no Indian data but scattered case reports abound and it is likely that many patients with EGPA might be missed and labeled "tropical eosinophilia". The disease occurs in all ages from 15 years to 70 years with a mean age of approximately 38 years. Several case reports and small series describe EGPA in pediatric populations as well. EGPA is slightly more common in males.

Pathophysiology

EGPA is an ANCA-associated granulomatous small-vessel vasculitis. It is an idiopathic disorder though recent reports have reported this condition secondary to a number of agents.

The report that has excited the greatest attention is the association of EGPA with the use of leukotriene receptor antagonists. These cases initially led to a general warning on the possible link between EGPA and leukotriene receptor antagonists. However, careful analysis of all reported cases suggests that EGPA develops primarily in those patients taking these medications who almost certainly had an underlying eosinophilic disorder, which was being masked by corticosteroids. Administration of the leukotriene receptor antagonists improved asthma control, permitted steroids to be tapered and stopped, and hence served to unmask the underlying EGPA.

The same reasoning helps to explain the link reported in small series with inhaled corticosteroids. Again, it is believed that the inhaled steroids improved asthma control sufficiently to permit reduction/withdrawal of systemic steroids thus unmasking the active vasculitis. These links between leukotriene antagonists and inhaled corticosteroids merely emphasize the importance of monitoring patients carefully when severe asthma is controlled with any substance allowing withdrawal from systemic steroids.

Other drugs believed to be implicated in EGPA include mesalazine, propylthiouracil, and freebase cocaine.

Clinical Features

The EGPA has three phases:

1. *Prodromal phase*—of allergic rhinitis and asthma
2. *Eosinophilic phase*—of infiltrative disease such as eosinophilic pneumonia or gastroenteritis
3. *Vasculitic phase*: Systemic small-to-medium–vessel vasculitis with granulomatous inflammation.

The three phases are not seen in all patients and do not necessarily appear in this order.

Asthma is a cardinal feature of EGPA, being present in 98% of patients. In general, asthma precedes the vasculitis by 3–10 years and may be well-controlled and even forgotten by the time the vasculitic phase announces itself. Less frequently, asthma may coincide with the appearance of the vasculitis. The asthma in EGPA is usually persistent and hence these patients are often on maintenance doses of steroids for their "persistent and chronic asthma". This might mask other features of the syndrome.

Sinusitis: Paranasal sinusitis is a feature in around 60% of patients with EGPA. Allergic rhinitis is also frequent. Unlike GPA, necrotizing and destructive lesions of the upper airways are not seen. In a few patients, long-standing sinusitis may take the place of asthma as the background or presenting feature of EGPA.

Pulmonary: In addition to asthma, important pulmonary manifestations include transient peripherally placed lung infiltrates, hemoptysis secondary to alveolar capillaritis, and pleural effusions, which are typically eosinophilic. Consolidation and cavitation have also been reported. Pulmonary involvement occurs in over 38% of cases.

Skin manifestations: These are frequent in the vasculitic phase and include nodules, palpable purpura, urticarial rash, livedo reticularis, necrotic bullae, digital ischemia, skin necrosis, and gangrene.

Rheumatological manifestations: Joint pains are common but arthritis is rare.

Renal: Renal involvement takes the form of a pauci-immune glomerulonephritis, which is seldom as frequent or severe as that observed in GPA.

Gastrointestinal: Symptoms related to vasculitis of the GI tract are distinctive and include abdominal pain and bloody diarrhea. Abdominal crisis as in Henoch-Schonlein purpura (HSP) may occur and the skin and GI manifestations of these two vasculitides are similar.

Peripheral neuropathy: Mononeuritis multiplex occurs in as many as 77% of patients, and, like polyarteritis nodosa (PAN), this vasculitis is an important cause of neuropathy.

Cardiac manifestations: These are important causes of morbidity and mortality in this condition. Myocarditis and myocardial infarction can be fatal. Pericarditis has also been reported.

Investigations/Laboratory Workup

Blood and biochemistry: Peripheral eosinophilia is always seen. The levels vary from a minimum of 10% to strikingly high-eosinophil counts. Mild anemia, elevated ESR, and C-reactive protein (CRP) are inevitably found. Immunoglobulin E (IgE) levels are usually elevated. Serum creatinine must always be checked along with routine urine microscopy for proteinuria, casts and microscopic hematuria. ANCA is positive in approximately 40% of patients with EGPA. The pattern of staining is usually perinuclear-ANCA (p-ANCA) positive (antimyeloperoxidase antibodies).

Radiology

Pulmonary infiltrates chiefly peripherally placed are found in up to 75% of cases of EGPA. Transient infiltrates, which are often bilateral, are common. Localized nodular or patchy opacities may be seen, which may cavitate on occasion. Extensive air-space consolidation should suggest intra-alveolar hemorrhage, especially if this is accompanied by drop in hemoglobin levels and hemoptysis. Eosinophilic pleural effusions are observed in 10–30% **(Fig. 7)**.

Other organ-specific tests that may be needed depending on the organ involved include—electromyography and

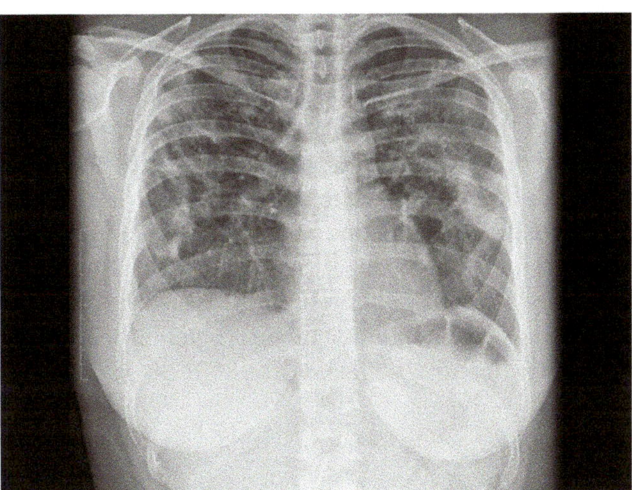

Fig. 7: Churg-Strauss syndrome: X-ray demonstrates ill-defined hazy ground-glass densities in both lung fields.

nerve conduction studies, ECHO and Holter monitoring for cardiac involvement, and GI endoscopy for GI bleeding.

Biopsy Proof

Pathological proof through a biopsy is helpful but not essential in confirming the diagnosis. Depending on the site of organ involvement, biopsies can be taken from skin, lung (ideally VATS or open-lung biopsies), kidney, nerves, or muscle. The characteristic pathological findings include small, necrotizing granuloma, and vasculitis affecting the small arteries and venules. The granulomas have an eosinophilic center and are surrounded by epithelioid giant cells and macrophages. Kidney biopsies usually reveal a focal and segmental glomerulonephritis.

Differential Diagnosis

The EGPA must be considered in the differential diagnosis of any asthmatic with more than the expected peripheral eosinophilia. If vasculitic manifestations occur in any asthmatic when oral steroids are tapered or stopped, often with the aid of inhaled steroids or leukotriene antagonists, EGPA must be the first disorder to be considered. It must be considered in any asthmatic with any evidence of multiorgan involvement or when asthma is accompanied by transient pulmonary shadows. Allergic bronchopulmonary aspergillosis (ABPA) and chronic eosinophilic pneumonias are close differentials. Other causes of pulmonary eosinophilia, especially hypereosinophilic syndromes and drug-induced eosinophilias must be distinguished from EGPA. Other vasculitis syndromes like GPA and microscopic polyangiitis must also be distinguished. When the GI system is primarily affected, the differential includes HSP, mesenteric ischemia, and eosinophilic gastroenteritis. Other causes of acute glomerulonephritis including PAN and Goodpasture's syndrome must be considered when the kidneys are primarily affected. Multisystem diseases like infective endocarditis, SLE, and essential cryoglobulinemia may share a few features with EGPA.

Treatment

Steroids are the drug of choice in EGPA and are usually the sole immunosuppressive therapy needed. They are usually given orally in a dose of 1 mg/kg/day of prednisolone. Life-threatening organ involvement like alveolar hemorrhage should be treated initially with a pulsed dose of 1 g IV methyl prednisolone daily for 3 days followed by oral prednisolone. No more than 20% of patients with EGPA will need additional immunosuppressive. The presence of vasculitis involving one or more organs necessitates the use of immunosuppressants. The regime for immunosuppression in the presence of systemic involvement due to any one of three primary small-vessel ANCA-associated vasculitis is the same and has been outlined in detail in the chapter on GPA.

Prognosis and Outcome

The 5-year survival in untreated EGPA is 25%. Treatment with systemic steroids improves survival rates to 70% at 5 years. The most common cause of mortality in EGPA is myocarditis and myocardial infarction secondary to coronary arteritis. Other causes of death reported in some series include alveolar hemorrhage, renal failure, GI bleeding, and status asthmaticus.

Microscopic Polyangiitis

Microscopic polyangiitis (MPA) was for several decades been grouped together with polyarteritis nodosa (PAN). It was only in 1944, that the Chapel Hill Consensus Conference recognized MPA as an entity in its own right, distinguishing it from PAN and GPA, the diseases with which it had been confused over the years and with which it has considerable overlap. MPA affects small and medium-sized vessels and is a disease of middle-aged patients. It is the most common cause of pulmonary renal involvement. Pulmonary involvement takes the form of DAH secondary to pulmonary capillaritis and occurs in approximately 12% of patients with MPA. Renal involvement occurs in more than 80% and results in glomerulonephritis with distinctive RBC casts in urine. The necrotizing vasculitis of MPA leads to a crescentic glomerulonephritis indistinguishable from that observed in patients with GPA. GI involvement is much more common in MPA than in GPA where it is rare. General nonspecific symptoms like fever, malaise, and weight loss are common as are skin lesions (palpable purpura,) arthralgia, myalgias, and peripheral neuropathy, which occur in 60% of cases. The histology is indistinguishable from GPA except that granulomatous inflammation is not a feature. The ANCA is usually positive and is of the p-ANCA variety, reacting with MPO. Treatment is as for GPA.

Table 4 describes the distinguishing features of MPA, GPA, and PAN.

Table 4: Distinguishing features of microscopic polyangiitis (MPA), granulomatosis with polyangiitis (GPA), and polyarteritis nodosa (PAN).

	MPA	GPA	PAN
Blood vessel size	Small	Small	Medium
Blood vessel type	Arterioles to venules	Arterioles to venules	Muscular arteries
Granulomatous inflammation	No	Yes	No
Lung symptoms	Yes	Yes	No
Glomerulonephritis	Yes	Yes	No
Renal hypertension	No	No	Yes
Mononeuritis multiplex	Common	Occasional	Common
Skin lesions	Yes	Yes	Yes
GI symptoms	Yes	No	Yes
Eye symptoms	Yes	Yes	No
ANCA-positivity	75% (p-ANCA)	65-90% (c-ANCA)	No
Constitutional symptoms	Yes	Yes	Yes
Necrotizing tissue	Yes	Yes	Yes
Microaneurysms	Rarely	Rarely	Typical

(ANCA: Antineutrophil cytoplasmic antibodies; c: Cytoplasmic; p: Perinuclear)
Source: John Hopkins Vasculitis Center, rheumatology@jhmi.edu.

■ OTHER PULMONARY VASCULITIDES

Takayasu's Arteritis

This is a large-vessel vasculitis predominantly affecting the aorta and its major branches. It results in intimal fibroproliferation of the aorta, great vessels, pulmonary arteries, and renal arteries and results in segmental stenosis, occlusion, dilatation, and aneurysmal formation in these vessels. Of the four types of Takayasu's arteritis, the most common is Type III, which is found in as many as 65% of patients. The most commonly involved vessels include the left subclavian artery (50%), the left common carotid artery (20%), the brachiocephalic trunk, and the renal arteries. The pulmonary arteries are affected in significant numbers of patients with Takayasu's arteritis. This leads to pulmonary hypertension and pulmonary stenosis. Fistula formation between branches of the pulmonary artery and bronchial arteries has been reported as has nonspecific interstitial lung disease. The link with mycobacterial infection remains unproven. Steroids have been tried with variable results. There are recent reports of anti-TNF agents being useful.

Giant Cell Arteritis

Giant cell arteritis is a vasculitis affecting large and medium-sized arteries. While the common symptoms are headaches, jaw pain, and blurred vision, respiratory symptoms are reported in a quarter of cases. Cough, hoarseness, and throat pain have all been reported and, on occasion, can be the presenting symptoms. Occasional cases of pleural effusion associated with giant cell arteritis have been reported. A strikingly high ESR is common and the response to steroids is generally dramatic.

Behcet's Disease

Behcet's disease is an immune complex vasculitis that affects arteries and veins of all sizes. It is characterized by aphthous oral and genital ulcers in combination with uveitis, arthritis, thrombophlebitis cutaneous nodules or pustules, and meningoencephalitis. The distinctive feature when the lungs are affected is hemoptysis. This can be massive and even fatal, and occurs secondary to rupture of pulmonary artery aneurysms that some of these patients develop.

Idiopathic Pauci-immune Pulmonary Capillaritis

This condition is diagnosed when the patient presents with alveolar hemorrhage and the biopsy shows capillaritis in the absence of any other detectable systemic disorder. It is a diagnosis of exclusion and the histology is indistinguishable from that of an ANCA-positive vasculitis. Treatment is with immunosuppressives as for GPA.

■ SUGGESTED READING

1. Cartin-Ceba R, Golbin JM, Keogh KA, et al. Rituximab for remission induction and maintenance in refractory granulomatosis with polyangiitis (Wegener's): ten-year experience at a single center. Arthritis Rheum. 2012;64:3770-8.
2. Craven A, Robson J, Ponte C, et al. ACR/EULAR-endorsed study to develop Diagnostic and Classification Criteria for Vasculitis (DCVAS). Clin Exp Nephrol. 2013;17: 619-21.
3. Frankel SK. Update in the diagnosis and management of pulmonary vasculitis. Chest. 2006;129(2):452-65.
4. Frankel SK. Vasculitis: Wegener's granulomatosis, Churg-Strauss syndrome, microscopic polyangiitis, polyarteritis nodosa, and Takayasu arteritis. Crit Care Clin. 2002;18(4):855-79.
5. Gómez-Puerta JA. Antineutrophil cytoplasmic antibody-associated vasculitides and respiratory disease. Chest. 2009;136(4):1101-11.
6. Jayne D. The diagnosis of vasculitis. Best Pract Res Clin Rheumatol. 2009;23:445.
7. Jennette JC, Falk RJ, Bacon PA, et al. 2012 revised International Chapel Hill Consensus Conference Nomenclature of Vasculitides. Arthritis Rheum. 2013;65:1.
8. Keogh KA. Churg-Strauss syndrome: clinical presentation, antineutrophil cytoplasmic antibodies, and leukotriene receptor antagonists. Am J Med. 2003;115(4):284-90.
9. Polychronopoulos VS. Airway involvement in Wegener's granulomatosis. Rheum Dis Clin North Am. 2007;33(4): 755-75, vi.
10. Stone JH, Merkel PA, Spiera R, et al. Rituximab versus cyclophosphamide for ANCA-associated vasculitis. N Engl J Med. 2010;363:221.

CHAPTER 51

Pulmonary Hypertension

INTRODUCTION

The pulmonary circuit is embedded in the matrix of the lung and interposed between the two sides of the heart. Though it plays a pivotal role in gas exchange and oxygen transport it is not the exclusive domain of either the cardiologist or the pulmonologist and hence has been relatively ignored by both sets of specialists. Tremendous advances have occurred in the last few decades in our understanding of the pathogenesis of pulmonary hypertension (PH) and its treatment which have served to redress the centuries of neglect in this field. Primary idiopathic pulmonary hypertension (IPH) is a devastating disease often. The treatment, even today is palliative, but not curative. The disease is often rapidly progressive and inevitably fatal. Indeed the outlook for a patient with primary PH and NYH 4 (breathless at rest) is worse than that for a patient with lung cancer, with a median survival of nine months.

DEFINITION

Pulmonary hypertension is defined as an increase in mean pulmonary artery pressure greater than 25 mm Hg at rest as assessed by right heart catheterization. The normal pulmonary artery pressure at rest is 14 ± 3 mm Hg with an upper limit of no more than 20 mm and the level of 25 mm Hg has been chosen to maintain consistency in all trials and registries of PH.

MILESTONES IN THE HISTORY OF PULMONARY HYPERTENSION

The pulmonary circulation was first described in the 16th century but it took another 400 years for the first clinical description of PH. In the 1950s this coincided with the advent of cardiac catheterization. In the 1960s an epidemic of PH secondary to appetite suppressants (fenfluramine) helped rekindle interest in the disease and this culminated in the first World Health Organization (WHO) meeting on PH in Geneva in 1975. In 1981, the National Institutes of Health (NIH) began a registry on all patients with PH in the US, so data on their natural history and course became available. Two further landmark WHO meetings on PH took place over the next few years in Evian and Venice. The current classification of PH was established at the Venice meeting in 2003. In terms of therapy, exciting developments were also occurring. After centuries of neglect, in 1991, the first Food and Drug Administration (FDA)-approved drug epoprostenol emerged and it was only after 2000 that sildenafil and its derivatives and the endothelin receptor blockers (bosentan) were developed.

ETIOLOGY

A wide range of common and rare disorders can result in PH. Primary PH is now called idiopathic pulmonary arterial hypertension (IPAH). This is a prototype of PH but is a diagnosis of exclusion. Other broad headings the chest physician should always exclude before labeling a patient "idiopathic" include: PH secondary to left heart disease, PH secondary to lung diseases and hypoxia and pulmonary veno-occlusive disease (PVOD). Chronic thromboembolic disease is a rare but surgically reversible cause of PH which should always be actively considered and ruled out. It results from recurrent thromboemboli or thrombi in the pulmonary vasculature, leading to increasing obliteration of the pulmonary vasculature. PH with right ventricular hypertrophy and failure are the presenting features, the true cause of which is often missed. Finally, PH could be secondary to a number of rarer hematological, systemic and metabolic disorders which should be considered before labeling a patient as IPH.

A detailed classification based on the Dana Point Consensus is given in **Table 1**.

The World Health Organization (WHO) has classified PH based upon etiology into the following five groups:

- *Group 1*: Pulmonary arterial hypertension (PAH). This group includes patients with idiopathic and heritable PAH, PAH due to drugs and toxins, PAH due to connective tissue diseases, HIV, PAH due to congenital heart diseases, schistosomiasis.
- *Group 2*: PH due to left heart disease
- *Group 3*: PH due to chronic lung disease
- *Group 4*: PH due to chronic thromboembolic disease
- *Group 5*: PH due to multifactorial causes.

A new disorder was added to group 5 is known as segmental PH which refers to PH in segments of the lung rather than the entire lung [*Ref: Simonneau G, Gatzoulis MA, et al. Updated clinical classification of pulmonary hypertension. J Am Coll Cardiol. 2013;62(25 Suppl):D34*].

Table 1: Updated classification of pulmonary hypertension.

1. Pulmonary arterial hypertension
1.1 Idiopathic PAH
1.2 Heritable PAH
1.2.1 BMPR2
1.2.2 ALK-1, ENG, SMAD9, CAV1, KCNK3
1.2.3 Unknown
1.3 Drug and toxin-induced
1.4 Associated with
1.4.1 Connective tissue disease
1.4.2 HIV infection
1.4.3 Portal hypertension
1.4.4 Congenital heart diseases
1.4.5 Schistosomiasis
1'. Pulmonary veno-occlusive disease and/or pulmonary capillary hemangiomatosis
1". Persistent pulmonary hypertension of the newborn (PPHN)
2. Pulmonary hypertension due to left heart disease
2.1 Left ventricular systolic dysfunction
2.2 Left ventricular diastolic dysfunction
2.3 Valvular disease
2.4 Congenital/acquired left heart inflow/outflow tract obstruction and congenital cardiomyopathics
3. Pulmonary hypertension due to lung diseases and/or hypoxia
3.1 Chronic obstructive pulmonary disease
3.2 Interstitial lung disease
3.3 Other pulmonary diseases with mixed restrictive and obstructive pattern
3.4 Sleep-disordered breathing
3.5 Alveolar hypoventilation disorders
3.6 Chronic exposure to high altitude
3.7 Developmental lung diseases
4. Chronic thromboembolic pulmonary hypertension (CTEPH)
5. Pulmonary hypertension with unclear multifactorial mechanisms
5.1 Hematologic disorders: chronic hemolytic anemia, myeloproliferative disorders, splenectomy
5.2 Systemic disorders: sarcoidosis, pulmonary histiocytosis, lymphangioleiomyomatosis
5.3 Metabolic disorders: glycogen storage disease, Gaucher disease, thyroid disorders
5.4 Others: tumoral obstruction, fibrosing mediastinitis, chronic renal failure, segmental PH

Source: Simonneau G, Gatzoulis MA, et al. Updated clinical classification of pulmonary hypertension. J Am Coll Cardiol. 2013;62(25 Suppl):D34.

PATHOGENESIS OF PULMONARY HYPERTENSION

Idiopathic PH has a complex etiology. Of singular importance is the excessive vasoconstriction these individuals develop due to abnormal expression of potassium channels in the smooth muscle cells and due to endothelial dysfunction. Endothelial dysfunction leads to impaired production of vasodilator and anti-proliferative agents like nitric oxide (NO) and prostacyclin. This is accompanied by overexpression of vasoconstrictor and proliferative substances such as endothelin-1. As a consequence vascular remodeling and proliferation occur. Prothrombotic abnormalities have also been demonstrated and small distal thrombi in pulmonary arterioles are known.

When PH occurs in a familial context mutations in the bone morphogenetic protein receptor 2 gene have been detected in 70% of cases. Mutations of this gene have been detected in around 10–40% of cases, with apparently sporadic cases thus representing the major genetic predisposing factor for PH.

Pulmonary hypertension due to lung disease: A number of pathophysiological factors are involved in this group including hypoxic vasoconstriction, mechanical stress of hyperinflated lungs, loss of capillaries and inflammatory and toxic effects of cigarette smoke. Endothelium-derived vasoconstrictor-vasodilator imbalance may also contribute. Serotonin gene polymorphism may determine the severity of PH in hypoxemic patients with chronic obstructive pulmonary disease (COPD).

PREVALENCE OF PULMONARY HYPERTENSION

Pulmonary arterial hypertension is not a common disease. Data from recent registries in Europe and

Scotland show the prevalence of PH and IPH are 16 and five cases per million respectively. In the French registry 39% of patients had IPAH of which around 4% had a family history of PH. PH secondary to chronic lung disease and hypoxia is of course much more common. The incidence of significant PH in COPD patients with at least one prior admission for acute exacerbation is around 20%. In advanced COPD, PH is highly prevalent (around 50%). In interstitial lung disease (ILD) the prevalence of PH is around 30–40%. In the subset of patients with a combination of emphysema and ILD the prevalence and severity of PH is even higher. There is no available data on the prevalence or epidemiology of PAH from India but with the ready availability of some of the newer drugs there are growing calls for maintenance of a national drug registry.

CLINICAL FEATURES

The clinical features of IPH may be subtle and nonspecific and the earliest symptom is often an unexplained dyspnea on exertion. This may indeed be the sole symptom in the first few years of presentation and patients often visit multiple doctors before the diagnosis is made. In a young patient this is often passed off as secondary to physical deconditioning or even anxiety and hyperventilation. Other early nonspecific symptoms include fatigue and palpitation. In more advanced cases, syncope (usually exertional), anginal pain, edema of the feet and free fluid in the abdomen may be noticed.

The earliest physical sign is also subtle and easily missed. It is an accentuation of the pulmonary component of the second heart sound. As the PH worsens the patient may develop a pansystolic murmur of tricuspid regurgitation often with an accompanying right-sided S3 gallop. A diastolic Graham Steele murmur of pulmonary regurgitation may also be heard. In advanced cases the patient presents with right heart failure with distended neck veins, congestive hepatomegaly and ascites and/or edema of the feet **(Table 2)**.

Examination should include attempts at determining other possible causes of PH. Thus gross clubbing may denote congenital cyanotic heart disease; telangiectasia and sclerodactyly point to scleroderma as the cause of PH. If PH is secondary to COPD there is obvious evidence of airflow limitation; the fine Velcro-like dry crackles of ILD causing PH may be missed unless carefully auscultated for.

DIAGNOSING PULMONARY HYPERTENSION (TABLE 3)

Once PH is suspected from history or examination it is incumbent on the clinician to:

- Confirm the diagnosis of PH
- Determine its severity
- Check for an underlying secondary cause before labeling the patient IPAH.

The following tests are useful:

- *Chest radiograph*: In the early stages the chest radiograph may be normal but in 90% of patients with IPAH the chest radiograph is abnormal at the time of diagnosis. Findings include central pulmonary artery dilatation, peripheral pruning and evidence of right atrial and ventricular enlargement **(Figs. 1 and 2)**. If present, radiographic features of ILD or emphysema may give a clue to secondary causes of PH.
- *Electrocardiography*: The electrocardiography (ECG) has insufficient sensitivity (55%) and specificity (70%) to be a screening tool for diagnosing PH. However, evidence of RV hypertrophy and strain may be seen in advanced cases. Atrial fibrillation if present carries a bad prognosis and invariably leads to further clinical deterioration.
- *Pulmonary function test*: A mild to moderate reduction in the diffusion capacity may be the sole abnormality directly due to the PH itself. The main role of

---

Table 2: Clinical features of pulmonary hypertension.

- Early unexplained dyspnea on exertion
- Syncope (usually exertional), anginal pain, accentuated P2 with progression of the disease
- Right ventricular enlargement
- Dilated PA
- Tricuspid incompetence
- Graham Steele murmur of pulmonary incompetence
- JVP +; prominent "a" wave
- Edema feet, free fluid in the abdomen
- Enlarged tender liver

Table 3: Investigations of pulmonary hypertension.

- Chest radiograph
- ECG
- Pulmonary function testing
- Arterial blood gases
- Polysomnography
- Echocardiography
- Ventilation/perfusion scanning
- CT chest
- Pulmonary angiography and right heart catheterization

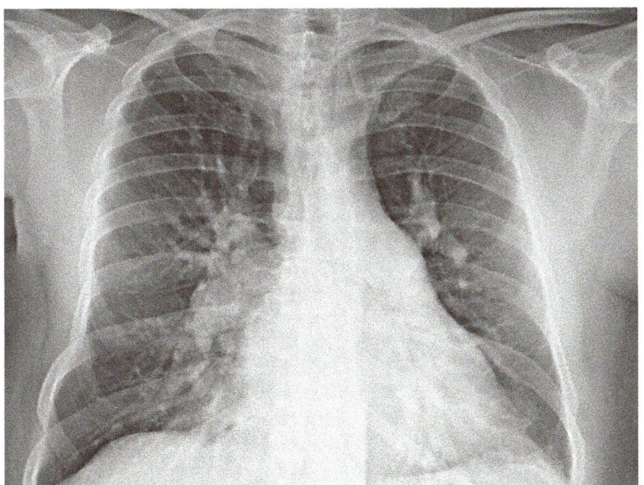

Fig. 1: Pulmonary hypertension. X-ray chest reveals a markedly dilated main pulmonary artery visualized as a well-defined opacity in the left paracardiac region just below the aortic arch. The right pulmonary artery is also dilated as seen by the prominence of the right hilum.

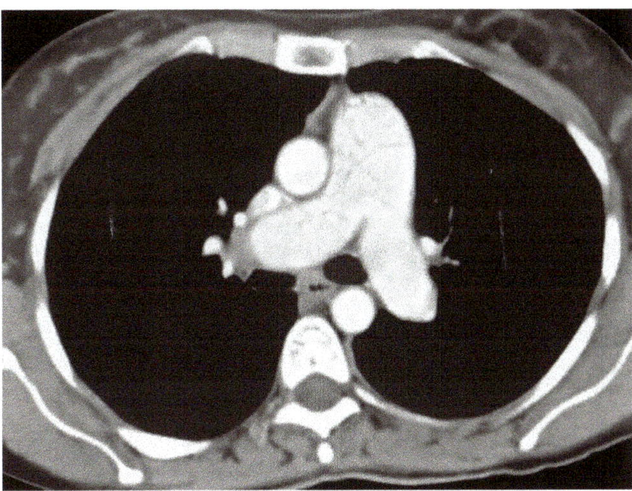

Fig. 2: Pulmonary hypertension. Computed tomography (CT) chest reveals markedly dilated main and right/left pulmonary arteries.

pulmonary function test (PFT) is to rule out an airway or an interstitial cause of PH.

- *Arterial blood gas* (ABG): Arterial blood gas (ABG) analysis is usually normal till advanced PH sets in. It may however show a mild hypoxia, and desaturation after exercise is a subtle and sensitive (but not specific) pointer to PH. Hypocapnia is often present secondary to alveolar hyperventilation. If COPD is the cause of the PH patients may have hypercapnia.
- *Polysomnography*: A history of snoring and excessive daytime sleepiness must be enquired from every patient with PH. Obstructive sleep apnea may present with PH and right heart failure and can only be diagnosed by overnight polysomnography.
- *Echocardiography* is an indispensable test to determine the presence and severity of PH. It may also be of value in picking up a hitherto undetected cardiac shunt responsible for the PH. The pulmonary artery pressure can be estimated based on the peak velocity of the tricuspid regurgitation jet. When tricuspid regurgitation is difficult to measure or cannot be measured, contrast echocardiography with agitated saline significantly increases the Doppler signal allowing proper measurement of peak tricuspid regurgitation velocity. Pulmonary artery measurements on echocardiography cannot be made for mild cases and do not always correlate with degree of PH determined on pulmonary angiography. A study based on echocardiographic screening of a tricuspid regurgitant jet in symptomatic

patients with scleroderma determined that 45% of patients with echocardiographic diagnosis of PH were actually falsely positive. Exercise echocardiography has been used in patients with PH to assess the heart's response to stress or exercise.

- *Ventilation/perfusion scanning*: The ventilation/perfusion (V/Q) scan is a good screening test for chronic thromboembolic PH and ideally should be performed on all patients before labeling them idiopathic. A normal or low-probability V/Q scan effectively rules out chronic thromboembolic PH with a sensitivity of 90–100% and a specificity of 94–100%.
- *CT scanning*: High-resolution computed tomography (HRCT) scanning is a useful way to rule out ILD or emphysema as a cause of PH. Pulmonary veno-occlusive disease also has a specific HRCT appearance with interstitial edema, central ground-glass opacification and thickening of interlobular septa. Contrast CT of the pulmonary artery helps determine if there is evidence of surgically amenable chronic thromboembolic pulmonary hypertension (CTEPH). CT features of CTEPH include blockages, webs, bands, and intimal irregularities **(Figs. 3A to C)**.
- *Pulmonary angiography and right heart catheterization*: This is an underutilized procedure, chiefly because of fears of safety in patients with severe PH. When performed in an experienced center, it carries a morbidity of not more than 1% and mortality of 0.05%. Pulmonary angiography remains the gold standard

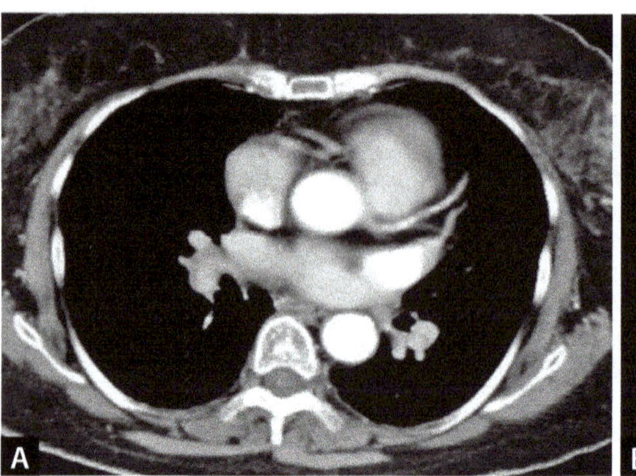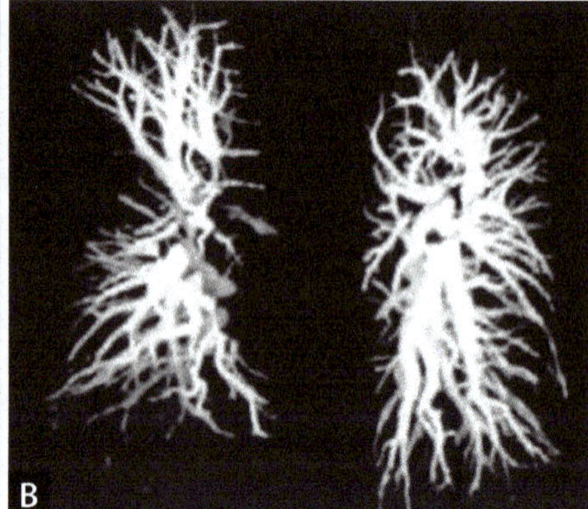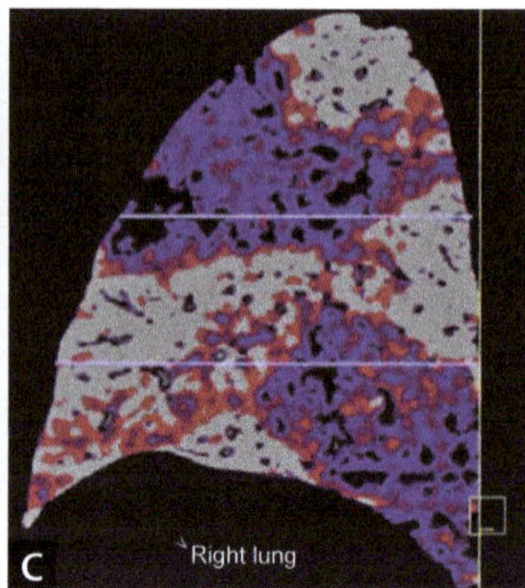

Figs. 3A to C: (A) Computed tomography (CT) angiography demonstrates linear bands in the descending left pulmonary artery indicating chronic pulmonary emboli; (B) Maximum intensity projection (MIP) of CT pulmonary angiography demonstrates a large wedge-shaped area of no vascularity in the right upper zone due to segmental occlusion; and (C) Dual-energy CT pulmonary angiogram perfusion image demonstrates multiple wedge-shaped areas of reduced perfusion indicative of chronic pulmonary embolism.

when it comes to diagnosing PH and assessing the severity of the hemodynamic derangement it produces. Right heart catheterization is also useful to test the vasoreactivity of the pulmonary circulation. Vasoreactivity testing is again seldom performed but invaluable to determine which patients with PH will respond to long-term therapy with calcium channel blockers. It should ideally be performed at the same time as right heart catheterization. The agents currently used in vasoreactivity testing are inhaled NO, intravenous epoprostenol or intravenous adenosine. An acute responder is defined as one whose mean pulmonary artery (PA) pressure declines more than 10 mm Hg to reach an absolute value of less than 40 mm Hg with an increased or unchanged cardiac output. Unfortunately, only around 10% of patients with IPAH will meet this definition of acute responders. These acute responders are the only ones likely to show a sustained response to long-term calcium channel blockers and these are the only patients in whom these drugs may safely be used in large doses. Only 50% of patients who are acute responders are likely to have a sustained long-term response to these drugs and these are the only patients in whom they should be continued.

Evaluation of Severity (Table 4)

A number of parameters predict poor survival.

- *Clinical parameters*: WHO class III or IV, extremes of age, syncope, hemoptysis or RV failure, are all clinical markers of severity.

Table 4: Estimating severity of pulmonary hypertension.	

- *Clinical parameters*: WHO class III or IV, extremes of age, syncope, hemoptysis or RV failure
- Echocardiographic markers like pericardial effusion, indexed right atrium area, and RV Doppler index
- Right heart catheterization parameters like PA oxygen saturation, right atrial pressure, pulmonary vascular resistance and cardiac output
- 6 minute walk test (6MWT)
- Brain natriuretic peptide (BNP) levels, pro-BNP levels and cardiac troponin levels

- *Echocardiographic markers* of poor survival include pericardial effusion, indexed right atrium area, and RV Doppler index. Interestingly, estimated systolic pulmonary arterial pressure (PAP) is not prognostic.
- *Right heart catheterization parameters* are also useful in determining prognosis. These include PA oxygen saturation, right atrial pressure, pulmonary vascular resistance and cardiac output. PAP is less reliable, as with the advent of right ventricular failure in the advanced stage of the disease, pulmonary artery pressure falls.
- *Six-minute walk test (6MWT)* is an inexpensive, reproducible, and well-standardized test. Walking distance less than 250 m and desaturation more than 10% indicate poor prognosis in PH.
- *Biochemical markers*: Over the last decade a number of biochemical markers have emerged. Brain natriuretic peptide (BNP) levels, pro-BNP levels and elevated cardiac troponin T levels have all been shown in several studies to correlate with survival.

Exact cut-off points of each of these markers have not been established as yet. Increases or decreases in these markers when serially measured over time also correlate well with response or lack of response to treatment. Newer markers like H-FABP and GDF-15 are also being looked at.

It is impossible in a single chapter to discuss the numerous causes of PH listed in **Table 1**—pulmonary hypertension due to left heart disease, PH secondary to pulmonary disease, and recently reported features of PVOD have been briefly discussed here.

Pulmonary Hypertension due to Left Heart Disease

An important diagnostic challenge is to distinguish between PH due to left heart failure with preserved ejection fraction and IPH. The demonstration of a pulmonary artery wedge pressure or a left ventricular (LV) end-diastolic pressure more than 15 mm Hg is proof that PH is secondary to LV failure. A frequent diagnostic error is to diagnose IPH when the actual cause of PH is heart failure. Noninvasive methods may help to make the distinction as well. Noninvasive parameters including medical history, LV hypertrophy on ECG and most importantly left atrial size on an ECHO study. An enlarged left atrium should point to heart failure as the cause of PH. When there is doubt, it becomes imperative to perform invasive tests to determine the wedge pressure or the LV end-diastolic pressure.

In a recent study it was shown that sildenafil did not reduce pulmonary artery pressure, did not improve the hemodynamic or clinical parameters in heart failure with preserved ejection fraction and in predominantly isolated postcapillary PH.

Pulmonary Hypertension due to Pulmonary Disease

Pulmonary hypertension in different types of lung diseases is associated with a poor outcome. Whether PH is the cause of death or to what extent it contributes to a fatal outcome is not defined. Pulmonary hypertension due to COPD is well known and requires no explanation (*see* chapter on COPD). Pulmonary hypertension in advanced ILD is explained by the strangling of the pulmonary vasculature by fibrous tissue. A study on ILD associated with mild to moderate lung volume restriction showed that severe PH is rare in IPF. It was also shown that ambrisentan

and bosentan were ineffective with regard to improving hemodynamics, symptoms and functional capacity in patients with idiopathic interstitial pneumonia and PH. It is also noteworthy that though phosphodiesterase inhibitors may reduce pulmonary artery pressure and improve cardiac output in COPD, this did not lead to improvement in functional exercise capacity. It needs to be determined whether vasodilators could help in a subgroup of patients with pulmonary disease who show very severe hypertension.

Pulmonary Veno-occlusive Disease

Several causes of PVOD have been recently identified—these include genetic predisposition, drugs and effects of radiation. The discovery of EIF2AK4 (eukaryotic translation initiation factor 2 alpha kinase 4) mutation in familial PVOD and pulmonary capillary hemangiomatosis (PCH) is bound to stimulate further research. Identification of this gene allows one to make the diagnosis of PVOD or PCH without the need for a histological diagnosis. Possible relation between the drug mitomycin and drug interferon and PVOD has also been recently commented upon.

Prognosis

Pulmonary hypertension (PH) is progressive, and often fatal. The prognosis depends upon the etiology and severity of PH.

Those with Group 1 PAH (WHO Classification) have worse survival than Groups 2 to 5. Chronic thromboembolic hypertension (CTEPH) has the best survival rate if surgically correctible.

The 5-year survival rate in Group 1 PAH following the time of diagnostic right heart catheterization is 57%.

Patients with severe PAH (mean PA pressure >35 mm Hg) and/or evidence of right heart failure have a poor prognosis.

■ THERAPY OF PULMONARY HYPERTENSION (TABLE 5)

The last decade has seen great advances in the treatment of PH. A position of helplessness with no drug options has been transformed to one of hope with the current availability and regulatory approval of eight drugs and further molecules at trial stage in the pipeline. Although PH remains a chronic disease without a cure, modern drug

Table 5: Therapy for pulmonary hypertension.

- Lifestyle changes
- Supportive therapy with oral anticoagulants, diuretics and digoxin
- Calcium channel blockers—nifedipine, diltiazem, and amlodipine
- Prostanoids—epoprostenol, iloprost, treprostinil, and beraprost
- Phosphodiesterase type-5 inhibitors—sildenafil and tadalafil
- Endothelin receptor antagonists—bosentan, sitaxsentan, and ambrisentan
- Combination therapy with prostanoids, endothelin receptor antagonists, and phosphodiesterase inhibitors
- Balloon atrial septostomy
- Pulmonary embolectomy
- Transplantation—heart-lung or bilateral-lung transplantation.

therapy leads to significant improvement in the patients' symptomatic status and a slower rate of clinical decline. Therapeutic options include:

General Measures

Once diagnosed the patient with IPH is advised about certain lifestyle changes that must be made. These patients are generally young: strenuous activity and pregnancy must be avoided. Pregnancy carries a 30–50% mortality in patients with PH. Barrier methods of contraception are to be preferred to hormonal methods like contraceptive pills. Travel should be curtailed unless essential and the need for supplemental oxygen on flights must be clarified.

Supportive Therapy

Oral anticoagulants are advised in all patients with IPH unless there is a specific contraindication. Diuretics and digoxin are useful if there is evidence of a decompensated right ventricle. Oxygen is required in many patients with severe PH who are hypoxemic at rest or with exertion. It should be titrated to maintain SaO_2 more than 90%. Long-term oxygen has been shown to partially reduce the progression of PH in COPD.

Calcium Channel Blockers

Only a small fraction of patients with PAH will benefit from calcium channel blockers. As discussed earlier, these should ideally be identified by acute vasodilator challenge testing at the time of right heart catheterization. The drugs used include nifedipine, diltiazem, and amlodipine. Relatively high doses are needed for them to be effective (120–240 mg for nifedipine and 240–720 mg for diltiazem).

This underscores the importance of not using them in patients who have not undergone a vasoreactivity study or have a negative study because of the potential of major side effects like hypotension and syncope.

Prostanoids

A number of prostacyclin derivatives have been used in the treatment of PH. These include epoprostenol, iloprost, treprostinil, and beraprost. Epoprostenol has a very short half-life (3–5 minutes) and is stable at room temperature for only 8 hours. It is therefore administered by means of a syringe pump via a permanent tunneled catheter. This is not practical on a long-term basis and this drug is usually reserved as a bridge to transplant. Iloprost is available by the intravenous, oral and inhaled routes and is well tolerated, though oral iloprost has been associated with flushing and jaw pain. Treprostinil is usually given by continuous subcutaneous infusion by a microinfusion pump and a small subcutaneous catheter. Infusion site pain is a limiting side effect. Beraprost is the first chemically stable and orally active prostacyclin derivative and recent studies have shown an improvement in exercise capacity that unfortunately persists for only 6 months. None of the drugs in this group are available in India.

Phosphodiesterase Type-5 Inhibitors

Since the pulmonary vasculature contains substantial amounts of phosphodiesterase type-5, the potential benefit of these agents in PH has been studied. Sildenafil and tadalafil, both drugs used to treat erectile dysfunction have been shown to cause significant vasodilatation with peak effects observed after 60 minutes and 90 minutes respectively. A number of smaller uncontrolled studies first reported the favorable effects of sildenafil in PH in IPH, PH secondary to connective tissue disease, in congenital cyanotic heart disease-associated PAH and in CTEPH. A large randomized controlled trial (RCT) of 278 PH patients treated with sildenafil called the SUPER-1 trial confirmed its favorable effects at different doses on symptoms, exercise capacity and hemodynamics. The approved dose is 20 mg three times a day but doses as high as 80 mg three times a day have been safely used. Side effects are mild and are mainly linked to vasodilatation (headache, flushing, and epistaxis). Tadalafil has the convenience of a once daily dose. A recent RCT called the PHIRST study on 406

PH patients showed good effects on symptoms, exercise capacity, hemodynamics and time to clinical worsening using the largest dose which was 40 mg once a day.

Endothelin Receptor Antagonists

Activation of the endothelin system has been consistently demonstrated in plasma and lung tissue of patients with PH. Endothelin exerts its effect by binding endothelin A and B receptors. Bosentan is an oral active dual endothelin-A and B receptor antagonist. It represents a breakthrough in PH because it is the first molecule in a new class of drugs specifically designed to treat this disorder. Its effect was established in five RCTs that have each shown improvement not just in functional class and exercise capacity, but also in hemodynamic and echocardiographic variables. Between them these studies have established its use in not just IPH but also PH secondary to connective tissue disease, cyanotic heart disease and CTEPH. Bosentan is initiated in a dose of 62.5 mg twice a day orally and then increased if tolerated to 125 mg twice a day after 4 weeks. Elevation of hepatic transaminases occurs in a dose-dependent manner in up to 10% of patients on this drug and hence monthly monitoring of liver function is mandatory. Sitaxsentan and ambrisentan are two other molecules in the same class that are also in use. Both cause less frequent elevation of liver transaminases compared to bosentan.

Combination Therapy

Combination therapy has become the standard of care in many centers. More than one PH-specific class of drugs are used in conjunction. These include prostanoids, endothelin receptor antagonists and phosphodiesterase inhibitors. The choice of combination agents, the optimal timing, when to switch and when to combine are all unclear and should prove fertile research opportunities for clinicians in the field.

The ambrisentan and tadalafil in patients with pulmonary arterial hypertension (AMBITION) trial showed that in comparison to monotherapy, combination therapy resulted in a significant lower risk of treatment failure.

Balloon Atrial Septostomy

The creation of an inter-atrial right to left shunt can decompress the right heart chambers, and increase LV preload and cardiac output. In addition this improves systemic oxygen transport despite arterial oxygen desaturation. The recommended technique is graded balloon atrial septostomy. This is often a last resort measure in patients on transplant lists, buying them some time while they await their transplant.

Pulmonary Endarterectomy

Surgical pulmonary endarterectomy is the treatment of choice for patients with CTEPH. Patients should be carefully selected and surgery should be done in a center with experience in this form of surgery. In India, Narayana Hrudayalaya Health City in Bengaluru has had the maximum experience, with excellent results with surgical removal of thromboemboli from blocked pulmonary vessels in patients with CTEPH. The pathogenesis of CTEPH requires further study. Though the disease has been considered to be precapillary in its location, human and experimental studies show that it is at least partly due to postcapillary remodeling. There is also evidence of bronchial artery to pulmonary venous shunting in CTEPH. This is the only form of PH where one can talk of cure. Surgery can transform a patient disabled by breathlessness, on continuous oxygen and in right heart failure into normalcy. A dramatic fall in pulmonary vascular resistance and near normalization of hemodynamics can occur in even the most severe cases if properly selected and operated on by an experienced surgeon.

In inoperable cases, the use of the drug Riociguat (as observed in Chest-2 study 2015) [*Ref: Simonnea G, D'Armini AM, Ghofrani HA, et al. Riociguat for the treatment of chronic thromboembolic pulmonary hypertension: a long-term extension study (CHEST-2). Eur Respir J. 2015;45(5):1293-302*] showed that there was sustained benefit in exercise and functional capacity for a year.

Another treatment modality in inoperable cases is the use of balloon pulmonary angioplasty. Fauci and colleagues showed a marked improvement in right ventricular end-diastolic and end-systolic volume index, together with significant improvement in functional capacity in 20 inoperable CTEPH patients treated by balloon angioplasty. The changes were similar to those observed with pulmonary endarterectomy.

Transplantation

Transplantation is a real option in patients with severe PH who fail to respond to all available medical measures.

Some forms of PH like PVOD have a worse prognosis and these patients should be referred to a transplant center as soon as they are diagnosed. Currently, either heart-lung or bilateral lung transplantation are offered for PH. The overall 5-year survival following transplantation for IPH stands at 50% in the best centers. Indications for lung transplantation are given in **Table 6**.

Table 6: Indications for lung transplantation.

- NYHA functional Class III or IV despite a trial of at least 3 months of combination therapy including prostanoids
- Cardiac index of <2L/min/m^2
- Mean right atrial pressure of >15 mm Hg
- 6 minutes walk test of <350 m
- Development of significant hemoptysis, pericardial effusion, or signs of progressive right heart failure.

(NYHA: New York Heart Association)
Source: Sunder T, Ramesh TP, Kumar KM, et al. Lung transplant: the Indian experience and suggested guidelines—Part 1 selection of the donor and recipient. J Pract Cardiovasc Sci. 2018;4:88-95.

■ SUGGESTED READING

1. Austin C, Alassas K, Burger C, et al. Echocardiographic assessment of estimated right atrial pressure and size predicts mortality in pulmonary arterial hypertension. Chest. 2015;147:198-208.
2. Brown LM, Chen H, Halpern S, et al. Delay in recognition of pulmonary arterial hypertension: factors identified from the REVEAL Registry. Chest. 2011;140:19-26.
3. Delcroix M, Naeije R. Optimising the management of pulmonary arterial hypertension patients: emergency treatments. Eur Respir Rev. 2010;19:204-11.
4. Galie N, Corris PA, Frost A, et al. Updated treatment algorithm of pulmonary arterial hypertension. J Am Coll Cardiol. 2013;62:D60-72.
5. Hoeper MM, Bogaard HJ, Condliffe R, et al. Definitions and diagnosis of pulmonary hypertension. J Am Coll Cardiol. 2013;62:D42-50.
6. Simonneau G, Gatzoulis MA, Adatia I, et al. Updated clinical classification of pulmonary hypertension. J Am Coll Cardiol. 2013;62:D34-41.

CHAPTER 52

Pulmonary Embolism

■ INTRODUCTION AND IMPORTANCE

Pulmonary embolism (PE) is the third most common cause of mortality after coronary artery disease and stroke. It is the most common cause of death in the puerperium and postoperative period. Despite its importance it remains underdiagnosed and hence in a sense neglected. Indeed, up to 80% of pulmonary emboli found at autopsy have not been suspected antemortem. This must be one of the most staggeringly poor diagnostic rates for any disease in all of medicine. Despite all the advances in diagnosis this appalling diagnostic rate has not changed over the last four decades. Sadly, physicians cannot diagnose what they do not suspect and this is the crux of the problem with PE as we shall discuss later in the chapter.

PE is believed to affect 600,000 patients annually in the US. Of these, 200,000 die from their PE. It is responsible for at least 15% of all hospital deaths in some hospital mortality series from the US. Its true incidence is unknown because its many nonspecific clinical features make it one of the most difficult diagnostic challenges in all of medicine. A study by Stein and colleagues in the mid-nineties from the Henry Ford Heart and Vascular Institute in Detroit showed PE occurred with an incidence of 1% of 51,000 hospitalized patients over a 21-month period. It, however, accounted for 14% of all autopsies, thus emphasizing the fact that most cases were only being diagnosed postmortem.

■ EPIDEMIOLOGY IN INDIA, CHINA, AND SOUTH-EAST ASIA

India

A study from a large private hospital in Mumbai showed that only 0.14% of 42,000 in-patients were given the diagnosis of PE. This does not mean that PE is uncommon in India; it is just a reflection of the extent of underdiagnosis. In one of our critical care units, the incidence of PE was very close to that in the West.

In Chandigarh (North India), of 700 autopsies performed between 1964 and 1980, the incidence of PE was 3.1%, lower than the West and similar to the low incidence in Africa. Yet in 2006, Kapadia SR and colleagues from Sir Ganga Ram Hospital, New Delhi noted that PE occurred in as many as 40% of 1,552 consecutive Indian patients with symptomatic deep vein thrombosis (DVT); 47% of patients with PE in this study (judged from a high-probability lung perfusion scan) were asymptomatic *[Ref: Parakh R, Kapadia SR, Sen I, et al. Pulmonary embolism: a frequent occurrence in Indian patients with symptomatic lower limb venous thrombosis. Asian J Surg. 2006;29(2):86-91].* Considering that many patients with DVT are asymptomatic, the incidence of both DVT and PE would be much higher than is apparent today. Increasing awareness will perhaps provide a much clearer idea about the prevalence of venous thromboembolism in India, which is certainly much higher than what is generally believed.

China and South-East Asia

There have been several reports on DVT and PE in the Chinese population in the recent years; they cite a prevalence of DVT of 2.6–17%. A similar figure has been reported from Malaysia and Thailand. Data from a study performed in Hong Kong between 1990 and 1994 showed an increased prevalence of 4.7% of pulmonary thromboembolism (PTE) *(Ref: Chau KY, Yuen ST, Wong MP. Clinicopathological pattern of pulmonary thromboembolism in Chinese autopsy patients: comparison with Caucasian series. Pathology. 1997;29:263-6).* These figures are within the lower range of the prevalence of PTE in Caucasian patients; reported rates of significant PTE from all autopsies are 3.4–9.0% in the United States and 12.8% in the United Kingdom.

Irrespective of the exact numbers, the impact of PE is considerable. PE has been described as the most important preventable cause of hospital deaths. In a recent study of 13,000 admissions to six trauma centers, 17% of preventable deaths were caused by PE.

■ SOURCES OF PULMONARY EMBOLISM

The two main sources of embolism are venous thrombosis in the lower limbs, thrombi within the right atrium in patients with atrial fibrillation, and other supraventricular arrhythmias. Thrombi within the right ventricle causing PE can occur following septal infarction or a right ventricular (RV) infarction.

■ ETIOLOGY

Link between DVT and PE

Pulmonary embolism and DVT are intimately related. The perils posed by DVT are most sharply forced into focus when it culminates in a life-threatening PE. Dissimilar at first sight, they are in reality, two sides of the same coin, twin partners in crime, part of the same pathological process. DVT is by far the most common cause of PE. Indeed, PE is not a disease, but most often a complication of DVT. Exploring the link further, 40% of DVT patients without symptoms of PE will have positive (high probability) ventilation/perfusion (V/Q) scans. From another angle, 30% of PE patients without symptoms of DVT will have a positive venous Doppler. DVT is not more universally found in patients with PE, because leg thrombi have often already embolized and Doppler as a screening test has limitations.

Venous thromboembolism is a multigenic disease. Virchow's triad of venous stasis in the lower limbs, a hypercoagulable state and damage to the venous endothelium still hold good today though they were formulated at the end of the 19th century.

Venous thrombi in the legs leading to thromboembolism are most frequent in the popliteal veins above the knee, and in the femoral vein within the thigh. Rarely, thrombi within the pelvic veins may also lead to PE. Deep vein thrombosis in the calves is common; generally, these thrombi extend upward into the popliteal veins before thromboembolism occurs.

■ Risk Factors for DVT and PE

Risk factors for DVT in the lower limbs include trauma to a limb, generalized trauma, immobilization of a limb, complete bed rest, sitting for long periods, as in air, train or vehicular travel, congestive heart failure, recent surgery, pregnancy, pelvic disease and recent myocardial infarction. Femoral and popliteal vein thromboses with thromboembolism are important complications of total hip or knee replacement surgery. Both oral contraceptives and postmenopausal hormone replacement therapy increase the risk of venous thromboembolism. The pulmonologist must not forget that chronic obstructive pulmonary disease (COPD) is an important risk factor both for DVT and PE. Cancer promotes the production of procoagulant factors and is an important risk factor in venous thrombosis and thromboembolism. Occasionally, venous thrombi in the legs and thromboembolism are manifestations of an occult cancer, in particular, cancer of the pancreas, ovary and a primary cancer of the liver. Any acute critical illness requiring intensive care may perhaps be associated with an increased incidence of venous thrombosis. Current data have identified heavy smoking and hypertension as new independent risk factors for DVT **(Table 1)**.

■ GENETIC DETERMINANTS

There have been major advances in our knowledge of the molecular markers of thrombophilic states. The two most important are the Leiden mutation of Factor V, which confers a resistance to activated protein C and the G20210A mutation of prothrombin. Both these occur in about 4% of the Caucasian population. Other rarer genetic defects include: antithrombin deficiency (0.02%), protein C deficiency (0.2%), and protein S deficiency (0.1%). Similar data from Indian populations are needed but at present lacking. Intriguingly, the Leiden mutation of factor V and the gene mutation of prothrombin are stronger risk factors for DVT than Protein C or S deficiency. Occasional patients are heterozygous for two of these anomalies and then carry a much greater thrombotic risk. Conversely, certain genetic traits offer protection. These include: the O blood group which appears to reduce the risk of DVT

Table 1: Environmental and acquired risk factors.

- Acquired thrombophilia:
  - Lupus anticoagulant
  - Antiphospholipid antibody syndrome
- Surgery:
  - Major abdominal, pelvic surgery
  - Hip, knee surgery
- Trauma:
  - Fractures
  - Spinal cord injury
- Immobilization:
  - Hemiplegia
  - Paraplegia
- Obstetrics:
  - Pregnancy
  - Puerperium
- Hormonal treatment:
  - Oral contraceptives
  - Hormone replacement therapy
  - Tamoxifen, raloxifene
- Cardiorespiratory:
  - Congestive cardiac failure
  - Myocardial infarction
  - Chronic obstructive pulmonary disease (COPD)
- Malignancy:
  - Abdominal, pelvic
  - Advanced, metastatic
  - Concurrent chemotherapy
- Inflammatory bowel disease
- Nephrotic syndrome

even in carriers of Factor V Leiden. Elevated levels of homocysteine are also independent risk factors though the genetics of transmission are not as yet clear. A detailed genetic prothrombotic screen should be mandatory in patients with a history of DVT or PE occurring without any other traditional risk factor, in those with a positive family history, those with recurrent episodes of thrombosis, patients with their initial thrombotic episode at a young age, and in patients with arterial and venous thrombosis or thrombosis in unusual sites.

■ PATHOPHYSIOLOGY

The clinical features of PE are due to three possible pathophysiological changes:

1. *Acute circulatory compromise* due to an obstructed pulmonary circulation. This occurs with massive embolism or when numerous thromboemboli block a large cross-section of the pulmonary circulation (>60–70% of the circulation). This circulatory compromise is characterized by pulmonary hypertension (PH), RV dilatation and dysfunction, right-sided heart failure and a low cardiac output, which when marked leads to cardiogenic shock. The dilated right ventricle causes a septal shift to the left, resulting in underfilling of the left ventricle, a decreased systemic cardiac output, and myocardial ischemia from reduced coronary perfusion.

2. *Gas exchange abnormalities* generally characterized by a low PaO_2 with a lowered $PaCO_2$. High ventilation-perfusion (V/Q) areas are responsible for increased dead space ventilation. Tachypnea and an increased minute ventilation allow a normal, and often a lower than normal $PaCO_2$ to be maintained. If the dead space is markedly increased, and the minute ventilation does not increase proportionately, the $PaCO_2$ may rise. The alveolar PCO_2 is characteristically slightly lower than the arterial $PaCO_2$.

Normal arterial blood gases do not exclude PE. In fact, arterial hypoxemia is generally never marked, except in massive embolism associated with a shock-like state. The PaO_2 is rarely less than 55 mm Hg. A lowered PaO_2 is due to V/Q mismatch resulting from atelectasis, and to redistribution of pulmonary blood flow, which causes a fall in the V/Q ratio in areas of the lung that are unobstructed by pulmonary emboli.

3. *Pulmonary infarction* may occur but is not commonly observed in PE. Patients with congestive heart failure are more prone to develop pulmonary infarction because of preexisting raised pulmonary venous pressure.

The clinical manifestations of thromboembolism often appear to be far more serious than what is expected from the degree of vascular occlusion. In critically ill patients in the ICU, this could be due to two causes: (i) a poor preexisting cardiopulmonary reserve; (ii) release of vasoactive and bronchoconstrictive mediators from platelets and perhaps from other sources, following embolism. This potentiates PH, accentuates V/Q disturbances, and adds to the already existing tachypnea.

The PE Spectrum

The outcome following a PE is a function of the size of the PE and the underlying cardiopulmonary status. A small PE may be poorly tolerated and tip the balance in a patient with advanced COPD while an otherwise fit young person might tolerate the effects of a larger PE without compromise. There is a spectrum in the severity of the PE, from mild to massive. At one end, the patient with mild PE may remain asymptomatic with the PE detected incidentally. In the Prospective Investigation of Pulmonary Embolism Diagnosis (PIOPED) study, there were 20 such patients who had mild PE which was not initially diagnosed and hence not treated. The mortality in these patients, untreated, was only 5%. At the other end of severity is a massive PE which can cause almost immediate cardiorespiratory arrest. A massive PE is one that results in hemodynamic instability. Overall, these PEs are rare; in the PIOPED series, only 10% of all PEs could be classified as massive. The mortality in this group was however 3–7% higher. The majority of PEs fall in between these two groups. This category includes submassive PE. These are patients with a sizeable clot burden, no hemodynamic instability when they first present, but show echocardiographic evidence of right heart dysfunction. These patients will be discussed in more detail later.

■ CLINICAL FEATURES: PULMONARY EMBOLISM SYNDROMES

The symptoms of PE are nonspecific and include dyspnea, chest pain, fever, cough, hemoptysis and apprehension.

The signs are equally nonspecific and include: tachypnea, tachycardia, crackles, a pleural rub, and an accentuated pulmonary component of the second heart sound. Evidence of an associated DVT must be carefully looked for, though this is often not clinically obvious. Because the symptoms and signs are nonspecific, attempts have been made to combine them into scoring systems. The best validated is that of Wells which can immediately be applied at the bedside when first seeing a patient **(Table 2)**. It gives the patient points based on: previous PE/DVT, heart rate more than 100/min, recent surgery or immobilization, clinical signs of DVT, alternative diagnosis less likely than PE, hemoptysis, and cancer. This scoring system can be applied to inpatients and outpatients and has recently been externally validated. Adding on D-dimer further increases the accuracy of this clinical prediction system.

The following pulmonary syndromes should be kept in mind **(Table 3)**.

1. *Pulmonary infarction syndrome:* This occurs due to peripheral pulmonary emboli causing pulmonary infarction. The hallmark of this syndrome is pleuritic chest pain and hemoptysis. Radiologically, the classic wedge-shaped pleural-based shadow is seen. Only about 20% of all PEs will present in this fashion.

Table 2: Wells' clinical prediction rule for pulmonary embolism (PE)*.

Clinical features	Points
• Clinical symptoms of DVT	3
• Other diagnosis less likely than PE	3
• Heart rate greater than 100 beats per minute	1.5
• Immobilization or surgery within past 4 weeks	1.5
• Previous DV or PE	1.5
• Hemoptysis	1
• Malignancy	1
Total	

(DVT: Deep venous thrombosis; PE: Pulmonary embolism)
*Risk score interpretation (probability of PE):
• >6 points: high risk (78.4%)
• 2 to 6 points: moderate risk (27.8%)
• <2 points: low risk (3.4%).

Table 3: Syndromes associated with pulmonary embolism.

• Pulmonary infarction syndrome
• Isolated dyspnea syndrome
• Syndromes associated with massive pulmonary embolism manifesting as:
  – Sudden death
  – Shock and/or prolonged syncope
  – Acute right heart failure
  – Acute respiratory failure
  – Severe bronchospasm and pulmonary edema
  – Combination of II, III, IV, V
• Subtle features like unexplained tachycardia, increasingly unstable circulatory state, supraventricular tachycardia, unexplained tachypnea, postural hypotension or syncope

2. *Isolated dyspnea syndrome:* A high index of suspicion is needed if this form of PE is not to be missed. It is often misdiagnosed and mislabeled as asthma or anxiety-related hyperventilation. An accompanying tachycardia may often be present. Another clue may be that these patients though having a normal SaO_2 at rest often desaturate when made to walk for a few minutes or climb a flight of stairs.

3. *Syndromes associated with massive PE:* The following manifestations singly or in combination may be observed:

  A. Sudden death—this may occur without apparent reason or typically follows straining over a bedpan.

  B. Shock and/or prolonged syncope—shock characterized by hypotension, tachycardia, sweating, and cold clammy extremities with or without substernal chest pain is a feature of massive

PE. The clinical picture may be indistinguishable from an acute myocardial infarct.

C. Acute right heart failure may be the presenting feature, with engorged neck veins, a prominent "a" wave in the neck, a right ventricular diastolic gallop and an accentuated pulmonary component of the second heart sound. The liver may be palpable and tender.

D. Acute respiratory failure with tachypnea, hypoxia associated at times with cyanosis and dyspnea.

E. Rarely, severe bronchospasm and pulmonary edema have also been reported. We have witnessed the former but not the latter.

F. Features of B, C, D, E are often combined in massive PE—various combinations are observed depending on the interval after acute embolism. Shock often predominates in the earlier phase and is associated with a raised central venous pressure, hypotension and hypoxemic respiratory failure. If recovery ensues, features of PH are more evident.

Pulmonary embolism, particularly small often multiple emboli occurring in already critically ill individuals may show very subtle features. These include any one or more of the following: unexplained tachycardia, increasingly unstable circulatory state, supraventricular tachycardia, unexplained tachypnea, postural hypotension or syncope, unexplained low-grade fever, icterus, and a marked rise in the erythrocyte sedimentation rate (ESR). There may be an unexplained fall in the PaO_2 or an increase in an already existing hypoxia. Sometimes a rapid deterioration in the clinical state is related to a silent PE. All these features described earlier, lack specificity and sensitivity. They could well be related and interpreted as being due to the critical illness per se, rather than to complicating pulmonary emboli rendering a correct diagnosis doubly difficult.

■ DIAGNOSTIC TESTS (TABLE 4)

1. *Chest radiograph:* The chest radiograph can be normal though this is rare with massive PE. In the PIOPED series of massive PE, only 16% of patients had a normal chest radiograph. Focal oligemia, if carefully looked for, will be noted in 40–80% of patients. Plate-like atelectasis, basal wedge-shaped shadows **(Figs. 1 and 2)** and pleural effusions are other distinctive but nonspecific radiological manifestations. The presence

Table 4: Diagnostic tests for pulmonary embolism (PE).
• Chest radiograph
• ECG
• D-dimer
• Lower limb venous compression ultrasonography
• Arterial blood gases
• Echocardiography
• Ventilation/perfusion lung scintigraphy
• Helical CT pulmonary angiography
• Pulmonary angiography

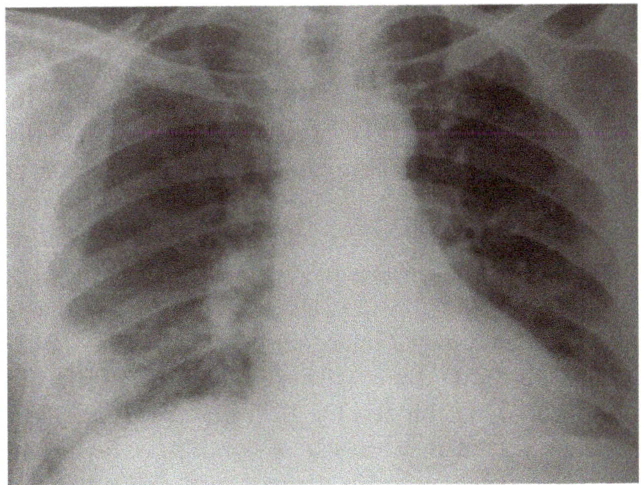

Fig. 1: Chest X-ray demonstrates a wedge-shaped opacity in the right lower zone with its apex pointing to the hilum representing a pulmonary infarct. Note the enlarged and prominent right pulmonary artery (Westermark sign).

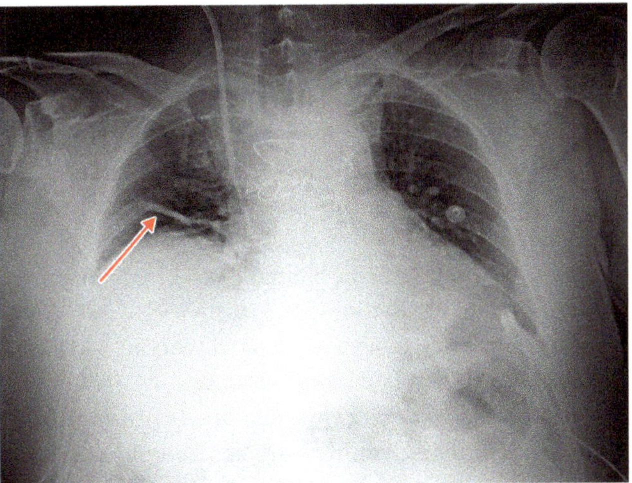

Fig. 2: Pulmonary infarct. Chest X-ray demonstrates a linear band in the right lower zone with an elevated right dome of diaphragm. The linear band represents an infarct with elevation of the right dome due to underlying volume loss.

of preexisting cardiopulmonary disease makes appreciation of these features even more difficult. The chest radiograph is also invaluable in patients with PE for differential diagnosis of other conditions like pneumonia, left ventricular failure (LVF) or pneumothorax.

2. *Electrocardiogram (ECG):* The ECG is usually normal in smaller PE. In massive PE a normal ECG is uncommon but did occur in as many as 30% of PIOPED patients with major PE. Transient ST-T changes are the most common ECG manifestation and may occur in 50–70% of patients. A $S_1Q_3T_3$ pattern may be seen, along with transient right bundle branch block (RBBB) or atrial fibrillation. Anterior lead T wave inversion is the pattern that best correlates with the severity of the PE, occurring in 90% of massive compared to 20% of nonmassive PE.

3. *D-dimer:* It is a breakdown product of cross-linked fibrin and is a sensitive marker of acute thrombosis. A normal D-dimer in a low clinical probability setting is an accurate way of ruling out PE. On the other hand, though the D-dimer is very specific for fibrin, the specificity of this test for PE is poor because fibrin is produced in a variety of conditions including inflammation, infection, necrosis, and cancer. Hence a D-dimer above 500 µg/L has a poor positive predictive value for PE and cannot reliably rule in the disease. But a D-dimer level below this cut-off value reliably rules it out, especially in a low probability setting. Nuclear scanning or spiral CT angiography may not be needed in this group. There are presently four different assays available and it is important to use the highly sensitive enzyme-linked immunosorbent assay (ELISA) or automated turbidimetric assay to get the most sensitive results. Results are generally available at the bedside in an hour, making this a cost-effective and useful screening test.

4. *Biomarkers:* A rise in the biomarkers—brain natriuretic peptide (BNP). N-terminal Pro-BNP (NT-pro BNP) and troponin has been associated with an increased mortality or PE related complications.

5. *Lower limb venous compression ultrasonography:* In studies using venography as the gold standard for detecting proximal DVT, lower limb venous compression ultrasonography, an entirely noninvasive test, had a sensitivity of 97% and a specificity of 98% for symptomatic, proximal DVT.

The absence of full compressibility of the deep vein on applying pressure through the ultrasound probe is the single best validated diagnostic criterion. The advantage of this test is that it is noninvasive and can be performed at the bedside. The finding of DVT by ultrasonography in a patient with suspected PE is sufficient evidence to commence anticoagulant therapy without any further testing. Approximately 50% of PE suspects will have evidence of DVT on ultrasonography and further invasive and costly tests are not required in these patients. The exact position of ultrasonography in the diagnostic algorithm of PE is still being refined.

6. *Arterial blood gases:* Hypoxia is usual but not universal following a major PE. Approximately 20% of patients with proven PE will have a normal arterial oxygen pressure and alveolar-arterial oxygen gradient.

7. *Echocardiography:* It is an enormously useful test to detect the presence and severity of right ventricular (RV) pressure overload. RV dysfunction (RV dilatation, dyskinesia) on ECHO helps in stratification of these patients. If present it denotes more than 30% obstruction to the pulmonary circuit. Other echocardiographic findings include: increased RV/LV diameter ratio, paradoxical septal motion, pulmonary artery dilatation and evidence of tricuspid regurgitation. The sensitivity of these signs which are often combined is between 40% and 70% in patients with clinically suspected PE and their specificity approaches 90%. Thus, echocardiography has emerged as a first-line test in patients with suspected massive PE. It is extremely useful in the differential diagnosis of shock due to massive PE from cardiogenic shock, cardiac tamponade, valvular heart disease, and aortic dissection. Indeed, absence of PH and/or right ventricular dilatation and hypokinesia makes PE as the cause of shock unlikely. In a small subset of patients with PE, transthoracic echocardiography allows a direct visualization of the clot in the right heart chambers or in the right main pulmonary artery.

8. *V/Q lung scintigraphy:* The landmark PIOPED study showed us that V/Q scanning retains its importance. The perfusion scan is done by injection of albumin macroaggregates labeled by technetium-99m. The macroaggregates are trapped in approximately 0.1% of the pulmonary capillary circuit and may

be imaged by a gamma camera. Any disease that narrows the airways or fills the alveoli will result in hypoxic pulmonary vasoconstriction, hence this pattern is not highly specific for PE. If the perfusion defect is large or segmental it makes the diagnosis more likely. The addition of ventilation scintigraphy by xenon-133 or aerosolized technetium-99m further increases the specificity. This so-called mismatched defect, i.e. perfusion defect with normal ventilation, is highly predictive of PE. Based on revised data from the PIOPED study, lung scans are currently classified into normal, high probability and nondiagnostic. The high negative predictive value of a normal lung scan has been confirmed by several studies including a large outcome study. Equally useful is the positive predictive value of a high probability scan (around 90%) and this is sufficient evidence to rule in PE and proceed with treatment without subjecting the patient to further testing. Recent evidence suggests that a chest radiograph may replace the ventilation scan and be combined with a perfusion scan to give excellent overall agreement of 88% and positive predictive value of 86% for a scintigraphic mismatch. Unfortunately, in the latest study from Wells and his group, only 41% of all V/Q scans fell into the normal or high probability group. The majority were nondiagnostic. These scans carry a 30% likelihood of PE and hence the majority (around 60%) of patients who undergo V/Q scanning will need to undergo further tests to rule in or rule out suspected PE.

9. *Helical CT pulmonary angiography (Figs. 3 to 8):* This noninvasive test offers excellent imaging of the pulmonary vasculature. It has by and large replaced V/Q scanning as a diagnostic modality for PE and has well-nigh completely eliminated the need for invasive pulmonary angiography. It is the quickest and surest way of clinching the diagnosis and cuts short the need for many of the diagnostic tests described above.

Newer and still evolving technology used in helical CT pulmonary angiography has further increased the sensitivity and specificity for detecting PE, the sensitivity ranging from 83% to 100% and specificity from 89% to 97%. This sensitivity and specificity favors comparably with that observed in invasive pulmonary angiography.

The advantages of CT angiography when compared to V/Q screening and invasive pulmonary angiography are summarized here:

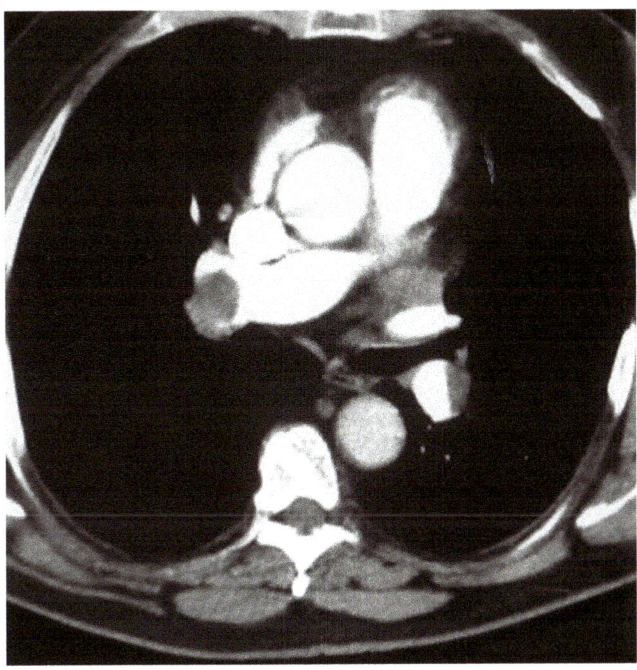

Fig. 3: Bilateral pulmonary emboli. CT angiography demonstrates pulmonary emboli in both pulmonary arteries.

- CT angiography is noninvasive, convenient and can be performed safely and quickly in critically ill patients, particularly those in shock and/or in acute right heart failure.
- Studies comparing CT angiography to V/Q scanning suggest that CT angiography is a better test because of more frequent definitive confirmation of pulmonary emboli.
- In a critically ill individual, there is often a large differential diagnosis to PE. A CT angiography offers evidence of other causes as well as that of PE, which neither a V/Q scan nor invasive pulmonary angiography can provide.
- CT angiography of the legs and pelvis could be performed with the same contrast injection used to image the pulmonary vasculature. Detection of DVT in the femoropopliteal veins is as accurate as with ultrasonography. This procedure can also detect clots in the iliac, renal and caval veins, which are ultrasonographically inaccessible.

The major limitation of helical CT pulmonary angiography is the inability to diagnose subsegmental branch emboli, with sufficient certainty. However, invasive pulmonary angiography also has significant limitations in detecting isolated subsegmental emboli.

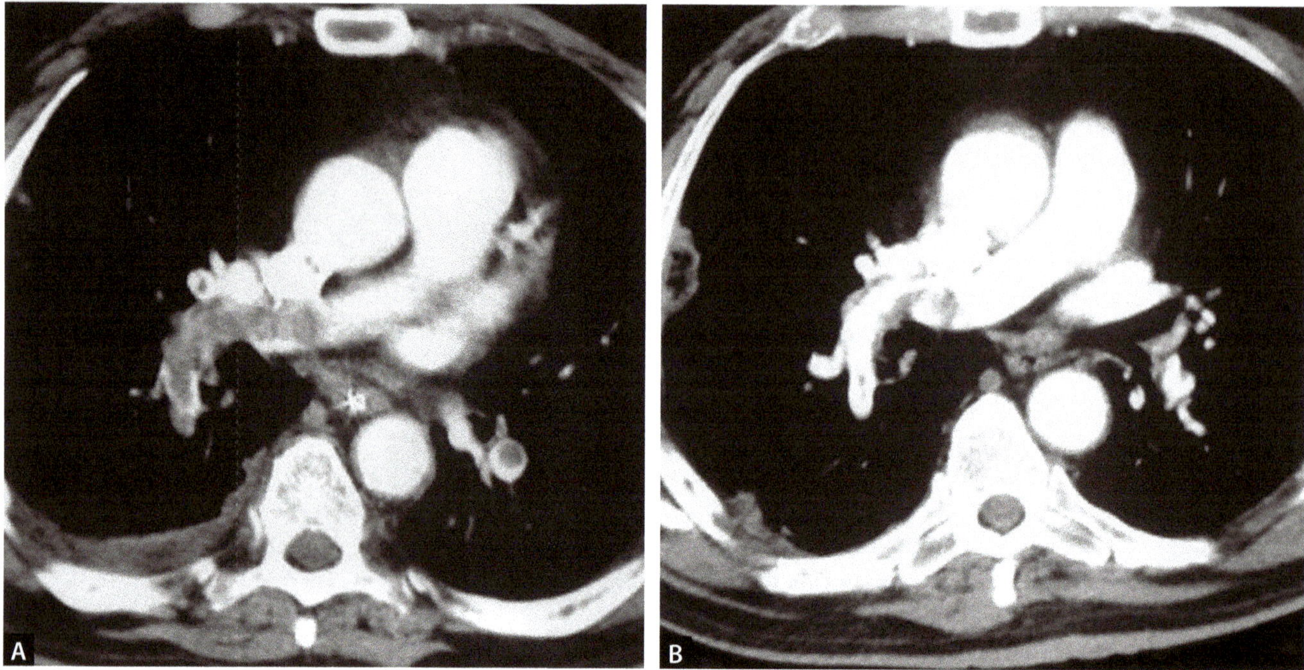

Figs. 4A and B: Pulmonary emboli. (A) CT angiography demonstrates a large embolus in the right pulmonary artery and a smaller embolus in the left pulmonary artery. (B) CT angiography following anticoagulation therapy demonstrates considerable resolution in the thrombi.

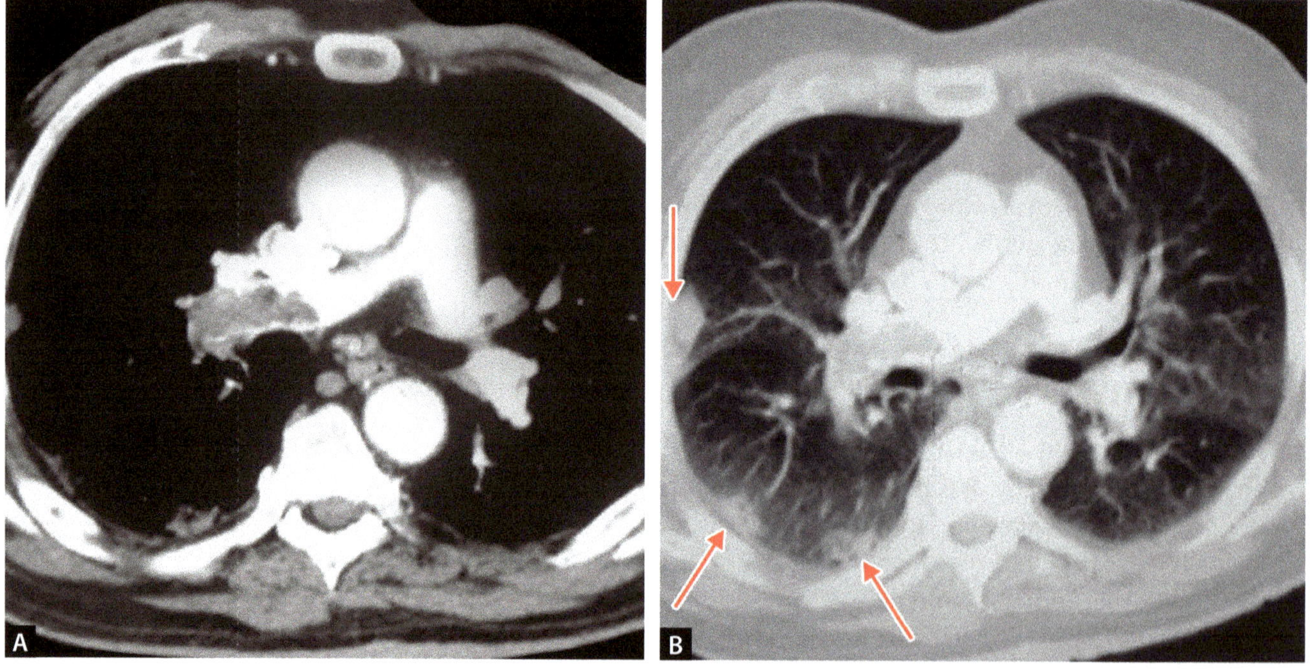

Figs. 5A and B: Pulmonary emboli with pulmonary infarcts. (A) CT angiography demonstrates a large embolus in the right pulmonary artery. (B) Lung window setting demonstrates multiple wedge-shaped subpleural soft tissue density lesions representing pulmonary infarcts.

The only other major limitation of helical CT pulmonary angiography compared to V/Q scanning is the need to use contrast material, precluding its use in patients with renal failure and in patients allergic to the dye.

It is also inadvisable to use this modality in pregnant women.

10. *Pulmonary angiography:* The role of pulmonary angiography in the diagnosis of PE is now sharply

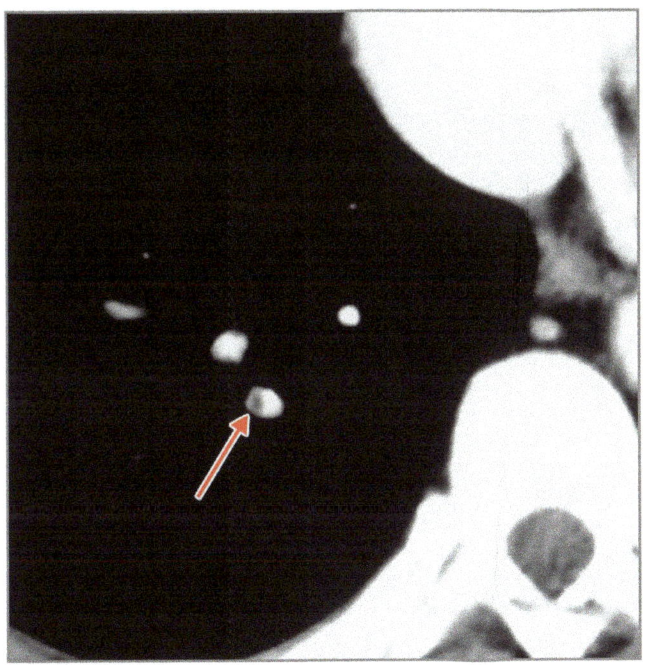

Fig. 6: Subsegmental pulmonary embolus. CT angiography demonstrates a small embolus in subsegmental pulmonary arteries.

reduced and almost extinct. Perhaps a helical pulmonary CT angiography might miss out on subsegmental pulmonary emboli which an invasive CT angiography would detect. But is it necessary to diagnose with certainty subsegmental emboli? Data from three large studies suggests that underdiagnosing subsegmental emboli by avoiding pulmonary angiography does not affect the clinical outcomes of recurrent embolism or death. A clinical outcome approach is as safe as the PIOPED approach, less expensive, more convenient, less fraught with immediate risks to the patient, and more acceptable to the patient and the physician.

■ RISK STRATIFICATION OF PATIENTS WITH ACUTE PE

It is important to be aware of the diagnostic tests listed earlier. Some are simple and cheap enough to be available to almost all hospitals in poor countries; others may not be available in the poorer parts of the developing world. It is equally important to perform a risk stratification of patients admitted for a suspected PE. A risk stratification allows a quick triage of patients arriving at a hospital and enables the physician to deliver optimal treatment according to current knowledge.

Thus for example, patients of PE who have sustained hypotension, unresponsive to vasopressors and who are in cardiogenic shock are at the highest risk for death. Advanced age, underlying cancer, comorbid cardiac or respiratory disease, sustained tachycardia, hypotension, right ventricular dysfunction, and hypoxemia are the main factors which determine the outcome of PE. The abovementioned features have been summarized in the pulmonary embolism severity index (PESI) and its simplified version (sPESI) **(Table 5)**.

Patients classified as PESI I and II or sPESI less than 1 can be reliably excluded from having an increased risk of a 30-day mortality. However, in the absence of hypotension, the above clinical assumption has a low predictive value for the risk of death or other PE complications.

Two other factors not included in PESI or sPESI also contribute to increased risk in acute PE. They are the presence of right ventricular dysfunction (RVD) and the presence of elevated cardiac biomarkers BNP, NT-Pro BNP and troponin. In *normotensive patients* elevated biomarkers and an echocardiography positive for RV dysfunction have been shown to be associated with an increased risk of death due to PE, cardiogenic shock and recurrent PE. In a cohort of 688 normotensive patients with PE it was confirmed that elevated biomarkers and echocardiography showing RV dysfunction have independent prognostic value.

According to the recent guidelines of the European Society of Cardiology, *patients with hypotension are high-risk patients.* Among normotensive patients those with PESI I-II or sPESI less than 1 are considered low risk without further risk stratification. Normotensives with a sPESI more than 1 or those with either RVD or elevated cardiac biomarkers are classified as intermediate low risk patients, and normotensives with sPESI more than 1 with both RVD and elevated cardiac biomarkers are classified as intermediate high risk patients **(Table 6)**.

Mortality of Pulmonary Embolism

The International Cooperative Pulmonary Embolism Registry (ICOPER) enrolled 2,454 consecutive PE patients from 52 hospitals in seven countries with the specific purpose of establishing the 3-month all-cause mortality rate and to identify factors associated with death **(Table 7)**. The results are important enough to discuss here. The all-cause mortality rate was 17.4% at 3 months. Importantly, most patients who

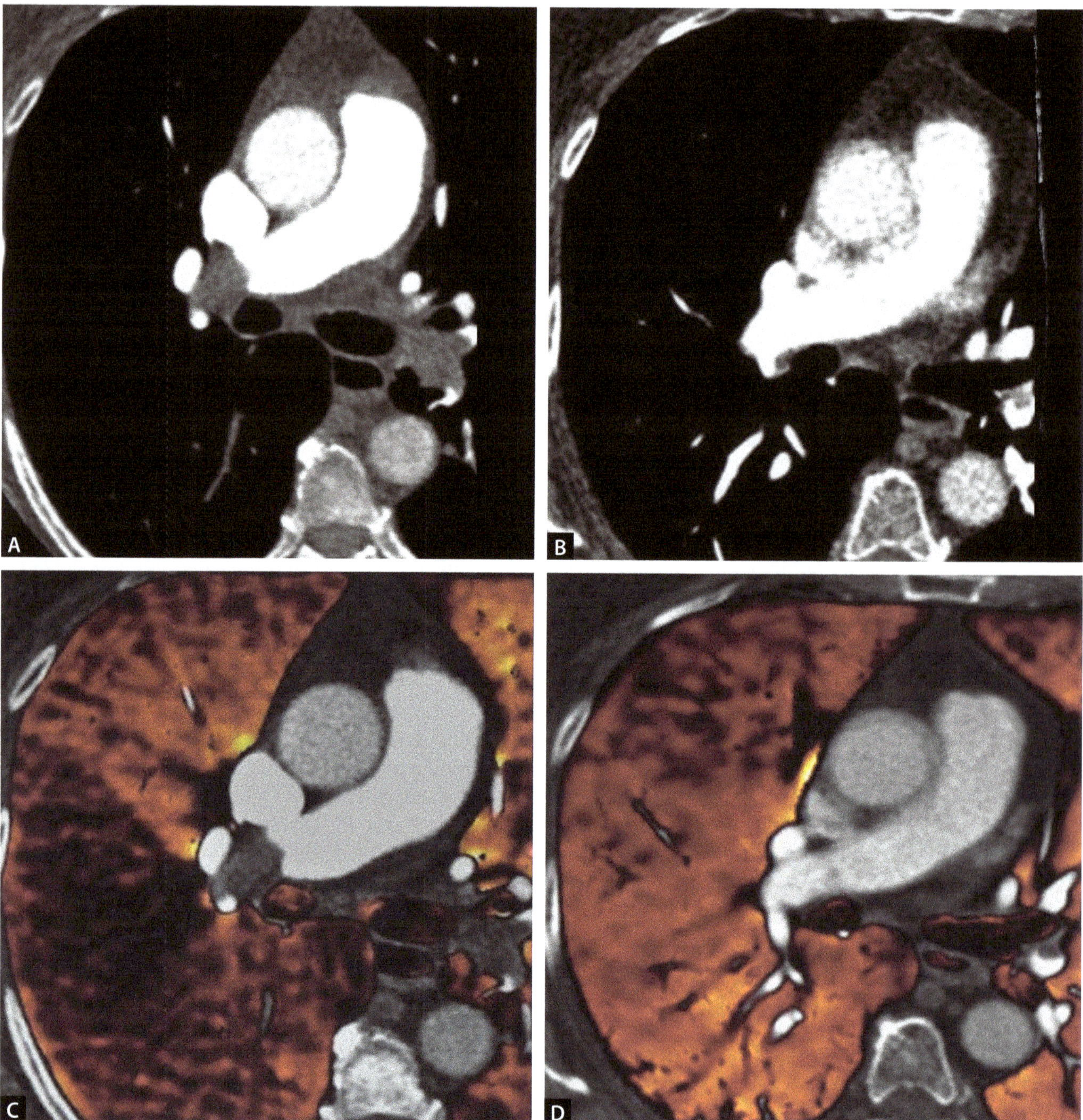

Figs. 7A to D: Pulmonary embolism. (A) CT angiography demonstrates a thrombus in the right pulmonary artery. (B) Dual-energy CT angiography reveals perfusion defect secondary to thrombus. (C and D) Follow-up CT angiography after thrombolysis reveals resolution of thrombus in right pulmonary artery, corresponding dual-energy CT angiography reveals resolution of perfusion defect.

succumbed died of their PE, not of other comorbidities like cancer. Age greater than 70 years increased the likelihood of death by 60%. Other risk factors which independently increased the likelihood of death by 2–3 fold included cancer, congestive cardiac failure (CCF), COPD, hypotension (systolic BP <90 mm Hg), tachypnea (respiratory rate >20/min) and evidence of right ventricular hypokinesia on echocardiogram. *The*

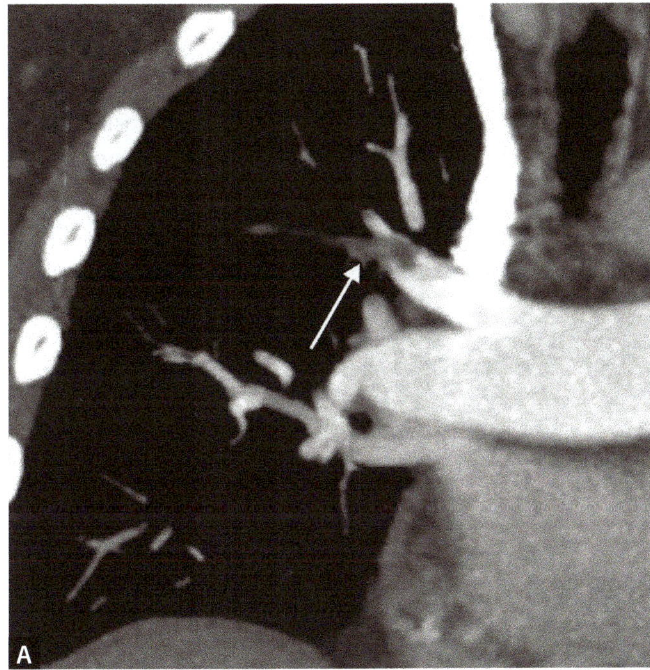 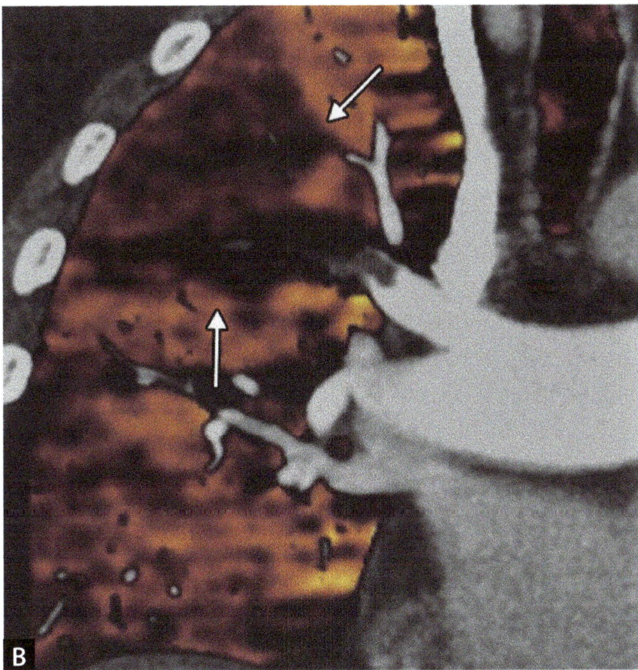

Figs. 8A and B: (A) CT angiography reveals a segmental embolus, in the right upper lobe pulmonary arterial branch. (B) corresponding dual-energy CT perfusion images reveal a segmental perfusion defect.

Table 5: Simplified pulmonary embolism severity index (sPESI).

Variables	Point
• Age > 80 years	1
• History of chronic cardiopulmonary disease	1
• History of cancer	1
• Pulse >110 beats/min	1
• Systolic BP < 100 mm Hg	1
• SaO_2< 90	1

Table 6: Risk stratification of patients with pulmonary embolism (PE) according to European Society of Cardiology (ESC).

Condition	Risk
PESI I–II or sPESI < 1	Low risk
sPESI >1 or with RVD/elevated cardiac biomarkers	Intermediate low risk
sPESI > 1 with both RVD and elevated cardiac biomarkers	Intermediate high risk
Patients with hypotension	High risk

(RVD: Right ventricular dysfunction; sPESI: Simplified pulmonary embolism severity index)

mortality rate of patients with sustained hypotension or cardiogenic shock due to acute cor pulmonale ranges from 35% to 68%.

Table 7: Predictors of poor prognosis in PE.

- Age more than 70 years
- Shock
- Hypotension
- SaO_2 < 90
- Right ventricular dysfunction (clinically or on ECHO)
- Right ventricular thrombus
- Tachypnea (respiratory rate >20/min)
- Cancer
- COPD
- Elevated BNP and NT—Pro BNP
- Elevated troponin I, T-levels

Recurrence

The rate of recurrence is reported to be 8% at 6 months [*Ref: Kyrle PA, Rosendaal FR, Eichinger S. Risk assessment for recurrent venous thrombosis. Lancet. 2010;376(9757): 2032-9*]. The rate is higher in patients who have suffered an unprovoked PE and in those with risk factors such as cancer, COPD. Chronic thromboembolic pulmonary hypertension is perhaps not as uncommon as is believed. It generally occurs within 2 years of PE; its presenting feature is breathlessness on exertion.

The following section first discusses the pharmacological agents used to treat acute PE, chiefly anticoagulants and thrombolytic agents, as well as measures necessary to provide cardiorespiratory support. It then briefly discusses surgical embolectomy and finally proposes clinical strategies in the management of acute PE.

■ MANAGEMENT OF PULMONARY EMBOLISM (TABLE 8)

1. *Anticoagulation with unfractionated or low molecular weight heparin (LMWH):* LMWH has several pharmacokinetic and practical advantages over unfractionated heparin. These are summarized as follow:
   - Ease of use without need for routine monitoring of prothrombin time or international normalized ratio (INR).
   - More predictable anticoagulant response.
   - Standard dose irrespective of weight apart from chronic renal failure (CRF) and morbid obesity.
   - Longer half-life which permits once or twice daily dosing.
   - Facilitates earlier discharge and in some stable patients even home treatment.
   - Lower risk of heparin-induced thrombocytopenia (HIT).
   - Less binding to osteoblasts hence less osteopenia.

   A meta-analysis of over 3,000 patients who participated in DVT treatment studies showed that those receiving LMWH had lower mortality rates, less recurrence and suffered fewer complications including reduced HIT. All this was achieved at lower cost compared to unfractionated heparin. A pivotal study by Levine showed that enoxaparin, a LMWH administered twice daily reduced mean hospital stay from 6.5 days to 1.1 days with fewer deaths and fewer bleeding complications. As a result of this and similar trials, the FDA has approved enoxaparin (1 mg/kg twice a day) and tinzaparin (175 units/kg once daily) for outpatient or home treatment for patients who present with symptomatic DVT with or without associated PE. As opposed to this data, there is as yet no data to suggest that out-patient treatment can be safely recommended in patients with PE alone.

Whether LMWH or unfractionated heparin is used, it serves as a bridge for 5–7 days till anticoagulation with warfarin takes over.

2. *Oral anticoagulation:* Oral anticoagulation with warfarin is the mainstay of treatment and the dose is adjusted according to the prothrombin time. This is standardized by reporting results as the INR with a target INR of 2–3 being aimed for. In patients with recurrent PEs or underlying thrombophilic states the target INR is raised to 3–4. Warfarin is not reliably effective for at least 5 days after it has been commenced. During this period patients are especially vulnerable to thrombosis hence concomitant heparin must be administered. If warfarin is used as monotherapy without heparin it will paradoxically result in hypercoagulability by decreasing the level of Protein C, resulting in a higher rate of recurrent venous thromboembolism.

   Warfarin interacts with a number of commonly used drugs and even with the Vitamin K in green leafy vegetables resulting in wide fluctuations of INR. In addition some patients (2–3% of the general population) have a genetic defect (polymorphisms in the cytochrome P450 CYP2C9) which makes them slow metabolizers and prone to major bleeding complications with even lower doses of warfarin.

   The current American College of Chest Physicians (ACCP) guidelines on optimal duration of anticoagulation after a DVT/PE is ideally three months, if the patient had an underlying precipitating factor which is no longer applicable. In patients with a first episode of idiopathic DVT/PE a 6–12 month initial period of anticoagulation is recommended. A study called the PREVENT trial showed that after 6 months of warfarin, lower intensity dosing, so as to target an INR of 1.5–2 resulted in a further significant reduction in the risk of recurrences by 64%. In patients who have documented antiphospholipid antibodies or an underlying thrombophilic state, indefinite anticoagulation therapy is recommended.

   Recurrent thrombosis: The 5-year incidence of recurrent venous thromboembolism off anticoagulants is approximately 30%. Well-documented factors for recurrent thrombosis include an initial unprovoked DVT or PE, advancing age, male sex, race (higher in blacks), presence of active cancer, obesity, an elevated serum d-Dimer prior to stopping warfarin or 2 months after stopping warfarin, and ongoing immobility.

Table 8: Management of pulmonary embolism.

- Anticoagulation with unfractionated or low molecular weight heparin (LMWH)
- Oral anticoagulation
- Thrombolysis
- Cardiorespiratory support
- Surgical embolectomy or catheter-directed embolectomy

Complications of warfarin include bleeding, skin necrosis, alopecia, and rashes. When patients present with very high INRs as a result of warfarin, the majority will be asymptomatic even with INR values > 5. Most can be managed with fresh frozen plasma if they are bleeding or low oral doses of Vitamin K. The usual injectable dose of 10 mg of Vitamin K will result in patients being resistant to further anticoagulation with warfarin for at least a week and hence should be avoided. Major contraindications to anticoagulant therapy are listed in **Table 9**.

3. *Thrombolysis:* Thrombolysis can be a potentially lifesaving measure in patients with massive PE. Thrombolytic agents such as TPA act on plasminogen by cleaving the peptide bond between arginine at position 560 and valine at position 561, thereby converting plasminogen to plasmin and dissolving the embolus. They help dissolve the clot at source in the pulmonary vessels and perform a "medical embolectomy", preventing the downward spiral into right heart failure. They may also help in dissolution of clot at its source in the pelvic and deep veins of the leg.

Besides recombinant tissue plasminogen activator (rTPA) other thrombolytic agent in use is alteplase (FDA approved) 100 mg given once in 2 hours. Tenecteplase is a more recent thrombolytic agent, with the advantage of being administered in a single bolus dose of 30–50 mg over 2 hours. Streptokinase continues to be used in poor countries and is perhaps as effective than the more expensive alteplase. It is given in a loading dose of 250,000 U over 30 minutes and then 100,000 units over 24 hours. *Thrombolytics can be administered within a 2-week time window from the onset of PE*; and dramatic results have been reported in patients with massive PE, even in patients with shock and circulatory arrest. In patients with PE who present with hemodynamic compromise and therefore are at a high risk, there is no doubt that thrombolysis is indicated and can dramatically reduce mortality. The beneficial hemodynamic effects of thrombolysis far outweigh the risk of bleeding and the only

contradiction to thrombolytic therapy in these patients is active uncontrolled bleeding.

The use of thrombolytic therapy in acute PE who are at intermediate risk is a bit controversial and we need to consider three studies with regard to the subject. The first was the landmark randomized double-blind controlled study by Konstantinides (NEJM 2003) on 256 patients of PE who had RVD on echocardiography. The patients were randomized to heparin + rTPA and to heparin + placebo. Though there was no difference in overall mortality in the two arms of the study, the clinical deterioration was significantly greater in those who did not receive rTPA. The 30-day event free period was also significantly greater in those receiving the thrombolytic agent. It was therefore proposed that thrombolytic therapy be used in this group of patients.

Recently the PEITHO study randomized 1,000 normotensive PE patients with both RVD + elevated troponin to receive either heparin and telectaplase or placebo and heparin. The main clinical composite endpoints of death from any cause or hemodynamic decompensation occurred in 2.6% of the telectaplase group and 5.6% of the placebo group. This increased efficacy in the telectaplase group was however associated with an increase in major bleeding and intracranial hemorrhage (2.4%) as compared to the heparin group (0.2%).

Finally a recent systematic review analyzed for the first time results of thrombolytic therapy in intermediate risk patients. Here again, thrombolytic therapy resulted in a significant reduction in PE related deaths but at the expense of a significant increase in the risk of major bleeding and fatal intracranial hemorrhage.

The current guidelines from the European Society of Cardiology suggest that the use of thrombolytic therapy is not recommended in all patients with intermediate risk PE but should be considered if clinical features of hemodynamic decompensation appear. This occurs in 5% of intermediate risk PE patients at a medium delay of 1.8 days after admission. These guidelines need not however be followed blindly. Clinical judgment is important particularly in patients who fall in high intermediate risk group.

4. *Cardiorespiratory support:* This is imperative in major or massive PE. Shock should be promptly treated. An intravenous (IV) infusion of isoproterenol (1–2 mg in 500 mL dextrose) is very useful as it dilates the pulmonary vasculature. If possible, the patient should

Table 9: Contraindications to anticoagulant therapy.

- Recent major surgery/ocular surgery/neurosurgery
- Diastolic BP > 110 mm Hg
- CNS hemorrhage
- Recent trauma/head injury
- Recent cerebrovascular accident/transient ischemic attack
- GI bleeding or other hemorrhagic diathesis
- Concomitant hepatic/renal failure

have a central venous line inserted and it is advisable to keep the central venous pressure (CVP) between 12 mm Hg and 14 mm Hg in order to ensure an adequate right ventricular stroke volume. This is best achieved by infusing 500 mL Dextran or Haemaccel, which besides raising right atrial pressure, also expands the pulmonary vascular bed, and thereby reduces pulmonary vascular resistance. If the patient does not respond to isoproterenol, or has marked tachycardia to start with, it is best to use dobutamine. Dopamine may need to be used in addition to dobutamine. The use of digoxin is disappointing, but it may be used in a dose of 0.25 mg intravenously to start with, and repeated 6-hourly till a digitalizing dose of 1 mg is given over 24 hours.

Oxygen is administered at 6–8 L/minute. Ventilator support is invariably required in the presence of acute cardiorespiratory failure. Morphine or pethidine is used for the relief of pain and/or restlessness.

An important question to answer is—What if thrombolytic therapy fails? The optimal therapy in this situation is unclear. Possible options include—repeat systemic thrombolysis, catheter-directed thrombolysis, catheter or surgical embolectomy. The choice is probably dependent on the expertise of individuals in an institution.

A catheter-directed thrombus removal with or without thrombolysis can also be tried in certain situations—those at high risk of bleeding if systemic thrombolysis is used, those with shock who would likely die before systemic thrombolysis can take effect (that is within hours).

Surgical embolectomy: Open surgical embolectomy is the most effective procedure for emergent removal of large amounts of thrombus due to acute PE. Surgery is especially useful in those in whom thrombolysis is contraindicated and who have not yet deteriorated to the point of cardiorespiratory arrest or shock. In this setting, when used in patients with anatomically extensive PE and concomitant moderate to severe RV dysfunction, Goldhaber and colleagues report impressive 89% survival rates. Impressive survival rates have been reported even in patients taken up *in extremis* after suffering cardiopulmonary arrest following massive PE.

Catheter-directed modalities: Several modalities are available but none clearly superior to the other. The modalities include—ultrasound-assisted thrombolysis, rheolytic embolectomy, rotational embolectomy, suction embolectomy, thrombus fragmentation. None of these

modalities is without risks. These include perforation of the pulmonary artery with resulting pericardial hemorrhage and cardiac tamponade, life-threatening hemoptysis, infection, cardiac arrest. The simultaneous use of thrombolytic therapy increases the risk of hemorrhagic side effects.

Management Strategies for Acute PE

Probable PE—hemodynamically unstable (hypotension, shock) **(Flowchart 1)**:

- *Resuscitate*:
    - Volume load of 500 mL to expand and dilate the pulmonary circulation.
    - IV noradrenaline infusion to raise blood pressure and improve right ventricular function. Maintain MAP > 65 mm Hg.
    - Inotropic support preferably with dobutamine 5–10 µg/kg.
    - In extreme shock and hypoxia, ventilate using low tidal volumes and keeping low plateau pressures.
- If sufficiently resuscitated to allow transfer to imaging department—CT pulmonary angiography. Thrombolyze if result is positive. If negative search for other causes of hypotension, shock.
- If CT pulmonary angiography not possible, do a 2D ECHO. If ECHO shows evidence of right ventricular dysfunction, thrombolyse.
- If during resuscitation a Doppler of the leg veins show thrombosis of the popliteal, femoral, iliac veins, thrombolyse without waiting for a CT pulmonary angiography or a 2D ECHO. Both these can be done later once the patient is stable.
- Thrombolysis should be followed by IV heparin; do not give thrombolytic therapy and heparin at the same time.
- If thrombolytic therapy is for any reason contra-indicated, surgical or catheter-directed embolectomy plus IVC filter insertion.

Probable PE—hemodynamically stable **(Flowchart 2)**.

■ PREVENTIVE MEASURES

Prevention of venous thrombosis, with the associated risk of PE, is a major objective in the management of critically ill patients in the intensive care unit (ICU). These patients often form a high-risk group as a consequence of bed rest, serious infections, or trauma.

Flowchart 1: Algorithm for hemodynamically unstable patients with suspected PE (also *see* text).

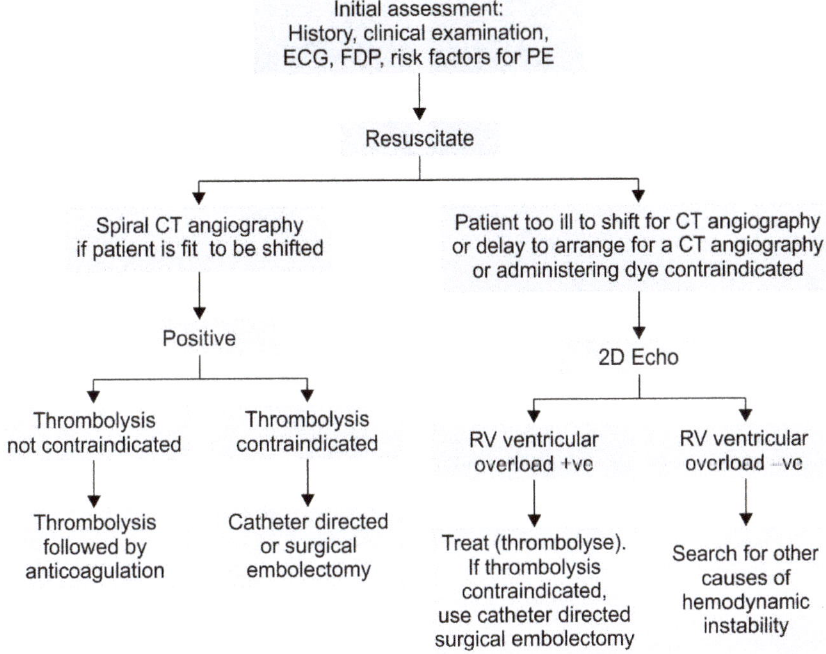

Flowchart 2: Algorithm for hemodynamically stable patients with suspected PE.

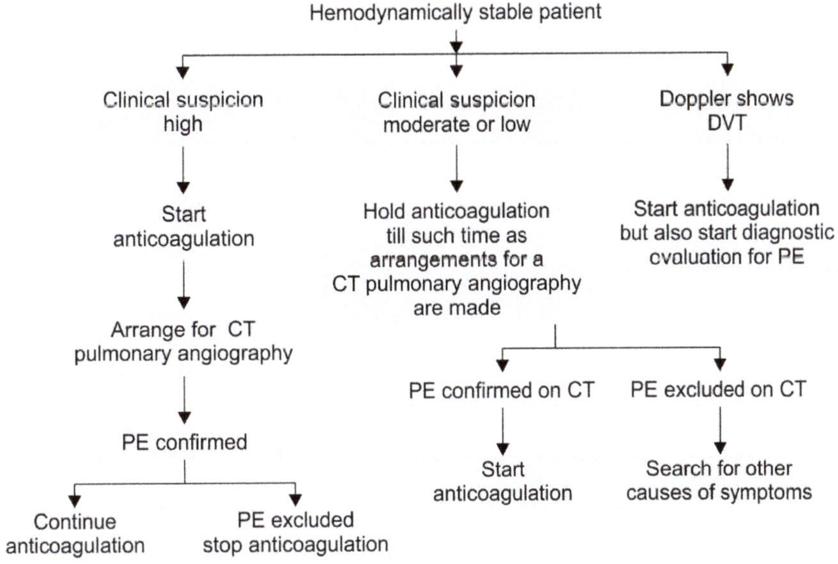

Note : 2D echo is preferably done in all PE confirmed patients. If right ventricular load is present a decision should be made on 'Yes' or 'No' to thrombolytic therapy depending on clinical background severity. If 'Yes' hold anticoagulants, thrombolyse and restart anticoagulation, if 'No' continue to anticoagulation.

Prevention of venous thrombosis in high-risk patients reduces morbidity. High-risk patients include the old and obese, those who are poorly mobile or are confined to bed, patients with myocardial infarction or a stroke, or those with atrial fibrillation and congestive heart failure. Postoperative patients are also at high risk, particularly after orthopedic surgery (particularly hip replacement or hip fracture), gynecological surgery, and other major

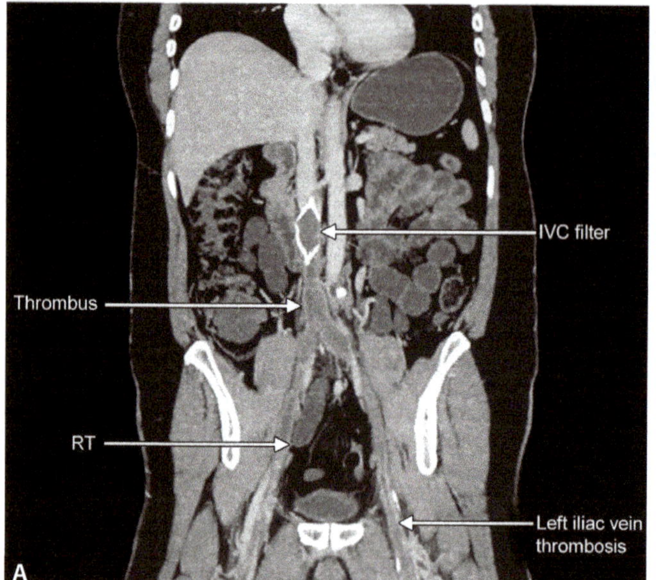

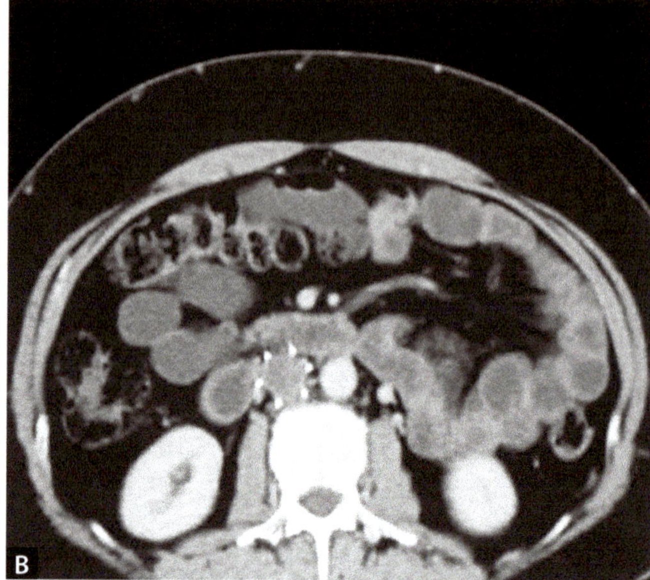

Figs. 9A and B: IVC filter: CT angiography following placement of IVC filter demonstrates IVC filter in situ with extensive thrombosis of IVC and iliac veins distal to the IVC filter.

surgery. Low molecular weight heparin like enoxaparin given in a dose 40 mg or 60 mg (depending on body weight and renal function) once daily offers good prophylaxis against DVT. Compression stockings over lower limbs, movement of the lower limbs at the ankles and knees, pneumatic compression of the lower limbs, all help to prevent DVT. Any form of heparin is contraindicated in certain patients—as after trauma, following surgery on the brain and spinal cord, or in patients with an acute peptic ulcer or a bleeding diathesis. In this group one can only offer pneumatic compression of the lower limbs, with active and passive movements at the ankles and knees as prophylaxis.

Once venous thrombosis is detected low molecular weight heparin in a dose of 40 or 60 mg of enoxaparin twice daily is given. Warfarin is started on the same day. It takes about a week of warfarin to take effect; heparin should be continued till such time as the INR is more than 2. As mentioned earlier, a 6–12 month period of anticoagulants is advised after the first episode of DVT/PE for which there is no apparent cause.

Transvenous Insertion of a Filter in the Inferior Vena Cava (Figs. 9A and B)

This is achieved by the placement of a filter in the inferior vena cava generally below the renal veins. The procedure

Table 10: Specific indications for vena caval interruption.
• Pulmonary embolism in patients in whom anticoagulants are absolutely contraindicated
• Recurrent thromboembolism in spite of adequate anticoagulation
• Hemodynamically unstable patients who have survived a massive embolism
• Patients with septic pulmonary embolism
• Prophylaxis in high risk patients

is done by a vascular surgeon or an interventional radiologist through the transvenous route. The filter stops emboli from the lower limb or pelvic veins from reaching the lungs. Specific indications for vena caval interruption include the following **(Table 10):**

- Pulmonary embolism in patients in whom anticoagulants are absolutely contraindicated—as in the neurosurgical patient, or in those with active bleeding.
- Recurrent thromboembolism in spite of adequate anticoagulation.
- Patients who have survived a massive embolism, but who are hemodynamically unstable, and in whom the risk of a fresh embolism is ever present.
- Patients with septic pulmonary embolism from thrombi in the lower limbs or pelvis, who have shown an unsatisfactory response after 48 hours of antibiotic plus anticoagulant therapy.

- *Prophylaxis in high-risk patients, as in:*
  - Extensive or progressive venous thrombosis;
  - In conjunction with catheter-based or surgical pulmonary embolectomy;
  - In patients with active cancer with extensive venous thrombosis of the pelvic or leg veins.

Vena caval interruption in the last four groups should be accompanied by the use of heparin in the dosage recommended earlier.

Though IVC filters reduce the incidence of short-term embolic recurrence and reduce short-term (90 days) mortality, this benefit may be lost over a prolonged period of time. In fact there appears to be a long-term increase in the incidence of venous thromboembolism following the use of IVC filters. For this very reason, retrievable IVC filters have been introduced. However, since these filters are endothelialized at the point of vascular contact retrievability may be difficult after a lapse of time.

■ FAT EMBOLISM

Fat embolism is a dramatic form of embolism which occurs when neutral fat gains entry into the vascular system. The precipitating factor is a fracture of a long bone, the incidence increasing with multiple fractures. Fat embolism has been also noted to occur after orthopedic procedures and rarely following liposuction. It generally occurs 24–72 hours after these precipitating factors.

Pathophysiology

Fat embolism produces two effects:
1. Blockage of vessels by neutral fat.
2. The release of fatty acids due to the action of lipase on neutral fat. Liberated fatty acids cause a vasculitis with increased permeability of pulmonary, cerebral, and other vascular beds.

Clinical Features

The clinical picture is characterized by the sudden onset of dyspnea, increasing hypoxemia and mental confusion. Acute lung injury or acute respiratory distress syndrome (ARDS) may occur as a result of increased permeability of pulmonary capillaries. Seizures or even focal signs may be present. About 30–50% have petechiae on the skin, chiefly on the upper half of the body.

There is no test which is diagnostic of fat embolism. Fat may be present in the serum of patients with fat embolism.

Treatment

Treatment is generally supportive as no specific treatment has proved effective. Ventilatory support is invariably necessary. Use of corticosteroids in the prevention of fat embolism following an inciting factor is controversial.

■ AIR EMBOLISM

An important form of nonthrombotic embolism is venous air embolism. The possibility of air embolism has increased with numerous invasive medical and surgical procedures in practice today. These include the use of central venous catheters, surgery on the neck, thorax, and use of positive pressure ventilation with high positive end expiratory pressure (PEEP). Two important causes are allowing a large bolus of air to enter a central vein by failing to notice that an infusion through the vein is over, and removing the central venous catheter in the sitting position.

Air bubbles enter the pulmonary vascular bed, blocking it; some bubbles go through microvascular pulmonary shunts to enter the systemic circulation.

Clinical Features

Clinical features include severe chest pain, dyspnea, hypoxia, syncope. Pulmonary edema and altered sensorium are observed if death has not already occurred. Symptoms are related to widespread blockage of the pulmonary circulation and of systemic capillaries by air and by platelet fibrin aggregates causing diffuse microthrombi.

Treatment

Treatment consists of:
- Placing patient in the Trendelenburg position with the left side down.
- Removing air through a central venous catheter or direct needle aspiration, thereby promoting blood flow.
- Cardiorespiratory resuscitation.
- Promoting absorption of air by using 100% oxygen and when possible hyperbaric oxygen.

■ OTHER FORMS OF EMBOLISM

These include tumor embolism, septic thromboembolism, catheter embolism (a cut-off segment of a central venous catheter) and thrombotic complications caused by IV use of drugs meant to be taken orally, as is met with in some drug addicts.

■ SUGGESTED READING

1. Bounameaaux H, de Moerloose P, Perriwer A, et al. D-dimer testing in suspected venous thromboembolism. QJ Med. 1997;90:437-42.
2. Cummings KW. Multidetector computed tomographic pulmonary angiography: beyond acute pulmonary embolism. Radiol Clin North Am. 2010;48(1):51-65.
3. Goldhaber SZ. Thrombolysis in pulmonary embolism: a debatable indication. Thromb Haemost. 2001;86:444-51.
4. Goldhaber SZ, Viani L, De Rossa M. Acute pulmonary embolism: clinical outcomes in the International Cooperative Pulmonary Embolism Registry (ICOPER). Lancet. 1999;353:1386-9.
5. Kabrhel C, Rosovsky R, Channick R, et al. A multidisciplinary pulmonary embolism response team: initial 30-month experience with a novel approach to delivery of care to patients with submassive and massive pulmonary embolism. Chest. 2016;150:384.
6. Konstantinides S, Geibel A, Heusel G, et al. Heparin plus alteplase compared with heparin alone in patients with submassive pulmonary embolism. N Engl J Med. 2002;347(15):1143-50.
7. Konstantinides SV, Torbicki A, Agnelli G, et al. 2014 ESC guidelines on the diagnosis and management of acute pulmonary embolism. Eur Heart J. 2014;35:3033.
8. Konstantinides SV. Trends in incidence versus case fatality rates of pulmonary embolism: Good news or bad news? Thromb Haemost. 2016;115:233.
9. Konstantinides SV, Vicaut E, Danays T, et al. Impact of thrombolytic therapy on the long-term outcome of intermediate-risk pulmonary embolism. J Am Coll Cardiol. 2017;69:1536.
10. Kuriakose J. Acute pulmonary embolism. Radiol Clin North Am. 2010;48(1):31-50.
11. Mullins MD, Brecker DM, Hagspiel KD, et al. The role of spiral volumetric computed tomography in the diagnosis of pulmonary embolism. Arch Intern Med. 2000;160:293-8.
12. The PIOPED Investigators. Value of the ventilation-perfusion scan in acute pulmonary embolism. JAMA. 1990;263:2753-9.

Principles of Critical Care

CHAPTER 53

Acute Respiratory Failure in Adults

■ GENERAL CONSIDERATIONS

Acute respiratory failure is an important and frequently encountered problem in intensive care units (ICUs) all over the world. The usual or traditional definition of respiratory failure is the inability of the respiratory system to maintain the normal homeostasis of arterial blood gases, so that the oxygen tension in arterial blood (PaO_2) is less than 60 mm Hg, and/or the carbon dioxide tension in arterial blood ($PaCO_2$) is 50 mm Hg or greater.

Respiratory failure may be acute or chronic depending on the onset and duration of the failure. An acute exacerbation may at times prevail on a background of chronic respiratory failure (acute on chronic failure).

Respiratory failure is mainly of two types. Type I or hypoxemic respiratory failure is due to a failure of oxygenation with a $PaO_2 < 60$ mm Hg; Type II or hypercapnic respiratory failure (ventilatory failure) is due to hypoventilation and is characterized by a $PaCO_2 > 50$ mm Hg. Hypoxemic and hypercapnic respiratory failure may both occur in the same patient. Some intensivists also consider Type III and Type IV failure.

Type III respiratory failure is that occurring perioperatively and is largely due to basal atelectasis. Cardiothoracic surgery and/or major upper abdominal surgery splint the diaphragm and induce an abnormal mechanics of the abdominal muscles. These factors cause a fall in the functional residual capacity and an increase in the closing volume of the lungs. The end result is increasing atelectasis of the dependent alveoli, "small lungs" with a high diaphragm, respiratory distress, and hypoxemia.

Type IV respiratory failure is that associated with shock—a poorly functioning circulatory system with a low cardiac output is the main cause of hypoxemic failure in this situation. Both Type III and Type IV failure merely constitute hypoxemic failure or both hypoxemic and hypercapnic failure occurring against specific background conditions.

The above traditional definition of acute respiratory failure evolved when measurements of arterial pH and arterial blood gas tensions were first introduced into clinical medicine. This definition is useful in that (1) it focuses attention on abnormalities of gas exchange due to disturbances in lung function; (2) it stresses the importance and need for a laboratory diagnosis of respiratory failure; and (3) it emphasizes the difficulty and often the impossibility of either diagnosing acute respiratory failure or gauging its severity on clinical grounds. Yet, this traditional definition ignores the role of the cardiovascular system in gas exchange, and above all in oxygen transport to tissues. In a critical care setting, this is of particular concern. It is vital to look upon the circulatory and respiratory systems as a single interrelated unit whose purpose is to supply oxygen to the tissues.

A broad definition of respiration would be an exchange of oxygen and carbon dioxide between man and his environment. It can be divided into the following sequential steps:

- *Ventilation*: In which an exchange of oxygen and carbon dioxide occurs between the lungs and the atmosphere.
- *Gas exchange*: This occurs across the alveolar-capillary membrane within the lungs, mixed venous blood being oxygenated, and carbon dioxide being removed during its transit through the lungs.
- *Gas transport*: The transport of oxygenated arterial blood to the tissues, and of venous blood (with a high carbon dioxide content), to the lungs.

- *Gas exchange within the tissues*: Release of oxygen, oxygen uptake and utilization by the tissues, and release of carbon dioxide by the cells for transport back to the lungs.

In critical care medicine, it is a great advantage to look upon acute respiratory failure as an acute impairment of any one or more of the steps described above. We shall briefly consider (1) acute ventilatory failure; (2) acute failure in gas exchange or acute hypoxemic failure; (3) a combination of (1) and (2); (4) a failure of oxygen transport; and (5) a failure of tissue oxygenation.

ACUTE VENTILATORY FAILURE

Definition

Acute ventilatory failure occurs when alveolar ventilation (V_A) cannot adequately remove the carbon dioxide produced by cell metabolism, via the lungs.

Relation between PaO$_2$ and PaCO$_2$ in Ventilatory Failure

Ventilatory failure always results in a rise in $PaCO_2$ and a fall in PaO_2, and as mentioned earlier is also termed hypercapnic respiratory failure. The relation between PaO_2 and $PaCO_2$ is defined by the alveolar gas equation

$$P_AO_2 = P_IO_2 - PaCO_2 \times \frac{1}{R}$$

where, P_AO_2 is the alveolar oxygen tension, P_IO_2 the inspired oxygen tension corrected for water vapor, and R is the respiratory exchange ratio (*see* section on Lung Physiology). Once the P_AO_2 is calculated from the above equation, the PaO_2 can be determined if the alveolar-arterial oxygen gradient is known. In ventilatory failure due to central nervous system (CNS) causes or due to neuromuscular disease, the alveolar-arterial gradient is normal (i.e. 10–20 mm Hg), so that the PaO_2 is 10–20 mm Hg less than the P_AO_2. The oxygen-carbon dioxide diagram **(Fig. 1)** gives the value of P_AO_2 and PaO_2 for any given value of $PaCO_2$. The arterial blood gas tensions of oxygen and carbon dioxide fall on this line in pure or isolated ventilatory failure.

Pathophysiology of Ventilatory Failure

The carbon dioxide produced by tissue metabolism ($\dot{V}CO_2$) is removed by the lungs. Normally, the alveolar carbon dioxide tension (P_ACO_2) and the $PaCO_2$ are maintained around 40 mm Hg by adjusting V_A to balance the $\dot{V}CO_2$.

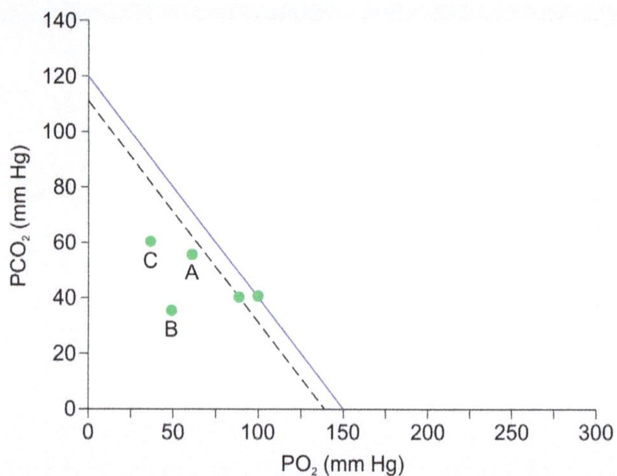

Fig. 1: O$_2$-CO$_2$ diagram. The continuous line represents the relation between alveolar PO$_2$ and alveolar PCO$_2$ with an RQ of 0.8 and when breathing air (PIO$_2$ = 149 mm Hg). The circle marked on this line represents the normal P$_A$O$_2$ and P$_A$CO$_2$. The broken line represents the normal relation between PaO$_2$ and P$_A$CO$_2$ (or PaCO$_2$) when breathing air. It takes into consideration the slight venous admixture occurring in normal lungs so that the PaO$_2$ may be 10–15 mm less than P$_A$O$_2$. The circle marked on the broken line represents the normal PaO$_2$ and PCO$_2$. Points A, B, and C illustrate blood gas readings in different types of respiratory failure: **A.** Ventilatory failure: PaCO$_2$ 60 mm Hg; PaO$_2$ 65 mm Hg. The point falls on or is very close to the broken line. **B.** Hypoxemic failure: PaCO$_2$ 38 mm Hg; PaO$_2$ 45 mm Hg. The point is markedly to the left of the broken line. The large alveolar-arterial gradient is chiefly due to a ventilation-perfusion imbalance and/or an increase in the true venous admixture. **C.** Hypoxemic and ventilatory failure: PaCO$_2$ 70 mm Hg. Note high PaCO$_2$ indicating ventilatory failure and PaO$_2$ less than what can be predicted from the PaCO$_2$ reading. The point is again to the left of the broken line.
Source: Udwadia FE. Diagnosis and Management of Acute Respiratory Failure. Mumbai: Oxford University Press; 1979.

Thus, an increase in the latter is met by a proportionate increase in V_A. The relationship between P_ACO_2, $\dot{V}CO_2$, and V_A, can be stated as follows:

$$P_ACO_2 = PaCO_2 = \frac{\dot{V}CO_2}{\dot{V}_A} \times \text{a constant (0.86)}$$

The $\dot{V}_A$ is the difference between minute ventilation ($\dot{V}_E$) and the physiological dead space ventilation ($\dot{V}_D$) within the lungs—i.e. the ventilation that does not participate in gas exchange. The above equation can thus be rewritten:

$$P_ACO_2 = PaCO_2 = \frac{\dot{V}CO_2}{\dot{V}_E - \dot{V}_D}$$

Thus, a rise in $PaCO_2$ due to ventilatory or hypercapnic respiratory failure can occur under the following conditions: (1) A fall in $\dot{V}_A$—this could be due to (a) a fall in $\dot{V}_E$ or (b) a rise in physiological $\dot{V}_D$, without a concomitant increase in $\dot{V}_E$. (2) A rise in carbon dioxide production ($\dot{V}CO_2$) without a proportionate increase in $\dot{V}_A$.

Important Causes of Acute Ventilatory or Hypercapnic Respiratory Failure in an Intensive Care Unit

1. *Hypoventilation in lungs which are normal to start with*: This occurs in patients with a depressed ventilatory drive or in neuromuscular disease. A depressed ventilatory drive is observed in poisonings with narcotics, sedatives, antidepressants, coma from other causes, in head injuries, encephalitis, increased intracranial tension, and other pathologies depressing the respiratory center. Important neuromuscular diseases causing hypoventilation include acute poliomyelitis, acute infective polyneuritis (Guillain-Barre syndrome), tetanus, myasthenia gravis, botulism, and snakebite poisoning. Other causes of respiratory muscle weakness and/or decreased respiratory muscle endurance include severe myopathy, amyotrophic lateral sclerosis, polymyositis, critical illness polyneuropathy/myopathy, malnutrition, severe electrolyte disturbances, notably hypokalemia, hyperkalemia, hypomagnesaemia, prolonged ventilator dependence, disorders of the phrenic nerve, and respiratory muscle fatigue from any cause.

2. Rarely, hypoventilation can occur following large airways obstruction. In an ICU setting, this is chiefly observed in tracheal or subglottic stenosis, when an artificial airway has been in place for many weeks or has been incorrectly managed. Upper airways obstruction with hypoventilation can also occur in children with acute epiglottitis, in obstructive sleep apnea, vocal cord paralysis, and foreign bodies including dentures, clots, secretions, soft tissue tumors or inflammation, and obstructing the upper airway.

3. Poor expansion of the thoracic cage with ventilatory failure can occur following trauma to the thorax (as in flail chest), in patients who are severely obese, or have marked kyphoscoliosis, or in those with well-marked pleural disease (as in bilateral pleural effusion or pneumothorax).

It is important to realize that in most of the above mentioned conditions, the lungs are normal to start with. However, if hypoventilation is not promptly recognized and correctly managed (and this is most important in hypoventilating comatose patients), secretions accumulate within the large and small airways producing areas of atelectasis. As a result of secondary changes within the lungs, gas exchange due to ventilation-perfusion imbalance is further impaired.

4. Hypoventilation can also occur in lungs which are abnormal. This is most frequently seen in severe airways obstruction—either acute severe asthma or an acute crisis in chronic bronchitis emphysema. In these patients hypoventilation is due to a decrease in $\dot{V}_E$ and/or an increase in physiological dead space. Extensive thromboembolic disease within the lungs can rarely produce a sufficient rise in $\dot{V}_D$, so as to cause a fall in $\dot{V}_A$. Severe late (almost terminal) stage restrictive disease can also be associated with hypoventilation and hypercapnic respiratory failure.

5. Increase in carbon dioxide production, at times cannot be countered by an increase in $\dot{V}_A$. Marked increase in carbon dioxide production can occur in high fever, hypermetabolic critical illnesses, severe hyperthyroidism, frequent seizures, and uncontrolled tetanus. In patients with respiratory muscle fatigue or in those with mechanical limitations to breathing [as in chronic obstructive pulmonary disease (COPD)], $\dot{V}_A$ cannot keep pace with carbon dioxide production and hypercapnic respiratory failure is observed. Hyperalimentation with increased caloric intake through carbohydrates or a high-carbohydrate diet given by the enteral route also results in an increase in $\dot{V}CO_2$. An increase in $\dot{V}_A$ is imperative if this excess CO_2 is to be removed. In critically ill patients, carbon dioxide retention may occur as respiratory muscle fatigue may prevent a proportionate rise in $\dot{V}_A$.

The important causes of hypercapnic respiratory failure are listed in **Table 1**.

■ HYPOXEMIC RESPIRATORY FAILURE

Acute hypoxemic respiratory failure results from poor gas exchange of oxygen within the lungs leading to a low PaO_2. The $PaCO_2$ may be normal or even less than normal.

Pathophysiology

The normal $\dot{V}_A$ is about 4–5 L, and the normal perfusion (Q) around 5 L, the $\dot{V}_A/Q$ ratio being approximately 0.8–1 L. Even in the normal lung, there are regional differences in ventilation-perfusion ratios, but by and large the ventilation-perfusion ratios are even and range from 0.8 L to 1.2 L. For explanatory purposes, the lung can be compartmentalized into the following divisions **(Figs. 2A to F)**:

- Alveoli with normal ventilation and perfusion—normal V/Q ratios.
- Alveoli with increase in ventilation-perfusion ratios, the V/Q ratios being more than 1. The capillaries leaving these alveoli have a normal or slightly increased PaO_2, but a reduced $PaCO_2$.

> **Table 1:** Important causes of hypercapnic respiratory failure in the intensive care unit.
>
> - Patients with normal lungs to start with (decrease in V_E)
>   - Depressed ventilatory drive:
>   - Poisoning, e.g. narcotics, antidepressants, sedatives
>   - Head injury, encephalitis, increase in intracranial tension
>   - Neuromuscular diseases:
>   - Acute poliomyelitis, acute infective polyneuritis, polymyositis, critical care neuropathy/myopathy, amyotrophic lateral sclerosis
>   - Tetanus, myasthenia gravis, botulism
>   - Snakebite poisoning
>   - Respiratory muscle weakness or fatigue from any cause
>   - Large airways obstruction:
>   - Tracheal/subglottic stenosis, obstructive sleep apnea, vocal cord paralysis, foreign bodies
> - Patients with abnormal lungs (decrease in V_E and/or increase in V_D)
>   - Acute severe bronchial asthma
>   - Acute crisis in chronic bronchitis, emphysema
>   - Extensive thromboembolic disease
>   - Severe terminal stage restrictive lung disease
> - Patients with increased production of CO_2
>   - High fever, hypermetabolic critical illness
>   - Frequent seizures, uncontrolled tetanus
>   - Hyperalimentation with increased carbohydrate intake

(V_D: Dead space ventilation; V_E: Minute ventilation)

- Alveoli with a decrease in ventilation-perfusion ratios; blood after perfusing these alveoli has a lowered PaO_2 and an increased $PaCO_2$. The lower the V/Q ratio, the lower the PaO_2 of the blood leaving these alveoli.
- Alveoli that are ventilated, but have no perfusion. The V/Q ratio is infinity and such alveoli contribute significantly to increased physiological dead space.
- Alveoli which are atelectatic, but continue to be perfused. These alveoli contribute to a right to left shunt within the lungs. The blood leaving the alveoli has the same PaO_2 as mixed venous blood, i.e. 40 mm Hg.
- Alveoli which are neither ventilated nor perfused. These are "resting" alveoli, and probably come into physiological action only when ventilatory or respiratory demands increase.

Acute hypoxemic respiratory failure occurs when: (1) there is a ventilation-perfusion mismatch characterized predominantly by low ventilation-perfusion ratios in the lungs; (2) there is a significant increase in the right to left shunt due to perfusion of atelectatic alveoli; (3) both the above factors are present; and (4) there is a marked decrease in the diffusion of oxygen across the alveolar capillary membrane.

Low Ventilation-perfusion (V/Q) Ratios

Alveoli which have a perfusion in excess of ventilation (i.e. low $\dot{V}_A/Q$ ratios), will have a reduced P_AO_2, and therefore

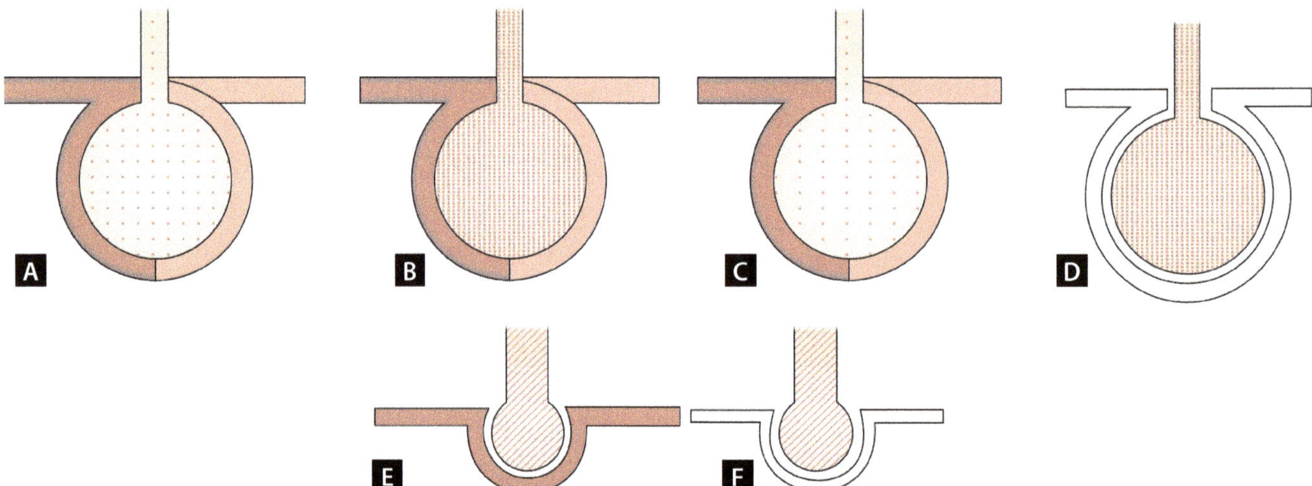

Figs. 2A to F: Various gas exchange units in the lung. (A) Normal unit-alveoli with normal V/Q ratios. (B) Hyperventilated unit-alveoli with increase in V/Q ratios (>1). (C) Hypoventilated unit-alveoli with decrease in V/Q ratios. (D) Dead space unit-alveoli are ventilated, but have no perfusion. (E) Shunt unit-alveoli are atelectatic, but have good perfusion. (F) Silent unit-alveoli are neither ventilated nor perfused.
Source: Udwadia FE. Diagnosis and Management of Acute Respiratory Failure. Mumbai: Oxford University Press; 1979.

a reduced PaO_2, as well as a reduced oxygen content of blood leaving the alveoli. When the poorly oxygenated blood mixes with the blood perfusing the alveoli that have $\dot{V}_A$, which is normal in proportion to the perfusion, or $\dot{V}_A$ even in excess of the perfusion, the resultant blood stream has a lower oxygen content and a lowered PaO_2. Increased V/Q ratios in some alveoli cannot therefore compensate for sharply lowered V/Q ratios in other alveoli. After all, the oxygen saturation of arterial blood in the presence of normal V/Q ratios is close to 100%. A further increase in the V/Q ratio may increase both the P_AO_2 and the PaO_2, but because of the plateau shape of the upper part of the oxygen-hemoglobin dissociation curve, there will be no appreciable increase in oxygen saturation or content, of blood leaving such alveoli. This is illustrated in **Figure 3**.

Increase in Right to Left Shunt within the Lungs

A shunt refers to the proportion or fraction of venous blood that enters the systemic arteries without coming into contact with gas exchanging areas of the lungs. The present discussion is not concerned with right to left shunts in the heart or the larger vessels due to congenital defects or anomalies. Right to left shunts within the lungs due to perfusion of atelectatic alveoli constitute

the most important cause of refractory acute hypoxemic respiratory failure. It is to be remembered that there is a small right to left shunt even in normal lungs. This is because of bronchial venous blood draining directly through pulmonary veins into the left atrium and a small amount of coronary venous blood that drains via the thebesian veins directly into the left ventricle. The normal shunt averages not more than 5%. In patients with a right to left shunt due to perfusion of atelectatic alveoli, the shunt fraction may be as high as 30–50%. The higher the right to left shunt within the lungs, the greater the degree of hypoxemia, and lower the PaO_2.

The effect of a right to left shunt within the lungs is illustrated in **Figure 4**.

Combination of Low V/Q Ratios and Increased Shunt

Most lung diseases causing acute respiratory failure are characterized by a pathology in which there are areas of low V/Q ratios, high V/Q ratios, and increase in the right to left shunt. Patients in whom disturbance in gas exchange is predominantly due to an increase in the shunt have the gravest prognosis.

Impairment in Diffusion of Oxygen

A diffusion abnormality does exist in several lung diseases, but it almost never is the chief cause of a low PaO_2 at rest.

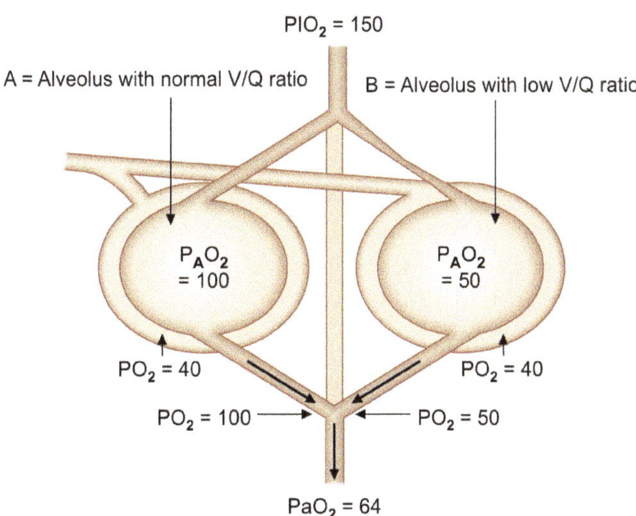

Fig. 3: The PaO_2 of blood leaving A (alveolus with normal V/Q ratio) is normal; the PaO_2 of blood leaving B (alveolus with reduced V/Q ratio) is reduced. When this poorly oxygenated blood mixes with well-oxygenated blood from alveoli with normal or high V/Q ratios, the resultant PaO_2 is still lower than normal. This shows that increased V/Q ratios in some alveoli cannot compensate for markedly lowered V/Q ratios in other alveoli.

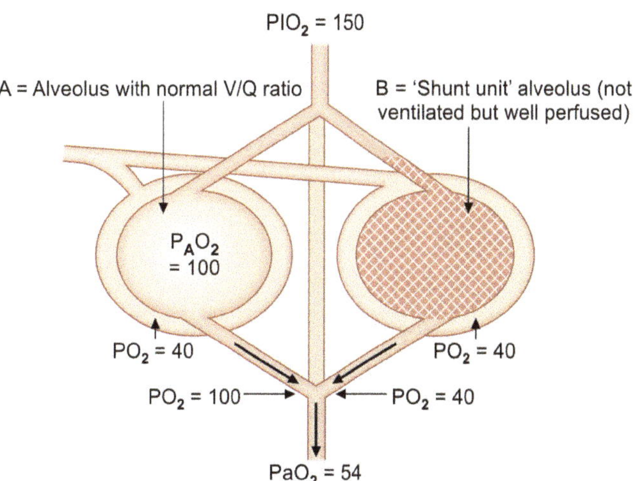

Fig. 4: The PaO_2 of blood leaving A (alveolus with normal V/Q ratio) is normal. The mixed venous blood perfusing B (shunt unit alveolus) is not oxygenated at all. When this blood mixes with well-oxygenated blood perfusing a normal alveolus, the resultant PaO_2 is still very low.

All patients with diffusion abnormalities have regional variations in compliance resulting in uneven and low ventilation-perfusion ratios.

Effect of an Increasing Fraction of Inspired Oxygen Content on V/Q Abnormalities

Increase in the fraction of inspired oxygen (FiO_2) rapidly produces an increase in the PaO_2 and the oxygen content of blood leaving the alveoli with low V/Q ratios. The hypoxemia of acute respiratory failure in patients with low V/Q ratios is thus easily corrected. The improvement in PaO_2 depends upon the degree of perfusion to areas with poor ventilation. Except where the V/Q ratios are extremely low, a satisfactory PaO_2 of about 60 mm Hg, with an oxygen saturation of 90% is achieved by using an FiO_2 of less than 0.6. Even in alveoli with extremely low V/Q ratios, as long as there is some ventilation present, an FiO_2 of 100% will always produce a marked increase in the PaO_2 of blood leaving such alveoli. This is illustrated in **Figure 5A**.

Effect of an Increased Fraction of Inspired Oxygen on the Shunt

It is obvious that the treatment of hypoxemia due to a severe right to left shunt within the lungs is difficult, because increasing the FiO_2 improves the oxygen content to a very slight extent. The greater the shunt, the poorer the response in PaO_2 to a rise in FiO_2 **(Fig. 5B)**. Fortunately, acute hypoxemic respiratory failure solely due to a marked increase in the right to left shunt within the lungs is rare. Even in patients with severe acute respiratory distress syndrome (ARDS), though there are many areas of shunt which do not respond to an increase in FiO_2, there are some areas of V/Q mismatch which respond to such an increase.

Clinical Problems causing Acute Hypoxemic Respiratory Failure

These can be broadly divided into three groups:

1. *Those characterized chiefly by airways' obstruction causing uneven ventilation and V/Q inequalities*: An acute crisis in chronic bronchitis emphysema and acute severe asthma are classic examples. In some of these patients there is an element of acute ventilatory failure in addition to hypoxemic respiratory failure. This is due to mechanical limitations which prevent increased ventilatory demands from being adequately met, due to alveolar hypoventilation consequent to a marked increase in physiological V_D or due to a diminished respiratory drive. One or more of these factors may contribute to an associated ventilatory failure.
2. *Restrictive lung diseases*: Examples of these include acute pulmonary edema, acute pulmonary infections, acute lung injury (ARDS), and major atelectasis within the lungs.
3. *Acute thromboembolic lung disease*: This is characterized by V/Q inequalities and increase in the dead space resulting in acute hypoxemic respiratory failure.

The important causes of acute hypoxemic respiratory failure are listed in **Table 2**.

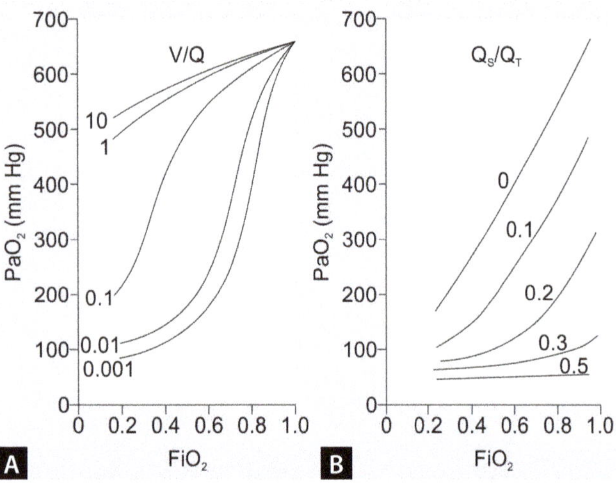

Figs. 5A and B: (A) PaO_2 improves with increasing fraction of inspired oxygen (FiO_2) in patients with a V/Q mismatch. When the FiO_2 is increased to 1 (100%), the PaO_2 reaches 600 mm Hg even if the V/Q ratio is very low. (B) Note that with increase in Q_s/Q_T beyond 0.3, increasing FiO_2 has little or no effect on the PaO_2.
Source: Albert RK. Physiology and management of failure of arterial oxygenation. In: Fallat RJ, Luce JM (Eds). Cardiopulmonary Critical Care Management. New York, United States: Elsevier Inc.; 1988. pp. 37-59.

Table 2: Important causes of acute hypoxemic respiratory failure.

• Obstructive airways disease:
  – Acute exacerbation of chronic obstructive pulmonary disease (COPD)
  – Acute severe bronchial asthma
• Restrictive lung disease:
  – Acute pulmonary edema
  – Acute pulmonary infection
  – Acute respiratory distress syndrome (ARDS)
  – Major pulmonary atelectasis
• Trauma to the chest
• Acute thromboembolic lung disease

■ COMBINATION OF ACUTE VENTILATORY AND HYPOXEMIC RESPIRATORY FAILURE

This is seen in intensive care medicine in four groups of patients.

1. Acute severe asthma.
2. Acute on chronic respiratory failure due to a respiratory crisis in patients with chronic airways obstruction.
3. Muscle fatigue involving muscles of respiration in patients with acute respiratory failure due to severe lung disease.
4. Advanced or late stage interstitial lung disease.

■ FAILURE OF OXYGEN TRANSPORT

A satisfactory gas exchange at the alveolar level must be accompanied by an adequate transport of oxygenated blood to the tissues. This requires an adequate cardiac output, a normal oxygen content of arterial blood, and good tissue perfusion. A low output state or shock from any cause can also indirectly lower the PaO_2 in the following ways:

- A low cardiac output results in increased oxygen extraction from the blood by the tissues. This leads to a fall in the mixed venous oxygen pressure (PvO_2). The lowered PvO_2 in the mixed venous blood reaching the alveoli will lead to a lowered PaO_2. This can be even more marked if the cardiac output falls in a patient who already has a right to left shunt within the lungs **(Fig. 6)**.
- A low output state leads to a low pressure of perfused blood in the pulmonary vessels; perfusion is more in the dependent alveoli of the lungs. This results in an increase in the physiological dead space involving nondependent alveoli and in low V/Q ratios within the dependent alveoli of the lungs, thereby contributing to a fall in PaO_2.
- Respiratory muscle fatigue is an important factor in low output states. Hypotension and shock lead to poor perfusion of respiratory muscles, and quick and easy fatigability. Respiratory muscle fatigue can cause hypoventilation, can increase ventilation-perfusion inequalities, and can thereby further reduce the PaO_2.

Respiratory Muscle Fatigue

The importance and role of muscle fatigue in acute respiratory failure (also *see* section on Lung Physiology)

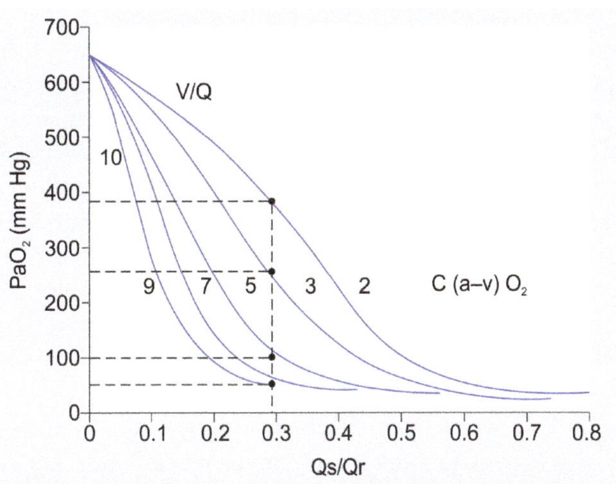

Fig. 6: Dependence of PaO_2 on the oxygen extraction C (a–v) and the shunt fraction. If the shunt fraction is 30%, the PaO_2 varies from 100 mm Hg to 400 mm Hg, as the C (a–v) O_2 narrows. The patient may have a high PaO_2 if he has a high cardiac output and a decreased C (a–v) O_2 of 3, even if his shunt fraction is as high as 0.3. However, if the patient's oxygen consumption increases without a corresponding increase in the cardiac output, the C (a–v) O_2 widens to 9, and the PaO_2 falls to 50 mm Hg.
Source: Albert RK. Physiology and management of failure of arterial oxygenation. In: Fallat RJ, Luce JM (Eds). Cardiopulmonary Critical Care Management. New York, United States: Elsevier Inc.; 1988. pp. 37-59.

in critically ill patients cannot be overemphasized and is best considered at this stage. As with other muscle groups in the body, excessive work performed by the muscles of respiration leads to fatigue. Increasing fatigue results in increasingly poor function and hypoventilation; ultimately the patient literally stops breathing. Increasing respiratory fatigue explains the abrupt stoppage of breathing with resulting disaster in patients with acute severe asthma or in patients with a very low pulmonary compliance due to acute alveolar edema. Difficulties in weaning patients off ventilator support are also frequently related to respiratory muscle fatigue brought on by the inability to cope with the work of breathing.

The second major factor predisposing to respiratory muscle fatigue is the gravity or critical nature of an illness. The more critically ill patient, the easier and quicker fatigue arises in respiratory muscles. Tachypnea and an unstable circulation, hypotension with poor perfusion of the respiratory muscles, and electrolyte disturbances, probably all play a role in muscle fatigue in these individuals.

The clinical recognition of respiratory muscle fatigue is difficult, and may occasionally be impossible to detect till the patient very nearly has a respiratory arrest. A voiced complaint by an ill patient that he or she is tired and cannot continue to breathe for long should always be taken seriously, particularly in a patient with severe airways' obstruction. Tachypnea with a rate more than 35/min, always predisposes to fatigue, particularly in obese individuals or very ill patients. Poor chest excursions, irregular breathing, and above all apneic spells, all point to fatigued respiratory muscles. Respiratory alternans, in which intercostal muscles and diaphragmatic contractions alternate, is also observed at times. Fatigued muscles also occasionally cause a paradoxical respiratory movement, with the lower part of the chest and the upper abdomen being drawn in, instead of being pushed out during inspiration.

Objective measurements are also of use. As a rough guide, spontaneous breathing can be easily sustained if the effort involved in each spontaneous breath is less than one-third of the maximal respiratory effort that can be achieved. The maximum inspiratory pressure (MIP) is a good guide to the respiratory muscle power. An MIP of less than 30 cm H_2O generally denotes muscle fatigue. Similarly a tidal volume (measured by a Wright's spirometer) of less than 300 mL, or a vital capacity (VC) less than three times the tidal volume, suggests respiratory muscle fatigue under appropriate clinical conditions. A V_E > 10–12 L/min is difficult to sustain indefinitely in critically ill individuals, and often ultimately leads to hypoventilation from respiratory muscle fatigue. The objective measurements stated above when judged against an appropriate clinical background can give only indirect evidence of probable respiratory muscle fatigue. It has to be admitted that unequivocal direct evidence of contractile fatigue has not yet been demonstrated. The major determinants of respiratory muscle fatigue are inspiratory muscle strength, mean inspiratory pressure, and the duration of inspiration, which when combined form the tension time index (TTI). However, interpretation of the TTI is difficult and often misleading. Recent work suggests that the magnetic stimulation of the phrenic nerve (a procedure far less painful than electrical stimulation) can detect diaphragmatic fatigue, and measuring changes in the esophageal twitch pressure can detect ribcage muscle fatigue. Magnetic stimulation of the phrenic nerve is however a research procedure in our setting. *Medicine need not always be evidence-based.* For the present we should act on the premise that respiratory muscles (particularly if they are weak) can, like other skeletal muscles, experience fatigue if subjected to excessive work for a prolonged period of time.

The clinical features of respiratory muscle fatigue are listed in **Table 3**.

Respiratory muscle fatigue causing or contributing to acute respiratory failure should be managed by resting the respiratory muscles by mechanical ventilation. During the period of rest, the acutely depleted glycogen stores of the respiratory muscles are replenished, and lactic acid and other metabolites associated with muscle fatigue are washed out. Aminophylline is believed to preserve muscle strength and contraction of the diaphragm; however, it is doubtful if this drug has a clinical role in patients with severe respiratory muscle fatigue.

Failure of Oxygen Release

This occurs in the presence of exposure to carbon monoxide (CO). The commonest cause of CO poisoning is inhalation of smoke following a fire accident. CO has a far greater affinity for hemoglobin (Hb) (240 times) than oxygen, so that a good proportion of Hb is converted to carboxy Hb instead of oxyhemoglobin. Oxygen release may therefore be grossly impaired leading to tissue hypoxia.

A rarer cause is in patients with methemoglobinemia and sulfhemoglobinemia. Here again oxygen release is reduced resulting in tissue hypoxemia.

Failure of Oxygen Utilization

Despite good ventilation, normal exchange of blood gases at the alveolar level and good oxygen transport, oxygen uptake may be deficient at the tissue level. The main purpose of the cardiorespiratory system is then defeated. Thus, cyanide poisoning is characterized by an arrest of intracellular respiration due to the inactivation of an intracellular enzyme and cytochrome oxidase. A patient with cyanide poisoning has a normal PaO_2, SaO_2, CaO_2, and oxygen transport, but cannot utilize oxygen at the

Table 3: Features of respiratory muscle fatigue.
• Complaint of fatigue in relation to breathing
• Respiratory rate > 35/min
• Poor chest excursions, irregular breathing, apneic spells
• Respiratory alternans, paradoxical respiratory movements
• MIP < 30 cm H_2O
• TV < 300 mL; VC < 3 × TV; MV > 10–12 L/min

(MIP: Maximum inspiratory pressure; MV: Minute ventilation; TV: Tidal volume; VC: Vital capacity)

tissue level. Blood after perfusing tissues shows severe lactic acidosis and has a high PvO_2 and mixed venous oxygen saturation (SvO_2). The patient literally dies of "strangulation" or hypoxia at the tissue level.

The most important clinical problem associated with failure of oxygen uptake is septic shock, often associated with ARDS. To many physicians it may seem inappropriate to consider failure of oxygen uptake by tissues in acute respiratory failure. Yet, it is ultimately the oxygen supply to, and oxygen uptake by tissues (in particular tissues of vital organs), which are of crucial importance. In the final analysis, acute cardiorespiratory failure is a failure to adequately oxygenate the tissues.

■ CLINICAL FEATURES OF ACUTE RESPIRATORY FAILURE

In the presence of a background disease known to cause acute respiratory failure, the only sure way to diagnose the latter is by estimating the arterial blood gases. One should never rely only on clinical features to diagnose acute respiratory failure. Clinical features may, however, be present. These include the presence of disease known to cause acute respiratory failure and the features associated with hypoxia and hypercapnia. Many, though not all patients, also show respiratory distress.

Hypoxia

Hypoxia is the basic underlying feature in every patient with acute hypoxemic respiratory failure. Increasing hypoxia depresses cell function, induces metabolic acidosis, and if marked and unrelieved leads to cellular death. It may be impossible to detect hypoxia on clinical grounds in critically ill patients. The only sure way of detecting hypoxia is by measuring the arterial PaO_2. The importance of this fact cannot be overemphasized.

The only pathognomonic manifestation of hypoxia is central cyanosis. Nevertheless, well-marked arterial hypoxemia may exist in the absence of clinical cyanosis, so that to await the development of cyanosis before diagnosing acute respiratory failure, is to court disaster. Cyanosis can only be clinically evident if the mean capillary concentration of reduced Hb exceeds 5 g/dL. It is evident that a patient with severe anemia (Hb < 7 g/dL), may die of severe arterial hypoxemia before cyanosis can become clinically manifest. A hypermetabolic state with a hyperdynamic circulation characterized by a quick blood flow through the peripheries, also renders the

clinical recognition of cyanosis difficult. The presence of anemia together with a quickened circulatory flow therefore constitutes a formidable combination which prevents the clinical appearance of cyanosis in spite of marked hypoxia.

Mental confusion, restlessness, and acute anxiety are early manifestations of hypoxia. The ghastly pitfall of dubbing the anxiety and restlessness of early hypoxia in acute respiratory failure as "functional" should be guarded against.

Compensatory Mechanisms Induced by Hypoxia

Hypoxia triggers compensatory mechanisms which are easily recognized, and are therefore of diagnostic value. The main compensatory mechanism is sympathetic stimulation, which causes tachycardia and hypertension. Increase in the respiratory rate is another compensatory mechanism produced by stimulation of the chemoreceptors in the carotid body and aorta. Increase in the respiratory rate will not occur if the respiratory center is markedly depressed or if there is weakness or paralysis of the respiratory muscles. However, tachycardia and hypertension are important signs of hypoxia. They should be sought for, and their significance recognized in situations that can lead to acute respiratory failure. These signs depend on the integrity of the sympathetic nervous system. In the old and feeble, in diabetics with a neuropathy involving the sympathetic nerves, or in patients who have received drugs affecting the autonomic nervous system, sympathetic response to hypoxia may be absent or feeble. With severe increasing hypoxia, the clinical hallmarks are progressive bradycardia, hypotension, lactic acid acidosis, arrhythmias, circulatory failure, and death.

The myocardium has no oxygen reserve so that hypoxia depresses myocardial function, and increases ectopic irritability. Bradycardia and hypotension result from the direct depressant effect of hypoxia on the myocardium. Arrhythmias arise due to increased ectopic irritability. Atrial flutter and fibrillation are often observed; severe hypoxia ultimately results in ventricular tachycardia, fibrillation, and arrest.

Hypercapnia

Hypercapnia may also be impossible to detect on clinical grounds. The $PaCO_2$ should therefore always be estimated in any disease which can conceivably produce carbon dioxide retention.

Carbon dioxide has a local depressant effect on the cardiovascular system. It thus produces generalized vasodilatation except in the pulmonary circulation. Generalized vasodilatation manifests as *cutaneous flushing, warmth, sweating, and a bounding pulse.*

The depressant effect of carbon dioxide on the CNS leads to confusion, disturbance in behavior, a reversal in the sleep rhythm, and increasing drowsiness that may lead to deep coma (carbon dioxide narcosis). Carbon dioxide narcosis is an important metabolic cause of coma and can be often missed if the $PaCO_2$ is not measured. Wing flap tremors of the outstretched hands are often observed with CO_2 retention. They are indistinguishable from those observed in hepatic failure. Wing flap tremors are not consistently present. At times, even a slight rise in the $PaCO_2$ induces wing flap tremors; at other times, a marked rise in $PaCO_2$ may not be associated with "flaps". However, increasing levels of $PaCO_2$ produce increasing disturbance of consciousness. Marked confusion and drowsiness occur by the time $PaCO_2$ rises to between 80 mm Hg and 100 mm Hg, and the patient is generally unconscious when the $PaCO_2$ is well over 100 mm Hg. Coma in CO_2 narcosis is associated with loss of the deep reflexes and urinary incontinence. The plantars are generally not elicitable or are flexor; rarely, they may be extensor.

High levels of $PaCO_2$ can produce headache, muscle twitching, seizures, and papilledema. The combination of drowsiness, headache, and papilledema closely simulates an intracranial tumor.

An increasing $PaCO_2$ stimulates the respiratory center, producing an increase in the respiratory rate and tidal volume. Nevertheless, a depressed center or a center with a reduced or absent sensitivity to increasing $PaCO_2$ will not permit an increased respiratory drive to materialize.

Hypercapnia also produces a central stimulation of the sympathetic nervous system, resulting in tachycardia and hypertension. The pattern of symptoms in a patient will depend on the balance between the depressant action on the cardiovascular system and the stimulant effects on the sympathetic nervous system.

Respiratory Distress or Dyspnea

Many patients in acute respiratory failure are uncomfortably aware of a difficulty in breathing. This unpleasant awareness of respiration and difficulty in breathing is termed as dyspnea. Dyspnea is a subjective phenomenon, and its correlation with the degree of respiratory failure is difficult. In fact, breathlessness and respiratory failure are not synonymous. Many patients who are breathless are not in respiratory failure, and a number of patients in respiratory failure are not breathless. Nevertheless, in a patient with chronic lung disease, increasing impairment of lung function and increasing respiratory failure are invariably associated with increasing dyspnea.

The important clinical features of hypoxia and hypercapnia are listed in **Table 4**.

■ COMPLICATIONS OF ACUTE RESPIRATORY FAILURE

- The most important complication is nosocomial infection. This is more common if the patient has an artificial airway (endotracheal tube or a tracheostomy tube) and even more so if the patient is on a mechanical ventilator.
- Patients with acute respiratory failure on invasive ventilatory support may suffer complications associated with this support (*see* Mechanical Ventilation).
- Fluid electrolyte disturbances, acid-base disturbances, and hemodynamic instability may be observed depending on the nature and extent of the underlying disease causing acute respiratory failure.
- Segmental or even lobar atelectasis may occur in patients with excessive tracheobronchial secretions particularly if there is hypoventilation.
- Ileus and dilatation of stomach may occur particularly when acute respiratory failure complicates pulmonary infection such as severe pneumonia.

Table 4: Important clinical features of hypoxia and hypercapnia.	
Hypoxia	*Hypercapnia*
Cyanosis	Flushing, warmth, sweating, bounding pulse
Mental changes, restlessness, anxiety	Headache, wing flap tremors
Tachycardia, hypertension	Drowsiness, confusion, coma
Rhythm disturbances	Muscle twitching, seizures, papilledema
Metabolic acidosis	
Bradycardia, hypotension, circulatory failure, when hypoxia is marked	

MANAGEMENT OF ACUTE RESPIRATORY FAILURE (TABLE 5)

A number of diseases produce acute respiratory failure for which there is no specific cure. The patient then needs respiratory care and support till such time as the disease resolves. There are other diseases producing acute respiratory failure for which specific therapy is available. Prompt diagnosis and specific treatment in such instances can quickly reverse respiratory failure. The general principles involved in the management of acute respiratory failure include: (1) maintenance of a clear airway; (2) maintenance of adequate ventilation; (3) use of oxygen; (4) treating the cause of acute respiratory failure, in so far as this is possible; and (5) the use of ventilatory support, when indicated—if the cause of acute respiratory failure cannot be treated, or if despite treatment the patient is hypoxemic or hypercapnic, ventilatory support is indicated.

Maintenance of a Clear Airway

Obstruction of the airways due to retained secretions, mucus plugs, or foreign matter (invariably food particles) worsen respiratory failure. Secretions obstructing airways can lead to hypoventilation with a further fall in the PaO_2. Mucus plugs within the airways contribute to uneven and poor distribution of inspired gas to the alveoli within the lungs, and also produce areas of atelectasis. Uneven ventilation accentuates V/Q inequalities, while increasing areas of atelectasis worsen or produce a right to left shunt within the lungs. The net effect is increasing hypoxia and worsening respiratory failure. Undrained secretions or mucus plugs also form a nidus for infection, which may

Table 5: Management of acute respiratory failure.

- Maintenance of clear airways
  - Clear secretions:
    - Liquefy secretions
    - Promote cough—good physiotherapy
    - Suctioning of secretions
    - Use of an airway—oropharyngeal airway, other airways, endotracheal intubation/tracheostomy
- Maintenance of adequate ventilation
  - Artificial ventilation with AMBU bag in emergency, till mechanical ventilator support is organized
  - Use of respiratory stimulants (in rare situations)
- Use of oxygen
- Treat cause of acute respiratory failure whenever possible
- Use mechanical ventilator support if cause cannot be treated, or if patient hypoxemic or hypercapnic despite above measures

ultimately lead to pneumonia or bronchopneumonia. Maintaining a clear airway is therefore vital. This is often lost sight of in a comatose patient who may have normal lungs to start with, but who develops a quickly worsening respiratory failure due to undrained secretions plugging the airways.

Methods to Clear Secretions

- *Liquefy secretions*: Undrained secretions can dry and form crusts, which obstruct the airways. Such crusted secretions can be removed only with great difficulty; therefore drying of secretions should be prevented and their liquefaction promoted by:
  - *Proper hydration of the patient, if necessary with intravenous fluids*: A severely ill, distressed, and breathless patient generally does not drink enough water on his own.
  - *Humidification of inspired gas*: This is of utmost importance when the nasal and upper respiratory passages are bypassed and the patient is breathing through an endotracheal or tracheostomy tube. Lack of humidification in such patients besides causing drying and crusting of secretions in the trachea, the large and the small airways, can also result in inspissated secretions that block the endotracheal or tracheostomy tube with disastrous consequences.
  - *Use of normal saline*: We often instil normal saline (2–5 mL at a time) through an endotracheal or tracheostomy tube, to help liquefy inspissated mucus secretions. This is particularly of value in patients with acute severe asthma on ventilator support.

  Acetylcysteine is also a good liquefactant of inspissated mucus, but is a strong irritant. It can produce severe bronchospasm even in a dose as small as 0.5 mL. The drug can also markedly increase the volume of secretions in the tracheobronchial tree, necessitating very frequent suction. We use this drug very rarely in our unit.
- *Promotion of cough*: Cough in a patient with acute respiratory failure should always be assisted and promoted, and never suppressed. When pain prevents cough (as after thoracic, open-heart or upper abdominal surgery, or in crush injuries), analgesics need to be given, taking care to use a dose that does not produce respiratory depression. Physiotherapy is vital to enable secretions to be brought up and coughed

out. The patient may need to be postured to drain his secretions. *In critically ill patients who retain secretions within the respiratory tract, good physiotherapy often spells the difference between survival and death.*

- *Removal of secretions by suction*: When secretions gather in the mouth and the upper respiratory passages, and the patient is too ill to spit or cough them out, frequent suction should be done to keep the upper airways patent and to prevent the possibility of aspiration of the secretions into the lungs. Secretions around the larynx can be sucked with the aid of indirect laryngoscopy. Suction stimulates cough in an obtunded patient, and this is of added help. It is important never to roughly touch or "hit" the tip of the catheter to the pharynx or larynx during suctioning, as this can traumatize the pharyngeal or laryngeal mucosa, induce bleeding and sloughing, and further worsen the problem of maintaining a clear airway. The tip of the suction catheter should lie on the posterior portion of the tongue, preferably not touching the pharynx during suctioning. The floor and sides of the mouth should be suctioned; the nasal cavity and the pharynx can also be conveniently suctioned through a catheter inserted through the nares.

- *Endotracheal intubation (also see chapter on Airway Management)*: If the upper airway cannot be kept clear and open by the methods indicated above, or by the use of a simple oropharyngeal or nasopharyngeal airway, the patient should be intubated. Endotracheal intubation is an invaluable aid to maintain a clear airway as it allows easy access to secretions in the trachea and the large airways.

The main indication for endotracheal intubation is upper airways obstruction and the inability of the patient to handle upper respiratory secretions. The latter feature is frequently observed in unconscious patients and is invariably so in comatose patients. It also occurs when the cough reflex is poor or the patient is just too ill or feeble to cough. Paralysis of the palate and pharynx will also prevent the patient from handling his upper respiratory secretions because of difficulty in swallowing. This could lead to aspiration of accumulated secretions, as also to aspiration of regurgitated stomach contents. The four common conditions in critical care medicine wherein an endotracheal tube serves to maintain an open airway are (1) poisoning by respiratory depressants, (2) cerebrovascular accidents, (3) coma from any cause, and (4) following major surgery. Endotracheal intubation is also indicated when the patient is to be put on mechanical ventilator support.

Maintenance of Adequate Ventilation
Artificial Ventilation

When respiration is feeble or the patient is apneic, immediate resuscitation is aimed at ensuring adequate ventilation. Initially mouth-to-mouth respiration may be necessary, followed within seconds by a mask fitted to an AMBU or anesthetic bag, fed with 100% oxygen. This should be quickly followed by endotracheal intubation, mechanical ventilation being carried out either through an AMBU bag, or by a mechanical ventilator.

Use of Respiratory Stimulants in Acute Respiratory Failure

The role of respiratory stimulants in acute respiratory failure in ICUs is very limited and to many nonexistent. No respiratory stimulant acts specifically and solely on the respiratory center; all such drugs in addition to stimulating the respiratory center, also act as analeptics, in that they awaken the patient, and thereby enable him to ventilate and cough better. In fact, almost certainly the analeptic effect is clinically more important than the specific stimulating effect on the respiratory center. Good physiotherapy should always be given during an analeptic phase, so that secretions within the lungs are mobilized, and either coughed up or removed through suction. Unfortunately, all respiratory stimulants and analeptics frequently produce vomiting as a side effect, and if the dose is large or the drug is administered rapidly, localized twitchings or generalized seizures can result. *If alveolar hypoventilation due to a depressed respiratory center is sufficiently severe to produce well-marked hypoxia and hypercapnia, it is far better to use noninvasive ventilation or to intubate and ventilate the patient, rather than waste time in administering respiratory stimulants.* We have stopped using respiratory stimulants in our units.

Perhaps the only valid uses of respiratory stimulants are (1) to tide over a critical period in a patient with acute respiratory failure, while he awaits transfer to an ICU and (2) in patients with hopelessly crippling COPD who on balance, are not given ventilator support. Respiratory stimulants could then be tried along with the other far more important conservative measures.

The respiratory stimulant with probably the least side effects is doxapram. It is given intravenously at a rate of 1–3 mg/min and can be continued till a maximum dose of 600 mg is reached. The risk of seizures is low with doxapram. The infusion can however cause hypertension and cardiac arrhythmias as the drug can stimulate the release of epinephrine from the adrenals. It should therefore be avoided in hypertensive patients and in those with ischemic heart disease.

Use of Oxygen

The prompt administration of oxygen is crucial in the management of acute respiratory failure. This is considered in a separate section (*see* section on "Airway Diseases").

Treatment of the Cause of Acute Respiratory Failure whenever Possible

Treatment is individualized depending upon the etiological factor operating in a patient. The following examples are illustrative and worthy of mention:

- *Treatment of infection*: This is the commonest cause that precipitates acute respiratory failure in patients with chronic lung disease. Infection can also occur later as a complication in the natural history of acute respiratory failure due to other causes.
- Removal of air in a tension pneumothorax and tapping of a massive unilateral pleural effusion or moderate-sized bilateral effusions.
- Removal of a foreign body obstructing the larynx, trachea, or a large bronchus.
- Expanding an atelectatic lobe or lung with physiotherapy or bronchoscopic suction.
- Use of prostigmine in myasthenia gravis, and of antivenin in snakebite poisoning.
- Use of naloxone in narcotic poisonings.
- Use of nebulized beta2-agonists, intravenous aminophylline, and oral or intravenous corticosteroids in acute severe asthma.

There are many situations where the cause of acute respiratory failure cannot be promptly treated. This particularly holds true for the numerous conditions which produce ARDS, severe tetanus, severe head injuries and other CNS problems, and poisonings due to sedatives and tranquillizers. The doctor in charge of the ICU has then to rely on the general principles of management outlined above, till such time as the illness causing acute respiratory failure resolves over a period of time.

Ventilator Support

When well-marked and in particular life-threatening hypoxia and/or hypercapnia are uncorrected by the general principles above, the patient needs ventilator support to aid in more effective gas exchange within the lungs. Ventilator support can be noninvasive as with the use of a bilevel positive airway pressure (BiPAP) or continuous positive airway pressure (CPAP) machine or invasive when given by a mechanical ventilator. This is dealt with in a separate chapter.

■ SUGGESTED READING

1. Davidson AC, Banham S, Elliott M, et al. BTS/ICS guideline for the ventilatory management of acute hypercapnic respiratory failure in adults. Thorax. 2016;71 Suppl 2:ii1-35.
2. Hill NS. Noninvasive ventilation in acute respiratory failure. Crit Care Med. 2007;35(10):2402-7.
3. MacIntyre NR. Current issues in mechanical ventilation for respiratory failure. Chest. 2005;128(5 Suppl 2):561S-7S.
4. UpToDate. (2017). Noninvasive ventilation in acute respiratory failure in adults. [online] Available from https://www.uptodate.com/contents/noninvasive-ventilation-in-acute-respiratory-failure-in-adults/print [Accessed July 2018].

CHAPTER 54

Airway Management

■ ESTABLISHING THE AIRWAY

Nothing is more critical in emergency respiratory care than ensuring a patent airway and then maintaining it. An obstructed airway can lead to death within a few minutes. In patients with cardiac arrest, inability to secure a patent airway generally renders all efforts at cardiopulmonary resuscitation ineffective.

■ UPPER AIRWAYS OBSTRUCTION

Upper airways obstruction may result from "soft tissue" obstruction or from laryngeal obstruction.

"Soft tissue" obstruction is probably the most common airway emergency. It results from the encroachment on the patency of the upper airway by soft tissues of the pharynx or by tissue in close relation to the pharynx. Upper airways obstruction is thus seen in comatose patients when the pharynx loses it tone or in patients with lower cranial nerve palsies when the pharynx is paralyzed. It also occurs in angioneurotic edema, inflammation, retropharyngeal abscess and can be caused by bleeding and soft tissue tumors within that area. Foreign bodies, dentures, vomitus, blood clots, thick oropharyngeal secretions can also block the upper airway. The common factor underlying all these causes of upper airways obstruction is the absent or the markedly diminished patency between the base of the tongue and the pharyngeal wall.

Obstruction at the larynx can be caused by laryngeal spasm as in tetanus, by bilateral vocal cord abductor palsy, by inflammatory or neoplastic lesions above or within the larynx or by laryngeal edema. A foreign body or food (such as a piece of meat) may also obstruct the larynx and cause severe asphyxia and death.

Partial upper airways obstruction is characterized by noisy breathing, akin to snoring. Partial upper airways obstruction can be easily missed, particularly in comatose patients who in addition often hypoventilate due to a depressed respiratory center. Laryngeal or tracheal obstruction gives rise to a high-pitched inspiratory sound termed "stridor".

Complete or almost complete airways obstruction results in marked inspiratory efforts with little or no movement of air into the lungs. There is severe retraction of the intercostal spaces, the sternum and epigastrium, together with strong contraction of the accessory muscles of respiration during inspiratory efforts. The patient, to start with, is extremely distressed, restless, anxious, and becomes increasingly cyanosed. Tachycardia or a bradyarrhythmia is related to hypoxia. Death ensues if hypoxia is unrelieved.

Management

The treatment obviously is to relieve soft tissue obstruction by simple basic maneuvers.

Neck Extension with Forward and Upward Chin Thrust

This should be the first maneuver to be attempted as it can promptly relieve mild to moderate obstruction by increasing the patency between the back of the tongue and the pharynx **(Fig. 1)**.

Careful suction of secretions, blood, and vomitus from the pharynx may be necessary, as also the removal of dentures or a foreign body that may be obstructing the airway.

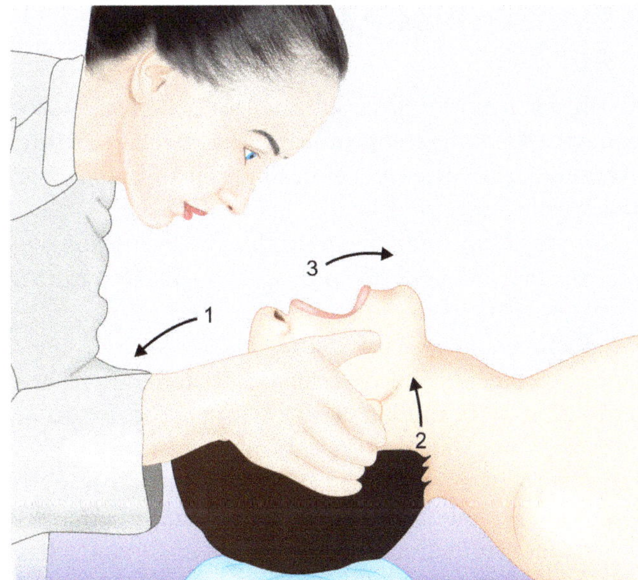

Fig. 1: Maintaining a clear airway by triple airway maneuver: (1) Tilt head backward; (2) Lift mandible forward; (3) Open the mouth and try to remove any foreign body.

Oropharyngeal Airway

This device is a conduit inserted along the top of the tongue until the teeth or gums limit its insertion. It is positioned between the base of the tongue and the pharynx (separating the two) thereby maintaining a patent airway. The airway should be inserted with its curve up initially and rotated into position when the end reaches the base of the tongue. It is designed to permit a suction catheter to pass through it, and allow suction of secretions in the pharynx and upper larynx.

An oropharyngeal airway is chiefly suited for comatose patients and that too for limited periods of time. As it rests at the base of the tongue, it stimulates the gag reflex, and can induce excessive salivation, vomiting, and even laryngospasm in the conscious patient.

■ ARTIFICIAL AIRWAYS

An artificial airway is a conduit or tube inserted into the trachea bypassing the pharynx and larynx which no longer form part of the total airway. In essence, this means endotracheal intubation or tracheostomy.

Indications

- Hypoxia and/or hypercapnia (due to acute respiratory failure) severe enough to necessitate invasive

ventilator support through an endotracheal tube or a tracheostomy is the prime indication for the insertion of an artificial airway.

In certain circumstances noninvasive ventilator support is preferred to invasive ventilator support at least to start with. When noninvasive ventilator support fails or is contraindicated invasive ventilator support is mandatory. Noninvasive ventilator support, its indications and contraindications have been discussed later in this section.

- To maintain an open airway in the presence of obstruction to the pharynx or larynx. If the obstruction is such that it is technically impossible to do an endotracheal intubation one has no option other than to perform a tracheostomy.
- To protect the airway in a patient whose protective reflexes are poor.

The pharynx, vocal cords, and the epiglottis play an important role in protecting the airway from aspiration of secretions, foreign matter, food or regurgitating gastric contents. The reflexes that normally protect the airways are: (1) the pharyngeal reflex, which normally includes the gag and swallowing reflexes; (2) the laryngeal reflex, which is a vagal reflex and is responsible for the apposition of the vocal cords, and closure of the epiglottis on stimulation of the larynx by secretions or by foreign matter; (3) the tracheal reflex, which is a vagal reflex causing cough when the trachea is stimulated by some irritant or foreign matter; (5) the carinal reflex, which is a vagal reflex causing cough on irritation of the carina.

The protective reflexes are generally obtunded from above downwards, irrespective of whether the cause of obtundation is due to drugs, disease or a deepening state of unconsciousness. When these reflexes return in a recovering patient, they recover from "below" "up". The preservation of the pharyngeal reflex (gag reflex) therefore suggests preservation of the laryngeal and tracheal reflexes. However, the gag reflex is believed to be diminished or inelicitable in 10% of the normal population. Therefore, absence of this reflex does not always indicate absence of other protective reflexes. Clinically, the inability to handle secretions in the upper airway and to swallow in a coordinated manner denotes a loss of protective airway reflexes and necessitates the establishment of an artificial airway. In such patients, the artificial airway also seals the respiratory from the alimentary tract, thereby preventing aspiration of gastric contents into the tracheobronchial tree.

- To facilitate suction of secretions (from within the tracheobronchial tree), which the patient is incapable of coughing up and expectorating. This could be because the secretions are copious, the cough reflex is poor, or the patient is just too feeble to cough and expectorate. Although it is possible to insert a suction catheter through the vocal cords for suctioning tracheal secretions, it is not advisable to do so except on rare occasions. Laryngeal edema and obstruction, and precipitation of fatal arrhythmias in critically ill patients can occur following such attempts. The establishment of an artificial airway allows easy, safe, and direct suctioning of the tracheobronchial tree **(Table 1)**.

Disadvantages of Artificial Airways

The establishment and maintenance of an artificial airway (endotracheal intubation or tracheostomy) has its hazards and complications depending on the expertise with which it is established, the quality of after care, and the nature and degree of the critical illness in the patient. These complications are dealt with later. However, there are some inherent universal drawbacks of artificial airways which need to be considered.

- An artificial airway bypasses the normal defense mechanisms which counter bacterial contamination of the airways. The airways and lungs are more prone to nosocomial infection.
- An endotracheal tube removes the effectiveness of cough because the vocal cords are nonfunctional; a tracheostomy bypasses the cords.
- An artificial airway prevents the patient from communicating vocally. This can be frustrating and frightening, and it is important, in a conscious patient, to provide a pad and a pen to help the patient communicate in writing.
- In a conscious patient, there is often a feeling of a loss of dignity and a loss of control over one's self due to tubes which prevent the patient from speaking or breathing normally.

Table 1: Indications for artificial airway.
• Acute respiratory failure necessitating invasive ventilator support • To maintain an open airway in the presence of obstruction to the pharynx or larynx • To protect the airway when protective reflexes are lost • To facilitate suction of secretions within the tracheobronchial tree which the patient is unable to cough up and expectorate

ESTABLISHING AN EMERGENCY AIRWAY

An emergency airway is one that must be established immediately, with utmost urgency, as it involves a matter of life and death. The chief indications for an "immediate" airway are:

- Severe life-threatening upper airways obstruction
- Cardiac or respiratory arrest—or impending cardiorespiratory arrest
- Fulminant pulmonary edema.

The emergency airway of choice is an oral endotracheal intubation, with the aid of direct laryngoscopy. In an intensive care unit (ICU) or in any setting where the expertise and the necessary equipment is promptly available, oral endotracheal intubation can be performed in a matter of minutes. However, emergency endotracheal intubation may prove difficult even in experienced hands, and at times, may fail. In such circumstances, an alternative airway needs to be established urgently.

OTHER EMERGENCY AIRWAYS

Laryngeal Mask Airway

The laryngeal mask airway (LMA) can secure the airway in an emergency, in a situation where endotracheal intubation fails, or in a situation where experienced personnel to intubate are unavailable **(Fig. 2)**. A properly placed LMA not only secures the airway, but allows ventilatory support and reduces the risk of gastric aspiration. A standard adult LMA consists of a 12 mm internal diameter tube fused at a 30° angle to an elliptical spoon-shaped cuff with an inflatable rim. The cuff is soft and when inflated adapts to

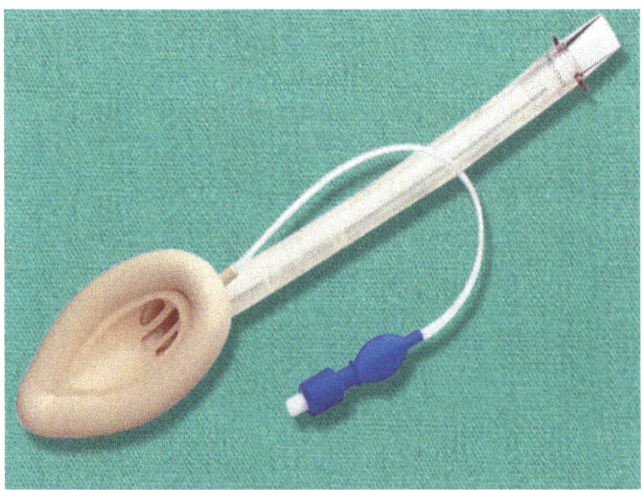

Fig. 2: Laryngeal mask airway.

the shape of the larynx forming an airtight seal over it. The tube opens into the concavity of the cuff ellipse through a fenestrated aperture. The LMA should be placed with the patient placed in sniffing position—neck flexed and head extended. The cuff is deflated and lubricated prior to insertion. The patient's mouth is opened and with the distal aperture of the cuff positioned anteriorly, the tip of the cuff is applied against the hard palate and advanced by the index finger of the right hand over the back of the tongue till it meets resistance when it abuts on the upper esophageal sphincter. The cuff is inflated with 30 mL air so that the cuff centers on the laryngeal inlet. Studies show that the procedure is easily learnt by nurses and that adequate ventilation could be provided in 87% of the cases. Studies in mannequins suggest that the LMA decreased gastric distension compared to the AMBU and could be more easily placed than the combitube.

Intubating Laryngeal Mask Airway

The standard LMA can allow intubation with the aid of a fiberoptic bronchoscope. This requires heavy sedation. However, the size of the endotracheal tube that can be inserted through the LMA is necessarily small. The intubating LMA consists of an anatomically curved rigid tube with a metal-guided handle and a distal silicone laryngeal cuff. The floor of the cuff aperture has an epiglottis-elevating bar and guiding ramp which permits a specially designed endotracheal tube (8 mm in diameter) to be directed toward the glottis and inserted blindly into the trachea. The intubating LMA can be placed without moving the patient's head or neck. This is of definite advantage to patients who have sustained an injury to the cervical spine or to those who have an unstable cervical spine—situations where spinal flexion is best avoided.

The major concerns in the use of the LMA are: (1) the risk of gastric aspiration; (2) the possibility of ineffective ventilation because of suboptimal positioning over the larynx; (3) the inability to generate high inflation pressures in patients with increased airway resistance or low lung compliance.

Cricothyroidotomy

A cricothyroidotomy with insertion of a tube or a conduit into the trachea may serve as a life-saving temporary emergency procedure. A cricothyroidotomy should be replaced by an appropriate airway as soon as possible (**Figs. 3A to D**).

Emergency Tracheostomy

An emergency tracheostomy can be performed by an experienced surgeon in 15 minutes.

Percutaneous Tracheostomy (*see* Section on "Diagnostic and Therapeutic Procedures")

A percutaneous tracheostomy can be carried out by an experienced intensivist or surgeon in perhaps even lesser time.

Till such time as an emergency airway is ultimately secured, it is vital to continue to ventilate the patient with a bag-mask using 100% oxygen and to ensure that at least the upper airway (above the vocal cords) is patent.

Endotracheal Intubation (*see* Section on "Diagnostic and Therapeutic Procedures")

Endotracheal intubation is often performed electively and in less emergent situations (**Figs. 4 and 5**). It can be performed:

- *With the patient awake*: This is very unpleasant for the patient but has the great advantage that it allows the patient to ventilate and oxygenate himself or herself. It is preferred particularly in patients with difficult airways. The approach may be a blind nasotracheal intubation or endotracheal intubation using topical anesthesia and direct laryngoscopy to visualize the larynx, or endotracheal intubation through the use of a fiberoptic bronchoscope.
- *With the patient sedated*: Sedative agents such as midazolam or propofol are administered. The patient though sedated, maintains spontaneous ventilation. Endotracheal intubation is then done with the aid of direct laryngoscopy, or if needs be with the help of a laryngoscope or a bronchoscope. If an LMA has been introduced earlier, intubation can be done via a fiberoptic bronchoscope passed through the larynx.
- *After inducing neuromuscular paralysis*: This is the method most frequently used when performing endotracheal intubation with the aid of direct laryngoscopy. Muscle paralysis with relaxation of the masseters and paralysis of the pharynx generally allows a good view of the larynx with the aid of a laryngoscope and allows quick intubation. However, respiratory muscle paralysis abolishes spontaneous

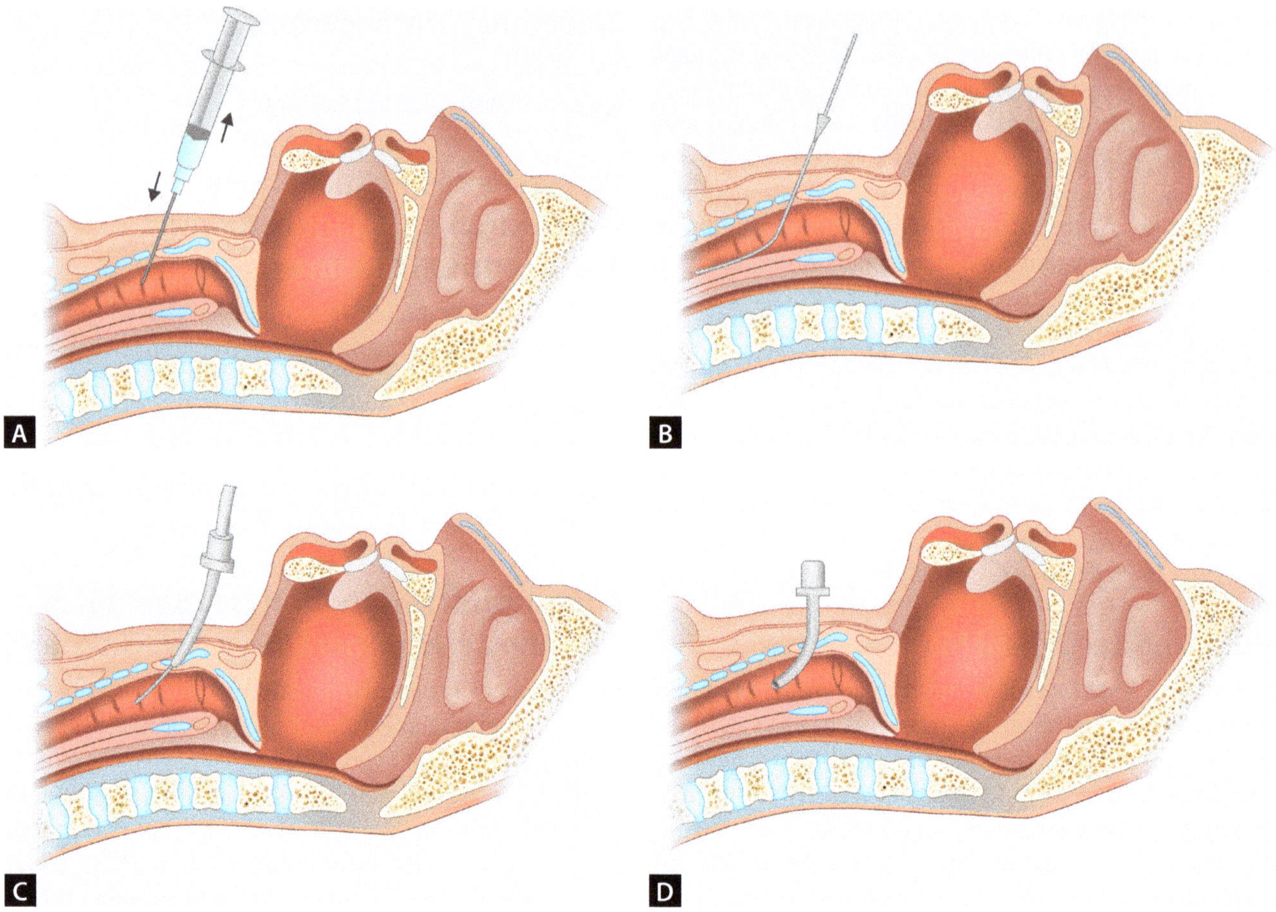

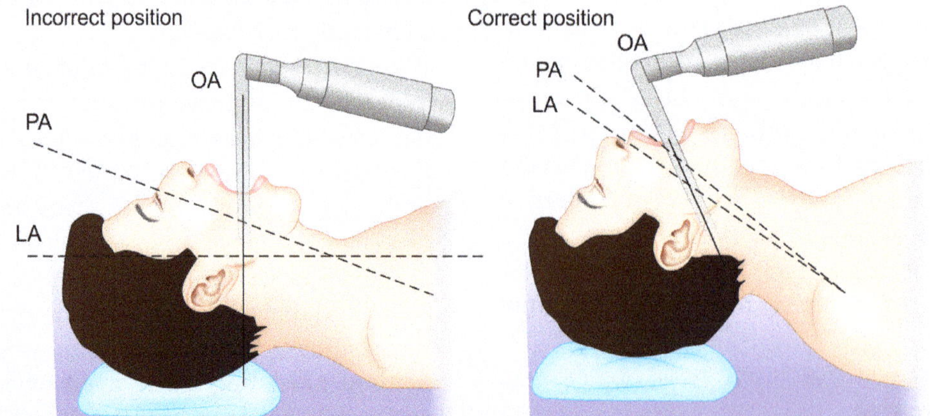

Figs. 3A to D: Procedure for cricothyroidotomy. (A) Pass needle through cricothyroid membrane; (B) Insert guide wire through the needle; (C) Jointly advance dilator and tracheostomy tube over guide wire; (D) Tracheostomy tube in place.

Fig. 4: The position of the head and neck for endotracheal intubation. (LA: Laryngeal axis; OA: Orax axis; PA: Pharyngeal axis)

ventilation and the physician must therefore obtain immediate airway control or failing this ensures effective bag-mask ventilation till spontaneous ventilation returns. Also, in a difficult intubation, the larynx if situated anteriorly may not be visualized even after neuromuscular paralysis, so an alternative

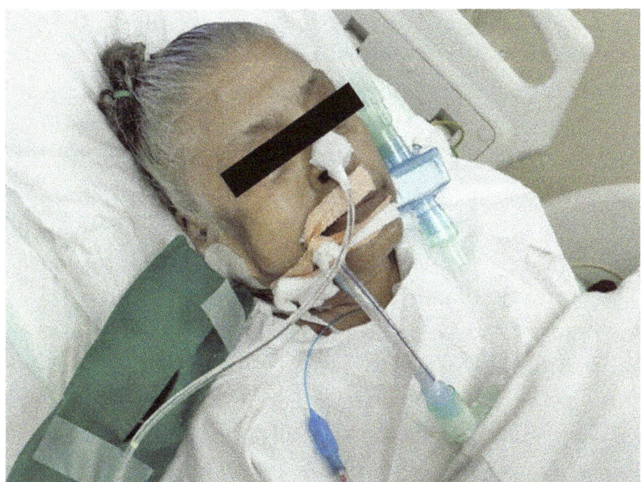

Fig. 5: Endotracheal Intubation.

plan to secure the airway and maintain ventilation should be promptly available.

A standard rapid sequence method is followed when using neuroparalytic agents prior to endotracheal intubation in patients at risk for aspiration of gastric contents.

- The patient is oxygenated with 100% oxygen for some minutes through a bag and full-face mask.
- A sedative (midazolam) is administered as a bolus followed immediately by the administration of a short-acting neuroparalytic agent like succinylcholine.
- At the same time an assistant exerts pressure on the cricoid using the Selick's maneuver which occludes the esophagus and reduces the risk of aspiration.
- Endotracheal intubation is quickly performed; the pressure on the cricoid being relieved only after the airway has been secured.

The major disadvantage of neuromuscular paralysis is that effective spontaneous respiration may not return for several minutes so that a failed intubation can turn into a disaster.

The procedure for endotracheal intubation has been described in the section on "Diagnostic and Therapeutic Procedures".

Management of Aspiration during Bag-Mask Ventilation

Danger of aspiration is significant in high-risk patients—those with a full stomach, patients with a hiatus hernia or gastroesophageal reflux, obese individuals, and in pregnancy. Aspiration should be countered by maintaining pressure over the cricoid cartilage (thereby closing the esophageal lumen), putting the patient promptly in the Trendelenburg position and suctioning the gastric contents. If possible intubation should be prompt with the help of direct laryngoscopy. The airway should be secured and the cuff of the endotracheal tube inflated before resuming positive-pressure ventilation.

■ DIFFICULT AIRWAY

A difficult airway is a clinical situation in which an anesthesiologist or an intensivist experiences difficulty with mask ventilation, or difficulty with tracheal intubation or both. Difficult mask ventilation implies an inability to maintain an O_2 saturation more than 90% using 100% oxygen and positive-pressure mask ventilation. Difficult intubations are those requiring three or more attempts using conventional laryngoscopy. In an ICU setting, a difficult-to-intubate airway may be apparent on a preintubation evaluation or becomes manifest only on attempted intubation. A markedly receding jaw, prominent incisors, macroglossia, soft tissue lesions obstructing the oropharynx or the entrance to the larynx, a rigid spine as in ankylosing spondylitis or a very anteriorly placed glottis can make intubation difficult or impossible.

Mallampati assessed the ability to perform a direct laryngoscopic endotracheal intubation by noting the degree of visibility of the faucial pillars and the uvula, with the patient seated, mouth wide open and the tongue fully protruded. Patients were classified into three classes according to the difficulty experienced in intubation.

- *Class I*—clearly visible fauces and uvula, with a wide oropharynx—easy intubation.
- *Class II*—less clearly visible fauces and uvula, with a smaller opening of the oropharynx—intubation not as easy as in Class I.
- *Class III*—poorly visible fauces and uvula, with a small oropharynx, encroached upon by the above structures—intubation could prove difficult. This preintubation evaluation correlated with the laryngoscopic visualization of the larynx—in Class I the larynx being well visualized and in Class III, the larynx being poorly visualized. Samson and Young added a Class IV to Mallampati classification.
- *Class IV*—is characterized by the inability to see the fauces, uvula, and the oropharyngeal opening (patient seated, tongue protruded, mouth wide open). The vocal

cords are not visualized on direct laryngoscopy, and intubation in these patients is generally unsuccessful.

In an emergency setting in the ICU, there is no time for elaborate preintubation evaluation. Patients requiring intubation are often hypoxic, restless, uncooperative, and hemodynamically unstable. The simplest predictor of a likely successful intubation at the bedside in an emergency is the "Rule of Threes". If the intensivist can place three finger breadths (6–7 cm) between the upper and lower teeth, between the mandible and the hyoid bone and between the thyroid cartilage and the sternal notch, intubation is usually successful.

Difficult Intubation in the Critical Care Unit

It is important not to make several attempts at intubation as this traumatizes the pharynx, larynx, and makes a subsequent successful intubation doubly difficult. More than two attempts are associated with increased morbidity and an increased risk of cardiac arrest. Patients who are hypoxic are rendered even more hypoxic with all the attendant risks. Patients who to start with are hypotensive, hemodynamically unstable, or are in shock from any cause, or who are on vasopressors to maintain perfusion are at grave risk from preintubation death following repeated failed attempts at intubation. Sudden fluctuations in blood pressure and heart rate consequent to repeated attempts at intubation are dangerous in patients with aneurysms or in patients with unstable angina or myocardial infarction.

The management of failed endotracheal intubation attempts in a critical care setting should be considered under two heads.

1. Failed intubation attempts in patients in whom securing an airway and establishing effective ventilation is a matter of extreme urgency, a matter of life and death, e.g. cardiac arrest, respiratory arrest, and extreme obstruction to the airway **(Flowchart 1)**.

The following emergency measures need to be followed:

- Call for help
- Continue bag-mask ventilation with 100% oxygen. Two individuals can perform this more effectively than one. One individual ensures that the mask fits tightly over the nose and mouth, preventing any air leak; the other squeezes the AMBU bag fed with 100% oxygen. The intensivist or physician should note whether the

bag-mask ventilation is effective, as judged by good breath sounds over both lungs and by oxygen saturation more than 90%. Difficulties in bag-mask ventilation are likely if any two of the following are present—age more than 55 years, edentulous patient, obesity (body mass index >30 kg/m^2), beard, and history of snoring.

- If a bag-mask ventilation fails or is ineffective, the situation is indeed very critical ("cannot intubate–cannot ventilate" scenario).

Insert an LMA or even better (if available), an intubating LMA (I-LMA) and ventilate the patient via this airway. If the intubating LMA is in place, attempt to intubate blindly using the specially designed endotracheal tube that goes with the I-LMA. *Intubation (with a small-sized endotracheal tube) can also be attempted through a plain LMA with the aid of a fiberoptic bronchoscope.*

If effective ventilation through an LMA fails, and intubation via the LMA or via the I-LMA is unsuccessful, the quickest way of securing ventilation and preventing death from hypoxia is by performing a cricothyroidotomy. A cricothyroidotomy should be promptly followed by an emergency percutaneous tracheostomy or by an emergency formal tracheostomy.

- Even if either bag-mask ventilation or ventilation through an LMA is successful, a more permanent and secure artificial airway is mandatory if spontaneous effective breathing has not returned. This is achieved either by a percutaneous tracheostomy or a formal tracheostomy. In expert hands, this can be performed within 10–15 minutes.
- If a preintubation clinical evaluation suggests that bag-mask ventilation or LMA ventilation cannot possibly be successful (as in extreme obstruction to the oropharynx, facial, neck injuries), proceed straight to a cricothyroidotomy, or a percutaneous tracheostomy, or a formal tracheostomy depending on the degree of the urgency of the situation.
- Transtracheal jet ventilation (TTJV) is an alternative to a surgical airway in a "cannot intubate-cannot ventilate" situation. After stabilizing the larynx, a 12–16-gauge catheter-over-needle (attached to a syringe particularly filled with saline) is directed caudally through the cricothyroid membrane into the trachea. Tracheal entry is confirmed by aspiration of air bubbles. The catheter is now advanced (up to the hub), over the needle into the trachea with the aid of a small skin incision. The placement is confirmed by aspiration of air. The hub of the catheter is connected

Flowchart 1: Algorithm for the management of difficult airway and ventilation (in the ICU) in a life and death emergency.

(LMA: Laryngeal mask airway; TTJV: Transtracheal jet ventilation)
Source: Reproduced with permission from: The Difficult Airway Course™: Emergency. In: Walls RM, Murphy MF (Eds). Manual of Emergency Airway Management. Philadelphia: Lippincott Williams & Wilkins; 2008, 4th edition, 2012.

to a jet ventilation system. Care should be taken to stabilize the catheter and prevent any air leak at the incision site. We are not familiar with TTJV but it has been performed in all age groups and is the preferred surgical airway in children below 12 years. Airway obstruction below the larynx or complete upper airway obstruction can render expiration impossible and is a contraindication to TTJV. Complications with TTJV include subcutaneous emphysema, esophageal puncture, bleeding, and barotraumas. TTJV is an emergency measure and is continued only till such time as a definitive airway has been secured.

2. Failed intubation attempts in situations which are emergent but which still allow some time to the intensivist for establishing an airway **(Flowchart 2)**.

In the above circumstance, the intensivist should use one or more of the other intubation techniques:

- Direct laryngoscopy with topical or local anesthesia (if topical anesthesia has not been already used)
- Use of a stylet, preferably a lighted one, to help guide the endotracheal tube into the trachea
- A flexible fiberoptic scope to aid nasal or oral intubation
- Blind nasal intubation
- Intubation through an LMA
- Retrograde intubation (in very rare circumstances).

Retrograde intubation is attempted by first puncturing the cricothyroid membrane with an 18 gauge introducer needle with catheter. A guide wire is threaded through the needle cephalad into the oropharynx and is then pulled out under vision using Magill's forceps. The guide wire is then placed directly in the lumen of the endotracheal tube. The latter is then guided along the guide wire through the glottis into the trachea. The guide wire is now pulled out through the proximal end of the endotracheal tube and the endotracheal tube fixed in proper position. This procedure requires practice and is more difficult than it appears; we have as yet never attempted retrotracheal intubation in our units.

Flowchart 2: Algorithm for the management of difficult airway and ventilation (in the ICU) in failed laryngoscopic attempts in less emergent situations.

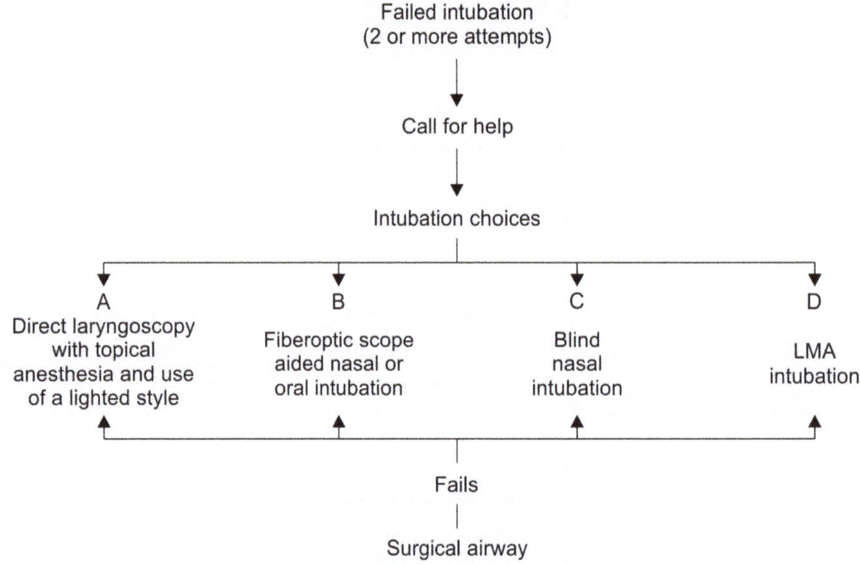

(LMA: Laryngeal mask airway)
Source: Reproduced with permission from: The Difficult Airway Course™: Emergency. In: Walls RM, Murphy MF (Eds). Manual of Emergency Airway Management. Philadelphia: Lippincott Williams & Wilkins; 2008, 4th edition, 2012.

■ TRACHEOSTOMY

A tracheostomy is in our opinion the most satisfactory artificial airway, particularly when the airway needs to be maintained for over 7–10 days. It completely bypasses the upper airway and the glottis, thus preventing any potential complications in that area. It causes less resistance to airflow (vis-a-vis the endotracheal tube), reduces dead space, allows easy and efficient suction of the tracheobronchial tree, and is easy to fix and stabilize. The conscious patient can eat freely, is not bothered by oropharyngeal secretions commonly observed with endotracheal tubes and tolerates the tracheostomy without undue discomfort. When performed by a skilled, experienced surgeon, the overall mortality (procedural with the tube in situ, or after removal) is around 1.5% (range 0–5%). This holds even when the procedure is done in critically ill patients.

Endotracheal Tube versus Tracheostomy

There is still a controversy as to when to continue with an endotracheal tube and when to opt for a tracheostomy. The decision to do a tracheostomy or persist with the endotracheal tube rests on the intensivist's perception of optimal patient care, available nursing care and the unit's experience, and record of complications with each of the two artificial airways.

We prefer to do an elective tracheostomy after first intubating the patient, whenever we are convinced that the disease will necessitate the use of an artificial airway for more than 7 days. If it is difficult to gauge the time duration required for the artificial airway, we persist with the endotracheal tube for about 7–10 days, and then change over to a tracheostomy. Probably each unit has its own preferences. We base our preferences on the fact that our unit has had few complications with tracheostomies, and that tracheobronchial toilet with suction of secretions is far easier through a tracheostomy than through an endotracheal tube. We have also noticed a significant incidence of subglottic edema and stenosis whenever an endotracheal tube has been in place for more than 7–10 days, prompting us to switch to a tracheostomy if we feel that an artificial airway is required beyond that period of time. However, there are many units in the West who persist with an endotracheal tube for as long as 3 weeks without encountering significant complications.

Complications (Figs. 6A to F)

The inability to secure a patent airway or the inability to perform bag-mask ventilation so as to provide oxygenation can lead to cardiac arrest with hypoxic brain damage.

Endotracheal intubation can lead to damage to teeth, to the mucosa of the airways, and to the larynx,

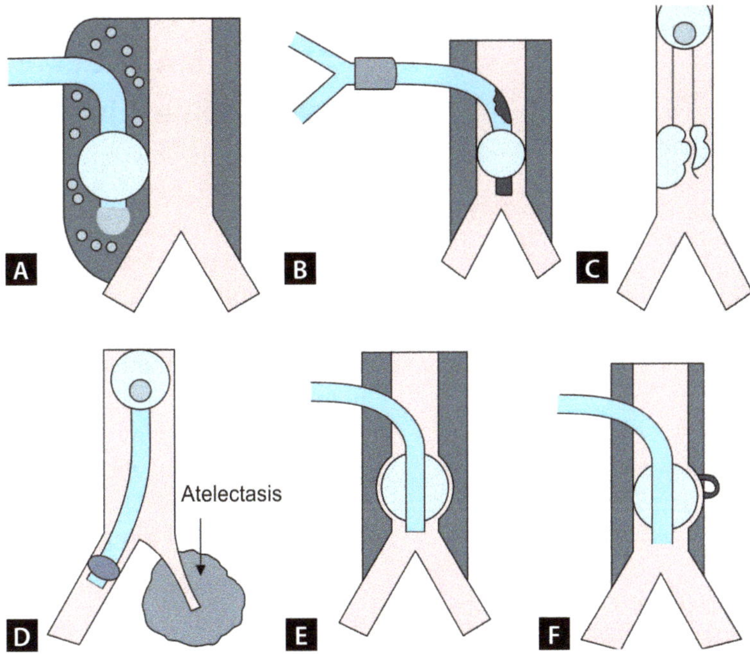

Figs. 6A to F: Complications of tracheostomy: (A) Tube in pretracheal fascia resulting in surgical emphysema of face and neck and sometimes of the mediastinum; (B) Blocked tube; (C) Overinflated cuff slipping over the end and blocking it; (D) Tube slipping into right main bronchus, preventing ventilation to the left lung; (E) Damage to trachea, either due to a very tight-fitting tube with an overinflated cuff, or injury to the posterior wall-end result, dilatation (as in the figure) or stricture; (F) Erosion of the posterior wall of the trachea, and rarely erosion of the innominate artery.
Source: Udwadia FE. Diagnosis and Management of Acute Respiratory Failure. Mumbai: Oxford University Press; 1979.

sometimes causing life-threatening hemorrhage. These risks are increased in patients with coagulopathy and in those with markedly inflamed mucosa of the air passage. The tracheotomy tube may be misplaced outside the trachea causing severe subcutaneous emphysema and life-threatening hypoxemia. Similarly, an endotracheal tube may be misplaced in the esophagus; attempts at ventilation would then cause acute gastric dilation and worsening of pre-existing hypoxia.

The endotracheal tube instead of being above the carina may lie in the right main bronchus resulting in ventilation of the right lung and collapse of the left. Position of endotracheal and tracheostomy tubes should be checked by an X-ray to ensure correct placement.

Tracheostomies can lead to bilateral pneumothorax because of the proximity of the apices of the lungs. Damage to neck veins during the surgical procedures can cause uncontrollable hemorrhage.

■ MAINTAINING THE ARTIFICIAL AIRWAY

It is not enough to establish and secure the airway. It is equally important to maintain, manage, and care for the artificial airway, if the hazards and complications involving the use of artificial airways are to be minimized.

Tracheostomy Care

A high tracheostomy is always preferable as it enables the tip of the tube to lie well above the carina. It is best to use the largest tube that can be comfortably accommodated by the trachea. Small tubes should be avoided as they tend to get blocked, and they offer resistance to airflow. This is particularly unwelcome in those patients with acute respiratory failure who have well-marked airways obstruction, or who have a low compliance due to "stiff lungs". The tube should have an even inflated cuff. High residual volume (low-pressure) cuffs should be always used; high-pressure cuffs have no place in modern respiratory care. Even when using high-volume, low-pressure cuffed tubes, the cuff pressure should be checked daily and kept within acceptable limits. Excessive cuff pressures can induce tracheal injury and subsequent stenosis, particularly if the tracheostomy has been in use over several days or weeks **(Fig. 7)**. Salient points in tracheostomy care are given in **Table 2**.

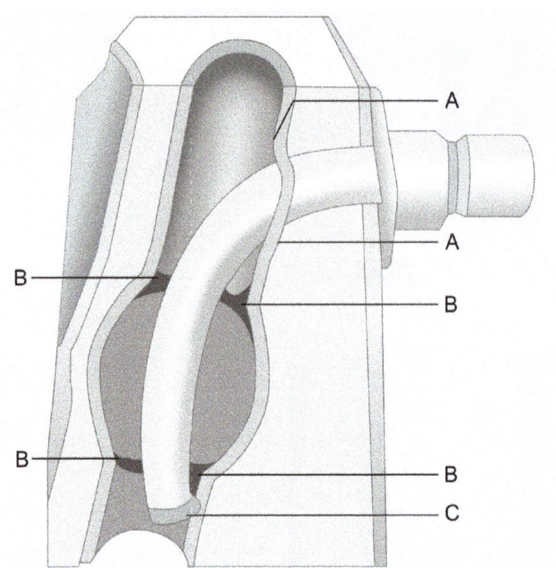

Fig. 7: Sites for occurrence of postextubation tracheal stenosis. [A: Site of tracheostomy; B: Cuff site (most common); C: Where tip irritates tracheal wall].

Table 2: Salient points in tracheostomy care.

- Use sterile gloves for handling tracheostomy tube
- Care of cuff:
  - Use minimal occluding volume for inflating cuff—minimal leak techniques
  - Measure cuff pressure daily, and keep this within acceptable limits (14–24 cm H_2O)
  - Deflate cuff periodically, except when this is contraindicated for specific reasons
- Care over suction of secretions:
  - Use "no-touch" sterile technique
  - Preoxygenate (with high FiO_2) a hemodynamically unstable patient before suction
  - Do not suck for more than 10 seconds
  - Do not use a very large bore catheter for suction
  - If possible, suck through an adaptor so that ventilator support on high-flow oxygen is not interrupted
  - Stop suction if bradycardia or hypotension occur
  - Increase FiO_2 to 100% for a short time
  - Liquefy viscid secretions; use physiotherapy
  - Humidify inspired gas
- Care of tracheostomy tube:
  - Ensure that tube is central in position and does not tilt and slip into one bronchus
  - Ensure that tube does not get blocked
  - Change tube every 4–7 days
- Care of tracheostomy wound:
  - Use sterile dressing and antibiotic ointment
  - Be alert to possible complications of tracheostomy

(FiO_2: Fraction of inspired oxygen)

SPECIAL CONSIDERATIONS IN AIRWAY MANAGEMENT

Cervical Spine Injury

A patient with polytrauma, who requires intubation, should be presumed to have a cervical spine injury. In the absence of severe maxillofacial trauma or cerebrospinal rhinorrhea, a nasal intubation can be attempted. However, if urgent intubation is required as in the apneic or hypoxic patient, oral intubation should be done. During oral endotracheal intubation, a colleague or assistant should hold the neck in position, ensuring axial stability and preventing any flexion or anterior movement of the neck for fear of damaging the spinal cord.

Increased Intracranial Tension

Intubating patients with head injury who have a rise in intracranial pressure may be difficult for several reasons—change in mental state, difficulty in opening the mouth, associated facial trauma. Further rise in intracranial pressure should be avoided as far as possible during intubation. Also, cervical spine trauma should always be suspected in a patient with head injury. The anesthetic agent used for intubating these patients should ideally preserve cerebral perfusion and lower cerebral blood volume while maintaining hemodynamic stability. Thiopental offers neuroprotection but cerebral hypoperfusion may result from its depressant effect on the myocardium and because of peripheral vasodilatation. Etomidate is preferred in hemodynamically unstable patients. If a neuroparalytic agent needs to be used for intubation, vecuronium (0.25 mg/kg) or rocuronium (1.2 mg/kg) is to be preferred.

In patients with polytrauma including head injury with raised intracranial pressure, it may at times be impossible to perform a laryngoscopic endotracheal intubation. The airway may need to be secured by alternative means.

SUGGESTED READING

1. Blanda M. Emergency airway management. Emerg Med Clin North Am. 2003;21(1):1-26.
2. Brown CA 3rd, Bair AE, Pallin DJ, et al. Techniques, success, and adverse events of emergency department adult intubations. Ann Emerg Med. 2015;65:363.

3. Doyle DJ, Hagberg CA, Marianna Crowley. Supraglottic devices (including laryngeal mask airways) for airway management for anesthesia in adults. [online] Available from https://www.uptodate.com/contents/search?search=Supraglottic%20devices%20(including%20laryngeal%20mask%20airways)%20for%20airway%20management%20for%20anesthesia%20in%20adults&x=0&-y=0 [Accessed July 2018].

4. Mace SE. Challenges and advances in intubation: rapid sequence intubation. Emerg Med Clin North Am. 2008;26(4):1043-68, x.

5. Marco CA. Airway adjuncts. Emerg Med Clin North Am. 2008;26(4):1015-27, x.

6. The Difficult Airway Course™: Emergency. In: Walls RM, Murphy MF (Eds). Manual of Emergency Airway Management. Philadelphia: Lippincott Williams & Wilkins; 2008, 4th edition, 2012.

7. Vissers RJ. The high-risk airway. Emerg Med Clin North Am. 2010;28(1):203-17, ix-x.

8. Walz JM. Airway management in critical illness. Chest. 2007;131(2):608-20.

9. Wittels KA. Basic airway management in adults. [online] Available from https://www.uptodate.com/contents/search?search=Basic%20airway%20management%20in%20adults&sp=0 &source=USER_INPUT& searchOffset=1 &autoComplete=false&language=en&max=10&index= &autoCompleteTerm= [Accessed July 2018].

CHAPTER 55

Mechanical Ventilation

■ INTRODUCTION

Mechanical ventilation as a therapeutic intervention was first widely used during the poliomyelitis epidemic in Europe and the United States in the 1940s and 1950s. Since then there have been great advances in technology, so that negative-pressure ventilators that were used originally in the 1940s and 1950s have been replaced by increasingly sophisticated positive-pressure machines.

The purpose of mechanical ventilation is to provide ventilation support partially or fully by an external device to patients who cannot maintain an adequate gas exchange, as for example in acute respiratory failure. Ventilator support also reduces the oxygen cost of breathing. Mechanical ventilator support, however, has its own hazards; these include ventilator-induced lung injury, barotrauma, adverse hemodynamic changes, and the potential for serious nosocomial infection.

Ventilator support to any critically ill individual requires expertise and round-the-clock supervision and care. Life in many such patients is totally dependent on the efficient working of a machine. A mechanical failure, accidental disconnection of the machine from the patient, or a sudden obstruction of the airway, are all potential disasters which can lead to sudden death or brain damage from protracted hypoxia. A patient on mechanical ventilator support must therefore, never be left unattended even for a minute. Thus, the optimal and safe use of mechanical ventilation is only possible in intensive care units (ICUs). Though the standard of critical care (which includes ventilator support) has improved and continues to improve significantly at least in the large metropolitan cities of India, care provided in large public and district hospitals in India and many other developing countries leaves much to be desired. In fact, critical care units in the poor countries of the world are often mere apologies of what they ought to be, or are nonexistent. In the absence of a full-fledged ICU, the next best option is to use ventilator support in a patient who needs it, in a special or even a general ward, provided that the medical registrar and nurses are well trained in ventilator management. We managed to do this at one of the large public teaching hospitals in Mumbai, and salvaged a number of very ill patients who would otherwise have died. The need for all medical registrars (at least in the large hospitals of India and other developing countries) to be familiar with the use of mechanical ventilators is thus imperative. It is the duty of the medical and administrative staff of such hospitals to provide basic facilities, and train a team of doctors and nurses who can manage critically ill patients on ventilator support, even in the absence of well-equipped ICUs.

This chapter to start with briefly tabulates the physiological effects of mechanical ventilation. It then proceeds to discuss the indications and criteria for ventilator support, types of ventilators for intermittent positive-pressure ventilation (IPPV), and the management of ventilatory support. This is followed by a description of the different modes of ventilator support, and the use of positive end-expiratory pressure (PEEP) as an adjunct. Then comes a section on the complications of mechanical ventilation, followed by a discussion on weaning from ventilator support. The chapter ends with a discussion on noninvasive ventilator support and of respiratory monitoring during mechanical ventilation.

■ INDICATIONS FOR MECHANICAL VENTILATION (TABLE 1)

In many ICUs in Mumbai and India, there is yet a certain hesitation and trepidation observed regarding the use of mechanical ventilation in patients who need ventilator support. In other words, mechanical ventilation is started much later than it should have been in the natural history of a disease requiring ventilatory support. The other equally common misconception and error is to be in a tearing hurry to remove ventilator support in a critically ill patient. Such a premature withdrawal of ventilator support is love's labor lost—the patient regresses from near recovery to a critical state, which again necessitates the use of the ventilator.

Established Acute Respiratory Failure

Early ventilator support is now initiated by all good units in patients with acute respiratory failure. The criteria and timing for initiating support depend on

Table 1: Indications for mechanical ventilation.

A. *Established acute respiratory failure*:
- Primary ventilatory failure where lungs are normal to start with, e.g. poisonings that depress the CNS, CNS and neuromuscular disorders (poliomyelitis, infective polyneuritis, myasthenia), snake bite, and severe tetanus
- Hypoventilating comatose patients
- Acute pulmonary disease, e.g. fulminant pneumonia, acute lung injury (ARDS)
- Fulminant pulmonary edema
- Major or massive pulmonary embolism
- Major or massive atelectasis
- Patients with COPD in acute crisis, unresponsive to conventional therapy
- Patients with acute severe asthma unresponsive to conventional therapy
- Patients with severe respiratory muscle fatigue

B. *Incipient respiratory failure*:
- Patients with excessive ventilatory demands
- Obese patients who have undergone upper abdominal surgery, or poor-risk surgical patients
- Patients with acute/fulminant parenchymal lung disease with rapidly progressive impairment of pulmonary function and reserve
- Respiratory muscle fatigue in critical illnesses

C. Low-output states—shock of any etiology

D. *Purposeful hyperventilation*:
- To decrease intracranial tension in patients with head injury associated with increased intracranial tension
- To reduce cerebral edema after CPR or massive CVA

(ARDS: Acute respiratory distress syndrome; CNS: Central nervous system; COPD: Chronic obstructive pulmonary disease; CPR: Cardiopulmonary resuscitation)

the etiological agent producing acute respiratory failure, and above all, on the rate at which respiratory function is observed to deteriorate. Different diseases producing acute respiratory failure present their own special problems with regard to initiating mechanical ventilation, technicalities in maintaining ventilation, and difficulties in weaning the patient from ventilator support. It is therefore, best from the practical point of view to consider the indications in acute respiratory failure, with reference to the different groups of diseases frequently encountered in the ICU.

Ventilator Support in Primary Ventilatory Failure

The most common indication for mechanical ventilation is acute primary failure of ventilation. Ventilatory failure occurs commonly in poisonings that depress the central nervous system (CNS), in acute inflammatory and other diseases involving the CNS, in some patients with head injury, increased intracranial tension, poliomyelitis, acute infective polyneuritis, and myasthenia gravis. Severe tetanus is an important cause of ventilatory failure in India. Neuromuscular paralysis following a krait or cobra bite is particularly common in South India. The lungs are normal to start with, but changes within the lungs (chiefly increasing widespread atelectasis), almost always occur if treatment is delayed. In many patients with neuromuscular disease, deterioration can occur suddenly, almost precipitously, with disastrous consequences. It is therefore, wise to start early ventilatory support in these patients.

Ventilator Support in a Hypoventilating Comatose Patient

Deep coma is an indication for securing the airways with an endotracheal tube or a tracheostomy. Hypoventilation in such patients may be due to depressed respiratory drive or secretions causing obstructed airways or patchy atelectasis. Hypoxia and hypercapnia resulting from hypoventilation may further impair the conscious state, which in turn may further depress ventilation. Unless the patient is clearly hyperventilating, a deeply comatose patient is safer on mechanical ventilation.

Ventilator Support in Acute Pulmonary Disease

These patients are hypoxic due to hypoxemic acute respiratory failure. Typical examples are acute respiratory distress syndrome (ARDS), and fulminant pneumonia. Patients with acute pulmonary disease are difficult to ventilate. They have a strong respiratory drive, are often severely hypoxic, and "fight" the ventilator. An inability to maintain a PaO_2 > 55 mm Hg while on oxygen at a flow rate of 6–8 L/min, is an indication for initiating ventilator support. Other criteria for starting mechanical ventilation in these patients are dealt with later.

Ventilator Support in Fulminant Pulmonary Edema

Acute pulmonary edema, if fulminant, literally chokes the patient at the level of the alveoli. Mechanical ventilation is life-saving not only because it allows the maintenance of an adequate partial pressure of arterial oxygen (PaO_2), but perhaps because the high inflation pressures used to ventilate the lungs reduces the transudation of fluid from the alveolar capillaries into the alveoli. Ventilator support buys time during which diuretics like furosemide has a chance to act, and other corrective measures to treat the underlying cause of acute pulmonary edema may be profitably undertaken.

Ventilator Support in Acute Thromboembolic Lung Disease

Ventilator support is indicated if the PaO_2 is less than 60 mm Hg on supplemental oxygen, particularly in the presence of shock.

Ventilator Support in Acute on Chronic Respiratory Failure in Patients with Chronic Airways Obstruction

Many patients in this group are used to a low PaO_2 less than 65 mm Hg, and a high $PaCO_2$ more than 50–60 mm Hg. Ventilator support should not be used unless all other modalities of treatment have been of no avail, clinical deterioration is evident, and there is a further deterioration in the arterial blood gases and arterial pH. In such patients, ventilatory support is fraught with difficulty, and requires experience and expertise.

Ventilator Support in Acute Severe Asthma

Acute severe asthma is probably one of the most difficult problems for effective mechanical ventilation. Yet ventilator support is life-saving in those cases of acute severe asthma not responding to corticosteroids, nebulized bronchodilators, and other medical therapy.

Ventilator Support in Patients with Severe Muscle Fatigue

Severe muscle fatigue (involving the muscles of respiration), is an increasingly recognized and important cause of hypoventilation and respiratory failure. Muscle fatigue can occur in patients with primary neuromuscular disease involving the respiratory muscles. It occurs much more frequently in lung disease and in any condition (not necessarily involving the lungs), where ventilatory demands are excessive. The timing of initiating ventilator support in these patients is a matter of fine judgment. Altered blood gases or feeble ventilatory efforts are of course an immediate indication. Irregular breathing patterns, or the presence of a respiratory paradox in which the abdominal muscles move inward rather than outward during inspiration, point to excessive muscle fatigue. Respiratory alternans is characterized by alternate excursions involving the diaphragm and the intercostals, and is also a pointer to muscle fatigue. Another important pointer to impending disaster is the presence of apneic spells which are often forerunners of prolonged respiratory arrest. It is better to ventilate such patients even if the arterial blood gases are not significantly distorted, rather than wait for disaster to occur.

Factors which precipitate and contribute to respiratory muscle fatigue are hypoperfusion of the muscles, hypermetabolic states leading to an increased workload on the muscles of respiration, hypoxia, electrolyte and acid-base disturbances, poor nutrition as in alcoholics or those with chronic liver or renal diseases, and in old, feeble, debilitated patients.

Incipient Respiratory Failure

Mechanical ventilation is increasingly being used in patients in whom some degree of respiratory failure is anticipated. Perhaps the most important group comprises patients who have to meet increased ventilatory demands, and who therefore, sooner or later show evidence of respiratory muscle fatigue. This is typically seen in acute severe asthma, but can occur in numerous medical and surgical problems. It is difficult for a seriously ill patient to sustain a ventilatory rate of more than 35–40/min or a minute ventilation (VE) more than 10–12 L/min for any prolonged period of time without increasing muscle fatigue and the danger of impending sudden respiratory failure.

There is a special category of surgical patients who frequently require ventilator support for impending or insidious respiratory failure. These are obese individuals who have undergone upper abdominal surgery. This often leads to "fixed" or "splinted" domes of the diaphragm resulting in a loss of volume in both lower lobes. These patients are markedly tachypneic, particularly in the presence of fever and infection; their VE is often as high as 12–15 L/min, and their respiratory rates between 35/min and 45/min. They maintain their arterial blood gases within the normal range for some length of time, but not uncommonly these patients go into sudden respiratory failure, deteriorate sharply, and pose problems in emergency intubation and ventilation. A quick anticipation of worsening problems calls for early intubation and ventilator support before such a disaster occurs.

Other susceptible patients in whom hypoventilation is a likely sequel include poor-risk surgical patients whose recovery from surgery or trauma is hindered by obesity, chronic lung disease, old age, debility, and electrolyte imbalance. In all these patients, postoperative ventilatory support is merely an extension of surgical care in the operation theater. They may require mechanical ventilation for a period varying from a few hours to a few days, and are weaned off ventilator support when they can maintain adequate gas exchange on spontaneous breathing.

Similarly, in acute or fulminant parenchymal lung disease where the tempo of impairment of respiratory reserve and respiratory function is very rapid, it is best to anticipate events in advance to allow for elective intubation and ventilatory support.

Low-output States and Septic Shock

Ventilator support is now always indicated in low cardiac output states as in cardiogenic shock, or for that matter in shock from any etiology. It is often used in septic shock, at times quite early in the natural history, when the march of events signifies a rapidly evolving dangerous clinical state. In shock from any cause, and in low-output states of any etiology (for example, in advanced liver cell failure or multiorgan failure), tissue perfusion is inadequate in relation to tissue oxygen needs. Also, a low cardiac output is generally associated with a low mixed venous oxygen tension (PvO_2), which in turn is responsible for a low PaO_2.

Shock of any etiology which results in low pulmonary artery pressure and diminished perfusion of the lungs lead to an increase both in the VD/VT ratio, as well as to a V/Q imbalance. Ventilator support helps in two ways: (1) with an increase in fraction of inspired oxygen (FiO_2) (if needs be to 70–80%), the PaO_2 increases, and therefore, both the arterial oxygenation and the arterial oxygen content rise; (2) the muscles of respiration are rested once the ventilator takes over the function of ventilation. This prevents incipient respiratory failure from progressing to frank ventilatory failure, and even ventilatory arrest. In patients who breathe excessively, the oxygen cost of breathing is considerably increased. At rest, the normal work of breathing accounts for 2–3% of total oxygen consumption. This can increase in acute respiratory failure to as high as 35–40%. In low-output states, resting the overworked respiratory muscles through mechanical ventilation sharply reduces the oxygen cost of breathing and allows more oxygen to be diverted to vital organs starved of their oxygen supply. However, in critically ill patients, it is equally important to control fever, shivering, constant movement, and restlessness, as these can all contribute to increased oxygen consumption, and thereby reduce the already meager available oxygen supply to the vital organs.

Mechanical Ventilation for the Specific Purpose of Hyperventilation

A comparatively rare indication for mechanical ventilation is to hyperventilate patients with head injury, when associated with increased intracranial pressure. Hyperventilating these patients reduces the $PaCO_2$ which leads to reduction in the cerebral blood flow, and hence in the intracranial pressure. Hyperventilation is generally combined with sedation and muscle paralysis to prevent coughing and clashing with the ventilator, as these could lead to a rise in intracranial pressure. Clinicians often prefer to manage unconscious neurological and neurosurgical patients with increased intracranial pressure, with controlled mechanical hyperventilation. The same approach is sometimes used to counter cerebral edema following resuscitation after a cardiopulmonary arrest or in patients with cerebral edema consequent to a massive cerebrovascular accident. However, the efficacy of hyperventilation in all the abovementioned situations is temporary (generally not exceeding 48 hours) and debatable.

OBJECTIVE CRITERIA FOR INITIATING VENTILATOR SUPPORT IN ADULTS

The criteria enumerated in **Table 2** are mere guidelines, and not sacrosanct rules. It is crucial to take the clinical picture, the evolution of the disease in a given patient, and the trend and rate of change in the parameters outlined here, into consideration.

The parameters given in **Table 2** apply to patients in ventilatory failure, and to respiratory failure occurring with acute lung disease; they are not applicable to patients with chronic obstructive airways disease. These patients even under normal or basal conditions may have a PaO_2 of 60 mm Hg, and a $PaCO_2$ between 55 mm Hg and 60 mm Hg. They are used to hypoxia and hypercapnia, and tolerate both rather well.

TYPES OF VENTILATORS FOR INTERMITTENT POSITIVE-PRESSURE VENTILATION (TABLE 3)

Ventilators in ICUs are either volume-cycled or pressure-cycled or time-cycled.

A volume-cycled, i.e. a volume-targeted ventilator, delivers a preset volume and continues to do so regardless of a change in the patient's airway resistance or lung compliance.

A pressure-cycled, i.e. a pressure-targeted ventilator, cycles to expiration after a specified preset pressure has been attained. Thus, gas flows into the lungs until a preset pressure limit is reached. The volume delivered will

Table 2: Criteria for initiating ventilator support in adults.

- Respiratory rate more than 35/min
- VC less than 10–15 mL/kg
- MV more than 10–12 L/min over a prolonged period
- Maximum inspiratory force less than –20 cm H_2O
- PaO_2 less than 60 mm Hg on nasal oxygen at 6–8 L/min and/or $PaCO_2$ more than 55 mm Hg
- Alveolar-arterial oxygen gradient more than 300–350 mm Hg on FiO_2 of 1
- VD/VT more than 0.6
- Visible excessive work of breathing in critically ill or debilitated patients
- Clinical evidence of respiratory muscle fatigue:
  - Poor chest excursions
  - Tachypnea
  - Respiratory muscle paradox, "respiratory alternans"
  - Apneic spells

(FiO_2: Fraction of inspired oxygen; PaO_2: Partial pressure of arterial oxygen; VT: Tidal volume)

Table 3: Comparison between volume-controlled (volume-targeted) and pressure-controlled (pressure-targeted) ventilation.

	Volume-targeted	*Pressure-targeted*
Rate	Set or variable	Set or variable
Tidal volume (VT)	Set	Variable
Peak airway pressure	Variable	Set
Peak alveolar pressure	Variable	Set
Peak flow	Set	Variable
Inspiration-expiration (I:E) ratio	Variable	Set

therefore, change if the airway resistance and/or the lung compliance change.

In a time-cycled ventilator, the inspiratory phase ends when a predetermined time has elapsed. This time remains fixed, and is controlled by a timing mechanism within the ventilator, which is unaffected by conditions in the patient's lungs.

Volume-targeted ventilatory support is more flexible, easier to learn, and easier to manage than pressure-targeted or time-cycled ventilator support. All modern ventilators are capable of delivering adequate VE and of varying the oxygen concentration (FiO_2) from 25% to 100%.

Most modern ventilators incorporate within a single unit, mechanisms that allow either volume-targeted or pressure-targeted ventilatory support, the use of PEEP, and the choice of several modes of ventilator support, detailed later. Adjustment of VE, respiratory rates, flow rates, and inspiratory-expiratory ratios are also possible. The ventilator is fitted with a series of alarms for better patient care, and can be fitted with modules that can monitor and display lung mechanics (compliance, airway resistance, waveforms, and flow-volume loops) and the end-tidal partial pressure of carbon dioxide (pCO_2).

From the clinical viewpoint, neither volume-targeted, nor pressure-targeted ventilation offers a distinct advantage with regard to gas exchange, hemodynamic stability, and pulmonary mechanics.

The major advantage of volume-targeted ventilatory support is its ease of application, and the provision of a fixed tidal volume (VT) in spite of changing airway resistance or pulmonary compliance.

The main advantage of pressure-cycled or pressure-targeted ventilation is that gas is delivered at a fixed preset pressure; if there is increased impedance to ventilation (either due to increased airways resistance or to a lowered pulmonary compliance), the VT delivered falls. Overstretching of the alveoli with resulting volutrauma, barotraumas, and biotrauma is thus prevented. Pressure-control ventilation may also be able to answer the high inspiratory flow demands of some critically ill patients.

■ MANAGEMENT OF MECHANICAL VENTILATION

Initiating Ventilation—Basics of Initial Ventilator Setup

There are a number of ventilator modes available to help ventilate a patient. We generally initiate ventilator support with volume-controlled or volume-targeted ventilation using the assist-control mode. In assist-control ventilation, the patient triggers the inspiration by a spontaneous effort which is enhanced by the ventilator. In this mode, if for some reason, the patient fails to trigger the machine, the machine takes over, initiates inspiration, and takes over full ventilatory support. Most patients with different respiratory problems can be adequately ventilated by the volume-targeted, assist-control mode.

Tidal Volume

The VT for an individual patient should be set between 5 mL/kg and 10 mL/kg body weight. Selection of VT in a given patient is influenced by the nature of the disease, the approximate VE requirement, pulmonary compliance, airway resistance, airway pressure, PaO_2, and $PaCO_2$.

Very low VTs result in atelectasis, hypoventilation, and hypoxemia. On the other hand, very high VTs can cause respiratory alkalosis, decrease cardiac output by reducing venous return, and predispose to barotrauma, volutrauma, and biotrauma. There is definite evidence that overstretch of alveolar walls through very large VTs can induce lung "injury".

In patients with normal lungs to start with (as in neuromuscular disease causing respiratory failure, CNS disease, coma, poisoning, and immediate postoperative conditions), the VT is set at 10 mL/kg.

In patients whose lungs are stiff because of abnormal respiratory mechanics (as in ARDS, pneumonia) VTs are set at 5–7 mL/kg. A convenient algorithm is to start with 10 mL/kg, stabilize the patient, and then progressively reduce the VT to 5–7 mL/kg so that the plateau pressure does not exceed 30 cm H_2O.

Respiratory Rate

The rate is generally set between 10 breaths/min and 14 breaths/min, if the patient is clinically stable. Higher rates may be required (20–25/min) in patients with stiff lungs (e.g. ARDS), so as to match the machine to the spontaneous breathing pattern of the patient. Lower rates may be necessary in chronic obstructive pulmonary disease (COPD) patients where VE needs to be restricted. If the respiratory rate is too high, respiratory alkalosis, auto-PEEP, and barotrauma can result. If too low, hypoventilation, hypoxemia, and patient discomfort are observed.

Minute Ventilation

Minute ventilation is set according to the approximate ventilatory requirements of a patient and to start with is set at 5–10 L/min. The VE decided upon is also influenced by the nature of the disease and the altered respiratory mechanics for which ventilatory support is offered.

Inspiration-expiration Ratio (I:E ratio)

The I:E ratio to start with, is set at 1:3 to allow sufficient time for expiration.

Oxygen Concentration

If the patient is hypoxic, the FiO_2 to start with should be 1.0. After 15–20 minutes, this is gradually reduced to a level which allows a PaO_2 more than or equal to 60 mm Hg, and an O_2 saturation more than or equal to 90%.

Inspiratory Flow Rate

The inspiratory flow rate is usually set at 40–60 L/min in volume-targeted ventilation. This can be increased to 60–100 L/min in patients with high inspiratory demands. However, higher inspiratory flow rates would cause an increase in the peak inspiratory pressure. Lower flow rates can be used to decrease peak inspiratory pressure in patients who to start with have high peak inspiratory pressures (as in ARDS). Lowering inspiratory flow rates would increase inspiratory time, but decrease expiratory time—this could lead to air trapping, auto-PEEP, patient discomfort, and barotrauma.

Positive End-expiratory Pressure

Positive end-expiratory pressure may need to be used if the O_2 saturation is less than 90% or a FiO_2 more than 0.5 (see subsequent section on PEEP.)

It needs to be stressed that the VT, respiratory rate, VE, I:E ratio, and inspiratory flow rates are so adjusted as to enable good exchange of gases and yet maintain a plateau pressure less than 30 cm H_2O. This lung protection strategy minimizes the risk of barotrauma and volutrauma.

All alarms on the ventilator provided both for patient safety and as indicators of proper functioning of the ventilator should be activated—in particular, the high pressure, low pressure alarm, and the apnea alarm.

Problems at Initiation of Ventilator Support (Table 4)

- The major and the most common problem is difficulty in synchronizing the patient's respiration with the ventilator. In an unconscious or apneic patient, this presents no difficulty. The problem is also easily surmountable in patients with respiratory failure due to poisoning, neuromuscular disease, or other

---

Table 4: Common problems encountered during initiation of ventilator support.

A. *Difficulty in synchronizing patient's respiration with the ventilator*:
- Reassure patient and use tranquillizers (diazepam 5–10 mg IV)
- Use adequate alveolar minute ventilation to maintain $PaCO_2$ at 35–40 mm Hg
- Use high FiO_2 temporarily to ensure there is no hypoxia
- Increase TV and RR beyond patient's spontaneous rate. Once patient is taken over by machine, setting gradually lowered to desired values
- Use high FiO_2 temporarily to ensure there is no hypoxia
- Recognize and treat other factors contributing to "clash" between machine and patient
- If in spite of earlier measures, asynchrony between patient and machine persists (as in patients with severe parenchymal disease producing stiff lungs), sedate and depress respiration by 2–4 mg IV morphine, or IV diazepam or IV midazolam, IV fentanyl or IV propofol or induce neuromuscular paralysis by 4 mg IV bolus of pancuronium

B. *Other problems*:
- Malposition of endotracheal tube
- Aspiration of stomach contents
- Hypotension

(IV: Intravenous; FiO_2: Fraction of inspired oxygen)

CNS problems. The following points are helpful in management:

- Allay, anxiety, and fright in the patient by explaining the situation in a gentle and confident manner, and by the use of a tranquillizer. Diazepam, 5–10 mg intravenously is of great help.

- The most common cause of difficulty in synchronizing is inadequate alveolar VE. The VE selected should result in a $PaCO_2$ between 35 mm Hg and 40 mm Hg. Ordinarily, a VT of 10 mL/kg with a respiratory rate of 12–15/min is adequate. However, many patients with lung disease require higher VEs than that stated earlier.

- If the patient continuously clashes with what appear to be reasonable ventilator settings, it is advisable to proceed as follows:

  - Use a high FiO_2 temporarily to ensure that there is no hypoxia—this can be easily checked by noting the oxygen saturation on the pulse oximeter.

  - If a very strong respiratory drive is responsible for asynchrony between the patient and the machine, the VT is increased, and the respiratory rate increased to well beyond the patient's spontaneous rate. Once the patient is taken over by the machine, the settings are gradually lowered and modified to the desired values. Generally, if alveolar ventilation is adequate, and if other causes contributing to restlessness and increased respiratory drive are looked into and taken care of, the patient does not fight the machine and is relaxed. The only way to determine whether the alveolar ventilation is adequate is by monitoring the $PaCO_2$. A $PaCO_2$ more than 45 mm Hg denotes alveolar hypoventilation; that less than 35 mm Hg, alveolar hyperventilation. Hyperventilation in the initial stages reduces the respiratory drive and helps the machine to take over. Once this is achieved, VE is adjusted so that the $PaCO_2$ is maintained around 35 mm Hg, and preferably not less than 30 mm Hg.

  - In tachypneic patients with a strong respiratory drive, the patient's inspiratory flow rate is generally higher than the usual 40–60 L/min set on the machine. Increasing the inspiratory flow rate appropriately, or decreasing the I:E ratio, prevents "clashing" and allows smoother ventilatory support in these patients.

- Manual control of ventilation by using 100% oxygen for 5 minutes is a useful method for abolishing the patient's respiratory effort, by ensuring oxygenation, and proper alveolar ventilation.

- Besides a strong respiratory drive chiefly related to altered mechanics of the lungs, there are other contributory factors which increase the degree of "clash" between the machine and the patient. These may be present at the very outset, or may evolve during the critical care of a patient. They are briefly discussed later, and should be recognized and treated for more efficient ventilator support.

– Asynchrony between the machine and the patient may persist, however, in spite of appropriate ventilator settings, the use of corrective measures, and despite all attempts to match the machine to the patient. This generally happens in patients with severe parenchymal lung disease producing very stiff lungs, tachypnea, and severe hypoxia. In many of these patients, the spontaneous respiratory rate is more than 40/min. It is unwise to even attempt to "match" the machine to this spontaneous respiratory rate. What is more, these patients are critically ill, often with multiorgan failure and cardiovascular instability. It is important that the respiratory muscles are rested in such circumstances. Effective ventilation can be achieved only by depressing respiration, or by inducing neuromuscular paralysis. The respiration can be depressed by the use of 2–4 mg morphine, or 0.2–0.4 mg buprenorphine intravenously, repeated as and when necessary. An alternative is to use 10 mg intravenous diazepam or 2.4 mg midazolam intravenously or an intravenous combination of midazolam and fentanyl titrated to produce the desired effect. The main disadvantage of morphine is hypotension, which should be countered by vasopressors or by a volume load. In patients where morphine or a morphine derivative or diazepam or midazolam or fentanyl is unsuitable or ineffective, particularly in ventilating patients with severe lung injury, it is necessary to use intravenous pancuronium or an intravenous bolus dose of vecuronium 0.08–0.1 mg/kg. After an intravenous bolus dose, vecuronium is given as a 0.8–1.2 mg/kg/min continuous infusion, to induce neuromuscular paralysis and thereby abolish or sharply reduce spontaneous ventilatory support. Pancuronium is given as an intravenous bolus dose of 0.06–0.1 mg/kg and repeated as and when necessary to allow smooth takeover by the machine. It is unwise and often unnecessary to produce total paralysis with curare-like drugs.

- *Other important problems* occurring within the first few minutes or hours of initiating ventilator support are: (i) malposition of the airways; (ii) aspiration of stomach contents; and (iii) hypotension. These are dealt with at length under complications of ventilator support.

OBJECTIVES OF VENTILATOR SUPPORT

- Regulate gas exchange
- Overcome mechanical problems
- Increase lung volumes—particularly in conditions in which the functional residual capacity (FRC) is reduced.

Regulate Gas Exchange

Oxygenation

- Most patients requiring ventilator support have uneven ventilation and disturbed ventilation-perfusion ratios. Only a small minority on ventilator support can be adequately oxygenated with room air or 20% oxygen; most require an increased concentration of oxygen in the inspired air.

- It is best to use an inspired oxygen concentration (FiO_2) sufficient to maintain an O_2 saturation more than 90% and a PaO_2 more than 60 mm Hg. In severe lung disease, high oxygen concentrations are necessary; oxygen concentrations more than 70% for a prolonged period are a hazard as they contribute to lung injury. In very severe lung injury, a FiO_2 of 100% may be necessary to prevent death from hypoxia. If this is indeed so, 100% oxygen should be used, notwithstanding the fear of oxygen toxicity.

- *Use of positive end-expiratory pressure*: Positive end-expiratory pressure is indicated when the PaO_2 is less than 60 mm Hg despite inspired oxygen concentrations exceeding 50%.

Carbon Dioxide Elimination and Regulation

The physiological dead space in patients with lung disease is often increased. The increase in dead space in relation to VT may in fact be so large, that in some patients on ventilators 50–70% or even more of the VT becomes dead space ventilation. It is therefore, important to note the following points:

- It is impossible to predict the ventilation requirements of patients on ventilatory support as most patients have an increase in physiological dead space. Their ventilation requirements are invariably in considerable excess of that predicted by standard nomograms.
- The only certain way to ensure adequate ventilation is to measure the $PaCO_2$ and to adjust volume exchange so that the $PaCO_2$ is close to normal.
- It needs to be stressed that a disturbance in ventilatory exchange may be as much due to a fault in the pulmonary circulation as to a fall in alveolar ventilation.
- Ventilator support can also be manipulated so as to purposely induce hyperventilation (with a low $PaCO_2$) in patients with raised intracranial pressure, or to purposely settle for hypoventilation (permissive hypercapnia) in certain clinical situations (ARDS and airways obstruction).

Overcome Mechanical Problems

Mechanical ventilation is of use to rest fatigued respiratory muscles, to overcome the abnormal mechanics of the thoracic cage in flail chest, and to prevent or treat atelectasis.

Increase in Lung Volumes in Patients with a Low Functional Residual Capacity

Use of PEEP improves ventilation-perfusion ratios and reduces the right-to-left shunt within the lungs.

■ SUMMARY OF VENTILATORY PATTERNS IN DIFFERENT GROUPS OF RESPIRATORY DISEASES REQUIRING VENTILATOR SUPPORT

- *In patients with normal lungs*: Tidal volumes of 10 mL/kg with respiratory rates between 10/min and 14/min, a flow rate of 40–60 L/min, and an I:E ratio of 1:2–1:3 are recommended.

- *Patients with trauma to the chest wall causing a flail chest, and often hematoma or injury to the lung*: These patients may need controlled ventilation for which sedation or neuromuscular paralysis becomes necessary. VTs of 10 mL/kg, with a respiratory rate between 12/min and 14/min are recommended. The VE is adjusted to maintain a $PaCO_2$ between 30 mm Hg and 40 mm Hg.

- *Acute hypoxemic respiratory failure due to severe lung disease, e.g. ARDS, pneumonia*: The principle is to avoid as far as possible high inflation pressures and to use small VTs of 5–7 mL/kg. In mild to moderately severe cases, smaller VTs of 6–8 mL/kg with a higher respiratory rate of 20–25/min are used to match the patient's breathing pattern. The inspiratory flow rates are adjusted to between 40 L/min and 60 L/min. An increased FiO_2 and the use of PEEP are necessary. If adequate or efficient ventilation is not possible, particularly so in severely hypoxic, tachypneic, critically ill individuals, heavy sedation, or even muscle paralysis with controlled ventilation becomes necessary, the principle again being not to exceed a plateau pressure of 30 cm H_2O as far as possible, even if this entails a rise in $PaCO_2$ (permissive hypercapnia). If pressure-controlled or pressure-targeted ventilator support is given to these patients, the peak inspiratory pressure should as far as possible not exceed 30 cm H_2O. PEEP is used in all patients. Inverse ratio ventilator support is occasionally tried when gas exchange remains unsatisfactory with the usual volume-targeted or pressure-targeted ventilatory support. The inverse ratio in our opinion should not be increased to more than 1:1.

- *Acute on chronic respiratory failure in patients with chronic airways' obstruction*: Small VTs of 6 mL/kg with a respiratory rate and VE enough to allow a $PaCO_2$ between 45 mm Hg and 55 mm Hg are adequate. These patients are used to a high $PaCO_2$ and it is unwise to aim at a $PaCO_2$ of 40 mm Hg, as their $PaCO_2$ even under ordinary conditions is significantly elevated. Sedation or at times induced paralysis is often necessary for ventilator support to be effectively maintained. Moderately low inspiratory flow rates (50 L/min), an I:E ratio of 1:3, and avoidance of high inflation pressures by using a low VT are recommended. Hypoxia is countered by an appropriate increase in the FiO_2.

- *Acute severe asthma*: These patients also require low VTs (350–400 mL), and comparatively low VE (often

< 5 L/min) to prevent hyperinflation of the lungs. A rise in $PaCO_2$ does not matter as long as hypoxia is relieved by an appropriate increase in the FiO_2. Ventilation in these patients can at times prove extremely difficult.

Lung protection strategies (outlined in the chapter on ARDS) should always be kept in mind in the management of mechanical ventilator support.

It is constant practice that allows the clinician to adjust ventilatory requirements to the need of each individual patient so as to allow adequate gas exchange and yet prevent as far as possible the hazards of mechanical ventilator support. We recommend that every patient in the ICU on ventilator support should have a chart of ventilator settings and blood gases as illustrated in **Table 5**.

Three more points need to be stressed:

1. Hypovolemia contributes to poor gas exchange, and accentuates or precipitates hypotension in patients on mechanical ventilation. It is therefore, important to ensure normal circulatory volume, good pump function, a normal blood pressure, and an adequate hemoglobin concentration.
2. Humidification of inspired gas, aseptic suction of secretions through the tracheobronchial tree at frequent intervals, and good chest physiotherapy are all vitally important. Good physiotherapy often spells the difference between life and death in critically ill patients on ventilator support.
3. Efficiently carried out mechanical ventilation can only ensure a satisfactory gas exchange. More often than not, a critically ill patient on ventilator support in the ICU has numerous other complications that pose potential hazards to life. Circulatory failure, renal dysfunction, gastrointestinal bleeding, acid-base disturbances, overwhelming sepsis, and in our country, a poor nutritional state, singly or in combination with other factors, can be dangerous enough to cause death. Therefore, to concentrate solely on the correct and efficient working of a machine and on a single aspect of deranged physiology, constitutes bad medicine. An overall perspective should never be lost sight of in the management of a critically ill patient.

■ MODES OF INVASIVE VENTILATOR SUPPORT

The most common modes in use are volume-controlled ventilation (VCV) mode, pressure-controlled ventilation (PCV) mode, synchronized intermittent mandatory ventilation (SIMV) support, and pressure support ventilation (PSV) **(Table 6)**. These modes and the use of PEEP are considered to start with in this section, followed by a brief explanation of the more recent modes. It is very important for the clinician or the intensivist to be thoroughly familiar with the basic modes of ventilator support before attempting familiarity with the numerous other modes that modern ventilators are able to provide.

Table 5: Chart of ventilator settings and blood gases in the ICU.

Name of patients: _________________   Bed number: _________________

Date	Time	Rate	MV	Tidal volume	FiO_2	Peak pressure	Pause pressure	PEEP	pH	$PaCO_2$	PaO_2	Standard bicarbonate	Base excess/ deficient	O_2 saturation

(FiO_2: Fraction of inspired oxygen; ICU: Intensive care unit; PaO_2: Partial pressure of arterial oxygen; PEEP: Positive end-expiratory pressure)

Volume-targeted Support (Figs. 1 and 2)

Controlled Mode

In CMV, the ventilator completely controls the patient's ventilation, delivering a set VT (or a preset peak pressure) at a set frequency. It is indicated in individuals who are apneic, or in those with respiratory muscle paralysis. It is also indicated in patients who are heavily sedated or those paralyzed with neuromuscular agents so that ventilatory support is mandatory—a classic example of this situation is fulminant tetanus. Patients receiving CMV cannot increase their VE voluntarily; their ventilator needs should therefore be closely monitored, and changing needs should be met by suitable adjustments on the machine.

Assist/Control Mode

This is the most commonly used mode. The machine delivers a preset volume (or pressure) in response to a patient-initiated breath. To prevent the patient from

> **Table 6:** Conventional modes of ventilator support.
>
> - Controlled mode (CMV)
> - Assist/control (A/C) mode
> - Pressure-controlled ventilation (PCV)
> - Synchronized intermittent mandatory ventilation (SIMV)
> - Pressure support ventilation (PSV)
> - Continuous positive airway pressure (CPAP)
> - Volume-controlled inverse ratio ventilation (VC-IRV) and pressure-controlled inverse ratio ventilation (PC-IRV)

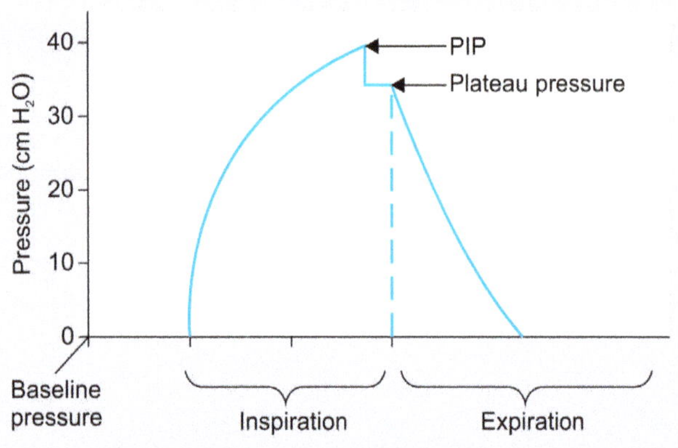

Fig. 1: The airway pressures (peak and plateau) during a positive pressure breath. Pressure rises during inspiration to peak inspiratory pressure (PIP). With a breath hold, the plateau pressure can be measured. Pressures fall back to baseline during expiration.
Source: Reproduced with permission from Pilbeam SP. Mechanical Ventilation, Physiological and Clinical Applications. Mosby: Elsevier; 1992.

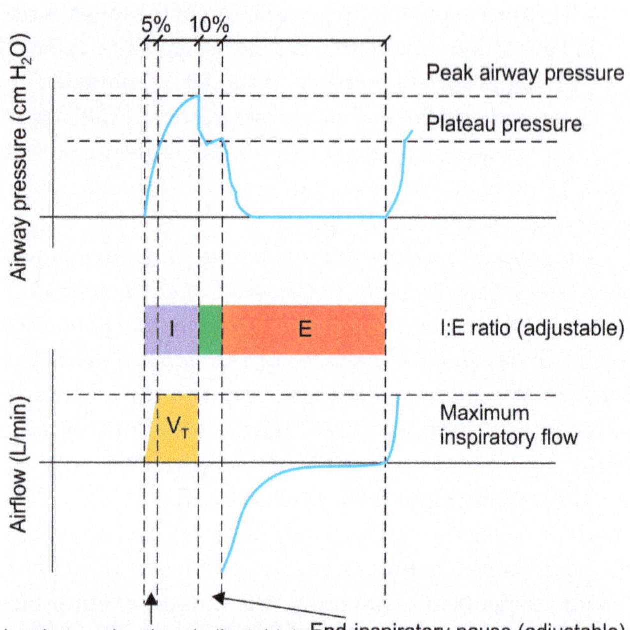

Fig. 2: Volume-targeted ventilation. Tidal volume is preset and the machine delivers the preset tidal volume regardless of change in compliance or airway resistance. Pressure rises during inspiration to peak inspiratory pressure (PIP). With a breath hold, the plateau pressure can be measured. Pressures fall back to baseline during expiration. (I:E: Inspiration-expiration)

being totally dependent on "triggered" breaths, a backup minimum respiratory rate is set. The requisite VE can then be provided even if for some reason or the other the patient fails to trigger the machine. The main advantage of this mode is that the patient can increase his VE by increasing his respiratory rate. The disadvantages include the production of respiratory alkalosis and of dynamic hyperinflation (particularly in COPD patients), if the machine is triggered too frequently, and the possibility of asynchrony between the ventilator and the patient. Initial ventilator settings are a VE of 8–10 L/min, respiratory rate at 10–14/min, and a sensitivity of –2 cm usually. If the patient triggers the machine too frequently, the sensitivity is set at –2 to –6 cm and the patient is sedated to reduce his respiratory drive. Most ventilators allow adjustment of the inspiratory flow rate or the I:E ratio, the inspiratory rise time, end-inspiratory pause time, and the flow pattern during inspiration.

Pressure-controlled Ventilation (Fig. 3)

In this mode, the maximum peak pressure is preset, so that the ventilator increases the pressure to this preset level with each inspiratory breath. The VT obtained depends

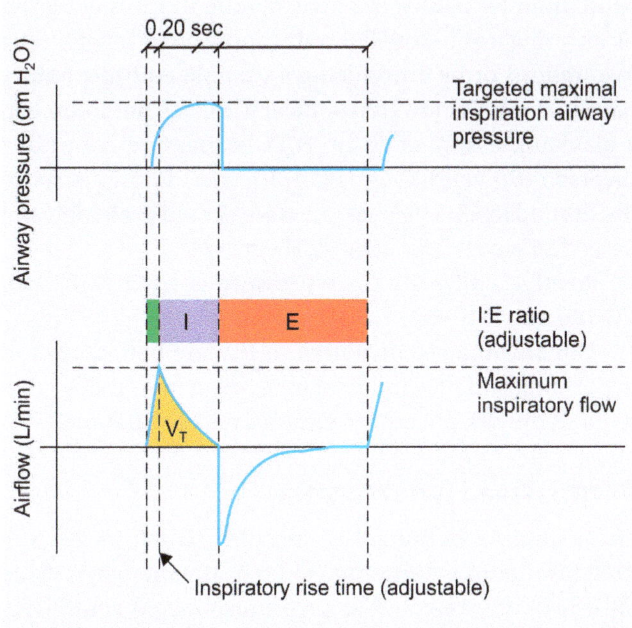

Fig. 3: Pressure-targeted ventilation. The maximum inspiratory pressure is preset and the tidal volume will depend upon lung compliance and airway resistance. I:E ratio and the inspiratory rise time are adjustable. (I:E: Inspiration-expiration; VT: Tidal volume)

on the preset pressure (the higher the preset pressure, the higher the VT), the stiffness of the lungs (greater the stiffness, the lower the VT for a preset pressure), and resistance to airflow (the greater the resistance, the lower the VT). The adjustable parameters are preset pressures delivered by the ventilator and the inspiratory time. The flow pattern is decelerating, in that the flow is high to start with but decreases as the preset pressure is about to be reached.

Synchronized Intermittent Mandatory Ventilation

In this mode, the ventilator delivers synchronized breaths at a set rate at either a preset VT or a preset pressure, in addition to allowing the patient to breathe spontaneously. The VT and rate are determined by the patient. If for any reason, the patient does not breathe for a predetermined period, a machine breath is delivered. SIMV can be used with pressure support for spontaneous breaths. PEEP can be introduced in this mode, in which case the machine breaths will be combined with PEEP and the spontaneous ones with continuous positive airway pressure (CPAP).

The advantages claimed for the SIMV mode are as follows:
- Decreased asynchrony with the machine and less sedation requirements
- Less chances of hyperventilation as compared to the assist/control (A/C) mode
- Greater patient comfort
- Continued use of respiratory muscles, which is believed to prevent respiratory muscle dysfunction
- Reduced mean airway pressure even with the simultaneous use of PEEP, because many respiratory cycles are related to spontaneous breaths. This minimizes the cardiovascular effects of mechanical ventilation and is less likely to cause a fall in cardiac output or in arterial blood pressure.

In our opinion, the advantages ascribed to SIMV with or without PEEP are theoretical, and except in occasional instances, most patients are more comfortably and more satisfactorily ventilated with the A/C mode of ventilator support. In fact, the more ill the patient, greater the necessity to rest the respiratory muscles rather than exercise them. The VO₂ by overworked respiratory muscles can be as high as 15–40% of the total oxygen consumption and this is certainly undesirable. The SIMV mode cannot also respond to changes in the patient's condition, and therefore, needs close monitoring **(Fig. 3)**.

The chief uses of this mode in our opinion are stated here:
- In patients who develop hypotension while on the A/C mode or CMV mode with PEEP. The use of SIMV in such patients is associated with a lower mean airway pressure and this may restore cardiovascular stability.
- In patients on the A/C mode who develop respiratory alkalosis. This can be countered by either sedation or by changing to the SIMV mode.
- To prevent auto-PEEP in certain situations.
- In patients with respiratory failure and a bronchopleural fistula. In this situation, one would desire the lowest mean airway pressure that does not adversely affect ventilation and gas exchange, yet allows the bronchopleural fistula to heal and get sealed. Low VTs with increased respiratory rates to allow for adequate VE, the avoidance of PEEP, and the use of the SIMV mode may be ideally suited to these patients. This should be combined with the smallest effective chest drainage tube suction.
- For weaning purposes.

Initial Setting

Settings to deliver a VE of 6–10 L/min or a preset pressure (sufficient to allow a VE of 6–10 L/min) with 10–12 mandatory breaths.

Pressure Support Ventilation

In this mode, a patient inspiratory effort triggers a response from the ventilator. The ventilator delivers a preset positive pressure to the airways, reducing the work of breathing, and helping in patient comfort. Once the predefined percentage of the maximal inspiratory flow is reached, the ventilator stops inspiration and opens the expiratory valve. The respiratory rate and inspiratory flow rate are determined by the patient. This mode cannot be used in an apneic patient or in one who lacks an adequate spontaneous respiratory drive. It is chiefly used in selected COPD patients and as a weaning procedure.

Initial Setting

Set a pressure of 10–12 cm of H_2O, ensuring a VT of 7–10 mL/kg. The pressure support is gradually decreased to 5–7 cm H_2O provided an adequate VT is maintained. Once this occurs, the patient can be weaned and allowed to breathe spontaneously.

Continuous Positive Airway Pressure

Continuous positive airway pressure is a mode of spontaneous breathing in which the airway pressure is maintained at levels greater than the ambient pressure throughout the entire respiratory cycle. A PEEP may be added as an adjunct to CPAP. All modern volume ventilators incorporate CPAP as a ventilatory mode. The ventilator does not provide any machine-generated breaths, but its humidification and alarm systems are available for use. Special CPAP systems without a ventilator are also available.

Inverse Ratio Ventilation

Inverse ratio ventilation (IRV) can be volume-targeted or pressure-targeted. Whereas the normal I:E ratio is 1:3 or 1:2, in IRV, the I:E ratio is 1:1 or even less. Ordinarily, one hesitates to go beyond 1:1.

This is used in patients with ARDS, pneumonia, atelectasis, and who show refractory hypoxemia (O_2 saturation < 90% or a FiO_2 > 60% on A/C mode in spite of suitable PEEP). In volume-controlled inverse ratio ventilation (VC-IRV), the inverse ratio of I:E is achieved by lowering inspiratory flow rate (and thereby lengthening inspiration) or by introducing a suitable end-inspiratory pause. The VT is lowered sufficiently so as not to exceed a plateau pressure of 30 cm H_2O. In pressure-controlled inverse ratio ventilation (PC-IRV), the I:E ratio is set to the desired level. The peak pressure should preferably not exceed 30 cm H_2O, or at most 35 cm H_2O.

Positive end-expiratory pressure is used with both VC-IRV and PC-IRV.

The advantages attributed to IRV are better relief of hypoxemia and promotion of lung protection strategy that reduces the risk of both barotrauma and volutrauma.

Permissive Hypercapnia

The principle behind this approach is to protect the lung from both volutrauma and barotrauma when using either volume-targeted or pressure-targeted ventilatory support. Small VTs (5–7 mL/kg) are used in certain groups of patients in volume-targeted ventilatory support, so that plateau pressures do not exceed 30 cm H_2O. When pressure-targeted ventilator support is used, peak pressures are generally set to not more than 30 cm H_2O. This lung protection strategy can lead to hypoventilation and thereby hypercapnia. The hypercapnia is generally well tolerated by the patient and is permissible as an offshoot of the lung protection strategy stated earlier.

Use of Positive End-expiratory Pressure

The use of PEEP is a valuable adjunct to every mode of volume-targeted ventilatory support, pressure-targeted ventilatory support, PSV, and to the SIMV support. The effects of PEEP are listed in **Table 7**.

Indications for Use of Positive End-expiratory Pressure (Table 8)

Positive end-expiratory pressure is indicated in patients with severe hypoxic respiratory failure who have poorly compliant lungs and a large degree of ventilation-perfusion mismatch so that hypoxia persists despite using a FiO_2 of 50–60% or more to ventilate the lungs.

It is invariably indicated in patients with ARDS, severe pneumonia, in patients with pulmonary edema who require ventilatory support, and in hypoxemic respiratory failure due to flail chest and marked obesity. All these patients have a reduced FRC leading to alveolar and small airways collapse thereby causing a ventilation-perfusion mismatch with a right-to-left shunt within the lungs. In these patients, PEEP increases the FRC, opens

---

Table 7: Physiological effects and complications of PEEP.

A. *Physiological effects:*
- *On lungs*:
  - Opening up of fluid-filled atelectatic alveoli, with increase in FRC and TLC
  - Decrease in shunt causing increase in PaO_2
  - Increase in VA/Q units
  - Increase in dead space and VD/VT ratio
  - Increase in compliance up to a point; later fall in compliance
- *On heart*: Decrease in cardiac output; this can decrease shunt, and thereby increase PaO_2. Thus, rise in PaO_2 may also result from a fall in cardiac output, and not necessarily from improvement in lung function

B. *Complications:*
- *Barotrauma*: Pneumothorax, pneumomediastinum, and interstitial emphysema
- *Fall in cardiac output*: Hypotension, poor oxygen transport with inadequate tissue perfusion
- Fall in PaO_2 due to overdistension of compliant alveoli, and increase in V/Q abnormalities
- Increase in intracranial pressure
- Water retention

(FRC: Functional residual capacity; PEEP: Positive end-expiratory pressure; TLC: Total lung capacity; VT: Tidal volume)

Table 8: Practical guidelines for the use of PEEP.

- PEEP only helps to counter hypoxia in acute hypoxemic respiratory failure due to lung injury; it does not alter the natural history of acute lung pathologies requiring ventilator support
- PEEP should not be used as a preventive measure, except after open heart surgery to prevent mediastinal bleeding, or to open up atelectatic segments chiefly present in the lower lobes
- It is not necessarily indicated if conventional ventilator support with FiO_2 of 50–60% maintains PaO_2 more than 60–65 mm Hg
- Start with PEEP levels of +5 cm H_2O, gauge effect, and then increase; do not exceed levels of +15 cm H_2O in Indian patients as barotrauma invariably results
- Use the lowest PEEP that allows a PaO_2 of 60 mm Hg on FiO_2 less than 0.6. Ascertain that the rise in PaO_2 following the use of PEEP is not associated with a fall in CO as this will lead to poor oxygen transport and poor tissue oxygenation
- If hypotension or decrease in CO is associated with use of PEEP, the PEEP level should be reduced, or even discontinued. The BP and CO are raised with volume load and/or inotropic support, and PEEP may then be better tolerated
- PEEP may rarely cause a fall in PaO_2—it then needs to be reduced, or even discontinued
- PEEP should be gradually tapered off, before discontinuing ventilator support

(BP: Blood pressure; CO: Cardiac output; FiO_2: Fraction of inspired oxygen; PaO_2: Partial pressure of arterial oxygen; PEEP: Positive end-expiratory pressure)

---

up collapsed alveoli, particularly in the dependent lung regions, prevents derecruitment of opened alveoli during expiration, redistributes fluid within the alveoli, and is believed to protect surfactant. The overall effect is to improve the ventilation-perfusion mismatch, reduce the absolute right-to-left shunt (also termed the true venous admixture) within the lungs, thereby increasing PaO_2, O_2 saturation, so that need for high FiO_2 is reduced. The danger of oxygen toxicity caused by prolonged use of high FiO_2 in these patients is thus obviated. The prevention of derecruitment or collapse of alveoli during expiration with PEEP allows breathing to occur in the favorable range of the pressure volume curve, reducing the work of breathing **(Fig. 4)**.

At one time, PEEP was strictly contraindicated in patients with respiratory failure due to severe asthma or following an acute exacerbation of COPD requiring ventilator support. Many of these patients have dynamic hyperinflation of the lungs. The FRC is high and the alveolar pressure at the end of expiration exceeds atmospheric pressure, resulting in auto-PEEP or intrinsic PEEP. Also, because of dynamic hyperinflation, this

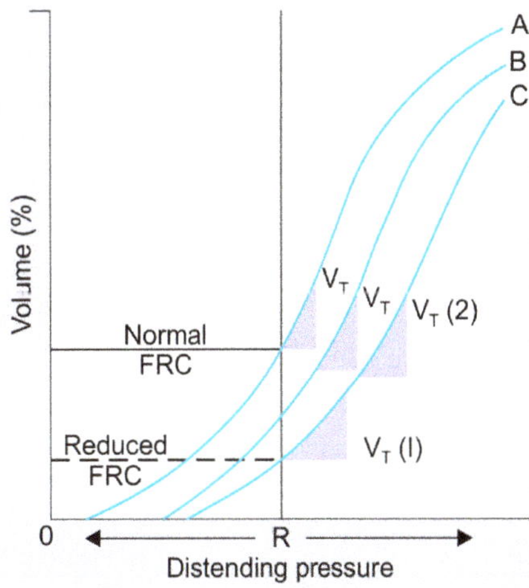

Fig. 4: Effect of positive end-expiratory pressure (PEEP) on functional residual capacity (FRC) in patients with reduced compliance, e.g. acute lung injury (ARDS). Curve A represents a normal pressure-volume curve, wherein a relatively small distending pressure is required to achieve a given tidal volume (VT). Curve C represents a pressure-volume curve in a patient with reduced compliance (as in ARDS) with decreased FRC. This is a more flattened curve and requires a greater distending pressure to achieve the same VT (1). With the addition of PEEP, the FRC may be improved along the same abnormal compliance curve (2) or would shift to curve B, so that lesser distending pressures are required to achieve the same VT, but the absolute value of the distending pressure is still greater than that required for curve A.

auto-PEEP progressively increases. A high auto-PEEP increases the inspiratory work of breathing and ultimately leads to respiratory muscle fatigue that can progress to respiratory arrest. The principle of ventilatory support is to use small VTs with an I:E ratio of 1:3 and a rate preferably not more than 12–14/min to help reduce dynamic hyperinflation. The application of extrinsic PEEP is also indicated in patients with severe airways obstruction who are on ventilatory support and develop a high auto-PEEP. The proper application of external PEEP will then counter the effect of auto-PEEP on the work of breathing, chiefly in relation to inspiratory effort. It is important, however, to set the level of extrinsic PEEP below that of the auto-PEEP observed in the patient.

In the past, the main focus of attention in the use of PEEP was to improve oxygenation by reducing ventilation-perfusion mismatch and right-to-left shunt within the lung. *An equally important concept on the use of PEEP today is that it prevents the concertina-like opening and closing of alveoli during inspiration and expiration, keeps the alveoli open all through the respiratory cycle, thereby reducing the sheer forces acting on the alveoli and hence reducing ventilator-induced injury.*

Selection of the Degree of Positive End-expiratory Pressure Used

A variety of methods have been used to determine the optimal level of PEEP. In busy ICUs, the simplest, safest, and most practical method is to use the lowest level of PEEP which maintains the PaO_2 equal to or more than 60 mm Hg, on a FiO_2 equal to or less than 0.6.

Other methods of selecting an optimum level of PEEP include the following:

- *Optimal oxygenation*: It is wrong to aim at an ever increasing PaO_2 by increasing the levels of PEEP. A high PEEP can cause an increasing rise in the PaO_2 and yet can result in a sharp drop in the cardiac output. This fall in cardiac output further reduces oxygen transport to the tissues, in spite of the increase in the PaO_2; this can have disastrous consequences.
- *Maximal oxygen transport*: Adjusting the PEEP so as to obtain maximal oxygen transport (i.e. the product of arterial oxygen content and the cardiac output), takes the PaO_2, the hemoglobin, and the cardiac output into consideration. Nevertheless, frequent measurements of cardiac output often pose problems in critically ill individuals.

- *Best compliance*: With the use of PEEP, the reduced FRC increases, and the compliance increases up to a point. If static compliance is measured with a graded increase in PEEP, a level of PEEP which produces an optimal increase in the compliance can be arrived at. Further increase in PEEP beyond this point now leads to a fall in static compliance pointing to overdistension of the alveoli. An optimal compliance produced by a particular level of PEEP in any particular patient, is generally associated with an optimal rise in the PaO_2.
- *Lowest QS/QT*: As long as the level of PEEP does not significantly reduce the cardiac output, the optimal level of PEEP correlates with the lowest level of QS/QT. Many workers aim at reducing the shunt fraction to 15%, or aim at a PaO_2/FiO_2 ratio of 300 or more.
- *Lowest VD/VT and lowest PaCO$_2$-PETCO$_2$*: The lowest VD/VT ratio and the lowest $PaCO_2$-end-tidal carbon dioxide ($PETCO_2$) gradient are other parameters used by some workers to arrive at an optimal PEEP setting.

Complications of Positive End-expiratory Pressure

The three major complications are: (1) barotrauma, (2) a fall in cardiac output, and (3) at times a fall instead of the expected rise in PaO_2. PEEP used over a number of days, can result in an increase in intracranial tension, and to an increase in water retention, and a decrease in renal and portal blood flow.

1. *Barotrauma*: The risk of barotrauma depends on the end-inspiratory airway pressure and regional overinflation of parts of the lung (**Figs. 5A and B**). End-inspiratory pressure is a function of the VT, the FRC, the inspiratory flow rate, the total compliance of the lungs, and the level of PEEP used. High VTs, high inspiratory flow rates, and high levels of PEEP, in association with a reduced FRC and compliance, potentiate the risk of barotrauma. Even in severely diseased lungs, there are some regional areas which are more compliant than others. With high levels of PEEP, these alveoli get enlarged and overdistended, and have a lower recoil pressure than the smaller, poorly compliant alveoli. High alveolar pressures in such distended alveoli predispose to rupture. On the other hand, the smaller, poorly compliant alveoli have a larger recoil pressure, and can therefore, withstand high alveolar pressures and are less liable to rupture.

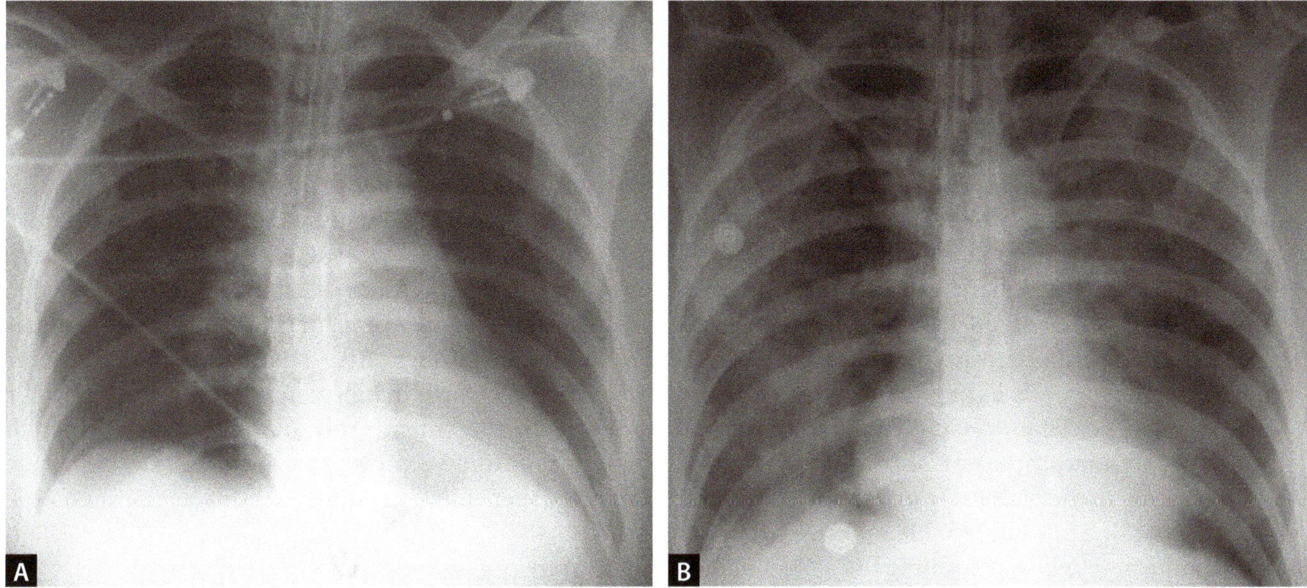

Figs. 5A and B: Positive end-expiratory pressure (PEEP) effect. Chest X-ray; (A) demonstrates overinflated lungs with a tubular-shaped heart; (B) Chest X-ray after removal of PEEP. The lungs are not inflated as much as with PEEP, the heart is not tubular. The apparent clearing of opacities on the X-ray (A) is a PEEP effect.

Alveolar rupture can lead to interstitial emphysema, pneumothorax, mediastinal emphysema, and surgical emphysema of the soft tissues which may involve the neck, face, and trunk. Pneumothorax or high levels of PEEP are a disaster which often leads to death.

2. *Fall in cardiac output:* High levels of inflation pressure and PEEP are transmitted to the pleural space. The rise in the intrapleural and intrathoracic pressures leads to a fall in the venous return to the right heart, and a poor filling of the left heart due to a decrease in the transmural pressure across the left ventricular wall. Overinflation of the alveoli also increases the pulmonary vascular resistance with right heart strain, which further reduces the cardiac output. Also, right ventricular strain produces a shift of the interventricular septum to the left, thereby distorting and diminishing the size of the left ventricular cavity, and further impairing left ventricular filling and cardiac output. A sharp fall in the cardiac output leads to hypotension, poor oxygen transport, and inadequate tissue perfusion. A volume load together with dopamine support may be necessary in some patients to restore the cardiac output and oxygen transport to desired levels.

3. *Fall in partial pressure of arterial oxygen:* A paradoxical fall in the PaO_2 is sometimes observed with PEEP. This occurs when there are regional areas of normally compliant or overcompliant lung in patients with hypoxemic respiratory failure due to parenchymal lung disease. Overdistension of compliant alveoli leads to a decrease in the blood flow to these alveoli, and a shift of blood flow to the nonventilated, noncompliant areas of the lung. This causes a further increase in the shunt and a fall in the PaO_2. Ventilatory settings and PEEP levels should be adjusted to allow less distension of the compliant alveoli, and better distribution of inspired gas to the poorly compliant portions of the lungs.

Open Lung Concept

The "open lung concept" is being increasingly used in some critical care units in ARDS and in postoperative atelectasis (*see* chapter on ARDS). The principle behind this concept is to "open" the lung and keep it "open" with the least changes in pressure so as to minimize alveolar shear forces. This serves to improve gas exchange and serves as a lung protection mechanism by avoiding the concertina-like opening of the alveoli during inspiration and their collapse and closure during expiration.

Sequential settings in a patient with ARDS on whom the open lung concept is used are given here:

- *Use pressure control and set upper pressure limit to 50 cm H_2O:* Set PEEP at 10–15 cm H_2O. Set pressure control level above PEEP to a value which gives a VT of 10–15 mL/kg. Set respiratory rate at 15/min. Inspiratory time 50% or I:E 1:1.

- *Determine opening pressure*: Raise peak inspiratory pressure stepwise by 2 cm H_2O at a time, allowing 10–15 breaths at each stepwise increase, till the lung is fully "open". This generally requires a rise in the peak inspiratory pressure to 40–60 cm H_2O. The features that signify a fully "open" lung are a sudden and sustained jump of the PaO_2, so that the PaO_2/FiO_2 more than 400, and also the sharp disproportionate increase in VT in relation to the stepwise increase in peak pressure.
- *Determine closing pressure of the lung*: Decrease in peak inspiratory pressure stepwise by 2 cm H_2O, allowing a few breaths for each setting to enable a stabilized reading. The "closing pressure" is that pressure at which the alveoli collapse or close. This is signified by an abrupt fall in the high PaO_2 and a sharp decline in VT. Note "closing pressure" **(Table 9)**.
- *Reopen the lung fully* by repeating the steps outlined in II.
- *Keep the lung open*: Slowly, stepwise, reduce the peak inspiratory pressure once more to a level which is 1–2 cm above the closing pressure. Now the lung has been opened and is being *kept open*. The VT should remain stable, and the arterial blood gases are good and constant **(Table 9)**.

Table 9: Open lung procedure.

Open lung and determine the "opening pressure"	• Use pressure control mode; rate 15/min, I:E 1:1, and PEEP 10–15 cm H_2O • Raise PIP stepwise to 40–60 cm H_2O to open the lung • Allow 10–15 breaths for each stepwise increase in PIP
	Open lung—signified by a sharp sustained jump of PaO_2, PaO_2/FiO_2, and disproportionate increase in tidal volume. Note PIP for opening lung
Determine "closing pressure"	• Lower PIP stepwise 2 cm at a time (allowing a few breaths at each reduction) till alveoli again start to close • This is signified by a sharp fall in PaO_2 and in tidal volume
Reopen lung	Reopen lung as described above
Now set PIP to just above closing pressure so that lung which has been opened is kept open	• Stepwise reduce PIP to a level just above closing pressure to keep lung open. Check PaO_2, PaO_2/FiO_2, and tidal volume • Adjust respiratory rate for adequate ventilation

(FiO$_2$: Fraction of inspired oxygen; I:E: Inspiration-expiration; PaO$_2$: Partial pressure of arterial oxygen; PEEP: Positive end-expiratory pressure; PIP: Peak inspiratory pressure)

Positive-end expiratory pressure is generally set at 10–15 cm H_2O. Some units prefer to set PEEP at higher levels of 15–25 cm H_2O. It is, however, not known if this high PEEP is necessary. Therefore, the same procedure as described earlier to determine ideal peak inspiratory pressure is now performed to find the lowest level of PEEP. After once again opening the lung, the peak inspiratory pressure and the PEEP are adjusted to just above closing pressures, so that the lungs remain "open".

Avoid unnecessary ventilatory disconnects, or changes in ventilator settings. If ventilator disconnects occur or there is a change in lung condition to suggest further atelectasis, the whole procedure described earlier to reopen lung and keep it open is repeated. Describes the stepwise open lung procedure.

■ NEWER MODES OF VENTILATOR SUPPORT

The conventional modes that assist spontaneous ventilation have been described earlier. They deliver a fixed, uniform, and predetermined degree of assist, without taking into account the variability of the breathing pattern present in different individuals in different situations and at different times in the same patient. Therefore, ideal synchrony between the patient and the ventilator is often absent. Asynchrony between the patient and ventilator can result in an increase in the workload on respiratory muscles, an undesirable event in critically ill patients. New technologies have therefore, been developed that allow the ventilator to provide assistance in proportion to the patient's demand, which may vary from breath to breath. These newer modes of ventilator support are briefly considered here **(Table 10)**.

Airway Pressure Release Ventilation

This ventilatory mode comprises CPAP that is intermittently released to allow a brief expiratory interval. The advantage is a lower mean alveolar pressure as compared to that during positive pressure ventilation. It has been used in patients with ARDS, and postoperatively in some patients, and has been found to be effective in providing adequate oxygenation.

Proportional Assist Ventilation

The ventilator in proportional assist ventilation (PAV) has the ability to sense every inspiratory effort breath by

Table 10: Newer modes of ventilatory support.
• Open lung concept • Airway pressure release ventilation (APRV) • Proportional assist ventilation (PAV) • Pressure-regulated volume control (PRVC) and volume support (VS) • Neurally adjusted ventilatory assist (NAVA) • High-frequency ventilation (HFV) • Bilevel positive airway pressure (BiPAP) • Differential lung ventilation • Extracorporeal membrane oxygenation (ECMO)

breath and adjust ventilator support accordingly. It does this by delivering positive pressure throughout inspiration in proportion to inspiratory airflow and volume generated by the patient. In conventional ventilatory modes, peak inspiratory pressures and VTs are relatively constant. In PAV, there is a direct constant relationship between the inspiratory effort of the patient and the peak inspiratory pressure generated by the ventilator from breath to breath. The VT and peak inspiratory pressure are thus dependent variables. The PAV mode necessitates that the patient is capable of performing a portion of the respiratory work. It demands that the ventilator should be able to determine the elastance and resistance of the respiratory system in spontaneously breathing patients.

Pressure-regulated Volume Control and Volume Support

In the pressure-regulated volume control (PRVC) mode, a pressure-targeted ventilation is used to achieve a desired VT. In the volume support (VS) mode, a pressure support is given by the ventilator to achieve a predesigned VT. This is done from breath to breath. The major concerns with both these assist modes is that if because of inspiratory respiratory demands (for example, fever or increased metabolism from any cause), there results an increased effort in breathing, the level of assistance offered by the ventilator will paradoxically decrease. Also, the machine delivers a predesigned VT; however, in spontaneously breathing patients, the VT is not constant and may vary from breath to breath.

Neurally Adjusted Ventilatory Assist

This mode uses the electrical activity of the diaphragm (Edi) to control the ventilator. It is based on the concept that electrical activity of the diaphragm (triggered through the phrenic nerve) is representative of the overall neural respiratory effort both in timing and amplitude. In neurally adjusted ventilatory assist (NAVA), positive pressure generated by the ventilator is in direct proportion to the amplitude of the electrical activity of the diaphragm, sensed by the ventilator. The patient's respiratory control mechanisms including feedback from various receptors adjust the electrical activity of the diaphragm thereby regulating both VT and the peak inspiratory pressure. NAVA has been tried out in specialized ICUs, and has been shown to enhance ventilator-patient synchrony, provide adequate gas exchange, and unload respiratory muscles without alteration in circulatory hemodynamics, both during invasive and noninvasive ventilatory support.

We have no experience with either the PAV or the NAVA ventilator modes and would rather wait for more clinical trials to define their optimum use.

Bilevel Positive Airway Pressure

In bilevel positive airway pressure (BiPAP) ventilation, two levels of continuous positive pressure are used, the patient being allowed to spontaneously breathe at both pressure levels. Assistance to spontaneous breathing can be given optimally at the low pressure level, high pressure level, or at both levels. The change from low pressure level to high pressure level is coordinated by the patient's breathing effort. The BiPAP mode has its chief use in noninvasive ventilator support rather than in the invasive form.

High-frequency Ventilation

Several modes of high-frequency ventilation (HFV) have been employed. The basic feature in common is the use of VTs which are smaller than the dead space volume. Gas exchange does not occur through convection as in conventional ventilatory modes, but by molecular diffusion, nonconvective mixing, and by other mechanisms. The two important modes of HFV are high-frequency oscillatory ventilation, and high-frequency jet ventilation. The advantages claimed for HFV include a decreased risk of barotrauma, and efficient gas exchange. This mode is believed to be best suited for healing of bronchopleural fistulae. Controlled trials, however, have shown no distinct benefit with this mode as compared to other conventional modes. The risk of complications is also significant.

Differential Lung Ventilation

Patients in respiratory failure due to severe asymmetrical lung disease may fail to be adequately ventilated by conventional ventilatory modes. In such patients, adequate gas exchange can be provided by differential lung ventilation.

Clinical examples include patients with bronchopleural fistulae, unilateral trauma, scoliosis, or marked asymmetrical degree of parenchymal inflammatory disease in each lung (one lung being grossly affected, and the other only slightly so). When there is a large difference in compliance, resistance, or both parameters between the two lungs, a larger proportion of each tidal breath (using conventional ventilatory modes), is distributed to the comparatively unaffected lung. This results in a mismatching of ventilation and perfusion, an increase in the shunt, and poor gas exchange.

The initiation of differential lung ventilation requires the patient to be intubated with a double-lumen endotracheal tube (Carlen, Robert-Shaw, Univent, or Broncho-Cath). Different VTs, flow rates, VE, and if necessary even PEEP, are set for each lung. Differential lung ventilation can be through two asynchronous ventilators each with its own circuit and its own settings, or through two synchronized ventilators which deliver tidal breaths to both lungs through two independent circuits. The VTs, FiO_2, and other ventilatory settings for each lung are independently adjustable.

Extracorporeal Membrane Oxygenation

More than a decade ago a multicenter trial using ECMO came to the conclusion that in ARDS patients there was no reduction in mortality in the ECMO treated group, rather there was a significantly greater number of complications in this group of patients. This does not hold true today. Improvement in equipment, greater experience has led to improving results. ECMO is now considered to be an established life support system of great value in the care of children and adults with serious cardiac and pulmonary dysfunction, refractory to conventional treatment.

ECMO is a form of cardiopulmonary life support in which blood is drained from the vascular system, circulated outside the body by a mechanical pump through an oxygenator and reinfused into the circulation. While outside the body, the hemoglobin becomes fully saturated with oxygen and carbon dioxide produced by the body is removed.

Indications for ECMO

Cardiac support: Patients eligible for ECMO are those with a low cardiac output (less than 2 $L/min/m^2$), severe hypotension leading to poor tissue perfusion, despite adequate volume replacement and large doses of inotropic support and the use of aortic balloon pump.

Refractory cardiogenic shock from any cause, inability to wean from cardiopulmonary bypass after cardiac surgery, severe cardiomyopathy, as a bridge to either a longer term ventricular assist device, or as a bridge to cardiopulmonary transplant, and post-transplant graft failure are the main indications for providing cardiac support using ECMO.

Respiratory support: ECMO can be used in severe respiratory failure from any cause—classically in patients with ARDS. It is responsible for proper oxygenation and carbon dioxide removal, rests the lung, giving it time to recover. It can also be used in the management of advanced respiratory disease from any cause or as a bridge to a lung or a heart-lung transplant.

Technique: The details of this technique are beyond the scope of this book.

Veno-venous (VV) ECMO: When a single cannula is used, blood is withdrawn by a cannula from the superior vena cava or right atrium, circulated and returned fully oxygenated to the right atrium. If a double venous cannula system is used, blood is withdrawn via a cannula in the femoral vein and returned fully oxygenated to the internal jugular vein or the femoral vein.

Veno-arterial (VA) ECMO: In this technique the blood bypasses both the heart and the lungs. Blood is withdrawn from the superior vena cava via a cannula and returned to the arterial system via a cannula either in the carotid, or femoral or axillary artery.

Complications

Bleeding: The most frequent complication during ECMO is hemorrhage. Bleeding may occur at the cannula site, at the surgical site of a prior surgical procedure or at any other site within the body—intrathoracic, intrapulmonary, intra-abdominal, retroperitoneal and intracerebral. Bleeding is increased because of heparinization, platelet dysfunction, clotting factors hemodilution.

Systemic thromboembolism: Systemic thromboembolism is due to thrombus formation within the extracorporeal circuit.

Neurological complications: Neurological complications include seizures, cerebral infarction, cerebral hemorrhage.

Hypertension: Hypertension is a dangerous complication because of the risk of stroke or an intracerebral bleed.

Sepsis: Sepsis and or multiorgan failure is one of the most dreaded complication of this procedure.

Mechanical complications: Clots in the circuit are the most frequent mechanical complication.

Specific complications related to VA – ECMO:
- Cardiac thrombosis is a possible complication whenever the femoral artery and vein are used for cannulation due to retrograde blood flow in the ascending aorta.
- When fully saturated blood is returned from the ECMO circuit to the femoral artery, there will be preferential circulation to the lower extremities and abdomen compared to circulation to the head and chest. Cerebral hypoxia and poor coronary perfusion could result.

Conclusion: ECMO is now a recognized efficient life support in patients with refractory cardiac or respiratory failure. In centers of excellence, it has been shown that 75% of patients with severe ARDS required ECMO. Of those that required ECMO, 60–70% survived. Similar good results were obtained following the use of ECMO in patients with severe H1N1 related acute respiratory distress syndrome. The mortality was 23.7%, compared to 52.5% in patients treated with conventional ventilator support.

According to data from the annual International ELSO registry report through January 2015, 65,171 patients received extracorporeal life support (ECLS). Among these, 70% were weaned and 59% were discharged or transferred.

Finally it must be recognized that ECMO is a supportive therapy and not therapy that modifies the natural history of a disease, or eradicates its cause. ECMO should only be performed by clinicians who are well trained and experienced. This is particularly important in developing countries where the lure and use of new technology not backed by training can do more harm than good.

■ COMPLICATIONS OF MECHANICAL VENTILATION (TABLE 11)

Alveolar Hyperventilation

A $PaCO_2$ of less than 20 mm Hg can be dangerous. Respiratory alkalosis results in cramps, tetany, reduced cerebral blood flow, and hypotension. Electrolyte

Table 11: Common complications encountered during mechanical ventilation.

- Alveolar hyperventilation resulting in $PaCO_2$ less than 25 mm Hg. This causes respiratory alkalosis (with decreased cerebral blood flow, tetany, hypotension), shift in K^+ from extracellular to cellular compartment causing arrhythmias, and difficulties in weaning
- *Atelectasis*: Segmental, lobar, or massive/diffuse airspace collapse
- Uneven compliances in different areas of the lung resulting in uneven distribution of inspired gas and difficulty in mechanical ventilation
- Occurrence of auto-PEEP
- Nosocomial infection
- *Hypotension*: Initially ventilator-related due to high inflation pressures; later, usually unrelated to ventilator support
- *Barotrauma/volutrauma/biotrauma*: Pneumothorax, pneumomediastinum, interstitial emphysema, and damage to alveolar walls
- "Clashing" with the machine
- *GI complications*: Paralytic ileus, gastric dilatation, and GI bleeds
- Water retention

(GI: Gastrointestinal; PEEP: Positive end-expiratory pressure)

disturbances characterized by a sudden shift of potassium from the extracellular to the cellular compartment can trigger dangerous arrhythmias like ventricular tachycardia, or ventricular fibrillation. Prolonged alveolar hyperventilation makes weaning difficult as the respiratory center gets used to a low arterial carbon dioxide tension, and cannot tolerate a rise of $PaCO_2$ to even normal levels.

Atelectasis

This may be of two kinds: (1) segmental, lobar, or even massive; (2) diffuse airspace collapse or atelectasis.

Lobar or massive atelectasis is easy to detect clinically as well as on X-ray. It produces distress with a rise in the static compliance (a rise in both peak and plateau pressures is observed). A slipping of the endotracheal tube into the right main bronchus is an important cause of collapse of part or whole of the left lung.

Diffuse airspace atelectasis is characterized by a collapse of very many scattered alveoli in both lungs, so that both the clinical examination, and the chest X-ray are essentially normal. It is at times observed when VTs less than 10 mL/kg are used to ventilate the lungs. The use of VTs of 10 mL/kg is the best prophylactic measure for this complication. Diffuse airspace atelectasis is suspected when there is a fall in the compliance, with an increase in the alveolar-arterial oxygen gradient, and a normal chest

X-ray. When due to an increase in the water content of the lungs, the condition can be corrected by the prompt use of a diuretic like furosemide.

Uneven Compliances within Different Areas of the Lung

These produce uneven distribution of inspired gas. When some areas of the lung are normal or overcompliant, while others show a marked decrease in compliance, the problem in mechanical ventilation is immense. Inspired gas overventilates the compliant lung, and often fails to "open" or ventilate the stiff or noncompliant parts of the lung. Overdistension of the compliant areas leads to increase in the physiological dead space, increasing zone I conditions especially when large VTs are used. The capillary perfusion in these areas is severely diminished, with blood being shunted to the less compliant, poorly ventilated areas. This produces an increased right-to-left shunt with a fall in the PaO_2. Lower VTs with a judicious adjustment of PEEP are necessary, but the difficulties in providing adequate gas exchange are not always solved.

Autopositive End-expiratory Pressure

An increase in PEEP occasionally occurs in patients on mechanical ventilation (auto-PEEP), even when PEEP is not used as an adjunct to ventilator support. Auto-PEEP (occult PEEP, intrinsic PEEP) is defined as an unintentional PEEP that occurs when a new inspiratory breath is delivered before expiration has ended, in patients on ventilator support. A progressively increasing auto-PEEP results in a "dynamic hyperinflation" of the lung, which is merely another expression for increasing air-trapping within the lung. Auto-PEEP and dynamic hyperinflation are most commonly seen in patients with COPD, where narrowed obstructed airways lead to prolonged expiration and air trapping. Other factors that predispose to the occurrence of auto-PEEP are: (a) VE equal to or more than 10 L/min; (b) patients more than 60 years of age; (c) use of a small-sized endotracheal tube; (d) increase in VT specially in patients with COPD; (e) increase in compliance; (f) increase in respiratory rate with increase in risk of air trapping, particularly when inspiratory time equals expiratory time; and (g) reduced inspiratory flow rate with shorter expiratory time.

Measurement of Autopositive End-expiratory Pressure

During normal mechanical ventilation, the auto-PEEP present in the patient's lungs at end-expiration is not registered on the ventilator manometer, as in most ventilators pressures during exhalation are measured internally on the inspiratory side of the machine. Also normally, the expiratory valve is open to the atmosphere during exhalation. Auto-PEEP can be measured by occluding the expiratory limb of the circuit just before the next positive pressure breath. When the exhalation valve is occluded, the manometer measures the pressure in the patient's airway as the pressure equilibrates with the circuit. This method of measuring auto-PEEP requires a quiet patient on controlled ventilation **(Fig. 6)**.

Some ventilators like the Siemens Servo 900C and the Ohmeda Advent have end-expiration pause buttons or controls. They are microprocessor ventilators that can time the closing of the exhalation valve. They close this valve just before the next positive breath is due, delay the next breath, and then measure the pressure in the circuit.

Effects of Autopositive End-expiratory Pressure

Effects of auto-PEEP are the same as those of PEEP used on purpose as an adjunct to ventilatory support. Deleterious

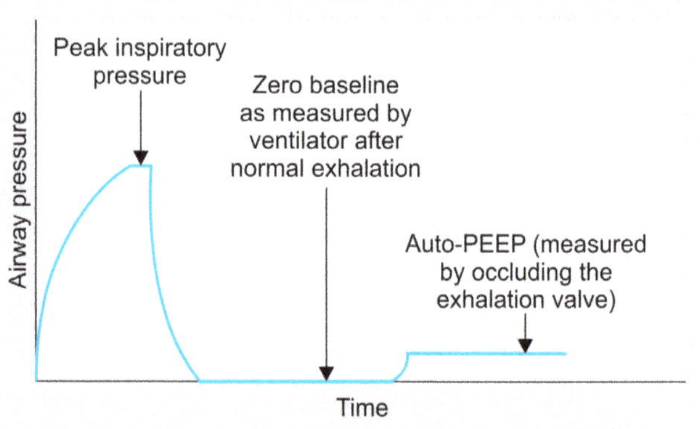

Fig. 6: The airway pressures (peak and plateau) during a positive pressure breath. Pressure rises during inspiration to peak inspiratory pressure (PIP). With a breath hold, the plateau pressure can be measured. Pressures fall back to baseline during expiration. Auto PEEP measured by occluding the exhalation valve.
(PEEP: Positive end-expiratory pressure)
Source: Reproduced with permission from Pilbeam SP. Mechanical Ventilation, Physiological and Clinical Applications. Mosby: Elsevier; 1992.

effects include barotrauma, hypotension, and a fall in PaO_2.

Methods of Reducing Autopositive End-expiratory Pressure

Auto-PEEP can be reduced by the use of: (a) higher inspiratory flow rates, thereby shortening the inspiratory time and allowing longer time for expiration; (b) increased expiratory time by using smaller VT and reduced respiratory rates; (c) low-resistance exhalation valves and large-bore endotracheal tubes to reduce air trapping; and (d) low compressible volume ventilator patient circuit.

It must be mentioned that the occurrence of auto-PEEP is not confined to patients on ventilator support. It is frequently observed in spontaneously breathing patients who have severe airways obstruction that leads to air-trapping.

Infection

Nosocomial infection is an important complication and the following preventive measures are enumerated here:

- Cleanliness in the patient's room with scrupulous attention to avoiding cross-infection. Washing hands prior to examining the patient is important.
- Care of the tracheostomy wound—spraying the wound with an antibiotic spray is useful.
- Aseptic suction of secretions through the tracheostomy/endotracheal tube—this should be done as often as is necessary.
- Meticulous attention to prevention of atelectasis by physiotherapy and postural drainage. Prompt treatment of atelectasis and diffuse airspace collapse is mandatory.
- Frequent sterilization of humidifiers, tubing is essential.
- Tracheostomy tubes should be changed every 4 days under aseptic conditions.
- Proper nutrition, oxygenation, and perfusion should be well maintained, so as to increase resistance to infection.

In patients on ventilator support, growth of gram-negative organisms (chiefly *Pseudomonas* strains and *Klebsiella*) is frequently observed on culture of tracheal secretions. A positive culture by itself does not indicate infection, and does not warrant treatment (see chapter on Nosocomial Pneumonia).

Hypotension

This is an important complication of mechanical ventilation. When it occurs soon after initiating ventilation, it is very likely to be related to the effects of the ventilator. In the presence of high-inflation pressures, the use of PEEP, or in patients with overcompliant lungs as seen in emphysema, there may be a marked rise in intrapleural pressure. This reduces venous return and cardiac filling and induces a fall in blood pressure. Hypotension is often marked in hypovolemic patients. The treatment in such patients is to reduce inflation pressures, reduce or go off PEEP totally (if this has been used), and give a volume load to expand the circulating volume. Hypotension can also result from barotrauma, for example, a pneumothorax induced by ventilator support. This may occur at the time of initiation of ventilator support or at a later period.

When hypotension occurs later during mechanical ventilation (the patient having been hemodynamically stable for several days), the cause is generally unrelated to the ventilator. Severe hypoxia and hypocapnia should be looked for, as they can induce a fall in blood pressure. If the blood gases are normal, hypotension may be due to shock, blood loss, fluid or electrolyte imbalance, sepsis, metabolic acidosis, or poor pump function. Only if all these factors have been excluded, should the possibility of a ventilator-induced hypotension be considered.

Barotrauma, Volume Trauma, and Biotrauma

Barotrauma and volume trauma (volutrauma) are the most important and dreaded complications of mechanical ventilation. Probably, both high inflation pressures and high VTs, particularly when PEEP is also used, contribute to barotrauma. It is generally the more compliant parts of the lungs, and not the poorly compliant areas, that are susceptible to barotrauma. Barotrauma classically takes the form of pneumothorax—tension pneumothorax occurs when high VTs are used with high inflation pressures. Unless promptly recognized, it causes cardiorespiratory collapse and death. Interstitial emphysema, mediastinal emphysema, and surgical emphysema of the soft tissues of the neck, spreading upward to the face and downward to the chest, may occur in the absence of pneumothorax.

A more subtle form of trauma to the alveolar walls can be caused by high VTs (volume trauma or *volutrauma*). High VTs are as important in producing alveolar damage as high alveolar pressures. The overstretched alveolar walls are damaged, so that alveoli (even those which were reasonably normal), are now thickened, distorted, and poorly compliant, thus adding to the overall stiffness and poor compliance of the lungs, and setting off a vicious cycle, which perpetuates respiratory failure to a point of no return. Overstretch of alveoli with high VTs is also believed to result in the production of cytokines that further injure the lung and perhaps also increase injury to other organs (biotrauma). The "opening" and "closing" of poorly compliant alveoli during inspiration and expiration results in shear forces that induce further lung injury (see chapter on Acute Lung Injury and ARDS).

Clashing with the Machine

This can occur at any time during mechanical ventilation, though it is most commonly observed during initiation of ventilator support. Clashing or fighting with the machine can be due to several causes, and each should be carefully evaluated prior to taking any decision on the management of the patient.

- Alveolar hypoventilation as stated earlier, is an important cause; if present, it should be corrected by increasing the VE.
- Obstructed tracheostomy/endotracheal tube or obstructed airways due to bronchospasm or mucus plugging is an important cause of distress, leading to a "clash" with the machine. A rise in peak pressure, with a fall in the dynamic compliance and a marked difference between the peak and pause pressures should point to the earlier cause.
- Atelectasis, pneumonia, and pneumothorax are very important causes of a clash with the machine. Distress and high peak pressures with a fall in the compliance are observed.
- Blood loss [as in bleeding within the gastrointestinal (GI) tract], shock from any cause, electrolyte imbalance, metabolic acidosis, high fever, pain, a distended bladder or colon, or a dilated stomach are other causes that aggravate difficulties in synchronization with the machine.
- A strong respiratory drive due to altered mechanics within diseased lungs may defy all efforts to match the machine to the patient. It is in this group that controlled ventilation after inducing neuromuscular paralysis or after depressing respiration with intravenous diazepam or morphine is mandatory.

Gastrointestinal Complications

Gastric dilatation and paralytic ileus are observed at times, particularly at the start of mechanical ventilation. The cause is obscure. Treatment is through gastric aspiration via a nasogastric tube, stopping all oral feeds, and using intravenous fluids till such time as gut motility returns. The maintenance of fluid and electrolyte balance in such patients is precarious. Hypokalemia tends to aggravate the ileus, and needs to be carefully corrected by potassium replacement through intravenous infusions.

Gastrointestinal bleeding occasionally occurs as a complication in patients on ventilator support. This is due to acute erosive gastroduodenitis in critically ill patients, particularly in those receiving corticosteroids. GI bleeding is particularly common with acute on chronic respiratory failure secondary to infection in patients with chronic bronchitis. These patients generally have a well-marked acidosis. Antacids and H2-receptor antagonists, or sucralfate reduce gastric acidity, and thereby help stop bleeding. At times, laser therapy or endoscopic cauterization of bleeding points may be necessary. The blood loss should be replaced by transfusions.

Water Retention

Patients on prolonged ventilator support may retain water even in the clinical absence of left heart failure, or of a rise in venous pressure. Increase in the water content of the lungs may cause some degree of pulmonary edema. This produces impaired gas exchange, and fluffy shadows in the lung on a chest X-ray. The problem is managed by restricting fluids to 1,000 mL in 24 hours, and by the use of diuretics like furosemide.

■ WEANING FROM VENTILATOR SUPPORT

Patients on mechanical ventilation should be weaned from ventilator support and extubated at the appropriate time. An unnecessary delay in weaning increases the patient's risk of nosocomial infection, trauma to the airways, adverse effects of prolonged sedation, and health care costs. Yet premature weaning can lead to reintubation with the enhanced risk of nosocomial pneumonia, increased morbidity and mortality.

There are a number of patients who are electively intubated and mechanically ventilated for brief periods of time for reasons other than respiratory failure. These include those ventilated briefly after major surgery as an extension of intraoperative and postoperative surgical care, or those intubated for airway protection. An abrupt termination of ventilator support and often quick extubation is generally possible in such patients, if the following criteria are satisfied:

- The patient is awake, alert and can breathe well spontaneously. He should have a good 'blast' through the endotracheal tube, and if needs be, his tidal volume can be checked by connecting a spirometer to the endotracheal tube.
- The clinical reason for ventilatory support no longer exists, or has resolved.
- The airways are free of secretions through proper suction or spontaneous coughing, and the patient is capable of protecting the airways from aspiration.
- The patient's chest X-ray is normal, and shows no atelectasis or pulmonary shadowing.
- In patients ventilated after open heart surgery or following major surgical procedures, the arterial blood gases and arterial pH should be normal or near normal, both during ventilator support, and after discontinuing support.
- The patient should remain under intensive care so that respiratory care can be continued in the form of humidification of inspired gas, nebulization therapy, physiotherapy, and if necessary, reintroduction of ventilator support.

The weaning parameters stated below are generally not required to be followed in these patients. When however postoperative pulmonary complications produce respiratory failure, or the presence of infection, bleeding or other complications lead to an increasingly critical state, the decision to wean is necessarily delayed. Clinical considerations together with the respiratory parameters discussed below, help to decide the appropriate time to commence weaning from ventilatory support in these patients.

Patients who require ventilator support for long periods of time, extending for weeks or even months, are not easy to wean. Prolonged mechanical ventilation is often necessary in severe or fulminant tetanus, prolonged severe ARDS, neurological problems such as acute infections, polyneuritis, poliomyelitis, injury to the cervical chord. It is also often necessary in fulminant *Plasmodium falciparum* infections, in other fulminant tropical infections such as leptospirosis, in severe sepsis, septic shock, and in multiorgan failure from any cause. In a number of critically ill patients, elective intubation and ventilatory support is offered at a point in time when arterial blood gases are not markedly deranged. The decision to wean such patients from ventilator support should first and foremost be a clinical one, based on clinical considerations. Parameters for weaning are useful, but they should support or supplement a clinical decision, and never be used as a substitute for it.

Clinical Considerations towards the Initiation of Weaning from Ventilator Support

As a general principle, mechanical ventilatory support can only be withdrawn when the reasons for initiating it are no longer present. This usually means that the underlying disease, whether it involves the lungs or not, has been cured or has markedly improved.

In 2008, the American College of Chest Physicians recommended (on the basis of a multisociety sponsored task force study) that every patient on ventilator support should be assessed each day with a "wean screen" to determine when the process of weaning should be initiated. The recommended wean-screen is given in **Table 12.**

We agree with this 'weaning screen' (if one wishes to use this label). The parameters in this 'screen' are invariably 'screened' and carefully noted on an ICU round often more than once every day. We however feel that the recommended 'screen' takes notice solely of the relevant parameters in the cardiorespiratory system, ignoring the fact that serious involvement of other organ systems (present in many critically ill individuals) may impinge on the function of the cardiorespiratory system. Ignoring the above fact leads to premature weaning, a relapse into cardiorespiratory dysfunction, necessitating reintubation with a return of ventilator support—procedures which enhance morbidity, mortality and health costs.

Guidelines are important, and should be understood. Yet they should never be blindly followed; clinical consideration and judgement should never be sacrificed at the altar of recommended guidelines when caring for an individual patient.

Besides cardiorespiratory parameters mentioned in the "weaning screen", the following conditions should be carefully assessed before initiating weaning **(Table 13):**

Table 12: Wean screen criteria used to identify patients ready for a trial of spontaneous breathing.

Criteria	Description
Reversal of respiratory failure	Evidence for some reversal of underlying cause of respiratory failure
Adequate oxygenation	PaO_2/FiO_2 ratio > 150–200 PEEP ≤ 5–8 cm H_2O FiO_2 ≤ 40–50% pH ≥7.25
Hemodynamic stability	Absence of myocardial ischemia Absence of clinically significant hypotension No vasopressors or dopamine/dobutamine <5 µg/kg/min
Respiratory drive	Capability to initiate an inspiratory effort

Table 13: Clinical considerations for weaning patient from ventilator support.

- Mechanical ventilator support should be withdrawn only when the underlying disorder (pulmonary or extrapulmonary) is completely resolved, or has improved markedly
- Patient should maintain normal arterial blood gases on FiO_2 of 0.4 (except in patients with COPD whose basal $PaCO_2$ values are raised and PaO_2 is around 60 mm Hg)
- There should be no significant pulmonary infection, pulmonary edema, atelectasis or airways obstruction
- Acid-base and electrolyte disturbances should be corrected prior to weaning
- The patient should generally be alert, co-operative and mentally prepared to be weaned; he must be hemodynamically stable and preferably off inotropic support
- General nutritional state and neuromuscular status must be clinically assessed as to whether patient can cope with work of breathing
- In presence of high fever, seizures, gastric dilatation, paralytic ileus, GI bleeds, hepatic or acute renal failure, weaning should not be attempted
- On T-tube breathing, there should be no significant change in pulse rate, BP, no tachypnea or respiratory distress, should maintain normal blood gases and a tidal volume of 5–7 mL/kg

- Blood gases as stated in the screen should be satisfactory before initiating the weaning process. An important exception to this are patients with chronic airways obstruction who are being ventilated for acute on chronic respiratory failure. These patients are used to a PaO_2 of < 60 mm Hg and to a high $PaCO_2$ even under normal conditions.
- The lungs should be free of infection, major atelectasis or edema, as far as possible. Airways obstruction, either from mucus plugging or bronchospasm should be significantly relieved, as these factors significantly increase the work of breathing.
- Disturbances in acid-base balance should be corrected before weaning is commenced. Metabolic acidosis can increase the work of breathing significantly, while alkalosis can result in mental obtundation, and depress respiration.
- A clinical judgment should be made whether the patient in the immediate future can withstand or cope with the demands imposed by the work of breathing. The general nutritional state and the neuromuscular status should be given careful consideration. Poor nutrition, electrolyte abnormalities, hypomagnesemia, hypokalemia and hypophosphatemia lead to difficulties in weaning. Severely catabolic states like tetanus result in marked weight loss and loss of muscle mass in spite of providing a large caloric and protein intake. High carbohydrate diets lead to an increase in carbon dioxide production with increasing demands on ventilation, particularly in debilitated individuals, or in those with pre-existing lung disease. In such patients, less carbohydrates and more fats should be used for nutrition.

  Patients with severe liver cell dysfunction, complications caused by renal failure, chronic alcoholics, and those who have weathered a prolonged critical illness, often pose great difficulties in weaning, chiefly because of their poor nutritional state, and their inability to cope with the work of breathing.

  Even when cardiorespiratory parameters are satisfactory, weaning is frequently unsuccessful in the presence of severe multiorgan failure involving other organ systems.
- Ventilator support should be continued and weaning delayed in the presence of high fever, seizures, or when complications such as gastric dilatation, ileus, GI bleeding, or acute renal failure exist.
- The patient should be awake, alert and cooperative, though there are exceptions to this consideration. The patient should also be prepared, indoctrinated and motivated to go off the ventilator.

The Process of Weaning

Weaning is established in two stages:

1. To free the patient of mechanical ventilator support so that he or she breathes spontaneously through an artificial airway.

2. Extubation (removal of the artificial airway) of the patient.

Indices to Predict Weaning Outcome

Many respiratory indices have been proposed in order to predict weaning outcomes. These include:

- Assessment of ventilatory parameters **(Table 14)**
- Oxygenation and $PaCO_2$ levels
- Respiratory muscle strength
- Work of breathing
- Central respiratory drive
- Pattern of spontaneous breathing in relation to tidal volume (V_T) and respiratory rate (f) or f/V_T
- Peak expiratory flow rate > 60 L/min.

Yang and Tobin studied the predictive power of several respiratory weaning indices and showed that the rapid shallow breathing index (f/V_T) had the best predictive value. The other indices listed above had relatively poor positive and negative predictive values. The f/V_T screening test has a high sensitivity and is useful to predict success in weaning when the test is positive ($f/V_T < 105$), and failure to wean when the test is negative ($f/V_T > 105$). However it must be stressed that the f/V_T test though sensitive has a low specificity (i.e. there is a large proportion of weaning failure patients in whom the test is positive).

Methods of Weaning

1. In the past the following methods were utilized:
   a. Weaning through lowering the number of ventilator assisted breaths in a patient on intermittent mandatory ventilation.
   b. Weaning through gradually reducing the level of inspiratory pressure support in a patient on pressure support ventilation (*see* below).
   c. Keeping the patient 'on' and 'off'; ventilator support, and progressively increasing the 'off' periods and reducing the 'on' periods so that the patient breathes spontaneously first all through the day and ultimately all through the night.

It is now accepted that weaning with IMV, significantly delays removal of ventilator support.

2. The currently accepted weaning strategy to free the patient from mechanical ventilator support is to allow a daily **spontaneous breathing trial** through a T-tube during which the patient is observed for signs of respiratory failure **(Table 15)**. If there is no respiratory or cardiac distress, nor any evidence of respiratory failure over a period of 120 minutes, prompt successful extubation can generally be achieved. If the spontaneous breathing trial is unsuccessful, the patient is put back on the ventilator and the spontaneous breathing trial is repeated each successive day till the test is judged to be successful. The patient is then kept off mechanical ventilator support and in most cases is ready for extubation.

In a multicenter randomized trial, Esteban et al. compared four methods of weaning from mechanical ventilation and noted that patients managed with daily spontaneous breathing trials were extubated three times more quickly as those managed with pressure support.

Ely et al. showed that patients managed with a two-step weaning protocol including a daily "wean screen" followed by a spontaneous breathing trial were extubated 1.5 days earlier than when managed with physician-directed weaning.

Esteban et al. subsequently evaluated the effect of the duration of the spontaneous breathing trial in a randomized trial. They found that patients who

Table 14: Objective respiratory parameters for weaning.
1. *Ventilatory parameters*: • RR < 30/minute • VE < 8 L/minute, and not > 10 L/minute • VT of minimum 5–7 mL/kg • VC of minimum 800–1000 mL • Maximum inspiratory force > – 20 cm H_2O • VD/VT < 0.6 • Alveolar-arterial oxygen gradient on FiO_2 of 1 < 250 mm Hg
2. *Arterial blood gases*: • pH 7.35–7.45 • PaO_2 70–100 mm Hg on FiO_2 of 0.4 • $PaCO_2$ 35–45 mm Hg

Table 15: Spontaneous breathing trial failure criteria.	
Criteria	*Description*
Increased work of breathing	Respiratory rate > 35 per min or < 8 per min for at least 5 minutes Two or more signs of respiratory distress, including tachycardia, bradycardia, accessory muscle use, abdominal paradox, diaphoresis or marked dyspnea
Inadequate oxygenation	SaO_2 < 88% for at least 5 minutes
Hemodynamic instability	Acute cardiac dysrhythmia
Neurological instability	Abrupt change in mental status

were extubated after successfully completing a 30-minute trial of spontaneous breathing had similar reintubation rates to those who were not extubated until they completed a 120 minute trial. Even so, most intensivists use a 120 minute trial in patients who fail multiple daily spontaneous breathing trial, before proceeding to extubation.

3. *Pressure-support ventilation*: This is the most common technique used to withdraw mechanical ventilator support when a patient repeatedly fails to pass the spontaneous breathing trial. During weaning the patients pressure support is reduced by 2 to 4 cm twice or thrice daily. If the patient tolerates and is comfortable with a pressure support of 5–8 cm without PEEP, he or she is given a spontaneous breathing trial for 120 minutes and if this is successful, then the patient is ready to be extubated.

   When a patient is on PSV it is important to ensure that there is no asynchronous breathing nor an ineffective respiratory effort. High levels of pressure support should be avoided as this can lead to high tidal volumes and alkalosis causing inefficient triggering with ventilator-patient asynchrony. Clinical experience suggests that the optimal initial levels of pressure support in PSV should be at a level that provide of respiratory rate of 25–30/min.

4. *The role of noninvasive ventilator support*: Non-invasive ventilator support has been used in three different scenarios:
   (i) If after successful extubation in a patient weaned off mechanical ventilation, the patient develops 'de novo' respiratory failure after a lapse of time, the intensivist has two options—to reintubate and reintroduce mechanical ventilation, or to use non-invasive ventilator support to help tide over the crisis.

   Two studies that have tried to assess the value of NIV in the above setting suggest that the use of NIV is of no help. We feel that each patient should be assessed separately not withstanding the result of these studies. If NIV is used it should not be persisted with if there is no clear improvement of respiratory failure after a lapse of 4–6 hours. Reintubation and mechanical ventilator support should not be unduly delayed.

   (ii) NIV is at times used as a preventive measure in high risk patients who have been weaned and extubated. If the patient is considered to be a high risk for reintubation he or she is put on NIV immediately after the endotracheal tube has been removed. Patients who fall in this category are generally old feeble patients, patients who remain hypercapnic at the end of the weaning test, those who have persistent cardiac problems and those who have presented difficulty in weaning. Of the two studies carried out one showed a reduction in extubation rate when NIV was given post-extubation and the other showed in addition a decrease in mortality.

   (iii) Rarely NIV is used as a substitute for invasive mechanical ventilation in some patients with chronic respiratory failure who are difficult to wean and who really do not fully meet the weaning criteria. They refuse a tracheostomy or are at high risk for a tracheostomy. Weaning can be successful through NIV in some patients that fall into this category.

5. *Newer modalities*: A number of newer weaning modalities have been tried with which we are unfamiliar. The use of closed loop PSV is one such modality that provides continuous ventilator assistance to patient's needs 24 hours a day. The above modality as also others in use are tried in the hope of reducing weaning trials compared to conventional methods.

Tracheostomy: Tracheostomy becomes necessary if ventilator support is necessary for over 10–12 days. It has both advantages and disadvantages (*see* Airway Management).

Unsuccessful Weaning from the Ventilator

Perhaps the commonest reason is wrong judgment in deciding to wean the patient. This will happen if the intensivist is solely protocol driven and has ignored clinical considerations. Potentially reversible reasons for a prolonged ventilator support are:

- Inadequate respiratory drive;
- Inability of the lungs to carry out gas exchange either because of infection, atelectasis, stiff lungs (very low compliance) or airways obstruction;
- Inspiratory muscle fatigue;
- Elevated diaphragm from a dilated stomach, marked ileus or a severely distended colon;
- Incipient undetected cardiac failure **(Table 16)**.

Table 16: Reasons for prolonged ventilation 'difficult to wean'.
• Inadequate respiratory drive • Inability of the lungs to carry out gas exchange either because of infection, atelectasis, stiff lungs (very low compliance) or airways obstruction • Inspiratory muscle fatigue • Elevated diaphragm from a dilated stomach, marked ileus or a severely distended colon • Incipient undetected cardiac failure

Table 17: Causes of extubation failure.
• Patient unable to protect the airway • Difficulty clearing secretions • Excessive endotracheal secretions • Mentally obtunded either due to neurological problems or to sedation • Poor cough reflex • Respiratory muscle fatigue • Incipient (often undetected) cardiac failure • Associated serious comorbid conditions

Extubation: Removal of the Artificial Airway

In a number of patients, extubation (removal of the artificial airway) is successful if the patients have passed the spontaneous breathing test for a period of 2 hours. This signifies total freedom from ventilator support. Nevertheless, there are situations where the patient may not need ventilatory support but still needs an artificial airway for a further length in time varying from hours to days. This is likely if the patient is unable to protect the airway, has difficulty clearing secretions or is mentally obtunded either due to neurological problems or to sedation. A normal or near-normal mental status is important for successful weaning. Salam et al. carried out a study on patients who were extubated after passing a spontaneous breathing trial. They found that patients who were unable to complete four simple tasks were more than four times likely to require reintubation as compared to patients who completed the tasks. A poor cough reflex, excessive endotracheal secretions are also features which should prompt the intensivist to delay extubation even when the patient has passed the spontaneous breathing test.

Sedation, though important in the management of many patients in the ICU who are on ventilator support can result in obtundation, so that both disconnecting the ventilator and/or extubation is delayed. Interruption of all sedation at the time a patient is given the spontaneous breathing trial ("wake up and breathe") leads to both quicker release from ventilator support and quicker extubation. It has been observed that patients who were made to "wake up and breathe" were discharged earlier from the ICU. There was also a 14% absolute reduction in the risk of death in one year when the above policy was followed.

Extubation Failure (Table 17)

Extubation failure is defined as the reintroduction of ventilator support within 24–48 hours of extubation. The extubation failure rate is the number of patients requiring the reintroduction of mechanical ventilator support divided by the total number of extubated patients. It is important to realize that extubation failure is associated with a significant increase in patient mortality and morbidity. The underlying pathology in a patient with extubation failure may well influence outcome. Patients requiring reintubation because of respiratory failure had a mortality of 30% compared to a mortality of 7% in patients reintubated because of upper airways obstruction.

The Role of Inspiratory Muscle Fatigue in the Weaning Process

Inspiratory muscle fatigue is often responsible for a patient failing the spontaneous breathing trial. Even more important, it is an important reason for reintubation once the patient has been extubated. Inspiratory muscle fatigue should be suspected if the respiratory rate is > 30–35/min on disconnection from the ventilator, if the respiratory excursions are poor, if there are periods of spontaneous apnea or irregularity in the breathing pattern, or if there is paradoxical breathing. Not uncommonly the only manifestation of inspiratory muscle fatigue is a failed spontaneous breathing test.

We have given an evidence based protocol driven approach to weaning from mechanical ventilator support—both in relation to disconnecting the ventilator and extubation. Evidence presented in Western literature suggests that if the patient "passes" the weaning screen, he should be given a daily spontaneous breathing trial through a T tube for 2 hours. If he passes this trial (in that he shows no respiratory or cardiovascular distress or failure) he is fit to go off ventilator support and in most cases fit to be extubated.

We now need to give a critical appreciation and add a few caveats to the above.

1. A protocol driven weaning program if divorced from clinical judgment has a significant chance to fail. The "weaning screen" (as proposed by the ACCP) which takes into consideration just cardiorespiratory parameters is not sufficient for a correct judgment in the suitability of initiating the weaning process. The overall criticality of the patient in relation to other organ functions and other complications prevailing in a particular critically ill patient must be given due consideration before considering the patient fit for weaning.

2. The evidence in relation to the spontaneous 120 minute breathing trial is from Western countries. There is no large prospective trial in India leave aside a multi-centered randomized trial. We need to gather our own evidence. There is a difference in ethnicity between the West and India and other South-east Asian and African countries. More importantly, there is in all probability a difference in the case-mix of patients on mechanical ventilator support in the ICUs of the West and the East. Also the case-mix in tertiary private hospitals in large metropolitan cities of India is different from the comparatively poor patient population in the ICUs of large government and municipal hospitals of these cities. It is important to accept the fact that the standard of intensive care both in relation to intensivists and particularly in relation to the nursing staff varies in the different ICUs in our country and also in other developing countries.

3. We have noticed that in our ICU even when a patient has passed the 120 minute spontaneous breathing test, he may fail to breathe well after 6–10 hours, necessitating a return to ventilator support. The more critically ill the patient is or has been, the more frequently is this observed. A premature extubation would have certainly resulted in a reintubation in these patients with the added increase in morbidity and mortality.

4. The nutritional state of many patients in our ICUs is often poor. Perhaps a 120 minute spontaneous breathing trial is too short for such patients.

5. Evidence not withstanding, the reintubation rates in the West are significant. Vallverdu et al. in a study of 217 medical and surgical patients noted an overall reintubation rate of 15%, ranging from 36% in neurological patients to 0% in COPD patients. Data by Estaban et al. show a reintubation rate of 13–19%. What would be the reintubation rate in our ICU? We feel for various reasons (some of which are mentioned above) that it would be more than the rates reported in the West.

6. The role of protocols in hastening the weaning process has been questioned. Krishnan et al. in a prospective controlled trial in a closed medical ICU compared protocol-based weaning to usual physician directed weaning and did not observe any improvement in clinical outcomes with protocols.

7. The two-hour spontaneous trial method of weaning invariably fails in patients who have been on ventilator support for several weeks or months. We have successfully managed to wean most of these patients by giving spontaneous breathing trial for progressively longer intervals, so that hours off the machine are gradually increased. The patient is then first weaned off support during the day and then slowly weaned off support during the night. Pressure support breathing is of help in these patients. Spontaneous breathing trials should be started when the patient breathes comfortably through a tracheostomy collar or a T-tube with a pressure support of 10–15 cm of H_2O.

■ CONCLUSION

Once the patient is judged (this is a clinical and judgmental decision) to be ready for weaning he should be given a daily spontaneous breathing trial for 120 minutes. On the day he passes the trial a decision needs to be taken about extubation. Should it be immediate or should one wait for some hours or even a few more days. If the duration of ventilator support has been short (<10 days) and there is nothing to suggest any contraindications to extubation the patient should be extubated promptly but watched closely. In our conditions the decision to extubate is not to be taken by the nursing staff but by the intensivist. We have seen disasters if this dictum is not followed.

If however there is any risk in prompt extubation (after a successful 120 minute spontaneous breath test), or if for any reason it is felt that through the patient has passed the spontaneous breathing test over 2 hours, he could well show cardiorespiratory distress later (this again is a judgemental decision), it is better to delay extubation than risk the possibility of a reintubation, as the latter in our opinion carries with it greater morbidity and mortality. Also if the airway is in place the patient can be reintroduced to ventilator support if after a lapse of time he shows evidence of cardiorespiratory distress.

Patients who have received prolonged ventilator support extending for weeks or months need a different approach in weaning—a gradual withdrawal of ventilator support as has been stated in clause 7.

NONINVASIVE POSITIVE PRESSURE VENTILATION

A number of critical care units attempt, in suitable patients, to offer ventilatory support through a nasal mask or through a fitting orofacial mask rather than through an endotracheal tube. The major advantage of noninvasive positive pressure ventilation (NIPPV) is the reduced incidence of nosocomial pneumonia and of other complications associated with endotracheal intubation.

The use of NIPPV has been standard therapy in patients with obstructive sleep apnea and in many patients with central sleep apnea. Other indications for NIPPV in acute respiratory failure are as follows **(Table 18):**

- Acute crisis in chronic airways obstruction. This is dealt with at length in the chapter on Acute Crisis in Chronic Airways Obstruction.
- In some patients with mild to moderate cardiogenic or noncardiogenic pulmonary edema. The more severe forms need intubation and ventilatory support.
- Community-acquired pneumonia with acute respiratory failure.
- In acquired immunodeficiency syndrome (AIDS) with *Pneumocystis carinii* infection or with other forms of disseminated pulmonary infection.
- Hypercapnic respiratory failure due to progressive chronic airways obstruction, or due to the obesity hypoventilation syndrome.
- Postoperative respiratory failure (chiefly due to atelectasis).

It is obvious that if NIPPV fails to effect efficient gas exchange, or cannot be tolerated by the patient, prompt intubation with ventilator support becomes necessary.

Noninvasive positive pressure ventilation is contraindicated under the following conditions **(Table 19):**

- In patients with a respiratory arrest or need for immediate intubation.
- Inability to protect the airway.
- In the presence of copious respiratory secretions.
- Hemodynamic instability or persistent hypotension (systolic < 90 mm Hg).
- Occurrence of dangerous or persistent arrhythmia.
- Inability to cooperate or tolerate either the nasal or facial mask.
- In the presence of facial injuries.

Noninvasive positive pressure ventilation is also occasionally used after extubation in patients with marginal weaning criteria. NIPPV offers a transition from intubation to spontaneous breathing.

Different modes of ventilator support have been used with NIPPV. These include volume A/C, pressure control, pressure support, and the CPAP modes.

The major danger with NIPPV is the risk of aspiration of gastric contents. It is best not to exceed positive inspiratory peak pressures of 20–25 cm H_2O as gastric dilatation with fear of aspiration can become a major problem. The setting should allow a VT of 7–10 mL/kg.

Bilevel pressure ventilators (BiPAP machine) should generally be used for long term or chronic application of NIPPV as in patients with obstructive sleep apnea or patients with chronic hypercapnic respiratory failure due to COPD. The expiratory positive airway pressure (EPAP) is set at 3–8 cm H_2O and the inspiratory airway pressure (IPAP) to +10 to +20 cm H_2O to provide effective ventilation. A backup assist rate should be set during sleep.

RESPIRATORY MONITORING DURING MECHANICAL VENTILATION

Monitoring of respiratory mechanics is only possible during VCV, a ventilatory mode perhaps most often used

Table 18: Indications of NIPPV.
- Obstructive sleep apnea - Acute crisis in chronic airways obstruction - Mild to moderate cardiogenic or noncardiogenic pulmonary edema - Community-acquired pneumonia with acute respiratory failure - AIDS with *Pneumocystis carinii* infection or any other infection - Hypercapnic respiratory failure due to chronic airways obstruction or the obesity hypoventilation syndrome - Postoperative respiratory failure (chiefly due to atelectasis)

(AIDS: Acquired immunodeficiency syndrome; NIPPV: Noninvasive positive pressure ventilation)

Table 19: Contraindications of noninvasive positive pressure ventilation (NIPPV).
- Respiratory arrest or need for immediate intubation - Inability to protect the airway - Presence of copious respiratory secretions - Hemodynamic instability or persistent hypotension - Persistent arrhythmia - Inability to cooperate or tolerate either the nasal or facial mask - Presence of facial injuries

in most ICUs at least at the start of invasive ventilatory support. The discussion here is limited to patients on volume-preset ventilation. Determining respiratory mechanics at the start and during mechanical ventilation is an important and necessary aspect of ventilatory management. It is important to note the peak pressures, the pause pressures, the V_{Ts}, the PEEP, both extrinsic and intrinsic (if present), and to determine from these observations the dynamic compliance, static compliance, and the resistance of the airway.

Airway Pressure and Positive End-expiratory Pressure Measurement

Measurements are reasonably accurate when the patient is relaxed (preferably sedated) on volume-preset ventilatory support. The inspiratory airway pressure (P_{aw}) has three components—First, to overcome resistance of the airways during inspiration, the second, to overcome elastic recoil of the alveoli and expand them, the third, equal to end-expiratory alveolar pressure (PEEP) if this is present.

$$P_{aw} = P_R + P_{stat} + PEEP$$

where P_{stat} = static elastic pressure
            P_R = resistive pressure component

$$P_{aw} = VI \times R + V_T \times E + PEEP$$

where   VI = inspiratory flow
            R = resistance of airways
            E = elastance of the airways

The individual components of P_{aw} when separated provide significant diagnostic and therapeutic information. PEEP can be measured by the end-expiratory occlusion method. Most ventilators now provide an expiratory pause switch which allows a direct read-out of the PEEP. An error may creep into the measurement of intrinsic PEEP by this method if there is a leak around the endotracheal tubing or around the endotracheal tube cuff or when there is continuous nebulization with bronchodilators at the time of measurement, so that there is gas flow into the circuit, or if the patient is not completely taken over by the machine, and is not relaxed. Extrinsic PEEP is measured as set by the machine. Once PEEP has been measured, the remainder of the airways pressure (AP = Ppeak – PEEP) can be apportioned between the pressure needed to overcome airways resistance (P_{res}) and pressure needed to overcome elastic recoil (P_{es}). This is done by stopping flow at end-inspiration and allowing the P_{aw} to drop to a plateau level (P_{plat}).

The difference between the peak pressure and the plateau pressure is a measure of the airway resistance. The greater the difference between the peak pressure and the plateau pressure, the greater the airways resistance.

If the inspiratory flow rate (VI) is 60 L/min or 1 L/s, the airways resistance during inspiration (P_{res}) is between 4 cm H_2O and 10 cm H_2O. A rise in airways resistance denoted by an increase in the difference between peak airway pressure and plateau pressure is observed with bronchospasm, obstruction of the large airways or mucus plugging of the bronchi, bronchioles, and small airways. An increase in airways resistance (increased difference between the peak and plateau pressures) also occurs if there is obstruction of the endotracheal tube or tracheostomy tube or the trachea. In patients with bronchospasm, the airways resistance may fall after nebulization with a bronchodilator and this is evinced by a narrowing of the gap between the peak pressure and the plateau pressure.

There now remains the need to determine the resistance offered by the elastic recoil of the lungs. This is indirectly determined by computing the compliance of the lung.

Dynamic compliance = Tidal volume/peak pressure – PEEP (if present)
Static compliance = Tidal volume/plateau pressure – PEEP (if present)

A significant fall in compliance (the causes of which are listed earlier) will cause a sharp rise in both peak and pause pressures, pointing thereby to stiff lungs but no increase in the airways resistance (since there will be no increase in the difference between peak and pause pressure).

Therefore increased elastic recoil of the lungs, i.e. stiff lungs, is associated with an overall reduction in both dynamic and static compliance. A reduced compliance is seen in pulmonary fibrosis, pulmonary edema, atelectasis, ARDS and consolidation. Compliance is also reduced when a patient on the ventilator develops pneumothorax or has a collapsed lobe or lung or when there is increased stiffness of the chest wall or in the presence of abdominal distension.

An increased compliance is observed in emphysema in which there is a loss of elastic recoil within the lungs. If the cause of ventilatory failure in a patient is undetermined at the time of intubation, an assessment of the peak and plateau pressure and of the compliance will help to determine the nature of the problem. A normal peak and plateau pressure in a patient intubated and ventilated for ventilatory failure should make the physician suspect an impaired central drive to breathe or neuromuscular weakness as the underlying cause of ventilatory failure.

■ SUGGESTED READING

1. Brochard L, Rauss A, Benito S, et al. Comparison of three methods of gradual withdrawal from ventilatory support during weaning from mechanical ventilation. Am J Respir Crit Care Med. 1994;150(4):896-903.
2. Courey AJ, Hyzy RC. Overview of mechanical ventilation. [online] Available from https://www.uptodate.com/contents/overview-of-mechanical-ventilation. [Accessed July, 2018].
3. Dojat A, Touchard D, Laforest M, et al. Evaluation of a knowledge-based system providing ventilatory management and decision for extubation. Am J Respir Crit Care Med. 1996;153(3):997-1004.
4. Dojat M, Harf A, Touchard D, et al. Clinical evaluation of a computer-controlled pressure support mode. Am J Respir Crit Care Med. 2000;161(4 Pt 1):1161-6.
5. Ely EW, Baker AM, Dunagan DP, et al. Effect on the duration of mechanical ventilation of identifying patients capable of breathing spontaneously. N Engl J Med. 1996;335:1864-9.
6. Epstein SK, Ciubotaru RL. Independent effects of etiology of failure and time to reintubation on outcome for patients failing extubation. Am J Respir Crit Care Med. 1998;158(2):489-93.
7. Epstein SK, Ciubotaru RL, Wong JB. Effect of failed extubation on the outcome of mechanical ventilation. Chest. 1997;112(1):186-192.
8. Epstein SK, Walkey A. (2017). Methods of weaning from mechanical ventilation. [online] Available from https://www.uptodate.com/contents/methods-of-weaning-from-mechanical-ventilation. [Accessed July, 2018].
9. Esteban A, Alia I, Gordo F, et al. Extubation outcome after spontaneous breathing trials with T-tube or pressure support ventilation. The Spanish Lung Failure Collaborative Group. Am J Respir Crit Care Med. 1997;156(2 Pt 1):459-65.
10. Esteban A, Alia I, Tobin MJ, et al. Effect of spontaneous breathing trial duration on outcome of attempts to discontinue mechanical ventilation. Am J Respir Crit Care Med. 1999;159:512-8.
11. Esteban A, Frutos F, Tobin MJ, et al. A comparison of four methods of weaning patients from mechanical ventilation. Spanish Lung Failure Collaborative Group. N Engl J Med. 1995;332(6):345-50.
12. Esteban A, Frutos-Vivar F, Ferguson ND, et al. Noninvasive positive-pressure ventilation for respiratory failure after extubation. N Engl J Med. 2004;350(24):2452-60.
13. Ferrer M, Esquinas A, Arancibia F, et al. Noninvasive ventilation during persistent weaning failure: a randomized controlled trial. Am J Respir Crit Care Med. 2003;168(1):70.
14. Ferrer M, Sellares J, Valencia M, et al. Noninvasive ventilation after extubation in hypercapnic patients with chronic respiratory disorders: randomised controlled trial. Lancet. 2009;374(9695):1082-8.
15. Girard TD, Kress JP, Fuchs BD, et al. Efficacy and safety of a paired sedation and ventilator weaning protocol for mechanically ventilated patients in intensive care (Awakening and Breathing Controlled trial): a randomised controlled trial. Lancet. 2008;371:126-34.
16. Hyzy RC. Physiologic and pathophysiologic consequences of mechanical ventilation. [online] Available from https://www.uptodate.com/contents/physiologic-and-pathophysiologic-consequences-of-mechanical-ventilation. [Accessed July, 2018].
17. Keenan SP, Powers C, McCormack DG, et al. Noninvasive positive-pressure ventilation for postextubation respiratory distress: a randomized controlled trial. JAMA. 2002;287(24):3238-44.
18. Krishnan JA, Moore D, Robeson C, et al. A prospective, controlled trial of a protocol-based strategy to discontinue mechanical ventilation. Am J Respir Crit Care Med. 2004;169(6):673-8.
19. Lee KH, Hui KP, Chan TB. Rapid shallow breathing (frequency-tidal volume ratio) did not predict extubation outcome. Chest. 1994;105(2):540-3.
20. Nava S, Ambrosino N, Clini E, et al. Noninvasive mechanical ventilation in the weaning of patients with respiratory failure due to chronic obstructive pulmonary disease. A randomized, controlled trial. Ann Intern Med. 1998;128(9):721-8.
21. Nava S, Gregoretti C, Fanfulla F, et al. Noninvasive ventilation to prevent respiratory failure after extubation in high-risk patients. Crit Care Med. 2005;33(11):2465-70.
22. Ramnath VR. Conventional mechanical ventilation in acute lung injury and acute respiratory distress syndrome. Clin Chest Med. 2006;27(4):601-13.
23. Salam A, Tilluckdharry L, Amoateng-Adjepong Y, et al. Neurologic status, cough, secretions and extubation outcomes. Intensive Care Med. 2004;30:1.
24. Santanilla JI. Mechanical ventilation. Emerg Med Clin North Am. 2008;26(3):849-62.
25. Vallverdu I, Calaf N, Subirana M, et al. Clinical characteristics, respiratory functional parameters, and outcome of a two-hour T-piece trial in patients weaning from mechanical ventilation. Am J Respir Crit Care Med. 1998;158(6):1855-62.
26. Yang KL, Tobin MJ. A prospective study of indexes predicting the outcome of trials of weaning from mechanical ventilation. N Engl J Med. 1991;324(21):1445-50.

Section 15

Acute Respiratory Distress Syndrome

CHAPTER 56

Acute Respiratory Distress Syndrome

■ GENERAL CONSIDERATIONS

The acute respiratory distress syndrome (ARDS) is an important condition characterized by noncardiogenic increased permeability, inflammatory pulmonary edema, with diffuse alveolar damage; it leads to hypoxemic respiratory failure necessitating ventilator support and prolonged intensive care.

The first description of what probably was ARDS was given by Osler in his Textbook of Medicine in 1927. He wrote of "uncontrolled septicemia leading to pulmonary edema" and went on to describe the clinical features and autopsy findings very nearly as we know them today. In 1967, Ashbaugh, Bigelow and Petty reported in the *Lancet* the occurrence of noncardiogenic pulmonary edema and acute respiratory failure in a number of diverse pathologies not directly involving the lungs. They termed this condition the adult respiratory distress syndrome. Semantically speaking, this was an unfortunate term. The syndrome can occur at all ages and is not related in its pathogenesis and pathology to the respiratory distress syndrome of the newborn. Also, the connotation of "respiratory distress" is both vague and common to numerous other unrelated pathologies in cardiorespiratory medicine. The syndrome is now termed the acute respiratory distress syndrome (ARDS). Semantic confusion would have been avoided if from the very outset the condition had been termed acute lung injury (ALI). Since 1967, the syndrome has been reported from many countries, including India. The precipitating factors have been recognized and the pathology of the lung has been elucidated. However, the pathogenesis after more than 40 years of research remains unclear and the mortality in spite of expert intensive care, even today is as high as 30–60%.

■ EPIDEMIOLOGY

The incidence of ARDS even in Western countries has not been clearly established. The National Heart, Lung and Blood Institute sponsored ARDS Network of 20 hospitals estimated that the incidence could be as high as 64 cases per 100,000 population. The prevalence in developing countries including India is unknown. ARDS constituted a little over 4% of ICU admissions in our unit over a 5-year period. It is unquestionably a problem that is likely to be encountered with increasing frequency by all physicians who look after critically ill patients.

■ DEFINITION AND CONCEPT

Acute respiratory distress syndrome is characterized by:

- An antecedent history of a precipitating condition.
- Respiratory distress and refractory hypoxemia not responding satisfactorily to supplemental oxygen and invariably necessitating the use of mechanical ventilatory support.
- Radiographic evidence of newly evolving bilateral pulmonary infiltrates, and
- Pulmonary artery occlusion pressure (PAOP) less than 18 mm Hg in the presence of a normal colloid oncotic pressure.

The physiological changes underlying the above clinical definition include a reduced functional residual capacity (FRC), stiff lungs (reduced pulmonary compliance), increased ventilation-perfusion inequalities, an increase in the right to left shunt within the lungs, and an increase in the extravascular water content of the lungs with, as already mentioned, a normal PAOP. *The underlying pathological abnormality is damage to the alveolar capillary membrane with increased capillary permeability, leading to edema, inflammation, and subsequent fibrosis.*

The American-European Consensus Conference in 1994 clinically defined and distinguished between acute lung injury (ALI) and acute respiratory distress syndrome (ARDS), so as to avoid semantic confusion. The American-European consensus definition of ALI and ARDS is given in **Table 1**.

The ARDS definition proposed by the American European Consensus Conference in 1994 was internationally accepted but has now been replaced by the recent Berlin Definition proposed by the ARDS Definition Task Force.

Berlin Definition

Acute respiratory distress syndrome can be diagnosed once cardiogenic pulmonary edema and alternative causes of acute hypoxemic respiratory failure and bilateral pulmonary infiltrates have been excluded. The Berlin definition of ARDS requires that all of the following criteria be present to diagnose ARDS.

- Respiratory symptoms must have begun within 1 week of a known clinical insult, or the patient must have new or worsening symptoms during the past week.

- Bilateral opacities consistent with pulmonary edema must be present on a chest radiograph or CT of the chest. These opacities must not be fully explained by pleural effusion, lobar collapse, lung collapse or pulmonary nodules.

- The patient's respiratory failure must not be fully explained by cardiac failure or fluid overload. An objective assessment (e.g. echocardiography) to exclude hydrostatic pulmonary edema is required if no risk factors of ARDS are present.

- A moderate to severe impairment of oxygenation must be present as defined by the ratio of arterial oxygen tension to fraction of inspired oxygen (PaO_2/FiO_2). The severity of the hypoxemia defines the severity of the ARDS.
  - Mild ARDS: The PaO_2/FiO_2 is > 200 mm Hg but < 300 mm Hg
  - Moderate ARDS: The PaO_2/FiO_2 is > 100 mm Hg but < 200 mm Hg
  - Severe ARDS: The PaO_2/FiO_2 is < 100 mm Hg on ventilator settings that include positive end-expiratory pressure (PEEP) > 5 cm H_2O.

As mentioned earlier the Berlin Definition of ARDS (2012) replaces the American European Consensus Conference Definition (1994). The major changes in the Berlin Definition are:

- The term acute lung injury (ALI) has been eliminated.
- The pulmonary capillary wedge pressure (pulmonary artery occlusion pressure) are no longer considered.
- Minimal ventilator settings have been added.

The PaO_2 is to be measured by a blood gas machine and the FiO_2 as a decimal between 0.1 and 1. If for some reason arterial blood gas estimation is difficult or not possible then the ratio of the oxyhemoglobin saturation to the FiO_2 can be a reasonable substitute. It has been shown in a study that an SpO_2/FiO_2 of 315 predicted a PaO_2/FiO_2 of 300 (the threshold for ARDS) with a sensitivity of 91% and a specificity of 56%.

Though there is a definite advantage in an internationally accepted definition certain limitations and lacunae need to be considered for a balanced perspective of the syndrome.

- *The Berlin definition, like all other previous definitions, does not include any etiology or responsible risk factors. Perhaps this is because there are many (and a growing number of) background risk factors—some common and others uncommon. Also there may be more than one responsible factor in a patient.*

- Though ARDS signifies non-cardiogenic pulmonary edema, patients with a background of left ventricular dysfunction and raised left atrial pressure may fortuitously suffer from a risk factor such as sepsis which could further evolve into ARDS. Both ARDS and cardiogenic pulmonary edema may thus coexist. This is uncommon, but has been observed in our intensive care unit. Again, in the natural history of ARDS due to severe sepsis, cardiac function is often seriously

Table 1: The American-European consensus definition of acute lung injury (ALI) and acute respiratory distress syndrome (ARDS).

Acute lung injury	**Acute respiratory distress syndrome**
Acute onset respiratory failure	Acute onset respiratory failure
Bilateral chest infiltrates on frontal radiographs	Bilateral chest infiltrates on frontal radiographs
$PaO_2/FiO_2 < 300$	$PaO_2/FiO_2 < 200$
Absence of elevated left heart filling pressure (PAOP < 18 mm Hg)	Absence of elevated left heart filling pressure (PAOP < 18 mm Hg)

compromised with a sharply reduced ejection fraction and raised filing pressures. When a patient is seen for the first time at this juncture, diagnosis is difficult.

- Bilateral "chest infiltrates" have been taken as a surrogate marker for the increased permeability inflammatory pulmonary edema that characterizes ARDS. Meade and colleagues have shown that the specificity of a chest radiograph in indicating inflammatory edema is questionable. Similar infiltrates on a chest radiography can occur from other causes. It may be difficult (at least to start with) to distinguish these infiltrates from "infiltrates" due to ARDS.

- An expanded concept of ARDS should include not only the severity, but also the background factor causing or precipitating the syndrome, and most importantly the associated or evolving dysfunction of organ systems. *Most investigators consider ARDS as merely one facet of the multiple organ dysfunction syndrome.*

- The diagnostic accuracy of the different definitions of ARDS has been assessed using as a reference or gold standard, the finding of diffuse alveolar damage at autopsy. The earlier accepted criteria for the diagnosis of ARDS as stated by the American-European Congress Conference showed an acceptable sensitivity (83%) but a poor specificity (51%).

In spite of the present Berlin definition of ARDS, it is possible that some patients (particularly when mild) could be missed. More importantly some patients who do not have ARDS may have pulmonary shadows and hypoxemia from other conditions, the cause of which to start with may not be evident. This could lead to an improper enrollment of patients in trials, which in turn could lead to biased and misleading results.

■ ETIOLOGY

A variety of clinical disorders and risk factors can lead to ALI and ARDS. The incidence of various risk factors in relation to ARDS will depend on the geographical areas and the population that is studied. In India and in other tropical developing countries in addition to the risk factors observed in the West, there are special important risk factors chiefly confined to tropical poor countries.

The various clinical disorders that can lead to ALI or ARDS may do so by directly involving the lung (direct injury), or may involve the lung indirectly (indirect injury). Our experience on ARDS with regard to etiology

and mortality in relation to each etiological factor is summarized in the **Table 2**.

In 187 patients of ARDS studied over several years in our intensive care unit, "direct injury" was the etiological factor in 67 patients; "indirect injury" was the causative factor in 68 patients; and 51 patients developed ARDS due to fulminant infections and problems peculiar to the tropical and developing countries of the world. For convenience, these 51 patients were categorized under ARDS due to tropical problems. The first two groups of patients, for convenience, were categorized under non-tropical problems, i.e. problems more or less common to the whole world. Though the exact incidence of various clinical disorders causing ALI/ARDS in different critical care units in India may vary for several reasons, the nature of risk factors is by and large common to critical care units in the large metropolitan centers of the country.

The most important cause of direct injury perhaps all over the world is acute pulmonary infection (chiefly bacterial or viral pneumonia). Aspiration pneumonia is also an important risk factor, both aspirated gastric acid and enzymes contributing to lung injury. After aspiration, lung injury may take some hours to evolve and manifest. Direct trauma to the chest with contusions within the lung is an important cause, particularly in trauma units. Polytrauma even when not directly involving the chest is an even more important cause and is probably due to inflammatory mediators released from trauma sites acting on the lungs.

Sepsis is unquestionably the most important cause of ALI/ARDS all over the world. In sepsis ALI and ARDS form merely one facet of the multiorgan dysfunction syndrome. The incidence of ALI and ARDS in severe sepsis or septic shock is over 25%. Sepsis not only initiates ALI but also perpetuates it. Even when ARDS is caused by a direct injury or insult to the lung, sepsis may subsequently supervene as a major complication and can worsen lung injury and cause multiple organ dysfunction. When sepsis is the indirect cause of ARDS, the source of sepsis is most frequently intra-abdominal. On the other hand, when sepsis is a supervening complication in a patient suffering from acute lung injury due to any other etiology, the source of sepsis is most frequently within the lung itself.

Acute pancreatitis, burns, poisoning (in particular organophosphorus poisoning) are other important causes of ARDS. There are some other causes of ARDS reported in literature which are not included in **Table 2**.

Table 2: The etiology of acute respiratory distress syndrome (ARDS) as observed in our unit with observed mortality for each etiological factor. Note the difference in mortality between ARDS [and multiple-organ dysfunction syndrome (MODS)] in "tropical problems" and "non-tropical problems".

ARDS	Total	Expired	Mortality
Total number of patients	187	91	49%
Patients with tropical problems	52	14	27%
Patients with non-tropical problems	135	77	57%
Patients with non-tropical problems (n = 135)			
1. Direct injury			
Acute pulmonary infection	33	23	70%
Aspiration pneumonia	18	11	61%
Direct trauma	7	2	29%
Noxious	5	0	0%
Pulmonary vasculitis	4	0	0%
Total	67	36	54%
2. Indirect injury			
Severe sepsis	36	24	67%
Pancreatitis	9	5	56%
Burns	4	3	75%
Extrathoracic injury	4	0	0%
Poisoning	2	0	0%
Miscellaneous	13	8	62%
Total	68	41	60%
Patients with tropical problems			
Tetanus	9	4	44%
OP poisoning	10	1	10%
Cerebral malaria	10	3	30%
Gram negative sepsis			
from contaminated food	5	0	0%
Miliary/disseminated hematogenous tuberculosis	8	3	38%
Amebiasis	5	2	40%
Salmonella infections	3	0	0%
Rabies	1	1	100%
Leptospirosis	1	0	0%
Total	52	14	27%

These include:
- Lung and hemopoietic stem-cell transplantation—primary graft failure following two to three days of lung transplant surgery can lead to ARDS . This has been attributed to poor preservation of the transplanted lung.

Hemopoietic stem cell transplant patients are at risk for ARDS due to a variety of infectious and non-infectious causes. The latter include the idiopathic pneumonia syndrome and the engraftment syndrome.

- Drugs implicated in causing ARDS include aspirin, cocaine, opioids, phenothiazines, nitrofurantoin and a few chemotherapeutic agents.

There are a number of other varying miscellaneous causes being reported with increasing frequency from different parts of the world. Among these, multiple blood transfusions head the list. ARDS following multiple blood transfusion has been reported in both trauma patients as also in nontrauma patients, such as patients transfused following massive GI bleeds. In trauma patients, systemic inflammatory mediators may perhaps play a greater or equal role as multiple blood transfusion in causing ARDS. Current evidence suggests that the risk of lung injury increases with the duration of stored blood.

Transfusion-related acute lung injury (TRALI) resembles ARDS, yet is not the same. This form of injury can be caused by transfusion of even small quantities of whole blood or any blood product. The cause is believed to be due to passively transfused antibodies that act as leukoagglutinins attaching to antigens on the recipient leukocytes, thereby causing lung injury. TRALI manifests with breathlessness during or after transfusion of whole blood or a blood product accompanied by shadows in the mid and lower zones of both lung fields.

Tachycardia and a fall in oxygen saturation are often observed. TRALI is often mistaken for acute left ventricular failure.

Among the miscellaneous causes, the important ones include cardiothoracic surgery, smoke inhalation, acute liver cell failure, eclampsia, poisoning.

■ TROPICAL INFECTIONS AND PROBLEMS

It is pertinent and important to briefly outline tropical problems causing ARDS. These, in our experience, include fulminant *P. falciparum* infections, severe tetanus, severe typhoid infections, fulminant gram-negative infections following ingestion of contaminated food, acute miliary tuberculosis, acute disseminated hematogenous tuberculosis, fulminant amebic infections of the liver and large bowel, fulminant leptospirosis, hemorrhagic fevers, and rabies. Severe organophosphorus poisoning is the most frequently encountered poisoning causing ARDS in western India. In the north, aluminum phosphide (added generally for the preservation of food grains) poisoning is an important cause of severe ARDS which invariably ends fatally. Each of these tropical problems can lead not only to ARDS, but to progressive multiple organ failure and death. The most important of these causes are fulminant *P. falciparum* infections, tetanus, acute miliary tuberculosis, acute hematogenous disseminated tuberculosis, leptospiral infections and fulminant *B. typhosus* infections **(Figs. 1 to 3)**.

The following clinical forms of ARDS have been noted in relation to severe *P. falciparum* malaria:

- Acute pulmonary edema due to hyperpyrexia (temperature > 107°F).

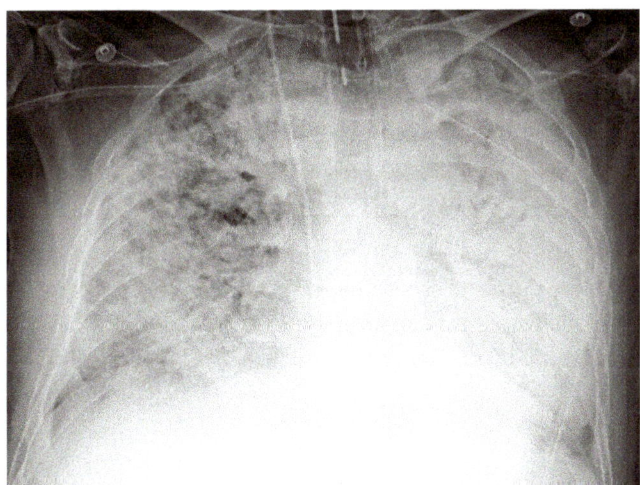

Fig. 1: Acute respiratory distress syndrome (ARDS) in typhoid, note extensive bilateral shadowing.

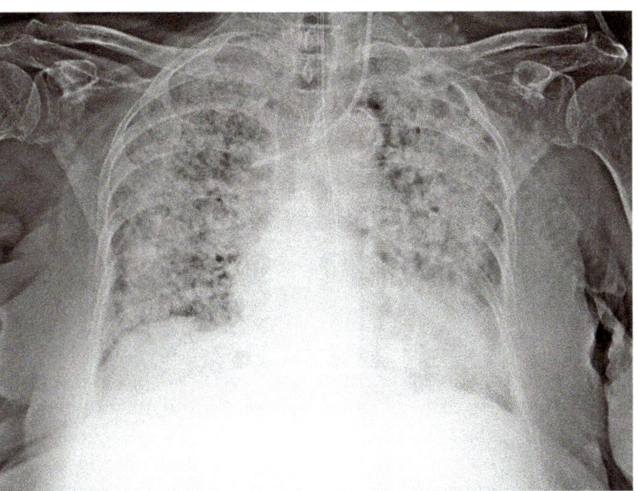

Fig. 2: Acute respiratory distress syndrome (ARDS) in tetanus.

- Progressive bilateral shadowing within the lungs characterized physiologically by marked ventilation-perfusion inequalities, but by only a slight increase in the right to left shunt within the lungs—recovery is possible with good management.
- Progressive bilateral fluffy shadows characterized physiologically by a marked increase in the right to left shunt—prognosis of patients in this category is grim.
- ARDS caused by disseminated intravascular coagulopathy complicating falciparum infection.
- ARDS due to aspiration of gastric contents in obtunded patients.

The time from the original insult (direct or indirect), to the development of full-blown ARDS has been studied in many large series. In Petty's original group it ranged from 1 hour to 96 hours. In a comprehensive, recent epidemiological study, 80% of patients had developed ARDS within 48 hours of the initial insult, and 90% by 80 hours. This latent period offers a window of opportunity for therapeutic interventions, when effective blockers of the inflammatory process can be identified. Indeed, today there is a massive search for circulating markers of ARDS which can be identified in the serum or bronchoalveolar lavage (BAL) fluid.

■ PATHOLOGY

The work of Gattinoni and his colleagues on computed tomography (CT) scans in ARDS has brought forth important new concepts. The first of these concepts is that the lung in ARDS is not homogeneously affected.

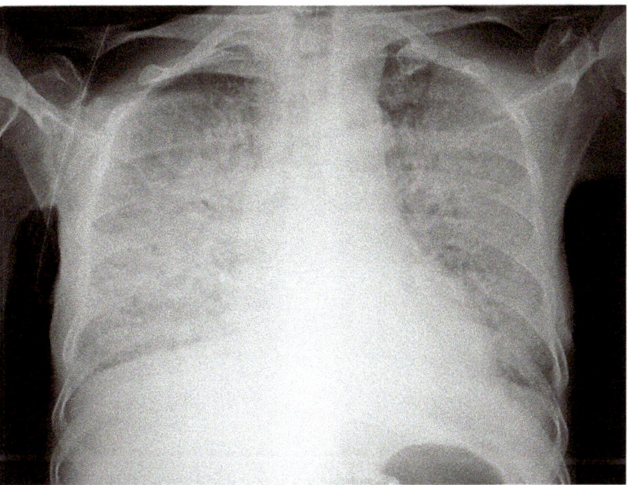

Fig. 3: Acute respiratory distress syndrome (ARDS) in malaria, showing extensive bilateral fluffy shadows.

The most affected part of the lung is the most dependent portion. This dependent area is consolidated and represents "core" disease, generally constituting about 24% of lung weight. The part or zone above this dependent portion is "collapsed lung", the collapse being due to the weight of inflammatory edema which is the hallmark of ARDS; still above the zone of inflammatory edema is the zone of normally aerated, or even overventilated lung **(Figs. 4 and 5)**. The extent of the zone constituting collapsed lung varies. Of importance is the fact that this collapsed lung is capable of being opened up, that is to say it is recruitable by ventilatory measures (raising inspiratory pressure from + 5 to 45 cm H_2O). The greater the recruitability, the greater the inflammatory edema, the more severe the disease and worse the prognosis. The lesser the recruitability, the lesser the inflammatory edema; the disease is then milder and the prognosis better.

The above views put forth by Gattinoni not only allow a better conceptualization of ARDS, but also better prognostication, and perhaps most importantly may further guide ventilatory strategies in the management of this syndrome.

The basic pathological feature is damage to the alveolar capillary membrane leading to an increased permeability, inflammatory interstitial and alveolar edema, alveolar atelectasis, consolidation, and diffuse alveolar damage. Three overlapping phases are observed:

1. Exudative phase in which there is an alveolar exudate with hyaline membrane formation along the alveolar ducts and within the alveoli.
2. Proliferative phase in which there is a proliferation of inflammatory cells, lymphocytes, and Type 2 pneumocytes. Organization of the inflammatory exudate, combined with damage to the surfactant leads to obliteration of air spaces, atelectatic alveoli and a poorly compliant lung.
3. Fibrotic phase which follows soon upon the proliferative phase, and is characterized by fibroblasts laying down fibrous tissue that strangles alveoli, and further reduces pulmonary compliance.

Severe lung injury distorts the pulmonary vasculature. Distortion with remodeling of the vasculature is due to fibrous tissue formation, thromboembolism, and increased muscularization with thickening and intimal fibrosis of the larger arteries. Thrombi may be present in the microcirculation and in the larger vessels. They may form *in situ*, or may have an embolic source. The end-result is an obstructed, distorted pulmonary circulation with increased pulmonary vascular resistance, causing pulmonary hypertension.

■ PATHOGENESIS

The pathogenesis of ARDS continues to remain unclear. Even so, current research allows a better comprehension of what transpires in this syndrome at a cellular and molecular level. Research into molecular genetics has

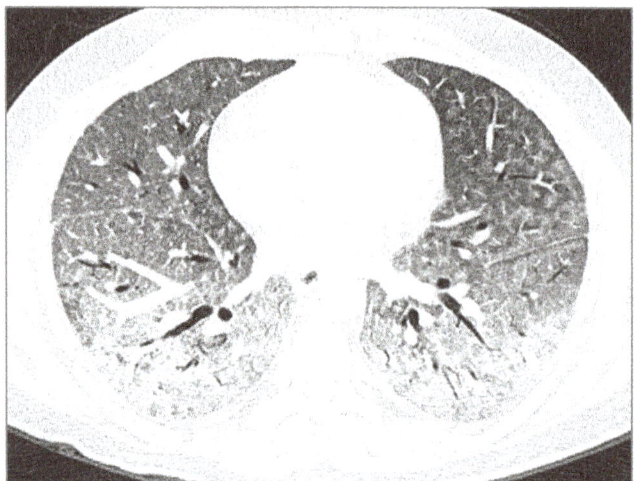

Fig. 4: High-resolution computed tomography (HRCT) of the chest in acute respiratory distress syndrome (ARDS). The most dependent part of the lung is dense and consolidated; above this is inflammatory edema; right at the top is normally aerated lung.

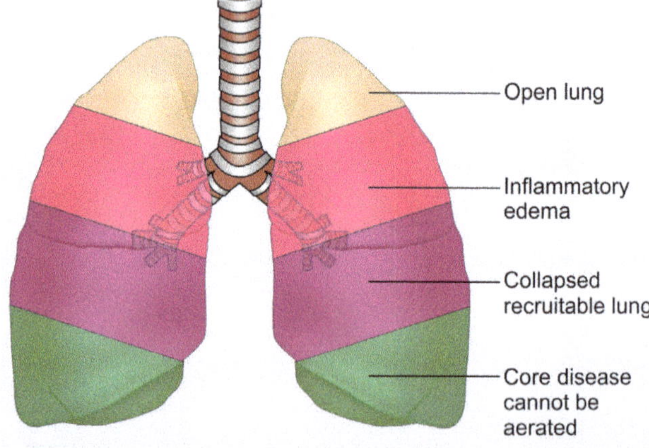

Fig. 5: A schematic representation of "zones" within the lungs in acute respiratory distress syndrome (ARDS). The most dependent zone is consolidated lung which cannot be aerated; above this is collapsed but recruitable lung; still above is the zone of inflammatory edema, the weight of which is responsible for the zone of collapsed recruitable lung; right at the top is normally ventilated or even hyperventilated lung.

revealed a complex network of interacting factors at the cellular level. It is clear that the cascade of mediators is far more complex than we thought, and many of yesterday's putative mediators are in reality modulators and regulators that fine-tune the inflammatory cascade, rather than cause it. **Flowchart 1** illustrates the basic steps in the pathogenesis of ARDS.

Role of Cytokines, Neutrophils and the Coagulation System

Cytokines, which are cell-derived peptide compounds, are the main mediators. Recombinant cDNA technology has permitted identification of the existence, structure, and function of several cytokines. The cytokine on which most attention is currently focused is the tumor necrosis factor (TNF). This cytokine has a molecular weight of 17 kD and is released from macrophages in response to gram-negative bacterial endotoxin. TNF is one of the main mediators of the septic state. After injection of endotoxin into animals or humans, TNF can be detected in the serum, the levels peaking at 2 hours. When TNF is infused into the sheep model, ARDS is produced. Three other cytokines of importance mediating inflammatory response include neutrophil activating peptide (NAP),

interleukin (IL)-6, IL-8 and macrophage inflammatory proteins (MIP 1 and 2). The neutrophil plays a vital role in the inflammatory response, and TNF is the chief mediator that promotes adherence of the neutrophils to the vascular endothelium and together with interleukin-8 causes and enhances neutrophil activation. The primed neutrophils degranulate, releasing proteases, reactive oxygen species, leukotrienes, all harmful to lung structure and function. The lipid mediators and platelet-activating factors also enhance inflammation.

The activation of the coagulation and complement systems promotes coagulation and decreases fibrinolysis. Endothelial damage results in pulmonary edema with a disturbance in pulmonary microcirculation. The end result is increasing respiratory failure with an increasing poverty of gas exchange, often leading to death. As mentioned earlier, *changes in the lung often form just one facet of similar changes in other organs of the body.*

There is a complex, poorly understood interaction at the molecular and cellular level as the syndrome continues to evolve. This interaction and inter-relation will continue to be the subject of future research.

Unfortunately, there is no definite biomarker which can reliably identify patients at risk, or assess the prognosis in ARDS. IL-6 and IL-8 can be found in alveolar fluid

Flowchart 1: Pathogenesis of acute respiratory distress syndrome (ARDS) due to sepsis.

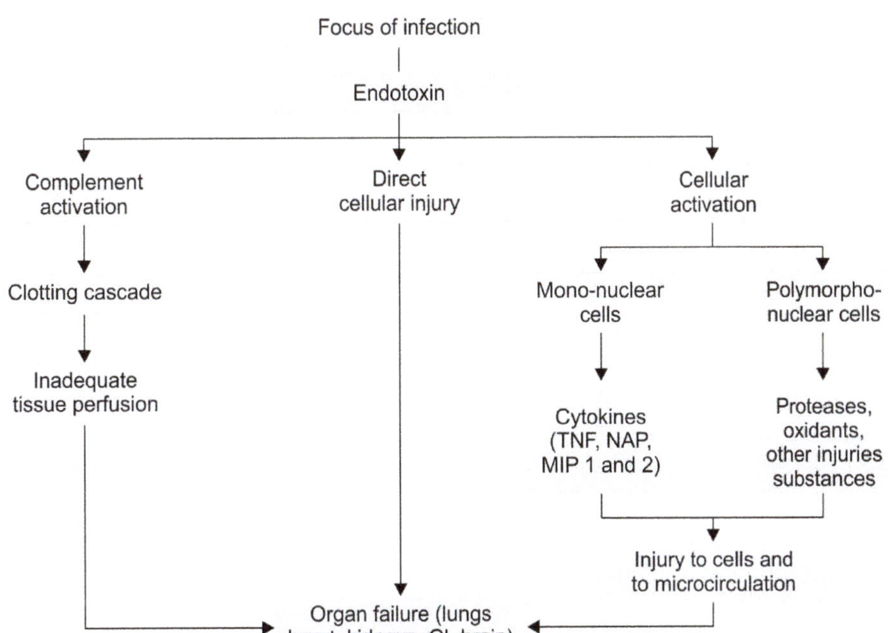

(TNF: Tumor necrosis factor; GI: Gastrointestinal)

and in plasma but these are nonspecific markers of lung inflammation. The ARDS network trial showed that high levels of IL-6 and IL-8 were associated with increased morbidity and mortality and that the strategy of using low tidal volumes attenuated the inflammatory response of the disease, suggesting that alveolar stretch is linked to and perhaps worsens the inflammatory response.

Alterations in Cardiopulmonary Physiology

The pulmonary edema, atelectasis, proliferation of inflammatory cells and increasing fibrosis occurring as a result of "injury", produce a fall in the total lung capacity (TLC) and FRC by 50%. The low lung recoil pressure at FRC leads to early closure of the small airways, with further alveolar collapse, necessitating high inflation pressures to expand or reinflate the lungs. The physiological consequences are an increase in the right to left shunt within the lungs due to perfusion of atelectatic alveoli, increased ventilation-perfusion inequalities, increase in dead space, and increasingly non-compliant or stiff lungs. "Injury" as stressed earlier, may be mild, moderate or severe. Of equal importance is the fact that even in severe injury, the lungs are not evenly or homogenously affected. Computerized tomography, as mentioned earlier, has demonstrated a three-zone model of the lung—the most dependent consolidated area representing core disease, above which is an atelectatic area caused by the weight of inflammatory edema. This zone is recruitable lung, i.e. can be opened up by ventilatory measures; finally there is the least dependent zone of normal or even overinflated alveoli.

Severe lung injury is sooner or later associated with increasing pulmonary hypertension. The latter is due to hypoxia and an obstructed, distorted pulmonary circulation. The resultant increase in right ventricular afterload can not only lead to right heart failure, but also cause a shift of the septum to the left. The septal shift can significantly reduce left ventricular filling and stroke volume.

Myocardial dysfunction is an important feature of ARDS. It is contributed to by a circulating myocardial depressant factor (probably the same as TNF) in patients with sepsis. A significant fall in cardiac output is frequently observed in these patients, particularly when the mean pulmonary artery pressure exceeds 35 mm Hg. A fall in cardiac output, particularly when combined with a low oxygen tension in arterial blood, can cause a significant reduction in oxygen transport to the tissues. A decreased oxygen transport in

association with a possible abnormality of oxygen uptake by the tissues, so frequently observed in ARDS, invariably spells disaster.

CLINICAL FEATURES

Against a background of one of the etiologies mentioned earlier, the patient with ARDS presents with rapidly worsening dyspnea and restlessness. On examination, such a patient has tachycardia, tachypnea, and increasing hypoxemia despite supplemental oxygen. Auscultation reveals scattered crackles and occasionally a wheeze. The condition may evolve rapidly over a few hours, or may take a few days to reach its maximum intensity. Respiratory distress is obvious, and the accessory muscles of respiration are active. Cyanosis may occur, but is not always evident in spite of severe hypoxemia.

In the early stages, a slight but disproportionate tachypnea may be the only warning sign of early ARDS, and in an appropriate setting this must never be ignored, even in the absence of auscultatory crackles, and with a normal chest X-ray. An important warning diagnostic feature in the early phase is a slight fall in the PaO_2 and an increased alveolar-arterial oxygen gradient.

As the respiratory failure worsens, one or more other organ systems may show signs of dysfunction and failure. This is in keeping with the current concept that ARDS is a multisystem disease, with the changes in the pulmonary endothelium mirroring widespread endothelial damage in other organs.

Patients who survive the initial course and have not succumbed to complications show improvement in their oxygenation and a clearing of the alveolar opacities. Some patients however continue to experience severe hypoxemia and need ventilator support for weeks. The fibroproliferative phase of ARDS is characterized by a reticular pattern with fibrosis best seen on a CT of the chest. Persistent hypoxemia, a low lung compliance and ventilator dependence are features of this phase. Complications often ensue. If the patients survive this phase, there now follows a phase of resolution and repair. Cardiopulmonary function starts to improve but may take 6 months or more to do so after the initial lung injury. Patients who have survived very severe ARDS may show some degree of impaired lung function, cognitive impairment and muscle weakness.

■ DIFFERENTIAL DIAGNOSIS

The lack of specificity in the radiological picture and in the diagnostic features proposed by the American-European Congress Conference has already been commented upon. The differential diagnosis includes:

- Other causes of air space consolidation—multiple pulmonary infarcts, multiple areas of atelectasis (as after major upper abdominal or cardiothoracic surgery), pneumonia, atypical pneumonia, Legionnaire's disease, alveolar hemorrhage, alveolar proteinosis, acute eosinophilic pneumonia and bronchiolitis obliterans organizing pneumonia (BOOP). Acute fibrinous organizing pneumonia is a rare alveolar filling disease either idiopathic or following organ transplantation. It can only be distinguished pathologically from ARDS by a lung biopsy.
- Acute exacerbation of previously unrecognized interstitial lung disease, or acute interstitial pneumonia, (Hamman-Rich syndrome). The Hamman-Rich syndrome may be impossible to distinguish from ARDS. Both show severe alveolar damage on histopathology. The only difference is that ARDS generally has a precipitating risk factor, while the Hamman-Rich syndrome has none.
- *Cardiogenic pulmonary edema*: Cardiac enlargement, the presence of more centralized edema, Kerley's lines, help in radiological differentiation. Clinical history and examination of the cardiovascular system are of critical importance. A significantly raised brain natriuretic peptide (BNP) and an echocardiography showing poor diastolic compliance of the left ventricle and/or poor left ventricular systolic function point to cardiogenic edema. As has been already mentioned patients with left heart disease and failure who develop sepsis from any cause could possibly have cardiogenic edema plus the inflammatory edema of ARDS.

In difficult problems, a Swan-Ganz catheter may be used to determine PAOP. It is to be noted that in intra-abdominal pathologies, the rise in intra-abdominal pressure may cause a rise in the PAOP and mislead the clinician.

Other pathologies that may need to be considered depending on the clinical background and other features include pulmonary vasculitis (SLE, Granulomatosis with polyangiitis (GPA), formerly known as Wegener's granulomatosis, Eosinophilic granulomatosis with polyangiitis (EGPA), formerly called Churg-Strauss syndrome (CSS), Goodpasture's syndrome and disseminated malignancy.

■ COMPLICATIONS

Death is uncommon from severe refractory hypoxia, provided the patient receives good ventilator support. In our unit it occurs in not more than 10% of patients.

Nosocomial Pneumonia

This is an extremely important complication. The incidence of this complication in severe acute lung injury (ARDS) varies in different units, and in our ICU is about 15%. The incidence increases with the length of time on ventilator support, and in our experience, is most marked when ARDS is due to severe abdominal sepsis. It is less than 10% when ARDS is caused by a direct insult, e.g. inhalation of noxious fumes, near-drowning, chest trauma, even when ventilator support is prolonged for weeks.

The lung injury per se, together with improper ventilatory management (such as use of high inflation pressures, high tidal volumes, high FiO_2), and the prolonged use of PEEP, also probably impair local immune and other defense mechanisms within the lung, and predispose to iatrogenic infection and sepsis. Background illnesses which impair immune function, and malnutrition, either present before ARDS, or occurring during the evolution of the syndrome, are other important predisposing factors. Colonization of the upper respiratory tract and of the gastrointestinal tract by gram-negative organisms remains an important source of infection.

The diagnosis of nosocomial pneumonia is difficult in the presence of shadows caused by atelectasis and edema. We have missed a good-sized lung abscess causing an empyema in a patient with ARDS due to severe tetanus, the diagnosis being apparent only at autopsy. Suspicion of a nosocomial infection should prompt a CT of the chest which may reveal an abscess or an empyema undetected on an X-ray. The choice of antibiotics in the management of nosocomial pneumonia is empiric, and will depend on the nature of bacteria causing nosocomial pneumonia and their sensitivity to antibiotics in a critical care unit.

Nosocomial blood stream infection chiefly through central venous catheters can also occur and worsen the situation.

Multiple Organ Dysfunction

The better and more intensive the care offered to the patient, and hence the longer he is kept alive, the more often is the complication of multiple organ dysfunction observed. It occurs early and most frequently when sepsis is the cause of ARDS. It can however complicate the course of ARDS from any cause.

In our experience, renal dysfunction occurs in 30–40% of patients, cardiovascular dysfunction necessitating inotropic support in 50–70% of patients, and liver cell dysfunction occurs in about 50% of patients. Complications and dysfunction involving the gastrointestinal tract are observed in 20–30% of patients. There is an obvious inter-relation between various organ systems, so that impairment of one organ system induces, amplifies and modulates impairment in other organ systems.

Translocation of bacteria from the lumen of the gut to the lymphatics, peritoneal cavity and even the bloodstream, plays an important role in perpetuating the inflammatory cascade that underlies multiple organ dysfunction. This is observed when the protective barrier normally provided by the wall of the gut is breached. The problem is markedly worsened in the presence of associated liver cell dysfunction. In fact when ARDS occurs against the background of liver cell failure, death invariably results.

GI bleeds from stress ulcers, deep vein thrombosis and pulmonary embolism can also complicate the problem.

Barotrauma

Complications related to ventilator support include pneumothorax, mediastinal emphysema, surgical emphysema of the soft tissues of the neck, and at times of the upper body. Tension pneumothorax is a disastrous complication. A pneumothorax requires prompt chest tube drainage.

Critical illness, polyneuropathy and myopathy are frequent in patients with ARDS receiving prolonged ventilator support.

■ INVESTIGATIONS

Chest X-ray (*see* Figs. 1 to 3)

The chest radiograph shows interstitial edema in the early stages, and full-blown pulmonary edema in established cases. The pulmonary edema causes bilaterally symmetrical shadowing, but the shadowing may initially be predominantly unilateral, depending on the position of the patient. The absence of cardiomegaly, of Kerley's lines

and of vascular redistribution toward the upper lobes, help distinguish the pattern from cardiogenic pulmonary edema. The absence of lobar consolidation helps differentiate it from infection. Having said this, cardiac failure, pneumonia, and pulmonary emboli may all cause diagnostic confusion. ARDS does not necessarily involve both lungs symmetrically; one lung may be considerably more involved than the other. This adds to the problem of effective ventilation. A CT chest can detect well marked pulmonary edema better than a chest X-ray. In advanced late stage ARDS, CT chest shows increasing evidence of pulmonary fibrosis.

Arterial Blood Gases

Blood gas estimation is essential in the initial diagnosis and subsequent monitoring of ARDS. In the initial stages, varying degrees of hypoxia are seen with hypocapnia. In late stages, hypercapnia may be seen. The pH disturbances range from respiratory alkalosis in the initial stages, to respiratory acidosis and metabolic acidosis in the later stages. The hypoxia is refractory to supplemental oxygen, indicating that in addition to ventilation-perfusion mismatch, increased right to left shunt and dead space ventilation also play major roles

Pulmonary Compliance

Lung compliance is usually decreased to less than 30 mL/cm H_2O. Compliance can easily be measured in patients on mechanical ventilator support.

Routine Tests

Tests for evidence of other organ dysfunction, e.g. renal, hepatic, hematological parameters, should be done.

Full Bacteriological Screen

This should include blood culture, cultures of tracheal aspirates, and in some patients with nosocomial pneumonia, culture of BAL fluid or culture of protected brush samples obtained bronchoscopically, to determine the nature of the infecting organism. Cultures of urine and other body secretions and discharges are often necessary **(Table 3)**.

Further diagnostic tests or procedures may be necessary to exclude one or more pathologies that may mimic ARDS. These include relevant blood studies, bronchoscopy,

Table 3: Investigations in acute respiratory distress syndrome (ARDS).

- Chest X-ray; CT chest if deemed necessary
- Arterial pH and blood gases
- Hemodynamic measurements using a Swan-Ganz catheter in selected cases
- Pulmonary compliance
- Routine biochemistry to evaluate other organ dysfunction
- Full bacteriological screen:
    - Blood culture
    - Urine culture
    - Culture of tracheal aspirates
    - Culture of BAL
    - Culture of any other secretions/discharges
- Other relevant tests or procedures to exclude a suspected differential diagnosis

(BAL: Bronchoalveolar lavage; CT: Computed tomography)

BAL study and when very rarely indicated, a lung biopsy.

Bronchoscopy and BAL studies are indicated in specific conditions:

- When there is a suspicion of bilateral pneumonia. Bilateral pneumonia is an important cause of ARDS, as also a mimic of ARDS.
- Select pathologies, e.g. alveolar hemorrhage, acute eosinophilic pneumonia, granulomatosis with polyangiitis , disseminated lung malignancy.
- To identify culprit organisms not found on a sputum study or a study of an endotracheal aspirate.

Bronchoscopy should only be undertaken after weighing the procedural risk in a ventilated hypoxemic individual against the diagnostic sensitivity of the condition suspected. The diagnostic sensitivity is good in alveolar hemorrhage, acute eosinophilic pneumonia, acute infections (before administration of antibiotics). It is poor in interstitial lung disease and vasculitis.

■ MORTALITY AND PROGNOSIS

Some studies suggest a fall in mortality figures in ARDS compared to earlier years. But mortality depends on the population under study. Even in the ARDS network study of 861 patients, the mortality of 31% in the group using lung protection measures (6 mL/kg TV) is significantly underestimated, because severely ill patients were excluded—those with advanced liver disease, bone marrow transplant, severe chronic respiratory disease, burns more than 30% BSA and those not expected to live more than 6 months.

Mortality remains quite high in population-based studies. Several multicenter studies in France, Sweden, Australia, Argentina defined mortality and prognostic variables in observational population-based studies rather than clinical trial participants. Mortality varied—32% in mild ARDS to 58–60% in severe ARDS. The highest mortality, close to 60%, was seen in the French study.

In other studies, mortality was highest in sepsis (43%), intermediate in pneumonia (36%) or aspiration (37%), and lowest in multiple trauma (11%). Low tidal volumes were effective in reducing mortality across all cases of ARDS.

Four factors determine prognosis in ARDS:

1. Severity of the lung injury (judged by PaO_2/FiO_2 ratio).
2. Nature and severity of the precipitating factor.
3. Presence and degree of dysfunction of other organ systems.
4. Background or associated disease.

In our experience, prognosis depends less on the severity of ARDS and more on the other three factors listed above. Uncontrollable sepsis, particularly uncontrollable intra-abdominal sepsis, has a hopeless prognosis with 100% mortality. Severe sepsis even when controlled can set into motion a chain of events that may carry a mortality of more than 60%. Prognosis is worse in the presence of septic shock. On the other hand, direct injury to the lungs as in drowning, inhalation of noxious fumes, mild to moderate aspiration of gastric contents has a mortality of less than 20%, provided there is no nosocomial infection and no other major complication. Severe nosocomial pneumonia occurring in ARDS has a mortality of about 30%.

In the West, the reported mortality for single organ failure is 15–30%, for two-organ failure it is 45–55%, and for three or more organ failure lasting for more than 4 days, more than 85%. In our experience we have found this true only for gram-negative sepsis. These figures are unnecessarily pessimistic and are not true when multiple organ failure complicates fulminant *P. falciparum* infection, fulminant tetanus and other severe tropical infections. Fulminant tetanus with excellent intensive care has a mortality of less than 10%, and in fulminant *P. falciparum* infection the mortality even with severe prolonged multiple organ dysfunction is below 30%.

■ MANAGEMENT

Despite the many recent advances in intensive care, severe ARDS continues to carry an overall mortality of 30–60%. As mentioned earlier, patients with ARDS do not usually die of respiratory failure (only 16% of all deaths in one large series were due to refractory hypoxemia and hypercapnia). The majority of patients die of sepsis and multiple organ failure. Intensive care is mandatory for efficient management. The important management principles are discussed here.

Treatment of the Underlying Condition

This should be identified promptly and treated aggressively. Unfortunately, the treatment of many diseases causing ARDS is largely supportive. Sepsis is an important exception and should be promptly recognized and treated. *Studies have shown that the prompt use of an appropriate antibiotic or antibiotics significantly improves morbidity and mortality.* Surgical drainage of an abscess and prompt surgery for abdominal sepsis are mandatory. Specific therapy for fulminant tropical problems causing ARDS should be immediate—in particular the use of artemisinin for severe *P. falciparum* infections.

Respiratory Support

This forms the cornerstone in the management of ARDS. Yet it needs to be stressed that mechanical ventilation is purely supportive, allowing the lungs time to recover from the acute insult. Mechanical ventilation in patients with severe acute lung injury (ARDS) presents complex problems and difficulties. To be effective, the intensivist must be aware of the changes in cardiorespiratory physiopathology, the interaction between the heart and the lungs, the importance not only of effective gas exchange but of efficient oxygen transport and the dangers and complications of ventilator support.

Initiating Ventilator Support

There are two important indications for initiating ventilator support in an evolving ARDS. The first is progressive hypoxemia not responding to oxygen inhalation; the second is a marked, unsustainable increase in the work of breathing, as when the respiratory rate is more than 35–40/minute and the minute volume exceeds 12 L/minute. Lowered lung compliance adds even more to the work of breathing. Under the above circumstances, it is best to electively intubate and initiate ventilatory support even if the PaO_2 is greater than 60 mm Hg on supplemental oxygen. Elective intubation and ventilatory support is also preferred in the presence of hemodynamic instability and

if for any reason the patient is unable to maintain and protect the airway.

Noninvasive Ventilator Support

Severe ARDS always needs intubation and mechanical ventilation. A small subset of patients with mild ARDS may however be adequately oxygenated with the help of continuous positive airway pressure (CPAP) or by the use of a BiPAP ventilator, using a tight-fitting face mask. A multicenter observational study has reported the merits of NIV in early ARDS from three ICUs in Italy and Spain. One-third of the patients were given NIV (the remaining two-thirds were already intubated and ventilated). The NIV patients had less ventilator-associated pneumonias and a lower mortality. This was not a RCT and though the study showed that NIV was effective in early cases, no definite conclusions are possible.

If NIV is decided upon, CPAP levels are kept between 10 cm of H_2O and 12 cm of H_2O. In order to maintain intrathoracic pressure at the required level of CPAP throughout the respiratory cycle, high gas flows in excess of 70 L/min are required. With a BiPAP machine, reasonable initial ventilator settings are EPAP of 7–10 cm H_2O and IPAP of around 15–18 cm, the settings being adjusted both for patient comfort and for providing and maintaining an SaO_2 of greater than 90%. Noninvasive mechanical ventilation in patients with mild ARDS recruits collapsed alveoli, increases the FRC and lung compliance, thereby unloading the respiratory muscles and reducing the work of breathing. A good response to noninvasive positive pressure ventilation is generally observed within 30 minutes of its initiation and is characterized by improved oxygen saturation, a fall in respiratory rate and less patient distress. An inability to maintain SaO_2 to more than 90% or the presence of hemodynamic instability, or a worsening clinical state are indications for intubation and mechanical ventilation.

Dangers of Endotracheal Intubation in ARDS

The major danger during intubation is a severe increase in hypoxia, in an individual who is already hypoxic to start with. Hemodynamic instability and the danger of gastric aspiration form additional risks during intubation.

Endotracheal intubation should therefore be performed by an expert, preferably with the patient awake, using mild sedation with a benzodiazepine or a narcotic.

In an acute crisis, succinylcholine along with intravenous (IV) propofol may be used.

Changing of the endotracheal tube in a patient with ARDS following rupture of the cuff, or due to obstruction of the tube is also risky. A sudden loss of PEEP during this procedure may cause rapid desaturation with dangerous sequelae.

Principles of Mechanical Ventilation

The last several years have seen the evolution of two *fundamental concepts in the ventilatory support of patients with ARDS. First is the prevention of overdistension of the alveoli by limiting tidal volume and the pause pressure. Second is to choose a level of PEEP which is sufficiently high to prevent derecruitment of the alveoli at end expiration. The fundamental concepts that guide ventilator support in ARDS are these two lung-protection goals.* Avoidance of oxygen toxicity to the lungs and prevention of hemodynamic instability of the cardiovascular system are two other important conditions guiding ventilator support in these patients.

Limiting Tidal Volume

The lung protection strategies have been firmly established following the result of the landmark ARDS Clinical Trials Network (ARDS net). In this large prospective RCT, patients were randomly assigned to receive a tidal volume (V_T) of 6 mL/kg of predicted body weight or 12 mL/kg of predicted body weight. The plateau pressure (the airway pressure under no flow conditions maintaining the tidal volume) was not to exceed 30 cm H_2O. If it did so, the tidal volume was further reduced to 5 mL/kg of predicted body weight or even to a minimum of 4 mL/kg of predicted body weight. Patients receiving lower tidal volume had a lower mortality (31%) compared to those receiving higher tidal volume (mortality 40%). There was relative reduction in mortality of 22%.

Protocol for ventilatory support in ARDS:

- Initial tidal volume at 8 mL/kg of predicted body weight (PBW) and initial respiratory rate set to meet patient's ventilatory requirement.
- Over the next 1–3 hours reduce tidal volume to 7 mL/PBW and then to 6 mL/PBW. Plateau pressure less than 30 cm H_2O.
- Increase respiratory rate as tidal volume is decreased to a maximum of 35 breaths/minutes so as to deliver patient's minute ventilation.

- Permissive hypercapnia is expected and acceptable
- Adjust FiO_2 and PEEP to maintain a reasonable oxygenation goal—a PaO_2 of 60–80 mm Hg and O_2 saturation of 90–95%. Do not exceed PEEP more than 15–16 cm H_2O. At times severe ARDS may necessitate the use of FiO_2 close to 100% to counter severe hypoxia. An attempt must be made over time (which may vary) to reduce the FiO_2 to not more than 50 to 60% so as to keep a PaO_2 close to 60 mm Hg and an oxygen saturation close to 90%. High FiO_2 (>60%) can induce lung damage.
- If in spite of the above measures, refractory hypoxemia occurs, adjust I:E to 1:2 or at most 1:1.

The ventilatory strategy of using low tidal volumes and limiting plateau pressure to 30 cm H_2O using a volume regulated mode prevents overdistension of alveoli and undue increase in intra-alveolar pressure. In fact large tidal volumes (10–15 mL/kg) in patients with ARDS are dangerous. It is accepted that overdistension of alveoli in these patients can cause an amplification of the already existing lung injury (volutrauma), presumably by increasing edema and pulmonary cytokine production. In addition to "volutrauma", high intra-alveolar and inspiratory pressures can lead to an increased incidence of barotraumas. The concept of barotrauma is not new, but its spectrum includes not just pneumothorax, but also pneumomediastinum, interstitial emphysema, subcutaneous emphysema, and pulmonary hemorrhage. A frequent consequence of a limitation of the tidal volume in the above manner is a rise in the $PaCO_2$ to above 40 mm Hg. The $PaCO_2$ is allowed to rise—a condition called permissive hypercapnia.

This difference in mortality between the low tidal volume group and the high tidal volume group in the ARDS network trial was related to a greater reduction in IL-6 levels in patients with low tidal volumes. Ranieri and coworkers have also shown lower levels of TNF, IL-1, IL-6, and IL-8 in the BAL fluid of patients treated with the "lung protective" ventilatory strategies, when compared to patients treated with the more conventional ventilatory techniques. These cytokines can produce further lung injury; they also gain entry into the bloodstream and produce "injury" at distant sites, perhaps contributing to multiple organ dysfunction and multiple organ failure.

Use of PEEP

Positive end-expiratory pressure is not a new ventilatory strategy but a mainstay of oxygenation in ARDS ever since the original description of the syndrome. It acts by recruiting collapsed alveoli, restoring FRC to normal, thus increasing compliance. It also causes redistribution of lung water within the alveolar space, improving V/Q mismatch, and decreasing the shunt and venous admixture. By improving oxygenation, PEEP allows the oxygen concentration delivered to the patient to be reduced, thus decreasing the chances of oxygen toxicity, which in itself can worsen lung injury.

Of interest, is the likelihood that PEEP, if properly adjusted, also prevents further lung injury during mechanical ventilation of patients with ARDS. How does it do so? The concertina effect of opening of the alveoli during the inspiratory phase of mechanical ventilation, followed by well-nigh total closure of alveoli during the expiratory derecruitment, generates strong shear forces that worsen and perpetuate lung injury. Choosing the exact level of PEEP that can prevent the derecruitment of alveoli during mechanical ventilation is a difficult but an important "lung protection" goal in patients with ARDS. In the ARDS network trial, the level of PEEP and FiO_2 were adjusted with a predetermined PaO_2/FiO_2 ratio in a stepwise fashion, so as to keep the PaO_2 and SaO_2 at a satisfactory desired range. Ideally, PEEP should be individualized for each patient. One can attempt to do so by plotting the pressure volume curve in a given patient, noting the upper and lower inflection points, and adjusting the PEEP level at 1–2 cm above the lower inflection point. There is however often an observer difference in determining the exact lower inflection point (which is a slope rather than a point). Again the pressure volume curve relates to the whole of the lung but does not reflect regional differences (some alveoli are overdistended, others collapsed or consolidated). It is obvious that PEEP is more likely to be useful in patients with ARDS where a good proportion of the affected lungs are "recruitable". On the other hand if in a patient the "recruitable lung" is very small, PEEP will be of little use. In fact it may be harmful as it may only serve to overdistend alveoli, thus contributing to lung injury. Gattinoni determined the degree of recruitability of lungs through CT studies, a luxury denied to most ICUs in the developing world. Perhaps the simplest approach is to use the least PEEP that provides adequate oxygenation at an FiO_2 of less than 0.6, starting with a PEEP of 10 cm and not exceeding 15 cm, as the risk of barotrauma, particularly in Indian patients is then significant. If oxygenation does not improve as judged by the PaO_2/FiO_2 ratio, and if there is no increase in compliance, PEEP should be reduced and not allowed to exceed 5 cm H_2O.

Three large randomized control trials (ARDS network trial, LOVS study, Express study) have compared the effects of higher PEEP to lower PEEP levels. All demonstrated increased oxygenation in the higher PEEP group, but there was neither a decrease in mortality nor in ventilator-free days. This suggests that the use of modest PEEP levels is to be generally preferred and is adequate to prevent ventilator-induced lung injury. High PEEP may perhaps open more atelectatic alveoli but overdistend normal alveoli, contributing further to lung injury.

Ventilator Modes

There are a large number of modes offered by currently available ventilators. These include pressure control ventilation, airway pressure release ventilation, high-frequency oscillatory ventilation, and open-lung ventilation. Whichever mode one uses, the focus should be on preventing alveolar overdistention, countering alveolar derecruitment, minimizing cardiovascular instability and avoiding oxygen toxicity. The volume-controlled mode (with lung protection strategies) was used in the ARDS network trial and remains the one most commonly adopted. There is no evidence to suggest that any of the other ventilatory modes are superior to the volume-controlled mode in the management of ARDS. Many units use pressure-controlled mode; it is important when using this mode to ensure low tidal volumes (6 mL/kg body weight) and not to exceed a peak pressure of 30 cm H_2O. Inverse ratio respiration has been used generally with pressure-controlled ventilatory support. The inspiration-expiration ratio should be preferably 1:2 or 1:1 and not lower. The increased inspiratory time may allow better oxygenation in these patients.

High frequency oscillating ventilation (HFOV) theoretically should offer lung protection as the tidal volumes delivered are very small (less than the dead space) and at a high frequency, gas exchange being promoted by diffusion. Its efficacy as a ventilatory mode in children is generally accepted. It remains to be established whether it reduces morbidity and mortality in ARDS when compared to the lung protection strategies adopted with the volume-controlled mode.

Use of Prone Posture

It was not until an original report by Piehl and Brown in 1976, that the benefits of a switch from the supine to the prone position were appreciated. The improvement in oxygenation may be dramatic, occurring soon after the patients are made prone. In their initial series, five patients of Piehl and Brown with ARDS showed a mean rise in PaO_2 of 47 mm Hg. The question at issue is whether ventilating a patient with ARDS in the prone position improves either morbidity or mortality. Till recently there was no evidence to suggest this. A large multicenter RCT from Italy compared patients with ARDS ventilated and nursed in a supine position to those in the prone position for 6 hours in the day. Though oxygenation improved in the prone position, there was no benefit in the ultimate outcome. However two subsequent studies suggest that the use of the prone position given over a longer period of time does help reduce mortality in ARDS. Nursing and other problems to enable a prone position to be maintained sufficiently long may prove insurmountable in most units in our country.

The generally accepted explanation for improved oxygenation in the prone position is improved perfusion to less damaged portions of the lung. The disadvantages of this method are the great difficulty in nursing such patients in the prone posture, the danger of disconnection of life-supporting lines, of obstruction to the airway, the occurrence of facial-dependent edema and even pressure sores. Even so, the prone position should be utilized when conventional modes of ventilator support do not result in adequate oxygenation.

Permissive Hypercapnia

When patients with ARDS are ventilated with the lung protection goal of low tidal volumes and pressure-limited ventilation, alveolar hypoventilation frequently occurs, causing a rise in $PaCO_2$ to 60–70 mm Hg or even more. Increasing $PaCO_2$ with respiratory acidosis can have potential adverse physiological effects such as arrhythmias, cardiovascular and central nervous system depression. However, these effects are not generally encountered in clinical practice. In fact, high $PaCO_2$ levels seem to be very well tolerated in adequately sedated patients. Most clinicians and intensivists favor permissive hypercapnia to the injurious effects of overdistended alveoli and high inspiratory inflation pressures. The $PaCO_2$ in permissive hypercapnia should preferably be allowed to rise slowly at the rate of 10 mm Hg/hr. Hypercapnia needs correction only if there is a significant fall in the pH. In the ARDS network trial, if the pH fell to less than 7.30, the respiratory rate was increased till the pH was more than 7.30 or the

respiratory rate equaled 35/min. If the pH was less than 7.3 in spite of the respiratory rate being increased to 35/min, an IV bicarbonate infusion was administered. Intravenous (IV) bicarbonate may temporarily correct the pH but could add substantially to the CO_2 that needs to be excreted by the patient via the lungs. Intravenous sodium bicarbonate could also lead to volume overload and potassium depletion in critically ill patients who already have an increase in intrapulmonary extravascular water content.

The Open Lung Ventilation (OLV)

The open lung concept though described first by Lachmann in 1977 has been adopted as a ventilatory strategy for ARDS over a little more than the last decade. Gattinoni and coworkers showed that patients with ARDS had multiple areas of atelectasis chiefly in the dependent lung regions, due to reduced volume of the aerated lung. The ventilatory strategy of an open lung opens up the atelectatic areas and keeps them open. Thereby the cyclic shear forces of alveolar opening and closing are minimized and optimal gas exchange is achieved (PaO_2 > 450 mm Hg on an FiO_2 of 1). The "open lung" procedure is always attempted using pressure-controlled ventilation with a I:E ratio of 1:1 and with an FiO_2 of 1. To start with PEEP is applied at 15–20 cm H_2O in patients with ARDS, and the lung is opened with slow progressive increase (by 2 cm at a time) in the peak inspiratory pressure up to 40–60 cm H_2O. The "opening pressure" is the peak inspiratory pressure at which the lung is "opened". The success of recruitment of closed alveoli is gauged either by noting the sudden sharp increase in PaO_2 more than 450 mm Hg when the lung fully "opens up" or by the proportional increase in tidal volume following increase in the peak inspiratory pressure. The peak inspiratory pressure and PEEP are now adjusted to the lowest pressure which keeps the lung open. This lowest pressure is realized when the tidal volumes are stable and the arterial blood gases continue to show a high constant PaO_2. The ideal pressure is generally 15–30 cm H_2O less than the required recruitment "opening" peak pressure. After opening the lung and finding the lowest pressure to keep it open, the resultant pressure amplitude is minimized and gas exchange maximized. The ventilatory strategy described above enables a reduction in FiO_2 and protects the lung from further injury. It is possible that an open lung is less likely to produce cytokines injurious to itself as also to other organ systems.

How beneficial is open long ventilation (OLV) in ARDS? Some clinical trials indicate that open lung ventilation may improve mortality, oxygenation and other clinical outcomes. However these trials had important methodological flaws *(Ref: Amato MB, Barbas CS, Medeiros DM, et al. Effect of a protective-ventilation strategy on mortality in the acute respiratory distress syndrome. N Engl J Med. 1998;338:347; Villar J, Kacmarek RM, Pérez-Méndez L, et al. A high positive end-expiratory pressure, low tidal volume ventilatory strategy improves outcome in persistent acute respiratory distress syndrome: a randomized, controlled trial. Crit Care Med. 2006;34:1311).* Although the earlier clinical trials were not associated with clinically adverse outcomes, a recent well-conducted randomized trial (Alveolar Recruitment for ARDS trial, ART (*Ref: Lu J, Wang X, Chen M, et al. An open lung strategy in the management of acute respiratory distress syndrome: a systematic review and meta-analysis. Shock. 2017;48:43)* reported harm in patients given OLV. Patients managed with the open lung strategy in this trial had a significantly higher 28 day mortality, and a higher 6-month mortality. In addition the open lung group had a higher risk of barotrauma.

In conclusion, the data so far suggests that OLV confers no conclusive benefit and possible harm. The current recommendation is that one should avoid OLV as an initial strategy in patients with ARDS. In rare cases when conventional ventilator support is for any reason unsuccessful, OLV may be given a try. However, the open lung strategy requires experience, close attention to ventilator settings and extra care. It is possible that the chief benefit of OLV may be more related to low tidal volumes rather than in opening the lungs.

Recruitment Maneuvers

A recruitment maneuver consists of a brief application of a high continuous positive pressure of 40 cm H_2O for 40 seconds, with the idea of opening up of collapsed alveoli. There is no consensus on the best level of continuous positive pressure, its duration or frequency. The maneuver improves oxygenation but its overall use in ARDS is undetermined. Perhaps it is of maximum benefit when a patient for whatever reason has been briefly disconnected from the ventilator, because this can result in marked alveolar collapse.

The important possible adverse effects of the recruitment maneuver are hypotension and desaturation.

These effects are generally self limited and without serious consequences. If however the recruitment maneuver is carried out for a longer duration, there is a risk of cardiac arrest and barotrauma.

Refractory Hypoxemia

Refractory hypoxemia may occur when FiO_2 and PEEP are optimized. In these patients increasing the I:E ratio by prolonging inspiratory time may improve oxygenation. The I:E ratio should first be set to 1:2 or at most 1:1. This allows more time for the 'stiffer' areas of the lungs to open up and hence improve oxygenation. The potential dangers of this procedure are auto-PEEP, barotrauma, hemodynamic instability and poor oxygen delivery. These patients not only require heavier sedation but also neuromuscular blockade. An inverse ratio ventilation with high applied PEEP should be given a try before the use of other rescue interventions.

The most important rescue intervention when conventional modes of ventilator support described above fail, is the use of extracorporeal membrane oxygenation (ECMO). The use of ECMO has been given in the chapter on Mechanical Ventilation to which the reader is referred.

Other Measures
Sedation

Sedation is invariably necessary in patients with ARDS on ventilator support. It allows efficient ventilation and decreases oxygen consumption. It may be necessary for several days and at times for many weeks. Narcotics may be used to relieve pain or suppress respiratory drive, benzodiazepines to relieve anxiety. Continuous sedation may be necessary if patients require repeated doses to achieve a sedative effect. A protocol that routinely wakes patients every day should be followed. The ideal degree of sedation is one that allows efficient ventilator support and yet allows the patient to be awakened easily. This is possible in mild to moderate patients of ARDS; severe ARDS necessitates deep sedation.

Use of Paralytic Agents

Use of paralytic agents can help improve oxygenation through more efficient ventilator support and yet can have undesirable side effects by prolonging neuromuscular weakness. A multicenter trial on 340 patients with severe ARDS ($PaO_2/FiO_2 < 120$ mm Hg) showed that the use of a continuous infusion of cisatracurium besylate for 48 hours resulted in a non-statistically significant lower ICU and hospital crude mortality rate when compared to placebo. These findings need to be replicated before using neuroparalytic agents as a routine measure in ARDS. However, current evidence suggests that use of these agents in severe ARDS with very low PaO_2/FiO_2 ratio is acceptable, reasonably safe and probably beneficial.

Fluid Balance

It is important not to overhydrate the patient as this worsens pulmonary edema. In established ARDS we have always preferred to keep filling pressures of the left ventricle on the lesser side of normal (PAOP <8 mm Hg), central venous pressure (CVP) ≤4 mm and not more than 6 mm Hg provided perfusion of vital organs is satisfactory. The ARDS Network Fluid and Catheter Treatment trial has recently shown that a conservative fluid management strategy increased the mean number of ventilator-free days (14.8 vs 12.1). There was a 2.9% reduction in mortality rate in the conservative arm but this was not statistically significant. This study showed that the conservative fluid strategy did not increase the incidence of renal failure or shock.

The above strategy applies to patients who are not in shock or whose shock has been effectively countered with appropriate fluid management. Unquestionably, a patient in shock will require emergency fluid resuscitation measures.

Other Fluid Management Strategies

In the particular setting of hypoproteinemia and ARDS, the combination therapy of albumin and frusemide may be useful in improving pulmonary physiology. There is however no evidence that outcome is favorably influenced. Hypoproteinemia is a documented risk factor in the development of ARDS as also for poor outcome in critical illness in general. This in our opinion is reason enough to counter hypoalbuminemia with infusions of albumin in patients with ARDS.

Hemodynamic Monitoring

In a trial concerning 1,000 patients with ARDS, hemo-dynamic monitoring with a central venous catheter (CVC) was compared with a pulmonary artery catheter (PAC) to guide management. Patients with ARDS were randomly assigned to a CVC or a PAC. There was no difference in mortality, lung function, ventilator free days, organ failure free days or ICU free days at day 28. Rates of hypotension, dialysis and vasopressor use were same in both groups. However the PAC group had a twofold increase of catheter related complications, in particular catheter related arrhythmias. The above study suggests that the PAC should not be used routinely in the management of patients with ARDS.

Notwithstanding these findings, hemodynamic monitoring through PA catheter may be of help under exceptional circumstances for individual patients. We very occasionally use the PA catheter in our unit to obtain specific answers to specific diagnostic problems, e.g. assessing the adequacy of volume resuscitation, titrating inotropic support, assessing left ventricular dysfunction, or assessing oxygen delivery in difficult complicated problems.

Circulatory Support

It is important to ensure adequate oxygen transport or delivery to the tissues. Oxygen transport or delivery (DO_2) is not only dependent on an adequate PaO_2, but is also dependent on cardiac output and the hemoglobin (Hb) concentration. The Hb concentration should be kept around 10 g/dL with a hematocrit of 35%. Inotropic support is often necessary in patients with severe lung injury. Dobutamine is preferred if the cardiac output is low as it generally does not induce tachycardia. If the systolic blood pressure is less than 90 mm Hg, or if the systemic vascular resistance is low, dopamine is to be preferred. Norepinephrine is often necessary in hypotensive patients.

Supramaximal oxygen transport (cardiac index > 4.5 $L/min/m^2$ and oxygen delivery above 600 $mL/min/m^2$), was earlier thought to reduce oxygen debt in the tissues, prevent hypoxic injury and organ system failure. This is however by no means certain, and there are a number of conflicting studies that support or refute this suggestion. It is possible that increasing oxygen delivery to supramaximal levels reduces mortality in just a subgroup of patients, such as high-risk surgical patients. In our experience and in the experience of most critical care units, supramaximal oxygen delivery does not reduce mortality in ARDS. Volume-loading patients with ARDS to maintain PAOP at upper normal limits (15–18 mm Hg) in an attempt to raise the cardiac output, invariably does harm by potentiating the lung injury.

Support to Other Organ Systems

All organ systems often need support, in particular the kidney. Ultrafiltration or dialysis may be necessary to treat volume overload or renal failure.

Nutritional Support

Good nutrition is vital, particularly when ARDS is due to excessively catabolic states as in fulminant tetanus, burns or severe sepsis. Severely catabolic states require a caloric intake of 2,500 or more calories/day, and this could lead to excessive fluid intake in a clinical situation which often necessitates fluid restriction. Under these circumstances, nutritional requirements are sacrificed on a short-term basis to allow fluid restriction. The alternative is to remove additional water by the use of loop diuretics if renal function is good or by the use of ultrafiltration if renal function is impaired. Enteral feeding is always to be preferred. In the presence of ileus, and abdominal sepsis, parenteral feeding becomes necessary.

Glucose Control

It is generally accepted that hyperglycemia should be prevented, the blood glucose levels being preferably kept between 120 mg/dL and 150 mg/dL.

DVT Prophylaxis

There is always a high rise of DVT and pulmonary embolism in patients with ARDS. Prolonged immobility, trauma, sepsis, the underlying illness, activation of coagulation pathway are all contributing risk factors. DVT prophylaxis is therefore of utmost importance.

GI Bleed Prophylaxis

Patients on ventilator support are more prone to GI bleeding from stress ulcers. Stress ulcer prophylaxis should always be instituted.

Measures to prevent nosocomial pneumonia and iatrogenic sepsis are of crucial importance.

Treatment of Complications

These can involve any organ system, they should be promptly diagnosed and treated. Iatrogenic sepsis and nosocomial pneumonias are of ominous significance.

Role of Corticosteroid in ARDS

The role of corticosteroids in ARDS is controversial. Results of randomized trials and meta-analysis demonstrate that glucocorticoids are not beneficial and may be harmful when given >14 days after the onset of ARDS. However the Society of Critical Care Medicine/European Society of ICU Medicine state that methylprednisolone 1 mg/kg/day may be administered to those with early (<14 days) moderate-to-severe ARDS (PaO_2/FiO_2 <200) *(Ref: Annane D, Pastores SM, Rochwerg B, et al. Guidelines for the diagnosis and management of critical illness-related corticosteroid insufficiency (CIRCI) in critically ill patients (Part I): Society of Critical Care Medicine (SCCM) and European Society of Intensive Care Medicine (ESICM) 2017. Intensive Care Med. 2017;43:1751).* We follow this recommendation; though there are many units who do not follow it awaiting better proof of its efficacy. The story of the use of corticosteroids in ARDS is unfortunately still buried under controversy.

Nitrous Oxide, Prostacyclin

Inhaled nitrous oxide or prostacyclin are not routine therapy in adult ARDS because even though they improve oxygenation, there is no improvement in mortality, duration of mechanical ventilation and ventilator free days.

■ SUGGESTED READING

1. Amato MB, Barbas CS, Medeiros DM, et al. Effect of a protective-ventilation strategy on mortality in the acute respiratory distress syndrome. N Engl J Med. 1998;338: 347.
2. Avecillas JF. Clinical epidemiology of acute lung injury and acute respiratory distress syndrome: incidence, diagnosis, and outcomes. Clin Chest Med. 2006;27(4):549-57.
3. Barr J, Fraser GL, Puntillo K, et al. Clinical practice guidelines for the management of pain, agitation, and delirium in adult patients in the intensive care unit. Crit Care Med. 2013;41:263.
4. Bercker S, Weber-Carstens S, Deja M, et al. Critical illness polyneuropathy and myopathy in patients with acute respiratory distress syndrome. Crit Care Med. 2005;33:711.
5. Brower RG, Matthay MA, Morris A, et al. Acute respiratory distress syndrome network, ventilation with lower tidal volumes as compared with traditional tidal volumes for acute lung injury and the acute respiratory distress syndrome. N Engl J Med. 2000;342:1301.

6. de Hemptinne Q. ARDS—a clinicopathological confrontation. Chest. 2009;135(4):944-9.

7. Ferguson ND, Fan E, Camporota L, et al. The Berlin definition of ARDS: an expanded rationale, justification, and supplementary material. Intensive Care Med. 2012;38:1573.

8. Gattinoni L. The role of CT-scan studies for the diagnosis and therapy for acute respiratory distress syndrome. Clin Chest Med. 2006;27(4):559-70.

9. Girard TD. Mechanical ventilation in ARDS: a state-of-the-art review. Chest. 2007;131(3):921-9.

10. Grissom CK, Hirshberg EL, Dickerson JB, et al. Fluid management with a simplified conservative protocol for the acute respiratory distress syndrome. Crit Care Med. 2015;43:288.

11. Herridge MS, Tansey CM, Matte A, et al. Functional disability 5 years after acute respiratory distress syndrome. N Engl J Med. 2011;364:1293.

12. Jia X. Risk factors for ARDS in patients receiving mechanical ventilation for > 48 hours. Chest. 2008;133(4):853-61.

13. Martin GS, Moss M, Wheeler AP, et al. A randomized, controlled trial of furosemide with or without albumin in hypoproteinemic patients with acute lung injury. Crit Care Med. 2005;33:1681-7.

14. Mikkelsen ME, Christie JD, Lanken PN, et al. The adult respiratory distress syndrome cognitive outcomes study: long-term neuropsychological function in survivors of acute lung injury. Am J Respir Crit Care Med. 2012;185:1307.

15. Prin S, Chergui K, Augarde R, et al. Ability and safety of a heated humidifier to control hypercapnic acidosis in severe ARDS. Intensive Care Med. 2002;28:1756.

16. Putensen C, Theuerkauf N, Zinserling J, et al. Meta-analysis: ventilation strategies and outcomes of the acute respiratory distress syndrome and acute lung injury. Ann Intern Med. 2009;151:566.

17. Rice TW, Wheeler AP, Bernard GR, et al. Comparison of the SpO_2/FiO_2 ratio and the PaO_2/FiO_2 ratio in patients with acute lung injury or ARDS. Chest. 2007;132:410.

18. Silversides JA, Major E, Ferguson AJ, et al. Conservative fluid management or deresuscitation for patients with sepsis or acute respiratory distress syndrome following the resuscitation phase of critical illness: a systematic review and meta-analysis. Intensive Care Med. 2017;43: 155.

19. The ARDS Network. Ventilation with lower tidal volumes as compared with traditional lung volumes for acute lung injury and acute respiratory distress syndrome. NEJM. 2000;342:1301-8.

20. The National Heart, Lung, and Blood Institute Acute Respiratory Distress Syndrome (ARDS) Clinical Trials Network. Efficacy and Safety of corticosteroids for persistent acute respiratory distress syndrome. N Engl J Med. 2006;354:1671-84.

21. The National Heart, Lung, and Blood Institute Acute Respiratory Distress Syndrome (ARDS) Clinical Trials Network. Pulmonary-artery versus central venous catheter to guide treatment of acute lung injury. N Engl J Med. 2006;354:2213-24.

22. The National Heart, Lung, and Blood Institute Acute Respiratory Distress Syndrome (ARDS) Clinical Trials Network. Higher versus lower positive end-expiratory pressures in patients with the acute respiratory distress syndrome. N Engl J Med. 2004;351:326-33.

23. The National Heart, Lung, and Blood Institute. Acute Respiratory Distress Syndrome (ARDS) Clinical Trials Network. Comparison of two fluid-management strategies in acute lung injury. N Engl J Med. 2006;354: 2564-75.

24. Vincent JL. New management strategies in ARDS. Immunomodulation. Crit Care Clin. 2002;8(1):69-78.

25. Wheeler AP, Bernard GR, Thompson BT, et al. National Heart, Lung, and Blood Institute Acute Respiratory Distress Syndrome (ARDS) Clinical Trials Network, Pulmonary-artery versus central venous catheter to guide treatment of acute lung injury. N Engl J Med. 2006;354:2213.

Section 16

Pulmonary Manifestations of Systemic Diseases

CHAPTER 57

Pulmonary Manifestations of Connective Tissue Disorders

■ GENERAL CONSIDERATIONS

Connective tissue disorders are a group of diseases characterized by an abnormality in the collagen or elastic framework of the body. There is a disturbance in immune function leading to the formation of autoimmune bodies in these diseases. Connective tissue disorders (also termed as collagen disorders) consist of rheumatoid arthritis (RA), systemic sclerosis (SSc), systemic lupus erythematosis (SLE), dermatomyositis (DM), polymyositis (PM), mixed connective tissue disease (MCD), Sjogren's syndrome (SS), ankylosing spondylitis and relapsing polychondritis.

Pulmonary involvement is commonly observed in connective tissue disorders. This involvement is more frequent than is clinically apparent and affects all components of the respiratory system. The airways, the alveoli, the interstitium, pulmonary vasculature and the pleura may all be involved singly or in various combinations depending on the nature of the connective tissue disorder.

Pulmonary disease has emerged as a major cause of death in collagen vascular disease. In SSc and DM/PM, pulmonary disease is now the most common cause of death.

The prevalence rate of pulmonary complications in connective tissue disorders varies in different studies. No estimate is available for India. Any estimate will depend on the geographical area and the population studied and more so perhaps on the investigational methods used to detect abnormalities within the respiratory system. Thus for example, dyspnea on exertion is a common symptom in SSc but some patients because of musculoskeletal involvement in SSc may not be able to exercise sufficiently to report dyspnea. Conversely, patients with RA or PM may be breathless secondary to increased work of locomotion, secondary to arthritis or myositis. Chest radiography is also an imprecise tool when it comes to diagnosing interstitial lung disease (ILD) in these patients. Studies which involve computed tomography (CT) of the chest, lung biopsies and autopsy studies will unquestionably show a much higher prevalence rate when compared to mere clinical studies coupled with a basic radiological examination of the chest.

Due to lack of evidence, it is impossible to compare the incidence of connective tissue disorders in India vis-a-vis the West. Pulmonary complications are however frequently encountered, their incidence in connective tissue disorders being probably similar to that in the West.

Interstitial pneumonia is perhaps the most important form of pulmonary involvement in most connective tissue disorders stated above. Systemic sclerosis has the highest prevalence rate of interstitial pneumonia which more often is of the nonspecific type. Autopsy studies in the West show that close to 75% of patients with SSc show some degree of pulmonary fibrosis and 30% show some degree of vascular involvement. Yet overt disease is reported in just 5% of these patients. Rheumatoid disease and DM/PM also show a high prevalence rate of interstitial pulmonary fibrosis on autopsy studies, though overt disease again is about 5%. The interstitial pneumonia that complicates RA and DM/PM is more frequently a usual interstitial pneumonia (UIP) and organizing pneumonia.

Pleural disease is perhaps the most frequent and common pulmonary manifestation of connective tissue disorders, particularly of SLE and RA. A rough estimate of the relative frequency of different pulmonary manifestations in different connective tissue disorders is given in **Table 1**.

Table 1: Relative frequency of different pulmonary manifestations in various connective tissue disorders.

Pulmonary manifestations	RA	SSc	DM/PM	SLE
Interstitial pneumonia	++	+++	++	+
Pleural involvement	+++			+++
Pulmonary hypertension		+++	+	++
Alveolar hemorrhage	**			+
Constrictive bronchiolitis	+		**	**

(+++: Common; ++: Fairly frequent; +: Occasional; **: Rare)
Source: Modified from Spiro SG, Albert RK, Jett JR. Clinical Respiratory Medicine, 3rd edition. St Louis: Mosby Inc.; 2008.

Currently, genetic risk factors are being studied in relation to pulmonary complications of connective tissue disorders. A number of genes have been shown to be associated with pulmonary complications in SLE and RA. Thus, the carriage of HLA-DRB1* 11 (04) and DPB1* 1,301 alleles is believed to be associated with lung fibrosis and that of DRB1*04 and DRB1*08 with pulmonary hypertension, which is linked to the presence of anticentromere antibodies (ACAs). The ACAs are associated with the carriage of a functional tumor necrosis factor (TNF) variant which may perhaps exert a pathological role in SSc. In RA there is an association between obliterative bronchiolitis and the histocompatibility antigens HLA-B40 and DR1. As yet, these and other genetic studies do not necessarily have clinical implications; further work in genetic and molecular biology may perhaps clarify this issue.

CLINICAL FEATURES OF RHEUMATOID ARTHRITIS

Pulmonary disease generally occurs in patients with well-marked RA. Occasionally, it may precede clinical evidence of joint disease by several months. A strongly positive RA factor in the serum of these patients may however suggest the link with rheumatoid disease. Pulmonary manifestations in RA may form the sole overt systemic complication or involvement. On the other hand, pulmonary manifestations may be associated with other extra-articular complications, notably rheumatoid nodules and occasionally with digital vasculitis.

Pleural Effusion

Pleural effusion is the most common respiratory manifestation of rheumatoid disease. At autopsy, histological evidence of pleural disease is present in 50% of patients. The majority are clinically silent. Clinically significant effusions occur in about 5% of RA patients, the majority resolving spontaneously. It is most often asymptomatic but may be associated with pleuritic pain and breathlessness. The effusion is generally small; it may however be moderate and in rare instances large in size. It may precede RA by several months in which case the diagnosis is often underdetermined. The main differential diagnosis is from tuberculosis and malignancy. A diagnostic pleural tap should always be done. A rheumatoid effusion is an exudate with a high protein content, low glucose (<60 mg/dL), a pH often less than 7.2 and a high lactate dehydrogenase (LDH); the cell count generally shows a lymphocytosis, though a significant number of polymorphs may also be present. The RA factor is positive in a high titer in the pleural fluid. In fact, the immunoglobulin M (IgM) rheumatoid factor may be higher in the pleural fluid than in the serum suggesting local pleural production of this factor by mononuclear cells.

A pleural biopsy (preferably a thoracoscopic biopsy) is often necessary, particularly when the pleural effusion precedes the joint pains and joint swellings of rheumatoid disease. Video-assisted thoracoscopy may reveal granular pleural surfaces. Histological examination in typical cases shows granulomatous inflammation with mesothelial pleural cells being replaced by palisading histiocytes. Unfortunately, more often than not, pleural biopsy merely shows nonspecific inflammatory changes with accompanying fibrosis. A pleural biopsy does however help to exclude other diseases, notably malignancy. A CT of the chest may reveal pulmonary nodules or subpleural nodules not visible on plain radiography; these findings may suggest the correct diagnosis.

Most pleural effusions, particularly when small, resolve spontaneously. Larger effusions may persist and may require paracentesis. Response to corticosteroids is unpredictable. Rarely, pleurodesis is necessary to prevent recurrence of the effusion particularly if it is large enough to cause symptoms.

Occasionally, a pleural effusion in rheumatoid disease becomes secondarily infected resulting in an empyema. Fever with chills, leukocytosis, and marked polymorphonuclear leukocytosis of the pleural fluid is observed. The empyema is treated on conventional lines—systemic antibiotics, pleural aspiration, and if this is unsuccessful, tube drainage or rib resection and tube drainage.

Interstitial Pneumonia (Figs. 1 and 2)

The prevalence of interstitial lung disease in rheumatoid arthritis (RA) is between 10% and 50% depending on the study. In India, the prevalence reported is near 15%. Risk factors for RA-ILD include older age, severe RA, male gender, a strongly positive RA and anti-CCP antibody test and cigarette smoking.

The histopathology of ILD associated with RA includes (a) usual interstitial pneumonia (UIP) which is the same as that observed in idiopathic pulmonary fibrosis; (b) nonspecific interstitial pneumonia (NSIP); (c) organizing pneumonia; (d) lymphocytic interstitial pneumonia; (e) desquamative interstitial pneumonia; (f) diffuse alveolar damage which clinically is characterized by acute interstitial pneumonia. The most frequent histological types are UIP and NSIP.

The clinical, imaging features, pulmonary functions and histopathological details in RA-ILD are similar to those observed in idiopathic interstitial pneumonia and bear no repetition (*see* chapter on ILD—Idiopathic Interstitial Pneumonia). A few features in relation to RA-ILD however need emphasis. The clinical presentation of RA-ILD to an extent depends on the underlying pathology. Exertional dyspnea may occur later in natural history of the disease because of exercise limitation due to the joint disease. For this reason patients with RA and UIP become symptomatic late in the natural history of UIP when widespread fibrosis is present. Though bibasilar crackles are present in over 80% patients, physical signs may be absent in early RA-ILD. Clubbing is frequently present when ILD in RA is of the UIP variety, but is much less common in patients with other patterns of RA-ILD. In rare cases, RA-ILD presents with a fulminant onset and fatal outcome, resembling the Hamman-Rich type syndrome.

The differential diagnosis of RA-ILD includes chiefly drug-induced lung toxicity, opportunistic infections, hypersensitivity pneumonitis, heart failure and frequent aspiration, chiefly into the lower lobes of both lungs.

Drug induced lung toxicity has been observed with most of the medications used to treat RA. These drugs include the nonsteroidal inflammatory drugs (NSAIDs), methotrexate, leflunomide, penicillamine, gold and biological agents—chiefly tumor necrosis factor inhibitors, such as rituximab. Development of sarcoid-like lesions within the lungs have been reported with infliximab, etanercept, adalimumab. Stopping the anti-TNF drug leads to resolution of these granulomas over a period of a few months *(Ref: Lake FR. Interstitial lung disease in rheumatoid arthritis.www.uptodate.com).*

Opportunistic infections are known complications of immune suppressive therapy used to treat RA. The important opportunistic infections are pneumocystis (jirovecii) infection, mycobacterial tuberculous and non-tuberculous infections and fungal infections.

Chronic hypersensitivity pneumonitis has imaging features closely resembling the UIP pattern of RA-ILD.

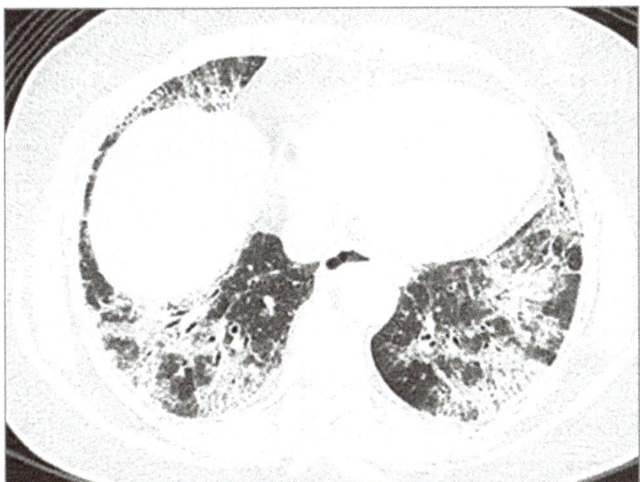

Fig. 1: Rheumatoid arthritis (RA) with NSIP HRCT demonstrates ill-defined reticular opacities and ground-glass densities in both lung bases in a subpleural and peribronchovascular location. This pattern is of NSIP as significant fibrosis and honeycomb changes are absent. UIP would demonstrate fibrosis, honeycomb cysts and architectural distortion.

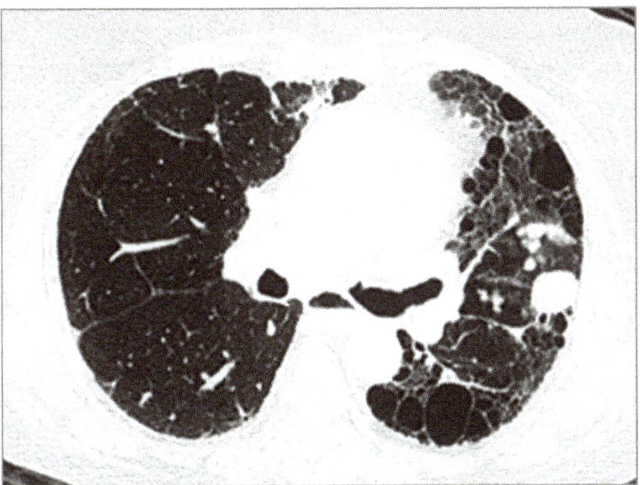

Fig. 2: Rheumatoid arthritis. HRCT chest in a patient with rheumatoid arthritis demonstrating subpleural interstitial thickening with honeycomb changes due to UIP. Additionally noted are well-defined rheumatoid nodules within the lung parenchyma.

Heart failure is generally excluded by physical examination and appropriate investigations.

Aspiration pneumonia should be particularly considered in patients with difficulty in swallowing.

Treatment

Treatment is influenced by the patient's age, symptomatology, histopathological serotype of ILD and rapidity of progression. Better response is observed in the younger age group < 60 years than in the older and in those with radiographic evidence of NSIP, OP or lymphocytic pneumonia than UIP. Rapid progression of the disease is an indication for prompt therapy. Cigarette smokers should be strongly advised to stop smoking.

Asymptomatic patients and those with very mild RA-ILD require no specific treatment. They can be monitored clinically, by imaging and by lung function tests at three to six monthly intervals or sooner if symptoms develop or worsen. Progression of the disease merits treatment. Similarly patients with a UIP pattern and stable disease as judged by symptoms, PFT and HRCT are best not given specific therapy as no treatment has been shown to improve this pattern of lung disease. These patients generally are in the older age group and are unresponsive to glucocorticoid or other immunosuppressive drugs. Some physicians are however prompted to treat younger patients with UIP whose disease is recent and who show a deteriorating lung function, in the possible hope that the outlook is better in RA-UIP than in IPF.

In symptomatic patients of RA-ILD with progressive respiratory impairment and with features that favor treatment response (e.g. NSIP, OP), prednisolone should be started in a dose of 0.5 mg/kg, not exceeding 60 mg/day. We prefer not to exceed 40 mg/day. A clinical response is generally observed in 3 to 4 weeks following which the drug is tapered over weeks or months to a maintenance dose of preferably not more than 10 mg/day. If there is a failure to respond to the drug, or if when the drug is being tapered there is a 'flare' of the disease, a second immunosuppressive drug is added. Possible choice should include either mycophenolate, azathioprine or cyclophosphamide. Mycophenolate mofetil given in a dose of 250 mg twice daily increasing very gradually to 1.5 to 2 g/day. The major side effects of this drug are bone marrow depression, increase in liver enzymes and gastrointestinal disturbances. If azathioprine is used it should be given to start with in a dose of 50 mg/day increased very gradually every 2 to 3 weeks by 50 mg to a total dose of 2 mg/kg/day. We generally do not exceed this dose. Considering the toxicity of cyclophosphamide, the drug should be reserved for severe or refractory cases.

A small number of patients with RA-ILD present with or develop acute interstitial lung disease resembling the Hamman-Rich syndrome and have or soon develop acute respiratory failure. These patients are treated with IV methyl prednisolone 1 g daily for 4 to 5 days. Many physicians prefer to add an immunosuppressive agent such as cyclophosphamide or azathioprine. After the course of methylprednisolone is over, the patient is started on 40–60 mg prednisolone, the dose being gradually tapered to a maintenance dose of 10–15 mg/day.

Methotrexate in patients with RA-ILD is best avoided because of the increased risk of lung toxicity from this drug. The role of pirfenidone and nintedanib in RA-ILD with a UIP pattern is not known and awaits study.

Patients with RA-ILD require careful clinical monitoring; lung functions should be done at periodic intervals as also imaging studies of the lung when necessary.

Monitoring for Side-effects of Immunosuppressive Drugs

Close monitoring for hematological toxicity is imperative. Toxicity of azathioprine is closely related to a deficiency of the enzyme thiopurine methyltransferase (TPMT) which normally metabolizes the drug. An analysis of this TPMT gene prior to the administration of the drug may predict those patients at risk for severe toxicity. Deficiency of this enzyme is however very rare. It is therefore perhaps best to start and persevere with a small dose of 50 mg/day for 2 to 3 weeks and stop the drug if hematological toxicity develops. Liver functions and renal functions should also be periodically monitored every 3 to 4 weeks.

Lung transplantation may be an option in end-stage RA-ILD. The potential role of rituximab and anti-TNF alpha regimes in RA-ILD is as yet unknown.

Prognosis

Prognosis depends on the severity of respiratory impairment and the histological pattern. It is poor in RA-UIP than in RA-NSIP. In a retrospective review of 84 patients with RA-UIP monitored for 33 months, respiratory abnormalities remained stable in about 50%, progressed in 30% and deteriorated rapidly in 17%. The stable group remained stable for a median of 45 months *(Ref: Song*

JW, Lee HK, Lee CK, et al. Clinical course and outcome of rheumatoid arthritis-related usual interstitial pneumonia. Sarcoidosis Vasc Diffuse Lung Dis. 2013;30:103). In a number of patients with RA-ILD the pulmonary disease does not progress and may remain subclinical.

Pulmonary Nodules

Rheumatoid nodules may occur within the lungs or may be subpleural in position. They are most frequently found in a peripheral or subpleural distribution. They are similar to the subcutaneous rheumatoid nodules with which they may be associated. The prevalence of rheumatoid nodules in the lung depends on whether chest X-ray is used to identify them (1%) or HRCT. In an HRCT study of 77 patients with RA, 22% of patients had rheumatoid nodules. Pulmonary nodules in RA are invariably silent and are discovered fortuitously on an X-ray chest. They may remain unchanged, increase in size or may even disappear. Rarely, they cavitate and then may cause hemoptysis. Their proximity to the pleural surface accounts for some of their rare complications including pneumothorax, pleural effusions, and bronchopleural fistula. The main difficulty is in differentiating them from other pulmonary pathologies. A cavitating nodule needs in particular to be distinguished from tuberculosis and from a squamous cell carcinoma. Sputum examination, bronchoscopy, BAL and a CT-guided biopsy may all help in the diagnosis. Even so, the diagnosis at times is uncertain and is made only after a lobectomy.

Kaplan's Syndrome

This syndrome develops in patients with RA who develop coal workers' pneumoconiosis or other pneumoconiosis. It is characterized by the appearance of nodules within the lung on an X-ray chest. They occur in crops; at times the nodules fuse to give the appearance of progressive massive fibrosis. The nodules may cavitate and cause problems in diagnosis. The pathogenesis of this syndrome is unclear; it could be related to an overactive response of the hyperimmune rheumatoid lung to the coal dust or other dust particles within it. Histologically, the nodules in Kaplan's syndrome resemble the subcutaneous necrotic nodules of rheumatoid disease; in addition the lesions contain coal dust particles. Amazingly, similar nodules are found in the lungs of coal-miners who are seropositive for rheumatoid disease but who have no arthritis. The diagnosis can pose problems, with the need to consider

both inflammatory and neoplastic pathologies in the differential diagnosis. No treatment is necessary.

Airway Disease

Some patients with rheumatoid disease develop arthritis of the cricoarytenoid joints. This leads to hoarseness, dyspnea, cough and supraglottic stenosis. An indirect laryngoscopy together with a flow-volume loop determination will enable an accurate diagnosis. At times a tracheostomy becomes necessary to keep the airway patent. A rare but dangerous airway complication in rheumatoid disease is *obliterative bronchiolitis (Fig. 3)*. Pathologically, it is characterized by inflammation of the walls of the small airways with the formation of obliterative scar tissue. The patient gets progressively breathless and may die within some months from respiratory failure due to increasing unremitting obstruction of small airways. There may be no physical signs at all and the diagnosis of functional breathlessness may be made in the early stages of this disease if the patient is not carefully evaluated. In some patients there is an audible inspiratory squeak together with a few crackles during end-inspiration. The lung functions show small airways obstruction with increased residual volumes and total lung capacity, but a preserved transfer factor of the lung for carbon monoxide (TLCO). Radiological examination of the chest shows overinflated lungs. CT scan shows areas of decreased attenuation and vascularity and areas of increased attenuation and vascularity (mosaic pattern) which

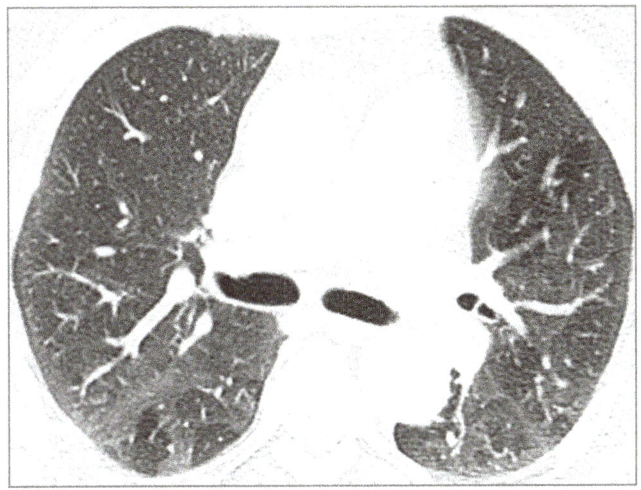

Fig. 3: Obliterative bronchiolitis, marked areas of mosaic perfusion due to air trapping seen in a patient with rheumatoid disease.

is brought out best in expiratory scans. Treatment is generally ineffective and prognosis poor. Young patients with severe progressive disease should be considered for lung transplant surgery.

There are some who attribute *obliterative bronchiolitis* in RA to the use of penicillamine. This may be so in rare instances but *obliterative bronchiolitis* has occurred in rheumatoid patients who have not been given penicillamine. Also, this complication has not been observed when penicillamine has been used for the treatment of biliary cirrhosis or Wilson's disease.

Follicular Bronchiolitis

Follicular bronchiolitis is a disorder of unknown etiology with lymphoid follicles being reported in airway walls. It is a rare entity most commonly found in RA. It may mimic ILD but is more steroid-responsive than obliterative bronchiolitis or RA-related ILD.

Pulmonary Infections

Pulmonary infections appear to occur more frequently in rheumatoid disease. There is also an increased incidence of both *bronchitis* and *bronchiectasis.* Perhaps this may be related to immune suppression caused both by the disease and its treatment. Poor local host defenses and difficulty in coughing and expectorating because of increasing debility and arthritic pain are other contributing factors. Finally, a very small minority of patients with rheumatoid disease develop relapsing polychondritis.

Pulmonary Hypertension

Very rarely, pulmonary hypertension has been reported as an isolated pulmonary complication of rheumatoid disease. There is widespread intimal fibrosis in the medium-sized pulmonary vessels observed on histopathological studies. Pulmonary hypertension when present is more often related to severe interstitial pulmonary fibrosis than to direct vascular involvement.

Drug Toxicity

Added to the pulmonary manifestations produced by rheumatoid disease are the toxic effects of the drugs used in the treatment of this disease. Gold is known to produce pulmonary fibrosis, in addition to other toxic effects on other systems. Penicillamine has been reported to cause *obliterative bronchiolitis* and has been suspect for causing alveolar hemorrhage. Aspirin and nonsteroidal anti-inflammatory drugs can exacerbate asthma in patients with bronchial hypersensitivity. Methotrexate lung occurs in about 5% of patients receiving this drug for their RA. This condition carries a mortality of up to 20%. A BAL lymphocytosis of up to 68% of the total cell count together with an increase in CD_4 lymphocytes is observed.

Clinical features of methotrexate lung are breathlessness and cough. X-ray chest shows bilateral shadows which become extensive and diffuse if the correct diagnosis is delayed. HRCT chest shows increasing fibrosis in both lungs. Methotrexate should promptly be stopped once a methotrexate lung is strongly suspected.

■ SYSTEMIC LUPUS ERYTHEMATOSUS

Systemic lupus erythematosus (SLE) often involves many organ systems. Pleuropulmonary manifestations are common, being more frequent when compared to any of the other connective tissue disorders. They occur both in the spontaneously occurring form as well as in the drug-induced form (**Fig. 4**).

Pleural Disease (Fig. 4)

Pleural effusion is the most common pulmonary manifestation of SLE. Clinically or radiologically overt

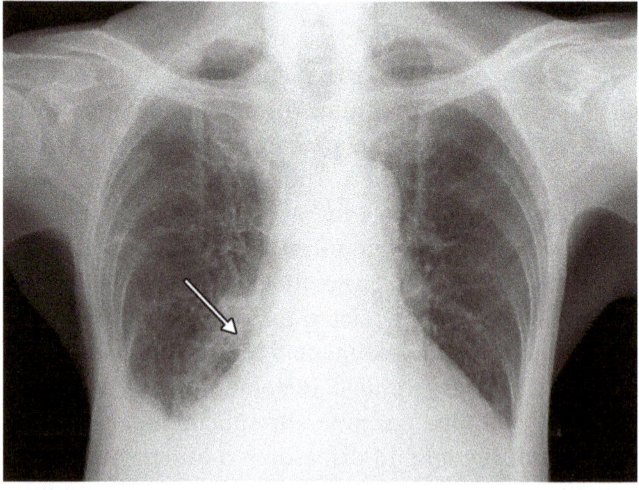

Fig. 4: Systemic lupus erythematosus (SLE). Chest X-ray demonstrates bilateral pleural effusions with a pericardial effusion in a patient with SLE.

pleural involvement is found in 20% of newly diagnosed SLE. In fact it is often the presenting feature. Pleurisy may be dry, but more often there is pleurisy with effusion, which may be small, moderate and rarely, large. Pleuritic pain, breathlessness, and fever are the presenting clinical features. The effusion may be unilateral, is bilateral in close to 50% of cases, and at times is consecutive, involvement of one pleural space being followed after a lapse of days or weeks by involvement of the other. The differential diagnosis (particularly in patients where a pleural effusion is the presenting feature) is chiefly from tuberculosis. Even though tuberculosis is rife in India, in our experience bilateral pleural effusion in young females with no parenchymal lung lesion on imaging is more frequently due to SLE than due to tuberculosis. Pleural effusion may be accompanied by pericardial effusion so that there is an enlargement of the cardiac silhouette on an X-ray chest. *Other conditions which need to be considered in the differential diagnosis are nontuberculous infections, drug-induced pleuritis, heart failure, nephrotic syndrome, uremia.*

Pleural fluid examination shows sterile lymphocytic exudates. In the early stages neutrophilic exudates may occur and a preponderance of mononuclear cells has been reported in studies where pleural aspiration has been done after one week. A pH of more than 7.33 and a normal glucose content distinguish this exudate from that seen in rheumatoid disease. The antinuclear antibody (ANA) factor in the pleural fluid may be strongly positive, LE cells may be present and the complement level may be low. Fibrothorax is a rare complication of lupus pleuritis, leading to breathlessness on exertion by hindering expansion of the affected lung.

Pleural effusion in SLE responds dramatically to corticosteroids, in contrast to pleural effusion in RA where the response is not predictable.

Pulmonary Involvement

Atelectasis is frequently observed in SLE. It takes the form of a plate atelectasis (about 2–4 cm in length), a little above the diaphragm and it may be associated with pleurisy **(Fig. 5)**. Restriction of breathing because of pain coupled with poor diaphragmatic movements probably explains the atelectasis, though an abnormality in surfactant has also been postulated. The differential diagnosis is chiefly from pulmonary embolism and infarction.

Shrinking Lung Syndrome (Fig. 6)

The shrinking lung syndrome observed in SLE is characterized by shrinkage of both lungs in size and volume with a progressive rise in the level of both domes of the diaphragm. This syndrome and the related rise in the diaphragm are due to progressive weakness and fibrosis of the muscles of diaphragmatic leaflets. The syndrome when advanced is characterized by dyspnea, orthopnea (in the late stages), episodic pleuritic chest pain with pulmonary function tests showing a progressive decrease in lung volumes. The CO diffusion capacity for

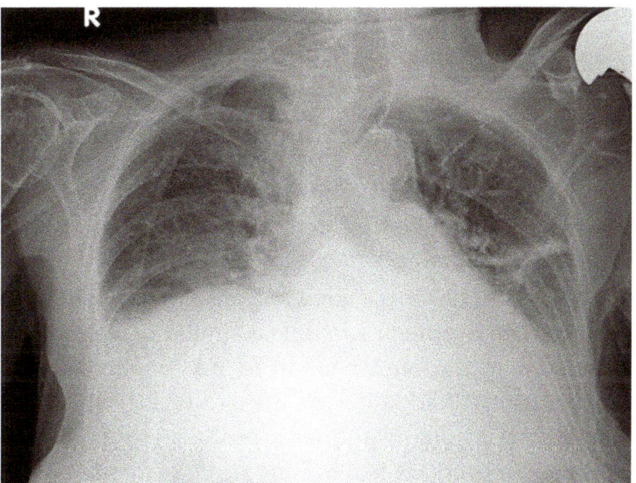

Fig. 5: Systemic lupus erythematosus (SLE). Chest X-ray shows plate atelectasis above the left dome of the diaphragm and bilateral pleural effusions in a patient with SLE.

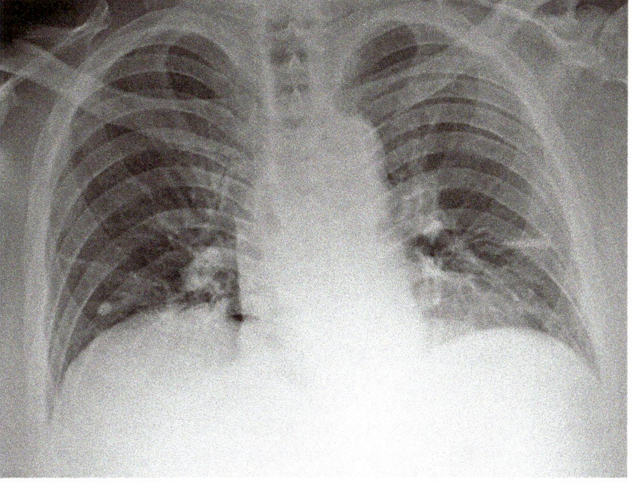

Fig. 6: X-ray chest reveals bilateral basal atelectasis in a case of shrinking lung syndrome.

unexplained reasons may also be reduced. There is also no evidence of pleural or interstitial lung disease on CT imaging of the chest. On fluoroscopy the movements of the diaphragm are markedly restricted. The FVC in the supine posture may be significantly lower (20%) compared to the upright sitting posture and this simple test when present may be an early pointer to diaphragmatic weakness.

The syndrome may remain stable or may be characterized by exacerbations with progressive increase in breathlessness which only partially responds to corticosteroids.

Interstitial Pneumonia

Interstitial pneumonia is less common in SLE compared to all other connective tissue disorders. Nonspecific interstitial pneumonia is the most frequent form of ILD observed **(Fig. 7)**. However UIP, organizing pneumonia, lymphocytic interstitial pneumonia, follicular bron-chiolitis, and nodular lymphoid hyperplasia have all been reported in SLE.

NSIP, OP, LIP show a good response to glucocorticoid therapy. The treatment schedule is similar to that already discussed in the management of RA associated ILD. If response is inadequate or if there is a 'flare' of the ILD during gradual withdrawal of the steroid, another immunosuppressant like azathioprine, mycophenolate,

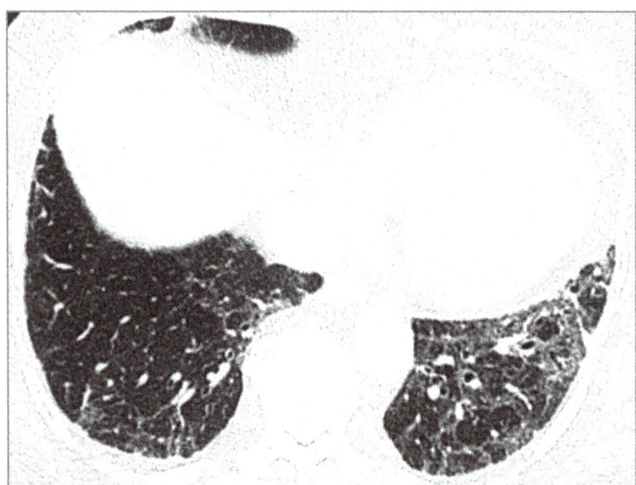

Fig. 7: Systemic lupus erythematosus (SLE) with NSIP. HRCT demonstrates bilateral basal posterior interstitial thickening essentially in a peribronchovascular and subpleural location. The peribronchovascular location is well-demonstrated as the bronchi are seen well-surrounded by the interstitial thickening. There are no honeycomb changes or fibrosis to suggest UIP pattern.

cyclophosphamide should be introduced since long term corticosteroids use has significant side effects, the maintenance dose of corticosteroids should be reduced to a minimum of 5 to 10 mg by using a steroid sparing immunosuppressant such as azathioprine or mycophenolate.

In patients who have a marked 'flare' of the ILD or when the ILD is severe, progressive, causing rapid impairment of pulmonary function, of if there is respiratory failure, IV methyl prednisolone (1 g IV daily for 3 days) followed by oral prednisolone 60 mg/day should be initiated. Cyclophosphamide intravenously is also used, which later can be replaced by azathioprine. Here again the treatment is similar to that already discussed in the management of severe ILD in RA.

In refractory ILD associated with SLE where corticosteroids and other immunosuppressants have proved ineffective rituximab may be given a try.

Treatment of UIP, Fibrotic NSIP

No specific treatment is likely to benefit patients with UIP or fibrotic NSIP. The prognosis in these patients is decidedly worse compared to cellular NSIP and the other interstitial pneumonias.

Three important points need to be stressed:
1. One needs to exclude pulmonary infections, drug toxicity and heart failure before diagnosing SLE associated ILD.
2. A thorough clinical examination, radiological study, lung function tests and if needs be a histological study should be done to determine the type of idiopathic interstitial pneumonia, the severity of the disease and the degree of its progression.
3. In patients with mild, stable fibrotic disease, close observation without specific therapy is advisable. Worsening disease is an indication for specific treatment.

Clinical features include breathlessness, clubbing of fingers, basal velcro crackles, restrictive lung function pattern and the presence of nodular and reticular basal shadows. An HRCT determines both the presence of ILD and the pattern of ILD.

Acute Lupoid Pneumonia

Acute lupoid pneumonia is an uncommon manifestation of SLE. It can present as a pneumonic consolidation of a lobe of one lung, indistinguishable radiologically from the usual pneumonia due to an infective etiology **(Fig. 8)**. It can also present with diffuse bilateral alveolar shadowing involving chiefly the mid and lower zones of both lung fields, resembling acute respiratory distress syndrome (ARDS) or idiopathic acute interstitial pneumonia. The clinical manifestations are acute onset fever, dry cough, and dyspnea. Hemoptysis may be present. The patient is tachypneic, has tachycardia and may desaturate. Crackles are generally heard over both lung bases. Increasing hypoxic respiratory failure may cause death if the condition is not correctly diagnosed.

Diagnosis

An acute infective etiology must be excluded by all possible tests including a study of the BAL fluid. An ANA test and an anti-DNA test should be performed on any patient who presents as an "acute infective pneumonia" but who fails to respond to empiric antibiotic therapy. Patients diagnosed as acute idiopathic interstitial pneumonia and patients diagnosed as ARDS for which there is no obvious cause should also have serological tests for SLE performed.

Differential Diagnosis

It includes ARDS, idiopathic interstitial pneumonia, infective pneumonia, aspiration pneumonia, diffuse alveolar hemorrhage, drug-induced lung toxicity.

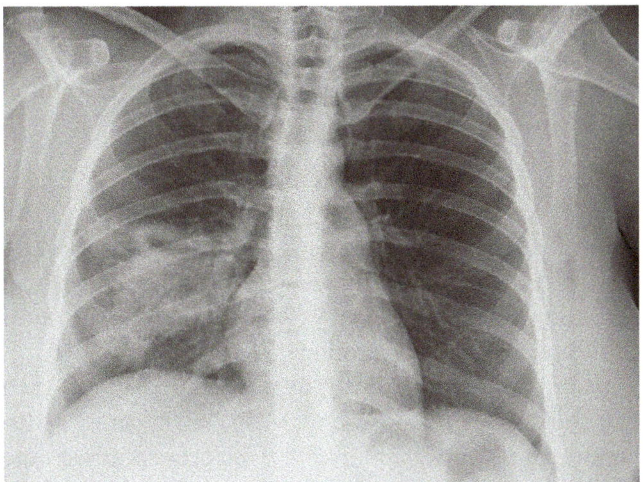

Fig. 8: Lupoid pneumonia. Chest X-ray shows an ill-defined area of consolidation in a patient with systemic lupus erythematosus (SLE) demonstrating a lupoid pneumonia. There was prompt resolution after the use of corticosteroids.

Pathology

The lung pathology is characterized by diffuse alveolar damage, alveolar edema, hyaline membrane formation, and mononuclear inflammation. Immunoglobulin and complement may be deposited in the alveolar membrane.

Imaging

CT chest reveals ground glass opacities chiefly in the mid and lower zones with patchy areas of consolidation. A unilateral consolidated lobe may also be occasionally observed.

Treatment

Prompt use of IV corticosteroids is imperative. Methylprednisolone 1g IV daily for 3 days is followed by 40 mg TDS for 4–7 days, followed by adequate doses of oral prednisolone gradually tapered over 2 weeks. Cyclophosphamide, IV immunoglobulins and rituximab are also used in severe cases. Initially a broad spectrum antibiotic cover is warranted till a definite diagnosis is made. Inhalation of oxygen and at times ventilator support needs to be given.

Pulmonary Vascular Involvement

Pulmonary vascular involvement in SLE may take two forms: (1) alveolar hemorrhage and (2) pulmonary hypertension. Alveolar hemorrhage is related to an underlying pulmonary capillaritis. We have seen this very rarely as a presenting feature of SLE. Acutely evolving breathlessness, tachypnea, increasing hypoxia, and bilateral alveolar shadows that may be mistaken for ARDS. Tachycardia and hypotension may be present and there is a fall in the hemoglobin. Hemoptysis may or may not be present, though a BAL study shows bloodstained fluid with macrophages filled with hemosiderin. The differential diagnosis is from other causes of intra-alveolar hemorrhage, notably from Wegener's granulomatosis, and in our country, from leptospirosis. Pulsed doses of methylprednisolone 1g IV daily for 3 days followed by prednisolone given orally 1 g/kg daily slowly tapered over weeks is the treatment of choice. Cyclophosphamide can be used in conjunction with steroids. Rituximab has been tried successfully in patients who do not tolerate cyclophosphamide. Factor VIIa has been given with good effect in the presence of torrential bleeding not responding to the above therapy.

Intubation and mechanical ventilatory support is needed in severe intra-alveolar hemorrhage.

Pulmonary hypertension is caused by intimal fibrosis and sclerosis involving medium and small-sized vessels within the lungs. Though rare in our study, it has been reported in 4–14% of patients in the West with an overall mortality of 20–50% at 2 years from the time of diagnosis. It occasionally dominates the disease and rarely may be its presenting feature. Breathlessness, evidence of right ventricular hypertrophy, and right-sided heart failure are observed. X-ray chest shows clear lung fields; the pulmonary function tests may be normal. It needs to be stressed that a diagnosis of idiopathic pulmonary hypertension in a young girl should not be accepted without doing relevant tests for SLE. Echocardiography may demonstrate right ventricular hypertrophy with pulmonary hypertension only when the disease is well advanced. In the few cases studied in our unit we noticed a definite response to corticosteroids. Perhaps this is observed only when steroids are used in the early part of the natural history of this complication. Vasodilator therapy with Bosentan, Sildenafil and prostacyclin may benefit some patients with pulmonary hypertension. When severe irreversible pulmonary hypertension is the dominant feature of SLE, a lung transplant should be considered.

Thromboembolic Disease

Patients with SLE are at greater risk for thromboembolic disease.

Antiphospholipid Antibody Syndrome

The antiphospholipid antibody syndrome shows positivity for lupus anticoagulant and the antiphospholipid antibody test. It is characterized by a tendency to thrombosis, chiefly in the veins but also in the smaller arteries. Clinical features consist of a history of multiple abortions, Raynaud's phenomenon, thrombotic episodes in veins and arteries, thrombocytopenia and a prolonged partial thromboplastin time. Thrombotic episodes in pulmonary vessels can lead to pulmonary hypertension. This syndrome is often associated with SLE.

Besides lung involvement due to the direct effects of SLE on the lungs, respiratory manifestations and pleuropulmonary complications may result from: (1) pulmonary infections to which these patients are very prone; (2) drugs used in the treatment of SLE; (3) lung complications secondary to SLE involvement of other organ systems, e.g. cardiac involvement, renal involvement, and thrombocytopenia.

Pulmonary Infections

Patients with SLE are at a great risk of pulmonary infections—bacterial, viral and opportunistic because of defects in immune responses resulting from disease and the use of immunosuppressant drugs.

Pulmonary hypertension in SLE can also be caused by hypoxemia due to severe ILD, thromboembolic disease, due to myocardial dysfunction and very rarely due to veno-occlusive disease.

■ SYSTEMIC SCLEROSIS

Involvement of the skin which may be localized or diffuse is generally the presenting feature of SSc. Nevertheless the disease often involves other organ systems, notably the heart, kidneys and the lungs. Pulmonary involvement is an important cause of morbidity and mortality. Pulmonary involvement is more likely in the presence of Scl 70 antibodies. In contrast the presence of anti-centromere antibodies (ACAs) is generally associated with limited disease without pulmonary involvement. The two main pulmonary manifestations of SSc are interstitial pneumonia and pulmonary hypertension (**Figs. 9A and B**). Other manifestations include aspiration pneumonia when there is involvement of the lower end of the esophagus in the sclerodermatous process and alveolar hypoventilation caused by very thickened tight scleroderma-affected skin over the thorax which acts as cuirass sharply restricting respiratory movements.

Interstitial Pneumonia

Interstitial pneumonia is most frequently observed in SSc—much more frequently than in any other connective tissue disease. Patients dying of SSc invariably have clinical or autopsy evidence of pulmonary fibrosis.

ILD is more frequently observed in patients with diffuse skin involvement (about 50%) than in patients with limited skin involvement. ILD may be present at the time of recognition of SSc or soon after; it may also develop later in the natural course of the disease. Rarely, it precedes the recognition of SSc by several months.

The symptoms and signs are similar to those detailed earlier. Pulmonary involvement should be suspected whenever the CO diffusion is impaired or lung functions show a mildly restrictive pattern. Lung function changes may be observed even in the presence of a normal X-ray chest. CT studies are far more sensitive in revealing interstitial pneumonia **(Figs. 9A and B)**.

In most patients with scleroderma (SSc) who develop ILD, the lung injury has the histopathological pattern of NSIP. This pattern consists of some degree of inflammation which is responsible for ground glass opacities on an HRCT of the chest and some degree of fibrosis which is evident on reticular shadowing on an HRCT chest. Some patients have a predominantly inflammatory pattern (cellular NSIP) and some a predominantly fibrotic pattern (fibrotic NSIP). Patients with fibrotic NSIP have a worse prognosis compared to those with cellular NSIP.

A UIP pattern is however observed in a minority of patients. In a study of 80 patients with SSc-ILD who had undergone an open lung biopsy, only six showed a UIP pattern. The prognosis is worse when this pattern is observed in patients SSc-ILD.

Treatment is generally unsatisfactory as immuno-suppressive drugs have a poor or modest effect and may cause significant toxicity.

Asymptomatic patients should be monitored clinically, as also by periodic lung function tests and imaging without using specific therapy.

Patients who are symptomatic, have declining pulmonary functions with clear evidence of ILD on imaging and no evidence of infection should be offered immunosuppressive therapy. The drugs used are mycophenolate mofetil (MMF), cyclophosphamide and azathioprine. The recommendation is to initiate treatment with mycophenolate in preference to cyclophosphamide because the former can be given on a long-term basis and has a better safety profile *(Ref: Mahler DA, Weinberg DH, Wells CK, et al. The measurement of dyspnea. Contents, interobserver agreement, and physiologic correlates of two new clinical indexes. Chest. 1984;85:751).* The duration of MMF therapy is generally about 2 years or even more depending on the patient's response.

As an alternative to MMF, cyclophosphamide may be used either intravenously once monthly for 6 monthly or orally daily for close to year with monitoring of the urine, CBC and renal function. After the above course, MMF or azathioprine is given as maintenance therapy till the disease stabilizes or improves. Once the improvement has leveled, gradual withdrawal of therapy should be initiated.

Role of Corticosteroids

Prednisolone 30–40 mg/day may be of temporary benefit in patients showing well-marked ground glass densities on an HRCT of the chest. Current opinion suggests that

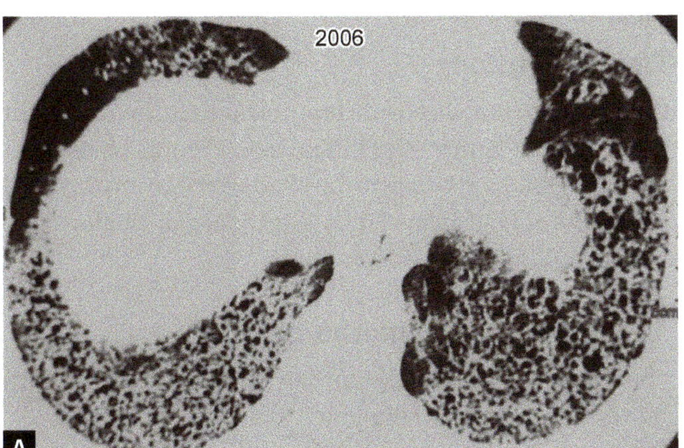
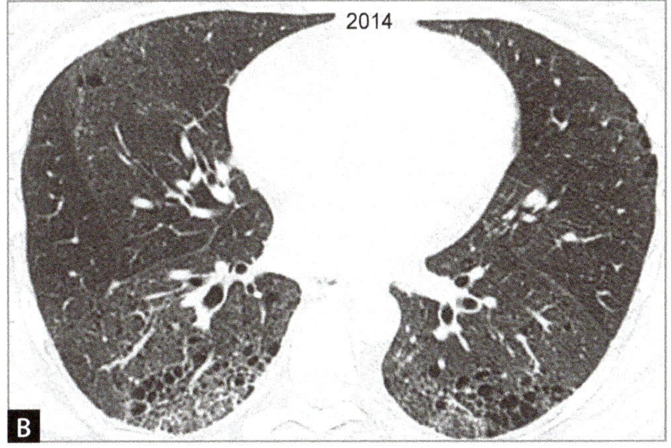

Figs. 9A and B: Systemic sclerosis. Interstitial pneumonia in a patient with systemic sclerosis. (A) There is extensive reticular thickening with honeycomb cysts and bronchiolectasis in both lung bases posteriorly. (B) Resolution of interstitial pneumonia following treatment with corticosteroids, the previously visualized extensive reticular opacities have resolved now with only residual honeycomb cysts.

corticosteroids may be used in a smaller dose (5 to 10 mg) as an adjuvant to the immunosuppressive therapy described above rather than as a primary drug.

The patient is monitored clinically as also with regard to exercise tolerance and pulmonary functions every 3 months. HRCT chest may be required as and when necessary.

Patients who are unresponsive to the above treatment may be offered a trial with rituximab. Experimental modalities for SSc-ILD include the use of pirfenidone, nintedanib and hematopoietic stem cell transplantation. Lung transplantation is the last resort in refractory patients, provided they meet the necessary requirements for lung transplant surgery.

Pulmonary Vascular Disease

Pulmonary hypertension is the most common feature. Pulmonary thromboembolism and rarely pulmonary hemangiomatosis and pulmonary veno-occlusive diseases are also observed.

Pulmonary Hypertension

Pulmonary hypertension (like interstitial pneumonia) is more frequently associated with SSc than with any other connective tissue disease. It is estimated to occur in 10–15% of scleroderma patients. Patients with long-standing scleroderma are at greater risk as also those with localized skin involvement, in particular patients with the CREST (calcinosis, Raynaud's phenomenon, esophageal dysmotility, sclerodactyly, and telangiectasia) syndrome. It is of interest that there is histological evidence of pulmonary vasculopathy in 65% of patients with limited SSc although about 10% develop overt pulmonary hypertension for life.

Pulmonary arterial hypertension due to disease localized to the small muscular pulmonary arterioles is indistinguishable in clinical features, natural history, and prognosis from idiopathic pulmonary hypertension. Dyspnea on exertion is the most common symptom, but early PAH may be asymptomatic.

Pulmonary hypertension in patients with SSc may be associated independently with ILD. The severity of ILD in these patients is not enough to cause hypoxia vasoconstriction and pulmonary hypertension.

Pulmonary hypertension can also result from hypoxemia caused by severe ILD as also secondary to scleroderma related myocardial dysfunction. Pulmonary vascular disease, hypoxemia from ILD and scleroderma induced myocardial dysfunction may all exist in different combinations in the same patient. Advanced pulmonary hypertension is characterized by right ventricular angina, increasing breathlessness and syncope on exertion. Clinical and ECHO evidence of right ventricular hypertrophy is present.

Finally, very rarely pulmonary hypertension with centrilobular nodular ground glass opacities may have pulmonary veno-occlusive disease and/or pulmonary capillary hemangiomatosis (*see* below).

Survival rates of SSc in patients with pulmonary hypertension due to vascular disease involving pulmonary arterioles is the same as in patients with idiopathic pulmonary hypertension (a 2-year survival rate of 50%).

Pulmonary Thromboembolic Disease

In a large cohort study, pulmonary thromboembolism was shown to be significantly more frequent in patients with SSc compared to the healthy adult population.

Pulmonary capillary hemangiomatosis (PCH) and pulmonary veno-occlusive disease are rare complications in SSc. Perhaps these two diseases form a spectrum of the same disease than two separate entities. They should be suspected when in a patient with pulmonary edema the pulmonary artery pressure is high and pulmonary capillary wedge pressure is normal or low.

Other Pulmonary Complications of Systemic Sclerosis

Pleural Effusion

Pleural effusion due to sclerodermatous involvement of the pleura is rare—less than 10%. Pleural effusion in scleroderma can however be secondary to myocardial dysfunction (LVF) caused by scleroderma, pneumonia, PCH-PVOD and lung cancer.

Spontaneous Pneumothorax

Spontaneous pneumothorax can occur in patients with ILD due to rupture of subpleural blebs.

Recurrent Aspiration

Esophageal dysmotility and gastroesophageal reflux disease (GERD) are present in many patients with scleroderma. This can lead to aspiration of gastric and pharyngeal contents resulting in aspiration pneumonia. Small frequent recurrent aspirations may lead to centrilobular fibrosis, thereby worsening ILD caused by scleroderma.

Hypercapnic Respiratory Failure

When the skin over the thorax is thick and tight because of sclerodermatous involvement, respiratory movements may be markedly restricted. Alveolar hypoventilation with hypercapnic respiratory failure may follow.

Airways Disease

Airflow limitation, bronchiolitis obliterans, follicular bronchiolitis (usually a minor feature in patients with interstitial pneumonia) and bronchiectasis are all less common features in SSc.

Lung Cancer

The risk of lung cancer is increased in patients with SSc, particularly in those patients who have ILD. This risk is independent of the risk associated with cigarette smoking.

■ DERMATOMYOSITIS, POLYMYOSITIS

This is an inflammatory connective tissue disorder involving the skin and the muscles. There is generally symmetrical skeletal muscle weakness. Difficulty in swallowing is due to weakness of pharyngeal muscles and this may precede, accompany or follow weakness of the proximal muscles of the upper and lower limbs. In about 10% of patients, PM and DM present as a paraneoplastic syndrome consequent to an underlying malignancy within the body. Autoantibodies are frequently present in this connective tissue disorder. Antisynthetase (anti-Jo) antibodies when present are often associated with interstitial pneumonia. Pulmonary complications are chiefly due to muscle weakness and to interstitial pneumonia leading to interstitial pulmonary fibrosis.

Complications due to Muscle Weakness

Weakness of pharyngeal muscles causes difficulty in swallowing with a risk of aspiration pneumonia. In fact, dysphagia may be the very first symptom of polymyositis, prompting repeated upper GI scopies until the true cause of dysphagia is finally identified. The patient may be unable to protect the airway; when this is well-marked a tracheostomy may be necessary to keep the airway patent and prevent aspiration. When muscle weakness involves the intercostal muscles and occasionally the diaphragm there is risk of hypoventilation causing both hypoxia and hypercapnia (hypercapnic respiratory failure). An increase in respiratory rate, a progressive fall in the tidal volume, in the vital capacity and in the maximal inspiratory force, are pointers to impending danger. Hypercapnic respiratory failure may develop in up to 5% of patients with DM/PM due to respiratory muscle weakness from muscle inflammation.

Interstitial Pneumonia

Interstitial pneumonia is commonly observed, particularly in the presence of antisynthetase antibodies. It is critical to note that interstitial pneumonia may be the first manifestation of DM or PM and may precede skin manifestations and/or muscle weakness by months or rarely by a few years. This happens in about 20% of patients with this connective tissue disorder. In these circumstances the interstitial pneumonia is often diagnosed as idiopathic or cryptogenic **(Fig. 10)**. The presence of autoantibodies and in particular of antisynthetase antibodies should forewarn of the future evolution of skin or muscle manifestations. The pattern of ILD in PM/DM is heterogeneous with a recent study of 22 biopsied patients demonstrating NSIP in the majority (82%) with the remainder having diffuse alveolar damage or organizing pneumonia. Many other series have confirmed a significant prevalence of organizing pneumonia in PM/DM.

Rarely, the interstitial pneumonia presents acutely or subacutely with cough, rapidly progressive dyspnea, rapidly evolving crackles all over the lungs and with increasing hypoxemic respiratory failure. The clinical features resemble an acute interstitial pneumonia and more often than not the course is inexorably downhill, unresponsive to all therapy.

Treatment

Patients with DM or PM who are asymptomatic and have very little disturbance in lung function should be carefully monitored and not given specific treatment.

Those who develop symptomatic ILD with significant and deteriorating lung function are given prednisolone 1 mg/kg body weight per day. We generally prefer not to

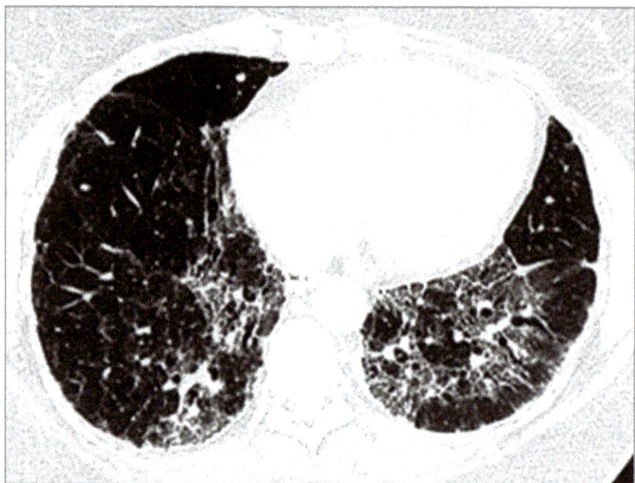

Fig. 10: Dermatomyositis. HRCT chest demonstrates ill-defined areas of ground-glass densities in both lung bases with subpleural and peribronchovascular interstitial thickening; there is also traction bronchiectasis secondary to the peribronchial interstitial thickening. There are also areas of air trapping interspersed between the areas of interstitial thickening.

exceed 40 mg/day, though one could increase the dose to a maximum of 60 mg/day. If the response to corticosteroids is poor or if a 'flare' occurs on a slow reduction of the dosage, another immunosuppressive drug is added, either azathioprine or mycophenolate. Some physicians prefer to add a second immunosuppressive agent from the very onset in symptomatic patients with significant impairment of respiratory function. If in the above situation there is no response to glucocorticoids and azathioprine or mycophenolate, tacrolimus may be substituted as the second agent in place of azathioprine or mycophenolate.

Patients with rapidly progressive disease or those who present with a fulminant acute interstitial pneumonia (of the Hamman-Rich type) should be given IV methyl prednisolone 1 g daily for 3 to 5 days followed by 60 mg prednisolone orally till the disease is controlled. Many prefer to add a second immunosuppressive, preferably cyclophosphamide in the above situation.

When ILD in DM or PM is refractory to glucocorticoid plus either azathioprine or mycophenolate, rituximab should be given in place azathioprine or mycophenolate. Alternatively IV immunoglobulins can be added to glucocorticoid therapy.

Patients receiving more than 20 mg/day of prednisolone plus another immunosuppressive agents should receive prophylaxis against pneumocystis jirovecii infection. *This*

holds not only for patients with DM, PM but for all patients with any connective tissue disease with ILD who receive the above mentioned immunosuppressants.

All patients with connective tissue disease with ILD should be vaccinated against the pneumococcus (once in 6 years) and with the influenza vaccine every year.

■ MIXED CONNECTIVE TISSUE DISEASE

As the name signifies this connective tissue disease partakes of more than one of the connective tissue disorders discussed above. It is also termed the "overlap syndrome". Thus, features of SLE may be associated with those of SSc and/or DM or PM. It is therefore difficult to semantically label such patients as belonging to one single connective tissue disorder. Mixed connective tissue disease is generally characterized by antibodies in high titer to nuclear ribonucleoprotein antigen.

Pulmonary manifestations are common in the overlap syndrome. Pleural involvement takes the form of pleural effusion. Pulmonary involvement is chiefly characterized by interstitial pneumonia, generally NSIP. Organizing pneumonia with or without involvement of the respiratory bronchioles though rare may also occur. Intra-alveolar hemorrhage due to pulmonary capillaritis (as in SLE) has also been observed. Perhaps the most dreaded complication is of rapidly progressive pulmonary hypertension due to intimal fibrosis and medial hypertrophy affecting medium-sized pulmonary arterioles. The clinical features and course of pulmonary hypertension are indistinguishable from idiopathic pulmonary hypertension. Increasing interstitial fibrosis may contribute to or may itself be responsible for pulmonary hypertension in some patients. Mixed connective tissue disease which has features of SLE may be associated with antiphospholipid antibodies. Pulmonary thromboembolic complications can then occur, and if extensive can lead to crippling pulmonary hypertension.

Interstitial lung disease in patients with mixed connective tissue is treated primarily with corticosteroids as outlined under dermatomyositis and polymyositis. A poor response or a flare of the disease on attempted reduction of corticosteroids merits the added use of azathioprine or mycophenolate.

Rarely in the presence of a very rapid deterioration of respiratory function as in acute interstitial pneumonia of the Hamman-Rich type, IV methyl prednisolone 1 g daily for 3 to 5 days followed by 60 mg prednisolone daily becomes necessary. A second immunosuppressive agent, as for example cyclophosphamide is also added to achieve better control. Opportunistic infections and toxic effects of the drugs used are often encountered in these patients.

SJÖGREN'S SYNDROME

This autoimmune disorder may occur as a primary disorder or is secondary to any one of the other connective tissue disorders. It affects the exocrine glands at different sites within the body, causing diminished glandular secretions and a drying of the mucosa. It typically involves the lacrimal glands leading to dry eyes which fail to secrete tears, and the salivary glands leading to a diminished salivary secretion. This may be so marked as to cause difficulty in swallowing. Upper and lower airways involvement may take the form of nasal mucosal infiltration with dryness (rhinitis sicca), lymphocytic infiltration of the tracheobronchial submucosal glands (xerotrachea) and lymphocytic subepithelial bronchial and bronchiolar infiltration. Tracheal disease is one of the most common respiratory manifestations in Sjögren's syndrome. It usually takes the form of xerotrachea, with loss of mucous secretions secondary to atrophy of tracheobronchial mucous glands. Patients present with a dry irritating cough and endobronchial inflammation on bronchoscopic biopsy. This dryness also predisposes these patients to recurrent bronchial infections which occur in about 20% of patients.

Pulmonary parenchymal manifestations have been reported in the primary and secondary forms of the disease. They include the different forms of interstitial pneumonia and lymphocytic interstitial pneumonia. Lymphoproliferative disorders may take the form of lymphomatoid granulomatosis or B-cell non-Hodgkin's lymphoma **(Fig. 11)**. In secondary Sjögren's syndrome, the pulmonary manifestations are influenced by the coexisting connective tissue disorders.

Treatment includes the use of glucocorticoids, hydroxychloroquine, conventional DMARDS like methotrexate, azathioprine, leflunomide and also drugs like cyclophosphamide and rituximab.

ANKYLOSING SPONDYLITIS

Ankylosing spondylitis is a seronegative spondyloarthritis involving the sacroiliac joints, the spine and the large joints, chiefly of the lower limbs. The majority of patients with this disease are HLAB27-positive though the incidence of

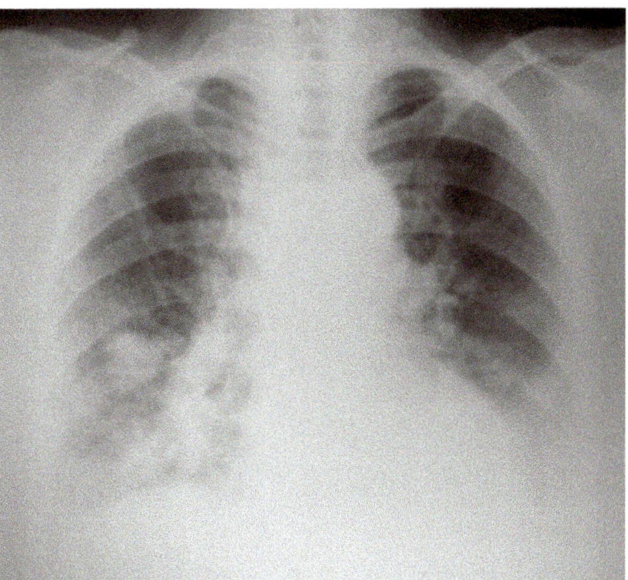

Fig. 11: Sjögren's syndrome (B-cell lymphoma). Chest X-ray demonstrates a well-defined mass lesion in the right lower zone which on CT-guided biopsy revealed a lymphoma.

this positivity in Indians is not as high as is reported in the West. The disease is also characterized by the occurrence of uveitis in 20%, aortic incompetence (in 10%), and a symptomatic inflammation of the thoracic aorta (10–15%).

Pulmonary complications take the form of bilateral upper lobe fibrosis with upward retraction of the hila. Bullous areas or cavities may be associated with the upper lobe fibrosis, so that a wrong diagnosis of pulmonary tuberculosis is often made. A fungal ball, chiefly an aspergilloma may be present in a bulla or a cavity. The aspergilloma may be silent or cause hemoptysis. Rarely, the hemoptysis is exsanguinating and can result in death **(Fig. 12)**.

In advanced ankylosing spondylitis chest excursions are markedly restricted due to fusion of the costovertebral joints and ankylosis of the thoracic spine; this leads to alveolar hypoventilation and hypercapnic respiratory failure. The limited chest movements, together with restricted cough also predispose to atelectasis and pulmonary infection.

There is no treatment for upper lobe fibrosis; corticosteroids are generally ineffective. The use of NSAIDs is suggested only when the disease is symptomatic. The use of DMARDs is not generally recommended. However some studies from South Korea have shown that TNF α inhibitors (infliximab, etanercept) have been used in advanced cases, although the ASAS guidelines recommend their use

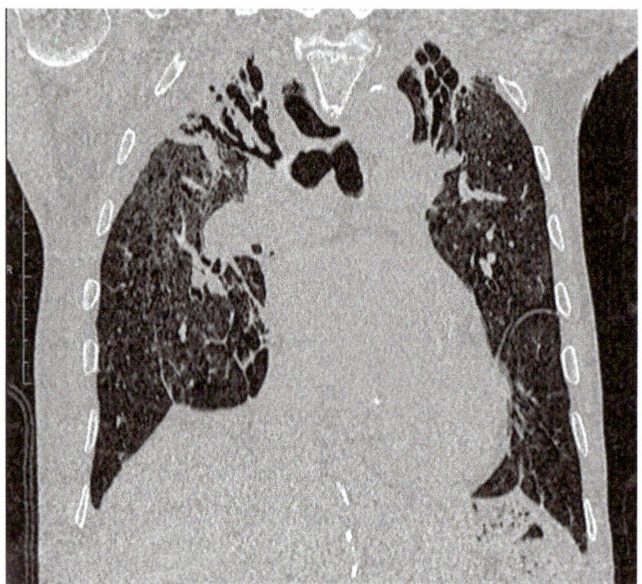

Fig. 12: Ankylosing spondylitis with fibroelastosis: Coronal CT chest demonstrates bilateral apical pleural thickening associated with fibrosis and consequent traction bronchiectasis and upward hilar retraction.

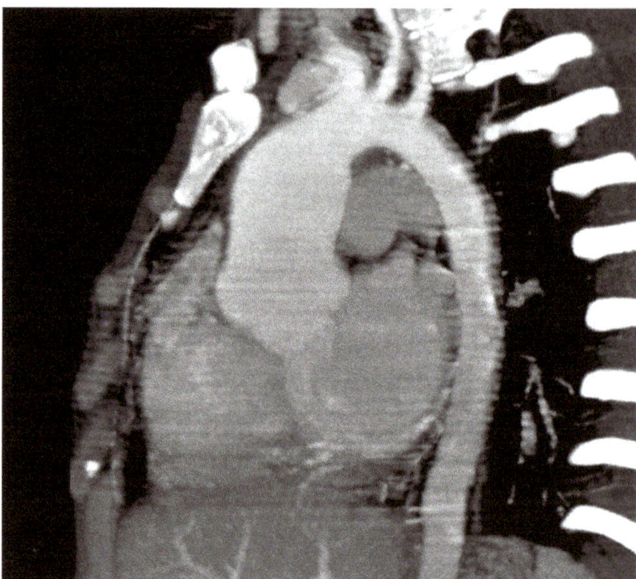

Fig. 13: Ascending aortic aneurysm in a patient with Behçet's disease.

in early disease [*Ref: Braun J, van den Berg R, Baraliakos X, et al. 2010 update of the ASAS/EULAR recommendations for the management of ankylosing spondylitis. Ann Rheu Dis. 2011;70(6):896-904*]. Hemoptysis resulting from an aspergilloma is best treated conservatively. When severe, bronchial embolism is the treatment of choice, and if this fails one may be forced into surgery, which more often than not takes the form of a lobectomy. Surgery, however, carries a high mortality and morbidity.

Hypercapnic respiratory failure may require ventilatory support; noninvasive ventilatory support is generally possible and is to be preferred.

■ BEHÇET'S DISEASE

Behçet's disease is classified by some as a form of connective tissue disorder. It is an inflammatory disorder of unknown etiology affecting blood vessels of all sizes and therefore can manifest with involvement of a number of organ systems. It is more prevalent in the Mediterranean zone and in the Far East, but is also observed in India occurring generally in the 20–30 years age group. It is often associated with HLA B5 antigen.

Its typical features are orogenital ulcers, ocular manifestations (chiefly anterior or posterior uveitis, retinitis), arthralgias and arthritis involving the large joints chiefly of the lower limbs and venous thrombophlebitis. Central nervous system involvement is fairly frequent, manifesting chiefly with headache, meningoencephalitis, cranial nerve involvement, peripheral neuropathy and seizures. Skin involvement takes the form of various forms of rashes, the disease often being first recognized in the skin department of hospitals.

Pulmonary involvement is rare and is characterized by pulmonary artery aneurysm or thromboembolic disease affecting pulmonary vessels. Chest pain, dyspnea, hemoptysis are the main symptoms. The pulmonary artery aneurysm is due to an inflammatory weakening of the vessel wall. Thromboembolic disease is due to inflammation of the pulmonary arterioles, leading to multiple pulmonary thrombi with pulmonary infarction. Thromboembolic disease requires the use of anticoagulants; the latter can however lead to catastrophe in patients with a pulmonary artery aneurysm. Corticosteroids and immunosuppressants form the mainstay of therapy. Just as involvement of the pulmonary artery wall can lead to an aneurysmal dilatation of the pulmonary artery, involvement of the aortic wall can lead to an aneurysm of the aorta **(Fig. 13)**.

The Hughes-Stovin syndrome is considered by some to be a variant of Behçet's disease. It is characterized by the presence of a pulmonary artery aneurysm, systemic venous thrombosis often involving the vena cava and causing a rise in the intracranial pressure, but no other extrapulmonary features generally associated with Behçet's disease.

■ SUGGESTED READING

1. Andrade C, Mendonca T, Farinha F, et al. Alveolar hemorrhage in systemic lupus erythematosus: a cohort review. Lupus. 2016;25:75.
2. Carrera GL, Hernan BG. Pulmonary manifestations of collagen diseases. Arch Bronconeumol. 2013;49: 249.
3. Kim EJ. Rheumatoid arthritis-associated interstitial lung disease: the relevance of histopathologic and radiographic pattern. Chest. 2009;136(5):1397-405.
4. Kim JS, Lee KS, Koh EM, et al. Thoracic involvement of systemic lupus erythematosus: clinical, pathologic, and radiologic findings. J Comput Assist Tomogr. 2000;24:9.
5. Massey H, Darby M, Edey A. Thoracic complications of rheumatoid disease. Clin Radiol. 2013;68:293.
6. Munoz ML, Gelber AC, Houston BA. Into thin air: shrinking lung syndrome. Am J Med. 2014;127:711.
7. Navarro-Zarza JE, Alvarez-Hernandez E, Casasola-Vargas JC, et al. Prevalence of community-acquired and nosocomial infections in hospitalized patients with systemic lupus erythematosus. Lupus. 2010;19:43.
8. Parambil JG. Diffuse alveolar damage: uncommon manifestation of pulmonary inolvement in patients with connective tissue disease. Chest. 2006;130(2):553-8.
9. Vij R, Strek ME. Diagnosis and treatment of connective tissue disease-associated interstitial lung disease. Chest. 2013;143:814.
10. Huh WJ. Two distinct clinical types of interstitial lung disease associated with polymyositis-dermatomyositis. Respir Med. 2007;101(8):1761-9.
11. Woodhead F. Pulmonary complications of connective tissue diseases. Clin Chest Med. 2008;29(1):149-64, vii.

CHAPTER 58

Pulmonary Manifestations of Hepatobiliary and Pancreatic Diseases

■ CHRONIC HEPATIC DISEASES

The pulmonary complications of chronic liver disorders may involve the pleura, the pulmonary vasculature or the pulmonary parenchyma.

Pleural effusions particularly in the right pleural space are common. They are secondary to ascites present in liver cirrhosis. Fenestrations within the domes of diaphragm (in particular the right dome) allow ascitic fluid entry into the pleural space. The pleural effusion is a transudate; it could be mild, moderate or massive. Hypoalbuminemia present in liver cell dysfunction reduces plasma oncotic pressure and contributes to the formation of the transudate.

The Budd-Chiari syndrome characterized by hepatic vein thrombosis is a rare but often missed cause of a recurrent pleural effusion. The effusion is a transudate, large, often right-sided and recurs quickly on being tapped. The diagnosis is occasionally stumbled upon when liver functions show some degree of derangement. The TIPS (transjugular intrahepatic portosystemic shunt) procedure, if successfully performed is the treatment of choice. The portosystemic shunt decongests the systemic veins and thereby stops accumulation of fluid within the pleural space.

The most dangerous though infrequent complications in chronic liver disease are the hepatopulmonary syndrome (HPS) and portopulmonary hypertension.

■ HEPATOPULMONARY SYNDROME

This syndrome is observed in patients with cirrhosis of the liver with portal hypertension. It can occur in all forms of cirrhosis including Wilson's disease. It has also been reported in non-cirrhotic portal hypertension, chronic active hepatitis, biliary cirrhosis and primary biliary atresia. The HPS is believed to be present in a quarter of patients with cirrhosis.

Clinical Features

There is a background of liver disease, both clinically and on liver function tests. Spider nevi are invariably present and are markers of spider nevi in the lungs and on the pleural surface, known to be present in these patients.

Breathlessness on exertion is the cardinal symptom. It is related to hypoxia which in some patients is so marked as to cause clinically evident central cyanosis. Clubbing is an early feature and in advanced cases is severe. Interestingly, these patients suffer from platypnea, the patient being increasingly breathless in the standing position and less in the supine position. Another characteristic finding in the HPS is orthodexia which is defined as a significant decrease in the PaO_2 ($PaO_2 < 3$ mm but often up to 30 mm Hg) when the patient moves from the supine to the standing posture. For reasons to be shortly explained, inhalation of oxygen does not bring complete relief and in severe cases hypoxia persists even when oxygen is delivered at high flow rates. Death occurs from hypoxic respiratory failure.

Not all cases are very severe and probably not all cases get progressively worse. Also, not all patients with this syndrome are so severely hypoxic as to be clinically cyanosed. *The combination of cirrhosis of the liver with a PaO_2 less than 55 mm Hg should suggest a HPS. The association of portal hypertension, cutaneous spider nevi and clubbing is also suggestive of the HPS and should necessitate further tests.*

Pathology

The typical feature of the HPS (seen at autopsy) is a marked dilatation of pulmonary precapillary and capillary vessels as also a marked increase in the number of dilated vessels. A few pleural and pulmonary arteriovenous shunts may also be observed.

Pathogenesis

The reasons for the dilatation of the pulmonary vessels are a subject of research. Two mechanisms causing pulmonary dilatation have been proposed.

- Increased bacterial translocation in patients with cirrhosis and portal hypertension may stimulate the release of vasoactive mediators like nitrous oxide (NO) and tumor necrosis factor-α (TNF-α) resulting in pulmonary dilatation and angiogenesis.
- Failure of a damaged liver to clear circulating vasodilators added perhaps failure to inhibit circulating vasoconstrictors.

Pathophysiology

The hypoxia and the associated breathlessness in the HPS are due to several factors of which the first two listed below are the most important.

- *Ventilation/perfusion abnormality*: This syndrome is characterized by a marked hyperdynamic circulation with marked dilation of the precapillary and capillary vessels perfusing the alveoli. The perfusion is both quick (hyperdynamic) and excessive in relation to ventilation so that there is fall in the ventilation/perfusion (V/Q) ratio of alveoli so perfused. In fact, the hemodynamics in the HPS is characterized by tachycardia, increased cardiac output, reduced pulmonary vascular resistance and a normal or low pulmonary artery pressure.
- Some patients with this syndrome develop new vessels within the lungs which shunt the unoxygenated blood to the left without allowing it to perfuse the alveoli— this results in an intrapulmonary right to left shunt, proven by the inability of 100% oxygen to abolish the alveolar arterial oxygen gradient. On 100% oxygen many patients with the HPS will have a PaO_2 of less than 300 mm Hg.
- The syndrome is also known to be associated at times with a thickening of the walls of the dilated pulmonary vessels, causing a diffusion defect that adds to hypoxia.
- One other reason for hypoxia is a diffusion-perfusion defect. With the increased dilatation and width of precapillary vessels, oxygen molecules have a difficult

time reaching the center of the mixed venous stream. Mid-stream erythrocytes fail to oxygenate, leading to a varying degree of hypoxia.

- Finally, hypoxemia may be increased by the decreased transit time of blood through the hyperdynamic pulmonary circulation, not allowing enough time for oxygen to reach the mid-stream *red blood cells* (RBCs) within the pulmonary capillaries.

Pulmonary Functions

Pulmonary function tests should be done to help exclude other causes of hypoxia (for example, COPD). In the HPS the lung functions are normal except for a CO diffusion which is mildly, moderately or even severely reduced. However, a normal CO diffusion does not exclude the diagnosis.

Imaging

X-ray chest, HRCT chest are of no help in diagnosis, but may help to exclude other pathologies that could cause hypoxia.

Diagnosis

The diagnosis of HPS can be made if all of the following criteria have been fulfilled and other etiologies have been excluded.

- The presence of liver disease with or without portal hypertension
- Proof of impaired oxygenation (hypoxia)—a lowered PaO_2 and an increase in the alveolar-arterial oxygen gradient as is described below
- Proof of pulmonary vascular abnormalities (**Figs. 1 and 2**).

Impaired Oxygenation (Hypoxia)

The definition of hypoxia varies with different authors. We would consider a PaO_2 less than 70 mm Hg breathing room air as hypoxia.

Many western experts have given the following criteria for hypoxia.

- A PaO_2 less than 80 mm Hg; a PaO_2 less than 70 mm Hg in those more than or equal to 65 years
- An alveolar arterial gradient more than 15 mm Hg. In patients more than or equal to 65 years; an alveolar arterial gradient more than 20 mm Hg or more than age adjusted value is also acceptable.

Blood gases are estimated with the patient in the sitting posture on room air. A careful estimation of PaO_2

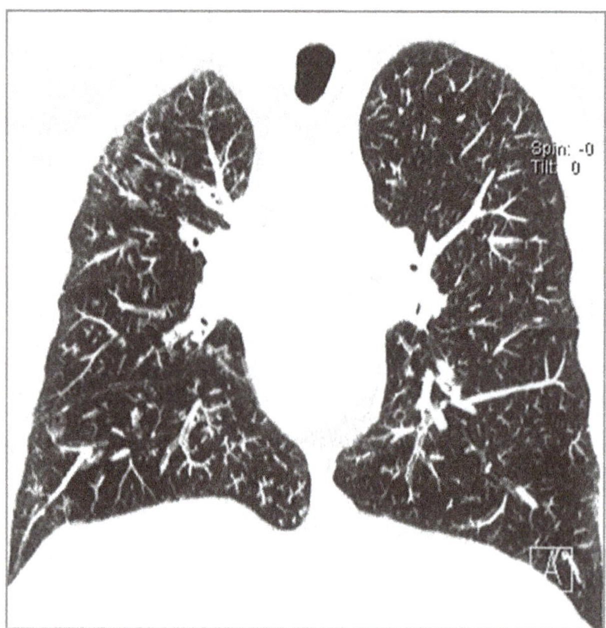

Fig. 1: Patient with hepatopulmonary syndrome.
Note: Vessels extending up to the subpleural space due to arteriovenous (AV) shunting.

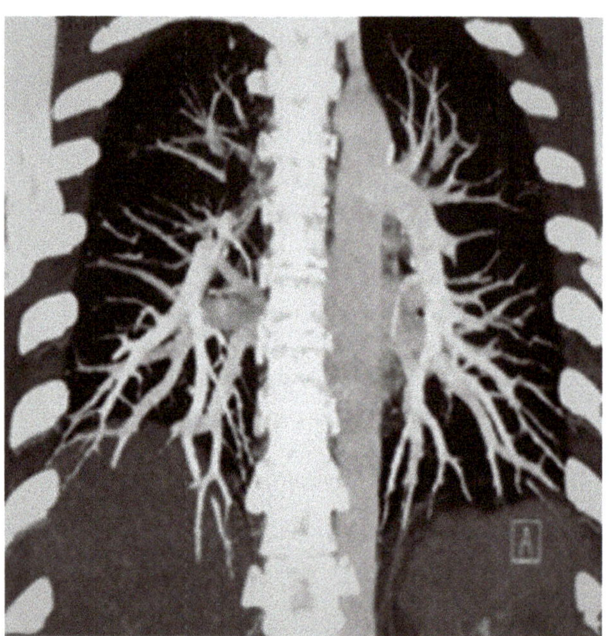

Fig. 2: Patient with hepatopulmonary syndrome.
Note: Vessels extending to the subpleural space due to arteriovenous (AV) shunting.

in the supine and standing posture could help prove the presence or absence of orthodexia.

Pulse oximetry is useful in evaluating patients with HPS with a reported sensitivity and specificity of 100% and 80% respectively when a cutoff less than 96% is used.

Pulmonary Intravascular Abnormalities

- The simplest and the most reliable method of proving the presence of intrapulmonary shunts due to changes in pulmonary vasculature in the HPS is by performing a *transthoracic contrast echocardiography (TTCE)*. This test is performed by injecting contrast (usually agitated saline) intravenously during echocardiography. Under normal circumstances the contrast opacifies only the right atrium and ventricle because it is filtered by the pulmonary capillary bed. However in the presence of a right to left pulmonary shunt or a right to left atrial shunt, the contrast opacifies the left heart chambers, appearing in the left heart three to eight beats after its appearance in the right atrium in the presence of an intrapulmonary shunt (as in the HPS) and appearing in the left atrium within one cycle of its appearance in the right atrium if there is an intracardiac shunt.

- A perfusion scan using Technetium-labeled macroaggregated albumin reveals an increased uptake in the brain (>6%) after lung perfusion. This again points to a quickened dilated pulmonary circulation with an intrapulmonary shunt.

- Pulmonary angiography may delineate the vascular abnormalities in this syndrome. Two angiographic patterns have been reported. Type 1 diffuse vascular abnormalities which may be mild or marked; and type II focal vascular abnormalities.

Pulmonary angiography may however miss small arteriovenous malformations that are indirectly demonstrated by contrast-enhanced echocardiography and technetium macroaggregated albumin perfusion scans.

Once a diagnosis of HPS has been made the severity of the disease should be graded. The following grading system has been recommended.

In patients with an alveolar-arterial gradient more than 15 mm Hg (>20 mm Hg in those > 65 years) the disease is considered

Mild: $PaO_2 \geq 80$ mm Hg, breathing room air

Moderate: $PaO_2 \geq 60$ mm Hg and < 80 mm Hg, breathing room air

Severe: $PaO_2 \geq 50$ mm Hg and < 60 mm Hg, breathing room air

Very severe: $PaO_2 < 50$ mm Hg breathing room air or a $PaO_2 < 300$ mm Hg while breathing 100% oxygen.

Management

The only definitive treatment is a liver transplant. One could embolize some of the right to left shunts provided these could be demonstrated by pulmonary angiography and provided they do not show a very diffuse distribution.

■ PORTOPULMONARY HYPERTENSION

Portopulmonary hypertension is characterized by an obstruction to the pulmonary vasculature caused by extensive intimal fibrosis and by medial hypertrophy of the pulmonary arterioles. Portosystemic and portopulmonary collaterals could transport vasomotor factors like, for example, endothelin-1 to the pulmonary circulation causing pulmonary vasoconstriction. Thrombosis occurring in situ within the pulmonary vessels adds to pulmonary hypertension. Clinically, the pulmonary second sound is loud, a right ventricular heave is present, and a wave in the jugular pulse is prominent. Right ventricular failure is the end result.

Transthoracic Doppler echocardiography should identify pulmonary hypertension. Increased right ventricular systolic pressure more than 50 mm Hg suggests the diagnosis. A right heart catheter study is generally performed for confirmation. A mean pulmonary artery pressure more than 25 mm Hg and pulmonary vascular resistance more than 240 dyn-s/cm^5 are definitive criteria for pulmonary hypertension.

Calcium channel blockers, ambrisentan (a selective endothelium antagonist) and phosphodiesterase type 5 inhibitors such as sildenafil and tadalafil are currently in use with some degree of temporary relief. Prostacyclin analogs (epoprostenol) are given IV continuously. Treprostinil is available for subcutaneous or inhalational administration.

The prognosis in patients with cirrhosis of the liver and portopulmonary hypertension is grim. In selected cases liver transplantation has restored liver function and reduced significantly the associated portal hypertension.

Pulmonary Hypertension in Liver Disease

Pulmonary hypertension can exist in three forms:
1. Passive pulmonary hypertension which is a feature of the generalized hyperdynamic circulation in a number of patients with cirrhosis of the liver.
2. Passive pulmonary hypertension which is marked, in association with the HPS.
3. Obstructive pulmonary hypertension due to widespread intimal fibrosis of the pulmonary vessels. This form is rare and indistinguishable from idiopathic pulmonary hypertension.

Portosystemic anastomosis: A marked portosystemic anastomosis in patients with cirrhosis can cause clinically detectable cyanosis with clubbing of nails.

Hepatic Hydrothorax

Hepatic hydrothorax (HH) is the accumulation of more than 500 mL fluid in patients with liver disease (generally liver cirrhosis) in the absence of cardiac or pulmonary disease. It is observed in close to 10% of patients with end-stage liver disease and is due to defects in the diaphragm that allow fluid within the peritoneal cavity to enter the pleural space helped perhaps by the negative pressure within the intrapleural space.

It occurs generally in the right pleural space, occasionally in the left and rarely in both spaces. The fluid is a transudate. Though usually associated with ascites, occasionally HH is a presenting feature without any ascites. This happens if there is a large defect in the diaphragm (generally the right dome) which allows fluid formed within the peritoneal space to quickly enter the pleural space. The correct diagnosis is missed if the relation of the pleural fluid to hepatic dysfunction is not realized. In these patients fluid may be large in quantity and rapidly reaccumulates after repeated thoracocentesis.

A diagnostic tap should be performed if there is fever, pleural pain or if there is suspicion of a possible other diagnosis—notably malignancy or pleural tuberculosis. Presence of a mild coagulopathy should not delay diagnostic testing.

Spontaneous Bacterial Empyema

Spontaneous bacterial empyema (SBEM) results when an existing hydrothorax becomes infected. The transudate now becomes an exudate which in a few patients turns to frank pus. The diagnosis is made if the pleural fluid has a positive culture and the polymorph count is more than 250 cells/cm^3, or if the culture is negative and polymorph count is more than 500 cells/mm^3.

The incidence of SBEM in Western literature is a little over 10% in hospitalized patients with a pleural effusion. In our experience, the incidence is much less and SBEM is only occasionally observed. The organisms commonly identified in SBEM are *Escherichia coli, Klebsiella pneumoniae, Enterococcus* species, *Streptococcus* species. Cefotaxime should be used till culture data are available. Repeated thoracocentesis may be necessary. A chest tube drainage is best avoided unless frank pus is present in the pleural space. This is because chest tube drainage is associated with serious complications from this procedure in these patients. SBEM carries a significant morbidity and a mortality of about 20%.

Management of Refractory Hydrothorax

Medical measures of salt restriction, furosemide and spironolactone may not suffice to counter both ascites and hydrothorax in more than 20–25% of patients. Refractory hydrothorax should be treated with repeated thoracocentesis. We prefer not to remove more than 1.5 L at a time and use IV albumin during the procedure, particularly in patients who to start with have a low systolic BP of less than 100 mm Hg. Large volume thoracocentesis may become imperative in patients with respiratory distress, the danger of reexpansion pulmonary edema always being present.

As mentioned earlier, tube thoracotomy is best avoided for fear of procedural complications. These include hemothorax, pneumothorax, empyema, electrolyte abnormalities, and hepatorenal failure.

Transjugular Intrahepatic Portocaval Shunt

Transjugular intrahepatic portocaval shunt (TIPS) reduces portovenous pressure by creating a shunt between the portal and hepatic veins and is believed to be the treatment of choice for refractory HH. TIPS however does not influence long-term survival rates which are determined by the severity of the liver disease. TIPS should not be advised on all patients with refractory HH. It can lead to liver cell failure in patients with hepatic decompensation and may further compromise patients with right heart failure and pulmonary hypertension. Contraindications include a MELD more than 18, pulmonary hypertension, portal vein thrombosis, hepatic encephalopathy, and elderly patients (age > 70 years).

Complications following TIPS can only be met by offering the patient a liver transplant. This should be discussed with the patient before the procedure.

Surgical Procedure

Large opening within the diaphragm, if identified have been repaired by a VATS procedure. This is often followed by pleurodesis.

Liver Transplantation

In many centers dealing with liver diseases, liver transplantation is the primary choice for the management of a large refractory hepatic hydrothorax.

■ PULMONARY PARENCHYMAL INVOLVEMENT IN PRIMARY BILIARY CIRRHOSIS

Primary biliary cirrhosis has been known to be associated with pulmonary granulomas, lymphocytic interstitial pneumonia and rarely with organizing pneumonia. Alpha-1 antitrypsin deficiency (ZZ or SZ type) can cause both liver cirrhosis and pulmonary emphysema. When either one or the other is found in a younger age group with no obvious risk factor, this genetic defect should be kept in mind.

Autoimmune hepatitis has been associated with interstitial pneumonia (UIP or NSIP).

■ FULMINANT HEPATIC FAILURE

Fulminant hepatic failure, acute hepatic failure, and acute on chronic hepatic failure are characterized chiefly by encephalopathy, coagulation defects and hyperbilirubinemia. Multiple organ failure follows, chiefly involving renal, pulmonary, cerebral, and hematological systems. Fulminant hepatic failure is associated with a hyperdynamic circulation evidenced by tachycardia, a high pulse pressure, an increased cardiac output with a low systemic vascular resistance and a low pulmonary vascular resistance. There may be a fair degree of passive pulmonary hypertension. Hypoxia is frequently present and has many causes. It could be caused by pulmonary infection, by bleeding into the lungs, by aspiration in a comatose patient, and by pulmonary edema caused by overhydration. Perhaps the most dreaded pulmonary complication is the development of acute respiratory distress syndrome (ARDS) related to increased capillary permeability. Severe ARDS occurring against the background of fulminant hepatic failure has a dreadful prognosis and is generally fatal. The pulmonary complications of hepatopulmonary disease have been listed in **Table 1**.

Table 1: Pulmonary complication in hepatobiliary diseases.

I. *Complications in association with liver cirrhosis:*
- Hydrothorax
- Spontaneous bacterial empyema
- Hepatopulmonary syndrome
- Portopulmonary hypertension
- Portosystemic shunt causing cyanosis and clubbing
- Emphysema and cirrhosis related to alpha-1 antitrypsin deficiency
- Frequent pulmonary infections
- Interstitial pneumonia (associated with chronic active hepatitis)

II. *Complications in fulminant hepatic failure or acute on chronic hepatic failure:*
- Pulmonary infections
- Aspiration pneumonia
- Pulmonary edema
- Intra-alveolar hemorrhage
- Acute respiratory distress syndrome (ARDS)

III. *Complications associated with primary biliary cirrhosis:*
- Fibrosing alveolitis
- Lymphocytic interstitial pneumonia
- Pulmonary granulomas
- Organizing pneumonia
- Bronchiectasis

◼ ACUTE PANCREATITIS

Respiratory complications are frequent in acute pancreatitis and are responsible for 50–70% of deaths. The end-result of these complications is hypoxia of varying degree. In fact, the severity of the hypoxia reflects the severity of the disease.

The respiratory features of acute pancreatitis can be classified into three groups:

Group I—Hypoxemia with a normal chest X-ray: Hypoxemia is a common and important presenting feature even in the absence of radiological shadows. The PaO_2 may fall even below 60 mm Hg. The severity of the hypoxia is directly related to the prognosis—the more severe the hypoxia, the worse the prognosis. The hypoxia is obviously related to pancreatic inflammation as it is not generally present in other similar acute abdominal conditions. The hypoxia is partly due to V/Q abnormalities and partly to an increased shunt. Though the pathogenesis is not clear, inflammatory mechanisms are responsible for causing microvascular leaks and alveolar filling. Inflammatory agents include pancreatic enzymes and elastase liberated into the systemic circulation, as also cytokines, such as IL6, TNF-α, platelet activating factor. NO-related endothelial damage has also been reported to occur. Fatty acids liberated from the inflamed pancreas may not only damage pulmonary capillaries but may shift the oxygen dissociation curve to the left, worsening hypoxia.

Group II—Hypoxemia with pleural effusion and localized abnormalities on X-ray chest: Localized radiological abnormalities are common and occur in 30–40% of patients. The more severe the pancreatitis, the more likely are local radiological abnormalities within the chest. The most common abnormality observed is a pleural effusion, generally left-sided but at times bilateral. This is invariably associated with a raised diaphragm involving chiefly the left dome, but at times to a lesser extent the right as well, so that the lung volumes seem small. A pleural effusion is a marker of the severity of the disease. It occurs in 84% of patients with severe disease and in only 8.6% of patients with mild disease. The pleural fluid on tapping is a hemorrhagic exudate with a high neutrophil count and markedly raised amylase content. The amylase in the pleural fluid is far higher than in the serum. Other radiological abnormalities include basal, segmental or even lobar atelectasis.

A rare complication is a pancreatic-pleural fistula. It occurs when the pancreatic duct or pseudocyst opens into the retroperitoneum. The fluid tracks up the mediastinum and ruptures into the pleural space causing a massive pleural effusion. The effusion requires to be tapped and will cease to recur only when the anatomical defect is surgically corrected.

Localized alveolar shadows and interstitial shadows probably reflect pulmonary edema **(Fig. 3)**. The

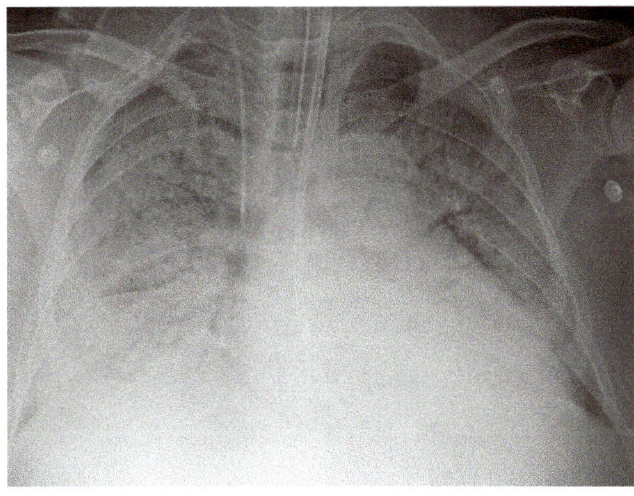

Fig. 3: Patient with acute pancreatitis having acute lung injury.

mechanism of pleural effusion as also of the pulmonary shadows is unclear. It is most likely related to the transport of the pancreatic inflammatory exudates through the diaphragm into the chest.

Group III—Hypoxemia with diffuse bilateral pulmonary shadows due to ARDS: In our unit, 15–20% of patients with acute pancreatitis develop ARDS within 3–7 days of the onset of the disease. The pathogenesis is complex and is discussed elsewhere. Perhaps liberation of pancreatic trypsin, lipase and fatty acids together with kinins may play a special role in causing the increased permeability inflammatory pulmonary edema that characterizes the syndrome. Ventilatory support is mandatory and the mortality is significantly increased in spite of good critical care **(Fig. 3)**.

■ SUGGESTED READING

1. Arguedas MR. Hepatopulmonary syndrome. Clin Lever Dis. 2005;9:733-46.
2. Golbin JM. Portopulmonary hypertension. Clin Chest Med. 2007;28:203-18.
3. Heller SJ, Noordhoek E, Tenner SM, et al. Pleural effusion as a predictor of severity in acute pancreatitis. Pancreas. 1997;15:222-5.
4. Krowka MJ, Fallon MB, Kawut SM, et al. International Liver Transplant Society Practice. Guidelines: Diagnosis and management of hepatopulmonary syndrome and portopulmonary hypertension. Transplantation. 2016;100(7):1440-52.
5. Layden TJ. Hepatic manifestation of pulmonary disease. Clin Liver Dis. 2002;6:969-79.
6. Pastor CM. Pancreatitis-associated acute lung injury: new insights. Chest. 2003;124:2341-51.
7. Polyzogopoulou E, Bikas C, Danikas D, et al. Baseline hypoxemia as a prognostic marker for pulmonary complications and outcome in patients with acute pancreatitis. Dig Dis Sci. 2004;49:150-4.
8. Raghu MG, Wig JD, Kochhar R, et al. Lung complications in acute pancreatitis. JOP. J Pancreas (Online). 2007;8(2):177-85.
9. Rockey DC, Cello JP. Pancreaticopleural fistula. Report of 7 patients and review of the literature. Medicine (Baltimore). 1990;69:332-44.
10. Zhou MT. Acute lung injury and ARDS in acute pancreatitis: mechanisms and potential intervention. World J Gastroenterol. 2010;16:2094-9.

CHAPTER 59

Pulmonary Manifestations of Renal Disease

■ INTRODUCTION

Pulmonary manifestations in renal disease may be related to renal disease per se or to the treatment of renal disease such as the use of peritoneal dialysis, hemodialysis or following a renal transplant. These pulmonary manifestations deserve serious consideration (**Table 1**).

■ PLEURAL EFFUSION

This is probably the most frequent association with renal disease. The effusion is generally a transudate and several factors may contribute toward it. In the nephrotic syndrome, a pleural transudate, often bilateral is due to

Table 1: Pulmonary associations of renal disease.	
Pulmonary manifestations	**Disease**
Pleural effusion (transudate)	Nephrotic syndrome Acute glomerulonephritis Acute renal failure Chronic renal failure (CRF) Peritoneal dialysis
Pulmonary edema	All of the above, hemodialysis
Pleural exudates	Uremic pleural inflammation
Uremic lung	CRF Long-term hemodialysis
Respiratory infections, tuberculosis, bacterial, viral, opportunistic	CRF Hemodialysis Peritoneal dialysis Renal transplant
Pulmonary alveolar hemorrhage	Pulmonary-renal syndrome
Non-Hodgkin's lymphoma	Renal transplant
Pulmonary calcification	Hemodialysis Renal transplant CRF

hypoalbuminemia resulting in a lowered oncotic pressure. Both acute and chronic renal failure and end-stage renal disease may be associated with pleural transudates caused by congestive cardiac failure and/or hypervolemia. Peritoneal dialysis is occasionally complicated by a large pleural effusion, the pleural fluid chemically resembling the peritoneal dialysate. In these cases, structural defects in the diaphragm are responsible for allowing the peritoneal dialysate to enter the pleural spaces. If the effusion is large the peritoneal dialysis should be stopped. Pleural fluid may need to be tapped. The abdominal catheter should be left in place as it helps drainage of pleural fluid. Invariably peritoneal dialysis will need to be discontinued.

Pleural exudates may also be occasionally encountered. These are due to "uremic" pleural inflammation. The effusions are generally bilateral, hemorrhagic and are often associated with pleuritic pain and a pleural rub. "Uremic'" effusions generally resolve spontaneously after some weeks. They may, however, result in pleural thickening with well-marked pleural fibrosis.

Uremic Lung

An important respiratory association of uremia is *uremic lung*—pulmonary edema with or without pneumonitis. The pulmonary edema is central; giving a typical "bat-wing" appearance on a radiological examination of the chest. The periphery of the lung remains translucent. This appearance is not specific for a uremic lung; it is also observed in chronic left ventricular failure which is a fairly frequent accompaniment of chronic renal disease and in early pulmonary edema caused by hypervolemia.

There are probably several factors responsible for the typical radiological picture of uremic lung:

- Possible fluid overload.
- Increased pulmonary artery occlusion pressure, which may also be associated with an increased right atrial pressure.
- Hypoproteinemia, more often related to poor nutrition in end-stage renal disease rather than to loss of protein in the urine.
- Impaired myocardial function.
- Increased capillary permeability.

The last factor may indeed play a major pathogenic role if hemodynamic pressure studies show normal right and left atrial pressures. Pulmonary edema fluid in some patients with uremic lung has high protein content, and increased capillary permeability to technetium-labeled diethylene triamine penta-acetic acid (DTPA) has been demonstrated in these patients.

The alveoli to start with contain fibrinous edema with swollen alveolar cells and edematous interlobular septa. If the edema persists, a fair degree of interstitial fibrosis results. The characteristic distribution of the "bat wing" edema is not well understood. It has been thought to result from diversion of blood flow to the more central parts of the lung due to peripheral vasoconstriction of the longer peripheral pulmonary vessels.

"Uremic" lung is also observed in patients on hemodialysis, particularly in patients on chronic hemodialysis. Failure to comply with fluid restriction is an important cause in these patients. If this cause is excluded the uremic lung is either related to persistent elevation of left atrial or left and right atrial pressure or due to increased capillary permeability.

Uremic lung may be associated with uremic pleurisy or with a hemorrhagic pleural exudate.

Urinoma

Ureteric rupture (from whatever cause) or a percutaneous nephrostomy may result in a retroperitoneal collection of urine which may track into the pleural space (urinothorax). Pleural fluid has an ammoniacal smell; the creatinine content is the same as in the urine and higher than in the blood.

Pulmonary Infections

Renal failure is associated with an increased risk of pulmonary infections. This is related to immune suppression from poor host defenses in patients with chronic renal disease. Besides usual bacterial and viral infections, there is an increased prevalence of tuberculosis which has a 15 times higher incidence than in the general population.

Pulmonary Complications following Renal Transplantation

Pulmonary complications may occur in as many as 15–20% of kidney allograft recipients. They are classified as being noninfectious or infectious in etiology. The most common noninfectious complication is pulmonary edema due to allograft dysfunction, generally occurring within the first month after the transplant. An increased frequency of B-cell non-Hodgkin's lymphoma which may affect the lungs has been reported in transplant patients after prolonged immunosuppressive therapy. Finally, pulmonary thromboembolism is more frequent in the post-transplant period when compared to pretransplant renal failure.

Infections are responsible for the large majority of pulmonary complications in the post-transplant period. Bacterial and cytomegalovirus infections are more frequent in the immediate post-transplant period. Opportunistic infections occur later—these include viral, nocardial, fungal infections, and infection due to *Pneumocystis*. The occurrence of pulmonary tuberculosis is several times greater than in the general population. It should be noted that renal dysfunction results in poor elimination of ethambutol and could thus add to its toxicity. Rifampicin when used in the treatment of tuberculosis may be the cause of renal dysfunction as it increases steroid catabolism and reduces the bioavailability of cyclosporin A.

■ PULMONARY HEMORRHAGE COMPLICATING RENAL DISEASE

This is often termed the pulmonary-renal syndrome and is characterized by alveolar hemorrhage and glomerulonephritis. Goodpasture's syndrome related to antiglomerular basement membrane antibodies (anti-GBM disease) is one cause of the pulmonary-renal syndrome. *The most common causes however are systemic vasculitides associated with positive antineutrophilic cytoplasmic antibodies (ANCA-positive).* These vasculitides include granulomatosis with polyangiitis (formerly called *Wegener's granulomatosis*), *microscopic polyangiitis*, and eosinophilic granulomatosis with polyangiitis (formerly called *Churg-Strauss syndrome*). Other rare systemic vasculitides (not associated with positive ANCA) have been reported to cause both pulmonary hemorrhage and glomerulonephritis. Pulmonary-renal syndrome can also occur in vasculitis associated with connective tissue disorders such as SLE, mixed connective tissue disease, scleroderma and rarely in rheumatoid disease.

Intra-alveolar bleeds have also been reported to occur in rapidly progressive glomerulonephritis and crescentic glomerulonephritis not associated with antibodies to glomerular basement membrane. Finally, drugs such as penicillamine/hydralazine have also been known to cause the pulmonary-renal syndrome.

A pulmonary-renal syndrome is suspected when there is a combination of hemoptysis due to alveolar hemorrhage and hematuria due to glomerulonephritis. The alveolar hemorrhage is confirmed radiologically by bilateral diffuse pulmonary shadows. Hypoxia, tachypnea invariably result in patients with severe intra-alveolar hemorrhage. Hemoptysis is not always present, but bronchoscopy reveals hemorrhagic fluid which on microscopy shows macrophages laden with hemosiderin. The glomerulonephritis is confirmed on a urine examination and by a renal biopsy. *In our part of the world fulminant leptospiral infection is an important cause of the pulmonary-renal syndrome* (**Table 2**).

Goodpasture's syndrome and the various ANCA-positive causes of the pulmonary-renal syndrome have been dealt with in a separate chapter.

■ METASTATIC CALCIFICATION

Metastatic calcification is commonly found at autopsy on patients with chronic kidney disease (CKD) who have been on dialysis. However, patients are generally asymptomatic. Metastatic calcification in CKD patients are due to: (1) chronic metabolic acidosis which draws out calcium and phosphorus from the bones; (2) secondary parathyroidism which draws out calcium and phosphorus from the bones. Deposition of calcium phosphate within the lungs is generally benign. The MDP bone scintigraphy can identify calcified foci within the lung.

Treatment consists in reducing the calcium phosphate product through medication and dialysis.

Very rarely extensive metastatic calcification within the lung can cause dyspnea, a restrictive physiopathology, hypoxemia, respiratory failure, and death.

■ PULMONARY HYPERTENSION

Pulmonary hypertension (PH) can complicate renal disease. The incidence of PH in CKD varies from 10–50%. Patients undergoing peritoneal dialysis have a lesser incidence of PH.

The presence of PH in CKD is associated with increased morbidity and mortality.

■ SUGGESTED READING

1. Bolton WK. Pulmonary renal syndrome and emergency therapy. Contrib Nephrol. 2010;165:166-73.
2. Conger ID, Hammond WS, Alfrey AC, et al. Pulmonary calcification in chronic dialysis patients. Clinical and pathologic studies. Ann Intern Med. 1975;83(3):330-6.
3. Kotloff RM. Noninfectious pulmonary complications of liver, heart, and kidney transplantation. Clin Chest Med. 2005;26(4):623-9, vii.
4. Papiris SA, Manali ED. Bench-to-bedside review: pulmonary-renal syndromes—an update for the intensivist. Crit Care. 2007;11(3):213.
5. Uchida M, Maeda T, Ikeda Y, et al. Acute progressive and extensive metastatic calcifications in a nephrotic patient following chronic hemodialysis. Am J Nephrol. 1995;15(5):427-30.
6. Vandermarliere A. Mycobacterial infection after renal transplantation in a Western population. Transpl Infect Dis. 2003;5(1):9-15.
7. Yigla M, Fruchter O, Aharonson D. Pulmonary hypertension is an independent predictor of mortality in hemodialysis patients. Kidney Int. 2009;75(9):969-75.
8. Zocacali C. Pulmonary hypertension in dialysis patients: a prevalent, risky but still uncharacterized disorder. Nephrol Dial Transplant. 2012;27(10):3674-7.

Table 2: Pulmonary-renal syndrome with alveolar hemorrhage.

- Goodpastures syndrome (positive for anti-GBM antibodies)
- Rapidly progressive glomerulonephritis, crescentic glomerulonephritis
  (both are negative for anti-GBM antibodies)
- Connective tissue disorders:
  - Systemic lupus erythromatosis
  - Mixed connective tissue disease
  - Scleroderma, rheumatoid disease
- Systemic vasculitides:
  - Wegener's granulomatosis
  - Microscopic polyangiitis
  - Churg-Strauss syndrome
  - Cryoglobulinemia
  - Henoch-Schönlein purpura
  - Behçet's disease
- Severe leptospiral infection
- Drug induced:
  - Penicillamine

CHAPTER 60

Pulmonary Manifestations of Inflammatory Bowel Disease

■ INTRODUCTION

Extraintestinal complications of ulcerative colitis and Crohn's disease have been known for several years. They include erythema nodosum, pyoderma granulosum, uveitis, sacroiliac arthritis, ankylosing spondylitis, hepatitis and sclerosing cholangitis. To these can now be added a number of pulmonary complications that are being increasingly reported. Both ulcerative colitis and Crohn's disease are being met with increasing frequency in our country though their incidence is not high as in the West. Pulmonary complications are rare but it is important to be aware of their possible occurrence.

Pulmonary complications have been reported much more frequently with ulcerative colitis (85%) when compared to Crohn's disease. These complications in most cases (80%) follow the inflammatory bowel disease (IBD) **(Table 1)**. Occasionally, they have been concomitant with the disease and in less than 10% of patients they may precede the bowel disease. Though pulmonary complications invariably produce overt manifestations, studies have shown the occurrence of subclinical

Table 1: Pulmonary complications in inflammatory bowel disease (IBD).

- Inflammation of the airways:
  - Upper airways-glottis
  - Tracheobronchitis
  - Bronchial stenosis
  - Bronchitis; purulent bronchitis
  - Small airways
- Bronchiolitis
- Organizing pneumonia
- Interstitial pneumonia (fibrosing alveolitis)
- Necrobiotic nodules
- Pulmonary eosinophilia (drug induced)
- Thromboembolic disease

abnormalities. These include a reduced forced expiratory volume in one second (FEV_1), small airways obstruction, and a reduced carbon monoxide transfer factor (TLCO). A subclinical lymphocytic alveolitis similar to that in sarcoidosis has been observed in Crohn's disease. Perhaps more extensive studies on the lungs in IBD may reveal the actual incidence of subclinical involvement and the natural history of this involvement.

■ INFLAMMATORY AIRWAY DISEASE

Inflammation of the airways is the most common complication of IBD. Inflammation may involve the glottis, epiglottis area, the large airways or the small airways. Rarely, the whole tracheobronchial tree is involved. Involvement of the upper airways produces cough, noisy breathing, stridor and may lead to asphyxia necessitating tracheostomy. Tracheobronchial involvement causes chronic cough which is dry or associated with mucopurulent sputum. Chronic inflammation of the airways can lead to bronchiectasis. Small airways may also be involved resulting in a diffuse inflammatory obstruction of the airways. Endoscopy reveals erythema and edema of the mucosa. Biopsy shows granulation tissue with many neutrophils together with a lymphocytic and plasma cell infiltrate. When inflammation is marked it leads to tracheal or bronchial stenosis. The histology described earlier bears a resemblance to the histology of the bowel lesion in ulcerative colitis, suggesting that a common antigen target is shared by the gut and the lung.

Bronchiolitis and Organizing Pneumonia

These are rare associations which however cannot be ignored. Bronchiolitis causes increasing breathlessness, air-trapping, a fall in the FEV_1 and a poor response to corticosteroids. Organizing pneumonia presents with fever, cough, breathlessness, and a high erythrocyte sedimentation rate (ESR) with radiological opacities. These shadows are multiple, peripherally placed and subpleural in location. The histology on biopsy is similar to organizing pneumonia observed in other conditions and the response to corticosteroids is excellent, though relapses do occur on withdrawal of steroids.

Interstitial Pneumonia (Fibrosing Alveolitis) and Vasculitis

Fibrosing alveolitis of the pattern of desquamative interstitial pneumonia is a rare but reported association of inflammatory bowel disease. The response to steroids is satisfactory. Withdrawal of sulfasalazine used in the treatment of IBD is recommended as these drugs are known to cause interstitial pneumonia in some instances.

Vasculitic lesions have been reported in ulcerative colitis. These include necrobiotic nodules within the lung with a histology resembling pyoderma gangrenosum. Patients present with fever, chest pain, dyspnea with multiple rounded parenchymal opacities on imaging. The nodules may cavitate and then resolve, leaving a residual scar. Lung nodules may be associated with necrotic ulcerating nodules within the dermis (**Fig. 1**).

■ DRUG-RELATED LUNG DISEASE

Inflammatory bowel disease patients receive several drugs for long periods of time. These can cause pulmonary complications which may be difficult to distinguish from pulmonary complications directly caused by IBD.

Sulfasalazine and mesalamine can cause eosinophilic pleuritis, eosinophilic pneumonia. Other lung pathologies related to the use of these compounds are interstitial lung disease and bronchiolitis obliterans. Patients present with dyspnea, cough, chest discomfort, and radiographic abnormalities. Asymptomatic lung injury may also be produced by these drugs. Adverse reactions generally occur 2–6 months after use, but may occur earlier. The drug reactions described earlier are reversed on withdrawal of the drug. Drug reactions to methotrexate and azathioprine have been described in a separate section.

Biologic therapy with drugs such as infliximab, adalimumab, and certolizumab are significant advances in the treatment of IBD. However, serious complications can occur. The most important is the reactivation of tuberculosis. Physicians should carefully determine any evidence of recent tuberculosis in a patient. If so, biologic therapy is contraindicated. Infliximab, other related anti-tumor necrosis factor (anti-TNF-α) drugs have been associated with pneumocystis infection as well as other infectious diseases. These include nocardiosis, aspergillosis, actinomycosis, and listeriosis, particularly in elderly patients. Histoplasmosis and coccidioidomycosis have been noted as complications in areas where these diseases are endemic. Close observation of patients treated with TNF inhibitors is warranted.

Pleuritis, Pericarditis

Western literature reports a serositis in as many as 30% of patients. The effusion is small, is an exudate and responds well to corticosteroids.

Thromboembolic Disease

The risk of thromboembolism is believed to be greater in patients with IBD. It has already been mentioned that sulfasalazine used in the treatment of IBD can by itself produce various pulmonary complications. To separate the effects of the disease per se from complications caused by drugs used to treat the disease may at times be impossibly difficult [*Ref: Xiao-Qing J, Li-Xia W, De-Gan L. Pulmonary manifestations of inflammatory bowel disease. World J Gastroenterol. 2014;20(34):13501-11*].

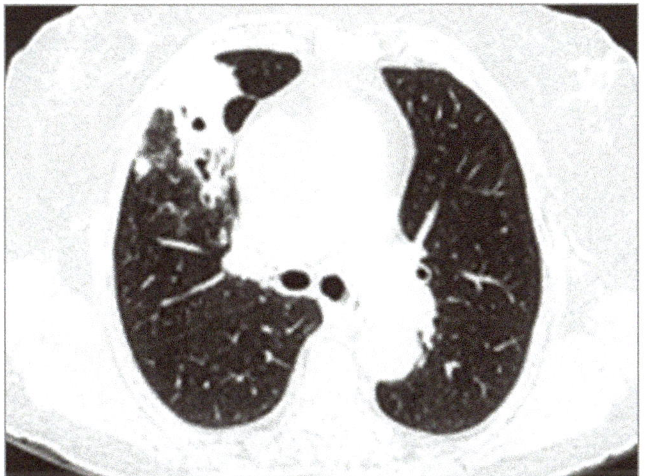

Fig. 1: CT chest demonstrates an ill-defined consolidation with cavitation representing necrobiotic nodules in a patient with Crohn's disease.

■ DIAGNOSIS AND MANAGEMENT

An acute awareness that pulmonary symptoms in IBD are often related to the latter is vital. Clinical examination and endoscopies with biopsies in patients with upper airways and tracheobronchial involvement will prove the inflammatory nature of the lesions. Imaging which should include computed tomography (CT) chest reveals parenchymal lesions of ILD, organizing pneumonia and necrobiotic nodules. Transbronchial or CT-guided biopsies may further clinch the diagnosis.

Steroids form the mainstay of management. Airways inflammation is chiefly tackled by the use of inhaled steroids. Acute inflammation may necessitate a course of oral prednisolone therapy. Parenchymal lesions within the lung respond well to oral corticosteroids. Drug toxicity should be borne in mind. Withdrawal of the offending drug leads to reversal of drug toxicity.

■ SUGGESTED READING

1. Abu-Hijleh M, Evans S, Aswad B. Pleuropericarditis in a patient with inflammatory bowel disease: a case presentation and review of the literature. Lung. 2010;188:505-10.
2. Black H, Mendoza M, Murin S. Thoracic manifestations of inflammatory bowel disease. Chest. 2007;131:524-32.
3. Foster RA, Zander DS, Mergo PJ, et al. Mesalamine-related lung disease: clinical, radiographic, and pathologic manifestations. Inflamm Bowel Dis. 2003;9:308-15.
4. Mahadeva R, Walsh G, Flower CD, et al. Clinical and radiological characteristics of lung disease in inflammatory bowel disease. Eur Respir T. 2000;15:41-8.
5. Songur N. Pulmonary function tests and high-resolution CT in the detection of pulmonary involvement in inflammatory bowel diseases. J Clin Gastroenterol. 2003;37(4):292-8.
6. Xiao-Qing J, Li-Xia W, De-Gan L. Pulmonary manifestations of inflammatory bowel disease. World J Gastroenterol. 2014;20(34):13501-11.

CHAPTER 61

Pulmonary Manifestations in Obstetric and Gynecological Conditions

■ PHYSIOLOGICAL CHANGES IN THE RESPIRATORY SYSTEM IN PREGNANCY

Breathlessness is a frequent complaint in the first trimester. It is due to hyperventilation caused by an increased ventilatory drive due to the increased concentration of progesterone. An awareness of hyperventilation is translated into a feeling of breathlessness. A degree of hyperventilation persists throughout pregnancy so that $PaCO_2$ is low and the pH may be a little on the alkaline side. The PaO_2 is normal or may show a small rise.

In the last trimester of pregnancy breathlessness is related to the effects produced by the enlarging uterus which leads to increased intra-abdominal pressure and a significant rise in the diaphragm. There is no change in the vital capacity, there is a 25% reduction in the functional residual capacity (FRC) chiefly related to a fall in the expiratory reserve volume. These changes may be observed by the sixth month of pregnancy. Expiratory flow rates are unaffected but chest wall and total pulmonary compliance are reduced in the third trimester. The T_{LCO} increases slightly during the first and second trimester; it then returns to normal in spite of changes in hemoglobin concentration and in the circulatory volume.

Though the PaO_2 as mentioned above is generally normal or slightly raised, at full term, particularly when the uterus is very large, there could be mild hypoxia with an increased alveolar-arterial O_2 gradient. When the patient is supine, this is related to premature closure of the small airways related to the reduced FRC. Oxygen consumption is increased during pregnancy being 25–30% above the normal at full term. The combination of increased oxygen consumption and reduced FRC diminishes oxygen reserve so that any emergency or catastrophe that causes apnea or alveolar hypoventilation can render both the mother and fetus dangerously hypoxic.

During labor there is further increase in tachypnea and minute ventilation (due to increased muscular effort coupled with anxiety) so that there is increasing respiratory alkalosis. Alkalosis can reduce uterine blood flow because of vasoconstriction, thereby adversely affecting fetal oxygenation. This may be of importance if fetal blood flow is already jeopardized for other reasons.

In some patients, pain during and after delivery or after cesarean section may lead to rapid shallow breathing with resultant areas of atelectasis within the lungs, leading to some degree of hypoxia. This is particularly observed in obese older women. Physiotherapy and providing adequate pain relief during and after labor corrects this problem easily. Lung function changes during pregnancy start reverting to normal soon after delivery and reach baseline values within a few weeks.

■ DYSPNEA DUE TO PATHOLOGICAL CONDITIONS ARISING DURING PREGNANCY, LABOR OR THE POSTPARTUM PERIOD

Though breathlessness is a frequent complaint during normal pregnancy, dyspnea is also an important symptom of an underlying pulmonary pathology. When acute and severe, it invariably points to the presence of a life-threatening emergency. The following pregnancy-related conditions should come to mind— pulmonary thromboembolism, pulmonary edema due to preeclampsia or eclampsia, aspiration pneumonia, amniotic fluid embolism, pneumomediastinum, cardiomyopathy of pregnancy, and acute respiratory distress syndrome (ARDS) related to eclampsia and drug-induced pulmonary edema.

Progressively increasing dyspnea could also be the early manifestation of sepsis unrelated to pregnancy or related to complicated labor, to impending liver cell failure in a pregnancy-related hepatic pathology, or to the coincidence of an acute respiratory infection such as pneumonia occurring around this period.

A few pregnancy-specific problems causing pulmonary complications will now be considered.

■ PULMONARY THROMBOEMBOLIC DISEASE

Venous thromboembolic disease in our experience is the most frequent respiratory emergency related to pregnancy and the postpartum period. The incidence is four to five times greater in the postpartum period (particularly in early postpartum) than in pregnancy. Deep vein thrombosis involving the lower limbs results from a hypercoagulable state of the blood related to pregnancy, a hormone-related venous stasis in the lower limbs combined with pressure effect of the enlarged uterus on the inferior vena cava.

Clinical Diagnosis

Though the clinical features are the same as in nonpregnant women, it is amazing how often this diagnosis is missed in clinical practice. This is probably because the symptoms of breathlessness, vague unease, and chest discomfort are often associated or confused with anxiety symptoms, which may also be present. Even the slightest suspicion of this potentially fatal condition necessitates investigation. A venous Doppler may occasionally give false positive results because of venous obstruction due to an enlarged uterus. A Doppler ultrasound may be more revealing. A d-dimer test is useful, as a negative test is a point against thromboembolic disease. If there is no immediate life-threatening emergency and if facilities are available, a lung perfusion scan with less than 50 mrad exposure to the fetus may help. In an emergency and for definite specific evidence, a CT pulmonary angiography should be done with less fetal exposure. Notwithstanding the danger of teratogenicity to the fetus, (an increased incidence of childhood leukemia has been reported with as low a radiation exposure as 2–5 rad) a definite diagnosis of pulmonary embolism is a must because of the hazard to the mother's life if correct treatment is not instituted,

as also because of the potential hazard of unnecessary treatment of pulmonary embolism if pulmonary embolism is not present.

Treatment

Warfarin should not be used, as it can cause embryopathy and central nervous changes during the second or third trimester. Low-molecular heparin does not cross the placental barrier, is effective and does not need monitoring in relation to clotting parameters.

In patients who are hemodynamically very unstable or in shock, streptokinase or urokinase or tissue plasminogen activator should never be withheld. There should be no hesitation to use an inferior vena cava filter. Placement may be difficult because of possible dislodgment due to the dilated vena cava and increased pressure within the venous system during labor.

Women who have had thromboembolism before or those with known hypercoagulable states should receive heparin prophylaxis during pregnancy.

■ PULMONARY EDEMA IN PREECLAMPSIA

Preeclampsia is characterized by hypertension, edema, albuminuria, hypoalbuminemia, together with some degree of liver cell and renal dysfunction. Pulmonary edema is uncommon in preeclampsia because patients with preeclampsia are more often than not volume-depleted. More than one factor is generally responsible when pulmonary edema does occur. More often than not, well-marked hypertension during or even before pregnancy, is present. Systolic cum diastolic myocardial dysfunction is an important cause of pulmonary edema. When edema occurs in the immediate postpartum period it is often precipitated by over-vigorous intravenous infusion of fluids during labor. A background of diastolic myocardial dysfunction caused by hypertension worsens matters. Hypoalbuminemia when present is another contributory cause. Increased capillary permeability is another factor that has been incriminated, particularly in the presence of associated sepsis and multiple blood transfusions.

Clinical Features

Tachypnea, respiratory distress, hypoxia, crackles over the bases and the radiological features of pulmonary edema are present. Tachypnea with a slight fall in oxygen saturation are early signs that are of ominous significance.

Treatment

Treatment consists of fluid restriction, use of oxygen, use of diuretics and in severe cases the initiation of ventilatory support. Inotropic support needs to be given in the presence of poor cardiac function. Vasopressor support is rarely necessary, diuretic therapy needs to be given cautiously, for if the patient becomes hypovolemic it could worsen renal function, reduce cardiac output and jeopardize placental perfusion. We have generally managed patients with a central venous catheter monitoring central venous pressure, without using a pulmonary artery catheter. Ultimately, urgent delivery of the fetus as soon as is feasible is probably the best treatment of both preeclampsia and eclampsia.

■ AMNIOTIC FLUID EMBOLISM

Amniotic fluid embolism is a rare disastrous obstetric emergency which is very often fatal. In our experience we have witnessed it about once every 8–10 years. Western figures give the incidence between 1 in 8,000 to 1 in 80,000 live births with a mortality of 10–80%. This complication in the West is believed to account for 10% of all maternal deaths.

Amniotic fluid embolism occurs classically during labor and delivery. Rarely, it occurs in the early postpartum period. Amniotic fluid contains cell debris, cells, and humoral factors. When perhaps purely by chance this fluid gains entry into the venous circulation through enlarged uterine venous sinuses or through small or large uterine tears, disaster strikes. The cellular debris together with the amniotic fluid and its contents result in two major disturbances. The first is obstruction together with severe vasoconstriction of the pulmonary vasculature leading to sudden severe pulmonary hypertension. The other is an anaphylactic reaction caused by sensitivity to the amniotic fluid debris and to the humoral factors within the fluid.

Clinical Features

Clinical features are characterized by sudden severe dyspnea, progressive profound hypoxemia coupled with cardiovascular collapse. Hypotension, tachycardia, an imperceptible pulse and increasing metabolic acidosis occur; seizures may supervene. In severe cases death occurs within minutes or a few hours from cardiac arrest, allowing very little time for resuscitative efforts. In fact when amniotic fluid embolism occurs at or immediately after cesarean section, cardiovascular collapse and arrest occur very often on the table.

Not all cases are as severe. The ones we have witnessed and who have recovered had sudden onset breathlessness, hypoxia, hypotension, tachycardia and developed within 6–8 hours the clinical features of ARDS. Coagulation abnormalities in the form of a raised prothrombin time and partial thromboplastin time were observed.

Differential Diagnosis

Myocardial infarction, left ventricular failure, pulmonary thromboembolism, and tension pneumothorax can all simulate amniotic fluid embolism. ARDS from aspiration or sepsis needs to be considered in the differential diagnosis in the presence of pulmonary edema.

Management

Urgent cardiorespiratory resuscitation is important for survival. Central venous pressures as also filling pressure of the left heart need to be measured and monitored for optimum fluid therapy. Inotropes and vasopressors are both necessary. Immediate intubation and ventilatory support with a high fraction of inspired oxygen (FiO_2) are mandatory. The occurrence of ARDS will need optimal ventilatory support for several days. Coagulation abnormalities if present should be appropriately corrected.

■ PERIPARTUM CARDIOMYOPATHY

Peripartum cardiomyopathy is an important cause of dyspnea before, during or after delivery. Cardiac failure in the absence of preexisting cardiac disease is either due to hypertension of pregnancy or cardiomyopathy.

It is important to exclude preexisting causes of cardiac disease (e.g. valvular heart disease, ischemic cardiomyopathy) before making a diagnosis of peripartum cardiomyopathy. Besides tachycardia and dyspnea, orthopnea, dry cough, epigastric discomfort and vomiting are important symptoms. The heart is enlarged on clinical examination. A diastolic third heart sound at the apex, a systolic murmur of functional mitral incompetence (due to a dilated mitral annulus) and an accentuated pulmonary second sound are often audible. Basal crackles are invariably present. The jugular venous pressure is elevated and the liver though difficult to feel may be palpable and tender. Edema over the feet may or may not be present.

Two-dimensional (2D) echocardiography shows the presence of a dilated cardiomyopathy with an ejection fraction which may be as low as 15–20%. A radiographic examination of the chest shows an enlarged heart with pulmonary congestion or even pulmonary edema.

During labor and immediately after, the exertion and the increased demand on the heart often triggers severe left ventricular failure with pulmonary edema. Pulmonary thromboembolic complications are frequent.

Management

Diuretics and reducing the after-load on the heart are both important. However angiotensin-converting enzyme inhibitors should not be used during pregnancy as these drugs cause fetal renal dysfunction. Aldactone, the judicious use of carvedilol, and digoxin are recommended in appropriate doses. Patients with severe pump dysfunction should be tided over with inotropic support using both dopamine and dobutamine. Low-molecular weight heparin should be used in all patients.

Over 50% of patients gradually improve with regard to cardiac function over 6 months after delivery. A significant proportion, however, remains unchanged or may even worsen. Even in those who improve, future pregnancy is fraught with danger as cardiomyopathy may recur as the pregnancy progresses. Cardiac transplantation may be offered to patients with severe persistent cardiomyopathy.

■ DRUG-INDUCED PULMONARY EDEMA (TOCOLYTIC PULMONARY EDEMA)

Beta-agonists in particular terbutaline are often used to reduce uterine contractions in premature labor. In pregnancy, a rather unique complication of β-agonist therapy is pulmonary edema. The frequency of this complication varies in reported studies between 1% and 9%. It is postulated that terbutaline used over a prolonged period causes both myocardial dysfunction and increased capillary permeability. Intravenous infusion of large quantities of fluid and reduced oncotic pressure due to hypoalbuminemia aggravate the edema. Corticosteroids often administered to these patients also worsen the problem.

Clinical Features and Diagnosis

Sudden onset of dyspnea in the setting described above points to pulmonary edema. Tachypnea, basal crackles, a fall in oxygen saturation and the radiological presence of shadows consistent with pulmonary edema confirm the diagnosis.

Treatment

The β-agonist is promptly stopped following which pulmonary edema resolves. Diuretics need to be given; over-diuresis is dangerous as this may reduce placental flow with further danger to the fetus. With gross pulmonary edema, mechanical ventilation support is given. This is however rarely necessary if the condition is promptly recognized.

■ TROPHOBLASTIC DISEASE IN PREGNANCY

A benign hydatidiform mole can rarely lead to trophoblastic embolism, particularly during evacuation of the mole in the last trimester of pregnancy. Pulmonary hypertension and pulmonary edema indistinguishable from ARDS result. Choriocarcinoma may be associated with a hydatidiform mole and can lead to pulmonary or mediastinal metastasis and/or to malignant pleural effusion.

There are four other conditions in obstetrics and gynecology practice which can lead to pulmonary complications. These are the ovarian hyperstimulation syndrome, Meigs' syndrome, and catamenial pneumothorax with or without thoracic endometriosis. Meigs' syndrome has been described in the section on "Diseases of the Pleura".

■ OVARIAN HYPERSTIMULATION SYNDROME

The increasing practice of *in vitro* pregnancy has led to awareness of the increasing frequency of this syndrome. It is caused by the artificial induction of ovulation, being observed in about 1% of these cases. The syndrome evolves following the use of follicle-stimulating hormone and human menopausal gonadotropin together with pituitary suppression with leuprolide acetate. It is characterized by massive ovarian enlargement (often felt as abdominal masses), and by increased capillary permeability leading to volume depletion, massive edema, ascites, and pleural transudates. Pulmonary edema similar to that observed in ARDS occurs. Oliguria, renal, and liver dysfunction may be present. Breathlessness, crackles over both lungs, hypoxia and hypotension are frequent. In severe cases, death occurs from hypotension or multiple organ failure.

Management consists of paracentesis of ascites and pleural fluid, volume repletion with crystalloids and colloids, use of oxygen and ventilator support if there is marked pulmonary edema. When ovarian enlargement is very large, drainage of the ovarian cyst helps. Diuretics are useful and hypotension may need to be corrected by inotropes and vasopressors. Once diuresis starts recovery generally ensues. The pathogenesis of this syndrome is unclear but is believed to be caused by high plasma rennin-like activity and increased capillary permeability mediated by vasoactive substances of ovarian origin releasing cytokines such as TNF, interleukin (IL)-6, and endothelial growth factor.

■ CATAMENIAL PNEUMOTHORAX

This is rare and is suspected if pneumothorax occurs within 48 hours of menstruation. Recurrence of pneumothorax occurring with the menstrual cycle is well-nigh diagnostic. Catamenial pneumothorax generally occurs in women over 30 years, is most often right-sided but may occur on the left side as well. The mechanism of catamenial pneumothorax has been described in the chapter on "Pneumothorax" in the section on "Diseases of the Pleura". A contraceptive pill to suppress ovulation is the treatment of choice for catamenial pneumothorax, but if this is contraindicated or if pregnancy is desired, surgical advice is sought. At thoracotomy, diaphragmatic defects or pores may be identified and repaired; areas of pleural and diaphragmatic endometriosis if present can be surgically removed.

■ ACUTE RESPIRATORY DISTRESS SYNDROME IN PREGNANCY

A number of pregnancy-specific or pregnancy-associated problems render a pregnant woman at risk. The most important of pregnancy-specific diseases causing ARDS in our part of the world is *eclampsia*. ARDS may also occur in preeclamptic states. The term eclampsia is applied to grand mal seizures in a patient with preeclampsia in whom the seizures could not be attributed to any other cause. Seizures are not necessarily related to the degree of hypertension but to microangiopathic changes in cerebral vessels. ARDS, disseminated intravascular coagulopathy, and multiple organ failure result in severe disease and have a high mortality.

Acute respiratory distress syndrome also results from amniotic fluid embolism, from the rare occurrence of trophoblastic embolism and from the administration of multiple transfusions to counter severe postpartum hemorrhage. In our part of the world, the most common cause of ARDS with multiple organ failure in pregnancy is fulminant sepsis following septic abortion or following sepsis after full-term delivery. Aspiration of gastric contents particularly during labor is an important cause of aspiration pneumonia, followed by ARDS. Pregnancy predisposes to aspiration because of lowered tone of the esophageal sphincter, increased abdominal pressure, and the supine position during delivery.

Clinical Features and Diagnosis

The clinical history and diagnostic features are the same as in nonpregnant patients; these have been discussed in an earlier section.

Management

Management is no different when compared to nonpregnant patients. When administering drugs it is important to consider effects not only on the mother but also on the fetus. Alkalosis during ventilator support should be avoided as alkalosis reduces placental flow. Delivery of the fetus in our experience helps the mother and perhaps even the child. This is particularly so in patients with eclampsia.

A few important conditions not directly related to the pregnant or peripartum state but which occur fortuitously during this state need brief consideration.

■ BRONCHIAL ASTHMA AND PREGNANCY

Asthma is the most common respiratory disorder encountered in pregnancy. The severity of a preexisting asthma is unchanged in one-third of pregnant patients, is reduced in one-third and worsens in one-third.

Exacerbations are generally observed between 17 weeks and 32 weeks. Poorly controlled asthma may negatively influence maternal and fetal outcome. Miscarriage, antepartum and postpartum hemorrhage, anemia are often seen in these women. There is also a reported increase in eclampsia, preeclampsia, gestational diabetes, and preterm birth. Studies have also shown an increased risk of preterm birth, small for gestational age, and low birthweight, if the mother is actively asthmatic.

Management

Current drugs, both inhaled and oral used to treat asthma in the general population are safe for pregnant women. Inhalers containing short or long acting β_2-agonist are safe as also are inhaled steroids. Acute exacerbations of asthma may necessitate the systemic use of corticosteroids. Uncontrolled or acute several asthma poses a far greater risk than the risk of steroid therapy in these patients.

If for any reason severe asthmatics require general anesthesia, Ketamine and halogenated anesthetic drugs are preferable because they may have a bronchodilatory effect.

Oxytocin and prostaglandins E_2 can be used safely for including labor. Other prostaglandins and morphine should be avoided as they can increase bronchospasm.

■ COMMUNITY ACQUIRED PNEUMONIA

Pneumonia is believed to be one of the leading causes of non-obstetric maternal deaths in the United States. We have no statistical data on this subject in India or other Asian countries. The risk of pneumonia is increased in pregnant mothers with comorbid states like asthma, HIV infection, and substance abuse.

Treatment with antibiotics should be prompt and empirical pending microbiological confirmation. During the influenza season, particularly in epidemics, oseltamivir should be started empirically on suspicion of an H1N1 infection. The use of antibiotics must be tempered with circumspection especially with regard to their effects on the fetus or the neonatal child. Ventilator support when indicated should not be delayed, even if this warrants intubation and mechanical ventilator support.

■ TUBERCULOSIS IN PREGNANCY

Though we have no statistics to offer, pulmonary tuberculosis (TB) must be fairly frequent in pregnant women in our country. In sub-Saharan Africa, TB is the third leading cause of maternal death, following sepsis and hypertensive disorders of pregnancy.

The diagnosis of TB may at time be difficult as fatigue, malaise present in early TB may be considered as a feature of the pregnant state.

It is believed in the West that pregnancy does not adversely affect the course of pulmonary TB. This may not hold true in poor third world countries. Also the presence of HIV infection in these countries poses a great risk for spread or reactivation of TB.

Management

- Treatment is similar to that of treatment in *nonpregnant patients*. Rifampicin, INH, ethambutol have been reported to be safe in pregnancy and not reported to cause human fetal abnormalities.
- The use of pyrazinamide has been debated. The WHO believes its use in pregnancy is justified, yet the CDC advises against its use.
- INH does carry an increased risk of hepatitis particularly when used with rifampicin.
- Second line drugs are more toxic but may need to be used in drug resistant cases.
- Streptomycin, kanamycin, amikacin should be avoided for fear of fetal ototoxicity.

Finally any illness occurring in the community could also occur during pregnancy or the peripartum state. These should be treated appropriately (as one would treat them in the community) with due care not just for the mother but also for the unborn fetus or the neonate.

■ SUGGESTED READING

1. Bandi VD. Acute lung injury and acute respiratory distress syndrome in pregnancy. Crit Care Clin. 2004;20:577-607.
2. Moore J. Amniotic fluid embolism. Crit Care Med. 2005;33:S279-85.
3. Namazy J, Schatz M. The treatment of allergic respiratory disease during pregnancy. J Investig Allergol Clin Immunol. 2016;26(1):1-7.
4. Pereira A. Pulmonary complications of pregnancy. Clin Chest Med. 2004;25:299-310.

Diseases of the Pleura

CHAPTER 62

Pleural Effusions, Empyema

GENERAL CONSIDERATIONS

The pleura is a thin double-layered membranous structure lining the inner thoracic surface as also the whole lung. It is lined by mesothelial cells, which secrete a surfactant that enables the pleural surfaces to glide smoothly over each other during respiration. The parietal pleura is connected to the chest wall by a thin endothoracic fascia which fixes the pleura to the chest and provides it blood supply.

In healthy individuals the pleural space contains 10–30 mL of pleural fluid. This is a plasma ultrafiltrate across the pleural surface formed at the rate of 0.3–0.5 mL/kg/day with a protein content of 0.9–1.2 g/dL. There is an equivalent daily clearance of this fluid by lymphatics draining the visceral and parietal pleura, chiefly the latter.

The pleural space which is approximately 10–20 microns in width and lined by a single layer of mesothelial cells comprises a surface area of approximately 2,000 cm^2 in a 70 kg man.

Functions of the pleura: The pleurae are absent in some mammalian species raising the question of what their exact function is in humans. They serve as a "coupling organ" between the lungs and the chest wall. Their lubricant action allows for smooth movement of the lungs in the thoracic cage. Also, they may serve as a convenient "drip pan" in patients who develop pulmonary edema.

EPIDEMIOLOGY

It is estimated that close to 30% of diseases affecting the respiratory system involve the pleura. This involvement invariably takes the form of a pleural effusion. It has also been estimated that 30–40% of all pleural effusions are due to systemic diseases such as heart failure, liver, and renal disease in which the pleura per se is uninvolved and normal. There are indeed numerous causes of pleural effusion. The relative frequency of these causes will depend on the geographic areas and the population under study. In India, Pakistan, South East Asia, China, and developing countries such as Africa the most important causes are congestive heart failure, pneumonia, tuberculosis, and malignancy. Western countries would include viral infection in this list though viral infections are difficult to prove. Tuberculous pleural effusions do occur in the West but not with the same frequency.

In the US, about 1 million pleural effusions occur a year. There is no such available data from India, so a look at the incidence of effusions in the West is informative. In order of decreasing frequency these would be as follows **(Table 1)**.

A glaring difference from India is that tuberculosis would be, by far, the most common cause of a pleural exudate in this country.

PATHOPHYSIOLOGY

Pleural effusion can occur under two situations:
1. When there is an increase in the hydrostatic filtration pressure and/or a decrease in the plasma oncotic pressure. This leads to the formation of a transudate.
2. When the pleura is involved in a pathological process, which increases capillary permeability leading to the formation of a pleural exudate.

Pleural pathology may be primary but is more often secondary to pulmonary disease. It could arise from pathology within the mediastinum (e.g. esophageal perforation) or from a subdiaphragmatic pathology (e.g.

Table 1: Causes of pleural effusion in the US, according to a study.

Type	Incidence
CCF	500,000
Parapneumonic	300,000
Neoplastic	200,000
PE	150,000
Viral	100,000
Cirrhosis or GI	100,000
CABG	50,000
TB	2,500
Mesothelioma	2,300

(CABG: Coronary bypass graft surgery; CCF: Congestive cardiac failure; PE: Pulmonary embolism; GI: Gastrointestinal; TB: Tuberculosis)
Source: Light RW. Pleural Effusion. N Engl J Med. 2002;346:1971-7.

a liver abscess). Pleural effusion could also occur from abnormal communication or blockage of the thoracic duct and its main draining channels (chylothorax), or from communication transdiaphragmatically with peritoneal fluid, or from communication with the pancreas or the kidney (urinothorax).

CLINICAL FEATURES

The main clinical symptom is dyspnea; at times cough is an important symptom. The degree of dyspnea depends not just on the size of the effusion but the speed at which the pleural space is filled. Therefore a very slow accumulation of even a liter of fluid may not be subjectively noted by the patient unless the clinical presentation is determined by the underlying cause of the pleural effusion such as pneumonia or cardiac failure. Dyspnea is generally perceived when half the hemothorax is filled with fluid. It occurs with smaller effusions when they are bilateral.

There needs to be at least 300 mL of fluid in the pleural space before it is detected on clinical examination. With a small-to-moderate pleural effusion, the important physical findings are a stony dull note over the fluid on percussion, diminished breath sounds, and diminished vocal fremitus. Decreased chest movements over the lower chest on the affected side may afford a valuable clue.

With larger effusions, there may be bulging of the intercostal spaces with marked diminution of chest movements on the affected side, a shift of the apex beat and the trachea to the opposite side, stony dullness over the fluid with absent breath sounds and diminished vocal fremitus.

Large unilateral pleural effusions or moderate-sized pleural effusions if bilateral will cause tachypnea and hypoxic respiratory failure. Massive unilateral pleural effusions produce a severe mediastinal shift to the opposite side. There is a reduced return of venous blood flow into the heart due to raised intrapleural pressure leading to a low cardiac output, hypotension, and alveolar hypoventilation with increasing hypoxic plus hypercapnic respiratory failure.

DIAGNOSTIC APPROACH

- Clinical evaluation—the first step in the evaluation of a patient with pleural effusion is a detailed history and a complete physical examination. This is because the cause of a pleural effusion may well lie outside the thorax; also, examination of the pleural fluid does not necessarily point to a specific cause. In fact even imaging findings or pleural biopsy may be noncontributory unless viewed in an overall perspective with the history and clinical findings.
- Imaging—a radiographic examination (postero-anterior view) of the chest shows a fairly dense shadow on the side of the effusion; the upper border may be slightly concave rising upwards toward the axilla **(Fig. 1)**. Large effusions push the heart and trachea to the opposite side. Very small effusions show a blunting of the costophrenic angle. The same effect can also be produced by pleural fibrosis and pleural adhesions in that area. Walled-off effusions over the anterior or lateral pleural surfaces are easily evident, but loculated effusions behind the heart or along the mediastinum as also subpulmonic effusions are difficult to diagnose.

Ultrasonography can detect even small pleural effusions; it has a sensitivity of nearly 100%. It is an invaluable mode to detect pleural effusion in critically ill patients in the intensive care units where basal shadows within the lung may be due to various factors—atelectasis, consolidation, fluid, or may result from a combination of one or more of the above factors. Ultrasound also distinguishes fluid from pleural thickening and is useful

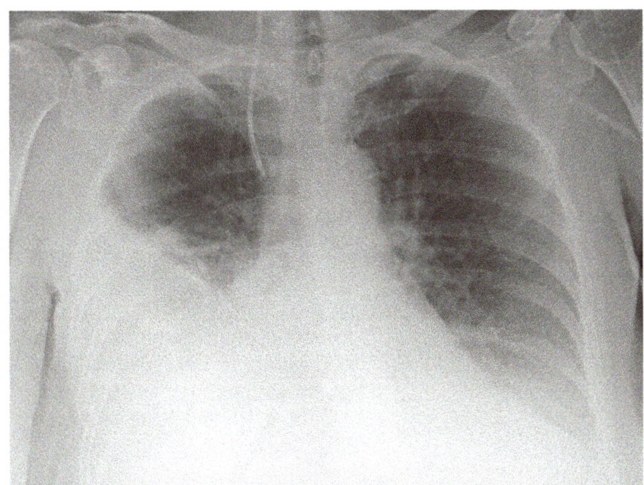

Fig. 1: Pleural effusion—chest X-ray reveals a well-defined homogenous opacity in the right hemithorax.

to demonstrate loculations and septa within the pleural fluid.

High-resolution computed tomography (HRCT) of the chest with pleural phase contrast enhancement provides better detection of pleuropulmonary pathologies. It may reveal, for example, an underlying pneumonia, a lung abscess, tuberculosis, mediastinal disease, or a subdiaphragmatic pathology that may be responsible for a pleural effusion.

Pleural Fluid Examination

A diagnostic thoracocentesis with an examination of the pleural fluid is a must in the investigation of a pleural effusion where the diagnosis is even in the slightest doubt. A thoracocentesis is generally safe. Complications include a vasovagal syncope, bleeding due to injury to a vessel, and pneumothorax. Removal of large quantities of pleural fluid can cause re-expansion pulmonary edema. The procedure should be promptly stopped, if the patient complains of chest pain or develops cough.

Appearance of the Pleural Fluid

Pleural fluid can be straw-colored, turbid, blood-tinged, or frankly hemorrhagic. Frank pus drawn from the pleural space points to an empyema. Milky fluid suggests a chylothorax or pseudochylothorax. Food particles in the fluid point to an esophageal perforation. An ammoniacal smell suggests an urinothorax.

Distinguishing a Pleural Transudate from an Exudate

After noting the appearance of the pleural fluid, the next step is to determine whether it is a transudate or exudate. A transudate points to systemic disease, the three most important and common being—(1) congestive heart failure, (2) cirrhosis of the liver, and (3) the nephrotic syndrome. Patients with severe hypoalbuminemia from any cause, those on peritoneal dialysis, patients with myxedema or with superior vena caval obstruction may also develop pleural transudates. The focus then is on the treatment of these systemic diseases.

If the pleural fluid is an exudate it could arise from diseases within the thorax or from subdiaphragmatic causes or from other systemic causes. The diagnostic focus is to determine which of these several possible causes has produced a pleural pathology.

Pleural exudates are traditionally defined by Light's criteria rule, wherein if any one of the three features mentioned below is positive, the fluid is considered to be an exudate:

1. The total protein in the pleural fluid divided by the total serum protein is more than 0.5;
2. The lactate dehydrogenase (LDH) of the pleural fluid divided by the serum LDH is more than 0.6;
3. The LDH of the pleural fluid is greater than two-thirds of the upper limit of the normal LDH in blood.

Combining two or more of these criteria instead of relying only on one makes the Light's criteria rule more sensitive, but less specific. The increased sensitivity is useful, in that it enables the physician not to miss out on pleural exudates, which require different management when compared to transudates.

Light's criteria have stood the test of time and remain the most robust biochemical criteria for distinguishing a transudate from an exudate. They retain a high sensitivity of 98%, specificity of 83%, and overall accuracy of 95% in achieving this crucial distinction. The only occasional drawback of Light's criteria is that they sometimes falsely label a transudate an exudate, especially in patients with congestive cardiac failure (CCF) who are on diuretics. This important clinical pitfall of Light's criteria was elegantly demonstrated by Chako et al. (Chest 1989) where thoracocentesis was performed before and after 6 days of diuretics in patients with CCF. The diuresis resulted in significant increase in protein and LDH so that 30% of all transudates were now falsely classified as "exudates".

This occurs because diuresis causes water to leave the pleural space faster than protein and LDH. The longer the patient is on diuresis, the more likely that this will occur. Combining Light's criteria with this knowledge of when "transudate by etiology" turns "exudate by biochemistry" render these criteria well-nigh perfect. Light's criteria maximize sensitivity over specificity. It is better to occasionally misdiagnose a transudate as an exudate than vice versa.

Other newer criteria have been looked at to see if these have greater sensitivity and specificity when it comes to differentiating a transudate from an exudate. Given below are proposed two criteria, three criteria diagnostic rules which require one criterion to be met to make the diagnosis of an exudate.

- *Two-test rule*:
  - Pleural fluid cholesterol more than 45 mg/dL
  - Pleural fluid LDH more than 0.45 times the upper limit of the lab's LDH.

  Three-test rule:
  - Pleural fluid protein more than 2.9 g/dL
  - Pleural fluid cholesterol more than 45 mg/dL
  - Pleural fluid LDH more than 0.45 times the upper limit of the lab's LDH.

None of these have been shown to have greater superiority over Light's criteria.

Differential Leukocyte Count (Table 2)

A neutrophilic or predominantly neutrophilic exudate is seen in a parapneumonic effusion, in an empyema, or soon after pulmonary infarction. A lymphocytic exudate is often due to tuberculosis, malignancy, and in other systemic disorders like connective tissue diseases. Tuberculous pleural effusions, particularly in the early part of their natural history, may show a predominance of polymorphs. An increase in the eosinophil count (>10% of cells) is observed following a hemothorax, long-standing tuberculous effusions, drug-induced pleural disease, Churg-Strauss syndrome, and eosinophilic pneumonia.

Chemical Analysis

- *Proteins:* A significant rise in the protein concentration of pleural fluid vis-a-vis the serum protein characterizes pleural exudates. Transudates generally have a protein concentration less than 3 g/dL.

  As mentioned earlier, in patients on diuretics (as in patients with CCF), the protein concentration of pleural fluid may rise due to an increased loss of water, so that

Table 2: Differential leucocyte counts in relation to the etiology of pleural exudates.

Pleural diseases	Remarks
Polymorphonuclear leucocytosis	
Complicated parapneumonic effusion; empyema	In chronic empyema there may be a significant lymphocytosis
Pleural fluid lymphocytosis (> 80%)	
Tuberculosis	Lymphocytes predominate (85–95% of lymphocytes). In early exudative phase polymorphs may constitute 1/3–1/2 of the leukocyte count
Malignancies	In over 50% of cases, but generally < 80% lymphocytes
Rheumatoid disease	–
Lymphoma	95–100% lymphocytes
Chylothorax	Fluid has milky appearance
Sarcoidosis	A very rare cause of pleural effusion, > 90% lymphocytes
Pleural fluid eosinophilia (>10%)	
Pneumothorax	Most common cause when a pneumothorax is associated with an effusion—due to blood
Hemothorax	Occurs some days after the event
Previous thoracocentesis	Related to bleeding caused by needle trauma
Parasitic disease	Generally seen
Pulmonary embolism	Hemorrhagic fluid
Lymphoma	Rare occurrence in Hodgkin's disease
Drug-induced	–
Churg-Strauss syndrome	Eosinophilia in blood and in pleural exudate
Tuberculosis	Rarely seen in old tuberculous effusions

the transudate may be mistaken for an exudate. Even then, these patients will have a difference between the serum and pleural fluid albumin values of more than 1.2 g/dL or a protein gradient more than 3.1 g/dL, which point to such effusions as transudates.

- *Glucose:* A low pleural fluid glucose concentration (< 60 mg/dL) or a pleural fluid/serum glucose ratio less than 0.5 is observed in tuberculous pleural effusion, empyema, pleuritis in systemic lupus erythematosus (SLE) and rheumatoid disease, in malignant effusions, and in esophageal rupture causing a pleural effusion. Lowest fluid glucose concentrations (when compared to other causes) have been observed in empyema and rheumatoid pleural effusions **(Table 3)**.

Table 3: Diseases often associated with low pH (<7.3) and low glucose (< 60 mg/dL) in the pleural exudate.

- Empyema, complicated parapneumonic effusion
- Malignant effusion
- Tuberculosis
- SLE involving the pleura
- Rheumatoid disease involving the pleura
- Chylothorax

(SLE: Systemic lupus erythematosus)

All other pleural exudates have a glucose concentration similar to blood. A significantly higher glucose concentration in pleural fluid will occur with a misplaced central venous catheter through which glucose is infused into the pleural space, or glucose rich peritoneal dialysis fluid entering the pleural space through pores within the diaphragm.

The reason for low blood glucose concentrations in the conditions mentioned above are either a decreased diffusion of glucose from the blood into the pleural fluid as in rheumatoid effusions and malignant pleurisy or increased utilization of glucose within the pleural fluid by bacteria (as in an empyema) or by malignant cells.

- *pH:* The pH of the pleural fluid (measured by a blood gas machine) as lowered less than or equal to 7.3 in all pleural exudates, which have a low blood sugar. The lowered pH is due to increased acid production by bacteria (as in an empyema) or due to a low H^+ ion efflux from the pleural space as in malignant and rheumatoid pleural effusions.

In malignant pleural effusions, a lowered pH is believed to relate to more extensive pleural involvement, a greater chance of positive cytology, a lowered success rate for pleurodesis, and a poorer prognosis.

- *Lactate dehydrogenase:* The LDH level is an important distinguishing feature between an exudate and a transudate. Particularly high LDH levels (>1000 IU/L) have been observed in malignant pleural effusion, empyema, and also in pleural paragonimiasis.

Pleural effusions due to pneumocystis are characterized by a pleural fluid/serum LDH ratio more than 1 and a pleural fluid protein/serum protein ratio of less than 1.

- *Cholesterol and triglycerides:* A significant elevation of the cholesterol concentration in pleural fluid may be present in chronic pleural effusions due to degenerating cells and to increased vascular permeability.

A cholesterol content more than 250 mg/dL is considered a pseudochylous or chyliform effusion.

A pleural triglyceride concentration more than 110 mg/dL points to a chylothorax. A level less than 50 mg/dL excludes the diagnosis; levels between 50 mg/dL and 110 mg/dL necessitate a lipoprotein analysis of the pleural fluid.

- *Adenosine deaminase:* The importance of adenosine deaminase (ADA) estimation in pleural fluid with reference to the diagnosis of tuberculous pleurisy has been discussed separately later in this chapter.
- *Amylase:* Pleural fluid amylase concentration is raised in acute pancreatitis, chronic pancreatitis that causes pleural effusion, esophageal rupture, and malignancy. In the last two conditions the rise in amylase is largely related to salivary enzymes; in pancreatic pathology the amylase in pleural fluid is due to pancreatic isoenzymes.

Specific tests: These depend on the disease causing pleural effusion and are detailed later under specific diseases. They include (among many others) relevant tests for an infective etiology (bacterial, viral, fungal, and tubercular), cytology for suspected malignancy, cytogenic studies to characterize chromosomal markers of suspected hematolymphoid and mesenchymal malignancies, and flow cytometry for the rare involvement of the pleura in lymphoma.

Pleural biopsy: If in spite of the above tests, the diagnosis of a pleural effusion is in doubt a pleural biopsy becomes necessary. The histological examination of the pleura together with other tests on the pleural tissue may help in a difficult diagnosis. A pleural biopsy can be done as a blind procedure using Abrams needle or a CT or ultrasound-guided biopsy, or done under direct vision through a thoracoscope or following a thoracotomy. With the advent of video-assisted thoracoscopy, thoracotomy as a diagnostic procedure is rarely necessary. Percutaneous blind biopsies using Abrams needle have a fair yield in the diagnosis of diseases causing a diffuse involvement of the pleura. CT-guided or ultrasound-guided biopsies are particularly useful to target focal lesions within the pleura (e.g. malignancy) revealed through imaging studies. The biopsy of choice, however, in most undiagnosed pleural disease is a video-assisted thoracoscopic biopsy. This is because a thoracoscopy is a simple procedure in expert hands, performed most often under local anesthesia. It has few complications even when carried out on critically ill patients. It gives a full visualization of the entire pleural surface allowing multiple biopsies from appropriate sites. Diagnosis of malignancy involving the pleura can be made with well-nigh 100% accuracy. It has one added advantage—drainage of pleural fluid and (if indicated) pleurodesis can be performed in the same procedure.

Tissue obtained through a biopsy should be submitted for histopathological examination, appropriately stained to detect infections, and should also be cultured, particularly when there is suspicion of tuberculosis. A diagnostic algorithm for a pleural effusion is given in **Flowchart 1**.

■ SPECIFIC DISEASES ASSOCIATED WITH PLEURAL EFFUSION

Conditions Associated with Pleural Transudates (Table 4)

Congestive cardiac failure is the most common and most frequent cause of pleural transudates all over the world.

The effusion is generally bilateral; if unilateral it occurs more frequently in the right than in the left pleural space. Left ventricular failure causes a rise in the end-capillary pressure. There is increased filtration of a transudate into the interstitial tissue of the lung which then seeps through the visceral pleura into the pleural space. Though pleural transudates are more common in congestive heart failure, they are also observed frequently in isolated left heart failure.

The diagnosis rests on the clinical features of left heart failure or CCF, the frequent presence of an enlarged heart with clinical and radiological evidence of pulmonary congestion. Transudative pleural effusions also occur in veno-occlusive disease and in constrictive pericarditis.

Management consists in the treatment of congestive heart failure. Pleurodesis may be of help in some patients with persistent pleural effusion.

Flowchart 1: Diagnostic flowchart for a pleural effusion.

Table 4: Causes of pleural transudate.
Common causes:
• Congestive heart failure
• Cirrhosis of liver
• Nephrotic syndrome
• Hypoalbuminemia from any cause
• Continuous peritoneal dialysis
Uncommon causes:
• Superior vena cava obstruction
• Constrictive pericarditis
• Hypothyroidism
• Atelectasis
• Urinothorax
• Budd-Chiari syndrome

It is to be remembered that a patient with congestive heart failure could also have an exudative pleural effusion due to a separate pathology. If the pleural effusion does not clear with successful treatment of congestive heart failure or if the effusion is large (or particularly if large and unilateral) a pleural fluid examination with other relevant tests are necessary.

Hepatic Disease

Pleural effusions due to hepatic disease are due to two causes:

1. Transdiaphragmatic migration of ascitic fluid;
2. A lowered oncotic pressure associated with hypo-albuminemia. Most pleural transudates due to hepatic disease are right-sided because of the frequency of "pores" in the right dome of the diaphragm which allow ascitic fluid to seep into the right pleural space. Ascites is generally present but is not an absolute prerequisite. Large diaphragmatic defects can lead to large pleural effusions, the significance of which is missed, particularly if there is little or no ascites.

Management is directed toward the treatment of hepatic disease—the use of diuretics, low-sodium diet, and treatment of portal hypertension. Symptomatic relief may be often necessary through repeated paracentesis. Pleurodesis may also be tried. Transjugular hepatic portovenous shunting (TIPS) when indicated for relief of portal hypertension has been noted to reduce the hydrothorax. A liver transplant when indicated is followed by disappearance of the hydrothorax.

Renal Diseases

Hydrothorax is typically observed in the nephrotic syndrome, due to hypoalbuminemia causing a lowered oncotic pressure. It can also occur in glomerulonephritis and in patients on peritoneal dialysis. Dialysis fluid generally seeps through communications (pores) in the right dome of the diaphragm into the right pleural space. Examination of the pleural fluid resembles dialysis fluid.

An urinothorax is a rare occurrence when there is renal obstruction with consequent retroperitoneal urine collection, which then seeps into the ipsilateral pleural space. The pleural fluid has an ammoniacal smell. An urinothorax should always be suspected when a pleural transudate has a low pH. The pleural fluid has a high creatinine content (greater than the creatinine level in the blood).

Diseases Associated with Pleural Exudates (Table 5)

Parapneumonic Pleural Effusions

Parapneumonic pleural effusions are pleural exudates associated with pneumonia, lung abscess, or infected bronchiectasis. They occur in 20–50% of patients with pneumonia and constitute one of the most common causes of a pleural exudate.

The pleural effusion is due to inflammation of the visceral pleura contiguous to a pneumonic patch. Increased permeability of the pleural vessels secondary to inflammation leads to formation of the exudate. To start with the fluid appears serous, has a low white blood corpuscle (WBC) count, a low LDH, a normal glucose content, and pH greater than 7.3; the protein content is high, however, pointing to an exudate. There are no organisms in the pleural fluid and the fluid culture is negative. The above description is that of an "uncomplicated" parapneumonic effusion. A diagnostic thoracocentesis is essential to confirm the sterile nature of a pleural exudate (an uncomplicated parapneumonic effusion) whenever there is clinical and/or radiological evidence of a significant pleural effusion in a patient with pneumonia.

If the underlying pneumonia is correctly treated with appropriate antibiotics, the pleural effusion generally resolves and requires no drainage. If an uncomplicated parapneumonic effusion is large or recurs, a therapeutic tap with a syringe and needle perhaps hastens resolution. This will also help to determine whether the effusion remains uncomplicated or whether it has progressed. If, however, the pneumonia is untreated or there is a delay

Table 5: Causes of pleural exudate.
• *Infections:*
– Tuberculosis
– Other infections
– Bacterial
– Viral
– Nocardial
– Fungal
– Parasitic
• *Malignancies:*
– Pleural metastasis
– Lymphoma
– Pleural mesothelioma
• *Vascular:*
– Pulmonary embolism
– Vasculitides
• *GI diseases:*
– Pancreatitis
– Pancreatic pseudocyst
– Perforation of the esophagus
– Intrahepatic or subphrenic abscess
• *Inflammatory (noninfectious):*
– Asbestosis
– Radiation
– Uremic
– Post-thoracotomy
– Post-transplant
• Connective tissue diseases
• Iatrogenic, traumatic (including hemothorax)
• *Miscellaneous:*
– Lymphangioleiomyomatosis
– Meigs' syndrome
– Yellow nail syndrome
– Chylothorax

(GI: Gastrointestinal)

in treatment, there is a strong chance of the development of an infected pleural effusion, also called a complicated parapneumonic effusion. A point to note is that pleural infection with microorganisms can occur in spite of adequate therapy in patients with severe pneumonia, particularly in the presence of comorbid factors. Recent genetic studies suggest that a variant of the protein tyrosine phosphatase (PTPN 22 Trp 620) is associated with increased susceptibility to invasive pneumococcal disease and empyema.

The exudate in a complicated parapneumonic effusion is often turbid; it will show a significant polymorphonuclear leukocytosis, generally over $100/mm^3$, at times over $1000/mm^3$. Besides a high protein content, the pleural fluid has a glucose less than 60 mg/dL, a raised LDH, pH less than 7.2. The pleural fluid culture is often positive. However, pleural fluid culture may be negative if antibiotics are in use.

Repeated paracentesis with strict aseptic precaution in the hope of keeping the pleura dry, together with appropriate antibiotic therapy may still effect resolution of the effusion, but unfortunately this is not always so. At this point in the natural history of the disease, fibrin begins to be laid down, compartmentalizing the effusion into several pockets, some large, and others small. Effective paracentesis with a syringe and needle is then impossible. A tube thoracostomy then becomes essential for adequate treatment. The tube should be positioned under CT guidance in the most dependent portion of the effusion. Additional chest tubes may be needed, if there is more than one large pocket requiring drainage. If the patient fails to improve or if the loculated effusion fails to respond to tube drainage, a thoracoscopically performed open-tube drainage, together with breaking of fibrinous loculi with decortication (depending on the thickness of the visceral pleura) should be performed.

The incidence of parapneumonic effusion depends on the case-mix of a study and the organisms involved. Complicated parapneumonic effusions are more frequent in immunocompromised patients and in those with associated comorbid factors such as diabetes, chronic lung disease, rheumatoid disease, and alcohol or other substance abuse.

Streptococcus pneumoniae is the most common cause of community-acquired pneumonia and leads to a parapneumonic effusion in 30–50% of patients. Yet pneumococci are grown from the pleural fluid in less than 10%. In contrast, parapneumonic pleural infections related to pneumonia due to *Klebsiella* or *Pseudomonas* or Staphylococci often show organisms in the pleural fluid on culture. Other gram-negative infections causing infected pleural effusions include *Escherichia coli* and the Enterobacteriaceae species. A study of 263 consecutive patients admitted to the Hinduja Hospital in 2005 showed that tuberculosis was the cause of 75 of these effusions (29%). Malignancies followed in 46 patients (17%) and infections (pneumonias) in 33 patients (13%).

It is important to differentiate community-acquired pleural infections from nosocomial pleural infections. The latter are generally due to pneumonia caused by *Pseudomonas*, *Klebsiella*, *Acinetobacter*, and occasionally by other gram-negative organisms. Methicillin-resistant *Staphylococcus aureus* is responsible for more than a quarter of hospital-acquired pleural infections in some countries of the West; it is fortunately comparatively less common in India. The mortality and morbidity of pleural infection in nosocomial infections is far worse than in community-acquired pleural infections.

EMPYEMA

Empyema is a suppurative pleural effusion leading to pus within the pleural space. When the pus is localized within the pleura, it forms an intrapleural abscess. Empyema can occur at any age but is most frequent in the middle-aged and elderly. Though the most common cause of an empyema is an underlying bacterial pneumonia, other important causes need to be kept in mind. A lung abscess or infected bronchiectasis may occasionally cause an empyema. Tuberculosis involving the lung may lead not just to a tuberculous pleural effusion but also a tuberculous empyema. An empyema can also result from infection distal to a bronchus obstructed by a foreign body or by a bronchogenic carcinoma. It can occur as a postoperative complication of cardiothoracic surgery, following penetrating or blunt trauma or an esophageal tear. A subdiaphragmatic abscess may involve the pleura either directly or via the lymphatics. A liver abscess, in particular an amebic liver abscess can rupture into the pleura, or into the lung (from where infection spreads into the pleura) or into the lung and pleura. The empyema that then follows is not bacterial in origin but is due to *Entamoeba histolytica*. Primary direct pleural infection causing empyema must indeed be very rare. It may occur in bacteremic or pyemic states. Even here, the possibility of a small subpleural abscess rupturing into the pleura rather than a direct pleural infection remains a possibility **(Table 6)**.

Predisposing Factors

Comorbid states associated with empyema have been mentioned under "Parapneumonic effusions". In Western

Table 6: Causes of empyema.

• *Pulmonary infection:*
  – Bacterial pneumonia
  – Tuberculous infection
  – Pneumonia due to other microorganisms (including fungi)
  – Lung abscess and infected bronchiectasis
  – Infection distal to an obstructed bronchus—bronchogenic carcinoma and foreign body
• Postoperative complication of cardiothoracic surgery
• Penetrating or blunt trauma to the chest
• Esophageal perforation
• Subdiaphragmatic abscess
• Hepatic abscess—pyogenic or amoebic
• Primary pleural involvement—bacteremic or pyemic state

studies, alcoholism is the most important risk factor and is present in 20–40% of cases in some studies. In our part of the world, diabetes, immunocompromised states [in particular acquired immune deficiency syndrome (AIDS)], neurological disorders favoring aspiration, and underlying chronic lung disease are the important predisposing factors.

Bacteriology

Gram-positive cocci, in particular *S. pneumoniae*, other streptococcal species, *Haemophilus influenzae*, staphylococci, and anaerobic infections from aspiration pneumonia are the important community-acquired causes of pneumonia that can lead to empyema. Empyema due to *Legionella* infection is rare in our experience; perhaps it is being missed. Empyemas due to nosocomial pneumonias are chiefly due to *Pseudomonas*, *Klebsiella*, Acinetobacter, and enterobacteria. Nosocomial staphylococcal infection is rare compared to its incidence in Western countries.

In a study of 60 consecutive cases in one of our units in Mumbai, over 5 years from 2001–2006, the three most common etiologies of empyema based on pleural culture were; *S. pneumoniae, S. aureus,* and *M. tuberculosis.*

Natural History and Pathogenesis

The natural history of empyema complicating pneumonia is a sequence of events or stages. The first stage is the formation of a sterile pleural exudate with few leukocytes. This stage graduates within a few days into an intermediate stage of infective pleurisy characterized by increased quantities of turbid pleural fluid, marked leukocytosis with many bacteria, a characteristic biochemical profile of the pleural fluid (described under complicated parapneumonic effusion), and by the formation of fibrous septa that loculate the pleural fluid into several compartments. The final stage is the presence of frank pus, which is generally loculated. The whole collection within the pleura may be walled off from the rest of the pleural space forming thereby an intrapleural abscess with several loculations. Different locations in which an empyema may be encysted within the pleural space are illustrated in the accompanying figure **(Fig. 2)**.

If death has not occurred from pleuropulmonary infection the empyema becomes chronic. Fibrous tissue is laid down in peels, at times encircling the lung in a tight vice (fibrothorax) rendering it well-nigh functionless. A

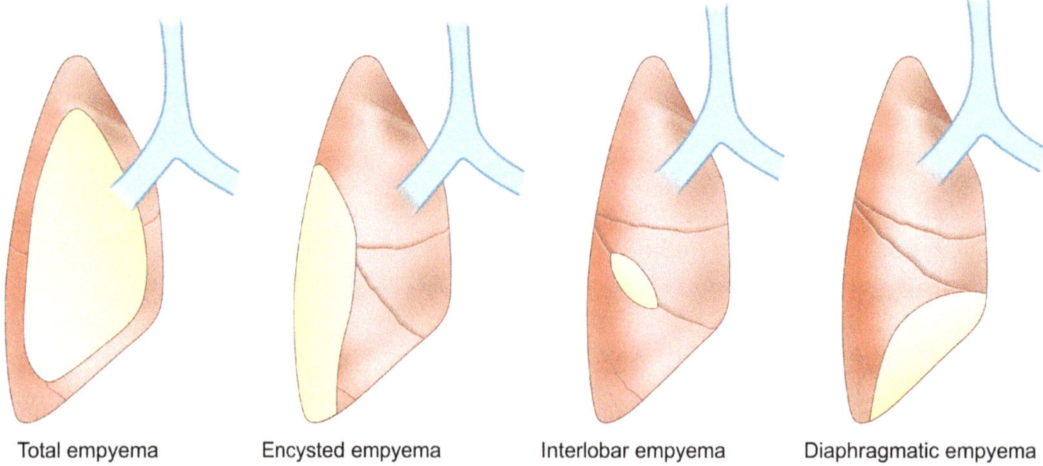

Fig. 2: Different locations of an empyema.

walled-off empyema, particularly situated anterolaterally within the thorax may point outwards causing an empyema necessitatis. A bulge is observed over the chest; there is an impulse over the bulge on coughing, and the bulge may be seen to pulsate. An "empyema necessitatis" may open outside leading to a purulent discharge.

Clinical Features

An acutely evolving empyema is characterized by fever with chills, tachycardia, and tachypnea if the pleural effusion is large or if an underlying pneumonia still persists. There is a well-marked leukocytosis. If undetected and not appropriately drained, all the features of increasing sepsis with progressive multiorgan dysfunction will appear. Hypotension and septic shock are of ominous significance. Pneumonia is an important cause of the acute respiratory distress syndrome (ARDS). An empyema in a patient with ARDS may be impossible to detect clinically or on a routine X-ray of the chest. A CT of the chest can, however, detect loculated fluid in ARDS; CT chest is indicated when a patient with ARDS fares poorly or when a patient with pneumonia fails to respond to therapy.

Not uncommonly, an empyema presents in a subacute or chronic form. In the subacute form, the patient apparently recovers from a lower respiratory tract infection but continues to run a low-grade evening fever. Some degree of leukocytosis is present. At times, the patient is afebrile for a few days or even weeks and then again runs low-grade or high fever. The relation of this fever to a recent lower respiratory tract infection may be missed. If the empyema is posteriorly placed, signs of fluid are apparent. If it is tucked away anteriorly and laterally physical signs are difficult to elicit. The empyema is, however, apparent on imaging—both on a posteroanterior (PA) and lateral X-ray and always on a CT chest.

A patient with chronic empyema generally presents with pyrexia of unknown origin (PUO). Leukocytosis and a raised C-reactive protein are generally present but not always so. In fact the WBC count may be normal in about 20% and some patients with chronic empyema may be afebrile (silent empyema). At times there are periods of low-grade fever followed by afebrile periods, the clinical pattern closely mimicking a Pel-Ebstein type of pyrexia. There may be no physical signs in the chest; even an X-ray chest may be reported as normal if the empyema is tucked away in the paravertebral space behind the heart. A CT of the chest is essential in all patients with a PUO, if a loculated walled-off empyema tucked away in the chest is not to be missed.

In summary, an empyema should be suspected under the following conditions:
- Pneumonia unresponsive to treatment or unexplained fever after the patient has received adequate treatment with resolution of the pneumonia
- Persistent leukocytosis and raised erythrocyte sedimentation rate (ESR) after pneumonia
- In a patient with PUO

- In an ill patient who has had cardiothoracic surgery, esophageal surgery or any other procedure (such as a thoracocentesis) where an empyema is a possible complication
- In the presence of a foul malodorous at times feculent sputum suggestive of a bronchopleural fistula
- Imaging findings that strongly suggest an empyema.

Imaging Studies

Ultrasound imaging of the chest, radiography of the chest, and an HRCT of the chest are important in the evaluation and management of both a complicated parapneumonic effusion and an empyema. Ultrasonography can identify free or loculated pleural effusions and distinguish between loculated effusions and solid masses. It is perhaps as sensitive or even more sensitive than a chest X-ray but less sensitive than an HRCT of the chest.

X-ray Chest

A routine chest X-ray may show a convex border to the fluid in the pleural space pointing to walled-off fluid rather than to the typical concave crescent of free fluid in the pleural cavity **(Fig. 3)**.

The CT chest reveals thickened parietal and visceral pleura, multiloculated effusion with multiple fibrin strands within the walled-off pleural fluid. These features distinguish an empyema from an exudative pleural effusion. Multiloculation occurs in more than 80% of empyemas. It is a fairly sensitive criterion but not very specific, because it is observed with equal frequency in untreated and improperly treated tuberculous pleural effusions. There may be an air-fluid level within the empyema if there is a bronchopleural fistula, or if the empyema is caused by anaerobic organisms, or if air has been inadvertently introduced during paracentesis.

An empyema with an air-fluid level may closely resemble a lung abscess on imaging studies. The differentiation is critical from the point of view of management. The following imaging features on a contrast CT of the chest may help in the differential diagnosis **(Figs. 4 to 6)**.

An empyema often has the following features:
- Thickened visceral and parietal pleurae separated ("dissected") by the fluid
- Compression of the adjacent lung
- Formation of a blunt angle with the chest wall
- No vessel markings within the opacity

A peripherally situated lung abscess often has the following features **(Fig. 6)**:
- A rounded opacity
- Absence of compression of adjacent lung
- Walls not smooth (as with an empyema) but often irregular and thickened (except in some patients with a staphylococcal lung abscess)

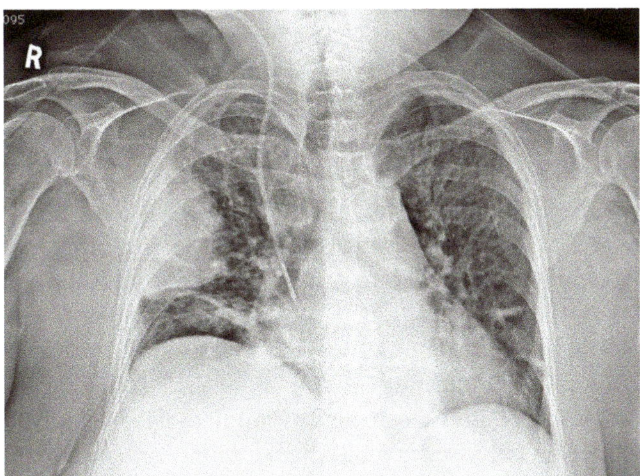

Fig. 3: Empyema—Chest X-ray reveals ill-defined homogenous opacity along the right chest wall representing an empyema.

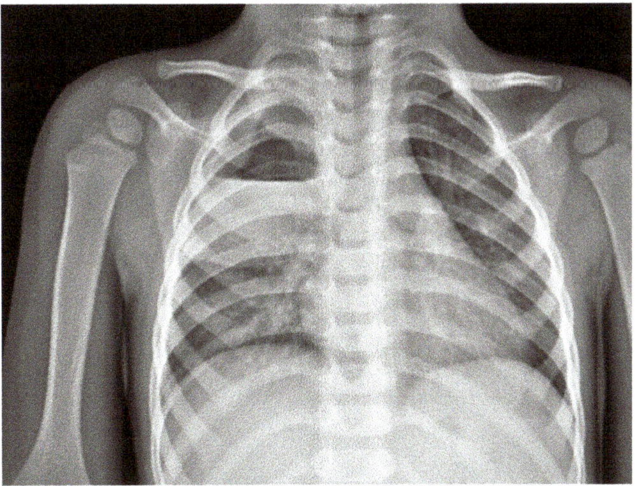

Fig. 4: Empyema—X-ray chest demonstrates a homogenous opacity in the left hemithorax with an air-fluid level. The differential diagnosis for this would be between an empyema and lung abscess. The lesion is not spherical, the diameters are unequal, as well as the angles the lesion makes with the chest wall are obtuse indicating an empyema.

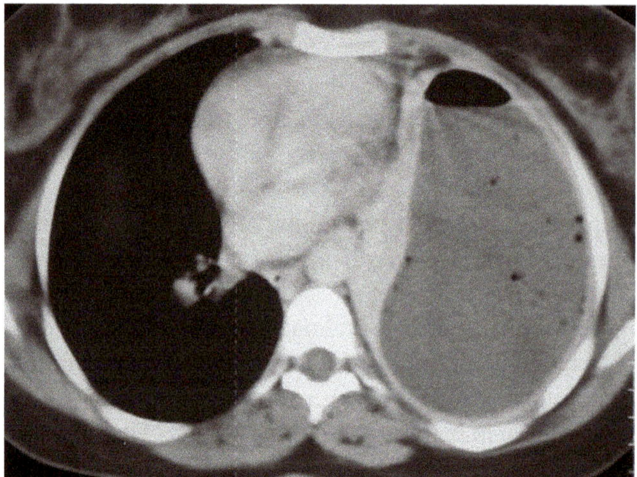

Fig. 5: Empyema—computed tomography chest demonstrates a well-defined and thick walled rounded opacity in the left pleural cavity with hyperdense contents with an air fluid level and air specks within, indicating an empyema.

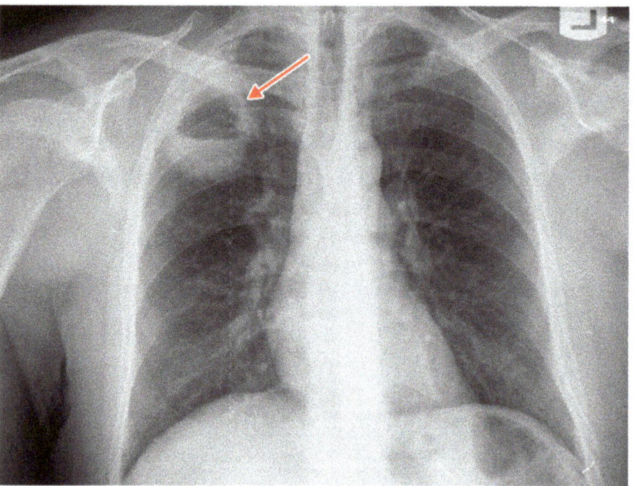

Fig. 6: Lung abscess: PA view of chest reveals thick walled cavitatory lesion with air-fluid level in right upper zone. The diameters are equal, as well as angles are acute indicating a lung abscess.

- Presence of vasculature around the abscess—if present this is sure proof of a suppurative lung abscess, rather than an empyema
- A sharp angle with the chest wall.

Pleural Fluid Examination

A suspicion of empyema necessitates a prompt thoracocentesis. The presence of pus in the pleural aspirate confirms empyema. A foul odor points to a likely anaerobic infection. When an empyema is loculated, it is extremely important to sample more than one location because the thoracocentesis may occasionally reveal clear fluid in one loculus and frank pus in a neighboring loculus. This is because the fibrinous partition may prevent bacteria crossing from one loculus A to the neighboring loculus B, so that the latter will have no or few pus cells, even though loculus A will have multiplying bacteria and numerous pus cells. The actively metabolizing bacteria in loculus A will cause a sharp fall in the glucose content of the fluid and CO_2 produced by active metabolism will cause a sharp fall in the pH of the fluid. Though bacteria may not penetrate into loculus B, glucose and CO_2 may do so. Thus fluid in loculus B may be sterile yet have a lowered glucose content and a lowered pH.

Light's criteria give the characteristics of the pleural fluid in an uncomplicated parapneumonic effusion and in both a complicated parapneumonic effusion and a frank empyema, helping to distinguish one from the other. Complicated parapneumonic effusion and empyema are characterized by a low pH (7.1) a low glucose (<40 mg/dL), a raised LDH (>1000 IU/L) and an elevated WBC count. The presence of an elevated amylase in a pleural exudate points either to the possibility of a pancreatic etiology to the fluid or an esophageal perforation.

Light's criteria have important clinical significance in the management of bacterial pleural exudates. Uncomplicated parapneumonic pleural effusions almost always resolve spontaneously following appropriate antibiotic therapy; complicated parapneumonic effusions and empyema require drainage.

Cultures are invariably positive in untreated patients with empyema but may be negative in those who have received antibiotics. While gram-positive cultures predominate in empyema due to community-acquired pneumonias, gram-negative cultures are far more frequent in empyemas consequent to nosocomial pneumonia. Gram-negative cultures are increasingly observed in elderly patients or in immunocompromised patients with empyema complicating community-acquired pneumonia. Anaerobic organisms are also encountered particularly in empyema following aspiration pneumonia or consequent to a lung abscess. Multiple infections have been reported in the Western literature but are uncommon in our experience.

When an empyema in an untreated patient is negative for bacterial infection, the possibility of a tuberculous infection should be kept in mind. Cultures for acid-fast bacilli (AFB) should always be done.

Sputum cultures and cultures of bronchoalveolar lavage (BAL) fluid may be of help in identifying organisms responsible for an empyema. Occasionally, in a tuberculous empyema, BAL cultures are positive for AFB even though the empyema fluid is sterile.

Bronchoscopy is useful in the following conditions:

- To determine obstruction to a bronchus by a foreign body or a tumor. A bronchogenic carcinoma is an important underlying cause of an empyema. In our country, an aspirated betel nut or "supari" (of which the patient has no recollection) is also an important cause of a necrotizing pneumonia with an empyema.
- To perform a microbiological study on the BAL fluid in a pneumonic consolidation complicated by an empyema.
- To determine the presence, exact location of a bronchopleural fistula or an esophageotracheobronchial fistula.
- To aspirate bronchial secretions in those with excessive secretions or in those who are unable to cough up secretions.

Management

The principles of management are:

- Use of appropriate antibiotic therapy
- Efficient drainage of the pleural cavity
- Use of tissue plasminogen activator (TPA) plus deoxyribonuclease (DNase) intrapleurally
- Surgery under certain select circumstances.

Antibiotic Therapy

In severely ill septic patients, the sooner antibiotics are given the better. Empiric antibiotic therapy should preferably be started after the pleural fluid is sent for microbiological examination and culture but should never await the result of a laboratory report. Antibiotics used in critically ill patients should cover gram-positive infections, gram-negative infections, and also anaerobes if there is reason to suspect anaerobic infection. A protocol followed in our unit is the use of a combination of amoxycillin and piperacillin tazobactam in the appropriate dosage. If anaerobes are suspected, clindamycin or metronidazole is added; some units use an antibiotic cover for anaerobic infection routinely. The regime is altered if necessary after culture sensitivity reports are available.

Instillation of antibiotics into the pleural space is not recommended for two reasons—(1) the risk of introducing fresh infection, and (2) because when the pleura is inflamed many studies have shown concentrations of antibiotics well above the minimal inhibitory concentration in the empyema fluid.

The duration of antibiotic therapy depends on clinical response, the degree and duration of drainage, and radiographic regression and resolution of the empyema. It may be necessary in many patients to administer antibiotics for about 4–6 weeks.

Drainage

Tube drainage of purulent fluid is imperative for cure. Four questions need to be answered with regard to drainage of an empyema.

1. When should one drain?
2. How should one drain?
3. Where should one drain?
4. How long should one drain?

1. *When should one drain?* (1) Drainage is always indicated when there is localized frank pus in the pleural cavity; (2) in an acutely forming empyema when the patient is septic and when fluid is large in quantity, more than 1.5 L, or when fluid rapidly refills after more than one or two paracentesis; (3) when there is a bronchopleural fistula (air-fluid level in the pleural space); and (4) following an assessment of pleural fluid examination by Light's criteria. Drainage should be done early. In the words of Stephen Sahn and Richard Light in 1989, "The sun should never set on a parapneumonic effusion—because time is of the essence".

The American College of Chest Physicians suggests that drainage of the pleural fluid should be done if pH is less than 7.2. This is not really applicable in our country because of technological difficulties and lack of expertise in many hospitals.

For all practical purposes, the presence of turbid pleural fluid with a high neutrophilic and WBC count and a high protein content (as in a complicated parapneumonic effusion), or in the presence of pus (as in an empyema) warrants drainage; even though no organisms may be seen on smear or grown on culture.

2. *How should one drain?* Drainage through a fair-sized drainage tube of 20-Fr size inserted through the appropriate intercostal space suffices in the formative, maturing stage of an empyema (as in a complicated parapneumonic effusion), or in an empyema when the pus is not too thick. Smaller tubes may get blocked if the fluid becomes increasingly viscous. Patency can be maintained by periodic flushing with sterile normal saline. Thick pus is best drained (particularly in a chronic empyema) by an appropriate rib resection followed by insertion of a large drainage tube.

3. *Where should one drain?* The drain is inserted at the most dependent portion of the empyema. Imaging studies (CT scan) can easily identify the most dependent portion. In poor countries, or in areas where CT scan facilities are not available, PA and lateral X-ray of the chest helps. A few drops of an iodine dye injected into the pleural space will sink to the bottom of the empyema and thus helps localize the site of tube insertion.

4. *How long should one drain?* Drainage is continued till the empyema cavity closes and there is next to no fluid drainage. The lung as it expands approaches the chest wall so that the tube is well-nigh pushed out into the dressing. This may take weeks or a few months.

Use of Fibrinolytic Agents

The principle of evacuating infected pleural fluid was established 2,000 years ago. The formation of multiple fibrinous septae in an empyema is thought to contribute to chest drain failure. Intrapleural thrombolytics have been investigated as potential agents to increase fluid drainage thereby potentially decreasing mortality and the need for surgery. Breaking down loculations to allow complete evacuation of pleural pus is traditionally considered the key to successful treatment. Fibrinolytics have gained popularity and are regarded as part of standard treatment. Successful intrapleural fibrinolysis can reduce the need for surgery and benefit patients in countries with limited surgical facilities and patients too sick for surgery.

The value of fibrinolytic agents has been shown in a few prospective trials. Even so, there are a number of units, which avoid their use. Instillation of streptokinase (SK) or urokinase is indicated in the presence of thick pus or the presence of many loculations; 200,000–250,000 IU SK or 30,000–100,000 IU of urokinase is instilled into the pleural space daily for 5–6 days. Occasionally, the instillation may be continued for longer—10–12 days. Some units use large-volume irrigation of the empyema cavity through a large drainage tube with the option of instillation of a fibrinolytic drug as well.

Fibrinolytic therapy with or without irrigation of the empyema cavity is not always successful. Failure of therapy is manifested by persistence of the empyema, persistence of loculations within the empyema cavity as judged by ultrasound or CT imaging and by persisting clinical features. Failure ratios vary from 15% (in those experienced in the use of fibrinolytics) to 30%.

Fibrinolytic therapy is contraindicated in patients with bronchopleural fistula (liquefied pleural secretions may then flood the lungs), in patients allergic to SK, in septic patients with a deranged coagulation profile (for fear of excessive bleeding) and in patients with coagulation disorders.

Evidence for and against Fibrinolytic Therapy

Many case reports, several small series and four small randomized trials have confirmed the important impact fibrinolytics have in empyema. However, the results of the landmark Multicenter Intrapleural Streptokinase Study (MIST 1) published in 2005 *[Ref: Maskell NA, Davies CWH, Nunn AJ; First Multicenter Intrapleural Sepsis Trial (MIST1), et al . Intrapleural streptokinase for pleural infection. N Engl J Med. 2005;352:865-74]*, failed to show significant benefit following the use of SK in empyema. This study, by far the largest in the field, enrolled 454 patients with empyema, with 226 randomly assigned to SK and the rest to placebo. The dose of intrapleural SK was 250,000 units twice a day for three days. The primary end points assessed were mortality and need for surgery while secondary end points were duration of hospital stay, lung function, and radiographic clearing. Rather surprisingly, the MIST 1 trial concluded that SK offered no therapeutic benefits over placebo in terms of need for surgical intervention, mortality or length of hospital stay. Possible explanations for the negative results of the MIST 1 study are that an older population of patients was enrolled and sonography or CT was not used to define loculations.

A prospective study in 2012 on 108 patients with complicated parapneumonic effusion showed that compared to placebo, intrapleural administration of 25 mg alteplase was more effective and led to better treatment outcomes.

Side effects of intrapleural administration of fibrinolytics include fever, chest pain, allergic reactions, and pleural hemorrhage

Use of Fibrinolytic Agents + Deoxyribonuclease (DNase)

The unsatisfactory results following the use of fibrinolytic therapy and the observation that DNase within the pleural fluid was responsible for its viscosity led to the assumption that the use of a mucolytic agent like deoxyribonuclease might reduce this viscosity and thereby allow proper drainage. The combination of intrapleural TPA (5–10 mg) twice daily for 3 days together with DNase (5 mg) twice daily for 3 days in a recent clinical study on 210 patients resulted in a greater reduction in radiographic pleural opacity, lesser rate of surgical reference and a shorter hospital stay compared with placebo.

The above combination therapy is being advocated as "rescue therapy" for patients with on-going signs of infection, poorly draining loculated empyemas, who have failed antibiotic therapy and conventional drainage and who would otherwise need surgical debridement. It is too early to determine the exact niche this therapy will assume in the management of empyema.

Surgical Treatment

Indications for surgery are—failure of medical treatment and failure of tube drainage to close the empyema cavity. Failure is generally due to incorrect drainage (too small a tube for proper drainage or tube inserted at the wrong site), multiple loculations within the empyema cavity, and a persistent underlying cause for the empyema—for example a bronchogenic carcinoma, a foreign body such as a "supari" aspirated within the bronchus, a persistent bronchopleural fistula or due to an esophageotracheobronchial fistula. A chronic empyema cavity may persist and remain unclosed, if there is thick fibrous tissue over the visceral pleura that prevents the lung from expanding. Surgery may take several forms.

- Rib resection with insertion of large-bore drainage tube at the appropriate site has already been mentioned.
- A video-assisted thoracoscopic approach that breaks loculations within the empyema so that proper

drainage now becomes possible through a large tube thereby promoting healing.

- A thoracoscopic approach which not only breaks loculations but allows decortication of the lung surface followed by drainage through a large-bore tube. A rib resection to allow insertion of the large-sized drainage tube may well be necessary.
- An open thoracotomy for a full decortication of the lung, breaking down loculi within the empyema, a pleural toilet, followed by adequate drainage through a tube.

To conclude, 2,400 years ago, in Hippocratic times the mortality from an empyema was 100%. To quote Hippocrates; "If an empyema does not rupture, death will occur". Today, in the modern antibiotic era, the mortality is closer to 15% but this is still a high rate for an infection. In the years to come, early diagnosis and appropriate treatment can bring down mortality further.

■ UNCOMMON PLEURAL INFECTIONS

Fungal infections are rare causes of pleural exudates. Invasive aspergillosis (due to *Aspergillus fumigatus*) may invade the pleural cavity causing pleural effusion. Pulmonary aspergillosis occurs under specific clinical settings—immunocompromised patients, human immunodeficiency virus (HIV) infections, long-standing bronchopleural fistulas, and chronic empyemas treated repeatedly with broad-spectrum antibiotics. The typical hyphae of *A. fumigatus* can be seen on smear and grown on culture. Amphotericin B is used systemically and can be used for local antifungal irrigation. Voriconazole is safer than and probably as effective as amphotericin B.

Histoplasmosis, coccidioidomycosis infections of the lung causing pleural effusions occur against an epidemiological setting where these diseases are endemic, as for example in the American continent. Fungal pleural effusions resemble tuberculous pleural effusions in relation to fluid examination. Primary pleural infection or secondary infection related to a parenchymal lung pathology are both possible. Routine fungal cultures confirm diagnosis. Specific therapy includes azole therapy or amphotericin B.

Pleural effusions due to *Cryptococcus neoformans* are rare and occur only in immunocompromised patients, in particular AIDS. The disease may be localized to the lungs and pleura or be disseminated.

Rarely, *Actinomyces israelii* causes a pleural effusion. The diagnosis is suspected when there are multiple sinuses leading from the pleural cavity discharging on to the skin. The organism can be detected in the granules present in the discharge and can be cultured as well. Penicillin is the drug of choice.

Atypical mycobacterial infection of the lung is increasingly encountered in our country but pleural effusions are rare and, if present, are small collections. Growth of atypical mycobacteria from pleural fluid should always arouse suspicion of contamination.

Nocardial *(Nocardia asteroids)* pleural effusions result from a spread of nocardial parenchymal lung disease, which may present as nodules or as small or large abscesses. These occur in immunedeficient states and in immunocompromised patients. One also encounters this infection in patients with long-standing chronic airways obstruction who have received corticosteroids and broad-spectrum antibiotics. Cotrimoxazole, doxycycline, and rifampicin are effective drugs. Pleural effusions if they occur are always small in size.

Viral infections due to influenza virus, cytomegalovirus, coxsackie virus, adenovirus, and other viruses can produce small acute pleural effusions. They remain unidentified because of difficulties in diagnosis. Perhaps quite a few small pleural effusions of undetermined etiology are due to viruses, or due to *Chlamydiae pneumoniae,* and *Coxiella burnetii.* Diagnostic proof that this is indeed so in our part of the world is often lacking.

Parasitic pleural involvement is seen in defined epidemiological circumstances. Important parasitic pleural effusions are due to echinococcus (where this infection is endemic) and paragonimiasis (common in South-East Asia). Amebic involvement of the pleura is extremely common in India and several other countries. It is considered in the section on "Tropical Infections Involving the Lung".

■ TUBERCULOUS PLEURAL EFFUSION

Though in the West, tuberculosis accounts for less than 5% of all pleural effusions, in India and in poor developing countries where tuberculosis is rife, it remains perhaps the most common and important cause of a pleural exudate. In India, it is a disease of young adults, the mean age being between 15 years and 30 years. In contrast, the mean age in the West lies between 47 years and 56 years.

Tuberculous pleural effusions generally occur in the primary or in the postprimary phase of the disease. It is believed that rupture of a small subpleural tuberculous

focus into the pleura leads to a marked exudative pleural reaction. Mycobacterial antigens within the pleural space elicit an intense immune response characterized initially by neutrophils and macrophages, followed by interferon-producing T helper cell (Th) type I lymphocytes sensitized to tuberculous antigen. This results in a lymphocytic predominant exudative pleurisy. A recent study has shown that cells of an alternative T cell profile CD4 + CD25 + FOXP3 + regulatory T cells are also increased in tuberculous pleural effusion. The role of these cells remains unclear.

Clinical Features

The onset may be insidious, subacute, or occasionally acute. When acute, pleuritic pain is associated with fever ranging from 102° F to 104° F and with severe constitutional symptoms. Dry cough and dyspnea are invariably present. When the onset is insidious the patient may have a low-grade fever, weight loss with very few respiratory symptoms. The effusion may be detected on a routine X-ray chest. Pleural effusion in tuberculosis may be small, moderate, or massive. Bilateral pleural effusions though uncommon, can occur and often cause severe dyspnea with respiratory failure. Large pleural effusions are invariably observed in the postprimary phase of tuberculosis. Imaging findings may reveal associated tuberculous mediastinal adenopathy but an obvious parenchymal lesion within the lung is often not observed.

Another form of tuberculous pleural effusion in the postprimary phase is caseous tuberculous involvement of the pleura. There are many who believe that caseous diffuse granulomatous involvement in the postprimary phase is the usual manifestation of pleural tuberculosis. This form of pleural involvement can produce severe pleural damage. A fibrous thickened pleura with calcification may envelop the lung resulting in a fibrothorax.

Tuberculous pleural effusion can also occur in reactivation tuberculosis with obvious parenchymal disease. Such tuberculous pleural effusions are generally small or at the most moderate in size—never large as at times observed in the postprimary phase of the disease. It is indeed a wonder why a patient with severe bilateral cavitative fibrocaseous tuberculosis involving the greater part of both lungs has generally little or no pleural involvement.

Miliary tuberculosis very often (though not necessarily) a postprimary event may have a pleural exudate, but again the effusion is generally small or moderate in size.

A tuberculous cavity within the lung may occasionally open into the pleura—the result is tuberculous pyopneumothorax. Tuberculous pleural effusion also occurs in HIV-related resurgence of tuberculosis. Pleurisy, however, occurs in the early stage of immune suppression with CD4 counts more than 200 cell/dL, suggesting that a reasonably preserved immune competence is required for an exudative pleural response to occur.

Finally, tuberculous pleural exudates may evolve into pus leading to a tuberculous empyema. Tuberculosis should figure in the differential diagnosis of any empyema where the pus is reported to be sterile on routine aerobic and anaerobic cultures.

Diagnosis

The pleural exudate shows an increase in leukocytes, at times as high as 500–750 cells/mm^3. There is a lymphocytic predominance though in the early stage polymorphs may form more than a third or half of the cellular count. The pH of the fluid may be low and the glucose content is often less than 60 mg/dL. The pleural fluid is either straw-colored or turbid and rarely, blood-tinged.

Acid-fast bacilli are almost never found in the pleural exudate on smear. Positive cultures for AFB are rare, being found in not more than 5% of patients. A positive polymerase chain reaction (PCR) for tuberculosis in the pleural fluid is of help but should never be relied upon for a definite diagnosis.

The Mantoux test is generally strongly positive. In the early phase of the natural history of a tuberculous pleural effusion, particularly in a postprimary effusion the Mantoux test may be negative. But it is invariably positive after 6–8 weeks of a pleural exudate.

Nonspecific Inflammatory Markers in the Diagnosis of Tuberculous Pleural Effusion

Adenosine deaminase released by activated lymphocytes and macrophages is a nonspecific marker of inflammation. The ADA levels are found to be invariably raised in tuberculous pleural effusions. A convincingly raised ADA (>50 U/L) in the pleural fluid has a very high sensitivity (close to 100%) and good specificity (close to 90%) for a tuberculous pleural exudate. The higher the pleural fluid ADA level, the more likely the diagnosis of tuberculosis. In fact, low ADA levels in pleural fluid negate the diagnosis of tuberculosis. However, raised ADA levels have also been observed in parapneumonic empyemas, malignancies, lymphomas, uremic pleuritis, and rarely in rheumatoid and other connective tissue diseases. Even so, in countries where tuberculosis is endemic (high-prevalence settings), a positive ADA test provides a 99% post-test probability of tuberculosis. On the other hand, in countries with low or intermediate tuberculosis incidence, a positive ADA test does not have the same strong predictive value as in countries where tuberculosis is endemic. This illustrates the fact that the predictive value of a test is highly dependent on the prevalence of the disease.

Adenosine deaminase occurs in two different isoenzymes—(1) ADA 1 and (2) ADA 2. Whilst the former is found in all cells, ADA 2 is present only in monocytes. The majority of ADA in tuberculous pleural effusion is ADA 2. Although the use of ratios of ADA 1 to ADA 2 have been advocated as a way of increasing the diagnostic value of the test in the diagnosis of tuberculous pleural effusions, the extra effort and cost does not justify the extra yield.

Other nonspecific inflammatory markers whose levels are found to be raised in tuberculous pleural effusion include *neopterin*, *leptin*, and *lysozyme*. They lack the sensitivity and specificity of ADA and are of no clinical importance.

The only cytokine in the pleural fluid which if raised is of diagnostic significance is *interferon-γ* (*IFN-γ*). A raised *IFN-γ* has a sensitivity of 89% and a specificity of 97% for a tuberculous pleural exudate. It is a difficult test to perform, extremely expensive, and can never replace the easy-to-perform, cheap ADA test in countries where tuberculosis has a high prevalence rate.

Detection of Tuberculosis Nucleic Acid Sequences by Amplification Test

The detection of *Mycobacterium tuberculosis* nucleic acids from pleural fluid has a sensitivity of 62% but a very high specificity of 97%; the test therefore is not useful in excluding the disease.

In summary, a good history and clinical examination, imaging studies, and examination of pleural fluid which should include ADA levels and AFB culture of the fluid suffice in the majority of cases to allow a diagnosis of tuberculous pleural effusion.

Pleural Biopsy

In the absence of a positive AFB culture of the pleural fluid, a confirmed diagnosis of tuberculosis can only be made by a pleural biopsy. A blind biopsy using Abram's needle is often negative and when malignancy is an important differential diagnosis a thoracoscopic biopsy is warranted.

Is a pleural biopsy mandatory for a diagnosis of a tuberculous pleural effusion when the fluid is negative for AFB culture? Not so. In a young individual with a pleural exudate compatible with tuberculosis, with raised ADA level, a positive Mantoux test, and no obvious lung pathology, the probability of tuberculosis is well-nigh certain. However, in an individual past 40 years, or in a heavy cigarette smoker, or when the ADA in the pleural fluid is marginally raised or when there is no response to specific antituberculosis drugs, a definite diagnosis is necessary, because the characteristics of a malignant pleural effusion are very similar to tuberculous pleural effusion. Imaging studies, studies on the BAL fluid and on the cytology of the pleural fluid may help but not always so. A video-assisted thoracoscopy, which enables the thoracoscopist to view the pleural cavity and takes multiple biopsies, will enable the physician to arrive at a correct diagnosis.

Spontaneous resolution is not uncommon in tuberculous pleural effusions. A follow-up of untreated patients over a 5-year period reveals a high rate of recurrence of tuberculosis, chiefly in the lungs but occasionally at extrapulmonary sites.

Large pleural effusions may require to be tapped more than once for symptom relief. The usual antituberculosis drugs need to be given for a period of 6–9 months. A course of corticosteroids starting with 30 mg prednisolone daily for a week and slowly tapered over a period of 6 weeks hastens resolution of a pleural effusion.

Untreated or incompletely treated pleural effusions may become loculated with thickened parietal and visceral pleura. Resolution and full expansion of the lung is possible in some of these patients only after thoracoscopic surgery which involves decortication and proper drainage of the fluid contents through a correctly placed drainage tube.

■ MALIGNANT PLEURAL EFFUSION

It is estimated that about one-third of all malignancies will develop a pleural effusion at some stage in their natural history. A malignant pleural effusion may be the initial presenting feature of underlying malignant disease.

Except for pleural mesothelioma, which is a primary malignancy of the pleura, all other pleural involvement is caused by secondaries from a primary situated elsewhere within the body **(Fig. 7)**. The most common primary sites giving rise to pleural metastasis and malignant pleural effusion are the breast, lung, stomach, and the rest of the gastrointestinal tract. These account for 60% of malignant pleural effusions. Nevertheless, primaries from almost any site are known to produce pleural metastasis. The pleura may be involved by direct spread (from the lung as an example), by hematogenous spread, or through lymphatics as in lymphoma. Non-Hodgkin's lymphoma involves the pleura far more frequently than Hodgkin's disease.

Pleural effusions (in patients with underlying malignancy) that show no detectable invasion of the pleura by malignant cells are often termed paramalignant effusions. These effusions may be due to tumor-related problems such as pneumonia, atelectasis, pulmonary embolism, lymphatic obstruction due to a malignant mediastinal adenopathy, radiation-induced pleural inflammation or may be transudative in nature due to hypoproteinemia, or associated cardiac, hepatic, or renal disease. Distinction from a malignant pleural effusion is important as paramalignant pleural effusions do not negate surgical resection of a malignant tumor.

Pleural fluid in malignant involvement of the pleura is often hemorrhagic but not always so. It invariably reaccumulates after paracentesis. The pleural fluid cytology is positive in about 50–70% of patients. Absence

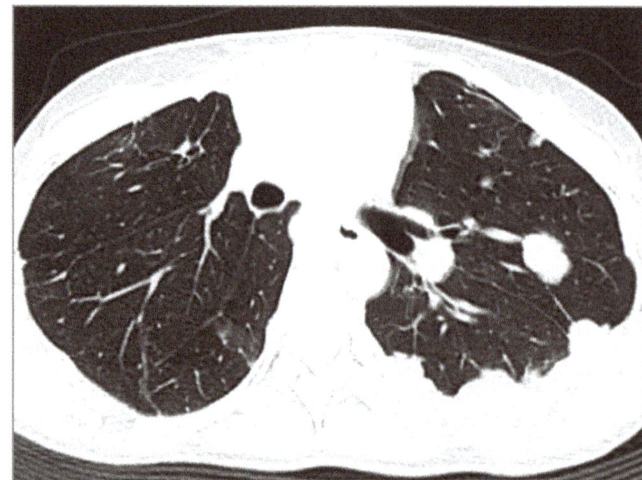

Fig. 7: Pleural metastases—CT chest demonstrates multiple nodular lesions within left lung field and along the left pleural surface posteriorly in a patient with a renal cell carcinoma. These represent pleural metastases.

of malignant cells in the pleural fluid should never exclude the diagnosis of malignancy.

Pleural biopsy either through a video-assisted thoracoscopy or a CT-guided biopsy, if a lesion is clearly visible on imaging studies is absolutely necessary for a confirmed diagnosis.

A malignant pleural effusion in our country is often mistaken for a tuberculous pleural effusion. The mistake is often compounded, if the PCR for tuberculosis is found positive in the pleural fluid and is relied upon to make a diagnosis of tuberculosis. A CT-guided or a thoracoscopic biopsy is a must for the confirmation of either tubercle or malignancy, particularly in pleural effusions occurring in those over 40 years of age.

Except in patients where pleural involvement is due to a lymphoma (which can respond to chemotherapy), cure of the underlying malignancy is not possible once pleural involvement is confirmed. Management is then palliative and directed toward improving the quality of the patient's life.

PLEURAL EFFUSION IN GASTROINTESTINAL DISEASE

Acute pancreatitis is the most common gastrointestinal disease causing a pleural exudate. The reported rate of a pleural effusion in acute pancreatitis is 3–17%. The effusion is left-sided in over two-thirds of patients because of the proximity of the pancreatic tail to the left dome of the diaphragm. The left dome is often elevated and immobile and examination of the pleural fluid reveals a raised amylase content often exceeding serum values. The effusion is generally small-to-moderate in size and clears as the pancreatitis subsides. Persistence of fluid over 2 weeks of therapy suggests a pancreatic pseudocyst, a pancreatopleural fistula, or a pancreatic abscess. A pancreatopleural fistula is characterized by a direct sinus tract between the pancreas and the pleura, resulting at times in a massive pleural effusion. Pancreatic ascites due to communication of the pancreatic duct with the peritoneal cavity is also associated with pleural effusion, which is often bilateral.

Pleural effusion occurring after major abdominal surgery should suggest a subphrenic or intrahepatic abscess. Pleural effusions are observed in 80% of subphrenic abscesses. The pleural effusion though an exudate is invariably sterile (sympathetic pleural effusion) and rarely leads to an empyema except when a subphrenic abscess breaches the diaphragm and opens into the pleura.

Pleural effusions are common in amebic abscesses of the liver. The subject is dealt with in the section on "Tropical Infections Involving the Lung".

Esophageal perforation whatever be the cause produces a left-sided and occasionally, bilateral pleural exudates with a raised amylase content. Apart from the typical history, imaging findings and analysis of the pleural fluid with the raised amylase (of salivary origin on enzyme study) confirm the diagnosis. A pleural exudate following esophageal perforation soon becomes an empyema.

PULMONARY EMBOLISM, PLEURAL EFFUSION FOLLOWING CORONARY BYPASS GRAFT SURGERY, AND DRUG-INDUCED PLEURISY

Pulmonary Embolism

This is an important frequently missed cause of pleural effusion. The diagnosis rests on a keen awareness of this possibility particularly in specific clinical settings, as for example in critically ill patients under intensive care. The possibility of pulmonary embolism as a cause of a pleural effusion should always be considered where the etiology of a pleural exudate remains undetermined. The effusion is often bloody but not always so. The presence of eosinophils in the pleural exudate should also arouse suspicion of an underlying pulmonary embolism.

Sickle cell crisis can lead to pleuritic chest pain with pleural effusions which may contain blood.

Postcoronary Bypass Graft Surgery

Pleural effusion following coronary bypass graft surgery (CABG) occasionally persists for weeks or months. The pathogenesis of such persistent effusions is unclear. They generally resolve after repeated paracentesis or drainage through an intercostal drain. Occasionally, pleurodesis becomes necessary.

Drug-induced Pleurisy

Drug-induced lupus, or hypersensitivity reactions leading to a pleural exudate has been reported with isoniazid, nitrofurantoin, methysergide, bromocriptine, procainamide, amiodarone, phenytoin, and dantrolene. Drug-induced lupus is generally associated with antinuclear antibodies not only in the blood but also in the pleural exudate. Histone antibodies are considered to be specific for drug-induced lupus. Treatment consists in withdrawing the drug (even if there is a suspicion of drug hypersensitivity) and the use of a 3–6-week course of corticosteroids. Thoracocentesis is necessary; eosinophils are often present in the pleural exudate. Failure to recognize drug-induced pleural effusion can lead to well-marked pleural fibrosis.

Hypersensitivity pleural exudates due to drugs can be associated with fever, well-marked constitutional symptoms, and with peripheral eosinophilia. This is particularly observed in hypersensitivity reactions to nitrofurantoin.

Ovarian Hyperstimulation Syndrome

Ovarian hyperstimulation syndrome (OHSS) is seen in 3–5% of women undergoing therapeutic ovarian stimulation through administration of ovarian hormones. The use of these hormones forms part of current reproductive techniques that help women to conceive. The syndrome is characterized by marked ovarian enlargement, the ovaries being often felt on palpating the abdomen. There is a marked increase in capillary permeability leading to depletion of intravascular volume. This results in hypotension, oliguria and the presence of edema, ascites, and at times massive hydrothorax. The pathogenesis of this syndrome is unclear. Treatment is supportive and is directed toward increasing intravascular volume through use of colloids and crystalloids.

■ HEMOTHORAX

Hemothorax is characterized by a markedly blood-stained pleural effusion. The diagnosis of hemothorax, however, requires a pleural fluid hematocrit more than 50% of that in the peripheral blood. This is important because many serosanguinous pleural effusions which appear as hemothorax may have hematocrits much lower than that stated above.

Etiology

Chest trauma (blunt or penetrating chest injury) is the single most important cause of hemothorax. Important medical causes include malignancy, severe forms of dengue, pulmonary infarction, rupture of an aortic aneurysm, in particular rupture of a dissecting aneurysm of the aorta. Hemothorax is also observed in bleeding disorders, coagulopathies, and as a complication of anticoagulation therapy. Rarely, a spontaneous pneumothorax is followed by a small to moderate-sized hemothorax due to a rupture of a vessel within the tear. Finally, iatrogenic causes include cardiothoracic surgical procedures, pleural or lung biopsies, perforation of the subclavian vein or superior vena cava by a central venous catheter, and perforation of a pulmonary vessel by a Swan-Ganz catheter.

A small hemothorax has the usual signs of a pleural effusion. A large hemothorax besides causing cardiorespiratory embarrassment is associated with pallor, severe hypovolemic shock, and a progressive fall in the hemoglobin.

Treatment

A large or moderate-sized hemothorax should be drained by insertion of a large-bore drainage tube. This allows the collapsed lung to expand, enables an estimation of continuing blood loss and prevents clotting of blood within the pleural cavity. Clots within the pleural space can get infected and lead to empyema. Organization of clots leads to fibrosis with an unexpanded lung.

Surgical intervention is indicated under the following conditions:

- Massive hemothorax, when the greater part of the hemothorax is opacified with blood;
- When bleeding exceeds the rate of 200 mL/h continuously for 3 consecutive hours via the drain;
- If a liter or more of blood is evacuated after insertion of the drainage tube; and
- The presence of hypovolemic shock even when the quantity of blood loss through the drain is not excessive. This point is of great importance. Blood gathered within the pleural space may occasionally not find egress through the drainage tube for several reasons, chiefly because of intrapleural clot formation and/or blockage of the drainage tube, so that the clinician gets a wrong impression of the quantum of blood loss.

It is advisable to administer broad-spectrum antibiotics to a patient with hemothorax to prevent infection or treat infection if it occurs. Infection often promotes fibrothorax—a lung trapped by a tight fibrous peel, which sharply restricts its movement. Amazingly, even large blood clots within the pleural space, if uninfected, often resolve spontaneously, leaving behind very little pleural fibrosis.

CHYLOTHORAX

Chylothorax is a rare disorder characterized by chyle within the pleural exudate. The pleural fluid is milky and remains milky on centrifugation. Chyle in a milky pleural effusion is confirmed by the presence of triglycerides above 110 mg/dL on analysis and in doubtful cases by the demonstration of chylomicrons on lipid electrophoresis.

A chylous pleural effusion is due to injury to the thoracic duct with spillage of chyle through the mediastinal pleura into the pleural space. Besides surgical and nonsurgical trauma, the two most important causes are malignancies which disrupt the thoracic duct and lymphomas. Tuberculosis (a tuberculous adenopathy) is another cause, particularly in countries where tuberculosis is rife. Even so, it is a rare cause, and if imaging demonstrates adenopathy along the course of the thoracic duct, it is necessary to exclude a lymphoma through a biopsy before considering tuberculosis as the causative disease. Blockage of the thoracic duct by an adult filarial parasite (generally *Wuchereria bancrofti)* should be considered in regions of the world where filariasis is endemic. Lymphedema, fever with chills and demonstration of microfilaria in the peripheral blood are pointers to a filarial etiology **(Table 7)**.

A rare but important cause of chylous pleural effusion is lymphangioleiomyomatosis; chylothorax occurs in about 20% of these patients. Not uncommonly in quite a few patients, the cause of a chylothorax, in spite of all investigations, remains obscure.

Clinical Features

A chylothorax invariably occurs on the right side because of the anatomical course of the thoracic duct. Escape of chyle into the pleural space leads to loss of nutrients, chiefly fats but also proteins. This can lead to severe inanition, weight loss, and depressed immune function.

Table 7: Causes of chylothorax.
• *Trauma:*
– Chest injury (blunt or penetrating)
– Rarely following forceful vomiting and cough
– Iatrogenic
– Surgery and radiation
• Malignancy
• Lymphoma
• Tuberculosis
• Filariasis
• Sarcoidosis
• Lymphangioleiomyomatosis
• Yellow nail syndrome

Diagnosis

Imaging, thoracoscopy, and biopsy studies of manifest lesions may give the diagnosis of a lymphoma, malignancy, or tuberculosis. The site of the leak is best determined by lymphangiography. A radioactive dye, injected into the web between two toes in both feet is carefully followed to determine the site of obstruction.

Treatment

Treatment for the underlying disease (such as a lymphoma, malignancy, tubercle, or any other treatable cause) is mandatory. A low-fat diet with medium chained triglycerides is necessary as this reduces the production of chyle substantially. In patients who have become malnourished through the loss of chyle, parenteral nutrition is advised, thereby reducing the flow of chyle to a minimum; this may help to seal a leak in the thoracic duct, particularly in traumatic chylothorax.

Local measures are often necessary to prevent further weight loss and inanition. Chemical pleurodesis and pleuroperitoneal shunt have their advocates, but the results are poor. Octreotide, a somatostatin analog has been tried (combined with a low-fat diet stated above) to reduce chyle production and help in closure of the leak. It may be of help, particularly in post-traumatic chylothorax. Ligation of the thoracic duct a short distance above the diaphragm through a video-assisted thoracoscopy is usually effective. It obviates the often difficult task of locating the leak. There are no long-term effects observed after ligation of the thoracic duct. When expertise is available, a lymphangiography should be done to determine the site from which chyle is observed to leak. This site can then be plugged through a catheter using lipcodol + glue in proper proportions (1 : 1 or 1 : 2).

PSEUDOCHYLOTHORAX

The term pseudochylothorax implies that the pleural fluid resembles chyle but in fact is not so. It results from accumulated cholesterol (>200 mg/dL) or lecithin globulin complexes in a long standing, often loculated pleural effusion. There are no chylomicrons within the fluid, distinguishing it from a true chylothorax. The most common cause is a long-standing tuberculous or post-traumatic effusion in which the pleura is fibrosed and at times calcified. Treatment is for the underlying disease.

■ MISCELLANEOUS CONDITIONS

Dressler's Syndrome

Dressler's syndrome is characterized by an aseptic inflammation chiefly of the pericardium but at times also involving the pleura. It can occur from 10 days to 6 weeks after a myocardial infarction or after cardiac surgery. The patient has precordial pain, fever, leukocytosis, and a raised ESR, often as high as 100 mm/h. A pericardial rub may be present; pericardial effusion is often observed on a 2D-Echo study and on imaging studies. Small pleural effusions may occur. They are often left-sided, at times bilateral; the pleural aspirate is often bloody and may contain eosinophils. Cultures of both pericardial and pleural fluid are sterile.

Dressler's syndrome soon following upon a myocardial infarct is often misdiagnosed as a second infarct or as an increase in size of the previous infarct. When the syndrome occurs later (6 weeks after an infarct or after cardiac surgery) its significance is often missed and a wrong diagnosis is entertained. The pathogenesis of Dressler's syndrome is uncertain; it is believed to be related to antibodies being developed against the patient's myocardial cells.

Nonsteroidal anti-inflammatory drugs are generally effective. If they fail to resolve the problem, steroids always do so. Effusions may, however, return after steroids are withdrawn. Recurrences occasionally occur even after repeated courses of corticosteroids. Very rarely a pericardiectomy becomes necessary.

Vasculitis

Vasculitides involving the lung such as Wegener's granulomatosis or Churg-Strauss syndrome are rare causes of exudative pleural effusions. Parenchymal lesions within the lungs are invariably present. The exudate is inflammatory in nature often with a mixture of neutrophils and mononuclear cells; expectedly the protein level is raised. The pH of the fluid may be low. Eosinophils are characteristically high in the pleural aspirate in Churg-Strauss syndrome. Antineutrophilic cytoplasmic antibodies (ANCAs), if present, are specific and of diagnostic significance. Pleural effusions in vasculitis are generally small and resolve with the use of corticosteroids.

Acquired Immune Deficiency Syndrome

Pleural effusion in AIDS may be due to specific infections or due to neoplastic diseases like Kaposi's sarcoma and non-Hodgkin's lymphoma. At times, the effusion is nonspecific and of undetermined origin.

Organ Transplants

Organ transplantation is also at times followed by pleural effusion due to various specific infectious or noninfectious causes. The frequency of pleural effusion varies greatly. It is very high (>80%) in chronic rejection of a lung transplant. A specific lesion in patients with chronic rejection is due to pleural involvement by a lymphoproliferative disorder.

Rheumatoid Disease, SLE, and Other Connective Tissue Diseases

Pleural effusions in these diseases are discussed in a separate chapter.

Uremic Pleurisy

This is a rare complication of uremia in chronic renal failure. Unlike the transudative effusion encountered in renal failure, there occasionally occurs an inflammatory exudate which may be blood-stained and which may lead to significant pleural fibrosis. The exudate resolves with the correction of uremia.

Meigs' Syndrome

Meigs' syndrome consists of an ovarian tumor (generally, a fibroma but also includes tumors with low-grade malignancies), associated with ascites and pleural effusion. The effusion is an exudate but is nonmalignant. Fluid produced is derived directly from the tumor. Ascites occurs to start with; the ascitic fluid then seeps into one or both pleural spaces through pores within the diaphragm. The polyserositis disappears after removal of the ovarian tumor.

Yellow Nail Syndrome

Unilateral or bilateral lymphocytic pleural exudates in this syndrome are due to generalized hypoplasia of the lymphatics. Pleural effusions may be chylous in nature.

The syndrome in addition is characterized by yellow discoloration of the nails and peripheral lymphedema. All these features may not occur simultaneously, but may occur one after the other, so that diagnosis may be difficult when the syndrome has not evolved in its entirety. Pleural effusions may be massive and may require pleurodesis.

Asbestosis

Exudative pleural effusion is a feature of asbestosis, and has been discussed in a separate chapter.

Sarcoidosis

Pleural effusions are very rare in sarcoidosis. They may be due to direct pleural involvement. Obstruction to lymphatic pathways can also lead to a pleural effusion, which then is a transudate. Sarcoid glands can obstruct and disrupt the thoracic duct leading to a chylous pleural effusion.

Familial Mediterranean Fever

The diagnosis of this entity is suggested when transient small (at times recurrent) pleural effusions associated with fever occur in Sephardic Jews, Turks, Armenians, and Arabs (Mediterranean communities). This entity is also associated with arthritis and recurrent attacks of abdominal pain occurring during bouts of fever.

■ SUGGESTED READING

1. British Thoracic Society Standards of Care Committee. BTS guidelines for the management of pleural disease. Thorax. 2003;58(Suppl II):1-59.
2. Chakko SC, Caldwell SH, Sforza PP. Treatment of congestive heart failure. Its effect on pleural fluid chemistry. Chest. 1989;95:798-802.
3. Chapman SJ, Davies RJ. Recent advances in parapneumonic effusion and empyema. Curr Opin Pulm Med. 2004;10:299-304.
4. Choi BY, Yoon MI, Shin K, et al. Characteristics of pleural effusions in systemic lupus erythematosus: differential diagnosis of lupus pleuritis. Lupus. 2015;24:321-6.
5. Kim HJ, Lee HJ, Kwon SY, et al. The prevalence of pulmonary parenchymal tuberculosis in patients with tuberculous pleuritis. Chest. 2006;129:1253-8.
6. Liam CK, Lim KH, Wong CM. Causes of pleural exudates in a region with a high incidence of tuberculosis. Respirology. 2000;5:33-8.
7. Light RW. The undiagnosed pleural effusion. Clin Chest Med. 2006;27(2):309-19.
8. Majid A, Kheir F, Folch A, et al. Concurrent intrapleural instillation of tissue plasminogen activator and DNase for pleural infection. A single-center experience. Ann Am Thorac Soc. 2016;13:1512-8.
9. Martinez-Garcia MA, Cases-Viedma E, Cordero-Rodriguez PJ, et al. Diagnostic utility of eosinophils in the pleural fluid. Eur Respir J. 2000;15:166-9.
10. Maskell NA, Davies CWH, Nunn AJ; First Multicenter Intrapleural Sepsis (MIST1) Group, et al. UK Controlled trial of Intrapleural Streptokinase for Pleural Infection. N Engl J Med. 2005;352:865-74.
11. Piccolo F, Pitman N, Bhatnagar R, et al. Intrapleural tissue plasminogen activator and deoxyribonuclease for pleural infection. An effective and safe alternative to surgery. Ann Am Thorac Soc. 2014;11:1419-25.
12. Porcel JM. Diagnostic approach to pleural effusion in adults. Am Fam Physician. 2006;73(7):1211-20.
13. Sahn SA, Huggins JT, San Jose E, et al. The art of pleural fluid analysis. Clin Pulm Med. 2013;20:77-96.
14. Scarci M, Abah U, Solli P, et al. EACTS expert consensus statement for surgical management of pleural empyema. Eur J Cardiothorac Surg. 2015;48(5):642-53.
15. Svigals PZ, Chopra A, Ravenel JG, et al. The accuracy of pleural ultrasonography in diagnosing complicated parapneumonic pleural effusions. Thorax. 2017;72:94-5.

CHAPTER 63

Pneumothorax

■ INTRODUCTION

Pneumothorax signifies air within the pleural space. Pneumothorax may be traumatic or spontaneous. Spontaneous pneumothorax can be either primary or secondary. Primary pneumothorax, also called benign spontaneous pneumothorax, occurs in apparently healthy individuals with no obvious evidence of lung disease. Secondary pneumothorax is secondary to an underlying lung pathology, the most common of which is chronic obstructive pulmonary disease (COPD).

■ PRIMARY SPONTANEOUS PNEUMOTHORAX (BENIGN SPONTANEOUS PNEUMOTHORAX)

Primary spontaneous pneumothorax (PSP) usually occurs in young males between 20 years and 40 years of age. It is fairly common in India though its exact incidence is not known and would probably be very difficult to establish. The reported incidence in the USA is 7.4 per 100,000 population per year and 37 per 100,000 per year in the UK. The incidence is much less in women—1.2 per 100,000 population per year in USA and 13.4 per 100,000 per year in the UK. The reason for this difference in males and females is not known.

Risk Factors for Primary Spontaneous Pneumothorax

Risk factors include smoking, family history, homocystinuria, Marfan's syndrome, and thoracic endometriosis.

Smoking is the most important risk factor. The risk increases with the number of cigarettes smoked. Compared to nonsmokers the relative risk of PSP is seven times greater in those smoking 1–12 cigarettes a day, 21 times greater in those smoking 13–20 cigarettes a day and over 100 times greater in heavy smokers (those smoking more than 21 cigarettes per day).

Family history—PSP has been known to occur in certain families. This clustering in some families can be due to autosomal dominant, autosomal recessive, polygenic, and X-linked recessive mechanisms.

The Birt-Hogg-Dubé syndrome is autosomal dominant and is characterized by benign skin tumors and renal cancer. It is associated with an increased incidence of PSP. The gene responsible for this syndrome has been mapped to chromosome 17p11.2.

However, other mutations have been observed to be associated with spontaneous pneumothorax and bullous lung diseases without the oncologic manifestations of the Birt-Hogg-Dubé syndrome.

Other Risk Factors

Primary spontaneous pneumothorax is more frequent in patients with Marfan's syndrome, homocystinuria, and thoracic endometriosis. There are reports of PSP in patients with anorexia, probably related to malnutrition causing defects in pulmonary architecture.

Pathophysiology

Primary spontaneous pneumothorax is believed to be due to rupture of small subpleural blebs or bullae ("emphysematous-like changes") into the pleural space. A bleb is a small air-filled space between the visceral pleura and the lung parenchyma. A bulla is a small air-filled space within the parenchyma. When close to the visceral pleura, it could rupture through the pleura and produce a pneumothorax. These subpleural blebs and superficial small bullae have been observed in more than 75% of patients undergoing thoracoscopic treatment for PSP. They are of course not apparent clinically or on imaging so that the lungs outwardly are healthy. The blebs may well be due to an underlying bronchiolitis with rupture of a few alveolar walls due to nonspecific infection, which is more common in smokers. Air may then travel outwards along interstitial tissue planes to form a subpleural bleb. Damage to alveolar walls at the very periphery of the lung could result in small peripherally placed bullae. There is a clear tendency for PSP to occur in tall thin individuals (this includes patients with Marfan's syndrome), who have a high transpulmonary pressure at the lung apex. Ordinarily, primary pneumothorax is independent of intrathoracic pressure changes. Interestingly, emphysematous like changes have been identified in close to 25% of control subjects; they do not necessarily lead to pneumothorax. A recent concept in the pathogenesis of primary pneumothorax is the role played by increased lung porosity identified by fluorescein-enhanced autofluorescence techniques. Leakage from these porous areas can lead to air within the pleural space.

Clinical Features

The presenting features of a PSP are dyspnea and pleuritic chest pain. A dry cough may be present in over a third of patients. Exceptionally, a primary pneumothorax may be virtually silent.

Physical findings over the chest depend on the size of the pneumothorax. Typically, there is diminished movement over the affected side, with perhaps a slight bulging of the intercostal spaces. The trachea and the apex beat may be pushed to the opposite side. The percussion note on the affected side is hyperresonant; the breath sounds and vocal resonance are diminished. *When the pneumothorax is small, the only reliable sign that may alert a discerning physician is the presence of diminished breath sounds on the affected side.*

■ TENSION PNEUMOTHORAX

Tension pneumothorax may occur either in primary or secondary pneumothorax. It is characterized by air entering the pleural space during inspiration but because of a check valve mechanism at the site of rupture, little or no air can gain egress back into the lung and thence to the outside during expiration. The intrapleural pressure continues to increase and causes rapid cardiorespiratory collapse. The patient is tachypneic, breathless, cold, clammy, extremely distressed, and gasping for air. The markedly increased intrapleural pressure together with the marked mediastinal shift hinders venous return. Hence, there is increasing tachycardia and hypotension. The total collapse of the lung together with preservation of a fair degree of blood flow through it leads to a large right-to-left shunt within the collapsed lung so that there is increasing hypoxia, cyanosis, and increasing respiratory failure. The markedly increased intrapleural pressure on the affected side is transmitted to an extent to the contralateral pleural space so that lung function of the contralateral side is also adversely affected. Ultimately, if the tension pneumothorax is not promptly relieved, there is well-nigh stoppage of venous return because of a tamponade-like effect on the heart. A cardiac arrest often associated with an electromechanical dissociation on the electrocardiogram (ECG) is the end result.

Diagnosis (Figs. 1A and B)

An X-ray of the chest confirms the clinical diagnosis. An X-ray chest after full expiration is more sensitive in picking up a small pneumothorax. Mediastinal displacement to the opposite side is seen when the pneumothorax is of sufficient size. About 10% of patients may have an associated small pleural effusion.

A computed tomography (CT) of the chest is generally unnecessary unless one suspects an underlying disease in the lung on the plain X-ray. CT may reveal a small cyst or bulla not visible on an X-ray. In a young non-smoking female, it may reveal the subtle presence of diffuse cystic lung disease, seen for example in lymphangioleiomyomatosis. It may also help to distinguish between a large bulla and a pneumothorax, and help to confirm a suspected localized pneumothorax. A CT is generally advised in dealing with a persistent air leak as also in a patient with recurrent pneumothorax.

The volume of a pneumothorax is quantified by the volume of the hemithorax the pneumothorax occupies and can be estimated by Light's index

$$\% \text{ of pneumothorax} = 100 - \frac{(\text{Diameter of collapsed lung})^3}{(\text{Diameter of hemithorax})^3} \times 100$$

The differential diagnosis of PSP involves the exclusion of the many underlying lung diseases known to cause a secondary pneumothorax **(Table 1)**.

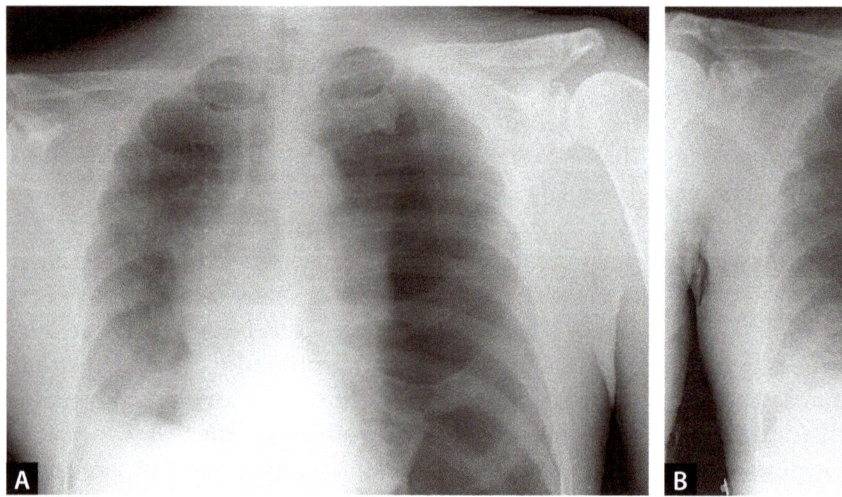

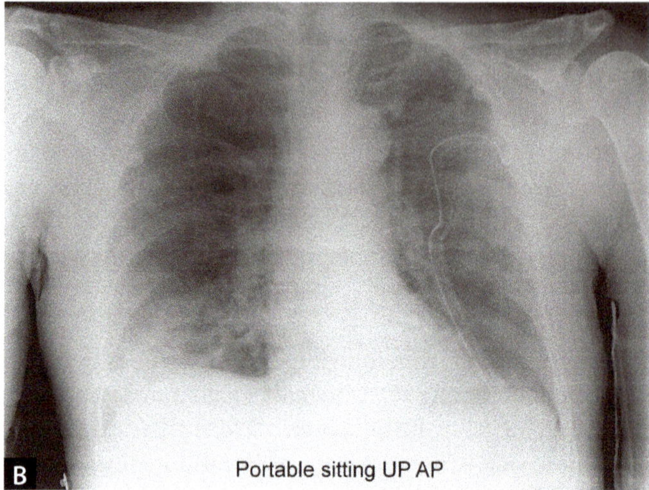

Figs. 1A and B: Tension pneumothorax. (A) Chest PA view reveals a translucency in left hemithorax due to a large pneumothorax. There is a mediastinal shift to right. These are features of a tension pneumothorax; (B) After intercostal drainage (ICD) tube insertion there is expansion of lung with return of mediastinal structures to their normal position.

Table 1: Causes of pneumothorax.
Primary spontaneous pneumothorax
Traumatic: • Penetrating and nonpenetrating chest injury
Secondary spontaneous pneumothorax: • Chronic obstructive airways disease • Asthma • Cysts and bullae within the lung • Tuberculosis • Interstitial lung disease • Pneumatoceles in Staphylococcal pneumonia • Whooping cough • Esophageal perforation • *Pneumocystis jirovecii* infection • Langerhans cell histiocytosis • Lymphangioleiomyomatosis • Lung malignancy • Necrotizing bacterial pneumonia • Cystic fibrosis
Iatrogenic: • Aspiration of pleural fluid • Intercostal tube insertion • Pleural or lung biopsy • Transbronchial biopsy • Central venous catheter insertion • Pacemaker insertion • Positive pressure ventilation • External cardiac massage

Management

Small pneumothoraces less than or equal to 3 cm with minimal symptoms and a stable cardiorespiratory system require only observation. The rate of spontaneous resorption of air from the pleural space is about 1.23% every 24 hours. This is of course obtained only if the tear in the visceral pleura has sealed. Oxygen administration at high flow rates is advantageous as it helps air resorption by reducing the partial pressure of nitrogen in the blood. It is to be noted that partial pressure in the alveolar air and in the pneumothorax equates with arterial blood and is 760 mm Hg, whereas the total partial pressure of venous blood is 706 mm Hg. There is therefore a driving force of 54 mm Hg promoting resorption of air from the pleural space.

In a symptomatic pneumothorax or in a large pneumothorax (>3–4 cm), air needs to be withdrawn from the pleural space. The current trend is to do this by simple aspiration. This succeeds in over 60% of patients. Aspiration may be repeated once or twice.

If re-expansion of the lung is good, though not complete, the patient may just require further observation to ensure that the pneumothorax slowly resolves and does not increase.

If aspiration is unsuccessful, or if the patient is markedly symptomatic, intercostal tube drainage is necessary. Small tube drains (10–14 Fr) are adequate, the drain being connected to an underwater seal. Gentle suction may be used to help re-expansion but should be avoided for the first 48 hours to reduce the risk of re-expansion edema. Once the lung has expanded and the tube in the underwater seal ceases to bubble the tube is clamped for 24 hours and a radiographic examination of the chest is repeated to ensure that there is no slow air leak. The tube is then removed **(Fig. 2)**.

If the air leak persists for more than 3 days in spite of chest tube drainage, surgical therapy (see below) is advised. In many small centers in our country, this may not be possible, in which case a chemical pleurodesis should be done while the intercostal tube drain is in place.

Surgical Treatment

Surgery is indicated when air leak persists in spite of tube drainage. This happens when the edges of the tear in the pleura and the lung beneath remain open so that air continues to have free egress into the pleural space. A persistent open tear may be due to a fibrotic thickened pleura in that area or a pleural adhesion holding the edges of the tear apart as shown in **Figure 3**.

Surgery is also indicated with the recurrence of a unilateral pneumothorax or following the occurrence of a first contralateral pneumothorax or the occurrence of bilateral synchronous pneumothorax. Surgery is also indicated in patients whose jobs (airline pilots and deep sea divers) demand that a recurrence is avoided as best as possible.

Video-assisted thoracoscopic surgery (VATS) allows stapling of blebs and small bullae through the use of an endostapler, laser ablation, or electrocoagulation. Following this, pleurodesis can be accomplished mechanically with pleural abrasion or partial pleurectomy or chemically through talc insufflation. Recurrence rates after the above procedures are very low (<5%). The new technology (not available in India) of fluorescence-enhanced autofluorescence thoracoscopy may help identify lesions not visible at routine thoracoscopy.

Prevention of Recurrence

The risk of a recurrence in a primary pneumothorax is about 30%; this risk is greatest in the first year. The recurrence rate is about 50% after one recurrence and over 80% after a third pneumothorax. The risk of a contralateral pneumothorax is about 10–15% after a primary event. Recurrence rate is higher in smokers and is believed to be also higher in tall thin individuals.

All patients with PSP who suffer a recurrence should undergo an intervention to prevent a future recurrence once the air leak has sealed and the lung has fully expanded. This is preferably through VATS as outlined above or at least thorough chemical pleurodesis, through a tube thoracotomy placed at the time of drainage.

■ SECONDARY PNEUMOTHORAX

A pneumothorax is considered to be secondary when it occurs in patients with underlying lung disease. The incidence depends on the population under study. Secondary pneumothorax is observed in an older age group, the highest rate being in men over 70 years. Many lung diseases can cause a pneumothorax. The most common (perhaps in over 40–60% of cases) is COPD, followed by bronchial asthma. Most patients with COPD have well-marked impairment of lung function before the

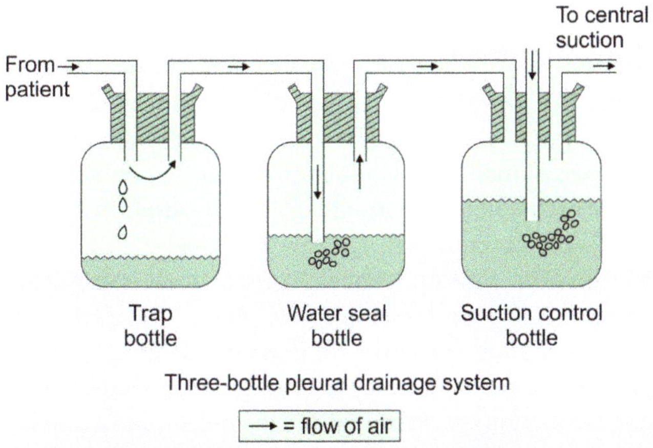

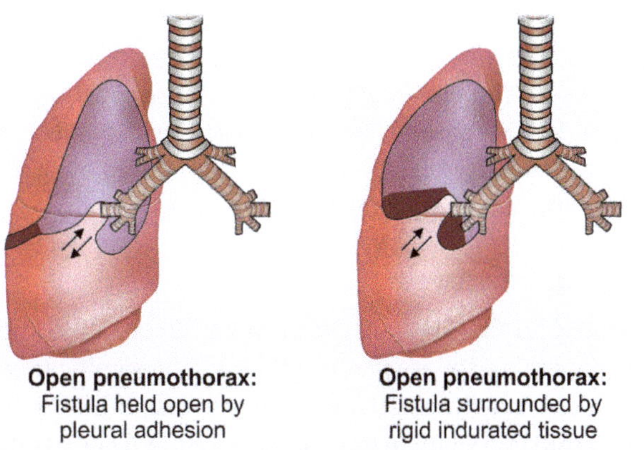

Fig. 2: Three-bottle pleural drainage system.

Fig. 3: Open pneumothorax.

event, with reduced forced vital capacity (FVC) and forced expiratory volume in the first second (FEV1) or FVC less than 40%. Pneumothorax may result from rupture of a subpleural bulla or the opening of a large bulla into the pleural space. It could also result from rupture of pleural adhesions, which tear and lay open the surface of an over-distended lung. A hemothorax may be associated because of bleeding from ruptured adhesions. Hyperdynamic inflation in patients with acute severe asthma may lead to alveolar rupture and pneumothorax.

Interstitial lung disease is another important underlying risk factor. Pneumothorax can also occur with tuberculosis, particularly in countries with a high prevalence rate. It is due to a rupture of a pleural adhesion allowing an air leak into the pleural space. It can be associated with either active tubercle or with old healed fibrotic tuberculosis. *Pneumocystis carinii* infection in acquired immune deficiency syndrome (AIDS) is another risk factor as are acute respiratory distress syndrome (ARDS) and aspiration pneumonia. Bilateral pneumothorax is not uncommon in ARDS and in *P. carinii* infection. Rare diseases like Langerhans' cell histiocytosis and lymphangioleiomyomatosis may present with spontaneous pneumothorax or with recurrent pneumothorax. An unusual type of secondary pneumothorax is catamenial pneumothorax characterized by recurrent pneumothorax (generally on the right side) occurring in young women 48–72 hours after the onset of menstruation. It is due to the cyclic loss of cervical mucus plug during menstrual flow allowing air from outside to gain access through the uterus and fallopian tubes into the abdomen. This air may gain access to the pleura through pores generally present in the right dome of the diaphragm.

Pneumothorax can occur in advanced cystic fibrosis, a disease common in the West but less common in India. It is a marker of end-stage disease because most patients with an FEV1 less than 30% are at risk. The list of diseases causing secondary pneumothorax observed in our unit is given in the accompanying table.

Clinical Features

The clinical features are often more severe than those observed in a primary pneumothorax. The significance of symptoms may be missed in patients with COPD as they may be attributed to an exacerbation of COPD rather than to a complicating pneumothorax. *Any patient admitted to hospital with an exacerbation of asthma or COPD should have an X-ray chest done to ensure that a pneumothorax is not responsible for worsening symptoms.* Even a shallow pneumothorax in these patients may prove dangerous; the over-inflated lung may fail to deflate even when the pressure in what appears as a small pneumothorax is significantly high. It therefore requires prompt drainage.

Diagnosis

Clinical diagnosis may be impossibly difficult in patients with COPD because of an over-inflated chest and also because unequal and reduced breath sounds are often heard in these patients even when there is no pneumothorax.

X-ray chest generally gives the diagnosis though it may be difficult to distinguish a large bulla from a pneumo-thorax. CT of the chest should help in differentiating one from the other.

Difficulties in diagnosis arise under the following conditions:

- Localized or mediastinal pneumothorax
- Anteriorly located pneumothorax which requires CT imaging for recognition
- Pre-existing bullous or generalized emphysema. The contour sign may help to distinguish a pneumothorax from a bulla. A lung contour convex toward the chest wall suggests a pneumothorax; a concave edge suggests a bulla
- Small pneumothorax in a patient with consolidated lobe or lung
- Air-fluid level in a pneumothorax may be confused with an intrapulmonary cavity
- Pneumothorax in ARDS is often missed on a routine radiological examination and is evident only on a CT of chest.

Complications of Pneumothorax

These are more often observed in secondary pneumo-thorax (an overall complication rate of 60%) though they may occasionally be also seen in primary pneumothorax (an overall complication rate of 10%). Complications are listed in the accompanying **Table 2**.

Tension pneumothorax is the most dangerous complication and has already been discussed. As an emergency measure, temporary drainage of the pneumothorax is done by inserting a large-bore needle into the pleural space through the second intercostal space. Then as quickly as possible the pneumothorax needs an intercostal tube drain connected to an underwater seal.

Table 2: Complications of pneumothorax (primary and secondary).

Complications	Remarks
Tension pneumothorax	An emergency requiring prompt aspiration of air, followed immediately by insertion of an intercostal tube drain
Mediastinal emphysema and surgical emphysema of soft tissues of neck, chest, and upper limbs	Almost always clears with time
Bilateral pneumothorax	An emergency—requires tapping
Bronchopleural fistula	May require special treatment—is difficult to close
Persistent alveolar leak	Generally closes with time, if pneumothorax is adequately drained
Chronic pneumothorax	Determine the cause and treat it—generally due to a bronchopleural fistula or a persistent alveolar leak
Loculated pneumothorax	Leave alone if small, drain if large
Pyopneumothorax	Requires drainage of pus and air—use of appropriate antibiotics
Re-expansion edema	Avoid immediate suction after a pneumothorax. Slow withdrawal of air

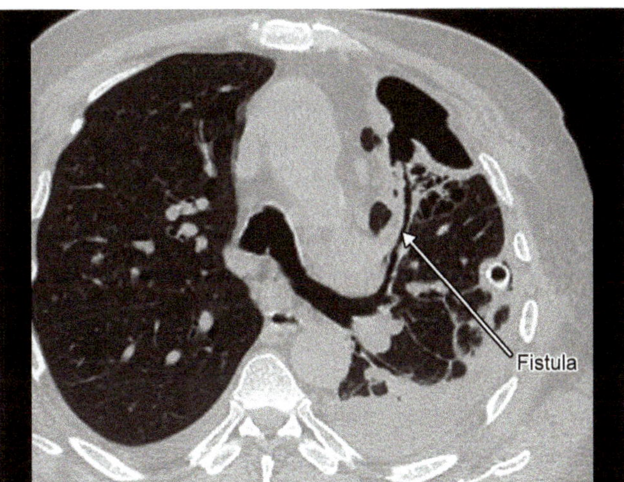

Fig. 4: Bronchopleural fistula. Axial image reveals an abnormal communication between the left bronchus leading to the pleura as evidenced by the fistulous tract. Posteriorly an intercostal drainage (ICD) tube is noted. Hence in a case of a persistent pneumothorax or hydropneumothorax in spite of an ICD tube in situ, the possibility of a bronchopleural fistula should always be thought of.

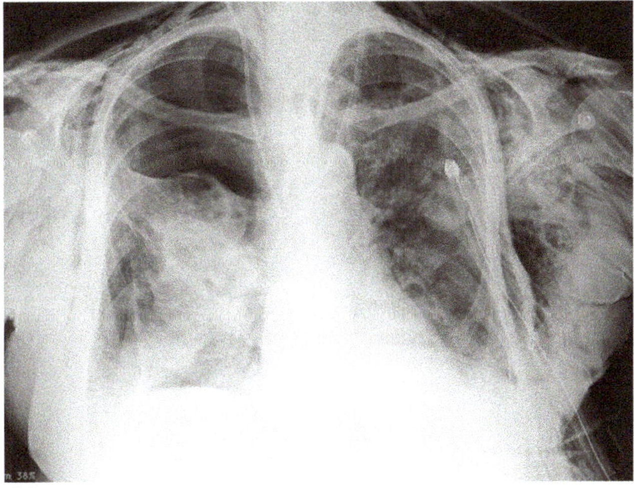

Fig. 5: X-ray chest demonstrating a pneumothorax with extensive surgical and mediastinal emphysema.

Use of high-flow oxygen together with cardiorespiratory resuscitative measures is often necessary. Resuscitation is possible even in extreme cases with cardiac arrest and electromechanical dissociation, provided the pneumothorax is promptly and adequately drained.

Severe respiratory failure PaO_2 less than 50 mm Hg, $PaCO_2$ more than 50 mm Hg may be precipitated in patients with secondary pneumothorax.

Bilateral pneumothorax is a rare but dangerous complication and is observed particularly in AIDS, ARDS, and in polytrauma.

Bronchopleural fistulas are difficult to heal, particularly in critically ill patients on ventilator support **(Fig. 4)**. They are caused by underlying pleural or lung disease, which keep the tear in the lung open, allowing the pleural space to communicate with a bronchiole or bronchus. Alveolar leaks are a nuisance and almost always heal on their own if the pneumothorax remains adequately drained.

Mediastinal Emphysema (Fig. 5)

Air from the alveoli may track along the interstitial tissue planes, breach the mediastinal pleura, and produce mediastinal emphysema followed by surgical emphysema of varying extent in the neck, upper limbs, and chest wall. Mediastinal emphysema and surgical emphysema of the soft tissues almost always resolve on their own. Extremely rarely, it may be massive enough to produce a cardiorespiratory emergency. Decompressive measures are then indicated.

Hemothorax

Rupture of a pleural adhesion may result not only in a pneumothorax but also cause bleeding into the pleural space.

Management

Secondary pneumothorax must be drained, even if the pneumothorax is small. An intercostal tube drain should be promptly inserted. Aspiration should be considered only in asymptomatic small pneumothoraces. Air leaks often persist in a secondary pneumothorax so that the lung may take more than 6 days to expand even with adequate drainage. Surgical intervention is necessary, if the leak persists. VATS is generally well tolerated except in patients with very poor respiratory reserve due to underlying lung disease. Chemical pleurodesis through the intercostal drainage tube is then an alternative approach. If chemical pleurodesis fails, a Heimlich flutter valve can be inserted with good success rates **(Flowchart 1)**.

Management of a pneumothorax with a bronchopleural fistula is summarized in **Table 3**.

Prevention Strategies

The recurrence rate in secondary pneumothorax is close to 40%. It is about 60% after the first recurrence and about 80% after the third. Preventive strategies should therefore be seriously considered even if the lung has fully expanded and the air leak sealed. Chemical pleurodesis through an intercostal tube carries the least risk. Video-assisted thoracoscopy with pleural abrasion or surgical talc pleurodesis is the procedure of choice; it is more effective with a much lesser degree of recurrence. Open thoracotomy with pleurectomy has the lowest recurrence rate but is invariably unsuitable in patients with well-marked underlying pulmonary disease.

Postdischarge Precautions

Patients should be instructed not to fly until radiography demonstrates complete resolution of a pneumothorax. Conventionally, air travel should be avoided for 6 weeks. It is also advisable to do a CT chest on these patients to ensure that a localized pneumothorax which can be missed on an X-ray chest, does not exist. Diving should be prohibited permanently unless a surgical procedure such as pleural abrasion with pleurodesis or pleurectomy has been performed. The patient should be advised strongly against smoking.

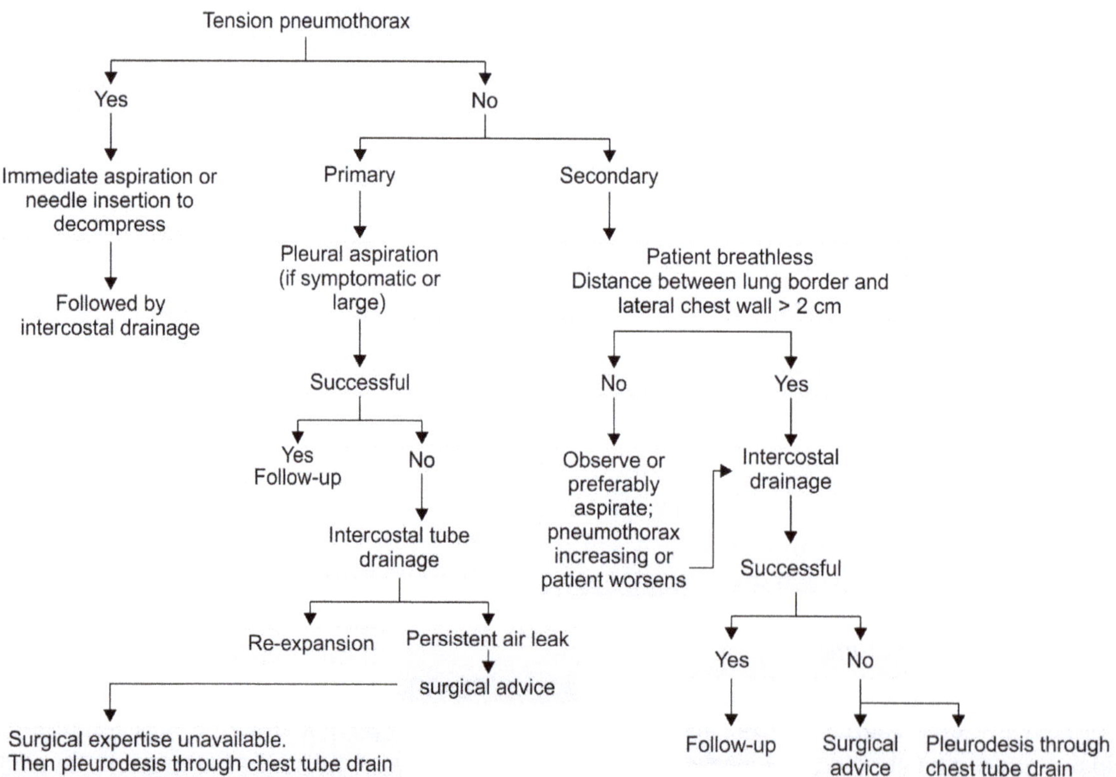

Flowchart 1: Management of spontaneous pneumothorax.

<table>
<tr><td style="background:#b5643c;color:white">Table 3: Management of pneumothorax with a bronchopleural fistula.</td></tr>
<tr><td>

- Drain pneumothorax with a large-bore drain—avoid suction or use very soft suction—else air leak will increase.
- Reduce "steal flow" (which is the difference between inspired volume and expired volume) by keeping the diseased lung in dependent position.
- Monitor "steal flow".
- *If on ventilator support:*
  - Reduce tidal volume, go off positive end expiratory pressure (PEEP), reduce inspiratory time
  - If possible allow spontaneous respiration, using BiPAP or CPAP.
- If air leak is not reduced over time, attempt to seal site of leak with a fibrin seal through a bronchoscope.
- *If the above measures fail:*
  - Surgery if patient's condition allows
  - Double lumen intubation for single lung or differential ventilation.

</td></tr>
</table>

(BiPAP: Bilevel positive airway pressure; CPAP: Continuous positive airway pressure)

Traumatic Pneumothorax

Traumatic pneumothorax may be due to direct injury or indirect injury (as in a bomb blast) or may be iatrogenic. Direct injury may be penetrating resulting in what is termed an "open pneumothorax" or a blunt injury. Traumatic pneumothorax does not require fracture of the rib or penetration of the pleura. It may result from compression of the chest leading to shear-force-related alveolar, bronchial rupture, or even a rupture involving a main bronchus. Tachypnea and respiratory distress in a trauma patient without evidence of a sharp penetrating injury should promptly raise suspicion of a pneumothorax, hemothorax, or massive lung contusion. A pneumothorax in a trauma patient can in time develop into a tension pneumothorax and may be simultaneously associated or followed by hemothorax and pulmonary contusion. Insertion of a chest tube drain in a symptomatic traumatic pneumothorax or hemothorax is imperative. A close follow-up is warranted.

■ IATROGENIC PNEUMOTHORAX

Iatrogenic pneumothorax results from procedures such as central venous catheterization, thoracocentesis, transbronchial biopsies, pleural biopsies, and CT-guided biopsies. It is an important cause of pneumothorax in critical care units. Iatrogenic pneumothorax is an important complication in patients on ventilator support. If not promptly recognized, tension pneumothorax results. Respiratory distress, clashing with the machine, deterioration of pulse, blood pressure, and oxygenation together with a marked rise in both peak and pause pressures are important pointers to a possible underlying pneumothorax. Pneumothorax in patients on ventilator support is due to inhomogeneity of the lung pathology, some alveoli being more compliant and some having a very low compliance. More gas from the machine reaches the over-compliant alveoli which therefore have a greater chance of rupture. Volutrauma together with barotrauma plays a role in causing a ventilator-induced pneumothorax.

A chest tube drain should be inserted, the tidal volume reduced as also the peak pressure and the inspiration time. PEEP is contraindicated, fraction of inspired oxygen may be increased to maintain an oxygen saturation of more than 90%. Some degree of hypercapnia must needs be tolerated. Ventilatory support should be removed as soon as feasible.

■ SUGGESTED READING

1. Baumann MH. Management of spontaneous pneumothorax. Clin Chest Med. 2006;27(2):369-81.
2. Hopkins TG, Maher ER, Reid E, et al. Recurrent pneumothorax. Lancet. 2011;377:1624.
3. Korom S, Canyurt H, Missbach A, et al. Catamenial pneumothorax revisited: clinical approach and systematic review of the literature. J Thorac Cardiovasc Surg. 2004;128(4):502-8.
4. Light RW. Pleural Diseases, 6th edition. Philadelphia: Lippincott, Williams and Wilkins; 2013.
5. Marquette CH, Marx A, Leroy S, et al. Simplified stepwise management of primary spontaneous pneumothorax: a pilot study. Eur Respir J. 2006;27(3):470-6.
6. Noppen M, De Keukeleire T. Pneumothorax. Respiration. 2008;76:121-7.
7. Ricci ZJ, Haramati LB, Rosenbaum AT, et al. Role of computed tomography in guiding the management of peripheral bronchopleural fistula. J Thorac Imaging. 2002;17(3):214-8.
8. Tschopp JM, Rami-Porta R, Noppen M, et al. Management of spontaneous pneumothorax: state of the art. Eur Respir J. 2006;28(3):637-50.
9. Varoli F, Roviaro G, Grignani F, et al. Endoscopic treatment of bronchopleural fistulas. Ann Thorac Surg. 1998;65:807-9.

CHAPTER 64

Malignant Pleural Mesothelioma

■ INTRODUCTION

Malignant mesothelioma is a rare, insidious, but highly malignant neoplasm with a very poor prognosis. It arises from the lining mesothelial cells of the pleura and peritoneal cavities, although rarely it can arise from the mesothelial cells of the pericardium and tunica vaginalis testis. Pleural mesothelioma is much more common than the peritoneal form. The ratio between the two varies in different studies from entirely pleural to 2:1 in favor of pleural mesothelioma. The pleural tumor may be localized to a well-defined area, may be multifocal or may involve the pleura as a continuous sheet. Pleural mesothelioma has been proven to be related to asbestos exposure. In 1960, Wagner and colleagues described 33 cases of pleural mesothelioma and all but one had been exposed to crocidolite. Several subsequent studies have confirmed the association between asbestos exposure and pleural mesothelioma.

■ ETIOLOGY

It is believed that even trivial exposure to asbestos carries the future risk of mesothelioma. The situations associated with nonindustrial mild exposure include domestic contact with contaminated clothing or working in an office with a deteriorating crumbling asbestos ceiling or neighborhood contact in an area which has asbestos factories. It must be noted that mesothelioma reported following nonoccupational exposure occurred among a very large population at risk, so that risk associated with low-level exposure though present, is probably small. In people with heavy exposures as in asbestos factory workers, or with recurrent exposure the risk of mesothelioma is high. The West has taken stringent measures against occupational asbestos exposure and the coming decades will witness a further fall in the incidence of asbestos-related mesotheliomas. In India, stringent antiexposure measures are absent or not enforced, so the incidence of asbestos-related pleural mesothelioma will continue to rise.

Many studies support the view that the greater the concentration of asbestos to which a patient is exposed and the greater the duration of exposure, the greater is the future risk of pleural mesothelioma. Also, each brief period of exposure following the first causes an addition to the total, proportionate to the dose of asbestos received.

The average latent period between the first exposure to asbestos and death from pleural mesothelioma is 20–40 years. It is unlikely that the tumor grows during this latent period, as this would mean that the tumor has a very long doubling period. This would in turn imply a prolonged survival once clinical manifestations are observed. It is difficult to surmise the period between the start of growth of the mesothelioma and death. An indirect surmise is by a comparison with lung cancer.

It has been calculated that the period between the start of growth of a lung cancer and its clinical manifestation and death in both lung cancer and pleural mesothelioma is between 12 months and 18 months. On this analogy, a pleural mesothelioma probably starts to grow 10 years before clinical manifestations appear.

Asbestos Fiber Type Involved

Evidence from various studies suggests that amphiboles are more potent than chrysolite, and among amphiboles, crocidolite is more potent than amosite in causing a mesothelioma.

Observations of differing incidence of mesothelioma in different industries involving exposure to asbestos suggest that the risk of mesothelioma is related to the fiber size and that fine fibers appear to be more dangerous. This has been substantiated by estimating the fiber content of lung tissue.

Nonindustrial mesothelioma has been reported from Turkey, Cyprus, and Greece caused by naturally occurring asbestos minerals including tremolite and perhaps chrysolite. Endemic mesothelioma was first reported in 1978 from Karan, a remote village in central Turkey. Many deaths occurred in middle-aged adults, but deaths were also reported in a 12-year-old boy and 15-year-old girl suggesting exposure to a carcinogenic agent from birth. The responsible agent was a fibrous zeolite called erionite. Other asbestos minerals including tremolite were found in the volcanic tuff, which was quarried and used for building.

Pleural Mesothelioma in the Absence of Asbestos Exposure

Although exposure to asbestos is the main association and risk factor for a pleural mesothelioma, patients with pleural mesothelioma with no exposure to asbestos are not uncommon. An important causal factor (other than asbestos) is radiation exposure. In one reported series, five patients with Hodgkin's disease who received radiotherapy developed malignant pleural mesothelioma, the average interval from radiotherapy to the diagnosis of the disease being 15 years. The simian virus (SV40) has also been implicated in the etiology of malignant pleural mesothelioma. This virus produces the disease in 100% of hamsters when injected intrapleurally. Also, using polymerase chain reaction (PCR) analysis SV40 deoxyribonucleic acid (DNA) sequences have been detected in 40–60% of malignant mesotheliomas in humans. The role of this virus however remains controversial.

It is of interest that the risk for mesothelioma is unrelated to smoking. The relative risk is not dependent on the age at which exposure begins, but the absolute risk is greater with earlier exposure merely because it provides more time for a mesothelioma to occur.

■ PATHOGENESIS

Inhaled asbestos fibers go through the lung to reach the visceral pleura. They reach the parietal pleura either through lymphatics or perhaps through direct penetration of the visceral pleura. The exact mechanism of malignant transformation of the mesothelium of the pleura is not clear, but evidence suggests chromosomal damage including chromosomal depletion. Studies suggest a depletion of genetic material in the short arms of chromosomes 1, 3, and 9 and the long arms of chromosomes 6, 15, and 22. Some of these regions contain suppressor genes. It is believed that the large T antigen of SV40 is capable of inactivating suppressor genes and may well be responsible for inducing the chromosomal changes described above. Perhaps SV40 alone does not cause pleural mesothelioma; it may act as a cocarcinogen with asbestos. Epidemiological data from Turkey suggest that genetic predisposition may play a role in increasing the susceptibility to pleural mesothclioma though no specific gene or genetic alteration that identifies this susceptibility has been found as yet.

■ PATHOLOGY

The tumor can arise from either the parietal or visceral pleura. It occasionally presents as a localized mass, but more commonly is characterized by multiple nodules studding the pleural surface or by a continuous sheet of thickened neoplastic tissue which spreads by continuity to partially or completely encase the lung with retraction of the chest wall. Pleural effusion is often present. With advancing disease the pleural space may be obliterated and spread occurs through continuity and contiguity to involve the lung, chest wall, mediastinum, pericardium, and diaphragm. The contralateral pleura may also be involved. Blood-borne distant metastases are also observed.

The histological appearance is varied. The main forms are epithelial, sarcomatous, and mixed. The epithelial form resembles an adenocarcinoma and is characterized by tubule formation; the sarcomatous form consists of spindle-shaped cells with collagen deposition. The mixed form combines elements of each of the above in varying proportions. Pleural effusions are observed in about 70% of epithelial and mixed forms, but in 16% of sarcomatous form. Distant metastasis is most often observed in the sarcomatous form, but can occur in the other forms as well.

■ CLINICAL FEATURES

Malignant pleural mesothelioma is more common in men (more than 70% of cases), perhaps due to their greater frequency of exposure to asbestos. Though most common between the fifth to the seventh decade, the disease may occur at any age.

The presenting features are dyspnea, dry cough, and a dull chest pain of insidious onset. The dyspnea is due to pleural effusion. The effusion invariably recurs when tapped. It is often blood-stained, but may be serous and may continue to be so right up to the end. Chest pain is dull but is sometimes severe and pleuritic.

General systemic features include a low-grade fever, night sweats, tiredness, and weight loss. Symptoms may be present for many months before a diagnosis is made.

At times, presenting symptoms are related to involvement of mediastinal and other intrathoracic structures. In rare instances, the presentation may be acute as with involvement of the brachial plexus causing neuritic pain, impingement of the superior vena cava causing the superior vena caval syndrome, or spread into the abdomen through the diaphragm causing symptoms of bowel obstruction.

Clinical examination often reveals the usual physical signs of a pleural effusion. Dullness over the base with diminished breath sounds may be present even in the absence of fluid because of markedly thickened pleura. Chest wall retraction is observed when the tumor encases the lung like in a cuirass. Chest movements and breath sounds are diminished over the whole affected chest and there is a restrictive ventilatory defect. Tumor tissue may infiltrate needle tracts caused during pleural paracentesis or following a pleural biopsy.

Infiltration of the pericardium can cause constriction; involvement of the mediastinum, diaphragm, peritoneum, and the chest wall may occur with advancing disease.

Death occurs chiefly from respiratory failure. Constrictive pericarditis, cardiac failure, and cardiac arrhythmias due to pericardial and cardiac invasion can also cause death. Extension of the pleural mesothelioma to involve the peritoneum can cause abdominal complications, chiefly intractable small bowel obstruction. Blood borne distant metastases are rare and may involve the bone, liver, or the central nervous system.

Paraneoplastic syndromes have been reported in patients with malignant mesothelioma. These almost always occur in patients with advanced disease and include disseminated intravascular coagulopathy, migratory thrombophlebitis, thrombotic thrombocytopenic purpura, hypoglycemia, peripheral neuropathy, cerebellar degeneration, and hypercalcemia.

■ INVESTIGATIONS

Imaging

An initial X-ray of the chest should be followed by a high-resolution computed tomography (HRCT) of the chest as the chest X-ray has a limited sensitivity and specificity when compared to a computed tomography (CT) chest **(Figs. 1 and 2)**.

The following imaging findings are commonly observed.

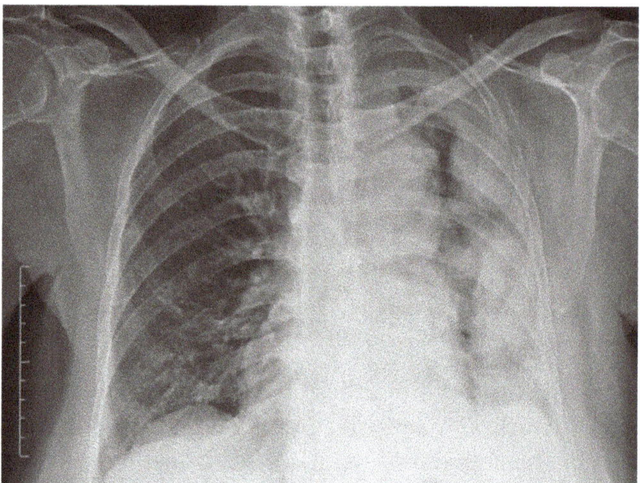

Fig. 1: Chest X-ray reveals extensive nodularity of the left pleura associated with loss of lung volume and mediastinal shift to the left, biopsy of the left pleura showed a mesothelioma.

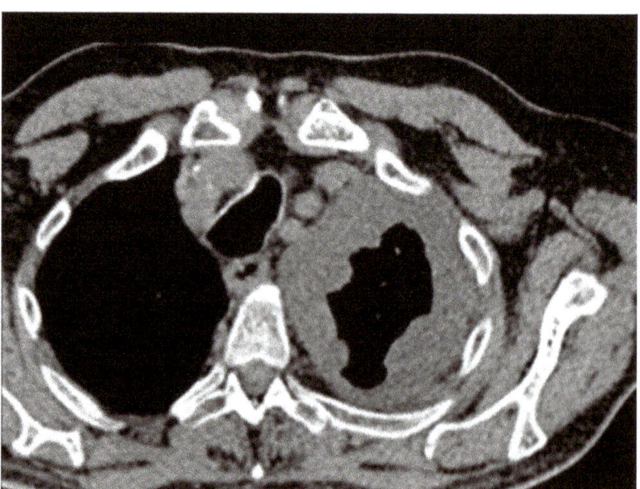

Fig. 2: Mesothelioma. Chest computed tomography (CT) reveals considerable thickening of the left pleura encasing the left lung with extension to the mediastinum encasing the mediastinal vasculature, as well as the left main bronchus. There is a right pleural effusion. Biopsy showed a mesothelioma.

- A unilateral, generally large pleural effusion, which recurs on tapping.
- A lobulated pleura, or a pleural mass, or a diffusely thickened pleura in the absence of a pleural effusion. Tapping the fluid of a pleural effusion when present and then imaging the chest (CT) may reveal the above mentioned changes.
- Pleural plaques with or without calcification.
- In advanced cases, encasement of the lung by a thick fibrotic ring with shift of the mediastinum to the same side, marked contraction of the affected hemithorax and a marked reduction in the lung volumes.
- Extension of the tumor into the chest wall, lung, pericardium, mediastinum, and peritoneum can be demonstrated on CT chest.
- Magnetic resonance imaging of the chest using multidimensional planer is superior to CT scans for evaluating the relationship of the tumor to the great vessels if surgery is needed.

Positron Emission Tomography Scan

The positron emission tomography (PET) scan is useful under the following circumstances:
- To distinguish benign from malignant pleural lesions. A positive PET scan needs pathological confirmation, but a negative scan lends reassurance and may permit close observation and follow-up without biopsy in a number of patients.
- As a pretreatment evaluation in patients with a pleural mesothelioma.
- To identify distant metastasis in patients who are to undergo pleuropneumonectomy.
- To assess response or lack of response to systemic treatment.

Non-immunohistochemistry Biomarkers

Three tumor markers reported recently in relation to pleural mesothelioma are soluble mesothelin related protein (SMRP), osteopontin and hyaluronan. SMRP has been reported in 84% of patients with pleural mesothelioma and 2% of patients with other malignant tumors. Mesothelin levels may also be useful to evaluate response to treatment.

Osteopontin is a glycoprotein expressed in many cancers. Osteopontin levels have been reported to be significantly higher in patients with pleural mesothelioma compared to a group with exposure to asbestos, but who did not have pleural mesothelioma. At an osteopontin value of 48 ng/mL the sensitivity and specificity at diagnosis was 78% and 86%, respectively. The efficacy of the marker as a screening test is under investigation.

■ EVALUATION

Though imaging findings may lead to a strong suspicion of a malignant mesothelioma, a tissue diagnosis is imperative.

Pleural Aspiration

Examination of an aspirate (when pleural effusion is present) should be the next investigative step after an X-ray of the chest. The pleural fluid is an exudate; it is often blood-stained but not always so. Cytological examination may reveal malignant cells in 30–60% of cases depending on the expertise of the pathologist. It is difficult to distinguish reactive from malignant mesothelial cells. Even if malignant cells are present it may be difficult to determine whether they represent a pleural mesothelioma or pleural metastasis.

Pleural Biopsy

A closed CT guided pleural biopsy generally does not provide sufficient tissue to definitely establish the diagnosis of a malignant pleural mesothelioma and especially to distinguish it from an adenocarcinoma. It is best therefore to use video-assisted thoracoscopic surgery (VATS) biopsy to enable definite histological diagnosis. This procedure allows direct visualization of the pleura and the taking of biopsies from different sites.

A study of 188 consecutive patients evaluated between 1973 and 1990 has illustrated the difficulties in establishing the diagnosis of a mesothelioma. Thoracocentesis and pleural fluid cytology yielded a diagnosis in 26%, thoracocentesis plus a closed pleural biopsy gave the diagnosis in 39% of cases. However VATS was diagnostic in 98% of cases. It is therefore best to proceed to VATS after evaluating imaging findings in these patients.

Bronchoscopy

Most units, particularly when surgery is contemplated, advise a bronchoscopy as an endobronchial lesion is not seen in a mesothelioma and its presence is against the diagnosis of a mesothelioma. In addition endobronchial ultrasound (EBUS) guided biopsies of mediastinal, pleural lesions, subcarinal lesions, and hilar lymph nodes, both ipsilateral and contralateral to the primary site help to provide staging of the mesothelioma.

■ TISSUE DIAGNOSIS

As mentioned under pathology, malignant pleural mesotheliomas fall into any of the three types: (1) epithelioid, (2) sarcomatous, and (3) mixed. However, morphology alone may be insufficient to make the diagnosis in many cases. Hence, the need to use immunohistochemical markers to evaluate the tissue further **(Figs. 3 and 4)**. At least two immunoreactive and two nonimmunoreactive markers have been recommended to definitely establish the diagnosis of a mesothelioma.

■ DIFFERENTIAL DIAGNOSIS

The differential diagnosis includes benign and other malignant pathologies.

Benign Pathologies

The single most important benign condition that can mimic a mesothelioma is a chronic empyema, which can cause a marked thickening of the parietal and visceral pleura together with a pleural effusion. Histological examination shows stromal invasion in a mesothelioma, but no such invasion in an empyema.

Malignant Pathologies

Pleural metastasis from a peripheral lung adenocarcinoma, as also pleural metastasis from other organs such as the breast, stomach, kidney, ovary, and prostrate may both grossly and histologically resemble mesothelioma.

■ STAGING SYSTEM

The generally used staging system is the tumor, node, and metastasis (TNM) staging system. In the TNM staging system which relies on imaging, stage I and II have pleural involvement and may involve diaphragmatic muscle and pulmonary parenchyma, but neither involve lymph nodes nor show distant metastasis.

Stage III mesothelioma includes locally advanced disease, which is potentially resectable, including cases of regional lymph node involvement.

Stage IV includes locally advanced unresectable disease, contralateral lymph node involvement, supraclavicular lymph node involvement, or distant metastasis.

Besides HRCT of the chest, PET scan + bronchoscopy, and results of endoscopic ultrasound assisted biopsies help in proper staging.

■ PROGNOSIS

The prognosis is poor. The median survival rate is between 9 months and 17 months after diagnosis. Fewer than 20% survive for more than 2 years. Patients with an epithelial

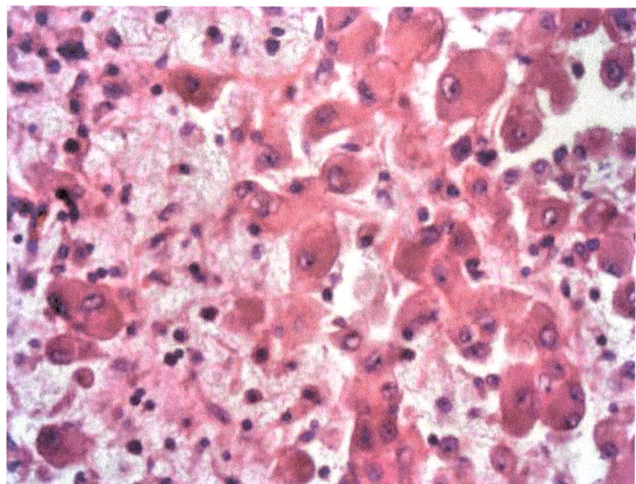

Fig. 3: Malignant mesothelioma (H&E 40×). Plump atypical mesothelial cells with enlarged nuclei are seen. Prominent nucleoli are also visible.

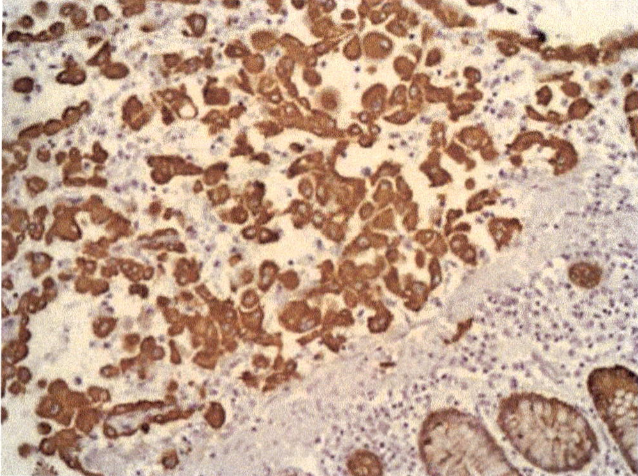

Fig. 4: Immunohistochemistry. Strong positivity for mesothelial marker, calretinin.

histopathology fare better than the others. Poor prognostic factors arrived at by the Cancer and Leukemia Group and the European Organization for the Research and Treatment of Cancer include nonepithelial histology, age less than 75 years, chest pain, male gender, white blood cell (WBC) less than 8.3×10^4/L, platelets less than 400,000 μL, and lactate dehydrogenase (LDH) less than 500 units/L.

■ TREATMENT

Treatment of pleural mesothelioma is unsatisfactory and produces little or no change in morbidity and mortality. The role of surgery is controversial. Surgical resection may take the following forms:

- *Extrapleural pneumonectomy (EPP)*: En bloc resection of the parietal and visceral pleura with the ipsilateral lung, pericardium, and diaphragm. If the pericardium and diaphragm are not involved they are left intact.
- *Extended parietal and visceral pleurectomy (P/D)*: P/D to remove all gross tumor with resection of the diaphragm and pleura if these are involved.
- *Parietal and visceral pleurectomy*: P/D to remove all gross tumor without touching the pericardium and diaphragm.
- Partial pleurectomy of parietal and/or visceral pleura for diagnostic or palliative purposes leaving gross tumor behind, because of impossibility of full resection.

Even in patients where surgery is feasible, there has been no significant increase in survival except in isolated instances. Surgery therefore should perhaps only be reserved for those with by and large localized tumors.

Recent trials include a three-pronged attack-starting with chemotherapy, followed by extrapleural pleuropneumonectomy and then by radiation. After induction chemotherapy, EPP has been feasible in over 70% of patients in many series with a surgical mortality of 0–7% per unit. Chemotherapy is given both prior to and as an adjuvant after surgery.

Patients with stage I and stage II expectedly fared better than those with stage III disease. No single chemotherapeutic agent has proved very effective. Combination chemotherapy has been found to be superior to the use of a single agent though a number of chemotherapeutic agents are being tried. At present the standard combination therapy is pemetrexed and cisplatin.

Palliative Therapy

In most patients the disease is too advanced for specific treatment. Pleural effusion produces increasing breathlessness. Repeated thoracocentesis brings temporary relief, but the fluid continues to refill and ultimately gets loculated. It is best to advise thoracoscopy with pleurodesis or chest tube drainage with chemical pleurodesis. A risk of thoracoscopy or tube drainage with pleurodesis is that after the pleural space is emptied, the lung if encased by tumor tissue would fail to expand (trapped lung). Pleurodesis would then be unsuccessful. It is only when the pleural space is obliterated after drainage that talc pleurodesis is possible. Currently, tunneled pleural catheters with drainage by the patient, nurse or any caregiver into disposable bags affords relief. Pleurodesis often occurs (without the use of talc) with time, following which the catheter is removed. Control of pleural effusion by this method is satisfactory and affords symptomatic relief. Pain relief is of great importance with advancing disease. Supportive treatment adds to patient comfort.

■ SUGGESTED READING

1. Hollevoet K, Reitsma JB, Creaney J, et al. Serum mesothelin for diagnosing malignant pleural mesothelioma: an individual patient data meta-analysis. J Clin Oncol. 2012;30(13):1541-9.
2. Husain AN, Colby TV, Ordóñez NG, et al. Guidelines for pathologic diagnosis of malignant mesothelioma: 2012 update of the consensus statement from the International Mesothelioma Interest Group. Arch Pathol Lab Med. 2013;137(5):647-67.
3. Munoz A, Barcelo R, Lopez-Vivanco G. Malignant mesothelioma. N Engl J Med. 2006;354:305-7.
4. Musk AW, Olsen N, Alfonso H, et al. Predicting survival in malignant mesothelioma. Eur Respir J. 2011;38(6):1420-4.
5. Ray M. Malignant pleural mesothelioma: an update on biomarkers and treatment. Chest. 2009;136(3):888-96.
6. Richards WG. Recent advances in mesothelioma staging. Semin Thorac Cardiovasc Surg. 2009;21:105-10.

Section 18

Diseases of the Mediastinum

CHAPTER 65

Diseases of the Mediastinum

■ GENERAL CONSIDERATIONS

The mediastinum is the vertical region within the middle of the thorax, between the two pleural cavities, thereby separating the lungs. It is bounded superiorly by the thoracic inlet, inferiorly by the diaphragm, posteriorly by the vertebral column and laterally by the mediastinal pleural reflections. The main structures within the mediastinum are the heart and great vessels, the trachea, the two main bronchi and the esophagus. The phrenic and vagus nerves course through it; the sympathetic trunks lie one on each side of the vertebral column. These vital structures are all closely connected to one another by loose connective tissue. Hence, air or infection can spread rapidly within the mediastinal space. Also fascial planes within the neck, mediastinum and retroperitoneum have both continuity and contiguity. Infection or air can

therefore find easy egress from any one of these sites to the other. The mediastinum is rich in lymphatics and lymph glands, permitting both the dissemination of infection and neoplastic disease within it.

Traditionally, the mediastinum is divided into anterior, middle and posterior compartments based on the lateral chest X-ray (**Fig. 1**).

This is not an actual anatomical division but is conceptualized to help in the differential diagnosis of mediastinal tumors and masses since different mediastinal tumors, masses or cysts have generally a distinct predilection for one or the other of these compartments (**Table 1**). In fact, there is no consensus between clinicians on the boundaries of these compartments. The compartmental boundaries adopted for this book are as follows (**Fig. 2**).

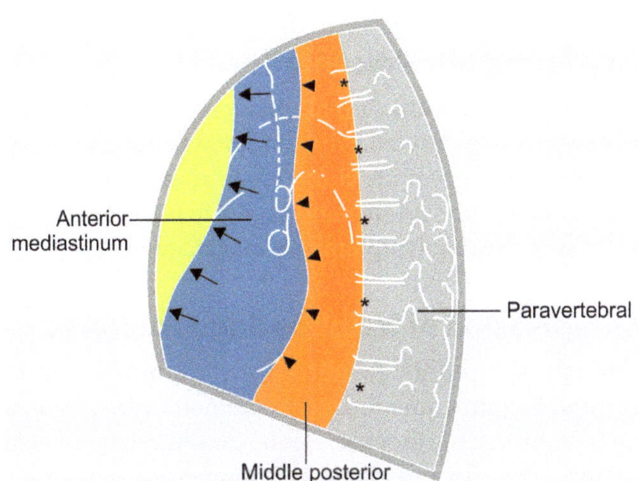

Fig. 1: Illustration of mediastinal compartments as seen on lateral chest radiography.

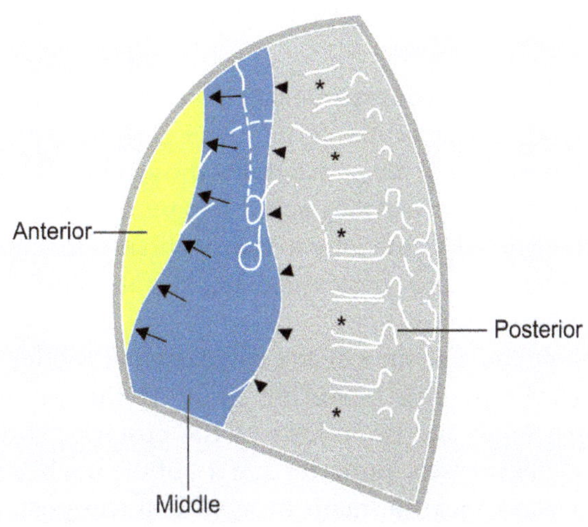

Fig. 2: Illustration of mediastinal compartments according to this book.

Table 1: Mediastinal masses in relation to the anterior, middle and posterior mediastinal compartments.

Anterior mediastinum	**Thymoma**
	Thymic hyperplasia
	Thymic carcinoma
	Germ cell tumors
	Teratoma
	Seminoma
	Intrathoracic goiter
	Aneurysm of the ascending and root of aorta
	Thymolipoma
	Thymic cyst
	Thymic carcinoid
	Nonseminomatous germ cell tumors
	Parathyroid adenoma
	Pericardial cyst
	Mesenchymal tumors
Middle mediastinum	**Benign mediastinal lymphadenopathy**
	Lymphoma
	Metastatic lymphadenopathy
	Bronchogenic cyst
	Enterogenous cyst
Posterior mediastinum	**Schwannomas, neurofbromas**
	Esophageal carcinoma
	Aneurysm of descending aorta
	Hiatus hernia
	Pott's disease with a paravertebral cold abscess
	Enterogenous cyst
	Achalasia of the cardia
	Nerve sheath tumors
	Malignant peripheral nerve tumors
	Ganglioneuromas
	Neuroblastomas
	Paragangliomas
	Extramedullary hematopoiesis

Note: "Masses" in **dark** font are those more frequently encountered in our units.

The anterior compartment is bounded anteriorly by the inner surface of the sternum and posteriorly by the anterior surface of the pericardium, the great vessels and the anterior surface of the trachea. Superiorly it extends to the thoracic inlet, inferiorly to the diaphragm. It contains the thymus gland, pericardial fat, lymph glands and connective tissue.

The middle or the visceral compartment is bounded anteriorly by the posterior limit of the anterior compartment and posteriorly by the posterior surface of the great vessels, posterior surface of the trachea and its division into the main bronchi and the posterior pericardial surface, extending upward to the thoracic inlet and downward up to the diaphragm. It contains the pericardium, heart, aorta and the great vessels, the superior vena cava (SVC) and the large veins draining into it, the pulmonary vessels, the trachea, major bronchi, the phrenic nerve and lymph glands.

The posterior compartment extends from the posterior aspect of the middle compartment to the anterior surface of the vertebral bodies including the paravertebral sulci. It contains the descending aorta, esophagus, sympathetic trunk on each side of the vertebral column, the azygos, hemiazygos veins, the thoracic duct and intercostal nerves.

Some authors conceptualize the middle or visceral compartment as extending posteriorly right up to the anterior surface of the vertebral column. The esophagus would then fall into the middle compartment. In this division, the posterior compartment would include only the sympathetic trunk, thoracic duct, intercostal nerves, azygos and hemiazygos veins. Whichever of the two conceptualizations of mediastinal compartments one follows, the three compartments appear approximate to one another in the superior portion of the mediastinum.

A large study between January 1993 and June 2003 from Jaipur, India showed that among the 106 patients who underwent surgical treatment of a mediastinal mass, the male to female ratio was 1.9:1. Histopathologically, 39% patients had thymic pathology, 29% had lymphoma, 13% had germ cell tumors, 11% had neurofibroma, 4% had ganglioneuroma, and 2% had bronchogenic cyst (*Ref: Shrivastava CP, Devgarha S, Ahlawat V. Mediastinal tumors: a clinicopathological analysis. Asian Cardiovasc Thorac Ann. 2006;14:102-4*).

■ CLINICAL FEATURES OF MEDIASTINAL MASSES

Asymptomatic Presentation

Approximately one-third to half of patients with mediastinal masses are asymptomatic; the condition being discovered on a routine X-ray of the chest. Interestingly, only 15% of asymptomatic masses are malignant, whereas close to 60% of those producing symptoms are malignant.

Compression of Neighboring Structures

Though symptoms produced by compression of surrounding structures are more common with malignant tumors and masses, they may also be caused by large benign tumors. The site and extent of compression symptoms depend on the nature of the mediastinal mass and its situation within the mediastinum. The most common symptoms of compression include cough, breathlessness and vague chest pain. Specific compression symptoms and signs depend on the anatomic structures compressed by a mediastinal mass. They are briefly detailed here **(Table 2)**.

- Pressure on the SVC leads to the superior vena caval syndrome, characterized by increasingly distended jugular veins; pulsations in the veins are not evident, unlike the pulsatile engorged jugular veins seen in congestive heart failure. Subtle signs of venous engorgement include slight puffiness of the face, particularly around the eyes with chemosis of the conjunctiva in the early morning, a flushed feeling due to congestion of the face and neck on bending or stooping to pick up an object from the floor or when tying a shoelace.
- Compression of the trachea, major bronchus compression of the trachea could lead to stridor; compression of the main bronchus could cause a unilateral monophonic wheeze; increasing pressure on the bronchus could cause atelectasis of a lobe or lung.
- Pressure on the esophagus could cause dysphagia.
- Compression of the left recurrent laryngeal nerve could cause hoarseness of the voice due to abductor paralysis of the left vocal cord.
- Cardiac compression or pericardial invasion may lead to palpitations, pain and rhythm disturbances.
- Pressure on the sympathetic nerve trunk will cause Horner's syndrome, and is invariably due to a malignant tumor.

- Compression of the intercostal nerves as they emerge from their vertebral foramina will lead to intercostal neuralgia; intraspinal extension of the mass could cause pressure on the spinal cord leading to varying neurological deficits.
- Pressure with erosion of the vertebra or ribs could cause bone pains and tenderness over the affected area.

A point of clinical importance is that however large a mediastinal tumor or cyst it does not obliterate an arterial pulse. Unequal pulses or an absent pulse in one or the other upper limb in the presence of a mediastinal mass is invariably due to an aortic aneurysm. The position of a mediastinal mass within the mediastinum, its size and the direction of expansion will determine as to which organ or structure is subject to compression.

Other Systemic Features

- Mediastinal masses when malignant may metastasize outside the mediastinum. A complete clinical examination is therefore important. One should particularly look out for pleural involvement (pleural effusion), lymphadenopathy (particularly in the neck and axilla) and hepatosplenomegaly. These features may provide a clue to a clinical diagnosis or allow an easy access for a biopsy procedure that establishes a diagnosis.
- Specific clinical features may also occur depending on the nature of the mass. Thus, myasthenia gravis may be the presenting feature in a thymoma, gynecomastia in a germ cell tumor, and a Pel-Ebstein fever in a patient with a mediastinal lymphoma.
- Nonspecific clinical features include low-grade fever, weight loss, and lassitude. Various paraneoplastic syndromes that may be encountered with different tumors and masses have been shown in **Table 3**.

■ INVESTIGATION OF MEDIASTINAL MASSES (TABLE 4)

- A good clinical history and a complete physical examination are vital. A careful search for compression syndromes, in particular the superior vena caval syndrome, is helpful. A recurrent laryngeal nerve palsy or a Horner's syndrome due to a mediastinal mass invariably points to a malignancy. Paraneoplastic syndromes should be carefully sought for, particularly

Table 2: Clinical features due to compression of neighboring structures by mediastinal masses.

Site of compression	Features
Superior vena cava	Distended jugular veins, flushing and puffiness of face on bending (SVC syndrome)
Trachea	Stridor
Main bronchus	Unilateral monophonic wheeze, atelectasis of lobe/lung
Esophagus	Dysphagia
Left recurrent laryngeal nerve	Hoarseness of voice
Cardiac compression, pericardial invasion	Cardiac pain, palpitations, arrhythmias
Sympathetic trunk	Horner's syndrome
Intercostal nerves	Intercostal neuralgia
Vertebra	Pain over affected area

Table 3: Paraneoplastic syndromes and other special features observed with different mediastinal masses.

Diseases	Features
Thymoma	Myasthenia gravis, acquired hypogammaglobulinemia, red cell hypoplasia
Thymic carcinoid	Cushing's syndrome, SIADH
Germ cell tumors	Gynecomastia, Klinefelter's syndrome
Intrathoracic goiter	Hyper/hypothyroidism
Pheochromocytoma	Hypertension
Autonomic ganglion tumors	Horner's syndrome, diarrhea, hypertension
Sarcoidosis	Hypercalcemia

Table 4: Investigation of mediastinal masses.

A good clinical history and examination	
Imaging studies	X-ray chest—PA and lateral view, HRCT chest, MRI if necessary
Radionuclide studies (when necessary)	^{131}I uptake points to—substernal goiter, ^{131}I-metaiodobenzylguanidine uptake points to pheochromocytoma Gallium scan—may help to distinguish thymoma from a lymphoma; gallium can also be picked up by an inflammatory mass or by a bronchogenic carcinoma Tc-99m sestamibi—parathyroid adenoma
Biochemical markets	AFP, β-HCG and CEA in anterior mediastinal masses; antibodies to acetylcholine receptors, metanephrines and nor-metanephrines estimation in blood and urine in suspected pheochromocytoma
Biopsy procedures	CT-guided, fine-needle or trucut biopsy, endobronchial biopsy (EBUS), mediastinoscopic biopsy, thoracoscopic biopsy (VATS)

in masses known to cause them. An X-ray chest is considered part of the basic examination and gives a clue to the possible diagnosis.

- High-resolution computed tomography (HRCT) has revolutionized accurate diagnosis of mediastinal masses. At times the appearances are so typical as with a pericardial cyst or an aortic aneurysm that further diagnostic proof may not be necessary. A computed tomography (CT) scan also forms the most appropriate guide for a CT-guided fine-needle biopsy or a core biopsy of a mediastinal mass.

- Magnetic resonance imaging (MRI) as an imaging technique is particularly useful under the following circumstances:
  - To determine invasion of vascular and neural structures or infiltration of tissue planes in malignant lesions. This information is of special significance if surgery is to be performed.
  - T1 and T2 images may help to clearly delineate mediastinal masses from surrounding soft tissues.
  - The difference between Tl and T2 values for bronchogenic carcinoma and inflammatory lesions is significant and may help in diagnosis.
  - Lesions close to the thoracic inlet are better outlined with an MRI study as infiltration of the brachial plexus and the vertebral foramina are better visualized.

- An ultrasound examination of the scrotum is important in a suspected germ-cell tumor.

- Positron emission tomography–CT (PET-CT) is useful in few situations. It may be performed on a mediastinal mass suspected to be a lymphoma. It may help identify a preferred biopsy site in those tumors found to be PET avid on an initial study. A PET study may also in some patients help monitor response to treatment. However, fluorodeoxyglucose (FDG)-PET imaging may be misleading because of the high incidence of false-positive results observed in noninvasive thymomas and neurofibromas. *This modality should be used therefore only in selected instances* and interpreted with caution.

Radionuclide Studies

Uptake of ^{131}I points to a substernal goiter while uptake of ^{131}I-metaiodobenzylguanidine (MIBG) can identify a pheochromocytoma either in the adrenals or in the mediastinum or other rare ectopic sites. Gallium scan (though not specific) may help in the identification of a lymphoma. It may help to distinguish a lymphoma in the anterior mediastinum from a thymoma, since a lymphoma picks up gallium avidly while a thymoma generally does not pick up gallium. Gallium is also picked up by any inflammatory mass or by a bronchogenic carcinoma. Carcinoids and germ cell tumors may or may not pick up gallium. Radioactive selenomethionine is picked up by a parathyroid adenoma and is therefore of particular help in the diagnosis of an ectopic mediastinal parathyroid adenoma.

Biochemical Markers

Antibodies to acetylcholine receptors should be a necessary investigation in a patient with a suspected thymoma. All patients with an anterior mediastinal mass should have a determination of the alpha-fetoprotein (AFP), human chorionic gonadotropin (β-HCG) and the carcinoembryonic antigen (CEA). Serum levels of β-HCG, AFP or both rise in the presence of nonseminomatous malignant germ cell tumor. Increased catecholamine secretion can be detected in pheochromocytomas through estimation of metanephrines and nor-metanephrines in the blood and urine. Paragangliomas and neuroblastomas may occasionally secrete epinephrine and norepinephrine.

Biopsy Procedures

Histological proof is very often (though not always) a sine qua non for a correct diagnosis. It should however not be performed in a well-capsulated mediastinal mass suggestive of a thymoma for fear of spillage of tumor cells that could hinder curative resection. It is also contraindicated in suspected vascular tumors and in a suspected pheochromocytoma. A tissue diagnosis through a biopsy procedure is however necessary in patients with mediastinal masses with raised AFP, β-HCG or CEA levels. This is because the treatment for patients with nonseminomatous germ cell tumor is primarily chemotherapy followed by resection of residual disease.

Biopsy procedures include the following:

- A CT-guided trucut biopsy is preferred to a fine-needle biopsy. A trucut core biopsy is however inadequate when tissue obtained is needed for immunohistochemistry and flow cytometric studies as is so necessary with lymphomas.
- An endobronchial ultrasound-guided (EBUS) biopsy should be considered when a mediastinal mass is adjacent to an airway. Lesions in these locations are difficult to approach even with CT guidance because of proximity to major vessels.
- Surgical biopsy techniques used are:
  - An anterior mediastinoscopy (Chamberlain's procedure) for lesions that are substernal, as also a cervical mediastinoscopy for sampling tissue in the middle mediastinum. A cervical mediastinoscopy allows adequate sampling of the paratracheal and subcarinal glands.
  - Video-assisted thoracoscopic surgery (VATS): This procedure allows an excellent view of structures within the thorax and also allows adequate tissue biopsy under vision of pathologies within the mediastinum, adjacent structures, and the pleura. The procedure usually requires general anesthesia but may be performed under local anesthesia with sedation.

◼ ANTERIOR MEDIASTINAL MASSES

Thymoma

A thymoma consists of a neoplastic proliferation of thymic epithelial cells interspersed with mature (non-neoplastic) lymphocytes. It is the most common primary mediastinal neoplasm in adults and the most frequent neoplasm of the anterior mediastinum. It can occur at any age but generally affects adults over 40 years of age with no gender predilection. A thymoma is generally situated in front of the root of the aorta but may occasionally be found anywhere within the anterior mediastinum between the thoracic inlet and the diaphragm.

A thymoma may be totally confined within a surrounding capsule. It is then termed benign or noninvasive. On the other hand, a thymoma may break through the capsule and may further invade surrounding structures. It is then termed malignant or invasive. It is impossible on histopathological study to determine whether the cells comprising a thymoma are benign or malignant, hence, it is more appropriate to use the terminology of noninvasive and invasive rather than benign and malignant when describing a thymoma. Most thymomas (about 70%) are well-capsulated or noninvasive; the remaining break through the capsule to invade surrounding structures.

Clinical Features

A thymoma may be asymptomatic, particularly when small, capsulated and noninvasive. Invasive thymomas as also large, noninvasive thymomas are often symptomatic, causing cough, vague chest pain and breathlessness. Pressure symptoms and signs are generally related to compression of the SVC. Pressure on the recurrent laryngeal nerve causes hoarseness of the voice. These pressure symptoms generally occur with invasive thymomas. Invasive thymomas can produce symptoms and signs due to invasion of neighboring structures. These include the mediastinum, the pericardium, the heart, the pleura and the pulmonary vessels. Pleural invasion may result in a pleural effusion or may spread to encase the lung on one side, entrapping the lung and mimicking a mesothelioma.

Paraneoplastic Manifestations

- Myasthenia gravis. Myasthenia is observed in one-third of patients and is the most frequent paraneoplastic disorder associated with a thymoma. It is estimated that 10% of patients with myasthenia gravis have a thymoma.
- Red cell aplasia is observed in 5% of patients with thymoma.
- Hypoglobulinemia causing recurrent infections, diarrhea and lymphadenopathy is seen in 10% of patients.
- Thymoma-associated multiorgan autoimmunity. This paraneoplastic syndrome is very similar to graft-versus-host disease and is characterized by various combinations of skin rash, diarrhea and liver cell dysfunction.
  Associated clinical disorders are:
- Collagen vascular diseases, such as systemic lupus erythematosus (SLE), polymyositis, scleroderma are reported to be rare associations.
- Nonthymic malignancies including thyroid carcinoma, bronchogenic carcinoma and lymphoma have also been reported.

Imaging Studies (Figs. 3 and 4)

The location of the tumor in the anterior mediastinum generally in front of the aortic root, suggests the diagnosis. On cross-sectional HRCT imaging, the tumor is seen as a homogeneous soft tissue mass. Large neoplasms may show heterogeneity due to necrosis, cystic changes or hemorrhage. Invasive thymomas, together with the nature and extent of invasion can generally be detected by CT scans. MRI scans are more effective in detecting vascular invasion. This is of importance before attempting surgical excision of invasive thymomas. Certain proof of invasiveness or noninvasiveness even in what appears to be a capsulated tumor can however only be judged at the time of surgical excision and by the demonstration of an unbroken capsule on histological study (**Figs. 5 and 6**). Besides direct invasion, "drop" metastasis leads to implantation of tumor seedlings into the ipsilateral pleura and pleural space. Imaging studies of pleural involvement

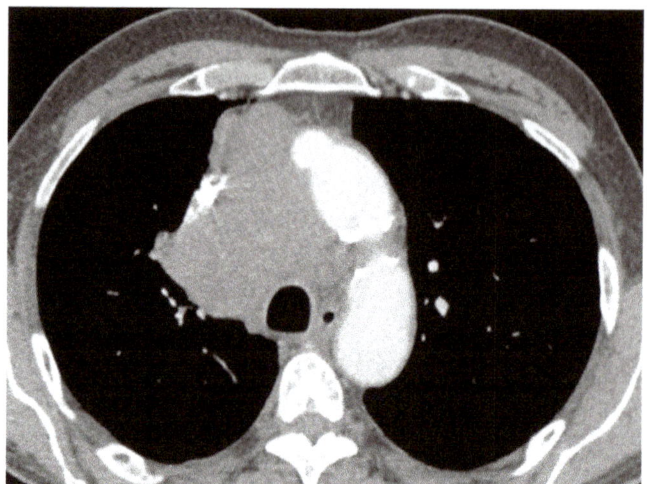

Fig. 3: CT scan demonstrates an anterior mediastinal mass lesion in the midline displacing SVC to the right and great vessels to the left. At surgery, this mass lesion was an invasive thymoma.

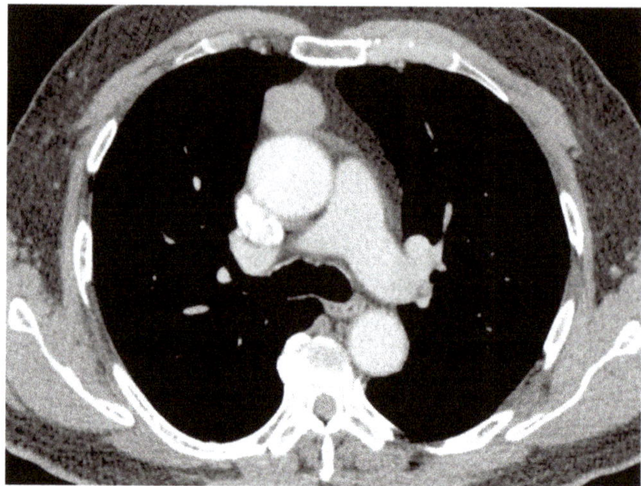

Fig. 4: Noninvasive thymoma. Chest CT shows a well-defined mass lesion in the anterior mediastinum to the right of the midline. At surgery, it was completely resectable with no invasion of surrounding structures nor any break in the capsule.

are characterized by solid tumor tissue encasing the ipsilateral lung or by an ipsilateral pleural effusion.

Diagnosis

Clinical and imaging features of an anterior mediastinal mass already described allow of a strong suspicion of a thymoma. The presence of any one of the paraneoplastic syndromes described above in association with an anterior mediastinal mass clinches the diagnosis. The presence of myasthenia gravis in association with an

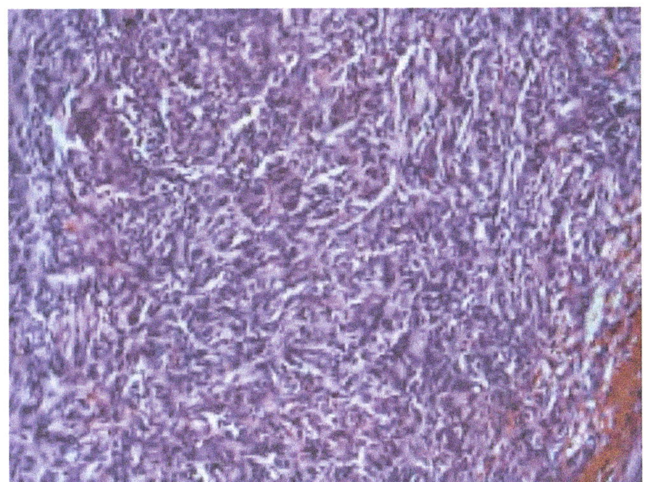

Fig. 5: Microscopic picture of Type A thymoma. Spindle tumor cells in a vague fascicular arrangement, some cells being haphazardly distributed.

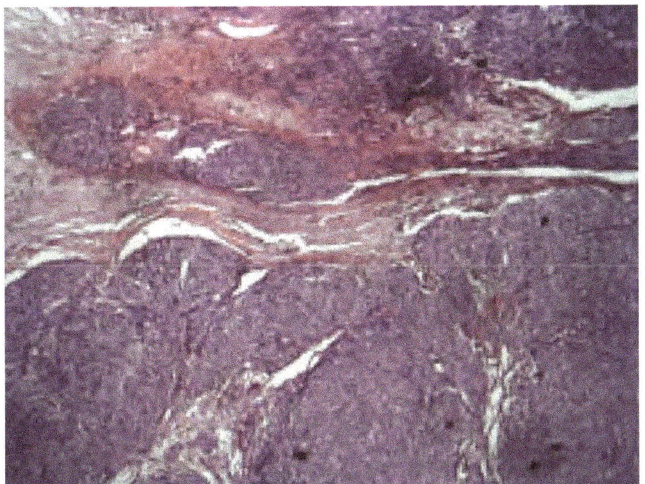

Fig. 6: Microscopic picture of Type A thymoma. Multiple lobules separated by fibrous septa. This is the characteristic appearance of a thymoma.

anterior mediastinal mass is diagnostic of a thymoma. It is to be noted that acetylcholine receptor antibodies are present in 60% of patients who have a thymoma without neurological features. Therefore, an estimation of these antibodies should always be done in a patient with an anterior mediastinal mass even in the absence of neurological features. A positive test confirms the presence of a thymoma.

Once the diagnosis of thymoma is suggested, the tumor should be resected without preliminary biopsy for reasons already stated earlier. A definite tissue diagnosis is only indicated when a presumed thymoma appears

Stage	Description	10-year survival (%)
I	Encapsulated tumors without gross or microscopic invasion	85–100
II	Capsular or pleural invasion	60–84
III	Macroscopic invasion of lung, pericardium, vena cava or aorta	21–77
IVA	Disseminated disease within the chest	26–47
IVB	Distant metastasis	Unknown

Table 5: Staging of thymic malignancies.

Source: Adapted with permission from Masaoka A, Monden Y, Nakahara K, et al. Follow-up study of thymoma with special reference to their clinical stages. Cancer. 1981;48:2485-92.

so advanced that it is best treated nonoperatively by chemotherapy, or radiotherapy, or by both, or when a lymphoma is very strongly suspected. We feel that a VATS should best be avoided when thymoma is a differential diagnosis for fear of pleural spread.

All patients with a suspected thymoma should undergo a thorough neurological evaluation for myasthenia gravis. If detected this disease should be treated first to prevent postoperative complications related to myasthenia.

Staging and Prognosis (Table 5)

The most frequently used classification scheme for thymoma is that proposed by Masaoka, based on the local invasiveness of the tumor. This classification also has prognostic value and helps stratification of use of neoadjuvant chemotherapy.

Recently the World Health Organization (WHO) has proposed a histological grading system that has helped to distinguish between a thymoma, a thymic carcinoma and a thymic carcinoid. The Masaoka staging system considered together with the WHO grading system provide a reasonably accurate prognostic guide for overall and disease-free survival.

Treatment

Treatment is by excision of the thymic tumor mass **(Fig. 7)**. Excision of invasive tumor may involve resection of adjacent structures such as pericardium, part of the lung, major veins and the pleura. Radiotherapy is reserved for the unresectable invasive thymomas; chemotherapy involving protocols containing cisplatin may provide palliative relief.

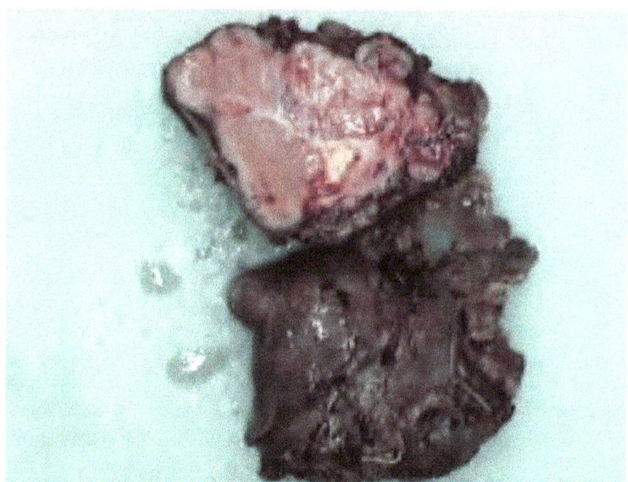

Fig. 7: Gross section of a thymoma. External surface is smooth and bosselated. Cut surface appears fleshy lobulated with fibrous septa.

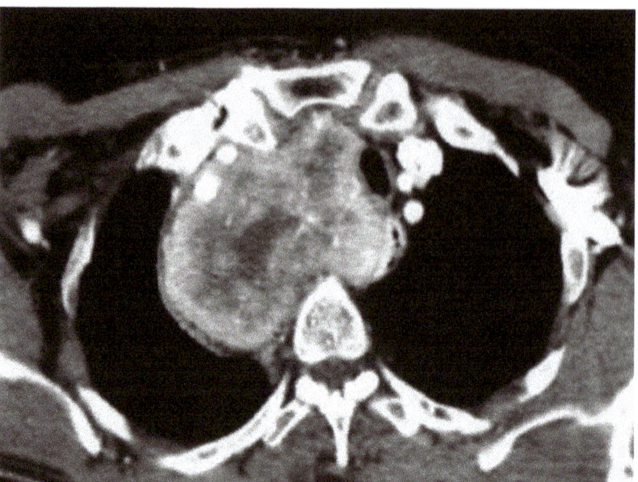

Fig. 8: CT scan demonstrates a large heterogeneous mass lesion in the anterior mediastinum displacing the trachea to the left and displacing and encasing the great vessels. The encasement is a strong sign of malignancy as benign lesions will displace and not encase. On biopsy, this was a thyroid carcinoma.

The role of thymectomy in paraneoplastic syndromes related to thymomas is uncertain. In selected patients with myasthenia gravis (young patients with progressive symptoms), thymectomy is of use in the absence of a thymoma. There is complete remission in over one-third of patients and an improvement in more than half. Clinical improvement of myasthenia gravis is less likely in the presence of a thymoma. Thymectomy in patients with red cell aplasia leads to 40–50% remission rates. Thymectomy is of no use in patients with hypogammaglobulinemia.

Thymic Carcinoma (Fig. 8)

Thymic carcinomas are malignant epithelial tumors of the thymus (type C of the revised WHO classification of thymic epithelial tumors) which are locally invasive and metastasize to distant sites. These tumors are distinct from thymomas with local invasion. Histopathologically, thymic carcinomas contain different cell types—squamous cell, lymphoepithelioma-like carcinoma, basaloid, mucoepidermoid, clear cell and sarcomatoid. Unlike thymomas, thymic carcinomas have the histological features of malignancy, some high grade and some low grade, and manifest as large anterior mediastinal masses with local infiltration, spread to lymph glands and to the lungs as also to distant sites.

Surgical resection (if possible) is the treatment of choice. Adjuvant radiotherapy plus cisplatin-based chemotherapy may help. The prognosis is poor even when total resection is possible, the 5-year survival being less than 30%.

Thymic Carcinoids (Fig. 9)

Thymic carcinoids are aggressive neuroendocrine tumors, locally invasive with distant metastasis. They rarely produce the carcinoid syndrome but may be associated with the multiple endocrine neoplasia syndrome. Adenomas may be present in the parathyroids, adrenals and pituitary giving rise to hyperparathyroidism, Cushing's syndrome, or the inappropriate antidiuretic hormone secretion syndrome. Surgical treatment is advised in the absence of distant metastasis or extensive local invasion.

Thymolipoma

These are benign lipomatous tumors which may attain a large size but may have few or no compressive symptoms because of their softness. The HRCT of the chest shows a lobulated tumor of fat density. Surgical excision is necessary to establish a definite diagnosis and to prevent compressive symptoms.

Thymic Cysts

A thymic cyst is a benign rounded or ovoid cystic mass with sharply defined walls which may show calcification on an X-ray chest or on a CT examination. Thymic cysts usually occur in children; they are asymptomatic and hardly ever produce compressive symptoms. They should be excised to establish a definite diagnosis so as not to miss out on a thymoma with cystic changes.

Thymic Hyperplasia

The thymus is relatively large in the newborn and the infant. It grows progressively up to puberty and then begins to involute so that it may be difficult to discern on imaging in the middle and older age group. If therefore the thymus gland appears larger than the range for a particular age group, and in particular if it is shown to progressively increase in size, it should be removed to exclude a thymoma. Thymic hyperplasia is the most common histopathology found in thymic glands excised for myasthenia gravis. Thymic hyperplasia may also occur following chemotherapy for malignancies both in children and adults.

Mediastinal Germ Cell Tumor

Germ cell tumors generally originate in the testis or ovary; the most common extragonadal site of this tumor is the anterior mediastinum. Mediastinal germ cell tumors are derived from primitive germ cells that fail to migrate during embryogenesis. They constitute about 15% of all mediastinal tumors in adults. It is always important to ensure that what appears to be a primary mediastinal germ cell tumor truly arises from the mediastinum and is not a metastatic lesion from an occult gonadal tumor. The latter

may not always be clinically evident. A careful clinical and ultrasound examination of the testicles is imperative. A careful work-up also involves a CT of the abdomen in addition to the chest. Germ cell tumors are classified into teratomas, seminomas and nonseminomatous malignant germ cell tumors.

Mediastinal Teratoma (Fig. 10)

A mediastinal teratoma is invariably a benign tumor (mature teratomas or dermoid). It is the most frequent of germ cell tumors (over 50% of all cases) and consists of tissue from at least two of the three primitive germ cell layers. Ectodermal tissues generally predominate and include skin, hair, tooth, and sebaceous glands. Sebaceous secretions (when present within teratomas) are extremely irritant and result in a severe surrounding inflammatory reaction. Mesodermal tissue when present includes cartilage, bone, and smooth muscle. Tissues derived from the endoderm include respiratory and intestinal epithelium. Very rarely, teratomas are immature or malignant and are then classified as malignant teratomas or teratosarcomas.

Mature (benign) teratomas are histologically well-defined and benign. Though occurring at any age they typically occur in children and young adults. Patients are frequently asymptomatic, though large teratomas may produce pressure symptoms—notably cough, dyspnea and vague chest pain. Rarely, a teratoma may open into

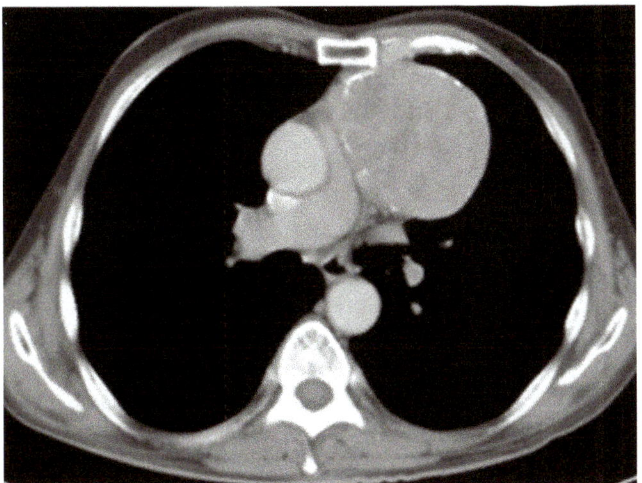

Fig. 9: Thymic carcinoid. CT chest reveals a well-defined anterior mediastinal mass lesion with multiple well-defined nodular areas of enhancement within. Histopathology revealed this to be a thymic carcinoid.

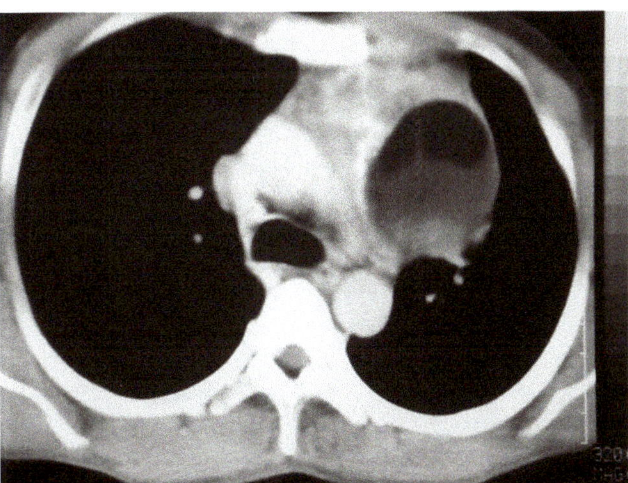

Fig. 10: Teratoma. Chest contrast CT reveals an anterior mediastinal mass lesion to the left of the midline displacing vascular structures posteriorly. The mass contains solid as well as fat-density components. Histopathology showed teratoma.

a bronchus and the patient may cough up its contents, which may include clear or viscid fluid or even hair (trichophytosis).

There have been reports of paraneoplastic encephalitis due to N-methyl-D-aspartate receptor antibodies in patients with benign mediastinal or ovarian teratomas. AFP is normal with teratoma.

Radiologically, teratomas present as well-defined spherical or lobulated anterior mediastinal masses which may show calcification of the wall or within the mass. Teeth and bone can occasionally be seen on imaging. A CT often shows multiloculation within the mass with fat attenuation.

Treatment of a teratoma is complete surgical excision, following which the prognosis is excellent. If the imaging features are convincing, a biopsy before excision is not necessary.

Mediastinal Seminoma (Fig. 11)

Seminomas typically occur in adult males between the third and fifth decades and constitute 40–50% of malignant mediastinal germ cell tumors. It presents as a large lobulated homogeneous anterior mediastinal mass, often causing dyspnea, cough, and substernal pain. Gynecomastia may be a presenting feature. Low-grade fever and weight loss may be the only symptoms, the mediastinal mass being detected as an investigative

finding. A CT-guided percutaneous core biopsy is generally needed to confirm the diagnosis. Tumors may sometimes grow as large as 20–30 cm before pressure symptoms develop. About 10% of patients present with a superior vena caval syndrome. Seminomas are not associated with a rise in AFP levels, but a slight elevation of β-HCG may be found. Invasion of mediastinal or intrathoracic structures can occur particularly with large tumors; the tumor may spread to the lymph nodes and metastasize to the bones.

Cisplatin-based chemotherapy alone has led to a 90% disease-free survival rate. Additional radiation therapy offers only a slight further advantage in survival. Patients treated with radiation alone have a much higher rate of recurrence.

In patients with advanced disease, chemotherapy should be followed by excision of residual disease. These tumors are usually FDG avid; A PET study may be useful to monitor response to therapy.

Mediastinal Nonseminomatous Germ Cell Tumor (Fig. 12)

These tumors are highly malignant and occur typically in young males invariably producing symptoms, either related to pressure on neighboring structures or to local

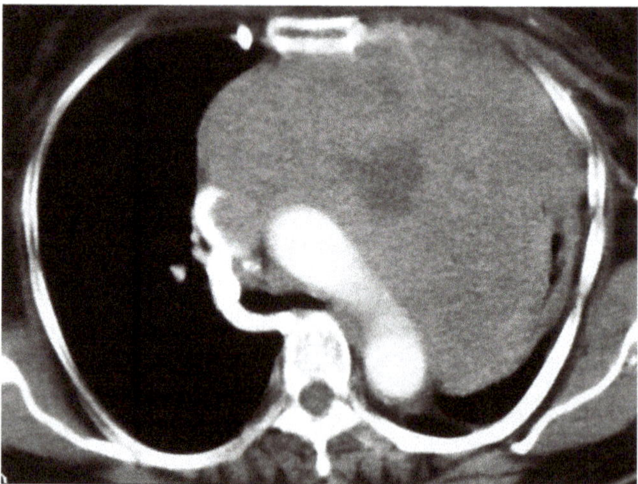

Fig. 12: Malignant germ cell tumor of the nonseminomatous variety. A young man, 30 years old, presented with vague chest pain and shortness of breath. Chest X-ray showed a large mass involving the greater part of the left hemithorax. CT scan showed a large heterogeneous anterior mediastinal mass displacing vascular structures posteriorly as well as occupying a greater part of the left hemithorax. At surgery, the entire mass was removed. Histopathology revealed a malignant germ cell tumor of the nonseminomatous variety.

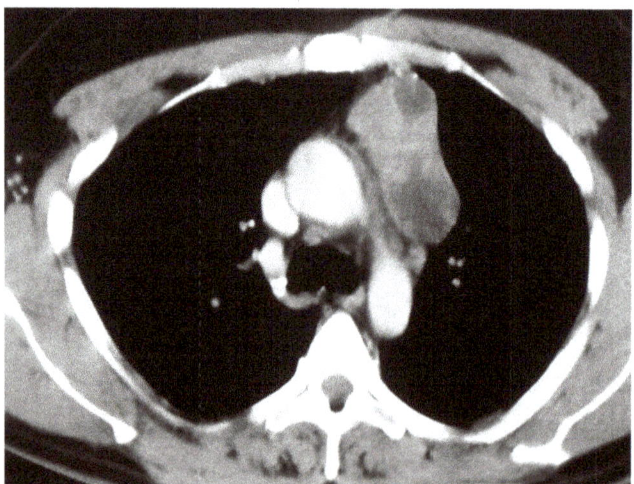

Fig. 11: Malignant germ cell tumor. Chest CT with contrast demonstrates an anterior mediastinal mass to the left of the midline with internal areas of necrosis. Histopathology revealed a malignant germ cell tumor of the seminomatous variety. β-HCG was markedly elevated.

or distant spread. Constitutional symptoms include fever, weight loss and increasing weakness. They are classified as choriocarcinoma, embryonal carcinoma, endodermal sinus (yolk sac) tumor and mixed germ cell tumor. Tumor markers AFP and β-HCG are significantly elevated in choriocarcinoma, while AFP is significantly high in embryonic carcinoma. Nonseminomatous germ cell tumors may be associated with hematological disorders such as acute leukemia and the myelodysplastic syndrome. Klinefelter syndrome is another association in 20% of patients. Radiologically, these tumors manifest as large nonhomogeneous masses with areas of necrosis, hemorrhage, together with enhancing nodular soft tissue. Local invasion may lead to pericardial effusion and tamponade as also to pleural effusion. Lymph node and distant metastasis are frequently observed.

Treatment consists of courses of cisplatin-based chemotherapy.

After completion of chemotherapy, a restaging should be done through CT imaging and measurement of tumor markers. Residual disease is invariably present. Even if the tumor markers are not elevated the presence of residual disease on imaging warrants surgical removal of remnant tumor. This can lead to a cure in a significant number of patients.

The prognosis is worse when compared to a seminoma. The overall 5-year survival being 48% compared to 86% in patients with seminomas.

Lymphomas

Lymphomas are best classified into Hodgkin's disease and non-Hodgkin's lymphoma. Lymphomas constitute 10–15% of all mediastinal masses in adults; they occur in the anterior and/or middle mediastinal compartment but are rarely found in the posterior compartment. Approximately 20% of anterior mediastinal masses and 20% of middle mediastinal masses are lymphomas.

Mediastinal lymphomas are usually associated with generalized disease, lymph node involvement being present in one or more sites as well. Primary mediastinal lymphoma presenting as a solitary anterior mediastinal mass is uncommon comprising about 10% of all lymphomas.

The three most common forms of mediastinal lymphomas are the nodular sclerosing subtype of Hodgkin's disease, the large B-cell lymphoma and lymphoblastic lymphoma (subtypes of non-Hodgkin's lymphoma).

Mediastinal lymphomas may be asymptomatic in about 25% of patients even when the glandular mass is fairly large. Symptomatic patients have systemic symptoms and/or present with pressure effects or with features of local invasion. Systemic features include fever, often of the Pel-Ebstein type, weight loss, pruritus, anemia and a significantly elevated erythrocyte sedimentation rate (often over 80 mm/hr). Local symptoms include chest discomfort, cough, and breathlessness. The superior vena caval compression syndrome may occur but is uncommon. Pressure on the trachea, bronchi can cause stridor, wheezing and dyspnea.

Hodgkin's Disease

The age distribution of patients with Hodgkin's disease is bimodal affecting individuals between 20 years and 30 years of age or greater than 50 years of age. The nodular sclerosing subtype accounts for 90% of patients with Hodgkin's disease involving the mediastinum. Of these close to 50% have only mediastinal disease and the rest have involvement of other sites as well. The chest X-ray typically shows a superiorly placed mass in the anterior mediastinal compartment and/or in the middle compartment. Most often glands (prevascular and paratracheal) first appear in the anterior compartment and then spread by contiguity to the nodes of the middle compartment, to the hilar nodes and then invade the lung. CT chest demonstrates this contiguous spread of disease. Skip involvement of lymph glands should prompt one to search for another diagnosis.

Though systemic features are common in Hodgkin's disease, local invasion of the pleura, pericardium, and lungs generally occurs only when the mediastinal mass has reached a very large size.

The accompanying **Table 6** gives the Ann Arbor classification of Hodgkin's disease. In stages IA and IIA, radiotherapy generally suffices, though many centers now use limited chemotherapy. For advanced disease, stages III and IV, chemotherapy is combined with radiotherapy. Cure rates of 90% are achieved in stage I and stage IIA. Even in patients with advanced disease, stages III and IV, cure rates as high as 60% have been observed. Patients who relapse may benefit from stem cell transplant.

Non-Hodgkin's Lymphoma (Fig. 13)

Non-Hodgkin's lymphoma involves cervical nodes, abdominal lymph nodes and lymphoid tissue of Waldeyer's rings far more often than the mediastinal nodes. Only 5% of non-Hodgkin's lymphoma present with a mediastinal mass. Thoracic lymphadenopathy can occur anywhere within the mediastinum and may involve unusual sites. Anterior mediastinal lymph node enlargement does

Table 6: Ann Arbor staging system with Cotswolds modification for Hodgkin's disease.
Stage
I   Involvement of 1 lymph node region or one extranodal organ or site
II   Involvement of 2 or more lymph node regions on the same side of the diaphragm, or localized involvement of an extranodal site or organ and one or more lymph node region on the same side of the diaphragm
III   Involvement of lymph node regions on both sides of the diaphragm, potentially accompanied by localized involvement of an extranodal organ or site, spleen, or both
IV   Involvement of extranodal site other than one contiguous or proximal extranodal site
Modifying features
A   No symptoms
B   Presence of at least one of: unexplained weight loss >10% baseline during 6 months prior to staging; recurrent unexplained fever; recurrent night sweats
X   Bulky disease (mass > 10 cm in diameter)
E   Extranodal extension or single isolated site of extranodal disease

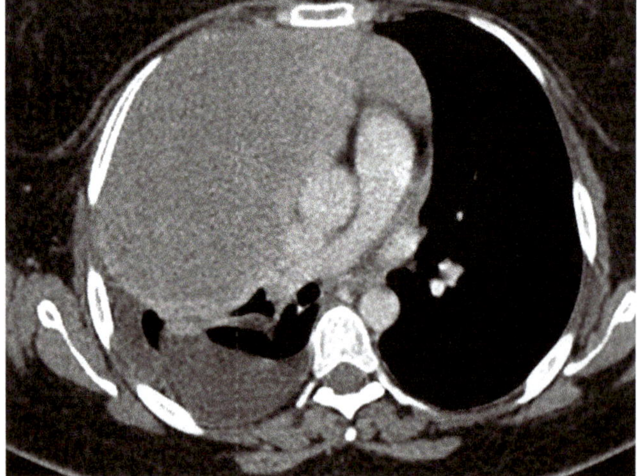

Fig. 13: Non-Hodgkin's lymphoma. Chest CT reveals large hypoenhancing mass lesion in the anterior mediastinum, extending into the right hemithorax. There is loss of fat plane with the ascending aorta. Mild right sided pleural effusion is noted. CT-guided biopsy showed large B cell lymphoma.

occur but is less common than in Hodgkin's disease. These lymphomas are extremely aggressive so that pleural effusion, pericardial effusion and involvement of the lung parenchyma are commonly observed. Lymphoblastic lymphoma is commonly associated with an acute lymphoblastic leukemia. Mediastinal spread (unlike in Hodgkin's disease) is typically noncontiguous and may occur in unusual sites, for example, in the posterior mediastinal, retrocrural sites. Non-Hodgkin's lymphomas consist of T-cell, B-cell, diffuse large cell lymphomas, and lymphoblastic lymphomas. According to the European American Classification of lymphoid neoplasms, non-Hodgkin's lymphomas are classified as indolent, aggressive or highly aggressive. Indolent lymphomas are more often associated with nodal disease; aggressive lymphomas are associated with extranodal involvement. Although untreated aggressive lymphomas have a poor prognosis, their potential for cure with chemotherapy is, remarkably enough, greater than indolent lymphomas. The treatment of indolent lymphomas depends on the stage of the disease and is often palliative.

Diagnosis: Histological proof is imperative for a definite diagnosis. When the lymphoma is solely confined to the mediastinum, histological proof is best provided by a video-assisted thoracoscopic biopsy, or a biopsy through mediastinoscopy or through an anterior mediastinotomy. A CT-guided needle core biopsy generally does not provide sufficient material to make both a correct histopathological diagnosis and typing of the lymphoma through immunohistochemical studies. Treatment consists of high-dose conventional chemotherapy plus in selected cases radiation to localized area of disease. Relapses are common and the diagnosis is worse compared to Hodgkin's lymphoma.

Lymphadenopathy within the mediastinum can be due to several other causes besides lymphoma. These must be considered in the differential diagnosis. Other causes of lymphadenopathy both benign and malignant are discussed in the section on masses in the middle mediastinum.

Intrathoracic Thyroid Masses

The most common thyroid mass is an intrathoracic goiter resulting from an extension of a cervical goiter into the anterior superior mediastinum. Rarely, an ectopic mediastinal thyroid goiter without any connection with a normally situated thyroid in the neck may also occur. Finally, cancer of the thyroid may extend into the anterior mediastinal compartment. A retrosternal goiter may be asymptomatic or if sufficiently large may compress the trachea causing dyspnea, stridor, cough, or the superior vena caval syndrome **(Fig. 14)**. Dysphagia results from pressure on the esophagus. The significance of a loud wheeze produced by pressure on the trachea has been occasionally missed and wrongly diagnosed as asthma. The wheeze is monophonic and though audible over both sides of the chest is best heard over the trachea and the manubrium.

Radiography of the chest in a patient with intrathoracic goiter demonstrates a cervicothoracic mass. CT demonstrates a well-defined lobular mass in the anterior-superior mediastinum, contiguous with the lower pole of the thyroid within the neck. The mass may be heterogeneous because of cystic changes or hemorrhage within it, is anterior to the trachea and generally to the right. Rarely, an intrathoracic goiter descends lateral to the trachea and may come to lie posterior to it. Pressure on the trachea if present is easily observed.

Marked enhancement of the mass generally follows after the administration of intravenous contrast. Isotope scans (^{131}I or technetium-99m) if positive are diagnostic. However, a retrosternal goiter may be nonfunctioning; negative isotope scans do not therefore exclude a thyroid origin of a mass in the anterosuperior mediastinum.

If a thyroid mediastinal mass is symptomatic, it should be excised. Even if asymptomatic and particularly if it is large, excision is advisable, as sudden hemorrhage into the gland can produce severe upper airways obstruction.

Parathyroid Masses

A parathyroid mass may be an adenoma of one of the inferior parathyroid glands extending by continuity into the anterior mediastinum: It could also be due to an ectopic functioning parathyroid adenoma which is generally situated anteriorly in the mediastinum close to the thymus gland **(Fig. 15)**. It presents as a small encapsulated mass which is missed on an X-ray chest and often mistaken for a lymph node in a CT of the chest. Localization is achieved by radioisotope studies using ^{99m}Tc. Localization through radioisotopes should be correlated with CT or MRI. An ectopic parathyroid mass should be assiduously sought in patients with features of hyperparathyroidism who show neither an adenoma nor hyperplasia of the gland in the neck, or in patients in whom features of hyperparathyroidism persist even after removal of a parathyroid adenoma within the neck. A functioning parathyroid adenoma should be excised.

Pericardial Cysts (Figs. 16A and B)

These are termed spring-water cysts because of the clear fluid contents. They are asymptomatic, most often found

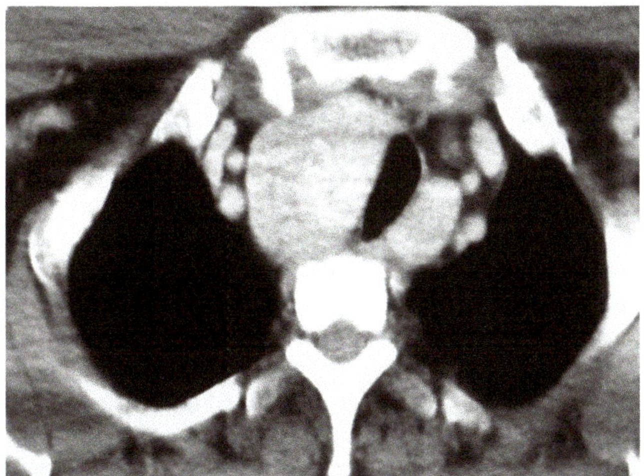

Fig. 14: Retrosternal goiter. CT chest demonstrates a homogeneously enhancing mass lesion in the prevertebral region displacing the trachea to the left and compressing it. This is a retrosternal goiter.

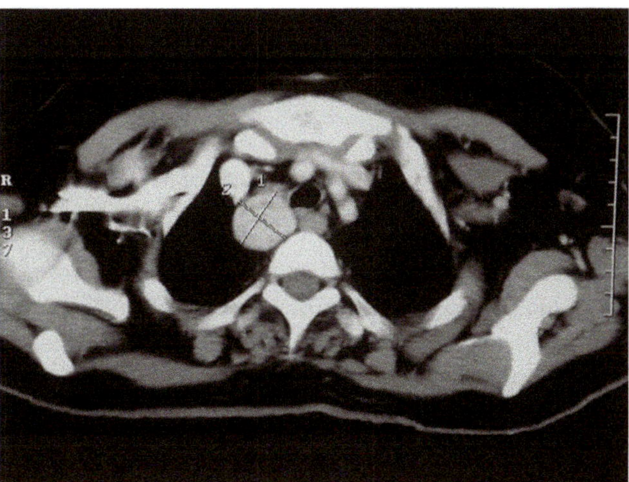

Fig. 15: Parathyroid adenoma. Well-defined homogeneously enhancing mass lesion in right paratracheal region. Excision biopsy showed parathyroid adenoma.

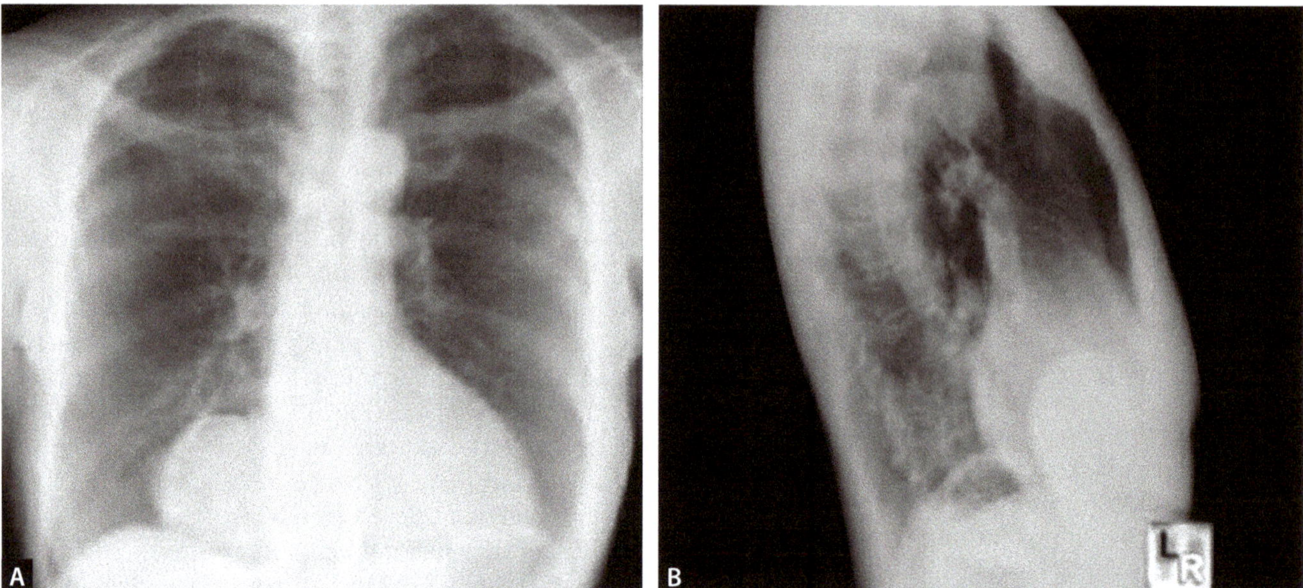

Figs. 16A and B: Pericardial cyst. (A) X-ray chest PA and (B) lateral demonstrate a well-defined homogeneous opacity in the right paracardiac region with peripheral calcification representing a pericardial cyst.

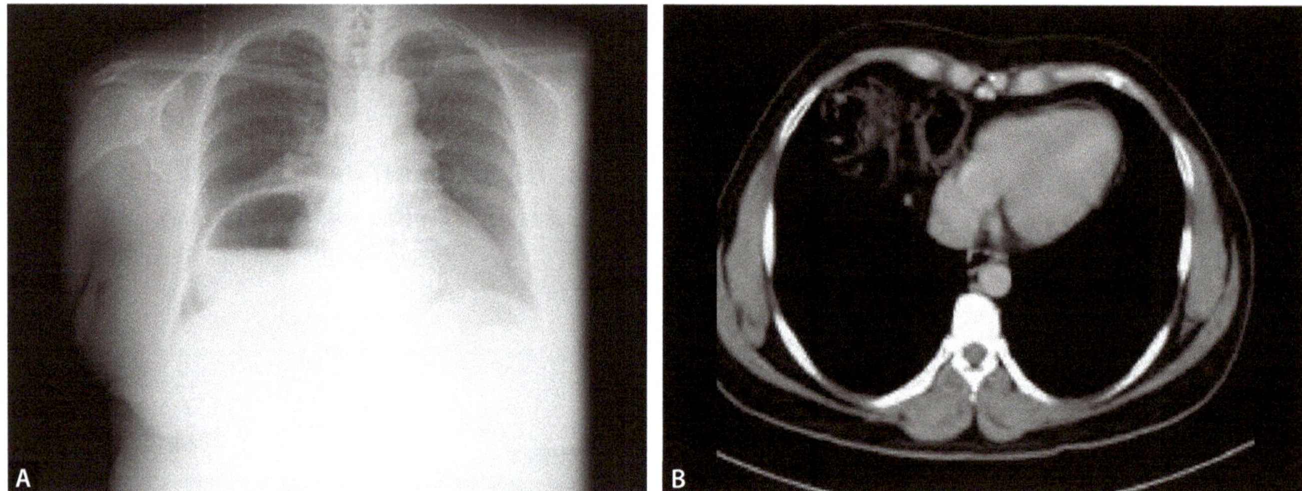

Figs. 17A and B: Morgagni's hernia. (A) X-ray demonstrates bowel loops in the right paracardiac region. These loops are anterior as there is no silhouetting with the diaphragm; (B) This is confirmed on the CT and represents a Morgagni's hernia.

in middle-aged adults, and are discovered on a routine X-ray of the chest. A pericardial cyst is a developmental lesion typically found in the right cardiophrenic angle. CT demonstrates a nonenhancing cystic mass lesion of water attenuation, with a very thin barely perceptible cyst wall. It generally requires no treatment.

Morgagni's Hernia (Figs. 17A and B)

Hernia through the foramen of Morgagni presents as a fairly large mass within the anteroinferior aspect of the anterior mediastinum. It generally includes the large bowel and omentum, but other viscera may also be found. A barium study may disclose the contents of the hernia. A CT is diagnostic, revealing the fat attenuation produced by omentum and the pockets of air within the herniated gut. Surgery is necessary to reduce the contents of the hernia and to repair the defect through which herniation occurred.

Rare Mediastinal Tumors

An example of a rare anterior mediastinal tumor is a lipoma which can attain a huge size producing severe

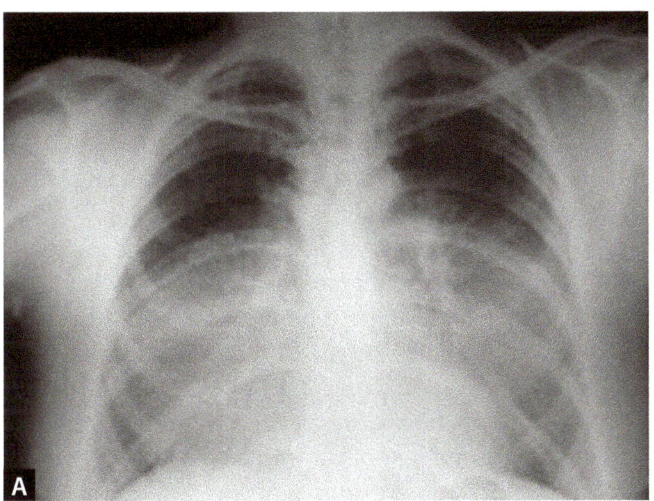
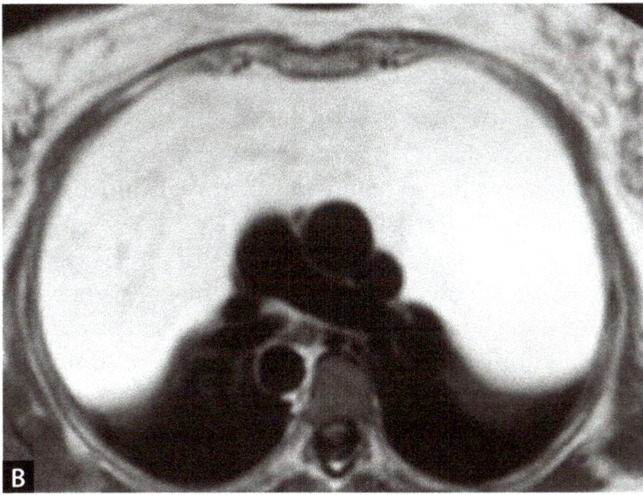

Figs. 18A and B: Mediastinal lipoma. Chest X-ray and T1 axial chest MRI demonstrate large hyperintense mass of fat intensity occupying the anterior lower half of thorax. This was a mediastinal lipoma in a young 36-year-old lady who complained of marked breathlessness over some years. It was resected but postoperatively, she went into cardiorespiratory failure resistant to all support.

compression of the mediastinum, great vessels, heart and lungs (**Figs. 18A and B**).

MASSES IN THE MIDDLE MEDIASTINUM

Mediastinal Cysts

Congenital foregut cysts represent 12–20% of mediastinal masses. When related to the trachea or major bronchi, they are termed bronchogenic cysts and when related to the esophagus in its cervical or mediastinal course, they are termed gastroenteric and neuroenteric cysts.

Bronchogenic Cysts (Fig. 19)

These are formed during embryonic development following abnormal ventral budding of the foregut. A bronchogenic cyst is most commonly found in the subcarinal or paratracheal region and is lined with pseudostratified columnar epithelium. It contains bronchial mucus-secreting glands, cartilage and smooth muscle within its wall and is filled with serous fluid or mucus. Bronchogenic cysts can occur at any age but are most frequently seen in young adults. They often are asymptomatic but may produce symptoms, especially when large and in children. The most common pressure symptoms are cough and breathlessness. Large cysts, particularly in children, can compress an airway causing air-trapping, atelectasis and infection in the atelectatic area.

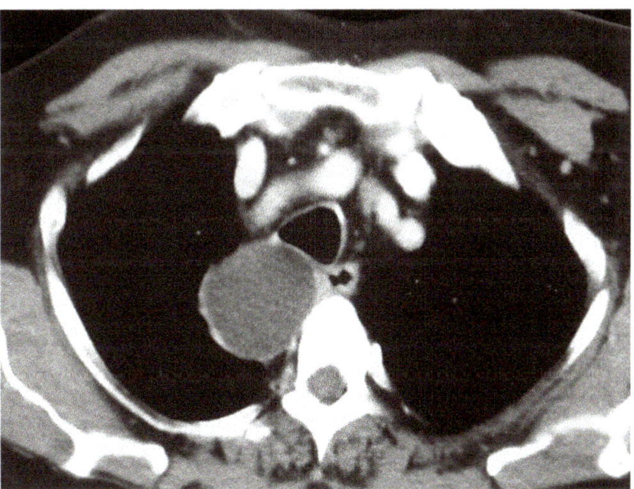

Fig. 19: Bronchogenic cyst. Chest CT with contrast demonstrates a well-defined homogeneous fluid-density lesion along the right paracardiac surface in the middle mediastinum causing compression of the adjacent lung. Surgery revealed a bronchogenic cyst.

Infection of the cyst contents converts the cyst into an abscess, causing fever with other systemic features of infection. When a bronchogenic cyst communicates with a bronchus, an air-fluid level is observed. Radiography reveals a well-defined spherical middle mediastinal mass, sometimes extending toward the posterior mediastinum. On CT, these cysts are homogeneous, without loculi and with varying attenuation, depending on the cyst contents. The cyst wall may show calcification;

though generally nonenhancing, it may rarely enhance following the administration of contrast. An MRI may help to differentiate the lesion from other masses. A tissue diagnosis for a definite diagnosis can be made by tracheobronchial, CT-guided or a thoracoscopic needle aspiration. Aspirated fluid typically reveals mucus and bronchial epithelial cells.

Surgical excision is the treatment of choice. Small asymptomatic cysts with a confirmed diagnosis may be followed up clinically and by imaging studies, as surgery is not without some risk. In poor-risk symptomatic patients, the cyst can be drained through a CT-guided, transbronchial or thoracoscopic approach.

Enterogenous Cysts (Figs. 20A and B)

Enterogenous cysts originate from the dorsal foregut and are located either in the middle or posterior mediastinum, more often in the latter. They are lined by squamous or enteric epithelium and may contain gastric or pancreatic tissue. Esophageal duplication cysts are located in or are attached to the esophageal wall and are associated with gastrointestinal malformations in 12% of cases.

Enterogenous cysts typically manifest in childhood as spherical well-defined cystic masses. Radiological features are indistinguishable from a bronchogenic cyst. Though often asymptomatic, hemorrhage or rupture may occur when gastric epithelium or pancreatic tissue is present.

Surgical excision is the treatment of choice. The prognosis after removal is excellent.

Aneurysm of the Major Vessels

Aneurysm of the ascending aorta, the arch of the aorta and of any of the vessels arising from the arch may mimic a mediastinal mass within any compartment of the mediastinum. Thus, an aneurysm of the ascending aorta, the aortic root or of the sinus of Valsalva may appear as an anterior mediastinal mass; an aneurysm of the arch may point anteriorly or extend into the posterior mediastinum while an aneurysm of the innominate or carotid vessels lies within the confines of the superior mediastinum and can extend in any direction.

Aneurysm of the ascending aorta is most often due to atherosclerosis but may occur with dissection of the aorta, syphilis or Marfan's syndrome. Aortic regurgitation may be an associated feature. A dissecting aneurysm involving the aorta proximal to the origin of the left subclavian needs surgery in spite of the hazard involved. An expanding aneurysm of the ascending or arch of the aorta may also require surgery.

Aneurysms of the pulmonary artery or its major branches also occupy the middle mediastinum.

A cardiac aneurysm following a myocardial infarction may arise from the anterolateral aspect or posterior aspect of the heart.

An aneurysm should be suspected when a mediastinal lesion or mass is adjacent to major vessels. CT with contrast enhancement of the involved vessel is diagnostic. Arteriography may still be necessary both for accurate diagnosis and planned treatment.

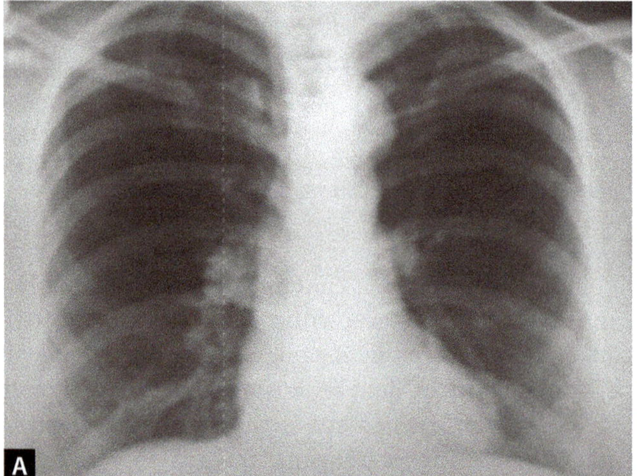
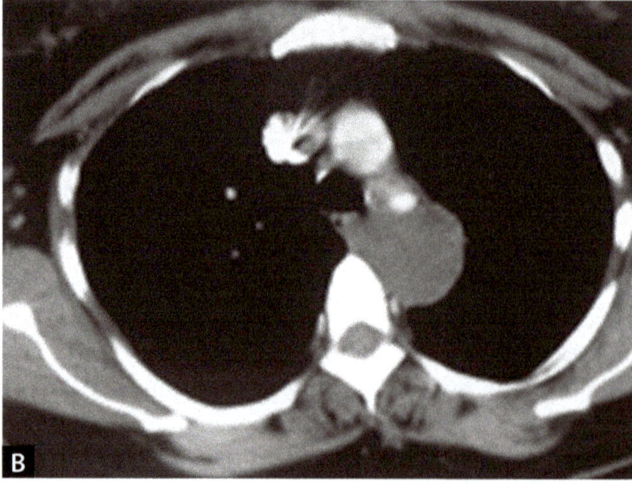

Figs. 20A and B: Enterogenous cyst. (A) Chest X-ray reveals a well-defined homogeneous mass on the left side just above the aortic arch; (B) CT reveals that the opacity seen on the chest X-ray is a well-defined homogeneous cystic mass in close relation to the esophagus representing an enterogenous cyst.

Benign Mediastinal Lymphadenopathy

Tuberculosis is unquestionably the most common cause of infectious granulomatous mediastinal lymphadenopathy in our country and in most developing countries of the world. Areas of necrosis and liquefaction within the glands almost always point to tuberculosis **(Fig. 21)**. Histoplasmosis and coccidioidomycosis may cause granulomatous mediastinal lymphadenopathy in countries where these fungal infections are endemic. Bacterial and viral infections may rarely cause a benign lymphadenopathy. The viral infection to particularly bear in mind is an Epstein-Barr virus infection. Invariably, mediastinal adenopathy in this viral infection is associated with adenopathy elsewhere, in particular the cervical region.

The most important noninfectious granulomatous disease, perhaps all over the world including India is sarcoidosis. It typically produces bilateral hilar adenopathy with or without mediastinal adenopathy **(Fig. 22)**. Unilateral hilar adenopathy is uncommon and should prompt one to seek other causes. Bilateral hilar adenopathy can also occur in tuberculosis and occasionally in lymphomas. Though an elevated serum angiotensin-converting enzyme (SACE) level may help, it is not specific for sarcoidosis and is also observed in tuberculosis and lymphoma. Silicosis can also cause both hilar and mediastinal adenopathy. Egg shell calcification is not specific to silicosis; it can occur in sarcoidosis and in tuberculosis.

Other causes of benign masses in the middle mediastinum include drugs such as phenytoin, and Castleman's disease (angiofollicular lymphoid hyperplasia).

Castleman's disease is an uncommon lymphoproliferative disease which may be unicentric (unicentric Castleman's disease) or multicentric (multicentric disease). The unicentric disease involves just one location, the most common site being the anterior and middle mediastinum. Though generally asymptomatic it can cause pressure symptoms. Multicentric Castleman's syndrome is characterized by fever, weight loss, peripheral lymphadenopathy and hepatosplenomegaly. Some of these patients also develop mediastinal and abdominal lymphadenopathy. Human herpes virus has been implicated in the pathogenesis of multicentric but not of unicentric disease.

Histological studies show two cell types: (1) hyaline vascular and (2) plasma cell. It is more often the centricity of the disease rather than the histological cell type which determines prognosis. Unicentric disease should be surgically excised. This is associated with 95% survival and 80% disease-free survival over a 5-year period. Multicentric disease can be rapidly progressive and is often fatal.

Metastatic Lymphadenopathy

Metastatic lymph node involvement is a common and important cause of mediastinal lymphadenopathy involving the middle mediastinal compartment. The common sites of a primary neoplasm are the lung, breast,

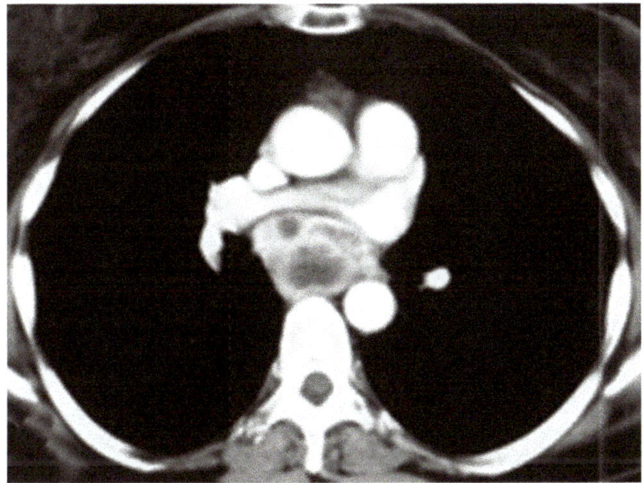

Fig. 21: Tuberculous subcarinal lymphadenopathy. Note multiple areas of necrosis indicating a tubercular etiology.

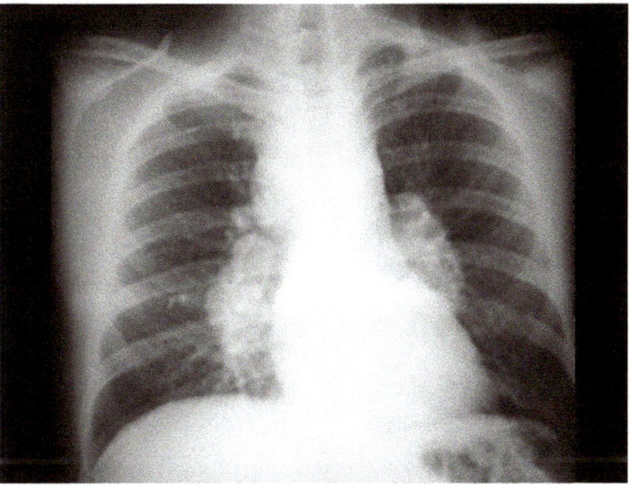

Fig. 22: Sarcoidosis. Chest X-ray demonstrates large hilar and paratracheal adenopathy. Biopsy revealed sarcoidosis.

gastrointestinal tract, kidney and prostate. Melanomas also metastasize to the mediastinum as do germ cell tumors arising within the testis or ovary. The secondaries in the mediastinum may involve just one group of glands or cause multifocal involvement.

Metastatic mediastinal lymphadenopathy should always enter the differential diagnosis of any mass within the mediastinum. A primary source if not evident should be assiduously sought. The diagnosis needs to be confirmed by a biopsy.

POSTERIOR MEDIASTINAL TUMORS

Neurogenic Tumors (Figs. 23A and B)

Neurogenic tumors arise from the tissue of the neural crest, including cells of the peripheral, autonomic and paraganglionic nervous system. They are classified according to cell type and constitute 12–20% of adult and 40% of all pediatric mediastinal tumors. Over 95% of these occur in the paravertebral region. Neurogenic tumors occurring in adults are most often benign; 50% of neurogenic tumors in the pediatric age group are malignant. Approximately 50% of patients affected are asymptomatic.

Nerve Sheath Tumors

Tumors arising from nerve sheaths are benign slowly-growing tumors comprising 40-60% of neurogenic mediastinal masses and are either schwannomas or neurofibromas **(Figs. 24A to C)**. The latter may be associated with von Recklinghausen's neurofibromatosis. Both schwannomas and neurofibromas are generally asymptomatic and are discovered incidentally. Large tumors may however cause erosion and deformity of the ribs and vertebral bodies. Ten percent of these tumors grow through the intervertebral foramina and create a dumb-bell-shaped appearance on imaging studies.

Radiologically, schwannomas and neurofibromas appear as spherical, sharply outlined, occasionally lobular masses extending one to three rib spaces. They could however attain a large size. Benign pressure erosion of one or more ribs, vertebral body or neural foramina may be observed. CT shows a sharply defined paravertebral mass which may be heterogeneous and show punctate calcification. An MRI should always be done to determine if there is an intraspinal extension of the growth. The treatment is surgical resection.

Malignant Peripheral Nerve Tumors

These are the malignant counterparts of schwannomas and neurofibromas. They are rare and occur equally in men and women between 30 years and 50 years of age. Nearly half of mediastinal neurofibromas occur in patients with neurofibromatosis. The incidence of malignant change in neurogenic tumors in patients with neurofibromatosis is close to 5%.

Increasing pain due to pressure on the ribs and vertebrae are the usual symptoms. Intraspinal extension

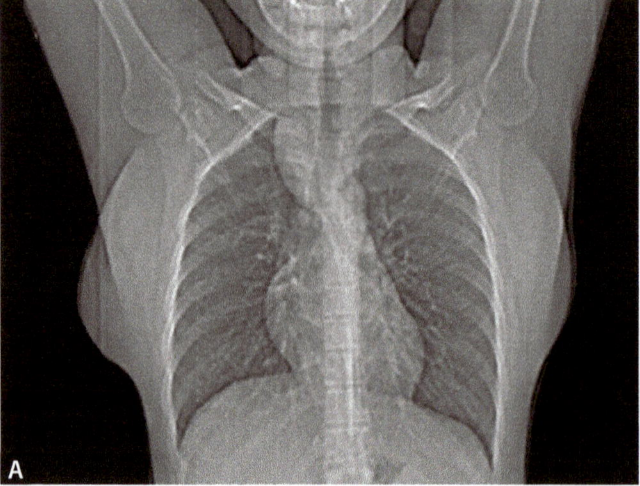
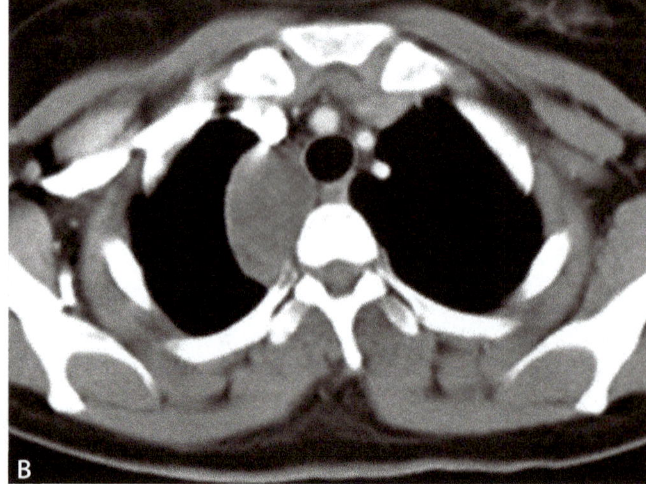

Figs. 23A and B: Neurogenic tumor. (A) X-ray demonstrates well-defined homogeneous mass in right paratracheal region; (B) Axial CT of the same patient demonstrates right paravertebral mass lesion representing a neurogenic tumor.

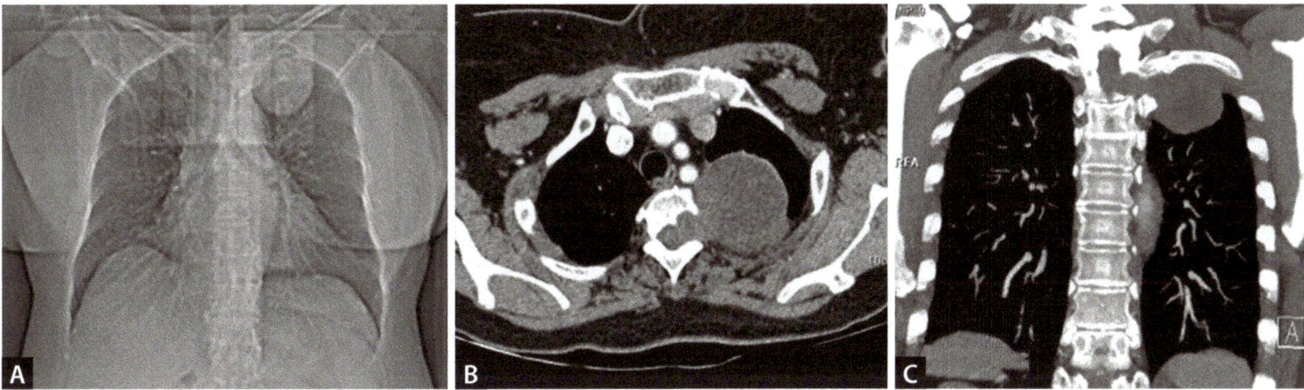

Figs. 24A to C: Neurofibroma. (A) Scanogram demonstrates a well-defined mediastinal mass in the left paravertebral region; (B) This is well seen on the axial images in the left paravertebral region extending into the spinal canal widening the neural foramen, scalloping the posterior surface of the vertebral body and compressing the dorsal cord, giving rise to long tract signs; (C) Similar features are seen on the coronal reconstructions. This was a neurofibroma extending through the neural foramen compressing the cord.

can result in pressure on the spinal cord. Radiologically on a CT, they may appear sharply defined fast-growing tumors often with manifest erosion of ribs and vertebral bodies.

Sympathetic Ganglion Neoplasms

Sympathetic ganglion neoplasms arise from the sympathetic ganglia in the paravertebral region. They affect both children and young adults; in children they are frequently malignant.

Ganglioneuromas

Ganglioneuromas are benign tumors affecting males and females equally. They are usually diagnosed in the second and third decade of life and are the most common neurogenic tumors occurring in childhood. Pain from rib or vertebral erosion and intraspinal extension occurs in 50% of patients. Radiologically, they form well-defined, large paravertebral masses extending over three to five vertebrae. Though generally asymptomatic, large tumors may cause cough, chest pain, dyspnea and pressure effects such as dysphagia and Horner's syndrome. MRI is necessary to determine the presence and extent of intraspinal extension which occurs far more frequently than with benign nerve sheath tumors. Surgical resection is the treatment of choice.

Ganglioneuroblastoma

Ganglioneuroblastomas are malignant neoplasms, generally occurring in children less than 10 years of age. Symptoms result from erosive pressure on neighboring

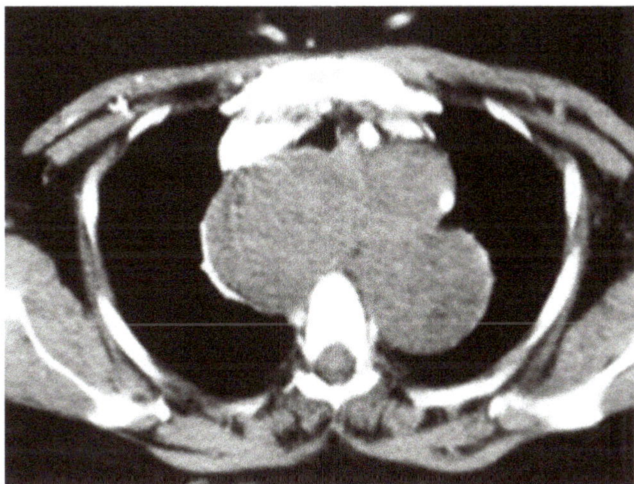

Fig. 25: Neuroblastoma. Axial CT demonstrates a large lobulated mass in the posterior mediastinum displacing the trachea and vascular structures anteriorly, representing a neuroblastoma.

structures or from local and distant metastasis. Staging and treatment are as for a neuroblastoma. Prognosis however is more favorable when compared to neuroblastoma.

Neuroblastoma (Fig. 25)

Neuroblastoma is a tumor occurring in young children, with 95% of them occurring below 5 years of age. It is a highly aggressive, nonencapsulated, posterior mediastinal tumor that spreads locally and metastasizes quickly. The tumor on a macroscopic examination often shows necrosis, hemorrhage and cystic degeneration. Microscopically, it consists of mitotic small round cells arranged in sheets or rosettes.

Patients are invariably symptomatic either because of local spread and pressure effects or because of distant metastasis.

Pain due to erosion of vertebrae, cough and respiratory distress are commonly encountered. The tumor can invade and infiltrate through the foramina causing pressure and involvement of nerve roots and the spinal cord. Neurological deficits include paraplegia and Horner's syndrome. Neuroblastomas have a propensity to produce vasoactive substances like catecholamines and vasoactive intestinal peptides. The former result in tachycardia and hypertension; the latter cause flushing and severe watery diarrhea. Radiologically, a neuroblastoma appears as a large paraspinal mass impinging on adjacent structures, crossing the midline, causing skeletal erosion and neurological damage. On a CT scan, 80% of these tumors show calcification; the tumors are heterogeneous because of hemorrhage and necrosis. An MRI should always be done to determine the presence and extent of intraspinal extension.

Neuroblastomas should be treated if possible by surgical resection. Chemotherapy and radiation may either follow resection to deal with residual disease, or may form primary therapy following which resection may be attempted.

The prognosis is poor and depends on the age at diagnosis, the size, the stage of the tumor and the histological differentiation.

Paraganglionic Neoplasms

Pheochromocytoma

Paragangliomas are pheochromocytomas that most often arise from the adrenal glands. Two percent of pheochromocytomas arise within the thorax, radiologically evident as enhancing well-localized posterior mediastinal masses. Pheochromocytomas occasionally occur as part of the multiple endocrine neoplasia type 2 (MEN2) syndrome. Symptoms are due to excessive catecholamine secretion or due to pressure on adjacent structures. Paroxysmal hypertension, hypertension with diabetes, hypermetabolic syndrome, and acute hypertension following anesthesia for a surgical procedure are common presenting features due to excessive catecholamine secretion. Diagnosis is made by measuring blood and urine catecholamines and their metabolites, in particular noting elevated levels of metanephrines and nor-metanephrines in the blood and urine. The diagnosis can be clinched if a tumor mass anywhere within the abdomen or thorax picks up the radioactive isotope, ^{131}I-MIBG.

Treatment consists of the use of alpha- and beta-blockers for a couple of weeks before excision.

Paragangliomas

Paragangliomas are rare tumors of paraganglion cells. They are benign, nonfunctioning, well-localized tumors situated in the posterior mediastinum in the paravertebral area or the middle mediastinum adjacent to the aorta or pulmonary artery. They show marked enhancement after contrast administration due to their vascularity. Treatment is by excision.

Esophageal Cancer

An esophageal cancer may extend outward and produce a posterior mediastinal mass. Dysphagia is the prominent symptom. The relation of this mass to the esophagus is easily determined by a CT study and also by esophagoscopy. Surgery is the treatment of choice. In extensive disease, chemotherapy is given to start with; residual disease can then be tackled whenever possible by surgery.

Other Posterior Mediastinal Masses

Aneurysm of the Descending Aorta

An aneurysm of the descending aorta is generally due to atherosclerosis or a dissection of the aorta which may extend below the origin of the subclavian artery to a varying extent. An aneurysm of the descending aorta often causes persistent pain over the thoracic spine due to erosion of one or more vertebrae. A systolic bruit may be heard over the spine generally to the left of the midline. The aneurysm may mimic a posterior mediastinal tumor mass but its relation with the aorta is easily determined by cross-sectional CT imaging. Whenever possible and particularly when symptomatic surgery is advised.

Paravertebral Tubercular Abscess

A paravertebral cold abscess should always be considered in the differential diagnosis of a posterior mediastinal mass. It could arise from tubercle involving the spine, or it could be due to tuberculosis involving the posterior end of the ribs or rarely from tuberculosis of the lymph glands in the posterior mediastinum. Spinal tuberculosis is evident on radiography and CT imaging of the spine. Erosion of endplates of adjacent vertebrae with involvement of the discs between vertebrae with soft tissue paravertebral shadows are the diagnostic features. Pain in the back as also neurological symptoms and signs due to pressure on nerve roots or the spinal cord may be observed. Systemic symptoms of fever and weight loss are often seen and may precede local signs of pain in the back by weeks or even months. Bed rest for 3–6 weeks with the use of antituberculosis drugs for a year invariably effects a cure. Large paravertebral cold abscesses need to be aspirated. Cord compression always necessitates surgical intervention.

Hiatus Hernia

A large herniation of the stomach through the esophageal hiatus into the chest manifests as a large retrocardiac posterior mediastinal mass. Diagnosis is confirmed by visualizing the stomach or other abdominal contents on a cross-sectional CT of the chest. Small or moderate-sized hernias can be managed conservatively. Symptomatic or large hernias need surgery.

Extramedullary Hematopoiesis

Extramedullary hematopoiesis can present as a large posterior mediastinal mass. It produces no symptoms and is discovered on imaging. It develops only in those with abnormal bone marrow function and should be particularly considered in patients with thalassemia. A fine-needle aspiration biopsy is pathologically characteristic; resection is not indicated.

Mesenchymal Tumors

Mesenchymal tumors are rare but constitute about 6% of all mediastinal tumors and are generally present in the posterior and superior mediastinum. These include soft tissue tumors (lipomas), hemangiomas, fibrous tissue tumors, smooth muscle tumors, skeletal muscle tumors, osseochondrous tumors. Large lipomas are usually present in the anterior mediastinum. Over half these lesions are malignant. Treatment consists of surgical excision whenever possible.

■ MISCELLANEOUS DISORDERS OF THE MEDIASTINUM

Acute Mediastinitis (Table 7)

Acute mediastinitis carries significant morbidity and mortality. The mediastinum contains loose connective tissue enclosing and connecting organs and structures within. This allows an easy spread of infection within

Table 7: Etiology of acute mediastinitis.

- Postoperative following trans-sternal operative procedures
- Esophageal perforation:
  - Mallory-Weiss syndrome
  - Iatrogenic
  - Tumor or foreign body
- Descending necrotizing mediastinitis
- An upward extension of a subdiaphragmatic infection
- Direct extension of infection from a necrotizing pneumonia
- Penetrating injuries of the chest
- Anthrax mediastinitis

a mediastinal compartment as also spread from one compartment to the other. Acute infection may take the form of diffuse cellulitis or a mediastinal abscess.

Acute mediastinitis is due to the following causes:

- Postoperative following trans-sternal operative procedures—chiefly cardiac procedures.
- Esophageal perforation—a tear with perforation of the esophagus can be due to forceful vomiting (Mallory-Weiss syndrome), a tumor, a foreign body, or due to instrumental procedures such as endoscopy. Attempts at stenting an obstructed segment, or at dilatation of an esophageal stricture or of an achalasia can result in an esophageal tear. It can also occur after variceal sclerosis or following tube placements (Sengstaken-Blakemore tube and very rarely a nasogastric tube).
- A descending infection originating in the oral cavity, pharynx or cervical tissue. This infection can spread by continuity and contiguity along tissue planes, resulting in a necrotizing mediastinitis.
- An upward extension of a subdiaphragmatic infection into the mediastinum chiefly by way of tissue planes connecting the retroperitoneal space with the mediastinum.
- A direct extension of infection from a necrotizing pneumonia into the mediastinum causing a mediastinitis is occasionally observed, particularly in immunocompromised patients.
- Penetrating injuries of the chest close to the midline can also result in acute mediastinitis.
- Anthrax mediastinitis.

Esophageal Perforation

This is the most common cause of acute mediastinitis in medical intensive care units through causes listed above. The Mallory-Weiss syndrome and instrumental procedures are the most common of these causes. Increasing substernal and upper abdominal pain is often associated with tachypnea, tachycardia, dysphagia and shock in severe cases. An important symptom often observed with a large perforation of the distal esophagus is inability of the patient to lie down because of unbearable increase in severity of pain. Increasing tachypnea and desaturation is observed in these patients when they attempt to lie flat. The patient therefore sits leaning forward.

Two radiological criteria are helpful in diagnosis. The first is the presence of a pleural effusion—left-sided when the distal esophagus is involved and right-sided when there is a perforation in the mid- or proximal esophagus. At times a distal esophageal perforation is associated with bilateral pleural effusion. The second radiological sign is the presence of pneumomediastinum. The air in the mediastinum may track up the tissue planes into the neck causing surgical emphysema with a crepitus on palpation. It is advisable never to perform an endoscopy to locate a tear as this can produce further trauma. A water-soluble contrast dye when swallowed generally outlines the tear but may fail to do so if the perforation is small. A CT of the chest is the best modality for diagnosis of a perforated esophagus **(Figs. 26A to C)**.

A bedside differential diagnosis of an esophageal perforation includes a perforated ulcer, acute pancreatitis, aortic dissection, acute myocardial infarction, pulmonary embolism.

Small perforations with normal homeodynamics and absence of sepsis may be treated conservatively with antibiotics, drainage of pleural fluid and with stoppage of all oral feeds. If symptoms worsen or there is increasing sepsis with mediastinitis, surgical repair is advised.

In patients who are severely symptomatic, show evidence of mediastinal sepsis with moderately large pleural effusions or who are hemodynamically unstable, surgery should be prompt. Early surgical management is critical for survival. Patients coming late into critical care after the onset of symptoms following a large tear in the esophagus, have increased morbidity and mortality in spite of surgery. Esophageal stenting may be offered to patients who are too frail or unfit for definitive surgery.

Descending Necrotizing Mediastinitis

A descending necrotizing mediastinitis is a complication of pharyngeal, tonsillar, retropharyngeal or cervical abscess. Infections can be due to beta-hemolytic streptococci, staphylococci, bacteroides or anaerobic streptococci. If these infections spread, are not drained, or remain uncontrolled in spite of treatment, they spread downward along tissue planes into the mediastinum. Clinical features consist of neck swelling and pain, substernal discomfort, dyspnea, fever and inflammation of the oropharynx. Over half the patients have comorbidities associated with immunosuppression. A CT scan best demonstrates spread of infection from the neck to the mediastinum. If uncontrolled, severe sepsis, multiorgan failure and death result.

The principles of management are:
- A broad-spectrum antibiotic cover against gram-positive, gram-negative and anaerobic organisms.
- Surgical drainage of the primary source—generally a cervical or retropharyngeal or odontogenic abscess. A review CT of the chest may help to decide whether

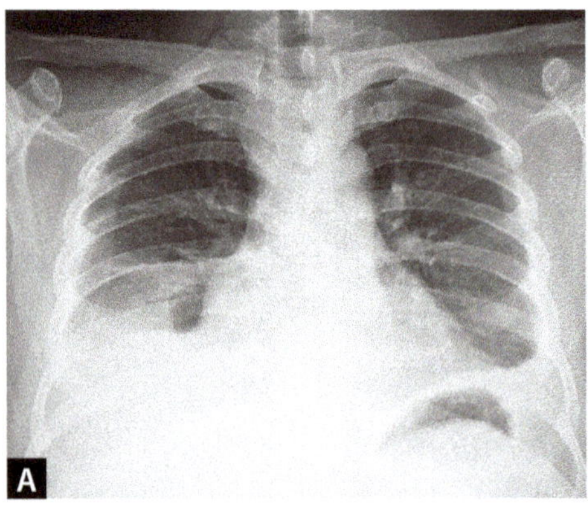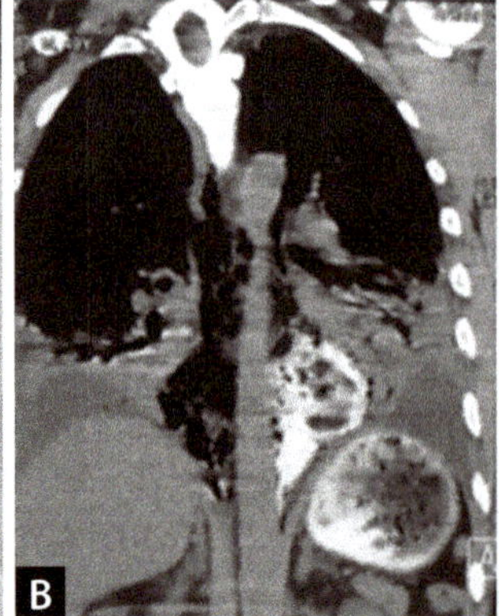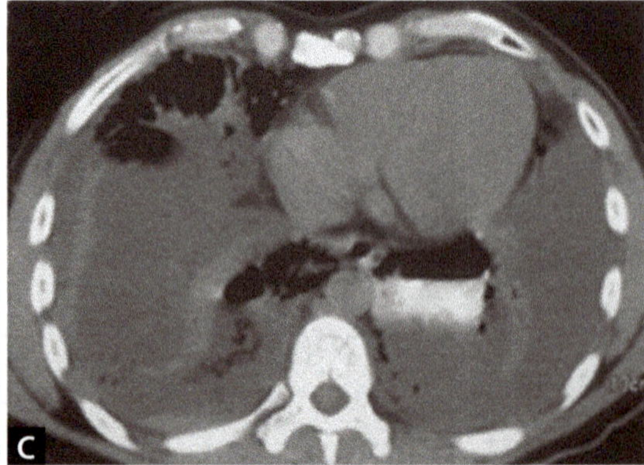

Figs. 26A to C: Young man with a bad esophageal tear (Mallory-Weiss syndrome) due to forceful vomiting. (A) Chest X-ray reveals bilateral pleural effusion. Pleural fluid aspiration revealed a markedly elevated amylase; (B and C) Coronal and axial CT shows a leak from the esophagus, pleural effusion, mediastinal and surgical emphysema. Total esophagectomy was necessary as two attempts at repair of the esophagus were unsuccessful.

more extensive drainage of the mediastinum is necessary. A localized mediastinal abscess must need be drained. Surgical expertise from a thoracic and/or a cardiothoracic surgeon is vital for survival.

- A tracheostomy becomes necessary only if there is a great deal of cervical inflammatory edema that compromises the airway. A tracheostomy can however be treacherous even after the airway is secured as it further opens tissue planes in the neck that communicate with mediastinal tissue planes and thereby can perhaps worsen the mediastinitis.

The prognosis is grim in severe necrotizing mediastinitis which has a mortality of close to 50%. Death occurs from increasing sepsis with multiorgan failure, or from erosion of large vessels causing exsanguinating bleeds. Early diagnosis and prompt medical and surgical treatment are critical for survival.

Direct Extension from the Retroperitoneal Space

Mediastinitis can occur from a spread of infection along the retroperitoneal space in patients with suppurative, necrotizing pancreatitis. Pancreatic pseudocysts can extend into the mediastinum. Pleural effusion and occasionally pericardial effusion with high amylase content are noted. A pseudocyst should be drained into the stomach at the appropriate point in the natural history of pancreatitis.

Mediastinitis Following Sternotomy

Infection of the sternum is occasionally seen as a postoperative complication after surgery. Such infections heal poorly because of the poor vascularity in this area and are invariably associated with a varying degree of anterior compartment mediastinitis. When healing does not occur, surgeons prefer to do a wide sternal excision of dead or infected tissue, closing the dead space with transposed gastrocolic omentum. This is a vascular viable graft that promotes healing.

Anthrax Mediastinitis

At one time anthrax was endemic in South India. It is rare today but may well return in the West and other parts of the world following the advent of bioterrorism. Anthrax spores when inhaled gain entry into the lungs and from there are transported to the regional lymph nodes. There ensues a necrotizing hemorrhagic mediastinitis with death within a few days. Ciprofloxacin, doxycycline, plus other antibiotics effective against the anthrax bacillus should be promptly used.

Fibrosing Mediastinitis

This is a rare disease characterized by the proliferation of dense fibrous tissue within the mediastinum. The extensive fibrosis compresses and strangles vital structures within the mediastinum. In most cases, the etiology is unknown. The two known infective causes are: (1) tuberculosis and (2) histoplasmosis.

Out of the six cases encountered by our unit one was proven to be due to *Histoplasma capsulatum* (in an Indian patient living in the United States but visiting India). The rest were of unknown etiology. It is postulated that fibrosing mediastinitis results from a delayed hypersensitivity reaction to fungal, mycobacterial or other antigens. This remains a postulate. The disease has been however reported in association with autoimmune disorders and has been reported following the use of the antimigraine drug methysergide. Mediastinal fibrosis may be associated with retroperitoneal fibrosis. Either one could precede the other.

Pathologically, dense fibrosis is seen to compress the trachea, bronchi, the veins in the superior mediastinum, the hila, extending into the vessels (in particular the pulmonary vessels) and even infiltrating into the lungs.

Clinical Compression Syndromes

These depend on the site of the mediastinal fibrosis. Mediastinal fibrosis predominating in the superior mediastinum causes the *superior vena caval syndrome*. Though malignancy or large mediastinal tumors are the most important cause of this syndrome, fibrosing mediastinitis though infrequent, should be kept in mind as an important cause of this syndrome. Patients complain of puffiness of face and eyes with edema of the neck and upper arms. Headache and visual disturbances are also observed. Symptoms worsen on bending or stooping to pick up an object. Clinical examination reveals a puffy plethoric face, puffy eyes; edema may extend into the upper arms. Collaterals are observed over the upper chest and arms. The jugular veins are nonpulsatile and engorged—in severe cases, right up to the angle of the jaw even in the sitting posture. Contrast CT or venography not only proves the diagnosis but also demonstrates the site and extent of blockage of contrast within the SVC. It also helps to exclude pressure from a neoplasm as the cause of the superior vena caval syndrome.

In symptomatic patients, stenting of the stenosed SVC may afford relief. Surgical bypass is offered to patients who have severe symptoms. It is done by connecting the unobstructed brachiocephalic vein to the right atrial appendage either through a saphenous vein graft or a prosthetic graft.

Hilar compression: At times mediastinal fibrosis starts or remains confined to the hilar areas causing compression of one or more bronchi with resultant atelectasis or pressure on branches of the pulmonary vessels. When unilateral, the appearance is that of a large hilar mass indistinguishable from a neoplasm. In fact, it is often misdiagnosed as a bronchogenic carcinoma. A thoracoscopic or an open-lung biopsy is often necessary for a definite diagnosis. Localized unilateral hilar fibrosis can compress the pulmonary arterial branch to the ipsilateral lung leading to an oligemic lung with diminished vascular markings.

Compression within the Middle and Posterior Mediastinal Compartment

- Increasing fibrosis could involve the tracheobronchial tree and lead to dyspnea, wheezing, cough and compression atelectasis of a lobe. Bronchoplastic procedures or the placement of stents into the trachea and/or main bronchi may keep the large airways patent.
- Mediastinal fibrosis around the pulmonary artery could lead to pulmonary hypertension, signs of right heart failure. If the fibrosis involves the pulmonary veins, the clinical picture resembles mitral stenosis or veno-occlusive disease, with cough, dyspnea and attacks of pulmonary edema. Constriction of the pulmonary veins at times produces a continuous murmur over the precordium, often also heard over the back. Constricted pulmonary veins could sharply reduce venous return to the left heart, the patient presents with fatigue, dyspnea and angina on effort.
- Mediastinal fibrosis starting or restricted to the posterior mediastinum constricts the esophagus chiefly in the middle third. The fibrosis generally also

involves the carina with compression of the main bronchi.

The diagnosis of mediastinal fibrosis is evident on an HRCT of the chest. It is even better visualized with an MRI **(Figs. 27A to D)**. A histopathological diagnosis through a biopsy is advised as far as possible. The tissue should be stained for possible tubercular and fungal infections and should also be cultured.

We have found corticosteroids useful in two patients. There was significant regression of fibrosis on imaging and marked relief of symptoms. The use of azathioprine, methotrexate and cyclophosphamide has also been advocated; these drugs are however of unproven efficacy.

Pneumomediastinum

The most common cause of pneumomediastinum is barotrauma causing alveolar rupture in patients on ventilator support. Spontaneous pneumomediastinum can also be due to rupture of alveoli because of increased intrathoracic volume and pressure in asthma or following trauma. Straining against a closed glottis as in vomiting, coughing or exercising can also lead to alveolar rupture. Obstruction to a large airway as with a foreign body or tumor can also increase alveolar volume and pressure leading to rupture. Pneumomediastinum has resulted from alveolar rupture during an epileptic fit. Following alveolar rupture, air dissects along the peribronchoalveolar tissue planes into the mediastinum and then frequently ascends upward into the tissue planes of the neck. Air from alveolar rupture could also move toward the parietal pleura, break through it and cause pneumothorax. High peak airway pressures, significant autopositive end-expiratory pressure (PEEP) and "clashing with the machine" are predisposing factors. A pneumomediastinum under the above circumstances may well be associated with a tension pneumothorax which dominates the clinical picture.

Pneumomediastinum if not severe may be asymptomatic being discovered as translucent air streaks along the cardiac borders. If marked, it causes substernal pain which may be also felt in the neck or the back. Dyspnea, dysphagia and dysphonia may present singly or in combination. Examination often reveals subcutaneous emphysema in the neck. Auscultation reveals a crunching clicking sound heard in systole and diastole (Hamman's

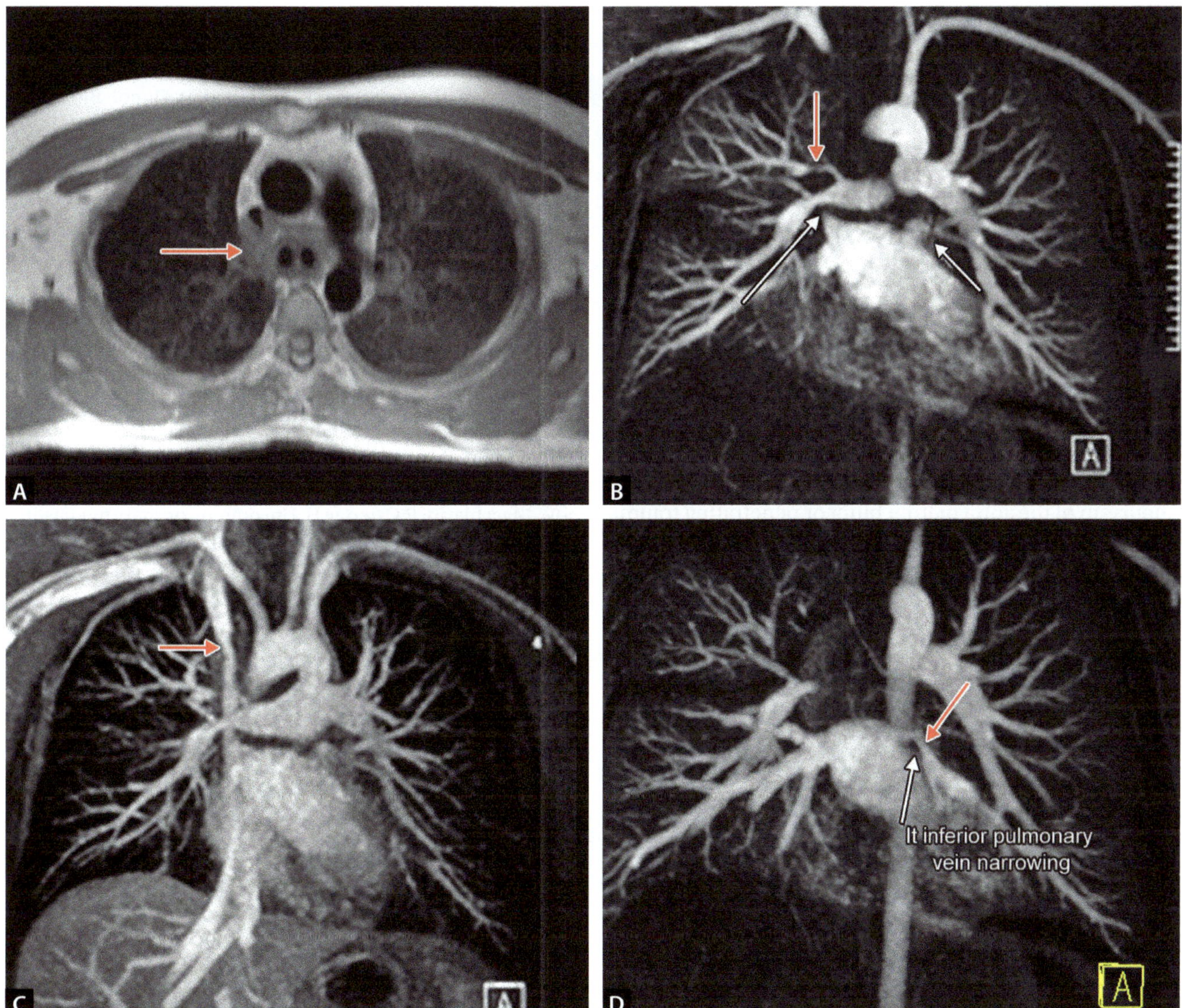

Figs. 27A to D: Mediastinal fibrosis. A 21-year-old man with dyspnea on exertion and marked angina on exertion. Clinical examination revealed a soft continuous murmur over the bases of the lung, also heard over the back. (A) Axial MRI demonstrated soft tissue encircling carina and extending to posterior surface of SVC; (B to D) MR angiography revealed a long segment narrowing of the SVC, as well as focal narrowing of right and left superior pulmonary veins. His coronary angiography was normal, the angina was due to a severe diminishment of blood flow to the left heart due to a tight constriction of pulmonary veins leading to markedly reduced cardiac output with decreased coronary flow. After treatment with steroids, the soft tissue as well as vascular compression were significantly reduced.

sign). Nonspecific ST-T changes may be present leading to a wrong diagnosis of myocardial infarction.

An X-ray chest reveals a translucent air streak most often along the left heart border and the left border of the mediastinum. CT defines the air with more clarity. There is often imaging evidence of air in the subcutaneous tissue of the neck and chest.

Treatment: When pneumomediastinitis results during mechanical ventilator support, it is important to reduce tidal volume thereby reducing both peak and pause pressure. An associated pneumothorax needs an intercostal drain. It is important to insert an intercostal drain even if the pneumothorax is shallow as the propensity for the patient to develop a sudden tension pneumothorax is significantly high. Some physicians prefer to insert intercostal drains in both pleural spaces prophylactically (even in the absence of pneumothorax) in patients who develop pneumomediastinum.

Treatment of spontaneous pneumomediastinum with surgical emphysema is directed at pain relief and at treating the cause. Oxygen may be administered in dyspneic patients. Needle aspiration or skin incisions to relieve subcutaneous emphysema are almost never necessary. Air is fairly quickly absorbed over a period of a few days.

Mediastinal Hemorrhage

Hemorrhage into the mediastinum can occur following rupture of an aneurysm, rupture or leak from a dissecting aneurysm of the aorta or from blunt or penetrating trauma or following invasive medical procedures. Spontaneous mediastinal hemorrhage has been reported but is indeed very rare.

Severe blood loss can cause hypovolemic shock. Dyspnea, chest pain and desaturation are observed. A CT chest will reveal a dissecting aneurysm if this is the cause of the bleed, or a hyperdense area within the mediastinum or in the area of partial tear of the aortic wall (following blunt trauma as in a car crash). It could also reveal extravasated blood in the mediastinum, pericardium or pleura. Treatment is surgical and depends on the cause and site of the bleed.

■ SUGGESTED READING

1. Aquino SL, Duncan G, Taber KH, et al. Reconciliation of the anatomical, surgical, and radiographic classification of the mediastinum. J Comp Assist Tomogr. 2001;25:489-92.
2. Aroor AR, Prakasha SR, Seshadri S, et al. A study of clinical characteristics of mediastinal mass. J Clin Diagn Res. 2014;8(2):77-80.
3. Casey EM, Kiel PJ, Loehrer PJ Sr. Clinical management of thymoma patients. Hematol Oncol Clin North Am. 2008;22(3):457-73.
4. Duwe BV, Sterman DH, Musani AI. Tumors of the mediastinum. Chest. 2005;128(4):2893-909.
5. Eng TY, Fuller CD, Tagirdar T, et al. Thymic carcinoma: state of the art review. Int J Radiat Oncol Biol Phys. 2004;59:654-64.
6. Falkson CB, Bezjak A, Darling G, et al. The management of thymoma: a systematic review and practice guideline. J Thorac Oncol. 2009;4:911-9.
7. Holty JE, Kim RY, Bravata DM. Anthrax: a systematic review of atypical presentations. Ann Emerg Med. 2006;48(2):200-11.
8. Kawahara K, Miyawaki M, Anami K, et al. A patient with mediastinal mature teratoma presenting with paraneoplastic limbic encephalitis. J Thorac Oncol. 2012;7:258-9.
9. Limaiem F, Ayadi-Kaddour A, Djilani H, et al. Pulmonary and mediastinal bronchogenic cysts: a clinicopathologic study of 33 cases. Lung. 2008;186(1):55-61.
10. Macchiarini P, Ostertag H. Uncommon primary mediastinal tumours. Lancet Oncol. 2004;5(2):107-18.
11. Reeder LB. Neurogenic tumors of the mediastinum. Semin Thorac Cardiovasc Surg. 2000;12(4):261-7.
12. Stover DG, Eisenberg R, Johnson DH. Anti-N-methyl-D-aspartate receptor encephalitis in a young woman with a mature mediastinal teratoma. J Thorac Oncol. 2010;5:1872-3.
13. Strollo DC, Rosado de Christenson ML. Primary mediastinal malignant germ cell neoplasms: imaging features. Chest Surg Clin North Am. 2002;12:645-58.
14. Strollo DC, Rosado de Christenson ML, Jett JR. Primary mediastinal tumors. Part I. tumors of the anterior mediastinum. Chest. 1997;112:511-58.
15. Strollo DC, Rosado de Christenson ML, Jett JR. Primary mediastinal tumors. Part II. tumors of the middle and posterior mediastinum. Chest. 1997;112:1344-57.
16. Takeda S, Miyoshi S, Ohta M, et al. Primary germ cell tumors in the mediastinum: a 50-year experience at a single Japanese institution. Cancer. 2003;97(2):367-76.
17. Tormoehlen LM, Pascuzzi RM. Thymoma, myasthenia gravis, and other paraneoplastic syndromes. Hematol Oncol Clin North Am. 2008;22(3):509-26.
18. Whooley BP, Urschel JD, Antkowiak JG, et al. Primary tumors of the mediastinum. J Surg Oncol. 1999;70(2): 95-9.

Occupational and Environmental Lung Diseases

CHAPTER 66

Common Occupational Lung Diseases

■ INTRODUCTION

Occupational lung disease is any of a group of unusual problems in the lungs caused by breathing dusts, fumes, gases, or vapors in a place where a patient works.

Many types of work are associated with health hazards. Very few places in either industry or agriculture are completely free from gases, vapors, mists, fumes or dust and hence a great number of workers are exposed to air contaminants. As a major portal to the environment, the lung often bears the brunt of these toxic exposures.

Occupations especially at risk are: coal miners, farmers, asbestos workers, workers with epoxy resins or isocyanates. Other jobs associated with an increased risk of occupational lung disease include: construction, carpentry, baking, soldering, laboratory work, hairdressing, bird breeding, drug manufacture, processing textiles, forestry, horticulture, and metal-working.

The physical properties of inhaled substances predict the site of deposition; irritants will produce symptoms at these sites. Large particles (10–20 µm) deposit in the nose and upper airways, smaller particles (5–10 µm) deposit in the trachea and bronchi, and particles less than 5 µm in size may reach the alveoli. Particles less than 0.5 µm are so small they behave like gases. Toxic gases deposit according to their solubility. A water-soluble gas will be adsorbed by the moist mucosa of the upper airway; less soluble gases will deposit more randomly throughout the respiratory tract.

Many host and environmental factors serve to modify the effects of inhaled chemicals, and the ultimate response is the result of their interaction. The main host factors are:

- Age—older people with chronically reduced cardiovascular and respiratory function
- Poor health status
- Poor nutritional status
- Immunological status
- Sex and other genetic factors, for example, enzyme-related differences in biotransformation mechanisms
- Psychological state, for example, stress, and anxiety
- Smoking—cigarette smoking may affect normal defenses or may potentiate the effect of other chemicals.

■ OCCUPATIONAL LUNG DISEASES— BURDEN IN INDIA

The prevalence of occupational lung diseases in developed countries is not high and deaths due to such exposure are low when compared to developing countries.

The common occupational lung diseases in India include silicosis, asbestosis, byssinosis, bagassosis, and coal workers' pneumoconiosis (CWP). Extrinsic allergic alveolitis and occupational asthma (OA) have been less well documented, and probably missed on account of lack of diagnostic facilities.

Silicosis in the unorganized sector has been reported to be as high as 25% among stone cutters, 22% in quarry workers, 16.7% in glass workers, 15.1% in ceramic workers, 27.2% in non-mechanized foundry workers, 28.7% in agate grinders, and 54.6% in slate pencil workers. In studies conducted in Ahmedabad, Mumbai, and Delhi the prevalence of byssinosis among textile workers was estimated at 7–8%.

The National program for control and treatment of occupational diseases (National Institute of Health and Family Welfare, Government of India) estimates the following prevalence of occupational lung diseases in India **(Table 1)**.

Table 1: Prevalence of occupational lung diseases in India.

Occupational lung disease	Prevalence
Silicosis in mica miners	6.2–34%
Silicosis in manganese miners	4.1%
Silicosis in slate pencil workers	54.6%
Silicosis in lead and zinc miners	30.4%
Asbestosis	3% of miners and 21% in mill workers
Byssinosis	28–47%

Source: http://inihfw.nic.in/ndc-nihfw/html/Programmes/National Programme For Control Treatment.htm.

■ CLASSIFICATION OF OCCUPATIONAL LUNG DISEASES (TABLE 2)

Occupational lung diseases can be classified according to exposure to various agents.

Occupational lung diseases also depend on the toxicity potential of various compounds. Agents which are capable of causing lung toxicity after low to moderate exposure include the following as given in **Tables 3 and 4**.

■ DIAGNOSIS OF AN OCCUPATIONAL LUNG DISORDER

The diagnosis of occupational lung disorders is usually based on a proven history of exposure to known agents, clinical evaluation as well as specific tests including lung function tests, chest X-ray and computerized tomography (CT).

An investigation which can be done on-site with appropriate training is to conduct the lung function tests which can be carried out to determine the condition of the lungs. The resultant spirogram can be analyzed to determine if the pulmonary functions have been compromised due to exposure to various substances at the workplace. The normal subdivisions of lung functions are depicted in **Figure 1**.

Lung function testing is an accepted way of diagnosing various conditions depending on the following parameters. The common deviations observed in occupational lung diseases include either a restrictive or an obstructive airway defect, or in many cases a combination of a restrictive cum obstructive defect depending on the type of exposure.

Although silicosis and CWP are becoming less common, hypersensitivity pneumonitis is increasingly

Table 2: Classification of occupational lung diseases.

General agent	Examples	Disorder
Mineral dusts	Asbestos Silica Coal	Pneumoconiosis
Metal dusts	Iron Tin Barium Vanadium Cadmium Nickel Chromic salts Platinum salts Cobalt Beryllium	"Inert dust" pneumoconiosis "Inert dust" pneumoconiosis "Inert dust" pneumoconiosis Irritant bronchitis Bronchitis, pneumoconiosis Asthma Asthma Asthma Asthma, giant cell pneumonitis Granulomatous pneumonitis
Biological dusts	Spores Mycelia Bird droppings	Hypersensitivity pneumonitis
Toxic fumes	NO_2 SO_2 Chlorine Ammonia	Airways inflammation, ARDS ARDS, bronchiolitis obliterans Airways inflammation Airways inflammation
High molecular weight (asthmatic agent)	Flour Dander	Asthma Asthma
Low molecular weight (asthmatic agent)	Isocyanates Epoxy resins	Biphasic asthma Asthma
Infections	Viral Bacterial Fungal	Specific infection Specific infection Specific infection
Carcinogens	Asbestos Arsenic Chromium Coke oven Fumes Nickel Halo ethers Radon prodigy	Lung cancer and mesothelioma Lung cancer—copper smelting Lung cancer—smelting process Lung cancer—steel making Lung cancer—smelting processing Lung cancer—engineered out the process Lung cancer—uranium mining

Source: Repoduced with permission from Dr Gary R Epler. Environmental and Occupational Lung Disease. http://www.epler.com/occu_tab.html#1.

recognized as an occupational lung disease with new antigens being introduced annually.

Imaging, particularly high-resolution CT (HRCT), is central to the management of occupational lung disease and is useful in diagnosis, assessment of disease activity, and evaluating response to therapy.

Table 3: Interpretations of various conditions depending on the mentioned parameters.

Condition	FEV$_1$	FVC	FEV$_1$/FVC	Interpretation
Silicosis, coal workers' pneumoconiosis, asbestosis, extrinsic allergic alveolitis (Farmer's lung, bagassosis, bird-handler's lung), beryllium disease	↓	↓	Normal/reduced	Restrictive or obstructive airways defect or a combination of both
Byssinosis, exposure to diisocyanates, COPD (asthma, chronic bronchitis, emphysema)	↓	↓	↓	Obstructive airway defect

Other important diagnostic tools include bronchoalveolar lavage (BAL). A predominance of lymphocytes could point to certain conditions like hypersensitivity pneumonia or beryllium disease. Characteristic multinucleated giant cells may be seen in those exposed to heavy metals. Transbronchial lung biopsies may also help in arriving at the diagnosis of the condition.

Figures 2 to 5 depict the histopathology of a few occupational lung diseases.

■ DIFFERENTIAL DIAGNOSIS

Exposure to silica and coal mine dusts may result in pulmonary scarring, with a ventilatory pattern that mimics

Table 4: Various agents causing lung toxicity.

Compound	Source of exposure	Toxicity
Arcolein	Plastics, textiles, pharmaceutical manufacturing, combustion products	Diffuse airways and parenchymal injury
Antimony trichloride; antimony pentachloride	Alloys, organic catalysts	Pneumonitis, noncardiogenic pulmonary edema
Cadmium	Alloys with zinc and lead, electroplating, batteries, insecticides	Tracheobronchitis, pulmonary edema (often delayed onset over 24–48 hours), kidney damage: tubule proteinuria
Chloropicrin	Chemical manufacturing, fumigant components	Upper and lower airways inflammation
Chlorine	Bleaching, formation of chlorinated compounds, household cleaners	Upper and lower airway inflammation, pneumonitis and noncardiogenic pulmonary edema
Hydrogen sulfide	Natural gas wells, mines, manure	Ocular, upper and lower airway irritation, delayed pulmonary edema, asphyxiation from systemic tissue hypoxia
Lithium hydride	Alloys, ceramics, electronics, chemical catalysts	Pneumonitis, noncardiogenic pulmonary edema
Methyl isocyanate	Pesticide synthesis	Upper and lower respiratory tract irritation, pulmonary edema
Mercury	Electrolysis, ore and amalgam extraction, electronics manufacture	Ocular and respiratory tract inflammation, pneumonitis, CNS, kidney, and systemic effects
Nickel carbonyl	Nickel refining, electroplating, chemical reagents	Lower respiratory irritation, pneumonitis, delayed systemic toxic effects
Nitrogen dioxide	Silos after new grain storage, fertilizer making, arc welding; combustion products	Ocular and upper airway inflammation, noncardiogenic pulmonary edema, delayed onset bronchiolitis
Nitrogen mustards, sulfur mustards	Military agents, vesicants	Ocular and respiratory tract inflammation, pneumonitis
Paraquat	Herbicides (ingested)	Selective damage to type-2 pneumocytes leading to RADS, pulmonary fibrosis; renal failure, GI irritation
Phosgene	Pesticide and other chemical manufacture, arc welding, paint removal	Upper airway inflammation and pneumonitis; delayed pulmonary edema
Zinc chloride	Smoke grenades, artillery	Upper and lower airway irritation, fever, delayed onset pneumonitis

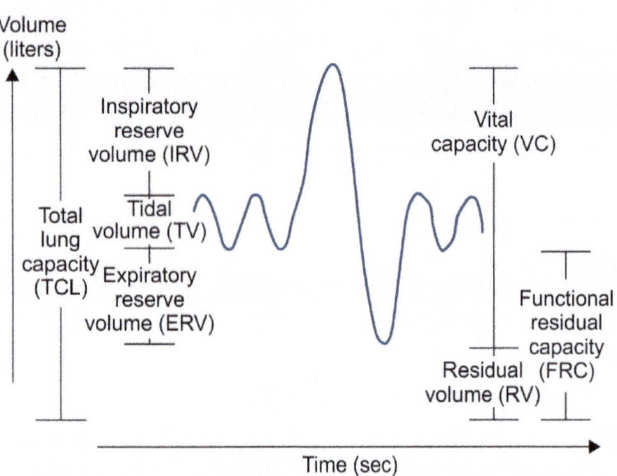

Fig. 1: Spirogram labeled to show the subdivisions of the total lung capacity inflammation.
Source: Ulf Ulfvarsoa and Monica Dahlqvist. Lung function examination in Encylopedia of occupational health and safety. Fig. 10.10 page 10.10. 4th edition. Geneva: International Labour Office; 1998.

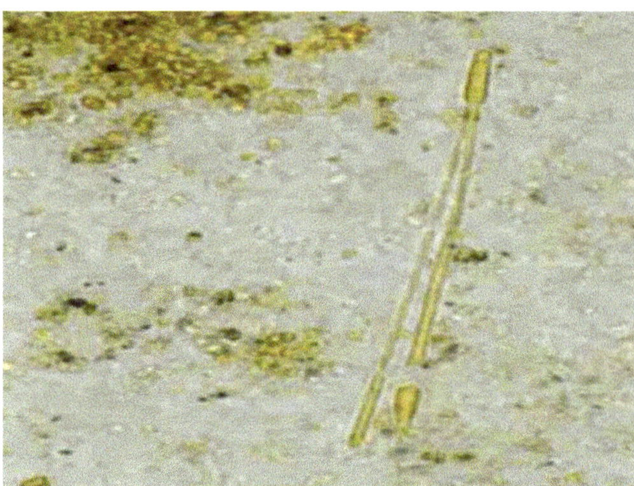

Fig. 3: Asbestosis. Asbestos fibers (seen as parallel vertical yellowish streaks) inhaled deep into the lung parenchyma induce diffuse alveolar and interstitial fibrosis. Fibrosis is first evident in the respiratory bronchioles and this progresses to involve the alveolar walls. The subpleural portions of the lower lobes are first involved.

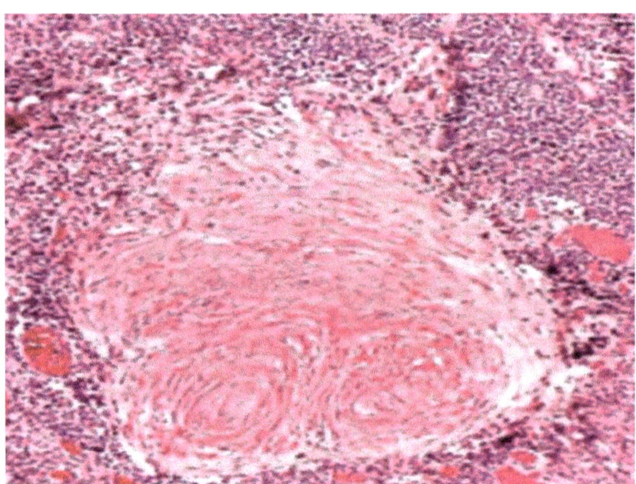

Fig. 2: Silicosis. The lesion is characterized by a cell-free central area of concentrically arranged, whirled collagen fibers, surrounded by cellular connective tissue with reticular fibers.

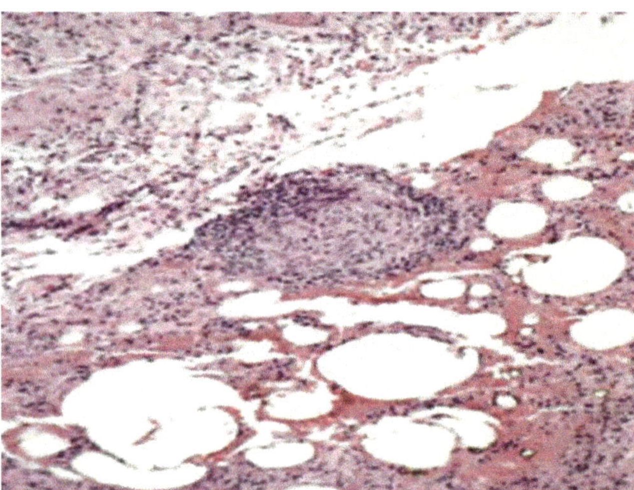

Fig. 4: Chronic beryllium disease. The histopathology of the lung is indistinguishable from that observed in sarcoidosis. Non-caseating granulomas are observed (in the center) together with some degree of fibrosis.

idiopathic pulmonary fibrosis. Clinical features may at times be indistinguishable from chronic obstructive pulmonary disease (COPD). Coal mine and silica dust may therefore result in restrictive, obstructive, or mixed patterns of impairment on pulmonary function testing.

■ COMMON OCCUPATIONAL LUNG DISEASES PNEUMOCONIOSIS

The International Labour Organization (ILO) has defined pneumoconiosis as "the accumulation of dust in the lungs and the tissue reactions to its presence". For the purpose of this definition, "dust" is meant to be an aerosol composed of solid inanimate particles.

Primary pneumoconiosis includes silicosis, CWP, and asbestosis. They are caused by inhalation of silica dust, coal mine dust and asbestos fibers. Other forms of pneumoconiosis caused by inhalation of dusts containing aluminum, antimony, barium, graphite, iron, kaolin, mica, talc, among other dusts are encountered by the physician infrequently.

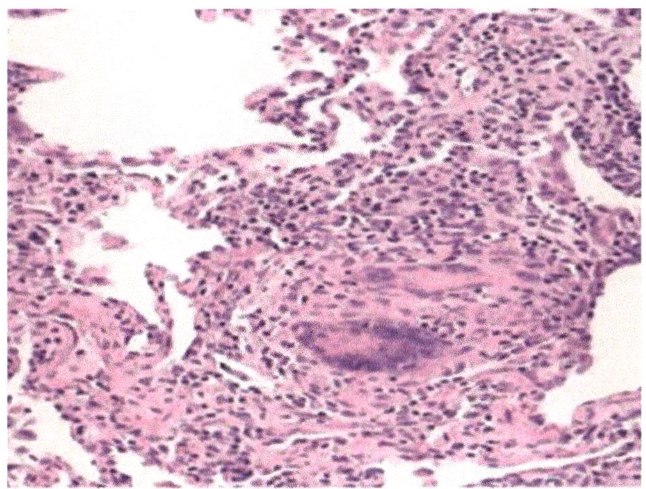

Fig. 5: Hypersensitivity pneumonitis. The presence of non-caseating granulomas with giant cells, together with alveolitis, lymphocytic infiltration of bronchial walls and laying down of fibrous tissue is observed.

Byssinosis is another pulmonary disease caused by exposure to cotton dust and is sometimes included under pneumoconiosis, although its pattern of lung abnormality is different.

Etiopathogenesis of Pneumoconiosis

Studies have shown four basic mechanisms in the etiology of CWP and silicosis: (1) Direct cytotoxicity of coal dust or silica, resulting in lung cell damage, release of lipases and proteases, and eventual lung scarring; (2) Activation of oxidant production by pulmonary phagocytes, which overwhelms the antioxidant defenses and leads to lipid peroxidation, protein nitrosation, cell injury, and lung scarring; (3) Activation of mediator release from alveolar macrophages and epithelial cells, which leads to recruitment of polymorphonuclear leukocytes and macrophages, resulting in the production of proinflammatory cytokines and reactive species and further lung injury and scarring; (4) Secretion of growth factors from alveolar macrophages and epithelial cells, stimulating fibroblast proliferation and eventual scarring. Results of in vitro and animal studies provide a basis for proposing these mechanisms for the initiation and progression of pneumoconiosis. Data obtained from exposed workers lend support to these mechanisms.

The exposure regimen seems to determine the time course of events. There is some indication that sufficiently low exposure regimens can, in most cases, limit the lung reaction to nonprogressive lesions with no disability or impairment.

Typically, these three diseases [(1) CWP, (2) silicosis, and (3) asbestosis] take many years to develop and manifest, although in some cases, in silicosis, particularly, rapidly progressive forms can occur after only short periods of intense exposure. When severe, the diseases often lead to lung impairment, disability, and premature death.

Clinical Manifestations and Diagnosis

Pneumoconiosis may be asymptomatic with only radiological abnormalities. Symptoms when they appear include cough (with or without expectoration), wheezing and shortness of breath, especially during exertion.

If pneumoconiosis causes severe lung fibrosis, breathing can become extremely difficult. Very advanced disease is associated with respiratory failure and right ventricular hypertrophy with congestive heart failure (cor pulmonale).

Pneumoconiosis is typically detected in individuals through the use of radiological imaging. Traditionally, this has been the chest X-ray, taken on film, but now increasingly being acquired through digital computer technology. The ILO provides guidelines for the systematic scientific classification of radiographs of pneumoconiosis.

A simplified format of the ILO classification of chest radiographs is given in **Table 5**.

Medical surveillance and screening have always been part of the strategies for the prevention of pneumoconiosis. In this context, the possibility of detecting some early lesions is advantageous.

Increased knowledge of pathogenesis paved the way for the development of several biomarkers and for the refinement and use of "nonclassical" pulmonary investigation techniques such as the measurement of the clearance rate of deposited 99 technetium diethylenetriamine-pentaacetate (99 Tc-DTPA) to assess pulmonary epithelial integrity, and quantitative gallium-67 lung scan to assess inflammatory activity.

Several biomarkers were considered in the field of pneumoconiosis: sputum macrophages, serum growth factors, serum type III procollagen peptide, red blood cell antioxidants, fibronectin, leukocyte elastase, neutral metalloendopeptidase and elastin peptides in plasma, volatile hydrocarbons in exhaled air, and tumor necrosis factor (TNF) release by peripheral blood monocytes. Biomarkers are conceptually quite interesting, but

Table 5: Chest radiograph classification format as per International Labour Organization (ILO) classification.

Film quality	Grade 1–4			
	Comment made (y/n)			
Small opacities	Profusion	R	L	
	Shape and size			
Large opacities	Presence (y/n)			
	Size (A, B, C)			
Pleural thickening Chest wall Circumscribed presence (y/n)		R	L	
	Face on (y/n)			
	Width (a, b, c)			
	Extent (1, 2, 3)			
Pleural thickening Chest wall diffuse Circumscribed presence (y/n)		R	L	
	Face on (y/n)			
	Width (a, b, c)			
	Extent (1, 2, 3)			
Pleural thickening (diaphragm)	Presence (y/n)			
	R	L		
Costophrenic angle obliteration	Presence (y/n)			
	R	L		
Pleural calcification	Presence (y/n)			
Chest wall Diaphragm Other Extent (1, 2, 3)	R	L		
Symbols	Used (Y/N)			
Comments	Made (Y/N)			

many more studies are necessary to assess their precise significance. This validation effort will be quite demanding, since it will require investigators to conduct prospective epidemiological studies. Such an effort was carried out recently for TNF release by peripheral blood monocytes in CWP. TNF was found to be an interesting marker of CWP progression. Besides the scientific aspects of the significance of biomarkers in the pathogenesis of pneumoconiosis, other issues related to the use of biomarkers must be examined carefully, namely, opportunities for prevention, impact on occupational medicine and ethical and legal problems.

The impact of newer understanding of the cascade of events in the pathogenesis of pneumoconiosis has not modified the traditional approach to workers' surveillance, but has significantly helped physicians in their capacity to recognize the disease (pneumoconiosis) early, at a time when the disease has had only a limited impact on lung function. It is indeed workers in the early stage of disease who should be recognized and withdrawn from further significant exposure if prevention of disability is to be achieved by medical surveillance.

■ SILICOSIS

Silicosis is the most common and one of the most serious occupational diseases. It is an irreversible fibrosis of the lungs caused by inhalation, retention and pulmonary reaction to free silica dust. It is estimated that about 3 million people working in various types of mines, ceramics, potteries, foundries, metal grinding, stone crushing, agate grinding, slate pencil industry, etc. are occupationally exposed to free silica dust and are at potential risk of developing silicosis. Silica exposure also predisposes to development of pulmonary tuberculosis, which is an important public health problem in India.

In India, a prevalence of 55% was found in one group of workers, many of them very young, engaged in the quarrying of shale sedimentary rock and subsequent work in small, poorly ventilated sheds. Studies on silicotic pencil workers in central India demonstrated high mortality rates; the mean age at death was 35 years and the mean duration of the exposure was 12 years.

Occupational exposure to silica particles of respirable size (aerodynamic diameter of 0.5–5 µm) is associated with mining, quarrying, drilling, tunneling and abrasive blasting with quartz-containing materials (sandblasting). Silica exposure also poses a hazard to stonecutters, and pottery, foundry, ground silica and refractory workers. The true prevalence of the disease is unclear.

Forms of Silica and Mechanism of Toxicity

Silica (silicon dioxide) exists in two forms— (1) crystalline and (2) amorphous. The amorphous form when inhaled is relatively nontoxic. Crystalline silica (quartz, cristobalite, and tridymite) when inhaled leads to a variety of pulmonary diseases. Quartz is the most common type of crystalline silica and is present in rock, granite, slate, and sandstone. Granite contains about 30% free silica, slate about 40% and sandstone is almost pure silica. Cristobalite and tridymite are formed when quartz or amorphous silica are subjected to high temperatures.

The toxicity of silica is related to its interaction with aqueous media to form free oxygen radicals and to injure target cells within the lung parenchyma, such as the alveolar macrophages. This leads to the production and liberation of inflammatory cytokines such as interleukast and TNF-β by the target cells. The end-result is the production of areas of inflammation and necrosis within the lung parenchyma. Free silica is unbound to other minerals. Silicates are compounds in which silica is bound to other minerals. Silicates commonly used in industry are asbestos (hydrated magnesium trisilicate) talc and kaolinite, a major component of kaolin.

Pathology

The pathologic hallmark of the chronic form is the silicotic nodule. The lesion is characterized by a cell-free central area of concentrically arranged, whorled hyalinized collagen fibers, surrounded by cellular connective tissue with reticulin fibers (*see* **Fig. 2**).

The susceptibility of silicotic workers to infections, such as tuberculosis and *Nocardia asteroides*, is likely related to the toxic effect of silica on pulmonary macrophages. Active tuberculosis in silicotic workers may exceed 20% when community prevalence of tuberculosis is high. Again, people with acute silicosis appear to be at a considerable higher risk.

Clinical Manifestations and Diagnosis

Acute silicosis can occur within a few weeks to 2 years after massive exposures to dust in unregulated environments.

It is characterized by severe dyspnea, hypoxemia, weight loss, cough, fever, and pleuritic pain.

These symptoms may precede radiological findings which initially show features identical to simple silicosis, but which progress in quick time (2–5 years) to progressive massive fibrosis (PMF). Clinical examination often reveals crackles on auscultation.

Chest X-ray: In acute silicosis the chest radiograph shows diffuse ground glass opacities in the lower zones. These progress over time to large coalescent opacities in both lungs involving chiefly the lower and midzones. These "mass like" opacities though bilateral are not necessarily symmetrical.

HRCT chest: High-resolution CT of the chest reveals numerous bilateral centrilobular nodular opacities, ground glass opacities and areas of consolidation. These appearances may be similar to the appearances in some patients with alveolar proteinosis. However, the crazy pavement appearance on imaging so frequently seen in the latter is not observed in acute silicosis.

Bronchoalveolar lavage: Bronchoalveolar lavage fluid in acute silicosis has a thick milky appearance, similar to that observed in alveolar proteinosis. On cytology, the macrophages in the BAL are foamy and the lipoproteinaceous material stains strongly positive with periodic acid-Schiff (PAS) reagent. If BAL shows milky lipoproteinaceous fluid one must rule out by history and investigation other conditions known to cause alveolar proteinosis.

BAL studies are generally done to exclude alveolar hemorrhage, eosinophilic pneumonia and infections—the three important conditions which enter into the differential diagnosis of acute silicosis.

1. *Histopathology*: The histopathology is different from chronic silicosis or accelerated silicosis. Silicotic nodules are rarely seen and if present are not well-defined. Proteinaceous fluid fills the alveoli. Desquamated pneumocytes, macrophages and silica particles are present in alveolar spaces. The interstitium shows the presence of inflammatory cells and the alveoli are lined by large type II pneumocytes. Little or no fibrosis is observed.
2. *Prognosis*: The prognosis is poor. Death results from respiratory failure and cor pulmonale. Survival is generally not more than 4 years. Bacterial, mycobacterial, and fungal infections may complicate the course of the disease.
3. *Treatment*: Complete avoidance of further exposure is important. Corticosteroids and whole lung lavage (as for alveolar proteinosis) have been tried but not proven to be of use. Lung transplantation remains an option.

Chronic silicosis occurs after 15–20 years of exposure to moderate to low levels of silica dust. Chronic silicosis itself is further subdivided into simple and complicated silicosis. This is the most common type of silicosis. Patients with this type of silicosis may not have obvious symptoms, so a chest X-ray is necessary to determine if there is lung damage. It presents as a radiographic abnormality with small (<10 mm), rounded opacities predominantly involving the upper lobes. Latency period of 15 years or more is quite common **(Fig. 6)**.

It is important to note that radiological appearances of silicosis may occur many years after leaving a job associated with exposure to silica. The progressive coalescence of silicotic nodules leads to what has been termed complicated or conglomerate silicosis, more commonly termed as PMF. In this condition, the conglomerated silicotic nodules replace the parenchyma of the upper lobes. There is a fibrotic retraction of the upper lobes and air trapping and emphysema in the lower lobes.

Clinical features: The patient may be totally asymptomatic, the only finding being an abnormal chest radiograph. If symptomatic, cough and dyspnea are observed; these become more marked when radiographic changes progress. 35% of workers exposed to silica have chronic cough and sputum production due to silica-induced chronic bronchitis, though cigarette smoking in smokers is undoubtedly a contributory factor.

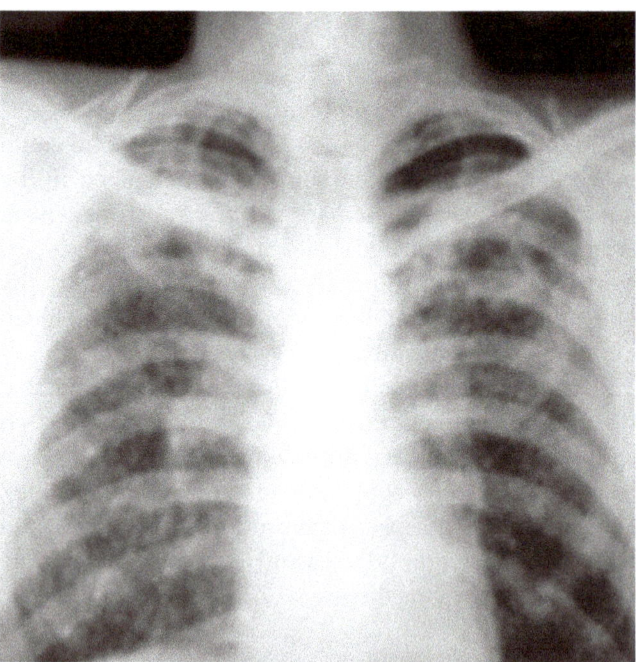

Fig. 6: Chest X-ray of a subject who worked in an underground tungsten metal mine for 18 years as a laborer, rock drilling operator and material feeding helper involving exposure to silica dust. A known smoker for 25 years—the radiograph shows r/r type of small regular pneumoconiotic opacities in all zones with profusion 3/2 (category 3). There is also evidence of healed tuberculosis in the upper zones. A few pneumoconiotic opacities show calcification and there is enlargement of the hilar lymph nodes.

Physical examination may be noncontributory in many patients. In some, crackles and wheezes may be heard on auscultation.

Progressive massive fibrosis is associated with increased dyspnea and cough and is frequently associated with decreased breath sounds over the upper lobes. Digital clubbing does not occur and if present should make one search for another or an associated pathology. Severe PMF results in chronic respiratory failure and cor pulmonale.

Pulmonary functions: Pulmonary functions may be normal in simple or chronic silicosis. They generally worsen pari passu with worsening radiographic abnormalities. The abnormality is typically characterized by a mixed picture of restrictive lung disease + airways obstruction. The forced vital capacity (FVC) is reduced; as is the FEV_1 and the FEV_1/FVC ratio with a decreased DLCO. Arterial hypoxemia may be present.

Imaging: X-ray chest in chronic or simple silicosis shows numerous small rounded opacities (<10 mm in diameter) in both upper lobes, and in line with the ILO classification of radiographs are usually the "q" and "r" type of opacities. Hilar node enlargement may be present; eggshell calcification of the nodes may also be observed. The latter is not peculiar to silicosis and can be observed with other granulomas as well. PMF occurs when these opacities conglomerate to form upper and midzone opacities more than 10 mm in diameter, which are classified by the ILO into categories A, B, and C. These opacities enlarge and are associated with a retraction of both hila and a hyperinflation of the lower lobes. The fibrotic masses may cavitate particularly if there is a superadded mycobacterial infection. The opacities of PMF though bilateral are not necessarily symmetrical **(Fig. 7)**.

HRCT: High-resolution CT is more sensitive than a chest X-ray. The typical findings in chronic silicosis are bilateral, symmetrical, centrilobular nodules with sharp margins. These nodules calcify in 10–20% of patients. Pleural effusions are rare, but pleural thickening is at times observed.

FDG-PET scan: The FDG-PET scan is often used to distinguish benign from malignant lesions. However, the FDG-PET scan is positive in PMF in the absence of malignancy.

Flexible bronchoscopy and BAL studies: Bronchoscopy is generally not indicated. BAL may be used for cytology and microbiological studies if infection or malignancy are considered in the differential diagnosis.

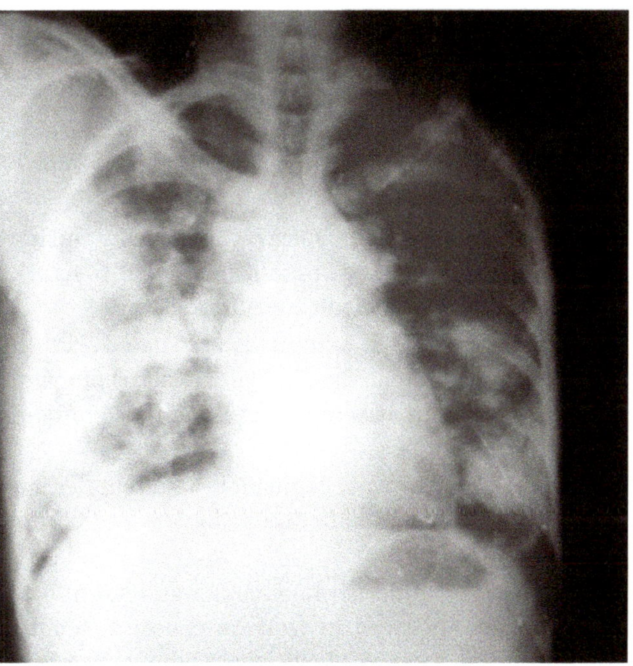

Fig. 7: Chest X-ray of a 25-year-old woman with complaints of breathlessness and cough. X-ray revealed egg-shell calcification of the hilar lymph nodes in addition to bilateral fibrocaseous tuberculosis. She had a history of exposure to silica as a child when she used to play around a glass factory where the quartz-rich stone was manually crushed. Her X-ray reveals classical features of silicosis and tuberculosis.

Clinical diagnosis: A clinical diagnosis is based on a history of exposure to silica, an appropriate latent period following which clinical features compatible with silicosis are observed.

Radiological features compatible with silicosis.

Absence of any other diagnosis more likely to be responsible for the clinical and radiological abnormalities.

Differential diagnosis: Diseases causing similar radiological appearances are tuberculosis, fungal infections, and Langerhans' cell histiocytosis. PMF may mimic the radiological appearances of malignancy.

Complications and Associated Diseases

- *Pulmonary tuberculosis*: As mentioned earlier, tuberculosis (TB) is the most important and most frequent complication in patients with silicosis. It should be suspected in the presence of constitutional symptoms, worsening respiratory functions or hemoptysis. All microbiological techniques should be used to prove the diagnosis since silicosis can mask the radiographic features of active TB. Treatment for TB in these patients should be extended to 9 months.

- Nocardial and other bacterial infections.
- *Chronic necrotizing aspergillosis*: Some cases of chronic necrotizing aspergillosis have been reported in patients with PMF.
- *Lung cancer*: Crystalline silica is carcinogenic and lung cancer can occur as a complication of silicosis. The diagnosis may be difficult and often delayed.
- *Rheumatic diseases*: Silicosis is associated with the production of autoantibodies like ANA and rheumatoid factor, and with systemic sclerosis and rheumatoid arthritis.
- *Chronic kidney disease*: Population-based studies have shown an association between silicosis and chronic kidney disease.
- *Chronic bronchitis*: Chronic cough and sputum are frequently observed in workers exposed to silica, even in the absence of silicosis. There is also more than expected decline in spirometric values in these patients.

Accelerated silicosis: Accelerated silicosis is distinguished from chronic silicosis by a more rapid development (within 10 years) following a high-level exposure to silica. Affected patients may be asymptomatic, the only manifestation being an abnormal X-ray chest. Symptomatic patients have cough, worsening dyspnea; rhonchi, and crackles may be present on auscultation. Patients who develop accelerated silicosis are at a greater risk for the development of PMF and at a greater risk for complications.

Treatment

No specific measures are available for treating silicosis. General measures are similar to those commonly used in the management of airway obstruction, infection, pneumothorax, hypoxemia, and respiratory failure complicating other pulmonary disease. Coexisting tuberculosis should be evaluated and treated with multidrug therapy.

Prevention

Prevention should focus on improved ventilation and local exhaust, process enclosure, use of wet techniques, personal protection including the proper selection of respirators, and where possible, industrial substitution of agents less hazardous than silica. The education of workers and employers regarding the hazards of silica dust exposure and measures to control exposure are also important.

■ COAL WORKERS' LUNG DISEASE

Exposure to coal mine dust may cause pneumoconiosis, chronic bronchitis and COPD.

In the developed countries, regulations have brought about a reduction in dust levels resulting in a substantial drop in disease prevalence since the 1970s.

■ COAL WORKERS' PNEUMOCONIOSIS (BLACK LUNG DISEASE)

Coal workers' pneumoconiosis is a distinct pathologic entity resulting from the deposition of coal dust in the lungs. The tissue reactions to deposits of dust include the *coal macule* and the *coal nodule* (simple CWP), and PMF (complicated CWP).

Etiopathogenesis

Alveolar macrophages engulf the dust, release cytokines that stimulate inflammation, and collect in the lung interstitium around bronchioles and alveoli (coal macules). Coal nodules develop as collagen accumulates, and focal emphysema develops as bronchiolar walls weaken and dilate. Fibrosis can occur but is usually limited to areas adjacent to coal macules **(Fig. 8)**. Distortion of lung architecture, airflow obstruction, and functional impairment are usually mild but can be highly destructive in some patients.

Two forms of CWP are described: (1) simple, with individual coal macules and (2) complicated, with coalescence of macules and PMF.

Patients with simple CWP develop PMF at a rate of about 1–2%. In PMF, nodules coalesce to form black, rubbery parenchymal masses usually in the upper posterior fields **(Fig. 9)**. The masses may encroach on and destroy the vascular supply and airways or may cavitate. PMF can develop and progress even after exposure to coal dust has ceased. Despite the similarity between coal-induced PMF and conglomerate silicosis, the development of PMF in coal workers is unrelated to the silica content of the coal.

Usually, CWP which is associated with mining coal takes about 10 years to develop and often much longer when exposures are less. However, over a period of

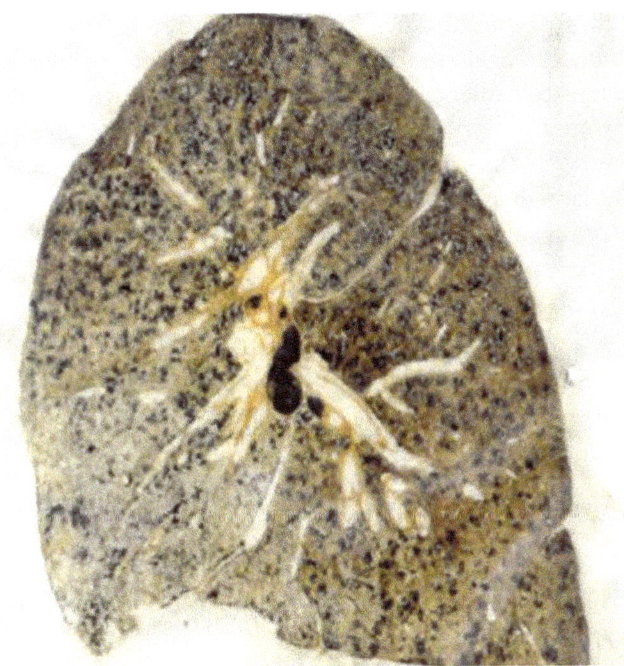

Fig. 8: Simple coal workers' pneumoconiosis. Gross specimen shows that the lung is studded with nodules representing simple coal workers' pneumoconiosis. Focal areas of emphysema in relation to these nodules are clearly visible.
Source: Image reprinted with permission from eMedicine.com, 2009. [online] Available from http://emedicine.medscape.com/ article/297887-overview. Copyright with eMedicine. Com [Accessed July, 2018].

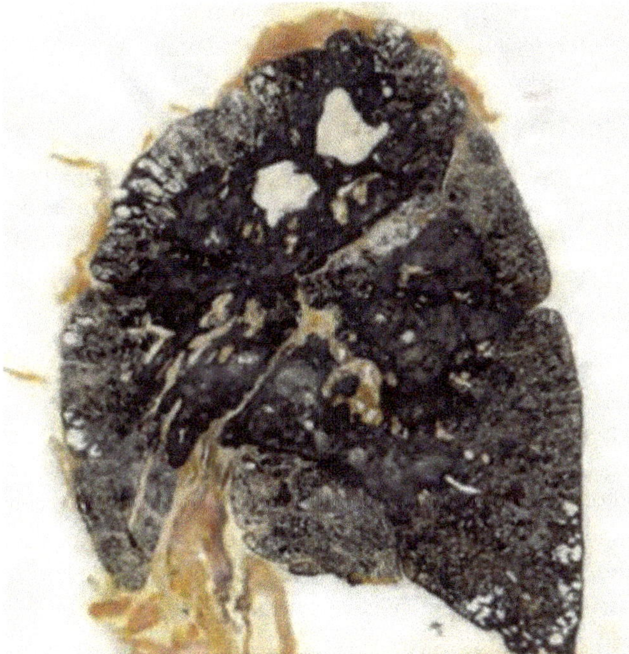

Fig. 9: Progressive massive fibrosis. Gross specimen shows that in addition to nodules studding the lung surface, there are two conglomerate masses which characterize progressive massive fibrosis. *Note* thickened pleura over the apex and upper lobe and the increased density of nodules subpleurally and along the fissure.
Source: Image reprinted with permission from eMedi-cine.com, 2009. [online] Available from http://emedicine.med-scape.com/article/297887-overview. Copyright with eMedicine.com [Accessed July, 2018].

time the disease could progress to massive pulmonary fibrosis.

Clinical Aspects

Coal workers' pneumoconiosis does not usually cause symptoms. Most chronic pulmonary symptoms in coal miners are caused by other conditions, such as industrial bronchitis from coal dust or coincident chronic airways obstruction from smoking. Cough can be chronic and problematic in patients even after they leave the workplace, even in those who do not smoke.

Progressive massive fibrosis causes progressive dyspnea. Occasionally, patients cough up black sputum (melanoptysis), which occurs as a result of rupture of PMF lesions into the airways. PMF often progresses to pulmonary hypertension with right ventricular and respiratory failure.

Diagnosis

Diagnosis depends on a history of exposure and chest X-ray or chest CT appearance. In patients with CWP, X-ray

or CT reveals diffuse, small, rounded opacities or nodules. The finding of at least one opacity more than 10 mm suggests PMF. The specificity of the chest X-ray for PMF is low, because up to one-third of the lesions identified as being PMF turn out to be cancers, scars, or other disorders. Chest CT is more sensitive than chest X-ray for detecting coalescing nodules, early PMF, and cavitation.

Pulmonary function tests are nondiagnostic but are useful for characterizing lung function in patients in whom obstructive, restrictive, or mixed defects may develop. Because abnormalities of gas exchange occur in some patients with extensive simple CWP and in those with complicated CWP, baseline and periodic measures of diffusing capacity of the lungs for carbon monoxide (DLCO) and arterial blood gases at rest and during exercise are recommended.

Because patients with CWP often have had exposure to both silica dust as well as coal dust, surveillance for tuberculosis is usually done. Patients with CWP should have annual tuberculin skin testing. In those with positive test results, sputum culture, and cytology, CT, and bronchoscopy with microbiological examination of BAL together with a gene expert test on both BAL fluid and sputum may be needed to confirm tuberculosis.

Treatment

Treatment should be geared toward symptom management and prevention of infectious complications of the affected miners. Miners should stop smoking. Treatment is usually for acute bronchitis, congestive cardiac failure and for complications arising out of respiratory failure.

Prevention

The key to prevention is the minimization of dust exposure. Various dust control methods include provision of ventilation, use of water sprays and modern mining methods. Respiratory use should be the final resort and not the primary way of managing exposures. Ongoing health surveillance is also effective in monitoring the respiratory health of miners.

■ PROGRESSIVE MASSIVE FIBROSIS

Diagnosis

Progressive massive fibrosis following exposure to silica or coal dust is characterized by the presence of one or more large fibrotic lesions (whose definition depends on the mode of detection) present in one or both lungs. PMF often becomes more severe over time, even in the absence of additional dust exposure. It can also develop after dust exposure has ceased, and may often cause disability and premature death.

Etiopathogenesis

Despite extensive research, the actual cause of PMF development remains unclear. Over the years, various hypotheses have been proposed, but none is fully satisfactory. One prominent theory was that tuberculosis played a role. Indeed, tuberculosis is often present in miners with PMF, particularly in developing countries. However, PMF has been found to develop in miners in whom there was no sign of tuberculosis, and tuberculin reactivity has not been found to be elevated in miners with pneumoconiosis. Despite investigation, consistent evidence of the role of the immune system in the development of PMF is lacking.

Progressive massive fibrosis lesions may be unilateral or bilateral, and are most often found in the upper or middle lobes of the lung. The lesions are formed of collagen, reticulin, coal mine dust, and dust-laden macrophages, while the center may contain a black liquid which cavitates on occasion. US pathology standards require the lesions to be 2 cm in size or larger to be identified as PMF entities in surgical or autopsy specimens.

Clinical Aspects

Each individual miner with large chest opacities must be appropriately evaluated. Miners with progressive symptoms, risk factors for other disorders (e.g. tuberculosis), or atypical clinical features should undergo a thorough appropriate examination before being diagnosed as PMF.

Dyspnea and other respiratory symptoms often accompany PMF, but may not necessarily be due to the disease itself. Congestive heart failure (due to pulmonary hypertension and cor pulmonale) is an infrequent complication. PMF leads to premature death.

Radiology

Large opacities (>1 cm) on the radiograph, coupled with a history of extensive coal mine dust exposure, are taken to imply the presence of PMF. However, other diseases such as lung cancer, tuberculosis and granulomas should also be considered. Large opacities are usually seen on a background of small opacities, but development of PMF from category 0 profusion has been noted over a 5-year period **(Fig. 10)**.

Treatment

Medical care should be organized around ameliorating the condition and associated lung illnesses, while protecting against infectious complications. Although maintaining functional stability may be more difficult in patients with PMF, in other respects, management is similar to simple CWP. The incidence and rate of CWP progression is related to the amount of respirable coal dust to which miners were exposed during their working lifetime. Early pneumoconiosis can be asymptomatic, but advanced disease often leads to disability and premature death.

Prevention

Avoidance of dust exposure is the only way to prevent PMF. Since the risk of its development increases sharply with increasing category of simple CWP, a strategy for secondary

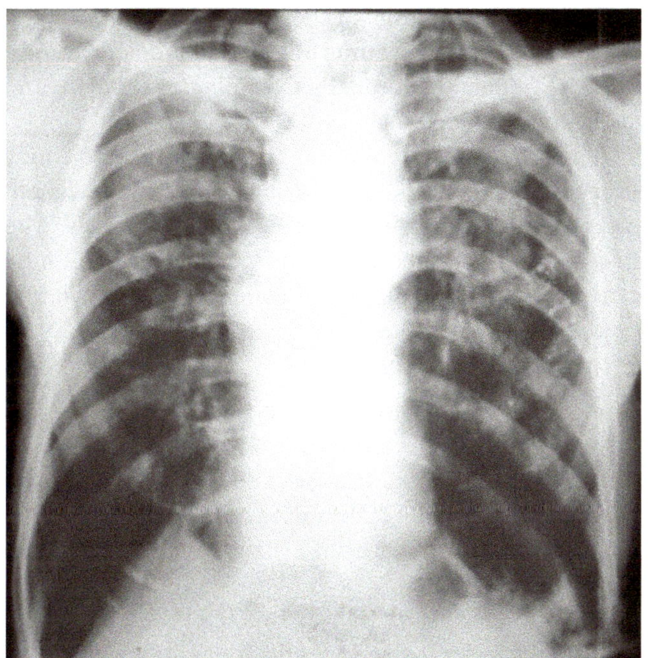

Fig. 10: The radiograph shows r/r type of small regular pneumoconiotic opacities in all zones with profusion of 3/2 (category 3). There is coalescence of pneumoconiotic opacities in both right upper zones; one opacity (80 × 30 mm) in the right upper zone, and another large opacity with dimensions of 50 × 40 mm mainly in the left upper zone indicate progressive massive fibrosis (PMF).

prevention of PMF is for miners to undergo periodic chest X-rays and to terminate or reduce their exposure if simple CWP is detected. Although this approach appears valid and has been adopted in certain jurisdictions, its effectiveness has not been evaluated systematically.

Legal exposure limits in India (coal dust): 2 mg/m^3, respirable dust fraction containing less than 5% quartz.

■ ASBESTOSIS

Definition and History

Asbestosis is a disease resulting in interstitial pneumonitis and fibrosis caused by inhalation of asbestos fibers.

Asbestos is the name given to a group of six naturally occurring fibrous silicate minerals that have been widely used in commercial products. Asbestos is composed of silicate chains bonded with magnesium, iron, calcium, aluminum, and sodium or trace elements to form long, thin, separable fibers. These fibers are often arranged in parallel or matted masses. Asbestos occurs naturally but much of its presence in the environment stems from mining and commercial uses.

There are two classes of asbestos, viz. (1) serpentine and (2) amphibole **(Table 6)**.

Asbestos was widely used commercially until the 1970s. Mining and milling of the raw material and production of asbestos has declined since the early 1970s, but asbestos is still used in some construction materials. Asbestos fibers are released into the air and dust when asbestos-containing materials are loose, crumbling, or disturbed. Until the 1970s, asbestos was widely used in the construction, shipbuilding, and automotive industries, among others. For example, asbestos was formerly used in the following items: boilers and heating vessels, cement pipes, clutch, brake, and transmission components, conduits for electrical wire, corrosive chemical containers, electric motor components, heat-protective pads, laboratory furniture, paper products, pipe covering, roofing products, sealants and coatings, insulation products, and textiles (including curtains).

Today, asbestos is still used in brake pads, automobile clutches, roofing materials, vinyl tile and imported cement pipe and corrugated sheets. Other occupations at risk include those in the construction industry, auto mechanics, demolition workers, refinery, and shipyard workers.

Although asbestos is no longer used in many products, it will remain a public health concern well into the 21st century.

Exposure to Asbestos

Exposure to asbestos can occur when asbestos-containing material (man-made or natural) is loose, crumbling or disturbed, releasing asbestos fibers into the air and dust **(Fig. 11)**.

The primary route of asbestos entry into the body is inhalation of air or dust that contains asbestos fibers. Asbestos can also enter the body via ingestion. With dermal exposure, asbestos fibers may lodge in the skin.

Table 6: Classes of asbestos.	
Serpentine: long, flexible fibers	*Amphiboles*: Brittle, rod or needle-shaped
Member: Chrysotile	*Members*: Crocidolite, amosite, anthophyllite, tremolite, actinolite, winchite, and richterite
Accounts for 93% of world's commercial, purposeful use of asbestos	Accounts for 7% of commercial, purposeful use of asbestos

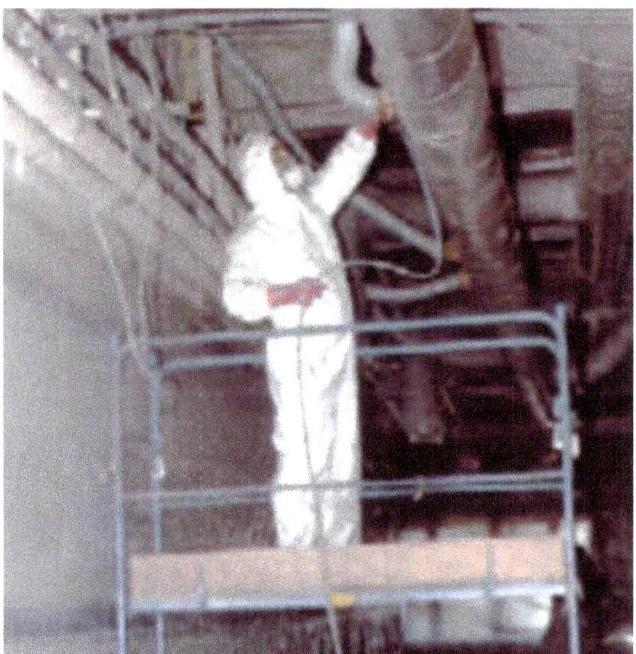

Fig. 11: Building demolition presents an asbestos hazard when the insulation is disturbed.
Courtesy: Picture Dr GK Kulkarni.

Inhalation: Inhalation is the most important route of exposure to asbestos, and the route that most commonly leads to illness.

Ingestion: Swallowing material removed from the lungs via tracheociliary clearance by a person who had inhaled asbestos fibers into the lungs.

Drinking water contaminated with asbestos, for example, from erosion of natural land sources, discarded mine and mill tailings, asbestos cement pipe, or disintegration of other asbestos-containing materials transported by rain.

Dermal: Today, dermal contact is rare. In the past, handling asbestos could result in heavy dermal contact and exposure. Asbestos fibers could become lodged in the skin, producing a callus or corn, but not any more serious health effects.

Asbestos-related Lung Diseases

The inhalation of asbestos fibers may lead to a number of respiratory diseases, including asbestosis, lung cancer, pleural plaques, benign pleural effusion, and malignant mesothelioma. Although exposure is now regulated, patients continue to present with these diseases because of the long latent period between exposure and clinical disease. Nonmalignant asbestos-related disease refers to the following conditions: asbestosis, pleural thickening or asbestos-related pleural fibrosis (plaques or diffuse fibrosis), "benign" (nonmalignant) pleural effusion, and airflow obstruction.

The prognosis depends on the specific disease entity. Asbestosis generally progresses slowly, whereas malignant mesothelioma has an extremely poor prognosis. The treatment of patients with asbestos exposure and lung cancer is identical to that of any patient with lung cancer.

Etiopathogenesis

Some of the inhaled asbestos fibers are deposited on the surface of the larger airways where some of them are cleared by mucociliary transport and swallowing. Other fibers are deposited further in the lung, especially in the bifurcations of the tracheobronchial tree and eventually in the alveolar sacs.

The dimensions of the asbestos fiber determine how easily and how far it penetrates the lungs and how quickly it is cleared. Wide fibers (diameter greater than 2–5 μ) tend to be deposited in the upper respiratory tract and cleared. Long thin asbestos fibers reach the lower airways and alveoli and tend to be retained in the lungs. However, it is important to remember that asbestos fibers of all lengths can induce pathological changes and cannot be excluded as contributors to asbestos-related disease.

The mechanisms by which asbestos causes disease are not fully understood. Currently, there are three hypotheses to account for asbestos's pathogenicity—(1) direct interaction with cellular macromolecules, (2) generation of reactive oxygen species, and (3) other cell-mediated mechanisms (especially inflammation).

Clinical Features and Diagnosis

Depending on the level of exposure, inhalation of asbestos fibers can cause different diseases such as parenchymal asbestosis, asbestos-related pleural abnormalities, lung carcinoma, and pleural mesothelioma.

Any combination of these syndromes (or all four of them) can be present in a single patient labeled as parenchymal asbestosis.

Parenchymal asbestosis is a diffuse interstitial fibrosis resulting from inhalation of asbestos fibers. Asbestos fibers inhaled deep into the lung parenchyma become lodged in the tissue, resulting in diffuse alveolar and interstitial fibrosis (*see* **Fig. 3**). The fibrosis first occurs in the respiratory bronchioles, particularly the subpleural portions of the lower lobes. The fibrosis can progress to include the alveolar walls. Fibrosis tends to progress even after exposure ceases. This fibrosis leads to a restrictive lung pathology, characterized by reduced lung volumes, diminished compliance, reduced CO diffusing capacity and impaired gas exchange. There is absence of airways obstruction on spirometry. The earliest lung function abnormalities are a reduction in the DLCO and pulmonary compliance, and the presence of arterial hypoxemia. Initially arterial hypoxemia occurs only on exertion but later persists even on rest. With progression of the disease, dyspnea on exertion, insidious in onset, is the prominent symptom. Advanced cases may lead to respiratory failure and to cor pulmonale with features of right heart failure.

Parenchymal asbestosis is characterized by the following radiographic changes: fine, irregular opacities in both lung fields (especially in the bases) and septal lines that progress to honeycombing and sometimes, in more severe disease, to obscuration of the heart border and hemidiaphragm, the so-called shaggy heart sign. Radiographic changes depend on the duration, frequency, and intensity of exposure. Patients with parenchymal asbestosis may have elevated levels of antinuclear antibody and rheumatoid factor and a progressive decrease in total lymphocyte count with advancing fibrosis.

Parenchymal asbestosis has no unique pathognomonic signs or symptoms, but diagnosis is made by the constellation of clinical, functional, and radiographic findings as outlined by the American Thoracic Society criteria (American Thoracic Society 2004). These criteria include sufficient history of exposure to asbestos, appearance of disease with a consistent time interval from first exposure, clinical picture such as insidious onset of dyspnea on exertion, bibasilar end-inspiratory crackles not cleared by coughing, lung function tests showing restrictive (occasionally obstructive) pattern with reduced diffusing capacity, characteristic X-ray appearance, exclusion of other causes of interstitial fibrosis or obstructive disease, such as usual interstitial pneumonia, connective tissue disease, and drug-related fibrosis.

Table 7 describes the natural history associated with parenchymal asbestosis.

Table 8 lists the asbestosis related pleural abnormalities. The imaging features of pleural involvement in asbestosis are illustrated in **Figures 12A to D**.

Differential Diagnosis

Differential diagnosis includes idiopathic pulmonary fibrosis, interstitial lung disease related to connective tissue

Table 7: Natural history associated with parenchymal asbestosis.	
Parameter	**Typical findings**
Sufficient exposures	Usually associated with high-level occupational exposures
Latency periods	Radiographic changes: <20 years. Clinical manifestation: 20–40 years. Asbestosis appears earliest in those with the highest exposure levels
Risk of asbestosis	Asbestosis develops in 49–52% of adults with occupational levels of asbestos exposure
Comorbid conditions	Increased risk for lung cancer and mesothelioma, though both can occur without parenchymal asbestosis
Mortality and morbidity	Severe asbestosis may lead to respiratory failure over 12–24 years. Many patients with asbestosis die of other causes such as asbestos-associated lung cancer (38%), mesothelioma (9%) and other causes (32%)

Table 8: Asbestos-related pleural abnormalities.			
Type of pleural change	**Appearance**	**Occurrence or frequency**	**Symptoms**
Pleural plaques	Well-circumscribed	Very common (58% in insulation workers)	Asymptomatic
Benign asbestos pleural effusions	Small unilateral pleural effusions—blood stained with mesothelial and various other cells	Earliest manifestation	Asymptomatic
Diffuse pleural thickening	Noncircumscribed fibrous thickening of the visceral pleura with adherence to the parietal pleura	10% of patients with asbestosis	Progressive dyspnea and chest pain
Rounded atelectasis (folded lung)	Rounded pleural mass with bands of lung tissue radiating outward	Least common	Asymptomatic

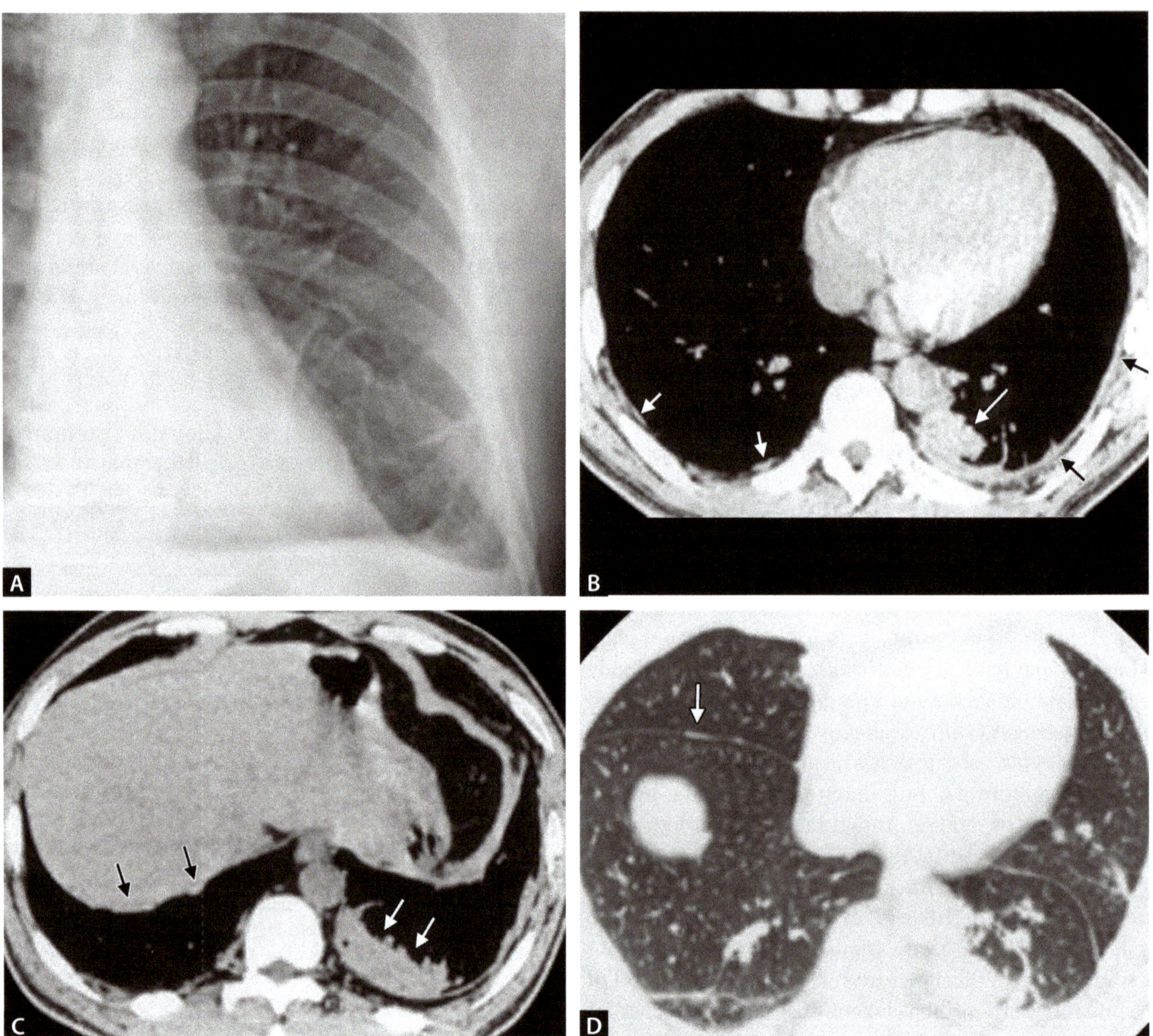

Figs. 12A to D: Pleural plaques, diffuse pleural thickening, rounded atelectasis, and asbestosis in a 50-year-old man with asbestos exposure from working in a brake lining production plant. (A) Chest radiograph shows diffuse thickening of the left pleura and curvilinear band opacities in the left lower lung zone; (B) High-resolution CT scan (mediastinal windowing) shows pleural plaques on the right side (small white arrows) and rounded atelectasis (large white arrow) with adjacent diffuse pleural thickening (black arrows) on the left side; (C) High-resolution CT scan obtained at a lower level than (B) demonstrates pleural plaques along the diaphragmatic contour (black arrows) and an irregular attenuation pattern, which is typical in rounded atelectasis (white arrows); and (D) High-resolution CT scan (lung windowing) obtained at the level of the liver dome shows a visceral pleural plaque in the right major fissure (arrow) and curvilinear bands of hyperattenuation in the posterior subpleural area. *Note* also the rounded atelectasis with posterior displacement of the left major fissure. The diagnosis of asbestosis was proved by open-lung biopsy.
Source: Reproduced with permission from Kim KI, Kim CW, Lee MK, et al. Imaging of Occupational Lung Disease, Radiographics. 2001;21:1371-91. The Radiological Society of North America (RSNA®).

disorders, drug-induced pneumonitis, hypersensitivity pneumonitis, and pulmonary fibroelastosis. The last two conditions can be generally excluded as they chiefly involve the upper lobes.

Bronchoalveolar lavage: Asbestos bodies in BAL studies are generally present in patients with asbestosis. However, the clinical utility of BAL for evaluation of asbestosis is limited. BAL study should be reserved only when imaging findings are not characteristic and infection or malignancy is being considered in the differential diagnosis.

Complications

The three main complications are respiratory failure, cancer of the lung and pleural mesothelioma. Respiratory failure occurs in a small minority due to increasing and progressive pulmonary fibrosis. Risk factors for progression are the degree of exposure, duration of exposure and fiber type—the crocidolite exposure being more likely to cause progressive fibrosis.

■ ASBESTOS AND LUNG CARCINOMA

Exposure to asbestos is associated with all major histological types of lung carcinoma (adenocarcinoma, squamous cell carcinoma, and small-cell carcinoma). It is estimated that 4–12% of lung cancers are related to occupational levels of exposure to asbestos. It is also estimated that 20–25% of heavily exposed asbestos workers will develop bronchogenic carcinomas. Whether asbestos exposure will lead to lung cancer depends on several factors—level, duration, and frequency of asbestos exposure (cumulative exposure), time elapsed since exposure occurred, age when exposure occurred, history of tobacco use, and individual susceptibility factors not yet determined **(Table 9)**.

Most asbestos-related lung cancers reflect the dual influence of asbestos exposure and smoking. Smoking and asbestos exposure have a multiplicative effect on the risk of lung cancer. Asbestos as the sole contributing factor for cancer in an individual patient can be difficult to prove especially when the patient has other risk factors for lung cancer. The presence of parenchymal asbestosis is an indicator of high-level asbestos exposure, but lung cancer can occur without asbestosis.

■ ASBESTOS AND PLEURAL MESOTHELIOMA (TABLE 10)

Pleural mesothelioma (*see* section Diseases of the Pleura) is a signal tumor for asbestos exposure; other causes are uncommon. The risk of mesothelioma does depend on the amount of asbestos exposure. All types of asbestos can cause mesothelioma, but some researchers believe that the amphibole form is more likely to induce mesothelioma than the serpentine form.

According to a Centre for Disease Control (CDC) report, during the period 1999–2015, a total of 45,221 deaths with malignant mesothelioma were reported in the United States, increasing from 2,479 deaths in 1999 to 2,597 in 2015.

Chest radiography in patients with malignant mesothelioma may show an effusion, pleural thickening, and as the tumor progresses, a more lobulated outline. CT can help identify the disease in its early stages. Asbestos-related cancers can occur anywhere in the lungs. Recognition of the clinical, radiological, and pathologic features of these diseases will be important for some years to come.

Clinical Evaluation of Patients with Asbestosis

Key Points

- Exposures to asbestos, smoking history, and other respiratory conditions
- The most typical abnormal finding on examination of patients with a history of asbestos exposure is bibasilar end-inspiratory rales on pulmonary auscultation. Patients with parenchymal asbestosis present to the

Table 9: Typical findings associated with lung carcinoma.

Typical exposures	Large cumulative exposure (short-term, high-level exposures or long-term, moderate-level exposures)
Latency periods	20–30 years
Clinical presentation	Only 5–15% of patients are asymptomatic when diagnosed. Most present with cough, hemoptysis, wheeze, dyspnea
Comorbid conditions	Asbestosis, other asbestos-related diseases
Mortality	Same as lung carcinoma from other causes—14% 5-year survival rate

Table 10: Typical findings associated with pleural mesothelioma.

Typical exposures	Short-term, high-level exposures or chronic low-level exposures, especially to amphibole asbestos; incidence increase in dose-related manner
Latency periods	10–57 years (30–40 years typical)
Clinical presentation	Frequently presents with chest pain accompanied by pleural mass or pleural effusion on chest X-ray
Mortality	High. The typical 1-year survival rate is < 30%. Average survival time is 8–14 months after diagnosis.

clinician with the chief complaint of fatigue, insidious onset of dyspnea on exertion

- Asbestos-related pleural abnormalities typically do not cause symptoms, although some patients experience progressive dyspnea and chest pain
- Lung cancer can be asymptomatic, but in the later stages patients experience fatigue, weight loss, chest pain, dyspnea, or hemoptysis
- Mesothelioma is typically asymptomatic until later stages, at which point patients have dyspnea and chest pain.

Pulmonary Function and Imaging Findings

Key Points

- Parenchymal asbestosis is associated with a reduction in FVC and restrictive patterns on spirometry. Signs of parenchymal asbestosis on chest X-ray include irregular opacities, interstitial fibrosis, and the "shaggy heart sign"
- On chest X-ray, pleural plaques appear as well-circumscribed areas of pleural thickening, sometimes with calcification, pleural effusions have a cloudy or bloodstained appearance, diffuse pleural thickening appears as a lobulated prominence and interlobar fissure thickening
- On chest X-ray, findings associated with rounded atelectasis appear as a rounded pleural mass with radiating bands of lung tissue
- Asbestos-associated lung cancer has the same appearance as lung cancer from other causes
- Chest X-ray findings associated with mesothelioma include pleural effusions or a pleural mass.

The HRCT findings often observed are as follows:

- Basilar lung parenchymal fibrosis with intralobar, intralobular, and peribronchial fibrosis
- Pleural plaques and fibrosis which helps to differentiate asbestosis from other interstitial lung fibrosis
- Subpleural linear densities parallel to the pleura
- Basal honeycombing in advanced disease.

Management of Asbestosis

Management is entirely symptomatic as there is no specific treatment available. Intercurrent respiratory infections should be appropriately treated. Patients should be given pneumococcal vaccine and influenza vaccine at intervals recommended by the CDC. Patients should be strongly counseled against smoking. Pulmonary rehabilitation may provide symptomatic relief. The degree of patient disability needs to be carefully assessed and clinical, radiological and lung function test follow-up should be maintained with specific reference to development of lung cancer and pleural mesothelioma.

■ OCCUPATIONAL ASTHMA

Definitions

Occupational asthma is asthma that is caused by environmental exposure at the workplace.

Work aggravated asthma is defined as concurrent or pre-existing asthma that worsens in the workplace.

Irritant induced asthma results from exposure to non-immunogenic irritant or irritants at a high level of intensity. It is a form of occupational asthma, though the airway histopathology is different from immunogenic occupational asthma.

Reactive airways dysfunction syndrome (RADS) is a variant of irritant-induced asthma triggered by exposure to a single nonimmunogenic stimulus. Asthmatic symptoms begin within minutes of exposure and on-going asthma with bronchial hyper-responsiveness persist for a prolonged period of time.

Occupational nonasthmatic eosinophilic bronchitis is an asthma variant that causes symptoms at the workplace which mimics asthma but is not associated with bronchial hyper-responsiveness.

Several hundred agents have been reported to cause occupational asthma (OA). Preexisting asthma or airway hyperresponsiveness, with symptoms worsened by work exposure to irritants or physical stimuli, is usually classified separately as work-aggravated asthma (WAA). There is general agreement that OA has become the most prevalent occupational lung disease in developed countries, although estimates of actual prevalence and incidence are quite variable. It is clear, however, that in many countries asthma of occupational etiology causes a largely unrecognized burden of disease and disability with high economic and noneconomic costs. Although occupational diseases such as asbestosis and silicosis may be eradicated with time because of better preventive measures, it is unlikely that OA will ever disappear, because of the constant introduction of new chemicals into workplaces. Much of this public health and economic burden is potentially preventable by identifying and controlling or eliminating the workplace exposures causing the asthma.

Magnitude of the Problem

Prevalence of asthma in adults generally ranges from 3% to 5%, depending on the definition of asthma and geographic variations, and may be considerably higher in some low-income urban populations. The proportion of adult asthma cases in the general population that is related to the work environment is reported to range from 2% to 23%, with recent estimates tending toward the higher end of this range.

Pathophysiology

Occupational asthma is the result of an interaction between environmental factors at the workplace and individual susceptibility. Genetic factors probably play a role. Most genetic studies suggest the importance of HLA class II polymorphisms in controlling the risk for sensitization in OA. Glutathione S-transferase protects cells from oxidative stress. It is believed to play an important role in OA caused by exposure to isocyanates. Over 200 agents (specific substances, occupations or industrial processes) have been reported to cause OA based on epidemiological studies and/or clinical evidence. In OA airways inflammation and bronchoconstriction can be caused by the following mechanisms:

- Immunological immunoglobulin E (IgE)-mediated
- Immunological non-IgE-mediated
- Nonimmunological
- Direct pharmacological action—an example of agents which do so are organophosphorous insecticides.

Immunological IgE-mediated Occupational Asthma (Table 11)

Many high molecular weight occupational agents, such as animal-derived allergens, flour, act as complete antigens and induce specific IgE antibody formation. Low molecular weight agents, for example tricyclic anhydride and other acid anhydrides may also induce specific IgE antibodies resulting in a type I hypersensitivity reaction. Some occupational agents give rise to IgG-specific antibodies. They act as haptens, bind with proteins to form complete antigens. These antigens are recognized by antigen-presenting cells and induce a CD4 response

Table 11: Agents causing immunologically mediated occupational asthma.

High molecular weight	Low molecular weight
Cereals	Isocyanates
Enzymes	Wood dusts
Gums	Anhydrides
Animal-derived allergens	Amines
Sea-foods	Sea-foods dyes
	Formaldehyde
	Metals
	Persulfate

resulting in production of specific IgE antibodies by B-cells stimulated by interleukin (IL)-4. The antigen-IgE antibody reaction leads to airways inflammation, mucosal edema, airways constriction, and increased bronchial hyperreactivity similar to what is observed in nonoccupational asthma. There is no pathogenetic difference in the mechanism operating in OA as compared to nonoccupational asthma.

Immunological Non-IgE-mediated Occupational Asthma

Many low molecular weight agents, notably isocyanates are known to cause OA without the presence of IgE antibodies. Specific IgG antibodies have been found to be associated with OA but their significance has not been exactly determined.

It has been suggested that T-lymphocytes may play an important role in the pathogenesis of OA. Bronchial mucosal biopsies show proliferation of activated T-cells. Cloning of cells from bronchial mucosal biopsy specimens show that most of the lymphocytes are of the CD8 phenotype. This is supportive of the possibility that CD8 lymphocytes play an important role in the pathogenesis of some forms of OA without the production of IgE antibodies.

The early asthmatic reaction in OA is characterized by constriction and mucosal edema related to the release of histamine, histamine-related substances and leukotrienes. The late asthmatic reaction is characterized by the influx of inflammatory cells. The eosinophil of course is the key cell in both OA and nonoccupational bronchial asthma. Current work also shows the importance of the neutrophils in the inflammatory response that characterizes asthma.

In fact eosinophils and neutrophil variants have been observed in cases of OA due to low molecular weight agents, especially isocyanates. Some low molecular weight agents, in particular isocyanates exert a variety of inflammatory effects to induce asthma. For example, isocyanates may block the β-adrenergic receptors and also stimulate sensory nerves to secrete substance P which inhibits endopeptides that are necessary for inactivation of neuropeptides. Neuropeptides are known to recruit inflammatory cells, cause mucosal edema and bronchial constriction.

Nonimmunological

The features that characterize the nonimmunologic form of OA are the absence of latency. Respiratory irritants often worsen symptoms in workers with preexisting asthma, and at high levels of exposure can cause new-onset asthma—termed reactive airways dysfunction syndrome (RADS) or irritant-induced asthma.

The exact mechanism of RADS is not known. The condition is characterized by extensive loss of mucosal epithelium of the airways leading to airways inflammation and hyperresponsiveness. Inflammation and hyperresponsiveness may well be due to exposure of nerve endings and nonspecific activation of mast cells with release of inflammatory mediators and cytokines. Airways remodeling is induced as a result of growth factors for epithelial cells, smooth muscle and fibroblasts. In the chronic form of RADS there is marked thickening of the bronchial walls **(Table 12)**.

Clinical Presentation

The symptom spectrum of OA is similar to nonoccupational asthma: wheeze, cough, chest tightness and shortness of breath. Patients sometimes present with cough-variant or nocturnal asthma. OA can be severe and disabling, and deaths have been reported. Onset of OA occurs due to a

Table 12: Agents responsible for reactive airways dysfunction syndrome.
• Acetic acid • Spray point • Ammonia • Bleaching agent • Chlorine • Isocyanates • Sulfur dioxide

specific job environment, so identifying exposures that occurred at the time of onset of asthmatic symptoms is the key to an accurate diagnosis. In WAA, workplace exposures cause a significant increase in frequency and/or severity of symptoms of preexisting asthma.

Several features of the clinical history may suggest an occupational etiology. Symptoms frequently worsen at work or at night after work, improve on days off, and recur on return to work. Symptoms may worsen progressively toward the end of the work week. The patient may note specific activities or agents in the workplace that reproducibly trigger symptoms. Work-related eye irritation or rhinitis may be associated with asthmatic symptoms. These typical symptom patterns may be present only in the initial stages of OA. Partial or complete resolution on weekends or vacations is common early in the course of OA, but with repeated exposures, the time required for recovery may increase to 1 or 2 weeks, or recovery may cease to occur. The majority of patients with OA whose exposures are terminated continue to have symptomatic asthma even years after cessation of exposure, with permanent impairment and disability. Continuing exposure is associated with further worsening of asthma. Brief duration and mild severity of symptoms at the time of cessation of exposure are good prognostic factors and decrease the likelihood of permanent asthma.

Several characteristic temporal patterns of symptoms have been reported for OA. Early asthmatic reactions typically occur shortly (less than 1 hour) after beginning work or the specific work exposure causing the asthma. Late asthmatic reactions begin 4–6 hours after exposure begins, and can last 24–48 hours. Combinations of these patterns occur as dual asthmatic reactions with spontaneous resolution of symptoms separating an early and late reaction, or as continuous asthmatic reactions with no resolution of symptoms between phases. With exceptions, early reactions tend to be IgE-mediated, and late reactions tend to be IgE-independent.

Increased nonspecific bronchial responsiveness (NBR), generally measured by methacholine or histamine challenge, is considered a cardinal feature of OA. The time course and degree of NBR may be useful in diagnosis and monitoring. NBR may decrease within several weeks after cessation of exposure, although abnormal NBR commonly persists for months or years after exposures are terminated. In individuals with irritant-induced OA, NBR is not expected to vary with exposure and/or symptoms.

Diagnosis and Evaluation of Occupational Asthma

Occupational asthma is the most prevalent form of work-related lung disease in industrialized nations. Increasing numbers of new chemicals are being produced and new manufacturing processes are being introduced. The variety of environments in which individuals may become exposed to respiratory sensitizers and irritants makes diagnosing and treating this illness even more challenging. Clinicians must first document the presence of asthma, and then establish a relationship between asthma and the workplace.

The adult patient's occupational history is the key diagnostic tool. In addition, lung function assessments that include spirometry and bronchial responsiveness are now often coupled with immunological assessment and an evaluation of inflammation in the investigation of OA. Evaluations may include serial peak expiratory flow rate (PEFR) measurements and nonspecific hypersensitivity challenges with histamine or methacholine. Serial PEFR monitoring while at work and away from work may be important in documenting whether asthma is work-related in selected people, work environment permitting. Information about workplace exposures to irritants and sensitizers may be useful. Specific challenge testing at tertiary referral centers providing specialized laboratories can also be helpful, but is rarely necessary.

Since asthma is an inflammatory disease, a measure of the degree of inflammation would be helpful in quantifying severity and titrating of anti-inflammatory therapy. There is evidence that monitoring eosinophils and neutrophils in induced sputum can help in the management of asthma.

Treatment and Prevention

The medical management of OA is similar to that for nonoccupational asthma. The key to managing OA is to ensure that the exposure which triggers asthma is optimally controlled. In many cases it may mean removal of a worker from the exposure source, especially in sensitizer-induced OA where the degree of symptoms could be disproportionate to the concentration of the sensitizer at the workplace. In some cases the employee may be able to continue in work with specific treatment and with lowering of the levels of the irritants at the workplace. It would be useful to institute a periodic follow-up of pulmonary functions along with a respiratory questionnaire to ensure appropriate follow-up.

Workplace environmental controls to avoid casual exposures and a system to record and deal with chemical spills can lead to prevention of sensitization of an employee. Substance-specific immunological tests can provide evidence of sensitization, although it is now accepted that sensitization is not the same as disease. In addition, the usual occupational health-related measures like substitution of the chemical, enclosure of processes, ensuring appropriate personal protective measures and employee education would all help in preventing OA at the workplace.

■ BYSSINOSIS

Byssinosis is an obstructive disease of the airways caused by prolonged exposure to cotton dust. It can also occur after similar exposure to jute, flax, hemp, and sometimes sisal dust. In fact the jute industry ranks second in importance after the cotton industry, especially in West Bengal, Andhra Pradesh, and Kerala.

China, USA, Russia, India, Pakistan, Egypt, and Brazil are among the largest cotton-producing countries in the world. The growing of cotton and the manufacture of cotton textiles is a major industry in India. Weaving cloth is also a cottage industry and there are several lakh cotton handlooms in the country employing several million people. The large number of people exposed to cotton dust in the work environment in India is therefore staggering.

Prevalence and Epidemiological Studies in India

Kamat and colleagues devised a 5-year prospective study of 1,241 textile workers from three mills in Mumbai to determine the incidence, pattern and course of byssinosis in India. The prevalence rate in the carding section was 14%, 10% in the spinning section, and 11% in the winding section. In these dusty sections, the prevalence of both byssinosis and bronchitis increased with longer duration of service.

Parikh and coworkers conducting a survey of 289 workers in four cotton gins in Gujarat noted that 39% of workers complained of work-related symptoms of chest tightness, cough, and breathlessness. The pulmonary function tests showed significant decline in the short-staple cotton gin workers, but not in the long-staple cotton gin workers. The difference in lung functions was attributed to a higher content of bract in the short-staple cotton.

Pathogenesis

All phases of textile manufacture pose a risk for cotton dust exposure, and byssinosis particularly occurs in workers in the gins and those in the carding department. Exposure to cotton dust causing disease constitutes exposure not only to cotton fiber but to a variety of other substances many of which are biologically active. The dust present in the air may thus include ground up plant matter, bacteria, fungi, and non-cotton contaminants that may accumulate during the growing, harvesting, and processing of cotton. Physical irritation of the airways by the cotton fiber, bacterial contamination with increased levels of endotoxin in the work environment and cotton dust and the direct release of histamine by cotton extracts may all play a role in the airways' obstruction that characterizes byssinosis.

Clinical Features

The clinical features are the same the world over. The classic symptom is chest tightness and work-related breathing difficulty typically occurring on Monday mornings during the first shift after a holiday weekend. The symptoms start 4–6 hours after the start of work, increase in severity over the rest of the shift and subside in the evening after leaving the work environment. In some workers symptoms develop within a few hours of starting work, increase by the end of the first half of the shift and then improve toward the end of the shift. Exposure over a number of years leads to chest tightness on all days of the work week with increasing breathlessness and cough not only in the work environment but also outside the work environment. Finally, the patient develops permanent incapacity characterized by increasing breathlessness on exertion, wheezing and cough.

The severity of byssinosis has been graded by Schilling and is given below **(Table 13)**.

Table 13: Schilling's classification.

Grade	Tightness
0	Chest tightness on the first day of some working weeks
1	Chest tightness on the first day of every working week
2	Chest tightness on the first and other days of the working week
3	Grade 2 symptoms along with evidence of permanent incapacity in the form of diminished effort tolerance and/or reduced ventilatory capacity

Lung function studies have shown lower values of forced expiratory volume in one second (FEV_1) associated with increasing grades of byssinosis, as well as more acute reduction in FEV_1 particularly in Monday shifts in patients with byssinosis.

Kamat and coworkers in their study on byssinosis noted that 54% workers had chest tightness, 56% had work-related and exertional dyspnea, 20% had wheezing, and 36% had cough. During a 5-year follow-up they noted that the atypical presentation of byssinosis with cough was more common in the carding department. The yearly decrease in FEV_1 in patients with work-related symptoms was 114 mL and was significantly higher than in those with nonspecific chest symptoms. The decrease in FVC and FEV_1 was greater with increased dust loads.

It is of interest that though chest tightness and decline in lung function are often associated in byssinosis workers, this is not always so. At times individuals with chest tightness do not have a measurable decline in lung functions and occasionally patients with decline in lung functions may not have chest symptoms.

Radiographic examination of the chest in severe byssinosis may show over-inflated lungs as in chronic airways obstruction, but the appearances are not specific. Hyperresponsiveness to methacholine is also often noted.

Treatment

Measures to avoid and reduce exposure of workers to cotton dust are of prime importance. Byssinosis is characterized by airways obstruction and airflow limitation. Inhaled β_2-agonists combined with inhaled corticosteroids as in asthma provide relief.

■ OCCUPATIONAL LUNG CANCER

The International Agency for Research on Cancer (IARC) has categorized certain substances as being human respiratory carcinogens. These include the following:

Individual Agents

- Asbestos
- Arsenic and arsenic compounds
- Beryllium and beryllium compounds
- Bis (chloromethyl) ether
- Cadmium and cadmium compounds
- Chlormethyl methyl ether

- Chromium (VI) compounds
- Nickel compounds
- Mustard gas
- Talc with asbestiform fibers.

Complex Mixtures

- Coal tars, coal tar pitches, soot, and tobacco smoke.

Other Occupations of Possible Risk

- Aluminum production
- Coal gasification and production
- Iron and steel founding
- Painters
- Radon and its decay products.

The signs and symptoms of lung cancer depend on the location of the tumor. The prognosis varies with the stage of the disease. In addition to the list enumerated above several agents which have been considered to be possible human carcinogens (IARC Group 2B) include inorganic lead compounds (IARC 1987), cobalt (IARC 1991b), man-made vitreous fibers (rockwool, slagwool and glasswool) (IARC 1988b) and welding fumes (IARC 1990c) (*see* Section on Lung Tumors).

■ EXTRINSIC ALLERGIC ALVEOLITIS

This subject has been dealt with in the Section on "Diffuse Lung Diseases".

■ SUGGESTED READING

1. Agnihotram RV. An overview of occupational health research in India. IJOWM. 2005;9:10-4.
2. American Thoracic Society. Diagnosis and initial management of nonmalignant diseases related to asbestos. Am J Respir Crit Care Med. 2004;170:691-715.
3. ATS. (2017). Environmental and Occupational Lung Diseases. [online] Available from https://www.thoracic.org/statements/environment-occupational-lung-disease.php [Accessed July, 2018].
4. Bang KM, Mazurek JM, Wood JM, et al. Silicosis mortality trends and new exposures to respirable crystalline silica—United States, 2001-2010. MMWR. 2015;64:117-20.
5. Banks DE. The health effects of silica and coal dust exposures. In: Schwarz MI, King TE Jr (Eds). Interstitial Lung Disease, 5th edition. Shelton, CT: People's Medical Publishing House; 2011. p. 499.
6. Bernstein IL, Bernstein DI, Chan-Yeung M, et al. Definition and classification of asthma in the workplace. In: Malo JL, Chan-Yeung M, Bernstein DI (Eds). Asthma in the Workplace, 4th edition. Boca Raton, FL: CRC Press; 2013. pp. 1-5.
7. Dodson RF, Atkinson MA, Levin JL. Asbestos fiber length as related to potential pathogenicity: a critical review. Am J Ind Med. 2003;44:291-7.
8. Kamat SR, Kamat GR, Salpekar VY, et al. Distinguishing byssinosis from chronic obstructive pulmonary disease. Results of a prospective five-year study of cotton mill workers in India. Am Rev Respir Dis. 1981;124:31-40.
9. Pande N, Khilnani GC. Indian Journal of Community Medicine. 1993;18(4):137. Respiratory research foundation of India.
10. Steele M, Schwarz DA. Asbestosis and asbestos-induced pleural disease. In: Schwarz MI, King TE Jr. (Eds). Interstitial Lung Disease, 5th edition. Shelton, CT: People's Medical Publishing House; 2011. p. 543.
11. Stellman JM. Encyclopedia of Occupational Health and Safety, 4th edition. Geneva: International Labour Office; 1998.
12. Tarlo SM, Lemiere C. Occupational asthma. N Engl J Med. 2014;370:640-9.

CHAPTER 67

Environmental Pollution*

DEFINITION

Pollution is the introduction of contaminants into an environment that causes instability, disorder, harm, or discomfort to the ecosystem, i.e. physical systems or living organisms.

FORMS OF POLLUTION

The major forms of pollution are listed below along with the particular pollutants relevant to each of them.

- Air pollution, the release of chemicals and particulates into the atmosphere. Common gaseous air pollutants include carbon monoxide, sulfur dioxide (SO_2), chlorofluorocarbons (CFCs), and nitrogen oxides produced by industry and motor vehicles. Photochemical ozone and smog are created as nitrogen oxides and hydrocarbons react to sunlight. Particulate matter or fine dust is characterized by their micrometer size PM_{10} to $PM_{2.5}$.

  In addition, there is the danger of atmospheric pollution caused by mines (coal, metals, and other substances), factories (manufacturing or processing asbestos, cotton, and numerous chemicals), and finally by dust, particularly in the hot Gangetic northern plains of India and in desert areas as in Rajasthan. Atmospheric pollution from factories, chemical plants, and mines pose not just a danger to workers but to people living environmentally close to these areas.

- Water pollution, by the release of waste products and contaminants on to the surface which run off into river drainage systems, leaching into the groundwater, liquid spills, waste water discharges, eutrophication, and littering.
- Soil contamination occurs when chemicals are released by spill or underground leakage. The most significant soil contaminants are hydrocarbons, heavy metals, herbicides, pesticides, and chlorinated hydrocarbons.
- Littering.
- Radioactive contamination, resulting from 20th century activities in atomic physics, such as nuclear power generation and nuclear weapons research, manufacture, and deployment.
- Noise pollution, which encompasses roadway noise, aircraft noise, industrial noise, as well as high-intensity sonar.
- Light pollution, includes light trespass, over-illumination and astronomical interference.
- Visual pollution, which can refer to the presence of overhead power lines, motorway billboards, scarred landforms (as from strip mining), open storage of trash, or municipal solid waste.
- Thermal pollution is a temperature change in natural water bodies caused by human influence, such as use of water as coolant in a power plant.

The major stress in this chapter will be on atmospheric pollution.

* Thanks are due to Dr HV Ravimohan, Specialist OH, Southern Region, Bengaluru, Hindustan Unilever Limited for background research on the topic of this paper.

I also thank Dr PK Sishodiya, Director, Institute of Miner's Health, Nagpur for according permission to use the chest radiographs dealing with silicosis and progressive massive fibrosis as well as Dr GK Kulkarni, CMO Siemens, India for providing a set of slides based on the ILO International Classification of Pneumoconiosis.

The United States Environmental Protection Agency (USEPA) calculates the air quality index (AQI) on the basis of five pollutants, viz. ozone, suspended particulate matter (SPM), carbon monoxide, SO_2, and nitrogen dioxide (NO_2). An AQI value of 100 generally corresponds to the national air quality standard for the pollutant **(Table 1)**.

ADVERSE EFFECTS OF POLLUTION

Health Effects

Adverse air quality can kill many organisms including humans. Ozone pollution can cause respiratory disease, cardiovascular disease, throat inflammation, chest pain, and congestion. The World Health Organization (WHO) estimates that about two million people die prematurely every year as a result of air pollution, while many more suffer from breathing ailments, heart disease, lung infections, and even cancer. Fine particles or microscopic dust from coal or wood fires and unfiltered diesel engines are rated as one of the most lethal forms or air pollution caused by industry, transport, household heating, cooking and ageing coal, or oil-fired power stations. Diseases caused by pollution were responsible for an estimated 9 million premature deaths in 2015—16% of all deaths worldwide—three times more deaths than from AIDS, TB and malaria combined and 15 times more than from all wars and form of violence (*Ref: Philip J, et al. The Lancet Commission on Pollution and Health. The Lancet. 19th Oct'17*).

In India, air pollution is believed to cause 527,700 fatalities a year. Studies have estimated that the number of people killed annually in the US could be over 50,000.

Table 1: Index of air pollution (air quality index).

Air quality index (AQI) values	Levels of health concern	Colors
When the AQI is in this range	Air quality conditions are	As symbolized by this color
0 to 50	Good	Green
51 to 100	Moderate	Yellow
101 to 150	Unhealthy for sensitive groups	Orange
151 to 200	Unhealthy	Red
201 to 300	Very unhealthy	Purple
301 to 500	Hazardous	Maroon

Environmental Effects

Pollution has been found to be widespread in the environment. Though increased concentration of SO_2, oxides of nitrogen, particulate matter, ozone, and smog have a direct effect on the respiratory system, it is of interest to note how they also contribute to pollution of the ecosystem in other ways. The need to control air pollutants is therefore of great importance.

The overall pollution of the ecosystem resulting from the increased concentration of atmospheric pollutants is summarized below:

- Sulfur dioxide and nitrogen oxides can cause acid rain, which lowers the pH value of soil.
- Nitrogen oxides are removed from the air by rain and fertilize land, which can change the species composition of ecosystems.
- Soil can become infertile and unsuitable for plants. This will affect other organisms in the food web.
- Smog and haze can reduce the amount of sunlight received by plants to carry out photosynthesis and leads to the production of tropospheric ozone which damages plants.
- Invasive species can out-compete native species and reduce biodiversity. Invasive plants can contribute debris and biomolecules (allelopathy) that can alter soil and chemical compositions of an environment, often reducing the competitiveness of native species.
- Carbon dioxide (CO_2) emissions cause ocean acidification, the ongoing decrease in the pH of the earth's oceans as CO_2 becomes dissolved.
- The emission of greenhouse gases lead to global warming, which affects ecosystems in many ways.

The Environmental Performance Index (EPI) gauges different countries on 25 parameters which fall into 10 categories that include environmental health, air quality, water resource management, biodiversity and habitat, forestry, fisheries, agriculture, and climate change.

Environmental Pollution in India

India ranks 123rd in pollution control according to the 2010 EPI, reflecting the strain that rapid economic growth imposes on the environment.

The WHO air quality guidelines recommend the following standards **(Table 2)**:

Table 2: The WHO air quality guidelines.	
PM$_{2.5}$	10 µg/m^3 annual means 25 µg/m^3 24-hour mean
PM$_{10}$	20 µg/m^3 annual mean 50 µg/m^3 24-hour mean
O$_3$	100 µg/m^3 8-hour mean
NO$_2$	40 µg/m^3 annual mean 200 µg/m^3 1-hour mean
SO$_2$	20 µg/m^3 24-hour mean 500 µg/m^3 10-minute mean

Source: WHO (2005). WHO Air quality guidelines for particulate matter, ozone, nitrogen dioxide and sulfur dioxide—global update 2005—summary of risk assessment. [online] Available from http://apps.who.int/iris/handle/10665/69477 [Accessed July 2018].

■ CAUSES OF ENVIRONMENTAL POLLUTION IN INDIA

Vehicular Growth in India

Air pollution and the resultant impacts in India could be broadly attributed to the emissions from vehicular, industrial, and domestic activities. Air quality has been, therefore, an issue of concern in the backdrop of various developmental activities. Due to uncontrolled urbanization in India, environmental degradation has been occurring very rapidly and causing shortages of housing, worsening of water quality, excessive air pollution, noise, dust and heat, and the problems of disposal of solid wastes and hazardous wastes. The situation in cities like Mumbai, Kolkata, Chennai, Delhi, and Bengaluru, is becoming worse year by year.

Following the trends of urbanization and population growth in Indian cities, people buying more vehicles for personal use have perpetuated an increase in vehicles that contribute to vehicular emissions containing pollutants such as SO$_2$, nitrogen oxides, carbon monoxide, lead, ozone, benzene, and hydrocarbons.

Air-borne emissions emitted from various industries are a cause of major concern. These emissions are of two forms, viz. solid particles (SPM) and gaseous emissions (SO$_2$, NO$_2$, CO$_2$, etc.). Heavy polluting industries were identified which are included under the 17 categories of highly polluting industries for the purpose of monitoring and regulating pollution from them.

The Ministry of Environment and Forests has developed standards for regulating emissions for various industries including thermal power stations, iron and steel plants, cement plants, fertilizer plants, oil refineries, pulp and paper, petrochemicals, sugar, distilleries, and tanneries.

Impressive growth in manufacturing (7.4% average over the past 10 years) is a reflection of growth trends in the fields of electronics and information technology, textiles, pharmaceuticals, basic chemicals, etc. These industries, belong to the "red category" of major polluting processes designated by the Central Pollution Control Board (CPCB), and have significant environmental consequences in terms of air emissions. The economic boom has also led to an increase in investments and activities in the construction, mining, and iron and steel sectors. This in turn, is causing a significant increase in brick-making units, sponge iron plants, and steel rerolling mills that involve highly polluting processes.

Domestic Sector: Indoor Air Pollution

A considerable amount of air pollution results from burning of fossil fuels. According to National Family Health Survey-3 (NFHS), more than 60% of Indian households depend on traditional sources of energy like fuel-wood, dung, and crop residue for meeting their cooking and heating needs. Burning of traditional fuels introduces large quantities of CO$_2$ in the atmosphere when the combustion is complete, but if there is an incomplete combustion followed by oxidation, then CO is produced, in addition to hydrocarbons.

Burning of wheat and rice straw and other agricultural residue has also contributed to loss of soil fertility, apart from causing air pollution.

Ambient Air Quality Trends in India (Figs. 1 to 4)

Annual average concentration of SO$_2$ levels are within the prescribed National Ambient Air Quality Standards (NAAQS) **(Table 3)**. During the last few years, a decreasing trend has been observed in NO$_2$ levels due to various measures taken for vehicular pollution control such as stricter vehicular emission norms. Vehicles are one of the major sources of NO$_2$ in the country. Annual average concentrations of respirable suspended particulate matter (RSPM) and SPM exceeded the NAAQS in most of the cities.

Environmental Impact

India is a fast-growing economy and has many future developmental targets, several of which are directly or indirectly linked to energy and therefore could lead to increased greenhouse gas emissions. Though the contribution of India to the cumulative global CO$_2$

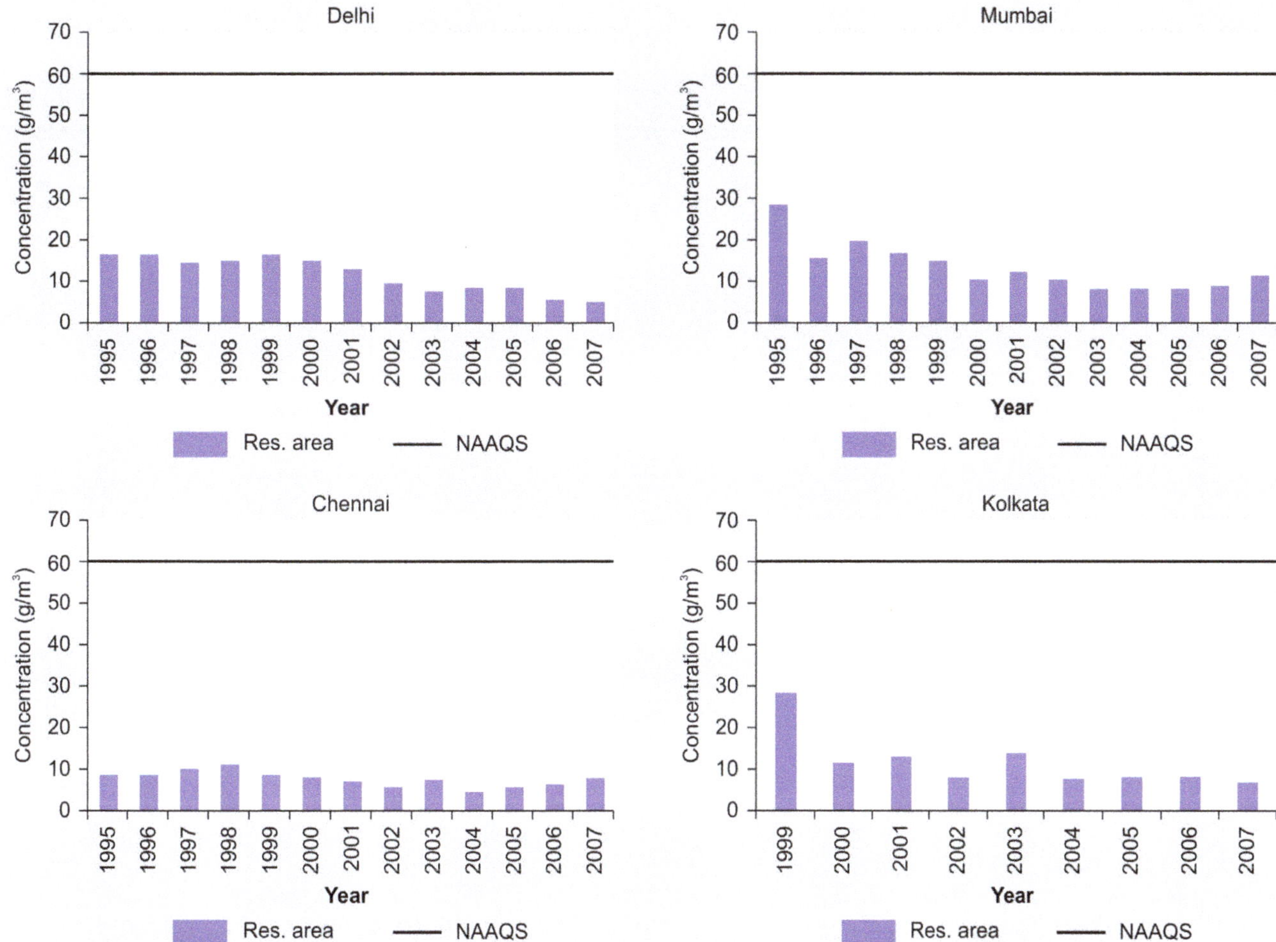

Fig. 1: Trends in annual average concentration of SO_2 in residential areas of Delhi, Mumbai, Chennai, and Kolkata. (NAAQS: National Ambient Air Quality Standards)
Source: Central Pollution Control Board, 2008.

emissions is only 5%, impacts could be severe at the local level.

Acid rain is the direct consequence of air pollution caused by gaseous emissions (CO, SO_2, and NO) from industrial sources, burning of fuels (thermal plants, chimneys of brick-kilns, or sugar mills), and vehicular emissions. The most important effects of acid rain are damage to freshwater aquatic life, vegetation, and damage to buildings and material. In India, the main threat of an acid rain disaster springs from our heavy dependence on coal as a major source of energy. Even though, Indian coal is relatively low in sulfur content, what threatens to cause acid rain in India is the concentrated quantity of consumption, which is expected to reach very high levels in some parts of the country by 2020.

Health Impact of Environmental Pollution

A study conducted by the All India Institute of Medical Sciences and CPCB in Delhi showed that exposure to higher levels of particulate matter contributed to respiratory morbidity *(Ref: Ministry of Environment and Forests Government of India. (2009). State of Environment Report India).*

Use of solid fuel (wood, animal dung, crop residue/ grasses, coal, and charcoal) exposes people to high levels of toxic air pollutants, which result in serious health consequences. NFHS found that 71% of India's urban households and 91% of rural households use solid fuels for cooking purposes.

There is a great deal of variation in the prevalence of tuberculosis (TB) according to the type of cooking fuel the

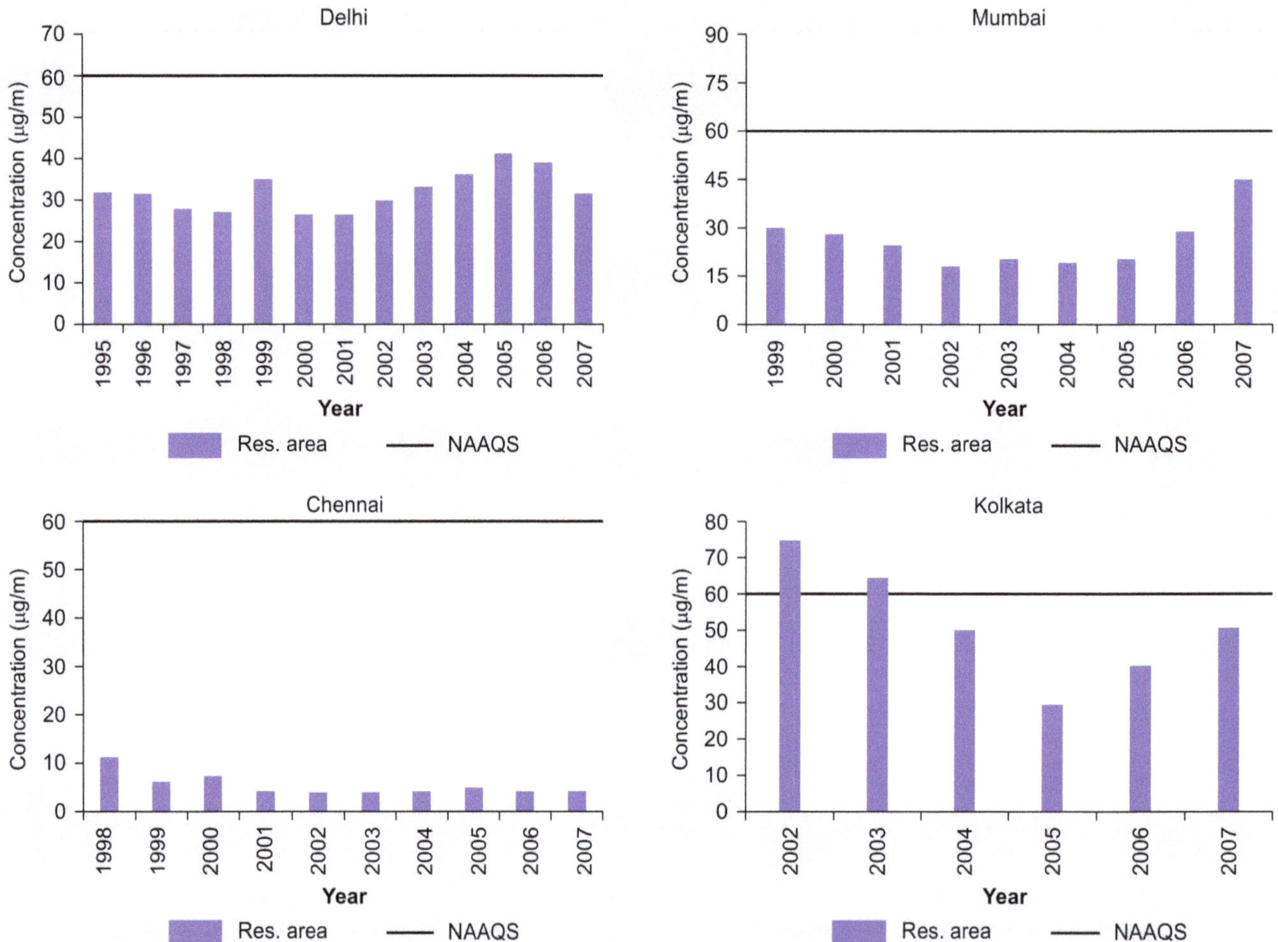

Fig. 2: Trends in annual average concentration of NO_2 in residential areas of Delhi, Mumbai, Chennai, and Kolkata. (NAAQS: National Ambient Air Quality Standards)
Note: Data for 2007 for Chennai, Kolkata, and Mumbai is the average of data available as on date.
Source: Central Pollution Control Board, 2008.

household uses. It ranges from a low of 217 per 100,000 residents (among households using electricity, liquid petroleum gas, natural gas, or biogas), to a high of 924 per 100,000 (among households using straw, shrubs, or grass for cooking). High TB prevalence is also seen amongst households using agricultural crop residue (703/100,000) or other fuels not specified.

Studies have found that besides TB, acute respiratory infections, chronic obstructive pulmonary disease, asthma, lung cancer, ischemic heart disease, and blindness can also be attributed to indoor air pollution.

Climate change may alter the distribution and quality of India's natural resources and adversely affect the livelihoods of its people. With an economy closely linked to its natural resource base and climatically sensitive sectors such as agriculture, water, and forestry; India may face a major threat because of the projected change in climate.

■ THE POLLUTION CONTROL APPROACH

Pollution control is a term used in environmental management. It means the control of emissions and effluents into air, water, or soil. Without pollution control, the waste products from consumption, heating, agriculture, mining, manufacturing, transportation, and other human activities, whether they accumulate or disperse, will degrade the environment. In the hierarchy of controls, pollution prevention and waste minimization are more desirable than pollution control.

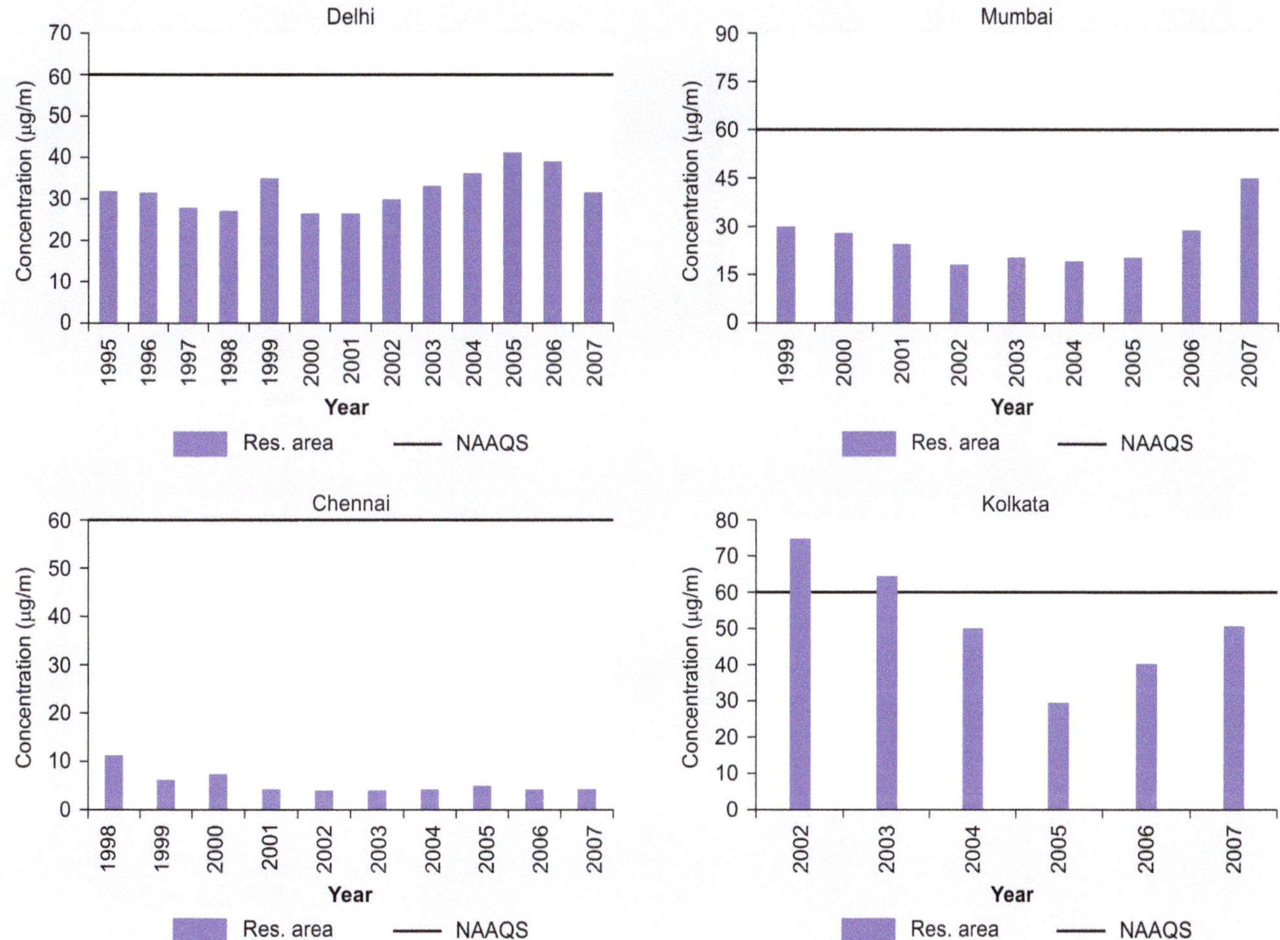

Fig. 3: Trends in annual average concentration of SPM in residential areas of Delhi, Mumbai, Chennai, and Kolkata. (NAAQS: National Ambient Air Quality Standards; SPM: Suspended particulate matter)

Note: Data for 2007 for Chennai, Kolkata and Mumbai is the average of data available as on date.

Source: Central Pollution Control Board, 2008.

Comprehensive Waste Management

Under the pollution control perspective, waste is regarded as an undesirable by-product of the production process, which is to be contained so as to ensure that soil, water, and air resources are not contaminated beyond levels deemed to be acceptable.

While the pollution control approach has achieved considerable success in producing short-term improvements for local pollution problems, it has been less effective in addressing cumulative problems that are increasingly recognized on regional (e.g. acid rain) or global (e.g. ozone depletion) levels.

The aim of a health-oriented environmental pollution control program is to promote a better quality of life by reducing pollution to the lowest level possible. Environmental pollution control programs and policies, whose implications and priorities vary from country to country, cover all aspects of pollution (air, water, land, and so on) and involve coordination among areas such as industrial development, city planning, water resources development, and transportation policies.

As environmental pollution control technologies have become more sophisticated and more expensive, there has been a growing interest in ways to incorporate prevention in the design of industrial processes with the objective of eliminating harmful environmental effects while promoting the competitiveness of industries. Among the benefits of pollution prevention approaches,

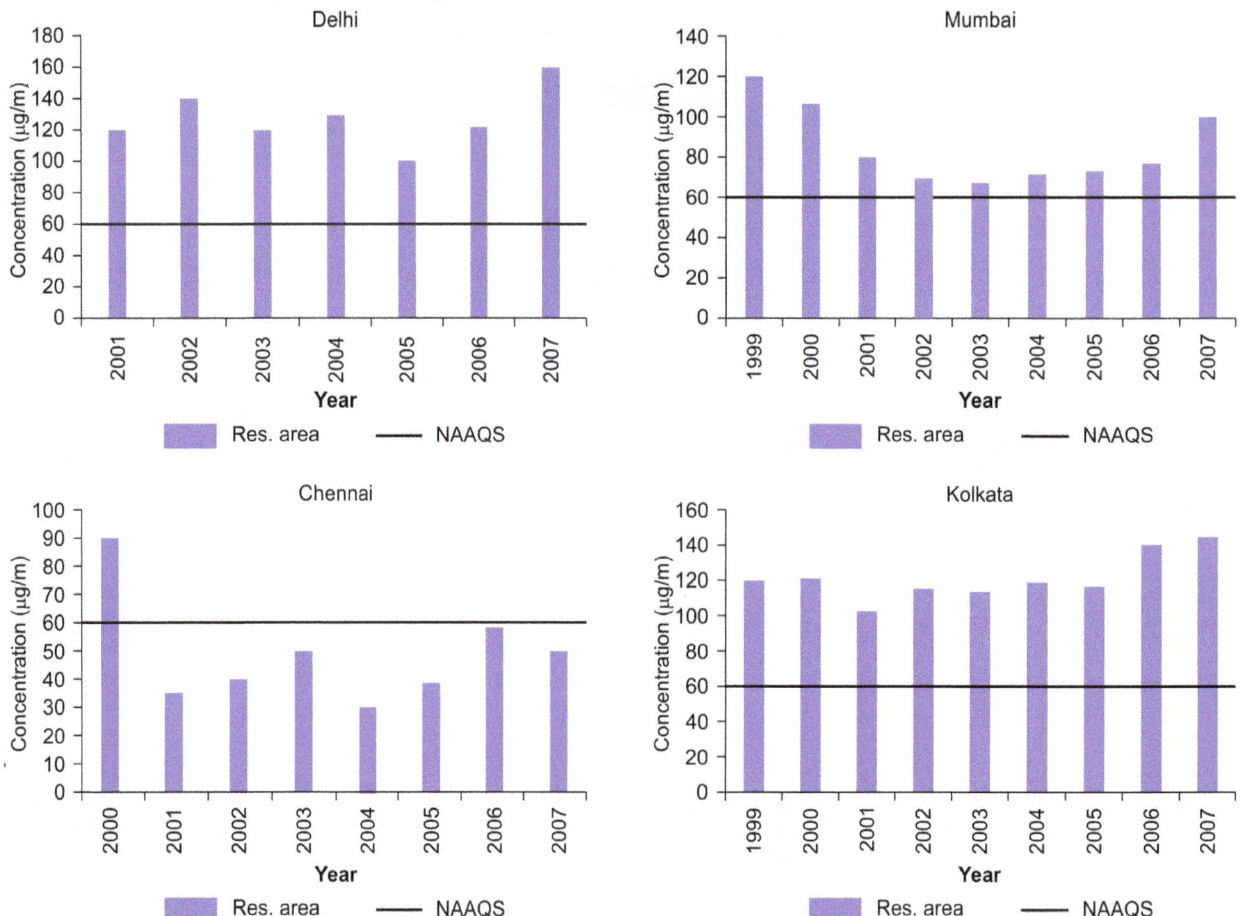

Fig. 4: Trends in annual average concentration of RSPM in residential areas of Delhi, Mumbai, Chennai, and Kolkata. (NAAQS: National Ambient Air Quality Standards; RSPM: Respirable suspended particulate matter)
Note: Data for 2007 for Chennai, Kolkata and Mumbai is the average of data available as on date.
Source: Central Pollution Control Board, 2008.

clean technologies, and reduction in the use of products or processes that lead to toxic pollutant effects would reduce worker exposure to health risks.

■ POLLUTION PREVENTION APPROACH

The pollution prevention approach focuses directly on the use of processes, practices, materials, and energy that avoid or minimize the creation of pollutants and wastes at source, and not on "addon" abatement measures. The corporate commitment plays a critical role in the decision to pursue pollution prevention.

As per the reports from the Ministry of Environment and Forests, spreading awareness and empowering people to take decisions at the local level is an effective way of dealing with the environmental problems of India.

Their decisions will enable initiatives that will benefit them as well as the local environment. It has been seen that solutions always emerge whenever governments involve people using a participatory approach to solve problems.

Community-based natural resource management initiatives, coupled with policy reforms, can prove to be an effective mechanism for improving access to, and productivity of, natural resources. The success of joint forest management and irrigation user groups in India provides enough evidence that social capital and participatory processes are as crucial to environmental protection as financial resources and development programs.

In the last few years, several measures relating to environmental issues have been introduced. They have

Table 3: Revised National Ambient Air Quality Standards (NAAQS—2009).

Schedule VII. Rule 3(3B) National Ambient Air Quality Standards, 16th Nov 2009, Ministry of Environment and Forests

| S. No. | Pollutant | Time weighted average | Concentration in ambient air | | Methods of measurement |
			Industrial, rural, and other area	Ecologically sensitive area (notified by govt. of India)	
1	Sulfur dioxide $\mu g/m^3$	Annual* 24 hr**	50 80	20 80	Improved West and Gaeke Ultraviolet (UV) fluorescence
2	Nitrogen dioxide $\mu g/m^3$	Annual* 24 hr**	40 80	30 80	Modified Jacob and Hochheiser (Na-Arsenite) Chemiluminescence
3	Particulate matter (Size less than 10 μm) $\mu g/m^3$	Annual* 24 hr**	60 100	60 100	Gravimetric TOEM Beta attenuation
4	Particulate matter (Size less than 2.5 μm) $\mu g/m^3$	8 hr* 1 hr*	40 60	40 60	Gravimetric TOEM Beta attenuation
5	Ozone $\mu g/m^3$	8 hr* 1 hr*	100 180	199 180	UV photometric Chemiluminescence Chemical method
6	Lead $\mu g/m^3$	Annual* 24 hr**	0.5 1.0	0.5 1.0	AAS/ICP method after sampling on EPM 2000 or equivalent filter paper ED-XRF using Teflon filters
7	Carbon monoxide $\mu g/m^3$	8 hr* 1 hr*	02 04	02 04	Nondispersive infrared (NDIR) spectroscopy
8	Ammonia $\mu g/m^3$	Annual* 24 hr**	100 400	100 400	Chemiluminiscence Indophenol blue method
9	Benzene $\mu g/m^3$	Annual*	05	05	Gas chromatography based continuous analyzer Adsorption and description followed by GC analysis
10	Benzo(a)pyrene particulate phase only $\mu g/m^3$	Annual*	01	01	Solvent extraction followed by HPLC/GC analysis
11	Arsenic (SO_2) $\mu g/m^3$	Annual*	06	06	AAS/ICP method after sampling on EPM 2000 or equivalent or filter paper
12	Nickel $\mu g/m^3$	Annual*	20	20	AAS/ICP method after sampling on EPM 2000 or equivalent or filter paper

*Annual arithmetic mean of minimum 104 measurements in a year at a particular site taken twice a week 24 hourly at uniform intervals.

**24 hourly or 8 hourly or 0.01 hourly monitored values as applicable shall be compiled with 98% of the time in a year, 2% of the time they may exceed the limits, but not on two consecutive days of monitoring. Note that whenever the monitoring results on two consecutive days of monitoring exceed the limit for the respective category, it shall be considered adequate reason to institute regular or continuous monitoring and further investigation.

(AAS: Atomic absorption spectrometry; ED-XRF: Energy dispersive X-ray fluorescence; GC: Gas chromatography; HPLC: High performance liquid chromatography; ICP: Inductively coupled plasma; TEOM: Tapered element oscillating microbalance)

targeted a significant increase in the capacity of renewable energy installations, improving the air quality in major cities (the world's largest fleet of vehicles fuelled by compressed natural gas has been introduced in New Delhi), and enhancing afforestation. Other similar measures have been implemented by committing additional resources and realigning new investments, thus steering economic development onto a climate-friendly path.

■ SUGGESTED READING

1. Badrinath KVS, Chand KTR, Prasad KV. Agriculture crop residue burning in the Indo-Gangetic Plains—a study

using IRS-P6 AWiFS satellite data. Current Science. 2006;91(8):1085-9.

2. Brunekreef B, Beelen R, Hoek G, et al. Effects of long-term exposure to traffic-related air pollution on respiratory and cardiovascular mortality in the Netherlands: the NLCS-AIR study. Res Rep Health Eff Inst. 2009;139:5-71.

3. Curtis L, Rea W, Smith-Willis P, et al. Adverse health effects of outdoor air pollutants. Environ Int. 2006;32(6): 815-30.

4. Health effects of outdoor air pollution. Committee of the Environmental and Occupational Health Assembly of the American Thoracic Society. Am J Respir Crit Care Med. 1996;153(1):3-50.

5. Khatri SB, Holguin FC, Ryan PB, et al. Association of ambient ozone exposure with airway inflammation and allergy in adults with asthma. J Asthma. 2009;46(8): 777-85.

6. Ministry of Environment & Forests Government of India. (2009). State of Environment Report India. [online] Available from http://www.envfor.nic.in/mef/State%20 of%20Environment%20Report_2009.pdf [Accessed July 2018].

7. Taylor-Clark TE, Undem BJ. Ozone activates airway nerves via the selective stimulation of TRPA1 ion channels. J Physiol. 2010;588 (Pt 3):423-33.

8. WHO. (2005). WHO Air quality guidelines for particulate matter, ozone, nitrogen dioxide and sulfur dioxide— global update 2005—summary of risk assessment. [online] Available from http://apps.who.int/iris/handle/ 10665/69477 [Accessed July 2018].

9. Zhao Z, Zhang Z, Wang Z, et al. Asthmatic symptoms among pupils in relation to winter indoor and outdoor air pollution in schools in Taiyuan, China. Environ Health Perspect. 2008;116(1):90-7.

CHAPTER 68

Inhalational Lung Injury

INTRODUCTION

Environmental pollution caused by smoke and the release of chemical gases, fumes and other noxious substances into the atmosphere can cause marked irritation and injury to the respiratory tract or could result in asphyxiation. Rarely, irritation and injury to the respiratory tract can occur several years after exposure, as with asbestos, an occupational hazard that not only involves asbestos factory workers, but also affects those living in the vicinity from environmental and atmospheric pollution with the asbestos fiber. Another example of a delayed prolonged effect on the respiratory and other systems related to atmospheric pollution is the Bhopal disaster following the leak of methyl isocyanate (MIC) gas from an industrial plant manufacturing a pesticide in early December 1984.

EPIDEMIOLOGY

Inhalation of smoke causing either death from asphyxiation or severe irritation of the respiratory tract constitutes the most common inhalational injury to humans. Smoke arises from fire and though domestic, industrial and other fires occur all over the world, they are most common in poor developing countries and affect far more people in these countries than in the Western countries of the world. This is because of inherent far greater fire-risks in dilapidated crowded houses and housing colonies and the comparatively poorer infrastructure which renders fire-fighting difficult and doubly dangerous. Hundreds of thousands in India and other poor developing countries of the world risk inhalation of smoke from domestic and other fires (as in unsafe cinema houses, bars, dance halls, etc.). Lung injury due to inhalation of smoke has been dealt with in greater detail at the end of this chapter.

The number of individuals exposed to dangerous pollutants in the world, particularly in India and other economically growing countries of the world such as China, Southeast Asian countries, South America and the African continent must perhaps run into several million. Why is this so? In India, the gross domestic product (GDP) per capita has increased from $1,000 in 1984 to about $2,700 in 2017 and it continues at a growth rate close to 8% per year. Rapid industrial development has contributed to this growth but it has been at the cost of great environmental degradation and a marked increase in public health risks. Chemical factories spout pollutants into the city atmosphere posing known and unknown hazards to people in the vicinity. Disaster, possibly very nearly akin to the Bhopal disaster, according to many environmentalists, waits just round the corner!

RISK FACTORS

Inhalation of smoke emanating from domestic fires to huge conflagrations as in wars, terrorist attacks, or fires in huge factories housing incendiary material are important examples. Inhalation of chemical fumes occurs particularly in poorly ventilated factories or when they escape the confines of a factory and pollute the atmosphere. Sources of occupational exposure to major chemicals causing injury to the respiratory tract are given in **Table 1**.

Factors that influence the toxic effects of chemicals include the inherent chemical toxicity of the substance, its particle size and concentration, its solubility and the duration of exposure. Water-soluble chemicals afflict the upper airways because they dissolve on reaching these sites. The less water-soluble chemical fumes reach the peripheral airways and exert maximum injury at these sites. The sources of inhalation exposure with regard to a few important noxious chemicals and gases are given in **Table 1**. The first six are examples of irritants and the last three of asphyxiants.

■ DIAGNOSIS

Inhalational injury produces either inflammation of the respiratory tract or asphyxia. Inflammation of the respiratory tract may involve the upper respiratory passage—the nose, sinuses, pharynx, larynx, trachea and the large bronchi. Inhalation injury may skip or mildly involve the upper respiratory passage and exert a major effect on the lower respiratory tract—the bronchioles, terminal bronchioles, respiratory bronchioles and the alveoli. Inflamed nasal passages, cough, hoarseness of voice, stridor may be present; rhonchi are often heard on auscultation **(Fig. 1)**.

Involvement of the lower air passages and alveoli leads to breathlessness, wheezing and crackles over the lungs on auscultation. Some chemical fumes such as ammonia, chlorine and the dreadful MIC gas in the Bhopal tragedy produce a chemical burn. This can lead to severe diffuse alveolar damage resulting in noncardiogenic pulmonary edema [acute respiratory distress syndrome (ARDS)] and severe bronchial and bronchiolar damage that over a period of time leads to bronchiolitis obliterans or severe progressive fibrosing bronchiolitis. Death can occur within a few hours or few days or the patient may be left with crippling sequelae characterized by well-marked pulmonary fibrosis with restrictive lung disease, or progressive bronchiolitis obliterans causing obstructive lung disease or a combination of both restrictive and obstructive lung disease. The extent of the injury and disease can be gauged clinically, by radiographic examination of the chest and by lung function tests. Routine spirometry, lung volumes, carbon monoxide (CO) diffusion tests will determine the presence of airways obstruction, involvement of small airways in the obstructive

Table 1: Exposure to industrial toxic gases.	
Gas	**Important sources**
1. Chlorine	Textile, paper, sewage treatment, swimming pools, chemical factories producing chlorine
2. Sulfur dioxide	Atmospheric pollution, chemical manufacture, smelting, power plants
3. Oxides of nitrogen	Air pollution, welding, agriculture, chemical and dye manufacture
4. Ammonia	Plastics, agriculture, manufacture of explosives
5. Hydrogen chloride	Manufacture of acid, fertilizer, textiles, dyes, rubber industry
6. Hydrofluoric acid	Insecticides, fertilizers, metal working, pharmaceuticals
7. Carbon monoxide	Smoke inhalation, smelters, miners, home fires
8. Hydrogen cyanide	Metallurgy, electroplating, plastics, polymethane manufactures
9. Smoke	Fires (as explained in the text) incomplete combustion of waste produces sought to be destroyed by fire

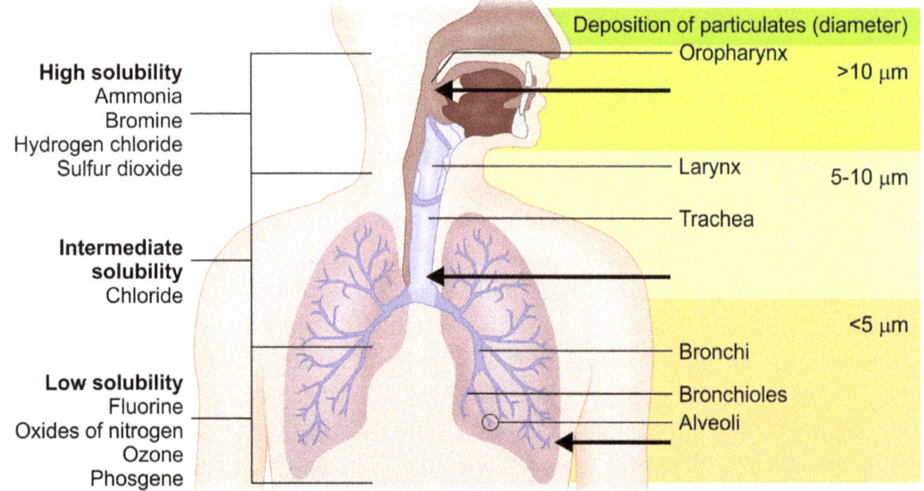

Fig. 1: Distribution of various gases and particulate matter in the respiratory tract.

pathology, as also the presence of restrictive lung disease. The lung functions will also enable the clinician to determine whether the patient has a combination of airways obstruction and restriction. High-resolution computed tomography (HRCT) of the chest (if facilities are available) will reveal more than a radiography of the chest—the nature of alveolar shadows, the presence of pulmonary edema as also the presence of air-trapping because of obstructed bronchi. The flow-volume loop will pick up large airways obstruction that may occasionally be the chief cause of breathlessness. Severe parenchymal injury to the lung in the form of diffuse alveolar damage, or ARDS will result in increasing hypoxemia necessitating not only the inhalation of oxygen but also ventilator support.

The presence of headache, dizziness, vomiting, and chest pain but with few physical findings in the chest suggests a systemic poisoning with something like cyanide or hydrogen sulfide. Cyanosis or a cherry pink color of the mucosa with a normal arterial pressure of oxygen (PaO_2) and normal O_2 saturation suggests cyanide poisoning. Hypoxemia (low O_2 saturation) with a normal PaO_2 points to CO poisoning. Both cyanide and CO poisoning are associated with a low pH and an increase in blood lactic acid.

Diagnosis of the nature of the compound inhaled is usually obvious as this is easily determined depending on how and where the poisonous gas originated, in relation to the manufacture of a particular chemical or product. At times this is difficult and may need to await the results of a careful investigation and analysis.

Some disasters may be associated with inhalation of toxic gases which injure the respiratory tract as also of asphyxiants such as smoke.

Individuals with persistent symptoms need a careful follow-up involving clinical examination, pulmonary function tests and imaging studies. Sequelae of some of the toxic irritant gases include pulmonary fibrosis which may be progressive, bronchiolitis obliterans causing obstructive lung disease or a combination of both. Severe sequelae can lead to persistent hypoxemia, varying degree of breathlessness and poor effort tolerance.

■ THE BHOPAL TRAGEDY—INHALATION OF METHYL ISOCYANATE

The Bhopal tragedy was and is one of the worst industrial accidents in history. On 2 December 1984 at 11 pm while most of the residents of Bhopal were asleep, there was a small leak of MIC gas and increasing pressure in the storage tank. Negligent events were direct contributing factors to the start of the disaster: (1) a safety device to neutralize toxic discharge from the MIC systems had been turned off; (2) a faulty valve allowed one ton of water to mix with 40 tons of MIC; (3) a refrigerating unit used to cool the MIC storage tank had been drained off its coolant for use in another part of the plant; (4) the gas flare safety system was out of order.

The pressure and heat from the marked exothermic reaction in the storage tank of MIC continued to build. At 1 am on 3 December, a loud reverberation arose as the safety valve gave way and the MIC gas escaped into the early morning air, and within a few hours the streets of Bhopal were littered with corpses of men, women, children and animals (cows, dogs) and birds. Three thousand eight hundred people died almost immediately (mostly in the slum colony adjacent to the Union Carbide factory). Estimates of the number of people killed in the first few days after the escape of MIC gas are as high as 10,000 with 15,000–20,000 premature deaths occurring in the subsequent two decades. More than 500,000 people were exposed to the gas and several epidemiological studies showed a marked increase in both morbidity and mortality in this exposed population. This is unquestionably an underestimate, as many exposed people left Bhopal soon after the tragedy, never to return and were lost to follow-up.

Immediate Respiratory Effects of Methyl Isocyanate (Tables 2 and 3)

Acute fulminant toxic chemical inflammation of the lower respiratory tract summarizes the immediate respiratory effects of MIC. These consisted of diffuse alveolar damage with noncardiogenic pulmonary edema (ARDS), pneumonitis and pneumothorax (observed in some patients). The chemical burn involved the bronchial mucosa, in particular the smaller bronchioles and the terminal and respiratory bronchioles causing an acute inflammatory bronchiolitis.

In patients with marked exposure, acute respiratory distress, severe hypoxemia and death occurred within a matter of hours. Those with lesser exposure developed ARDS, pneumonitis, bronchiolitis, increasing difficulty in breathing, and increasing hypoxemia within 24–72 hours. Some with ARDS who managed to be taken to the sparse (poorly equipped) critical care units in the city survived with ventilator support together with support to other systems.

Table 2: Early effects on the respiratory system (0–6 months) after exposure to MIC.

- Respiratory distress
- Diffuse alveolar damage, ARDS
- Pneumonitis, acute bronchiolitis
- Pneumonia
- Hypoxemia which may be severe enough to cause death
- Secondary pulmonary or bronchopulmonary infection.

Table 3: Early effects on the organ systems other than the respiratory system (0–6 months) after exposure to MIC.

Gastrointestinal system	Abdominal pain, anorexia, persistent diarrhea
Ocular	Chemosis, redness, photophobia, corneal ulcers
Psychological	Neurosis, anxiety states
Neurobehavioral	Impaired audio and visual memory, impaired vigilance and impaired response time, impaired reasoning and spatial ability, impaired psychomotor coordination
Genetic	Increased chromosomal abnormalities

Source: Broughton E. The Bhopal disaster and its aftermath: a review. Environ Health. 2005;4:6.

Table 4: Late effects on the respiratory system (6 months) after exposure to MIC.

1. Obstructive airways disease due to obliterative bronchiolitis	
Lung function tests	Airways obstruction
Imaging studies	Hyperinflated lungs on X-ray
	Air-trapping in many areas of the lung on CT chest causing a mosaic appearance of the lung fields
2. Restrictive airways disease due to pulmonary fibrosis	
Lung function tests	Restrictive pattern
Imaging studies	Pulmonary fibrosis
3. Combined airways obstruction + airways restriction	
Lung function tests	Combination of obstruction and restriction
Imaging studies	Features of air trapping, bronchial fibrosis, pulmonary fibrosis
4. Chronic hypoxemic respiratory failure or hypoxemic + hypercapnic respiratory failure in those severely afflicted.	

Late effects on the respiratory system consisted of increasing pulmonary fibrosis and airways obstruction due to obliterative bronchiolitis. Some developed more of the former, others more of the latter; many had a combination of both obstructive and restrictive lung disease as judged by imaging studies and by lung function tests **(Table 4)**.

The question that was asked soon after the tragedy was whether MIC gas was the sole toxic agent involved in the disaster. To start with, the immediate crisis was compounded by the ignorance of people and doctors as to what gas was involved and what were its immediate and long-term effects. At every turn, the Union Carbide Company which owned and ran the plant withheld scientific data from the doctors, authorities and people at large. When MIC is exposed to 200°C heat, it forms degraded MIC that contains the very deadly hydrogen cyanide (HCN). There was evidence that the storage tank temperature did reach 200°C or more. The corpses that littered the vicinity had a cherry red color of blood and of viscera at autopsy; many victims responded to the administration of sodium thiosulfate, an antidote to cyanide poisoning but not effective against MIC toxicity. Almost certainly cyanide poisoning was responsible for some of the very quick deaths occurring after escape of the overheated MIC gas.

Methyl isocyanate toxicity had far-reaching effects on other organ systems of the body which are briefly shown in **Table 5**. These include the induction of genetic chromosomal abnormalities, the effects of which may haunt the descendants of this tragedy for generations to come.

The reasons for briefly describing the genesis of the Bhopal disaster are:

- The inseparable links between the medical, human, social, moral and ethical aspects of this disaster. It is indeed incredible that the norms followed for workers and public safety by large international manufacturing companies in their own Western countries are set aside in poor developing countries. Such double standards betray a total lack of ethical, moral and social responsibility. In a settlement mediated by the Indian Supreme Court, the Union Carbide Company agreed to pay $470 million to the Indian government to be distributed to the claimants affected by this disorder as the final settlement. Edward Broughton believes that the liability of the same company in the United States would have exceeded $10 billion if a similar disaster had occurred in that country.
- Despite more stringent laws passed in India since the Bhopal disaster, many small-scale industries and large manufacturing establishments continue to produce

Table 5: Late effects on the organ systems other than respiratory system after exposure to MIC.

Ocular	Persistent watering of eyes, corneal opacities
Reproductive	Increased pregnancy loss, increased infant mortality, decreased fetal weight
Genetic	Increased chromosomal abnormalities
Neurobehavioral	Impaired associate learning, motor speed, precision

Source: Broughton E. The Bhopal disaster and its aftermath: a review. Environ Health. 2005;4:6.

toxic chemicals within city limits or just outside large heavily populated cities not only in India but in most poor developing countries of the world and in China. The world (and in particular the poorer countries of the world) has not yet learnt a lesson from the Bhopal disaster.

- The Bhopal tragedy emphasizes the dire need for improving public health infrastructure and planning for disaster management in India and other poor countries of the developing world.
- Economic growth and industrial development should not be at the cost of environmental degradation and public health risks, if a repetition of this great tragedy is to be averted.

■ OTHER CHEMICAL IRRITANTS

The effects of some important chemical irritants on the respiratory systems are now briefly described.

Chlorine

Chlorine is a soluble gas liberating chloride and oxygen free radicals when in contact with water. At low levels of exposure, it causes irritation of the conjunctiva and the mucosa of the upper respiratory passage. Higher exposure leads to pulmonary edema within 6–24 hours. Chemical inflammation of the airways leads to airflow obstruction. Breathlessness, wheezing and crackles are heard over the lungs. Imaging may reveal pulmonary edema or evidence of air-trapping. Clinical evidence of serious respiratory tract involvement (including the development of pulmonary edema) may occur 6–8 hours after exposure to the gas so that observation of the patient for a length of time is imperative.

Treatment is supportive; oxygen, nebulized salbutamol and ipratropium bromide for airways obstruction are of help. Intravenous corticosteroids are of use in patients with severe chemical injury to the airways. In some severe cases, pulmonary edema may necessitate ventilator support.

Sulfur Dioxide

Fossil fuel combustion leads to the formation of sulfur dioxide and sulfuric acid. Various industrial processes such as smelting, chemical manufacture, paper manufacture, metal refining lead to possible exposure to this noxious agent. Exposure to sulfur dioxide or fumes of sulfuric acid leads to burning of the eyes, conjunctivitis, corneal ulcers, cough, chest pain, chest tightness and breathlessness due to pharyngeal inflammation and chemical inflammation of the airways. Greater exposure leads to pulmonary edema. The chemical inflammation of the airways can lead to bronchiolitis obliterans. This leads to permanent airways obstruction and is particularly observed in smelter workers following overexposure to this agent.

Oxides of Nitrogen (NO, NO_2, N_2O_4)

Oxides of nitrogen can produce fatal respiratory injury to workers who come in contact with high concentration of this gas. Occupations at risk include welders using acetylene torches, exposure to fumes in the manufacture of dye, nitric acid and lacquers.

The most dangerous and important exposure to oxides of nitrogen occurs in silo-filler's disease. This occurs when corn is stored in silos so that it ferments. Fermented corn releases oxides of nitrogen which are strongly irritant to the respiratory system. In contact with water within the lung, oxides of nitrogen form nitric and nitrous acid. The dissociation of oxides into nitrates, nitrites and free radicals is strongly irritant to the mucosa of the airways and the lung parenchyma. Exposures greater than 150 ppm are generally fatal leading to death from pneumonia and pulmonary edema. A lesser degree of exposure leads to cough, breathlessness, tightness in the chest due to bronchiolitis and pneumonitis. An even lesser degree of exposure may just lead to irritation of the eyes, conjunctivitis and pharyngitis.

Symptoms after significant exposure may be delayed and relapses may occur after 3–6 weeks with symptoms of cough, breathlessness and tightness of the chest. Chronic bronchitis has been reported to occur in some patients.

Treatment is supportive, aerosolized bronchodilators and the use of corticosteroids for airways obstruction resulting from bronchiolitis may help.

Ammonia

Ammonia though a noxious gas is generally transported as a liquid. Fumes of ammonia in contact with water in the respiratory mucosa form a strong alkali, ammonium hydroxide. Acute irritation of the mucosa is followed by a chemical inflammation, sloughing of the mucosa of the larynx, trachea, bronchi and the smaller airways. Laryngeal edema causes stridor. Bronchial inflammation can lead to bronchiolitis and later to bronchiolitis obliterans. Parenchymal inflammation can lead to a chemical pneumonitis and ARDS. Treatment is with bronchodilators, and oxygen therapy. Intubation may be necessary to protect the airways form impending laryngeal obstruction due to progressive laryngeal edema.

Hydrogen Chloride

Hydrogen chloride (HCl) is a strong acid and when it comes in contact with the respiratory mucosa, it induces a severe inflammation of the airways. HCl exposure is encountered in the manufacture of textile, rubber, dye, and fertilizers. High levels of exposure cause airways obstruction due to mucosal edema, as also pneumonitis and pulmonary edema.

Hydrofluoric Acid

Hydrofluoric acid like other strong acids or alkalis is highly corrosive, even more corrosive than sulfuric acid or ammonia. Hydrofluoric acid is water-soluble, releases H^+ ions and has a strongly corrosive effect on the airways and lung parenchyma. There is rapid damage to the airways, parenchymal lung damage leading to pneumonia, bronchopneumonia, ARDS and death. ARDS may occur after a lapse of some hours after exposure.

■ CHEMICAL ASPHYXIANTS

Carbon monoxide, HCN, and hydrogen sulfide are examples of chemical asphyxiants which interfere with delivery and/or utilization of oxygen resulting in asphyxiation at the tissue level.

Carbon Monoxide Poisoning

Carbon monoxide is a colorless, odorless, tasteless gas produced by incomplete combustion of carbon and other organic materials. Inhalation of CO is an important cause of accidental and suicidal deaths all over the world.

Common sources of CO are car exhausts, and smoke from all types of fire. In the developing world, combustion of coal, wood and other biofuels is an important source of CO and an important cause of CO poisoning. Inhalation of methylene chloride (seen in paint strippers) can also lead to CO poisoning.

Mechanism of Toxicity

Hemoglobin (Hb) has 240 times greater affinity for CO than for oxygen. CO therefore avidly combines with Hb to form carboxyhemoglobin, thereby reducing the oxygen-carrying capacity of blood. Also, the oxygen dissociation curve shifts to the left and modifies oxygen binding sites. As a result, the affinity for remaining heme groups for oxygen is increased. The leftward shift and distortion of the oxygen dissociation curve results in a far greater tissue hypoxia than what would result from a reduced oxygen-carrying capacity of blood.

Carbon monoxide may also inhibit cellular respiration due to reversible binding to cellular cytochrome oxidase.

Clinical Features

Acute exposure leading to a carboxyhemoglobin concentration of 10% generally does not cause symptoms. Ten to thirty percent may produce headache, dyspnea and at times confusion. Symptoms are more prominent in the elderly; patients with cardiorespiratory disease are at greater risk. High concentrations of carboxyhemoglobin in the blood as after acute, prolonged or severe exposure to CO cause increasing confusion, agitation, seizures and coma. Hyperventilation, Cheyne-Stokes breathing, pulmonary edema and respiratory failure may occur. There is marked metabolic acidosis.

Neurological examination, besides revealing an altered mental state or an altered state of consciousness, is often characterized by hypertonia, hyperreflexia and bilateral extensor plantar responses. The condition is often mistaken for a brainstem infarct. Rarely, focal signs in the form of monoplegia or hemiplegia may be present.

Cardiovascular features include myocardial ischemia, and infarction, particularly in older patients with cardiovascular disease. Arrhythmias which include atrial fibrillation, ventricular asystole and various degrees of heart block can occur. ST depression and prolonged QT interval may be seen on the electrocardiograph (ECG).

Severe hypoxemia may result in a hearing loss due to ischemia to the cochlea. Acute renal failure is a known complication of severe CO poisoning, related to hypoxemic damage to renal tubule cells. Carboxyhemoglobin greater than 60% leads to coma, seizures and death from cardiorespiratory arrest. The important features of CO poisoning are listed in **Table 6**.

Diagnosis

The possibility of CO poisoning should always be kept in mind depending on the history and the situation in which the patient is discovered. The possibility of CO poisoning due to a gas leak and accidental poisoning from incomplete combustion of biofuel is often missed. Spectroscopic examination of blood for CO-Hb confirms the diagnosis. The presence of hypoxemia with low O_2 saturation in the presence of a normal PaO_2 also suggests the correct diagnosis (*see* injury due to smoke inhalation).

Delayed Effects (Table 7)

Following recovery from the effects of acute exposure to CO, delayed neuropsychiatric problems may develop insidiously over a matter of weeks. These include features of cerebral, cerebellar and midbrain damage. Cerebellar signs and spasticity are most often seen.

Impairment of higher functions may occur in the form of impairment of memory, intellectual deterioration, aggressive and abnormal behavior. Parkinsonism is a known sequel to CO poisoning.

Treatment

Treatment consists of removal of the patient from the site of exposure and inhalation of humidified 100% oxygen with a tight-fitting mask. Comatose patients, severely hypoxemic with poor respiration should be intubated and given mechanical ventilator support with 100% oxygen. Oxygen at high concentration should be continued till the carboxyhemoglobin is below 10%.

Hyperbaric oxygen if available may be used, leading to a quicker replacement of carboxyhemoglobin with oxyhemoglobin. Controlled studies have not shown a clear benefit with hyperbaric oxygen compared to endotracheal intubation and ventilator support using an FiO_2 of 100%.

Supportive treatment is important. Convulsions should be countered by intravenous diazepam. Intravenous corticosteroids and mannitol may be used for cerebral edema.

Hydrogen Cyanide

Fumes of HCN are released following combustion or pyrolysis of plastic and polyurethane. Individuals engaged in this occupation and exposed to the fumes are at grave risk of HCN poisoning. The fumes are absorbed through the skin and respiratory tract. Cyanide binds to the cytochrome oxidase, paralyzes the tricarboxylic acid cycle so that the utilization of oxygen by tissue cells and cellular respiration cease.

Clinical Features

Minor exposures (50 ppm) cause headache, tachycardia, tachypnea and tightness in the chest.

Major exposures (>100 ppm) cause dyspnea, tightness in the chest, confusion, seizures, pulmonary edema, ataxia, apnea, coma and death. Cardiac arrest, respiratory arrest and death can occur within minutes.

Diagnosis

Diagnosis rests on a history of relevant occupational or environmental exposure. The skin and blood may have a cherry pink color and a smell of almonds may be recognized by those with a good sense of smell.

Table 6: Features of acute CO poisoning.

- Headache, agitation, confusion, seizures
- Drowsiness, coma
- Cheyne-Stokes breathing
- Pulmonary edema, respiratory failure
- Metabolic acidosis
- Arterial hypoxemia with a normal PaO_2
- Spasticity, hyperreflexia, extensor plantar
- Myocardial ischemia, infarction
- Arrhythmia, atrial fibrillation, heart block, ST-T changes, prolonged QT on ECG
- Hearing loss
- Acute renal failure.

Table 7: Delayed effects of CO poisoning.

Neuropsychiatric complications:
- Changes in higher functions—intellectual deterioration, impairment of memory, aggressiveness, abnormal behavior
- Cerebral, cerebellar, midbrain damage
- Parkinsonism
- Hearing loss following ischemia to the cochlea.

The arterial blood gases show a metabolic acidosis, a normal PaO_2, a normal O_2 saturation and an increase in the blood lactate level.

Treatment

The patient should be removed from the site of exposure and given oxygen with a tight-fitting mask. If transported to the hospital alive, endotracheal intubation and ventilator support with an FiO_2 of 100% is recommended. Support to the cardiovascular and all other systems is of crucial importance.

Specific antidotes include cobalt salts (dicobalt acetate), sodium thiosulfate and sodium nitrite and hydroxocobalamin. Cobalt salts form inert salts with cyanide and constitute the treatment of choice. They are unavailable in most units.

Thiosulfate detoxifies by conversion of cyanide to thiocyanate; 12.5 g (25 mL of a 50% solution) is given intravenously over 15 minutes.

Sodium nitrite converts a portion of the Hb to the methemoglobin which binds cyanide. It is administered intravenously, 300 mg (10 mL of a 3% solution) over 3 minutes. Inhalation of amyl nitrite may be of some use.

Hydroxocobalamin—1 mole of hydroxocobalamin inactivates one mole of cyanide but on a weight-for-weight basis, 50 times more hydroxocobalamin is needed than cyanide. Concentrated hydroxocobalamin is unavailable in India and perhaps in most countries of the world. If available it is given in a dose of 5 g intravenously over 30 minutes. The dose may be repeated in severe poisoning.

Hydrogen Sulfide

Hydrogen sulfide is a colorless gas that smells of rotten eggs. The gas is found in mines and sewers so that workers in mining and with sewage may be exposed to it. It is also liberated from decomposing fish (a hazard to fishermen with decomposing fish in the hold of their boats) and from manure systems.

Mechanism of Action

It acts by inhibition of cytochrome oxidase within the cells thereby stopping cellular respiration, a mode of action similar to cyanide.

Clinical Features

Headache, drowsiness, sore throat, and blurred vision with colored halos around the light occur with lesser degree of exposure. Exposure to higher concentration leads to confusion, seizures, cyanosis, coma and death.

Treatment

The patient should be removed from the site of exposure (the rescuer must have appropriate breathing apparatus) and be given 100% oxygen through a tight-fitting mask. Intravenous sodium nitrite (as given in cyanide poisoning) is of help though its mechanism of action is not well understood.

■ SMOKE INHALATION INJURY

Smoke inhalation injury resulting from fire is an important and leading cause of death all over the world. In the United States an estimated 372,900 fires in residential buildings result in an average of 2,530 deaths, 13,125 injuries and $7 billion in property loss. Pulmonary complications following burns and smoke inhalation are responsible for close to 77% of the deaths, the majority of which are due to CO poisoning.

There is however no reliable study on the prevalence and incidence of pulmonary compilations following burns and smoke inhalation in India. It remains an incontrovertible fact that injuries caused by fire and smoke inhalation are frequent. Unfortunately, the infrastructure required to prevent and counter these accidents leaves much to be desired, and the facilities to treat the unfortunate victims need to be vastly improved.

Pathophysiology

Inhalation injury can affect the upper airway, the trachea, bronchial tree and the lung parenchyma. The site and severity of injury in the respiratory system depends on the source of the fire, the duration of the exposure to smoke, size of the particles in the inhaled smoke and the solubility of gases within the smoke.

To start with, excessive inhaled smoke within the airways is tantamount to very little oxygen within the air passages, so death could quickly occur from suffocation due to severe acute hypoxia. Direct toxic damage is also caused by the lower molecular weight constituents of smoke, because of their ability to form free radicals and reach the smaller airways and the lung parenchyma. Smoke inhalation-related injuries may also be associated with burns of the face and neck which complicate the issue, particularly in relation to management. The additional problems caused by the associated facial and neck burns are not considered in this chapter.

Smoke inhalation injury can be to the upper airway, tracheobronchial tree and the lung parenchyma.

Upper Airway Injury

The main injury to the upper airway is a thermal injury due to efficient heat exchange in the oropharynx and nasopharynx. The immediate injury results in erythema, edema and ulceration of the mucosa of the upper airway. Damage to the mucosa and its ciliary function increases the risk of bacterial infection which may persist for many weeks. The inflamed, edematous mucosa produces thick secretions which are often aspirated causing distal airway obstruction, atelectasis, infection and impaired gas exchange.

Tracheobronchial Tree

Injury to the tracheobronchial tree can be caused by the extreme heat generated by a nearby fire, but is mostly due to chemicals within the smoke. Smoke inhalation stimulates the sensory and vasomotor nerve endings resulting in the release of neuropeptides which cause bronchoconstriction, and induce the formation of nitric oxide synthase (NOS) and reactive oxygen species (ROS). Neuropeptides are responsible for causing an inflammatory response, bronchoconstriction, increased vascular permeability and vasodilation. Local cellular damage, in particular to the bronchial epithelium results, and there is a leak of proteins and fluid form the vascular compartment into the bronchioles and alveoli. This shift of protein-rich fluid results in exudate and cast formation within the airways leading to alveolar atelectasis. All of the above contribute to an increasing ventilation-perfusion mismatch resulting in progressively worsening hypoxia.

Lung Parenchyma

Injury to the lung parenchyma is characterized by atelectasis, alveolar cell damage, decrease in surfactant, loss of hypoxic vasoconstriction, an alveolar edema. There is in addition a decreased fibrinolytic activity, resulting in the deposits of fibrin within the airways. The overall result is an increasing ventilation-perfusion inequality with increasing hypoxia.

If the patient is on ventilator support, the degree of hypoxemia can be gauged by the PaO_2/FiO_2 ratio. It should be noted that damage to the lung parenchyma is a bit delayed after the initial injury. The time difference between the latter and a fall in the PaO_2/FiO_2 ratio correlates with the severity of the injury.

Systemic Toxicity

Direct systemic effects are caused by breathing toxic products formed by combustion or pyrolysis.

Carbon Monoxide

Carbon monoxide is the most common immediate cause of death following inhalation injury. It has a 200 times greater affinity for Hb when compared to oxygen. If also shifts the oxyhemoglobin dissociation curve to the left impairing both the release of oxygen to the tissues and its utilization by cell mitochondria.

Carbon monoxide poisoning should be suspected in all patients presenting with a smoke inhalation injury or in those rescued from a fire. *Pulse oximetry cannot screen for CO exposure as it does not differentiate between carboxyhemoglobin and oxyhemoglobin.* Carboxyhemoglobin levels need to be always measured with CO oximetry on arterial or venous blood.

Hydrogen Cyanide

Hydrogen cyanide is a colorless gas with the odor of almonds. Because of the high probability of its presence in smoke related to the outbreak of fire, cyanide toxicity should always be considered in victims of smoke inhalation. Treatment for cyanide toxicity is important. It should be promptly given in victims whose consciousness is depressed or those who suffer cardiac arrest or decompensation, even in the absence of laboratory confirmation.

History

Inhalation smoke injury should be suspected on a history of exposure to fire, heat, and smoke. Relevant information regarding duration and degree of exposure, exposure in an enclosed space, and a history of loss of consciousness is important.

Clinical Features

Clinical symptoms of upper airway injury include difficulty in breathing, cough, hoarseness of voice. Symptoms of lower airways injury include dyspnea, productive cough with black sputum because of the carbonaceous deposits of smoke within the airways.

Physical findings include singed nasal vibrissae, black soot in the nasal passages, oropharynx, and black carbonaceous sputum. Other physical findings of upper airway obstruction include stridor and hoarseness of voice. Upper airway obstruction may lead increased work of breathing which contributes to respiratory muscle fatigue and ventilatory failure.

Clinical features of lower respiratory tract injury include one or more of the above together with tachypnea, diminished breath sounds, rhonchi, crackles on auscultation, labored breathing with the use of accessory muscles of breathing.

Investigations

Blood should be sent for a routine blood count, creatinine, lactate level and a full toxicology screen. An arterial blood gas should be sent for CO oximetric measurement of the oxyhemoglobin saturation, the carboxyhemoglobin concentration and methemoglobin concentration. It needs to be restressed that CO oximetry is essential as standard pulse oximetry cannot distinguish between carboxyhemoglobin and oxyhemoglobin.

Imaging Studies

Chest X-ray has a low sensitivity for inhalation injury. Most patients on admission will have a normal chest X-ray to start with. Later when X-ray changes appear they invariably underestimate the degree of injury. The presence of pulmonary opacities in the initial chest X-ray always signifies severe injury and a poor prognosis.

Diagnosis

A diagnosis of smoke inhalation injury is based on the history, coupled with clinical findings in a setting of exposure to smoke. A confirmed or definitive diagnosis can be made by direct examination of the airways.

After the patient has been hemodynamically stabilized, a fiberoptic bronchoscopy allows examination from the oropharynx, larynx, trachea and the major bronchi. Bronchoscopic findings include erythema of the respiratory mucosa, blistering, ulcerations, charring, bronchorrhea and fibrin casts within the lower respiratory air passages.

Injury Severity Scoring

Bronchoscopic findings can help in predicting the risk and severity of lung injury. The Abbreviated Injury Score (AIS) grading scale using bronchoscopy correlates well with mortality as well as gas exchange.

The AIS grading of smoke inhalation injury by bronchoscopy is as follows:
- *0 (no injury):* Absence of erythema, edema, bronchorrhea or obstruction.
- *1 (mild injury):* Minor or patchy areas of erythema or carbonaceous deposits in the proximal or distal bronchi.
- *2 (moderate injury):* Moderate degree of erythema, carbonaceous deposits, bronchorrhea, or bronchial obstruction.
- *3 (severe injury):* Severe inflammation with friability, copious carbonaceous deposits, bronchorrhea or obstruction.
- *4 (massive injury):* Evidence of mucosal sloughing, necrosis, endoluminal obliteration.

Management

Management includes primarily proper airway stabilization and supportive care.

Once the airway is secured, either by endotracheal intubation or tracheostomy, treatment of systemic toxicity and airway inflammation is prime. Fluid balance and managing hypermetabolism is of crucial importance. In the late stages, recognition of ARDS should prompt appropriate management.

■ SUGGESTED READING

1. Broughton E. The Bhopal disaster and its aftermath: a review. Environ Health. 2005;4:6.
2. Miller K, Chang A. Acute inhalation injury. Emerg Med Clin North Am. 2003;21(2):533-57.
3. Mlcak RP. (2018). Inhalation injury from heat, smoke, or chemical irritants. [online] Available from https://www. uptodate.com/contents/inhalation-injury-from-heat-smoke-or-chemical-irritants. [Accessed July, 2018].
4. Niven AS, Roop SA. Inhalational exposure to nerve agents. Respir Care Clin N Am. 2004;10(1):59-74.
5. Parrish JS, Bradshaw DA. Toxic inhalational injury: gas, vapor and vesicant exposure. Respir Care Clin N Am. 2004;10(1):43-58.
6. Woodson LC. Diagnosis and grading of inhalation injury. J Burn Care Res. 2009;30(1):143-5.

CHAPTER 69

Clinical Disorders at High Altitude

■ PHYSIOLOGICAL CHANGES AT HIGH ALTITUDE

Ascent to higher altitude causes hypoxemia. The barometric pressure (P_B) at sea level is 760 mm Hg and the pressure of inspired oxygen (P_IO_2) is 150 mm Hg. With normal alveolar ventilation (VA) the partial pressure of carbon dioxide $PaCO_2 = 40$ mm Hg. Assuming that R = 1, the alveolar oxygen partial pressure (P_AO_2) is 110 mm Hg. This figure is evident from the equation

$$P_AO_2 = P_IO_2 - PaCO_2/R$$

The P_IO_2 at sea level being equal to (P_B – 47 mm Hg) × 0.21 = 150 mm Hg; where 21% being the concentration of oxygen in air breathed at sea level; 47 mm Hg being water vapor pressure.

Assuming a normal alveolar-arterial gradient of 10–15 mm Hg in a healthy individual the arterial partial pressure of oxygen (PaO_2) would be P_AO_2 – 10 mm Hg = 100 mm Hg.

As one ascends, the barometric pressure of air breathed decreases. The higher the altitude the lower the barometric pressure, the lower the P_IO_2, resulting in a proportionate decrease in the P_AO_2 and PaO_2. **Table 1** gives

Table 1: Approximate effect of reduced P_IO_2 at different altitudes.

Altitude (meters)	P_B mm Hg	P_AO_2 mm Hg	PaO_2 mm Hg
Sea level	760	150	100
1,620	620	120	70
3,500	500	95	55
8,848 (Mount Everest)	253	43	26

(P_AO_2: Alveolar oxygen partial pressure; PaO_2: Arterial partial pressure of oxygen; P_B: Barometric pressure; P_IO_2: Pressure of inspired oxygen).

an approximate effect of reduced P_IO_2 on PaO_2 at varying altitudes.

A PaO_2 of 26 mm Hg would be close to the lowest limit compatible with life, without breathing an increased concentration of oxygen. Yet there have been some amazing successful attempts at reaching the summit of Mount Everest without the use of supplemental oxygen.

■ ACUTE RESPONSE TO HYPOXIA

Hypoxia among several other effects increases the ventilatory rate, through stimulation of the peripheral chemoreceptors in the carotid and aortic bodies. The carotid body is composed of highly specialized aerobic tissue cells, which depend on mitochondrial oxidative phosphorylation for the production of adenosine triphosphate (ATP). The production of ATP is linked to oxygen consumption. Deprivation of oxygen as in hypoxemic states leads to the inability of mitochondria to produce ATP. Inhibition of mitochondrial function has been shown to stimulate afferent activity of the carotid body. Afferent nerve impulses travel via the carotid sinus nerve to reach the respiratory center in the brain; efferent discharge from the center leads to an increase in the respiratory rate.

There are two views with regard to the oxygen sensor responsible for the immediate and rapid response to hypoxia. One view holds that the oxygen sensor is mitochondrial cytochrome oxidase, which through oxidative phosphorylation transmits information to the rest of the cell. The other view holds that glomus cells within the carotid body have sensitive potassium channels, whose conductance is lowered with decreasing oxygen pressure. Perhaps both mitochondrial cytochrome oxidase and potassium ion channels act as sensors and are responsible for the sensitivity to change in oxygen pressure.

In the 1960s, Lahire and Milledge working at high altitudes in the Himalayas and Severinghaus and coworkers working in the South American high mountains with natives living at these altitudes noted that these subjects showed a diminished or blunted ventilatory response to an acute reduction in the inspired PO_2. It was uncertain whether this was related to genetic factors or whether this was an acquired trait related to exposure to chronic hypoxia. The conclusion was that the adaptive response to acute hypoxia was more due to environmental than genetic factors.

■ CHANGES IN THE PULMONARY CIRCULATION

The pulmonary circulation is a low-pressure, high-flow, and high-volume circulation which easily accommodates the whole cardiac output that passes through it, not only at rest but also at exercise. This is because of the very low vascular resistance of the pulmonary vessels compared to the high vascular resistance observed in the systemic circulation. Hypoxia observed at high altitude alters the hemodynamics of the pulmonary circulation. It causes vasoconstriction of the pulmonary vessels resulting in both systolic and diastolic pulmonary hypertension. The higher the altitude the more severe the pulmonary vasoconstriction, and the higher the pulmonary hypertension. This has been observed in several studies. Though the pulmonary vasculature is supplied by both sympathetic (vasoconstrictor) and parasympathetic (vasodilator) fibers, vascular tone is chiefly governed by the PO_2 and PCO_2 in the alveoli. A fall in the alveolar PO_2 leads to pulmonary vasoconstriction and a shunting of blood away from alveoli with a low P_AO_2 to those which have a normal P_AO_2. A rise in alveolar PCO_2 (P_ACO_2) also causes well-marked vasoconstriction of the pulmonary vessels and pulmonary hypertension, in strong contrast to dilatation of the systemic vessels when the $PaCO_2$ is raised.

Exercise at high altitude (as for example in climbers negotiating a steep slope) further increases pulmonary arterial pressure and pulmonary hypertension. The pulmonary hypertension caused by acute hypoxia lasting for just a few hours, regresses with a return to normal pulmonary artery pressures once acute hypoxia is relieved. If hypoxia continues for several weeks as in mountaineers

on a mountaineering expedition, pulmonary artery pressure does not decline quickly after return to lower altitudes or to sea level. It takes days, perhaps weeks before pulmonary vasoconstriction and muscularization of the pulmonary vessel walls regress and the pulmonary artery pressure returns to normal. Prolonged hypoxia (as in an expedition to the Himalayas) leads not only to pulmonary hypertension but right ventricular hypertrophy. The latter also regresses over time on a return to sea level.

■ EFFECTS OF LIVING AT HIGH ALTITUDE

People living at a high altitude (9,000–12,000 feet above sea level) have an increase in pulmonary artery pressure so that there is an appreciable increase in the gradient between the pulmonary artery diastolic pressure and the left atrial pressure (as judged by the capillary wedge pressure or the pulmonary artery occlusion pressure through a Swan-Ganz catheter). This may not be always evident at rest, but is promptly brought on at exercise. Chronic hypoxia in patients living at high altitude leads to increased levels of erythropoietin, which causes well-marked polycythemia. Chronic hypoxia also stimulates ventilation, thereby causing hypocapnia and a rise in arterial pH. There is also an increase in 2–3 diphosphoglycerate. The increased affinity of hemoglobin (Hb) for oxygen caused by respiratory alkalosis is balanced to an extent by the decreased affinity of Hb for oxygen caused by an increase in 2–3 diphosphoglycerate. As mentioned earlier, studies have shown that over time the increased ventilatory response to hypoxia is often blunted in people living at high altitudes.

■ CLINICAL DISORDERS OF HIGH ALTITUDE

Clinical disorders of high altitude include acute mountain sickness (AMS), high-altitude pulmonary edema (HAPE), high-altitude cerebral edema (HACE), and chronic mountain sickness (CMS). While these are generally observed at a height of 10,000 feet or greater, they may occasionally be observed at altitudes of just 8,000 feet. All these entities are of crucial importance to India for several reasons. There are a number of tourist resorts, places of tourist interest and religious temples on sites at altitudes more than 8,000 feet. These include Gulmarg, Khilanmarg, the Kolahoi glacier in Kashmir, religious sites as the Amarnath Caves (Kashmir) and Mount Kailash along Lake Mansarovar, which is at an altitude of 14,900 feet. Gangotri, another important pilgrim town on the Greater Himalayan range is at an altitude of 12,313 feet. Leh, the capital of Ladakh stands at an attitude of 11,483 feet. Tanglang La, probably the highest motorable pass travelled by lay people, tourists, and soldiers which connects Leh to Manali in Northeast India is as high as 17,469 feet.

Jawans of the Indian army live on and guard the Siachen glacier which is at an altitude of 18,875 feet. The recently fought Kargil war in which Pakistani soldiers were ferreted out successfully by Indian jawans was fought at high altitudes.

Finally, the largest numbers of climbing expeditions in the whole world are directed to reaching the formidable heights of Himalayans peaks. These include for example, Mount Everest, Mounts K2, Annapurna, Nanga Parbat, and several others.

Mountaineers also climb Alpine peaks and many of the high peaks in the Andes in South America, Kilimanjaro in Africa, as also mountain peaks in North America, Australia, and other high mountains.

Acute Mountain Sickness

Acute mountain sickness (AMS) affects healthy individuals who ascend too rapidly to high altitudes. AMS is uncommon below 2000 m but is quite common between 2000 and 3000 meters. The incidence depends on the rate of ascent and the altitude reached, the quicker the ascent and higher the altitude the greater the likelihood of AMS. Physical fitness nor youth confer protection against AMS. Obesity and heavy exertion after reaching high altitude are risk factors. The incidence of AMS has unquestionably increased with the sharp rise in tourist traffic and quicker modes of travel to high-altitude resorts and for other reasons already stated above. Among trekkers trekking to the Mount Everest base camp, the incidence was 43% at 4,300 meters and was noted to be higher in those who had flown to an airstrip at 2,800 meters compared to those who had trekked all the way up to the base camp.

Clinical Features

AMS usually occurs after 6 to 12 hours after arrival at high altitude but can occur within 1 to 2 hours or as late as 24 hours. Headache is the symptom which is required for the diagnosis of AMS by the most frequently used scoring system. However, about 5% of individuals with symptoms clearly due to AMS would be missed if headache was to be considered a compulsory symptom for diagnosis.

There is also an inability to sleep, sleep being disturbed by nightmares. Nausea, vomiting, lassitude, fatigue and malaise are often observed. There is usually no response to first-line antiemetics or analgesics. In mountaineers, a reduced or poor climbing ability is noted. This mild or benign form of AMS resolves in 3–5 days and then generally does not recur unless the individual goes on to an even higher height. In some individuals AMS takes on a very serious form and progresses to HACE. Unless promptly treated this condition is generally fatal. AMS and HACE are a continuum of one form of the same illness.

Pathogenesis

The pathogenesis of AMS is related to two factors. The trigger factor is unquestionably hypoxia due to high altitude. Yet AMS may occur 24 hours or even later after reaching a high altitude, and hypoxia should be maximum on immediately reaching a particular altitude. The reason for the delay in symptoms is therefore not easily explained. The second factor is cerebral edema. Symptoms in AMS are similar to those observed with increased intracranial pressure, notably the occurrence of headache and vomiting. Also, evidence of increased intracranial pressure has been observed in some patients with HACE. The current concept is that even in the usual AMS, subclinical interstitial pulmonary edema and a mild degree of cerebral edema are responsible for the presenting symptoms of the disease. The cerebral edema has been related to increased vascular permeability due to increased cerebral blood flow. Loss of autoregulation of intracranial pressure may well-contribute to this increase. Chemical factors may also play a role in increasing vascular permeability.

The exact pathogenesis of headache in AMS is unclear. Pain perception is present only in the large blood vessels and meninges through sensory fibers of the trigeminal ganglion, which convey pain sensation to the cortex. Connections of these pain carrying afferent fibers to vegetative centers in the brainstem can explain nausea and vomiting that accompany the headache. Possible mechanisms that stimulate pain receptors in AMS are cerebral edema or increased intracranial pressure or increased intravascular pressure leading to distension of large vessels within the skull or release of nociceptive substances. A recent sequential magnetic resonance imaging (MRI) study carried out over 24 hours showed the presence of white matter edema, as also increased inflow into the brain which preceded the formation of white mater edema.

The underlying susceptibility to AMS probably depends on the degree of hypoxia, the physiological responses of an individual to hypoxia (which need not be the same in all), and the interaction of these physiological responses with arterial inflow and venous out flow.

Prevention

Ascent should be gradual. It is advised that over 10,000 feet, ascent should not exceed 1,000 feet per day with a rest period of preferably 2–3 days. Some manifest AMS on further ascent even after the precautions; others can climb higher with lesser periods of acclimatization. If symptoms of AMS occur ascent should stop. If symptoms persist or become more severe, rapid descent to a lower altitude is advisable. Ataxia, disturbance in consciousness, lethargy, dyspnea at rest are indications for immediate descent.

Acetazolamide and dexamethasone are the two established drugs for prevention. Acetazolamide (250 mg twice daily) for several days after arrival may reduce headache, improve sleep, and reduce or abolish other symptoms. The drug may also be started as a preventive measure for AMS 2–3 days before arrival at a high altitude. Dexamethasone 4 mg, 6–8-hourly, is also of use, particularly in patients allergic to sulfa drugs. Acetazolamide and dexamethasone may well have an additive effect. Drug therapy should continue till acclimatization occurs after 2–4 days.

Treatment

Mild AMS is treated symptomatically, headache being relieved by paracetamol or by the use of nonsteroidal anti-inflammatory drugs such as ibuprofen. Acetazolamide and dexamethasone are the drugs to use if symptoms are bothersome or for rapidly evolving symptoms.

Oxygen at 1–3 L/minute given through nasal prongs effectively relieves symptoms and can serve as an alternative to descent. It is generally prescribed for 24 to 48 hours.

Hyperbaric Therapy

Portable light weight (<5 kg) manually inflated hyper-baric chambers are common in the West in mountain clinics and high altitude resorts. By increasing barometric pressure, hyperbaric bags can simulate a descent of 2500 m or more. Oxygen may be used in the chamber for increased effectiveness. We are not aware of any such facility in mountain resorts in India.

If features of HACE or HAPE develop, imminent descent is imperative.

High-Altitude Pulmonary Edema (HAPE)

In most individuals, AMS is a nuisance which resolves on its own in a few days. In a small minority of individuals ascending to high altitude, a potentially lethal complication is high-altitude pulmonary and/or HACEs. The frequency depends on the rate of ascent, the altitude reached, and the rest periods at lower level altitudes to allow for acclimatization. It is less likely to occur in those already living at higher altitudes compared to "lowlanders". Its prevalence ranges from less than 0.2% when an altitude of 4,000–5,000 m is reached in more than 3 days to 7% if this altitude is reached in a single day ascent.

Individuals who have experienced HAPE are at greater risk of developing high-altitude problems on a repeat ascent. Individuals who are acclimatized to high altitudes (for example, soldiers stationed at an altitude of 17,500 feet) lose their acclimatization when they descend to sea level. They remain at risk for HAPE or HACE if they are once again posted at that altitude. The crucial point to remember is that athletic fitness or prowess in no way influences or affords protection from HAPE. Men and women at all ages may succumb though younger individuals seem more at risk than others.

Clinical Features

Symptoms typically occur in young individuals who have ascended to a high altitude quickly (without a period of acclimatization) and who exert unduly or are very active on arrival. Symptoms of AMS may precede HAPE, but not necessarily so. Initial symptoms are breathlessness and cough. The cough is initially dry, then productive, the patient expectorating frothy sputum, often tinged with blood. Breathlessness increases rapidly and the patient shows evidence of central cyanosis. Tachycardia, tachypnea, and later hypotension occur. Auscultation reveals crackles starting at the bases and then involving the whole of both lungs. The jugular venous pressure is elevated. Palpation reveals a right ventricular heave, while auscultation reveals an accentuated pulmonary compo-nent of the second heart sound. Dependent edema may be present. The whole scenario may evolve with frightening rapidity, often within a matter of a few hours. Death occurs from gross pulmonary edema, severe hypoxemia, the patient often lapsing into coma towards the end.

Pathogenesis

It is now accepted that HAPE is not due to left ventricular failure, the pulmonary artery occlusion pressure being always reported as normal.

The accepted pathogenesis is that HAPE is caused by severe, quickly evolving hypoxic pulmonary vasoconstriction causing severe pulmonary hypertension. Catheter studies on the right heart have shown mean pulmonary pressures ranging from 35 mm Hg to 115 mm Hg. The hypoxic pulmonary vasoconstrictive response is uneven within the lungs. In areas where the vasoconstrictive response is very severe, the alveoli (in these areas) are protected from pulmonary edema. In areas where the pulmonary vasoconstriction though present is less marked, the increased blood flow is associated with pulmonary edema. Edema in these areas may be due to several causes—increased intracapillary pressure, flow-related damage to capillary walls, and sheer stress damaging capillary walls. Increased permeability of capillary endothelium due to kinins or cytokine release may also play a role.

It has however been shown that some mountaineers with severe hypoxic pulmonary hypertension at high altitudes do not develop HAPE. Studies suggest that other factors may contribute to the development of HAPE. These include an inflammatory pathogenesis, reduced sodium and water reabsorption by the hypoxic alveolar epithelial cells, and as already mentioned above, an unevenness of the pulmonary vasoconstriction within the pulmonary vascular bed.

Prevention

The prophylactic use of nifedipine 20 mg twice daily prior to ascent and then 20 mg thrice daily has been shown to reduce the incidence of HAPE. The mean pulmonary artery pressure is reduced. Surprisingly, nifedipine is of no use in the prophylaxis of AMS.

Inhaled β_2-agonists are also believed to reduce the risk of HAPE.

Treatment

The following are the principles of management:

- Recognition of the problem in its incipient stage. A dry cough and breathlessness portend disaster if the significance of these symptoms is not promptly realized.
- Immediate descent to a lower altitude.
- While arrangements for the above are made, supplemental oxygen should be administered at a high flow rate through a mask with a reservoir bag, so as to allow a fraction of inspired oxygen (FiO$_2$) more than 90%.
- Nifedipine 20 mg sustained release every 12 hours can be given both as preventive and treatment. Tadalafil 10 mg twice daily every 12 hours is also given both as preventive and treatment. Salmeterol 125 μg inhaled 12 hourly is administered as a preventive, but not for treatment.
- The use of intravenous (IV) furosemide in a titrated dose, to increase urine output and help reduce pulmonary edema may be of some help.
- Some well-equipped mountaineering expeditions include a portable hyperbaric chamber. If available, it should be used while awaiting arrangements for quick descent.

High-Altitude Cerebral Edema

High-altitude cerebral edema (HACE) in its early stage is characterized by persistent headache, nausea, vomiting, and is indistinguishable from AMS. In fact some patients progress from AMS to HACE with or without associated pulmonary edema. The occurrence of blurred vision and ataxia is a warning of a potentially lethal, quickly-evolving cerebral edema. Truncal ataxia (ataxia on sitting) is often a prominent symptom. Absence of concurrent or preceding headache does not exclude the diagnosis of HACE. Confusion, hallucinations, and obtundation progressing to an unconscious state occur. Plantars are often extensor and the fundus on examination reveals papilledema. There may be associated features of HAPE. If not promptly recognized and treated death preceded by coma is inevitable.

Pathophysiology

The pathophysiology is the same as that of AMS which when present may graduate in HACE. HACE is characterized by more severe hypoxia which accounts for greater progression. There is an increase in intracranial pressure, visible cerebral edema, and a leak in the blood-brain barrier with hemosiderin deposits in the brain.

Treatment

- Prevention as in AMS in the use of acetazolamide 125–250 mg every 12 hours and dexamethasone as in AMS.
- Swift descent to a low altitude or to sea level is (as in HAPE) of crucial importance. HACE often occurs in remote high altitude areas where immediate descent may not be feasible. Early recognition is therefore imperative, patients being evacuated to a lower altitude before they are too ill and unable to assist in their descent.
- Supplemental oxygen should be given as explained under HAPE at a flowrate of 6–8 L/min.
- Dexamethasone 8–12 mg, 4–6-hourly intravenously or intramuscularly is given in the hope of reducing cerebral edema. Dexamethasone is a critically important rescue drug and should be given at the first suspicion of HACE. The drug works well when given early, improves the patient's condition and his ability to help in the descent. Symptoms can recur if the drug is stopped and descent has not materialized.
- Mannitol IV 150–300 mL given as a quick infusion (if available) may also help.
- Portable hyperbaric chamber if available should be used while awaiting arrangements for descent.

Chronic Mountain Sickness

Chronic mountain sickness affects residents at a high altitude. It was first described by Carlos Monge who reported polycythemia in those living at high altitude in the Andes (Monge's disease).

Chronic mountain sickness is more common in males and occurs generally in middle and later life. Its main features are severe polycythemia with Hb concentration more than 20 g/dL and with hematocrits as high as 80%. The cause is chronic hypoxia operating over a long period of many years.

Patients generally have neuropsychiatric symptoms, consisting of headache, dizziness, inability to concentrate, fatigue, and poor effort tolerance. Symptoms characteristically disappear on descent to sea level, but reappear on a return to high altitude.

In severe CMS, the lips and mucosa appear cyanosed (because of the marked increase in reduced Hb), the conjunctiva shows marked congestion and the fingers are clubbed. Florid signs are particularly observed in Andes Indians who have the highest prevalence rate of CMS.

Milder forms of CMS (in those residing at not very high altitudes) may have few or even no symptoms, the problem being suspected in residents at high altitude who are discovered to have polycythemia. Patients with mild disease bear a close resemblance to patients with chronic obstructive pulmonary disease with hypoxemia and secondary polycythemia.

Treatment

The clinical features improve if those severely afflicted were to shift residence to sea level. But for many residing at high altitudes this is not practical. These patients should have repeated phlebotomies to lower the hematocrit if possible to less than 50% and the Hb less than 16 g/dL. This provides relief from many of the neuropsychiatric symptoms observed in severe cases. Supplemental oxygen is also of help.

The long-term use of respiratory stimulants such as medroxyprogesterone has been advocated as an alternative to phlebotomy. Acetazolamide is not as effective as in AMS, but may be used to increase O_2 saturation during sleep and perhaps reduce the hematocrit. The role of sildenafil and of newer drugs used for the reduction of pulmonary hypertension is yet to be evaluated.

■ SUGGESTED READING

1. Bartsch P, Mairbaurl H, Maggiorini M, et al. Physiological aspects of high-altitude pulmonary edema. J Appl Physiol. 2005;98:1101-10.
2. Basnyat B, Murdoch DR. High-altitude illness. Lancet. 2003;361(9373):1967-74.
3. Luks AM. Travel to high altitude with pre-existing lung disease. Eur Respir J. 2007;29(4):770-92.
4. Luks AM, Swenson ER, Bartsch P. Acute high-altitude sickness. Eur Respir Rev. 2017;26(143):16009.
5. Sartori C, Allemann Y, Duplain H, et al. Salmeterol for the prevention of high-altitude pulmonary edema. N Engl J Med. 2002;346:1631-6.
6. Singh I, Roy SB. High altitude pulmonary edema: Clinical, hemodynamic, and pathologic studies. In: Hegnauer A (Ed). Biomedical Problems of High Terrestrial Elevations. Springfield, Va: Federal Scientific Technical Information Service; 1962. p. 108.
7. Swenson ER, Bartsch P, Bailey DM. Acute Mountain Sickness and High-altitude Cerebral Oedema. In: Swenson ER, Bartsch P (Eds). High Altitude Human Adaptation to Hypoxia. New York: Springer; 2014. pp. 379-404.
8. Voelkel N. High-altitude pulmonary edema. N Engl J Med. 2002;346:1606-7.
9. Walmsley M. Continuous positive airway pressure as adjunct treatment of acute altitude illness. High Alt Med Biol. 2013;14:405-7.

Drug-induced Lung Injuries

CHAPTER 70

Adverse Drug Reactions on the Lung

■ INTRODUCTION

Almost all drugs which are therapeutically effective can produce adverse effects, some more than others. One is reminded of Osler's saying: "If all drugs in the pharmacopoeia were thrown into the sea, it would be bad for the fish and good for man". The pharmacopoeia has increased by geometric progression since Osler's time. More so today than in earlier years, the saying is a reminder to all physicians to use drugs only when indicated (easier said than done) with due circumspection and with a keen awareness of their adverse effects.

A large number of drugs produce adverse effects on the lungs and it is impossible to detail each of them in this chapter. Adverse reactions may involve the airways, the lung parenchyma, the pleura, the pulmonary circulation, and the mediastinum. Drugs can also cause a systemic adverse reaction, the reaction within the lung being just a part of this reaction. An example is drug-induced systemic lupus erythematosus (SLE) or drug-induced vasculitis which also involves the lung.

This chapter will go on to state the importance of recognizing an adverse drug-induced reaction on the lung and the difficulties in diagnosis; it then briefly gives the mechanisms involved in these adverse reactions. The patterns of clinical presentation of adverse reactions are then described, followed finally by adverse reactions caused by certain important frequently used individual drugs.

■ IMPORTANCE OF RECOGNIZING AN ADVERSE DRUG REACTION ON THE LUNG

Recognition is important for several reasons. These are as follows:

- It prevents further unnecessary diagnostic tests and further unnecessary use of extra drugs. Stopping the drug and observing the reversal or persistence of suspected adverse reactions would be the right approach.
- Recognizing the incriminating drug and stopping it would prevent further damage to the lung.
- Some adverse lung reactions to drugs are treatable; this can only happen if they are correctly recognized.

■ DIFFICULTIES IN DIAGNOSIS

Diagnosis of drug-induced lung disease even if one were keenly aware of this entity can be difficult for the following reasons (**Table 1**):

- Drug-induced lung toxicity may mimic clinical features of pulmonary involvement from the underlying disease.
- An important drug-induced lung toxicity is pneumonitis. An immunocompromised patient may develop pneumonitis due to an infective agent. There are no distinguishing features clinically or radiologically between these two forms of pneumonitis. The importance of excluding an infective etiology before considering drug-induced lung toxicity cannot be overstressed. Unfortunately, this may not always be possible.

Table 1: Diagnosis of drug-induced pulmonary toxicity.

- Awareness of possible pulmonary toxicity in related to drug use
- Pattern or nature of lung toxicity and whether it is associated with the drug in use
- Compatible clinical, lung function, and imaging features
- Exclusion of other pathologies in particular infective etiologies. Bronchoalveolar lavage (BAL) study is necessary in most cases
- Measurable effect of drug withdrawal

- Ill individuals are often given a number of drugs each of which may have potential adverse effects on the lung. To determine causality in relation to a specific drug may be impossibly difficult.
- A wrong diagnosis of drug-induced lung toxicity can have an adverse effect on the patient's recovery just because an effective and important drug is withdrawn when it should have been continued.

■ MECHANISM OF DRUG-RELATED LUNG TOXICITY (TABLE 2)

Underlying mechanisms are as follows:

- Adverse effect on the airways causing smooth muscle contraction, bronchospasm, and dyspnea.
- Increase in endothelial permeability resulting in pulmonary edema.
- Drug induced inflammation through a drug metabolite or drug + haptene; the inflammation could involve the lung parenchyma, the airways, or the pleura.
- Increased fibrinogenesis which can lead to pulmonary fibrosis, bronchiolitis obliterans, pulmonary hypertension, and veno-occlusive disease; the pathology and clinical features depending on the site of fibrinogenesis with resulting fibrosis.
- Severe bleeding within the lungs or pleural space caused either by anticoagulants or in rare instances by a drug-induced capillaritis.

Table 2: Nature and site of drug-induced lung toxicity.

- Parenchymal injury:
  - Hypersensitivity pneumonitis
  - Eosinophilic pneumonia
  - Diffuse alveolar injury
  - Granulomatous inflammation
  - Organizing pneumonia
  - Diffuse alveolar hemorrhage
  - Pulmonary fibrosis
- Airway injury:
  - Acute bronchospasm
  - Upper airways obstruction
  - Obliterative bronchiolitis
  - Cough
- Pleural injury:
  - Pleural effusion
- Injury to the pulmonary circulation:
  - Pulmonary hypertension
  - Obstruction to the pulmonary circulation through various causes
- Drug-induced systemic lupus erythematosus (SLE)
- Neuromuscular disorders

■ DRUG-INDUCED ADVERSE EFFECTS ON THE LUNG

Adverse Effects on the Lung Parenchyma

Hypersensitivity Pneumonitis

Hypersensitivity pneumonitis can be caused by a number of drugs, the important ones being nitrofurantoin, methotrexate, sirolimus, and gold.

Hypersensitivity pneumonitis can occur acutely as is seen with methotrexate or gold toxicity or it could be subacute as with adverse effects related to nitrofurantoin and sirolimus.

Systemic features include fever, malaise, and arthralgias. Respiratory symptoms which accompany or follow systemic features are dry cough with breathlessness. Pneumonitis is often bilateral though one lung may be more involved than the other. Severe forms of hypersensitivity pneumonitis as in methotrexate toxicity can lead to acute respiratory failure.

Radiography of the chest shows multiple shadows, the mid-zones, and bases being more involved. High-resolution computed tomography (HRCT) of the chest reveals multiple streaky linear interstitial shadows, intralobular shadows with ground-glass opacities.

The more acute cases often show areas of alveolar consolidation with air bronchograms; the alveolar shadows may be focal, diffuse or rarely, lobar in distribution.

The clinical and imaging findings are in no way specific for lung-induced toxicity. Similar findings occur with diverse lung infections. It is vital to exclude an infective etiology, particularly in patients who are immunosuppressed because of their background disease or because of immunosuppressant therapy or because of both. Bronchoalveolar lavage (BAL) study to detect a possible infectious etiology in addition to the clinical and imaging findings is almost always necessary in patients who have no sputum.

Histopathological confirmation through a trans-bronchial or thoracoscopic biopsy is usually not necessary. Biopsy studies when done show interstitial inflammation with a mononuclear infiltrate, the pathology resembling that of nonspecific interstitial pneumonia.

Treatment consists of withdrawal of the drug. Corticosteroids are unquestionably effective and should be used in the presence of breathlessness, hypoxia, and diffuse lung involvement. Most physicians would use corticosteroids on any patient who is symptomatic from interstitial pneumonia. Complete recovery ensues after drug withdrawal. The drug in question should never be exhibited again as drug toxicity towards the lung can be even more violent. This is particularly so with reference to methotrexate.

Diffuse Alveolar Damage

Diffuse alveolar damage (DAD) is a dangerous form of drug toxicity involving the lungs. It occurs acutely or subacutely and is a complication following the use of antineoplastic drugs in multidrug chemotherapeutic regimes. The condition is often termed as the "chemotherapy lung". Drugs incriminated in causing this adverse reaction are bleomycin, mitomycin C, busulfan, cyclophosphamide, chlorambucil, and melphalan. Many other antimitotic drugs are believed to have the potential to cause DAD. These include antimetabolites like azathioprine, methotrexate, and 6-metacaptopurine. Others in the category are the newer nitrosoureas like etoposide and the taxanes tyrosine kinase inhibitors such as gefitinib and imatinib, and the granulocyte monocyte colony-stimulating factors (so often used to counter severe leucopenia following the use of antimitotic drugs).

Diffuse alveolar damage is characterized by dyspnea, cough, and diffuse infiltrates which on radiographic examination of the chest cause a diffuse haze, and on computed tomography (CT) scan diffuse bilateral ground-glass opacities. In its most severe form, DAD manifests as acute respiratory distress syndrome (ARDS) with respiratory distress, increasing hypoxemia and total white-out lungs. Patients with solid tumors and a high tumor load are at risk after chemotherapy (particularly the first chemotherapy). They may develop the tumor lysis syndrome where lysis of tumor cells can result in DAD and even multiorgan failure.

The differential diagnosis of drug-induced DAD is from fluid overload, left ventricular failure, transfusion-related lung injury, alveolar hemorrhage, and infections. Infections could be bacterial, viral, fungal, or parasitic; opportunistic infections are especially important in patients with mitotic disease who are on antimitotic drugs.

Biopsy is generally not possible as these patients are very ill. Histopathology determined from autopsy studies shows varying degree of cellular inflammatory exudate, DAD, alveolar edema, and hyaline membrane formation.

Treatment is supportive. Ventilator support is often necessary. Corticosteroids may be used, but the response is unpredictable. The offending chemotherapeutic agent should never be used again.

Eosinophilic Pneumonia

Eosinophilic pneumonia is a classic and generally easily recognizable complication of drug therapy. The drugs known to cause eosinophilic pneumonia are minocycline, sulfa drugs, nonsteroidal anti-inflammatory drugs (NSAIDs), antiepileptics (like carbamazepine and phenytoin), antidepressants, and a few others. Eosinophilic pneumonia is characterized by fever, cough, breathlessness, eosinophilic pulmonary infiltrates, and peripheral eosinophilia. A BAL study is useful as the BAL fluid contains an excess of eosinophils.

The condition may be mild or even asymptomatic, being discovered on radiographic examination as a peripheral shadow which disappears after drug withdrawal, in 2–4 weeks (**Fig. 1**). On the other hand, the condition may be severe with diffuse pulmonary infiltrates causing dyspnea and respiratory failure. Eosinophilic pneumonia may be accompanied by an eosinophilic pleural effusion. The more serious forms of eosinophilic pneumonia are sometimes observed following use of minocycline and occasionally following use of nitrofurantoin.

A few patients (generally on minocycline or anticonvulsants), in addition to eosinophilic pneumonia, develop a severe cutaneous drug rash together with systemic symptoms probably related to the eosinophilic

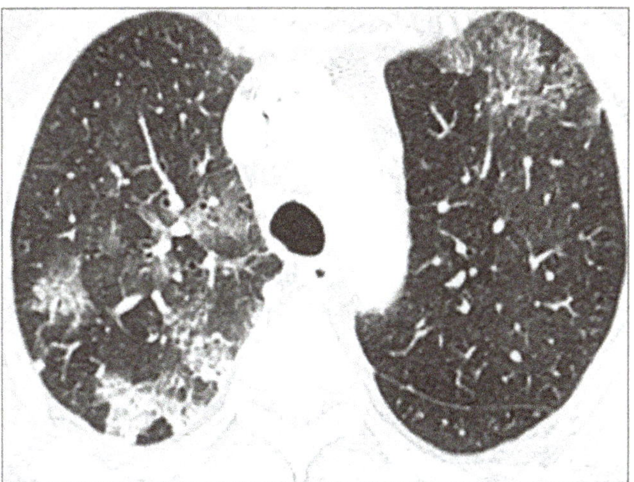

Fig. 1: Eosinophilic pneumonia following a sulpha drug. Computed tomography chest shows bilateral ill-defined areas of subpleural and peribronchovascular ground-glass densities posteriorly in right upper lobe and anteriorly in left upper lobe. The patient had well-marked eosinophilia. The shadows disappeared after stopping the drug.

involvement of other organ systems. This is the drug rash with eosinophilia and systemic symptoms (DRESS) syndrome. The syndrome should be promptly recognized; the offending drug should be stopped and treatment with corticosteroids instituted. The outcome of drug-induced eosinophilic pneumonia is good if promptly recognized and the offending drug is withdrawn. Corticosteroids hasten resolution and should always be used in symptomatic patients with diffuse pulmonary infiltrates.

Granulomatous Infiltrative Lung Disease

This is a rare pulmonary reaction observed with a few drugs, notably interferon α, β, etanercept, methotrexate, and sirolimus. The granulomatous inflammation manifests as micronodular or linear pulmonary infiltrates, which may be associated with hilar and mediastinal adenopathy. The picture bears a resemblance to sarcoidosis. The serum angiotensin-converting enzyme (SACE) level may be elevated. Transbronchial biopsy shows a granulomatous lesion suggesting the diagnosis.

Organizing Pneumonia

Organizing pneumonia (OP), also called bronchiolitis obliterans with OP is an uncommon reaction to drugs. It has been reported after treatment with amiodarone, nitrofurantoin, statins, and interferon α, β. The disease manifests as single or multiple opacities within the lung. The opacities may be migratory. Clinical, radiological, and histopathological features are the same as in idiopathic OP. OP responds well to drug withdrawal and corticosteroid therapy.

Diffuse Alveolar Hemorrhage

Diffuse alveolar hemorrhage (DAH) is characterized by bleeding into the alveoli. This causes dyspnea and when severe results in hypoxemic respiratory failure. Hemoptysis, at times exsanguinating, is often present, but not always so. A sharp drop in hemoglobin is observed. BAL studies show blood-stained fluid with hemosiderin-laden macrophages. DAH is seen in following:

- Use of anticoagulants, abciximab, fibrinolytic agents, clopidogrel, and sirolimus
- Drug-induced severe thrombocytopenia, e.g. following use of abciximab
- A capillaritis occurring in isolation or as part of a drug-induced micropolyangiitis as following use of penicillamine and hydrazaline.

Treatment: Besides drug withdrawal, severe DAH requires respiratory support. Pulsed doses of intravenous (IV) methyl prednisolone 0.5 g IV daily for 3 days are helpful when bleeding is related to capillaritis. Bleeding related to coagulation defects needs appropriate replacement of clotting factors, and that related to thrombocytopenia needs infusion of platelet concentrates.

Pulmonary Fibrosis

Pulmonary fibrosis is most often seen as a delayed reaction to antimitotic drugs. The drugs proven to cause pulmonary fibrosis are bleomycin (the most frequent cause), as also busulfan, chlorambucil, cyclophosphamide, and nitrosoureas: carmustine (BCNU) and lomustine (CCNU). Besides drugs used in oncology, the one other major drug known to result in pulmonary fibrosis is amiodarone.

Drug-induced pulmonary fibrosis can develop acutely with rapidly evolving fibrosis within the lung, or soon after drug therapy, or develop insidiously so as to manifest several months or even years after drug therapy.

Clinical features include progressive breathlessness, cough, and dry velcro crackles at bases. Severe fibrosis as with bleomycin toxicity or in a few patients with amiodarone toxicity can cause crippling breathlessness and hypoxic respiratory failure.

Chest radiography shows basal interstitial shadows. HRCT shows a reticulonodular pattern and subpleural fibrosis with honeycombing at the bases. Fibrosis induced by cyclophosphamide has a predilection for the apices with retraction of the chest wall over the upper lobes. Drug withdrawal is imperative. A varying degree of improvement with corticosteroids is observed if the problem is detected early. Advanced pulmonary fibrosis (the condition being undetected or detected late), shows no response to steroid therapy. Lung transplant is an option to be considered in these patients.

Pulmonary Edema

Pulmonary edema as a manifestation of drug toxicity is due to drug-induced increased capillary permeability. Drugs incriminated include antimitotic drugs docetaxel and gemcitabine; pulmonary edema occurs during or soon after use of these antimitotic agents. Pulmonary edema has also been observed after the use of salicylates, interleukin-2, high doses of IV beta agonists or following blood transfusion or transfusion of blood products [transfusion-related acute lung injury (TRALI)]. Drugs used for ovarian stimulation for purpose of in vitro fertilization can lead to dangerous pulmonary edema due to a pronounced capillary leak (ovarian hyperstimulation syndrome).

Clinical manifestations are cough, breathlessness, and in severe cases hypoxemic respiratory failure. Imaging appearances are those of diffuse bilateral shadowing as is seen with any form of pulmonary edema.

Treatment consists of drug withdrawal, use of oxygen, and in severe cases ventilator support.

Adverse Effects on Airways

Acute Bronchospasm

The three most common drugs causing acute bronchospasm are aspirin, NSAIDs, and beta blockers. Although acute bronchospasm with severe breathlessness can occur without warning in an individual who is not asthmatic, more often than not it occurs in those who have asthma or chronic obstructive pulmonary disease. These drugs should therefore be avoided in asthmatics. The triad of nasal polyposis, with nasal allergy, asthma often difficult to control, and intolerance to aspirin or NSAID is an established entity. Bronchospasm after inadvertent use of aspirin or NSAID in asthmatics may occur within minutes or after a few hours. If may be severe enough to cause death from asphyxia.

Beta blocker-induced bronchospasm in asthmatics may also cause severe airways obstruction which may be resistant to β_2-agonists because of the prevailing β-blockade.

Upper Airways Obstruction

Angiotensin-converting enzyme (ACE) inhibitors are known to occasionally cause angio-edema with upper airways obstruction. This may occur at any time in the course of therapy. Angio-edema results in swelling of the tongue and back of the throat with an obstructed upper airway.

Anaphylaxis from any drug to which a patient is severely allergic can cause upper airways obstruction together with severe bronchospasm and even seizures.

Treatment consists of promptly securing the airways, use of adrenaline, antihistamine, corticosteroids, and the use of resuscitative measures and supportive care.

Bronchiolitis Obliterans

Bronchiolitis obliterans is reported to be a rare complication following the use of penicillamine in rheumatoid arthritis. It causes progressive dyspnea and cough. Physical examination may be normal or there may be scattered auscultatory high-pitched squeaks or crackles. Chest radiography shows hyperinflated lungs. HRCT shows clear evidence of air trapping with a mosaic appearance. The pathology consists of narrowing of the smaller bronchioles through lymphocytic infiltration of the walls and fibrosis. Drug withdrawal should be prompt; use of corticosteroids may help.

Cough

Angiotensin-converting enzyme inhibitors produce a troublesome dry cough in about 30% of patients using the drugs. Angiotensin II receptor antagonists can also cause cough, but less frequently than the ACE inhibitors. Cough usually occurs within a month of therapy, but can occur much later as well. The pathogenesis is not clear. It is not generally associated with airways obstruction. Stopping the drug abolishes cough. It takes 2–3 weeks for symptoms to abate completely, though in some patients cough may persist for as long as few months.

Adverse Effects on the Pleura

Drugs causing an eosinophilic pneumonia described earlier can also cause an eosinophilic pleural effusion.

A pleural exudate may accompany the pulmonary toxicity of amiodarone, methotrexate, and nitrofurantoin.

Ergot compounds and methysergide may cause well-marked bilateral pleural thickening and fibrosis leading to fibrothorax, which may evolve gradually over months or years. Increasing dyspnea is the presenting clinical feature. Pleural pain may be accompanied by a pleural rub. Imaging studies (best visualized on CT) show extensive pleural thickening with underlying areas of rounded atelectasis. Lung function studies show a restrictive pattern.

Adverse Effects on the Pulmonary Circulation

Diffuse alveolar hemorrhage has been dealt with earlier. Pulmonary hypertension was the dreadful effect observed following the use of the anorectic drug aminorex. It took several years before this dangerous toxic effect was realized.

Newer anorectic drugs fenfluramine and dexfenfluramine also cause pulmonary hypertension.

Pulmonary veno-occlusive disease is a rare condition characterized by obliteration of pulmonary venules. It causes pulmonary edema and later, pulmonary hypertension. Progressive dyspnea and pulmonary congestion in the absence of cardiomegaly are the main features. The disease has been reported following use of a number of cytotoxic drugs, following radiation, or following marrow transplant.

Acrylate glue used to obliterate intracranial arteriovenous fistulas in the brain or elsewhere may spill into the systemic circulation and then go on to plug several pulmonary vessels, causing chest pain and dyspnea.

In the same manner, cement injected to stabilize a vertebral body involved in an osteoporotic fracture or fracture from metastasis or multiple myeloma, can result in pulmonary embolism.

Use of silicon injection for breast enlargement or for changing body shape can also cause vascular damage to the pulmonary circulation and result rarely in alveolar hemorrhage.

THE DRUG-INDUCED SYSTEMIC LUPUS ERYTHEMATOSUS SYNDROME

The SLE syndrome is known to occur after the use of some drugs, the most common being isoniazid, hydralazine, procainamide, and diphenylhydantoin. Interferon and tumor necrosis factor-α (TNF-α) antibody have also been reported to do so. The incidence of pleuropulmonary symptoms is high with drug-induced SLE, whereas renal and neurological involvement is rare. Antibodies to histones are believed to be present in drug-induced SLE. Withdrawal of the offending drug leads to a disappearance of SLE.

NEUROMUSCULAR ADVERSE EFFECTS

Aminoglycosides, muscle relaxants, neuroleptics, corticosteroids, and opiates either inhibit the neural drive or induce a neuromuscular blockade, or cause peripheral neuropathy or a myopathy. Hypoventilation with hypercapnic respiratory failure may follow.

SPECIFIC DRUGS

The drugs briefly discussed below are rather arbitrarily chosen. They however are in frequent use and therefore their adverse effects need to be always kept in mind.

Nitrofurantoin (Fig. 2)

This drug is very frequently used for treatment of urinary tract infection and as prophylaxis against urinary tract infection in certain circumstances. Even though adverse effects on the lung are rare (<1%), they should be recognized as and when they occur.

Two forms of lung toxicity occur. The first is an acute hypersensitivity pneumonitis, the clinical and radiological features of which have been already described. Pleural effusion may accompany the pneumonitis. Systemic symptoms in the form of fever, chest pain, arthralgia, and occasionally a macular rash may be present in association with cough and dyspnea. Peripheral eosinophilia is present in most cases.

The second form is one which is often missed. It can occur after months while on therapy and is characterized by cough and breathlessness on exertion. Systemic features and peripheral eosinophilia are generally absent. Chest radiography shows interstitial infiltrates; occasionally, patchy opacities in peribronchovascular distribution are observed. Antinuclear antibodies may be present in the chronic form.

The prognosis is good for hypersensitivity pneumonitis if the drug is withdrawn. The chronic form of pneumonitis may persist in a number of patients even after drug withdrawal. Corticosteroids may help, but their effect is not predictable.

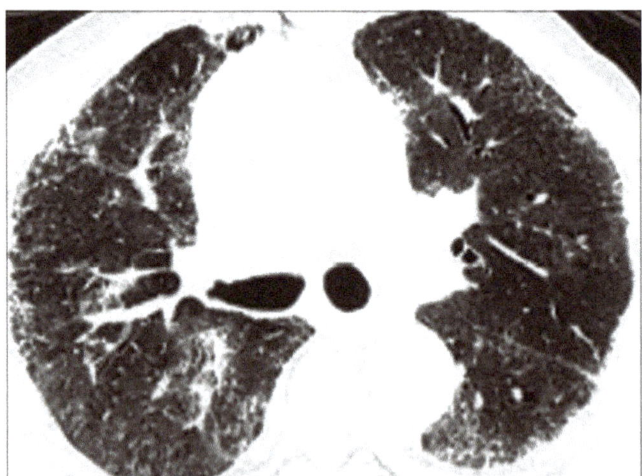

Fig. 2: Nitrofurantoin toxicity. Computed tomography chest shows ill-defined peribronchial areas of air-space opacification with ground-glass densities and mild prominence of the bronchi bilaterally.

Aspirin (Salicylates)

Severe aspirin-bronchospasm has already been described. Another adverse effect often missed is the occurrence of noncardiogenic pulmonary edema. This only occurs when salicylate levels are very high, generally more than 40 mg/dL, as in individuals who have taken an overdose of aspirin with a suicidal intent or in older individuals who have dosed themselves for long and perhaps indiscriminately on salicylates for effective pain control. The clinical features are confusion, tachypnea, auscultatory crackles more marked over the bases, together with metabolic acidosis and respiratory alkalosis. Chest radiography shows the presence of pulmonary edema. A lack of awareness will lead to a missed diagnosis or a late diagnosis. The combination of metabolic acidosis + respiratory alkalosis should always arouse suspicion of salicylate intoxication. Treatment consists of forced alkaline diuresis and supportive care. Pulmonary edema recedes once salicylate levels decline.

Sulfasalazine

Fever, rash and pneumonitis can occur as side-effects of this drug. A number of these patients present with the clinical syndrome of pulmonary infiltration and eosinophilia. Clinical improvement occurs after cessation of the drug.

Rarer pulmonary complications of sulfasalazine include non-specific interstitial pneumonia, organizing pneumonia, granulomatous lung disease. Very rarely pleural effusion may occur.

Nonsteroidal Anti-inflammatory Drugs (NSAIDs)

Several NSAIDs (ibuprofen, naproxen, diclofenac) have been reported to cause pulmonary infiltrates with eosinophilia. Resolution of the infiltrates follows withdrawal of the drug. In rare instances, if the infiltrates still worsen corticosteroids generally help.

Leflunomide

Leflunomide used in RA rarely causes interstitial pneumonia. Pneumonitis typically occurs within the first 20 weeks of therapy and may occur after stopping medication. The clinical presentation is with cough and breathlessness. HRCT of the chest shows reticular shadowing, ground glass shadows, bilateral nodular opacities and areas of consolidation. Corticosteroids should be used promptly; resolution generally results. Since leflunomide has a hepatobiliary circulation it has a long half-life, cholestyramine (8 g/day for 3 days) can be used to hasten its elimination.

Leflunomide is also associated with the appearance of accelerated progression of rheumatoid nodules within the lung. These may cavitate and may be associated with fever and cough. Withdrawal of the drug generally leads to resolution of the lung lesions.

Amiodarone (Fig. 3)

Amiodarone is perhaps the most frequently used antiarrhythmic drug today. Its adverse effects involve the eye, the liver, the thyroid gland, the skin, and most important of all, the lung. Pulmonary toxicity occurs in 5–15% of patients and is the major reason for drug withdrawal. Several forms of amiodarone lung toxicity are observed. The commonest adverse reaction in the lung is an interstitial pneumonia starting and progressing slowly after months of drug therapy. The higher the maintenance dose the greater the risk. Maintenance doses of 400 mg/day or more carry greater risk. The clinical features are cough, breathlessness, auscultatory crackles over lower lobes, restrictive lung function, and basal interstitial lesions on imaging studies.

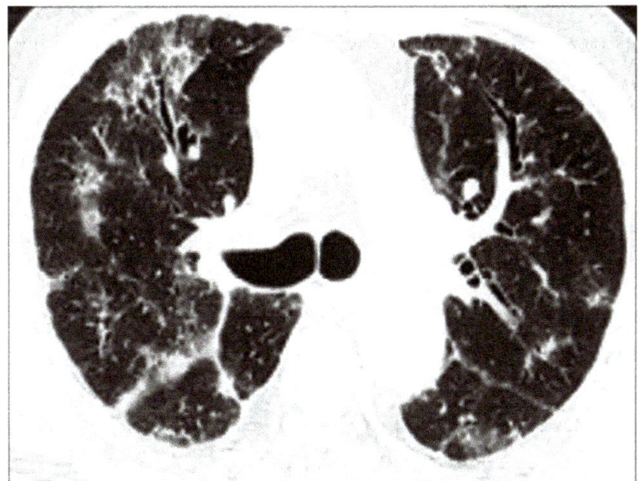

Fig. 3: Amiodarone toxicity. Computed tomography chest reveals ill-defined subpleural, reticular and peribronchovascular interstitial opacities with associated ground-glass densities. This patient was on amiodarone for several months and came with the history of increasing breathlessness. Pulmonary functions revealed a restrictive ventilatory pattern.

The second form of amiodarone toxicity is *an acute reversible pneumonia* in which one or more pneumonic patches in the lung are associated with fever, cough, chest pain, breathlessness, leukocytosis, and a raised erythrocyte sedimentation rate (ESR).

The third is the hyperacute life-threatening form producing the clinical and imaging features of ARDS. This form is rare, generally occurs after cardiac surgery when high doses of IV amiodarone are given to counter arrhythmias during and after surgery. It also occurs when high IV doses of the drug are given over several days in patients with cardiac disorders (most often acute myocardial infarction) to counter dangerous recurrent arrhythmias. We have seen this toxicity develop within 4–7 days of drug administration. The lung injury is perhaps aggravated in patients on ventilator support, particularly patients on large tidal volume, and high FiO_2. The ARDS picture may resolve or it may go on to a crippling irreversible pulmonary fibrosis, causing death. Occasionally, progressive pulmonary fibrosis occurs as an adverse reaction without the patient having experienced the acute drug toxicity just described. Amiodarone has also been reported to cause the clinical and radiological features of OP.

The usual slowly progressive chronic interstitial pneumonia caused by amiodarone is manifested on chest radiography by asymmetrical interstitial infiltrates, most marked over lung bases. In acute pneumonia there are both interstitial and alveolar shadows. The hyperacute form is characterized by bilateral fluffy shadows, which progress to the usual radiological appearance of white-out lungs seen in ARDS.

Organising pneumonia: When amiodarone produces the adverse effects of OP, radiological appearances take the form of infiltrates, nodules, or alveolar opacities that may be migratory in nature.

Eosinophilic pneumonia: A rare adverse effect of amiodarone on the lung is acute or chronic eosinophilic pneumonia. Clinical features are similar to those observed in idiopathic acute and chronic eosinophilic pneumonia. Treatment consists of withdrawal of the drug and the use of corticosteroids.

Diffuse alveolar hemorrhage: This again is a rare complication of amiodarone toxicity. It generally occurs within the first few days or months after starting therapy.

Clinical features consist of an acute onset of cough, fever, dyspnea and at times hemoptysis. Imaging studies show diffuse bilateral glass opacities with areas of alveolar consolidation. Confirmation of the diagnosis is by study of the BAL fluid which show large numbers of hemosiderin laden macrophages positive for Prussian blue staining.

Pulmonary nodules or masses: Solidary and multiple pulmonary nodules have been attributed amiodarone in a number of case reports and case series. In some patients stopping amiodarone and using prednisolone resulted in resolution of these nodules.

Gallium scans are positive in pulmonary toxicity following amiodarone and as mentioned earlier, lung function tests show restriction with a reduced CO diffusion.

■ PATHOLOGY AND RISK FACTORS

Pathology

The histopathology is that of a nonspecific interstitial pneumonia, characterized by a mononeuclear cell infiltrate, type II cell hyperplasia, interstitial edema and fibrosis. The presence of lipid laden foamy macrophages in the alveoli is a characteristic feature in all patients exposed to amiodarone. The foamy appearance is due to amiodarone-phospholipid complexes and is also seen in patients taking the drug in the absence of lung toxicity.

Pathogenesis

A direct toxic effect on the lung is believed to be the cause of interstitial pneumonia. A possible hypersensitivity is suggested by patients who had histopathological features of hypersensitivity pneumonitis.

Risk Factors

Risk factors include a daily dose > 400 mg/day, duration of therapy > 2 months, increased patient age, thoracic or nonthoracic surgery and pulmonary angiography. In a retrospective analysis, patients over 60 years of age, and those on amiodarone for 6–12 months carried the highest risk for drug toxicity. Pulmonary toxicity occurs more in relation to the total cumulative dose than in relation to serum drug levels. Hence, cordarone toxicity generally occurs 6–12 months after the initiation of therapy. There are however rare exceptions when severe progressive lung toxicity can set in within two to three weeks of therapy, particularly if large doses have been administered.

Diagnosis

The usual forms of pulmonary toxicity are generally recognizable provided the clinician is aware of their occurrence.

The principal features that help establish a diagnosis are:

- Increasing cough, dyspnea in a patient taking > 200 mg/day of the drug for more than 6 to 12 weeks
- Imaging features of ground glass opacities and reticular shadows on chest X-ray and HRCT chest
- Exclusion of heart failure clinically and on investigation and an absence of radiological improvement following diuresis produced by frusemide
- Exclusion of other lung diseases
- Clinical and radiological improvement after the withdrawal of the drug.

A lung biopsy is the confirmatory gold standard for diagnosis. It is rarely necessary.

The difficulty arises in recognizing the acute toxicity characterized by bilateral interstitial and alveolar opacities ultimately indistinguishable from ARDS. The difficulty is compounded in the presence of a critical illness following cardiac surgery or because of a primary cardiac problem. The differential diagnosis is between pulmonary edema due to left ventricular failure, pulmonary infection, and amiodarone toxicity. If good diuresis after furosemide produces no changes in the clinical and radiological picture, left ventricular failure is unlikely. Clinical examination and echocardiographic studies also help in the diagnosis of left ventricular dysfunction. It is indeed difficult to exclude nosocomial infection in these patients. Also, a patient may grow organisms from the endotracheal aspirate and yet have acute amiodarone toxicity. Presence of evolving fibrosis always points to amiodarone toxicity.

Once amiodarone toxicity is strongly suspected the drug should be withdrawn. This is particularly important if the acute or hyperacute forms of pulmonary toxicity are considered likely. Mere stoppage of the drug is not sufficient for resolution of the toxic effects on the lung, because the half-life of the drug is as long as 60 days. Corticosteroids 40–60 mg/day are given till resolution is observed and then slowly tapered over 3–4 months, else

pulmonary toxicity may return because of the long half-life of the drug.

Mortality is high in the hyperacute form or in patients with ARDS who progress to crippling pulmonary fibrosis. Overall mortality is believed to be around 10%.

Two less commonly used drugs considered below are gold and D-penicillamine; both used in the treatment of rheumatoid disease. D-penicillamine is also used in the treatment of Wilson's disease.

Oral and Parenteral Gold

Both oral and parenteral gold can cause pulmonary toxicity. The most common manifestation is acute hypersensitivity pneumonitis, but occasionally OP is also observed. Pulmonary toxicity generally occurs within 6 months of therapy. Clinical features include cough, breathlessness, and a skin rash; peripheral eosinophilia may also be present. Chest radiography shows bilateral diffuse reticular infiltrates. Drug withdrawal together with the use of corticosteroids is effective.

Features of gold-induced pneumonitis should be differentiated for underlying rheumatoid arthritis (RA) induced ILD. The chest X-ray in gold induced pneumonitis generally involves the upper lobes while that in RA generally involves the lower lobes. Fever, skin rash, eosinophilia as also occasionally liver cell dysfunction and proteinuria may be observed due to gold toxicity. In patients with fever and lung opacities without eosinophilia the possibility of infection should be kept in mind and excluded.

Fortunately, gold is rarely used today so that pulmonary toxicity following gold is not frequently observed.

D-penicillamine: This drug, like gold, is very rarely used today. It serves as an illustration of possible pulmonary toxicity encountered in clinical practice. Lung toxicity attributed to D-penicillamine takes two forms.

1. Obliterative bronchiolitis, which has been briefly described earlier and which is reported to occur only in patients with rheumatoid arthritis.
2. Pulmonary renal syndrome which resembles Goodpasture syndrome, only antiglomerular basement membrane antibodies are absent. Patients developing pulmonary renal syndrome have acute respiratory distress, diffuse intra-alveolar hemorrhage, and hemoptysis. Treatment is with corticosteroids the use of immunosuppressants like cyclophosphamide or azathioprine and the use of plasmapheresis.

Infliximab and Etanercept

These are monoclonal human antibodies directed against TNF-α. Excessive production of the latter is responsible for inflammatory reactions central to the evolution of a number of diseases, such as rheumatoid arthritis, ulcerative colitis, and Crohn's disease. Both infliximab and etanercept are capable of producing long-lasting remissions in severe forms of the above diseases. These drugs however have serious side-effects that can pose a danger to life.

Adverse Effects

Infection

A variety of infections have been noted. Infections are more common in patients with underlying COPD and when monoclonal antibodies are used together with glucocorticoids and other immunomodulatory drugs. An important and common infection is pneumonia due to the usual bacterial organisms but also at times caused by opportunistic infections such as Listeria monocytogenes, fungal infection, cytomegalovirus infection. In developing countries where tuberculosis is endemic, infection due to Mycobacterium tuberculosis would probably head the list of infections caused by these drugs. It is imperative to screen the patient carefully for underlying tuberculosis before using these drugs. They should not be used when there is a history of tuberculosis in the recent past, or if the tuberculin skin test is strongly positive. Tuberculosis when it occurs does so within weeks or months of starting therapy, suggesting reactivation of tuberculosis rather than fresh infection. Both pulmonary and extrapulmonary tuberculosis may occur and may be difficult to treat. Chemoprophylaxis with isoniazid or with isoniazid and rifampicin needs to considered in special circumstances.

Drug-induced ILD

Drug-induced ILD is an accepted complication of TNFα inhibitors, particularly, particularly in older individuals over 65 years in age and in those with pre-existing ILD. Drug withdrawal and use of corticosteroids result in improvement in most cases, but progression and death does occur in a small minority.

Granulomatous Lung Disease

Lung toxicity characterized by granuloma formation both necrotizing and non-necrotizing without evidence of mycobacterial or fungal infection has been reported in a number of case reports . Symptoms consist of fever, cough and dyspnea. Imaging features reveal single, multiple or cavitory nodules. The drug should be discontinued.

Antimitotic Cytotoxic Drugs

There has been a profusion of new and newer antimitotic cytotoxic drugs used as chemotherapy against cancer, solid tumors, lymphomas, and hematological malignancies. It is well-nigh impossible to keep track of their adverse effects including toxic effects on the lungs. Their use and the recognition of side effects on various organ systems including the lungs belong chiefly to the field of oncology, in particular to the medical oncologist. Problems that arise following chemotherapy should be jointly managed by the oncologist, the pulmonologist and the intensivist. The following section briefly describes the adverse effects on the lungs of a few commonly used antimitotic cytotoxic drugs.

Bleomycin (Figs. 4 and 5)

Bleomycin is used in chemotherapeutic regimes for a number of malignancies, particularly hematological malignancies. The drug is known to cause pulmonary fibrosis, the incidence of this toxicity being 5%. The incidence is 15% if subclinical toxicity as judged by lung function tests and HRCT is also taken into account. Though

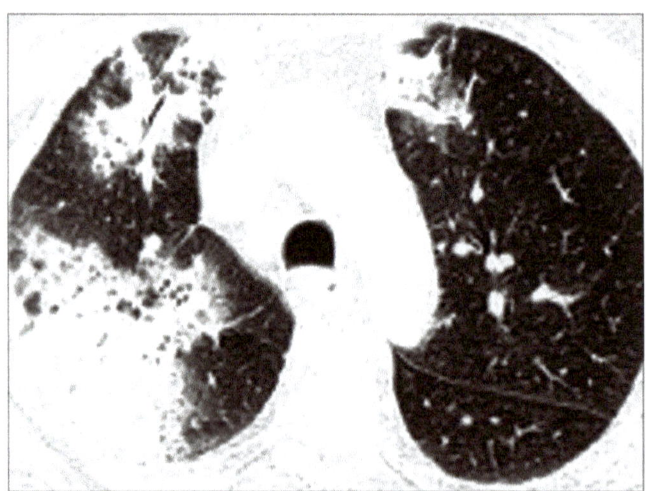

Fig. 4: Bleomycin toxicity. Computed tomography chest reveals ill-defined areas of subpleural and peribronchovascular air-space opacification with air-bronchograms representing an organizing pneumonia. Bleomycin can also give rise to well-marked bilateral interstitial pulmonary fibrosis.

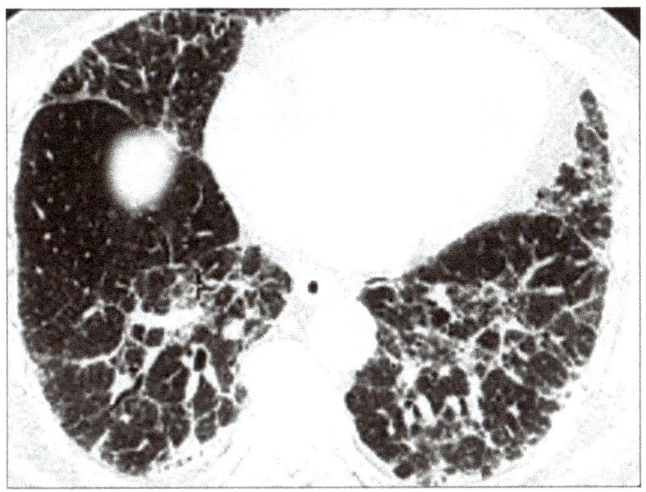

Fig. 5: Bleomycin toxicity. High-resolution computed tomography (HRCT) chest demonstrates thickening of the peribronchovascular and subpleural interstitium as a result of interstitial fibrosis induced by bleomycin.

lung fibrosis is the chief toxic effect, acute hypersensitivity pneumonitis may also be occasionally observed.

There are certain important risk factors governing the occurrence and severity of pulmonary fibrosis. These are age more than 70 years, rapid infusion instead of slow infusion of the drug, total dose of the drug received, the use of supplemental oxygen, and multidrug regimens. Although toxicity can occur with low doses, chances of toxicity increase with increasing dosage. Clinical features of pulmonary fibrosis include cough and increasing breathlessness. Auscultation reveals basal crackles. Severe fibrosis leads to hypoxemic respiratory failure. Chest radiography reveals diffuse interstitial infiltrates with small lung volumes. CT chest reveals subpleural fibrosis, interstitial thickening with fibrosis extending upwards to involve the greater part of the lungs. Alveolar shadows occur if the drug produces a hypersensitivity pneumonitis. CT changes may be seen even when the chest radiography is normal. Lung functions show a restrictive lesion with impaired CO transfer.

The mortality with bleomycin toxicity is around 10%. Patients who have received a large total dose have a higher mortality, severe fibrosis being associated with a mortality as high as 50%.

Treatment involves discontinuation of the drug, use of corticosteroids, and avoiding supplemental oxygen. Chest radiation therapy should not be given as a treatment for malignant disease of the breast or lung. Even with improvement in the lung condition, respiratory symptoms may persist to a lesser extent together with some degree of impaired lung function.

Cyclophosphamide

Cyclophosphamide is widely used to treat a variety of malignancies and autoimmune disorders. Pulmonary adverse effects are interstitial pneumonia and pulmonary fibrosis. The latter may be progressive, particularly when higher doses are used. Some patients with cyclophosphamide toxicity develop upper lobe fibrosis and pleural thickening with indrawing of the upper chest. The histopathology is characterized by interstitial edema, interstitial cellular infiltrates, alveolar damage, and fibrosis. The prognosis is generally poor; corticosteroids may offer some relief.

Methotrexate (Figs. 6A and B)

Methotrexate, besides being used in the treatment of lymphomas, leukemias, and other malignancies, is frequently used in the treatment of inflammatory disorders, particularly rheumatoid arthritis.

The most dangerous complication is hypersensitivity pneumonia termed as "methotrexate lung". Risk factors include its use in combination chemotherapy, some combinations being reported to be associated with a high incidence of methotrexate toxicity. "Methotrexate lung" is a subacute illness developing over a few weeks and is characterized by fever, malaise, dry cough, and breathlessness. Auscultatory basal crackles are often heard. The chest radiograph shows diffuse bilateral reticulonodular alveolar shadows. Peripheral eosinophilia may be present. Occasionally, there is progressive interstitial fibrosis. Overall mortality is approximately 10%.

Transbronchial lung biopsy reveals extensive infiltration with lymphocytes and loosely formed granulomas. BAL studies show the presence of T-helper cells and occasionally T-suppressor cells.

The drug should be promptly omitted. Reintroduction of the drug after recovery can cause a fatal relapse of hypersensitivity pneumonitis. The response to corticosteroids is good. There is a suggestion that methotrexate toxicity is immunologically mediated rather than due to a direct toxic effect on the lung.

Rituximab

Rituximab is a β-cell depleting anti-CD20 monoclonal antibody that has been primarily used for the treatment

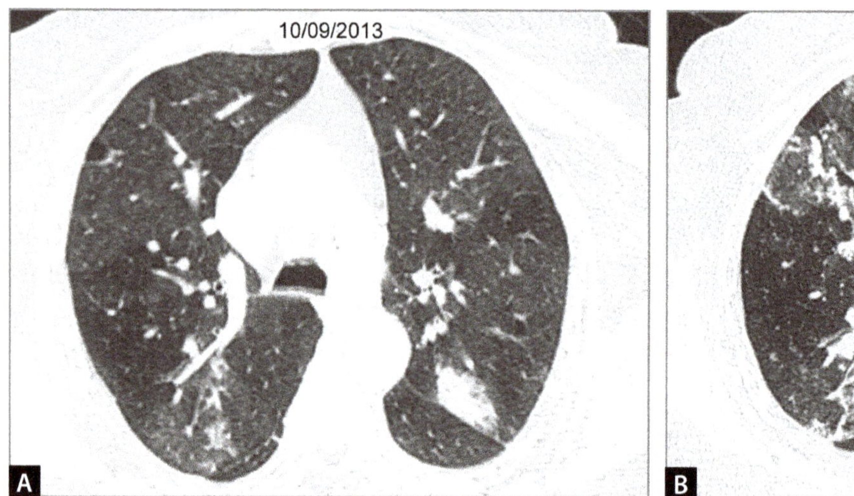
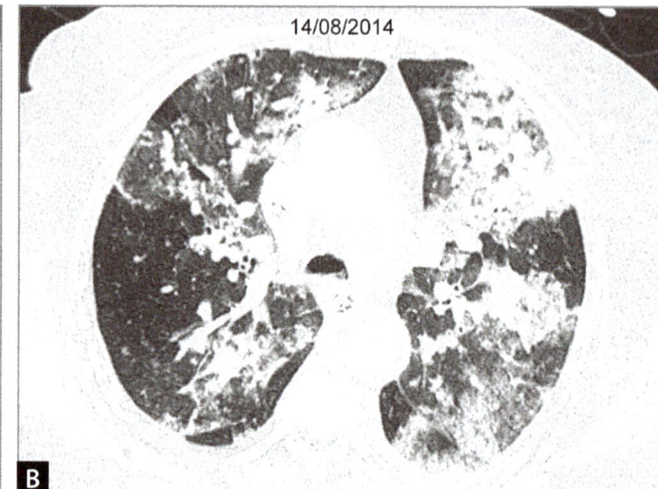

Figs. 6A and B: Methotrexate toxicity. (A) Computed tomography (CT) chest in a patient on methotrexate performed on 10/09/13 reveals diffuse ill-defined areas of ground-glass densities and consolidations in both lung fields. Follow-up CT; (B) performed on 14/08/14 revealed progression in disease process indicative of methotrexate toxicity.

of CD20 positive non-Hodgkin's lymphoma. There are however increasing indications for its use in rheumatology, inflammatory bowel disease and in Granulomatosis with polyangiitis (GPA) (formerly known as Wegener's granulomatosis).

A predictable and frequent side-effect is the reaction experienced by as many as 50% of patients during the first 15 to 30 minutes of the first exposure to the drug which is given by an IV infusion. The reaction is characterized by fever, chills, sweating, skin rash, dyspnea, hypotension, urticaria, angioedema of the throat. Bronchospasm may be observed. Rarely pulmonary edema may occur. Infusion reactions are much less common after subsequent infusions.

Interstitial pneumonia is an uncommon complication occurring in about 8% of patients receiving rituximab for non-Hodgkin's lymphoma. Clinical features consist of high fever often accompanied by dyspnea and cough. Treatment consists of corticosteroids in high doses slowly tapered, together with an antibiotic cover against the usual plus opportunistic organisms.

ILD is more common in patients who receive rituximab + CHOP therapy, than in those receiving CHOP alone. Treatment consists of discontinuing the drug and starting corticosteroids therapy. Though recovery generally occurs, death can occur from rituximab induced lung injury. If corticosteroids are used for rituximab induced ILD, it is mandatory to exclude an infectious etiology by appropriate culture which may include a BAL study. Empiric antibiotic therapy should be given to cover all likely pathogens while cultures and diagnostic procedures are performed.

Mitomycin

Mitomycin is one other drug like bleomycin which causes severe interstitial pneumonia and fibrosis, the incidence of pulmonary toxicity being approximately 4%.

When mitomycin is used with vinca alkaloids, it can cause acute pneumonitis with DAD. Clinically, this is characterized by episodes of severe respiratory distress several hours after this combination therapy is administered. In some cases, intubation and ventilator support is required. Radiography of the chest shows extensive bilateral infiltrates. Following the use of corticosteroids and supportive care, improvement generally occurs over some weeks. However, a number of these patients (close to 50%) are left with pulmonary fibrosis similar to that observed with use of mitomycin alone.

A rare mitomycin toxicity is mitomycin-induced microangiopathic hemolytic anemia with intra-alveolar hemorrhage. The condition is characterized by dyspnea, hypoxia, and diffuse pulmonary infiltrates. Treatment is with corticosteroids and plasmapheresis. Fortunately, the drug is now less frequently used in lung cancer.

Taxanes

Taxanes are newer antineoplastic drugs used for different cancers, notably cancers of the lung, breast, ovary, and cancers of the head and neck. Pulmonary toxicity takes the form of bronchospasm and dyspnea. Urticaria, skin rash, and hypotension may also be observed. Prior use of corticosteroids and H_2 blockers has reduced the incidence of these reactions.

Rarely, acute pneumonia has been observed as a dangerous toxic effect. Treatment consists of omission of the drug and the use of corticosteroids. Prognosis in general is good.

Cardiovascular Drugs Causing Adverse Pulmonary Effects

The incidence of diffuse parenchymal lung disease associated with cardiovascular drugs is rare, though cough, dyspnea and radiographic abnormalities can be caused by a number of drugs. Many adverse effects due to cardiovascular drugs have been mentioned in the earlier part of this chapter. A few more observations are pertinent.

- Treatment of ischemic heart disease with anticoagulants, antiplatelet medications and thrombolytic agents can cause diffuse alveolar hemorrhage (DAH). Clopidogrel and ticlopidine have rarely been associated with interstitial pneumonia.
- ACE inhibitors, beta blocker medications and statins have very rarely been reported to cause eosinophilic pneumonia. Organising pneumonia has been occasionally reported in association with statins and tocainide.
- Drug induced lupus has been caused by procainamide, hydrazide and quinidine. Pleuropericarditis is an important clinical feature of drug-induced lupus. The diagnosis is based on combination of clinical features, serological studies and complete response to the discontinuation of the drug.
- Procainamide and quinidine can cause respiratory muscle weakness, by unmasking or exacerbating an underlying myasthenia.
- Overdoses of nitrates can cause methemoglobinemia
- *Paclitaxel eluting stents*: Paclitaxel is an antineoplastic agent that is used to prevent restenosis following the placement of coronary stents. The drug is known to cause interstitial pneumonia when used for cancer. Case reports have reported interstitial pneumonia after placement of these stents. Clinical features consist of cough, dyspnea within few days of stent placement. X-ray chest shows diffuse bilateral opacities. Three reported patients died of progressive respiratory failure in spite of use of corticosteroids.

CONCLUSION

The diagnosis of pulmonary toxicity related to drugs is difficult because a number of diseases produce pulmonary manifestations similar to the pulmonary toxic effects of drugs used to treat these diseases. The simultaneous associations of pulmonary infection, progression of a mitotic lesion are compounding factors which make the diagnosis of pulmonary drug toxicity difficult. Unfortunately, radiographic findings are nonspecific and histopathologic studies are not always helpful. Invasive biopsy procedures carry a grave risk in very ill people. Nevertheless all possible investigations, in particular a BAL study, need to be done to ensure that an infective etiology is not missed, more so as many of the drugs detailed in the chapter are often used in immunocompromised patients.

The key diagnostic factor is awareness of pulmonary toxicity related to a number of drugs and a keen suspicion of their possible occurrence under certain circumstances.

Periodic lung function tests done on patients exposed to drugs with a potential for pulmonary toxicity may help early detection. A restrictive lesion with a fall in CO diffusion may well be a pointer to interstitial lung disease caused by drugs. Toxicity caused by bleomycin, mitomycin, and amiodarone is believed to be increased with the use of supplemental oxygen. Supplemental oxygen should be avoided with these drugs unless absolutely necessary.

SUGGESTED READING

1. Camus P, Bonniaud P, Fanton A, et al. Drug-induced and iatrogenic infiltrative lung disease. Clin Chest Med. 2004;25(3):479-519.
2. Costabel U, Uzaslan E, Guzman J. Bronchoalveolar lavage in drug-induced lung disease. Clin Chest Med. 2004;25(1):25-35.
3. Dhokarh R, Li G, Schmickl CN, et al. Drug-associated acute lung injury: a population-based cohort study. Chest. 2012; 142:845.
4. Epler GR. Drug-induced bronchiolitis obliterans organizing pneumonia. Clin Chest Med. 2004;25(1):89-94.
5. Huttner A, Verhaegh EM, Harbarth S, et al. Nitrofurantoin revisited: a systematic review and meta-analysis of controlled trials. J Antimicrob Chemother. 2015;70(9):2456-64.
6. Lee-Chiong T Jr, Matthay RA. Drug-induced pulmonary edema and acute respiratory distress syndrome. Clin Chest Med. 2004;25(1):95-104.
7. Leger P, Limper AH, Maldonado F. Pulmonary toxicities from conventional chemotherapy. Clin Chest Med. 2017; 38:209.

8. Limper AH. Chemotherapy-induced lung disease. Clin Chest Med. 2004;25(1):53-64.
9. Roubille C, Haraoui B. Interstitial lung diseases induced or exacerbated by DMARDS and biologic agents in rheumatoid arthritis: a systematic literature review. Semin Arthritis Rheum. 2014;43(5):613-26.
10. Schwarz MI, Fontenot AP. Drug-induced diffuse alveolar hemorrhage syndromes and vasculitis. Clin Chest Med. 2004;25(1):133-40.
11. Vahid B, Marik PE. Pulmonary complications of novel antineoplastic agents for solid tumors. Chest. 2008;133(2):528-38.

Trauma and Chest Wall Disorders

CHAPTER 71

Trauma to the Chest

INTRODUCTION

Trauma to the chest when severe can lead to significant morbidity and mortality. In civilian life, chest trauma is largely due to accidents chiefly road or rail, though violence, as in assault, riots and terrorist attacks are clearly on the rise all over the world. In most severe accidents, there is polytrauma when more than one organ system is involved. The morbidity and mortality worsen when trauma to the chest is associated with trauma to other systems. The mortality also worsens with age, especially after the sixth decade, particularly in the presence of comorbid disease involving the respiratory or cardiovascular systems.

PREVALENCE

The World Health Organization (WHO) report (Global Status Report on Road Safety) states that over 1.2 million people die in road accidents every year and 20–25 million suffer nonfatal injuries. India's record with regard to road vehicular accidents is dismal. Road fatalities increased between 2003 and 2008 from 84,000 in 2003 to 1.18 lakhs in 2008; 4.69 lakh people were injured in road accidents, nearly four times the total death toll. Current figures are equally disturbing. The total number of individuals killed in road accidents increased by 4.6% from 139,671 in 2014 to 146,113 in 2015; 400 deaths take place every day on Indian roads, which works out to a loss of 17 lives on an average, every hour. This is almost certainly an underestimation, many nonfatal accidents or even fatal accidents go unrecorded. Andhra Pradesh has the highest death rates due to road accidents (12%), followed by Maharashtra and Uttar Pradesh (11% each). In most fatal accidents, chest wall trauma was the main or contributory cause of death. The WHO states that India has topped the global list of deaths in road accidents, leaving behind the world's most populous country, China. This is particularly disturbing considering the comparatively low density of overall vehicular traffic in the country compared to many other countries in the world. India's vehicular population is just 5% of the world's, and yet, as has already been stated, the country has the highest incidence of road accidents, with over 1.5 lakhs fatalities and five or even perhaps 10 times that number injured or admitted to hospital. The increased incidence of accidents with injury to one or more organ systems in all developing countries (including India) is because of rapid urbanization and industrialization and the need for mechanized transport. Even in rural India, the impact of injuries and deaths caused by accidents is increasingly evident because of mechanization of agriculture and the increased use of vehicular transport.

In road traffic accidents, chest trauma is responsible for death in 30% of cases. Isolated chest trauma in good trauma centers in the Western world has a mortality close to 10%; the mortality is over 20% when two or more organ systems suffer injury.

Road, rail and aeroplane accidents are not the only causes of chest trauma. Even if we discount wars where trauma in all forms can be horrendous, one has to consider natural disasters like earthquakes, house collapse (so common in some countries), civil and political unrest, terror attacks as other important causes of chest trauma.

Care for trauma is ideally organized at two sites. The first and extremely important is the site of the accident, and next ideally, in the Emergency Medical Services (EMS) or ICU of a trauma center, or failing that Emergency Department or ICU of any reasonably well-equipped hospital.

Analysis shows that prompt attention to serious chest trauma after an accident significantly improves mortality. The first 1–6 hours are crucial and prompt attention at the site of accident is vital. Though this is possible in the developed countries of the West, it is well-nigh impossible in India and many other developing countries. Even in large cities like Mumbai and Delhi, it may take hours before accident victims find their way to a good hospital because of the traffic jams that are routine on all busy city roads. Helicopter service to send emergency medical teams to the site of the accident or to transport the victim to a well-equipped medical center is almost nonexistent in the poorer countries of the world.

APPROACH TO CHEST TRAUMA

Initial Assessment

A quick but careful examination of the patient is necessary to assess the extent and severity of injuries. *As with any emergency, immediate attention is focused on the airway, the breathing and the circulation.* Is the airway patent? If not, it should be rendered so. An unconscious patient generally requires an oropharyngeal airway; secretions and blood, should be aspirated from the oropharynx, and in emergency situations, endotracheal intubation may be necessary. The possibility of trauma to the cervical spine must always be kept in mind so that flexion of the cervical spine is avoided during intubation. If the airway is patent, is the breathing satisfactory? If not, respiration needs to be supported—mouth-to-mouth respiration, or when possible bag-mask respiration, and in an ICU, endotracheal intubation with ventilator support. Equally important is to determine with urgency whether the circulation is adequate. Most accident victims are hypovolemic. It is important to secure a venous line and start an intravenous infusion with normal saline or Ringer lactate, at the same time sending blood to the laboratory for all appropriate tests.

The heart and lungs combine to supply oxygen to the organs and tissues of the body. Serious injury to either results in hypoxemia. The most important question to determine in chest trauma is the presence and the degree of hypoxemia. This may indeed be difficult. Central cyanosis may be clinically difficult to determine even in the presence of severe hypoxemia, particularly so in a patient who is pale following blood loss, or in the presence of severe peripheral vasoconstriction due to shock.

Life-threatening hypoxemia in chest trauma can be due to either one or more of several causes—blocked airway, tension pneumothorax, hemothorax, lung contusions, fractures of the sternum and/or multiple ribs causing a flail chest, myocardial injury or hemopericardium. Each of these causes must be carefully looked out for and excluded **(Table 1)**. A tension pneumothorax can kill within a short time. Initially, there is marked tachypnea, tachycardia and hypotension. If not dealt with quickly, it leads to gasping breathing and cardiac arrest with an electromechanical dissociation. A hemothorax is suspected from signs of blood loss coupled with a stony dull note over the affected side of the chest. Lung contusions should be suspected

Table 1: Immediate complications of chest trauma.	
Complications	***Clinical features***
Obstruction to trachea or main bronchus	Stridor, tachypnea, indrawing of intercostal spaces, hypoxemia (if obstruction unrelieved and severe)
Tension pneumothorax	Severe increasing dyspnea, absent breath sounds over affected lung, displaced mediastinum, hyper-resonant note over the lung, cardiovascular collapse, typical X-ray chest
Hemothorax	Shock due to blood loss; stony dull note over affected chest. Chest X-ray shows fluid which on aspiration is blood
Cardiac tamponade	Tachycardia, hypotension with other features of low output state. Jugular venous pressure raised, or even normal in presence of hypovolemia or shock; enlarged cardiac silhouette on X-ray of the chest. Echocardiography reveals pericardial fluid
Lung contusion	Tachypnea, hypoxemia, hemoptysis, chest X-ray shows airspace consolidates of varying size
Flail chest	Unstable flail segment showing paradoxical motion, progressive dyspnea, hypoxemia
Rupture or tear of trachea or a large bronchus	Dyspnea, hemoptysis, stridor, subcutaneous emphysema
Rupture or tear of diaphragm	Chest pain, dyspnea, complications of herniation of abdominal contents into the pleural cavity.

when there is tachypnea and evidence of hypoxemia in spite of a patent airway and absence of pneumothorax or hemothorax. A flail chest is immediately evident as there is a sucking in of the flail segment on inspiration and a puffing outwards of the flail segment on expiration. The patient is dyspneic and in severe cases increasingly hypoxemic. Finally, hypoxemia may be related to injury to the myocardium, or to the hemopericardium causing a cardiac tamponade. A large contusion involving the myocardium is akin to an infarct and can lead to a low cardiac output and shock. Cardiac tamponade due to hemopericardium should always be suspected in a crush or penetrating injury to the chest. Clinical features of tension pneumothorax, hemothorax, lung contusions, flail chest, myocardial injury and hemopericardium causing cardiac tamponade are detailed later in this chapter.

Initial assessment as already stated should be at the site of injury or accident. Basic resuscitative measures before transport to a trauma center or hospital saves many lives. In fact, assessment and emergency measures in the first or first 2 "golden hours" in trauma patients is crucial for reduction in morbidity and mortality. At least a few of the emergency measures outlined below could be administered at the site of accident or injury if the necessary facilities are available.

Emergency Management

A patent airway, ventilatory support, oxygenation, and circulatory support as already mentioned are of prime importance.

If it has not been already done, a vein should be secured and an IV infusion of crystalloids started. Fluid resuscitation of patients in shock is imperative. Blood should be promptly grouped and matched. All necessary investigations should be carried out pari passu with emergency management. This should include arterial pH, blood gases and an X-ray chest. If the patient is conscious and is capable of standing, an X-ray chest should be done in the standing position. If not, a portable X-ray chest suffices.

Pneumothorax

Pneumothorax should be strongly suspected in any patient with either a blast injury, a penetrating injury or blunt trauma to the chest. Unilateral diminution of breath sounds suggests either pneumothorax or hemothorax.

Surgical emphysema in the neck or the chest wall is invariably associated with a pneumothorax, particularly so in penetrating injures. It is also a feature of injury to the trachea or major bronchi. The severity of symptoms and clinical signs even in a patient with a significant pneumothorax does not necessarily correlate with its size. Unless a pneumothorax is very shallow, it merits chest tube drainage.

Tension pneumothorax: Tension pneumothorax is characterized by severe respiratory and circulatory distress. Clinical findings include tachypnea, dyspnea, hypoxemia and hypotension; the jugular venous pressure is markedly increased, provided the patient is not hypovolemic due to severe blood or fluid loss. The chest is hyperresonant on the affected site, breath sounds are absent and the mediastinum shifted to the opposite side. Bag-mask ventilation becomes difficult; if the patient is on ventilator support, the peak pressure is very high and the patient clashes with the machine.

A tension pneumothorax can be easily overlooked in a patient with polytrauma, particularly in the presence of a severe head injury causing unconsciousness which precludes any complaint of pain or breathlessness. Bilateral simple pneumothoraces can produce serious cardiorespiratory embarrassment. This should be evident on an X-ray of the chest and should be treated by chest tube drains connected to underwater seals.

Tension pneumothorax should be actively looked out for and if present should be promptly relieved by the emergency insertion of a large-bore cannula needle, leaving the cannula in situ till an intercostal tube connected to an underwater seal has been introduced. An X-ray of the chest should confirm the presence of tension pneumothorax but in critical situations, the pneumothorax needs to be drained as an emergency procedure without awaiting an X-ray of the chest.

Hemothorax

Clinical examination supported by an X-ray chest should confirm the presence of a hemothorax. A small hemothorax can be treated by chest aspiration, but more often than not, catheter drainage through a USG or CT guided intercostal drain inserted through the sixth intercostal space in the mid-axillary line is necessary. Depending on the degree of injury, large quantities amounting to more than a liter of blood may be drained from the pleural space. Prompt blood replacement is necessary. Usually, the blood loss lessens with time, then ceases, and the patient continues to improve. If blood loss continues unabated, an emergency thoracotomy may be mandatory to control bleeding under vision.

Myocardial Injury or Contusion

Contusion involving the myocardium behaves like a myocardial infarct. The ECG may show nonspecific ST-T changes or show the typical features of an ST-elevated myocardial infarct. The cardiac enzymes are elevated. Myocardial contusion should be treated if necessary with adequate inotropic or vasopressor support, together with all the other care one takes in a patient with a myocardial infarct.

Lung Contusion

Lung contusions are common in chest trauma. Severe lung contusions in both lungs are most often seen after blast injuries and penetrating injuries caused by shotgun or high-velocity missile wounds. Blunt injury to the chest may also cause contusion of the underlying lung and this may occur without fractures of either the sternum or ribs.

Severe lung contusions are often associated with other major injuries involving multiple body systems. The mortality with severe lung contusions is indeed very high as they result in marked ventilation-perfusion disturbances and severe hypoxemic respiratory failure.

Mild contusion may only be detected on an X-ray chest; however, what appears to be mild in a very early X-ray may turn out to be much larger in subsequent radiographs of the chest. Patients with severe lung contusion (particularly involving both lungs) present with tachypnea and progressive hypoxemia. Radiographs of the chest show fluffy shadows, which may become confluent with time. Though mild contusion may be managed using a high-flow oxygen mask, severe contusion requires intubation and ventilator support, the fractional inspired oxygen (FiO_2) being adjusted so as to keep the O_2 saturation more than 90%. At times, it is impossible to keep a PaO_2 of even 40 mm Hg on an FiO_2 of 100%. The contused lung is easily prone to fluid overload which makes management of patients who are in shock doubly difficult. The potency of airways must be ensured and infection rigorously combated. Both inotropic and vasopressor support may be necessary. An ECG may show ST-T changes

of a nonspecific nature or show the typical features of ST-elevated myocardial infarction if there is associated myocardial contusion.

Cardiac Tamponade

Cardiac tamponade can kill quickly if not promptly recognized. Clinically, a low output state in the presence of a raised central venous pressure should point to a tamponade. In fact, chest trauma is one condition where significant tamponade may exist with a central venous pressure which is normal, or in the upper limit of normal. The normal or even low central venous pressure in the presence of tamponade is because of hypovolemia caused by associated blood loss, or because of shock due to trauma to other organ systems. A normal-sized cardiac silhouette on a chest X-ray does not exclude cardiac tamponade. An echocardiogram can be of immense diagnostic value. Careful aspiration of blood from the pericardial space is necessary. If bleeding recurs or continues, a surgical procedure entailing the insertion of a drain into the pericardial space through a pericardial window becomes necessary.

The Airways, Breathing and Circulation

The prime importance of attending to and securing these three vital features has already been stressed under "*Initial Assessment*". A few points need further consideration.

Airway patency is of great importance and an important decision is to decide on the need for tracheal intubation. However, immediate tracheal intubation of patients with cardiac tamponade or hemothorax or severe hypotension may cause cardiovascular collapse due to increased positive intrapleural pressure sharply reducing venous return.

Breathing: A quick percussion and auscultation can help diagnose a large pneumothorax, a tension pneumothorax and a hemothorax. All these conditions cause diminished breath sounds; a pneumothorax if sufficiently large is associated with a hyperresonant note, while a hemothorax has a stony dull note on percussion. *Physical examination however is not sufficient to rule out a pneumothorax or hemothorax caused by chest trauma. An X-ray chest is imperative.*

Oxygen is always necessary in severe trauma. Hypoxia as judged by an oxygen saturation well below 90% needs to be promptly accounted for and addressed.

Circulation: For patients with clinical features of hemorrhagic shock resuscitation with IV normal saline or Ringer lactate and blood products is necessary. The concept of "low volume resuscitation" or "controlled hypotension" is controversial. It entails the administration of minimal amount of fluid necessary to maintain adequate oxygenation and tissue perfusion while preventing the dilution of clotting factors, hypothermia, and the risk of pulmonary edema. However, much remains uncertain with regard to "low volume resuscitation" and one must await further research on this subject. Besides volume replacement, hypotension may necessitate the use of vasopressors and at times the use of inotropes.

Flail Chest

A severe flail chest causing dyspnea with life-threatening hypoxemia is dealt with promptly by intubation and positive pressure ventilator support. This complication is dealt with at greater length later in the chapter (*see* Table 1).

Replacement of Blood and Maintenance of Fluid Electrolyte Balance

Serious chest trauma is often accompanied by trauma to other organ systems, by blood loss, fluid loss and disturbance in electrolyte balance. These factors should be recognized and corrected pari passu with treatment of the life-threatening complications described earlier.

Polytrauma requires the attention and help of appropriate specialists. A protocol for priority of treatment should be agreed upon. Serious abdominal trauma may warrant an urgent laparotomy, an intracranial injury may require urgent craniotomy as a priority. If surgery for polytrauma is necessary, it is best to undertake as many procedures as possible in one anesthetic cumoperative session, with due regard to patient safety. In the presence of critical chest injury, fractures of long bones can be stabilized temporarily by skin traction; operative reduction, fixation can be done when the patient has a stable circulation and respiration.

Besides the immediate life-threatening emergencies mentioned earlier, it is important to bear in mind other lurking threats and complications associated with chest trauma. These include in the main, closed aortic rupture **(Figs. 1A and B)**, ruptured or torn trachea or bronchus, rupture esophagus and rupture diaphragm. These may not be immediately evident and may make their presence felt later. Some of these complications necessitate a thoracotomy, the timing of which should be decided upon by the treating team of physicians and surgeons.

Extended Focused Assessment with Sonography for Trauma (e-FAST)

Primary assessment and emergency management in all trauma, including trauma to the chest is significantly helped by the use of ultrasonography. Sonography

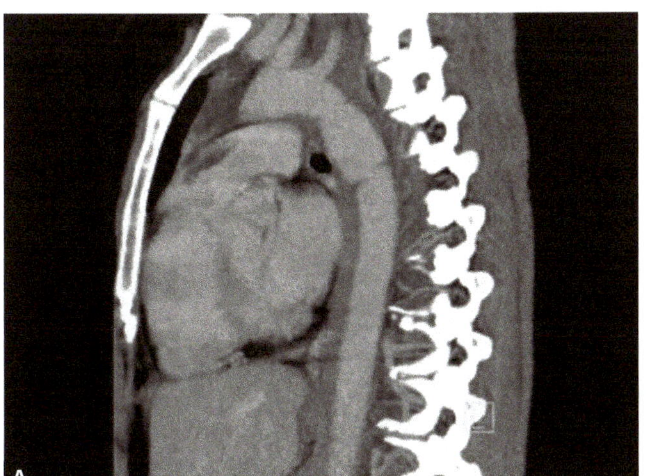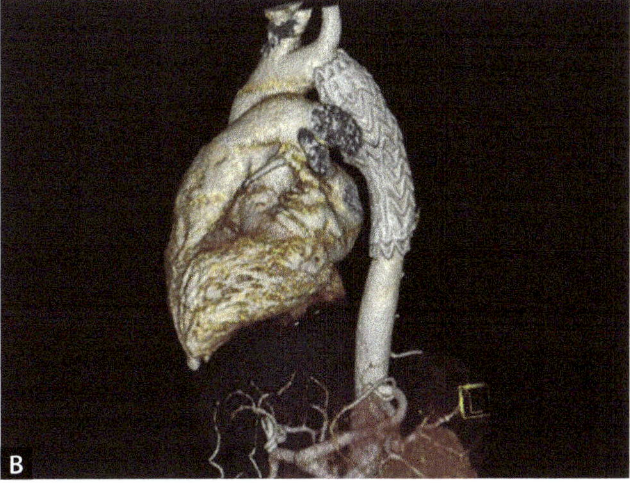

Figs. 1A and B: Aortic transection. (A) An 18-year-old girl riding pillion on a motorcycle was thrown off following a head-on collision. CT angiography revealed an aortic transection as evidenced by focal intimal tear in the descending aorta at the level of the aortic isthmus, a typical site for blunt aortic injury. (B) An aortic stent was placed across the isthmus intimal tear: This is a post-stent CT angiogram demonstrating the stent in situ.

accurately detects the presence of hemothorax, pneumothorax, hemopericardium and peritoneal fluid. It distinguishes a pleural shadow from a pulmonary parenchymal shadow. It should form a necessary aspect of emergency primary assessment and management of a trauma victim. It enables together with clinical examination a quick triage of trauma victims, so that whenever possible, patients with multiple severe injuries can be transported directly to a trauma center rather than remain in a community hospital.

Secondary Survey

Once a patient with chest trauma has been stabilized, a secondary survey consisting of a thorough complete re-examination should be performed to ensure that no complication has been missed out in the earlier assessment.

Imaging Studies

The radiography of chest and sonography of the thorax are always done. Echocardiography is a routine procedure in severe chest trauma to detect pericardial effusion, hemopericardium, cardiac tamponade, myocardial contusion.

High-resolution computed tomography of the chest is the gold standard to detect the nature and extent of injury to the thorax and intrathoracic structures, particularly if tracheobronchial, vascular or esophageal injury is suspected.

■ OTHER PULMONARY COMPLICATIONS

Lobar or Segmental Atelectasis

Lobar or segmental atelectasis is perhaps the most frequent complication occurring within 48 hours of chest trauma. It results from the inability of the patient to take deep breaths and inability to cough and keep the airways clear of secretions. Relief of pain and good physiotherapy generally suffices to open up the atelectatic lobe of the lung. If lobar atelectasis persists, bronchoscopic aspiration is warranted. Repeated bronchoscopy to aspirate secretions is undesirable and may do more harm than good.

Flail Chest

Double fractures of three or more contiguous ribs or a combination of fracture of the sternum and ribs causes a flail segment in the thoracic cage. As mentioned earlier, during inspiration the flail segment is sucked inwards rather than expanding outwards with the rest of the thoracic cage, while during expiration it is pushed outwards when the rest of the chest moves inwards **(Figs. 2A and B)**. The most common cause of a flail chest is trauma to the chest following automobile accidents or following other forms of crush injury. The next most important cause is fractures of the sternum and/or ribs caused by over-aggressive cardiopulmonary resuscitation. Rarely, multiple pathological fractures of contiguous ribs may also cause a flail chest.

Diagnosis

The diagnosis of flail chest is obvious from the nature of the paradoxical movement of the flail segment during spontaneous breathing. Chest radiography reveals multiple fractures of the ribs **(Fig. 3)**. A CT scan provides more information with regard to associated injuries to the lung, pleura and other mediastinal structures. In fact pulmonary contusion, pneumothorax and hemothorax occur in over 50% of patients with flail chest. Trauma serious enough to cause a flail chest is often associated with traumatic fracture of long bones, intra-abdominal injuries and rupture of the aortic arch or other vessels within the mediastinum. Patients with multiple traumatic injuries and lung contusions complicating flail chest have a mortality more than 50%.

Pathophysiology

The paradoxical movement of the flail segment is related to changes in intrapleural pressure during breathing.

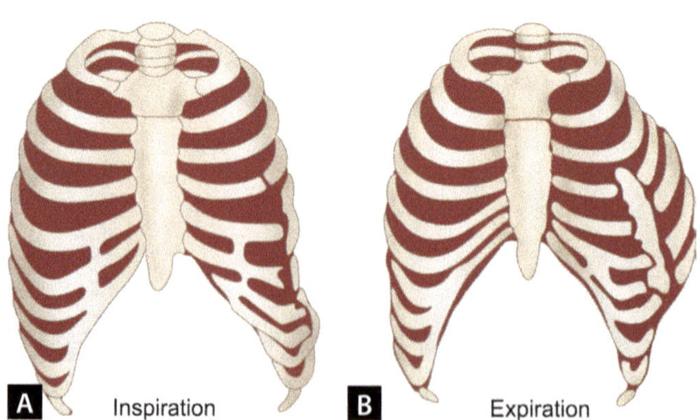

Figs. 2A and B: Diagram showing a flail segment. (A) sucked in during inspiration; and (B) pushed out on expiration.

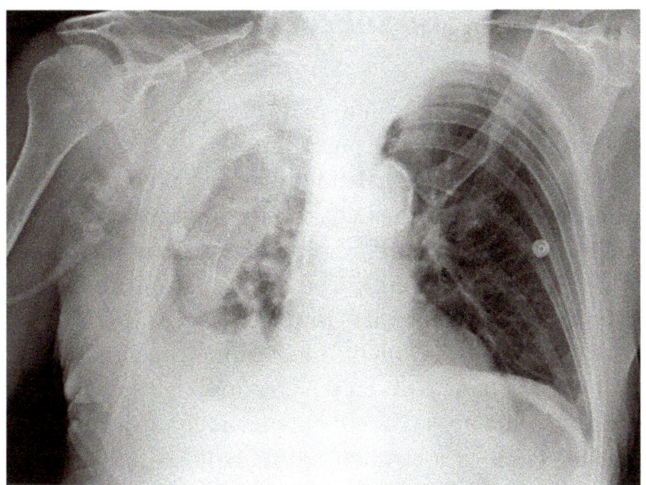

Fig. 3: Chest X-ray reveals multiple rib fractures involving right middle and lower ribs associated with right hemothorax.

During inspiration, the negative intrapleural pressure inflates the lungs but exerts a deflationary effect on the rib cage. In spite of this deflationary effect, normal rib cage expansion during inspiration occurs due to outward forces exerted by the insertions of the diaphragm as it descends during inspiration, due to the action of the upper intercostal muscles on the upper rib cage and to the outward recoil of the thoracic cage at high inspiratory lung volumes. Following contiguous double fractures of three or more ribs, the flail segment is uncoupled from the rest of the thoracic cage, so that the deflationary effect of increased intrapleural negative pressure during inspiration is no longer countered by factors that promote chest wall expansion. Therefore, the increase in the negative intrapleural pressure during inspiration sucks the uncoupled flail segment inwards. During expiration, the intrapleural pressure becomes more positive and the flail segment moves outwards. This paradoxical movement of the flail segment is worsened if there is obstruction to the airways which increases the negativity of the intrapleural pressure during inspiration, or in the presence of lung contusions which cause a decrease in lung compliance.

Most flail segments are laterally placed due to rib fractures of the lateral chest wall. Fractures separating the sternum from the ribs produce anteriorly placed flail segments; posterior flail chest segments occur with fractures of the posterior portion of the ribs. Posterior flail chest segments are associated with comparatively less paradoxical movement because of the splinting effect of the back muscles.

Table 2: Management of flail chest.

- Relief of pain—drugs, regional anesthesia, epidural anesthesia
- Oxygen
- Physiotherapy
- Ventilator support for respiratory failure:
    – Noninvasive support (CPAP)
    – Invasive ventilator support when indicated
- Surgical fixation of flail chest

The danger of a flail chest is that it sets into motion events that can lead to respiratory failure. This can be due to several causes:

- Reduction in vital capacity and functional residual capacity by as much as 50% occurring as a result of the paradoxical movement of the flail segment.
- Severe chest pain, which can lead to hypoventilation. Inability to cough and clear secretions from the airways because of pain leads to regional atelectasis over the flail segment and generalized microatelectasis due to poor inspiration and low tidal volumes. Hypoxemia results from ventilation-perfusion imbalance, and a vicious cycle of increasing hypoventilation and increasing hypoxemia is set into motion.
- The atelectatic areas within the lung increase the elastic load on the respiratory muscles.
- A further increase in the work of breathing is due to shortening of the muscles of inspiration because of the flail segment. These muscles therefore work at a mechanical disadvantage and are more prone to respiratory muscle fatigue. The oxygen cost of breathing is increased.

Thus, a combination of hypoventilation, hypoxemia due to ventilation-perfusion imbalance, respiratory muscle inefficiency, and respiratory muscle fatigue is responsible for progressive hypoxemic + hypercapnic respiratory failure.

Treatment (Table 2)

Control of pain is critical as it prevents both hypoventilation and atelectasis, which is central to the development of respiratory failure. Pain control allows the patient to cough, clear secretions and allows efficient physiotherapy. Narcotics need to be titrated with great care so as to prevent hypoventilation and excessive drowsiness. Intercostal nerve blocks can provide good analgesia. Epidural anesthesia can also be used in selected patients for pain relief.

Supplemental oxygen to keep oxygen saturation more than 90%, physiotherapy that allows an efficient bronchial toilet, and careful fluid replacement are all necessary. In patients where paradoxical movements of the flail segment are not marked and when the flail segment is not large, the above conservative management may successfully prevent or counter respiratory failure and promote recovery.

Mechanical ventilation is necessary: (a) when the flail segment is large with a marked paradoxical movement of the segment; (b) when respiratory failure is present or imminent in spite of the conservative therapy outlined earlier.

Noninvasive ventilation should be tried if the patient is breathing spontaneously; relief of pain through regional anesthesia or through other means is necessary. Noninvasive ventilation (CPAP) when appropriately used can effectively stabilize the flail segment and abolish its paradoxical movements during the respiratory cycle.

Positive pressure ventilatory support following endotracheal intubation or tracheostomy is advised when there are multiple large flail segments, when noninvasive ventilatory support fails, when there is well-marked hypoxemic + hypercapnic respiratory failure, or when there is associated shock, intracranial injury or associated intra-abdominal injury. Ventilatory support needs to be given till such time as the flail segment or segments are sufficiently stable to allow weaning **(Table 3)**.

Chest wall stabilization: The chest wall can be stabilized in selected patients by a number of surgical procedures such as external fixation of the chest wall with wires, staples or steel plates. Surgical fixation improves respiratory mechanics and reduces the duration of mechanical ventilatory support. Selection of patients for surgical fixation depends on the experience of the unit concerned. Large flail segments, multiple segments, and patients whose flail segments fail to stabilize on mechanical ventilator support are potential candidates for surgery.

Patients undergoing thoracotomy for intrathoracic injuries are often candidates for surgical stabilization of the flail segment at the time of thoracotomy.

Table 3: Indicators for invasive ventilatory support after endotracheal intubation or tracheostomy in flail chest.
• Failure of noninvasive ventilation support • Multiple or large flail segments • Well-marked hypoxemic + hypercapnic respiratory failure • Associated shock, intracranial injury, intra-abdominal injury

Mediastinal and Subcutaneous Emphysema

Mediastinal emphysema may be associated with a pneumothorax following blunt or penetrating injury to the chest. Severe mediastinal emphysema is often associated with a tear in the trachea or a rupture of a bronchus or the esophagus. Positive pressure ventilator support worsens mediastinal emphysema. The diagnosis is evident on a radiological examination of the chest **(Fig. 4)**.

Extension of air from the mediastinum occurs first into the neck and then to the face. A crepitus is felt on palpation of the face and neck. The subcutaneous emphysema when marked leads to a swollen "crepitus-filled face", the air then travelling subcutaneously to involve the chest, upper limbs and even the abdomen.

Treatment consists of dealing with the root cause of mediastinal emphysema and appropriate drainage of the pleural space in the presence of a pneumothorax, which is usually an association of mediastinal emphysema.

Rupture of the Trachea or Bronchus or Esophagus or any Combination of these Structures

Lacerations or rupture of the trachea or main bronchus leads to air within the mediastinum with surgical emphysema of the neck as also of the chest wall and upper

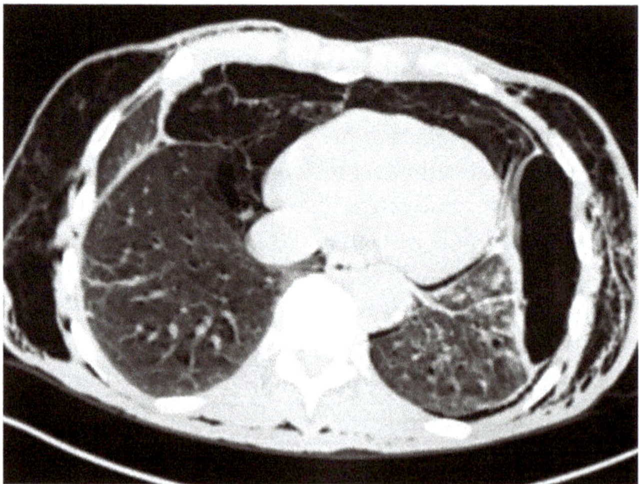

Fig. 4: Chest trauma. CT chest lung window demonstrates extensive subcutaneous emphysema on left side. Extensive mediastinal emphysema as evidenced by air in the mediastinum outlining the mediastinal vasculature. An ill-defined area of altered attenuation is seen in the left upper lobe representing a pulmonary contusion.

limbs. A crunching sound (Hamman's sign) may also be heard over the precordium. Air may rupture through the visceral pleura causing an associated pneumothorax. Hemoptysis is frequently observed. Rupture of the trachea or main bronchus needs expert surgical intervention and is associated with a high morbidity and mortality.

Rupture of the Diaphragm

Traumatic closed severe rupture of the diaphragm leads to the herniation of abdominal contents into the chest and requires surgical repair as soon as the diagnosis is made.

Traumatic Rupture of the Thoracic Duct

Traumatic chylothorax is rare, but should nevertheless be anticipated in severe crush injuries of the chest and in falls from a height which may involve hyperextension of the spine. Chylothorax becomes evident some days after the injury, manifesting as a large-sized pleural effusion which on aspiration is milky because of the presence of chyle.

Conservative treatment generally results in effectively reducing the flow of chyle into the pleural space. Chest tube drainage may be necessary. The reader is referred to the section on *"Diseases of the Pleura"*.

Acute Respiratory Distress Syndrome

Acute respiratory distress syndrome (ARDS) is indeed an important complication of chest trauma, particularly in the presence of lung contusion. It is characterized by increasing tachypneas, tachycardia, increasing hypoxemia, crackles over both lungs accompanied by fluffy shadows on a radiological examination of the chest. The patient is increasingly hypoxemic, the hypoxemia being uncorrected by high-flow oxygen therapy. Endotracheal intubation and ventilator support is vital. The subject is dealt with at length in a separate section.

■ IMPORTANT THERAPEUTIC MEASURES IN CHEST TRAUMA

These have been mentioned earlier but need to be doubly stressed. They include:

Relief of Pain

Relief of pain has already been touched upon. It is of vital importance as it enables the patient to cough, take deep breaths and permits efficient, effective physiotherapy. Usual analgesics generally fail to relieve pain and narcotics may relieve pain but depress respiration. An epidural block using 5–8 mL of 0.5% bupivacaine or an intravenous fentanyl drip or both together, may provide significant relief.

Table 4: Indications for thoracotomy.

- Rupture of trachea or main bronchus
- Uncontrolled hemothorax
- Severe cardiac tamponade due to a massive hemopericardium
- Closed rupture of the aorta (stenting the aorta if thought appropriate may suffice)
- Ruptured esophagus
- Ruptured diaphragm with herniation of abdominal contents into the chest
- Thoracoabdominal injury, e.g. injury involving the liver, spleen or other abdominal viscera; pleura and peritoneal taps reveal blood

Bronchoscopy, Endotracheal Intubation and Tracheostomy

Fiberoptic bronchoscopic aspiration of thick secretions helps to keep the airways patent. Repeated bronchoscopic aspiration however tends to cause or increase infection. When the airways are prejudiced, endotracheal intubation or tracheostomy becomes necessary. Suction of secretions then becomes easy; the patient can receive humidified oxygen and if needed be sedated and ventilated.

Physiotherapy

Expert physiotherapy to the chest often makes the difference between life and death. Effective physiotherapy is not possible without effective pain relief.

Thoracotomy

Thoracotomy may be considered necessary as an emergency measure or electively done at the appropriate time. Indications for thoracotomy are listed in **Table 4**.

■ SUGGESTED READING

1. Berg RJ, Karamanos E, Inaba K, et al. The persistent diagnostic challenge of thoracoabdominal stab wounds. J Trauma Acute Care Surg. 2014;76:418.
2. Burack JH, Kandil E, Sawas A, et al. Triage and outcome of patients with mediastinal penetrating trauma. Ann Thorac Surg. 2007;83:377.
3. Inaba K, Chouliaras K, Zakaluzny S, et al. FAST ultrasound examination as a predictor of outcomes after resuscitative

thoracotomy: a prospective evaluation. Ann Surg. 2015;262:512.

4. Karmy-Jones R, Jurkovich GJ. Blunt chest trauma. Curr Probl Surg. 2004;41:211.

5. Meredith JW. Thoracic trauma: when and how to intervene. Surg Clin North Am. 2007;87(1):95-118.

6. Miller LA. Chest wall, lung, and pleural space trauma. Radiol Clin North Am. 2006;44(2):213-24.

7. Ullman EA. Pulmonary trauma emergency department evaluation and management. Emerg Med Clin North Am. 2003;21(2):291-313.

8. Uptodate (2017). Initial evaluation and management of penetrating thoracic trauma in adults. [online] Available from https://www.uptodate.com/contents/initial-evaluation-and-management-of-penetrating-thoracic-trauma-in-adults. [Accessed July 2018].

CHAPTER 72

Chest Wall Disorders

■ SCOLIOSIS AND KYPHOSCOLIOSIS

General Considerations

Curvature of the spine is the most common deformity that results in a chest wall deformity. Scoliosis is characterized by a lateral curvature of the spine. Kyphosis is a backward curvature of the spine in the anteroposterior plane and lordosis, a forward curvature in the anteroposterior plane. Most patients with scoliosis have a crowding of the ribs on the side of the convexity, so that the condition is often mistakenly labelled as kyphoscoliosis. However, at times, scoliosis and kyphosis coexist, leading to a true *kyphoscoliotic spinal deformity.*

This chapter to start with, chiefly deals with kyphoscoliotic chest deformity and the effect of this deformity on the lungs and the respiratory system. It then goes on to very briefly consider other chest deformities encountered in clinical practice.

Prevalence

Scoliosis with more than 35° angle affects 1 in 1,000 of the population in the United States, an angle greater than 70° having a prevalence of 0.1 per 1,000. Females are more often affected with more severe scoliotic deformities compared to males.

An epidemiological study to determine the prevalence of scoliosis in schoolchildren in lower Assam revealed an incidence of 0.2% with a female to male ratio of 2.2:1. The idiopathic variety was the most common form of scoliosis which occurred mainly in the thoracic spine. The highest number of cases was observed between the ages of 11 years and 13 years and in over 70% of cases, the patients or their parents were unaware of the deformity *(Ref: Saikia KC, Duggal A, Bhattacharya PK, et al. Scoliosis: an epidemiological study of schoolchildren in lower Assam. Indian J Orthop. 2002;36:243-5).*

Etiology

- *Idiopathic*: In more than 80% of patients, the cause of scoliosis is unknown, the scoliosis being therefore considered as idiopathic. A proposed classification of idiopathic scoliosis is based on the age of onset of the lateral curvature of the spine—infantile (from birth to 3 years), juvenile (3–11 years) and adolescent (11 years and older). The angle of lateral curvature may vary from less than 30° to over 70°. Females are more often afflicted with significant scoliotic deformity compared to males and the defect is often observed to increase with age. Congenital scoliosis is generally related to developmental defects of the spine such as partial or fused vertebrae or hemi-vertebrae; or genetic syndromes such as the Klippel-Feil syndrome and spondylocostal dystonia.
- *Genetic:* The genetic basis of idiopathic scoliosis is uncertain. Perhaps, there is a genetic predisposition which is responsible for a different growth pattern in the spine. A possible genetic factor (among perhaps other multifactorial causes) is suggested by an increase in the incidence of scoliosis not only among first-degree relatives, but also to a lesser extent in second- and third-degree relatives as well.
- *Congenital scoliosis:* It is observed in association with congenital heart disease and congenital renal tract disease.
- *An association with neuromuscular disease:* Scoliosis is invariably associated with poliomyelitis which has affected the spinal muscles unequally. It is commonly observed in muscular dystrophy (particularly of the

Duchenne variety), in myopathies, syringomyelia and Friedreich's ataxia.

- *An association with other syndromes:* There are a number of syndromes or diseases known to be associated with scoliosis. The important ones include neurofibromatosis, Marfan's syndrome, osteogenesis imperfecta, Klippel-Feil syndrome, Ehlers-Danlos syndome and the rare various forms of mucopolysaccharidosis.
- *Disease or trauma:* An important cause of both kyphosis and kyphoscoliosis in India and other developing countries is tuberculosis of the spine (Pott's spine) which results in the formation of a kyphotic "gibbus", and at times also causes scoliosis. Trauma to the spine or surgery on the spine for whatever reason can also lead to a scoliotic deformity. Thoracoplasty for pulmonary tuberculosis was a frequently performed surgical procedure several decades ago. It often led to well-marked scoliotic deformity of the spine.
- *Tumors or granulomatous disease:* These are indeed rare causes of a lateral curvature to the spine; they include tumors such as large osteomas, chordomas and very rarely eosinophilic granuloma of the spine.

The causes of scoliosis are listed in **Table 1**.

■ KYPHOSIS

Kyphosis is invariably acquired and is often age-related, so that it is an accompaniment in many individuals past 60 years. Marked kyphosis sometimes results from osteoporotic fractures of the thoracic vertebrae, either related to age, use of corticosteroids or other causes. Tuberculosis involving multiple contiguous vertebrae

can lead to a pronounced "gibbus" resulting in a serious kyphotic deformity.

Pathophysiology

Marked chest wall deformity (whether scoliotic or kyphotic or kyphoscoliotic) always adversely affects cardiorespiratory function. A thoracic curve more than 70° imposes serious limits to ventilatory function. The effects of a severe scoliotic deformity are generally more marked than that of a pure kyphotic deformity. The ventilatory defect is of a restrictive nature. The vital capacity, the total lung capacity, inspiratory capacity and expiratory reserve volume are all reduced. In a pure scoliotic deformity, the residual volume though reduced is relatively better preserved. The forced expiratory volume in one second/forced vital capacity (FEVi/FVC) is generally also preserved but occasionally there is a degree of obstruction to the airways in adults with severe idiopathic scoliotic deformity. The obstructive element when present is due to the association of hyperreactive airways, smoking, occupation, environmental pollution or other factors. Factors which influence the degree of restrictive ventilatory defects are the number of vertebrae involved in the curve, involvement of the upper and mid-thoracic vertebrae rather than the lower dorsal vertebrae, severity of the kyphosis and Cobb angle (**Fig. 1**).

Table 1: Causes of scoliosis.
• Idiopathic
• Congenital
• Genetic
• *An association with neuromuscular disease*: Muscular dystrophy (particularly of the Duchenne variety), myopathies, syringomyelia and Friedreich's ataxia, poliomyelitis (among several others)
• *An association with other syndromes*: Neurofibromatosis, Marfan's syndrome, osteogenesis imperfecta, Klippel-Feil syndrome. Ehlers-Danlos syndrome and the rare various forms of mucopolysaccharidosis
• *Disease or trauma*: Pott's spine, surgery on the spine, thoracoplasty
• *Tumors or granulomatous disease*: Osteomas, chordomas and eosinophilic granuloma of the spine

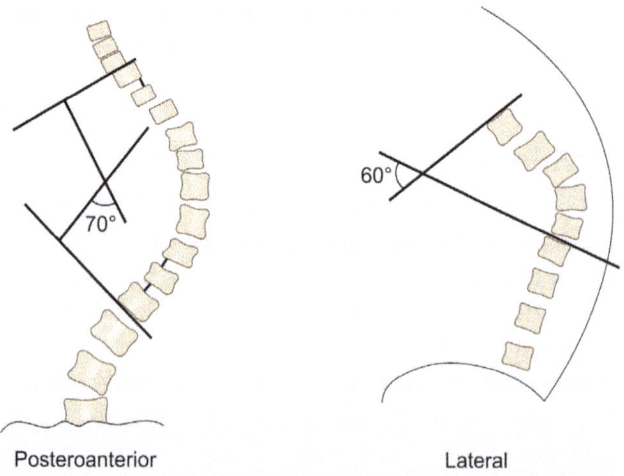

Fig. 1: Posteroanterior radiograph depicting the lines constructed to measure the Cobb angle of scoliosis and the lines drawn on the lateral radiograph to measure the Cobb angle of kyphosis.
Source: Based on data from Rochester DF, Findlay LJ. The lungs and neuromuscular and chest wall disorder. In: Murray JF, Nadel JA (Eds). Textbook of Respiratory Medicine. Philadelphia: WB Saunders; 1988.

Lung Compliance

Though there is no direct pathology within the lungs, the decrease in lung expansion because of the chest deformity and the ensuing hypoventilation produce a fall in compliance. As hypoventilation becomes more marked and as chest wall compliance decreases with increasing scoliotic or kyphotic deformity, cough becomes increasingly ineffective and areas of microatelectasis and segmental atelectasis ensue, causing a further fall in lung compliance. Atelectasis due to hypoventilation is even more frequent in scoliotic patients whose deformity is due to neuromuscular disease. Recurrent chest infections involving the airways (causing bronchospasm and increased respiratory secretions) introduce an element of airways obstruction, while involvement of the parenchyma (as in pneumonia) further reduces lung compliance setting off a vicious cycle terminating in increasing respiratory failure or causing acute or chronic respiratory failure.

Carbon monoxide diffusion or the transfer factor is reduced, yet the Krogh constant (KCO) [i.e. diffusion lung capacity for carbon monoxide (DLCO)/accessible alveolar volume] is increased. This is because the thoracic deformity and the ensuing stiffness of the chest wall squeezes more air out of the affected lung than blood, so that accessible alveolar volume is reduced **(Table 2)**.

Chest Wall Compliance

Chest wall compliance is reduced and the greater the deformity, the greater the fall in the chest wall compliance and greater the increase in the work of breathing.

Table 2: Pulmonary function tests in severe idiopathic thoracic scoliosis.	
Forced vital capacity (FVC)	Reduced
Forced expiratory volume in first second (FEV$_1$)	Reduced
FEV$_1$/FVC ratio	Generally normal, occasionally reduced
Total lung capacity	Reduced
Expiratory reserve volume	Reduced
Maximal inspiratory capacity	Reduced
Diffusion lung capacity for carbon monoxide (DLCO)	Reduced
KCO (DLCO/accessible alveolar volume)	Increased
Chest wall compliance	Reduced
Respiratory muscle strength	Reduced

As a consequence of the chest wall deformity, the respiratory muscles are shortened and work at a significant mechanical disadvantage. The effort required of the inspiratory muscles to meet the "load" (i.e. ventilatory demands) is ultimately inadequate so that hypercapnic respiratory failure ensues. There are some who believe that impaired central ventilatory drive contributes to hypoventilation; the center being less responsive to an increase in PaCO$_2$ because of chronic CO$_2$ retention. It is however more likely that in most patients the ventilatory load is far too much for the "effort" the mechanically disadvantaged respiratory muscles are capable of. This is the prime reason for ventilatory failure in patients with chest wall deformities. In fact, ventilatory drive is often increased in patients with scoliosis who develop hypoxemic + hypercapnic respiratory failure.

The ventilatory drive may however be primarily affected in brainstem disorders, amyotrophic lateral sclerosis or the ventilatory drive even if more than normal may fail to be translated into effective inspiratory muscle contraction in patients with neuromuscular disorders.

End Result

The end result as mentioned earlier is hypoxemic cum hypercapnic respiratory failure. Features of ventilatory failure in patients with well-marked scoliotic deformity generally first appear during sleep when loss of intercostal muscle tone further reduces the "effort" vis-a-vis the ventilatory "load". Ventilatory failure finally supervenes both during the day and night.

Pulmonary artery pressure increases with progressive hypoxemia and hypercapnia, with the final development of chronic cor pulmonale and right heart failure. Nocturnal dips in O$_2$ saturation during sleep are associated with a further rise in pulmonary artery pressure. Whether these dips with their associated rise in pulmonary artery pressure influence a gradual overall permanent increase in pulmonary artery pressure is undetermined. Death results either from progressive respiratory failure, chronic right-sided heart failure or from a complicating pulmonary infection. Chronic cor pulmonale is the most common cause of death.

Clinical Features

It is vital to ascertain that there is no other cause of a scoliotic, kyphoscoliotic or kyphotic deformity before dubbing it as idiopathic. Search should in particular include the clinical possibility of Marfan's syndrome, the presence of café au lait spots to suggest neurofibromatosis and a careful radiological study for the presence of hemivertebrae, a Klippel-Feil syndrome suggesting the presence of congenital scoliosis.

A full neurological examination is important. A careful cardiovascular examination in early onset scoliosis may reveal the presence of congenital heart disease which may be associated with congenital scoliosis.

Patients should be viewed in the standing position and also when bending forward to obtain an indication of the lateral deformity of the scoliotic, kyphotic or kyphoscoliotic spine.

Patients with symptoms related to chest wall abnormalities complain of progressive breathlessness on exertion, cough often with expectoration. With progression of the deformity, there is hypoventilation with features of hypoxemia and hypercapnia. A worsening of nocturnal hypoventilation during sleep, most marked during rapid eye movement (REM) sleep, causing a further rise in $PaCO_2$ is often responsible for nocturnal confusion, poor quality of sleep and early morning headache.

Right heart enlargement may be difficult to determine clinically but is evident on echocardiographic studies. Right-sided heart failure and progressive chronic hypercapnic respiratory failure constitute the end stage of the disease.

Most patients with chest wall deformities do not have cardiorespiratory problems. It is however important to determine which patients are likely to do so. Patients who have a vital capacity of less than 50% of predicted value at the time of presentation are more likely to progress to pulmonary and later cardiac decompensation compared to those with a higher vital capacity. It has also been shown that of the patients with cardiorespiratory symptoms related to scoliosis, 90% had an early onset scoliosis (before the age of 5 years). Finally, a fall in vital capacity more than 15% on assuming the supine position indicates weakness of the diaphragm.

High-risk patients require a careful follow-up. This should include:

- Clinical assessment—degree of breathlessness, chest expansion, symptoms of nocturnal hypoventilation, careful examination of the chest and cardiovascular system. Edema of the feet unless otherwise explained, is generally due to right heart failure.

- Lung function tests, in particular FVC and FEV1 using an office spirometer, and peak flow measurements through a peak flow meter.
- Arterial blood gas analysis at periodic intervals.
- Radiography of the chest and spine as and when deemed necessary.
- Periodic electrocardiography (ECG) and echo-cardiography for evidence of right ventricular hypertrophy and right ventricular systolic and diastolic dysfunction.

Management

Conservative Management

Conservative management consists in the use of specially fitted braces which help to create a normal thoracic kyphosis, extend the spine and derotate the scoliosis. The design and fit of the brace is individualized and is best left to the discretion of the orthopedic team. Conservative treatment is only possible if the spinal curvature is not marked and not progressive. The earlier the onset of scoliotic deformity, the greater the propensity for the deformity to progress.

Smoking should be strongly prohibited. Influenzal and pneumococcal vaccines are indicated, particularly in patients with limited ventilation. Exercise under supervision should be encouraged and these patients may perhaps benefit from a pulmonary rehabilitation program. Patients with Marfan's syndrome and associated scoliosis should avoid undue exercise and keep their blood pressure under close control, preferably with beta-adrenergic blocking drugs, as the risk of aortic dissection is significantly high in these patients.

Surgery

Surgery is indicated in marked deformity and to prevent progression. Thoracic scoliosis more than 50° is generally unacceptable; lesser degree of scoliosis may be associated occasionally with a greater degree of rotation of the ribs so as to result in an ugly deformity.

The current surgical approach provides rod instrumentation to stabilize the curve, and spinal fusion to prevent growth. The details of surgical procedure are beyond the scope of this chapter. Nevertheless fitness for surgery has to be decided by the physician. Preoperative investigations include lung functions, ECG, chest radiography, echocardiography, arterial blood gas analysis and the presence or absence of nocturnal hypoventilation. If nocturnal hypoventilation is present, a period of noninvasive ventilatory support before surgery is believed to help. Surgery unquestionably should be performed by experienced orthopedic surgeons in units which can provide excellent cardiorespiratory support.

Severe scoliosis accompanying Duchenne muscular dystrophy often presents special surgical problems. Surgery should be attempted only if FVC is not too compromised, preferably not less than 30% of predicted value. These patients generally need noninvasive ventilator support during the postoperative period, and excellent physiotherapy coupled with cough-assist devices.

Management of Ventilatory Failure

There is evidence to show that ventilatory failure caused by abnormalities of the chest wall or neuromuscular disease involving the muscles of respiration is successfully treated by the use of noninvasive ventilatory support (NIV). 5-year survivals in patients who receive NIV are as high as 80–100% in post-polio patients and in those with kyphoscoliotic deformity caused by tuberculosis of the spine. If NIV support is offered before the onset of pulmonary hypertension, patients have a normal or near normal life span and can often continue at work. In a retrospective study on patients with kyphoscoliosis receiving either long-term oxygen therapy (LOT) or NIV, those on NIV had a better survival rate at the end of 1 year and a greater improvement in $PaCO_2$ and PaO_2. A more recent Swedish study also showed that patients on NIV had a survival rate three times greater than those on LOT. Oxygen should be added to the NIV if the latter by itself does not increase O_2 saturation to more than 90% even when there is control over the $PaCO_2$. NIV support reduces discomfort and the feeling of breathlessness.

Pregnancy in scoliotic patients can be fraught with danger if the vital capacity is less than 1.25L or less than 50% of predicted value. This is observed chiefly in patients with early onset scoliosis starting at adolescence. Pregnancy is contraindicated in the presence of pulmonary hypertension and hypoxemia. If a ventilatory problem arises in pregnancy, labor or in the postpartum period, NIV should be used.

Other chest wall deformities are briefly considered below:

Congenital Deformities

The only chest wall congenital deformity that persists into adult life is pectus excavatum, also called funnel chest. This is an anterior chest wall deformity and is characterized by a concave depression in the form of a broad shallow defect or a narrow central depression. There is often a systolic bruit over the precordium. Though complaints of breathlessness and chest discomfort are common, the lung function tests are normal.

Ankylosing Spondylitis

Ankylosing spondylitis is a chronic inflammatory disease affecting joints of the axial system with fibrosis, calcification and even ossification of the ligamentous structures of the spine and rib cage. The serology is characterized by an HLA B27 positive in many but not in all patients.

The disease results in:

- Stiffness and ankylosis of the spine and the costochondral joints leading to what is termed a "bamboo spine". When marked it leads to poor inspiration, a slowly decreasing tidal volume, a reduced forced vital capacity culminating in ventilatory failure characterized chiefly by hypercapnia. When patients with ankylosing spondylitis require general anesthesia for any surgical procedure, endotracheal intubation may prove impossibly difficult. An endotracheal tube should be inserted with the help of a bronchoscope.
- *Pleuropulmonary disease:* Bilateral upper lobe fibrocystic disease is observed in a small proportion of patients who have suffered from this disease for over 15 years. Aspergillomas may form in one or more of these cystic spaces. The condition is often wrongly mistaken for tuberculosis. In rare cases the disease affects the cricoarytenoid joint, causing hoarseness and upper airway obstruction.
- Extra-articular manifestations of the disease include uveitis, aortic incompetence, aortic aneurysm, conduction abnormalities and peripheral arthropathy.

Treatment: Treatment is outside the scope of this book. Hypercapnic respiratory failure should be managed by noninvasive ventilatory support.

Flail Chest

Flail chest has been discussed in the section on Trauma to the Chest.

Thoracoplasty

The present use of thoracoplasty is for closure of a persistent pleural space. Prior to the 1950s it was the standard collapse therapy for cavitary pulmonary tuberculosis. Thoracoplasy consists of removal of a number of the posterior portions of the ribs (often from the third to the eight rib). The procedure results in a restrictive lung disease with decreased VC, FVC and total lung capacity. Breathlessness on exertion is the main symptom. The restrictive ventilatory defect may increase with time and age. Some patients may have a superadded airways obstruction, either related to healed underlying tuberculosis or to cigarette smoking. Hypercapnic respiratory failure may necessitie the use of noninvasive ventilatory support.

Fibrothorax

Fibrothorax results from fibrosis of the visceral pleura or to marked fibrosis (chiefly of the upper lobe of one or both lungs), generally consequent to old healed fibrotic tuberculosis.

Common pleural causes of a fibrothorax are an incorrectly treated pleural effusion or an empyema or an incorrectly treated hemothorax. Severe pleural fibrosis results in all these conditions. Lung functions show a restrictive lesion. Marked fibrothorax immobilizes one lung completely and can lead to hypoventilation with hypercapnic respiratory failure. Noninvasive ventilatory support becomes necessary in these patients. Open or video-assisted decortication is considered in some patients but is only of value if the underlying lung is healthy.

■ SUGGESTED READING

1. Crawford AH. Scoliosis associated with neurofibromatosis. Orthop Clin North Am. 2007;38(4):553-62.
2. Demetracopoulos CA. Spinal deformities in Marfan syndrome. Orthop Clin North Am. 2007;38(4):563-72.
3. Gonzalez C. Kyphoscoliotic ventilatory insufficiency: effects of long-term intermittent positive-pressure ventilation. Chest. 2003;124(3):857-62.
4. Good CR, Auerbach JD, O'Leary PT, et al. Adult spine deformity. Curr Rev Musculoskelet Med. 2011;4:159.
5. Gupta MC. Degenerative scoliosis. Options for surgical management. Orthop Clin North Am. 2003;34(2):269-79.
6. Hedequist DJ. Surgical treatment of congenital scoliosis. Orthop Clin North Am. 2007;38(4):497-509.
7. Kanathur N, Lee-Chiong T. Pulmonary manifestations of ankylosing spondylitis. Clin Chest Med. 2010;31:547.
8. Saikia KC, Duggal A, Bhattacharya PK, et al. Scoliosis: an epidemiological study of school children in lower Assam. Indian J Orthop. 2002;36:243-5.

CHAPTER 73

Central Nervous System and Neuromuscular Disorders Involving the Respiratory System

■ INTRODUCTION

A large number of central nervous system (CNS) and neuromuscular disorders are capable of involving respiratory muscles, causing hypoventilation, respiratory failure, or even respiratory muscle paralysis. A discussion of each of the very many would amount to writing a neurological textbook. Therefore, a brief description of important representative examples is given below together with a rather lengthy table so as to give an overall perspective of the problem. CNS and neuromuscular disorders involving respiratory muscles may be acute or chronic, though occasionally chronic disorders may have an acute presentation.

■ CENTRAL NERVOUS SYSTEM DISORDERS

Acute Disorders

The two major examples that need serious consideration are stroke and head or spinal cord injury.

Stroke

Brainstem strokes can disturb the pattern of breathing. Lesions of the dorsolateral medulla damage the respiratory center and can produce apnea that is soon fatal. If the dorsolateral position of the medulla is spared automatic or reflex breathing is preserved. Lateral medullary infarct arising from an occlusion of one of the distal vertebral branches is characterized by normal breathing or hypoventilation during waking hours and severe hypoventilation or even apnea during sleep—Ondine's curse. Rarely, Ondine's curse may occur as an isolated abnormality—a form of central sleep apnea.

Strokes affecting the cerebral hemisphere affect the voluntary pathway of respiration and also reduce movements of the contralateral diaphragm. Massive cerebral infarcts or cerebral hemorrhage is associated with marked cerebral edema that seriously jeopardizes respiration. Temporal herniation with pressure on the brainstem or a lateral shift or torsion of the brainstem can lead to hypoventilation apnea and death within a matter of minutes. Massive strokes can also cause pulmonary edema. Whenever respiration is jeopardized or the airway is obstructed as a result of secretions or because of palatal or pharyngeal paralysis, the patient needs prompt intubation and ventilator support. Intubation with induced hyperventilation through a positive pressure machine is often implemented to lower the arterial carbon dioxide tension ($PaCO_2$) to 25 mm Hg to help reduce cerebral edema in patients with massive strokes. Its effectiveness is generally limited to 24–48 hours.

Head and/or Spinal Cord Injury

Acute injury to the brain or spinal cord when severe can be associated with a total or near total loss of respiratory muscle function requiring prompt intubation and ventilator support. Other complications include:

- Ventilation-perfusion inequalities leading to progressive hypoxemia. Hypoventilation and partially obstructed airways are responsible for this event.
- Neurogenic pulmonary edema which is believed to result from an excessive β-adrenergic discharge, systemic hypertension, pulmonary vasoconstriction, and increased capillary permeability. This is indeed a form of acute respiratory distress syndrome (ARDS) and again needs intubation with ventilator support.

Incidentally subarachnoid hemorrhage can also cause neurogenic pulmonary edema. Occasionally, pulmonary edema is a presenting feature of subarachnoid hemorrhage, which can be missed if a careful CNS examination has not been done.

Spinal cord injury: Cervical cord injury causes quadriplegia. The latter also results from anterior spinal artery thrombosis or hematomyelia involving the cervical cord. In a transection, during the period of spinal shock the function of the intercostal muscles and the abdominal muscles is completely lost. Diaphragmatic paralysis results if the lesion is at C3 to C5 level. Diaphragmatic function is preserved if the lesion is below the above level. In these patients there is a paradoxical movement of the chest on inspiration, the upper chest being drawn in because of paralysis of the intercostal muscles. When the diaphragm is paralyzed there is a paradoxical movement of the abdomen and the patient is severely hypoxemic in the supine posture. Though ventilatory function improves after the initial period of spinal shock, high cervical cord injuries necessitate urgent intubation and ventilatory support.

Chronic Central Nervous System Disorders
Multiple Sclerosis

Multiple sclerosis is a demyelinating disease, very common in the West. It is not as uncommon as it was believed to be in India, being particularly observed in the Zoroastrian community of the country. Demyelinating plaques can occur anywhere within the CNS and/or spinal cord, symptoms and signs depend on the situation and size of these plaques. Rarely, plaques within the medulla may be so situated as to impair either reflex automatic breathing or voluntary breathing. More often, medullary involvement in multiple sclerosis leads to lower cranial nerve palsies with danger of aspiration pneumonia. A demyelinating plaque in the region of C3, C4, and C5 can cause diaphragmatic weakness or paralysis and multiple plaques within the thoracic segment of the spinal cord can result in a fair degree of respiratory muscle weakness. Acute respiratory failure may be precipitated if pulmonary infections complicate an exacerbation of the disease.

Parkinson's Disease

Parkinson's disease, common all over the world, has many respiratory complications. Aspiration of upper respiratory secretions or food or liquids is frequently observed in advanced disease due to difficulty in swallowing. This results in repeated episodes of aspiration pneumonia. Stiffness of the intercostal and other respiratory muscles together with abnormal control of breathing leads to dyspnea, tachypnea, reduced tidal volume, and reduced lung volumes. Patients with parkinsonism also have an instability of the large airways so that flow volume is saw-toothed both in the inspiratory and expiratory limbs. It is very important to bear in mind that the therapy with L-dopa can precipitate respiratory dysfunction in parkinsonian patients, sometimes within an hour of administrating a dose. Patients may develop tachypnea and dyspnea due to respiratory dyskinesia characterized by choreiform movements, and rigidity due to akinesia of the respiratory muscles.

Multiple System Atrophy or Shy-Drager Syndrome

Multiple system atrophy or Shy-Drager syndrome is characterized by parkinsonism coupled with autonomic nervous system disturbances—chiefly urinary retention and marked postural hypotension. Abnormalities in breathing patterns are also observed. These include abnormal control of breathing, irregular respiratory rate, Cheyne-Stokes breathing, central hypoventilation, and rarely apneustic breathing. The most dangerous complication that can cause death is bilateral abductor paralysis, which manifests as stridor, and obstructive sleep apnea.

■ DISEASES INVOLVING THE BRAIN AND/ OR ANTERIOR HORN CELLS

Rabies

Rabies, a fatal disease, still remains a grave problem in poor developing countries though a few cases continue to be reported in North America and very rarely in Western Europe as well. It is for all practical purposes a universally fatal disease caused by the rabies virus which gains entry through the bite of a rabid animal or through their lick over abraded skin. The incubation period varies from several weeks to several months, at times as long as a year. The reader is referred to a text in Medicine or Neurology for a detailed description of the disease. However, in 20% of cases, the inflammation the virus induces is initially confined to the spinal cord, where it produces a clinical picture indistinguishable from the Guillain-Barre syndrome (GBS). There is progressive, quickly evolving ascending paralysis with involvement of the respiratory muscles leading to respiratory arrest. If life is prolonged through ventilator and other supports, an encephalopathy with coma results.

Immediate treatment of the wound caused by bites or licks over abraded skin and postexposure prophylaxis is vital in subjects likely to be exposed to the virus. This consists of the prompt use of the rabies vaccine and of human rabies immunoglobulins.

Poliomyelitis

Poliomyelitis though extinct in many parts of the world is still reported from poor developing countries. Respiratory complications of the paralytic form of poliomyelitis are observed with extensive involvement of the anterior horn cells in spinal poliomyelitis or when there is involvement of the medulla. Respiratory involvement takes the form of respiratory paralysis. This may occasionally occur with frightening suddenness and rapidity. Rarely, it occurs as the first manifestation of the disease when limb power is normal and limb reflexes are still present. Extensive paralysis in these patients is then manifested over the next 24–48 hours. The gravity of the situation can be missed to start with, a ghastly mistake of dubbing the difficulty of breathing as "functional" being occasionally made.

Chronic Disorders

Amyotrophic Lateral Sclerosis

This progressive degenerative disorder is characterized by anterior horn cell involvement of the spinal cord and/or the motor nuclei of the cranial nerves together with lateral (pyramidal) tract involvement.

Respiratory involvement takes various forms. In many patients respiratory muscle strength is preserved even though the limbs are extensively paralyzed, the patient being wheelchair-bound or even bedridden. Motor neuron involvement is characterized by muscle weakness and fasciculations. Involvement of the motor nuclei in the brainstem is typically characterized by paralysis of muscles supplied by the 9th, 10th, and 11th nerves with fasciculations in the tongue. Long tract involvement is characterized by spasticity and extensor plantar responses. Aspiration pneumonia is a frequent accompaniment of medullary involvement. Paresis or paralysis of the abdominal muscles leads to weakness of expiratory muscles. Involvement of anterior horn cells of C3, C4, and C5 leads to diaphragmatic paralysis. These patients become hypoxemic when supine and need to be propped up in bed.

Very rarely, acutely involving respiratory paralysis may be the first manifestation of motor neuron disease due to involvement of the motor neurons of C3, C4, and C5. Again, a diagnosis of functional difficulty in breathing is mistakenly made. Fluoroscopy, however, reveals paresis or paralysis of the diaphragm. Basic lung function tests reveal reduced forced vital capacity (FVC) and a careful neurological examination will generally unearth a degree of muscle weakness, perhaps with evidence of muscle fasciculation. An electromyography (EMG) study will confirm the diagnosis.

Postpoliomyelitis Muscular Atrophy

About 20% of patients with previous poliomyelitis develop further muscle weakness as late as 20–40 years after the attack of poliomyelitis. This is due to denervation of regenerated motor units over a long period of time. This loss of muscle strength is gradual and if it involves respiratory muscles can cause respiratory failure. When kyphoscoliosis is an associated feature of poliomyelitis, further respiratory dysfunction due to hypoventilation results.

Spinal Muscular Atrophy

These are rare disorders only occasionally encountered by respiratory physicians. Spinal muscular atrophy (SMA) is of three types. Type I and Type II are also termed Werdnig–Hoffman disease. In Type I, SMA begins before 6 months of age and causes respiratory paralysis by the age of 2 years. Type II begins before the age of 2 years, is slower in evolution, and leads to respiratory failure in late childhood. The association of scoliosis or kyphoscoliosis worsens hypoventilation and respiratory failure. Type III also called Kugelberg-Welander disease begins before the age of 2 years and causes late respiratory failure due to respiratory muscle weakness and associated kyphoscoliosis. All forms of SMA cause more pronounced weakness in the lower limbs, most marked in the proximal muscles. The disease is an autosomal recessive one and arises from an anomaly on chromosome 5.

■ DISORDERS OF NERVE ROOTS AND/OR PERIPHERAL NERVES

Acute Disorders

Guillain-Barré Syndrome

The Guillain-Barré syndrome is characterized by extensive demyelinating polyradiculoneuropathy. Generally no proven etiology can be found though the disease has been reported due to the *Campylobacter, Epstein-Barr virus, Cytomegalovirus*, other viruses, and mycoplasmal infection. The condition has also rarely been reported to precede or be associated with Hodgkin's disease, non-Hodgkin's lymphoma, and other malignancies.

Muscle weakness commences in the lower limbs and ascends upwards with varying rapidity in many patients so as to involve the respiratory muscles. Proximal muscle weakness of the limbs is often more marked than the distal. Deep reflexes are lost starting with the lower limbs and then involving the upper limbs. Rarely, a descending variant of the disease may be observed. Sensory loss is minimal, generally affecting the distal lower limbs. Maximal muscle weakness takes place between 2 days and 2 weeks in a majority of patients. Motor cranial nerves may also be involved. A third nerve palsy associated with cerebellar signs is another variant of this syndrome (Miller Fisher variant). Autonomic dysfunction is observed in severe cases and is characterized by episodes of hypertension, hypotension, and rarely arrhythmias. Cerebrospinal fluid (CSF) examination shows a significant rise in proteins with perhaps a slight increase in lymphocytes.

Respiratory failure is chiefly due to respiratory muscle weakness. Aspiration causing atelectasis or aspiration pneumonia contributes to respiratory failure.

Ventilator support is necessary when there is respiratory muscle paresis. The tempo of the disease should be evaluated so that elective intubation with ventilator support can be offered without awaiting an emergency of well-nigh rapidly evolving apnea that could be disastrous.

Specific therapy consists of plasma exchange preferably followed by intravenous immunoglobulin. Most patients recover completely, but 15% are left with residual weakness and less than 2–5% develop relapsing episodes of demyelination.

Critical Care Polyneuropathy and Myopathy

Critical care polyneuropathy and/or myopathy are assuming increasing importance in patients under intensive care for several days or weeks. It is characterized by a subacute reversible axonal neuropathy giving rise to weakness of the lower limbs or all four limbs. Respiratory muscle paresis or paralysis is observed in severe cases and is an important cause for difficulty in weaning patients off ventilator support. Deep reflexes are generally absent. EMG points generally to an axonal neuropathy. Muscle biopsy shows changes of denervation and/or myopathic changes. CSF examination is normal. Complete recovery may take weeks and necessitates physiotherapy and prolonged rehabilitation.

Phrenic Nerve Injury

Damage or compression of the nerves induces bilateral diaphragmatic paralysis. The commonest cause of the injury is following open-heart surgery; other causes include massive intrathoracic surgery, mediastinal tumors, and severe mediastinal infection.

Bilateral diaphragmatic paralysis following open-heart surgery or intrathoracic surgery is characterized by inability of the patient to be weaned off ventilator support. The patient becomes extremely tachypneic and hypoxemic without ventilator support in the supine posture and improves when he sits upright. Recovery invariably occurs over time; we have seen complete recovery of diaphragmatic paralysis following open-heart surgery after as long as 6 months of ventilator support.

Rarer Neuritic Pathologies

Diphtheria due to *Corynebacterium diphtherias* causes an inflammatory membrane involving the tonsils and pharynx. Occasionally, the larynx is also involved causing life-threatening airways obstruction. Diphtheria toxin may occasionally affect the heart causing cardiomyopathy or arrhythmias and/or affect the peripheral nerves causing a peripheral neuropathy. A demyelinating polyneuropathy may develop 4–8 weeks after the initial infection, at times involving the respiratory muscles and causing respiratory failure. Neurological features, particularly those causing respiratory paralysis are indeed rare even in developing countries. They may take 12–36 weeks to resolve.

Herpes zoster is generally due to the reactivation of the varicella zoster infection. It causes a unilateral vesicular eruption involving one or two sensory nerve roots. The motor neuron of the root or roots affected may occasionally also be involved resulting in flaccid paralysis. Involvement of the motor neuron of either C3, C4, or C5 may result in hemidiaphragmatic paralysis. This may result in dyspnea, but does not cause respiratory failure. Occasionally, the eruption caused by herpes zoster is sparse and can be missed. Unexplained hemidiaphragmatic paralysis may at times be related to herpes zoster infection.

Metabolic Causes

Two important metabolic causes that cause respiratory muscle weakness and respiratory failure and that always need to be remembered include electrolyte disturbances in the form of hyperkalemia, hypokalemia, and hypomagnesemia. Hyperkalemia has many causes, the most important being acute or chronic renal failure. These patients can have acute hyperkalemia with acute respiratory paralysis and profound cardiac disturbances. Drugs such as angiotensin-converting enzyme (ACE) inhibitors and aldactone contribute to the sharp rise in serum potassium.

The second rare but important metabolic cause of acute respiratory paralysis is acute intermittent porphyria, which causes an axonal neuropathy, at times severe enough to involve the respiratory muscles and cause acute respiratory failure.

Toxic Causes

Rare toxic causes of acute neuropathy causing acute respiratory failure are toxins transmitted by fish— ciguatoxin produced by algae and transmitted by fish, saxitoxin transmitted by shell fish and tetrodotoxin produced by puffer fish. Thallium toxicity besides causing various organ system disorders can cause an axonal neuropathy that can result in respiratory failure.

■ DISORDERS INVOLVING THE NEUROMUSCULAR JUNCTION

Acute Disorders

Organophosphorus Poisoning

Organophosphorus poisoning is the most common cause of suicidal poisoning in India. Poisoning follows ingestion of organophosphorus insecticides. It can also occur from inhalation or absorption of the poison by the mucous membrane. Organophosphorus compounds are anticholinergic and initially cause a severe cholinergic crisis with marked pupillary constriction and involvement of major body systems. Severe hypotension and pulmonary edema together with bradyrhythms are observed. There is

widespread skeletal muscle weakness due to dysfunction at the postsynaptic neuromuscular level. The patient might appear to recover following full support to all systems and the use of pralidoxime, but after 2–4 days often manifests with cranial and proximal muscle weakness and respiratory failure. Specific therapy includes intravenous atropine, titrated to enable the pupil to return to and keep its normal size, and the intravenous use of pralidoxime. Ventilator support as also inotropic and vasopressor support is mandatory in all severe cases. Over-atropinization should be guarded against, as it causes serious problems.

Snakebite

The cobra and the krait are common snakes in India, Africa, Southeast Asian, and other developing countries. A bite from either of these snakes results in an injection of a neurotoxin which induces paralysis by preventing release of acetylcholine at the neuromuscular junction. Symptoms start within 1–12 hours of the bite. There is to start with ptosis, blurred vision, dysphagia, and a rapidly progressive descending paralysis which also involves the respiratory muscles causing acute respiratory failure. The patient invariably remains conscious to the very end.

Specific therapy consists of prompt use of polyvalent antivenom serum (4–6 vials as initial dose), prompt ventilatory support to counter respiratory paralysis, and support to organ systems as and when necessary. If death does not occur the paralysis regresses over 2–7 days. A bite from a king cobra can kill within less than 15 minutes to half an hour if the venom happens by chance to be directly injected into a vein.

Tick paralysis also follows a bite from a tick, which secretes a neurotoxin that blocks the release of acetylcholine. An ascending paralysis is observed after a latent period of 3–5 days. Respiratory muscle involvement leads to respiratory muscle paralysis and acute respiratory failure. Removal of the tick rapidly reverses the paralysis. Ventilator support is necessary till recovery ensues.

Botulism

Botulism is indeed a rare disorder in India. It is caused by the release of an exotoxin produced by *Clostridium botulinum*, a gram-positive spore-bearing anaerobe frequently and widely present in soil. The disease is chiefly caused by the consumption of improperly cooked food containing the exotoxin and spores. Canned food is particularly suspected when followed by symptoms described below. Rarely, botulism occurs from contamination of a wound by spores of the organism or by the exotoxin or from contaminated drugs given intravenously or intramuscularly. It has been reported to occur following colonization of the gastrointestinal (GI) tract by *C. botulinum* in the first 6 months of life. The exotoxin after hematogenous distribution, enters the neurons, binds irreversibly to calcium channels and blocks release of acetylcholine at neuromuscular junctions and at postganglionic parasympathetic nerve terminals.

After an incubation period of a few hours to a few days in food-borne disease, and up to about 2 weeks in wound botulism, symptoms become manifest. There is usually but not necessarily nausea and vomiting to start with, followed by blurred vision and a rapidly progressive descending paralysis. Respiratory muscle involvement leads to acute respiratory failure.

Botulism should always enter into the differential diagnosis of a GBS particularly when there is a descending paralysis instead of the generally expected ascending paralysis observed in the GBS. Blurred vision is another important differential feature; ptosis is frequent in botulism but occurs only in one of the variants of GBS. Extensive paresis or even paralysis of the GI tract and the bladder results from blockage of acetylcholine release at the postganglionic parasympathetic nerve terminals.

Diagnosis is by isolating the organism from contaminated food or from gastric aspirates in food-borne poisoning and from the wound and the serum in wound botulism.

Specific therapy consists of the use of specific antitoxin, which is unavailable in most countries outside America and Western Europe; penicillin in high doses and ventilatory support are necessary till the effect of the poison wears off.

Chronic Disorders

Myasthenia Gravis

Myasthenia gravis is the commonest chronic neuromuscular disorder met with in clinical practice. It is due to antibodies against acetylcholine receptors, so that though acetylcholine is secreted at the neuromuscular junction it cannot exert its effect.

The classic feature is increased fatigability and weakness following use of the affected muscles. The disease may be confined to causing a ptosis or diplopia, with features of a third nerve palsy being often noticed towards the evening or following a long stretch of reading. It could also be associated or solely confined to muscles innervated by the lower cranial nerves, or by involvement of skeletal muscles causing proximal muscle weakness, or the disease may be generalized and then presents with involvement of not only muscles supplied by the cranial nerves but also with skeletal muscle weakness. Occasionally, the only symptom is fatigability and at the time of examination muscle power may be passed off as normal. Notably, in all forms of presentation, including severe paralysis of limb muscles, the deep reflexes are preserved, and there is no sensory loss.

Involvement of respiratory muscles with respiratory failure occurs under the following circumstances:

- A slow progression of the disease involving skeletal muscles and/or muscles innervated by the cranial nerves, ultimately involving the respiratory muscles (intercostal and diaphragm).

- An acute myasthenic crisis can result in acute respiratory failure. A myasthenic crisis is characterized by worsening of symptoms generally related to a triggering factor. Triggering factors include intercurrent infections, surgery, stress, noncompliance in taking the anticholinesterase drug pyridostigmine, or the use of certain drugs in particular aminoglycosides which potentiate the disturbance in nerve conduction defect at the neuromuscular junction.

- At times, the disease presents as an emergency or in the intensive care unit (ICU) with rapidly evolving acute respiratory failure due to respiratory muscle paralysis in a patient who may have no preceding symptoms suggestive of myasthenia. *Myasthenia gravis should always enter into the diagnosis of acute respiratory failure when no obvious cause is found.*

Diagnosis rests on a clinical examination, presence of antibodies to acetylcholine receptors, and characteristic EMG findings pointing to increased fatigability of muscles on nerve stimulation. It is noted that in about 5% of patients the antibodies to acetylcholine receptors and antimuscle specific tyrosine kinase (MuSk) may not be present.

In an acute crisis occurring in an untreated patient, pyridostigmine 2–5 mg intravenously results in a prompt improvement of muscle weakness. An X-ray and computed tomography (CT) of the chest should always be done to determine the presence or otherwise of an enlarged thymus or a thymoma.

Treatment: Treatment consists of the use of anticholinesterases like pyridostigmine 60 mg thrice daily, prednisolone, starting with a low dose and increasing over a few weeks to 30–40 mg daily. Intravenous immunoglobulin and plasma exchange are also of help.

In an acute myasthenic crisis causing respiratory failure particularly after surgery, ventilator support becomes mandatory. It is best to omit pyridostigmine and to reintroduce it when the respiratory muscles have been rested and weaning is about to start.

In patients with chronic well-marked myasthenia which produces paresis of respiratory muscles (not needing ventilator support) standard therapy consists of the use of pyridostigmine orally, corticosteroids increased gradually over weeks to a dose of 100 mg on alternate days with azathioprine in a dose of 2 mg/kg body weight. The steroid is reduced by 5 mg every 3 weeks so that ultimately if possible the patient is maintained on azathioprine and pyridostigmine alone.

In spite of therapy some patients worsen over years and ultimately fail to respond to all therapy. Death is invariably due to respiratory failure, often worsened by intercurrent infection in the lungs or elsewhere.

■ DISORDERS OF THE MUSCLES

Acute Disorders

An important cause of rapidly evolving generalized muscle weakness is the use of high-dose corticosteroids, more so if these patients have in addition received neuromuscular blocking agents during ventilator support. This combination when continued for a length of time can be lethal, particularly in elderly patients. When the administration of steroids is considered imperative, it is wise to avoid neuromuscular blocking agents or limit their use, as these combinations can lead to grave problems in weaning, because of paresis of respiratory muscles. In the medical ICU this is most commonly observed in patients treated for acute severe asthma who have been given corticosteroids in large doses and have required both sedation and neuromuscular agents for effective ventilator support.

Chronic Disorders

Inflammatory Myopathies

The commonest disorders encountered in clinical practice giving rise to respiratory muscle weakness and hypoventilation are polymyositis, dermatomyositis, and inclusion body myositis. All these inflammatory myopathies are characterized by skeletal muscle weakness, more marked in the proximal muscles. Diagnosis is made by clinical examination, antibodies to $J0_1$ antigen, EMG studies, rise in creatine phosphokinase (CPK) levels, and by muscle biopsy. The reader is referred to the section on "Pulmonary manifestations of Systemic Diseases". The shrinking lung syndrome observed in systemic lupus erythematosus is due to atrophy with fibrosis of the diaphragmatic muscle.

Chronic Inherited Myopathies

These include Duchenne's muscular dystrophy, the facioscapulohumeral myopathy, and myotonic dystrophies. The reader is referred to a neurological text for a description of each of these neurological disorders.

Respiratory failure is seen most frequently in Duchenne's muscular dystrophy, most patients with this disease being wheelchair-dependent in their early teens. Tidal volumes as also lung volumes in these patients start to diminish by the age of 12. Though there is hypoventilation they may remain fairly stable for a decade or so. Initially there is nocturnal hypoxemia, followed by hypoxemia and hypercapnia during both day and at night during sleep. Scoliosis adds to the problems both in lung functions and chest wall mechanics. Death generally results from an acute respiratory crisis triggered by a chest infection. Noninvasive ventilator support should be considered early in the course of respiratory failure.

Respiratory failure in myotonia dystrophica occurs in advanced disease and is due to respiratory muscle weakness. Rarely, episodes of dyspnea are related to myotonia of the respiratory muscles which can be alleviated by antimyotonic treatment. Obstructive sleep apnea may add to the respiratory problem. These patients are extremely sensitive to anesthetic drugs and may require temporary postoperative ventilator support after a surgical procedure.

Congenital Myopathies

These are of several types and are characterized by typical abnormalities on muscle biopsy. The commonest form develops in infancy and childhood causing generalized muscle weakness and respiratory failure. The other less common forms of congenital myopathies are generally not associated with respiratory failure.

Metabolic Myopathies

Metabolic myopathies are indeed rare, but again should always be considered in the differential diagnosis of any patient with respiratory failure of obscure etiology.

Acid maltase deficiency (Pompe's disease) occurring in adults may present with respiratory failure, which is frequent and generally caused by dysfunction of the diaphragm.

Mitochondrial myopathies form a very rare group of systemic diseases due to various anomalies of deoxyribonucleic acid (DNA). We have never seen one but the following mitochondrial anomalies have been reported to be associated with respiratory failure, which is occasionally triggered by anesthetic agents or respiratory depressants, to which these patients are extremely sensitive. These mitochondrial myopathies are Kearns-Sayre syndrome, mitochondrial DNA depletion syndrome, and the syndrome which goes by the abbreviation MELAS—Mitochondrial myopathy, encephalopathy, lactic acid acidosis and stroke-like syndromes.

Pathophysiology

Neuromuscular disorders ultimately lead to poor respiratory muscle function, hypoventilation, and respiratory failure. In some disorders this is acute, in others, slowly evolving and chronic.

It needs to be kept in mind that even chronic neuromuscular disorders may occasionally present with acute respiratory failure as the initial event. It also needs to be mentioned that to start with there is no underlying lung pathology, but as hypoventilation and with it respiratory failure worsens, the risk of aspiration pneumonia increases. Once this transpires, a vicious cycle occurs leading to worsening respiratory failure unless appropriate measures are promptly taken.

Figure 1 illustrates the various points at which neuromuscular disorders may ultimately affect respiratory muscle function.

Diagnosis

The diagnosis of respiratory failure is easy in a patient with a previously known chronic neuromuscular disorder.

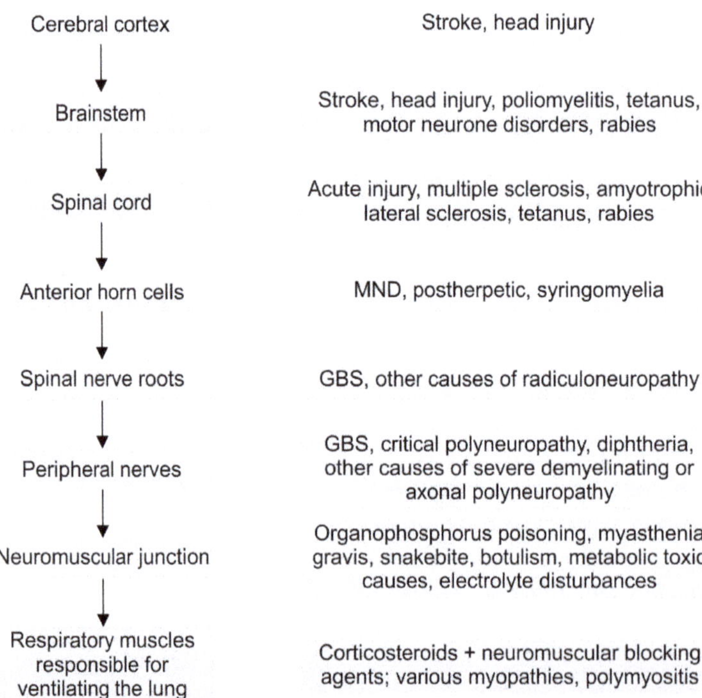

Fig. 1: The vertical column to the left illustrates the chain of nervous impulses that ultimately reach the respiratory muscles enabling them to ventilate the lung. The column to the right gives a few examples of disorders that act at various sites disturbing, slowing, or stopping this chain of nervous impulses. (GBS: Guillain-Barré syndrome; MND: Motor neuron disease)

However, it must be kept in mind that a smouldering chronic neuromuscular disorder may occasionally present with quickly evolving respiratory muscle paralysis and acute respiratory failure. Even if there is no past history of known neuromuscular disease, a careful history and physical examination is imperative. A history of fatigability on exertion, difficulty in getting up from a low chair or stool without the use of the upper limbs or a difficulty in swallowing are important clues. A history of ingestion of possible contaminated food (botulism) or of poisonous shell-fish (contaminated oysters, squid, and rarer fish), or of exposure to ticks should be sought. In the villages of India and in other poor tropical countries the possibility of snakebite should also be kept in mind. A history of dyspnea on exertion is obviously not specific for respiratory muscle involvement in neuromuscular disease. Dyspnea at rest is however a crucial clue if the lungs during examination are found to be clinically normal. Dyspnea at rest in a patient with neuromuscular disease is an indicator of acute respiratory failure or impending respiratory failure. Paralysis of both leaflets of the diaphragm causes orthopnea; the patient is unable to lie down supine, though for some inexplicable reason some of these patients are able to lie down on their side.

Paresis of respiratory muscles due to neuromuscular disease often leads initially to hypoventilation and hypercapnic respiratory failure at night, followed later by hypoxemic hypercapnic respiratory failure, both in the day and night.

Physical Examination

A meticulous examination of the central and peripheral nervous system should be done. Examination should particularly search for muscle weakness, whether more proximal or distal, presence of fasciculations, evidence for lateral column involvement, presence of atrophy or wasting, and presence or absence of deep reflexes. Wasting of the biceps in the presence of an exaggerated biceps tendon reflex is classically associated with amyotrophic lateral sclerosis, though compressive cord lesions at the C5 level could do likewise. Evidence of ptosis which becomes apparent only when the patient is made to fix his or her gaze upwards for a time is excellent evidence of underlying myasthenia. Poor gag reflex and poor movement of the palatal fold suggest involvement of either the lower cranial nerves, or is seen in polymyositis. The latter is at times

clinically unmasked only if the patient is observed to get up from a low stool, as this proves difficult without the use of the upper limbs.

Examination of the chest should be meticulously performed. The respiratory rate should be counted for a whole minute; presence or absence of the use of accessory muscles of respiration should be noted. The degree of chest expansion should be observed both on inspection and palpation. Diaphragmatic paralysis, besides being characterized by the inability to lie flat, is characterized by dyspnea, tachypnea, and paradoxical respiration, wherein the diaphragm is sucked inwards during inspiration and pushed out during expiration. Paresis of diaphragmatic leaflets is suggested by the absence of the outward movement of the diaphragm during inspiration. *A serial count of numbers at as fast a speed as possible after making the patient take a maximum inspiratory breath is an excellent bedside test to determine the presence and progress of respiratory muscle paresis or paralysis.* This of course holds true only if there is no underlying parenchymal lung disease, cardiac disease, or any other disease responsible for the difficulty in breathing.

In the differential diagnosis of neuromuscular disease causing acute respiratory failure often associated with paralysis of the skeletal muscles, one should consider GBS, acute myasthenic crisis, paralytic poliomyelitis, acute corticosteroid myopathy, critical illness polyneuropathy and myopathy, acutely evolving polymyositis, acute hypokalemic or hyperkalemic paralysis, botulism, cobra or krait snakebite, and acute intermittent porphyria. Poisoning with various known and perhaps lesser known toxins can also present in the same manner. A GBS may also rarely occur in association with concurrent malignancy (particularly a small cell lung cancer) and preceding or accompanying malignant lymphoproliferative disease.

The important chronic neuromuscular disorders which may occasionally present with an acutely evolving respiratory paralysis causing acute respiratory failure are myasthenia gravis, polymyositis or dermatomyositis, and rarely amyotrophic lateral sclerosis.

Acute diaphragmatic paralysis due to phrenic nerve involvement can cause isolated acute respiratory failure. This is observed after open-heart surgery and after major surgery on the thorax or mediastinal structures. Each of these conditions should be carefully excluded in patients presenting with acute respiratory paralysis causing acute respiratory failure.

Imaging

Elevation of the dome of the diaphragm can occur with diaphragmatic paralysis, but can also result from basal atelectasis. In diaphragmatic paralysis the sniff test reveals a paradoxical movement of the diaphragm, the diaphragmatic leaflets moving upwards during an inspiratory sniff instead of the usual brisk downward movement. A subpulmonic pleural effusion can give the appearance of a raised diaphragm. Imaging studies in particular an high-resolution computed tomography (HRCT) of the chest gives the correct diagnosis.

Arterial Blood Gas Studies

The distinguishing feature of hypoventilation causing respiratory failure is hypoxemic hypercapnic respiratory failure. To start with, respiratory failure occurs in sleep. Nocturnal hypercapnia manifests with sleepiness during the day, confusion at night, and early morning headaches.

Lung Function Tests and Tests to Assess Inspiratory and Expiratory Muscle Strength

Changes in Lung Studies

Lung volumes: Respiratory muscle weakness leads to a fall in vital capacity (VC), FVC, end-expiratory lung volume, the functional residual capacity (FRC), and the total lung capacity (TLC). The residual volume (RV) may be normal or even slightly increased. In the absence of lung or skeletal disease, a reduced VC should point to respiratory muscle weakness. The VC test is not a very sensitive test as respiratory muscle strength needs to be reduced substantially (by over 50%) to cause a significant fall in the VC. The RV/TLC ratio is increased, but this is not due to obstructive airways disease. The pressure volume curve in patients with respiratory muscle weakness is shifted to the right, so that a large increase in inspiratory pressure near TLC or a large increase in expiratory pressure close to RV produces comparatively small changes in lung volume.

Lung Compliance and Chest Wall Mechanics

In acute respiratory muscle weakness, the fall in lung volumes is associated with normal lung compliance. In chronic or longstanding respiratory failure the following changes in lung compliance and chest wall mechanics occur:

- Reduced lung compliance
- Reduced chest wall compliance
- Lung elastic recoil is higher than normal at any given lung volume
- Lung elastic recoil pressure in higher than normal at TLC which itself is significantly reduced.

The reduction of lung compliance is due to stiffening of the lung elastin tissue due to prolonged hypoventilation together with microatelectasis so often seen in poorly expanded lungs, as also the occurrence of segmental atelectasis related to shallow breathing and ineffective cough. The fall in chest wall compliance is believed to be related to the stiffening of the costosternal and costovertebral joints due to prolonged poor excursions of the chest wall. The low compliance of the lung and chest wall, in addition to lessened movement of the chest during the respiratory cycle because of respiratory muscle weakness, is responsible for the low TLC.

Flow-volume Loop

The flow-volume loop shows the following abnormalities:

- A reduction in the peak expiratory flow
- Delay in reaching the peak expiratory flow
- A sharp drop in expiratory flow rate towards end of expiration
- The forced inspiratory volume in first second (FIV_1) is less than the forced expiratory volume in first second (FEV_1) because of weakness of the inspiratory muscles.

Diffusion Capacity for Carbon Monoxide

The diffusion capacity for carbon monoxide (DLCO) is reduced, but as mentioned earlier the transfer coefficient (KCO) or DLCO/VA (alveolar volume) is typically increased. In patients with neuromuscular diseases, a sniff test below 30% of normal is generally associated with hypercapnic respiratory failure. If the maximum transdiaphragmatic pressure generated during a sniff test is less than 30 cm H_2O there is again a strong likelihood of hypercapnic respiratory failure.

Serial Number Counting Test after Taking a Deep Inspiration

This is an extremely useful test for inspiratory muscle strength particularly in acutely evolving respiratory weakness. The patient is asked to take as deep an inspiratory breath and is asked to number serially 1, 2, 3, as fast as possible. Most normal individuals can easily count up to 30 and much more in a single breath. Inability to go beyond 20 and in particular a falling number count when tested at intervals is a good guide to inspiratory muscle weakness.

Tests for Expiratory Muscles (see Chapter on Mechanics of Ventilation)

The PEmax is an index of expiratory muscle strength though values below normal are difficult to interpret.

Cough Test

It is best to gauge the strength of a patient's cough clinically at the bedside. The patient is requested to cough as loudly as possible after a deep inspiration. With a little practice one can judge whether the cough is weak or normal. Serial observations in patients with acutely evolving respiratory muscles weakness are of great help.

Reduced Muscle Strength and Function

Reduced lung volumes may occur in lung pathologies other than in patients with pure respiratory muscle weakness, so that direct measurement of muscle strength may be necessary. Strength of both inspiratory and expiratory muscles should be evaluated as the decline in respiratory muscle strength need not be necessarily the same. Inspiratory muscle weakness leads to dyspnea and hypoxemic cum hypercapnic respiratory failure. Expiratory muscle weakness is responsible for a poor ineffective cough that predisposes to aspiration, microatelectasis, and segmental atelectasis.

Tests for Inspiratory Muscles

The easiest test for inspiratory muscle strength is to determine the PImax. A PImax less than 50% of predicated is often associated with CO_2 retention. There are however fallacies that may enter in performing the test in patients with respiratory muscle weakness (e.g. air leak around the mouth piece) and difficulties in interpretation as some normal patients may also have a low PImax.

Sniff nasal inspiratory pressure test and the sniff diaphragmatic pressure test have been described in the chapter Respiratory Muscle Function Tests.

Management

Treatment of the Cause

This is possible in just a few of the neuromuscular disorders causing respiratory paresis and respiratory failure. In most patients with neuromuscular disorders there is no specific treatment and no adequate measure that can prevent respiratory failure in the natural history of the disease (see chapter on Acute Respiratory Failure in Adults).

Patients with chronic neuromuscular disease who develop over a period of observation slowly progressive chronic respiratory failure are managed comfortably on noninvasive ventilator support. Noninvasive ventilator support to start with may be necessary only at night. As respiratory failure worsens, support becomes necessary both during day and night. It is best not to delay noninvasive ventilator support once there is persistent hypercapnia.

In amyotrophic lateral sclerosis, noninvasive ventilator support should be introduced once hypercapnia occurs. When the brainstem is involved so that the patient is unable to swallow and cannot handle upper airways secretions, tracheostomy becomes necessary. Invasive ventilator support prolongs life, but the quality of life is indeed poor and the situation should be carefully explained to the patient as he or she has the right to make the choice—to ventilate invasively or not.

Functional Approach to the Management of Neuromuscular Diseases

The neuromuscular respiratory system has three main areas of function:
1. Ventilatory function, depending chiefly on the inspiratory muscles.
2. Effective cough, dependent on inspiratory, expiratory muscles, and on glottic function.
3. Airway protection, through integrity of muscles of deglutition and proper glottic function.

Any one of these three functions may be affected singly or in combination. Amyotrophic lateral sclerosis is an example where all three functions may be affected. Bilateral diaphragmatic paralysis involves chiefly an impairment of ventilatory function though cough would also be mildly impaired. GBS could again affect all these areas of neurorespiratory function. A practical approach would be to test appropriately (both clinically and by relevant tests) which one or more these areas of function are impaired in a given patient.

Ventilatory muscle dysfunction: The FVC is a measure of global respiratory muscle strength. The maximum inspiratory pressure and maximum expiratory pressure gauge inspiratory and expiratory muscle strength, respectively. Early bilateral diaphragmatic muscle weakness is judged by noting the significantly lower FVC in the supine position as compared to the upright sitting or standing position. The sniff inspiratory nasal pressure (SNIP) is a reliable measure of the strength of the inspiratory muscles. It has been shown to be an accurate predictor of the presence of nocturnal desaturation and respiratory failure in patients with amyotrophic lateral sclerosis.

Hypoventilation in neuromuscular disease to start with often presents at night in sleep, particularly during the rapid eye movement (REM) stage. Symptoms include frequent nocturnal awakenings, daytime hypersomnolence, morning headaches, and diminished daytime performance. Nocturnal measurement of oxygen saturation during sleep should prove the diagnosis. Polysomnography may be necessary in some individuals. Noninvasive positive pressure ventilation (NPPV) is the preferred treatment for hypoventilation due to neuromuscular disease. It is used at night to prevent nocturnal desaturation and if hypoventilation persists in the day ($PaCO_2 \geq 48$ mm Hg) NPPV is given during the day as well. NPPV has been extensively used in patients with acute myeloid leukemia (AML) and in demyelinating diseases (DMD). A number of nonrandomized studies have suggested increased survival in both amyotrophic lateral sclerosis and DMD following the use of NPPV. Tracheostomy ventilation may be necessary when bulbar involvement prevents use of noninvasive modalities, but is associated with many potential complications.

Ineffectual cough: An ineffectual cough is manifest when the patient is asked to cough; the cough is feeble and ineffective. The patient cannot expectorate respiratory secretions which continue to be retained within the chest. Cough function (i.e. the strength of a cough) can be assessed by measuring the peak cough flow (PCF). This can be measured with a usual asthma peak flow meter. Normal values ranges from 360 L/min to 906 L/min. A value below 150 L/min points to a very poor cough. Patients who to start with have a poor PCF may drop their peak flow to dangerous levels in the presence of a severe respiratory infection.

There are a number of cough augmentation methods in use to promote a stronger cough and help expectorate respiratory secretions.

Steam inhalation coupled with good conventional physiotherapy to the chest in our opinion is still of great value. An experienced physiotherapist has saved many lives in the ICU.

Lung recruitment measures that inflate the lung to the maximal insufflation capacity above the patients VC is achieved by "breath stacking". Extra breaths are delivered with a resuscitation bag, mouthpiece volume ventilator, mechanical insufflator-exsufflator (MI-E). The lung is thereby increased to a supramaximal lung volume. Lung volume recruitment improves compliance, increases elastic recoil, and allows a better cough with an increased PCF that allows clearance of respiratory secretions.

Devices that oscillate or vibrate the respiratory system may loosen mucus and thick respiratory secretions and thereby indirectly help in their removal.

Swallowing dysfunction: Swallowing dysfunction occurs in a number of neuromuscular disorders involving the nuclei of the 9th, 10th, and 11th cranial nerves, the trunk of the nerves, the neuromuscular junction, and the muscles involved in swallowing. Patients whose swallowing disturbance is due to neuromuscular disease can swallow semisolid better than liquids. Pseudobulbar palsy can also lead to difficulty in swallowing. The major risk is of aspiration pneumonia. If the patient constantly coughs on swallowing, it is better to feed him or her through a nasogastric tube. If the swallowing dysfunction is related to a cause which cannot be medically addressed a percutaneous endoscopic gastrostomy (PEG) insertion is advised through which nutrition can be given.

Irrecoverable Diaphragmatic Paralysis

Cervical cord lesions at C5, C6 level, or severe irrecoverable bilateral phrenic nerve damage as after open-heart or thoracic surgery, or patients with central alveolar hypoventilation, are indications for diaphragmatic pacing. The phrenic nerves are stimulated by intrathoracic implanted electrodes, the receiver being activated by radiofrequency waves generated by an external power source. The method is costly, requires special expertise; we have no experience in this field.

Physiotherapy

Physiotherapy is vital for survival both in acute respiratory failure and in chronic respiratory failure due to neuromuscular cause. The airways should be kept free of secretions through careful suction and gentle percussion and vibration to the chest. Frequent change of posture is essential. Cough must be encouraged. This may be impossible with severe respiratory muscle paralysis. Manual assistance to cough is given through squeezing of the chest and by a gentle yet sudden upper abdominal thrust timed with opening of the glottis. Mechanical insufflation followed by desufflation may help. It is done by first using a positive pressure insufflation followed by an abrupt negative pressure which causes desufflation. Cough assist devices are fairly popular abroad. In our opinion, the best method and the least inconvenient method to the patient who fails to cough and clear secretions in spite of expert physiotherapy is to perform a tracheostomy through which secretions can be sucked and the airways kept open.

■ SUGGESTED READING

1. Benditt JO, Boitano LJ. Pulmonary issues in patients with chronic neuromuscular disease. Am J Respir Crit Care Med. 2013;187(10):1046-55.

2. De Jonghe B, Lacherade JC, Durand MC, et al. Critical illness neuromuscular syndromes. Crit Care Clin. 2006;22(4):805-18.

3. Hemachudha T, Laothamatas J, Rupprecht CE. Human rabies: a disease of complex neuropathogenetic mechanisms and diagnostic challenges. Lancet Neurol. 2002;1(2):101-9.

4. Horowitz BZ. Botulinum toxin. Crit Care Clin. 2005;21(4):825-39.

5. Lambert DA, Giannouli E, Schmidt BJ. Postpolio syndrome and anesthesia. Anesthesiology. 2005;103(3):638-44.

6. Maramattom BV, Wijdicks EF. Acute neuromuscular weakness in the intensive care unit. Crit Care Med. 2006;34(11):2835-41.

7. Radunovic A, Annane D, Tewitt K, et al. Mechanical ventilation for amyotrophic lateral sclerosis/motor neuron disease. Cochrane Database Syst Rev. 2009;4:CD004427.

8. Simonds AK. Recent advances in respiratory care for neuromuscular disease. Chest. 2006;130(6):1879-86.

9. Trojan DA, Cashman NR. Post-poliomyelitis syndrome. Muscle Nerve. 2005;31(1):6-19.

10. Van Doorn PA, Ruts L, Jacobs BC. Clinical features, pathogenesis, and treatment of Guillain-Barre syndrome. Lancet Neurol. 2008;7(10):939-50.

11. Yazici Y, Kagen LJ. Clinical presentation of the idiopathic inflammatory myopathies. Rheum Dis Clin North Am. 2002;28(4):823-32.

Sleep-related Breathing Disorders

CHAPTER 74

Sleep-related Breathing Disorders

■ INTRODUCTION

We spend a third of our lives asleep but it is now clear that sleep is not always the tranquil resting state it is imagined to be. We now know, the lives of millions are disturbed and disrupted by the consequences of sleep-disordered breathing (SDB).

Sleep disorders involve any difficulties related to sleeping, including difficulty falling or staying asleep, falling asleep at inappropriate times, excessive total sleep time, or abnormal behaviors associated with sleep.

■ TYPES OF SLEEP DISORDERS

The International Classification of Sleep Disorders (ICSD), published in 2004 lists 85 sleep disorders, each presented in detail and with a specific diagnostic test. These have been classified as follows into the following eight major categories:

1. The insomnias
2. The sleep-related breathing disorders
3. The hypersomnias not due to a breathing disorder
4. The circadian rhythm sleep disorders
5. The parasomnias
6. The sleep-related movement disorders
7. Isolated symptoms, apparently normal variants and unresolved issues
8. Other sleep disorders.

This chapter will focus on obstructive sleep apnea (OSA) and central sleep apnea (CSA) as these are the two major sleep-related breathing disorders.

■ OBSTRUCTIVE SLEEP APNEA

History

What is so remarkable about OSA is that it should have been so obvious and common yet escaped recognition by the medical community till it was first described by Gastaut in a neurology journal in 1965. Yet, Charles Dickens, an astute observer of the human condition, must be given the credit for first describing this disorder, well over a century before its first medical report. Dickens was only 21 years at the time, yet he went on, in 1836, to describe in his first book, *The Pickwick Papers,* a textbook description of a person with OSA. In Joe, the fat boy, we see an uncannily accurate description of OSA almost 130 years before the world of medicine had acknowledged its existence. The snoring and the irresistible urge to fall asleep, the two cardinal symptoms of OSA are summed up when he has a character say:

"Asleep! He is always asleep. Goes on errands fast asleep, and snores as he waits at table."

Definition

Obstructive sleep apnea is defined as repetitive episodes of upper airway obstruction occurring during sleep, usually associated with a reduction in SaO_2, with features of snoring and daytime sleepiness. The apnea-hypopnea index is the most commonly used criterion to quantify the severity of OSA. According to the American Association of Sleep Medicine, OSA exists when the patient has five or more obstructed breathing events (apneas or hypopneas) per hour of sleep with an appropriate clinical presentation.

Epidemiology

Obstructive sleep apnea is a difficult disease to study, as the standard diagnostic test, polysomnography (PSG), is expensive and cumbersome. Until the American Academy of Sleep Medicine Task Force published recent guidelines in 1989, there was no clear consensus regarding diagnostic classification. Thus, worldwide there have been only a few good-quality epidemiological studies.

Global Epidemiology

Initial studies in the eighties and early nineties involved short case series or prevalence studies in selected cohorts rather than in the general population. These early studies sought to determine the "lower limit" of prevalence by conducting PSG in small subsets comprising only people with self-reported OSA symptoms selected from sample surveys and then assuming that all cases of OSA had been identified. Although such studies were undermined by the low sensitivity of screening questions, even these lower limits of prevalence established the importance of studying OSA further. Stradling analyzed these early epidemiological studies in a review and noted that the prevalence of OSA varied from 1–4% in adult males. Since then, studies on much larger population-based samples have shown an even higher prevalence. The landmark epidemiological study that brought OSA to the attention of physicians and the lay public was the Wisconsin Sleep Cohort Study in 1993 by Terry Young and colleagues. These authors showed that based on a sample of 625 adults, 9% of women and 24% of men had SDB with an average of at least five or more apneas and hypopneas per hour of sleep. OSA, defined as SDB plus the cardinal symptom of excessive daytime sleepiness (EDS), occurred in 2% of women and 4% of men. This study put OSA on the world map by demonstrating that it was a widely prevalent disorder. When one factored in the major cardiovascular impact of this potentially disabling condition, it became clear that undiagnosed OSA represented a potential public health hazard that had to be addressed. Since Young's study, there have been several other studies of prevalence from across the developing world but direct comparison is difficult due to considerable variations in methodology. Different studies have, for example, studied different patient populations, used different diagnostic tools, and

often used different definitions of OSA. These differences in methodology must be borne in mind when making comparisons. Many prevalence studies have had one or more methodological weaknesses including selection biases, varying definitions of OSA, failure to distinguish types of apneas, failure to control for confounding variables, and small sample sizes. These inherent weaknesses in the available studies have made direct comparisons difficult.

Asian Epidemiology

It had initially been perceived that OSA might not be common in the Asian populations due to the fact that obesity, the major risk factor for OSA, is less prevalent than in Western communities. However, this is not the case. Several studies comparing OSA in Asians and Caucasians have shown that Asian subjects have greater severity of illness, as indicated by higher respiratory disturbance indices compared to Caucasian patients matched for age, sex and body mass index (BMI).

A study by Ng looked at the prevalence of OSA in the three major ethnic populations in Singapore; Chinese, Malays and Indians. This study established that Indians living in Singapore had the highest prevalence rates (4.5%), significantly higher than the prevalence in Malays (3.7%) and Chinese (1.6%). This was the first study to suggest that Indians, as a race, had a predisposition to OSA. An important study by Hilloowalla hinted that Indian craniofacial anatomy might be the factor predisposing this race to OSA. He compared 75 skulls of Indian origin to 98 Tuscan skulls and noted important cephalometric differences. This pointed to a possible osteogenic etiology of OSA in Indians.

Indian Epidemiology

Obstructive sleep apnea is a disease that is strongly affected by racial factors and it seems vital to establish the prevalence in a country of 1.2 billion Indians. India also has amongst the largest populations with ischemic heart disease, diabetes and hypertension and the potential impact of untreated OSA on these subpopulations of Indians is clearly a cause for concern.

There is almost no data on the epidemiology of OSA from India. Possible reasons for this include lack of awareness and formal training in sleep medicine and the cost and lack of availability of PSG. Although the first sleep laboratory in the country was established only in 1991, there has been a rapid and exponential increase in the number of private and public sleep laboratories since then. The laboratories are mainly concentrated in the big metros and the numbers are still very limited for a country of 1 billion. An occasional study has looked at the prevalence of OSA in patients referred to and assessed at sleep clinics but an accurate idea of the prevalence of OSA in the general population was until recently lacking. A recent population-based study by Udwadia published in 2004 will be discussed in more detail here, as it was the first epidemiological attempt to study the prevalence of OSA in India.

The authors chose 700 consecutive healthy Indian male residents of Mumbai, aged 35–65 years coming as outpatients to the Hinduja Hospital for a routine health checkup between December 1999 and December 2000. None of these patients were coming to the hospital because of suspected sleep problems. Most were undergoing health checks as part of company policy or for insurance reasons.

A two-stage sampling scheme was designed to optimize the study's precision. In the first stage, subjects were given a specially designed comprehensive 32-part questionnaire adapted to local conditions and translated into local languages where needed. It sought detailed information on the cohorts sleep habits, snoring, daytime sleepiness, nocturnal choking and associated medical conditions. Physical examination was done thereafter with measurements of BMI, neck girth and blood pressure. All questionnaires were collected and analyzed by a doctor on the same day. Based on the responses, subjects were classified into habitual snorers and non-snorers. All (100%) snorers and 25% of non-snorers were contacted and offered a sleep study if they consented. The type of sleep study chosen was a limited, home-based, semi-supervised sleep study performed on a Compumedics P series 10-channel system. This was considered a more practical and economical approach than a full electroencephalogram-based PSG in the hospital. The home-based Compumedics system had been validated in several home-based studies and gave polygraphic recordings of nasal and oral airflow, electrocardiographic, thoracic and abdominal effort, tracheal sounds, limb movement, body position and oxyhemoglobin level by pulse oximetry.

The results of the study were as follows: 700 questionnaires were given out and 658 were completed and returned giving an initial response rate of 94%. All 171 snorers and 122 non-snorers (25% contacted) were asked if they would undergo sleep testing at home. A total of 254 subjects agreed (151 of the snorers and 103 non-snorers) giving a good participation rate of 87%. Habitual snoring was seen in 26% of the study population, nocturnal choking or witnessed apneas in 5% and daytime hypersomnolescence in 22% of the study population. The mean age of the sample was 47.84 years, and the mean BMI was 24.56. The mean Epworth score of snorers was 8.39 and that of non-snorers was 6.05.

The prevalence of SDB was 19.5% and that of obstructive sleep apnea-hypopnea syndrome was 7.5% in healthy urban Indian males between 35–65 years of age. These prevalence rates are among the highest reported from epidemiological studies across the globe and are higher than in most Western and Asian studies. In this study, BMI, neck girth, and a history of diabetes mellitus were significantly associated with SDB, and a history of snoring, EDS, nocturnal choking, recurrent awakening from sleep, unrefreshing sleep and daytime fatigue were all associated with OSA.

Reasons for Higher Prevalence Found in Indians

The exact causes of this unexpectedly high prevalence are unclear. It must first be pointed out that this data cannot be extended to the country as a whole as only urban Indian men in Mumbai were studied. The study population represents men that are better educated and employed, have higher incomes and are of better socioeconomic class than rural Indians. Also, urban Indian males are significantly more obese (BMI of 24) than their rural counterparts (BMI of 20). Obesity is a major risk factor for OSA in white populations. In this study, a higher BMI was a risk factor for SDB and OSA in Indian subjects as well. However, it is worth stating that 46% of our subjects with SDB had a BMI of less than 30, the Western cut-off for obesity whereas 27% of subjects with SDB had a BMI less than 27, which is the cut-off point for obesity in Asians. These observations suggest that a significant number of patients, though not obese by Western or Asian standards, still had SDB and OSA. This leads the authors to postulate that other craniofacial risk factors for SDB, such as oropharyngeal narrowing, retrognathia or micrognathia, and pharyngeal collapsibility, might assume greater pathogenic significance in Indian subjects and may be responsible for our higher prevalence rates.

In agreement with other Western studies, this study found neck girth to be an important predictor of OSA and found that the risk of SDB is 5.34 times higher for subjects with a neck girth of 17 inches or more.

Other subsequent Indian epidemiological studies: The only other epidemiological studies from India reported lower prevalence rates: The first by Sharma in 2006, reported a prevalence rate of 13.7% for SDB and 3.6% for OSA in a community-based prevalence study in a semi-urban community in Delhi. The second from Reddy in 2009 again from an urban Delhi population reported the prevalence of SDB to be 9.3% and that of OSA to be 2.8% (4% in males and 1.5% in females).

Conclusion

Thus, there is a divergence in the prevalence rates reported from India with higher prevalence rates in the study from Mumbai in western India, and lower rates from the two Delhi-based studies from northern India. These differences could be real differences as it is possible that different regions and populations in a country as diverse as India could have different prevalence rates. The other explanation could be methodological. The Mumbai study was performed only in men belonging to a higher socioeconomic status with a home-based system, which could have introduced an element of selection bias. The Delhi studies were in both sexes in a community-based setting and had fully supervised PSG performed in a sleep laboratory. Irrespective of which rates are more accurate, these studies have established that OSA is indeed at least as prevalent and possibly even more prevalent in India compared to the West. The high prevalence rates found in these studies might have major public health implications in a developing country with limited health resources. Indian men in this age group have among the highest rates of ischemic heart disease and hypertension worldwide. When compared to whites, blacks, Hispanics and other Asians, coronary artery disease rates among Indians worldwide are 2–4 times higher at all ages. India also has the largest population of individuals with diabetes (approximately 25 million) and the potential impact of untreated OSA on this population might be considerable. Further studies in populations from different races, in different communities (urban and rural) from all regions of this vast country are urgently needed before a clearer picture of OSA in India emerges. Finally, Indian cranial anthropometric studies are needed to determine if our facial structure uniquely predisposes Indians to a higher prevalence of OSA.

Clinical Features

The cardinal symptoms of OSA are disruptive snoring, EDS, nocturnal choking and witnessed apneas.

Snoring

Snoring is a cardinal symptom of OSA. It is defined as an inspiratory vibration of the soft tissue of the oropharynx. It denotes partial obstruction of the upper airway. Not all snorers have OSA of course; it is estimated that at least 60% of men over the age of 40 snore. The snoring of OSA is distinctive in its quality. It is often disruptively loud, loud enough to drive the spouse out of the bedroom and sometimes out of the house. In one study in the US, almost 50% of all patients slept in separate bedrooms from their partner. Its intensity is often noted to be more than 50 dB when measured by PSG. An astute partner will describe the snoring as intermittent, more in the supine than the lateral position, of a waxing and waning quality, and sometimes interrupted by long periods of ominous silence when it is felt the patient seems to have stopped breathing altogether. While snoring on its own has a low diagnostic accuracy for OSA, the pattern of snoring just described is very predictive of a positive sleep study. Most snorers are unaware that they snore and there is poor agreement between snorers and their bed-partners when it comes to this symptom. Women are less likely to admit to snoring and patients from poorer socioeconomic backgrounds are also less likely to complain of it or be questioned regarding their snoring habits. In any case, snoring is the most common complaint precipitating referral to a sleep laboratory. A patient and sometimes his spouse may not be forthcoming with a history of snoring hence asking each patient if they snore should be part of each and every medical history. OSA is one of the least diagnosed diseases and we must train ourselves and our medical students that it would be negligent not to enquire about snoring and sleepiness from every patient we encounter. This is even more important with the realization that snoring alone (i.e. even non-apneic snoring) may be an independent risk factor for hypertension, cardiovascular disease and cerebrovascular disease.

Excessive Daytime Sleepiness

Excessive daytime sleepiness is the second major symptom of OSA. Like snoring, it is a nonspecific symptom and occurs in a host of other conditions enumerated in **Table 1**. In OSA, it is often but not always present. In patients with severe OSA, it is an overwhelming urge to sleep in situations that the patient himself acknowledges are inappropriate. Thus, we have had patients who routinely fall asleep whilst driving, those who fall asleep whilst addressing a meeting, in the midst of signing a check and even, on one occasion, whilst climbing a ladder.

Nocturnal Choking

Nocturnal choking is another important but nonspecific symptom of OSA. It occurs in a few other conditions as outlined in **Table 2**. However, it is a frightening symptom and will often alert the patient and his spouse into consulting a doctor.

Witnessed Apnea

Witnessed apnea is the most specific symptom of OSA. Apneic episodes may be reported by as many as 75% of bed partners. Episodes of loud snoring often terminate in an apnea. A characteristic pattern observed in OSA is that of loud snoring or brief gasps that alternate with episodes of silence that typically last 20–30 seconds. An apnea is defined as complete cessation of breathing for a period of at least 10 seconds. Many apneas are longer, some stretching to almost 60 seconds or beyond. An apnea terminates in an arousal and these cycles of apnea and subsequent arousal fragment the patient's sleep resulting in sleep that is of very poor quality.

Table 1: Causes of excessive daytime sleepiness.
• Sleep deprivation • Obstructive sleep apnea • Narcolepsy • Idiopathic hypersomnolescence • Nocturnal myoclonus • Periodic limb movement disorder (PLMD) • Psychological (20% depressed patients) • Drugs and alcohol • Hypothyroidism • Postviral fatigue syndrome

Table 2: Causes of nocturnal choking.
• Pulmonary edema (paroxysmal nocturnal dyspnea) • Nocturnal asthma • Obstructive sleep apnea • Gastroesophageal reflux disease causing laryngeal spasm

Other Symptoms

A host of other symptoms and signs are reported in OSA. These include:
- Restless, nonrefreshing sleep
- Diaphoresis usually in the neck and chest area
- Nocturia, with one study reporting a third of all patients with OSA getting up 4–7 times at night to urinate
- Morning headaches, a study from a headache clinic found OSA to be the commonest cause of morning headaches. None of these patients had been previously investigated for OSA.
- Gastroesophageal reflux is common in patients with OSA and is believed to be due to the raised intra-abdominal pressure observed in patients with OSA related to increased breathing efforts during periods of apnea.

Clinical Presentations of Obstructive Sleep Apnea

The following are some of the clinical presentations we have encountered where OSA must be clinically suspected:
- Unexplained respiratory failure (pulmonologist)
- Unexplained pulmonary hypertension or cor pulmonale (pulmonologist)
- Unexplained polycythemia (hematologist)
- Confusional state (neurologist)
- Nocturnal seizure (neurologist)
- Nocturnal arrhythmia (cardiologist)
- Postanesthetic respiratory failure (anesthetist)
- Postextubation problems (anesthetist)
- Nocturia, enuresis (urologist)
- Impotence in a male (andrologist).

Thus, as can be seen, OSA can present to a wide range of specialists.

Diagnosing Obstructive Sleep Apnea

History

The cardinal symptoms mentioned earlier must be inquired about in the history. Clinical pointers or risk factors that increase the index of suspicion are obesity, male sex and age more than 65 years. A positive family history also increases the risk of OSA 2–4-fold. First-degree relatives of OSA patients have a 21–84% chance of having OSA themselves compared to 10% of the controls. This genetic predisposition is likely to be expressed through craniofacial anatomy, though obesity is also often genetic, and both these factors can explain why OSA often runs in families.

Physical Examination

Body mass index: Body mass index must always be measured. This is often used to define and quantify obesity and in one study, a BMI of more than 25 kg/m^2 had a sensitivity of 93% and specificity of 74% for OSA. Having said this, these Western figures may not translate to Indian populations. In Udwadia's study, 46% of subjects with OSA had a BMI less than 30, the Western cut-off for obesity, whereas 27% had a BMI less than 27, which is the cut-off for obesity in Asians. Thus, the important lesson emerging from these observations is that while obesity makes it more likely that the Indian patient has OSA, the absence of obesity does not rule it out.

Neck girth: Neck girth must always be measured. The importance of a larger neck girth in producing upper airway incompetence during sleep has been documented in patients with sleep apnea in a number of studies and the mechanism is presumably external compression of the pharynx by adipose tissue. In agreement with these Western observations, the study by Udwadia found that the risk of SDB is 5.34 times higher for subjects with a neck girth of 17 inches.

Upper airway examination: Upper airway examination should be part of the evaluation of any OSA suspect. This should include a look at the nose for any gross septal deviation, polyps or growths. Dentition must be checked especially the presence of retrognathia and dental overjet. The oropharynx should be examined for the presence of tonsillar hypertrophy, uvula size, length, and height. Edema or erythema of the uvula indicates repetitive vibration trauma from snoring. Macroglossia must also be checked for, as it is another cause of partial airway occlusion. It is rare to get an actual structural abnormality but patients with OSA have what can best be described as a "crowded" oropharynx. Finally, micrognathia and retrognathia can predispose to OSA and must always be checked for.

Clinical scales have been used for standardizing oropharyngeal clinical evaluation, the most frequently used scale being the Mallampati scale. Whether one uses a scale or not, routine visual examination of the upper airway and facial structure will allow the trained observer to suspect OSA in certain patients.

Nocturnal oximetry: Nocturnal oximetry has often been used as a "poor-man's sleep study". It may be an adequate screening test in a patient with a high pretest clinical suspicion of OSA. It will, however, miss OSA in significant numbers (almost a third) of patients; a study by Douglas showed that it diagnosed only 66% of all patients with OSA. Many of the patients missed by oximetry had moderately severe OSA and benefited from treatment.

Polysomnography (Figs. 1 and 2): Symptoms and signs alone are not reliable enough to make a definite diagnosis of OSA. A study showed them to have a combined sensitivity of around 60% and specificity of around 70% when diagnosing OSA. Routine tests like radiography, pulmonary function test (PFT) and arterial blood gas analysis add little to this. Hence, the only way to confirm

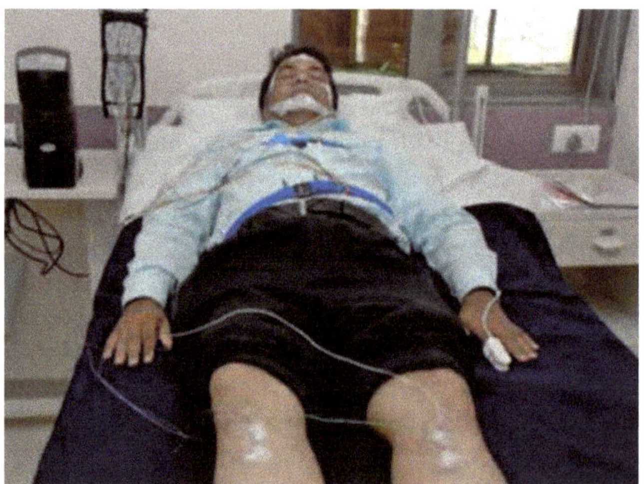

Fig. 1: Polysomnography being performed at a hospital.

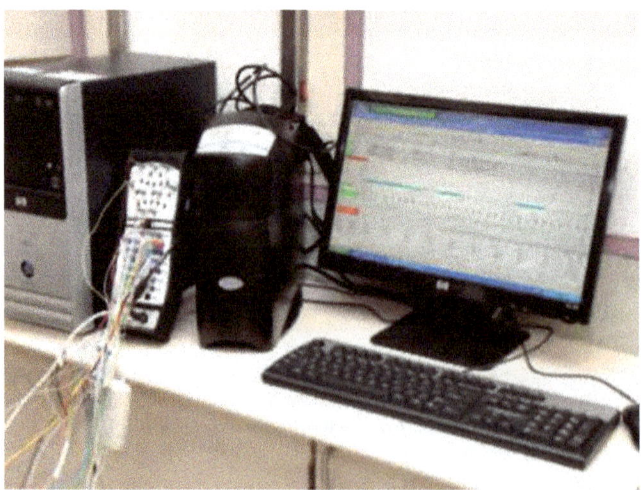

Fig. 2: Polysomnography monitoring equipment.

a clinical suspicion of OSA is by performing PSG. The nocturnal, laboratory-based PSG is the gold standard for the diagnosis of OSA. It also quantifies the severity of OSA and can grade it into mild, moderate or severe. A PSG involves recordings of airflow, ventilatory effort (chest and abdominal movements), oxygen saturation, body position, electrocardiography, electromyography, and electroencephalography (EEG). All these are measured dynamically, through the night. In the standard laboratory-based PSG, a technician is present throughout the night to monitor the patient for the entire study. There are a number of variations, however. In patients with obvious OSA diagnosed in the early part of the night, a "split-night" study can be performed with the continuous positive airway pressure (CPAP) titration being performed in the second half of the night. In some centers, a more limited study is performed without the EEG leads, as these are not crucial when it comes to diagnosing OSA. Sometimes, for reasons of manpower or financial constraints, a partially supervised study is done where the technician sets the patient up for the night and then leaves once the patient falls asleep, returning in the morning to disconnect him from the machine. Finally, with the pressure on beds in many hospitals, home sleep studies are being increasingly performed. Many patients often prefer this as they feel they would sleep more naturally in their own homes than in the artificial confines of a hospital. Modern, lightweight PSG machines are very portable and this has facilitated testing at home. Proponents of home sleep studies thus point out the increased accessibility, reduced cost, enhanced patient convenience and better sleep in a familiar environment. Critics point out that equipment problems cannot be sorted out leading to the occasional technical study failure, and that non-OSA disorders cannot be diagnosed. Irrespective of how or where the test is performed, it must be stressed that a doctor trained in sleep medicine must carefully interpret it.

Impact of Obstructive Sleep Apnea

Cardiovascular

The association between OSA and cardiovascular morbidity has been evident since the first patients with OSA were investigated in the laboratory. Normal sleep induces reduction in blood pressure, heart rate, stroke volume, cardiac output, peripheral resistance and sympathetic activity. OSA causes cyclical surges in all these variables due to exaggerated negative intrathoracic

pressure, hypoxia and recurrent arousals. Coincident with apnea termination is a surge in blood pressure well over 40 mm Hg, coupled with a rise in heart rate which is probably consequent upon the arousal-related. increase in sympathetic tone. It is believed that in patients with OSA, the initial step is absence of the normal nocturnal dipping, then nocturnal hypertension sets in, and sustained hypertension finally follows this.

Hypertension: Fifty to ninety-six percent of OSA patients have hypertension, and conversely, about 40% of hypertensive patients have occult OSA. If a population of patients with refractory hypertension is considered, this figure is even higher. Ample evidence has emerged, not just from animal studies but also from several well-designed longitudinal epidemiological studies, of the link between these two conditions. The landmark Wisconsin Sleep Cohort Study by Peppard, prospectively studied 709 participants for the development of hypertension. The authors found a linear dose-response relation between the severity of OSA and the odds of developing hypertension four years later, with an apnea-hypopnea index (AHI) of 5–15 conferring a 2.03 times odds ratio for the development of hypertension. More interestingly, even at a minor AHI of 1–4.9/h, a level that would not even be labeled OSA, the odds ratio already increased from 1 to 1.6 with further rise being exponential. A similar relationship between OSA and the risk of hypertension is seen in other studies. There is also evidence that successfully treating OSA with CPAP reduces blood pressure in patients with hypertension. Thus, the lessons to the physician, based on the cumulative research in the field, is to suspect OSA in every patient with hypertension, screen for it if there are other risk factors (obesity, snoring, thick neck) and treat with CPAP once it is confirmed. Indeed, CPAP should be added to exercise, salt reduction and weight reduction as a non-pharmacological measure to reduce hypertension.

Coronary artery disease: Several studies report a high prevalence of OSA in patients with coronary artery disease. While this connection may be indirect, because of shared comorbidities like obesity and hypertension, there is some evidence that there may be a direct link as well. OSA itself may promote atherogenesis. The evidence for this is based on the increased C-reactive protein (CRP) and endothelin levels seen in patients with OSA. Studies have shown that patients with OSA have a greater prevalence of increased carotid wall thickness and calcified carotid artery atheromas. A study by Hung from Australia of 101 consecutive men with myocardial infarction (MI) who consented to a sleep study 3 weeks after their infarction showed that an AHI more than 5.3 was a more powerful predictor of MI (RR 23.3), than the more traditional risk factors like hypertension (RR 7.8), or smoking (RR 11.1). In patients with established coronary artery disease, severe OSA may trigger acute nocturnal cardiac ischemia. A study by Franklin documented the presence of OSA in 9 of 10 patients with severe disabling nocturnal angina despite optimal drug therapy. Treatment with CPAP therapy abolished the nocturnal angina.

Cardiac arrhythmias: Sleep apnea is associated with an increased incidence of brady- and tachyarrhythmias, the majority of these arrhythmias recorded in patients with severe OSA and hypoxia, mainly in rapid eye movement (REM) sleep. Heart blocks with Stoke Adams syndrome have also been recorded in patients with severe OSA. CPAP therapy has been shown to be curative in a sample of patients primarily referred for pacemaker implantation for bradyarrhythmias in sleep, most of whom were subsequently diagnosed to have OSA. Atrial fibrillation (AF) is also seen more frequently in patients with OSA, with a study from the Mayo Clinic showing that 49% of patients with AF referred for cardioversion had OSA (OR 3.42), a rate significantly higher than in general cardiology clinic controls matched for age, sex, weight and diabetes.

Congestive cardiac failure: Sleep-disordered breathing is common in congestive cardiac failure (CCF). Several studies have looked at the prevalence of OSA in patients with systolic heart failure and found that as many as 50–60% of CCF patients have some form of SDB. This is most commonly CSA (Cheyne-Stokes breathing), but OSA and mixed obstructive and central apneas are also frequently seen. A single study looked at the incidence of SDB in isolated diastolic failure and reported that 50% of these patients had OSA as well. At the Hinduja Hospital, we prospectively studied 70 patients hospitalized for CCF. Sleep studies were performed on them prior to discharge and we found OSA to be present in 59% and CSA in 20% of these patients. The significance of the impact of SDB in CCF is considerable. SDB adds to the considerable fatigue that patients with CCF routinely face. It can also be considered a marker of severe CCF and sets up a worsening cycle of heart failure, predisposing these patients to arrhythmias and death. Indeed, Cheyne-Stokes respiration is recognized to be an independent

risk factor for mortality in CCF. Cheyne-Stokes respiration in CCF is associated with worse left ventricular ejection fraction (LVEF), higher pulmonary wedge pressures, more arrhythmias and significantly higher mortality and worse survival than in matched patients with CCF and normal nocturnal breathing. When it comes to treatment, there is good news. CPAP at a pressure of 5–12 cm H_2O can have a positive impact. Another noninvasive device used to treat CSA in patients with CCF is adaptive pressure support servo ventilation. This device provides varying amounts of ventilatory support during different phases of periodic breathing. In small studies, treating OSA or CSA with CPAP has been shown to substantially improve not just symptoms like dyspnea and fatigue but also substantially improve LVEF. Hence, the results of the much-anticipated 11-center CANPAP (Canadian CPAP study for patients with CSA and heart failure) study which showed that CPAP over 2 years in these patients ultimately failed to improve survival were disappointing and unexpected. Several criticisms have been made about the design of this trial including the fact that patients treated with CPAP did not receive a titration study but received CPAP at 5–10 cm H_2O. Another possible explanation is that this study was underpowered to conclude with certainty that CPAP is ineffective in this patient population. A post hoc subgroup analysis of this data revealed that patients on CPAP did have significant improvements in performances in the 6-minute walk test and LVEF, hence the last word on treatment with CPAP in this challenging group of patients has not been written.

Other cardiovascular features: Smaller studies have noted intriguing associations between cardiomyopathy and OSA and between aortic dissection and OSA. Finally, OSA has been linked to sudden cardiac death with a study showing an average SaO_2 of 93% and a lowest SaO_2 of 78% strongly predicting sudden cardiac death.

Neuropsychiatric

Stroke: Sleep-related breathing disorders are strongly associated with increased risk of stroke, independent of known risk factors. The mechanisms underlying this increased risk are multifactorial and include reduction in cerebral blood flow, altered cerebral autoregulation, impaired endothelial function and accelerated atherogenesis. There are also several overlapping risk factors for both diseases such as age, gender, hypertension, obesity, smoking and alcohol use that may contribute to the association between OSA and stroke. Perhaps the strongest epidemiological evidence of the association between SDB and stroke comes from the Sleep Heart Health Study, which explored the cross-sectional association between SDB and risk of cardiovascular disease in 6,424 individuals. This study found an odds ratio of 1.58 (1.02–2.46) for the association of stroke with SDB after adjusting for all other confounding risk factors. It is also being increasingly recognized that the association of OSA and stroke may result in unfavorable clinical outcomes after stroke including early neurological worsening, delirium, depression, poor functional status and impaired cognition. Results of CPAP treatment trials in patients with stroke have recently been published. These establish that CPAP is well tolerated and accepted in patients with stroke and OSA and this treatment may have a beneficial effect on wellbeing, depression and hypertension, post stroke. Larger treatment trials are clearly needed to determine whether treatment improves outcome after stroke and whether treatment may serve as secondary prophylaxis preventing the risk of recurrent stroke, or death. It is suggested that all patients with stroke or transient ischemic attack (TIA) should have a detailed sleep history enquiry with a low threshold for proceeding with PSG if there is any suspicion of OSA.

Psychiatric: Numerous studies have identified significant neuropsychological impairment in patients with OSA. These include impairments in general intellectual function, attention, memory and cognitive impairment. OSA has also been linked to depression, with a study by Mosko reporting that 58% of their OSA patients met the Diagnostic and Statistical Manual of Mental Disorders, third edition (DSM-III) criteria for major depression. Several studies have shown an improvement in many of these neuropsychiatric parameters and quality of life after treatment with CPAP.

Metabolic

Type 2 diabetes: It has long been felt that central obesity which is common in type 2 diabetes and OSA is the fundamental link between these disorders. However, rapidly accumulating data from both clinical and epidemiological studies suggest that OSA is independently associated with disturbances in glucose metabolism, and places patients at increased risk of developing type 2 diabetes. At least nine earlier studies have all found an association between OSA and alterations in glucose metabolism consistent with an increased risk of diabetes. Frequent habitual snoring, even in the absence of OSA has itself been linked with increased risk of development of diabetes. In the largest study till date, Meslier studied 595 men referred to a sleep laboratory for PSG and found that type 2 diabetes was present in 30% of OSA patients and 14% of non-apneic snorers. More importantly, blood sugar levels increased and insulin sensitivity decreased with rising severity of OSA, independent of BMI. Thus, while there is strong evidence to indicate that OSA and the risk of type 2 diabetes are associated, the evidence supporting a role for OSA in the development of type 2 diabetes is still limited. The direction of causality remains unclear; it is conceivable that diabetes may itself cause SDB as its autonomic neuropathy could indeed disturb the control of breathing. The effect of CPAP therapy on glucose metabolism has also been looked at. Several recent studies have shown that treatment with CPAP improves glucose levels and insulin sensitivity, at least when it is continued for a few months.

Thus, based on current evidence, it is noteworthy to urge clinicians to systematically evaluate the risk of OSA in type 2 diabetic patients, and conversely, to assess glucose tolerance in patients with known OSA. Further studies are needed to unravel the complex link between obesity, type 2 diabetes and OSA. This need is even more pressing in a country like India with among the highest prevalence of diabetes and of OSA. Unravelling this link could have important public health consequences in these ever-growing patient populations.

Metabolic syndrome: Many patients with OSA have features of the metabolic syndrome; central obesity, insulin resistance, hypertension and dyslipidemia. While the clustering of OSA with these risk factors may be explained by the common link with obesity, it is also postulated that OSA may provide a stress stimulus that triggers or aggravates these metabolic factors, thus conferring independent predisposition to atherosclerosis and cardiovascular disease. The combination of syndrome X (the metabolic syndrome) and OSA has been termed syndrome Z by Wilcox in 1998.

Motor Vehicular Accidents

Multiple studies have linked sleep apnea with an increased risk of having a motor vehicular accident. Such accidents are particularly dangerous because there is lack of reaction of a sleeping driver to an impending collision. These collisions are, as a consequence, often head-on and more likely to be fatal. Sleep-related accidents are most likely to occur early in the morning and late afternoon when there is a natural propensity to feel more sleepy. The risk of accidents in patients with OSA is estimated to vary from 2–7 times that of the general population. Even patients with mild sleep apnea have an increased risk of crashes in some studies, making a compelling case for treating patients with even mild OSA. It is now clear that OSA is an important preventable cause of motor vehicular accidents. Treating these patients with CPAP has been shown to reduce this accident rate. Screening and treatment for OSA has been recently recommended for commercial motor vehicle drivers in some parts of the developed world. This strategy has been shown to be cost-effective, with savings of over $6,000 in total health cost per treated driver.

Treatment of Obstructive Sleep Apnea

General Measures

The patient is encouraged to lose weight and sleep in the lateral position. Weight loss of 10% predicts a 25% reduction in the AHI. Instructions must be given to avoid sedatives, smoking and alcohol as these worsen sleep quality and may actually worsen OSA.

Continuous Positive Airway Pressure (Fig. 3)

Before the 1980s, the only effective treatment for OSA was a permanent tracheostomy; a highly effective but undesirable option. In 1981, an Australian pulmonologist

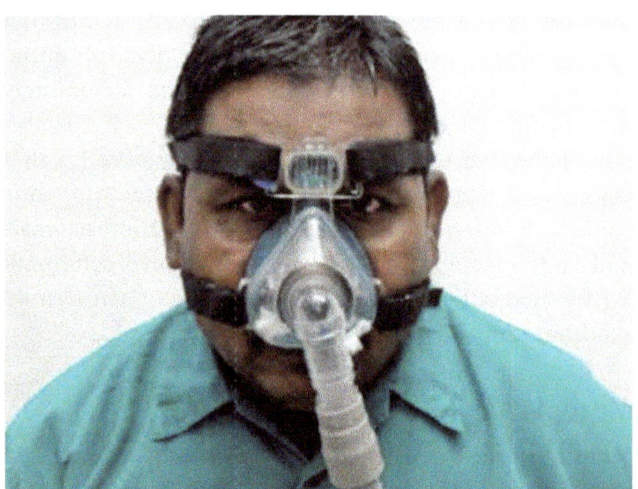

Fig. 3: A patient using the continuous positive airway pressure machine.

Colin Sullivan, in a brief report in the Lancet in 1981, described "reversal of OSA by CPAP applied through the nares in five patients with severe OSA. Like any new idea, this took several years to catch on, but this form of therapy eventually transformed not just the treatment of OSA but also the face of sleep medicine. CPAP is now the gold standard for moderate or severe OSA and at an appropriate pressure will be effective in almost all patients with this syndrome.

Benefits: Continuous positive airway pressure therapy is gratifying to use because its benefits are almost instantly obvious. Within a single night, it eliminates snoring, reverses desaturation, abolishes arousals and favorably affects EDS. When used regularly, it improves vascular risk, cognitive performance, and quality of life. In Young's cohort of 1,522 patients with OSA from Wisconsin, regular use of CPAP was shown to significantly reduce mortality. Several studies show that driving risk also significantly improves after regular CPAP. A study by Douglas showed that just the saving that accrued from reduced accidents over 5 years would far exceed the costs of the treatment.

Compliance: Since the benefits are so obvious to the patient, compliance, even with this cumbersome form of therapy is remarkably good. Patient-reported compliance runs at around 75%, while actual objective monitoring reveals a figure closer to 50%, which is still better than the measured compliance for asthma inhalers and anti-tuberculosis drugs. Compliance can be improved by improvements in technology, with auto-CPAP machines, bi-level CPAP and humidifiers all improving compliance.

Side effects: The side effects of CPAP are generally minor and include dry mouth, ocular irritation, conjunctivitis, nasal congestion, and abrasions and ulcers over the bridge of the nose due to a badly fitted mask. Advances in technology are constantly being developed to address this crucial issue of the interface between the patient and the CPAP machine. Some patients may feel very claustrophobic with a mask, and for such patients, nasal prongs or pillows may prove a more comfortable option. Rarely reported, more dangerous complications of CPAP include pneumothorax, massive epistaxis, pneumocephalus, increased intraocular pressure and tympanic membrane rupture. These are all very rare, constituting isolated case reports. It must be stressed again that, on the whole, CPAP is very safe.

Practical aspects: We have found that patient education goes a long way in alleviating the apprehensions most patients have regarding CPAP. A trial of CPAP for an hour or so in the daytime, prior to the first night of CPAP titration is also helpful. There is ample evidence that the patient's experience with the machine on the first night will influence his subsequent long-term acceptance (or rejection) of the treatment. This, in turn, can be affected by providing education, motivation and support to the patient.

Oral Appliances

These are established treatment options for snoring and mild OSA. They may also be considered in patients where CPAP has been tried and failed. There are two broad types of oral devices: (1) tongue repositioning devices; and (2) mandibular repositioning devices. These devices must be designed and fitted for each individual patient by the sleep physician in close consultation with a dentist. In a recent, comprehensive meta-analysis of oral appliances, 70% of the 304 subjects had a reduction in their AHI by at least 50% from the baseline.

Surgical Options

A variety of surgical approaches have been attempted in OSA. These are listed in **Table 3**. The only one that will be discussed in detail is uvulopalatopharyngoplasty (UPPP) as it is the best studied and most frequently performed. This surgery involves excising the uvula, distal soft palate, faucial muscles, tonsillar pillars and the mucosa of the pharynx. It eliminates snoring with almost 80% success, but a recent meta-analysis by Sher showed that the mean decrease in AHI across studies was around 55%. Overall, its success rate is approximately 50% and it is less effective in patients with a BMI more than 30 and in those with more severe OSA. The procedure is not without morbidity and major complications have been reported, including the

Table 3: Surgical options for obstructive sleep apnea.

- Uvulopalatopharyngoplasty (UPPP)
- Laser-assisted uvulopalatopharyngoplasty (LAUP)
- Septoplasty
- Tongue reduction
- Genioglossus advancement-hyoid myotomy and suspension (GAHMS)
- Maxillary and mandibular osteotomy (MMO)
- Tracheostomy
- Bariatric surgery

occasional fatality. Finally, relapses occur over time in as many as 50% of those who initially respond. Thus, this and other forms of surgery, should never be the first-line treatment for OSA. Surgery should only be performed in special referral centers, under the supervision of experienced ear-nose-throat (ENT) surgeons with a special interest in the field. They should only be offered to patients who have tried and failed CPAP or refuse a trial of CPAP.

■ NASAL EXPIRATORY POSITIVE AIRWAY DEVICES (nEPAP)

These are single use devices that are inserted into the nares with an adhesive to provide a seal at night. The nEPAP allows for low inspiratory resistance whilst increasing expiratory resistance to prevent upper airway collapse. There have been six clinical trials using nEPAP with all studies demonstrating a significant decrease (31–49%) in the AHI. Two studies showed a significant additional change in daytime sleepiness and sleep quality. Snoring, as expected also significantly reduced. These devices might be ideal for mild OSA and given the challenges of travelling with a CPAP machine might be good travel replacements for the frequent traveller. As with CPAP, adherence and tolerability remain an issue. However, considering ease of application, compact design, low cost, and availability without a prescription, these may emerge as important second line therapy in the patient with mild OSA.

■ ELECTRICAL STIMULATION

A new and promising form of treatment is hypoglossal nerve stimulation (HNS). In HNS, a silicone cuff with stimulating electrodes is placed around a unilateral hypoglossal nerve, which includes motor neurons innervating the protrusor and retractor muscles of the tongue. Stimulating leads are tunneled via the neck to a pacemaker like neurostimulator which is placed inferior to the clavicle. From the neurostimulator, sensory leads are tunneled subcutaneously to intercostal muscles to monitor respiration. The neurostimulator delivers either synchronous or continuous stimulation causing bulk muscle tongue protrusion. After patients are implanted, stimulus titration for the patient occurs by gradually adjusting stimulus intensity, frequency, and pulse width to tolerable levels that consistently abolish inspiratory flow restriction during sleep. HNS has been tested in five recent trials. In all five studies, AHI decreased by >50% with significant improvement in the oxygen desaturation index. This translated into significant symptomatic improvement in sleep quality, daytime sleepiness, mood, and quality of life.

HNS therapy though initially invasive and requiring surgery has the potential to change the way OSA is treated especially in patients who cannot tolerate or refuse to adhere to CPAP. Phenotyping of the airways can increase the probability of HNS success. However, larger scale clinical trials are needed to assess the long-term safety of this technique. It remains best suited to patients with BMI <40 and trials to assess its effectiveness in patients with higher BMIs are awaited.

◼ CENTRAL SLEEP APNEA

Central sleep apnea comprises a heterogeneous group of disorders characterized by momentary cessation of breathing in sleep due to a transient withdrawal of the respiratory drive to the muscles of respiration. Thus, in contrast to OSA, in which the respiratory drive continues during apnea, in CSA, no respiratory efforts or intrathoracic pressure swings are generated.

Etiology

These disorders are rare and may be idiopathic or secondary. Idiopathic central hypoventilation is called Ondine's curse after a character in Greek mythology who was cursed with having to voluntarily control his automatic body functions including respiration. Secondary causes include a range of neurological conditions that cause specific damage to the neurons in the respiratory center located in the medulla and pons. These include encephalitis, brainstem infarctions, radiation injury, bulbar poliomyelitis, multiple sclerosis and the Shy-Drager syndrome.

Clinical Presentation

Central hypoventilation syndromes can go unnoticed over the years until an episode of respiratory failure develops, usually in association with respiratory infection. Indeed, many patients may have several episodes of respiratory failure before the correct diagnosis is eventually made. The disorder may be discovered in childhood, but milder forms may go undetected into adult life. These patients demonstrate awake hypoxemia and hypercapnia but can normalize gas exchange by voluntary hyperventilation. Snoring may or may not be present and is not as prominent

as in patients with OSA. Morning headaches and daytime sleepiness are common. Patients may also manifest unexplained polycythemia or cor pulmonale, which are consequences of chronic hypoxemia. Pulmonary function tests and tests of respiratory muscle strength are usually normal unless the patient has coexisting lung disease or neuromuscular weakness. A further example is the obesity hypoventilation syndrome where the increased mechanical ventilatory load caused by morbid obesity may unmask an underlying weakness in the central respiratory drive resulting in alveolar hypoventilation and blood gas abnormalities that are very similar to those seen in patients with idiopathic central hypoventilation.

Impact of Sleep

Patients with central hypoventilation frequently develop severe respiratory insufficiency during sleep as a consequence of the reduction in the respiratory drive which normally occurs during sleep. The central feature is an abnormal increase in $PaCO_2$ during sleep, usually associated with severe hypoxemia. This may occur during all sleep stages but is particularly pronounced and severe during REM sleep. Apneas and hypopneas may occur in association with hypoventilation; however, central hypoventilation should only be diagnosed if the clinical sequelae can be attributed to hypoventilation distinct from the apneas and hypopneas.

Management

A number of pharmacological agents have respiratory stimulant properties. These include theophylline, progesterone and almitrine. The treatment of choice is noninvasive ventilation (NIV). This is generally delivered by a nasal or full-face mask. Several studies have reported an improvement in daytime blood gases after a night of NIV. Its mechanism includes resting of the respiratory muscles and a resetting of the respiratory drive at the chemoreceptor level. Electrophrenic pacing is an interesting form of treatment that has been in use for this condition for over two decades. The procedure involves implanting a pacing electrode around the phrenic nerve either in the cervical or high thoracic region. There are several reports of its utility in patients with central alveolar hypoventilation. Adults with central alveolar hypoventilation can often be successfully managed with a unilateral phrenic nerve pacemaker, while children generally require bilateral pacemakers by virtue of their chest wall being more compliant. Unilateral phrenic nerve pacing in children with CSA is inefficient as it results in paradoxical movement of the contralateral diaphragm and chest wall.

■ SUGGESTED READING

1. Bradley TD, Logan AG, Kimoff J, et al. Continuous positive pressure for central sleep apnea and heart failure. N Engl J Med. 2005;353:2025-33.
2. Kryger MH, Roth T, Dement WC. Principles and Practice of Sleep Medicine, 4th edition. St. Louis: Elsevier Saunders; 2005.
3. Mosko S, Zetin M, Glen S, et al. Self-reported depressive symptomatology, mood ratings, and treatment outcome in sleep disorders patients. J Clin Psychol. 1989;45:51-60.
4. Ng TP, Seow A, Tan WC. Prevalence of snoring and sleep breathing related disorders in Chinese, Malay and Indian adults in Singapore. Eur Respir J. 1998;12:198-202.
5. Peppard PE, Young T, Palta M, et al. Prospective study of the association between sleep-disordered breathing and hypertension. N Engl J Med. 2000;342:1378-84.
6. Reddy EV, Kadhivaran T, Mishra HK, et al. Prevalence and risk factors of obstructive sleep apnea among middle-aged urban Indians: a community-based study. Sleep Med. 2009;10:913-8.
7. Sahar E, Whitney CW, Redline S, et al. Sleep disordered breathing and cardiovascular disease: cross-sectional results of the Sleep Heart Health Study. Am J Respir Crit Care Med. 2001;163:19-25.
8. Schmidt-Nowara WW, Meade TE, Hays MB. Treatment of snoring and obstructive sleep apnea with a dental orthosis. Chest. 1991;99:1378-85.
9. Sharma SK, Kumpawat S, Banga A, et al. Prevalence and risk factors of obstructive sleep apnea syndrome in a population of Delhi, India. Chest. 2006;130:149-56.
10. Stradling JR. Obstructive sleep apnea: definitions, epidemiology, and natural history. Thorax. 1995;50:683-9.
11. Udwadia ZF, Doshi AV, Lonkar SG, et al. Prevalence of sleep disordered breathing and sleep apnea in middle-aged urban Indian men. Am J Respir Crit Care Med. 2004;169:168-73.
12. Weaver T, Calik M, Farabi S, et al. Innovative treatments for adults with obstructive sleep apnea. Nat Sci Sleep. 2014;6:137-47.
13. Young T, Palta M, Dempsey J, et al. The occurrence of sleep-disordered breathing among middle aged adults. N Engl J Med. 1993;328:1230-5.

Index

Page numbers followed by *f* refer to figure, *fc* refer to flowchart, and *t* refer to table.